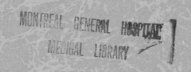

Surgery of the Liver, Biliary Tract, and Pancreas

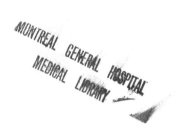

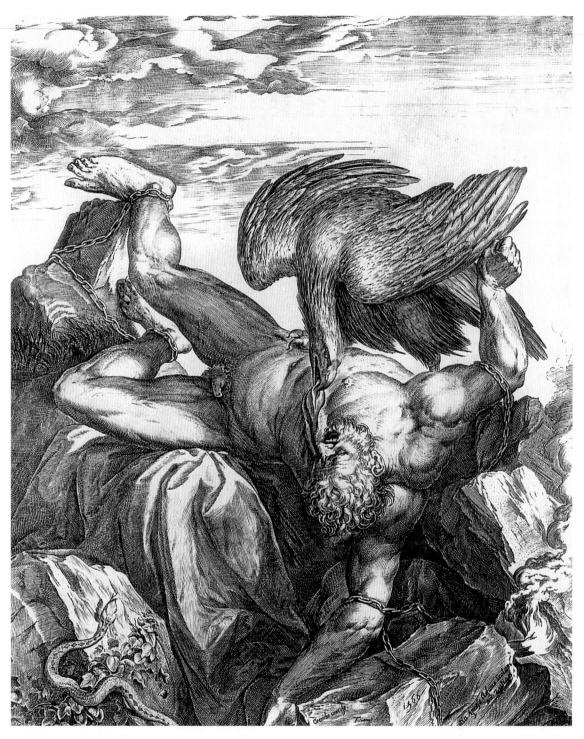

Prometheus, chained to the rocky Mount Caucasus, has his liver eaten by the eagle of Zeus. (Engraving, 1566, possibly after a work by Titian. Reproduced by permission of the Hulton Getty Picture Collection, London.)

Surgery of the Liver, Biliary Tract, and Pancreas

Fourth Edition

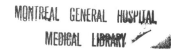
EDITOR-IN-CHIEF

Leslie H. Blumgart, BDS, MD, DSc (Hon), FACS, FRCS (ENG, EDIN), FRCPS (GLAS)

ASSOCIATE EDITORS

Jacques Belghiti, MD

William R. Jarnagin, MD, FACS

Ronald P. DeMatteo, MD, FACS

William C. Chapman, MD, FACS

Markus W. Büchler, MD

Lucy E. Hann, MD

Michael D'Angelica, MD

VOLUME 2

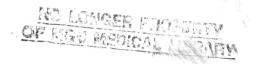
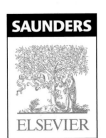

SAUNDERS

ELSEVIER

SAUNDERS
ELSEVIER

1600 John F. Kennedy Blvd.
Ste 1800
Philadelphia, PA 19103-2899

SURGERY OF THE LIVER, BILIARY TRACT, AND PANCREAS   ISBN-13: 978-1-4160-3256-4
Copyright © 2007, 2000, 1994, 1988 by Saunders, an imprint of Elsevier Inc.   ISBN-10: 1-4160-3256-8

Notice

Knowledge and best practice in this field are constantly changing. As new research and experience broaden our knowledge, changes in practice, treatment, and drug therapy may become necessary or appropriate. Readers are advised to check the most current information provided (i) on procedures featured or (ii) by the manufacturer of each product to be administered, to verify the recommended dose or formula, the method and duration of administration, and contraindications. It is the responsibility of the practitioner, relying on his or her own experience and knowledge of the patient, to make diagnoses, to determine dosages and the best treatment for each individual patient, and to take all appropriate safety precautions. To the fullest extent of the law, neither the Publisher nor the Editors assume any liability for any injury and/or damage to persons or property arising out of or related to any use of the material contained in this book.

The Publisher

Library of Congress Cataloging-in-Publication Data
Surgery of the liver, biliary tract, and pancreas / [edited by] Leslie H. Blumgart. —4th ed.
  p.; cm.
  Rev. ed. of: Surgery of the liver and biliary tract. 3rd ed. 2000.
  Includes bibliographical references and index.
  ISBN 1-4160-3256-8
  1. Liver—Surgery. 2. Biliary tract—Surgery. I. Blumgart, L. H. II. Surgery of the liver and biliary tract.
  [DNLM: 1. Liver—surgery. 2. Biliary Tract Surgical Procedures. 3. Pancreas—surgery.
WI 770 S9617 2006]
RD669.S87 2006
617.5'56—dc22   2005052682

Acquisitions Editor: Judith Fletcher
Developmental Editor: Deidre Simpson
Publishing Services Manager: Tina Rebane
Project Manager: Jodi Kaye
Design Direction: Karen O'Keefe Owens

Printed in China

Last digit is the print number: 9 8 7 6 5 4 3 2

*This book is dedicated to
the development of surgery of the liver, biliary tract,
and pancreas as a specialty.*

Editors

**Leslie H. Blumgart, BDS, MD,
DSc (Hon), FACS, FRCS (ENG, EDIN),
FRCPS (GLAS)**
Enid A. Haupt Chair in Surgery
Chief, Hepatobiliary Service
Department of Surgery
Memorial Sloan-Kettering Cancer Center
New York, New York

Jacques Belghiti, MD
Professor and Chairman
Department of Digestive and Transplant Surgery
Hospital Beaujon
Paris, France

William R. Jarnagin, MD, FACS
Associate Professor of Surgery
Weill Medical College of Cornell University
Attending Surgeon
Memorial Sloan-Kettering Cancer Center
New York, New York

Ronald P. DeMatteo, MD, FACS
Associate Professor of Surgery
Weill Medical College of Cornell University
Associate Attending Surgeon
Memorial Sloan-Kettering Cancer Center
New York, New York

William C. Chapman, MD, FACS
Professor and Chief
Section of Transplantation
Department of Surgery
Washington University in St. Louis School of Medicine
St. Louis, Missouri

Markus W. Büchler, MD
Professor and Chairman
Department of Surgery
University of Heidelberg
Heidelberg, Germany

Lucy E. Hann, MD
Professor of Radiology
Weill Medical College of Cornell University
Attending Radiologist
Memorial Sloan-Kettering Cancer Center
New York, New York

Michael D'Angelica, MD
Assistant Professor of Surgery
Weill Medical College of Cornell University
Assistant Attending Surgeon
Memorial Sloan-Kettering Cancer Center
New York, New York

Contributors

Eddie K. Abdalla, MD
Assistant Professor of Surgery
Department of Surgical Oncology
The University of Texas M.D. Anderson Cancer Center
Houston, Texas
Portal Vein Embolization: Preoperative Portal Vein Embolization—A Western Perspective

Ghassan K. Abou-Alfa, MD
Instructor
Weill Medical College of Cornell University
Assistant Attending Physician
Memorial Sloan-Kettering Cancer Center
New York, New York
Chemotherapy of Liver Tumors: Systemic Therapy for Hepatocellular Carcinoma; Chemotherapy of Liver Tumors: Systemic Therapy for Metastatic Colorectal Cancer

Reid B. Adams, MD
Associate Professor of Surgery
University of Virginia School of Medicine
Chief, Hepatobiliary and Pancreatic Surgery
University of Virginia Health System
Charlottesville, Virginia
Intraoperative Ultrasound of the Liver: Techniques for Liver Resection and Transplantation

N. Volkan Adsay, MD
Associate Professor of Pathology
Wayne State University School of Medicine
Pathologist
The Karmanos Cancer Institute
Harper University Hospital and Detroit Medical Center
Detroit, Michigan
Tumors of the Bile Ducts—Pathologic Aspects; Pathology and Classification of Pancreatic and Ampullary Tumors

Jatinder P. Ahluwalia, MD
Associate Professor of Internal Medicine–Gastroenterology
Southern Illinois University School of Medicine
Springfield, Illinois
Management of Ascites in Cirrhosis and Portal Hypertension

Timothy Akhurst, MBBS, MD, FRACP
Assistant Professor of Radiology
Weill Medical College of Cornell University
Assistant Attending
Memorial Sloan-Kettering Cancer Center
New York, New York
The Role of Nuclear Medicine in the Diagnosis and Management of Hepatobiliary and Pancreatic Diseases

Thomas D. Atwell, MD
Instructor of Radiology
Mayo Clinic College of Medicine
Consultant, Diagnostic Radiology
Mayo Clinic
Rochester, Minnesota
Metastatic Tumors: Hepatic Metastases from Primary Neuroendocrine Tumors

Mary T. Austin, MD, MPH
Resident Physician
Vanderbilt University School of Medicine
Resident Physician
Vanderbilt University Medical Center
Nashville, Tennessee
The Mesocaval Shunt: Technique

Claudio Bassi, MD
Associate Professor
University of Verona Faculty of Medicine
Verona, Italy
Definition and Classification of Pancreatitis

Christoph D. Becker, MD
Professor of Radiology
University of Geneva Faculty of Medicine
Head of Abdominal Radiology and Acting Chairman
Department of Diagnostic and Interventional Radiology
Geneva University Hospital
Geneva, Switzerland
Percutaneous Approaches to the Treatment of Gallbladder Disease

Ian J. Beckingham, MD
Section of Surgery
University Hospital, Queen's Medical Centre
Nottingham, United Kingdom
Postcholecystectomy Problems

Jacques Belghiti, MD
Professor and Chairman
Department of Digestive and Transplant Surgery
Hospital Beaujon
Paris, France
Benign Liver Lesions; Liver Resection for Benign Disease and for Liver and Biliary Tumors (Liver Resection in Living Related Donors); Vascular Isolation Techniques in Liver Resection

Thomas V. Berne, MD
Professor of Surgery
Keck School of Medicine of USC
Chief, Emergency (Non-Trauma) Surgery Service
Los Angeles County–USC Medical Center
Los Angeles, California
*Liver, Biliary, and Pancreatic Injury: Liver and Bile
Duct Injury*

Anton J. Bilchik, MD, PhD, FACS
Director, Gastrointestinal Surgical Oncology
Director, Gastrointestinal Program
Associate Director, Surgical Oncology
John Wayne Cancer Institute
Santa Monica, California
*Ablation of Liver Tumors: Radiofrequency Thermal Ablation
of Liver Tumors*

Kenneth F. Binmoeller, MD, FACG
Director
Interventional Endoscopy Service
California Pacific Medical Center
San Francisco, California
Interventional Endoscopy: Technical Aspects

Henri Bismuth
Professor and Head
Department of Surgery
Paul Brousse Hospital
Villejuif, France
Liver Transplantation in Patients with Fulminant Hepatitis

Martin J. K. Blomley, MD[†]
Professor of Radiology
Imaging Sciences Department
Imperial College School of Medicine
London, United Kingdom
Ultrasound of the Liver, Biliary Tract, and Pancreas

**Leslie H. Blumgart, BDS, MD, DSc (Hon),
FACS, FRCS (ENG, EDIN), FRCPS (GLAS)**
Enid A. Haupt Chair in Surgery
Chief, Hepatobiliary Service
Department of Surgery
Memorial Sloan–Kettering Cancer Center
New York, New York
*Historical Perspective; Surgical and Radiologic Anatomy of the
Liver, Biliary Tract, and Pancreas; Liver Blood Flow:
Physiology, Measurement, and Clinical Relevance; Liver
Hyperplasia, Hypertrophy, and Atrophy; Biliary-Enteric
Anastomosis; Stones in the Common Bile Duct—Clinical
Features and Open Surgical Approaches and Techniques;
Biliary Stricture and Fistula: Benign Biliary Strictures; Biliary
Stricture and Fistula: Biliary Fistula; Benign Tumors and
Pseudotumors of the Biliary Tract; Intrahepatic and
Extrahepatic Biliary Cancer; Hemobilia and Bilhemia; Liver
Resection for Benign Disease and for Liver and Biliary Tumors;
The Technique of Portacaval Shunt*

**P. C. Bornman, MBChB, MMed(Surg), FCS(SA),
FRCS(Ed)**
Professor of Surgery
University of Cape Town Health Sciences Faculty
Head and Chief Surgeon
Surgical Gastroenterology Unit
Groote Schuur Hospital
Cape Town, South Africa
*Endoscopic Therapy in the Management of Esophageal Varices:
Injection Sclerotherapy and Variceal Ligation*

Lynn Brody, MS, MD
Assistant Professor of Radiology
Weill Medical College of Cornell University
Assistant Clinical Radiologist
Memorial Sloan-Kettering Cancer Center
New York, New York
Percutaneous Biopsy

Christoph E. Broelsch, MD, PhD, FACS
Director of General Surgery and Transplantation
University of Duisburg-Essen
Duisburg, Germany
*Liver Resection for Benign Disease and for Liver and Biliary
Tumors (Computer-Assisted Operation Planning and Virtual
Liver Resection)*

Carlos V. R. Brown, MD
Assistant Professor of Surgery
Keck School of Medicine of USC
Los Angeles County–USC Medical Center
Los Angeles, California
Liver, Biliary, and Pancreatic Injury: Pancreatic Injury

Karen T. Brown, MD
Professor of Radiology
Weill Medical College of Cornell University
Member
Memorial Sloan-Kettering Cancer Center
New York, New York
*Intrahepatic and Extrahepatic Biliary Cancer (Interventional
Radiologic Techniques in Hilar and Intrahepatic Biliary
Strictures)*

Melissa L. Brown, MS, RD
Clinical Dietitian
University of Illinois at Chicago Medical Center
Chicago, Illinois
Preoperative and Postoperative Nutrition in Hepatobiliary Surgery

Jordi Bruix, MD
Associate Professor of Medicine
University of Barcelona School of Medicine
Senior Consultant
Barcelona Clinic Liver Cancer Group
Liver Unit Hospital Clinic
Barcelona, Spain
Hepatocellular Carcinoma; Liver Transplantation for Tumors

[†]Deceased

Elizabeth M. Brunt, MD
Professor of Pathology
Saint Louis University School of Medicine
St. Louis, Missouri
Cirrhosis and Portal Hypertension: Pathologic Aspects

Markus W. Büchler, MD
Professor and Chairman
Department of Surgery
University of Heidelberg
Heidelberg, Germany
Management of Acute Pancreatitis and Complications;
Pancreaticoduodenectomy, Distal Pancreatectomy, Segmental
Pancreatectomy, Total Pancreatectomy, and Transduodenal
Resection of the Papilla of Vater

Andrew K. Burroughs (Hon), ChB, MB, FRCP
Professor of Hepatology
Royal Free and University College Medical School
Consultant Physician and Hepatologist
Royal Free Hospital
London, United Kingdom
Medical Management of Bleeding Varices

Giovanni Butturini, MD, PhD
Consultant, General Surgery
Faculty of Medicine
University of Verona
Verona, Italy
Definition and Classification of Pancreatitis

Iain C. Cameron, MD, FRCS
Honorary Senior Clinical Lecturer
University of Sheffield Medical School
Consultant Hepatobiliary Surgeon
Royal Hallamshire Hospital
Sheffield, United Kingdom
Cholecystolithiasis and Stones in the Common Bile Duct:
Which Approach, When?

Alessio Carloni, MD
Clinic Assistant
Department of Digestive Surgery
University of Paris
Paris, France
Assistant Attending
Department of Digestive Surgery
Hospital Antoine Béclère
Paris, France

David L. Carr-Locke, MB, BCh, DRCOG, FRCP, FACG
Associate Professor of Medicine
Harvard Medical School
Director of Endoscopy
Brigham and Women's Hospital
Boston, Massachusetts
Stones in the Bile Duct: Endoscopic and Percutaneous Approaches

Charles Cha, MD, FACS
Assistant Professor
Departments of Gastrointestinal Surgery and Surgical Oncology
Yale University School of Medicine
New Haven, Connecticut
Liver Hyperplasia, Hypertrophy, and Atrophy

William C. Chapman, MD, FACS
Professor and Chief
Section of Transplantation
Department of Surgery
Washington University in St. Louis School of Medicine
St. Louis, Missouri
Orthotopic Liver Transplantation

Jin Wook Chung, MD, PhD
Professor of Radiology
Seoul National University College of Medicine
Seoul National University Hospital
Seoul, Korea
Embolization of Liver Tumors

Dania Cioni, MD
Assistant Professor of Radiology
Department of Oncology, Transplants, and Advanced
    Technologies in Medicine
Pisa University School of Medicine
Pisa, Italy
Ablation of Liver Tumors: Percutaneous Methods for Ablation
of Hepatic Neoplasms

Kevin C. Conlon, MD
Professor of Surgery and Head, Department of Surgery
Trinity College School of Medicine
National Children's Hospital Tallaght,
Dublin, Ireland
Intraoperative Diagnosis of Liver, Biliary, and Pancreatic Disease

Mauro M. Correia, MD
Professor of Surgery
University of Rio Grand School of Medicine
Consultant Surgeon
National Institute of Cancer Praça da Cruz Vermelha
Rio de Janeiro, Brazil
Radiotherapy of Liver Tumors: Selective Internal Radiation
Therapy for Liver Tumors

Carlos U. Corvera, MD
Assistant Professor
Department of Surgery, Division of General Surgery
University of California, San Francisco, School of Medicine
Staff Surgeon
Division of General Surgery
San Francisco VA Medical Center
San Francisco, California
Biliary Stricture and Fistula: Biliary Fistula

David O. Cosgrove, MA, MSc, FRCR, FRCP
Emeritus Professor
Imaging Sciences Department
Imperial College School of Medicine
Consultant Radiologist
Hammersmith Hospital
London, United Kingdom
Ultrasound of the Liver, Biliary Tract, and Pancreas

Anne M. Covey, MD
Assistant Professor of Radiology
Weill Medical College of Cornell University
Assistant Professor of Radiology
Memorial Sloan-Kettering Cancer Center
New York, New York
Percutaneous Biopsy

Michael D'Angelica, MD
Associate Professor of Surgery
Weill Medical College of Cornell University
Assistant Attending Surgeon
Memorial Sloan-Kettering Cancer Center
New York, New York
*Biliary-Enteric Anastomosis; Tumors of the Gallbladder;
Intrahepatic and Extrahepatic Biliary Cancer; Ablation of
Liver Tumors: Cryotherapy for Liver Tumors; Intra-arterial
Chemotherapy for Liver Tumors; Liver Resection for Benign
Disease and for Liver and Biliary Tumors (Addendum:
Laparoscopic Techniques)*

Michael Darcy, MD
Professor of Radiology and Surgery
Division of Diagnostic Radiology
Chief, Interventional Radiology Section
Washington University in St. Louis School of Medicine
St. Louis, Missouri

Brian D. Davison, MD, MS
Instructor in Radiology
Harvard Medical School
Chief
Division of Vascular and Interventional Radiology
Children's Hospital Boston
Boston, Massachusetts
Radiologic Hepatobiliary Interventions

Douglas R. DeCorato, MD
Clinical Assistant Professor of Radiology
Weill Medical College of Cornell University
Radiologist
New York Hospital–Cornell Medical Center
New York, New York
*Magnetic Resonance Imaging of the Liver, Biliary Tract,
and Pancreas*

Ronald P. DeMatteo, MD, FACS
Associate Professor of Surgery
Weill Medical College of Cornell University
Vice Chair
Department of Surgery
Associate Attending Surgeon
Hepatobiliary Service
Memorial Sloan-Kettering Cancer Center
New York, New York
*Liver Immunology; Metastatic Tumors: Noncolorectal
Non-neuroendocrine Metastases; Segment-Oriented Anatomic
Liver Resections*

Demetrios Demetriades, MD, PhD, FACS
Professor of Surgery
Keck School of Medicine of USC
Director of Trauma and Surgical Critical Care
Los Angeles County–USC Medical Center
Los Angeles, California
*Liver, Biliary, and Pancreatic Injury: Liver and Bile Duct Injury;
Liver, Biliary, and Pancreatic Injury: Pancreatic Injury*

Achilles A. Demetriou, MD, PhD
Executive Vice President and Chief Operating Officer
University Hospitals Health System
Cleveland, Ohio
Support of the Failing Liver

Niraj M. Desai, MD
Assistant Professor of Surgery
Washington University in St. Louis
School of Medicine
Director
Pancreas Transplant Program
Barnes-Jewish Hospital
St. Louis, Missouri
Whole Organ Pancreas and Pancreatic Islet Transplantation

Kiran K. Dhanireddy, MD
Senior Resident
Department of Surgery
Georgetown University Hospital
Washington, DC
Research Fellow, Transplantation Branch
National Institute of Diabetes and Digestive and
Kidney Diseases
National Institutes of Health
Bethesda, Maryland
Liver and Pancreatic Transplantation Immunobiology

Thomas Diamond, MD, FRCS
Consultant in Hepatobiliary and Pancreatic Surgery
Mater Hospital
The Queen's University of Belfast
Belfast, Northern Ireland
*Aneurysm and Arteriovenous Fistula of the Liver and Pancreatic
Vasculature*

Fabio F. Di Mola, MD
Department of Surgery
University of Heidelberg School of Medicine
Heidelberg, Germany
Specialist in General Surgery
Department of Abdominal Surgery
IRCCS Casa Sollievo Della Sofferenza
Foggia, Italy
Management of Chronic Pancreatitis: Conservative, Endoscopic, and Surgical

Pierluigi Di Sebastiano, MD
Privat-Docent of Surgery
University of Heidelberg School of Medicine
Heidelberg, Germany
Head
Department of Visceral Surgery
IRCCS Casa Sollievo della Sofferenza
Foggia, Italy
Management of Chronic Pancreatitis: Conservative, Endoscopic, and Surgical

Majella Doyle, MD
Clinical Fellow
Department of Surgery–Transplant Surgery,
Washington University in St. Louis School of Medicine,
St. Louis, Missouri
Intraoperative Diagnosis of Liver, Biliary, and Pancreatic Disease

Robert J. Eckersley, PhD
Research Associate
Imaging Sciences Department
Imperial College School of Medicine
Hammersmith Hospital
London, United Kingdom
Ultrasound of the Liver, Biliary Tract, and Pancreas

N. Joseph Espat, MD, MS
Associate Professor
Department of Surgery–Hepatobiliary Surgery
University of Illinois at Chicago Medical Center
Chicago, Illinois
Bile Secretion

Sheung-Tat Fan, MS, MD, PhD
Chair Professor
The University of Hong Kong
Chair Professor
Queen Mary Hospital
Hong Kong, China
Recurrent Pyogenic Cholangitis; Liver Resection in Cirrhosis of the Liver

Olivier Farges, PhD, MD
Professor of Surgery
Faculty of Medicine
University of Paris VII
Department of Surgery
Hospital Beaujon
Paris, France
Nonparasitic Cystic Diseases of the Liver and Intrahepatic Biliary Tree

Carlos Fernández-Del Castillo, MD
Associate Professor of Surgery
Harvard Medical School
Visiting Surgeon
Massachusetts General Hospital
Boston, Massachusetts
Periampullary and Pancreatic Tumors: Cystic Neoplasms of the Pancreas

Mary Fischer, MD
Associate Professor of Clinical Anesthesiology
Weill Medical College of Cornell University
Clinical Member
Memorial Sloan-Kettering Cancer Center
Attending Anesthesiologist
Memorial Hospital for Cancer and Allied Diseases
New York, New York
Anesthesia and Postoperative Intensive Care

Yuman Fong, MD
Professor of Surgery
Weill Medical College of Cornell University
Chief
Gastric and Mixed Tumor Service
Murray F. Brennan Chair in Surgery
Memorial Sloan-Kettering Cancer Center
New York, New York
Preoperative and Postoperative Nutrition in Hepatobiliary Surgery; Metastatic Tumors: Surgical Treatment of Hepatic Metastases from Colorectal Cancer

Helmut Friess, MD
Professor of Surgery and Vice-Chairman
Department of Visceral Surgery
University of Heidelberg School of Medicine
Heidelberg, Germany
Management of Chronic Pancreatitis: Conservative, Endoscopic, and Surgical; Pancreaticoduodenectomy, Distal Pancreatectomy, Segmental Pancreatectomy, Total Pancreatectomy, and Transduodenal Resection of the Papilla of Vater

Josep Fuster
Associate Professor
University of Barcelona School of Medicine
Senior Consultant and Professor of Surgery
Barcelona Clinic Liver Cancer Group
Liver Unit
Hospital Clinic
Barcelona, Spain
Liver Transplantation for Tumors

Nisha Garg, PhD
Associate Professor
Department of Microbiology and Immunology
University of Texas Medical Branch
Galveston, Texas
Amebiasis and Other Parasitic Infections

Hans Gerdes, MD
Professor of Clinical Medicine
Weill Medical College of Cornell University
Attending Physician and Director
GI Endoscopy Unit
Memorial Hospital for Cancer and Allied Diseases
New York, New York
Endoscopic Ultrasound: Endoscopic Ultrasound of the Pancreas

Philippe Gertsch, MD, FRCS, ICSHK, IHKAM(Surg)
Professor of Surgery and Chief
Department of Surgery
Oncology Institute of Southern Switzerland
Bellinzona, Switzerland
The Technique of Cholecystectomy

George Getradjman, MD
Associate Professor of Clinical Radiology
Weill Medical College of Cornell University
Clinical Director
Interventional Radiology Section
Department of Radiology
Memorial Sloan-Kettering Cancer Center
New York, New York
Direct Cholangiography

George K. Gittes, MD
Benjamin R. Fisher Chair of Pediatric Surgery
   and Surgeon-in-Chief
Children's Hospital of Pittsburgh
Pittsburgh, Pennsylvania
Biliary Atresia

Sean C. Glasgow, MD
Resident
Department of Surgery
Washington University in St. Louis School of Medicine
Barnes–Jewish Hospital
St. Louis, Missouri
Orthotopic Liver Transplantation

Gabriel E. Gondolesi, MD
Adjunct Associate Director
Liver Unit
Chief
Nutrition Rehabilitation
Favaloro Foundation
Buenos Aires, Argentina
Living Donor Liver Transplantation

John Goulis, MD
Lecturer in Medicine
Thessaloniki University
Faculty of Medicine
Thessaloniki, Greece
Medical Management of Bleeding Varices

Dirk J. Gouma, MD
Professor of Surgery
Academic Medical Center
University of Amsterdam
Amsterdam, The Netherlands
Palliation of Pancreatic and Periampullary Tumors

Neil A. Halpern, MD, FACP, FCCP, FCCM
Professor of Clinical Medicine and Professor of Medicine in
   Clinical Anesthesiology
Weill Medical College of Cornell University
Chief of Critical Care Medicine Service
Attending Critical Care Medicine Physician and Medical
   Director, Respiratory Therapy
Department of Anesthesiology and Critical Care Medicine
Memorial Sloan-Kettering Cancer Center
New York, New York
Perioperative Critical Care in Hepatobiliary Surgery

Lucy E. Hann, MD
Associate Professor of Radiology
Weill Medical College of Cornell University
Associate Attending Radiologist
Memorial Sloan-Kettering Cancer Center
New York, New York
*Surgical and Radiologic Anatomy of the Liver, Biliary Tract,
   and Pancreas*

Werner Hartwig, MD
Department of General and Visceral Surgery
Ruprecht–Karls University
University of Heidelberg
Heidelberg, Germany
Management of Acute Pancreatitis and Complications

Nancy Heffernan, RN, BSN
Clinical Research Nurse
Hepatobiliary Service
Chief of General Surgery
Memorial Sloan-Kettering Cancer Center
New York, New York
Quality of Life and Hepatobiliary Tumors

William Scott Helton, MD
University of Illinois at Chicago Medical Center
Chicago, Illinois
Preoperative and Postoperative Nutrition in Hepatobiliary Surgery

Alan W. Hemming, MD, MSc
Professor of Surgery
University of Florida College of Medicine
Director of Hepatobiliary Surgery
Shands Hospital at the University of Florida
Gainesville, Florida
Ex Vivo and In Situ Hypothermic Hepatic Resection

J. Michael Henderson, MD, FRCS
Professor of Surgery
Cleveland Clinic Lerner College of Medicine
Vice-Chairman
Division of Surgery
Cleveland Clinic Foundation
Cleveland, Ohio
The Place of Transjugular Intrahepatic Portosystemic Shunting;
Distal Splenorenal Shunt

Choon-Kiat Ho, MD
Consultant Surgeon
Department of General Surgery
Tan Tock Seng Hospital
Singapore
Pancreaticoduodenectomy, Distal Pancreatectomy, Segmental
Pancreatectomy, Total Pancreatectomy, and Transduodenal
Resection of the Papilla of Vater

Philippe Ichai, MD
Paul Brousse Hospital
Villejuif, France
Liver Transplantation in Patients with Fulminant Hepatitis

Hiroshi Imamura, MD, PhD
Lecturer
Division of Hepato-Pancreatic-Biliary Surgery
Department of Surgery
Tokyo University Graduate School of Medicine
Tokyo, Japan
Portal Vein Embolization: Place of Portal Vein Embolization

C. W. Imrie, BSc, MBChB, FRCS
Professor of Upper Gastrointestinal Surgery and Consultant
    Surgeon
Lister Department of Surgery
University of Glasgow
Consultant Surgeon
Royal Infirmary
Glasgow, United Kingdom
Etiology, Pathogenesis, and Diagnostic Assessment of Acute
Pancreatitis

James Jackson, MBBS, MRCP, FRCR
Honorary Senior Lecturer
Imperial College School of Medicine
Consultant Radiologist
Hammersmith Hospital
London, United Kingdom
Angiography

Piotr K. Janicki, MD, PhD
Professor of Anesthesiology
Vice-Chair of Research
Department of Anesthesiology
Penn State College of Medicine
Director of Solid Organ Transplantation Anesthesia
Milton S. Hershey Medical Center
Hershey, Pennsylvania
Liver Transplantation: Anesthesia, Perioperative Management,
and Postoperative Intensive Care

William R. Jarnagin, MD, FACS
Associate Professor of Surgery
Weill Medical College of Cornell University
Assistant Attending Surgeon
Memorial Sloan-Kettering Cancer Center
New York, New York
Intraoperative Diagnosis of Liver, Biliary, and Pancreatic Disease;
Biliary-Enteric Anastomosis; Biliary Stricture and Fistula:
Benign Biliary Strictures; Biliary Stricture and Fistula: Biliary
Fistula; Benign Tumors and Pseudotumors of the Biliary Tract;
Tumors of the Gallbladder; Intrahepatic and Extrahepatic
Biliary Cancer

Roger L. Jenkins, MD
Professor of Surgery
Tufts Medical School
Boston
Chief of Surgery
Division of Hepatobiliary Surgery and Liver Transplantation
Lahey Clinic Medical Center
Burlington, Massachusetts
Early and Late Complications of Liver Transplantation

Stefan Kahl, MD
Associate Professor
Department of Gastroenterology
Otto Von Guericke Medical School
University of Magdeburg
Magdeburg, Germany
Etiology, Pathogenesis, and Diagnosis of Chronic Pancreatitis

Junichi Kamiya, MD
Chief
General Surgery
Aichiken Koseiren Kamo Hospital
Toyota, Japan
Intrahepatic Stones

Cuneyt Kayaalp, MD
Associate Professor of Surgery
Gastrointestinal Surgery Department
Turkey Yuksek Ihtisas Hospital
Ankara, Turkey
Hydatid Cyst of the Liver

Colleen R. Kelly, MD
Fellow in Gastroenterology
Brown Medical School and Rhode Island Hospital
Providence, Rhode Island
Molecular Biology of Liver Carcinogenesis and Hepatitis

Nancy E. Kemeny, MD
Professor of Medicine
Weill Medical College of Cornell University
Attending Physician
Solid Tumor–GI Division
Memorial Sloan-Kettering Cancer Center
New York, New York
Intra-arterial Chemotherapy for Liver Tumors

Allan D. Kirk, MD, PhD
Associate Professor of Surgery
Uniformed Services, University of Health Sciences
F. Edward Hébert School of Medicine
Senior Investigator and Chief
Transplantation Branch
National Institute of Diabetes and Digestive and Kidney
  Diseases
National Institutes of Health
Bethesda, Maryland
Liver and Pancreatic Transplantation Immunobiology

Yuichi Kitagawa, MD
Staff Specialist for Surgery
National Center for Geriatrics and Gerontology
Obu, Japan
Intrahepatic Stones

Jörg Kleeff, MD
Consultant Surgeon
Department of Surgery
University of Heidelberg School of Medicine
Heidelberg, Germany
*Pancreaticoduodenectomy, Distal Pancreatectomy, Segmental
  Pancreatectomy, Total Pancreatectomy, and Transduodenal
  Resection of the Papilla of Vater*

David S. Klimstra, MD
Professor of Pathology and Laboratory Medicine
Weill Medical College of Cornell University
Attending Pathologist and Chief
Surgical Pathology
Memorial Sloan-Kettering Cancer Center
New York, New York
*Tumors of the Bile Ducts—Pathologic Aspects; Pathology
  and Classification of Pancreatic and Ampullary Tumors*

Stuart J. Knechtle, MD
Professor of Surgery and Ray D. Owen Professor of
  Transplantation
University of Wisconsin School of Medicine and Public Health
Madison, Wisconsin
The Place of Portosystemic Shunting

Hiroyuki Kobayashi, MD, PhD
Associate Professor
Department of Pediatric Surgery
Juntendo University School of Medicine
Tokyo, Japan
Biliary Atresia

Anil Kotru, MD, MS, MRCS(UK), FRCS(UK)
Fellow
Department of Organ Transplantation
Washington University in St. Louis School of Medicine
St. Louis, Missouri
*Orthotopic Liver Transplantation; Liver Transplantation in
  Children and Segmental Transplantation*

**Jake E. J. Krige, MBChB, FACS, FCS(SA),
FRCS(Ed)**
Associate Professor of Surgery
University of Cape Town Health Sciences Faculty
Head and Prinicipal Surgeon HPB Surgery Unit
Groote Schuur Hospital
Cape Town, South Africa
*Endoscopic Therapy in the Management of Esophageal Varices:
  Injection Sclerotherapy and Variceal Ligation*

Yonson Ku, MD, PhD
Professor and Chairman
Department of Liver Surgery and Transplantation
Kobe University Graduate School of Medical Sciences
Kobe, Japan
Isolated Hepatic Perfusion for Extensive Liver Cancers

Robert C. Kurtz, MD
Professor of Clinical Medicine
Weill Medical College of Cornell University
Chief
Gastroenterology and Nutrition Service
Department of Medicine
Memorial Sloan-Kettering Cancer Center
New York, New York
Direct Cholangiography

Douglas R. LaBrecque
Professor of Internal Medicine
University of Iowa Roy J. and Lucille A. Carver College
  of Medicine
Attending Surgeon
Department of Internal Medicine
Director of Liver Service
Division of Gastroenterology/Hepatology
University of Iowa Hospital and Clinics
Iowa City, Iowa
Management of Ascites in Cirrhosis and Portal Hypertension

Hauke Lang, MD
Professor of Surgery
University of Essen Medical School
Clinic for General, Gastrointestinal, and Transplantation
  Surgery
University of Essen Medical Center
Essen, Germany
*Liver Resection for Benign Disease and for Liver and Biliary
  Tumors (Computer-Assisted Operation Planning and Virtual
  Liver Resection)*

Michael P. La Quaglia, MD
Professor of Surgery
Weill Medical College of Cornell University
Cheif, Pediatric Surgery
Memorial Sloan-Kettering Cancer Center
New York, New York
Hepatic Tumors in Childhood

Nicholas F. LaRusso, MD
Professor of Medicine and Professor of Biochemistry
  and Molecular Biology
Mayo Clinic College of Medicine
Distinguished Investigator
Mayo Foundation
Rochester, Minnesota
Primary Sclerosing Cholangitis

K. N. Lazaridis, MD
Assistant Professor of Medicine
Mayo Clinic College of Medicine
Rochester, Minnesota
Primary Sclerosing Cholangitis

L. S. Lee, MD
Instructor in Medicine
Harvard Medical School
Associate Physician and Director, Women's GI Health
Brigham and Women's Hospital
Boston, Massachusetts
Stones in the Bile Duct: Endoscopic and Percutaneous Approaches

Riccardo Lencioni, MD
Associate Professor of Radiology
Department of Oncology, Transplants, and Advanced
  Technologies in Medicine
Pisa University School of Medicine
Pisa, Italy
*Ablation of Liver Tumors: Percutaneous Methods for Ablation
  of Hepatic Neoplasms*

**Kui Hin Liau, MBBS, MMed(Surg), FRCS(Edin),
FICS, FAMS(Surg), IHPBA, APHPBA**
Clinical Lecturer
The National University of Singapore,
  Yong Loo Lin School of Medicine
Consultant Surgeon and Chief of Hepatobiliary and Pancreatic
  Surgery
Department of Surgery, Digestive Disease Centre
Tan Tock Seng Medical Centre and Hospital
Singapore
Segment-Oriented Anatomic Liver Resections

Charles J. Lightdale, MD
Professor of Clinical Medicine
Division of Digestive and Liver Diseases
Columbia University College of Physicians and Surgeons
Attending Physician
Department of Medicine New York–Presbyterian
  Hospital/Columbia University Medical Center
New York, New York
Endoscopic Ultrasound: Endoscopic Ultrasound of the Biliary Tract

Keith D. Lillemoe, MD, FACS
Professor of Surgery
Indiana University School of Medicine
Attending Physician
University Hospital
Indianapolis, Indiana
Infections in Hepatic, Biliary, and Pancreatic Surgery

James Lin, MD
Resident
General Surgery
Mount Sinai Medical Center
New York, New York
*Endocrine Tumors of the Pancreas: Clinical Picture, Diagnosis,
  and Therapy*

David C. Linehan, MD
Associate Professor of Surgery
Washington University in St. Louis School of Medicine
Attending Surgeon
Barnes-Jewish Hospital
St. Louis, Missouri
Benign Tumors and Pseudotumors of the Biliary Tract

Pamela A. Lipsett, MD
Program Director, General Surgery
Professor of Surgery, Anesthesia, Critical Care and Nursing
Johns Hopkins University School of Medicine
Co-Director, Surgical Intensive Care Units
Johns Hopkins Hospital
Baltimore, Maryland
Cholangitis

Josep M. Llovett, MD
Associate Professor
Mount Sinai School of Medicine
New York, New York
ICREA Senior Researcher
Barcelona Clinic Liver Cancer Group
Liver Unit
Hospital Clinic
Barcelona, Spain
Hepatocellular Carcinoma

Jeffrey A. Lowell, MD
Professor of Surgery and Pediatrics
Washington University in St. Louis School of Medicine
Chief
Pediatric Transplant Surgery
St. Louis Children's Hospital
Associate Director, Transplant Surgery
Barnes-Jewish Hospital
St. Louis, Missouri
*Liver Transplantation in Children and Segmental
  Transplantation*

David C. Madoff, MD
Assistant Professor
Department of Diagnostic Imaging
Section of Interventional Radiology
The University of Texas M.D. Anderson Cancer
Houston, Texas
*Portal Vein Embolization: Preoperative Portal Vein
  Embolization—A Western Perspective*

Anirban Maitra, MBBS
Associate Professor of Pathology and Oncology
The Sol Goldman Pancreatic Cancer Research Center
Johns Hopkins University School of Medicine
Pathologist
Johns Hopkins Hospital
Baltimore, Maryland
Genetics and Molecular Biology of Pancreatic and Biliary Cancers

Ali W. Majeed, MD, FRCS
Honorary Professor of Surgery,
Sheffield Hallam University
Consultant Surgeon
Royal Hallamshire Hospital
Sheffield, United Kingdom
Clinical Investigation of Hepatopancreatobiliary Disease; Cholecystolithiasis and Stones in the Common Bile Duct: Which Approach, When?

Masatoshi Makuuchi, MD, PhD
Professor and Chairman
Department of Surgery
Hepato-Biliary-Pancreatic Surgery Division and Artificial Organ and Transplantation Division
University of Tokyo Graduate School of Medicine
Tokyo, Japan
Portal Vein Embolization: Place of Portal Vein Embolization

Peter Malfertheiner, MD
Professor of Medicine and Director
Department of Gastroenterology, Hepatology, and Infectious Diseases
Otto von Guericke Medical School
University of Magdeburg
Magdeburg, Germany
Etiology, Pathogenesis, and Diagnosis of Chronic Pancreatitis

Amadeo Marcos, MD
Professor of Surgery
University of Pittsburgh
Pittsburgh
Chief
Division of Transplant Surgery
University of Pittsburgh Medical Center
Pittsburgh, Pennsylvania
Techniques of Liver Replacement

James F. Markmann, MD, PhD
Associate Professor of Surgery
University of Pennsylvania School of Medicine
Director
Pancreas Transplant Program
Hospital of the University of Pennsylvania
Philadelphia, Pennsylvania
Whole Organ Pancreas and Pancreatic Islet Transplantation

Robert T. Mathie, BSc, PhD
Senior Lecturer in Surgical Physiology
Division of Surgery, Anaesthetics, and Intensive Care
Imperial College School of Medicine
Hammersmith Hospital
London, United Kingdom
Liver Blood Flow: Physiology, Measurement, and Clinical Relevance

Priscilla F. McAuliffe, MD, PhD
Resident
General Surgery
University of Florida College of Medicine
Shands Hospital
Gainesville, Florida
Endotoxin and Cytokines in Liver and Biliary Tract Disease

Colin J. McKay, MD, FRCS
Senior Lecturer and Consultant Surgeon
Lister Department of Surgery
Royal Infirmary
Glasgow, United Kingdom
Etiology, Pathogenesis, and Diagnostic Assessment of Acute Pancreatitis

Jose A. Melendez, MD
Associate Chair of Anesthesiology and Associate Professor of Anesthesiology
University of Colorado School of Medicine
Senior Medical Director of Perioperative Services
University of Colorado Hospital
Denver, Colorado
Anesthesia and Postoperative Intensive Care

Lyle L. Moldawer, PhD
Professor and Vice Chairman for Research
Department of Surgery
University of Florida College of Medicine
Gainesville, Florida
Endotoxin and Cytokines in Liver and Biliary Tract Disease

Damian J. Mole, BMedSc, MBChB, MRCS
Research Fellow and Specialist Registrar in General Surgery
Department of Surgery
The Queen's University of Belfast
Belfast, Northern Ireland
Aneurysm and Arteriovenous Fistula of the Liver and Pancreatic Vasculature

Klaus Mönkemüller, MD
Associate Professor
Otto von Guericke Medical School
University of Magdeburg
Director, Molecular Endoscopy
Magdeburg University Hospital
Magdeburg, Germany
Etiology, Pathogenesis, and Diagnosis of Chronic Pancreatitis

Masato Nagino, MD
Associate Professor
Division of Surgical Oncology, Department of Surgery
Nagoya University Graduate School of Medicine
Nagoya, Japan
Intrahepatic and Extrahepatic Biliary Cancer (Perihilar Cholangiocarcinoma with Emphasis on Presurgical Management)

Alexander Nagle, MD
Associate Professor of Surgery
Division of Gastrointestinal/Endocrine Surgery
Northwestern University Feinberg School of Medicine
Chicago, Illinois
Laparoscopic Cholecystectomy and Choledocholithotomy

David M. Nagorney, MD
Professor of Surgery
Mayo Clinic and College of Medicine
Rochester, Minnesota
Bile Duct Cysts in Adults; Surgical Management of Cystic Disease of the Liver; Metastatic Tumors: Hepatic Metastases from Primary Neuroendocrine Tumors

Eric K. Nakakura, MD, PhD
Assistant Professor of Surgery
University of California, San Francisco, School of Medicine
Staff Surgeon
UCSF Comprehensive Cancer Center
San Francisco, California
Periampullary and Pancreatic Tumors: Periampullary and Pancreatic Cancer

Attila Nakeeb, MD
Associate Professor of Surgery
Indiana University School of Medicine
Attending Surgeon
Indiana University Hospital
Indianapolis, Indiana
Biliary Tract Pathophysiology: Pathophysiology of Biliary Tract Obstruction

James Neuberger, DM, FRCP
Honorary Professor of Medicine
University of Birmingham School of Medicine
Consultant Physician, Liver Unit
Queen Elizabeth Hospital
Birmingham, United Kingdom
Liver Transplantation: Indications

Yuji Nimura, MD
Professor and Chairman
Division of Surgical Oncology, Department of Surgery
Nagoya University Graduate School of Medicine
Nagoya, Japan
Intrahepatic Stones; Intrahepatic and Extrahepatic Biliary Cancer (Perihilar Cholangiocarcinoma with Emphasis on Presurgical Management); Liver Resection for Benign Disease and for Liver and Biliary Tumors (Extended Resection for Biliary Tumors— An Alternative Approach)

Quentin M. Nunes
Surgical Registrar
University Hospital
Queens Medical Centre
Nottingham, United Kingdom
Postcholecystectomy Problems

John G. O'Grady, MD, FRCPI
Consultant Hepatologist
Institute of Liver Studies
King's College Hospital
London, United Kingdom
Management of Liver Failure

Risteard O'Laoide, MD
Department of Radiology
St. Vincent's University Hospital
Dublin, Ireland
Radiologic Hepatobiliary Interventions

Kim M. Olthoff, MD
Associate Professor of Surgery
University of Pennsylvania School of Medicine
Director
Liver Transplant Program
Hospital of the University of Pennsylvania
Philadelphia, Pennsylvania
Liver Regeneration

Evan S. Ong, MD, MS
Chief Surgical Resident
University of Illinois at Chicago Medical Center
Chicago, Illinois
Bile Secretion

Marshall J. Orloff, MS, MD
Distinguished Professor of Surgery
University of California, San Diego, School of Medicine
La Jolla
Staff Surgeon
UCSD Medical Center
San Diego, California
Budd-Chiari Syndrome and Veno-occlusive Disease

Mark S. Orloff, MD
Professor of Surgery
University of Rochester School of Medicine
Staff Physician
Division of Organ Transplantation
University of Rochester Medical Center
Rochester, New York
Budd-Chiari Syndrome and Veno-occlusive Disease

Susan L. Orloff, MD
Professor of Surgery and Molecular Microbiology and Immunology
Division of Liver and Pancreas Transplantation
Oregon Health & Science University School of Medicine
Portland, Oregon
Budd-Chiari Syndrome and Veno-occlusive Disease

Valérie Paradis, MD
Professor, Faculty of Medicine,
University Paris VII
Pathologist
Hospital Beaujon
Paris, France
Benign Liver Lesions

Steven D. Passik, PhD
Associate Professor of Psychiatry
Weill Medical College of Cornell University
Associate Attending Psychologist
Department of Psychiatry and Behavioral Sciences
Memorial Sloan-Kettering Cancer Center
New York, New York
Quality of Life and Hepatobiliary Tumors

Heinz-Otto Peitgen, PhD
President
MeVis—Center for Medical Diagnostic Systems and
   Visualization
Director
CeVis—Center for Complex Systems and Visualization
University of Bremen
Bremen, Germany
*Liver Resection for Benign Disease and for Liver and Biliary
   Tumors (Computer-Assisted Operation Planning and Virtual
   Liver Resection)*

Venu Pillarisetty, MD
General Surgery Resident
University of Massachusetts Medical School
Worcester, Massachusetts
Liver Immunology

C. Wright Pinson, MD, MBA
Chief Medical Officer, Associate Vice-Chancellor Clinical
   Affairs and Surgical Director
Vanderbilt Transplant Center
Vanderbilt University Hospital
Nashville, Tennessee
The Mesocaval Shunt: Technique

Henry A. Pitt, MD
Professor of Surgery and Vice Chairman for Academic Affairs
Indiana University School of Medicine
Attending Surgeon
Indiana University Hospital
Indianapolis, Indiana
*Biliary Tract Pathophysiology: Pathophysiology of Biliary Tract
   Obstruction; Cholangitis*

James J. Pomposelli, MD, PhD
Associate Professor of Surgery
Senior Staff Surgeon
Tufts Medical School
Boston
Division of Hepatobiliary and Liver Transplantation Surgery
Lahey Clinic Medical Center
Burlington, Massachusetts
Early and Late Complications of Liver Transplantation

Ronnie T. Poon, MBBS, MS
Associate Professor
Division of Hepatobiliary and Pancreatic Surgery
University of Hong Kong Medical Center
Associate Professor
Queen Mary Hospital
Hong Kong, China
Liver Resection in Cirrhosis of the Liver

Richard A. Prinz, MD
Helen Shedd Keith Professor and Chairman
Department of General Surgery
Rush Medical College
Chairman
Department of General Surgery
Rush University Medical Center
Chicago, Illinois
*Endocrine Tumors of the Pancreas: Clinical Picture, Diagnosis,
   and Therapy*

Florencia G. Que, MD
Associate Professor of Surgery
Mayo Clinic College of Medicine
Consultant
Department of Surgery
Mayo Clinic
Rochester, Minnesota
*Metastatic Tumors: Hepatic Metastases from Primary
   Neuroendocrine Tumors*

Layton F. Rikkers, MD
A. R. Curreri Professor of Surgery
Chairman
Department of Surgery
University of Wisconsin School of Medicine and Public Health
Madison, Wisconsin
The Place of Portosystemic Shunting

Brian J. Rowlands, MD, FRCS, FACS
Professor of Surgery
Section of Surgery
University Hospital, Queen's Medical Centre
Nottingham, England
Postcholecystectomy Problems

Margarita Sala, MD
Research Fellow
Barcelona Clinic
Liver Cancer Group, Liver Unit
Hospital Clinic
Barcelona, Spain
Hepatocellular Carcinoma

Pierre F. Saldinger, MD, FACS
Associate Professor of Clinical Surgery
New York Medical College
Valhalla, New York
Chairman
Department of Surgery
Carmen and Peter Buck Chair in Surgical Oncology
Danbury Hospital
Danbury, Connecticut
*The Natural History of Gallstones and Asymptomatic Gallstones;
Intra-arterial Chemotherapy for Liver Tumors*

Ali Salim, MS, MD
Assistant Professor of Surgery
Keck School of Medicine of USC
Staff Surgeon
Los Angeles County–USC Medical Center
Los Angeles, California
*Liver, Biliary, and Pancreatic Injury: Liver and Bile Duct Injury;
Liver, Biliary Tract, and Pancreatic Injury: Pancreatic Injury*

Leonard B. Saltz, MD
Professor of Medicine
Weill Medical College of Cornell University
Attending Physician
Memorial Sloan-Kettering Cancer Center
New York, New York
*Chemotherapy of Liver Tumors: Systemic Therapy for
Hepatocellular Carcinoma; Chemotherapy of Liver Tumors:
Systemic Therapy for Metastatic Colorectal Cancer*

Dimitrios N. Samonakis, MD
Clinical Research Fellow
Royal Free Hospital
London, United Kingdom
Medical Management of Bleeding Varices

Didier Samuel, MD
Professor of Hepatology
Paul Brousse Hospital
Villejuif, France
Liver Transplantation in Patients with Fulminant Hepatitis

Tsuyoshi Sano, MD, PhD
Chief
Department of Surgery
Ogaki Municipal Hospital
Ogaki-City, Japan
*Liver Resection for Benign Disease and for Liver and Biliary
Tumors: Extended Resection for Biliary Tumors —
An Alternative Approach*

Juan M. Sarmiento, MD
Assistant Professor of Surgery
Emory University School of Medicine Attending
Winship Cancer Institute and Veterans Affairs Medical Center
Atlanta, Georgia
Surgical Management of Cystic Disease of the Liver

O. Scatton, MD
Professor and Chairman
Department of Digestive and Transplant Surgery
Hospital Beaujon
Paris, France
Vascular Isolation Techniques in Liver Resection

Mark Schattner, MD
Assistant Professor of Surgery
Weill Medical College of Cornell University
Assistant Clinical Member and Assistant Attending Physician
Department of Medicine
Memorial Hospital for Cancer and Allied Diseases
New York, New York
Endoscopic Ultrasound: Endoscopic Ultrasound of the Pancreas

Christian Max Schmidt, MD, PhD, MBA, FACS
Assistant Professor of Surgery, Biochemistry and
Molecular Biology
Indiana University School of Medicine
Attending Physician
University Hospital Clarian Health Care System
Indianapolis, Indiana
Infections in Hepatic, Biliary, and Pancreatic Surgery

Richard D. Schulick, MD
Associate Professor of Surgery, Oncology, and Gynecology
and Obstetrics
Chief
Cameron Division of Surgical Oncology
John L. Cameron Endowed Chair in Surgery
Johns Hopkins Medical Institutions
Baltimore, Maryland
Assessment of Liver Function in the Surgical Patient

Lawrence H. Schwartz, MD
Vice Chairman for Technology Development
Director
Department of Radiology
Memorial Sloan-Kettering Cancer Center
New York, New York
*Magnetic Resonance Imaging of the Liver, Biliary Tract,
and Pancreas*

Myron E. Schwartz, MD
Professor of Surgery
Department of Magnetic Resonance Imaging
Mount Sinai School of Medicine
Director of Surgical Oncology and Associate Director of
Liver Transplantation
Department of Surgery
Mount Sinai Hospital
New York, New York
Living Donor Liver Transplantation

Ross W. Shepherd, MD, FRACP, FRCP
Professor of Pediatrics
Washington University in St. Louis School of Medicine
Medical Director, Liver Program
St. Louis Children's Hospital
St. Louis, Missouri
Portal Hypertension in Children

Nasir H. Siddiqi, MD
Instructor of Radiology
Harvard Medical School
Department of Radiology
Attending Interventional Radiologist
Brigham and Women's Hospital
Boston, Massachusetts
Radiologic Hepatobiliary Interventions

Samuel H. Sigal, MD
Assistant Professor
Center for Liver Disease and Transplantation
Division of Gastroenterology and Hepatology
Weill Medical College of Cornell University
Assistant Attending Physician
New York-Presbyterian Hospital and Weill Cornell
    Medical Center
New York, New York
Perioperative Critical Care in Hepatobiliary Surgery

C. Smajda, MD, PhD
Professor of Digestive Surgery
Department of Digestive Surgery
University of Paris
Hospital Antoine Béclère
Clamart, France
Operative Devascularization and Esophageal Transection

Aaron J. Small, BS
Medical Student (MMS III)
Mayo Clinic College of Medicine
Rochester, Minnesota
Primary Sclerosing Cholangitis

Andrew M. Smith, BSc, DM, FRCS
Honorary Senior Lecturer
Leeds University
Consultant Pancreatic and Hepatobiliary Surgeon
St. James' University Hospital
Leeds, United Kingdom
The Place of Transjugular Intrahepatic Portosystemic Shunting

Nib Soehendra, MD
Professor of Surgery
University of Hamburg Faculty of Medicine
Director
Department of Interdisciplinary Endoscopy
University Hospital Hamburg
Hamburg, Germany
Interventional Endoscopy: Technical Aspects

Nathaniel J. Soper, MD
Director
Minimally Invasive Surgery
Chief
Division of Gastrointestinal/Endocrine Surgery
Northwestern University Feinberg School of Medicine
Chicago, Illinois
Laparoscopic Cholecystectomy and Choledocholithotomy

Thomas E. Starzl, MD
Professor of Surgery
University of Pittsburgh Medical Center
Director Emeritus
Thomas E. Starzl Transplantation Institute
Pittsburgh, Pennsylvania
Techniques of Liver Replacement

Michael Steer, MD
Professor of Surgery, Anatomy, and Cellular Biology
Tufts University School of Medicine
Emeritus Professor of Surgery
Harvard Medical School
Chief
General Surgery and Associate Surgeon-in-Chief
Tufts–New England Medical Center
Boston, Massachusetts
Pancreatic Physiology and Functional Assessment

Peter D. Stevens, MD
Assistant Professor of Clinical Medicine
Columbia University College of Physicians and Surgeons
Chief of Endoscopy
New York–Presbyterian Hospital—Columbia University
    Medical Center
New York, New York
Endoscopic Ultrasound: Endoscopic Ultrasound of the Biliary Tract

Russell W. Strong, MBBS, FRCS, FRACS, FACS, FRACDS
Emeritus Professor of Surgery
Faculty of Medicine
University of Queensland
Emeritus Consultant Surgeon
Princess Alexandra Hospital
Brisbane, Australia
Pyogenic Liver Abscess

Richard S. Stubbs, MD, FRCS, FRACS
Director
The Wakefield Clinic
Wakefield Hospital
Wellington, New Zealand
*Radiotherapy of Liver Tumors: Selective Internal Radiation
    Therapy for Liver Tumors*

Tadatoshi Takayama, MD, PhD
Professor
Department of Digestive Surgery
Nihon University School of Medicine
Tokyo, Japan
Portal Vein Embolization: Place of Portal Vein Embolization

Rebecca Taylor, MD
Clinical Fellow
Memorial Sloan-Kettering Cancer Center
New York, New York
*Metastatic Tumors: Surgical Treatment of Hepatic Metastases from
    Colorectal Cancer*

Jerrold Teitcher, MD
Associate Professor of Clinical Radiology
Weill Medical College of Cornell University
Attending Radiologist
Memorial Hospital for Cancer and Allied Diseases
New York, New York
Computed Tomography of the Liver, Biliary Tract, and Pancreas

Onno T. Terpstra, MD, PhD, FRCS
Professor of Surgery
Leiden University Medical Center
Leiden, The Netherlands
Auxiliary Liver Transplantation

Sylvain Terraz, MD
Clinical Instructor
Department of Radiology
University of Geneva Medical School
Staff Radiologist
Department of Diagnostic and Interventional Radiology
Geneva University Hospital
Geneva, Switzerland
Percutaneous Approaches to the Treatment of Gallbladder Disease

Philip G. Thomas, MBBS, MS, FACS
Assistant Professor of Surgery
University of Texas Medical Branch
Transplant Surgeon
University of Texas Medical Branch Health Care and Affiliated
    Hospitals
Galveston, Texas
Amebiasis and Other Parasitic Infections

William E.G. Thomas, MS, FRCS
Honorary Senior Lecturer in Surgery
Sheffield University Medical School
Consultant Surgeon and Clinical Director of Surgery
Sheffield Teaching Hospitals, NHS Foundation Trust
Member of Council
Royal College of Surgeons of England
Sheffield, United Kingdom,
Clinical Investigation of Hepatopancreatobiliary Disease

James Toouli, MBBS, PhD, FRACS
Professor of Surgery
Flinders University Faculty of Medicine
Adelaide
Surgeon, Flinders Medical Centre
Bedford Park
South Australia, Australia
*Biliary Tract Pathophysiology: Function of the Biliary Tract and
    Factors in the Production of Biliary Pain*

Christos K. Triantos, MD
Clinical Research Fellow
Royal Free Hospital
London, United Kingdom
Medical Management of Bleeding Varices

Jennifer F. Tseng, MD
Assistant Professor of Surgery
University of Massachusetts Medical School
Surgeon
UMass Memorial Medical Center
Worcester, Massachusetts
*Periampullary and Pancreatic Tumors: Cystic Neoplasms
    of the Pancreas*

Eric Van Sonnenberg, MD
Chairman and Professor of Radiology
St. Joseph's Hospital and Medical Center
Phoenix, Arizona
Radiologic Hepatobiliary Interventions

Maria Varela, MD
Barcelona Clinic Liver Cancer Group
Liver Unit
Hospital Clinic
Barcelona, Spain
Liver Transplantation for Tumors

Deepak Varma, MD
Professor and Chairman
Department of Digestive and Transplant Surgery
Hospital Beaujon
Paris, France
Vascular Isolation Techniques in Liver Resection

Jean-Nicholas Vauthey, MD
Professor and Chief
Liver Service
Department of Surgical Oncology
The University of Texas M.D. Anderson Cancer Center
Houston, Texas
*Portal Vein Embolization: Preoperative Portal Vein
    Embolization—A Western Perspective*

Elizabeth C. Verna, MD
Internal Medicine Resident
New York–Presbyterian Hospital
New York, New York
*Endoscopic Ultrasound: Endoscopic Ultrasound of the Biliary
    Tract*

V. Vilgrain, MD
Professor of Radiology
Faculty of Medicine
University of Paris VII
Head
Department of Radiology
Hospital Beaujon
Paris, France
*Nonparasitic Cystic Diseases of the Liver and Intrahepatic Biliary
    Tree; Benign Liver Lesions*

Louis Voigt, MD, FCCP
Assistant Professor of Medicine
Weill Medical College of Cornell University
Assitant Attending Physician
Critical Care Medicine
Department of Anesthesiology and Critical Care Medicine
Memorial Sloan-Kettering Cancer Center
New York, New York
Perioperative Critical Care in Hepatobiliary Surgery

Raquel Wagman, MD
Attending Radiation Oncologist
St. Barnabas Medical Center
Livingston, New Jersey
*Radiotherapy of Liver Tumors: External-Beam Radiation Therapy
for Primary Hepatocellular Carcinoma and Biliary Disease*

Jack R. Wands, MD
Jeffrey and Kimberly Greenberg–Artemis and Martha
Joukowsky Professor in Gastroenterology and Professor of
Medical Science
Brown Medical School
Director
Division of Gastroenterology and Liver Research Center
Rhode Island Hospital
Providence, Rhode Island
Molecular Biology of Liver Carcinogenesis and Hepatitis

Han Lin Wang, MD, PhD
Associate Professor of Pathology
Washington University in St. Louis School of Medicine
St. Louis, Missouri
Cirrhosis and Portal Hypertension: Pathologic Aspects

Andrew L. Warshaw, MD
W. Gerald Austen Professor of Surgery
Harvard Medical School
Surgeon-in-Chief
Massachusetts General Hospital
Boston, Massachusetts
*Periampullary and Pancreatic Tumors: Cystic Neoplasms
of the Pancreas*

Kaare J. Weber, MD
Assistant Professor of Surgery
Mount Sinai School of Medicine
Surgeon
Mount Sinai Medical Center
New York, New York
*Endocrine Tumors of the Pancreas: Clinical Picture, Diagnosis,
and Therapy*

Sharon Weber, MD
Associate Professor
Department of Surgery
University of Wisconsin School of Medicine and Public Health
Chief of Surgery
William S. Middleton Veterans' Hospital
Madison, Wisconsin
Cholecystitis

Jürgen Weitz, MD, PhD
Head
Section of Surgical Oncology
Department of Surgery
University of Heidelberg School of Medicine
Heidelberg, Germany
Metastatic Tumors: Noncolorectal Non-neuroendocrine Metastases

Jens Werner, MD
Associate Professor
Department of General and Visceral Surgery
Ruprecht-Karls University of Heidelberg
Heidelberg, Germany
Management of Acute Pancreatitis and Complications

Anthony M. Wheatley, PhD
Professor of Physiology
University of Otago School of Medical Sciences
Dunedin, New Zealand
*Liver Blood Flow: Physiology, Measurement, and Clinical
Relevance*

Corinne Winston, MD
Assistant Professor of Radiology
Weill Medical College of Cornell University
Associate Attending Radiologist
Memorial Hospital for Cancer and Allied Diseases
New York, New York
Computed Tomography of the Liver, Biliary Tract, and Pancreas

Joseph J. Wizorek, MD
Chief Resident
Department of Surgery
Washington University in St. Louis School of Medicine
St. Louis, Missouri
Liver Transplantation in Children and Segmental Transplantation

John Wong, PhD
Professor and Chair
Department of Surgery
The University of Hong Kong, Faculty of Medicine
Head
Department of Surgery
University of Hong Kong Medical Centre
Queen Mary Hospital
Hong Kong, China
Recurrent Pyogenic Cholangitis

Charles J. Yeo, MD, FACS
Samuel D. Gross Professor and Chair
Department of Surgery
Jefferson Medical College of Thomas Jefferson University
Philadelphia
Chair of Surgery
Thomas Jefferson University and Hospital,
Philadelphia, Pennsylvania
*Genetics and Molecular Biology of Pancreatic and Biliary
Cancers; Periampullary and Pancreatic Tumors: Periampullary
and Pancreatic Cancer*

Chang Jin Yoon, MD, PhD
Assistant Professor of Radiology
Seoul National University College of Medicine
Seoul
Radiologist
Seoul National University Bundang Hospital
Sungnam, Korea
Embolization of Liver Tumors

Arthur Zimmerman, MD
Professor of Pathology
Institute of Pathology
University of Berne
Berne, Switzerland
Tumors of the Liver—Pathologic Aspects

Theresa G. Zogakis, MD
Assistant Professor of Surgery
The University of Texas Southwestern Medical School
Dallas, Texas
Ablation of Liver Tumors: Radiofrequency Thermal Ablation of Liver Tumors

Preface

The title of this text, *Surgery of the Liver, Biliary Tract, and Pancreas*, reflects the biggest change since the third edition of *Surgery of the Liver and Biliary Tract*, namely, the inclusion of pancreatic disease. However, there are other major changes—the principal of which is that I have now invited a number of associate editors to work with me in order to cover, in comprehensive fashion, the extraordinary accumulation of knowledge and advances that have taken place since the publication of the last edition.

The associate editors are all highly experienced, knowledgeable physicians in the field. Four work at Memorial Sloan-Kettering Cancer Center in New York. Dr. Lucy Hann has been involved with liver, hepatobiliary, and pancreatic radiology for many years and is one of the leading practitioners of diagnostic ultrasound in the United States. Dr. William Jarnagin has developed a national and international reputation in the surgical management of diseases of the biliary tract, including the gallbladder. Dr. Ronald DeMatteo is especially interested in the management of cancers of the liver and biliary tract, and he has a fine appreciation of the pathophysiology as well as the molecular and genetic determinants of hepatobiliary and pancreatic neoplasms. Dr. Michael D'Angelica has extensively edited the DVD that is an important accompaniment to the text. Dr. Jacques Belghiti, of Paris, France, is one of the leading hepatobiliary surgeons in the world and has made major recent contributions to the field. Dr. William Chapman, from St. Louis, Missouri, has a firm grounding in hepatobiliary disease and liver transplantation in particular. As one of the outstanding surgeons worldwide in the management of pancreatic disease, Dr. Markus Büchler, of Heidelberg, Germany, graciously accepted my invitation to undertake the difficult task of introducing a comprehensive section on diseases of the pancreas.

My colleagues and I have attempted to maintain the general format of covering all surgical aspects of the management of hepatobiliary and pancreatic disorders. The contributors are specialists in their own fields and have been asked to discuss the subject from the point of view of surgical management and to relate their views to the opinions of others. In many instances, authors with conflicting opinions have been chosen to allow the reader to assess the views of enthusiasts with different approaches to the same problem. In some instances, deliberate overlap between chapters has been encouraged: first, to allow each contribution to be an encapsulated account that stands on its own for the reader who wishes to consult the book as a reference and second, to allow the display of different nuances of approach to particularly difficult problems.

In addition to considering the pancreas in great detail, there have been very extensive modifications and additions throughout this text. There is a new chapter on the historical aspects of hepatobiliary and pancreatic surgery. Some chapters have been eliminated entirely, and others have been combined. An important feature is the inclusion of considerable technical detail so that major sections of this book can be used, in conjunction with the DVD, as an atlas of technique. All previous communications have been updated to take into account recent advances in the biologic understanding of disease processes and the newer diagnostic and therapeutic modalities.

The initial section of the book is devoted to the applied anatomy of the liver and biliary tract, including its radiologic demonstration. Throughout this edition, the anatomic contributions of Claude Couinaud are recognized and the liver anatomy and nomenclature of the various operative approaches are generally based on his descriptions.

Normal anatomy and physiology, together with their variations in the disease state, and reference to the molecular and genetic basis of liver regeneration and hepatobiliary disease are covered. Diagnostic approaches to hepatobiliary and pancreatic disease are extensively discussed, and important new techniques—both in diagnostic radiology and interventional radiologic and endoscopic techniques—are described in detail and compared with surgical approaches.

There are detailed discussions and illustrations of the operative approaches to biliary disease, with special emphasis on the management of gallstones, biliary strictures and fistulae, and biliary, ampullary, and pancreatic cancers. Hepatic and biliary infections due to pyogenic organisms and parasitic infestations are detailed. Hepatic and biliary cysts—and their surgical management—are fully described, as is the management of injuries to the liver and pancreas and associated biliary ducts, arteries, and veins. In particular, the entire section covering biliary tumors and primary and secondary hepatic tumors has been updated. The differences of approach in the Western World and Asia are extensively highlighted, with particular recognition of the major contribution of Japanese surgeons to the field of biliary cancer. In addition, there is a thorough description of the anatomy and of the diseases of the pancreas—including acute and chronic pancreatitis—as well as of pancreatic tumors.

In recent years, there has been extraordinary refinement in the operative techniques pertaining to hepatic, biliary, and pancreatic resection, and these are covered in special detail. Newly introduced approaches and the importance of conserving hepatic and pancreatic parenchyma is emphasized. The importance of minimizing blood loss in major liver resection and performing ultrasonographically guided operations is detailed.

Cirrhosis of the liver and the management of portal hypertension—including operative descriptive techniques for the control of variceal hemorrhage—are discussed extensively. Recent advances such as the role of radiologic intervention are included. The management of liver failure and the treatment of ascites and fulminant hepatic failure are covered. The entire section on liver transplantation and its complications and results has been expanded to cover new developments in the field.

In short, I have attempted to include all aspects of the anatomy, pathology, diagnosis, and surgically related therapeutic approaches to hepatobiliary and pancreatic disorders. The aim is to provide a text that will be of value not only to the trainee surgeon and the established surgeon but also to other physicians in related disciplines who are concerned with the management of diseases of the liver, biliary tract, and pancreas. I and my coauthors have attempted to enlist new contributors throughout the book, to give latitude to conflicting opinions and yet provide guidance to allow the reader to form an individual approach based on contemporary attitudes.

I express my sincere thanks to the coeditors who have collaborated with me in this endeavor and who join me in the hope that this book will prove of value not only as an account of the current "state of the art" in the surgical aspects of hepatobiliary and pancreatic disease but also as a stimulus to those interested in further study of the many unresolved problems that require investigation.

This book, in its fourth edition, has seen the establishment and maturation of the specialty of hepatobiliary and pancreatic surgery. The four editions span forty years of my personal endeavor in the subject, and I dedicate this work to the specialty and to the many excellent physicians who have contributed and continue to work in the field.

L.H. BLUMGART
New York, 2006

Acknowledgments

We are deeply grateful to all who have contributed to this publication. Our colleagues in surgery, internal medicine, radiology, gastroenterology, pathology, and anesthesiology all responded enthusiastically and conveyed the weight of their experience. We are especially grateful to them for adding the spice of differing opinion and the aroma of international practice to the basic flavor of this work. Particular thanks are due to the members of our staff in New York, St. Louis, Heidelberg, and Paris who have contributed and assisted in the preparation of this work.

In the first edition, the illustrative work was of a uniform character, and nearly all of the drawings were done by Mr. Doig Simmonds, medical illustrator at the Royal Postgraduate Medical School at Hammersmith Hospital, London. However, many of these illustrations have now been extensively modified and there are many new illustrations by Mr. Philip Wilson of London, who has once again produced a remarkable series of drawings.

Editorial assistance has been carried out by Ms. Maria Reyes, who has very efficiently undertaken the major task of coordinating with the publishers, the artists, and ourselves. We are extremely grateful to her for this major task, which she has accomplished with great expertise.

Finally, our thanks and appreciation is due to our esteemed publisher, Elsevier.

L. H. BLUMGART, New York
J. BELGHITI, Paris
M. W. BÜCHLER, Heidelberg
W. C. CHAPMAN, St. Louis
M. D'ANGELICA, New York
R. P. DEMATTEO, New York
L. E. HANN, New York
W. R. JARNAGIN, New York

Contents

SECTION 16:
LIVER AND PANCREATIC TRANSPLANTATION

Liver and Biliary Infection and Infestation

Cholangitis

P. A. LIPSETT AND H. A. PITT

Acute cholangitis in its most severe form is a life-threatening infection originating in the biliary tree. In 1877, Charcot first described the triad of jaundice, fever, and right upper quadrant pain that is the hallmark of cholangitis. Charcot conceived that "stagnant bile" caused cholangitis, and that gallstones and benign and malignant strictures were most often the underlying causes of biliary obstruction. The biliary tree is normally sterile, but biliary pathology is often associated with secondary bacterial colonization. The combination of obstruction and colonization leads to cholangitis, but neither obstruction nor colonization by itself is sufficient to cause disease.

Patients with acute cholangitis present with highly variable degrees of illness. Some patients are mildly ill, whereas a few present with hypotension and mental obtundation. About 5% of all patients with acute cholangitis present in shock. The presence or degree of purulence in bile does not define the severity of disease. The descriptive term of *suppurative cholangitis* is probably not helpful, and the use of the term *toxic cholangitis* is best.

Currently, the treatment of acute cholangitis is primarily supportive, with intravenous hydration and antibiotics being the mainstays. More recent studies have identified high-risk patients warranting early biliary decompression. Today, standard indications that warrant emergent biliary decompression include septic shock, clinical deterioration, and failure to improve with hydration and antibiotics. This chapter discusses the pathophysiology, etiology, clinical presentation, laboratory evaluation, and radiologic evaluation of the spectrum of patients with acute cholangitis. Treatment options are presented along with outcome data in patients with and without the toxic form of cholangitis.

PATHOPHYSIOLOGY

Acute cholangitis results from the combination of biliary tract obstruction and infection and does not result from obstruction without infection or from infection without obstruction (Fig. 58.1). In the early stages of biliary obstruction, normal hepatic bile secretion continues, and an increase in intraductal pressure ensues. As obstruction continues, biliary pressures approach the secretory pressure of bile (25-30 cm H_2O) (Jacobson et al, 1962). Normally, the biliary tree is sterile, in part because of the continuing flow of bile. When the biliary tree is obstructed, and flow is diminished, any bacteria present have time to proliferate. Although the exact mechanism of bacteremia is still unknown, systemic bacteremia can result from increased intrabiliary pressure when biliary bacteria reflux into hepatic veins and perihepatic lymphatics (Jacobson et al, 1962). In addition, the systemic release of inflammatory mediators, such as endotoxin, interleukin (IL)-1, and IL-6, can produce profound hemodynamic effects in the toxic form of cholangitis

(Kanazawa et al, 1997). In a rat model, acute obstructive cholangitis resulted in nuclear factor κB activation, release of proinflammatory cytokines, and mulitorgan dysfunction (Tu et al, 2003). Gallstones, parasites, and other foreign bodies all can cause obstruction and act as a nidus for increased bacterial overgrowth (Kaufman et al, 1989).

Obstruction

Obstruction to bile flow is an important component in the development of acute cholangitis. With normal conditions, biliary ductal pressures usually range from 7 to 14 cm H_2O (Mallet-Guy, 1952). Intraductal pressure can increase rapidly to 20 to 30 cm H_2O, however, with either partial or complete obstruction (Mallet-Guy, 1952). At biliary pressures greater than 15 cm H_2O, systemic reflux of radiolabeled biliary bacteria occurs (Jacobson et al, 1962). The reticuloendothelial system within the liver normally kills most bacteria that enter the liver, with an estimated 10% entering the systemic circulation. In a canine model, Huang and colleagues (1969) showed that blood cultures were sterile when the biliary pressure was less than 20 cm H_2O, but became positive when intraductal pressure exceeded 25 cm H_2O. Similarly, infected bile (10^5 organisms) does not produce bacteremia and illness unless biliary obstruction also is present (Flemma et al, 1967).

Csendes and coworkers (1988) documented that patients with toxic acute cholangitis had intrabiliary ductal pressures that were significantly higher than values in patients with gallstones but without common duct stones and patients with common duct stones but without cholangitis. Of patients, 24 had pressures greater than 20 cm H_2O, and 9 with pressures greater than 30 cm H_2O also had the absence of bilirubin, suggesting the absence of biliary secretion into the bile duct. Several studies have shown that the cause of obstruction (i.e., malignant versus benign) influences the development and outcome of cholangitis (Shinagawa et al, 1997; Thompson J, et al, 1994, Thompson JE et al, 1990). Patients with malignant biliary obstruction often have a high-grade obstruction, but may not have infected bile, whereas patients with gallstones may have a partial obstruction to bile flow, but more often have colonized bile.

The systemic signs of clinical cholangitis—fever, chills, and occasionally mental confusion and hypotension—are caused by bacterial toxin and inflammatory mediator release via cholangiolymphatics or cholangiovenous pathways. Patients with toxic cholangitis usually have systemic endotoxemia and high serum levels of tumor necrosis factor even in the absence of documented bacteremia (Kanazawa et al, 1997; Lau et al, 1996). Survival of patients with acute toxic cholangitis has been correlated with serum levels of nuclear factor κB, with higher levels being associated with nonsurvival (Gong et al, 2002).

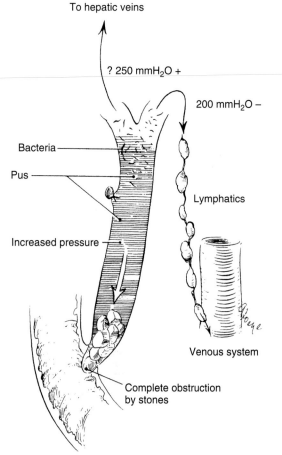

To hepatic veins

? 250 mmH₂O +

200 mmH₂O –

Bacteria

Pus

Lymphatics

Increased pressure

Venous system

Complete obstruction
by stones

Fig. 58.1. Cholangitis is caused by the combination of biliary obstruction, often related to distally impacted stones, and bactibilia. Bacteria reflux into the hepatic veins and perihepatic lymphatics, resulting in systemic bacteremia. (From Pitt HA, Longmire WP, 1980: Suppurative cholangitis. In Hardy JM [ed]: Critical Surgical Illness, 2nd ed. Philadelphia, Saunders, p. 380.)

Bacteria

In normal patients, the gallbladder and biliary tree are sterile (Csendes et al, 1975). In the presence of gallstones within the gallbladder or the biliary tree, positive cultures are seen in 15% to 50% and 70% to 90%, respectively (Lipsett & Pitt, 1990). Among patients with complete ductal obstruction secondary to malignancy, only 25% to 40% have positive cultures. In a study of patients with proximal cholangiocarcinoma, intraoperative bile cultures in patients who did not undergo preoperative endoscopic retrograde cholangiopancreatography (ERCP) were positive in 7 (37%) of 19 patients compared with 23 (55%) of 42 patients who did undergo preoperative ERCP. If a preoperative bile stent had not been placed, 14% of bile cultures were positive, whereas 69% of bile cultures were positive when a preoperative stent had been placed (Hochwald et al, 1999). The method of biliary decompression, percutaneous transhepatic cholangiography (65% positive) versus ERCP (100% positive), also made a difference in the presence of bactibilia. Advancing age also increases the likelihood of a positive bile culture; elderly patients frequently present with the more toxic form of cholangitis (Sugiyama & Atomi, 1997).

The organisms most often isolated (Table 58.1) are the gram-negative aerobes *Escherichia coli* and *Klebsiella pneumoniae*,

Table 58.1 Presentation of Biliary Bacteriology at Johns Hopkins Hospital

	PERCENTAGE OF PATIENTS		
Bile Culture	1976-1978 (n = 40)	1983-1985 (n = 48)	1986-1989 (n = 96)
Escherichia coli	55	55	39
Klebsiella spp.	41	32	54
Enterococcus spp.	41	55	34
Bacteroides spp.	28	9	15
Enterobacter spp.	0	33	34
Pseudomonas spp.	0	23	24

gram-positive enterococci, and the gram-negative anaerobe *Bacteroides fragilis* (Edlund et al, 1959; Muller et al, 1987; Pitt et al, 1983; Stewart et al, 1988). In a study of patients with brown pigment stones and paired bile cultures, 91% of bile and 99% of stone samples yielded positive cultures, with a total of 151 and 149 bacteria isolated from bile and stones, respectively (Leung et al, 2001). In 22 patients (33%), the bacteria isolated from the paired bile and stone samples were different. Even when bacteria were similar, they often had differing antibiotic sensitivities. Both observations suggest that time was a factor in the evolution of bacterial flora in stones and bile cultures. In 30% to 50% of patients, more than two organisms are present (Keighley et al, 1975, 1976; Lee et al, 1992; O'Connor et al, 1981; Pitt et al, 1982). In some series, anaerobes are present in 25% to 30% of patients, but these bacteria are rarely an isolated pathogen (Keighley et al, 1976; Lee et al, 1992; Pitt et al, 1982). Not only is the presence or absence of bacteria in the biliary tree important, but also the absolute concentration of organisms in the biliary tree is greater in patients with acute cholangitis than in patients with common duct stones or with gallstones (Csendes et al, 1996). More than 10^5 organisms are seen in 0% of normal patients, 3% of patients with symptomatic gallstones, 36% of patients with common duct stones but without cholangitis, and 85% of patients with acute cholangitis (Csendes et al, 1996).

The origin of biliary bacteria is unknown. Possible explanations include ascending infection from the duodenum, lymphatic spread, vascular spread from portal venous or hepatic arterial flow, and seeding from a chronically infected gallbladder (Scott & Kahn, 1967). Because the bacteriology of the duodenum and infected bile are similar, the ascending infection theory is plausible. The sphincter of Oddi normally prevents bacterial reflux into bile, however. Dineen (1964) showed that lymphatic flow is caudad from the liver to the duodenum; this mechanism of infection is unlikely. Hepatic arterial infection and resulting hepatic abscesses do occur, but in only a small percentage of patients with cholangitis. The degree of biliary tract obstruction and severity of disease is related to the proportion of patients with positive microorganisms in the hepatic parenchyma (Csendes et al, 1995). In this study, no correlation was observed between altered hepatic histology and the presence of bacteria in bile; however, all cases of acute cholangitis had bactibilia (Csendes et al, 1995).

Portal venous bacteremia results in bacterial infection, and the concentration of bacteria is related to the degree of biliary obstruction (Dineen, 1964). Portal venous bacteremia has been shown in patients with cholangiohepatitis. Not all patients with portal venous bacteremia are ill, however. One possible explanation for this observation is that the bacteria, its by-products, and inflammatory mediators are destroyed in the liver by an efficient hepatic reticuloendothelial system, which eliminates bacteria by excretion into the biliary tree and subsequent elimination in stool. The rate of decrease of bilirubin after percutaneous drainage correlates directly with IL-6 levels in bile, suggesting that this potent inflammatory mediator may have a role in maintaining illness after drainage (Akiyama et al, 1998; Kanazawa et al, 1997). Bile endotoxin levels decreased more slowly after percutaneous transhepatic biliary drainage in patients with acute cholangitis compared with patients with a remote history of cholangitis. In addition, these authors showed that both bile and serum levels of IL-1 receptor antagonist, IL-6, and IL-8 were higher in patients with acute cholangitis and even higher in patients with severe disease. Five hours after percutaneous transhepatic biliary drainage, serum IL-6 and biliary endotoxin levels were directly correlated, suggesting a direct role of biliary decompression in diminishing intraductal biliary pressure and systemic cytokine levels.

In a rat model (Raper et al, 1989), constant retrograde infusion of bacteria into the biliary tree resulted in an increase in intraductal pressure and a proportional increase in bacteremia. In this model, bacterial reflux into the bloodstream occurred via intracellular pathways, and preexisting biliary obstruction was not a major determinant of bacteremia. Although this model provides important information about obstruction and bacteremia, the rat does not have a gallbladder and is not equivalent to the human. The gallbladder is enormously efficient at absorption of water and may function to relieve some biliary pressure when distal ductal obstruction is present. An infected gallbladder itself can serve as a source of biliary infection.

ETIOLOGY

Biliary obstruction is most commonly caused by choledocholithiasis, benign strictures, postoperative anastomotic strictures, and malignant processes. In the past, 80% of all cases of biliary obstruction and cholangitis were caused by choledocholithiasis. Depending on hospital location and referral patterns, malignancy and congenital problems account for most problems at tertiary referral centers (Thompson et al, 1990). In addition, the more frequent use of endoscopic and percutaneous biliary stents has increased the incidence of bacterial infection.

At many institutions over the last 4 decades, a change has occurred in the microbiology and etiology of many surgical infectious diseases. This change can be explained partly by tertiary referral and differing treatment options, such as biliary stents

and aggressive chemoradiotherapy for biliary and pancreatic malignancies. At the Johns Hopkins Hospital from 1952 to 1978, choledocholithiasis was the most common cause of cholangitis (Table 58.2). In the last 2 decades, malignant obstruction and sclerosing cholangitis have been seen with increasing frequency (Csendes et al, 1975; Lipsett & Pitt, 1990).

More than 1 billion individuals worldwide are infected with *Ascaris lumbricoides,* an increasing cause of acute cholangitis in tropical and subtropical countries. *A. lumbricoides,* a roundworm, causes infection by ingestion of eggs that hatch in the duodenum, releasing the larva stage of this parasite. The larvae penetrate the small bowel mucosa and enter the venous circulation. On reaching the lungs, the larvae lodge in the alveoli and ascend into the bronchial tree. In the oropharynx, they are swallowed, and mature adult worms cause a wide variety of symptoms, including acute cholangitis, gallstone formation, cholecystitis, liver abscess, pancreatitis, and small bowel obstruction. In most cases of acute cholangitis secondary to ascariasis, the roundworms are located in the common bile duct (95%), with evidence of a damaged ampulla and worms seen on endoscopy (86%) (Sandouk et al, 1997).

CLINICAL PRESENTATION

The clinical presentation of patients with acute cholangitis can be extremely varied. About 5% of patients present with toxic cholangitis, which means that they are severely ill with evidence of septic shock (i.e., mental obtundation and hypotension). This severe form of cholangitis originally was described by Reynolds and Dargan (1959) and extended the previous clinical description of patients with cholangitis having the triad of jaundice, fever, and right upper quadrant pain proposed by Charcot (1877). Much as the etiology of cholangitis has changed over the last 50 years, so too has the clinical presentation.

Although many patients with acute cholangitis present in their 40s and 50s, more recent reports document patients presenting with acute cholangitis in their 90s (Hui et al, 2004). In a large series of patients with cholangitis presenting from Hong Kong, patients were febrile, with mild elevation of the white blood cell count (Hui et al, 2004). Patients may or may not be jaundiced. The fact that only two thirds of patients are jaundiced at presentation compared with the almost uniform presence of jaundice in the past is a distinct change (Table 58.3) (Csendes et al, 1975; Thompson et al, 1990). This change may be due partly to the increased number of patients with malignancy and indwelling biliary catheters (Fig. 58.2).

Table 58.2   Changing Etiology of Cholangitis at Johns Hopkins Hospital and in Hong Kong

Etiology	PERCENTAGE OF PATIENTS					
	1952-1974 (*n* = 76)	1976-1978 (*n* = 40)	1983-1985 (*n* = 48)	1986-1989 (*n* = 96)	1998-2003, age >90 (*n* = 69)	1998-2003, age <90 (*n* = 167)
Choledocholithiasis	70	70	32	28	65	74
Benign strictures	13	18	14	12	8	2
Malignant strictures	17	10	30	57	3	1
Sclerosing cholangitis	0	3	24	3	—	—
Normal	—	—	—	—	15	10

Table 58.3 Clinical Presentation of Cholangitis at Johns Hopkins Hospital

Symptom	PERCENTAGE OF PATIENTS		
	1952-1974 (*n* = 76)	1976-1978 (*n* = 40)	1983-1985 (*n* = 48)
Fever	65	98	92
Jaundice	79	90	67
Abdominal pain	79	78	42
Chills	79	63	65
Shock	5	5	4

The third component of Charcot's triad is abdominal pain, which, if present, is usually mild. The classic presentation for acute cholangitis of jaundice, fever, and right upper quadrant pain is not the most common presentation today. Most patients have two of the three components, but fever, which is nonspecific, is usually one of the components. Despite the varied clinical presentation of cholangitis today, the severe form of toxic cholangitis has remained constant at approximately 5% of all cases.

The physical examination of a patient, similar to the clinical presentation, varies. The combination of jaundice and mild right upper quadrant tenderness may be seen in two thirds of patients. The presence of severe tenderness on physical examination should prompt consideration of an alternative diagnosis, such as acute cholecystitis.

DIAGNOSIS

The diagnosis of cholangitis should be considered in any patient who presents with fever, jaundice, or right upper quadrant pain. The differential diagnosis of patients with these symptoms

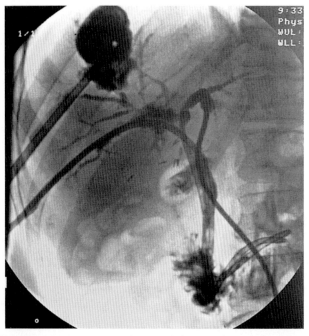

Fig. 58.2. Percutaneous transhepatic cholangiography and liver abscess drainage. Note right hepatic abscess drainage catheter in a patient with biliary obstruction secondary to a proximal cholangiocarcinoma.

and a history of gallstones, previous biliary reconstruction, or indwelling biliary catheters should include acute cholangitis. Virtually all patients with cholangitis have some abnormality in laboratory values. Most patients have an elevated white blood cell count greater than 10,000/mm^3 (Hui et al, 2004), often with a higher mean white blood cell count of greater than 19,000/mm^3 (Lai et al, 1990, 1992). In a few patients with overwhelming gram-negative sepsis and in patients with acquired immunodeficiency syndrome, leukopenia may be seen.

Abnormalities of liver function tests are common in patients with cholangitis. The pattern and degree of liver function abnormalities have been correlated to the cause of the biliary obstruction as noted by Thompson and associates (1990). In patients with a malignant obstruction, a higher elevation of alkaline phosphatase was observed (531 IU versus 278 IU; *P*<.05) compared with patients who had a benign biliary blockage. Patients with benign disease more often have elevations of transaminase values, which usually is secondary to an acute common duct obstruction. Hyperbilirubinemia (>2.2 mg/dL) has been correlated with clinical treatment failure in patients with acute cholangitis (Thompson et al, 1994). Although liver function abnormalities usually are seen in patients with acute cholangitis, many other disease processes have these nonspecific elevation in liver function values. Specifically, sepsis of any origin and hepatitis must be considered. Entirely normal liver function tests are unusual in patients with cholangitis.

Serum amylase also may be elevated in some patients with acute cholangitis (Lipsett & Pitt, 1990). A simple scoring system was developed to help identify patients with pancreatitis who also have acute cholangitis (Isogai et al, 2002). The scoring system consists of four predictive factors: (1) pyrexia (temperature ≥38°C), (2) elevated serum bilirubin (>2.2 mg/dL), (3) dilated bile duct (≥11 mm maximum diameter on ultrasound), and (4) bile duct stones detected on ultrasound. The scoring system predicts severe cholangitis with 92% sensitivity and 98% specificity in patients with scores of 3 or 4 points (Isogai et al, 2002). In patients with toxic cholangitis, additional systemic signs of sepsis, such as thrombocytopenia, prolongation of prothrombin time, and disseminated intravascular coagulation, may occur (Shimada et al, 1984). Patients with *E. coli* bacteremia secondary to acute cholangitis often developed septic shock (11 of 24) and had disseminated intravascular coagulation (10 of 24) (Wang et al, 2002). Although known as a tumor marker, CA 19-9 has been markedly elevated in patients with benign biliary obstruction and acute cholangitis, but with therapy the elevated values return to normal (Albert et al, 1988). As mentioned previously, endotoxin and inflammatory mediators have been measured and usually are elevated in patients with acute cholangitis (Akiyama et al, 1998; Kanazawa et al, 1997; Lau et al, 1996).

The diagnosis of acute cholangitis is not a radiologic diagnosis, even though multiple studies are employed and are necessary to help determine the cause and treatment plan. Radiographs of the abdomen, although often obtained, are rarely helpful in establishing this diagnosis. Occasionally, radiopaque gallstones may be seen, or, even more rarely, pneumobilia may be detected (Saharia & Cameron, 1976). Nuclide scans are helpful in establishing the diagnosis of acute cholecystitis, but not cholangitis. Ultrasound and computed tomography (CT) can visualize dilated biliary ducts or may show a potential cause of cholangitis, such as common duct stones or a pancreatic mass, but these studies do not establish a diagnosis of acute cholangitis. In a study of dynamic CT scans in patients with and without cholangitis, 11 (85%) of 13 patients with cholangitis showed nodular, patchy, wedge-shaped, or geographic inhomogeneous enhancement throughout the liver in the early phase on dynamic CT (Arai et al, 2003). In the control group, only 19 (5%) of 393 patients without cholangitis showed inhomogeneous enhancement in the early phase on dynamic CT. Follow-up dynamic CT performed after treatment for acute cholangitis showed decreased inhomogeneous enhancement or no inhomogeneous enhancement in seven (78%) of nine patients in the cholangitis group.

At some point in the patient's clinical course, either in acute treatment or in defining ultimate management, cholangiography is required. Direct cholangiography via the endoscopic or percutaneous route is equally informative. Generally, if common duct stones or a periampullary tumor is suspected, ERCP is preferred. If a perihilar tumor is expected, percutaneous transheptic cholangiography has some advantages. Cholangitis can be a complication of either procedure, but with appropriate attention to biliary pressures, a generally low incidence of 3% to 7% can be expected (Gould et al, 1985; Kadir et al, 1982; Lois et al, 1987). Another option that is becoming increasingly available and has the advantage of being noninvasive is magnetic resonance imaging (MRI) cholangiography. The MRI findings include the presence of biliary duct dilation, intraluminal filling defects owing to stones or sludge, bands of mucosal edema of the biliary ducts, intraperitoneal and retroperitoneal edema or fluid, and definition of the cause of obstruction (e.g., stones, stenosis or tumor).

The timing of cholangiography is important. With the exception of patients who have toxic cholangitis, invasive cholangiography should be delayed until fever has resolved. Ideally, ERCP should be delayed for 72 hours after the patient has defervesced when performed for diagnostic reasons alone (Lai et al, 1989). In some situations, MRI cholangiography has the advantage of establishing a diagnosis without aggravating sepsis. In patients who have a malignant obstruction or recent cholangitis, the incidence of ERCP-associated cholangitis is higher, and these patients warrant early elective biliary decompression (Davis et al, 1975).

MICROBIOLOGY

Bacteremia can result from the combination of biliary obstruction and infection. Systemic signs, such as high fever, rigors, and, particularly, hypotension, signify that gram-negative bacteremia is likely in patients with acute cholangitis. In a series from Johns Hopkins, 21% of patients with cholangitis had bacteremia, but E. coli and Klebsiella species represented a much smaller proportion of the total number of isolated organisms (Thompson et al, 1990). In comparing the clinical presentation and outcome of elderly versus younger patients, bacteremia was present in 63 of 134 patients (Sugiyama & Atomi, 1997). Although positive blood cultures were slightly more common in elderly patients (56% versus 44%), this difference did not achieve statistical significance. This observation suggests that the underlying obstruction and infection have a high tendency to result in bacteremia, regardless of the underlying medical and physical condition. Patients with E. coli bacteremia and acute cholangitis presented with septic shock apparently more often than is generally reported in patients with acute cholangitis and may be related to the presence of E. coli virulence factors (Wang et al, 2002).

The bacteriology of the biliary tree has changed over the last 5 decades (see Table 58.1). In most current series, bactibilia is confirmed in virtually all patients, and more than one pathogen is usually isolated (Gerecht et al, 1989; Hui et al, 2004; Lai et al, 1990, 1992; Lee et al, 1992; Sugiyama & Atomi, 1997; Thompson et al, 1990). The enteric gram-negative aerobes E. coli and Klebsiella and the gram-positive aerobes enterococci formally were the most common isolates. The more resistant gram-negative organisms Pseudomonas and Enterobacter are being seen with increasing frequency (Hui et al, 2004; Shinagawa et al, 1997; Thompson et al, 1990). Anaerobes, such as Bacteroides species, continue to play a small, but significant, role in biliary infection (Lee et al, 1992; Muller et al, 1987). Candida species are increasingly isolated from bile and blood cultures. In analyzing failures of therapy, isolation of Candida, panresistant bacteria, and more than two bacteria are associated with clinical treatment failures (Thompson et al, 1994).

TREATMENT

Patients with acute cholangitis have a wide spectrum of illness. A few patients with mild forms of acute cholangitis may be treated with oral antibiotics as an outpatient. An equally small number of patients with the toxic form of cholangitis may require intensive care unit admission, invasive monitoring, and use of vasoactive agents to support blood pressure. Maintenance of euvolemia is important to preserve organ function, and hydration usually is required. The selection of vasoactive agents depends on the individual hemodynamics of each patient. The routine use of renal dose dopamine remains unproven (Bellomo et al, 2000; Perdue et al, 1998).

Antibiotic Therapy

Antibiotics are the cornerstone of therapy for all patients with acute cholangitis. The specific agent selected for use is a matter of choice, however (Mazuski et al, 2002). In part, the antibiotics chosen should be based on an institutional experience with cholangitis. If the microbiology is unknown at a particular institution, broad empiric antibiotic selection must be used and should include coverage against gram-negative aerobes and enterococci.

The aminoglycosides have excellent activity against the gram-negative bacteria (Miyagawa, 1993; Parker & Davey, 1993). Great reluctance to use aminoglycosides continues, however, owing to perceived renal toxicity and ototoxicity, and a meta-analysis has questioned the effectiveness of aminoglycosides in patients with intra-abdominal infections (Bailey et al, 2002). Patients with the toxic form of cholangitis are critically ill. In these patients, aminoglycosides are even more difficult to use given that the volume of distribution is often markedly underestimated. Most typically, aminoglycosides frequently are underdosed with initial low peak levels (Miyagawa, 1993; Parker & Davey, 1993). The mortality from gram-negative sepsis when treated with aminoglycosides is directly related to (1) the time until a therapeutic peak level is reached and (2) low initial drug trough levels (Moore et al, 1984). The renal toxicity of aminoglycosides also is related to the trough level, and prolonged dosing intervals, with trough levels falling to at least less than 2 mg/dL, are recommended (Perdue et al, 1998).

To account for a larger volume of distribution, the initial loading dose for gentamicin and tobramycin in a critically ill patient is 4 to 6 mg/kg (Dorman et al, 1998). A peak serum level can be obtained to ensure initial adequate doses. If aminoglycosides are administered on a once-daily dosing schedule, a trough level is recommended at the second dose. Alternatively, it has been suggested that a "random" level be obtained between 6 and 14 hours after the initial 5 mg/kg dose of gentamicin or tobramycin, and a nomogram for the dosing schedule with this method is available (Nicolau et al, 1995). These methods ensure that the kidneys have cleared adequate drug to prevent renal toxicity. This method of administering aminoglycosides also ensures high initial serum levels with better concentration-dependent bacterial killing and allows for the postantibiotic effect of aminoglycosides to be used.

Aside from the aminoglycosides, gram-negative aerobes are well covered by third-generation cephalosporins, ureidopenicillins, carbapenems, and fluoroquinolones (Mazuski et al, 2002). Ureidopenicillins, such as piperacillin, offer the advantage of gram-positive coverage, including the enterococci, and of anaerobic coverage (Thompson et al, 1990). When combined with a β-lactamase inhibitor, such as tazobactam, piperacillin offers extended and improved coverage against organisms that have acquired resistance. In *Klebsiella* species, these extended spectrum β-lactamases are present in 25% of all organisms and cause resistance to usual agents, especially the penicillin derivatives. The carbapenems imipenem and meropenem also cover gram-negative aerobes, gram-positive aerobes, and anaerobes. These two agents have been used successfully as monotherapy for abdominal or unknown sepsis even in critically ill patients (Mazuski et al, 2002; Namias et al, 1998).

Most currently released fluoroquinolones do not have adequate antibiotic coverage for biliary organisms, and additional anaerobic coverage should be added. Because of the increased isolation of *Pseudomonas* from patients with biliary sepsis, in ill patients an empiric treatment regimen that covers *Pseudomonas* should be considered. This recommendation includes piperacillin; cefepime, a fourth-generation cephalosporin; the carbapenems; and select fluroquinolones. Although most experts agree that *Pseudomonas* should be treated with two drugs, this recommendation has never undergone rigorous study and is currently subject to substantial debate. The data supporting dual antibiotic coverage come from randomized controlled trials with monotherapy. Patients in whom *Pseudomonas* is isolated are statistically more likely to fail with monotherapy. Studies suggest that appropriate initial selection of empiric agents is linked to survival in critically ill patients (Alvarez-Lerma, 1996). This observation emphasizes the need to be familiar with the local microorganisms and resistance patterns.

Several randomized prospective trials for the antibiotic treatment of isolated acute cholangitis have been performed (Gerecht et al, 1989; Muller et al, 1987; Thompson et al, 1990). In a study done at the Mayo Clinic, mezlocillin, a ureidopenicillin, favorably compared with the combination of ampicillin/gentamicin (Gerecht et al, 1989). Twenty of 24 patients (83%) treated with mezlocillin were cured compared with only 9 of 24 (41%) patients treated with ampicillin/gentamicin. In addition, fewer toxic effects were seen in the mezlocillin arm. Aminoglycosides were administered in the traditional every-8-hour dosing schedule, however.

In a study from Johns Hopkins, the University of California Los Angeles, and the Olive View Medical Center, 96 patients were randomized to either piperacillin or ampicillin and tobramycin (Thompson et al, 1990). The cure rate of both treatment groups was similar, but the outcome was related to the cause of the obstruction (benign versus malignant) (Fig. 58.3). This observation has been confirmed, with patients with malignancy being less likely to respond (63%) to antibiotics than patients with benign disease (88%) (Shinagawa et al, 1997). The Surgical Infection Society released a comprehensive publication on antibiotic treatment of intra-abdominal sepsis (Mazuski et al, 2002).

Biliary Decompression

Initial therapeutic interventions for acute cholangitis, such as hydration and antibiotics, are successful in 80% to 85% of all patients. Twenty percent of patients with acute cholangitis require urgent biliary decompression, however, for the treatment of ongoing sepsis. Retrospective analysis and prospective randomized controlled trials have shown that urgent endoscopic drainage is an effective treatment for suppurative cholangitis and is superior to surgical drainage, with a better clinical outcome (Hui et al, 2002, 2003; Lai et al, 1989).

Nonoperative means for establishing biliary decompression are now available in most hospitals. Percutaneous transhepatic decompression is a well-established technique for biliary drainage in patients with obstructive jaundice (Gould et al, 1985; Kadir et al, 1982; Lois et al, 1987). In patients who are already ill, this technique may alleviate the need for general anesthesia and an operative intervention. Patients, especially elderly patients and patients who are critically ill, may require intubation and mechanical ventilation for any intervention where additional sedation may compromise an already depressed mental state (Sugiyama & Atomi, 1997). If a patient has a proximal perihilar obstruction or a previous biliary-enteric anastomosis, percutaneous drainage may be the preferred route of biliary decompression. Although highly variable rates for morbidity and mortality have been reported, in most series urgent percutaneous decompression in patients can be done with a morbidity of less than 10% and a mortality of 5% (Huang & Ker, 1988; Kadir et al, 1982; Pessa et al, 1987).

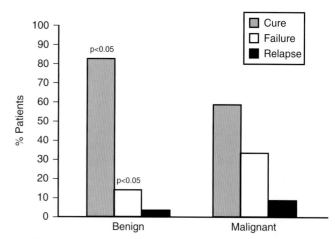

Fig. 58.3. Cure, failure, and relapse rates among 96 patients with cholangitis caused by either benign or malignant obstruction. Outcome was significantly worse with malignant obstruction.
(From Thompson JE Jr, et al, 1990: Broad spectrum penicillin as adequate therapy for acute cholangitis. Surg Gynecol Obstet 171:275.)

The specific subset of patients with acute toxic cholangitis secondary to choledocholithiasis was prospectively studied by Lai and colleagues (1992). In this seminal study, 82 patients with toxic cholangitis were randomized to receive either urgent endoscopic treatment or surgical decompression. Surgical decompression was associated with an increased need for ventilatory support, respiratory failure, and death (32% versus 10%; P<.05) compared with endoscopic decompression. This study suggests that if the expertise is available for urgent endoscopic decompression, this treatment is preferable for patients with toxic cholangitis secondary to choledocholithiasis. The addition of endoscopic sphincterotomy to biliary decompression for patients with severe acute cholangitis has been questioned. When endoscopic sphincterotomy is performed together with biliary stent insertion, the procedure is prolonged, and the patient is exposed to the risks associated with endoscopic sphincterotomy and extended sedation (Hui et al, 2002). Whether or not decompression of the bile duct is beneficial in patients with acute cholangitis and gallstones, but without evidence of common duct or intrahepatic stones, is unclear. Although ERCP and decompression can decrease the duration of acute cholangitis and reduce hospital stay, it does not affect the outcome of recurrent acute cholangitis (Hui et al, 2002). Endoscopic sphincterotomy is not routinely recommended because the short-term gains do not justify the increased complications and perhaps death that may result from unnecessary sphincterotomy in the absence of ductal stones.

In institutions where endoscopic or percutaneous biliary decompression is not available, operative drainage is a lifesaving intervention for seriously ill patients with acute cholangitis (Lai et al, 1990). It was shown that the outcome of 30 patients who were managed with operative decompression was not different from a similar group of patients who were resuscitated successfully before surgery (Lai et al, 1990). When nonoperative means of biliary decompression are unavailable, even patients who are severely ill with cholangitis can be managed successfully with timely and appropriate operative intervention. Among 100 patients undergoing urgent common bile duct exploration for obstruction, of whom 51 patients had severe cholangitis, preoperative endoscopic decompression had a beneficial effect on survival (mortality 9.4% versus 33%) (Koh et al, 2003).

The hemodynamic status of the patient in the operating room should guide the extent of the surgical procedure. In an unstable patient, cholangiography and choledochoscopy should not be performed. Operative drainage alone may be lifesaving. Biliary drainage alone was performed in 24 of the 44 patients in the series reported by Lai and colleagues (1992). Because the common bile duct is the site of biliary obstruction in most series, cholecystostomy is often inadequate treatment, and biliary ductal decompression of some type is required. Additional, and often definitive, therapy should not be performed at the same operative procedure when the indication for intervention has been toxic cholangitis, and the patient remains hemodynamically unstable during surgery.

The widespread availability of emergency endoscopic biliary services has largely negated the role of emergency common bile duct exploration. In acute cholangitis, emergency endoscopic biliary drainage significantly decreases mortality compared with open surgery. Even when endoscopic biliary drainage fails to abate sepsis adequately in cholangitis, subsequent emergency common bile duct exploration carries lower mortality. Emergency common bile duct exploration remains an indispensable lifesaving

procedure in the hands of the general surgeon when endoscopic biliary drainage fails and when complications arise from endoscopic procedures.

OUTCOME

As is true of any patient with severe sepsis or septic shock, high-risk patients with toxic cholangitis are at risk for considerable morbidity and mortality (Angus & Wax, 2001; Gigot et al, 1989; Thompson et al, 1994). Outcome is worse in cases of malignant obstruction (see Fig. 58.3) (Thompson et al, 1990). These high-risk patients are at particular risk for the development of end organ dysfunction or organ failure, and careful management is necessary to prevent the development of these complications. Gigot and coworkers (1989) retrospectively showed seven independent risk factors that predicted mortality after acute cholangitis: (1) acute renal failure, (2) liver abscess, (3) cirrhosis, (4) high malignant strictures, (5) percutaneous transhepatic cholangiography, (6) female gender, and (7) age. In a multiple regression formula with proportional weight given to the individual factors, a score of 0 to 27 could be obtained. If the score was less than 7, the predicted mortality was 1.8%; if the score was greater than 7, the predicted mortality was 49%. The development of renal dysfunction and renal failure is common in this group of patients and undoubtedly is related to the combination of altered hemodynamics and low effective circulating volume from the production of inflammatory mediators released by the severe infection. These inflammatory mediators can be found in high concentrations in the bile and the serum of these patients (Akiyama et al, 1998; Kanazawa et al, 1997; Lau et al, 1996).

Biliary drainage can diminish the concentration of these mediators in blood and bile, and this decrease in mediators has been linked to survival. Direct and indirect effects of hormonal and sympathetic control on renal blood flow can cause acute or relative renal ischemia. The maintenance of adequate intravascular volume is essential. In some cases in which hepatic and renal failure is present, circulating endotoxin has been documented and associated with the clinical features of acute cholangitis (Lau et al, 1996). In theory, therapies directed at decreasing absorption of endotoxin through the small bowel mucosa and decreasing levels in the portal bloodstream have been proposed. These methods include oral bile acids, lactulose, and internal bile drainage (Dawson, 1965, 1968; Koutelidakis et al, 2003; Pain et al, 1985). Although an animal model has shown that lactulose decreased tumor necrosis factor and improved survival (Koutelidakis et al, 2003), the general use of this drug has not been adopted.

A liver abscess is frequently seen in association with biliary pathology (Fig. 58.4) (see Ch. 59). The development of one or more liver abscesses considerably increases the morbidity and mortality of acute cholangitis. A liver abscess should be considered in any patient with cholangitis who is seriously ill or who fails to improve after initial therapy. If multiple small abscesses are present, biliary drainage and systemic antibiotics may be all that is required. If a large hepatic abscess is present, however, additional drainage usually becomes necessary. Drainage of a liver abscess can be managed percutaneously in most patients, but occasionally, operative drainage is necessary, particularly if concurrent intra-abdominal pathology is present. In most series, the overall mortality of patients with acute cholangitis is 5%.

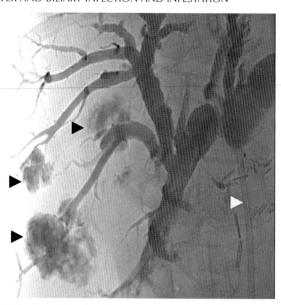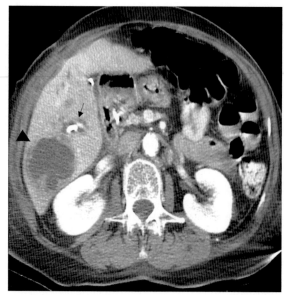

Fig. 58.4. Cholangitis and intrahepatic abscess in a patient with cholangitis. Transheptic cholangiography *(left)* shows marked dilation of the intrahepatic biliary tree, a nonfunctioning endoscopic stent *(white arrowhead)*, and multiple intrahepatic collections in communication with the bile ducts *(black arrowheads)*. Axial CT *(right)* shows a rim-enhancing collection in the posterior sector *(arrowhead)* consistent with an abscess and corresponding to the collection on the lower left portion of the cholangiogram. A percutaneous biliary drainage catheter is indicated by the *arrow*.

The highest mortality occurs in the small subgroup of patients who present with toxic cholangitis. Several authors have suggested additional risk factors for patients who present with acute cholangitis. As might be expected, concomitant medical disease, acute renal failure, and low serum albumin are additional risk factors (Gigot et al, 1989; Lai et al, 1990; Little, 1998; Thompson et al, 1994).

In the past, patients older than 80 years have had a poorer outcome of acute cholangitis, with a higher incidence of mental obtundation and shock (43%) compared with younger patients (25%) (Sugiyama & Atomi, 1997). In a large series of patients with cholangitis undergoing ERCP, including 64 patients older than 90 years, complication rates were 4.7% in the older group and 7.3% in the younger group (P = not significant) (Hui et al, 2001). Similarly, mortality was not different between the two groups (7.8% >90 years versus 4.2% <90 years; P = not significant). In patients with acute cholangitis, the underlying cause of the biliary obstruction does have prognostic importance (Thompson et al, 1990). In this study designed to evaluate antibiotic therapy, the benign or malignant nature of the biliary obstruction was an independent and important predictor of outcome. The initial cure rate of the patients with a benign obstruction was 83% compared with only 59% of patients with a malignant obstruction (P<.05). In this study, mortality was 5%, but all of these patients had end-stage malignancy, and many also had liver failure or renal failure or both. This finding has been validated in another study (Sugiyama & Atomi, 1997).

To date, only one study (Lai et al, 1992) has attempted a controlled trial to stratify management decisions in patients with acute cholangitis. Identification of the highest risk patient groups and proposing a management strategy that incorporates aggressive supportive measures combined with early intervention may improve prognosis in the highest risk patients.

REFERENCES

Akiyama T, et al, 1998: Serum and bile interleukin 6 after percutaneous transhepatic cholangio-drainage. Hepatogastroenterology 45:665-671.

Albert MA, et al, 1988: Elevated serum levels of tumor marker CA19-9 in acute cholangitis. Dig Dis Sci 33:1223.

Alvarez-Lerma F, 1996: Modification of empiric antibiotic treatment in patients with pneumonia acquired in the intensive care unit. ICU-Acquired Pneumonia Study Group. Intensive Care Med 22:387-394.

Angus DC, Wax RS, 2001: Epidemiology of sepsis: an update. Crit Care Med 7S:109-116.

Arai K, et al, 2003: Dynamic CT of acute cholangitis: early inhomogeneous enhancement of the liver. AJR Am J Roentgenol 181:115-118.

Bailey JA, et al, 2002: Aminoglycosides for intra-abdominal infection: equal to the challenge? Surg Infect (Larchmt) 3:315-335.

Bellomo R, et al, 2000: Low-dose dopamine in patients with early renal dysfunction: a placebo-controlled randomized trial. Australian and New Zealand Intensive Care Society (ANZICS) Clinical Trials Group. Lancet 356:2139-2143.

Charcot JM, 1877: Lecons sur les maladies du fore des voices biliares et des veins. Paris, Faculte de Medicine de Paris, Recueillies et Publices Par, Bourneville et Sevestre.

Csendes A, et al, 1975: Bacteriology of the gallbladder bile in normal subjects. Am J Surg 129:629.

Csendes A, et al, 1988: Common bile duct pressure in patients with common bile duct stones with or without acute suppurative cholangitis. Surgery 123:697-699.

Csendes A, et al, 1995: Bacteriological studies of liver parenchyma in controls and in patients with gallstones or common bile duct stones with or without acute cholangitis. Hepatogastroenterology 42:821-826.

Csendes A, et al, 1996: Counts of bacteria and pyocites of choledochal bile in controls and in patients with gallstones or common bile duct stones with or without acute cholangitis. Hepatogastroenterology 43:800-806.

Davis JL, et al, 1975: Septic complication following endoscopic retrograde cholangiopancreatography. Surg Gynecol Obstet 140:365-367.

Dawson JL, 1965: Acute postoperative renal function in obstructive jaundice: effect of mannitol diuresis. BMJ 5427:82-86.

Dawson JL, 1968: Acute postoperative renal failure in obstructive jaundice. Ann R Coll Surg Engl 42:163-181.

Dineen P, 1964: The importance of the route of infection in experimental biliary obstruction. Surg Gynecol Obstet 119:1001-1008.

Dorman T, et al, 1998: Impact of altered aminoglycoside volume of distribution on the adequacy of a 3 mg/kg loading dose. Surgery 124:73-78.

Edlund YA, et al, 1959: Bacteriologic investigation of the biliary system and liver in biliary tract disease correlated to clinical data and microstructure of the gallbladder and liver. Acta Chir Scand 116:461-476.

Flemma RJ, et al, 1967: Bacteriologic studies of biliary infection. Ann Surg 166:563-572.

Geier A, et al, 2000: Regulation of organic anion transporters in a new rat model of acute and chronic cholangitis resembling human primary sclerosing cholangitis. J Hepatol 36:718-724.

Gerecht WB, et al, 1989: Prospective randomized comparison of mezlocillin therapy alone with combined ampicillin and gentamicin therapy for patients with cholangitis. Arch Intern Med 149:1279-1284.

Gigot JF, et al, 1989: Acute cholangitis: multivariate analysis of risk factors. Ann Surg 209:435-438.

Glasgow R, et al, 2000: The spectrum and cost of complicated gallstone disease in California. Arch Surg 135:1021-1027.

Gong JP, et al, 2002: Nuclear factor κB activity in patients with acute severe cholangitis. World J Gastroenterol 8:346-349.

Gould RJ, et al, 1985: Percutaneous biliary drainage as an initial therapy in sepsis of the biliary tract. Surg Gynecol Obstet 160:523-527.

Hochwald SN, et al, 1999: Association of preoperative biliary stenting with increased postoperative infectious complications in proximal cholangiocarcinoma. Arch Surg 134:261-266.

Huang MH, Ker CG, 1988: Ultrasonic guided percutaneous transhepatic bile drainage for cholangitis due to intrahepatic stones. Arch Surg 123:106-109.

Huang T, et al, 1969: The significance of biliary pressure in cholangitis. Arch Surg 98:629-632.

Hui CK, et al, 2001: Acute cholangitis—predictive factors for emergency ERCP. Aliment Pharmacol Ther 15:1633-1637.

Hui CK, et al, 2002: A randomised controlled trial of endoscopic sphincterotomy in acute cholangitis without common bile duct stones. Gut 51:245-247.

Hui CK, et al, 2003: Does the addition of endoscopic sphincterotomy to stent insertion improve drainage of the bile duct in acute suppurative cholangitis? Gastrointest Endosc 58:500-504.

Hui CK, et al, 2004: Outcome of emergency ERCP for acute cholangitis in patients 90 years of age and older. Aliment Pharmacol Ther 19:1153-1158.

Isogai M, et al, 2002: Cholangitis score: a scoring system to predict severe cholangitis in gallstone pancreatitis. J Hepatobiliary Pancreat Surg 9:98-104.

Jacobson K, et al, 1962: Cholangiovenous reflux: an experimental study. Acta Chir Scand 123:316-321.

Kadir S, et al, 1982: Percutaneous biliary drainage in the management of biliary sepsis. AJR Am J Roentgenol 138:25-29.

Kanazawa A, et al, 1997: Concentrations of bile and serum endotoxin and serum cytokines after biliary drainage for acute cholangitis. Osaka City Med J 43:15-27.

Kaufman HW, et al, 1989: The role of bacteria in gallbladder and common duct stone formation. Ann Surg 209:584-591.

Keighley MR, et al, 1975: Antibiotic treatment of biliary sepsis. Surg Clin North Am 55:1379-1390.

Keighley MR, et al, 1976: Multivariate analysis of clinical and operative findings associated with biliary sepsis. Br J Surg 63:528-531.

Kimmings AN, et al, 2000: Systemic inflammatory response in acute cholangitis and after subsequent treatment. Eur J Surg 166:700-705.

Koh JS, et al, 2003: Outcomes of emergency common bile duct exploration: impact of preoperative endoscopic decompression. Aust N Z J Surg 73:376-380.

Koutelidakis I, et al, 2003: Systemic endotoxaemia following obstructive jaundice: the role of lactulose. J Surg Res 113:243-247.

Lai ECS, et al, 1989: Urgent biliary decompression after endoscopic retrograde cholangiopancreatography. Am J Surg 157:121-125.

Lai ECS, et al, 1990: Emergency surgery for severe acute cholangitis: the high-risk patients. Ann Surg 211:55-59.

Lai ECS, et al, 1992: Endoscopic biliary drainage for severe acute cholangitis. N Engl J Med 326:1582-1586.

Lau JY, et al, 1996: Endoscopic drainage aborts endotoxaemia in acute cholangitis. Br J Surg 83:181-184.

Lee RA, et al, 2003: Geographical difference of disease association in Streptococcus bovis bacteraemia. J Med Microbiol 52:903-908.

Lee W, et al, 1992: Surgery in cholangitis: bacteriology and choice of antibiotic. Hepatogastroenterology 39:347-349.

Leung JW, et al, 2001: Bacteriologic analyses of bile and brown pigment stones in patients with acute cholangitis. Gastrointest Endosc 54:340-345.

Lipsett PA, Pitt HA, 1990: Acute cholangitis. Surg Clin North Am 70:1297-1312.

Little JM, 1998: A prospective evaluation of computerized estimates of risk in the management of obstructive jaundice. Surgery 102:473-476.

Lois JF, et al, 1987: Risks of percutaneous transhepatic drainage in patients with cholangitis. AJR Am J Roentgenol 148:367-371.

Mallet-Guy P, 1952: Value of preoperative manometric and roentgenographic examination in the diagnosis of pathologic changes and functional disturbances of the biliary tract. Surg Gynecol Obstet 94:385-393.

Mazuski JE, et al, 2002: The Surgical Infection Society guidelines on antimicrobial therapy for intra-abdominal infections: an executive summary. Surg Infect (Larchmt) 3:161-173.

Miyagawa CI, 1993: Aminoglycosides in the intensive care unit: an old drug in a dynamic environment. New Horiz 1:172-180.

Moore RD, et al, 1984: Association of aminoglycoside plasma levels with therapeutic outcome in gram-negative pneumonia. Am J Med 77:657-662.

Muller EL, et al, 1987: Antibiotics in infections of the biliary tract. Surg Gynecol Obstet 165:285-292.

Namias N, et al, 1998: Empiric therapy of sepsis in the surgical intensive care unit with broad-spectrum antibiotics for 72 hours does not lead to the emergence of resistant bacteria. J Trauma 45:887-891.

National Institutes of Health, 2002: NIH state-of-the-science statement on endoscopic retrograde cholangiopancreatography (ERCP) for diagnosis and therapy. NIH Consens State Sci Statements 19:1-26.

Nicolau DP, et al, 1995: Experience with a once-daily aminoglycoside program administered to 2,184 adult patients. Antimicrob Agents Chemother 39:650-655.

Nomura T, et al, 1999: Bacteribilia and cholangitis after percutaneous transhepatic biliary drainage for malignant biliary obstruction. Dig Dis Sci 44:542-546.

O'Connor MJ, et al, 1981: Cholangitis due to malignant obstruction to biliary outflow. Ann Surg 193:341-345.

Pain ME, et al, 1985: Perioperative complications in obstructive jaundice: therapeutic considerations. Br J Surg 72:942-945.

Parker SE, Davey PG, 1993: Practicalities of once daily aminoglycoside dosing. J Antimicrob Chemother 31:4-8.

Perdue PW, et al, 1998: 'Renal dose' dopamine in surgical patients: dogma or science? Ann Surg 227:470-473.

Pessa ME, et al, 1987: The treatment of acute cholangitis: percutaneous transhepatic biliary drainage before definitive therapy. Ann Surg 205:389-392.

Pitt HA, Couse NF, 1990: Biliary sepsis and toxic cholangitis. In Moody FG (ed): Surgical Treatment of Digestive Disease, 2nd ed. Chicago, Year Book Medical Publishers, p 332.

Pitt HA, Longmire WP Jr, 1980: Suppurative cholangitis. In Hardy JM (ed): Critical Surgical Illness, 2nd ed. Philadelphia, Saunders, p 380.

Pitt HA, et al, 1982: Biliary bacteria: significance and alterations after antibiotic therapy. Arch Surg 117:445-449.

Pitt HA, et al, 1983: Consequences of preoperative cholangitis and its treatment on the outcome of surgery for choledocholithiasis. Surgery 94:447-452.

Poon RT, et al, 2001: Management of gallstone cholangitis in the era of laparoscopic cholecystectomy. Arch Surg 136:11-16.

Raper SE, et al, 1989: Anatomic correlates of bacterial cholangiovenous reflux. Surgery 105:352-359.

Reynolds BM, Dargan EL, 1959: Acute obstructive cholangitis: a distinct clinical syndrome. Ann Surg 150:299-303.

Saharia PC, Cameron JL, 1976: Clinical management of cholangitis. Surg Gynecol Obstet 142:369-372.

Sandouk F, et al, 1997: Pancreatic-biliary ascariasis: experience of 300 cases. Am J Gastroenterol 92:2264-2267.

Scott AJ, Kahn GA, 1967: Origin of bacteria in the bile duct. Lancet 2:790-792.

Sharma BC, et al, 1997: Endoscopic management of acute calculous cholangitis. J Gastroenterol Hepatol 12:874-876.

Shimada H, et al, 1984: Pathogenesis and clinical features of acute cholangitis accompanied by shock. Jpn J Surg 14:269-277.

Shinagawa N, et al, 1997: Efficacy and safety of sulbactam/cefoperazone for hepato-biliary infections. Jpn J Antibiot 50:862-870.

Silva AC, et al, 2004: MR cholangiopancreatography: improved ductal distention with intravenous morphine administration. Radiographics 24:677-687.

Stewart L, et al, 1988: Cholangiovenous reflux pathways as defined by corrosion casting and scanning electron microscopy. Am J Surg 155:23-28.

Suc B, et al, 1998: Surgery vs endoscopy as primary treatment in symptomatic patients with suspected common bile duct stones: a multicenter randomized trial. French Associates for Surgical Research. Arch Surg 133:702-708.

Sugiyama M, Atomi Y, 1997: Treatment of acute cholangitis due to choledocholithiasis in elderly and younger patients. Arch Surg 132:1129-1133.

Thompson J, et al, 1994: An analysis of infectious failures in acute cholangitis. HPB Surg 8:139-144.

Thompson JE Jr, et al, 1990: Broad spectrum penicillin as adequate therapy for acute cholangitis. Surg Gynecol Obstet 171:275.

Tu B, et al, 2003: Role of NF-κB in multiple organ dysfunction during acute obstructive cholangitis. World J Gastroenterol 9:179-183.

Wang MC, et al, 2002: The role of bacterial virulence and host factors in patients with *Escherichia coli* bacteremia who have acute cholangitis or upper urinary tract infection. Clin Infect Dis 35:1161-1166.

Wu ET, et al, 2001: Change: bacterial cholangitis in patients with biliary atresia: impact of short-term outcome. Pediatr Surg Int 17:390-395.

Pyogenic Liver Abscess

R. W. STRONG

Liver abscess was recognized in ancient times and through the centuries was invariably fatal. No progress was made until the seminal paper by Ochsner and colleagues in 1938. They reported a 62% survival rate for patients undergoing surgical drainage, and with the advent of antibiotic therapy, the combination of surgical drainage and antibiotics became standard treatment for the next 4 decades. Successful treatment was hampered, however, by the late diagnosis and the relative inaccuracy that was associated with palpation in identifying induration or fluctuation as the site of the lesion. The next landmark paper was in 1953, when McFadzean and coworkers first reported on percutaneous drainage, which was successful in 14 patients without a death. Percutaneous drainage remained relatively unheralded for several decades until the mid-1980s, when reports of patients successfully treated by percutaneous drainage and antibiotics were published (Bertel et al, 1986; Gerzof et al, 1985).

The development of ultrasound and computed tomography (CT) allowed earlier and more definitive diagnosis followed by percutaneous procedures using these modalities for accurate drainage. The major shift from open surgical treatment to percutaneous needle aspiration (PNA) or percutaneous catheter drainage (PCD), which accompanied the advances in radiology, has made a nonsurgical approach the first choice of treatment for single and multiple abscesses. The role of open operation in the treatment of pyogenic liver abscess (PLA) is limited to patients who fail nonoperative treatment or in whom operation is necessary for the cause of the abscess. Open operation as a primary mode of therapy may be indicated when there has been rupture of the PLA into the peritoneal cavity, or when there are multiple abscesses above an obstructed duct system that cannot be negotiated by nonoperative means.

ETIOLOGY AND INCIDENCE

Over the past 50 years, there has been a major shift in the etiology of PLA. PLA may be of biliary, portal, arterial, or traumatic origin (Table 59.1). Portal pyemia secondary to appendicitis, diverticulitis, or other intra-abdominal infective process has decreased markedly, owing to improved management of the primary condition through earlier diagnosis and evolution of antibiotic therapy. Patients with portal pyemia as an identifiable cause of PLA have been replaced by an increasing proportion of patients with complications of hepatobiliary pathology or its treatment. Ascending infection of the biliary tree secondary to obstruction is now the most identifiable cause of PLA. The etiology of the biliary obstruction has some geographic differences. Percutaneous or endoscopic instrumentation and stenting of an obstructed bile duct can introduce infection into the biliary system, and cholangitis, especially when associated with stent occlusion, has the propensity to cause PLA (see Ch. 58). In Western countries, this scenario is common in patients with underlying malignant

disease (Huang et al, 1996). In Asian countries, hepatolithiasis and its associated biliary strictures predominate in the identifiable etiology of PLA (Table 59.2).

Hematogenous spread of infection from sources other than the gastrointestinal tract may cause PLA. Bacterial endocarditis and intravenous drug abuse are classic examples. Immunocompromised patients, such as patients with underlying malignancy, acquired immunodeficiency syndrome, and chronic granulomatous disease, are prone to develop PLA. The treatment of some liver tumors can lead to the development of PLA. Chemoembolization for hepatocellular carcinoma may be complicated by the formation of a PLA, and this is more likely to occur when the tumor size is greater than 5 cm in diameter (Chen at al, 1997). Physical ablation therapy of a liver tumor occasionally is associated with liver abscess formation (De Baere et al, 1996).

Liver trauma (see Ch. 66) from penetrating or blunt injury may result in parenchymal necrosis, intrahepatic biloma, or hematoma, and these can become secondarily infected and give rise to a PLA. After liver transplantation, necrosis secondary to hepatic artery thrombosis invariably becomes infected by bacteria or fungi and, because of the distribution and magnitude of the process, frequently necessitates repeat transplantation (see Ch. 110).

Direct extension of infection into the liver from an adjacent organ may invoke a PLA, the most common neighboring site being the gallbladder. Gastric or duodenal perforation directly into the liver may give rise to a PLA—there have been numerous cases of PLA secondary to foreign body (mainly fish bone) perforation of the stomach or duodenum with penetration into the liver (Chan et al, 1999).

In some patients, no identifiable cause for or source of PLA is found. These cases are labeled as cryptogenic and account for 15% to 55% in various series, with the higher end of the spectrum being evident in Asian series. The routine use of ultrasound and CT is likely to rule out unrecognized biliary or other intra-abdominal sources of infection, and the question arises whether further invasive investigations are warranted when the etiology is presumed to be cryptogenic. Seeto and Rockey (1996) concluded that patients with an initial diagnosis of cryptogenic abscess, with a normal bilirubin and no duct dilation on imaging and without clinical or radiologic evidence of a possible source of pyelophlebitis, should not undergo aggressive random invasive evaluation of the biliary tree or gastrointestinal tract. It is advisable, however, to rule out an arterial source of infection (see Table 59.1).

The incidence of diabetes in patients with PLA varies, ranging from 6% to 65%. In Western countries, it has ranged from 6% to 17% (Barakate et al, 1999; Robert et al, 1992; Seeto & Rockey, 1996), whereas in Asian series, the incidence has been 45% (Chou et al, 1997), 65% (Wang et al, 1998), and 41% (Wong et al, 2002). In Malaysia, 40% of patients with cryptogenic PLA were diabetic, and *Klebsiella pneumoniae* was the most common organism cultured (Strong, 2005).

Table 59.1   Most Frequent Causes of Pyogenic Liver Abscess

Hepatobiliary
  Benign
    Lithiasis
    Cholecystitis
    Biliary-enteric anastomosis
    Endoscopic biliary procedures
    Percutaneous biliary procedures
  Malignant
    Common bile duct
    Gallbladder
    Ampulla
    Head of pancreas
Portal
  Benign
    Diverticulitis
    Anorectal suppuration
    Pelvic suppuration
    Postoperative sepsis
    Intestinal perforation
    Pancreatic abscess
    Appendicitis
    Chronic inflammatory bowel disease
  Malignant
    Colonic cancer
    Gastric cancer
Arterial
  Endocarditis
  Vascular sepsis
  Ear, throat, nose infection
  Dental infection
Traumatic
  Benign
    Open or closed abdominal trauma
  Malignant
    Chemoembolization
    Percutaneous ethanol injection or radiofrequency
Cryptogenic

Table 59.2   Causes of Pyogenic Liver Abscess in Different Areas of the World

| | HEPATOBILIARY | | | | |
	Benign	Malignant	Cryptogenic	Portal	Other
Western Series					
Giorgio et al, 1995 (n = 115)	38%	13%	28%	19%	2%
Huang et al, 1996 (n = 153)	18%	42%	15%	7%	18%
Seeto & Rockey, 1996 (n = 142)	29%	8%	40%	11%	12%
Barakate et al, 1999 (n = 98)	37%	10%	37%	—	16%
Asian Series					
Chu et al, 1996 (n = 83)	45%	6%	45%	1%	3%
Chou et al, 1997 (n = 483)	35%	2%	59%	—	4%

With the advent and development of improved antibiotics over the past 50 years, the incidence of PLA would be expected to have decreased. The incidence has not decreased, however, and may be increasing, as indicated by the studies of Branum and colleagues (1990) and Huang and associates (1996), in which there were 20 to 22 cases per 100,000 hospital admissions. These figures appear to be almost double those of the previous 2 decades. Over time, the increase in the age of patients with PLA is a reflection of the change in epidemiology. The median age of patients with PLA previously was in the 20s, but the population of patients with hematogenous spread from intra-abdominal infective foci has been decreased by effective treatment of the primary condition. There is now a growing population of older patients with biliary obstruction, malignant disease, and immunocompromised states. The median age of patients with PLA is now in the 50s and 60s (Chou et al, 1997; Rintoul et al, 1996; Wong et al, 2002).

CLINICAL PRESENTATION

Early symptoms during the onset of a PLA are nonspecific and include malaise, nausea, anorexia and weight loss, headaches, myalgia, and arthralgia. These prodromal symptoms may be present for many weeks before the appearance of more specific symptoms, such as fever, chills, and abdominal pain, although the pain is not always localized to the right upper quadrant. An abscess adjacent to the diaphragm may cause pleuritic-type pain, cough, and dyspnea, and when this presentation is associated with the above-mentioned nonspecific symptoms, it can cause diagnostic difficulty (Fig. 59.1). Septic shock may occur in a few patients, especially in the setting of an obstructed biliary tree. Although uncommon, some patients present with peritonitis after free rupture of an abscess into the peritoneal cavity.

DIAGNOSIS

Laboratory investigations show an elevated white blood cell count in most cases, and many patients are anemic because of the chronicity of the pathologic process, which also is manifested by hypoalbuminemia. Elevated transaminases may occur, and an increased alkaline phosphatase level is frequently present. Although clinical jaundice suggests, but is not diagnostic of, biliary tract disease, an elevated bilirubin without clinical jaundice may be present in PLA without underlying bile duct pathology. As indicated earlier, diabetes mellitus is being increasingly recognized in association with PLA. The finding of hyperglycemia may be the first indication that the patient is diabetic or, in the case of a known diabetic, that there is loss of control because of the septic process.

Plain abdominal and chest radiographs are usually too nonspecific to be diagnostic. Unless there are gas-forming organisms in the abscess, which may exhibit air or an air-fluid level, a plain abdominal x-ray does not have a significant role in diagnosis (Fig. 59.2A). On the chest film, an elevated right hemidiaphragm, pleural effusion, and basal atelectasis are likely to be present in about half of cases. Ultrasound is the most likely imaging modality to be used in the initial evaluation of the liver. The appearance on ultrasound varies according to the stage of evolution of the abscess (Saini, 1997). Initially, the abscess is hyperechoic and indistinct, but with maturation and pus formation,

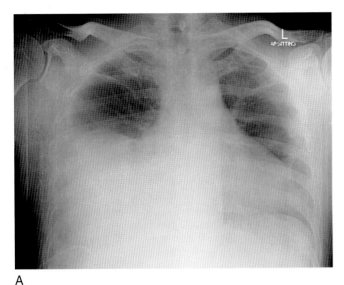

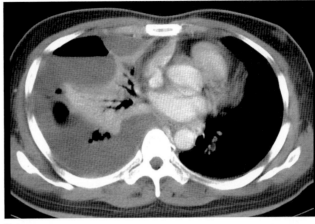

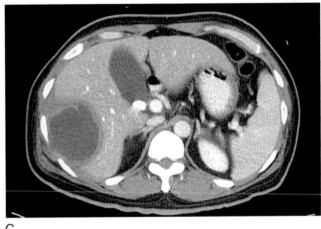

Fig. 59.1. A 42-year-old man presented with cough, fever, dyspnea, and right-sided pleuritic chest pain. Chest x-ray (**A**) showed a large pleural effusion and possible consolidation, and a diagnosis of pneumonia was made. A chest CT scan (**B**) showed collapse/consolidation and pleural effusion in the right hemithorax, whereas CT of the liver (**C**) revealed a PLA that involved the diaphragm. The PLA was treated successfully with antibiotics and percutaneous drainage, whereas the empyema of the right thorax required thoracoscopy and drainage.

it becomes hypoechoic with a distinct margin. When the pus is very thick, a fluid-containing lesion may be confused for a solid lesion on ultrasound. Ultrasound has a sensitivity of 75% to 95%, but has difficulty in detecting an abscess high in the dome of the right hemiliver and especially multiple small PLAs.

By showing gallstones, dilated bile ducts, and hepatolithiasis, ultrasound has the advantage of identifying biliary tract pathology.

A CT scan is more accurate than ultrasound in the differentiation of PLA from other liver lesions and is reported to have a sensitivity of approximately 95% (Saini, 1997). The portal venous

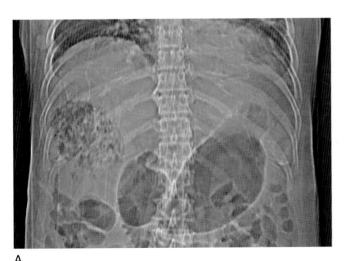

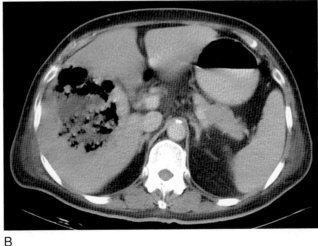

Fig. 59.2. A, Plain abdominal x-ray shows an air-containing cavity in the right upper quadrant of a 53-year-old woman who was diabetic and presented with fever, rigors, and right upper quadrant pain. **B,** CT scan showed the air-filled cavity in the right hemiliver. The PLA, which was caused by *Klebsiella,* was managed successfully by percutaneous drainage.

phase using intravenous contrast material gives the best differentiation between the liver and the abscess, with the periphery of the PLA having contrast enhancement as opposed to non-enhancement of the central portion. Abdominal CT may detect other intra-abdominal pathology, such as diverticulitis or appendicitis, and was reported by Seeto and Rockey (1996) to detect the primary cause of noncryptogenic PLA in almost 70% of cases. Gas-containing PLAs are uncommon (Ralls, 2002), but a high prevalence of gas-containing abscesses was reported in a series from Taiwan (Yang et al, 1993), where it was more common in diabetic patients (see Fig. 59.2B).

Magnetic resonance imaging does not seem to have any advantage over ultrasound and CT in the diagnosis of PLA. When biliary tract disease is suspected, however, magnetic resonance imaging cholangiography is a noninvasive method of identifying the nature and site of the biliary pathology and permits the clinician to plan the best method of intervention.

Liver abscess may be single or multiple. A single abscess is more likely to be cryptogenic in origin, whereas multiple abscesses have a higher incidence of biliary tract disease as the underlying cause (Chou et al, 1997; Perez et al, 2001). Single abscesses are usually larger than multiple abscesses and are located on the right side in about 70% of patients. Multiple PLAs occur on the right side in almost 50% of cases, on the left side in 10%, and on both sides in 40% (Chou et al, 1997). The reason for predilection for PLA to occur in the right hemiliver is unknown, but is most likely to be related to the greater liver mass.

A PLA that is less than 2 cm in diameter is described as a microabscess. Multiple microabscesses have been reported as having two distinct imaging characteristics—multiple, widely scattered lesions and a cluster pattern of microabscesses that appear to aggregate or coalesce focally (Fig. 59.3) (Ralls, 2002). The diffuse miliary pattern of pyogenic microabscesses is usually staphylococcal in origin, whereas the cluster pattern is associated with coliform and enteric organisms. Multifocal clustered abscesses occur in cholangitic abscesses secondary to biliary obstruction. It is probable that the clustering of pyogenic microabscesses is an early stage of an evolving pyogenic abscess cavity, and the tendency of coliform microabscesses to coalesce into a larger abscess with intercommunicating cavities explains the success of single catheter drainage of multiseptate PLAs.

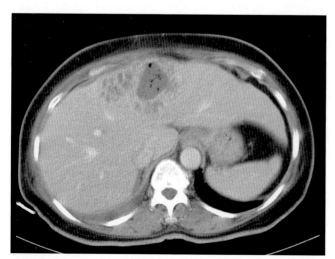

Fig. 59.3. Cluster pattern of microabscesses with coalescence in one portion. The PLA was treated successfully by percutaneous drainage of the larger abscess.

MICROBIOLOGY

The organisms that cause PLA are related to the underlying etiology of the abscess. Identification of the causative organisms may be made from blood culture or aspiration of pus from the PLA or both. A positive culture is less likely from the blood than the pus, but there are different positivity rates depending on the etiology. Patients with cryptogenic PLAs are more likely to have negative cultures from the blood, whereas patients with PLAs secondary to biliary tract disorders are more likely to have positive cultures from blood and aspirated pus (Seeto and Rockey, 1996).

The most common organisms isolated are the gram-negative aerobes *Escherichia coli* and *Klebsiella* species with *E. coli* being cultured most frequently in Western series (Perez et al, 2001; Seeto & Rockey, 1996) and *Klebsiella* in Asian series (Chou et al, 1997; Wang et al, 1998; Wong et al, 2002), although Chou and colleagues (1997) found *Klebsiella* more frequently in single abscesses and *E. coli* more frequently in multiple abscesses in the series from Taiwan. PLAs secondary to *K. pneumoniae* infections are associated with an increased risk of septic metastases and most notably of endophthalmitis (Lin et al, 2004). An abscess secondary to biliary tract disease or originating from a gastrointestinal source is more likely to be polymicrobial with aerobic gram-negative organisms and anaerobes; the latter have been isolated with greater frequency through improvements in collection and culture techniques. *Bacteroides* is the most common isolated anaerobic organism.

Liver abscess as a result of hematogenous spread from a nongastrointestinal source is usually monomicrobial, and staphylococci and streptococci are the most frequent bacteria. In children, *Staphylococcus aureus* PLA is most common and occurs in the setting of chronic granulomatous disease, disorders of granulocyte function, and hematologic malignancy. A liver abscess caused by the *Streptococcus milleri* group of organisms exhibits stellate necrosis with the abscess comprising a solid gelatinous substance and limited liquefaction; what pus does form is inspissated and often too thick to be adequately aspirated or drained percutaneously.

The spectrum of organisms that may be cultured in PLA is listed in Table 59.3. Negative cultures occur in 15% of cases (Perez et al, 2001). Although poor culture technique may be the reason in some cases, negative cultures also can be caused by the use of broad-spectrum antibiotics before cultures are obtained.

TREATMENT

The principles of treatment are to drain the pus, institute appropriate antibiotics, and deal with any underlying source of infection, if present. The advances in ultrasound and CT that have permitted earlier and more accurate diagnosis also have enabled these modalities to facilitate treatment through guided aspiration and drainage, shifting management away from open surgery to minimally invasive techniques. Percutaneous drainage combined with antibiotics has become the first line and mainstay of treatment for most PLAs.

Before obtaining positive cultures from the blood or pus, broad-spectrum antibiotics should be started to cover gram-negative and gram-positive aerobes and anaerobes. Initial therapy with amoxicillin, an aminoglycoside, and metronidazole or a third-generation cephalosporin and metronidazole generally covers the causative organisms most commonly found, although

Table 59.3 Spectrum of Microorganisms That May Cause Pyogenic Liver Abscess

Gram-Negative Aerobes

Escherichia coli
Klebsiella pneumoniae
Pseudomonas aeruginosa
Proteus spp.
Enterobacter cloacae
Citrobacter freundii
Others

Gram-Positive Aerobes

Streptococcus milleri
Staphylococcus aureus
Enterococcus spp.
Others

Gram-Negative Anaerobes

Bacteroides spp.
Fusobacterium spp.

Gram-Positive Anaerobes

Clostridium spp.
Peptostreptococcus spp.

this regimen may be varied according to geographic differences and antimicrobial treatment policies. When information obtained from cultures of blood or pus becomes available, modifications can be instituted. Initially, antibiotics should be administered parenterally, and after 2 weeks of systemic therapy, appropriate oral agents may be used for a further 4 weeks (Ng et al, 2002). In patients with multiple PLAs that are too small to drain, antibiotics may be the only treatment possible. The mortality is likely to be high; Chou and colleagues (1997) reported 29% mortality in their series. Efforts must be made to identify any underlying biliary obstruction, which needs to be overcome for the antibiotic therapy to succeed. Matoba and coworkers (2004) reported that when percutaneous drainage cannot be performed and intravenous administration of antibiotics is ineffective, intermittent hepatic artery antibiotic infusion therapy is a useful alternative.

Percutaneous drainage is performed under ultrasound or CT guidance. Aspiration of the PLA to confirm the diagnosis and obtain pus for culture should be accompanied by complete aspiration of the pus or insertion of a drain at the same time. Clinicians have questioned when should the primary treatment be aspiration alone and when should a percutaneous catheter drain be inserted. Giorgio and associates (1995) reported successful PNA in 98% of 115 consecutive patients with a PLA. Half the patients required only one aspiration, whereas the remainder needed two or three aspirations. These investigators attributed their high success rate to the patient population that they treated, rather than to any great technical expertise. Ch Yu and colleagues (1997) also reported a high success rate (97%) in patients treated by PNA with a similar percentage of patients requiring second or third aspirations to achieve success. Seeto and Rockey (1996) achieved a cure rate of 58% with PNA and 77% with PCD. Chu and coworkers (1996) reported rates of 89% for PNA and PCD. Rajak and colleagues (1998) reported a prospective randomized controlled trial comparing PNA and PCD for amebic and pyogenic abscesses. The trial showed a 100% success rate for PCD and 60% for PNA with the failures successfully treated by PCD. In contrast to other studies using PNA, repeat

aspirations were not performed, and this may account for the lower success rate with PNA. In a prospective randomized trial comparing PNA and PCD in the treatment of PLA, Yu and associates (2004) found that the PNA group had a higher treatment success rate, a shorter hospital stay, and a lower mortality rate, although this did not reach statistical significance. They concluded that intermittent PNA was as effective as PCD.

It can be concluded from the various studies that with a solitary PNA, some patients experience complete resolution, whereas others require repeat procedures. An abscess that is unilocular and less than 5 cm in diameter is most likely to respond, but even when completely evacuated, treatment is prone to failure when there is a thick, noncollapsible wall. Failure also occurs when the pus is too viscous to be aspirated through the needle and is likely when the PLA is multiloculated. When PNA fails, catheter drainage should be performed. Primary treatment by PCD is performed when the pus is too thick to be aspirated, when the PLA is greater than 5 cm in diameter, when the wall is thick and noncollapsible, and when the PLA is multiloculated.

The use of PCD is not precluded by the presence of multiple abscess cavities, but this does necessitate the placement of several catheters. Seeto and Rockey (1996) and Tazawa and colleagues (1997) found PCD was as effective for multiple abscesses as for a single PLA. Chou and coworkers (1997) found PCD procedures failed more frequently in multiple PLAs. These investigators believed that although PCD was indicated as initial therapy, there should be a low threshold to convert to open surgical treatment when early failure to respond becomes apparent.

Although highly successful, PCD fails in approximately 10% of patients. Incomplete or unsuccessful drainage may result from the catheter being too small to drain thick pus. Large drainage tubes are better at emptying highly viscous material, but are prone to iatrogenic complications, such as bleeding. Failure may be due to the position of the catheter not being conducive to adequate drainage. Repositioning of the catheter may rectify the situation. Early success with PCD may be negated unless the catheter is left for sufficient time, and premature removal may result in recurrence. Zenda and associates (2001) proposed that irrigation of the abscess cavity via the drainage tube may be advantageous. The chronicity of the PLA may cause a thick fibrous encasing structure, which is unable to collapse, leading to the failure of PCD. A cluster of abscesses may be misinterpreted as a multiloculated PLA on imaging, and the absence of communication results in incomplete drainage.

An abscess with biliary communication has been reported to be treated as effectively by PCD as a noncommunicating abscess, although the continuous output of bile leads to a prolonged period of abscess drainage (Bayraktar et al, 1996). In a study by Sugiyama and Atomi (2002), 70% of patients whose PLA communicated with the biliary tree and without obstruction were refractory to PCD alone and required an endoscopic stent to be effective. These authors found that in all cases when there was biliary obstruction with a communicating abscess, complete cure after PCD required additional treatment to relieve the obstruction. These biliary abscesses are a complication of cholangitis and are addressed in a separate chapter (see Ch. 58).

Although chronic granulomatous disease is rare, hepatic abscess is a common manifestation of the disease. It is an inherited primary immunodeficiency in which phagocytes cannot destroy catalase-positive bacteria and fungi. The most frequent organism cultured is *S. aureus*. The abscesses are dense, septate masses with a fibrous pseudocapsule and thick inspissated fluid and usually

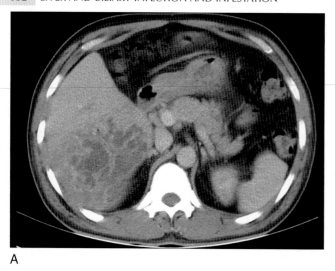
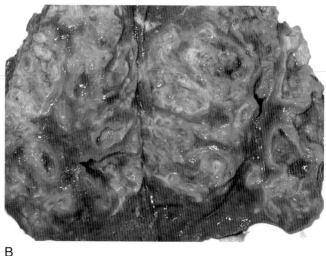

A   B

Fig. 59.4. CT scan (**A**) and resected specimen (segments VI and VII) (**B**) of a multiloculated PLA caused by *Klebsiella*. The PLA failed to resolve with antibiotics and attempted percutaneous aspiration and catheter drainage, which produced only a small amount of thick pus. The open resected specimen shows the solid components of the PLA with minimal liquefaction.

cannot be treated by PCD. Early excision and treatment with antibiotics against *S. aureus* is recommended (Lublin et al, 2002).

SURGICAL TREATMENT

Open operation is indicated when there is failure of nonoperative treatment and for complications of percutaneous drainage, such as bleeding or intraperitoneal leakage of pus. Surgery is required to treat any underlying causative disease if present, although the treatment of this primary abdominal pathology outside the hepatobiliary area may be delayed until percutaneous intervention of the PLA has been performed and resulted in defervescence (Farges et al, 1988; Stain et al, 1991). Primary surgical treatment of PLA is not indicated except in patients with an initial presentation with intraperitoneal rupture or in patients with multiple abscesses above an obstructed duct system that cannot be negotiated by nonoperative means.

The traditional surgical treatment of PLA has been to identify the abscess cavity and perform needle aspiration before blunt puncture of the abscess. Localization of the abscess and identification of any additional lesions can be aided by the use of intraoperative ultrasound. When the abscess cavity is opened and pus is evacuated, finger exploration is needed to break down any loculations and achieve loosening of debris from the wall. A large bore drainage tube or several drainage tubes should be inserted. Ideally, tubes should be positioned to maximize dependent drainage, but the site may make this difficult. Postoperative irrigation and suction of the cavity via the drainage tube is usually advantageous.

There have been isolated references to the use of hepatic resection in the treatment of PLA. In a report on the management of 125 PLAs, Balasegaram (1981) performed resection in 23 patients and had 3 deaths (13%). Chu and colleagues (1996) reported six liver resections for PLA, and all were secondary to hepatolithiasis. In a series of 483 PLAs, Chou and coworkers (1997) performed resection in 27 patients and had 1 death (3.7%). Liver atrophy and multiple PLAs above a long-standing biliary

obstruction from hepatolithiasis or intrahepatic biliary stricture is best treated by hepatic resection. Although the left liver is more frequently involved, hepatolithiasis and PLAs confined to the right hemiliver occasionally require similar treatment. When single or multiple abscesses have caused severe hepatic destruction, resection of the involved liver has been advocated by Chou and coworkers (1997). PNA or PCD is likely to be successful in 90% of liver abscesses. When percutaneous techniques have failed, and open operation is required, the PLA probably has different physical characteristics, such as a noncollapsible thick wall or inspissated pus that is of limited volume and associated with granulomatous or necrotic tissue that has not or is unable to liquefy. Under these circumstances, a different surgical approach may be required.

Lublin and associates (2002) strongly recommended resection of PLAs secondary to chronic granulomotous disease because the abscesses were dense septate masses with a fibrous pseudocapsule and thick inspissated pus and usually could not be treated with percutaneous drainage. Strong and colleagues (2003) reported on hepatic resection in 49 patients in whom the indications were failed medical treatment and complications of PCD (76%) or management of hepatobiliary pathology and the PLA (20%). There were two deaths (4%), which occurred after intraperitoneal rupture of the PLA. The causative bacteria in 72% of the cases of failed medical treatment were *S. milleri* and *K. pneumoniae*; these abscesses showed a solid granulomatous/gelatinous substance with limited liquefaction and histologically showed solid walls, stellate necrosis, and surrounding fibrosis (Figs. 59.4 and 59.5). These findings were similar to the findings with chronic granulomatous disease.

There is no single therapy that cures all cases. Antibiotics combined with percutaneous aspiration (which may need to be repeated) or PCD is successful in 90% of patients. Surgery is reserved for failure of or complications from nonsurgical methods, for intraperitoneal rupture, or for any underlying causative disease process that necessitates surgery. When open operation is required for failure of percutaneous methods, the physical characteristics of the PLA are likely to be different, and hepatic resection may be the most appropriate treatment.

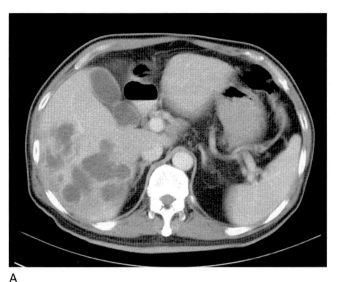
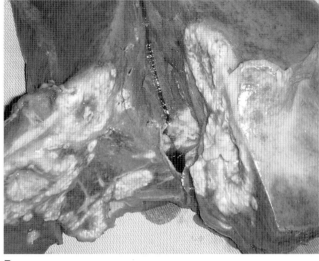

A   B

Fig. 59.5. CT scan (**A**) and resected specimen (segments V and VI) (**B**) of a multiloculated PLA caused by *Streptococcus milleri*. Attempted percutaneous aspiration and catheter drainage failed to obtain more than a minimal amount of thick pus. The open resected specimen shows the typical appearance of a PLA caused by *S. milleri* with solid granulomatous walls and limited liquefaction.

PROGNOSIS

After the introduction of surgical drainage and systemic antibiotics, the mortality of PLA was reduced to less than 50%. The development of ultrasound and CT brought about earlier diagnosis and facilitated percutaneous drainage methods so that by the 1990s, mortality had been reduced to less than 20% (Branum et al, 1990; Seeto & Rockey, 1996). The evolution of more effective treatment of PLA and improvements in supportive therapy resulted in a mortality of 2% for uncomplicated PLA in the series by Seeto and Rockey (1996). With modern treatment, the prognosis depends more on the underlying etiology and comorbid factors than the PLA itself, although delay in presentation and diagnosis contributes to a poor outcome.

The risk factors most commonly associated with mortality include septic shock, clinical jaundice, coagulopathy, leukocytosis, hypoalbuminemia, intraperitoneal rupture, and malignancy. The importance of the severity of underlying illness in the prognosis of PLA is reflected in the series by Mischinger and associates (1994) and Perez and colleagues (2001), who found that a high primary Acute Physiology, Age, and Chronic Health Evaluation (APACHE II) score was a significant factor contributing to a complicated clinical course and mortality. Rupture of a PLA was associated with a high mortality (43.5%) compared with nonruptured abscesses (15.5%) in the series reported by Chou and colleagues (1995). The mortality for patients with multiple PLAs (22%) was significantly higher than in patients with a single abscess (13%), with the former cases more often associated with serious underlying disease than the latter cases, which were more likely to be cryptogenic in origin (Chou et al, 1997).

In general, the prognosis of patients with PLA and underlying malignant disease has been poor. However, Yeh and associates (1998) reported on 53 patients with PLA and malignant disease, and found a discrepancy in mortality rates between patients with hepatopancreatobiliary malignancy (28%) and patients with other malignant disease (10%). In any individual series, the results of treatment of PLA are affected not only by the proportion of patients with malignancy, but also by the relative proportion of patients with hepatopancreatobiliary malignancy.

REFERENCES

Balasegaram M, 1981: Management of hepatic abscess. Curr Prob Surg 18: 282-340.

Barakate M, et al, 1999: Pyogenic liver abscess: a view of 10 years' experience in management. Aust N Z J Surg 69:205-209.

Bayraktar Y, et al, 1996: Percutaneous drainage of hepatic abscess: therapy does not differ for those with identifiable biliary fistula. Hepatogastroenterology 43:620-626.

Bertel C, 1986: Treatment of pyogenic hepatic abscess: surgical versus percutaneous drainage. Arch Surg 121:554-558.

Branum G, et al, 1990: Hepatic abscess: changes in etiology, diagnosis and management. Ann Surg 212:655-662.

Chan SC, et al, 1999: Hepatic abscess due to gastric perforation by ingested fish bone demonstrated by computed tomography. J Formos Med Assoc 98:145-147.

Chen C, et al, 1997: Clinical and microbiological features of liver abscess after transarterial embolization for hepatocellular carcinoma. Am J Gastroenterol 92:2257-2259.

Chou FF, et al, 1995: Rupture of pyogenic liver abscess. Am J Gastroenterol 90:767-770.

Chou FF, et al, 1997: Single and multiple pyogenic liver abscesses: clinical course, etiology and results of treatment. World J Surg 21:384-389.

Chu KM, et al, 1996: Pyogenic liver abscess: an audit of experience over the last decade. Arch Surg 131:148-152.

Ch Yu S, et al, 1997: Pyogenic liver abscess: treatment with needle aspiration. Clin Radiol 52:912-916.

De Baere T, et al, 1996: Liver abscess formation after local treatment of liver tumours. Hepatology 23:1436-1440.

Farges O, et al, 1988: Pyogenic liver abscess: an improvement in prognosis. Br J Surg 75:862-865.

Gerzof S, et al, 1985: Intrahepatic pyogenic abscess: treatment by percutaneous drainage. Am J Surg 149:487-494.

Giorgio A, et al, 1995: Pyogenic liver abscess: 13 years of experience in percutaneous needle aspiration with US guidance. Radiology 195:122-124.

Huang C, et al, 1996: Pyogenic hepatic abscess: changing trends over 42 years. Ann Surg 223:600-609.

Lin JC, et al, 2004: High prevalence of phagocytic-resistant capsular serotypes of *Klebsiella pneumoniae* in liver abscess. Microbes Infect 6:1191-1198.

Lublin M, et al, 2002: Hepatic abscesses in patients with chronic granulomatous disease. Ann Surg 235:383-391.

Matoba M, et al, 2004: Intermittent hepatic artery antibiotic infusion for pyogenic hepatic abscess. Acta Radiol 45:13-17.

McFadzean AJ, et al, 1953: Solitary pyogenic liver abscess treated by closed aspiration and antibiotics: a report of 14 consecutive cases with recovery. Br J Surg 41:141-152.

Mischinger H, et al, 1994: Pyogenic liver abscess: studies of therapy and analysis of risk factors. World J Surg 18:852-858.

Ng FH, et al, 2002: Sequential intravenous/oral antibiotics vs continuous intravenous antibiotics in the treatment of pyogenic liver abscess. Aliment Pharmacol Therap 16:1083-1090.

Oschner A, et al, 1938: Pyogenic abscess of the liver: an analysis of 47 cases with review of the literature. Am J Surg 40:292-319.

Perez J, et al, 2001: Clinical course, treatment and multivariate analysis of risk factors for pyogenic liver abscess. Am J Surg 181:177-186.

Rajak C, et al, 1998: Percutaneous treatment of liver abscesses: needle aspiration versus catheter drainage. AJR Am J Roentgenol 170:1035-1039.

Ralls PW, 2002: Inflammatory disease of the liver. Clin Liver Dis 6:203-225.

Rintoul R, et al, 1996: Changing management of pyogenic liver abscess. Br J Surg 83:1215-1218.

Robert J, et al, 1992. Critical review of the treatment of pyogenic hepatic abscess. Surg Gynecol Obstet 174:102.

Saini S, 1997: Imaging of the hepatobiliary tract. N Engl J Med 336:1889-1894.

Seeto R, Rockey D, 1996: Pyogenic liver abscess: changes in etiology, management and outcome. Medicine 75:99-113.

Stain S, et al, 1991: Pyogenic liver abscess: modern treatment. Arch Surg 126:991-995.

Strong RW, 2005: Unpublished data.

Strong R, et al, 2003: Hepatectomy for pyogenic liver abscess. HPB Surg 5:86-90.

Sugiyama M, Atomi Y, 2002: Pyogenic abscess with biliary communication. Am J Surg 183:205-208.

Tazawa J, et al, 1997: Solitary and multiple pyogenic liver abscesses: characteristics of the patients and efficacy of percutaneous drainage. Am J Gastroenterol 92:271-274.

Wang JH, et al, 1998: Primary liver abscess due to *Klebsiella pneumoniae* in Taiwan. Clin Infect Dis 26:1434-1438.

Wong WM, et al, 2002: Pyogenic liver abscess: retrospective analysis of 80 cases over a 10 year period. J Gastroenterol Hepatol 17:1001-1007.

Yang CC, et al, 1993: Pyogenic liver abscess in Taiwan: emphasis on gas-forming abscess in diabetes. Am J Gastroenterol 88:1911-1915.

Yeh TS, et al, 1998: Pyogenic liver abscesses in patients with malignant disease. Arch Surg 133:242-245.

Yu SC, et al, 2004: Treatment of pyogenic liver abscess: prospective randomized comparison of catheter drainage and needle aspiration. Hepatology 39:932-938.

Zenda T, et al, 2001: Irrigation of liver abscess: proposal of a novel method and possible indications. Hepatogastroenterology 48:847-850.

Amebiasis and Other Parasitic Infections

P. G. THOMAS AND N. GARG

AMEBIC LIVER ABSCESS

History

The first mention of blood and mucous diarrhea is found in the Sanskrit document *Bhrigu-samhita,* dated 3000 B.C. (Vaidya & Ray, 1982). The association of "ball-like" abdominal masses with this condition also has been recorded and is thought to be indicative of coexisting hepatic abscess. The occurrence of a similar syndrome in different parts of the Old World is recorded in the writings of Hippocrates (5th century B.C.), Roman physicians, and practitioners in the Middle Ages (Martinez Baez, 1986).

In 1818, Ballingall described a serendipitous cure of tropical liver abscess when during a duel in Madras (now called Chennai) between two British military officers one of them received a lucky shot that punctured his liver abscess. The pus drained, and he was cured of his malaise. Open drainage of liver abscesses with insertion of setons into the abscess cavity was advocated by Ballingall, but the technique fell into disrepute because of the high associated mortality owing to sepsis. Twenty-six such tropical abscesses in association with dysentery were described in an autopsy series in 1828 by Amesley in Bombay (Kapoor, 1979).

Lesch was the first to recognize amebae in colonic lesions accompanying acute dysentery. In his 1875 case report describing a fatal case of amebic colitis in a Russian peasant who migrated to St. Petersburg from within the Arctic Circle, Lesch found motile amebae in the mucous clots of the patient's feces and showed at autopsy that the terminal ileum and colon had submucosal invasion by amebae (Martinez Baez, 1986).

The debate about whether amebae were etiologic agents or secondary invaders in amebic colitis and liver abscess continued even as Kartulis in Greece (1886) reported 150 cases of amebic dysentery with 20 associated liver abscesses, and Osler in America (1890) reported a young physician who died of amebic hepatic abscess after an attack of dysentery while in Panama. The detailed study of Councilman and LaFleur (1891) at the Johns Hopkins Hospital established the pathogenic role of amebae and coined the terms *amebic dysentery* and *amebic liver abscess* (Martinez Baez, 1986).

Between 1849 and 1919, the different species of amebae found in the human host—*Entamoeba gingivalis, Entamoeba coli, Iodamoeba bütschlii,* and *Entamoeba hartmanni*—were discovered, and Schaudin in 1903 named the pathogenic species *Entamoeba histolytica* (Martinez Baez, 1986). The discovery of two distinct species of *Entamoeba* that are morphologically indistinguishable—*Entamoeba dispar* and *E. histolytica*—has shed more light on the *asymptomatic carrier state* commonly encountered all over the world. *E. dispar* is the more prevalent species and is associated only with an asymptomatic carrier state. The pathogenic species *E. histolytica* is associated with invasive disease (Ravdin, 1995).

Experimental inoculation of dogs and cats was achieved by Lesch (dogs) and Koch (cats), but the axenic culture of *E. histolytica* proved a much more difficult task and was not achieved until 1978 (Diamond et al, 1978).

Molecular phylogeny revealed that *Entamoeba* species (*E. histolytica* and *E. dispar*) are close to *Dictyostelium discoideum* on one of the lowest branches of the eukaryotic tree. Amebae previously were thought to lack organelles (e.g., mitochondria, endoplasmic reticulum, and Golgi apparatus). Sequencing of the genome and other studies provide evidence for the nuclear-encoded mitochondrial genes, a remnant mitochondrial organelle (Tovar et al, 1999). The detection of a calreticulin-like protein indicates that a system akin to the eukaryotic endoplasmic reticulum and the Golgi apparatus exists in amebae (Gonzalez et al, 2002).

Medical treatment for amebic colitis has been described since ancient times. A plant alkaloid called concessine, advocated in the *Ayurveda,* has been found to kill *E. histolytica* in culture (Vaidya & Ray, 1982). The first effective treatment known in the Old World came from Brazil in the 17th century in the form of ipecac—the active principle of the root of *Cephaelis ipecacuanha*—the curative powers of which were known to indigenous tribes of South America. Emetine was isolated from ipecac in the early 19th century, but was ignored until Rogers in 1912 showed its usefulness in the treatment of colonic and hepatic amebiasis. Although largely replaced by the imidazoles in the 1980s, it remains a useful drug today.

Epidemiology

Worldwide, amebiasis is the third most common parasitic cause of death (Li & Stanley, 1996). It is classically defined as infection with *E. histolytica* with or without overt clinical symptoms. *E. histolytica* was thought to be ubiquitous in distribution with an estimated 12% global incidence of infection (Davis & Pawlowski, 1985), and 50% of the population may harbor amebae in tropical and subtropical regions, including Mexico, Central and South America, India, Southeast Asia, and eastern and southern Africa (Ravdin, 1995). It is now recognized that many individuals may harbor *E. dispar* and not *E. histolytica.* Together, these two organisms are thought to infect 10% of the world's population, with *E. dispar* infection being 10-fold more common than *E. histolytica.* Among individuals infected with *E. histolytica,* 40 million develop invasive amebiasis (colitis and hepatic abscess) resulting in 40,000 deaths annually (Li & Stanley, 1996). Disease expression varies geographically; invasive disease in Egypt is predominantly amebic colitis, whereas in South Africa an excessive rate of amebic liver abscess is noted. Although amebic liver abscess has been encountered in epidemic form in temperate climates in the past, as in the water-borne epidemic of Chicago in 1933 (Munoz, 1986), it is at present a problem chiefly of the tropics and developing countries, where the disease is endemic and occurs in approximately 2% of adult patients (Sepulveda, 1982). In developed countries, it continues to be encountered sporadically and can pose considerable problems in the diagnosis and interpretation of physical and radiologic findings. High-risk groups include immigrants and travelers from endemic zones, members of low socioeconomic groups, residents of institutions (especially mentally retarded individuals), and promiscuous male homosexuals (Ravdin, 1995). Traveler's diarrhea is rarely caused by *E. histolytica,* which usually occurs only after a long stay (usually >1 month) in an endemic area. The observation that male homosexuals despite a high incidence of infection rarely get invasive disease in temperate climates is probably because the usual organism harbored is the morphologically indistinguishable *E. dispar* (Allason-Jones et al, 1988).

In the past, the highest reported incidence of invasive amebiasis came from Mexico, where seropositivity was found in 29% of the population tested by the indirect hemagglutination technique, which detects antibodies that persist for many years. The counterimmunoelectrophoresis test, which estimates recent infection, suggested an annual incidence of 5% (Walsh, 1986). Few population surveys of this size and quality are available from other developing countries, although prevalence rates of 50% are estimated in some developing areas, where cultural habits, crowding, and poor sanitation are responsible (Cabellero-Salcedo et al, 1994). In a study in Bangladesh, in the impoverished population, 55% of children acquired *E. histolytica* within the 2-year study period. Of these, 17% exhibited multiple infections as determined by polymerase chain reaction (PCR) for the gene-encoding serine-rich *E. histolytica* protein (Haque et al, 2002). Poverty facilitates infection because of deficiencies in sanitation and hygiene and suboptimal sewer systems, which facilitate ingestion of infective *E. histolytica* cysts.

Organism

The protozoan *E. histolytica* belongs to the subphylum Sarcodina (whose motility depends on pseudopodia), the superclass Rhizopoda, and the order Amoebida. The genus *Entamoeba* includes the species *E. histolytica, E. hartmanni* (a noninvasive "small race" with cysts <10 μm in diameter), *E. coli, E. polecki* (infects pigs), and *E. moshkovskii* (a free-living nonpathogenic form found in sewage) (Guerrant, 1986). Except for *E. histolytica,* the other species are regarded as nonpathogenic. With the discovery of *E. dispar,* the identification of *E. histolytica* on morphology has become unreliable. The presence of ingested erythrocytes is seen only with *E. histolytica.* The two species now have been characterized by the study of zymodemes (patterns of electrophoretic mobility of isoenzymes) and genetic differences using RNA and DNA probes and the use of PCR amplification (Tannich et al, 1989).

E. histolytica has two forms: trophozoite and cyst. The trophozoites are uninucleate, facultative anerobes with a double-layered limiting membrane surrounded by a fuzzy, external 20- to 30-μm glycocalyx. Using the electrophoretic patterns of amebic enzymes such as glucose-6-phosphate isomerase, L-malate dehydrogenase, nicotinamide adenine dinucleotide phosphate oxidoreductase, phosphoglucomutase, and hexokinase, 18 zymodemes of *E. histolytica* have been described from various parts of the world. Seven of these strains have been isolated from subjects with mucosal ulceration and hepatic abscesses and consequently are labeled as pathogenic (Sargeaunt et al, 1984).

Cysts of *E. histolytica* are quadrinucleate. These cysts, measuring 8 to 20 μm, are an important identifying feature and constitute the infective form of the organism. They are responsible for fecal-oral transmission via food, water, or direct person-to-person contact. After ingestion, the quadrinucleate cysts reach the intestinal tract, where they develop into a metacystic stage and undergo an additional nuclear division; eight new uninucleate trophozoites emerge to complete the life cycle (Guerrant, 1986). Cysts survive 45 minutes in fecal material lodged under the fingernails and 1 month in soil at 10°C. They remain infective in fresh water, seawater, and sewage, but are rapidly destroyed by drying, 200 ppm of iodine, and heat greater than 68°C. They are not killed by chlorination used to purify ordinary drinking water (Munoz, 1986).

Community Screening Procedures

The parasitologic protocol in practice includes the following: (1) microscopic examination of unfixed fecal samples that are unstained or stained with iodine; (2) Ritchie's fecal concentration of formalin-fixed samples; (3) trichrome staining of polyvinyl alcohol–fixed stools; (4) Robinson's in vitro culture; (5) screening with two stool antigen detection tests, one specific for pathogenic *E. histolytica* (*E. histolytica* II; TechLab, Blacksburg, VA) and one that cross-reacts with nonpathogenic *E. dispar* (Prospect *Entamoeba histolytica* Microplate Assay; Alexon-Trend, Ramsey, MN); (6) serologic analysis that includes indirect hemagglutination test, enzyme immunoassay, and indirect immunofluorescence test; and (7) starch gel isoenzyme electrophoresis of stool samples, which permits zymodeme identification.

Although direct microscopic examination is found to be more sensitive than the serologic tests, the sensitivity of both techniques is lower than Robinson's culture and zymodeme identification—the "gold standards" that together are highly sensitive and specific to distinguish *E. histolytica* from *E. dispar* (Gatti et al, 2002). The more recently developed DNA-based PCR technique is sensitive enough to detect a few (<5) cysts in the stool sample and in amebic liver abscess fluids, is rapid to perform, and selectively differentiates *E. histolytica* from *E. dispar* without the need for precultivation. PCR offers promise for accurate and reliable epidemiology of the two species (Rivera et al, 1998).

Host Factors

The human host represents the major reservoir, although cross-infection from animals—particularly monkeys and rodents—has been postulated. Interperson transmission occurs via flies and handlers and by sewage contamination of water sources. Male homosexuals also transmit the infection, but usually harbor nonpathogenic *E. dispar. E. dispar* infection occurs more frequently in females than in males. *E. histolytica* has an equal prevalence and incidence in males and females (Gatharim & Jackson, 1987). For reasons not completely understood, menstruating women are protected against invasive infection. Breastfed children also have a low incidence of invasion, and this has been postulated to be due to the presence of protective IgA in the immune mother's milk and to the low iron content of milk.

A high content of iron in the diet, often obtained from country liquor, predisposes to invasive amebiasis, as does a diet rich in carbohydrate. Young men of low socioeconomic status are the most commonly affected group (Gatharim & Jackson, 1987). A study of 8800 cases of amebic liver abscess found that men accounted for 86% of the cases (Wells & Arguedas, 2004). Elderly individuals with underlying diseases and patients with depressed immunity secondary to malnutrition or corticosteroid therapy also are prone to invasion by amebae. The natural resistance of menstruating women is lost in pregnancy (Guerrant, 1986). In the Mexican mestizo population, the presence of HLA DR3 and comploty pe SCO1 in adults and children constitutes a primary independent risk factor for the development of amebic liver abscess, regardless of age or sex (Arellano et al, 1996).

Pathogenesis

On infection, trophozoites infest the large intestine, where they actively feed on bacteria and fecal material. Invasive disease occurs when *E. histolytica* trophozoites, instead of remaining confined in the intestinal lumen, penetrate the intestinal mucosal barrier and establish extraintestinal infection throughout the portal vein radicles, most commonly in liver (Ravdin, 1995). Three virulence factors are currently thought to determine the course of disease: lectin (a parasite surface protein), amebapores, and cysteine proteases.

Adhesion of the trophozoite to colonic walls is mediated by the parasite surface galactose/*N*-acetylgalactosamine (GalNAc) lectin. This lectin is a complex heterodimer that comprises a 170-KD subunit joined to a 35/31-KD subunit via a disulfide bond and is associated with another 150-KD protein. If the parasite lectin attaches to host mucin glycoproteins lining the intestine, it results in persistent infection. Attachment of the lectin to a host cell surface glycoprotein leads to lectin-induced calcium concentration flux in the host cell, which results in caspase activation. Activation of caspase 3, a distal effector molecule in the apoptotic pathway, is a crucial step in cell killing and in the formation of abscess in vivo. Virulence may be directly proportional to the ameba's ability to cause apoptosis and phagocytize the dead cells (Huston et al, 2003).

Small peptides termed *amebapores* are inserted into the host cell by the trophozoite and have the capacity to puncture the lipid bilayer, disrupt the barrier function of the mucosal epithelium, and form a portal of entry into the host. The amebapore is similar to human complement and results in colloid osmotic lysis of the cell and is likely involved in pathogenicity (Leippe et al, 1991).

Cysteine proteases are important to the pathogenesis of *E. histolytica* because they contribute to degradation of the extracellular matrix proteins and disruption of cell monolayers (Que & Reed, 1997). Cysteine proteases are encoded by a family of approximately 20 genes. The differential expression of these 20 genes between *E. histolytica* and *E. dispar* possibly contributes to invasive characteristics of *E. histolytica* (Que & Reed, 1997). One could anticipate that antiamebic antibodies protective against invasive infection would block lectin binding, neutralize amebapore and cysteine proteases, or inhibit amebic receptors involved in endocytosis of apoptotic cells.

The hepatic infection occurs primarily from trophozoites entering the portal venous system. In experimental studies, extensive necrosis in the liver is associated with minimal inflammation. Polymorphonuclear neutrophils are particularly ineffective against *E. histolytica* and are readily lysed by the virulent strains; this could result in the release of toxic neutrophil enzymes, and such enzymes may increase further the local tissue destruction in amebic liver abscess. There is experimental evidence that liver cell necrosis is increased when neutrophils are present along with *E. histolytica*. Although small infarcts resulting from small vessel occlusion by amebae have been shown (Aikat et al, 1979), these may be only very early lesions.

Molecular Genetics

Molecular biology and genomics research is initiating revolutionary advances in medicine, and amebiasis research is no exception. The Institute for Genomic Research in Rockville, Maryland, and Sanger Institute in Cambridge, United Kingdom, are jointly involved in sequencing the complete *E. histolytica* genome and, for comparative purposes, partially sequencing four other closely related intestinal protozoa (*E. dispar, E. moshkovskii, Entamoeba terrapinae, Entamoeba invadens*). These efforts have identified that *E. histolytica* has a small (approximately 20 Mb) genome that is rich in adenosine-thymidine contents, is highly repetitive, contains densely packed coding sequences, and lacks introns (Mann, 2002). Although some regions of the genome encode highly conserved proteins, other areas exhibit high degrees of polymorphism (Haghighi et al, 2002). These polymorphic loci may assist geographic origin and transmission of the isolates. The comparative genome analysis would offer a potential opportunity to elucidate specific genes and proteins that differ between *E. dispar* and *E. histolytica* and may contribute to the pathogenicity of the latter.

Host Defense and Potential for Vaccine Development

Immunologic reactions to *E. histolytica* are humoral and cellular. Some immune components are effective in limiting the disease process, whereas others may exacerbate the pathologic sequelae of disease. The organism has developed multiple methods to evade the immune system. Although it has not been finally established as to which mechanism is responsible for limiting invasion by amebae, immunity against recurrent disease does develop. Recurrence of amebic liver abscess is rare (e.g., only 0.29% recurrence among 1021 patients followed for 5 years in Mexico) (Ravdin & Guerrant, 1982).

The first line of defense against *E. histolytica* is provided by innate mechanisms. The organism is susceptible to complement in the serum of healthy and immunocompromised individuals. Complement probably cannot prevent invasion, however, because it is absent from gut mucosal secretions. Strains resistant to complement have developed over time. Resistant strains express an epitope on the GalNAc lectin that has sequence similarity and antigenic cross-reactivity to the human CD59. This epitope prevents the assembly of the C5b-9 complement complex and makes the organism invisible to the host alternative complement system (Braga et al, 1992). Amebic cysteine proteases also degrade C3a and C5a complement components (Reed et al, 1995). Similarly, neutrophils fail in initial host defense because *E. histolytica* produces a chemoattractant for neutrophils that kills these cells on contact (Salata et al, 1989).

The second line of adaptive immune response constituted by activated lymphocytes and macrophages is the important effector mechanism against *E. histolytica* (Vohra et al, 2003). The cell-mediated response releases cytokines (e.g., interferon-γ, tumor necrosis factor-α, and interleukin-4) that are essential in the activation of macrophages, which kill *E. histolytica* trophozoites.

Noninvasive and invasive *E. histolytica* infection elicits mucosal IgA and serum IgG response to the lectin protein. The mucosal IgA response against a carbohydrate domain of the galactose/GalNAc lectin protein has been shown in Bangladeshi children to be protective against infection (Haque et al, 2002). In a prospective study of adult patients cured of amebic liver abscess, antilectin IgA antibodies were found to be protective against new infections (Abd-Alla et al, 2004). Molecular studies have identified that a cysteine-rich portion of the galactose-lectin heavy subunit is recognized as a main epitope to induce protective humoral (IgA) immunity (Mann et al, 1993). In addition, epitope-specific antibodies have been shown to inhibit adherence to target cells (Pillai et al, 1999). The galactose/GalNAc lectin isolates from three distinct areas of the world (Bangladesh, Georgia, and Mexico) retain remarkable sequence conservation (Beck et al, 2002), and galactose/GalNAc lectin is recognized as a potential vaccine target.

Serum IgG response to the lectin protein does not provide protection against infection and was associated with a higher likelihood of future invasive disease in Bangladeshi children (Haque et al, 2002). In prospective studies, 81% to 100% of adult patients with invasive colonic amebiasis were shown to develop specific circulating IgG antibodies, and this response lasted 2 to 11 years. There is no positive correlation, however, between this response and invasive infection. Amebae have been shown to aggregate, ingest, and shed human antibodies, and invasive amebiasis can recur in the presence of high titers (Salata & Ravdin, 1986).

Acquired immunity to *E. histolytica* is correlated with mucosal immune response. Amebic antigens that induce gut-associated lymphoid tissue are considered the primary vaccine candidates. Oral vaccines are known to be effective in inducing mucosal immune response. Studies have used live attenuated *Salmonella* (Mann et al, 1997) and *Yersinia* outer protein E (Lotter et al, 2003) to deliver orally the antigenic candidate (lectin). These reports show induction of significant antibody response to galactose-lectin and protection against amebic liver abscess in the gerbil model. Finally, codon-optimized DNA vaccine targeting a portion of the galactose-lectin heavy subunit also has been tested in a murine model and found useful in stimulating a lectin-specific type 1 cellular immune response and serum antibodies (Gaucher and Chadee, 2002). The process of screening and testing of the antigenic candidates and the development, processing, and testing of a vaccine is extraordinarily expensive and remains in its infancy.

Pathology

Regardless of the mechanism involved, trophozoites that successfully penetrate the colonic mucosal barrier cause invasive disease and enter into the portal system and travel to the liver. Direct extension to the liver and lymphatic spread are not thought to occur. Active colitis and amebic liver abscess rarely occur simultaneously, and as a rule the colonic lesions are silent. Liver cells undergo liquefaction necrosis starting in the center and spreading peripherally to produce a cavity filled with blood and liquefied liver tissue. The appearance of this pus typically is described to resemble anchovy sauce (Fig. 60.1); it has no odor and is sterile. There is little inflammation at the expanding edge of the abscess cavity. Amebae are known to lyse neutrophils, and the release of neutrophilic mediators may promote hepatocyte death and extension of the abscess. Amebae can be found at the edge of the lesion, but are not present in the pus. Secondary infection rarely occurs spontaneously, but may alter the color and consistency of the pus and certainly its odor. With centrifugal extension and a lack of fibrotic response by the surrounding tissue, the abscess soon extends to Glisson's capsule, which is resistant to the amebae.

Typically, the lesion is solitary and large and located in the right liver. Left lobe abscesses are less common, but because of the smaller volume of the left liver, abscesses in this location are more prone to rupture the capsule. The abscess cavity is crisscrossed by vascular and biliary portal structures, which, because of their intrahepatic covering of Glisson's capsule, are resistant to

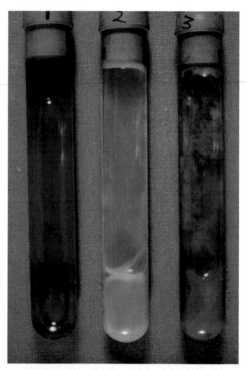

Fig. 60.1. Variable appearance of fluid aspirated from a single amebic liver abscess: (1) initial aspirate, straw-colored, but tinged with bile; (2) mid-aspirate, creamish in color; and (3) terminal aspirate, typical "anchovy pus."

the process of liquefaction necrosis. These structures can be mistaken for septa within the abscess cavity, and fracturing of these strands can lead to hemorrhage or biliary leak or can create a communication between the vascular and biliary channels resulting in hemobilia.

The abscess wall is typically ill defined with a minimal host response of fibrous tissue, but long-standing abscesses may develop a fibrous wall and even calcify. In treated cases, complete resolution is the rule, but may take 6 months to 2 years—longer usually than the time for pyogenic abscesses to resolve.

Clinical Presentation

Amebic liver abscess occurs 10 times more commonly in adults than in children and is 3 to 10 times more common in men (Sepulveda & Manzo, 1986). Although worldwide the peak incidence is between 20 and 60 years, it is predominantly a disease of young men. In population groups not commonly affected, such as children and especially neonates, pregnant women, and women in the postpartum period, there is increased risk of severe disease and death. Treatment with steroids, malignancy, and malnutrition are other risk factors for severe disease (Li & Stanley, 1996).

The time interval between penetration of colonic mucosa and damage to hepatic parenchyma is unknown. Less than 30% of patients have active diarrhea at any time before presentation, even though intestinal infection by *E. histolytica* must have occurred. Although standard stool microscopy is negative in most cases, in research studies cultures of stool are positive for *E. histolytica* in more than 75% of patients with amebic liver abscess (Irusen et al, 1992). A concomitant hepatic abscess is found in only a third of patients with amebic colitis.

The duration of symptoms is usually 10 days or less. In nonendemic regions, such as Western Europe and the United States, patients usually report travel to an endemic area in the last 2 to 5 months (median 3 months) (Wells & Arguedas, 2004). Although abdominal pain and fever are the cardinal symptoms of the disease and seen in 90% or more of patients, the signs and symptoms vary according to the gravity of the illness and the location of the abscess. Typically, the onset is abrupt, with pain located in the right hypochondrium being the chief complaint. The pain may radiate to the right shoulder and scapular area and increase with movements of coughing, deep breathing, and walking. If the abscess is located in the left lobe, the pain may be epigastric, precordial, or retrosternal and may radiate to the left shoulder. An abscess located on the inferior aspect of the liver may present similar to peritonitis resulting from any upper abdominal cause.

Fever typically is between 38°C and 40°C and is seen in virtually all patients. Other, less specific symptoms include anorexia, nausea, vomiting, and an acute colitic illness. Occasionally, the presentation is insidious, lasting 2 or more weeks, and in such patients significant weight loss may occur. One report suggested that amebic liver abscesses can be silent and asymptomatic (Blessman et al, 2003).

Physical examination reveals a painful, generalized, and soft hepatomegaly that usually is accompanied by overlying muscle guarding, intercostal tenderness, and, occasionally, increased warmth and cutaneous edema. Mild jaundice is seen often, although it is a prominent feature in only 5% to 8% of cases (Pitt, 1990). In the most common location—the right posterior-superior surface—amebic liver abscess always is accompanied by right basal lung signs. A pericardial rub may occur in association with a left-side abscess. Signs of hepatic failure, ascites, and splenomegaly are rare. Clinically, the usual differential diagnosis includes acute cholecystitis, hepatitis resulting from viral or other causes, and pyogenic liver abscess. With atypical presentation, hepatocellular carcinoma, hepatic hydatid cyst, or simple cyst may be considered.

Hematologic investigations in amebic liver abscess usually reveal leukocytosis (12,000-30,000 cells/mm³) without eosinophilia. Mild anemia, with hemoglobin typically around 12 g/dL, may occur in half of patients, although in young male alcoholics hemoglobin may be normal or increased. Liver function tests show moderate elevation of alkaline phosphatase. Typically, bilirubin is usually less than 3 mg/dL, and transaminases are less than three times above the normal range. The most common abnormality is an increased prothrombin time. Chest radiography typically shows elevation of the right dome of the diaphragm with an anterior bulge on the lateral view (Debakey & Ochsner, 1951), atelectasis of the right lung, and pleural effusion. The hepatic shadow on plain abdominal x-ray is diffusely enlarged and is usually featureless. Gas in the biliary tree or liver parenchyma is unusual, unless there is communication of the hepatic abscess cavity with the lung or hollow viscus.

Ultrasonography

Ultrasonography is simple, inexpensive, and quick to perform, with a diagnostic accuracy of 90% (Sepulveda & Manzo, 1986) (see Ch. 15). Interpretation of ultrasound findings against the clinical background and confirmation when necessary by serologic tests are required, however, to avoid major errors in diagnosis. Abscesses usually are located peripherally in contact with the liver capsule (Fig. 60.2) and vary from 2 to 21 cm in size (mean 7.75 cm).

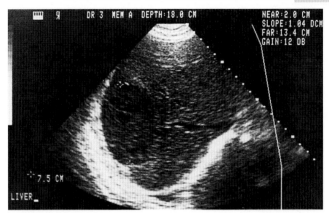

Fig. 60.2. Ultrasound showing a typical liver abscess in a 36-year-old man, peripherally located, 7.5 cm in diameter, with poor rim, internal echoes, and distal sonic enhancement.

The outline is round, oval, or lobulated. The abscess, although clearly defined from the surrounding normal liver parenchyma with distal sonic enhancement (Figs. 60.3 to 60.5), rarely has rim echoes that can be interpreted as an abscess wall (Ralls et al, 1979). The contents of the abscess cavity are usually hypoechoic and nonhomogeneous, with the internal echoes increasing at high gain and decreasing or almost absent at normal gain (Ralls et al, 1982). In 78% to 80% of cases, the abscess occurs singly and in the right lobe; 10% of abscesses are in the left lobe; and the remaining abscesses are multiple. In 6% of cases, the abscess may be located in the caudate lobe (Ralls et al, 1979).

Only 40% of patients have typical ultrasound features of amebic liver abscess, and 9% may have completely bizarre findings. Serial scanning tends to show no change in the ultrasound picture despite adequate treatment with amebicidal drugs or complete aspiration of the abscess or both (Ralls et al, 1979; Sukov et al, 1980). The mean resolution time is 7 months, and in 70% of patients, the ultrasound findings persist for 6 months or more; this must be taken into account when evaluating treatment responses. Serial scanning is unwarranted in patients with clinical improvement. The persistence of ultrasound signs also must be taken into account in evaluating patients with a focal lesion in the liver in whom a definite diagnosis of amebic liver abscess was not made before initiating treatment. Although pyogenic liver abscesses tend to resolve earlier, with 50% resolving

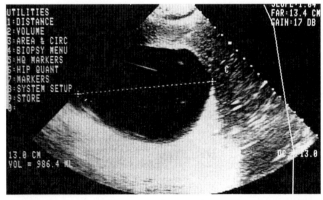

Fig. 60.3. Ultrasound showing an abscess with more liquid contents in a 25-year-old man. The distal sonic enhancement has resulted in a "white-out" of structures distal to the abscess cavity.

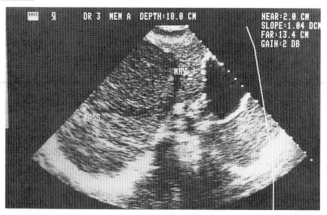

Fig. 60.4. Ultrasound from a 50-year-old woman with a right liver mass initially mistaken for amebic liver abscess, but which proved on further investigation to be a tumor. There is a mixed echo pattern with hyperechoic and medium-level echoes. There is no clear margin, and no distal sonic enhancement typical of an amebic abscess.

in 2 months and 90% within 4 months, amebic liver abscesses acquire a more echogenic and fibrous wall in 8 to 16 weeks and begin to resemble, but should be differentiated from, an encapsulated tumor (see Figs. 60.3 to 60.5). With time, resolution may be complete or result in a small residual cystic cavity that resembles a simple cyst of the liver (Ralls et al, 1983; Sheen et al, 1989).

Computed Tomography

Especially in the acute situation, a computed tomography (CT) scan does not add to the diagnostic accuracy of ultrasound except in the evaluation of imminent rupture of abscess. In an atypical or chronic case, CT may be of value; it shows better rim enhancement with contrast enhancement in pyogenic liver abscess and high density of the contents in necrotic liver tumors. Similarly, hydatid and simple cysts may be diagnosed more accurately if CT supplements ultrasound examination. Better delineation of organs in the vicinity of the liver is possible with CT (Radin et al, 1988).

Magnetic Resonance Imaging

Although current evidence shows that magnetic resonance imaging (MRI) is not significantly superior to CT in the diagnosis of amebic liver abscess, it may be useful in follow-up of a treated

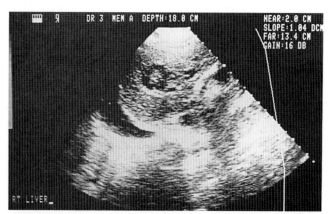

Fig. 60.5. Ultrasound showing a typical metastatic "target" deposit in a 45-year-old woman. The central location, smaller size, and poor distal enhancement differentiate it from an amebic abscess. The presence of ascites is visible.

case and in differentiating it from a hepatic neoplasm. Untreated amebic liver abscesses show up as heterogeneous abscess cavities that appear hypointense on T1-weighted and hyperintense on T2-weighted MRI. Incomplete hyperintense rings can be seen at the abscess margin. With successful treatment, the abscess cavity becomes homogeneous, and complete concentric rings develop caused by periabscess fibrosis and hemosiderin deposits. Reparative tissue changes are seen 4 days after treatment and indicate a favorable response. Evidence of hemorrhage would show up on MRI, but the iron deposition is not typically in the periphery as in the case of a hematoma.

Angiography

Although rarely required in the diagnosis of a straightforward amebic liver abscess, angiography may be necessary in a case in which a differential diagnosis of carcinoma is difficult to exclude. Typically, and in contrast to a neoplasm, angiography reveals a hypovascular or avascular mass displacing the hepatic artery branches. The venous phase images likewise may show displacement of the portal vein branches, but occasionally may show a block of the portal vein.

Gallium Scanning

Gallium scanning helps in the differentiation of amebic from pyogenic abscess. Amebic abscesses, lacking in neutrophils, appear as cold spots, whereas pyogenic lesions are seen as warm spots. Owing to the long time it takes to perform the scan, however, and the relative safety and speed of diagnostic aspiration, the role of gallium scanning is limited. It may be particularly useful in the differentiation between amebic and pyogenic abscess.

Amebic Serology

Patients with amebic liver abscess virtually always (90-95%) have serum antiamebic antibodies. These antibodies can be shown using indirect hemagglutination or counterimmunoelectrophoresis, which are similar in sensitivity. Enzyme-linked immunosorbent assay (ELISA) also is highly sensitive and widely available. More recent developments in ELISA (Sharma et al, 1988) have resulted in rapid and accurate diagnosis; the test can be completed in 35 minutes. Antibody response is directly related to the duration of illness and may be detectable 7 to 10 days after the onset of symptoms. Titers reach a peak by the second and third months, decreasing to lower, but still detectable levels by 9 months (Munoz, 1986). Problems with interpreting serology results occur in endemic areas, where widespread amebic colonic infection can result in high titers without invasive colonic or hepatic amebiasis. The chief value lies in differentiating amebic from pyogenic liver abscess and from hepatocellular carcinoma.

ELISA or indirect hemagglutination assay cannot differentiate acute from remote infection in endemic areas. Counterimmunoelectrophoresis and gel diffusion methods are less sensitive, but may be more helpful in diagnosing current infection in endemic areas because the results become negative 6 to 12 months after acute infection. Efforts are ongoing to identify antigens specific for acute infection (Ravdin, 1995).

Role of Aspiration

In the era before there was experience with ultrasound diagnosis, aspiration of the typical anchovy sauce pus from the liver was considered vital to confirm the diagnosis of amebic liver abscess (see Fig. 60.1). Nowadays, ultrasound-guided aspiration is often justified on the basis that the diagnosis would be "more certain," or that the abscess can be "aspirated to dryness" at the time of diagnostic aspiration. PCR is an important adjunct to the diagnostic armamentarium because it is able to detect the presence of *Entamoeba* in the fluid aspirated from the abscess (Roy et al, 2005). As the experience with the test increases, it might become the standard for diagnosis of amebic liver abscess. Currently, the controversy about routine aspiration of uncomplicated amebic liver abscess in which the diagnosis is confirmed by typical presentation and ultrasound and positive amebic serology in high titers remains unresolved. No randomized controlled trial has ever shown that aspiration is beneficial in survival, length of hospitalization, or time to becoming afebrile (Sharma et al, 1989; Stanley, 2003; Van Allan et al, 1992) compared with treatment with antiamebic drugs alone, and aspiration may only confuse the diagnosis by revealing atypical pus or blood. The belief that aspiration hastens clinical recovery and may not involve significant procedure-related morbidity is widespread in clinical practice, however. This approach is supported by a small prospective study (Tandon et al, 1997) and continues to be advocated in reviews (Haque et al, 2002). Clinical improvement invariably occurs with antiamebic therapy alone in an uncomplicated case. When the differential diagnosis in a given case includes operable neoplasm or hydatid disease, aspiration is risky and may be contraindicated.

Therapeutic aspiration is now regarded as generally superfluous in the management of amebic liver abscess (Ralls et al, 1982) and should be reserved for the following situations:

1. Amebic serology is inconclusive, delayed, or unavailable, and the main differential diagnosis is a pyogenic liver abscess.
2. A therapeutic trial with antiamebic drugs is deemed inappropriate (as in pregnancy).
3. There is suspicion of secondary infection of the liver abscess; this is estimated to occur in 15% of cases (McDermott, 1995).
4. When fever and pain persist for more than 3 to 5 days after starting appropriate therapy, aspiration may provide symptomatic relief.
5. Rupture is suspected to be imminent in an extremely large abscess, especially if pericardial rupture from a left lobe abscess appears likely.

Single aspiration may be sufficient for diagnostic purposes, but when performed as part of therapy, it is likely to be inadequate. When more than one aspiration is required, the placement of a percutaneous drain probably is indicated to reduce the risk of recurrence (McDermott, 1995).

Aspiration for diagnostic purposes is presently too inaccurate to recommend because the characteristic anchovy sauce may or may not be found. Subjecting the aspirated fluid to PCR testing for the amebic hemolysin may be a valuable adjunct to diagnosis in the future, but experience with this is limited at present.

Complications

Communication or extension of amebic liver abscesses occurs into neighboring cavities and organs—the peritoneum, viscera, and large vessels on one side of the diaphragm and the pleura, bronchi, lungs, and pericardium on the other.

Peritoneal and Visceral Involvement
Peritonitis associated with amebiasis is due to a rupture of amebic liver abscess in 78% of cases and perforated or necrotizing

amebic colitis in the rest (22%) (Monga et al, 1976). The two processes can occur simultaneously in a few cases, and this must be kept in mind while making therapeutic decisions for a given patient.

The incidence of spontaneous rupture of amebic liver abscess varies from 2.7% to 17% of cases (Eggleston et al, 1982; Monga et al, 1976; Sarda et al, 1989). Of all amebic liver abscess ruptures, 18% to 70% are into the peritoneal cavity (Ken et al, 1989). Adherence of the liver abscess to the diaphragm, anterior abdominal wall, omentum, and bowel tends to confine the area of contamination. Rupture into a hollow viscus, such as the stomach (Angel et al, 2000) or colon, may occur in this situation. Although such ruptures usually are encountered as isolated reports of rare cases, they probably are underreported in the literature. A hepatogastric, hepatoduodenal, or hepatocolonic fistula may result. Free rupture into the peritoneal cavity is uncommon and usually occurs in a nutritionally depleted and moribund patient. Patients present with abdominal pain and a mass or generalized distention. Sudden bloody diarrhea may occur in colonic rupture, and hematemesis may occur in patients with hepatogastric fistula. Signs of peritonitis along with tender hepatomegaly, intercostal tenderness, and right basal lung signs and clinical jaundice may lead to a suspicion of the diagnosis, which is confirmed on ultrasound. At times, the diagnosis may be made only at laparotomy, at which time the excessive bleeding resulting from decreased prothrombin levels can be difficult to manage.

Ultrasound and CT often show perihepatic fluid collection in cases of amebic liver abscess. It is impossible to tell by these imaging techniques if these collections are reactive or actual leaks from the abscess cavity (Radin et al, 1988), and the differentiation must be made clinically.

Various forms of management of an abscess that has extended into the peritoneal cavity have been advocated. The aggressive surgical approaches of the 1970s and early 1980s (Balasegaram, 1981; Eggleston et al, 1982) were associated with increased mortality and have now been replaced by increasingly successful attempts at percutaneous drainage of the liver abscess and the extravasated pus (Ken et al, 1989; Sarda et al, 1989).

Absolute indications for laparotomy include doubtful diagnosis, concomitant hollow viscus perforation with fistulization resulting in life-threatening hemorrhage or sepsis, and failure of conservative management. At laparotomy, the liver abscess, which usually appears as a tan-colored bulge on the surface, must be handled gently. Septa running across the cavity are usually blood vessels and bile ducts traversing the abscess cavity. Hemorrhage can be difficult to control, especially if the clotting is disordered, and postoperative bile leaks may result. Irrigation of the abscess cavity with saline usually is sufficient and may be followed by the installation for 3 to 5 minutes of a solution of 65 mg of emetine hydrochloride in 100 mL of normal saline. Tube drains are inserted and retained as necessary. Hollow viscus perforations must be dealt with on an individual basis, with exteriorization, proximal diversion, or serosal patch closure as indicated.

Postoperative antiamebic therapy in the form of intravenous metronidazole is combined with broad-spectrum antibiotics. Dehydroemetine is added if no cardiac contraindication exists. The mortality of this complication ranges from 12% to 50% (Sarda et al, 1989).

Thoracic and Pleuropulmonary Involvement
Thoracic complications associated with amebic liver abscess include a sympathetic straw-colored, right-sided effusion; rupture

of the abscess into the pleural cavity; and rupture of the abscess into the bronchial tree. Supradiaphragmatic signs and symptoms in abscesses located high on the right lobe are so common as to be part of the clinical syndrome of amebic liver abscess. Clinically, this condition manifests as dyspnea and a dry cough, which exacerbates the right hypochondriac pain caused by the hepatic lesion. Right basal crepitations are a frequent accompaniment to the abdominal signs. A pleural rub may be found, which decreases as signs of pleural effusion supervene. Chest radiography shows atelectasis and blunting of the costophrenic angle. Ultrasound and CT often detect the pleural effusion before it is clinically detectable. There are no ultrasound or CT features to differentiate between a sympathetic effusion and a transdiaphragmatic intrapleural rupture except that the former tends to be small and clinically insignificant. No treatment is required for this kind of pleural collection other than the treatment of the liver abscess.

Rupture of an abscess into the pleural cavity usually occurs suddenly and extends rapidly to collapse the right lung and fill up the right pleural space. Clinically, it manifests as the sudden onset of severe dyspnea. Radiography reveals a homogeneous opacification throughout the right hemithorax with displacement of the mediastinum to the opposite side. Ultrasonography reveals the liver abscess.

Treatment consists of thoracentesis. An important precaution to be observed in chest aspiration and establishment of intercostal tube drainage is to go in high on the right lateral side of the chest near the axilla because the right diaphragm is considerably elevated in these patients. The tube can be inserted easily across the diaphragm into the liver, where it would fail to evacuate the pleural collection and might keep the tract from the liver abscess from closing. Ineffective early drainage of the amebic empyema usually is complicated by secondary infection requiring more aggressive surgical procedures, such as pulmonary decortication, at a later date.

Rupture of the abscess into the bronchi is characterized by the sudden onset of coughing with expectoration of copious quantities of chocolate-colored sputum. Although this is a complication of amebic liver abscess, it almost always has a beneficial effect as the abscess drains itself (Guarner, 1986). Because the abscess usually is well walled off from the pleural and peritoneal cavities, surgical intervention is not required, and postural drainage, bronchodilators, and antiamebic drugs suffice. Lung abscess occurs rarely. In cases in which adhesions are not well formed, the liver abscess can rupture into the pleural space and bronchi simultaneously, and postural drainage of bronchial secretions must be combined with thoracentesis. Metronidazole used as a single drug is effective in the treatment of thoracic complications of amebic liver abscess, but emetine produces a more rapid response and may be required in cases in which metronidazole resistance occurs (Jain et al, 1990).

Pericardial Involvement

Abscesses of the left lobe of the liver are more prone to pericardial complications, which may range from asymptomatic pericardial effusion to cardiac tamponade from intrapericardial rupture of a left lobe abscess. Signs of pericardial effusion may be detected clinically or on chest radiography, but amebic liver abscess as the cause is often difficult to detect except on abdominal ultrasound.

Although left lobe abscesses resolve equally well with antiamebic drugs as do right-sided abscesses (Thompson et al, 1985),

the detection of pericardial thickening or a pericardial effusion on CT or ultrasound may constitute an indication for aspiration of a left-sided amebic liver abscess (Radin et al, 1988). In the presence of cardiac tamponade, aspiration of the pericardium by the subxiphoid route must be performed along with drainage of the liver abscess followed by antiamebic drugs, of which metronidazole is the drug of choice. Dehydroemetine is used with caution because of its propensity for cardiotoxicity.

Chemotherapy

Metronidazole

Metronidazole has been of proven use in amebic hepatic abscess since 1966 and is the drug of choice. The oral dose is 800 mg three times a day for 5 to 10 days in adults and 35 to 50 mg/kg in three divided doses for 10 days in children. Smaller doses also have been effective, and hepatopulmonary amebiasis was found to respond equally to doses of 400 and 800 mg three times daily given over 5 days (Jain et al, 1990). The intravenous route is highly effective in patients unable to take oral medication; the recommended dose is 500 mg every 6 hours, although in practice an 8- or 12-hour schedule is more commonly used.

Metronidazole reaches high concentrations in the liver, stomach, intestine, and kidney. It crosses the placenta and the blood-brain barrier. Its half-life is approximately 8 hours, and it is excreted in the urine. Its use is contraindicated in the first trimester of pregnancy, and it must be used cautiously in the second and third trimesters because the effect on fetal development is unknown. Likewise, because the drug is excreted in the milk, breastfeeding should be discontinued during its use.

Serious side effects are rare. The most commonly observed side effects are nausea, vomiting, a metallic taste in the mouth, and dark brown discoloration of the urine. It has a disulfiram (Antabuse) effect owing to inhibition of alcohol dehydrogenase. Although metronidazole is carcinogenic in animals, no such effects are seen in humans.

A favorable response to metronidazole usually is obtained by the third day of treatment. Over 5 days, an 85% cure rate is achieved; this may increase to 95% after 10 days (Guarner, 1986). Five percent to 15% of patients with amebic liver abscess may be resistant to metronidazole (Thompson et al, 1985), but this may not be a major clinical problem (Li & Stanley, 1996), and most reports of "drug resistance" equate this term with delayed resolution of either clinical symptoms or ultrasound findings and not a true resistance documented by the failure of the drug to kill amebae. Current opinion is that no resistance of amebae to metronidazole has been documented, although experimental resistance is known and may be related to inducing increased superoxide dismutase activity in vitro (Wells & Arguedas, 2004).

The timing of clinical response remains the most significant predictor of successful therapy; 94% of metronidazole responders show dramatic clinical improvement within 72 hours of therapy. Alternate medical therapy, percutaneous aspiration, or surgical intervention usually must be considered in patients who do not respond or show only modest improvement in 72 hours (Thompson et al, 1985).

Some newer imidazoles are worth mentioning. Reports from Brazil suggest that tinidazole can be used orally at 2 g daily for 5 days. Secnidazole has a longer half-life, and a single daily dose of 2 g for 5 days is effective (Salles et al, 2003).

Emetine Hydrochloride

Probably the oldest useful drug in amebiasis, emetine is more effective against trophozoites than cysts and reaches amebicidal concentrations in the tissues rather than in the intestinal lumen, being mainly concentrated in the liver. Emetine is administered by intramuscular or "deep subcutaneous" injection in a dose of 1 mg/kg/day (maximum 60 mg/day) for no more than 10 days. The patient must be confined to complete bed rest. Tissue levels persist for 40 to 60 days after termination of treatment, and readministration of the drug should be avoided for 6 weeks. The analogue dehydroemetine is less toxic and disappears earlier from tissues; the dose is the same.

Side effects include a regional myositis at the injection site presenting as muscular aching relieved by hot fomentation. Cardiovascular side effects are characterized by hypotension, tachycardia, chest pain, dyspnea, and abnormalities in the electrocardiogram, including T wave inversion and an increase in the Q-T interval. Blood pressure and pulse rate are monitored closely with the patient on complete bed rest, and at the first sign of persistent tachycardia the drug must be discontinued and electrocardiogram monitoring instituted. The drug is contraindicated in renal, cardiac, and muscular disease and must be used cautiously in children and elderly patients. Despite these side effects, emetine or dehydroemetine is valuable in the treatment of hepatic and hepatopulmonary amebiasis, either replacing or as an adjuvant to metronidazole, particularly in patients in whom a rapid clinical response is required or in whom metronidazole response is poor (Guarner, 1986; Jain et al, 1990; Thompson et al, 1985).

Chloroquine Phosphate

Chloroquine was first reported to be useful in 1948 in a patient whose amebic liver abscess was resistant to all other therapy. This antimalarial 4-aminoquinolone, although possessing less amebicidal activity than emetine, is often effective in patients with resistance to emetine. It is also effective in pulmonary amebiasis (Guarner, 1986). Chloroquine has practically no luminal amebicidal activity.

Chloroquine is administered orally in a dose of 1 g (600-mg base) per day for 2 days followed by 500 mg (300-mg base) per day for 2 to 3 weeks. It is contraindicated in patients with retinopathy and with active psoriasis. It has been used in pregnancy (Guarner, 1986). A short course has few side effects; the most common are gastrointestinal upset, headache, visual disturbances, and pruritus. Routine administration in all cases of amebic liver abscess is probably not justified. The principal value of chloroquine may be in recurrent and resistant cases.

Diloxanide Furoate

Diloxanide is used to treat amebic colitis and is effective in cyst passers and relatively ineffective in invasive amebiasis. Diloxanide is recommended for the treatment of asymptomatic carriers and may be required to treat family members and intimate contacts of patients with diagnosed amebic liver abscess. The recommended dose is 500 mg three times a day for 10 days. No serious side effects are reported; gastrointestinal upsets and flatulence are reported. Other luminal agents include paromomycin and iodoquinol, etofamide, and teclozan.

Therapeutic Strategy

Metronidazole is administered as a single drug after diagnosis, with concomitant correction of hypoprothrombinemia, hypoproteinemia, and anemia. The oral route is preferred.

If dramatic improvement in 48 to 72 hours is noted, no therapy other than the complete course of metronidazole is required. A luminal agent, such as diloxanide furoate (500 mg orally three times a day × 10 days) or paromomycin (30 mg/kg/day in three doses × 10 days), must be administered after metronidazole therapy for the eradication of intestinal infection as a part of the complete treatment (Irusen et al, 1992).

In patients who do not respond satisfactorily, emetine or dehydroemetine is added. Evidence of pulmonary, peritoneal, or pericardial extension is an indication for aspiration of the liver abscess with an intercostal tube or catheter drainage into a closed-circuit collection system. Failure to control the abscess adequately by these means, as shown by increasing signs of peritonitis, fistulization into a hollow viscus, or secondary infection with septicemia, constitutes an indication for laparotomy.

Prevention

Modern biologic techniques have helped to characterize amebic antigens that show great promise in the development of a vaccine. These antigens include (1) serine-rich *E. histolytica* protein, (2) a 170-KD subunit of Gal/Gal Nac binding lectin, and (3) a 29-KD cysteine-rich protein. Recombinant vaccines based on these antigens have been used successfully in animal models of amebiasis. Attempts are ongoing to fuse these antigens with the relevant subunits of cholera toxin and *Salmonella* species to develop an oral combination *enteric pathogen* vaccine (Stanley, 1997).

Prognosis

A meta-analysis of 3081 patients with amebic liver abscess showed that 114 (4%) died (Pitt, 1990). In comparison, the mortality rate for pyogenic liver abscess was 46%. In patients treated with amebicidal drugs alone, the mortality was 2%, and the addition of needle aspiration did not improve this result. Independent risk factors for mortality include serum bilirubin greater than 3.5 mg/dL, encephalopathy, hypoalbuminemia (defined as <2 mg/dL), and multiple abscess cavities (Sharma et al, 1996) or total volume of abscess greater than 500 mL (Wells & Arguedas, 2004).

There is widespread consensus on minimally invasive treatments being the standard of care, with ultrasound-guided or other image-guided aspiration and drainage effective in the management of severe or complicated cases. Patients treated with a strategy of early and aggressive surgery as advocated by some authors (Balasegaram, 1981; Eggleston et al, 1982) did not show a remarkable improvement in mortality, although in Balasegaram's series the hospital stay was probably reduced. Ruptured amebic liver abscess occurs in 2% to 17% of patients, with reported mortality 6% to 50%. These patients usually constitute a major risk for surgery and anesthesia, and the increasing use of minimally invasive techniques in management can be anticipated to improve survival.

LIVER FLUKE DISEASE

Humans are subject to infection with several species of liver flukes, of which the two major ones of clinical importance are *Fasciola hepatica* and *Clonorchis sinensis*. The flukes are digenetic trematodes and undergo sexual (in the definitive host) and asexual (in the intermediate host) reproduction. Although both have common features with respect to their structure and life cycle with accidental infection of humans, there are some epidemiologic differences. *F. hepatica* is found all over the world, most commonly in middle Europe and Western Europe, in South America, and in the Caribbean, occurring in small outbreaks in people who are fond of eating raw vegetables or watercress. Most physicians have never seen a case of human fascioliasis, although their veterinary counterparts in advanced countries are familiar with the disease, including its diagnosis in farm animals by sophisticated radiologic techniques.

With *C. sinensis,* human cases frequently are encountered because it is endemic in East Asia; in regions bordered by the South China Sea; and along the great rivers and streams of China, North Vietnam, and Korea. Disease results from eating contaminated raw freshwater fish. These areas also are endemic for viral hepatitis, and epidemiologic surveys of the population yield patients with common symptoms in whom the differential diagnosis has to be made (Wang et al, 2004). In addition to *Clonorchis, Opisthorchis viverrini* and *Opisthorchis felineus* are the other liver flukes transmitted by the consumption of raw freshwater fish. Infection rates may be more than 25%, but most cases are asymptomatic. The Western Hemisphere is free of the disease, but because of the long life span of the parasite (20 years), clinical manifestations may occur in natives of these areas several years after emigration to other countries. The first report of *C. sinensis* infestation was described in a Chinese carpenter residing in Calcutta (McConnell, 1875).

Fascioliasis

The trematode parasites *F. hepatica* (temperate) and *Fasciola gigantica* (tropical) are the causative agents of liver fluke disease (fascioliasis) in cattle and sheep. Human infections with *F. hepatica* are found in areas where sheep and cattle are raised and where humans consume raw watercress, including Europe, the Middle East, and Asia. Infections with *F. gigantica* have been reported, more rarely, in Asia, Africa, and Hawaii. Disease prevalence is particularly high in specific regions of Bolivia (65-92%), Ecuador (24-53%), Egypt (2-17%), and Peru (10%). In hyperendemic areas of Bolivia, 68% of children have evidence of infection; 11% of Ethiopians who emigrated to Israel also have evidence of infection. It is estimated that 2.4 million people are infected with liver fluke worldwide, and incidences apparently have increased since 1980 (Mas-Coma et al, 1999).

The parasite is found in temperate and tropical climates, in sheep- and cattle-rearing countries throughout the world. Although it has been known to decimate entire flocks with progressive liver disease, the incidence in humans is estimated to be only 1%, with most patients being encountered as sporadic cases or in small community outbreaks (Ashton et al, 1970).

Morphology and Life Cycle

F. hepatica is a flat, leaflike, hermaphrodite trematode 15 to 30 mm long, 10 mm thick, and 3 mm wide that inhabits the bile ducts and gallbladder of the host. Eggs laid in the bile ducts enter the intestine and, after being passed in the feces, hatch to form a motile ciliated miracidium, which penetrates the body of snails of the genus *Lymnae.* The snails excrete free-swimming, tadpole-like cercariae, which swim to aquatic vegetation and encyst as metacercaria on water plants. After ingestion of contaminated riverside plants or irrigated crops, the larvae are liberated and proceed to penetrate the intestinal wall. After traversing the peritoneal cavity, they penetrate the liver capsule and eat their way down to the bile ducts. The life cycle takes about 5 months for completion, of which 3 months are required for the journey through the human host, and the adult worms that develop in the bile ducts at the end of this period have a life span of 3 to 4 years. During migration, the parasite may invade other organs, such as the urinary tract, and cause hematuria. Ectopic fascioliasis also may affect the peritoneum, muscles, brain, and subcutaneous tissues (Jones et al, 1977).

Pathology

F. hepatica is a relatively large parasite. Hepatic lesions that occur first during the infection include white or gray nodules on the liver capsule, subcapsular tracts, and, rarely, a localized hepatic mass. Later the worm enters the biliary system. In the intrahepatic ducts, the worms move to and fro, and the spinous nature of the integument causes extensive destruction of the biliary epithelium. The presence of the parasite stimulates fibrosis in the bile duct wall (Fig. 60.6). Serious infection may be associated with hepatic and biliary fibrosis, hepatic necrosis and abscess formation, cholangiohepatitis, impaired nutrition, and death. A liver biopsy specimen may reveal only a nonspecific round cell infiltration of the portal tracts. Cholangiocarcinoma has been described in association with fascioliasis.

Clinical Features

Only 25% of patients may give a history of eating watercress. In the remaining patients, drinking contaminated water in an endemic area is the likely route of infection. The clinical presentation is best described as a combination of symptoms and radiologic findings.

In the acute phase, right upper quadrant pain, hepatomegaly, fever, vomiting, diarrhea, and allergic reactions may develop.

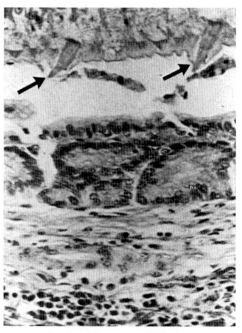

Fig. 60.6. Spines of *F. hepatica (arrows)* damaging the biliary epithelium. (Original magnification, ×500.)

This phase is caused by the migration of the immature fluke through the hepatic parenchyma and usually lasts 4 months. No motile echogenic images are seen on ultrasound examination of the intrahepatic and extrahepatic bile ducts (Saba et al, 2004). The findings in the liver parenchyma are nonspecific, although a suspicion of nodules or cavitary lesions might warrant further imaging. CT is the most useful imaging method for diagnosis. Findings on CT include peripherally located hypodense lesions, usually on the right lobe, with peripheral enhancement on contrast scans, arranged in a "tracklike" fashion with no coalescence into a larger abscess cavity as is seen in pyogenic abscesses. MRI usually adds nothing and cannot show the tracklike appearance of the lesions (Oto et al, 1999).

In the chronic phase (caused by the adult fluke within the biliary system), the symptoms persist more than 4 months, are more discrete, and reflect intermittent biliary obstruction and inflammation. Symptoms include recurrent episodes of biliary colic, cholangitis, and cholecystitis occurring with accompanying constitutional upset, jaundice, anemia, hypoproteinemia, and edema. Tender hepatosplenomegaly may be found. Motile echogenic images can be seen in the gallbladder and bile ducts on ultrasound during this phase. Biliary ductal dilation is common, and MRI cholangiography may show signal loss in the large bile ducts consistent with flukes or edema (LaPook et al, 2000).

Hematologic screening characteristically reveals eosinophilia, which may be 50% or more of the total white blood cell count (Hardman et al, 1970). Eosinophilia is seen regardless of the clinical stage of infection and may be seen in asymptomatic contacts of the patient who have latent infection (Saba et al, 2004). Anemia is usually present and has been attributed to ingestion of blood by the flukes and toxic suppression of the pituitary leading to a decrease in the rate of hematopoiesis (Bassiouny et al, 1991). Liver function tests show features of cholestasis. Hemoglobinuria is often present because the flukes can penetrate and lodge in the kidneys during their migration through the peritoneal cavity. Adult flukes and eggs are absent from the feces and bile during the acute phase because the parasites cannot produce eggs before invasion of the biliary tree, and even in the chronic phase, stool examination may not be diagnostic. A specific serologic test detecting IgG antibodies to crude fasciola worm antigen preparation has been found to be positive in 97% to 100% of patients (Maher et al, 1999).

The findings on imaging already have been described, and a differential diagnosis from necrotic hepatic neoplasms and liver abscesses has to be made. Liver biopsy specimens may be reported as eosinophilic hepatitis with centrilobular necrosis and cholangitis (LaPook et al, 2000). At laparoscopy or laparotomy, the characteristic features of hard, grayish white nodules on the liver surface with subcapsular channels may be seen in 55% to 75% of cases. Portal lymph nodes are often enlarged, and the common bile duct may be dilated.

The diagnosis of fascioliasis should be considered in patients with a history of fondness for raw watercress or other aquatic plants or who dwell in or have recently traveled to an endemic area, who develop prostration, cholangitis, hepatosplenomegaly, anemia, and eosinophilia. Diagnosis is difficult, particularly in the acute or parenchymal phase, and confirmation is obtained by serologic tests for fasciola. Detecting the ova in stool involves using a concentration technique or the filtration-ninhydrin method. The eggs are morphologically indistinguishable from those of *Fasciolopsis buski*. False fascioliasis (pseudofascioliasis) refers to the presence of eggs in the stool resulting not from an actual infection, but from recent ingestion of infected livers containing eggs. This situation (with its potential for misdiagnosis) can be avoided by having the patient follow a liver-free diet several days before a repeat stool examination.

Treatment

Medical treatment with emetine and chloroquine is usually successful in the short-term, but may confuse further a difficult clinical situation that eludes diagnosis. Recurrence is the rule because these drugs have no effect on the parasite. Fasciolae also usually are refractory to praziquantel. The drug of choice is triclabendazole, 10 mg/kg orally, repeated after 12 hours. It can be used even in the presence of biliary obstruction. Cure rates of 90% have been reported with no significant drug-related side effects. Bithionol is an alternative; available as 200-mg tablets, the daily dose is 30 mg/kg/day, to a total therapeutic dose of 150 mg/kg. The drug usually is administered on alternate days in three divided doses after meals. Adverse effects are frequent and include nausea, abdominal pain, diarrhea, and photosensitivity reactions. Clinical improvement is gradual and occurs over 2 to 3 weeks. Surgical treatment may be indicated for diagnosis or for cholangitis. Occasionally, a live worm may be found in the gallbladder or the bile duct, or the worm may find its way out through a T-tube placed at surgery (Nicholas, 1970).

Vaccine Development

Advances in proteomics and genomics have led to identification of molecules, including cathepsin L, glutathione S-transferase, leucine aminopeptidase, and fatty acid binding proteins (Dalton et al, 2003). Testing of these molecules as vaccine candidates has shown the feasibility of inducing protective responses in laboratory and large animals. The systemic analysis of the protective effector mechanism provided by different vaccine candidates, vaccine formulations, doses, and route of administration is required during the developmental stages of a commercial vaccine.

Clonorchiasis

Morphology and Life Cycle

C. sinensis is a flat trematode worm 10 to 25 mm long and 3 to 5 mm wide. The worms are pink and transparent when alive and appear as hard, friable, black bodies when dead (Hou, 1956). The adult worms inhabit the intrahepatic bile ducts, and although they may migrate or be carried down the common bile duct, they tend to die in the gallbladder. In association with heavy infestation, they may be found in the pancreatic duct, where they remain alive.

When the cysts from infected fish are digested by gastric juice, the larva emigrate from the duodenum into the common bile duct, traveling upward until they lodge in a bile duct too small to allow further passage. They travel against the flow of bile by means of their two large suckers, oral and ventral, which are their organs of fixation and locomotion. Eggs laid in bile ducts reach the intestine to be excreted in feces. The life cycle continues in fresh water, where the *Hydrobiid* snail is the intermediate host. In contrast to *F. hepatica*, an additional intermediate host, a cyprinoid fish—usually a grass or black carp—is involved. The cercarial forms that emerge from the snail in fresh water attach to and penetrate the fish, with encysted metacercariae developing in the muscles of this secondary intermediate host. Humans are definitive hosts, and infection is acquired by ingestion of raw fish. The duration of the life cycle is approximately 3 months. Other definitive hosts include dogs, cats, hogs, and rats.

Pathology

Biliary epithelium, in response to irritation by the worm, undergoes hyperplasia, which progresses to metaplasia and adenomatous hyperplasia. Periductal inflammation is mild in the initial stages and facilitates dilation of the small and medium-sized ducts in the periphery of the liver (Choi et al, 2004; Hou, 1956). Metaplastic changes in the biliary epithelium into mucin-producing cells occur early in the infection, resulting in highly mucinous bile. Stagnation of bile leads to bacterial infection, cholangitis, and cholangiohepatitis. These inflammatory conditions are unfavorable to the worms, eventually killing them. Ductal fibrosis and stricturing with formation of intrahepatic calculi occurs later in the course of the disease and is secondary to cholangitis (Choi et al, 2004).

Progression to biliary cirrhosis is unusual, but a greater incidence of cholangiocarcinoma is thought to result from the effects of *C. sinensis* infection (Choi et al, 2004; Flavell, 1981; Hou, 1956). The etiology of cholangiocarcinoma arising in association with the trematodes is multifactorial. Initially, a high turnover of hyperplastic biliary epithelium occurs in response to the parasite; this may be stimulated further by low protein intake in the diet. The hyperplastic and proliferating bile ducts may be susceptible to carcinogens present at levels insufficient to induce bile duct carcinoma in noninfected individuals. Infection also may alter the immunologic status of these patients (Flavell, 1981).

Associated stones are brownish yellow. Also called calcium bilirubinate stones or bile pigment calcium stones, they occur in the biliary ductal system and almost always are associated with infection. Organisms responsible for sepsis are *Escherichia coli* and anaerobic streptococci in 76% of cases (Fung, 1961). β-Glucuronidase present in these bacteria hydrolyzes conjugated bilirubin to liberate unconjugated bilirubin, which is highly insoluble in bile and tends to bind to the predominantly available biliary cation calcium. The colloid stability of the calcium bilirubinate salt now formed depends on the concentration of bile salts. Because this is low in hepatic bile compared with the gallbladder bile, the calcium bilirubinate tends to precipitate in the bile ducts, after which partial polymerization may occur, or it may complex with proteins and fatty acids (Tandon, 1988).

Relationship to Recurrent Pyogenic Cholangitis

There is little doubt that clonorchiasis is associated with recurrent episodes of cholangitis that conform to the syndrome of recurrent pyogenic cholangitis (see Ch. 62). There is now also a large and compelling body of evidence that clonorchiasis is etiologically associated with cholangiocarcinoma (Choi et al, 2004). Both conditions occur independent of *Clonorchis* infection in endemic regions, however. About half of patients with Oriental cholangiohepatitis are infected with *C. sinensis,* but infection also is common in individuals from the same area and culture who do not have recurrent pyogenic cholangitis clinically. Recurrent pyogenic cholangitis has been reported in India (Augustine et al, 1988; Tandon, 1988) from regions where *C. sinensis* endemicity is unknown, which would seem to support the theory that postulates portal bacteremia secondary to serious enteric infections as the etiology of recurrent pyogenic cholangitis (Teoh, 1963). For now, it seems prudent to investigate patients diagnosed with either cholangitis or cholangiocarcinoma who have been residing in an endemic area of the Far East, for evidence of *Clonorchis* infection because screening for latent infection may be appropriate in relatives and close contacts of patients who test positive for clonorchis.

Clinical Features

The severity of infection is graded by determining the number of eggs per gram of feces. Clinical features are independent of the severity of infestation, however, as shown by a population survey in an endemic area in which 86% of 1091 patients screened by stool examination were found to have clonorchiasis. Only one patient had intrahepatic stones, and the 8% incidence of gallbladder stones was related more to ethnicity than to infestation with *C. sinensis*. No correlation of mild, moderate, and serious infection with symptoms was found (Hou et al, 1989). The explanation for this phenomenon may lie in the observation that cholangitis kills the worm, and the eggs may disappear from the feces at the stage when symptoms are most prominent.

The classic symptom complex associated with clonorchiasis is the occurrence of recurrent pyogenic cholangitis. Acalculous clonorchiasis is rarely symptomatic. In a percentage of cases of recurrent cholangitis, however, the bile is sterile, and this is an indicator that *C. sinensis* is not merely a harmless commensal. Early symptoms include general malaise, abdominal discomfort, and diarrhea; these are often ignored or treated symptomatically alone. Screening investigations may show eosinophilia with fluctuating jaundice or elevated liver enzymes, which is seen in 40% of patients with low worm burden and no clinical cholangitis (Choi et al, 2004).

Males and females are equally susceptible and range in age from 3 to 72 years, with the peak incidence in the 20s and 30s (Fung, 1961). According to one study, men are more commonly affected because most consumption of raw fish nowadays is in association with the social consumption of alcohol at gatherings that women tend to avoid (Choi et al, 2004). All patients have pain in the right upper abdomen, and about half present with cholangitis. In 70% of patients, there is a history of recurrent attacks over a long time, usually about 10 years. Signs of anemia and hypoproteinemia are common. Right upper quadrant tenderness is seen in all patients, with a palpable tender liver and gallbladder occurring in one third. Jaundice varies in intensity. Progression to cirrhosis results in splenomegaly. The serum bilirubin level is 60 to 70 mmol/L, serum transaminase levels are only slightly elevated, and the alkaline phosphatase level is high. Evidence of pancreatitis may be found.

Plain films of the abdomen may reveal gas in the biliary tree. Stones are rarely visualized. Ultrasound and CT detect ductal dilation and calculi. Contrast imaging of the biliary tract is essential, however, to delineate the distribution of stones and strictures and to plan operative therapy. Hepatic ducts are usually dilated—the left more than the right. The common bile duct is dilated in supraduodenal and retropancreatic portions, tapering off abruptly at the sphincter of Oddi, which is almost always closed but patent, yielding readily to bougienage (Fung, 1961). Definite stenosis is seen only in 5%.

Cholangiocarcinoma attributed to *Clonorchis* infection is clinically indistinguishable from standard cholangiocarcinoma and may be peripheral (intrahepatic), hilar, or extrahepatic (Choi et al, 2004) (see Ch. 52). Diagnosis of clonorchiasis in patients with cholangitis depends on a high index of suspicion.

Elevated eosinophil counts warrant a search for the parasite. Demonstration of eggs in feces or duodenal aspirate gives a definitive diagnosis. In recent times, detection of specific antibodies (Lin et al, 1995) and circulating antigen by a Dot-ELISA test has been described (Wang et al, 2004).

Treatment

Praziquantel (Biltricide) is the drug of choice. The dosage schedule is usually 25 mg/kg/day for 1 or 2 days. Interventional procedures are required only in cases complicated by calculus formation and depend on the location of ductal stones and strictures. Endoscopic and minimally invasive techniques have affected the treatment choices in this area in keeping with universal trends and have the advantage over open surgery in reduced morbidity (Zhi et al, 2004). As is the experience with biliary strictures overall, however, these procedures are usually adequate only in relatively simple and easily accessible strictures, and patients referred to surgery are likely to be more complicated cases in whom multiple endoscopic procedures have failed to solve the problem. Operations ranging from T-tube drainage alone in an emergency situation to complex bile duct drainage procedures and access-loop hepaticojejunostomies continue to be required and are discussed in greater detail in Chs. 30 and 43.

BILIARY ASCARIASIS

Epidemiology

The roundworm *Ascaris lumbricoides* infects more than a quarter of the world's population and is particularly common in Asia, Africa, and Central America. Immigrants from these regions to countries in the Western Hemisphere constitute a sizable pool of potential patients; it is estimated 4 million individuals are infected in the United States (Khuroo, 2001). Clinical disease is restricted, however, to individuals with heavy worm load and occurs in an estimated 1.2 to 2 million cases with 20,000 deaths per year (Khuroo, 2001). Most of these cases occur in endemic areas, usually tropical and subtropical regions, where poor socioeconomic conditions along with fecal contamination of the soil around dwellings and farms have resulted in 30% of the adult population and 60% to 70% of children harboring the adult worm (Khuroo et al, 1989a; Louw, 1966).

Ascaris infestation when confined to the intestine is usually asymptomatic. When the worm enters the biliary tract, however, it always is symptomatic. In a study from urban Kashmir, an area where 30% of the adult population harbors *A. lumbricoides,* only 5 of 1104 individuals screened had ascarids in the biliary tract, and all 5 were having recurrent biliary symptoms (Khuroo et al, 1989a, 1989b). There is a similar incidence of gallstones in developing countries of the East and in developed countries of the West (Hou et al, 1989; Khuroo et al, 1989a); although recognizing that this is an additional problem in endemic areas, it is unnecessary to consider ascariasis as an etiologic factor in all patients diagnosed with gallstone disease who hail from an endemic area.

In humans, the adult worm inhabits the small intestine, where the fertilized female lays approximately 200,000 eggs a day. These ova are excreted in the host's feces and can survive adverse environmental conditions. In warm, moist soil, the ova undergo maturation and are able to infest humans if swallowed.

Mature ova hatch in the duodenum, releasing larvae that penetrate the mucosa of the proximal intestine to enter the portal venous blood, in which they are carried through the liver and via the right side of the heart to the pulmonary capillary bed. Here the larvae develop further before penetrating the alveoli to travel up the trachea, enter the esophagus, and return to the intestine. In the ileum, they mature to adulthood, reaching 20 to 30 cm in length, and have a life span of 1 to 2 years.

Pathology

The ability of *A. lumbricoides* to enter the common bile duct, especially when there is heavy duodenal infestation, is well known. Usually only one or two worms enter the biliary system, but massive infestation may occur. The worm moves head first through the ampulla of Vater, and because the length of the extrahepatic tree is only 4 to 10 cm, part of the worm may remain in the duodenum (Davies & Rode, 1982). The worm tends to move out of the biliary tract within 24 to 36 hours of inducing biliary or pancreatic symptoms, and the detection of live ascarids in the duodenal lumen is considered strong evidence of biliary ascariasis. The impacted worm causes spasm of the sphincter of Oddi, resulting in partial biliary obstruction and colicky pain.

Superimposed on the effects of mechanical obstruction, cholangitis can occur. Apart from causing chemical irritation of the bile duct mucosa, secondary infection by bacteria introduced by the worm results in suppurative cholangitis, which may extend to intrahepatic ducts causing multiple cholangiolitic liver abscesses. Acalculous cholecystitis, empyema of the gallbladder, and, less commonly, necrosis and perforation of the bile duct may occur (Chang & Han, 1966). Dead worms cannot leave the bile duct, and they disintegrate, providing a nidus for stones and provoking a chronic inflammatory response leading to ductal strictures.

Calculi associated with ascariasis are of the calcium bilirubinate type, similar to the primary ductal stones of recurrent pyogenic cholangitis of Asia (Khuroo et al, 1989b; Maki, 1966), with the exception that ascarid ova or debris usually can be identified in the calculus. *Escherichia coli,* the pathogen usually identified with calcium bilirubinate stones, is a frequently encountered organism in suppurative cholangitis caused by *A. lumbricoides.* Worm extract and *E. coli* possess high levels of β-glucuronidase and can cause bile pigment deconjugation (Maki, 1966). Studies of the eggs of various human parasites showed that fertilized ascarid eggs have the most stable shells, probably because of the second layer, which is thick, doubly refractile, and crystalline in structure. Another factor that may facilitate stone formation is the albuminoid membrane that covers most of the eggs and is not found in any other parasite.

Worms reaching the intrahepatic ducts may become impacted or invade the liver parenchyma forming nests of worms (Lloyd, 1982). Unable to extricate themselves, the worms die. The resultant cholangiolitic abscess may enlarge and present on the surface or rupture into the peritoneal cavity. Extension of the abscess through the diaphragm to cause bronchopleural fistula and lung abscess is a well-known and potentially fatal complication (Chang & Han, 1966; Lloyd, 1981). Based on the aforementioned pathologic features, biliary ascariasis has been classified as uncomplicated and complicated (Table 60.1). Previous biliary surgery increases the risk of complications in children and adults.

Table 60.1   Classification of Biliary Ascariasis

I. Uncomplicated biliary ascariasis

II. Complicated biliary ascariasis
   A. Early complications
      1. Acute cholecystitis
      2. Acute suppurative cholangitis
      3. Hepatic invasion with or without abscess
      4. Hemobilia
      5. Acute pancreatitis
   B. Late complications
      1. Biliary calculi
      2. Granulomatous strictures of the bile ducts
      3. Hepatic granuloma

Clinical Features

Biliary ascariasis in the pediatric age group is most commonly seen in children 2 to 8 years old. In endemic areas, adults are affected frequently, and the mean age at presentation is 35 years. For unknown reasons, women are almost three times more commonly affected than men; in children, a similar sex difference in incidence has not been noted. The mean duration of symptoms varies from 4 to 6 years, and 40% of patients may give a previous history of biliary surgery, usually cholecystectomy for acalculous cholecystitis. In one large series, 80% of patients had undergone either cholecystectomy or endoscopic sphincterotomy (Sandouk et al, 1997). Microscopic examination of stool and bile samples in these patients gives a positivity rate for *A. lumbricoides* of nearly 100% (Khuroo et al, 1990). Vomiting of worms is common, as is a past history of passing worms in the stool (Lloyd, 1981; Louw, 1966).

Uncomplicated Biliary Ascariasis

The most common presentation is usually a short, sharp illness, starting with the sudden onset of severe upper abdominal colic associated with tenderness and muscle guarding localized to the right upper quadrant or epigastrium. The gallbladder may be palpable. Fever, if present, is usually low grade, and jaundice, marked toxemia, and hepatomegaly are usually absent. The clinical picture merges with that of acute acalculous cholecystitis. The illness may stretch over 7 to 10 days, with persistence of the gallbladder mass clinically and on ultrasound. Worms are rarely seen in the gallbladder, and the ultrasound finding of distention, wall edema, and intraluminal sludge completely resolves, usually within 2 weeks. Endoscopic examination is difficult to perform and unnecessary in the acute phase, but if done it may show duodenal or ampullary worms.

Acute Suppurative Cholangitis

The next most common clinical presentation, seen in roughly one third of patients, has the usual features of right hypochondriac pain; high-grade fever (38-40°C); jaundice; tender hepatomegaly; pronounced leukocytosis; and increased serum bilirubin, alkaline phosphatase, and aminotransferase levels. Progressive apathy, hypotension, metabolic acidosis, and electrolyte disturbances signify a grave prognosis. Ultrasound may show worms in the biliary tree, and endoscopy may visualize pus or the worm itself emerging from the ampulla (Fig. 60.7).

Hepatic Ascariasis

No clinical features distinguish hepatic ascariasis from suppurative cholangitis. The diagnosis is usually made at ultrasonography, and aspirated pus might yield the ova of *A. lumbricoides*. The right lobe is more commonly affected, and rupture into the peritoneal cavity is a recognized complication.

Acute Pancreatitis

The character of the pain is different in that it is referred to the back. An associated increase in serum amylase confirms the diagnosis. Although encountered half as commonly as the purely biliary presentation (Louw, 1966), the condition is probably much rarer, being seen in only 31 of 500 patients in the series by Khuroo and colleagues (1990). In only one tenth of these

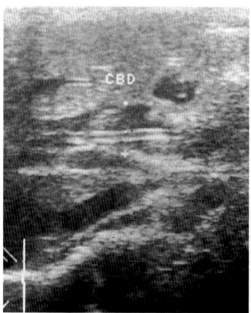

A

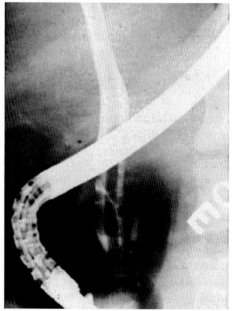

B

Fig. 60.7. A, Ultrasound of a 30-year-old woman with biliary colic of 7 days' duration, showing the dilated common bile duct with an echogenic tubular structure in the lumen. There is no distal shadowing. **B,** Endoscopic retrograde cholangiopancreatography in the same patient revealing the worm in the common bile duct and across the papilla.
(Courtesy of Professor M.S. Khuroo, Sher-I-Kashmir Institute of Medical Sciences, Srinagar, India.)

cases is the pancreatitis severe, with progression to hemorrhagic pancreatitis or pancreatic fluid collections.

Late Complications

Late complications include intraductal calculi and biliary strictures. There may be no evidence of ascariasis if the complications become manifest long after the precipitating infection, and the picture merges with that of recurrent pyogenic cholangitis (see Ch. 62).

Diagnosis

Laboratory Studies

Stool microscopy may show ascarid ova or remnants of dead worms. As in the case of other biliary parasites, detection by stool examination is usually possible and may approach 100% (Khuroo et al, 1990). In uncomplicated biliary ascariasis, the peripheral white blood cell count is usually normal. Leukocytosis greater than 12,000/mm^3 usually is associated with suppurative biliary and hepatic complications. The eosinophil count is seldom elevated more than 5%. Transient elevation of the serum bilirubin level may occur in uncomplicated biliary ascariasis. Bilirubinemia greater than 3.5 mg/dL is uncommon and occurs in association with biliary and hepatic complications (Lloyd, 1982). Elevation of the serum alkaline phosphatase and liver enzyme levels also may occur when cholangitis supervenes. The serum amylase level is usually normal or moderately elevated, but acute pancreatitis is suggested if the serum amylase is greatly elevated. Specific serologic tests are available and can be used to monitor successful eradication of the parasite after treatment (Santra et al, 2001), but are not commonly used in clinical practice.

Diagnostic Imaging

Abdominal radiographs may confirm the presence of intestinal worms in 90% of children. Occasionally, air is seen in the biliary tree or in hepatic or subphrenic abscesses (Lloyd, 1982). Ultrasound is highly accurate in showing dilated bile ducts containing linear or round areas of increased echogenicity representing worms. Real-time scanning may reveal the diagnostic movement of active worms within the biliary system. On transverse scanning, the biliary worm produces a bull's eye appearance (Cremin, 1982). Other characteristic appearances include single or multiple long linear echogenic strips within the bile duct without acoustic shadowing (Khuroo et al, 1987). A live worm in the gallbladder and edema of the pancreas also may be identified. Ultrasound is useful for identifying intrahepatic worms and abscesses and monitoring the response of these lesions to therapy. Ascarid liver abscesses characteristically contain echogenic worm debris. CT does not offer any significant advantage over real-time ultrasound.

Endoscopy and endoscopic retrograde cholangiopancreatography (ERCP) may reveal a worm in the duodenum, and occasionally a worm may be seen impacted in the ampulla of Vater. ERCP has been done safely even in the acute setting and shows worms in the extrahepatic and intrahepatic biliary tree, including liver abscesses (Lloyd, 1981). Biliary strictures can be studied, and endoscopic extraction of worms and biliary decompression may succeed in aborting an attack of severe cholangitis (Khuroo et al, 1990). Percutaneous transhepatic cholangiography has been used chiefly in adults to show intrahepatic abscesses and the abnormal biliary tree containing worms (Lloyd, 1982). Ova or worm debris may be identified in the aspirated bile.

Management

With appropriate nonoperative management, worms spontaneously return to the duodenum in 98% of children (Chang & Han, 1966; Louw, 1966) and 94% of adults (Khuroo et al, 1990). Parenteral antispasmodic drugs to relax the sphincter of Oddi, analgesics for the relief of biliary colic, nasogastric decompression, and intravenous fluids are recommended in the acute stage. Antihelminthics traditionally have been used after the acute stage has resolved to avoid killing the worms in the biliary tree. Successful elimination of an adult ascaris worm from the gallbladder 7 days after killing it with albendazole has been documented, however (Cha et al, 2002). Albendazole (400 mg/day for 1 day) or mebendazole (100 mg twice daily for 3 days) and pyrantel pamoate (single dose of 11 mg/kg to a maximum of 1 g) are the preferred agents, and cure can be achieved in nearly 100% of cases. The safety of these drugs in pregnant women and children younger than 2 years of age is not established, and in this situation piperazine is safe in a single dose of 75 mg/kg (maximum 3.5 g) on 2 consecutive days.

Follow-up after successful treatment of the acute stage involves stool examination to confirm eradication of the infestation and ultrasound to look for persistence of intraductal worms. Follow-up ERCP is recommended if symptoms or ultrasound abnormalities persist beyond 2 weeks. In endemic areas, antihelminthic therapy must be repeated every 2 months in patients who are cured to prevent reinfection (Khuroo et al, 1990).

Although uncomplicated biliary ascariasis is a relatively benign condition that resolves spontaneously, complications may be fatal, and it is imperative that they be recognized and treated early. The problem of reinfection of the bile ducts after operative or endoscopic removal of worms has led to important modifications in the interventional approach previously advocated (Chang & Han, 1966; Louw, 1966). Preoperative eradication of intestinal worms ideally should be done before endoscopic or surgical manipulation of the common bile duct.

Severe persistent pain not responding to antihelminthics is an indication for ERCP and endoscopic removal of intrabiliary worms. In an endemic area, multiple reinvasion of the bile ducts by worms is seen in patients who have undergone endoscopic sphincterotomy (Khuroo et al, 1990). In children especially, it would seem to be of paramount importance to preserve the sphincter of Oddi, and persistence of attempts at medical treatment for 10 days has met with success in this age group (Khuroo & Zargar, 1985; Khuroo et al, 1990).

Failure of response to conservative management with increasing jaundice may indicate coexisting stones in the common bile duct (Khuroo & Zargar, 1985; Khuroo et al, 1990). When skilled endoscopic intervention has either failed or is unavailable, these features constitute an indication for surgery—a situation more likely to occur in children than in adults (Hangloo et al, 1989).

Overall, 20% of patients with biliary ascariasis need surgery (Wani & Chrungoo, 1992). At surgery, an initial operative cholangiogram helps define the extent of the infection. Worms are removed through a longitudinal choledochotomy. Compression of the liver often propels intrahepatic worms toward the common bile duct. Choledochoscopy is valuable, especially if worms, debris, or stones are impacted in the intrahepatic ducts. The evacuated biliary tree is irrigated with saline and closed over a large-bore T-tube. Intraoperative cholangiography through the T-tube is done to identify residual worms. The liver may contain granulomatous nodules or abscesses, and worms under the liver capsule can be extracted by incision and drainage of the abscess.

Removal of all worms from the intestine via enterostomy is an important part of the operation to prevent biliary reinfestation, a serious complication that may require reoperation. Antihelminthics administered in the immediate postoperative period may not reach the small intestine, and merely milking worms into the colon does not prevent reinfestation. A broad-spectrum antibiotic is instituted postoperatively.

If worms are identified in the bile duct postoperatively, the initial treatment is expectant because the worm may return spontaneously to the intestine. Irrigation of the T-tube with saline may help. Antihelminthics should not be administered through the T-tube because this would kill the worm in the common bile duct, preventing spontaneous evacuation. Endoscopic extraction may be successful, or if the worm is impacted around the T-tube, it can be removed by applying suction to the T-tube and gently withdrawing it with the worm. If these measures fail, reoperation is necessary, preceded by oral antihelminthics.

Prognosis

Full recovery is usual in uncomplicated biliary ascariasis, with a mortality rate of 1% or less. Worm reinvasion after successful initial management is almost always symptomatic and in endemic areas may occur in 30% of cases (Khuroo et al, 1989b, 1990). Biliary lithiasis may occur on longer follow-up in 5% of patients. Such calculi usually are located in the intrahepatic and extrahepatic bile ducts, and the associated sepsis and biliary strictures would result in the picture merging with the syndrome of recurrent pyogenic cholangitis.

REFERENCES

Abd-Alla MD, et al, 2004: Identification of the *Entamoeba histolytica* galactose-inhibitable lectin epitopes recognized by human immunoglobulin A antibodies following cure of amebic liver abscess. Infect Immun 72:3974-3980.

Aikat BK, et al, 1979: The pathology and pathogenesis of fatal hepatic amoebiasis: a study based on 79 autopsy cases. Trans R Soc Trop Med Hyg 73:188-192.

Allason-Jones E, et al, 1988: Outcome of untreated infection with *Entamoeba histolytica* in homosexual men with and without HIV antibody. BMJ 297:654-657.

Angel C, et al, 2000: Gastric wall erosion by an amebic liver abscess in a 3-year-old girl. Pediatr Surg Int 16:429-430.

Arellano J, et al, 1996: Increased frequency of HLA-DR3 and complotype SCO1 in Mexican mestizo children with amebic abscess of the liver. Parasite Immun 18:491-498.

Ashton WL, et al, 1970: Human fascioliasis in Shropshire. BMJ 3:500-502.

Augustine P, et al, 1988: Recurrent pyogenic cholangitis (Oriental cholangiopathy) in Kerla. J Gastoenterol Hepatol 3:515.

Balasegaram M, 1981: Management of hepatic abscess. Curr Probl Surg 18:282-340.

Bassiouny HK, et al, 1991: Human fascioliasis in Egypt: effect of infection and efficacy of bithionol treatment. J Trop Med Hyg 94:333-337.

Beck DL, et al, 2002: *Entamoeba histolytica*: sequence conservation of the gal/galnac lectin from clinical isolates. Exp Parasitol 101:157-163.

Blessman J, et al, 2003: Hepatic ultrasound in a population with high incidence of invasive amoebiasis: evidence for subclinical, self-limited amoebic liver abscess. Trop Med Int Health 8:231-233.

Braga LL, et al, 1992: Inhibition of the complement membrane attack complex by the galactose-specific adhesion of *Entamoeba histolytica*. Arch Med Res 23:133.

Cabellero-Salcedo A, et al, 1994: Seroepidemiology of amebiasis in Mexico. Am J Trop Med Hyg 50:412-419.

Cha DY, et al, 2002: Successful elimination of *Ascaris lumbricoides* from the gallbladder by conservative medical therapy. J Gastroenterol 37:758-760.

Chang CC, Han CT, 1966: Biliary ascariasis in childhood. Chin Med J 85:167-171.

Choi BI, et al, 2004: Clonorchiasis and cholangiocarcinoma: etiological relationship and imaging diagnosis. Clin Microbiol Rev 17:540-552.

Cremin BJ, 1982: Real-time ultrasound in paediatric biliary ascariasis. S Afr Med J 61:914-916.

Dalton JP, et al, 2003: *Fasciola hepatica* cathepsin L-like proteases: biology, function, and potential in the development of first generation liver fluke vaccines. Int J Parasitol 33:1173-1181.

Davies MR, Rode H, 1982: Biliary ascariasis in children. Prog Pediatr Surg 15:55-74.

Davis A, Pawlowski ZS, 1985: Amoebiasis and its control. Bull World Health Organ 63:417-426.

Debakey ME, Ochsner A, 1951: Hepatic amebiasis: a 20-year experience and analysis of 263 cases. Surg Gynecol Obstet 92:209-231.

Diamond LS, et al, 1978: A new medium for the axenic cultivation of *Entamoeba histolytica* and other entamoeba. Trans R Soc Trop Med Hyg 72:431-432.

Eggleston FC, et al, 1982: Amoebic peritonitis secondary to amoebic liver abscess. Surgery 91:46-48.

Flavell DJ, 1981: Liver-fluke infection as an aetiological factor in bile-duct carcinoma of man. Trans R Soc Trop Med Hyg 75:814-824.

Fung J, 1961: Liver fluke infestation and cholangio-hepatitis. Br J Surg 48:404-415.

Gatharim V, Jackson TF, 1987: A longitudinal study of asymptomatic carriers of pathogenic zymodemes of *Entamoeba histolytica*. S Afr Med J 72:669-672.

Gatti S, et al, 2002: Amebic infections due to the *Entamoeba histolytica*–*Entamoeba dispar* complex: a study of the incidence in a remote rural area of Ecuador. Am J Trop Med Hyg 67:123-127.

Gaucher D, Chadee K, 2002: Construction and immunogenicity of a codon-optimized *Entamoeba histolytica* gal-lectin-based DNA vaccine. Vaccine 20:3244-3253.

Gonzalez EG, et al, 2002: Calreticulin-like molecule in trophozoites of *Entamoeba histolytica* HM1:IMSS (Swissprot: accession P83003). Am J Trop Med Hyg 67:636-639.

Guarner V, 1986: Treatment of amebiasis. In Martinez-Palomo A (ed): Amebiasis: Human Parasitic Diseases, No. 2. Amsterdam, Elsevier, pp 189-211.

Guerrant RL, 1986: Amebiasis: introduction, current status, and research questions. Rev Infect Dis 8:218-227.

Haghighi A, et al, 2002: Remarkable genetic polymorphism among *Entamoeba histolytica* isolates from a limited geographic area. J Clin Microbiol 40:4081-4090.

Hangloo VK, et al, 1989: Biliary ascariasis. Indian J Gastroenterol 8:265-266.

Haque R, et al, 2002: Innate and acquired resistance to amebiasis in Bangladeshi children. J Infect Dis 186:547-552.

Hardman EW, et al, 1970: Fascioliasis—a large outbreak. BMJ 3:502-505.

Hou MF, et al, 1989: The ultrasound survey of gallstone diseases of patients infected with *Clonorchis sinensis* in Southern Taiwan. J Trop Med Hyg 92:108-111.

Hou PC, 1956: The pathology of *Clonorchis sinesis* infestation of the liver. J Pathol Bacteriol 70:53-60.

Huston CD, et al, 2003: Apoptotic killing and phagocytosis of host cells by the parasite *Entamoeba histolytica*. Infect Immun 71:964-972.

Irusen EM, et al, 1992: Asymptomatic intestinal colonization by pathogenic *Entamoeba histolytica* in amebic liver abscess: prevalence, response to therapy, and pathogenic potential. Clin Infect Dis 14:889-893.

Jain NK, et al, 1990: Hepatopulmonary amoebiasis: efficacy of various treatment regimens containing dehydroemetine and/or metronidazole. J Assoc Physicians India 38:269-271.

Jones EA, et al, 1977: Massive infection with *Fasciola hepatica* in man. Am J Med 63:836-842.

Kapoor OP, 1979: Amoebic Liver Abscess. Bombay, SS Publishers.

Ken JG, et al, 1989: Perforated amebic liver abscesses: Successful percutaneous treatment. Radiology 170:195-197.

Khuroo MS, 2001: Hepatobiliary and pancreatic ascariasis. Indian J Gastroenterol 20:C28-32.

Khuroo MS, Zargar SA, 1985: Biliary ascariasis: a common cause of biliary and pancreatic disease in an endemic area. Gastroenterology 88:418-423.

Khuroo MS, et al, 1987: Sonographic appearances in biliary ascariasis. Gastroenterology 93:267-272.

Khuroo MS, et al, 1989a: Prevalence of biliary tract disease in India: a sonographic study in adult population in Kashmir. Gut 30:201-205.

Khuroo MS, et al, 1989b: Biliary and pancreatic ascariasis: a long-term follow up. Natl Med J India 2:4-7.

Khuroo MS, et al, 1990: Hepatobiliary and pancreatic ascariasis in India. Lancet 335:1503-1506.

LaPook JD, et al, 2000: Sheep, watercress, and the internet. Lancet 356:218-220.

Leippe M, et al, 1991: Pore-forming peptide of pathogenic *Entamoeba histolytica*. Proc Natl Acad Sci U S A 88:7659-7663.

Li E, Stanley SL Jr, 1996: Protozoa: amebiasis. Gastroenterol Clin North Am 25:471-492.

Lin YL, et al, 1995: Antibodies in serum of patients with clonorchiasis before and after treatment. Southeast Asian J Trop Med Public Health 26:114-119.

Lloyd DA, 1981: Massive hepato-biliary ascariasis in childhood. Br J Surg 68:468-476.

Lloyd DA, 1982: Hepato-biliary ascariasis in children. Surg Annu 14:277-297.

Lotter H, et al, 2003: Oral vaccination with recombinant *Yersinia* expressing hybrid type III proteins protects gerbils from amebic liver abscess. In EMBO Workshop on Pathogenesis of Amoebiasis: from Genomics to Diseases. Paris, Institut Pasteur, p 60.

Louw JH, 1966: Abdominal complications of *Ascaris lumbricoides* infestation in children. Br J Surg 53:510-521.

Maher K, et al, 1999: Parasite-specific antibody profile in human fascioliasis: application for immunodiagnosis of infection. Am J Trop Med Hyg 61:738-742.

Maki T, 1966: Pathogenesis of calcium bilirubinate gallstone: role of *E. coli*, beta-glucuronidase and coagulation by inorganic ions, polyelectrolytes and agitation. Ann Surg 164:90-100.

Mann BJ, 2002: *Entamoeba histolytica* genome project: an update. Trends Parasitol 18:147-148.

Mann BJ, et al, 1993: Neutralizing monoclonal antibody epitopes of the *Entamoeba histolytica* galactose adhesin map to the cysteine-rich extracellular domain of the 170-kilodalton subunit. Infect Immun 61:1772-1778.

Mann BJ, et al, 1997: Protection in a gerbil model of amebiasis by oral immunization with *Salmonella* expressing the galactose/N-acetyl D-galactosamine inhibitable lectin of *Entamoeba histolytica*. Vaccine 15:659-663.

Martinez Baez M, 1986: Historical introduction. In Martinez-Palomo A (ed): Amebiasis: Human Parasitic Diseases, No. 2. Amsterdam, Elsevier, pp 1-9.

Mas-Coma MS, et al, 1999: Epidemiology of human fascioliasis: a review and proposed new classification. Bull World Health Organ 77:340-346.

McConnell JFP, 1875: Remarks on the anatomical and pathological revelation of a new species of liver fluke. Lancet 2:271-273.

McDermott VG, 1995: What is the role of percutaneous drainage for treatment of amebic abscesses of the liver? AJR Am J Roentgenol 165:1005-1006.

Monga NK, et al, 1976: Amebic peritonitis. Am J Gastroenterol 66:366-373.

Munoz O, 1986: Epidemiology of amebiasis. In Martinez-Palomo A (ed): Amebiasis: Human Parasitic Diseases, No. 2. Amsterdam, Elsevier, pp 213-239.

Nicholas JL, 1970: Obstruction of the common bile-duct by *Fasciola hepatica*: occurrence in a boy of 12 years. Br J Surg 57:544-546.

Oto A, et al, 1999: Focal inflammatory diseases of the liver. Eur J Radiol 32:61-75.

Pillai DR, et al, 1999: The cysteine-rich region of the *Entamoeba histolytica* adherence lectin (170-kilodalton subunit) is sufficient for high-affinity Gal/GalNAc-specific binding in vitro. Infect Immun 67:3836-3841.

Pitt HA, 1990: Surgical management of hepatic abscesses. World J Surg 14:498-504.

Que X, Reed SL, 1997: The role of extracellular cysteine proteinases in pathogenesis of *Entamoeba histolytica* invasion. Parasitol Today 13:190-194.

Radin DR, et al, 1988: CT of amebic liver abscess. AJR Am J Roentgenol 150:1297-1301.

Ralls PW, et al, 1979: Gray-scale ultrasonography of hepatic amoebic abscesses. Radiology 132:125-129.

Ralls PW, et al, 1982: Sonographic findings in hepatic amebic abscess. Radiology 145:123-126.

Ralls PW, et al, 1983: Patterns of resolution in successfully treated hepatic amebic abscess: sonographic evaluation. Radiology 149:541-543.

Ravdin JI, 1995: Amebiasis. Clin Infect Dis 20:1453-1464.

Ravdin JI, Guerrant RL, 1982: A review of the parasite cellular mechanisms involved in the pathogenesis of amebiasis. Rev Infect Dis 4:1185-1207.

Reed SL, et al, 1995: The extracellular neutral cysteine proteinase of *Entamoeba histolytica* degrades anaphylatoxins c3a and c5a. J Immunol 155:266-274.

Rivera WL, et al, 1998: Application of the polymerase chain reaction (PCR) in the epidemiology of *Entamoeba histolytica* and *Entamoeba dispar* infections. Tokai J Exp Clin Med 23:413-415.

Roy S, et al, 2005: Real-time PCR assay for diagnosis of *Entamoeba histolytica* infection. J Clin Microbiol 43:2168-2172.

Saba R, et al, 2004: Human fascioliasis. Clin Microbiol Infect 10:385-387.

Salata RA, Ravdin JI, 1986: Review of the human immune mechanisms directed against *Entamoeba histolytica*. Rev Infect Dis 8:261-272.

Salata RA, et al, 1989: Chemoattractant activity of *Entamoeba histolytica* for human polymorphonuclear neutrophils. J Parasitol 75:644-646.

Salles JM, et al, 2003: Hepatic amebiasis. Braz J Infect Dis 7:96-110.

Sandouk F, et al, 1997: Pancreatic-biliary ascariasis: experience of 300 cases. Am J Gastroenterol 92:2264-2267.

Santra A, et al, 2001: Serodiagnosis of ascariasis with specific IgG4 antibody and its use in an epidemiological study. Trans R Soc Trop Med Hyg 95:289-292.

Sarda AK, et al, 1989: Intraperitoneal rupture of amoebic liver abscess. Br J Surg 76:202-203.

Sargeaunt PG, et al, 1984: Influence of geographical factors in the distribution of pathogenic zymodemes of *Entamoeba histolytica*: identification of zymodeme XIV in India. Trans R Soc Trop Med Hyg 78:96-101.

Sepulveda B, 1982: Amebiasis: host-pathogen biology. Rev Infect Dis 4:1247-1253.

Sepulveda B, Manzo NTG, 1986: Clinical manifestations and diagnosis of amebiasis. In Martinez-Palomo A (ed): Amebiasis: Human Parasitic Diseases, No. 2. Amsterdam, Elsevier, pp 169-187.

Sharma M, et al, 1988: A simple and rapid Dot-ELISA dipstick technique for detection of antibodies to *Entamoeba histolytica* in amoebic liver abscess. Indian J Med Res 88:409-415.

Sharma MP, et al, 1989: Needle aspiration of amoebic liver abscess. BMJ 299:1308-1309.

Sharma MP, et al, 1996: Prognostic markers in amebic liver abscess: a prospective study. Am J Gastroenterol 91:2584-2588.

Sheen IS, et al, 1989: Resolution of liver abscesses: comparison of pyogenic and amebic liver abscesses. Am J Trop Med Hyg 40:384-389.

Stanley SL Jr, 1997: Progress towards development of a vaccine for amebiasis. Clin Microbiol Rev 10:637-649.

Stanley SL Jr, 2003: Amebiasis. Lancet 361:1025-1034.

Sukov RJ, et al, 1980: Sonography of hepatic amebic abscesses. AJR Am J Roentgenol 134:911-915.

Tandon A, et al, 1997: Needle aspiration in large amoebic liver abscess. Trop Gastroenterol 18:19-21.

Tandon R, 1988: Pigment gallstones. Indian J Gastroenterol 7:5-6.

Tannich E, et al, 1989: Genomic DNA differences between pathogenic and nonpathogenic *Entamoeba histolytica*. Proc Natl Acad Sci U S A 86:5118-5122.

Teoh TB, 1963: A study of gall-stones and included worms in recurrent pyogenic cholangitis. J Pathol Bacteriol 86:123-129.

Thompson JE Jr, et al, 1985: Amebic liver abscess: a therapeutic approach. Rev Infect Dis 7:171-179.

Tovar J, et al, 1999: The mitosome, a novel organelle related to mitochondria in the amitochondrial parasite *Entamoeba histolytica*. Mol Microbiol 32:1013-1021.

Vaidya AB, Ray DK, 1982: Amoebiasis: the tropical scourge. Science Today 16:21-26.

Van Allan RJ, et al, 1992: Uncomplicated amebic liver abscess: prospective evaluation of percutaneous therapeutic aspiration. Radiology 183:827-830.

Vohra H, et al, 2003: Effective human defense against *E. histolytica*: high amoebicidal activity of lymphocytes and monocytes in amoebic liver abscess patients until 3 months follow-up. Parasitol Int 52:193-202.

Walsh JA, 1986: Problems in recognition and diagnosis of amebiasis: estimation of the global magnitude of morbidity and mortality. Rev Infect Dis 8:228-238.

Wang KX, et al, 2004: Clinical and epidemiological data of patients with clonorchiasis. World J Gastroenterol 10:446-448.

Wani NA, Chrungoo RK, 1992: Biliary ascariasis: surgical aspects. World J Surg 16:976-979.

Wells CD, Arguedas M, 2004: Amebic liver abscess. South Med J 97:673-682.

Zhi FC, et al, 2004: Treatment of severe *Clonorchis sinensis* by endoscopic nasobiliary drainage and oral praziquantel. World J Gastroenterol 10:2150-2152.

Hydatid Cyst of the Liver

C. KAYAALP

Hydatid cyst of the liver, a zoonotic parasitic disease, is caused most frequently by *Echinococcus granulosus* or *Echinococcus multilocularis*. The life cycle of *Echinococcus* has a definitive host, which is often a dog, and an intermediate host, which is commonly a sheep. Humans become accidental intermediate hosts when they get infected from dogs. The development of the cyst in the liver is often responsible for severe complications, including local infection, biliary fistula leading to biliary infection, and rupture into the peritoneum or chest. Diagnosis is easy with a good imaging technique. Surgery is the most effective treatment of complicated cases. The tendency to treat this benign lesion with a conservative approach is counterbalanced by a high rate of local postoperative complications, such as biliocutaneous fistula and infection of the residual cavity. Less morbidity and lower recurrence rates are obtained by a radical surgical approach, which requires an extensive experience in liver surgery. Uncomplicated cysts located anteriorly in the liver can be treated successfully through a laparoscopic approach. Medical treatment for definitive cure of univesicular cysts and adjuvant treatment with surgical and percutaneous techniques are promising. Percutaneous techniques are an important therapeutic advance for this disease, which is a public health problem in endemic areas. Increasing migration and world travel necessitates knowledge of this disease by clinicians, radiologists, and surgeons in developed countries. *E. multilocularis*, which causes alveolar echinococcosis, is discussed separately.

HISTORY AND TERMINOLOGY

Hydatid cyst infection is one of the oldest diseases in animals and humans. It was first described in the Talmud as "bladders full of water." Hippocrates described it as "the liver is filled with water." The animal origin of the disease was first recognized by Redi in the 17th century. The relationship between the adult tapeworm in the dog and the cystic form in the sheep was recognized in 1853 by Von Siebold. The life cycle of *E. granulosus* was clarified at the end of 19th century, and the clinical aspects of the disease became clear at the beginning of the 20th century.

PATHOGENESIS AND ETIOLOGY

Although 16 species and 13 subspecies originally were described in the genus *Echinococcus*, molecular epidemiologic studies led to recognition of only four clinically important species: *E. granulosus*, *E. multilocularis* (*Echinococcus alveolaris*), *Echinococcus oligarthrus*, and *Echinococcus vogeli* (Thompson, 2001). Characteristics of four *Echinococcus* species are summarized in Table 61.1. *E. granulosus* is the most common and constitutes the main topic of this chapter. *E. multilocularis*, a rare and aggressive form, is discussed separately at the end of the chapter.

The life cycle of *E. granulosus* requires two hosts (Fig. 61.1). The adult tapeworm lives in the intestine of the dog, which is the most common definitive host for *E. granulosus*. Worms release countless infected eggs that pass out with dog feces, and they contaminate the soil, water, and plants on the ground. Sheep, the most readily available intermediate host, and other animals, such as goats, marsupials, Bovidae, and pigs, acquire the larval stage by ingesting the egg from the contaminated materials (Fig. 61.2). After ingestion by the hosts, the embryos migrate through the intestinal wall and develop mostly in the liver. Sometimes the eggs penetrate the circulation and via the bloodstream may settle in any organ, including lung, spleen, kidney, brain, and bone. In the liver, the parasite develops into the larval stage, which is the hydatid cyst filled with fluid and contains hundreds to thousands of protoscoleces. For the life cycle to be completed, a canine host must ingest the hydatid cyst or its contents, which

Table 61.1 Characteristics of *Echinococcus* Species

	E. granulosus	*E. multilocularis*	*E. oligarthus*	*E. vogelii*
Geographic distribution	Worldwide	Limited to Northern Hemisphere	Central and South America	Central and South America
Definitive hosts	Dog, fox, wolf, dingo, jackal	Fox, dog, cat	Wild felines (e.g., jaguar, puma)	Bush dog
Intermediate hosts	Sheep, cattle, pig, goat, camel, buffalo, human	Rodent, pig, horse, human	Rodent, human	Rodent, human
Cyst structure	Typically unilocular, spherical in shape	Multivesicular	Polycystic	Polycystic
Infiltration or metastasis	No	Yes	No	No
Location of cysts	Visceral, primarily liver and lungs	Visceral, primarily liver	Peripheral, primarily muscles	Visceral, primarily liver
No. segments in worm (range)	3 (2-7)	5 (2-6)	3	3
Total length of worm (mm)	2-11	1.2-4.5	2.2-2.9	3.9-5.5

Modified from Thompson RCA, 2001: Echinococcosis. In Gillespie S, Pearson RD (eds): Principles and Practice of Clinical Parasitology. Chichester, England, John Wiley & Sons Ltd, pp 587-612.

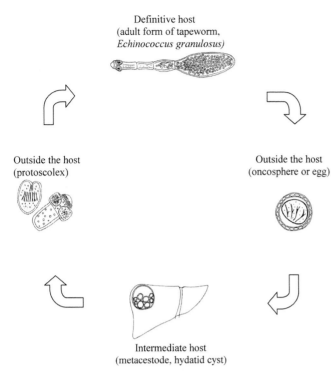

Definitive host
(adult form of tapeworm,
Echinococcus granulosus)

Outside the host
(protoscolex)

Outside the host
(oncosphere or egg)

Intermediate host
(metacestode, hydatid cyst)

Fig. 61.1. Life cycle of *E. granulosus.*

commonly occurs when infected sheep are slaughtered, and organs containing hydatid cysts are fed to the dogs.

EPIDEMIOLOGY

The disease occurs principally in sheep-grazing areas with a wide distribution influenced by the presence of dogs, especially if they are allowed to remain loose and are able to eat uncooked viscera. Echinococcosis is endemic in many Mediterranean countries, the Middle and Far East, South America, southern Australia, and East Africa. The incidence of disease in humans in endemic areas depends on the level of health care and veterinary control. The incidence of human hydatidosis often is established according to the number of surgically treated patients. The yearly incidence of human hydatidosis per 100,000 population ranged from 0.4 in Switzerland and Wales to 196 in Turkana, which is located in the northwest region of Kenya. The cause of this high incidence is a close relationship of the Turkana people and dogs. They sleep with their dogs for warmth at night, and dogs are kept as "nurses" to lick infants after they vomit or defecate (Richards, 1992; Watson-Jones & Macpherson, 1988).

In the Western Hemisphere, immigrants from endemic areas have a higher incidence of hydatid diagnosis than the native residents. Indigenous people in endemic areas are the primary risk group; less frequently aid workers and rarely tourists are at risk. Children playing with infected dogs may become infected early in life. As a result of slow growth, cysts usually become symptomatic a few years after infection, in adolescence or early adulthood. Infected adults may become symptomatic later in life. Host immunity may overcome infection, however, making the echinococcal cyst nonviable without ever becoming symptomatic.

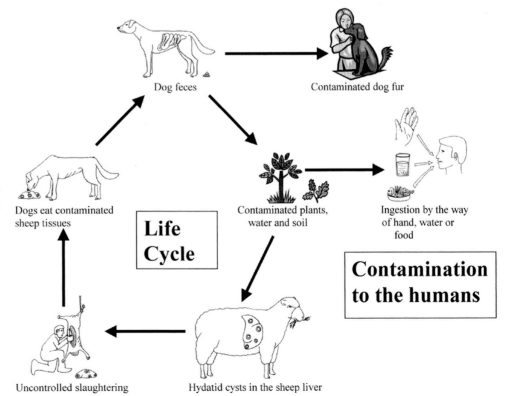

Fig. 61.2. Usual route of *E. granulosus* and contamination of humans during the life cycle.

Dog feces

Contaminated dog fur

Dogs eat contaminated sheep tissues

Life Cycle

Contaminated plants, water and soil

Ingestion by the way of hand, water or food

Contamination to the humans

Uncontrolled slaughtering

Hydatid cysts in the sheep liver

The origin of the patient should be asked during the evaluation of a cystic mass. Humans are a dead-end host; the disease is not transmitted from human to human.

DEVELOPMENT OF HYDATID CYST

When the parasite reaches the liver parenchyma, if it survives, it develops into a cyst, which is visible after 3 weeks and may measure 3 cm in diameter after 3 months. The mature cyst of *E. granulosus* consists of a layer of living tissue, which includes the germinal layer that surrounds the fluid-filled central hydatid cavity and the laminated layer. These two layers (germinative and laminated) form the *endocyst*. The compression of the host's tissue around the endocyst produces a fibrous layer, which is called *ectocyst* or *pericyst* (Fig. 61.3).

The germinal layer, also called the germinative membrane, is the living component of the parasite. Undifferentiated cells in the germinal layer produce invaginations toward the cyst cavity forming brood capsules, which are released into the cystic fluid. Germinal membrane has the absorptive function for nutrition of the cyst and secretes the hydatid cyst fluid into the cyst. Lastly, it is the source of daughter cysts. The presence of daughter cysts produces multivesicular cysts, which are more common in adults than in children. Daughter cysts have similar structures as the mother cysts, including laminated membrane, germinative membrane, cyst fluid, and brood capsules and protoscoleces. The only difference is the absence of an adventitial layer.

The thin germinal layer is supported externally by the most characteristic structural component of the parasite, known as the laminated layer or membrane. The laminated membrane, which is totally acellular and always separable from the pericyst, is usually 1 to 2 mm thick. Although the laminated membrane is permeable to water, potassium, chloride, calcium, and urea, it protects the cyst from host enzyme, bile, and bacteria. The formation of daughter cysts is known as the process of *endogenic vesiculation*. Ectogenic vesiculation occurs when there is a small rupture or defect in the laminated membrane, and the germinal layer passes through and creates a "satellite" hydatid cyst.

The pericyst or ectocyst is a fibrous capsule developed from host tissue against *E. granulosus* as an inflammatory reaction. The pericyst, initially composed of a thin connective lamina, subsequently tends to become thicker (up to 1 cm). This thick

fibrous layer is present in hydatid cysts in the liver and spleen, but is not present in pulmonary and brain hydatid cysts. Vascular structures and the bile ducts in the adventitial layer remain intact for a long time despite the development of the cyst. The compression induced by the cyst makes biliary duct fissures often not detectable, resulting in postoperative biliary leakage after partial pericystic resection. The blood supply of the adventitial layer is good resulting in an appearance of a hypervascular rim or halo around the cystic cavity on computed tomography (CT) scans with contrast injection. There are no cleavage planes between the adventitial layer and the surrounding normal host tissue, and it is not readily separable from the surrounding parenchyma. With time, the adventitial layer may calcify partially or totally. The calcification of the pericyst hinders the passage of nutrients and oxygen into the cyst. Partial calcification does not mean death of cysts.

The hydatid cyst fluid is secreted by germinative membrane. This fluid is characteristic for hydatid cysts, and an uncomplicated cyst typically contains a colorless, odorless fluid, clear as water. The levels of sodium, chloride, and bicarbonate concentrations are about the same as those of the patient's plasma, whereas potassium and calcium are lower. Bile-stained fluid is an indicator of cystobiliary communication. When there is an infection, the cyst fluid can become frankly purulent. In degenerated cysts, the fluid becomes turbid. In noncomplicated cysts, the fluid is bacteriologically sterile. Hydatid fluid pressure within a living hydatid cyst can reach 70 cm H_2O, which explains the risk of rupture after trauma or surgical manipulation. Intracystic pressure can predict the viability of the cysts as well. Yalin and coworkers (1992) measured the median intracystic pressure during the operation and found 35 cm H_2O for viable cysts and 0 for nonviable cysts located in the liver. The spillage of hydatid materials as a result of traumatic or iatrogenic rupture produces implantations of protoscoleces, and secondary cysts can occur on the viscera. These diseases in humans or animals are known as secondary hydatidosis. Any part of the liver can be the location of hydatid cysts. The location of hydatid liver cysts seems to be related to the respective volume of each part of the liver, with a higher involvement of the right lobe and within the right liver a higher involvement of segments VII and VIII (Kayaalp et al, 2003).

COMPLICATIONS

Symptoms of the cyst may result from direct pressure; from the inflammatory reaction around the cyst; from distortion of neighboring structures or viscera; or from rupture into physiologic channels (e.g., the biliary or bronchial tree), free body cavities (e.g., peritoneal, pleural, or pericardial), or adjacent organs (e.g., digestive tract).

Compression

While they are growing, cysts tend to enlarge toward Glisson's capsule, compressing the surrounding parenchyma and leading to compensatory hypertrophy of the remaining liver tissue. Frequently, an entire liver lobe can be replaced by an enormous cyst without clinical or biologic manifestations. Depending on the location, large cysts can cause compression of the adjacent bile ducts, portal vein, or hepatic veins or vena cava causing

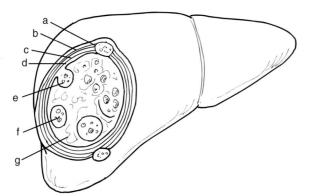

Fig. 61.3. Structure of hydatid cyst showing exogenous daughter cyst (a); pericyst membrane (b); laminated membrane, which is acellular (c); germinal membrane (d), from which the daughter cysts are formed (e); daughter cyst, which is getting detached from the germinal membrane (f); and hydatid cyst fluid (g).

obstructive jaundice, portal hypertension, or Budd-Chiari syndrome (Moreno Gonzalez et al, 1994).

Cyst Infection

Cysts may become infected after bacteremia or via communicating bile ducts, especially when endoscopic retrograde cholangiopancreatography (ERCP) has been performed. Patients present with high fever, sepsis syndrome, and tender liver. Similar to liver abscess, antibiotics and drainage are the principal methods of treatment.

Rupture into the Biliary Tract

Intrabiliary rupture is the most common complication of hydatid liver cysts (Iscan & Duren, 1991; Yilmaz & Gokok, 1990). Cystobiliary communications that occur after rupture of the cysts into the bile ducts can be minor or major. Minor communications are usually asymptomatic, revealed postoperatively by biliary leakage, whereas major communications cause obstructive jaundice and cholangitis. In histologic studies of the pericyst wall, numerous biliary ducts of various sizes communicating with the residual cavity were shown (Gahukamble et al, 2000), suggesting the existence of biliary communications in almost all hydatid cysts (Langer et al, 1984). The true incidence of cystobiliary communication is unknown; and the reported rates vary from 2.6% to 28.6% (Langer et al, 1984; Ozmen et al, 1992). In our studies, the incidence of cystobiliary communications was 37%, and the incidence of clinically apparent biliary leakage was 26% (Kayaalp et al, 2003). Incidence of cystobiliary communications depends largely on the criteria used for defining the communications. Morel and coworkers (1988) showed a 36% rate of biliary leak via routine intraoperative cholangiography.

Preoperative and intraoperative determination of biliary communication is important. Kayaalp and colleagues (2002a) found that the risk of biliary-cyst communication was higher in male patients (40.9% versus 10.4%; P<.01), in patients with abnormal preoperative serum alkaline phosphatase and gamma-glutamyltransferase (GGT), in patients with multiple cysts, in patients with multilocular (23.8%) and degenerated (24%) cysts compared with unilocular cysts (12.5%), and in patients with cysts near the biliary bifurcation and in the presence of bile-stained or purulent cyst contents compared with others

(61.9% versus 2%; P<.001) (Kayaalp et al, 2003). Although the size of the cyst did not seem to be significant in the occurrence of biliary leakage in the study by Kayaalp and colleagues, Atli and associates (2001) found that cyst diameter greater than 10 cm was an independent clinical predictor for the presence of intrabiliary rupture.

Major biliary communications were defined by a fistula greater than 5 mm diameter or by the presence of cystic communication into the main bile duct or both (Bourgeon, 1985). The incidence of major biliary-cyst communication ranged from 5% to 10% (Zaouche et al, 2001), especially when large segmental ducts are involved, leading to passage of cyst elements into the bile duct and causing obstructive jaundice or cholangitis or both. Serum alkaline phosphatase, GGT, and bilirubin levels are abnormal. Ultrasound and CT show a detached membrane in the cyst cavity associated with dilated intrahepatic bile ducts (Fig. 61.4). Endosonography also detects the cystic material in the extrahepatic bile ducts in some suspected cases. ERCP has proved to be a valuable tool for the diagnosis of frank rupture into the biliary tract (Fig. 61.5) (Ozaslan & Bayraktar, 2002).

Rupture into the Bronchial Tree

Bile-stained cysts located in the upper and posterior parts of the liver may induce inflammatory adhesions within the diaphragm and the pleural layer and with time can cause spontaneous erosion into the pulmonary parenchyma, leading to bronchobiliary fistula and causing serious injury to the bronchial tree (Gerazounis et al, 2002).

Rupture into the Peritoneum

Intraperitoneal rupture of hydatid cyst is an uncommon clinical presentation, even in endemic regions, with an incidence ranging from 1% to 8% (Sozuer et al, 2002). Rupture can occur spontaneously. Although this complication may be totally silent (Abdel Hameed & Abu Aisha, 1987), abdominal pain, nausea, vomiting, and urticaria are the most common symptoms, and all acute abdominal signs, such as guarding, rebound, and tenderness, are generally present. This complication should be included in the differential diagnosis of acute abdomen, especially in endemic areas. The release of brood cystic fluid into the peritoneal cavity leads to multiple cysts throughout the peritoneal

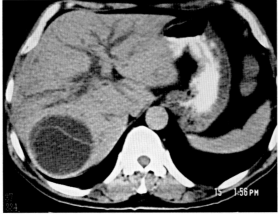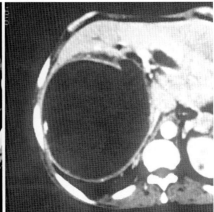

Fig. 61.4. Dilated intrahepatic bile ducts and detached cyst membrane indicate major cystobiliary communication. The patient was jaundiced because of biliary obstruction by hydatid material.

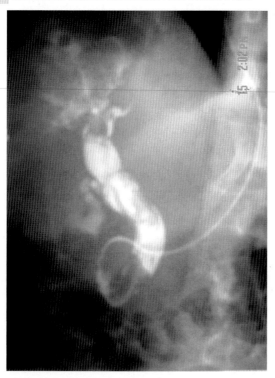

Fig. 61.5. Hydatid material in the common bile duct shown by cholangiogram through nasobiliary drainage after ERCP.

cavity with intestinal obstruction, gross abdominal distention, and ascites. Ultrasound and CT may be helpful for defining the cysts with detached membrane and the presence of intra-abdominal fluid in patients with perforated hydatid cysts (Fig. 61.6). Diagnostic peritoneal lavage also is a helpful and highly specific test for hydatid cyst perforation (Kurt et al, 2003).

Rupture into Other Cavities or Organs

Rupture into the gastrointestinal tract was observed with the stomach and the duodenum (Diez Valladares et al, 1998).

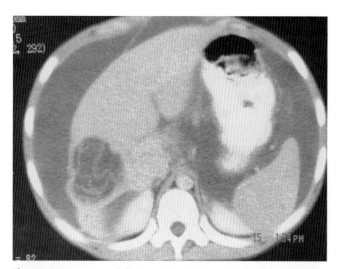

Fig. 61.6. Free peritoneal fluid and detached membrane indicate peritoneal perforation of hydatid liver cysts.

Isolated cases of rupture of liver hydatid cysts into the pericardium (Thameur et al, 2001) and into large vessels, including inferior vena cava, also have been described (Karunajeewa et al, 2002).

DIAGNOSIS

The diagnosis is based on history and geography, imaging, and serology. Parasitology of cyst contents confirms the diagnosis.

Symptoms

Small (<5 cm in diameter) and uncomplicated cysts are usually asymptomatic. Their incidence ranges from 8% to 75% (Barnes & Lillemoe, 1997; Milicevic, 1994). Small cysts can be detected incidentally during radiologic examinations of the right upper quadrant. The expansion of larger cysts or the inflammatory reaction around the cyst that irritates the adjacent parietal peritoneum may cause moderate pain in the right upper quadrant or in the lower chest. Acute abdominal pain usually indicates a purulent cyst (hydatid abscess) or rupture into the peritoneal cavity. When the antigenic cyst fluid is released into the circulation, especially after rupture into the peritoneal cavity, a variety of acute allergic manifestations (urticaria, anaphylactic attacks, or episodes of asthma) may occur (Vuitton, 2004). Extrusion of cyst contents into the biliary tree also can lead to sudden absorption of the hydatid antigen in sensitized patients resulting in similar allergic manifestations (Little, 1976). Clinical characteristics of rupture into the biliary tree are recurrent colicky pain and jaundice, with or without resultant fevers and chills, mimicking obstructing bile duct stones. Bronchobilia resulting from hepato-bronchial fistula and ascites resulting from pressure on hepatic veins or inferior vena cava or both (Budd-Chiari syndrome) are rare but possible clinical presentations.

Laboratory Tests (Except Serology)

Hydatid disease, even extremely large cysts, may not alter the liver function tests. Transaminase levels (serum aspartate and alanine transaminases) are usually normal. Cholestatic enzymes, such as alkaline phosphatase and GGT, can be mildly elevated in about one third of cases, however, especially in patients with biliary involvement (Kayaalp et al, 2002a). Elevated bilirubin levels (>1 mg/dL) with elevated alkaline phosphatase and GGT levels almost always are diagnostic of cystobiliary communications. White blood cell counts are elevated only if the cyst has become secondarily infected. Eosinophilia (>3%) occurs in 25% to 45% of patients with hydatid cysts in Western countries, but it is a nonspecific finding in endemic areas (Pitt et al, 1986). Serum immunoglobulin levels also may be elevated (31% of patients with hydatid liver cysts) (Kayaalp et al, 2002a).

Radiology

Ultrasound and Computed Tomography

Ultrasound and CT are suitable for diagnosis, percutaneous treatment, and post-treatment follow-up. Ultrasound is the preferred first-line imaging method for hydatid liver cysts followed by CT, which gives more precise information regarding the morphology

Table 61.2   World Health Organization Classifications of Hydatid Cysts

Cyst Type	Status	Ultrasound Features	Remarks
CL	Active	Signs not pathognomonic, unilocular, no cyst wall	Usually early stage, not fertile; differential diagnosis necessary
CE 1	Active	Cyst wall, hydatid sand	Usually fertile
CE 2	Active	Multivesicular, cyst wall, rosette-like	Usually fertile
CE 3	Transitional	Detached laminated membrane, water-lily sign, less round—decreased intracystic pressure	Starting to degenerate, may produce daughter cysts
CE 4	Inactive	Heterogeneous hypoechogenic or hyperechogenic degenerative contents; no daughter cysts	Usually no living protoscoleces; differential diagnosis necessary
CE 5	Inactive	Thick calcified wall, calcification partial to complete; not pathognomonic, but highly suggestive of diagnosis	Usually no living protoscoleces

(size, location, neighborhood, and number) of the cyst. CT shows exogenous daughter cysts and cysts in the other parts of the peritoneal cavity, suggests complications (common bile duct evaluation is indicated when there is a hydatid liver cyst with jaundice), and estimates the density of the cyst contents and the volume of the cysts. CT is not as operator dependent as ultrasound and gives the surgeon an accurate roadmap of the sites of the cysts in the liver.

Hydatid cysts are well-defined, circumscribed lesions with a clear membrane and do not infiltrate surrounding liver tissue. Cysts are staged according to the content patterns. Staging is important for employing a uniform nomenclature to allow more rational comparisons of different management strategies. Although most staging protocols were based on ultrasound findings in the past, CT findings can be adapted easily to these systems. Illustrations used in this chapter for this classification include CT scans. The World Health Organization (WHO) Informal Working Group on Echinococcosis (2003) described an ultrasound classification system, which was intended to follow the natural history of hydatid disease. Based on several studies and classifications, liver hydatid cysts can be divided into six types (Table 61.2) (Beggs, 1983; Gharbi et al, 1981; McCorkel & Lewall, 1985):

1. *CL* type, a well-circumscribed liquid image with a clearly defined wall, is often difficult to differentiate from simple biliary cyst and corresponds to an early stage of development.
2. *CE 1* type is characterized by a concentric hyperechogenic halo around the cyst (Fig. 61.7), which may contain free-floating hyperechogenic foci called "hydatid sand."
3. *CE 2* type includes multivesicular cysts that have the most characteristic appearance with the "daughter and granddaughter" cysts identified by "honeycomb," "rosette," "spoke wheel" or "cluster" images. They also can have some free cyst fluid within the main cavity or may be full of daughter cysts without any free fluid (Fig. 61.8).
4. *CE 3* type is characterized by a partial or total detachment of the laminated layer with floating undulated hyperechogenic membranes showing the "dual wall," "water lily," and "water snake" signs (Fig. 61.9).
5. *CE 4* type includes cysts that contain cystic and solid components together without visible daughter cysts.
6. *CE 5* type includes cysts with a matrix or amorphous mass with a solid or semisolid appearance. A limited amount of calcification in the rim of the host adventitial tissue is common.

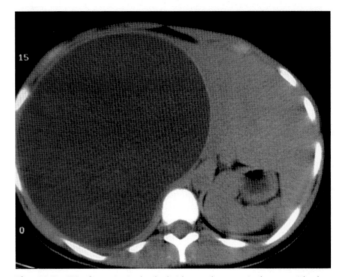

Fig. 61.7. CT of a univesicular hydatid cyst shows a single cyst with clear cyst contents.

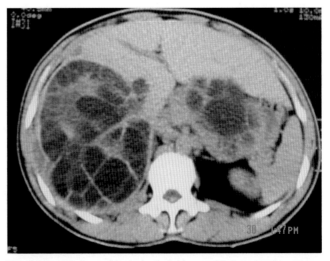

Fig. 61.8. CT of a multivesicular hydatid cyst with honeycomb or rosette appearance containing minimal fluid and filled with daughter cysts.

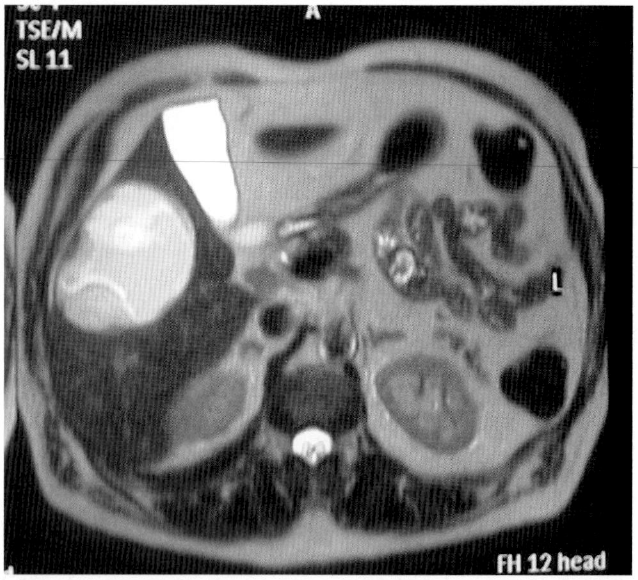

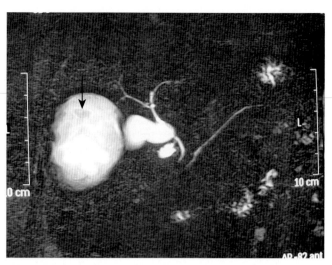

Fig. 61.11. MRI cholangiography shows the relationship of the biliary system and the cyst along with intracystic fat density *(arrow)* suggesting cystobiliary communication.

Fig. 61.9. MRI of hydatid liver disease. Transverse section shows the cyst with detached membrane showing water lily appearance.

This type of cyst is least typical and poses a diagnostic problem. It can be mistaken for a tumor, hepatic abscess, or hemangioma. Calcification in the cyst wall and hypoechogenic lacunar structures in the matrix do not mean that the cyst is dead. Completely calcified cyst (eggshell appearance) is accepted as a dead cyst (Fig. 61.10).

CL, CE 1, and CE 2 are considered as active fertile cysts. CE 3 is a transitional cyst, and it is thought to have begun degeneration. CE 4 is a degenerated cyst. CE 5 is a calcified cyst. The degree of calcification varies from partial to complete. CE 4 and CE 5 are accepted as inactive cysts.

Other Imaging Studies

Plain radiography of the abdomen is of limited value in the diagnosis of hydatid liver cysts. Plain film of the chest can reveal concurrent hydatid cysts of the lung, however. Scintigraphy and angiography has been mostly abandoned.

Hydatid liver cysts may have a low signal intensity rim on T2-weighted magnetic resonance imaging (MRI). This is a characteristic sign of hydatid disease that represents the outer, collagen-rich laminated membrane of the cyst. When present, daughter cysts are seen as cystic structures attached to the germinal layer that are hypointense relative to the intracystic fluid on T1-weighted images and hyperintense on T2-weighted images (Pedrosa et al, 2000). MRI is more specific than CT, especially if intracystic fat density is present, which suggests cystobiliary communication (Basaran et al, 2005). In cysts with biliary complications, MRI cholangiography can provide good visualization of the intrahepatic and extrahepatic biliary tree and its relationship with the hydatid cyst and cystobiliary communication (Fig. 61.11) (Little et al, 2002).

Serology

Serologic tests in hydatid disease can be used for (1) differential diagnosis of a liver cystic mass, (2) epidemiologic surveillance, and (3) post-treatment follow-up. Several serologic tests have been used in the diagnosis of human cases, and there are considerable differences in specificity and sensitivity among the various tests. Circulating *E. granulosus* antigens are small, and most of them are in the form of immune complexes. Detection of these antigens is less sensitive than antibody detection. At present, serologic tests usually are based on the reaction and precipitation between the test antigen and the circulating antibodies in the host. The sensitivity and specificity of the tests depend on the quality of antigens.

Immunoelectrophoresis

The diagnostic value of hydatidosis with immunoelectrophoresis was 91% to 94% for hepatic cysts and 69% to 70% for pulmonary cysts (Varela-Diaz et al, 1983). Immunoelectrophoresis is not suitable for epidemiologic surveillance. It can be used for post-treatment follow-up.

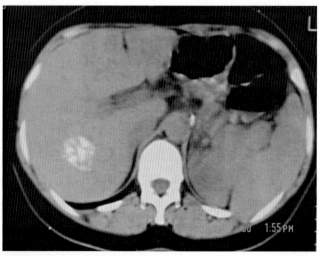

Fig. 61.10. CT of a calcified hydatid cyst.

Enzyme-Linked Immunosorbent Assay

Sensitivities for enzyme-linked immunosorbent assay (ELISA) vary from 64% to 100% depending on the antigens used (Coltorti, 1986; Iacona et al, 1980; Rickard, 1984). ELISA can be automatized for large-scale epidemiologic studies. It was reported that organ location does not affect the test results. Selected test antibodies affect its value on post-treatment follow-up. IgG assay still can be positive after 4 years of successful treatment, so it is not a suitable test for post-treatment follow-up. IgM assay has been reported negative after 6 months of successful treatment (Zhang et al, 2003).

Blotting

Blotting allows molecular weight analysis of the antigens detected by the patient's serum. Western blotting with purified antigens proved to be highly useful in the diagnosis and postsurgical monitoring of hydatidosis patients (Doiz et al, 2001). The Arc 5 antibody test is a specific precipitation during electrophoresis of blood of hydatid cyst patients with a specificity of 91%. Purification of antigens strongly affects the diagnostic value of the tests, however. Purified fractions enriched in antigens 5 and B and glycoprotein yield a sensitivity of 95% and specificity of 100% (Sbihi et al, 1996).

TREATMENT INDICATIONS AND METHODS

There are currently three treatment options for hydatid disease of the liver: surgery, which remains the most efficient treatment; percutaneous aspiration; and medical treatment. In general, hydatidosis is a public health problem, especially in developing countries, and the treatment often is selected depending on the social and medical professional's conditions. Since the 1990s, percutaneous treatment is increasingly used. Surgery remains the most effective treatment, which aims to treat concurrently the parasitic disease, the cavity, and often the biliary complications. Although surgery is technically demanding and often considered risky, the development of hepatic surgery permits safer performance of this therapeutic option.

No Indication for Treatment

Asymptomatic and small (<5 cm) CL type cysts could be followed up with a policy of "wait and see" with serial ultrasound examinations (Buttenschoen & Buttenschoen, 2003). Similarly, totally calcified hydatid cysts can be followed without any specific therapy because they are accepted as dead cysts.

Surgical Treatment

The literature on surgical treatment of hydatid liver disease contains many different techniques, ranging from simple evacuation to major liver resection. All these techniques can be subdivided into two groups—radical or conservative methods. The radical method involves total excision of the cyst, and the conservative method involves removal of the cyst contents and inactivation of protoscoleces. Although there is no prospective randomized study to compare radical and conservative surgery, some surgeons favor pericystectomy or hepatectomy whenever possible, and some surgeons, especially in endemic areas, prefer

conservative surgery in most cases. Advantages and disadvantages of radical surgery can be summarized as follows:

1. The total removal of the cysts, including all the exocysts, is associated with a reduced incidence of local recurrence (Tagliacozzo, 2003). Drug therapy is unnecessary after radical resections with closed removal of the cysts (Kayaalp et al, 2001).
2. The use of protoscolicidals is unnecessary during closed removal of the cyst.
3. Radical methods treat the invisible bile duct orifices and do not leave behind a cavity, reducing the chances of biliary fistula and cavity-related complications, which are common after conservative surgery.
4. Radical surgical methods usually require a surgical team experienced with liver resections and sometimes special surgical equipment. Hydatid cysts usually occur in rural areas, and most local hospitals do not have experienced liver surgeons and special costly equipment.
5. Radical surgery is not easy and suitable for every cyst. Cysts with adherence to major hepatic vasculature are difficult to treat by radical methods. Almost all hydatid liver cysts are suitable for conservative surgery. A general surgeon with standard surgical equipment can perform successful conservative surgery.

Surgical Incision, Exposure, and Protection

The surgical incision depends on the location of the cyst in the liver, presence of complications, and presence of extrahepatic cysts. Although thoracophrenolaparotomy was used frequently in the past, today a transthoracic approach can be selected only for combined right lung and liver hydatid cysts and when a one-stage procedure can be done successfully for both cysts (Sahin et al, 2003). Generally, a right subcostal incision with a midline extension or bilateral subcostal incision gives adequate exposure to cysts in all locations. Midline laparotomy is preferred in patients with cysts of the left lobe of the liver, abdominal hydatidosis, and perforated abdominal hydatid cysts.

Before evacuation, mobilization of the liver and the cyst should be minimal to avoid iatrogenic perforation. The area around the cyst is carefully isolated by gauze packs, a first layer soaked with normal saline and a second layer soaked with a protoscolicidal agent, which act as a mechanical and chemical barrier (Besim et al, 1998). An area of almost 2 cm in diameter on the most prominent part of the exposed pericyst is left uncovered by the packs for insertion and evacuation. Intraoperative ultrasound examination is helpful for identifying the extent of the cyst, especially for exogenous cyst identification and for planning resection if needed.

Conservative Surgery

Conservative surgery is performed to prevent spillage of cyst contents, inactivate protoscoleces, evacuate the cyst contents, suture the cystobiliary communications, and manage the residual cavity of the cyst. Prevention of intraoperative spillage of the hydatid cyst contents is one of the most important steps of the hydatid surgical procedure, for which several methods have been described. Cone techniques, first introduced by Saidi and Nazarian (1971) and later by Aarons and Kune (1983), permit opening of the cyst in a safe and controlled manner. Cones usually are not suitable on posterosuperior cysts, however. Opening and emptying of hydatid cysts should be in a closed system in modern hydatid surgery, and laparoscopic trocar insertion and evacuation is preferable. After the protection of the surgical area by protoscolicidal-soaked gauzes, cysts are entered at the most prominent point using a laparoscopic trocar, a high-pressure laparoscopic suction-irrigation apparatus is inserted into the cyst, and daughter cysts and membranes are broken into pieces by the suction followed by complete evacuation of cyst contents. The cyst is filled with the protoscolicidal agent through the gas hole of the trocar, and aspiration is continued until evacuation is complete (Kayaalp, 2002). The prominent part of the cyst roof is excised with electrocautery after complete evacuation.

Protoscolicidals are injected into the cyst if the aspirated contents are clear, but never in a case of bile-stained or purulent content for fear of caustic cholangitis. Although there is debate regarding the efficacy and safety of protoscolicidal solutions injected into the cyst cavity, it is generally believed that it is a mandatory step for conservative surgery to lessen the recurrence rate. Protoscolicidal agents include the following:

1. *Hypertonic saline.* This is probably the most widely used scolicidal agent in current practice (Kayaalp et al, 1999) because of its availability and effective scolicidal properties. Studies on different concentrations of hypertonic saline, ranging from 3% to 30%, have shown that the higher the concentration, the higher the scolicidal properties with a shorter contact time. In practice, 20% hypertonic saline is preferable, which has 100% scolicidal effect with an ideal contact time of 6 minutes (Besim et al, 1998).

2. *Cetrimide and chlorhexidine.* Half-percent cetrimide and 0.05% chlorhexidine combination (Savlex; Drogsan, Ankara, Turkey) for 5 minutes is an effective protoscolicidal agent in laboratory and clinical studies (Besim et al, 1998). Metabolic acidosis and methemoglobinemia were reported (Baraka et al, 1980; Momblano et al, 1984), but no caustic cholangitis.

3. *Absolute ethyl alcohol.* Nowadays, absolute alcohol is usually preferred by interventional radiologists for the percutaneous treatment of hydatid cysts, aimed at sclerosis of the cyst cavity (Akhan & Ozmen, 1999); it is not effective on protoscoleces inside daughter cysts (Karayalcin et al, 1999). It is effective in high concentrations, but very sensitive to dilution effects. Other disadvantages of absolute alcohol are the potential danger of caustic cholangitis and its flammable nature during surgical procedures when using electrocautery.

4. *Povidone-iodine.* Although povidone-iodine has been criticized because of an inappropriate animal model (Kolbakir & Erk 1992), Gokce and colleagues (1991) reported 1% povidone-iodine is superior to 20% saline. Landa Garcia and associates (1997) reported that 10% povidone-iodine was an effective agent for prevention of secondary hydatidosis in their in vivo study. The disadvantages of povidone-iodine are concentration dependency (Besim et al, 1998); reported caustic cholangitis cases (Castellano et al, 1994); and coloring of the cyst cavity, which makes it difficult to identify the cystobiliary communications. Other agents, such as silver nitrate and formalin, are no longer used because of their high propensity to induce caustic sclerosing cholangitis and unpredictable scolicidal effect.

One of the most controversial aspects of conservative surgery is the management of the residual cavity. A wide variety of techniques have been described for prevention of cavity-related complications.

External Tube Drainage.   Partial pericystectomy combined with external tube drainage, in which a tube drain is placed in the cavity and brought out through an external stab incision, is one of the most commonly used cavity management techniques. This easy and bloodless procedure was considered for decades as the first-choice cavity management technique in infected cysts and cysts with biliary communication (Balik et al, 1999; Sayek et al, 1980). High morbidity and prolonged hospital stay preclude its use in these circumstances, however (Balik et al, 1999; Sayek et al, 1980). At present, external tube drainage should be considered only in uncomplicated cysts. The incidence of biliary fistula and cavity infection is 3% and 10% in uncomplicated cysts, which increases to 29% and 36% in complicated cysts, respectively (Kayaalp et al, 2002b).

Capsulorrhaphy.   Capsulorrhaphy, in which the cyst wall is primarily closed after evacuation of its contents, has the risks of creation of a closed cavity and blockage of peritoneal absorptive capacity and the high risk of secondary endogenous infection. Capsulorrhaphy has only limited value in current hydatid cyst surgery (Rakas et al, 1990).

Capitonnage.   For capitonnage, after partial excision of the pericyst, approximation of the cyst walls is performed with successive, purse-string or mattress transfixing sutures from the depth to the surface. This procedure has the advantages of diminishing the size of the residual cavity and obliterating the potential bile duct orifices by closing the adventitial pericystic walls. This procedure, which should not be used in complicated cysts, is not possible for rigid or calcified cysts, for very large cavities, for intraparenchymal cysts, and for cysts lying close to the diaphragm or posterior surface of liver (Atalay et al, 1995).

Omentoplasty.   Omentoplasty, also called *omentopexy* or *omental packing,* is the only cavity management technique that has a preventive effect on postoperative biliary leakage, biliary fistula, and deep cavity abscess, as proved by prospective randomized studies (Dziri et al, 1999; Mentes et al, 1993). After unroofing the residual cavity, a pedunculated omental flap with a good blood supply is fashioned and drawn up into the cavity to obliterate the dead space, and the flap is maintained in position without tension with sutures to the pericystic wall (Fig. 61.12). Omentum has a natural absorptive capacity, which decreases the risk of infection and minimizes fistula formation.

Other Methods.   Other, less frequently used methods include the following:

1. *Internal collapse,* in which the anterior pericyst wall is sutured to the posterior wall with absorbable sutures (Filippou et al, 2004)

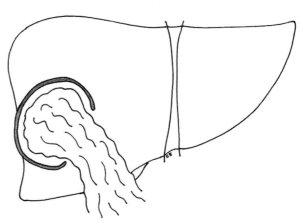

Fig. 61.12. Omentoplasty in hydatid liver cysts.

2. *Introflexion,* in which the wall of the cyst alone or together with the adjacent hepatic tissue covering the pericyst is folded inside the cavity

3. *Introflexion plus omentoplasty,* which combines these two procedures, but has not shown advantage over omentoplasty in randomized studies (Mentes et al, 1993)

4. *Myoplasty,* in which rectus abdominis (Dolatzas, 1978) or diaphragmatic muscle flap (Dosios et al, 2003) is used to fill the cavity, especially in patients with bronchobiliary fistula

5. *Cystojejunostomy or cystogastrostomy,* which has some anecdotal reports of success (Balik et al, 1999)

6. *Marsupialization,* in which the cyst wall is sutured to the skin, effecting open drainage of the cyst; this procedure is no longer used because of its high morbidity rates (Cirenei & Bertoldi, 2001)

Radical Surgery

Radical surgery for hydatid cyst ideally includes complete removal of the cyst along with the pericyst, including exocysts when present and some adjacent liver parenchyma. This approach, which requires experience in liver surgery, is the best treatment for all forms of hydatid cysts.

Anatomic and Nonanatomic Liver Resection

Anatomic and nonanatomic liver resection refers to removal of the total cyst with the surrounding normal liver tissue. This method is especially suitable for peripherally located cysts. Nonanatomic wedge resections sometimes can be better than pericystectomy if the cut surface of the liver after removal of the cyst is thought to be smaller with the wedge resection. This resection also prevents ischemic regions in the remaining peripheral liver tissue, which become pedunculated after pericystectomy. A formal hepatectomy is resection along the anatomic lines of the liver, including the hydatid cyst or cysts. The cyst is removed with its surrounding normal liver tissue. This procedure is indicated in case of large multilocular cysts localized in the right or left lobe, provided that the future remnant liver is hypertrophied, and in complicated cysts with large biliary fistulae. The liver resection allows closure of the bile duct, far from the area of biliary-cyst fistula. True anatomic resection is rarely feasible in the presence of large cysts, however. The development of the cyst distorts adjacent vessels and bile ducts, which necessitates leaving some portion of the pericyst along the resection plane. This remnant portion of the pericyst should not contain a biliary fistula or an exocyst. Incomplete excision, leaving behind a small portion of pericyst that is densely adherent to major vessels, also can be considered as radical hydatid surgery (Fig. 61.13).

Pericystectomy

Pericystectomy may be either closed or open. Closed pericystectomy is defined by a complete removal of the cyst by creating a surgical plane just outside the pericyst layer without opening the cyst. It also is called *radical cystectomy, capsulectomy, total pericystectomy,* and *cystopericystectomy.* The parasite and the adventitial layer are excised en bloc (Fig. 61.14). No such anatomic plane exists, however. The surgical approach of this plane does not differ from a classic liver parenchymal transection. The Cavitron ultrasonic aspirator is particularly useful in this disease, following the pericyst and isolating all the vessels and biliary ducts that

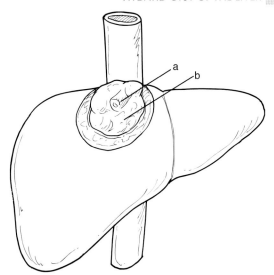

Fig. 61.13. Subtotal pericystectomy. a, The membrane of the pericyst is overlying the vena cava and right hepatic vein. b, Classic liver transection surface. The vena cava and the right hepatic vein are shown lying behind the unresected membrane.

are deviated and compressed by the cysts. The parenchymal transection allows the suture of these vessels and bile ducts within the liver parenchyma. The aspirator should be used away from the pericyst to avoid a fracture of the cyst, which can be responsible for spillage of the cyst contents. Manipulation of a large cyst during mobilization for radical resection may cause rupture. To reduce this risk, some surgeons recommend decompressing the cyst by preliminary needle aspiration or open evacuation, and subsequently they perform pericystectomy.

Intraoperative Management of Biliary-Cyst Communication

Careful inspection for cyst-biliary communications should be done from a wide opening on the pericyst and should be confirmed by leaving a dry pad on the inner surface of the cyst and applying gentle pressure on the gallbladder. In cases of suspected cyst-biliary communication, intraoperative cholangiography is preferable to identify the site of communication. After excision

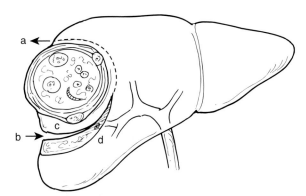

Fig. 61.14. Closed pericystectomy. a, Line of parenchymal section that passes close to the pericyst. b, Line of parenchymal section a little further from the pericyst; along the line, the liver parenchyma is shown as opened to some distance. c, Exogenous cyst just outside the pericyst layer. d, Suture of a biliary duct that communicated with the cyst.

of the cyst, a methylene blue test through a transcystic duct tube is helpful in identifying overlooked small biliary communication. Any obvious biliary orifices should be sutured to prevent postoperative biliary leakage, fistula, and cavity infections.

Radical surgery, whenever possible, in the form of total pericystectomy, subtotal pericystectomy, pericyst resection, or hepatic resection, would be the best choice for large biliary-cyst fistulae. Radical surgery has been shown to result in shorter hospital stays and less morbidity (Rohner, 1988). Because radical surgery requires great expertise, and hydatid cyst surgery is often performed in rural centers, these procedures are not possible in all circumstances. Conservative surgery with individualized management of biliary fistula is necessary. Direct suturing of the fistula orifice, with absorbable material, is indicated if the perifistulous cyst wall is not calcified or is not too fibrotic. All patients with large biliary-cyst communication should undergo operative cholangiography (Fig. 61.15), and exploration of the main bile duct is mandatory in cases of presence of common bile duct filling defects on cholangiography. T-tube drainage usually is added in case of the presence of hydatid debris in the common bile duct. In the presence of a rigid pericyst wall, suturing can be performed after a limited perifistulary pericystectomy to freshen up the edges. Suturing along with omentoplasty has been shown to decrease the rate of biliary fistula in a randomized controlled trial (Dziri et al, 1999). Direct suturing is contraindicated in cases of very large, lateral, or central fistulae (Zaouche et al, 2001). In such cases, intubation or directed fistulization, in which a catheter is introduced through the fistula orifice and is left in the intrahepatic biliary tree and is brought out through the skin along the shortest route, is indicated. This procedure can be considered only as a temporary method, however, in large multilocular cysts or cysts with a central fistula.

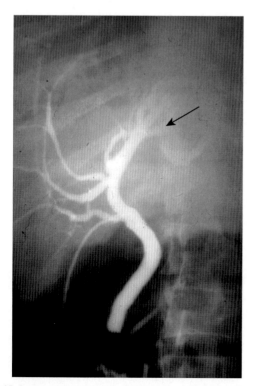

Fig. 61.15. Intraoperative transcystic cholangiogram, which is mandatory in all suspected cases of cyst-biliary communication, shows fistula in the left biliary system (*arrow*).

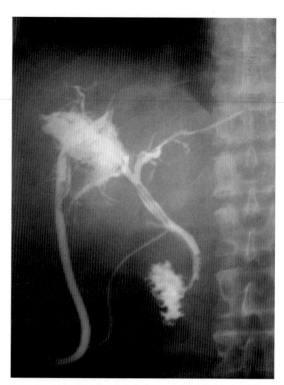

Fig. 61.16. Postoperative T-tube cholangiogram shows external biliary fistula drained by the abdominal drain.

Postoperative Complications

Biliary Fistula

Patients who had postoperative biliary drainage through the cavity drains are considered to have biliary leakage regardless of the amount of drainage. Patients who continued with persistent biliary drainage more than 10 days postoperatively are considered to have a fistula (Fig. 61.16) regardless of the drainage amount (Kayaalp et al, 2002a, 2003; Ozaslan & Bayraktar, 2002). The incidence of biliary fistula after hydatid liver surgery varies from 1% to 10% (Abu Zeid et al, 1998; Barros, 1978). Endoscopic treatment is the main approach, and the aim of endoscopic drainage for biliary fistulae is to reduce the bilioduodenal pressure difference to 0. The optimal endoscopic approach for managing external biliary fistulae resulting from hydatid liver disease is unknown. Sphincterotomy alone, stent or nasobiliary drain placement alone, or the combination of sphincterotomy and stent or nasobiliary drain has been used successfully for fistula healing. The overall success rate is 83.3% to 100%. Although closure time was reported to be 2 to 6 days, average length of drainage seems to be 2 to 4 weeks (Ozaslan & Bayraktar, 2002; Simsek et al, 2003).

Biliary Stricture

Postoperative biliary stricture after surgical treatment of hepatic hydatid disease is rare. The most dramatic form is caustic sclerosing cholangitis, which is caused by the scolicidal solution having passed from the cyst into the biliary tree (Belghiti et al, 1986). Diffuse caustic sclerosing cholangitis may result from the development of secondary biliary cirrhosis and portal hypertension causing ascites and bleeding esophageal varices, requiring a liver transplantation (Loinaz et al, 2001). Minor passage of the scolicidal solution could induce a localized biliary stricture, which may be asymptomatic if the bile duct confluence is not involved (Belghiti et al, 1986). The presence of a biliary stenosis within the biliary confluence often results from a large biliary fistula treated by conservative surgery. The size of the bile duct defect, the kind of repair applied for these defects, and the trauma to the bile duct during surgery are factors resulting in these strictures. Surgical repair is usually not feasible (Fig. 61.17), and long-term endoscopic stenting is a safe and effective method in these patients (Eickhoff et al, 2003; Yilmaz et al, 1998).

Recurrence

Recurrent disease is defined as the appearance of new active cysts after therapy of intrahepatic or extrahepatic disease (Sielaff et al, 2001). The failure to achieve permanent control of the primarily treated cyst is considered local recurrence, and newly developed cysts in the peritoneum are considered disseminated disease.

Radical surgical methods have a lower recurrence rate than conservative methods. The incidence of local recurrence is approximately 10% after conservative surgery (Table 61.3). Intraoperative spillage of the cyst contents, reduced effect of protoscolicidal agents, remnant cyst materials, and overlooked cysts all can lead to recurrence. Diagnosis of the recurrence requires a close follow-up program of at least 6 months' interval, which should include radiologic and serologic studies. Complement fixation test, immunoelectrophoresis, counterimmunoelectrophoresis, ELISA, and blotting are tests for the detection of recurrences. Blood titers may decrease slowly over months to years even with complete removal of disease. A positive serologic test during follow-up is not diagnostic of recurrence, but a rising titer is (Sielaff et al, 2001). Radical surgical methods should have a priority in the selection of the surgical methods of recurrent disease particularly after multiple local recurrences or peritoneal disseminations (Nardo et al, 2003).

Laparoscopy

Although the laparoscopic approach to this disease offers some advantages, laparoscopic hydatid surgery has not gained a wide acceptance. The disadvantages of the laparoscopic approach are

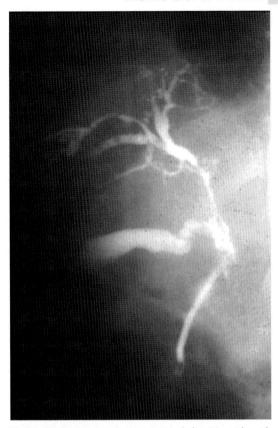

Fig. 61.17. Cholangiogram shows caustic cholangitis with widespread intrahepatic and extrahepatic strictures. Surgical management is often difficult in these situations.

the limited area for manipulation, difficulty in controlling spillage during puncture, and difficulty in aspirating the thick, degenerated cyst contents. There are no prospective randomized clinical trials comparing laparoscopic treatment with conventional open treatment, and it is still too early to report on recurrence rates with the laparoscopic approach (Table 61.4).

Pneumoperitoneum can put pressure on the hydatid cyst and increase the risk of hydatid fluid contamination during

Table 61.3 Results of Treatment of Recurrence According to the Surgical Method Used

		CONSERVATIVE SURGERY		RADICAL SURGERY	
Reference	Follow-Up (Yr)	n*	Recurrence (%)	n*	Recurrence (%)
Magistrelli et al, 1991	3	73	13 (18)	46	2 (4)
Karavias et al, 1992	3.5	32	3 (9)	—	—
Khuroo et al, 1997	1.4	25	0	—	—
Alfieri et al, 1997	6.9	—	—	72	1 (1.4)
Yol et al, 1999	1-7	55	0	—	—
Cirenei & Bertoldi, 2001	12.4	71	8 (11)	105	1 (1)
Yorganci & Sayek, 2002	2.7	32	8 (25)	10	NA
Nardo et al, 2003	4.4	—	—	33	0
Kayaalp, 2004[†]	4.5	19	0	—	—
Total		*307*	*32/307 (10.4)*	*266*	*4/256 (1.5)*

*Number of followed up patients.
[†]Long-term follow-up of reference Kayaalp, 2003.

Table 61.4 Results of Laparoscopic Operation for Hydatid Liver Disease in Series of More than 20 Patients

Reference	n	Conversion (%)	Morbidity (%)
Alper et al, 1995	22	6 (27)	4 (18)
Berberoglu et al, 1999	87	0	23 (28)
Seven et al, 2000	30	7 (23)	5 (17)
Khoury et al, 2000	83	3 (3.6)	9 (11)
Bickel et al, 2001	31	1 (3)	5 (16)
Ertem et al, 2002	48	2 (4)	3 (6)
Total	301	19 (6.4)	49 (16.3)

laparoscopic intervention. Bickel and colleagues (1998) examined the risk of spillage, however, and found that laparoscopy has no disadvantage in hydatid liver cysts. Berberoglu and coworkers (1999) used gasless laparoscopy for hydatid cyst surgery, but found no significant advantage over the pneumoperitoneum method.

A supraumbilical port is the most frequent entry for the telescope. The precise position of the trocars varies according to the position of the cyst. The puncture site of the cyst is protected with long pieces of gauze soaked in a protoscolicidal agent. Several authors have developed special tools or techniques for safer and more effective evacuation of the cyst contents. Some surgeons prefer puncture, aspiration, filling with a protoscolicidal agent, reaspiration, and evacuation of the cavity. During the procedure, the laparoscope can be introduced into the cyst cavity for magnified inspection and to ensure that no daughter cysts, laminated membranes, or biliary orifices are overlooked.

Some groups reported the use of a perforator-grinder and aspirator apparatus for insertion and evacuation (Alper et al, 1995; Saglam, 1996). An umbrella-shaped laparoscopic trocar for evacuation of the cysts has been used with the locking mechanism enabling the surgeon to suspend the cyst wall against the abdominal wall (Seven et al, 2000). Bickel and Eitan (1995) reported the use of a large, transparent cannula (12 mm) with a beveled tip for safe laparoscopic management of hydatid cysts of the liver. Suction is applied through the cannula to the surface of the cyst, enabling oblique contact. The cyst is aspirated through the cannula under a "vacuum," and it was claimed that spillage was less with this method (Bickel & Eitan, 1995). Some authors recommend washing the peritoneum with protoscolicidal solutions or creating a perihepatic protoscolicidal pool during laparoscopic hydatid surgery (Berberoglu et al, 1999; Palacios-Ruiz et al, 2002).

Percutaneous Treatment

Percutaneous aspiration and treatment of hydatid cysts has long been discouraged because of the risk of anaphylaxis and intraperitoneal seeding. Unintended percutaneous aspirations in a few sporadic cases were not associated with the expected side effects, however (McCorkell, 1984). These findings have encouraged interventional radiologists to aspirate and treat hydatid cysts of the liver with ultrasound guidance. Mueller and associates (1985) were the first to report successful percutaneous drainage of hydatid cysts, and since then several authors have reported successful percutaneous treatment of hydatid liver cysts. With the

increased experiences, successful percutaneous treatments of hydatid cysts for thorax, kidney, peritoneum, and orbital cavity have been reported as well (Akhan & Ozmen, 1999).

It now is generally accepted that the appearance of cyst contents on ultrasound and CT examination is an important determinant for percutaneous treatment. Indications for percutaneous treatment include univesicular cysts (WHO classification type CE 1), univesicular cysts with detached membrane (WHO type CE 3), and some multiple cysts (WHO type CE 2). It is contraindicated in cysts that are inaccessible to puncture, in cysts in which puncture may damage important vascular structures, and in peripheral cysts that do not have a sufficient layer of hepatic tissue that permits transhepatic puncture. There is no indication for percutaneous treatment of liver hydatid cysts ruptured into the bile ducts, peritoneum, or pleura. Recurrent cystic collections after surgery can be diagnosed and treated by percutaneous aspiration. Percutaneous treatment can be considered before other treatment modalities in pregnant patients with hydatid liver cysts (Menezes da Silva, 2003).

Three different techniques are used in percutaneous treatment of liver hydatid cysts. The first is the PAIR technique described by Ben Amor and associates (1986). *PAIR* is an acronym for *p*uncture, *a*spiration of cyst content, *i*njection of protoscolicidal solution, and *r*easpiration of the fluid. The patients are given mebendazole or albendazole before and after the procedure for prophylaxis. Under local anesthesia, the interventional procedure is performed with the presence of medical personnel from the intensive care unit, in case of anaphylaxis. A fine needle is inserted into the cystic cavity thorough the normal liver tissue, with ultrasound or CT guidance. Aspiration of the cystic fluid is performed as much as possible. A protoscolicidal agent is injected into the cavity. After 15 minutes, the maximal possible amount of fluid is reaspirated, and the needle is withdrawn. The most characteristic sonographic signs of involution at follow-up are (1) heterogeneous reflections of cyst content (3 months), (2) obliteration and pseudotumor aspect (5 months), and (3) loss of echogenicity and disappearance of cyst (9 months) (Bret et al, 1988; Khuroo et al, 1997). Direct microscopic examination of the aspirated fluid is done to identify protoscolices (Pelaez et al, 2000).

The second technique is the PAIR-catheterization technique described by Akhan and associates (1993) in an experimental study in sheep. A catheter is placed into the cavity by Seldinger technique, and similar to the PAIR technique, the cyst is aspirated, injected with a protoscolicidal agent, and reaspirated, but the catheter is not removed at the end of the procedure and left to free drainage for 24 hours. If there is no biliary fistula within 24 hours, it is accepted that there is no communication between the biliary system and the cavity; this also is confirmed by obtaining a cystogram under fluoroscopic guidance. If the amount of drainage in 24 hours is less than 10 mL and free of bile, absolute alcohol (95%) is injected into the cavity (approximately 25-35% of the volume), and after a waiting period of 20 minutes, all of the fluid is reaspirated, and the catheter is withdrawn. If the amount of drainage in 24 hours is more than 10 mL or contains bile, the catheter is kept in place until the daily amount of drainage is decreased to less than 10 mL. After that, cystogram and sclerosis are performed as already mentioned. Alcohol instillation in cysts having biliary communications is contraindicated. Some researchers suggest that all the liver hydatid cysts that are suitable for percutaneous technique should be treated by the PAIR technique. Others suggest that the cysts smaller than

6 cm in diameter (volume <100 mL) should be treated by PAIR technique, and cysts larger than 6 cm in diameter (volume >100 mL) should be treated by the catheterization technique (Akhan & Ozmen, 1999).

In the PAIR and the PAIR-catheterization techniques, the ruptured daughter cysts and laminated membranes remain inside the cavity; both techniques usually are advocated for uncomplicated univesicular cysts, but not for multivesicular, so-called mother and daughter cysts. Each daughter cyst has to be punctured separately, which is difficult and may be dangerous for the patient. Saremi and McNamara (1995) developed an alternative method called *PEVAC* (percutaneous *evac*uation of cyst content). As in the PAIR-catheterization technique, first the cyst is aspirated as much as possible, and the catheter is left in place for drainage. In a second session, the catheter is replaced with a 14-Fr to 18-Fr stiff sheath. A suction catheter is introduced into the cyst cavity through the sheath, and the cyst contents are evacuated by applying suction and directing the catheter toward the daughter cysts, endocyst, and nondrainable material. A special cutting instrument is used to fragment and evacuate daughter cysts and laminated membrane, while the cavity is continuously irrigated with protoscolicidals. After removal of the sheath, a catheter of the same French size as the sheath is placed into the cavity similar to the PAIR-catheterization technique (Schipper et al, 2002). The catheter is removed in the absence of bile leakage or any discharge.

Radiofrequency thermal ablation is an experimental technique that focuses on predominantly solid echinococcal cysts in the liver. It is suggested as an alternative treatment for PEVAC. So far, four patients have been treated with radiofrequency thermal ablation preceded by multiple courses of albendazole (Brunetti & Filice, 2001). The results are preliminary, and the efficacy of radiofrequency thermal ablation is not yet proved.

The effectiveness and safety of percutaneous treatment are proved by the results of more than 2500 cases carried out in several countries by different teams, with a low morbidity (4.1%) and mortality (0.08%) (Filice et al, 1999). The major risk of percutaneous drainage of hydatid cysts is spillage of hydatid fluid during the placement of the needle. With ultrasound or CT guidance, the route of the needle can be precisely monitored, and a transhepatic approach to the cyst, rather than a direct transperitoneal approach, can be used that minimizes the chance of spillage. Urticaria, itching, and hypotension are minor complications that may occur during or several hours after the procedure and can be treated with antihistamines. In some patients, fever (≤38.5°C) may be observed; this generally does not require any medication. Cavity complications, such as biliary fistula and infections, can be observed with an incidence of 10% (Akhan & Ozmen, 1999).

Chemotherapy

Benzimidazole carbamates (mebendazole and albendazole) are antihelminthic drugs that kill the parasite by impairing its glucose uptake. The first report on the successful treatment of four patients with hydatid liver cysts was in 1977 (Bekhti et al, 1977). Mebendazole was introduced first, but albendazole became the drug of choice because of its better absorption and better clinical results (Morris et al, 1983; Saimot et al, 1983). Benzimidazole treatment is contraindicated for patients with chronic liver diseases and in early pregnancy (Saimot, 2001).

Albendazole, in contrast to mebendazole, is better absorbed from the gastrointestinal tract. Albendazole absorption varies from person to person, however, and even within the same individual variability may be high. For clinical practice, albendazole should be administered in a dose of 10 mg/kg twice daily with a meal, and it is best not to coadminister it with drugs that reduce gastric acidity. Adverse events of this treatment were reported in 5% to 10% of patients treated (Schipper et al, 2000). General complaints are headache, nausea, anorexia, vomiting, abdominal pain, and itching. In the first weeks of treatment, a transient increase of liver enzymes may be observed. Leukopenia is rare. Complete hair loss, which is reversible when albendazole is stopped, may occur.

Although most studies were not well designed, not prospective, and not randomized, it has been shown that a success rate of 74% can be expected in patients with single cysts treated for 3 to 6 months (Franchi et al, 1999). Most relapses occurred within 2 years after the end of treatment. More prolonged monitoring showed, however, that a significant number of relapses could occur 2 to 8 years after treatment. A controlled study including 29 patients who received albendazole (400 mg twice a day in three cycles of 6 weeks with 2 weeks between cycles) or placebo showed that 82% of the patients in the treatment group experienced cure or improvement compared with 14% in the placebo group (Keshmiri et al, 2001).

Factors influencing the efficacy of benzimidazoles have not been well defined, but it is known that penetration of drug across the cyst walls depends on the nature of the cyst. Young cysts without particular pericystic fibrosis are more sensitive to drugs than thick, calcified cysts. Chemotherapy is less effective on daughter cysts within a mother cyst and in cysts with infection or biliary communication. Small cysts (<8 cm) and secondary cysts are mostly sensitive to chemotherapy, and chemotherapy seems to be more effective in young patients than older ones (Teggi et al, 1993; Todorov et al, 1990).

The efficacy of preoperative albendazole treatment was established by two studies. In the first study (Wen et al, 1994), cyst viability after 3 months of albendazole pretreatment was 8% at the time of surgery, significantly lower than in the control group (100%). In the other study, 1-month and 3-month preoperative courses of albendazole significantly reduced cyst viability to 28% and 6%. Although there are no published data on the efficacy of perioperative prophylaxis, it is generally advised at least 2 days before surgery. Similarly, postoperative treatment is recommended for 6 months in case of intraoperative hydatid spillage.

Treatment usually was administered in three or four courses lasting 4 weeks separated by a 14-day interval. Three courses are routinely recommended, in agreement with viability data suggesting that a maximum benefit is not reached with less than 3 months of therapy, and more than 6 months of treatment is rarely necessary (WHO Informal Working Group on Echinococcosis, 1996). This cyclic method of treatment was recommended because of the limited toxicology data available at the time of the first treatment attempts, but more recent data on uninterrupted treatment show that this approach could have better efficacy (Saimot, 2001). The use of continuous treatment has been followed without evidence of increased adverse events, but controlled comparisons with intermittent treatment have not been carried out. Preoperative treatment with a benzimidazole should begin at least 4 days before surgery (WHO Informal Working Group on Echinococcosis, 1996). A new albendazole formulation showed a 5-fold to 10-fold enhancement of bioavailability compared with classic albendazole (Rigter et al, 2004).

Medical treatment that is focused on killing of the protoscoleces and on destruction of the germinal layer cannot achieve the latter goal in all cases. Four different goals can be pursued with medical treatment: definite cure, reduction of cyst viability, preoperative treatment, and perioperative prophylaxis. Definite cure of univesicular cysts requires a 3- to 6-month course, which can achieve an 80% success rate and 25% relapse rate. Most relapses occur within 2 years after treatment. Lifelong follow-up is advised. Reduction of viability can be achieved in multivesicular cysts and preoperatively in univesicular cysts when percutaneous or elective surgery is planned. Perioperative prophylaxis should start 3 days before the procedure. Recommendations for post-treatment prophylaxis are 3 to 8 weeks for uncomplicated cases. In complicated cases with higher risk of spillage of cyst contents, 3 to 6 months is arbitrarily advised.

ALVEOLAR HYDATID DISEASE

All four species of *Echinococcus* are potentially zoonotic, but *E. alveolaris* or *E. multilocularis* is the most pathogenic, and unusual for a parasitic helminthic infection, it is a potentially fatal, chronically progressive hepatic infestation. The fatal outcome may occur in 95% of untreated patients within 10 years after the diagnosis. The parasite occurs within a large belt between the 40th and 45th degree of northern latitude (Ammann & Eckert, 1996). Surveys in central Europe have extended the known distribution of *E. multilocularis* from four countries at the end of 1980 to at least 11 countries in 1999 (Eckert & Deplazes, 1999). There is evidence of parasites spreading from endemic areas to previously nonendemic areas in North America, Japan, and China (Deplazes & Eckert, 2001). Control of the transmission of *E. alveolaris* is difficult because the definitive and intermediate hosts involved are usually wild animals. Risk factors for alveolar hydatid disease in endemic regions are complex and include seasonal fluctuations in the size of the fox population, the susceptibility and immunity of definitive hosts, and resistance of eggs to environmental factors (McManus et al, 2003).

The life cycle is similar to *E. granulosus*. After ingestion of an infected rodent, protoscoleces transform to tapeworms. Maturation of the tapeworms to adult forms takes 28 to 35 days in the jejunum of the fox. Adult tapeworms probably live for 6 to 12 months in the fox intestine. Eggs in the gravid proglottis are released with fox feces and contaminate the environment. Eggs may remain viable for months, even under extreme climatic conditions. When they are ingested by the intermediate host, they are released from their capsule, and an active six-hooked embryo (oncosphere) penetrates the mucosa of the small intestine. Similar to *E. granulosus,* the eggs pass to the portal vein and are carried to the liver, and when it is inoculated, it rapidly vesiculates. The laminated layer is secreted by the germinal layer of the parasite within 7 to 14 days after the postoncosphere period. About 98% of primary lesions occur in the liver. Humans can come into contact with the eggs accidentally (e.g., when skinning foxes). Ingestion of the eggs results in alveolar hydatid disease. The laminated membrane is very thin; brood capsules and protoscoleces rarely are formed in the human host (<10%). In most cases, germinal membrane is undetectable, or it appears as an isolated thin form. This tissue still has the potential for proliferation, however, and produces protoscoleces when

inoculated into a viable intermediate host (rodent). The growth rate of the alveolar hydatid disease in the liver is usually slow, and calculated median growth rate is 14.8 mL/yr (Luder et al, 1985).

The parasitic mass tends to be massive, infiltrating through the parenchyma of the liver. It proliferates and metastasizes similar to a malignant tumor. Satellite lesions are frequent, and multiple vesicles are formed in all directions. The parasitic lesion exhibits dense granulomatous infiltration and microcalcifications. The center of the cyst may become necrotic and takes the form of a spongy mass, consisting of small, irregular cavities filled with a gelatinous fluid. In addition, there is a risk of metastases in advanced alveolar echinococcosis, usually resulting in secondary lesions in the lungs or brain or both, forming large necrotic and cavitating masses.

The symptoms are similar to those of a slowly growing liver carcinoma. Clinical symptoms vary, but at the beginning of the disease there is a long asymptomatic period (5-15 years). Almost one third of the patients are diagnosed in this incubation period incidentally during the examination of a nonspecific symptom (fatigue, weight loss). One third of patients have primarily epigastric pain or dyspepsia, and another one third have cholestatic jaundice. Palpable abdominal mass and enlarged liver are the most frequent signs. Patients are usually in a well general condition. In advanced disease, jaundice, ascites, and hepatic failure can be encountered.

Routine laboratory tests do not yield specific findings. The blood sedimentation rate is elevated in most cases. Eosinophilia is usually mild or absent (Ammann & Eckert, 1996). Increased alkaline phosphatase or GGT levels are frequent, especially in advanced disease. Ultrasound or CT visualizes the lesions characterized by heterogeneous, hypodense masses with irregular contours (Fig. 61.18). A necrotic cavity in the center of the mass and lacking a well-defined wall is frequent. Pressure on the portal vein, hepatic veins, or inferior vena cava may occur. Calcifications are usual, and they are irregularly distributed clusters of microcalcifications or plaquelike foci (Fig. 61.19) (Czermak et al, 2001). MRI identifies central necrosis better than CT. MRI seemed to be less effective, however, in showing microcalcifications and small lesions. In most cases, T1-weighted images showed more clearly the margins of the lesions and extensions, especially of hepatic veins, vena cava, and perihepatic spaces,

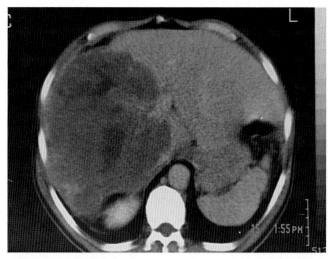

Fig. 61.18. Heterogeneous mass with irregular contours and necrotic cavity in the center in alveolar hydatid cyst.

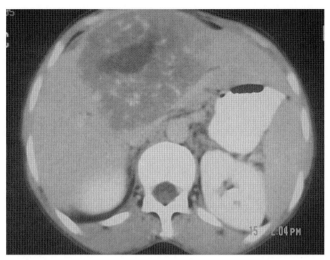

Fig. 61.19. Plaquelike calcifications on the liver mass in alveolar hydatid cyst.

Table 61.5 PNM Classification of Human Alveolar Echinococcosis

P—Hepatic Localization of Metacestode

PX	Primary lesion unable to be assessed
P0	No detectable hepatic lesion
P1	Peripheral lesion without biliary or proximal vascular involvement
P2	Central lesions with biliary or proximal involvement of one lobe
P3	Central lesions with biliary or proximal vascular involvement of both lobes or two hepatic veins or both
P4	Any lesion with extension along the portal vein, inferior vena cava, or hepatic arteries

N—Extrahepatic Involvement of Neighboring Organs

NX	Not evaluable
N0	No regional involvement
N1	Involvement of neighboring organs or tissues

M—Presence or Absence of Distant Metastasis

MX	Not completely assessed
M0	No metastasis on chest radiograph and CT brain scan
M1	Metastasis present

From Pawlowski I, et al, 2001: Echinococcosis in humans: clinical aspects, diagnosis and treatment. In Eckert J, et al (eds): WHO/OI Manual on Echinococcosis in Humans and Animals: A Public Health Problem of Global Concern. Paris, World Organisation for Animal Health, pp 20-71.

than did CT (Harman et al, 2003). Differential diagnosis for suspected alveolar hydatid disease images includes hepatocellular carcinoma, hematomas, and isolated calcifications (Bartholomot et al, 2002). Alveolar hydatid disease is characterized clinically by a discrepancy between the often large tumorlike lesions of the liver and the usually well general condition of the patient, which is in contrast to advanced malignancy.

Immunodiagnosis of alveolar hydatid disease is useful, effective, and more reliable than the diagnosis of cystic hydatid disease. The sensitivity in alveolar hydatid disease is 95% to 100%, and the specificity is very high if purified and specific antigens are used. Native Em2 antigen, alone or mixed with recombinant Em10, is highly specific for alveolar hydatid disease using ELISA, and only a few cystic hydatid disease cases are cross-reactive (Silas-Lucas & Gottstein, 2001). It has a diagnostic sensitivity of 97.1% and overall specificity of 98.9%. The reported sensitivity of the recombinant Em18-ELISA was 87% with 97% specificity (Ito et al, 2002; Sako et al, 2002).

Stage of the disease is the main prognostic factor similar to malignant tumors. A clinical staging system for alveolar hydatid disease is designated the PNM system (Tables 61.5 and 61.6) (Pawlowski et al, 2001).

Alveolar hydatid disease is much harder to treat than cystic hydatid disease. Early diagnosis is crucial, and new imaging and serologic techniques, progress in surgery, and the introduction of chemotherapy have improved the results of therapy. When alveolar hydatid disease is diagnosed, every patient should be planned for treatment regardless of whether the patient is symptomatic or asymptomatic. The two treatment modalities are surgery and chemotherapy.

Curative liver resection is the treatment of choice in localized lesions. Because of the frequent involvement of the biliary bifurcation, the liver resection often is associated with a biliary reconstruction using a Roux-en-Y jejunal loop. Most of the lesions are located in the right part of the liver, requiring, in many cases, an associated diaphragmatic resection. Palliative resection has been proposed in cases of large bilobar involvement with extension to the portal vein or to the vena cava. This approach, combined with medical treatment, can result in long-term survival. In contrast, surgical external biliary drainage of cyst cavities is associated with poor outcome. Liver transplantation should be

considered in patients who have unresectable disease, especially with massive involvement of the pedicle or coexisting chronic liver failure (Bresson Hadni et al, 2003). The frequent extrahepatic extension of the disease, including the hepatoduodenal ligament, the vena cava, the diaphragm, and sometimes the pericardium, makes total hepatectomy technically difficult. In addition, parasitic disease can recur even after liver transplantation (Bresson-Hadni et al, 1999). The therapeutic immunosuppression may allow proliferation of metastasis remnants or proliferation of previously inapparent metastases elsewhere (e.g., the brain) (Koch et al, 2003). Adjuvant chemotherapy with albendazole should be added to the post-transplant medications for prevention of recurrence (WHO Informal Working Group on Echinococcosis, 1996).

Albendazole (15 mg/kg/day) is probably the best currently available drug for alveolar hydatid disease. It is generally accepted that long-term albendazole therapy is primarily parasitostatic. Evidence of a parasiticidal effect of long-term albendazole has been reported, however, in a few cases (Ammann et al, 1998). More recent studies provide clear evidence that long-term chemotherapy of alveolar hydatid disease is effective. Oral albendazole resulted in an improved 10-year survival rate of 80% to 83% compared with 6% to 25% for untreated historical

Table 61.6 Staging of Alveolar Echinococcosis on the Basis of PNM Classification

Stage	P	N	M
I	P1	N0	M0
II	P2	N0	M0
IIIa	P3	N0	M0
IIIb	P1-3	N1	M0
	P4	N0	M0
IV	P4	N1	M0
	Any P	Any N	M1

controls (Craig, 2003). Nitazoxanide, a broad-spectrum antihelminthic, also has been tested for experimental alveolar hydatid disease. Nitazoxanide is much better absorbed than albendazole after oral administration, and it provides an attractive potential alternative for medical treatment (Stettler et al, 2003). Another study evaluated the antifungal agent amphotericin B; however, it could not be considered to be parasiticidal (Reuter et al, 2003).

REFERENCES

Aarons B, Kune GA, 1983: A suction cone to prevent spillage during hydatid surgery. Aust N Z J Surg 53:471-472.

Abdel Hameed AA, Abu Aisha H, 1987: Uneventful intraperitoneal rupture of a hepatic hydatid cyst: a case report. Trop Geogr Med 39:80-82.

Abu Zeid M, et al, 1998: Surgical treatment of hepatic hydatid cysts. Hepatogastroenterology 45:1802-1806.

Akhan O, Ozmen MN, 1999: Percutaneous treatment of liver hydatid cysts. Eur J Radiol 32:76-85.

Akhan O, et al, 1993: Percutaneous treatment of abdominal hydatid cysts with hypertonic saline and alcohol: an experimental study in sheep. Invest Radiol 28:121-127.

Alfieri S, et al, 1997: Radical surgery for liver hydatid disease: a study of 89 consecutive patients. Hepatogastroenterology 44:496-500.

Alper A, et al, 1995: Laparoscopic surgery of hepatic hydatid disease: initial results and early follow-up of 16 patients. World J Surg 19:725-728.

Ammann RW, Eckert J, 1996: Cestodes, Echinococcus. Gastroenterol Clin North Am 25:655-689.

Ammann RW, et al, 1998: Long-term mebendazole therapy may be parasitocidal in alveolar echinococcosis. J Hepatol 29:994-998.

Atalay F, et al, 1995: Surgery for hydatid cysts of the liver. Hiroshima J Med Sci 44:89-92.

Atli M, et al, 2001: Intrabiliary rupture of a hepatic hydatid cyst: associated clinical factors and proper management. Arch Surg 136:1249-1255.

Balik AA, et al, 1999: Surgical treatment of hydatid disease of the liver: review of 304 cases. Arch Surg 134:166-169.

Baraka A, et al, 1980: Cetrimide-induced methaemoglobinaemia after surgical excision of hydatid cyst. Lancet 2:88-89.

Barnes SA, Lillemoe KD, 1997: Liver abscess and hydatid cyst disease. In Zinner MJ, et al (eds): Maingot's Abdominal Operations, 10th ed. Stamford, Conn, Appleton & Lange, pp 1513-1546.

Barros JL, 1978: Hydatid disease of the liver. Am J Surg 135:597-600.

Bartholomot B, et al, 2002: Combined ultrasound and serologic screening for hepatic alveolar echinococcosis in central China. Am J Trop Med Hyg 66:23-29.

Basaran C, et al, 2005: Fat-containing lesions of the liver: cross-sectional imaging findings with emphasis on MRI. AJR Am J Roentgenol 184:1103-1110.

Beggs I, 1983: The radiological appearances of hydatid disease of the liver. Clin Radiol 34:555-563.

Bekhti A, et al, 1977: Treatment of hepatic hydatid disease with mebendazole: preliminary results in four cases. BMJ 2:1047-1051.

Belghiti J, et al, 1986: Caustic sclerosing cholangitis: a complication of the surgical treatment of hydatid disease of the liver. Arch Surg 121:1162-1165.

Ben Amor N, et al, 1986: Trial therapy of inoperable abdominal hydatid cysts by puncture. Ann Parasitol Hum Comp 61:689-692.

Berberoglu M, et al, 1999: Gasless vs gaseous laparoscopy in the treatment of hepatic hydatid disease. Surg Endosc 13:1195-1198.

Besim H, et al, 1998: Scolicidal agents in hydatid cyst surgery. HPB Surg 10:347-351.

Bickel A, Eitan A, 1995: The use of a large, transparent cannula, with a beveled tip, for safe laparoscopic management of hydatid cysts of liver. Surg Endosc 9:1304-1305.

Bickel A, et al, 1998: Laparoscopic approach to hydatid liver cysts: is it logical? Physical, experimental, and practical aspects. Surg Endosc 12:1073-1077.

Bickel A, et al, 2001: The laparoscopic approach to abdominal hydatid cysts. Arch Surg 136:789-795.

Bourgeon R, 1985: L'ouverture des kystes hydatiques aux voies biliaires intra-hépatiques. Lyon Chir 81:161.

Bresson-Hadni S, et al, 1999: Primary disease recurrence after liver transplantation for alveolar echinococcosis: long-term evaluation in 15 patients. Hepatology 30:857-864.

Bresson-Hadni S, et al, 2003: Indications and results of liver transplantation for Echinococcus alveolar infection: an overview. Langenbecks Arch Surg 388:231-238.

Bret PM, et al, 1988: Percutaneous aspiration and drainage of hydatid cysts in the liver. Radiology 168:617-620.

Brunetti E, Filice C, 2001: Radiofrequency thermal ablation of echinococcal liver cysts. Lancet 358:1464.

Buttenschoen K, Buttenschoen D, 2003: Echinococcus granulosus infection: the challenge of surgical treatment. Langenbecks Arch Surg 388:218-230.

Castellano G, et al, 1994: Sclerosing cholangitis: report of four cases and a cumulative review of the literature. Hepatogastroenterology 41:458-470.

Cirenei A, Bertoldi I, 2001: Evolution of surgery for liver hydatidosis from 1950 to today: analysis of a personal experience. World J Surg 25:87-92.

Coltorti EA, 1986: Standardization and evaluation of an enzyme immunoassay as a screening test for the seroepidemiology of human hydatidosis. Am J Trop Med Hyg 35:1000-1005.

Craig P, 2003: Echinococcus multilocularis. Curr Opin Infect Dis 16:437-444.

Czermak BV, et al, 2001: Echinococcus multilocularis revisited. AJR Am J Roentgenol 176:1207-1212.

Deplazes P, Eckert J, 2001: Veterinary aspects of alveolar echinococcosis—a zoonosis of public health significance. Vet Parasitol 98:65-87.

Diez Valladares L, et al, 1998: Hydatid liver cyst perforation into the digestive tract. Hepatogastroenterology 45:2110-2114.

Doiz O, et al, 2001: Western blot applied to the diagnosis and post-treatment monitoring of human hydatidosis. Diagn Microbiol Infect Dis 41:139-142.

Dolatzas TC, 1978: Myoplasty for the treatment of biliary fistulas due to remaining cavities after surgery for hydatid cyst of the liver. Am J Surg 136:638-639.

Dosios T, et al, 2003: Diaphragm myoplasty in the prevention of complications after surgery of hydatid disease of the liver. World J Surg 27:164-167.

Dziri C, et al, 1999: Omentoplasty in the prevention of deep abdominal complications after surgery for hydatid disease of the liver: a multicenter, prospective, randomized trial. J Am Coll Surg 188:281-289.

Eckert J, Deplazes P, 1999: Alveolar echinococcosis in humans: the current situation in Central Europe and the need for countermeasures. Parasitol Today 15:315-319.

Eickhoff A, et al, 2003: Endoscopic stenting for postoperative biliary strictures due to hepatic hydatid disease: effectiveness and long-term outcome. J Clin Gastroenterol 37:74-78.

Ertem M, et al, 2002: Laparoscopically treated liver hydatid cysts. Arch Surg 137:1170-1173.

Filice C, et al, 1999: Treatment of echinococcal cysts. Ultrasound Q 15:223-233.

Franchi C, et al, 1999: Long-term evaluation of patients with hydatidosis treated with benzimidazole carbamates. Clin Infect Dis 29:304-309.

Gahukamble DB, et al, 2000: Outcome of minimal surgery for hydatid cysts of the liver in children with reference to post-operative biliary leakage. Ann Trop Paediatr 20:147-151.

Gerazounis M, et al, 2002: Bronchobiliary fistulae due to echinococcosis. Eur J Cardiothorac Surg 22:306-308.

Gharbi HA, et al, 1981: Ultrasound examination of the hydatic liver. Radiology 139:459-463.

Gokce O, et al, 1991: Povidone-iodine in experimental peritoneal hydatidosis. Br J Surg 78:495-496.

Harman M, et al, 2003: MRI findings of hepatic alveolar echinococcosis. Clin Imaging 27:411-416.

Iacona A, et al, 1980: Enzyme-linked immunosorbent assay (ELISA) in the serodiagnosis of hydatid disease. Am J Trop Med Hyg 29:95-102.

Iscan M, Duren M, 1991: Endoscopic sphincterotomy in the management of postoperative complications of hepatic hydatid disease. Endoscopy 23:282-283.

Ito A, et al, 2002: Evaluation of an enzymed-linked immunosorbent assay (ELISA) with affinity-purified Em18 and an ELISA with recombinant Em18 for differential diagnosis of alveolar echinococcosis: results of a blind test. J Clin Microbiol 40:4161-4165.

Karavias DD, et al, 1992: Improved techniques in the surgical treatment of hepatic hydatidosis. Surg Gynecol Obstet 174:176-180.

Karayalcin K, et al, 1999: Effect of hypertonic saline and alcohol on viability of daughter cysts in hepatic hydatid disease. Eur J Surg 165:1043-1044.

Karunajeewa HA, et al, 2002: Hydatid disease invading the inferior vena cava: successful combined medical and surgical treatment. Aust N Z J Surg 72:159-160.

Kayaalp C, 2002: Evacuation of hydatid liver cysts using laparoscopic trocar. World J Surg 26:1324-1327.

Kayaalp C, 2003: Evacuation of hydatid liver cysts using laparoscopic trocar. World J Surg 27:1339-1340.

Kayaalp C, et al, 1999: Türkiye'de kist hidatik cerrahisinde skolisidal ve perioperatif benzimidazol kullanimi. Ankara Cerrahi Dergisi 4:201-207.

Kayaalp C, et al, 2001: Re: Gollackner, B et al: Radical surgical therapy of abdominal cystic hydatid disease: factors of recurrence. World J Surg 25:387-389.

Kayaalp C, et al, 2002a: Biliary complications after hydatid liver surgery: incidence and risk factors. J Gastrointest Surg 6:706-712.

Kayaalp C, et al, 2002b: Importance of cyst content in hydatid liver surgery. Arch Surg 137:159-163.

Kayaalp C, et al, 2003: Distribution of hydatid cysts into the liver with reference to cystobiliary communications and cavity-related complications. Am J Surg 185:175-179.

Keshmiri M, et al, 2001: Albendazole versus placebo in treatment of echinococcosis. Trans R Soc Trop Med Hyg 95:190-194.

Khoury G, et al, 2000: Laparoscopic treatment of hydatid cysts of the liver and spleen. Surg Endosc 14:243-245.

Khuroo MS, et al, 1997: Percutaneous drainage compared with surgery for hepatic hydatid cysts. N Engl J Med 337:881-887.

Koch S, et al, European collaborating clinicians, 2003: Experience of liver transplantation for incurable alveolar echinococcosis: a 45-case European collaborative report. Transplantation 75:856-863.

Kolbakir F, Erk MK, 1992: Povidone-iodine in experimental peritoneal hydatidosis. Br J Surg 79:373-375.

Kurt N, et al, 2003: Spontaneous and traumatic intra-peritoneal perforations of hepatic hydatid cysts: a case series. J Gastrointest Surg 7:635-641.

Landa Garcia JI, et al, 1997: Evaluation of scolicidal agents in an experimental hydatid disease model. Eur Surg Res 29:202-208.

Langer JC, et al, 1984: Diagnosis and management of hydatid disease of the liver: a 15-year North American experience. Ann Surg 199:412-417.

Little AF, et al, 2002: MR cholangiography in the evaluation of suspected intrabiliary rupture of hepatic hydatid cyst. Abdom Imaging 27:333-335.

Little JM, 1976: Hydatid disease at Royal Prince Alfred Hospital, 1964 to 1974. Med J Aust 1:903-908.

Loinaz C, et al, 2001: Long-term biliary complications after liver surgery leading to liver transplantation. World J Surg 25:1260-1263.

Luder PJ, et al, 1985: High oral doses of mebendazole interfere with growth of larval Echinococcus multilocularis lesions. J Hepatol 1:369-377.

Magistrelli P, et al, 1991: Surgical treatment of hydatid disease of the liver: a 20-year experience. Arch Surg 126:518-522.

McCorkell SJ, 1984: Unintended percutaneous aspiration of pulmonary echinococcal cysts. Am J Radiol 143:123-126.

McCorkell SJ, Lewall DB, 1985: Hepatic echinococcal cysts: sonographic appearance and classification. Radiology 155:773-775.

McManus DP, et al, 2003: Echinococcosis. Lancet 362:1295-1304.

Menezes da Silva A, 2003: Hydatid cyst of the liver/criteria for the selection of appropriate treatment. Acta Trop 85:237-242.

Mentes A, et al, 1993: Omentoplasty versus introflexion for hydatid liver cysts. J R Coll Surg Edinb 38:82-85.

Milicevic M, 1994: Hydatid disease. In Blumgart LH (ed): Surgery of the Liver and Biliary Tract, 2nd edition. Edinburgh, Churchill Livingstone, pp 1121-1150.

Momblano P, et al, 1984: Metabolic acidosis induced by cetrimonium bromide. Lancet 2:1045.

Morel P, et al, 1988: Surgical treatment of hydatid disease of the liver: a survey of 69 patients. Surgery 104:859-862.

Moreno Gonzalez E, et al, 1994: Liver transplantation for Echinococcus granulosus hydatid disease. Transplantation 58:797-800.

Morris DL, et al, 1983: Albendazole in hydatid disease. BMJ 286:103-104.

Mueller PR, et al, 1985: Hepatic echinococcal cyst: successful percutaneous drainage. Radiology 155:627-628.

Nardo B, et al, 2003: Radical surgical treatment of recurrent hepatic hydatidosis. Hepatogastroenterology 50:1478-1481.

Ozaslan E, Bayraktar Y, 2002: Endoscopic therapy in the management of hepatobiliary hydatid disease. J Clin Gastroenterol 35:160-174.

Ozmen V, et al, 1992: Surgical treatment of hepatic hydatid disease. Can J Surg 35:423-427.

Palacios-Ruiz JA, et al, 2002: Hypertonic saline in hydatid disease. World J Surg 26:1398-1399.

Pawlowski I, et al, 2001: Echinococcosis in humans: clinical aspects, diagnosis and treatment. In Eckert J, et al (eds): WHO/OI Manual on Echinococcosis in Humans and Animals: A Public Health Problem of Global Concern. Paris, World Organisation for Animal Health, pp 20-71.

Pedrosa I, et al, 2000: Hydatid disease: radiologic and pathologic features and complications. Radiographics 20:795-817.

Pelaez V, et al, 2000: PAIR as percutaneous treatment of hydatid liver cysts. Acta Trop 75:197-202.

Pitt HA, et al, 1986: Management of hepatic echinococcosis in Southern California. Am J Surg 152:110-115.

Rakas FS, et al, 1990: Omentoplasty or tube drainage for the management of the residual cavity following the removal of an hepatic hydatid cyst. Hepatogastroenterology 37:55-57.

Reuter S, et al, 2003: Effect of amphotericin B on larval growth of Echinococcus multilocularis. Antimicrob Agents Chemother 47:620-625.

Richards KS, 1992: Biology of Echinococcus and diagnosis of hydatid disease. In Morris DL, Richards KS (eds): Hydatid Disease: Current Medical and Surgical Management. Oxford, Butterworth Heinemann, pp 1-24.

Rickard MD, 1984: Serological diagnosis and post-operative surveillance of human hydatid disease: I. latex agglutination and immunoelectrophoresis using crude cyst fluid antigen. Pathology 16:207-210.

Rigter IM, et al, 2004: Relative bioavailability of three newly developed albendazole formulations: a randomized crossover study with healthy volunteers. Antimicrob Agents Chemother 48:1051-1054.

Rohner A, 1988: Traitement du kyste hydatique du foie. Ann Chir 42:635.

Saglam A, 1996: Laparoscopic treatment of liver hydatid cysts. Surg Laparosc Endosc 6:16-21.

Sahin E, et al, 2003: Single stage transthoracic approach for right lung and liver hydatid disease. J Thorac Cardiovasc Surg 126:769-773.

Saidi F, Nazarian I, 1971: Surgical treatment of hydatid cysts by freezing of cyst wall and instillation of 0.5 per cent silver nitrate solution. N Engl J Med 284:1346-1350.

Saimot AG, 2001: Medical treatment of liver hydatidosis. World J Surg 25:15-20.

Saimot AG, et al, 1983: Albendazole as a potential treatment for human hydatidosis. Lancet 2:652-656.

Sako Y, et al, 2002: Alveolar echinococcosis: characterisation of diagnostic antigen Em18 and serological evaluation of recombinant Em18. J Clin Microbiol 40:2760-2765.

Saremi F, McNamara TO, 1995: Hydatid cysts of the liver: long-term results of percutaneous treatment using a cutting instrument. AJR Am J Roentgenol 165:1163-1167.

Sayek I, et al, 1980: Surgical treatment of hydatid disease of the liver. Arch Surg 115:847-850.

Sbihi Y, et al, 1996: Serologic recognition of hydatid cyst antigens using different purification methods. Diagn Microbiol Infect Dis 24:205-211.

Schipper HG, et al, 2000: Effect of dose increase or cimetidine co-administration on albendazole bioavailability. Am J Trop Med Hyg 63:270-273.

Schipper HG, et al, 2002: Percutaneous evacuation (PEVAC) of multivesicular echinococcal cysts with or without cystobiliary fistulas which contain non-drainable material: first results of a modified PAIR method. Gut 50:718-723.

Seven R, et al, 2000: Laparoscopic treatment of hepatic hydatid cysts. Surgery 128:36-40.

Sielaff TD, et al, 2001: Recurrence of hydatid disease. World J Surg 25:83-86.

Silas-Lucas M, Gottstein B, 2001: Molecular tools for the diagnosis of cystic and alveolar echinococcosis. Trop Med Int Health 6:463-475.

Simsek H, et al, 2003: Diagnostic and therapeutic ERCP in hepatic hydatid disease. Gastrointest Endosc 58:384-389.

Sozuer EM, et al, 2002: The perforation problem in hydatid disease. Am J Trop Med Hyg 66:575-577.

Stettler M, et al, 2003: In vitro parasiticidal effect of nitazoxanide against Echinococcus multilocularis metacestodes. Antimicrob Agents Chemother 47:467-474.

Tagliacozzo S, 2003: Management of hydatid disease of the liver. In Poston GJ, Blumgart LH (eds): Surgical Management of Hepatobiliary and Pancreatic Disorders. New York, Martin Dunitz, pp 215-235.

Teggi A, et al, 1993: Therapy of human hydatid disease with mebendazole and albendazole. Antimicrob Agents Chemother 37:1679-1684.

Thameur H, et al, 2001: Cardiopericardial hydatid cysts. World J Surg 25:58-67.

Thompson RCA, 2001: Echinococcosis. In Gillespie S, Pearson RD (eds): Principles and Practice of Clinical Parasitology. Chichester, England, John Wiley & Sons Ltd, pp 587-612.

Todorov T, et al, 1990: Evaluation of response to chemotherapy of human cystic echinococcosis. Br J Radiol 63:523-531.

Varela-Diaz VM, et al, 1983: Immunodiagnosis of human hydatid disease: applications and contributions to a control program in Argentina. Am J Trop Med Hyg 32:1079-1087.

Vuitton DA, 2004: Echinococcosis and allergy. Clin Rev Allergy Immunol 26:93-104.

Watson-Jones DL, Macpherson CN, 1988: Hydatid disease in the Turkana district of Kenya. VI. man:dog contact and its role in the transmission and control of hydatidosis amongst the Turkana. Ann Trop Med Parasitol 82:343-356.

Wen H, et al, 1994: Albendazole chemotherapy for human cystic and alveolar echinococcosis in north-western China. Trans R Soc Trop Med Hyg 88: 340-343.

WHO Informal Working Group, 2003: International classification of ultrasound images in cystic echinococcosis for application in clinical and field epidemiological settings. Acta Trop 85:253-261.

WHO Informal Working Group on Echinococcosis, 1996: Guidelines for treatment of cystic and alveolar echinococcosis in humans. Bull World Health Organ 74:231-242.

Yalin R, et al, 1992: Significance of intracystic pressure in abdominal hydatid disease. Br J Surg 79:1182-1183.

Yilmaz E, Gokok N, 1990: Hydatid disease of the liver: current surgical management. Br J Clin 44:612-615.

Yilmaz U, et al, 1998: Management of postoperative biliary strictures secondary to hepatic hydatid disease by endoscopic stenting. Hepatogastroenterology 45:65-69.

Yol S, et al, 1999: Open drainage versus overlapping method in the treatment of hepatic hydatid cyst cavities. Int Surg 84:139-143.

Yorganci K, Sayek I, 2002: Surgical treatment of hydatid cysts of the liver in the era of percutaneous treatment. Am J Surg 184:63-69.

Zaouche A, et al, 2001: Management of liver hydatid cysts with a large biliocystic fistula: multicenter retrospective study. Tunisian Surgical Association. World J Surg 25:28-39.

Zhang W, et al, 2003: Concepts in immunology and diagnosis of hydatid disease. Clin Microbiol Rev 16:18-36.

Recurrent Pyogenic Cholangitis

S. T. FAN AND J. WONG

Recurrent pyogenic cholangitis (RPC) is a condition characterized by repeated attacks of bacterial infection of the biliary tree as a result of stones and strictures in the bile ducts, especially in the intrahepatic segments. Synonyms include *Oriental cholangiohepatitis* (Stock & Fung, 1962), *Hong Kong disease* (Mage & Morel, 1965), *intrahepatic stones* (Wen & Lee, 1972), *hepatolithiasis* (Nakayama et al, 1980), *primary cholangitis,* and *Oriental infestational cholangitis* (Seel & Park, 1983). RPC was first described in Hong Kong by Digby in 1930, and the name *recurrent pyogenic cholangitis* was first used by Cook and colleagues in 1954. Since then, reports of RPC occurring in many countries in Southeast Asia and the Far East have appeared (Balasegaram, 1972; Chang & Passaro, 1983; Maki et al, 1964; Nakayama et al, 1980; Ong, 1962; Seel & Park, 1983; Wen & Lee, 1972). With ease of travel and increasing migration from Asian countries, RPC is being encountered more frequently in Western countries, particularly in cities where Asian emigrants congregate (Harris et al, 1998). RPC should not be regarded as a curiosity peculiar only to Asia, but a disease that may affect Asians wherever they may be.

In contrast to gallstone disease seen in Western countries, RPC affects a younger age group of the lower socioeconomic classes, and males and females are equally susceptible. In the past, RPC was one of the most commonly encountered surgical emergencies, but the incidence has declined in recent years, particularly in urban centers (Nakayama, 1982). The overall incidence of RPC has decreased from 50% of biliary stones in the pre–World War II years to 20% in Japan (Nakayama et al, 1980) despite advances in diagnostic techniques. In Hong Kong today, 12% of cases of biliary stones are due to RPC (Fan et al, 1991a).

ETIOLOGY AND PATHOGENESIS

The exact etiology of RPC is unknown, but the likely initial event is the establishment of infection by bowel organisms in the small biliary radicles. Experimental and clinical studies (Nakayama et al, 1980; Ong, 1962) indicated that the organisms isolated from portal vein blood, common duct bile, and liver biopsy specimens are usually identical and are predominantly of bowel origin. Although bowel organisms may reach the liver under ordinary circumstances, clinical infection does not occur except when bowel infection is severe, the organism is of particular virulence, or the host defense (in the liver) is compromised. In RPC, numerous organisms may enter the portal vein during a serious attack of enteric infection, which is common in Asia. As this condition also affects the lower socioeconomic classes, malnutrition and perhaps infection by flukes and worms may reduce the capacity of the liver to clear enteric bacteria effectively.

When the organisms are established in the liver, infection begins in the cholangioles and subsequently involves the rest of portal triads. If the infection is severe, the hepatocytes show vacuolation and may undergo necrosis—hence the name

cholangiohepatitis. Hepatocellular damage is usually mild if the infection is confined to the cholangioles. If cholangiolitis spreads to the larger intrahepatic ducts and to the common bile duct, hepatocellular damage is severe. Resolution of infection in the early phases restores normal morphology, but more intense or repeated infection may result in fibrosis of intrahepatic ducts or cholangitic liver abscess formation.

Whether stones or strictures develop first is not clear. Endoscopic retrograde cholangiopancreatography (ERCP) of the bile ducts in RPC (Lam et al, 1978) suggests that structural changes may occur in the ducts before stones are demonstrable, and strictures often are seen at cholangiography in the absence of stones. Conversely, stones also are found in the intrahepatic ducts when no significant narrowing of the ducts is discerned. In advanced cases, strictures are associated with extensive formation of stones, which can fill the ducts throughout the liver. Cisternal dilation of a duct may not be associated with very tight stenosis, and the cavernous ducts do not contain many stones; perhaps a ball-valve mechanism is responsible for these changes. In some patients with acute attacks, stones are not found, but infected, viscous bile permeates the whole biliary tree, which may represent the early stages of precipitation of bile before discernible stones are formed. Whatever the sequence of development, repeated or severe infection leads to transmural inflammation of the ducts and results in stenosis in the larger ducts, forming weblike strictures, and in the smaller peripheral ducts, showing more tubular narrowings. As a result of obstruction, together with parenchymal damage to the adjoining liver, the rest of the ducts dilate.

The calculi formed in RPC are bilirubinate stones. Infection in the bile duct alters the bile from a supersaturated solution to an insoluble precipitate. It is postulated that β-glucuronidase derived from *Clostridium perfringens* and *Escherichia coli* splits the bilirubin diglucuronide to free bilirubin, and the ionized unconjugated bilirubin together with ionic calcium precipitates to form insoluble calcium bilirubinate, which with time coagulates and consolidates into stones (Leung et al, 2001; Maki, 1966; Nakayama et al, 1980).

Although positive bile cultures are commonly obtained in patients with Western-type stones that are lodged in the common duct, when the stones are confined to the gallbladder, the incidence of infection is low. In contrast, regardless of whether the stones are located in the gallbladder or the common duct, the incidence of positive bile cultures in RPC is high (Suzuki et al, 1984; Tabata & Nakayama, 1981), a finding that favors infection as the primary step in the etiology of RPC. It also has been shown that in affected intrahepatic ducts, there is an increased number of mucous glands in the epithelial lining (Nakanuma et al, 1988; Terada & Nakanuma 1988). The integrated role of bacteria and mucus in the lithogenesis of hepatolithiasis was shown in a study by Zen and coworkers (2002), who found that lipopolysaccharide could induce overexpression of gel-forming apomucin (MUC2 and MUC5AC) in biliary epithelial cells via synthesis of tumor necrosis factor-α and activation of protein kinase C. Mucin hypersecretion contributes to more stone formation by impeding bile flow and creating a nidus for pigment deposition (Sasaki et al, 1998). Augmented expression and secretion of trefoil factor family protein, which is a mucin-associated protein important for mucosal defense and repair, may play a role in lithogenesis together with gel-forming apomucin (Sasaki et al, 2004).

When nidation has started, the stones enlarge; where they finally reside depends on whether they can pass through existing strictures. When the stones are larger than the strictures, they are trapped proximally and increase in size because layers of calcium bilirubinate become encrusted on their surface. If the stones are small, they may pass into the common duct, then egress through the ampulla into the duodenum, or may be held in the common duct and enlarge. At any site, stones trapped in the liver or the common duct perpetuate infection and cause further inflammation and scarring of the duct wall.

An association with infection by *Clonorchis sinensis* and *Ascaris lumbricoides* has been implicated in the past (Fung, 1961) and is still regarded as causally significant (Seel & Park, 1983). In countries where clonorchiasis is absent, such as the Philippines, RPC remains prevalent, however, whereas in Japan, where clonorchiasis is endemic, RPC is on the decline. Other evidence against clonorchiasis as a causal factor is that *Clonorchis* ova are isolated from the stools of only 25% of patients with RPC (and ascariasis is present in only 5%) (Ong, 1962). It is indisputable that clonorchiasis is a serious infection that may cause structural changes in the bile ducts within and outside the liver (Hou, 1956). Although the cholangiographic changes of clonorchiasis are distinctly different from the changes of RPC (Choi et al, 1984), in that the terminal ducts are dilated rather than narrowed, the predominant and more severe changes are seen in the left duct. This occurrence corresponds to the distribution of RPC, a finding that still defies explanation.

Even if clonorchiasis and ascariasis are merely coincidental infections, they may become a nidus for stone formation (Teoh, 1963). Ascariasis probably plays no role in RPC except as a source of foreign bodies. Clonorchiasis may be a contributory factor in countries where RPC is endemic.

PATHOLOGY

The primary pathologic changes are infection and fibrosis with stricture and stone formation in the bile ducts, with other changes being consequences of these main events. The consequences of repeated infection are progressive biliary epithelial and hepatocellular damage, as discussed previously. Suggested sequential changes in the bile ducts in RPC have been documented in detail by Lam and associates (1978). These changes include loss of parallelism of duct walls, excessive branching, abrupt termination or "arrowhead" formation of smaller ducts, and development of strictures (Fig. 62.1).

Strictures may be found anywhere in the biliary tree, but are more common in the major hepatic duct branches, especially in the left liver, and in the intrahepatic ducts. When in the extrahepatic ducts, strictures are weblike, situated toward the lower end, and if the obstruction is severe, there is marked proximal dilation (Fig. 62.2). Strictures in the hepatic ducts also extend over a short distance and are usually intrahepatic, but may extend to the extrahepatic portion (Fig. 62.3). In the smaller

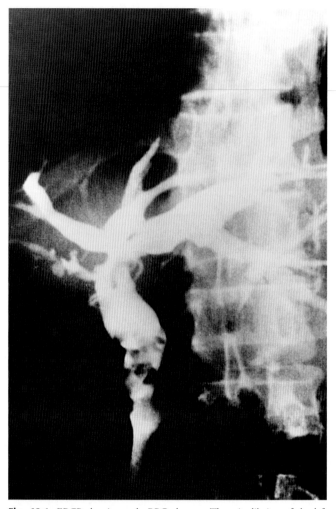

Fig. 62.1. ERCP showing early RPC changes. There is dilation of the left hepatic duct system and excessive branching of the intrahepatic ducts. Several small stones and some biliary debris are present in the intrahepatic duct and common duct.

intrahepatic ducts, the strictures are longer, and there may be a series of tubular narrowing over a length of duct (Fig. 62.4; see Fig. 62.1).

The left duct is more frequently and severely affected than the right. Left duct involvement alone is found in 40% of cases of intrahepatic disease, right duct involvement alone is found in 20%, and involvement of both ducts is found in 40%. No satisfactory explanation has been offered for this finding, but it has been suggested that the left duct is more horizontal, and bile in the left duct may not drain as well as bile in the right duct. On the right side, one would expect that the incidence of intrahepatic stones should be higher if the right posterior hepatic duct joins the left hepatic duct at a sharp angle. A detailed study of the confluence patterns of segmental hepatic ducts did not show a causal relationship, however (Kitagawa et al, 2003).

Proximal dilations behind the strictures are an expected secondary phenomenon. These dilations sometimes can be so large as to be called cisterns (Maki et al, 1964), and little liver parenchyma remains in such affected segments (Fig. 62.5). In these dilated ducts, relatively fewer stones are found (Fig. 62.6). Dilated segments taper toward the strictures, which are thick and fibrous. When operative plastic repair of such strictures is attempted, restenosis is common as a result of ongoing fibrotic

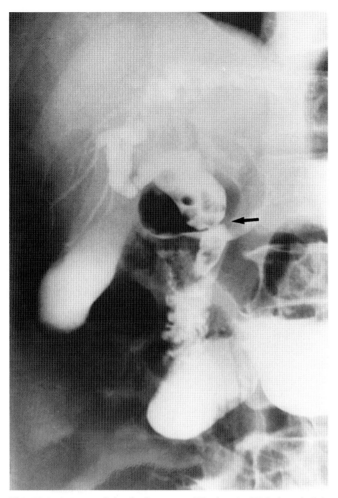

Fig. 62.2. Stricture of the distal common bile duct in RPC *(arrow)*. It is weblike, and there is proximal dilation with stones seen above and below the stricture. The gallbladder is normal.

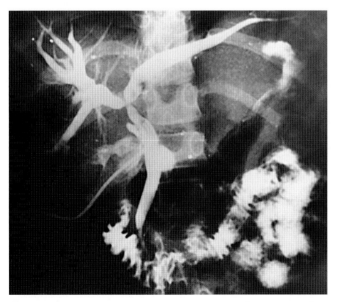

Fig. 62.3. T-tube cholangiogram shows tight strictures at the confluence of the left and right hepatic ducts and the common hepatic duct.

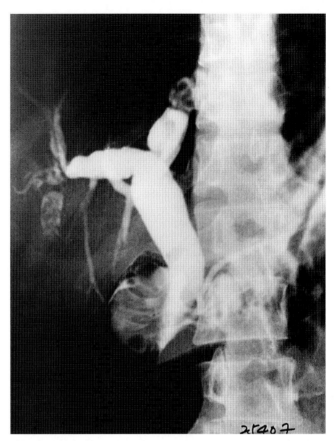

Fig. 62.4. RPC affecting only the intrahepatic ducts in both lobes of the liver. Many stones are present in the liver proximal to strictures.

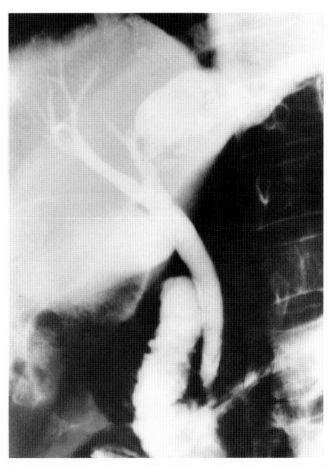

Fig. 62.5. The left lateral segmental duct is obstructed, and the proximal ductal system has become grossly dilated to form cisterns. Few stones are seen within the duct. The resected specimen is shown in Fig. 62.6.

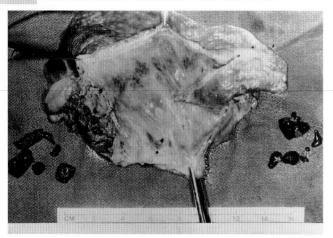

Fig. 62.6. Resected specimen of the left lateral segment (ERCP is shown in Fig. 62.5) showing saccular enlargement of the intrahepatic ducts with few stones. The surface is hemorrhagic, and the duct walls are thick. Little functional liver parenchyma remains.

changes in the diseased ductal tissues, and failure can be expected in most cases.

The gallbladder is diseased in about 20% of patients with RPC, but in many patients with extensive ductal disease, the gallbladder is normal (see Figs. 62.2, 62.17A, and 62.19). When stones are found in the gallbladder, disease is invariably present

elsewhere as well. In the acute attack, and when common duct obstruction is severe, the gallbladder may be grossly distended and develop empyema, gangrene, or perforation. When a normal gallbladder is left behind after drainage procedures to the common duct, however, the risk of developing a complication arising from the gallbladder requiring operation is small. It is justified, although perhaps not recommended, to leave an apparently normal gallbladder when an operation is performed for patients with RPC, when stones are found only in the bile duct.

All stones recovered in RPC patients are bilirubinate stones; these are soft, pigmented, earthy stones that are very friable and crumble when pressed between the fingers. Application of forceps to these stones leads to fragmentation, and the small pieces usually left behind can be flushed out with saline (Fig. 62.7). The stones are irregular in shape and conform to the configuration of the bile duct in which they reside; when packed together, some may have facets. Their size varies from greater than 4 cm to almost microscopic, and in a single patient there may be a continuum in size, in contrast to the stepwise size change in Western-type mixed stones (Fig. 62.8).

In the fresh state, the stone surface is covered with mucus or a film of viscous bile. In some stones, the outer color may be almost black from prolonged exposure to bile; in others, it is orange or green. Flakes of more recently deposited bile debris are separated from the surface when gently scraped, exposing a lighter colored interior, which may appear laminated. Some stones show no organized structure and, with slight compression,

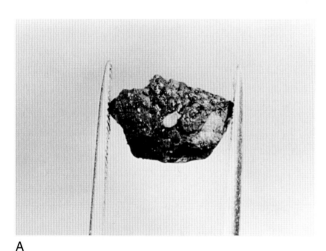

A

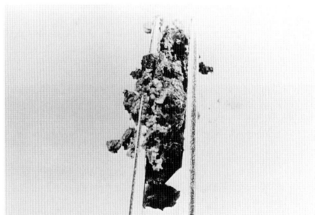

B

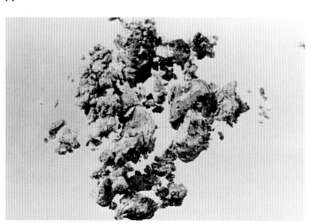

C

Fig. 62.7. RPC stone is placed between tissue forceps (**A**) and is crushed easily by gentle pressure (**B**), fragmenting into soft amorphous masses (**C**).

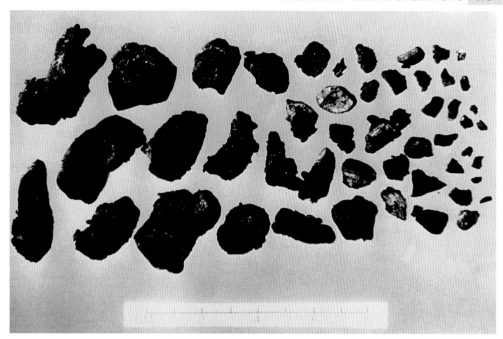

Fig. 62.8. Gradation of sizes of irregular RPC stones. The surfaces are bile stained, but the interior is lighter in color. The shape of the stones molds to the contours of the intrahepatic ducts.

disintegrate into irregular powdery clumps. A nidus sometimes may be identified, and microscopic examination of this area may show dead parasites or clumps of bacteria or cells (Teoh, 1963).

In about 10% of patients, stones are absent, and the bile duct is filled with biliary debris, termed *biliary mud*. This debris is composed of mucus, pus, parasites, altered bile products, microcalculi, and desquamated epithelium, all mixed to form a thick, porridge-like material that exudes from the duct when it is opened. This material also may coexist with stones. In an acute attack, this soft, infected material with or without stones is more commonly encountered.

At operation for an acute problem, the liver appears "cholangitic," or congested, bile stained, and soft, and bleeds easily.

In the quiescent phase, avascular adhesions are found between the surface of the liver and the parietal peritoneum, evidence of previous, resolved acute episodes. In long-standing cases, the adhesions are dense and vascular and contain pockets of pus, which are due to rupture of cholangitic liver abscesses into the peritoneal cavity. Scars on the liver surface indicating previous attacks and dilated bile ducts may appear prominently, especially from the undersurface of the left lobe (Fig. 62.9). When the left lobe is atrophic, there is compensatory hypertrophy of the right lobe. Conversely, in the rare situation of severe right lobe disease, the left lobe may be massive and the liver hilum anatomy grossly distorted (Fig. 62.10). Even when the external appearance is normal, intrahepatic disease may be extensive, and stones are easily palpable through the surface.

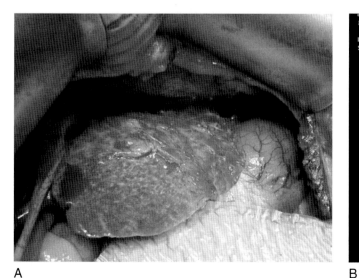

A

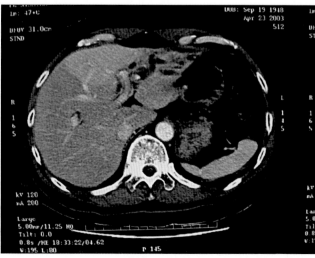

B

Fig. 62.9. A, At laparotomy, the left lateral segment appears cholangitic with scars, and dilated ducts are seen on the surface. Stones may be palpable in the dilated ducts through the atrophic liver parenchyma. **B,** CT scan of the same patient shows the typical features of this condition.

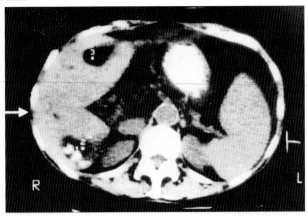

Fig. 62.10. CT scan of a patient with RPC shows right lobe atrophy and shifting of liver hilum toward the right side. Stones are located within the right duct. The *arrow* indicates the preferred incision (thoracoabdominal) for right hepatectomy in this situation.

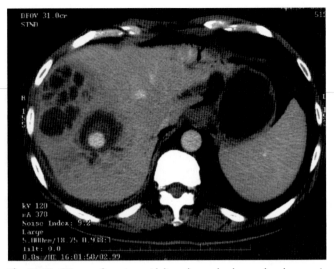

Fig. 62.11. CT scan of a patient with liver abscess that has produced a mycotic aneurysm.

Biliary cirrhosis and liver failure are possible complications (Jeng et al, 1989) and usually follow long-standing severe disease that has failed to improve with multiple operations, some of which may be associated with stricture of the biliary-enteric anastomosis. When cirrhosis has developed, portal hypertension and bleeding esophageal varices may ensue. Further corrective biliary surgery is feasible only after decompression by portosystemic shunting.

Stones at the lower end of the common bile duct may cause two additional complications in addition to biliary obstruction: choledochoduodenal fistula and acute pancreatitis. Choledochoduodenal fistula is not serious, but may be confusing to the endoscopist and the radiologist. Acute pancreatitis is an important potential consequence of RPC. In Hong Kong, in the past, acute pancreatitis was associated with RPC in approximately half of all patients (Ong et al, 1971), and in about 20% of patients with RPC, a high serum amylase level was recorded, although many cases were clinically silent.

Although rare, abscesses in the left liver may rupture into the pericardial cavity to cause cardiac tamponade (Fan & Wong 1997). Abscesses in the right liver may rupture to form a pleurobiliary or bronchobiliary fistula (Wei et al, 1982). These abscesses also may bleed into the abscess cavity (Fig. 62.11) or bile duct (Joo et al, 2003), rupture into the abdominal cavity or into adjacent hollow viscera, or extend into the subphrenic or subhepatic spaces.

A chronic abscess may be indistinguishable clinically, at operation or on contrast studies, from cholangiocarcinoma and may be identified as such only through detailed histologic examination after resection. An increased incidence of cholangiocarcinoma owing to clonorchiasis, as with hepatolithiasis, has been noted (Hou, 1956; Ohta et al, 1984). Whether cholangiocarcinoma is coincidental or etiologically related to RPC is controversial. Cholangiocarcinoma is found in 2% to 13% of patients with intrahepatic stones (Chen et al, 1989; Chu et al, 1997; Ohta et al, 1984, 1988). Autopsy studies suggest that recurrent cholangitis can induce progressive changes leading to atypical epithelial hyperplasia and cholangiocarcinoma (Ohta et al, 1984). The tumor may take the form of nodular or papillary growth. Stones may be found within the tumor mass or the ductal lumen with tumorous invasion (Fig. 62.12). Cholangiocarcinoma should be

suspected whenever a mass lesion is seen on imaging studies (Fig. 62.13). Inflammatory pseudotumor also is present in patients with RPC, however (Yoon et al, 1999). The imaging characteristics are nonspecific, however. Only resection and pathologic examination can reliably differentiate the two conditions.

Thrombophlebitis of major portal vein branches may develop when adjacent large biliary ducts are affected by RPC causing extensive periductal inflammation (Fig. 62.14). When the hepatic veins become thrombosed, pulmonary emboli may develop and, in rare instances, lead to pulmonary hypertension (Lai et al, 1968). Microscopically, the portal triads are infiltrated with inflammatory cells, and the cholangioles are filled with pus. In severe attacks, neutrophils also are seen in the sinusoids of the lobules, and adjacent hepatocytes undergo vacuolation. The larger bile ducts show acute inflammatory changes initially, but with repeated attacks the ducts become thickened. Surface mucosal lining is lost, and there is marked glandular proliferation into the thickened duct wall and beyond (Fig. 62.15). With repeated attacks, many of the glands undergo metaplasia. Fibrosis may extend far beyond the already thickened duct wall into the adjoining liver parenchyma, which undergoes degeneration and necrosis.

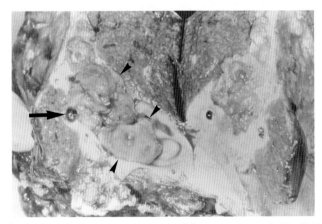

Fig. 62.12. Right hepatectomy specimen of the same patient as in Fig. 62.13 showing tumor mass *(arrowheads)* growing within the dilated bile duct; a black stone is seen within a branch of the bile duct *(arrow)*.

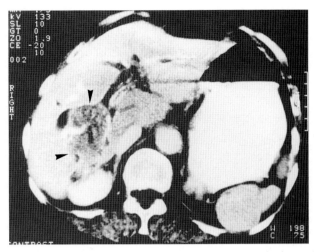

Fig. 62.13. CT scan of a patient with RPC shows a dilated right duct with a soft tissue mass within *(arrowheads)*.

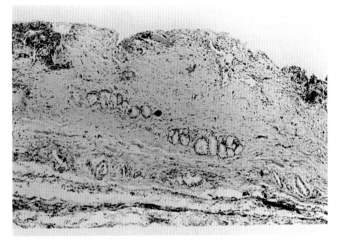

Fig. 62.15. Photomicrograph of a large intrahepatic duct affected by RPC. The wall is thick and fibrosed, the epithelial lining in the duct lumen is denuded, and there is glandular proliferation into the depths of the thickened duct wall. (Hematoxylin and eosin stain, ×67.)

CLINICAL FEATURES

In contrast to biliary calculous diseases seen in Western countries, RPC affects men and women equally, in a younger age group (20-40 years old), and there is a predilection for the lower socioeconomic classes. These features, together with the Asian origin of the patients and the presence of cholangitis, allow the

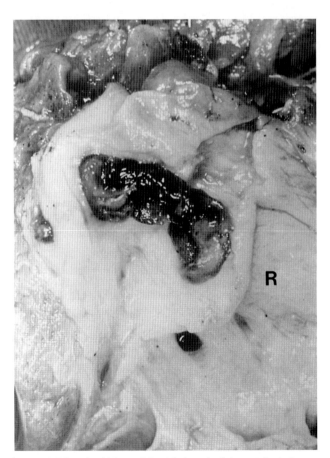

Fig. 62.14. Thrombophlebitis of the right branch of the portal vein in severe RPC affecting the right hepatic duct *(R)*. The vein wall is thickened with white fibrous tissue.

diagnosis of RPC to be made with near certainty. In Hong Kong today, with improved socioeconomic conditions, there are fewer new cases, however, and fewer young patients with RPC. In a survey, the median age of patients with RPC was 59.5 years, and 56% had previous biliary operations for biliary stone disease (Liu et al, 1998).

The symptoms of RPC are not in themselves distinctive and are characteristic of acute cholangitis: pain, fever, and jaundice (Charcot's triad). The pain is right hypochondrial or epigastric; it may be distending, sharp, gnawing, or cutting, with frequent radiation to the back. It is constant, seldom colicky, and lasts for hours. Nausea is common, but vomiting is unusual. Temperature is often less than 40°C. If the temperature is elevated, septicemia or liver abscess must be suspected. The temperature chart shows spikes rather than a continuous fever. Jaundice is seldom marked and may be just clinically perceptible, indicating incomplete obstruction. Pruritus is rarely a complaint, and the patient does not note pale stools. More typically, the patient is aware of the passage of tea-colored urine.

Physical examination in the acute attack reveals a restless patient, slightly jaundiced and unwell. The abdomen may bear the scars of previous surgery. Tenderness is elicited in the epigastrium or right hypochondrium, and there is guarding. The liver is enlarged in 60% of patients, but this may be masked by guarding. Similarly, a distended gallbladder may not be palpable. The spleen is enlarged in 25% of patients.

Should the abdominal signs deteriorate, indicating worsening peritonitis, or if generalized peritonitis is present, emergency operation or nonoperative intervention is mandatory. In elderly patients, abdominal signs may be minimal, even in septicemic patients, and reliance on physical findings alone may delay a decision to operate until the patient is in shock. Even when shock is present, there still may be a reluctance to operate on these elderly patients for lack of convincing abdominal signs. A transient increase in blood pressure in a patient with acute cholangitis may be a prelude to shock and must be regarded as a sign of impending deterioration, rather than a positive response to treatment. In between attacks, there are few, if any, significant clinical features. Recent weight loss in elderly patients known to have RPC should raise the suspicion of development of cholangiocarcinoma.

Cholangiocarcinoma also should be suspected during follow-up when a patient's serum alkaline phosphatase increases markedly (Kim et al, 2003) or when intrahepatic stones involving both lobes have not been completely cleared in the previous operations (Jan et al, 1996).

INVESTIGATIONS

Routine hematologic and biochemical tests are consistent for a patient with bacterial infection of an obstructed bile duct and do not distinguish patients with RPC from patients with other causes. Leukocytosis is present, and liver function tests show an obstructive picture with a moderate elevation of the bilirubin level and high serum alkaline phosphatase and gamma-glutamyltransferase levels. Occasionally, patients with RPC have completely normal liver biochemistry, even during an acute attack.

Imaging studies are important for the diagnosis of the disease, evaluation of the extent of involvement, and formulation of treatment plans for eradication of stones and strictures. Ultrasonography, computed tomography (CT), cholangiography, and magnetic resonance imaging (MRI) are complementary to each other in achieving such goals (see Chs. 15, 18, and 19).

When applied optimally, ultrasonography diagnoses the size of the common duct and intrahepatic ducts and the location of stones. It also shows liver abscesses, biloma, or tumor, if present. Color Doppler ultrasonography is useful in studying portal vein hemodynamics. Intrahepatic stones are readily identified if they cast sonic shadows (Fig. 62.16), but some stones found in RPC are isoechoic and may be isoechoic with respect to the surrounding tissue (Federle et al, 1982). This fact, combined with the propensity of these stones to form biliary casts, may lead to failure of ultrasonography to identify intrahepatic stones in some cases (Chau et al, 1987). Another deficiency of ultrasonography in this disease is related to pneumobilia, which may produce highly reflective echoes and acoustic shadowing simulating stones (Federle et al, 1982). Pneumobilia is a common finding in patients with RPC who have undergone biliary-enteric drainage procedures. In 30% of patients with RPC, prominent periportal echogenicity is found (Chau et al, 1987). These changes could represent pericholangitis and periportal fibrous

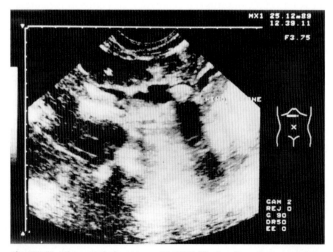

Fig. 62.16. Ultrasound of a patient with RPC. The intrahepatic stone produces an acoustic shadow, a feature not always demonstrable.

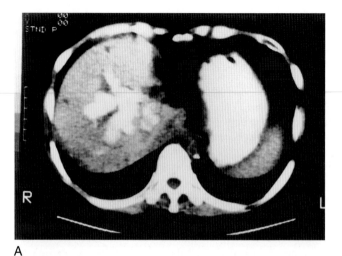

A

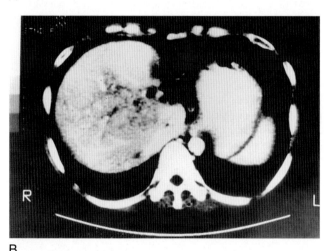

B

Fig. 62.17. A, CT scan shows obvious intrahepatic stones on a noncontrast film. **B,** CT scan shows the stones being masked by parenchymal contrast enhancement.

thickening found in advanced stages of RPC. The finding should prompt the ultrasonographer to search for other evidence of RPC.

CT is more expensive than ultrasound, but provides imaging that is largely free from observer bias and operator-dependent interpretation. In addition to providing the information offered by ultrasonography, it can differentiate accurately intrahepatic stones from pneumobilia, which may be confusing on ultrasound, and provide accurate topographic localization for drainage of liver abscess (Fan et al, 1990). In RPC, some stones may become less conspicuous on postcontrast scans, however, against the contrast-enhanced hepatic parenchyma (Fig. 62.17). It is mandatory to examine a noncontrast scan to avoid false negative interpretation. On CT scan, volumetric and contour alteration of the liver can be seen readily. Liver lobe atrophy, hypertrophy, and rotation of the liver hilum are present in long-standing cases (see Fig. 62.10). Parenchymal changes also can be detected. During an acute attack, persistent segmental enhancement is observed in 36% of patients (Chan et al, 1989), representing parenchymal suppuration analogous to the angiographic finding of diffuse hypervascularity and arteriovenous shunting described for the disorder (Freeny, 1980).

Ultrasound and CT are complementary examinations to cholangiography, which provides clear delineation of the ductal anatomy. In RPC, in which the pattern of ductal disease can be so diverse, detailed delineation of the entire biliary tract is essential. ERCP and percutaneous transhepatic cholangiography are the direct cholangiographic methods of choice for RPC. We generally prefer to perform ERCP first because the extrahepatic ducts, which affected in more than 50% of patients with RPC, are better visualized. Percutaneous transhepatic cholangiography is preferred when there has been a hepaticojejunostomy or choledochojejunostomy and when a stone or stricture located at the confluence of bile ducts prevents filling of the intrahepatic ducts. Ultrasonography can be useful in this instance by guiding percutaneous puncture of the targeted bile duct and by offering greater safety (Nakayama & Koga, 1984). On interpreting cholangiograms obtained in patients with this condition, care should be exercised in looking for missing segmental ducts, especially when there is paucity of intrahepatic filling (Fig. 62.18). Correlation with ultrasound or CT may yield useful information

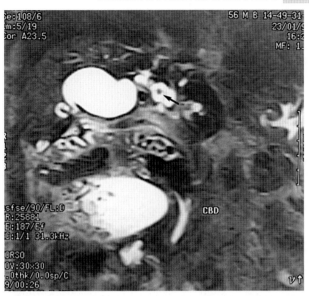

Fig. 62.19. MRI shows coronal plane of a patient with RPC. Cisternal dilation of intrahepatic ducts and stone *(arrow)* are seen, whereas the common bile duct (CBD) is normal in caliber.
(Courtesy of Dr. F. L. Chan.)

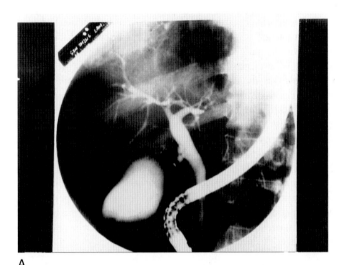

A

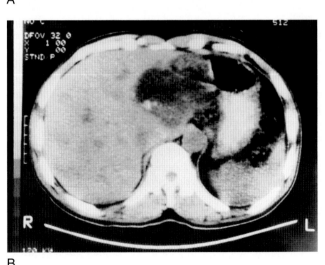

B

Fig. 62.18. A, ERCP shows an apparently normal cholangiogram. On closer examination, there is paucity of intrahepatic ductal filling on the left side. **B,** CT scan of the same patient shows that the absent intrahepatic filling is due to stricture of the left duct leading to cisternal dilation. Multiple stones are present inside the dilated duct.

in defining the cause of repeated attacks of cholangitis in patients who apparently have clearance of all stones.

Similar to CT and ultrasound, MRI is a sensitive modality for showing the volume and contour change in RPC. Contrast-enhanced T1-weighted MRI can show acute suppurative changes by enhancement of the ductal walls and parenchyma. Periportal inflammation is seen on MRI as an intermediate signal between that of the liver and bile on T2-weighted images (Chan et al, 1997). T2-weighted images are best for showing ductal dilation and stones because bile appears with high signal intensity, whereas stones (without free protons) are signal void and appear as an intraductal filling defect (Fig. 62.19). Compared with ultrasound and CT, MRI is slightly better in detecting intrahepatic stones, ductal dilation, and strictures (Kubo et al, 1995). The presence of pneumobilia, which is also signal void, may adversely affect the stone detection rate, however. Three-dimensional display of the biliary system by MRI cholangiography (see Ch. 19) is indicated when ERCP cannot be performed and may supplant direct cholangiography for diagnostic purposes (Fig. 62.20) (Soto et al, 1996). MRI cholangiography is more sensitive than ERCP in detecting intrahepatic stones because intrahepatic stricture inhibits filling of intrahepatic branches by contrast material in ERCP. MRI cholangiopancreatography may replace ERCP in situations in which a therapeutic procedure is not mandatory (Kim et al, 2002).

MANAGEMENT

Most patients present with an acute attack, which is often not their first. The acute attack settles in most patients with conservative treatment, then patients undergo radiologic investigation. In particular, the site of the strictures, location of stones, size of the ducts, volume of the liver parenchyma, and any associated complications can be ascertained before a decision is made regarding the need for or the type of operation to be performed.

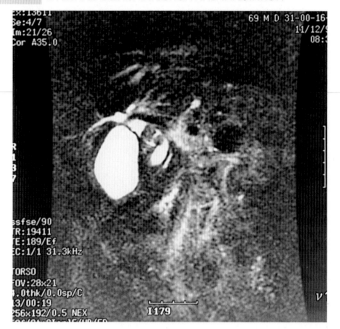

Fig. 62.20. MRI cholangiopancreatography shows large common bile duct stones and irregular caliber of intrahepatic ducts in a patient with RPC. The gallbladder does not contain stone. (Courtesy of Dr. F. L. Chan.)

Definitive operation usually is required. The only patients in whom operation is not recommended are the few who have minimal ductal changes and in whom stones are absent and the rare patients whose bile ducts are filled with *C. sinensis* and whose attack of cholangitis is presumably due to bacterial infection on top of a heavy infection by flukes.

Acute Attack

The goal of treatment of an acute attack is to provide energetic conservative measures. This phase of treatment is regarded as preoperative or preinterventional. Intravenous fluids, broad-spectrum antibiotics, and potent analgesics are given, and the gastrointestinal tract is rested. Antibiotics must cover gram-positive and gram-negative organisms, particularly *E. coli, Klebsiella* species, and anaerobes, especially in patients with previous biliary-enteric anastomosis (Sheen-Chen et al, 2000). Patients who present in shock or whose condition is unstable must receive surgical or nonsurgical intervention without delay.

Conservative treatment for an acute attack fails in about 30% of patients. Complications occur in about 35% of patients in this group, and operative mortality ranges from 12% to 17% (Chen et al, 1984; Fan et al, 1991b). Why conservative treatment fails in some patients but is successful in others is perplexing. A retrospective analysis suggested that failure of conservative treatment is more likely to occur when there is obstruction to the entire biliary tract by stones or strictures in the common duct than when the biliary obstruction involves an isolated segment only. In other words, sepsis involving the entire biliary tract seems to be more virulent than sepsis with segmental involvement. Factors such as age, incidence of concomitant medical diseases, previous surgery, positive blood culture, resistant bacterial strains to antibiotics used, and multiplicity of bacterial cultures seem to be less important determinants (Fan et al, 1991b).

Failure of conservative treatment is evidenced by persistent fever, mental obtundation, spreading peritonitis, tachycardia, oliguria, and hypotension. Urgent biliary decompression is required before the patient lapses into irreversible shock and mortality. Biliary decompression can be achieved by an endoscopic, radiologic, or operative approach.

Surgical Treatment during an Acute Attack

In an acute attack, operation is aimed at saving the patient's life by decompressing the obstructed bile duct and providing free biliary drainage. The usual approach is by exploration of the common bile duct through a choledochotomy and insertion of a large-bore T-tube. The common duct may be 10 cm (average 2.5 cm) and very thick walled. When the common bile duct is extremely large and fibrosed, the normal anatomy is distorted, and recognition may not be straightforward, especially if there has been a previous operation or operations. When the duct is opened, thick, infected biliary mud or pus exudes. After this material has been sucked away, stones within the duct are removed with forceps, which must be applied gently; otherwise, fragmentation occurs. A scoop is useful in retrieving these soft stones and thick mud.

Intrahepatic strictures and stones are not dealt with definitively at the emergency operation, but intrahepatic ductal infection must be relieved by dilation of strictures with graduated sounds. When tight strictures are dilated, a gush of infected bile emerges from the duct. To establish the drainage and decompression of the intrahepatic segmental ducts, a transhepatic tube can be inserted on the same principle as a percutaneous transhepatic biliary drain inserted by radiologic means (Fan & Wong, 1996). During exploration of the common bile duct, irrigation of the bile duct with warm saline solution must be done gently because syringing at high pressure may initiate or aggravate septicemia. For this reason, among others, choledochoscopic examination of the intrahepatic duct should not be performed. Choledochoscopy can be done for the lower end of the common bile duct, provided that the choledochotomy is large and allows free egress of saline.

After the common duct is cleared, patency of the lower end can be established by gently passing a biliary Fogarty catheter. Inflation of the Fogarty catheter without choledochoscopic guidance is not recommended because inflation of the balloon at the sphincter of Oddi may damage the sphincter or induce acute pancreatitis. Similarly, blind passage of a biliary sound is not recommended because it may create a false passage or damage the sphincter of Oddi. Digital exploration also is helpful to detect stones and strictures in the common bile duct and the proximal hepatic ducts, but it is not reliable in ascertaining complete clearance of stones.

When bile flow from both lobes of the liver is established, a T-tube of the largest size that can be accommodated in the bile duct is inserted. The choledochotomy is closed with absorbable sutures. The large-bore T-tube allows debris to pass unimpeded and, because residual stones are found in more than 30% of patients after emergency exploration, affords a large tract for percutaneous manipulation after operation.

Whether additional procedures are required depends on the presence of concomitant pathology and the condition of the patient. Cholecystectomy or cholecystostomy is not routinely performed, unless the condition of the patient is satisfactory; or there is acute cholecystitis, empyema, or gangrene of the gallbladder; or the gallbladder is extremely distended. The presence of stones in an otherwise normal gallbladder is not an indication for cholecystectomy during operation for the acute attack when the condition of the patient is not satisfactory. Palpable liver abscesses are drained externally. Smaller, multiple abscesses should resolve with adequate biliary drainage and antibiotics. If the cardiovascular condition of the patient is stable, hepatic resection can be performed safely for multiple liver abscesses in a destroyed left lateral segment (Fan et al, 1993a).

A stone impacted at the lower end of the common bile duct that cannot be extracted via a choledochotomy is left in situ if there is no associated acute pancreatitis. In the presence of acute pancreatitis, removal through a transduodenal sphincteroplasty is mandatory because pancreatitis may progress. This operation can be performed with low risk (Ong et al, 1979). Although it may be argued that such an impacted stone may be left for endoscopic removal, this strategy entails further intervention in the immediate postoperative period, a procedure that neither is without risk nor possesses the assured success of surgical removal at the same operation. The patient may lose a large volume of bile in the postoperative period leading to hyponatremia, hypokalemia, metabolic acidosis, and dehydration. An alternative to transduodenal sphincteroplasty for impacted stone at the lower end of the common bile duct is fragmentation of the stone using electrohydraulic lithotripsy (Fan, 1989). In experienced hands, this procedure is safe and quick, and transduodenal sphincteroplasty can be avoided.

Postoperatively, the patient's improvement is usually dramatic. Patients who undergo operation for septic shock may need a prolonged convalescence in the intensive care unit to recover from hepatic and renal dysfunction; temperature, pulse rate, and blood pressure may take some time to return to normal levels. Some of these critically ill patients remain in shock and subsequently die of multiple organ failure, sepsis, and generalized bleeding secondary to coagulation defects.

Patients with heavy *C. sinensis* infections may pass large volumes of thin bile through the T-tube despite demonstrated patency of the lower end of the common bile duct. The mechanism for this choleresis is unknown. Praziquantel should be given to eradicate the infestation, and adequate fluid and electrolyte replacement must be given to avoid complications.

Nonoperative Treatment of an Acute Attack
Biliary decompression can be achieved by endoscopic papillotomy (see Chs. 28, 37, and 40) and nasobiliary catheter or large-bore endoprosthesis insertion (Lam, 1984). Biliary decompression has the advantage of immediate relief of biliary obstruction if the site of obstruction is within the common bile duct, but it is not beneficial if the disease is mainly intrahepatic. In this situation, percutaneous transhepatic biliary drainage (see Ch. 29) of the obstructed segmental ducts under ultrasound guidance may be helpful (Huang & Ker, 1988). The drainage tubes used in these procedures are small (the lumen is even smaller), however, and can be blocked easily in the presence of thick, infected bile and soft stones (Takahashi et al, 1990). Because multiple strictures are often present inside and outside the liver, a single drain is inadequate in affording total decompression.

Careful assessment of the clinical condition after endoscopic or radiologic biliary decompression is necessary. If the patient's condition does not improve, further imaging is necessary to identify the location of sepsis. Sepsis locations may include empyema of gallbladder with perforation and bile peritonitis, one or more undrained segmental ducts, liver abscess, and blockage of the lumen of a previously placed drainage tube by thick bile. In this situation, prompt surgical intervention is indicated.

In the past, biliary decompression was performed when the patient's condition deteriorated or failed to improve after conservative treatment. The mortality of this approach is about 10% and is unacceptable. With the availability of emergency endoscopic service, we advocate emergency ERCP and endoscopic decompression within 24 to 48 hours of admission, hoping to avoid surgical intervention at the time of an unfavorable physiologic condition. ERCP is the best initial step because the pathology leading to failure of conservative treatment usually resides in the common bile duct (Fan et al, 1991a, 1991b), and adequate decompression can be achieved by the use of a large-bore endoprosthesis. With this approach, there is almost no hospital mortality for an acute attack (Liu et al, 1998). The condition of the patient must be meticulously observed, however. If a sign of immediate improvement is not apparent, the patient must be considered for surgical intervention.

Definitive Surgery

The goals of elective definitive surgery are to clear the biliary tract of stones, to bypass or enlarge the strictures, to provide adequate biliary drainage, and, where necessary, to provide percutaneous access to the biliary tract. Because the disease affects the biliary tract at different sites and with varying degrees of severity, many procedures have been developed to deal with the different circumstances. These procedures include common duct exploration, hepatotomy, partial hepatectomy, hepaticocutaneous jejunostomy, and strictureplasty. A complete and exact imaging study to outline the location of stones and strictures and the degree of segmental liver atrophy is mandatory in planning elective definitive treatment.

Generally, RPC can be arbitrarily divided into simple and complicated cases depending on the absence or presence of intrahepatic strictures. For simple cases, cholecystectomy, exploration of common duct, and choledochoscopy with or without hepaticojejunostomy suffice. For complicated cases, hepaticocutaneous jejunostomy, strictureplasty, and partial hepatectomy are additional procedures needed to circumvent intrahepatic ductal strictures and to eradicate impacted stones.

Approach to the Biliary Tract
Similar to the operations performed for an acute attack, a choledochotomy or hepaticodochotomy is made for initial exploration of the bile duct. In patients with predominantly intrahepatic involvement, the hepaticodochotomy can be extended up into the right or left duct. By such an extension, pathology located at the confluence involving the main right or left duct can be readily approached. The orifice of the right posterior sectoral duct, especially when it joins the left duct, can be exposed for removal of an impacted stone. If a stricture is found at this orifice, dilation or strictureplasty (Fan & Wong, 1996) can be performed. Exposure of the common bile duct is sometimes difficult, however, when it is obscured by dense adhesions as a result of previous operations or by a pericholedochal venous plexus related to portal vein thrombosis or portal hypertension. Occasionally, the common bile duct becomes posterior to the portal vein as a result of left lobe hypertrophy and right lobe atrophy (see Ch. 3) (Czerniak et al, 1986). In these situations, the biliary system can be approached by extraperitoneal mobilization of the duodenum

followed by transduodenal sphincteroplasty (Choi et al, 1982) or dissection of the left duct (Blumgart & Kelley, 1984) or the segment III duct (Dudley et al, 1979). Sometimes, dilated intrahepatic ducts with or without impacted stones are palpable on the surface of the liver or located by intraoperative ultrasound. In this situation, access to the intrahepatic ducts can be achieved by direct hepatotomy (Zhang et al, 1997). This method incurs little bleeding if the parenchyma is thin, but massive bleeding if the stones are deep-seated. Careful Doppler and ultrasound assessment must be done before a decision to proceed with direct hepatotomy is made.

Removal of Stones during Laparotomy

When the biliary tract is opened, stones can be readily removed by forceps, scoops, Fogarty catheter, or saline flushing. Intraoperative flexible choledochoscopy (see Ch. 23) is mandatory to discover and remove additional stones. Extraction of stones can be difficult, however, when they are impacted, situated behind strictures, or within sharply angulated ducts, such as the right posterior sectoral or segment IV ducts (Fan et al, 1991a; Jeng et al, 1994; Mahadeva et al, 2003). The difficulty can be circumvented by electrohydraulic lithotripsy (Fan et al, 1989). The technique involves introduction of an electrohydraulic probe through the working channel of a flexible choledochoscope. Under direct visual control, the probe is brought into direct contact with the stone, which is disintegrated by electric sparks generated by the electrohydraulic lithotripter. The electrohydraulic lithotripter should be applied cautiously because the probe in contact with the ductal wall may damage the wall leading to hemobilia. A holmium:yttrium-aluminum-garnet laser (Uchiyama et al, 2002) and a new design plasma shock wave lithotripter (Xu et al, 2002) may be viable alternatives because they do not damage the ductal wall and clear intrahepatic stones in almost 100% of cases.

Cholecystectomy

Cholecystectomy, as in the emergency operation, has been recommended by some authors only when gallbladder disease is present. This approach is justified on the grounds that a normal gallbladder left in situ has only rarely required subsequent removal for acute complications, it might act as a sentinel when there is distal obstruction in the bile duct, and it may be used for further biliary operation should the need arise. For RPC, these reasons are not compelling, however, and it is prudent to remove the gallbladder at the first opportunity in an elective situation.

Biliary Drainage Procedures

Additional drainage procedures, such as transduodenal sphincteroplasty and choledochojejunostomy or hepaticojejunostomy, are carried out when specific indications are present. For sphincteroplasty, these indications include stenosis at the ampulla of Vater or distal common duct, a stone impacted at the lower end, or residual small stones in the intrahepatic ducts. In addition, the duct wall should not be thickened. Transduodenal sphincteroplasty is performed in the standard manner (see Ch. 36). An extraperitoneal approach for this operation has been described (Choi et al, 1982) and is particularly useful for patients who have had multiple previous operations. A high transverse incision is used, and the duodenum is identified by its anterior relationship to the kidney. After the sphincteroplasty has been completed, the common duct is explored from below, and residual stones are extracted. Although a supraduodenal choledochoduodenostomy suffices for some of the indications listed, and the anastomosis allows passage of an endoscope for diagnosis or therapy, the disadvantage is the possible development of the sump syndrome and liver abscess because food debris may reflux into the partially obstructed segmental duct (Rumans et al, 1987). Conversion from choledochoduodenostomy to hepaticojejunostomy is required. Choledochojejunostomy or hepaticojejunostomy (see Ch. 30) is carried out most commonly for a stricture in the intrapancreatic portion of the common bile duct and a dilated thickened common bile duct that has lost its elasticity. It is performed with the hope that newly formed stones may pass into the bowel. In this instance, sphincteroplasty may not suffice because the common duct may act as an inert sac and drain inadequately.

Hepaticojejunostomy also is required when a stricture is present in the common hepatic duct. When the stricture involves the common hepatic duct at or near the confluence, biliary-enteric anastomosis to the left hepatic duct or segment III duct is necessary. When stricture involves the right and left ducts simultaneously in their immediate extrahepatic portion, the difficulty in treatment is increased (see Fig. 62.20). It may be possible to resect the strictures and to perform a bilateral hepaticojejunostomy (Figs. 62.21 and 62.22).

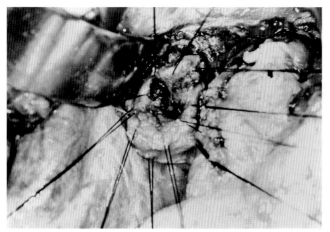

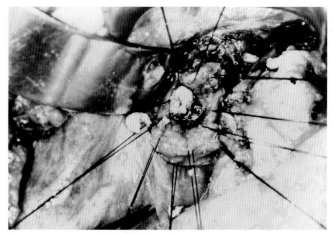

A   B

Fig. 62.21. A, Stricture of the right hepatic duct at the porta hepatis. A stone can be seen within the stricture. **B,** Application of forceps on the stone results in fragmentation, showing the paler interior of the stone.

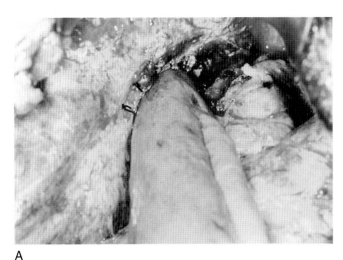

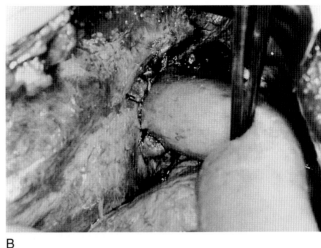

A   B

Fig. 62.22. A, Hepaticojejunostomy performed after the stricture shown in Fig. 62.21 had been excised and stones cleared from the intrahepatic duct. **B,** Posterior aspect of the hepaticojejunostomy showing the anastomosis is essentially intrahepatic.

Hepaticocutaneous Jejunostomy

Hepaticojejunostomy is constructed with the hope of providing adequate drainage to the biliary tract and unimpeded passage of newly formed intrahepatic stones. Intrahepatic strictures above the hepaticojejunal anastomosis, if present, prevent free drainage of bile and passage of stones, however. Reoperation for recurrence of stones after hepaticojejunostomy becomes increasingly difficult and hazardous. Percutaneous access to the biliary tract can be achieved by flexible choledochoscopy if the Roux-en-Y limb of the hepaticojejunostomy can be extended to the cutaneous level and opened as a stoma (see Ch. 30) (Fan et al, 1993b;

Fang & Chou, 1977). Via the stoma, it is possible to perform unlimited sessions of choledochoscopy until all stones are removed, and all strictures are adequately dilated (Figs. 62.23 to 62.25). The stoma is closed and buried under the skin. It may be reconstructed as a stoma for diagnostic and therapeutic purposes when recurrence of disease is suspected. The operative procedure of hepaticocutaneous jejunostomy is simple, but it is imperative to construct a relatively straight and short loop from the skin to the biliary-enteric anastomosis because choledochoscopy through a redundant loop of small bowel is difficult, and access to the intrahepatic branches may be impossible.

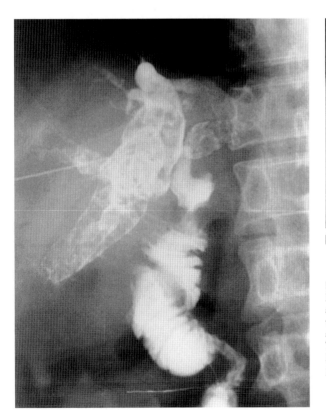

A

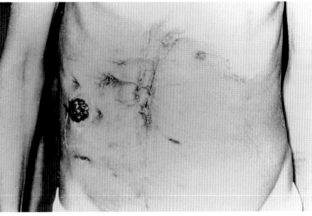

B

Fig. 62.23. A, Percutaneous transhepatic cholangiography of a patient who had undergone six previous operations for RPC, including a left hepatectomy, a choledochojejunostomy, and a hepaticojejunostomy. The right duct is packed with stones proximal to an intrahepatic duct stricture, and the enteric anastomosis is patent. **B,** Postoperative appearance of the abdomen of the same patient. The end of the right intrahepatic duct was anastomosed to the side of a jejunal loop, the proximal end of which was brought out as a cutaneous stoma for permanent access to the intrahepatic duct.

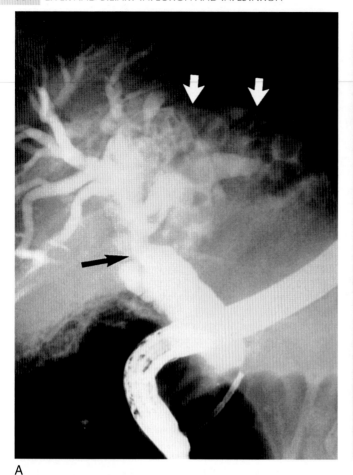 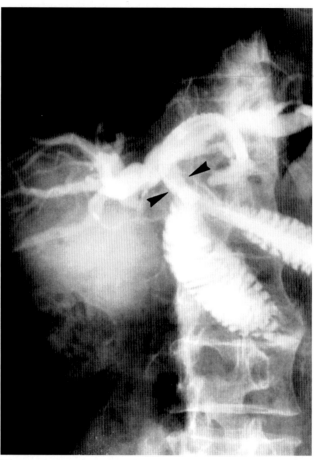

A   B

Fig. 62.24. A, Cholangiogram of a patient with stricture at the common hepatic duct *(black arrow)* and numerous stones inside dilated left ducts *(white arrows).* **B,** Hepaticojejunostomy is constructed at segment III duct *(arrowheads),* and a flexible choledochoscope is shown passing through the anastomosis deeply into peripheral branches of left ducts. All stones have been cleared.

There are a variety of methods for constructing hepaticocutaneous jejunostomy (Hutson et al, 1984). In patients with RPC and numerous abdominal operations, a simpler attachment of a part of the circumference of the long limb of the jejunal loop to the abdominal wall is possible (see Fig. 62.25D).

Postoperative Choledochoscopy and Extraction of Stones

During the definitive operation, intraoperative choledochoscopy is performed, and as many stones as possible are extracted. Complete clearance of stones is sometimes impossible because of the presence of a huge number of stones or because many more stones are discovered only on postoperative cholangiogram. Postoperative choledochoscopy via the T-tube tract or a cutaneous stoma is required. With numerous sessions of choledochoscopy, aided by electrohydraulic lithotripsy, complete stone clearance can be achieved in 90% of cases (Fan et al, 1991a). A similar complete stone clearance rate also can be achieved by choledochoscopy via a percutaneous transhepatic biliary drain (PTBD) tract, which is favored by some authors (Cheung et al, 2003; Huang et al, 2003; Lee et al, 2001; Pitt et al, 1994). The merits of choledochoscopy via a cutaneous stoma or PTBD tract are compared in Table 62.1. Generally, choledochoscopy via a cutaneous stoma is preferred for patients with many stones and strictures because introduction of the choledochoscope is not

painful, approach to the orifices of the segmental ducts is direct, extraction of stones from intrahepatic ducts is not limited, and there is no worry of loss of access. Bile may induce excoriation of skin, however, especially when the stoma adhesive cannot be applied properly. The location of the stoma has to be planned carefully before the operation to avoid scarred areas. On the contrary, bile leakage is not a major problem with PTBD, but the presence of the drainage tube can be a nuisance. Finally, creation of a PTBD pathway is less cumbersome than hepaticocutaneous jejunostomy, but it is not entirely free from serious complications, such as injuries to the hepatic artery and portal vein. Despite the pros and cons, the two routes of access should not be considered mutually exclusive, but complementary for complete clearance.

Choledochoscopic extraction of stones is generally effective, but occasional large stones may prove difficult and may defy fragmentation by electrohydraulic lithotripsy. Extracorporeal shock wave lithotripsy is an alternative. Stone fragments are extracted endoscopically or passed spontaneously (Adamek et al, 1999; Sackmann et al, 2001).

ERCP has been advocated as a sole modality in eradication of intrahepatic stones (Okugawa et al, 2002). With the aid of the "mother-baby" endoscope system, the complete stone removal rate is about 64%. Considering cost and efficacy, ERCP is considered as the only treatment only in patients who are unfit for surgery or supplementary to PTBD in difficult situations.

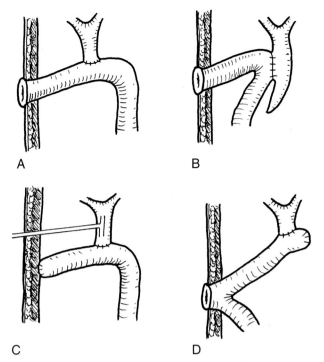

A   B

C   D

Fig. 62.25. Diagram showing the standard operation of hepaticocutaneous jejunostomy (**A**) and modifications in selected circumstances (**B-D**). Method B is employed when separation of the common bile duct from the portal vein is dangerous. Method C is employed when a stoma is not required immediately after the operation. Method D is employed when the patient has had a previous choledochojejunostomy (see Ch. 30).

Access to the biliary tract using the gastroscope via choledochoduodenostomy or interposition duodenojejunostomy has been considered (Cunha et al, 2002; Ramesh et al, 2003). Although these techniques have the advantage of having no cutaneous stoma or percutaneous tube, both have the disadvantage of poor access to the small intrahepatic ducts by the gastroscope. Food reflux into the intrahepatic duct with stenosis cannot return freely to the duodenum. The incidence of ascending cholangitis and liver abscess may be higher in these cases.

Table 62.1 Comparison of Data of Patients Treated in 2 Decades at Queen Mary Hospital

	1984-1989*	1991-1996[†]
No. patients	137	96
Age (median)	56	59.5
Intrahepatic strictures	46 (33.5%)	31 (32%)
Emergency ERCP	1 (0.7%)	61 (64%)
Partial hepatectomy	44 (32%)	55 (57%)
Hepaticocutaneous jejunostomy	19 (14%)	70 (73%)
Right hepatectomy	1 (0.7%)	5 (5%)
Stone clearance rate	114 (90%)	96 (100%)
Hospital mortality	4 (3%)	1 (1%)
Stone recurrence rate	18 (16%)	3 (3%)

*Fan et al, 1991a.
[†]Liu et al, 1998.

Hepatic Resection

Partial hepatectomy is indicated for destroyed liver segments, multiple cholangitic liver abscesses, and concomitant cholangiocarcinoma (Fan et al, 1993a; Jeng et al, 1996; Otani et al, 1999) (see Ch. 80). In the past, hepatic resection for RPC was confined largely to left lateral segmentectomy and occasionally left hepatectomy because intrahepatic stones are located mainly in the left intrahepatic ducts. Right hepatectomy was rarely performed and was considered dangerous and undesirable for a nonmalignant condition. With improved surgical technique and anesthetic care, however, more and more right hepatectomies are performed safely for RPC associated with impacted stones, an atrophic right lobe, or concomitant cholangiocarcinoma (Table 62.2 and Fig. 62.26; see Table 62.1 and Fig. 62.12) (Hung & Lin, 1997; Liu et al, 1998).

The technique of partial hepatectomy for RPC is not different from the standardized procedures (see Chs. 80 to 83). Modification is needed, however, when difficulty is encountered. When right hepatectomy is indicated for an atrophic right lobe, a thoracoabdominal approach may be indicated (see Fig. 62.10). If the inflow and outflow vascular dissection is difficult because of previous operation or infection, it may be wise to proceed to parenchymal transection directly and to achieve vascular control within the liver parenchyma. Adhesion of the left lateral segment to the adjacent viscera owing to repeated infection and rupture of liver abscess may predispose to injury to the vagus nerve, diaphragm, and the phrenic veins and a higher incidence of postoperative septic complications (Fan et al, 1993a). With advances in laparoscopic surgery technique, left lateral segmentectomy and even left hepatectomy could be performed in selected patients with atrophic segment using a hand-assisted device (Chen et al, 2004; Tang & Li, 2003). Such an approach is feasible generally for patients who have not undergone multiple operative procedures and without excessive perihepatic infection and adhesions, although with increasing experience even these patients are potentially amenable to a laparoscopic resection. Longer follow-up is needed, however, before laparoscopic resection can be considered a standard technique for RPC.

Treatment for Intrahepatic Duct Strictures

Strictures located in the extrahepatic bile duct may be treated or circumvented by hepaticojejunostomy performed proximal to the stricture (e.g., at the confluence, left hepatic duct, or segment III duct). Intrahepatic duct strictures associated with liver atrophy or numerous cholangitic abscesses are best treated by partial hepatectomy. If significant thickness of liver parenchyma is still present, the stricture is best treated by instrumental dilation (Cheng et al, 2000). After adequate dilation and removal of stones, however, such strictures may recur, and the stoma of the hepaticocutaneous jejunostomy, if present, has to be reopened for repeat dilation. Intrahepatic duct strictures have been treated by self-expanding metallic stents with a reported patency rate of approximately 60% (Jeng et al, 1999; Tsukamoto et al, 2004; Yoon et al, 1997). The use of self-expanding metallic stents for benign biliary stricture is still controversial. For patients who have refractory intrahepatic biliary strictures and who refuse surgery, self-expanding metallic stents are a potential option, but at present should be considered only as a secondary alternative in cases in which surgery is impossible.

Table 62.2 Comparison of Choledochoscopy via Percutaneous Transhepatic Biliary Drain versus Hepaticocutaneous Jejunostomy

	Via PTBD Route	Via Jejunal Loop
Choledochoscopy	Painful at skin entry site	Painless
Stone extraction	Stone fragments may be too large for the tract	No limitation
Approach to intrahepatic duct by choledochoscope	Difficult to bend over angulation into segmental ducts	Theoretically easy
Loss of access	Tract disruption after repeated use	Redundant loop
Wound complication	Granuloma around skin entry site	Skin excoriation by bile

RESULTS OF TREATMENT

Short-Term Results

The short-term result of the treatment of RPC is measured by mortality rate, stone clearance rate, and stone recurrence rate. The outcome depends on scrutiny for residual stone by various types of imaging and on the experience of the team, especially in choledochoscopy. The best results are achieved after good imaging studies, selection of the appropriate procedure for the individual case, and vigilant postoperative choledochoscopy before removal of a T-tube or closure of a cutaneous stoma. Our series indicate that the increasing use of aggressive treatment, such as partial hepatectomy, hepaticocutaneous jejunostomy, and diligent postoperative choledochoscopy, can lead to 100% stone clearance rate and 3% stone recurrence rate after a median period of follow-up of 26 months, for a mortality rate of only 1% (see Table 62.1).

Long-Term Results

The long-term result is best measured by the reappearance of stones and strictures after 5 years of follow-up and the occurrence of portal hypertension, bleeding esophageal varices, ascites, liver failure, and cholangiocarcinoma. With respect to location of the disease, patients with simple cases can be expected to do well in the long-term with drainage procedures, whereas patients with complicated diseases are expected to have a 30% recurrence of symptoms (Chijiiwa et al, 1995; Jan et al, 1996). Along with recurrence of stones and strictures, progressive liver damage leads to portal hypertension, liver failure, and cholangiocarcinoma. Ten percent to 20% of patients eventually may die of the disease. The occurrence of such complications is related to the failure to eradicate stones completely at the time of treatment (Jan et al, 1996).

Treatment of cases of RPC complicated by liver failure and portal hypertension is extremely difficult. Liver transplantation is perhaps the only way to salvage the patients. Liver transplantation in such patients is difficult, however, because of the presence of dense perihepatic vascular adhesion resulting from previous infection, multiple previous abdominal operations, and cholangitic liver abscesses rupturing into the perihepatic region. Torrential bleeding on mobilization of the liver may occur. This hemorrhage, together with the underlying sepsis, results in a much higher risk than in other patients submitted to liver transplantation. The number of patients with RPC having liver transplantation is small, and the hospital mortality rate has been reported to be 33% (Krissat et al, 1998). If liver transplantation is performed before multiple biliary procedures are performed, the outcome seems to be more satisfactory (Strong et al, 2002).

CONCLUSION

To achieve an optimal result in the management of RPC, a judicious choice of a combination of treatment modalities by a dedicated multidisciplinary team is necessary. Although it may not be possible to prevent recurrence of stones and strictures in all patients, the construction of a permanent percutaneous access to the biliary tract can facilitate the overall management and reduce the magnitude of any subsequent procedures. For simple cases, aggressive removal of all stones and dilation or bypass of all strictures combined with vigilant follow-up are mandatory to

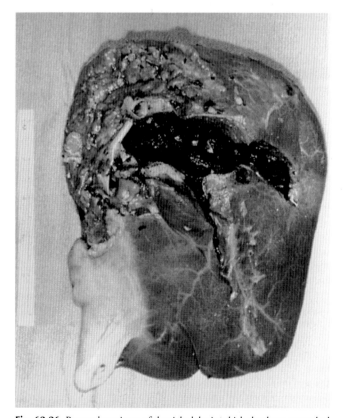

Fig. 62.26. Resected specimen of the right lobe in which the ducts are packed with stones. Despite a significant residual functional parenchyma, the frequency and severity of symptoms of RPC necessitated resection.

prevent progression of the disease. In complicated cases associated with liver failure, a decision for early liver transplantation must be made so that the operative risk is not excessively high.

REFERENCES

Adamek HE, et al, 1999: Treatment of difficult intrahepatic stones by using extracorporeal and intracorporeal lithotripsy techniques: 10 years' experience in 55 patients. Scand J Gastroenterol 34:1157-1161.

Balasegaram M, 1972: Hepatic calculi. Ann Surg 175:149-154.

Blumgart LH, Kelley CJ, 1984: Hepaticojejunostomy in benign and malignant high bile duct stricture: approaches to the left hepatic ducts. Br J Surg 71:257-261.

Chan FL, et al, 1989: Evaluation of recurrent pyogenic cholangitis with CT: analysis of 50 patients. Radiology 170:165-169.

Chan FL, et al, 1997: Modern imaging in the evaluation of hepatolithiasis. Hepatogastroenterology 44:358-369.

Chang TM, Passaro E Jr, 1983: Intrahepatic stones: the Taiwan experience. Am J Surg 146:241-244.

Chau EMT, et al, 1987: Recurrent pyogenic cholangitis: ultrasound evaluation compared with endoscopic retrograde cholangiopancreatography. Clin Radiol 38:79-85.

Chen HH, et al, 1984: Twenty-two year experience with the diagnosis and treatment of intrahepatic calculi. Surg Gynecol Obstet 159:519-524.

Chen MF, et al, 1989: Intrahepatic stones associated with cholangiocarcinoma: clinical analysis of 20 cases with particular reference to the possibility of its early diagnosis. Am J Gastroenterol 84:391-395.

Chen P, et al, 2004: Laparoscopic left hemihepatectomy for hepatolithiasis. Surg Endosc 18:717-718.

Cheng YF, et al, 2000: Treatment of complicated hepatolithiasis with intrahepatic biliary stricture by ductal dilatation and stenting: long-term results. World J Surg 24:712-716.

Cheung MT, et al, 2003: Percutaneous transhepatic choledochoscopic removal of intrahepatic stones. Br J Surg 90:1409-1415.

Chijiiwa K, et al, 1995: Current management and long-term prognosis of hepatolithiasis. Arch Surg 130:194-197.

Choi TK, et al, 1982: Extraperitoneal sphincteroplasty for residual stones: an update. Ann Surg 196:26-29.

Choi TK, et al, 1984: Cholangiographic appearance in clonorchiasis. Br J Radiol 57:681-684.

Chu KM, et al, 1997: Intrahepatic cholangiocarcinoma. World J Surg 21:301-306.

Cook J, et al, 1954: Recurrent pyogenic cholangitis. Br J Surg 42:188-203.

Cunha JE, et al, 2002: A new biliary access technique for the long-term endoscopic management of intrahepatic stones. J Hepatobiliary Pancreat Surg 9:261-264.

Czerniak A, et al, 1986: Liver atrophy complicating benign bile duct strictures: surgical and interventional radiologic appearances. Am J Surg 152:294-300.

Digby KH, 1930: Common-duct stones of liver origin. Br J Surg 17:578-591.

Dudley SE, et al, 1979: Biliary decompression in hilar obstruction: round ligament approach. Arch Surg 114:519-522.

Fan ST, 1989: Transduodenal sphincteroplasty for impacted stone made unnecessary by electrohydraulic lithotripsy. Surg Gynecol Obstet 168:363-364.

Fan ST, Wong J, 1996: Recurrent pyogenic cholangitis. In Carter D, et al (eds): Rob and Smith's Operative Surgery: Hepatobiliary and Pancreatic Surgery, 5th ed. London, Chapman & Hall Medical, pp 382-396.

Fan ST, Wong J, 1997: Recurrent pyogenic cholangitis. In Zinner MJ, et al (eds): Manigot's Abdominal Operations, vol II, 10th ed. Stamford, Conn, Appleton & Lange, pp 1771-1781.

Fan ST, et al, 1989: Electrohydraulic lithotripsy for biliary stones. Aust N Z J Surg 59:217-221.

Fan ST, et al, 1990: Role of computed tomography in the management of recurrent pyogenic cholangitis. Aust N Z J Surg 60:599-605.

Fan ST, et al, 1991a: Treatment of hepatolithiasis: improvement of result by a systematic approach. Surgery 109:474-480.

Fan ST, et al, 1991b: Acute cholangitis secondary to hepatolithiasis. Arch Surg 126:1027-1031.

Fan ST, et al, 1993a: Hepatic resection for hepatolithiasis. Arch Surg 128:1070-1074.

Fan ST, et al, 1993b: Appraisal of hepaticocutaneous jejunostomy in the management of hepatolithiasis. Am J Surg 165:332-335.

Fang K, Chou TC, 1977: Subcutaneous blind loop—a new type of hepaticocholedochojejunostomy for bilateral intrahepatic calculi. Chin Med J 3:413-418.

Federle MP, et al, 1982: Recurrent pyogenic cholangitis in Asian immigrants: use of ultrasonography, computed tomography and cholangiography. Radiology 143:151-156.

Freeny PC, 1980: Acute pyogenic hepatitis: sonographic and angiographic findings. AJR Am J Roentgenol 135:388-391.

Fung J, 1961: Liver fluke infestation and cholangiohepatitis. Br J Surg 48:404-415.

Harris HW, et al, 1998: Recurrent pyogenic cholangitis. Am J Surg 176:34-37.

Hou PC, 1956: The relationship between primary carcinoma of the liver and infestation with Clonorchis sinensis. J Pathol Bacteriol 72:239-246.

Huang MH, Ker CG, 1988: Ultrasonic guided percutaneous transhepatic bile drainage for cholangitis due to intrahepatic stones. Arch Surg 123:106-109.

Huang MH, et al, 2003: Long-term outcome of percutaneous transhepatic cholangioscopic lithotomy for hepatolithiasis. Am J Gastroenterol 98:2655-2662.

Hung CJ, Lin PW, 1997: Role of right hepatic lobectomy in the treatment of isolated right-sided hepatolithiasis. Surgery 121:130-134.

Hutson DG, et al, 1984: Balloon dilatation of biliary strictures through a choledochojejunocutaneous fistula. Ann Surg 199:637-647.

Jan YY, et al, 1996: Surgical treatment of hepatolithiasis: long-term results. Surgery 100:509-514.

Jeng KS, et al, 1989: Secondary biliary cirrhosis: a limiting factor in the treatment of hepatolithiasis. Arch Surg 124:1301-1305.

Jeng KS, et al, 1994: Coexisting sharp ductal angulation with intrahepatic biliary strictures in right hepatolithiasis. Arch Surg 129:1097-1102.

Jeng KS, et al, 1996: Reappraisal of the systematic management of complicated hepatolithiasis with bilateral intrahepatic biliary strictures. Arch Surg 131:141-147.

Jeng KS, et al, 1999: Are expandable metallic stents better than conventional methods for treating difficult intrahepatic biliary strictures with recurrent hepatolithiasis? Arch Surg 134:267-273.

Joo YE, et al, 2003: Hemobilia caused by liver abscess due to intrahepatic duct stones. J Gastroenterol 38:507-511.

Kim TK, et al, 2002: Diagnosis of intrahepatic stones: superiority of MR cholangiopancreatography over endoscopic retrograde cholangiopancreatography. AJR Am J Roentgenol 179:729-734.

Kim YT, et al, 2003: Factors predicting concurrent cholangiocarcinomas associated with hepatolithiasis. Hepatogastroenterology 50:8-12.

Kitagawa Y, et al, 2003: Intrahepatic segmental bile duct patterns in hepatolithiasis: a comparative cholangiographic study between Taiwan and Japan. J Hepatobiliary Pancreat Surg 10:377-381.

Krissat J, et al, 1998: Intrahepatic stones: a multidisciplinary approach. Hepatogastroenterology 45(suppl II):213.

Kubo S, et al, 1995: Case of hepatolithiasis diagnosed by magnetic resonance cholangiography. Osaka City Med J 41:25-30.

Lai KS, et al, 1968: Microembolic pulmonary hypertension in pyogenic cholangitis. BMJ 1:22-24.

Lam SK, 1984: A study of endoscopic sphincterotomy in recurrent pyogenic cholangitis. Br J Surg 71:262-266.

Lam SK, et al, 1978: Recurrent pyogenic cholangitis: a study by endoscopic retrograde cholangiography. Gastroenterology 74:1196-1203.

Lee SK, et al, 2001: Percutaneous transhepatic cholangioscopic treatment for hepatolithiasis: an evaluation of long-term results and risk factors for recurrence. Gastrointest Endosc 53:318-323.

Leung JW, et al, 2001: Expression of bacterial beta-glucuronidase in human bile: an in vitro study. Gastrointest Endosc 54:346-350.

Liu CL, et al, 1998: Primary biliary stones: diagnosis and management. World J Surg 22:1162-1166.

Mage S, Morel S, 1965: Surgical experience with cholangiohepatitis (Hong Kong disease) in Canton Chinese. Ann Surg 162:187-190.

Mahadeva S, et al, 2003: Endoscopic intervention for hepatolithiasis associated with sharp angulation of right intrahepatic ducts. Gastrointest Endosc 58:279-282.

Maki T, 1966: Pathogenesis of calcium bilirubinate gallstone: role of E. coli, β-glucuronidase and coagulation by inorganic ions, polyelectrolytes and agitation. Ann Surg 164:90-100.

Maki T, et al, 1964: Treatment of intrahepatic gallstones. Arch Surg 88:260-270.

Nakanuma Y, et al, 1988: Pathologic features of hepatolithiasis in Japan. Hum Pathol 19:1181-1186.

Nakayama F, 1982: Intrahepatic stones: epidemiology and etiology. In Okuda K (ed): Postgraduate course. Hong Kong, International Association for the study of the Liver/Asian Pacific Association for the Study of the Liver.

Nakayama F, Koga A, 1984: Hepatolithiasis: present status. World J Surg 8:9-14.

Nakayama F, et al, 1980: Hepatolithiasis in Japan: present status. Am J Surg 139:216-220.

Ohta G, et al, 1984: Pathology of hepatolithiasis: cholangitis and cholangiocarcinoma. Prog Clin Biol Res 152:91-113.

Ohta T, et al, 1988: Clinical experience of intrahepatic cholangiocarcinoma associated with hepatolithiasis. Jpn J Surg 18:47-53.

Okugawa T, et al, 2002: Peroral cholangioscopic treatment of hepatolithiasis: long-term results. Gastrointest Endosc 56:366-371.

Ong GB, 1962: A study of recurrent pyogenic cholangitis. Arch Surg 84:199-225.

Ong GB, et al, 1971: Acute pancreatitis associated with recurrent pyogenic cholangitis. Br J Surg 58:891-894.

Ong GB, et al, 1979: Acute pancreatitis in Hong Kong. Br J Surg 66:398-403.

Otani K, et al, 1999: Comparison of treatments for hepatolithiasis: hepatic resection versus cholangioscopic lithotomy. J Am Coll Surg 189:177-182.

Pitt HA, et al, 1994: Intrahepatic stones: the transhepatic team approach. Ann Surg 219:527-535.

Ramesh H, et al, 2003: Biliary access loops for intrahepatic stones: results of jejunoduodenal anastomosis. Aust N Z J Surg 73:306-312.

Rumans MC, et al, 1987: Hepatic abscesses as a complication of the sump syndrome: combined surgical and endoscopic therapy: case report and review of the literature. Gastroenterology 92:791-795.

Sackmann M, et al, 2001: Extracorporeal shock wave lithotripsy for clearance of bile duct stones resistant to endoscopic extraction. Gastrointest Endosc 53:27-32.

Sasaki M, et al, 1998: Expression of apomucins in the intrahepatic biliary tree in hepatolithiasis differs from that in normal liver and extrahepatic biliary obstruction. Hepatology 27:46-53.

Sasaki M, et al, 2004: Expression of trefoil factor family 1, 2, and 3 peptide is augmented in hepatolithiasis. Peptides 25:763-770.

Seel DJ, Park YK, 1983: Oriental infestational cholangitis. Am J Surg 146:366-370.

Sheen-Chen SM, et al, 2000: Bacteriology and antimicrobial choice in hepatolithiasis. Am J Infect Control 28:298-301.

Soto JA, et al, 1996: MR cholangiopancreatography after unsuccessful or incomplete ERCP. Radiology 199:91-98.

Stock FE, Fung JHY, 1962: Oriental cholangiohepatitis. Arch Surg 84:409-412.

Strong RW, et al, 2002: Liver transplantation for hepatolithiasis. Asian J Surg 25:180-183.

Suzuki Y, et al, 1984: Bacteriological study of transhepatically aspirated bile: relation to cholangiographic findings in 295 patients. Dig Dis Sci 29:109-115.

Tabata M, Nakayama F, 1981: Bacteria and gallstones: etiological significance. Dig Dis Sci 26:218-224.

Takahashi T, et al, 1990: Hepatolithiasis and clogged endoprosthesis after endoscopic retrograde biliary drainage. Am J Gastroenterol 85:1204-1205.

Tang CN, Li MK, 2003: Hand-assisted laparoscopic segmentectomy in recurrent pyogenic cholangitis. Surg Endosc 17:324-327.

Teoh TB, 1963: A study of gallstones and included worms in recurrent pyogenic cholangitis. J Pathol Bacteriol 86:123-129.

Terada T, Nakanuma Y, 1988: Morphological examination of intrahepatic bile ducts in hepatolithiasis. Virchows Arch A Pathol Anat Histopathol 413:167-176.

Tsukamoto T, et al, 2004: Self-expanding metallic stent for benign biliary strictures: seven-year follow-up. Hepatogastroenterology 51:658-660.

Uchiyama K, et al, 2002: Indication and procedure for treatment of hepatolithiasis. Arch Surg 137:149-153.

Wei WI, et al, 1982: Bronchobiliary fistula due to stones in the biliary tree: report of two cases. World J Surg 6:782-785.

Wen CC, Lee HC, 1972: Intrahepatic stones: a clinical study. Ann Surg 175:166-177.

Xu Z, et al, 2002: Clinical applications of plasma shock wave lithotripsy in treating postoperative remnant stones impacted in the extra- and intrahepatic bile ducts. Surg Endosc 16:646-649.

Yoon HK, et al, 1997: Benign biliary strictures associated with recurrent pyogenic cholangitis: treatment with expandable metallic stents. AJR Am J Roentgenol 169:1523-1527.

Yoon KH, et al, 1999: Inflammatory pseudotumor of the liver in patients with recurrent pyogenic cholangitis: CT-histopathologic correlation. Radiology 211:373-379.

Zen Y, et al, 2002: Lipopolysaccharide induces overexpression of MUC2 and MUC5AC in cultured biliary epithelial cells. Am J Pathol 161:1475-1484.

Zhang W, et al, 1997: Intraoperative ultrasound-guided transhepatic lithotomy. Arch Surg 132:300-303.

Biliary and Liver Cysts

Bile Duct Cysts in Adults

D. M. NAGORNEY

Bile duct cysts are typically a surgical problem of infancy or childhood (Altman, 1994). The diagnosis is delayed until adulthood, however, in nearly 20% of patients. Although clinically similar, the presentation and therapeutic strategies for bile duct cysts in adults may differ substantially from that of younger patients. In contrast to the pediatric experience, adults have an increased rate of cyst-related complications (Nagorney et al, 1984a; Powell et al, 1981; Rattner et al, 1983; Söreide et al, 2004; Visser et al, 2004), and they often present with complications of previous cyst-related procedures (Gigot et al, 1996; Ono et al, 1982; Nagorney et al, 1984a; Todani et al, 1984a). The surgical management of bile duct cysts in adults is complicated by associated hepatobiliary pathology and the added technical difficulties of repeat biliary surgery. Despite the heterogeneity of the disease and the absence of clinical trials, a consensus for the management of extrahepatic bile duct cysts has been established—excision. The management of intrahepatic bile duct cysts remains problematic, however, and the method of choice for re-establishing biliary-enteric continuity after excision is debatable. This chapter examines the spectrum of hepatobiliary pathology encountered in adults with bile duct cysts and describes the surgical alternatives for managing patients with bile duct cysts.

DIAGNOSIS

Classification

Bile duct cysts are classified on the basis of site, extent, and shape of the cystic anomaly of the ductal system. Although the term *choledochal cyst* often is used interchangeably for bile duct cysts, *bile duct cyst* is semantically more appropriate because cystic dilation can occur anywhere throughout the biliary ductal system and not just in the common bile duct (choledochus). The first coherent classification of extrahepatic bile duct cysts was proposed by Alonso-Lej and colleagues in 1959. Cysts were classified into three types: type I, a fusiform or saccular dilation of the common hepatic and common bile duct; type II, a supraduodenal diverticulum of the common hepatic or common bile duct; and type III, an intraduodenal diverticulum of the distal common bile duct or choledochocele. Although the classification of Alonso-Lej and colleagues (1959) did not include intrahepatic bile duct cysts, this simple and practical scheme has provided the basis for all other classification systems.

The recognition of intrahepatic bile duct cysts prompted modification of the Alonso-Lej classification system. In 1958, Caroli and associates described the entity of multiple intrahepatic bile duct cysts in the absence and presence of extrahepatic cysts. Although initially described as an entity of multiple saccular dilations of only the intrahepatic ducts, the term *Caroli's disease* has been applied broadly to describe any patient with intrahepatic bile duct cysts, regardless of the presence of extrahepatic bile duct cysts or shape of the intrahepatic cysts (Dayton et al, 1983).

Caroli's disease represents a spectrum of diseases, which may include such variants as cysts with congenital hepatic fibrosis or Grumbach's disease (Grumbach et al, 1954). Todani modified the classification system of bile duct cysts by combining the Alonso-Lej classification and the variants of Caroli's disease (Todani et al, 1977). The comprehensive Todani classification system is shown in Fig. 63.1. Matsumoto and colleagues (1977a) also modified the Alonso-Lej classification system based not only on the location of the cyst, but also on the configuration of cysts. To date, clinical management of bile duct cysts is dictated by cyst location, not configuration, and there is little clinical rationale for adoption of more detailed classification schemes (Komi et al, 1992; Matsumoto et al, 1977b).

Etiology

Multiple etiologic theories have been proposed for the origin of bile duct cysts. The most widely accepted hypothesis is that cystic dilation of the bile ducts is related to an anomalous arrangement of the pancreaticobiliary ductal junction (Babbitt, 1969; Komi et al, 1992; Okada et al, 1990; Todani et al, 1984b; Wiedmeyer et al, 1989). When the pancreaticobiliary junction is proximal to the sphincter of Oddi (Fig. 63.2) (Matsumoto et al, 2003; Nagata et al, 1986), the resultant long common channel allows reflux of pancreatic juice into the biliary tree, which causes inflammation, ectasia, and ultimately dilation. This postulate has been supported by biliary manometric studies (Craig et al, 2001; Guelrud et al, 1999; Iwai et al, 1986); high concentration of pancreatic enzymes in cyst fluid (Todani et al, 1990); and histopathologic studies of ductal epithelial hyperplasia, round cell infiltration, and marked ductal fibrosis (Oguchi et al, 1988). In experimental canine studies, pancreaticocholecystostomy and pancreaticocholedochostomy resulted in cystic dilation of the extrahepatic bile duct (Oguchi et al, 1988; Ohkawa et al, 1981).

Although damage and cystic degeneration of the bile duct caused by reflux of pancreatic juice through an anomalous pancreaticobiliary ductal junction (APBDJ) is an attractive hypothesis, not all patients with bile duct cysts have associated APBDJ, not all patients with APBDJ develop bile duct cysts. Anomalous pancreaticobiliary junction in the absence of bile duct dilation has been termed *forme fruste choledochal cyst* (Levy & Rohrmann, 2003). The prevalence of APBDJ and bile duct cysts varies from 21% to 90% (Komi et al, 1992; Nagata et al, 1986). Some patients with APBDJ have normal proximal bile ducts; an experimental study failed to cause cystic dilation of the bile duct despite reflux (Benhidjeb et al, 1994). These findings suggest other causes or at least other unidentified etiologic cofactors with APBDJ. Specifically, in contrast to bile duct cysts in neonates and children, bile duct cysts recognized later in life may be an acquired condition from sphincter of Oddi dysfunction (Craig et al, 2001). Presumably, the time of onset and degree and duration of sphincter dysfunction variably lead to the development

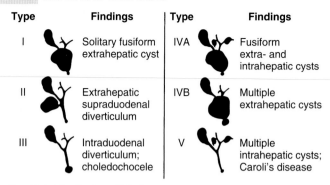

Type	Findings	Type	Findings
I	Solitary fusiform extrahepatic cyst	IVA	Fusiform extra- and intrahepatic cysts
II	Extrahepatic supraduodenal diverticulum	IVB	Multiple extrahepatic cysts
III	Intraduodenal diverticulum; choledochocele	V	Multiple intrahepatic cysts; Caroli's disease

Fig. 63.1. Classification of bile duct cysts.

of bile duct cysts, although few data support this hypothesis. The anatomic type of APBDJ may affect directional bile and pancreatic juice flow dynamics, which may influence the shape of the bile duct cyst and the clinical presentation (Fumino et al, 2002). Bile duct cysts also have been reported in association with incomplete or partial pancreas divisum (Dalvi et al, 1999; Matsumoto et al, 2003) (i.e., incomplete division of the ventral and dorsal pancreatic ductal system).

Reports of bile duct cysts in family members suggest that a hereditary factor may contribute rarely to their development (Iwafuchi et al, 1990; Iwata et al, 1998; Lane et al, 1999). Finally, oligoganglionosis in the distal neck of the cyst may account for some bile duct cysts. The reduction in ganglion cells in the narrow portion of the cyst wall may be a biliary equivalent of Hirschsprung's disease of the colon (Kusunoki et al, 1988).

Demographics

Bile duct cysts are an uncommon, although well-recognized condition (Flanigan, 1975; Powell et al, 1981; Yamaguchi, 1980). Estimates of actual clinical incidence range from 1 in 13,000 to 1 in 2 million patients (Olbourne, 1975). Biliary cysts account for approximately 1% of all benign biliary disease (Saxena et al, 1988). The estimated prevalence of bile duct cysts by type (Todani classification), based on a selective review of the literature, is shown

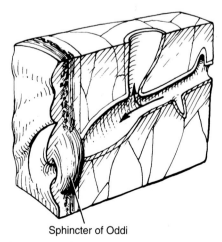

Sphincter of Oddi

Fig. 63.2. A long common channel, as shown in this figure of the pancreaticobiliary ductal confluence, is the most accepted cause of choledochal cysts.

in Table 63.1. The true prevalence of bile duct cysts by specific type is underestimated because classification schemes often are not detailed. The relative frequency of bile duct cysts in decreasing order is type I (79%), type IV (13%), type III or choledochocele (4%), and type II (2.6%). Multiple intrahepatic bile duct cysts without an extrahepatic component (Caroli's disease) occur in less than 1% of patients. The distribution of cyst types encountered in adults is similar to that in infants and children (Gigot et al, 1996; Ono et al, 1982; Söreide et al, 2004) except

Table 63.1 Literature Review of Prevalence of Bile Duct Cysts by Todani Classification

	CYST TYPE				
Reference	I	II	III	IV*	V
Alonso-Lej et al, 1959	86	4	4	—	—
Lee et al, 1964	86	2	5	—	—
Flanigan, 1975	659	23	42	19	—
Yamaguchi, 1980	682	18	12	166	—
Powell et al, 1981	255	7	13	60	—
Ono et al, 1982	21	—	—	1	—
Deziel et al, 1986	18	1	2	6	4
Nagata et al, 1986	21	—	1	5	—
Tan & Howard, 1988	31	0	1	2	1
Hopkins et al, 1990	5	—	—	2	—
Joseph, 1990	45	1	2	3	1
Lopez et al, 1991	15	2	5	1	—
Chijiiwa et al, 1993	26	2	—	18	—
Lipsett et al, 1994	22	1	2	17	—
Scudamore et al, 1994	8	—	1	14	—
Swisher et al, 1994	21	1	2	4	5
Hewitt et al, 1995	8	1	—	4	—
Stain et al, 1995	22	1	—	4	—
Chen et al, 1996	41	1	—	14	4
Gigot et al, 1996	19	1	—	11	—
Kouraklis et al, 1996	5	4	1	—	—
Benhidjeb et al, 1994	6	3	3	—	—
Chaudhary et al, 1997	9	—	—	7	1
Ishibashi et al, 1997	23	1	1	21	1
Jesudason et al, 1997	10	—	—	4	—
Belli et al, 1998	8	—	2	3	—
Lenriot et al, 1998	18	2		21	—
Bismuth & Krissat, 1999	22	1	1	8	16
Kabra et al, 2001	8	—		2	—
Liu et al, 2002	20	2	—	8	—
Durgun et al, 2002	10	1	—	1	—
Jan et al, 2002	55	—	1	29	4
Jordan et al, 2004	9	1	1	4	1
Nicholl et al, 2004	41	—	—	10	6
Visser et al, 2004	30	2	—	7	—
Total	*2365*	*83*	*102*	*457*	*28*
Percentage	*78*	*3*	*3*	*15*	*1*

*Subclassifications of type IV cysts generally not reported.

that type IV cysts are more frequent in adults (Todani et al, 1978, 1984a). A geographic population prevalence has been seen in Japan (Flanigan, 1975; Powell et al, 1981; Yamaguchi, 1980), from which more than one third of cases have been reported. Although the number of reported cases has increased, this finding probably reflects advances in diagnosis through improvements in hepatobiliary imaging rather than a true increase in incidence.

A female preponderance among patients with bile duct cysts is well known, regardless of cyst type. In Flanigan's (1975) collected series of 820 cases, 81% of the patients were female. A similar female-to-male ratio was found in adults (Powell et al, 1981). Current etiopathogenesis of bile duct cysts has yet to implicate sex hormones or intrauterine endocrine disturbances as possible factors. Bile duct cysts have been reported increasingly in adults, and adults often constitute the preponderance of patients reported (Jordan et al, 2004; Lenriot et al, 1998; Lipsett et al, 1994; Liu et al, 2002; Nicholl et al, 2004; Söreide et al, 2004).

Clinical Features

Bile duct cysts may remain asymptomatic indefinitely. Initial clinical presentation in adulthood (age >16 years) occurs in less than 20% of all patients with common duct cysts (Flanigan, 1975), but the increasing recognition of bile duct cysts in adults suggests that delayed presentation is frequent. Initial recognition may be incidental via hepatobiliary imaging studies for unrelated processes. When symptomatic, bile duct cysts usually present similar to calculous biliary tract disease, regardless of cyst type. Symptoms typically are intermittent. Recurrent epigastric or right hypochondrial pain, abdominal tenderness, fever, and mild jaundice are the most common presenting findings. The pain may radiate to the right infrascapular region or to the mid back and generally persists for hours. Abdominal pain or discomfort is often overshadowed by fever and rigors, which may occur repeatedly for several days. An abdominal mass is uncommon in adults, and if a mass is present, cyst-associated malignancy must be strongly suspected. Biliuria heralds the onset of clinical jaundice. Nausea, vomiting, and anorexia generally accompany the other symptoms. If cholangitis persists, jaundice deepens and overt signs of sepsis may evolve.

Approximately 15% of adults with common duct cysts present with overt evidence of cirrhosis or hepatic fibrosis from chronic biliary obstruction. Typically, such patients have had multiple operations for complications of type I or IVA cysts or Caroli's disease. Hepatomegaly and splenomegaly are common in patients with cirrhosis and portal hypertension. Hematemesis, melena, and ascites may accompany portal hypertension; however, cholangitis remains the most common presenting symptom complex in adults, whether or not cirrhosis is present. Other signs of chronic liver disease—muscle wasting, fatigue, spider angiomas, and pruritus—are uncommon. Liver failure may be seen late in Caroli's disease.

Clinical pancreatitis is present in 30% to 70% of patients with bile duct cysts (Nagorney et al, 1984a; Söreide et al, 2004). In contrast to patients with cholangitis, patients with pancreatitis have more intense and prolonged epigastric pain and vomiting. Fever and jaundice are less prominent. Weight loss, although unusual, is noteworthy because nearly 70% of adults with this finding harbor an associated bile duct malignancy.

Imaging

Accurate preoperative diagnosis can be achieved by the standard imaging modalities for other hepatobiliary diseases, including abdominal ultrasound, computed tomography (CT), percutaneous transhepatic cholangiography (PTC), endoscopic retrograde cholangiopancreatography (ERCP), and magnetic resonance imaging (MRI) cholangiopancreatography (Fig. 63.3) (see Chs. 15, 18, and 19). Current reviews of the diagnostic imaging modalities of bile duct cysts with representative images are referenced (Kim et al, 1995; Levy & Rohrmann, 2003; Savader et al, 1991a, 1991b). Although hepatobiliary scintigraphy has been useful in identifying bile duct cysts, its clinical value is limited because the information is functional and not anatomic and only complements direct cholangiography or dimensional imaging.

Ultrasonography is noninvasive and accurate and permits visualization of adjacent liver and pancreas to define cyst extent. The ultrasound features of bile duct cysts have been well defined for type I bile duct cysts and the variants of Caroli's disease (Akhan et al, 1994; Kim et al, 1995; Levy & Rohrmann, 2003; Todani et al, 1978). Ultrasound of type I cysts simply shows an irregular hypoechoic segmental dilation of the extrahepatic bile duct. Focal duct wall thickening or nodularity should arouse suspicion for cancer in an adult. Ductal stones within the cyst also can be identified by typical echogenic features and acoustic shadowing. The absence of septations on ultrasound distinguishes bile duct cysts from extrahepatic cystadenomas (Nagorney et al, 1984b). Although the sensitivity of ultrasound is excellent for cysts involving the bile duct proximal to the pancreas, ultrasound is limited in adults in identifying choledochoceles because of the frequency of bowel gas overlying the terminal common bile duct and the small size of these cysts.

Caroli's disease is clinically recognized by multiple cysts adjacent to the major intrahepatic bile ducts on ultrasound (Bruneton et al, 1983). Cysts may be unilobar or bilobar. Confirmation of communication of the intrahepatic cysts to the bile ducts can be confirmed by scintigraphy (Sty et al, 1978) or CT with biliary contrast medium (Musante et al, 1982). CT combined with intravenous cholangiography is useful for demonstration of cyst communication with the biliary tract (Hoglund et al, 1990). Intravenous cholangiography is performed 2 hours before abdominal CT. The sensitivity of CT allows for accurate identification of accumulated contrast material within the cyst if communication is present and accurate definition of the bile duct cyst.

Some form of cholangiography, with direct or indirect imaging (MRI cholangiopancreatography or CT), is required in all patients. Direct cholangiography is the preferred diagnostic modality for accurate classification of bile duct cysts (Matsumoto et al, 1977a; Todani et al, 1977). All bile duct cysts communicate with the ductal system. Direct cholangiography defines the pancreaticobiliary ductal anatomy, the configuration and extent of the cyst, stones within the biliary and pancreatic ducts, ductal strictures, and polypoid filling defects suggestive of malignancy. Direct cholangiography also provides good definition of the relationship between the distal bile duct and a type I cyst or the extrahepatic component of a type IVA cyst and the pancreatic duct. Typically, the bile duct cyst joins the pancreatic duct 2 to 4 cm proximal to the duodenum (Fig. 63.4), resulting in a long common channel (ampulla) (Jona et al, 1979; Komi et al, 1992; Ono et al, 1982; Rattner et al, 1983). The angle of fusion between the distal bile duct and pancreatic duct can vary

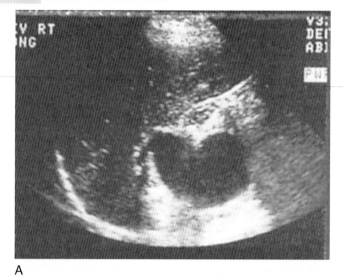

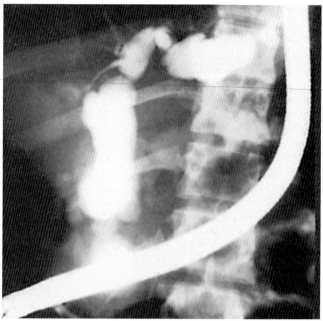

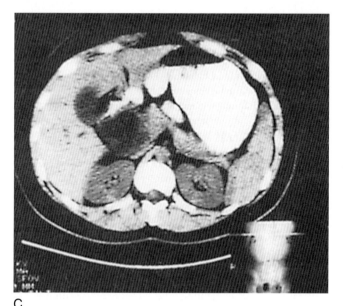

Fig. 63.3. Ultrasound (**A**), ERCP (**B**), and CT (**C**) showing a type IVA cyst with fusiform dilation of the common bile duct and the left intrahepatic ductal system.

widely and has led to a subclassification of cyst types (Komi et al, 1992). Anatomic definition of the pancreaticobiliary ductal junction is crucial as a guide during operative management of bile duct cysts to avoid intraoperative damage of the pancreatic duct during cyst excision, to recognize stones impacted within the common channel or junction, and to exclude distal tumors. Regardless of method, complete cholangiographic visualization of the entire biliary and pancreatic ductal systems is essential in these patients because failure to recognize segmental areas of dilation within the liver or pancreas may lead to sepsis, subsequent cholangitis, pain, pancreatitis, and eventual reoperation from otherwise occult pathology.

PTC and ERCP (see Ch. 20) have advantages and disadvantages in the diagnosis of bile duct cysts. Regardless of method, large volumes of radiographic contrast material may be required for complete visualization of the bile ducts. Adults without previous cystenterostomy probably are best evaluated by ERCP because it permits a focused view of the pancreaticobiliary ductal junction through the papilla (Komi et al, 1992; Savader et al, 1991b). Carcinoma can be confirmed by biopsy or brush cytology. Intracystic stones can be extracted after papillotomy to relieve

severe cholangitis before surgery. Cholangitis can be relieved with temporary endoscopic biliary stenting until definitive operation. Endoscopy also allows visualization of the esophagus and stomach to exclude signs of portal hypertension. The endoscopist should attempt to examine the ductal bifurcation and the lining of the cyst if a prior cystoduodenostomy allows introduction of the endoscope into the biliary tree. Endoscopically directed biopsy of an intracystic mass should be performed to exclude malignancy. Obstructing balloons should be available to ensure that complete radiographic filling of the biliary tree is possible, especially in patients with prior cystoduodenostomy. Endoscopy of the cyst through a cystenterostomy also may permit diagnosis of intraductal stenoses by membranes or septa at the confluence of the major bile ducts in patients with type IVA cysts (Ando et al, 1995). The procedure of choice for a type III cyst or choledochocele is ERCP because endoscopic papillotomy is potentially therapeutic (Sarris & Tsang, 1989; Venu et al, 1984).

PTC is an efficacious alternative to ERCP in the diagnosis of bile duct cysts, although its use has declined because of the versatility of ERCP. PTC is most advantageous in patients with a prior Roux-en-Y cystojejunostomy or hepaticojejunostomy

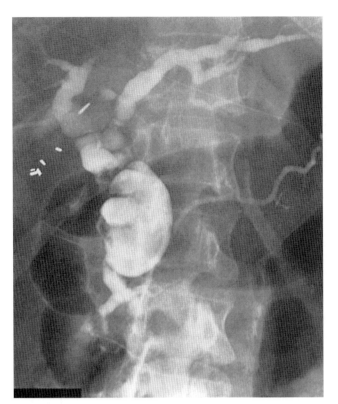

Fig. 63.4. ERCP shows the most frequent anomaly of the bile duct cyst and pancreatic duct anatomy with perpendicular fusion of the distal bile duct or cyst to the pancreatic duct and the presence of a long common channel.

because of limited endoscopic access depending on the length of the Roux-en-Y limb and in patients with type IV bile duct cysts in whom ductal strictures or tumor prevents complete visualization of intrahepatic cysts by ERCP (Savader et al, 1991b). Percutaneous biliary drainage may be performed after PTC for control of biliary sepsis or for stenting after surgical reconstruction. PTC is limited particularly in patients with a widely patent cystenterostomy, in whom runoff of the contrast precludes complete evaluation of the cyst, and in patients with huge extrahepatic cysts, in whom intracystic contrast material is superimposed over the pancreaticobiliary junction and obscures the radiographic definition.

MRI cholangiography (see Ch. 19) has provided equivalent or superior imaging of bile duct cysts compared with conventional cholangiography (Fulcher & Turner, 2002; Kim et al, 2000). MRI cholangiography has provided an accurate anatomic definition of bile duct cysts in neonates, infants, young children, and adults (Kim et al, 2002; Miyazaki et al, 1998) inclusive of Caroli's disease (Guy et al, 2002). MRI cholangiography application to adults can be anticipated because image acquisition in adults is not hindered by the technical difficulties posed by children. Early limitations of MRI cholangiography in defining the anomolous pancreaticobiliary junction have been reduced by improvements in MRI resolution. MRI lacks therapeutic capability, however, and biopsy of suspicious lesions is not possible.

Associated Hepatobiliary Pathology

Adults with bile duct cysts frequently harbor concurrent hepatobiliary or pancreatic pathology that complicates or confounds

clinical management (Gigot et al, 1996; Komi et al, 1984; Lenriot et al, 1998; Liu et al, 2002; Nicholl et al, 2004; Visser et al, 2004). Cystolithiasis, hepaticolithiasis, calculous cholecystitis, pancreatitis, cholangiocarcinoma, intrahepatic abscess, and cirrhosis with portal hypertension are potential problems that may precipitate or complicate treatment. Although spontaneous perforation of bile duct cysts has been reported in infants and children, the complication has not been recognized in adults (Ando et al, 1998). Studies in adults suggest that nearly 80% of adults with bile duct cysts have one or more cyst-related complications (Nagorney et al, 1984a; Ono et al, 1982), the incidence of which is decreased if excision is used routinely in infants and children (Gigot et al, 1996; Visser et al, 2004).

Cystolithiasis is the most frequent accompanying condition in adults with bile duct cysts. In contrast to the low prevalence of cystolithiasis in pediatric patients (Flanigan, 1975; Matsumoto et al, 1977a, 1977b; Rattner et al, 1983), the prevalence of intracystic stones ranges from 2% to 72% in adults (Chijiiwa & Koga, 1993; Lenriot et al, 1998; Nagorney et al, 1984a; Todani et al, 1988). Although the composition of intracystic stones has not been analyzed biochemically, most intracystic stones have been described as soft, earthy, and pigmented in appearance, supporting bile stasis as a primary etiologic factor (Matsumoto et al, 1977a, 1977b). Typically, these stones are associated with thick, viscous bile, which may form bile duct or cyst casts. Cystolithiasis frequently complicates anastomotic strictures after previous cystenterostomies, suggesting that stasis and infection are major factors contributing to the pathogenesis of these stones (Söreide et al, 2004; Uno et al, 1996). Stones can develop in a cyst remnant in the head of the pancreas after incomplete excision of the extrahepatic component of a type I or IVA bile duct cyst (Fig. 63.5). The composition of these stones is similar to pancreatic calculi and may cause recurrent pancreatitis or episodic abdominal pain.

Hepaticolithiasis has been recognized with increasing frequency with long-term follow-up and may occur with or without evidence of anastomotic stricture (Fig. 63.6) (Deziel et al, 1986; Gigot et al, 1996; Uno et al, 1996). Some patients have complete or partial stricture of the cyst-enteric anastomosis, and hepaticolithiasis develops as a consequence of proximal migration

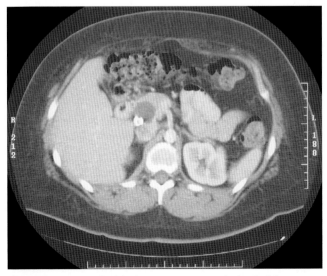

Fig. 63.5. CT scan of a bile duct cyst remnant in the head of the pancreas harboring a calcified stone.

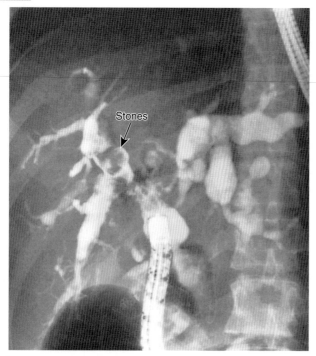

Fig. 63.6. ERCP of a type IVA bile duct cyst showing multiple intrahepatic stones and a patent choledochoduodenostomy.

of intracystic stones. Usually, hepaticolithiasis occurs in type IV bile duct cysts. A study has shown that more than 80% of type IV bile duct cysts are associated with a membranous or septal stenosis of the major lobar bile ducts near the confluence (Ando et al, 1995; Todani et al, 2003). Stenosis of the major ducts should be sought in all patients with hepaticolithiasis. Intrahepatic stones may be sequestered in segmental ducts, leading to further localized intrahepatic ductal dilation or subsequent intrahepatic abscess formation.

Gallbladder disease is a frequent complication of patients with bile duct cysts. Gallbladder disease can occur de novo leading to the incidental discovery of bile duct cysts or can evolve after treatment for bile duct cysts. In particular, a gallbladder that is not excised as part of the initial treatment for symptomatic bile duct cysts is frequently a subsequent source of biliary tract disease. Acute and chronic cholecystitis, with or without stones, has been recognized in these patients. Similar to cystolithiasis, cholelithiasis in patients with bile duct cysts is typically bilirubinate in appearance. Stasis is probably involved in the etiology of cholelithiasis in patients with bile duct cysts.

The association of pancreatitis with bile duct cysts is a well-recognized entity, particularly in adults. The prevalence ranges from 2% to 70% (Lipsett et al, 1994; Nagorney et al, 1984a; Okada et al, 1990; Rattner et al, 1983; Swisher et al, 1994). The true incidence of pancreatitis is difficult to determine because the diagnosis of pancreatitis is based on the clinical findings of epigastric pain, nausea and vomiting, and hyperamylasemia. Another clinical condition, the common channel syndrome (Jona et al, 1979) or pseudopancreatitis (Todani et al, 1990), may mimic these findings completely, overestimating the true incidence of pancreatitis. Whether differentiation between these two entities has clinical or therapeutic significance is unclear. Pancreatitis associated with bile duct cysts is typically mild. The pattern of pancreatitis is acute and often relapsing, but objective

pancreatic dysfunction seldom occurs. Chronic pancreatitis associated with bile duct cysts is rare.

The pathogenesis of pancreatitis in patients with bile duct cysts is related primarily to the anomalous pancreaticobiliary ductal anatomy and the presence of cystolithiasis or cholelithiasis. Numerous authors have confirmed that the base of the extrahepatic cyst or distal common bile duct in type I or IV cysts joins the main pancreatic duct more proximally than normal, resulting in a long common channel (Jona et al, 1979; Nagorney et al, 1984a; Ono et al, 1982; Rattner et al, 1983; Swisher et al, 1994). The type of anomolous pancreaticobiliary junction may influence the probability of developing pancreatitis. Two distinct anomolous pancreaticobiliary junctions have been described: type 1, in which the major pancreatic duct joins the side of the common bile duct, and type 2, in which the distal common bile duct joins the side of the main pancreatic duct. The type 2 anomalous junction is more likely to result in pancreatitis anatomically (Chiijiwa & Koga, 1993). Obstruction of the pancreatic duct at the pancreaticobiliary junction or distally in the common channel (ampulla) by stones is postulated currently as the precipitating factor. A few studies (Nagorney et al, 1984a; Rattner et al, 1983) have shown an association between biliary tract stones and bile duct cysts and pancreatitis. Stone impaction within the pancreaticobiliary junction may cause pancreatitis (Fig. 63.7). An alternative mechanism for pancreatitis is bile reflux into the pancreatic duct (Okada et al, 1983; Swisher et al, 1994). The anatomy of the pancreaticobiliary ductal system is conducive to bile reflux (Fumino et al, 2002). Despite the presence of APBDJ in most patients with pancreatitis, some patients with bile duct cysts and pancreatitis have a normal pancreaticobiliary anatomy (Swisher et al, 1994). Some patients with choledochoceles also may have recurrent acute pancreatitis (Martin et al, 1992; Masetti et al, 1996). Obstructive pancreatitis also has been described from mucus produced by metaplastic epithelia in a bile duct cyst (Dussaulz-Garin et al, 2000).

A significant association between bile duct cysts and hepatobiliary malignancies is well established (Bismuth & Krissat, 1999; Dayton et al, 1983; Fieber & Nance, 1997; Flanigan, 1977;

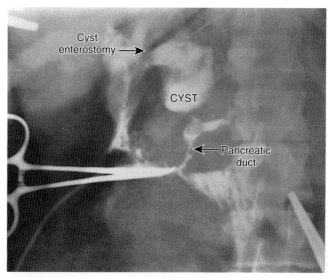

Fig. 63.7. Intraoperative cholangiopancreatography in a patient with clinical pancreatitis and a type I cyst shows a stone impacted in the anomalous junction of the distal common bile duct and pancreatic duct. Previous cystenterostomy also is identified.

Ishibashi et al, 1997; Komi et al, 1989; Rossi et al, 1987; Todani et al, 1979; Tsuchiya et al, 1977). The incidence of hepatobiliary malignancies associated with bile duct cysts has ranged from 2.5% to 28% (Fieber & Nance, 1997; Flanigan, 1975; Ono et al, 1982). Malignancies of the hepatobiliary tract arising in or associated with bile duct cysts have included cholangiocarcinoma or adenocarcinoma, adenoacanthoma, squamous cell carcinoma, anaplastic carcinoma, bile duct sarcoma, hepatoma, pancreatic carcinoma, and gallbladder carcinoma (Fieber & Nance, 1997; Ono et al, 1982; Todani et al, 1979, 1987; Tsuchiya et al, 1977). Cholangiocarcinoma is the most common malignancy associated with bile duct cysts, and its incidence is 20 to 30 times greater than the incidence of bile duct carcinoma in the general population (Flanigan, 1975; Söreide et al, 2004). The incidence of cyst-associated malignancy is age related, increasing from 0.7% in the first decade of life to greater than 14% after 20 years of age (Nicholl et al, 2004; Voyles et al, 1983). The mean age of patients with malignancies associated with bile duct cysts is 32 years (Ishibashi et al, 1997; Ono et al, 1982). Risk of malignancy remains high even after resection of the bile duct cyst (Ishibashi et al, 1997; Koike et al, 2002; Watanabe et al, 1999). These findings underscore the necessity for a high index of suspicion of carcinoma in adults.

Malignancies associated with bile duct cysts may arise within the cyst or elsewhere within the liver or pancreaticobiliary tract. Only 57% of tumors are intracystic (Fig. 63.8) (Flanigan, 1977) and may occur after cyst excision (Fig. 63.9) (Ishibashi et al, 1997; Watanabe et al, 1999). Malignancies may be associated with any type of bile duct cyst, although the prevalence of cancer is significantly greater in type I and IV cysts. Caroli's disease (type V cysts) also has been associated with an increased incidence of carcinoma (Dayton et al, 1983).

The etiology of cyst-associated malignancies is unknown. Bile stagnation with the development of intrabiliary carcinogens

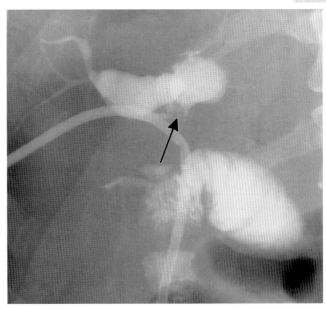

Fig. 63.9. PTC of a hilar cholangiocarcinoma *(arrow)* after excision of a type I bile duct cyst and Roux-en-Y hepaticojejunostomy.

leading to epithelial malignant degeneration is postulated as the most likely mechanism (Flanigan, 1977; Todani et al, 1979). Unconjugated deoxycholate and lithocholate have been associated with biliary metaplasia and mutagenicity, which may lead to neoplasia. Although secondary bile acids have been found in bile duct cysts with cancer (Reveille et al, 1990), neither their relative nor their absolute concentration in patients with bile duct cysts has differed in the presence or absence of cancer (Chijiiwa et al, 1993), suggesting other factors as primary carcinogens. Epithelia of dilated and nondilated bile ducts in patients with anomalous pancreaticobiliary junctions can exhibit k-*ras* and *p53* mutations and microsatellite instability (Matsubara et al, 2002; Nagai et al, 1999, 2002). An association between cystolithiasis and malignancy has not been established, although stasis and bacterial overgrowth associated with stones may lead to secondary bile acid formation. Long-term survival of patients with bile duct cysts and malignancy is rare. Delayed diagnosis, advanced stage of disease, and intra-abdominal seeding from previous operations and tumor multicentricity generally preclude curative resection. Whether primary prophylactic excision of cysts in childhood can reduce the incidence of malignancy is unknown (Ono et al, 1982; Voyles et al, 1983).

Rare hepatobiliary problems arising in adults with bile duct cysts include intrahepatic abscess, portal hypertension, and cyst rupture. The former conditions usually result from recurrent cholangitis and biliary obstruction after strictures of prior cystenterostomies. Large solitary hepatic abscesses represent an end stage of obstructive cholangitis and usually are completely obstructed, pus-filled intrahepatic cysts. These intrahepatic abscesses occur predominantly in the left intrahepatic duct (Mercadier et al, 1984; Ramond et al, 1984) and may be due in part to angulation of the left main duct. Adjacent liver parenchyma is fibrotic and atrophic and may harbor miliary abscesses within the periphery of the bile ducts.

Portal hypertension associated with choledochal cysts may be due to secondary biliary cirrhosis or fibrosis, portal vein thrombosis, or Caroli's disease with congenital hepatic fibrosis (Kim, 1981;

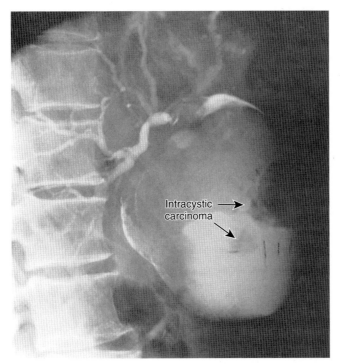

Intracystic carcinoma

Fig. 63.8. PTC of a type I choledochal cyst with a polypoid intracystic cholangiocarcinoma.

Martin & Rowe, 1979; Ono et al, 1982). Portal hypertension in adults generally is preceded by numerous operations for cyst drainage (Chaudhary et al, 1997; Hewitt et al, 1995; Lipsett et al, 1994; Nicholl et al, 2004). Portal hypertension in patients with bile duct cysts is manifested clinically by hepatosplenomegaly, hematemesis, melena, or ascites. Portal hypertension causes a hypervascularity of the hepatoduodenal ligament with prominent pericholedochal varices. Hepatic functional reserve deteriorates progressively, and hepatic coma and renal failure may be precipitated by recurrent cholangitis. Clinical suspicion or documentation of portal hypertension dictates careful angiographic evaluation before operative management.

Cyst rupture, albeit rare even in children and infants, can occur in adults. Pregnancy may be a predisposing factor (Bostanoglu et al, 2000; Hewitt et al, 1995).

TREATMENT

General Principles

The surgical management of adults with bile duct cysts is based on cyst type and the presence of associated hepatobiliary pathology. The aims of preoperative management are complete cholangiographic definition of the extent of the cystic process and associated ductal pathology and control of biliary infections. Specifically, in adults, any patient with recurrent symptoms after prior cyst-related operations must be evaluated for anastomotic

stricture, ductal stones, biliary tract malignancies, and cirrhosis and portal hypertension. Broad-spectrum antibiotics that are concentrated in bile and are effective against proximal enteric bacteria are preferred for control of biliary infections. Patients in whom sepsis fails to resolve with intravenous antibiotics require preoperative percutaneous or endoscopic drainage of infected bile duct cysts, which usually affords control of sepsis before definitive operation.

The definitive treatment of bile duct cysts is surgical. The therapeutic alternatives for the treatment of each type of bile duct cyst are shown in Fig. 63.10. In general, all bile duct cysts should be excised and bile flow re-established by mucosa-to-mucosa biliary-enteric anastomosis. If complete excision is not feasible, partial cyst excision and Roux-en-Y cystojejunostomy to an epithelial-lined portion of the cyst remnant is preferred. External drainage alone has no definitive role in the surgical management of bile duct cysts. Routine cholangioscopy is employed in adults to exclude retained ductal stones and ductal malignancies. Finally, long-term follow-up must be maintained in adults because of the age-related risk of malignancy and the frequency of late anastomotic strictures in patients treated without cyst resection.

Type I Cyst

The treatment of choice for type I bile duct cysts in adults is total cystectomy and Roux-en-Y hepaticojejunostomy. Cyst excision

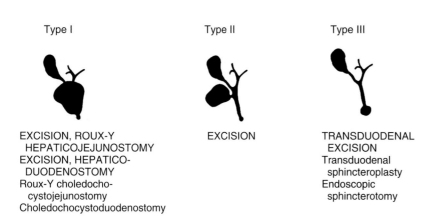

Type I

EXCISION, ROUX-Y
  HEPATICOJEJUNOSTOMY
EXCISION, HEPATICO-
  DUODENOSTOMY
Roux-Y choledocho-
  cystojejunostomy
Choledochocystoduodenostomy

Type II

EXCISION

Type III

TRANSDUODENAL
  EXCISION
Transduodenal
  sphincteroplasty
Endoscopic
  sphincterotomy

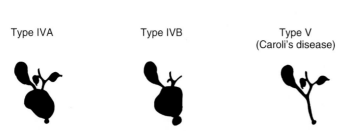

Type IVA

Extrahepatic component
EXCISION, ROUX-Y
  HEPATICOJEJUNOSTOMY
EXCISION, HEPATICO-
  DUODENOSTOMY
Intrahepatic component
Hepatic resection ±
  Roux-Y hepatico-
  jejunostomy
Transhepatic intubation

Type IVB

EXCISION, ROUX-Y
  HEPATICOJEJUNOSTOMY
  OR HEPATICO-
  DUODENOSTOMY
± transduodenal
  sphincteroplasty

Type V
(Caroli's disease)

HEPATIC RESECTION
Roux-Y intrahepatic
  cholangiojejunostomy
Transhepatic intubation
Orthotopic liver
  transplant

Fig. 63.10. Surgical options for treatment of choledochal cysts. Preferred treatment is capitalized.

eliminates the primary site of bile stasis and permits a biliary-enteric anastomosis of normal jejunum and epithelial-lined proximal bile duct. The theoretical advantages of this approach include a reduced incidence of anastomotic strictures, stone formation, cholangitis, and intracystic malignancy. The purported advantages of a mucosa-to-mucosa anastomosis have been extrapolated from similar biliary reconstructions for other biliary tract problems (i.e., benign strictures, common bile duct stones, and suppurative cholangitis). Reduction in risk of malignancy is based on the premises that (1) the potential carcinogenic effect of pancreatic secretions is eliminated because of total diversion from the biliary tract, (2) the production of mutagenic secondary bile acids is reduced because bacterial overgrowth in the bile is less frequent, and (3) abnormal cyst epithelium is excised.

The clinical results of cyst excision and Roux-en-Y hepaticojejunostomy have been excellent. Morbidity and mortality of excision have not been greater than that of drainage by Roux-en-Y choledochocystojejunostomy (Flanigan, 1975; Liu et al, 2002; Nagorney et al, 1984a; Nicholl et al, 2004; Ono et al, 1982; Rattner et al, 1983; Stain et al, 1995; Todani et al, 1978; Visser et al, 2004). Most reports with late follow-up have confirmed that most patients remain asymptomatic after excision (Chen et al, 1996; Chijiiwa et al, 1993; Gigot et al, 1996; Lenriot et al, 1998; Nagorney et al, 1984a; Ono et al, 1982; Rattner et al, 1983; Uno et al, 1996). Recurrent cholangitis from anastomotic strictures occurs in 10% to 25% of patients (Chijiiwa & Tanaka, 1994; Gigot et al, 1996; Ono et al, 1982; Rattner et al, 1983; Uno et al, 1996). Although reduction of malignancy by cyst excision has been suggested by some series (Todani et al, 1987), cancer has developed after cyst excision (Nagorney et al, 1984a; Watanabe et al, 1999; Yamamoto et al, 1996). Previous cystenterostomy does not preclude cyst excision (Chaudhary et al, 1997; Gigot et al, 1996; Ono et al, 1982; Todani et al, 1988). Although morbidity is increased, low mortality and excellent long-term functional results can be achieved in adults with previous cystenterostomy (Gigot et al, 1996; Kaneko et al, 1999; Nicholl et al, 2004; Söreide et al, 2004). Excision should be undertaken for recurrent symptoms. Biliary-enteric continuity can be re-established by hepaticoduodenostomy after cyst excision, although this method has been employed infrequently in adults (Todani et al, 1981). An advantage of hepaticoduodenostomy is that the residual biliary epithelium is partially accessible to direct visualization by endoscopy (Todani et al, 1988), although diversion of pancreatic juice is incomplete. Technical factors influencing choice of hepaticoenterostomy (Roux-en-Y hepaticojejunostomy versus hepaticoduodenostomy) include aberrant hilar ductal anatomy, ductal strictures, ductal size, and hilar arterial anatomy (Todani et al, 1998). Mobility of the duodenum may limit the use of the duodenum in some patients. In brief, a large ductal confluence without fibrous bandlike strictures favors hepaticoduodenostomy.

Cyst excision in adults differs technically from the approach generally advocated for pediatric patients (Altman, 1994; Lilly, 1979; Lipsett & Pitt, 2003). Most adults have had prior cyst drainage procedures that may result in dense subhepatic adhesions. Recurrent cholangitis may result in epithelial degeneration or ulceration, which can obscure or mimic malignancy, and regenerative epithelium may be densely adherent to the cyst wall. Although the vascularity of the pericholedochal tissue may increase, most often hypervascularity is limited to the ductal wall, unless portal hypertension is present. In contrast to reports in pediatric patients (Lilly, 1979), complete dissection of the

intracystic epithelium from the posterior cyst wall after excision of the anterior wall may be difficult. Because of the increased age-related incidence of cancer and its often occult operative and radiographic manifestations, total cyst excision to remove all intracystic epithelium is essential in adults. Only extensive hypervascularity from portal vein thrombosis or secondary biliary cirrhosis with portal hypertension would preclude excision.

Technically, cyst excision in adults can be accomplished by initially mobilizing the gallbladder from its bed to dissect the cyst away from the hilar structures. The portal vein is identified. Isolation and proximal control of the hepatic artery before dissection of the posterior cyst wall can be helpful, especially if hypervascularity and dense adhesions are encountered. Before division of the cyst, the distal cyst is dissected from the pancreas to identify the pancreaticobiliary ductal junction (Ando et al, 1996; Nicholl et al, 2004). The intrapancreatic portion of the cyst is separated from the pancreas along the loose areolar plane between these structures. Meticulous fine suture ligature of collateral vessels on the surface of the pancreas, rather than cautery coagulation, more reliably prevents postoperative hemorrhage. Preoperative definition of the ductal anatomy by cholangiopancreatography is important to avoid damage to the pancreatic ducts. The cyst is transected distally within the head of the pancreas, and the distal bile duct is ligated carefully just proximal to its junction with the pancreatic duct to prevent narrowing of the pancreatic duct. The cyst is mobilized proximally to the ductal confluence, the proximal cyst is transected, and the cyst is removed. Biliary-enteric flow is re-established through a wide mucosa-to-mucosa Roux-en-Y hepaticojejunostomy at the level of the hilum (see Ch. 30, Figs. 30.9 to 30.12) or hepaticoduodenostomy.

If a previous cystenterostomy has been performed, the same technique is used for excision after the cystenterostomy has been divided. An existing Roux-en-Y loop can be reused for the new anastomosis. Hepatic arteries should be positioned posterior to the cystenterostomy to reduce potential injury in case of reoperation (Fig. 63.11). Rarely, the extrahepatic component of the cyst is associated with a dense reactive pancreatitis, which may dictate pancreaticoduodenectomy for complete excision. The intrapancreatic portion of bile duct cysts should be excised to avoid a focus for future stone development.

Laparoscopic treatment of type I bile duct cysts has been reported (Chowbey et al, 2002; Shimura et al, 1998; Tanaka et al, 2001). Laparoscopically assisted and complete laparoscopic resection and Roux-en-Y hepaticojejunostomy have been performed successfully and warrant further evaluation.

Portal hypertension secondary to biliary cirrhosis and inflammatory adhesions from severe pancreatitis or past drainage procedures rarely preclude cyst excision. In these circumstances, Roux-en-Y choledochocystojejunostomy is the preferred alternative treatment for type I choledochal cysts. Perioperative morbidity and mortality are similar to that of cyst excision. Adequate long-term functional results from Roux-en-Y cyst drainage can be expected in 60% to 70% of patients (Lenriot et al, 1998; Nagorney et al, 1984a; Ono et al, 1982; Rattner et al, 1983). Long-term results are improved by partial cyst excision in an effort to ensure a mucosa-to-mucosa biliary-enteric anastomosis (Gigot et al, 1996). When either excision or Roux-en-Y drainage is performed, intraoperative choledochoscopy to exclude retained ductal stones and to obtain a biopsy specimen of the abnormal epithelium to exclude malignancy is advised. In patients with recurrent acute pancreatitis and unresectable cysts, intracystic

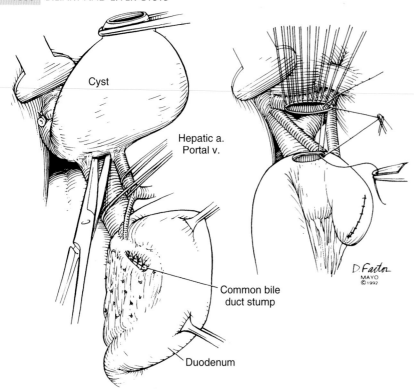

Fig. 63.11. Isolation of vascular structures, complete excision of the cyst with closure of the distal stump, and biliary-enteric reconstruction with hepaticojejunostomy with a Roux-en-Y loop.

closure of the base of the cyst proximal to its junction to the pancreatic duct or concurrent transduodenal sphincteroplasty should be employed to prevent further episodes of pancreatitis (Nagorney et al, 1984a; Ono et al, 1982; Rattner et al, 1983). Careful long-term follow-up is essential because of the late development of malignancies, recurrent ductal stones, and anastomotic stricture (Chijiiwa & Tanaka, 1994; Fieber & Nance, 1997; Todani et al, 1998; Uno et al, 1996).

Portal decompression may be required before biliary reconstruction in patients who develop portal hypertension (Nagorney et al, 1984a). Preoperative assessment of these patients should include hepatic arteriography and portography. In general, central splenorenal shunts are preferred because portal decompression can be performed in an area distant from the subhepatic pericystic inflammation. Generally, drainage is undertaken 6 to 12 weeks after portosystemic shunting. Alternatively, transjugular intrahepatic portosystemic stenting can be employed for preoperative portal decompression.

Type II Cyst

The treatment of choice for type II bile duct cysts is cyst excision (Flanigan, 1975; Powell et al, 1981). Because of the low incidence of type II cysts, however, experience is limited. Reported results after excision have been excellent (Kouraklis et al, 1996; Lopez et al, 1991; Nagorney et al, 1984a; Powell et al, 1981; Söreide et al, 2004). Technically, excision of type II bile duct cysts is similar to that of cholecystectomy. Depending on the size of the neck of the cyst at its junction with the common bile duct, the neck can be closed primarily or with T-tube decompression of the common duct. Excision with Roux-en-Y hepaticojejunostomy also has been successful. but has no clinical advantage to excision alone (Benhidjeb et al, 1994).

Type III Cyst (Choledochocele)

Choledochoceles are true cysts of the distal bile duct protruding into the duodenum. Patients present clinically with biliary colic, cholangitis, or pancreatitis (Masetti et al, 1996). Typically, choledochoceles are small (≤2 cm). A classification scheme for choledochoceles has been proposed (Sarris & Tsang, 1989). Until more recently, transduodenal cyst excision with or without sphincterotomy was the treatment of choice (Flanigan, 1975; Powell et al, 1981; Venu et al, 1984). Endoscopic sphincterotomy and cyst unroofing has become the treatment of choice (Chatila et al, 1999; Ladas et al, 1995; Martin et al, 1992; Masetti et al, 1996). The excellent long-term results with endoscopic treatment coupled with the diagnostic advantage of ERCP in defining the terminal pancreatic biliary anatomy favor the endoscopic approach. Although transduodenal excision eliminates the risk of malignancy, the fact that only three cases of carcinoma in choledochoceles have been documented confirms that the risk of cancer alone is inadequate to justify this surgical approach (Masetti et al, 1996).

Because damage to the major pancreatic duct is the major source of operative morbidity and mortality, identification of the duct of Wirsung is paramount before transduodenal cyst excision or sphincteroplasty because of numerous pancreatic biliary ductal variations (Komi et al, 1989, 1992). The pancreatic duct of Wirsung may enter the posterior wall of the choledochocele or enter normally into the duodenum at the inferior aspect of the major papilla adjacent to the choledochocele (Sarris & Tsang, 1989). Before cyst excision or sphincteroplasty, the pancreatic duct orifice must be identified at the papilla to avoid damage to the pancreatic duct. If the major pancreatic duct empties normally into the duodenum, the pancreatic duct should be left in situ and not transected during choledochocele excision. If the pancreatic duct enters into the posterior wall of the cyst, the distal common bile duct and the duct of Wirsung should be implanted separately into the duodenal mucosa after cyst excision (Powell et al, 1981).

Type IV Cyst

The treatment of choice for type IV bile duct cysts is cyst excision of extrahepatic cyst and Roux-en-Y hepaticojejunostomy (Mercadier et al, 1984; Nagorney et al, 1984a; Todani et al, 1984a). The extrahepatic component of type IVA and IVB cysts is approached as a type I bile duct cyst. Transduodenal sphincteroplasty and Roux-en-Y hepaticojejunostomy complete the treatment of type IVB cysts, which have a choledochocele component. Type IVA cysts require more selective management because of the wide range of problems associated with the intrahepatic component of these cysts (Ando et al, 1997; Chijiiwa & Tanaka, 1994; Nagorney et al, 1984a; Todani et al, 1984a; Uno et al, 1996). In patients with type IVA cysts in whom the intrahepatic bile duct cysts are not complicated by hilar or intrahepatic ductal strictures, intrahepatic stones, intrahepatic abscess, or malignancy, biliary-enteric continuity should be restored by a wide Roux-en-Y hepaticojejunostomy at the bile duct confluence (Todani et al, 1988, 1998). Additionally, the hepaticojejunostomy must incorporate any ductal anomaly. In patients with stones sequestered within the intrahepatic cysts, with refractory ductal strictures distal to the intrahepatic cysts, or with intrahepatic abscess secondary to chronic cholangitis, the abnormal hepatic segment should be resected. Bile flow is restored by Roux-en-Y hepaticojejunostomy. Lobar hepatic resection usually is required to eliminate the complicated unilobar intrahepatic cyst or lobar atrophy (Lipsett & Pitt, 2003). In addition to the hepaticojejunostomy at the hilus, Roux-en-Y cholangiojejunostomy incorporating the segmental bile duct of the resected segment may optimize intrahepatic bile drainage further. In patients with type IVA cysts, with complicated intrahepatic cysts involving both lobes of the liver or cirrhosis, transhepatic tubes can be added to the Roux-en-Y hepaticojejunostomy for access to the biliary tree for diagnosis and treatment.

The results of the treatment of type IVA cysts have been reviewed by several centers (Ando et al, 1997; Gigot et al, 1996; Lenriot et al, 1998; Liu et al, 2002; Nicholl et al, 2004; Todani et al, 1998; Uno et al, 1996). Although treatment varied widely because of the spectrum of pathology associated with these cysts, the results of cyst drainage alone without excision of either the intrahepatic or extrahepatic cystic components were considered satisfactory or good in less than 50% of patients (Todani et al, 1984a). In contrast, 90% of patients who had excision of the extrahepatic component of the type IVA cyst had good results, whether or not the intrahepatic component was resected, although late complications occurred in nearly 30% of patients (Lenriot et al, 1998). These findings suggest that adequate treatment of the extrahepatic component in these patients may provide effective prophylaxis for biliary problems associated with intrahepatic cystic disease; however, more recent studies (Ando et al, 1997; Todani et al, 1998, 2003) emphasize the importance of addressing the presence of variant ductal anatomy and stenoses at the hilus. If intrahepatic ductal stenosis or aberrant ducts are not recognized and addressed during extrahepatic cyst excision, subsequent reoperation often is necessary. Membranous or bridgelike stenoses should be excised circumferentially to their base. The long-term results of the treatment of type IVB cysts in adults are similar to those of type I choledochal cysts. Although patients with type IVA cysts and portal hypertension may be approached by proximal splenorenal shunts before cyst drainage, liver transplantation may provide a more durable solution. Resection of intrahepatic cysts in cirrhotic patients is associated with an increase in morbidity and mortality and generally is contraindicated.

Caroli's Disease

Treatment of Caroli's disease depends on the extent of the intrahepatic bile duct cysts and the presence of congenital hepatic fibrosis, secondary biliary cirrhosis, or carcinoma. Caroli's disease in adults may present in a localized form limited to one hepatic lobe or segment or a diffuse form involving the entire intrahepatic biliary tree (Fig. 63.12) (Barros et al, 1979; Dayton et al, 1983; Mercadier et al, 1984; Witlin et al, 1982). Most adults with Caroli's disease have a unilobar fusiform dilation of the intrahepatic ducts, most commonly involving the left ductal system (Mercadier et al, 1984; Ramond et al, 1984). In patients with Caroli's disease limited to one lobe of the liver without the presence of concurrent cirrhosis or hepatic fibrosis, hepatic resection, with or without Roux-en-Y cholangiojejunostomy, remains the treatment of choice. Cyst removal by hepatic resection provides the simplest solution to the recurrent problems of cholangitis, stone formation, and intrahepatic cancer (Mercadier et al, 1984; Todani et al, 1984a). Resection always is preferable to drainage if the liver parenchyma surrounding the cyst is atrophic. Segmental fibrosis and atrophy from complications

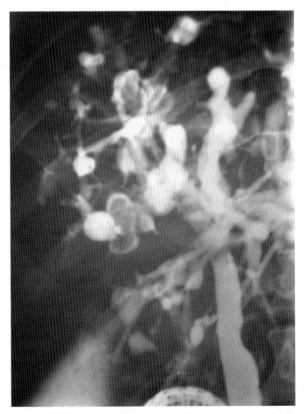

Fig. 63.12. ERCP of Caroli's disease and multiple saccular cysts of only the intrahepatic bile duct with intrahepatic stones.

of the underlying cyst is irreparable and does not respond to drainage and dictate segmental resection. Morbidity and mortality associated with hepatic resection for localized Caroli's disease has been minimal, and functional results have been good, although follow-up has been short (Mercadier et al, 1984; Ramond et al, 1984). Alternative approaches to localized intrahepatic Caroli's disease have included external T-tube biliary decompression or internal drainage via choledochoduodenostomy, Roux-en-Y choledochojejunostomy, or Roux-en-Y hepaticojejunostomy. These alternatives are often ineffective because ductal drainage is distal to the intrahepatic cysts (Witlin et al, 1982). In general, recurrent cholangitis, hepatic abscess formation, intrahepatic stone formation, and carcinoma eventually complicate these approaches. If resection in patients with localized Caroli's disease is not feasible, Roux-en-Y intrahepatic cholangiojejunostomy to the intrahepatic cyst is preferable (Mercadier et al, 1984). Long-term transanastomotic stents should be placed at operation to afford access to the biliary tree for future diagnostic and possibly therapeutic intervention.

The results of the treatment of Caroli's disease involving both lobes of the liver or associated with portal hypertension from congenital hepatic fibrosis or secondary biliary cirrhosis remain poor (Barros et al, 1979; Dayton et al, 1983; Mercadier et al, 1984). Most patients with diffuse Caroli's disease have chronic recurrent cholangitis, portal hypertension with variceal bleeding, and death secondary to liver failure or carcinoma. Long-term medical therapy, including antibiotics, analgesics, and litholytic agents, may improve but does not eliminate symptoms permanently. In selected patients with diffuse intrahepatic Caroli's disease but with dominant unilobar disease, extended hepatic resection has been advocated, but long-term benefit remains unproven (Mercadier et al, 1984). Long-term transhepatic decompression using bilobar silicone tubes has been successful in the management of recurrent cholangitis (Witlin et al, 1982). To date, the treatment of diffuse Caroli's disease remains disappointing, however. In light of the natural history of Caroli's disease (cirrhosis, variceal bleeding, and liver failure), hepatic transplantation offers the best chance of success. Orthotopic liver transplantation has been employed successfully for Caroli's disease (Scharschmidt, 1984). If the diagnosis of Caroli's disease is made, nonoperative medical treatment should be employed until the patient is considered a transplant candidate. Avoidance of numerous ineffective operative procedures reduces the technical risk of transplantation.

REFERENCES

Akhan O, et al, 1994: Choledochal cysts: ultrasonographic findings and correlation with other imaging modalities. Abdom Imaging 19:243-247.

Alonso-Lej F, et al, 1959: Congenital choledochal cysts, with a report of 2, and an analysis of 94 cases. Int Surg 108:1-30 (abstract).

Altman RP, 1994: Choledochal cyst. In Blumgart LH (ed): Surgery of the Liver and Biliary Tract, 2nd ed. Edinburgh, Churchill Livingstone, p 1177.

Ando H, et al, 1995: Congenital stenosis of the intrahepatic bile duct associated with choledochal cysts. J Am Coll Surg 181:426-430.

Ando H, et al, 1996: Complete excision of the intrapancreatic portion of choledochal cysts. J Am Coll Surg 183:317-321.

Ando H, et al, 1997: Operative treatment of congenital stenoses of the intrahepatic bile ducts in patients with choledochal cysts. Am J Surg 173:491-494.

Ando H, et al, 1998: Spontaneous perforation of choledochal cyst: a study of 13 cases. Eur J Pediatr Surg 8:23-25.

Babbitt DP, 1969: Congenital choledochal cysts: new etiological concept based on anomalous relationships of common bile duct and pancreatic bulb. Ann Radiol 12:231-240.

Barros JL, et al, 1979: Congenital cystic dilatation of the intrahepatic bile ducts (Caroli's disease): report of a case and review of the literature. Surgery 85:589-592.

Belli G, et al, 1998: Cystic dilatation of extrahepatic bile ducts in adulthood: diagnosis, surgical treatment and long-term results. HPB Surg 10:379-385.

Benhidjeb T, et al, 1994: Cystic dilatation of the common bile duct: surgical treatment and long-term results. Br J Surg 81:433-436.

Bismuth H, Krissat J, 1999: Choledochal cystic malignancies. Ann Oncol 10(suppl 4):S94-S98.

Bostanoglu S, et al, 2000: Ruptured choledochal cyst. HPB Surg 2:57-59.

Bruneton JN, et al, 1983: Congenital cysts of the liver in echography. J Radiol 64:471-476.

Caroli J, et al, 1958: La dilatation polykislique congenitale des voies biliaries intrahepatiques: essai de classification. Semnares des Hopitaux de Paris 34:488-495.

Chatila R, et al, 1999: Endoscopic resection of a choledochocele. Gastrointest Endosc 50:578-580.

Chaudhary A, et al, 1997: Reoperative surgery for choledochal cysts. Br J Surg 84:781-784.

Chen H-M, et al, 1996: Surgical treatment of choledochal cyst in adults: results and long term follow-up. Hepatogastroenterology 43:1492-1499.

Chijiiwa K, Koga A, 1993: Surgical management and long-term follow-up of patients with choledochal cysts. Am J Surg 165:238-242.

Chijiiwa K, Tanaka M, 1994: Late complications after excisional operation in patients with choledochal cyst. J Am Coll Surg 179:139-144.

Chijiiwa K, et al, 1993: Are secondary bile acids in choledochal cysts important as risk factors in biliary tract carcinoma? Aust N Z J Surg 63:109-112.

Chowbey PK, et al, 2002: Complete laparoscopic management of choledochal cyst: report of two cases. J Laparoendosc Adv Surg Tech 12:217-221.

Craig AG, et al, 2001: Sphincter of Oddi dysfunction associated with choledochal cyst. J Gastroenterol Hepatol 16:230-234.

Dalvi AN, et al, 1999: Incomplete pancreas divisum with anomalous choledochopancreatic duct junction with choledochal cyst. Arch Surg 134: 1150-1152.

Dayton MT, et al, 1983: Caroli's disease: a premalignant condition? Am J Surg 145:41-48.

Deziel DJ, et al, 1986: Management of bile duct cysts in adults. Arch Surg 121:410-415.

Durgun AV, et al, 2002: Choledochal cysts in adults and the importance of differential diagnosis. J Hepatobiliary Pancreat Surg 9:738-741.

Dussaulz-Garin L, et al, 2000: Obstructive pancreatitis due to mucus produced by metaplastic choledochal cyst epithelium. Gastrointest Endosc 52:787-789.

Fieber SS, Nance FC, 1997: Choledochal cyst and neoplasm: a comprehensive review of 106 cases and presentation of two original cases. Am Surg 63: 982-987.

Flanigan DP, 1975: Biliary cysts. Ann Surg 182:635-643.

Flanigan DP, 1977: Biliary carcinoma associated with biliary cysts. Cancer 40: 880-883.

Fulcher AS, Turner MA, 2002: MR cholangiopancreatography. Radiol Clin North Am 40:1363-1376.

Fumino S, et al, 2002: New insight into bile flow dynamics in anomalous arrangement of the pancreaticobiliary duct. Br J Surg 89:865-869.

Gigot JF, et al, 1996: Bile duct cysts in adults: a changing spectrum of presentation. J Hepatobiliary Pancreat Surg 3:405-411.

Grumbach R, et al, 1954: Maladie fibrokystique du foie avec hypertension portale chez l'enfant: deux observations. Archives d'Anatomie et de Cytologie Pathologique 74:30.

Guelrud M, et al, 1999: Sphincter of Oddi dysfunction in children with recurrent pancreatitis and anomalous pancreaticobiliary union: an etiologic concept. Gastrointest Endosc 50:194-199.

Guy F, et al, 2002: Caroli's disease: magnetic resonance imaging features. Eur Radiol 12:2730-2736.

Hewitt PM, et al, 1995: Choledochal cysts in adults. Br J Surg 82:382-385.

Hoglund M, et al, 1990: Computed tomography with intravenous cholangiography contrast: a method of visualizing choledochal cysts. Eur J Radiol 10:159-161.

Hopkins NFG, et al, 1990: Complications of choledochal cysts in adulthood. Ann R Coll Surg Engl 72:229-235.

Ishibashi T, et al, 1997: Malignant change in the biliary tract after excision of choledochal cyst. Br J Surg 84:1687-1691.

Iwai N, et al, 1986: Biliary manometry in choledochal cyst with abnormal choledochopancreatic ductal junction. J Pediatr Surg 21:873-876.

Iwafuchi M, et al, 1990: Familial occurrence of congenital bile duct dilatation. J Pediatr Surg 25:353-355.

Iwata F, et al, 1998: Familial occurrence of congenital bile ducts cysts. J Gastroenterol Hepatol 13:316-319.

Jan Y-Y, et al, 2002: Malignancy in choledochal cysts. Hepatogastroenterology 49:100-103.

Jesudason SRB, et al, 1997: Choledochal cysts in adults. Ann R Coll Surg Engl 79:410-413.

Jona JZ, et al, 1979: Anatomic observations and etiologic and surgical considerations in choledochal cyst. J Pediatr Surg 14:315-320.

Jordan PH Jr, et al, 2004: Some considerations for management of choledochal cysts. Am J Surg 187:434-439.

Joseph VT, 1990: Surgical techniques and long-term results in the treatment of choledochal cyst. J Pediatr Surg 25:782-787.

Kabra V, et al, 2001: Choledochal cyst: a changing pattern of presentation. Aust N Z J Surg 71:159-161.

Kaneko K, et al, 1999: Secondary excision of choledochal cysts after previous cyst-enterostomies. Hepatogastroenterology 46:2772-2775.

Kim M-J, et al, 2002: Using MR cholangiopancreatography to reveal anomalous pancreaticobiliary ductal union in infants and children with choledochal cysts. AJR Am J Roentgenol 179:209-214.

Kim OH, et al, 1995: Imaging of the choledochal cyst. Radiographics 15:69-88.

Kim SH, 1981: Choledochal cyst: survey by the surgical section of the American Academy of Pediatrics. J Pediatr Surg 16:402-407.

Kim SH, et al, 2000: Choledochal cyst: comparison of MR and conventional cholangiography. Clin Radiol 55:378-383.

Koike M, et al, 2002: Carcinoma of the hepatic hilus developing 21 years after biliary diversion for choledochal cyst: a case report. Hepatogastroenterology 49:1216-1220.

Komi N, et al, 1984: Nationwide survey of cases of choledochal cysts: analysis of coexistent anomalies, complications and surgical treatment in 645 cases. Surg Gastroenterol 3:69-73.

Komi N, et al, 1989: Choledochal cyst: anomalous arrangement of the pancreaticobiliary ductal system and biliary malignancy. J Gastroenterol Hepatol 4:63-74.

Komi N, et al, 1992: Does the type of anomalous arrangement of pancreaticobiliary ducts influence the surgery and prognosis of choledochal cyst? J Pediatr Surg 27:728-731.

Kouraklis GR, et al, 1996: Cystic dilatations of the common bile duct in adults. HPB Surg 10:91-95.

Kusunoki M, et al, 1988: Choledochal cysts: oligoganglionosis in the narrow portion of the choledochus. Arch Surg 123:984-986.

Ladas SD, et al, 1995: Choledochocele, an overlooked diagnosis: report of 15 cases and review of 56 published reports from 1984 to 1992. Endoscopy 27:233-239.

Lane GJ, et al, 1999: Different types of congenital biliary dilatation in dizygotic twins. Pediatr Surg Int 15:403-404.

Lee SS, et al, 1964: Choledochal cyst: a report of nine cases and review of literature. Arch Surg 99:19-28.

Lenriot JP, et al, French Association for Surgical Research, 1998: Bile duct cysts in adults: a multi-institutional retrospective study. Ann Surg 238:159-166.

Levy AD, Rohrmann CA Jr, 2003: Biliary cystic disease. Curr Prob Diagn Radiol 32:233-263.

Lilly JR, 1979: The surgical treatment of choledochal cyst. Surg Gynecol Obstet 149:36-42.

Lipsett PA, Pitt HA, 2003: Surgical treatment of choledochal cysts. J Hepatobiliary Pancreat Surg 10:352-359.

Lipsett PA, et al, 1994: Choledochal cyst disease: a changing pattern of presentation. Ann Surg 220:644-652.

Liu C-L, et al, 2002: Choledochal cysts in adults. Arch Surg 137:465-468.

Lopez RR, et al, 1991: Variation in management based on type of choledochal cyst. Am J Surg 161:612-615.

Martin LW, Rowe GA, 1979: Portal hypertension secondary to choledochal cyst. Ann Surg 190:638-639.

Martin RF, et al, 1992: Symptomatic choledochoceles in adults: endoscopic retrograde cholangiopancreatography recognition and management. Arch Surg 127:536-539.

Masetti R, et al, 1996: Choledochocele: changing trends in diagnosis and management. Surg Today 26:281-285.

Matsubara T, et al, 2002: K-ras and p53 gene mutations in noncancerous biliary lesions of patients with pancreaticobiliary maljunction. J Hepatobiliary Pancreat Surg 9:312-321.

Matsumoto Y, et al, 1977a: Clinicopathologic classification of congenital cystic dilatation of the common bile duct. Am J Surg 134:569-574.

Matsumoto Y, et al, 1977b: Congenital cystic dilatation of the common bile duct as a cause of primary bile duct stone. Am J Surg 134:346-352.

Matsumoto Y, et al, 2003: Pancreaticobiliary maljunction; pathophysiology and clinical aspects and impact on biliary carcinogenesis. Langenbacks Arch Surg 388:122-131.

Mercadier M, et al, 1984: Caroli's disease. World J Surg 8:22-29.

Miyazaki T, et al, 1998: Single-shot MR cholangiopancreatography of neonates, infants, and young children. AJR Am J Roentgenol 170:33-37.

Musante F, et al, 1982: CT cholangiography in suspected Caroli's disease. J Comput Assist Tomogr 6:482-485.

Nagai N, et al, 1999: Analysis of microsatellite instability, TGF-beta type II receptor gene mutations and hMSH2 and hMLH1 allele losses in pancreaticobiliary maljunction-associated biliary tract tumors. Anticancer Res 19:1765-1768.

Nagai M, et al, 2002: Clinical and genetic analysis of noncancerous and cancerous biliary epithelium in patients with pancreaticobiliary maljunction. World J Surg 26:91-98.

Nagata E, et al, 1986: Choledochal cyst: complications of anomalous connection between the choledochus and pancreatic duct and carcinoma of the biliary tract. World J Surg 10:102-110.

Nagorney DM, et al, 1984a: Choledochal cysts in adults: clinical management. Surgery 96:656-663.

Nagorney DM, et al, 1984b: Cystadenoma of the proximal common hepatic duct: the use of abdominal ultrasonography and transhepatic cholangiography in diagnosis. Mayo Clin Proc 59:118-121.

Nicholl M, et al, 2004: Choledochal cysts in Western adults: complexities compared to children. J Gastrointest Surg 8:245-252.

Oguchi Y, et al, 1988: Histopathologic studies of congenital dilatation of the bile duct as related to an anomalous junction of the pancreaticobiliary ductal system: clinical and experimental trials. Surgery 103:168-173.

Ohkawa H, et al, 1981: The production of anomalous pancreaticobiliary ductal union in canine models. Z Kinderchir 4:328-336.

Okada A, et al, 1983: Common channel syndrome: diagnosis with endoscopic retrograde cholangiopancreatography and surgical management. Surgery 93:634-642.

Okada A, et al, 1990: Congenital dilatation of the bile duct in 100 instances and its relationship with anomalous junction. Surg Gynecol Obstet 171:291-298.

Olbourne NA, 1975: Choledochal cysts: a review of the cystic anomalies of the biliary tree. Ann R Coll Surg Engl 56:26-32.

Ono J, et al, 1982: Surgical aspect of cystic dilatation of the bile duct—an anomalous junction of the pancreaticobiliary tract in adults. Ann Surg 195:203-208.

Powell CS, et al, 1981: Management of adult choledochal cysts. Ann Surg 193:666-676.

Ramond M-J, et al, 1984: Partial hepatectomy in the treatment of Caroli's disease: report of a case and review of the literature. Dig Dis Sci 29:367-370.

Rattner DW, et al, 1983: Abnormalities of the pancreatic and biliary ducts in adult patients with choledochal cysts. Arch Surg 118:1068-1073.

Reveille RM, et al, 1990: Increased secondary bile acids in a choledochal cyst: possible role in biliary metaplasia and carcinoma. Gastroenterology 99:525-527.

Rossi FL, et al, 1987: Carcinomas arising in cystic conditions of the bile ducts: a clinical and pathologic study. Ann Surg 205:377-384.

Sarris GE, Tsang D, 1989: Choledochocele: case report, literature review, and a proposed classification. Surgery 105:408-414.

Savader SJ, et al, 1991a: Choledochal cysts: classification and cholangiographic appearance. AJR Am J Roentgenol 156:327-331.

Savader SJ, et al, 1991b: Choledochal cysts: role of noninvasive imaging, percutaneous transhepatic cholangiography, and percutaneous biliary drainage in diagnosis and treatment. J Vasc Interv Radiol 2:379-385.

Saxena R, et al, 1988: Benign disease of the common bile duct. Br J Surg 75:803-806.

Scharschmidt BF, 1984: Human liver transplantation: analysis of data on 540 patients from four centers. Hepatology 4:95S-101S.

Scudamore CH, et al, 1994: Surgical management of choledochal cysts. Am J Surg 1167:497-500.

Shimura H, et al, 1998: Laparoscopic treatment of congenital choledochal cyst. Surg Endosc 12:1268-1271.

Söreide K, et al, 2004: Bile duct cysts in adults. Br J Surg 91:1538-1548.

Stain SC, et al, 1995: Choledochal cyst in the adult. Ann Surg 222:128-133.

Sty JR, et al, 1978: Hepatic scintigraphy in Caroli's disease. Radiology 127:732.

Swisher SG, et al, 1994: Pancreatitis associated with adult choledochal cysts. Pancreas 9:633-637.

Tan KC, Howard ER, 1988: Choledochal cyst: a 14-year surgical experience with 36 patients. Br J Surg 75:892-895.

Tanaka M, et al, 2001: Laparoscopically assisted resection of choledochal cyst and Roux-en-Y reconstruction. Surg Endosc 15:545-551.

Todani T, et al, 1977: Congenital bile duct cysts: classifications, operative procedures, and review of thirty-seven cases including cancer arising from choledochal cyst. Am J Surg 134:263-269.

Todani T, et al, 1978: Management of congenital choledochal cyst with intrahepatic involvement. Ann Surg 187:272-280.

Todani T, et al, 1979: Carcinoma arising in the wall of congenital bile duct cysts. Cancer 44:1134-1141.

Todani T, et al, 1981: Hepaticoduodenostomy at the hepatic hilum after excision of choledochal cyst. Am J Surg 142:584-587.

Todani T, et al, 1984a: Congenital choledochal cyst with intrahepatic involvement. Arch Surg 119:1038-1043.

Todani T, et al, 1984b: Anomalous arrangement of the pancreaticobiliary ductal system in patients with a choledochal cyst. Am J Surg 147:672-676.

Todani T, et al, 1987: Carcinoma related to choledochal cysts with internal drainage operations. Surg Gynecol Obstet 164:61-64.

Todani T, et al, 1988: Reoperation for congenital choledochal cyst. Ann Surg 207:142-147.

Todani T, et al, 1990: Pseudopancreatitis in choledochal cyst in children: intraoperative study of amylase levels in the serum. J Pediatr Surg 25:303-306.

Todani T, et al, 1998: Co-existing biliary anomalies and anatomical variants in choledochal cyst. Br J Surg 85:760-763.

Todani T, et al, 2003: Classification of congenital biliary cystic disease:special reference to type Ic and IVA cysts with primary ductal stricture. J Hepatobiliary Pancreat Surg 10:340-344.

Tsuchiya R, et al, 1977: Malignant tumors in choledochal cysts. Ann Surg 186:22-28.

Uno K, et al, 1996: Development of intrahepatic cholelithiasis long after primary excision of choledochal cyst. J Am Coll Surg 183:583-588.

Venu RP, et al, 1984: Role of endoscopic retrograde cholangiopancreatography in the diagnosis and treatment of choledochocele. Gastroenterology 87:1144-1149.

Visser BC, et al, 2004: Congenital choledochal cysts in adults. Arch Surg 139:855-862.

Voyles CR, et al, 1983: Carcinoma in choledochal cysts—Age-related incidence. Arch Surg 118:986-988.

Watanabe Y, et al, 1999: Bile duct cancer developed after cyst excision for choledochal cyst. J Hepatobiliary Pancreat Surg 6:207-212.

Wiedmeyer D, et al, 1989: Choledochal cyst: findings on cholangiopancreatography with emphasis on ectasia of the common channel. AJR Am J Roentgenol 153:969-972.

Witlin LT, et al, 1982: Transhepatic decompression of the biliary tree in Caroli's disease. Surgery 91:205-209.

Yamaguchi M, 1980: Congenital choledochal cyst. Am J Surg 140:653.

Yamamoto J, et al, 1996: Bile duct carcinoma arising from the anastomotic site of hepaticojejunostomy after the excision of congenital biliary dilatation: a case report. Surgery 119:476-479.

64

Nonparasitic Cystic Diseases of the Liver and Intrahepatic Biliary Tree

O. FARGES AND V. VILGRAIN

Nonparasitic cystic diseases of the liver and intrahepatic biliary tree include entities that differ in etiology, prevalence, manifestations, and severity, but have two common characteristics. First, these diseases result from a congenital malformation, inherited or not inherited, of the intrahepatic bile ducts. Second, the basic lesion consists of macroscopic or microscopic cysts. Macroscopic cysts are recognized easily by ultrasonography or computed tomography (CT), which are the main diagnostic imaging procedures. Microscopic cysts are shown only by histologic examination.

SIMPLE CYST OF THE LIVER

Simple cysts of the liver are cystic formations, containing serous fluid, not communicating with the intrahepatic biliary tree. Numerous terms have been used to designate this lesion, including *biliary cyst, nonparasitic cyst of the liver, benign hepatic cyst, congenital hepatic cyst, unilocular cyst of the liver,* and *solitary cyst of the liver* (the last designation is inappropriate because, as mentioned later, simple cysts are often multiple). Simple cysts occur frequently in the general population. Most simple cysts are less than 3 cm in diameter, are easily identified by ultrasound, and are asymptomatic. Symptoms, when present, usually are related to intracystic bleeding that changes the morphologic appearance of the cyst, which may mimic cystadenoma or hydatid disease.

Pathology and Pathogenesis

Macroscopically, a simple cyst of the liver has a spherical or ovoid shape. The diameter ranges from a few millimeters to 20 cm or more. The cyst does not communicate with the intrahepatic bile ducts. Small cysts are surrounded by normal hepatic tissue. Large cysts produce atrophy of the adjacent hepatic tissue; a huge cyst may result in complete atrophy of a hepatic lobe with compensatory hypertrophy of the other lobe. Atrophy respects the large bile ducts and blood vessels, which appear to be abundant in the atrophic tissue in contact with the cyst. Large bile ducts and blood vessels persisting after atrophy may protrude and form folds over the inner surface of the cyst. There is no septation; the cysts are unilocular. The cystic fluid is usually clear; however, intracystic bleeding is relatively common, and the fluid may be brownish. Even when a simple cyst is apparently unique, imaging studies disclose the presence of one or more small additional cysts in most patients. In a few cases, simple cysts are multiple, resembling the liver cysts of adult polycystic kidney disease.

Microscopically, the cysts appear to be bordered by a single layer of cuboid or columnar epithelial cells, resembling biliary epithelial cells. The cells are uniform, without any atypia. Stroma is absent in small cysts and reduced to a thin layer of connective tissue in large cysts.

Simple cysts of the liver are regarded as a congenital malformation. An aberrant bile duct would have lost communication with the biliary tree and would dilate progressively. Liver cyst epithelial cells retain differentiated secretory function; they secrete fluid and generate a positive luminal pressure that may be greater than 30 cm H_2O. The composition of the fluid, which contains water and mineral electrolytes without bile acids and bilirubin, is close to that of the normal secretion of the epithelium of the bile ducts. It is not toxic for the peritoneum, which is the rationale for cyst fenestration (see later).

Prevalence and Etiology

Simple cysts have long been considered rare. By 1971, only 350 cases had been reported (Flagg & Robinson, 1967; Moreaux & Bloch, 1971), and early estimates from autopsy studies were less than 1% (Larsen, 1961). The development of imaging techniques revealed, however, that simple cysts are much more frequent. Prevalence in ultrasound studies is 3% to 5% (Caremani et al, 1993; Gaines & Sampson, 1989) and was 18% in a more recent spiral CT study of an adult population (Carrim & Murchison, 2003). These discrepancies are explained by the usual small size of most cysts, which are discovered only with accurate imaging techniques.

The incidence of simple cysts is age and gender related. Simple cysts are uncommon before age 40, and their incidence increases sharply thereafter. Simple cysts also are larger in adults older than 50 than in younger individuals (Larsen, 1961). The female-to-male ratio is 1.5:1 for asymptomatic simple cysts shown at necropsy or on ultrasound. The female-to-male ratio is 9:1 in symptomatic or complicated simple cysts, however (Moreaux & Bloch, 1971). Huge cysts affect women older than 50 almost exclusively. An association between simple hepatic cysts and simple renal cysts has been documented (Carrim & Murchison, 2003), but is unexplained.

Manifestations and Diagnosis

In most cases, simple cysts—all small cysts, but also most large cysts—are asymptomatic and fortuitously shown by ultrasound or CT. Only some large cysts produce abdominal pain or discomfort. Because of the high prevalence of simple cysts in adults, the fortuitous coincidence of this lesion and another hepatic or extrahepatic disease is common. The causal relationship between abdominal pain or discomfort and a simple cyst of the liver must be admitted with caution and accepted only if the cyst is large and the other possible causes of the symptoms have been excluded. At clinical examination, only large cysts can be palpated as spherical tumors. In most cases, the fluid content of the tumor can be suspected. In some cases, the cyst is so tense that it may be taken for a solid tumor. The condition of individuals with simple cyst of the liver is good. Liver function tests are normal; abnormal liver function tests in a patient with simple cyst of the liver are not related to the cyst and are caused by another liver disease except when the cysts compress bile ducts.

Ultrasonography (see Ch. 15) is the best procedure for recognizing simple cysts. A simple cyst is a circular or oval, totally anechoic lesion, with sharp, smooth borders and strong posterior wall echoes, indicating a well-defined tissue-fluid interface (Spiegel et al, 1978). There is accentuation of the echoes beyond the cyst compared with echoes at a similar depth transmitted through normal adjacent liver tissue (Fig. 64.1) (Spiegel et al, 1978). Accentuation of the echoes beyond the cyst, so-called acoustic posterior enhancement, which indicates that the lesion is fluid-filled, is observed only when the deep tissue transmits ultrasound and is not seen when a total reflector, such as gas or bone, lies behind the cyst. In some patients, because of intracystic bleeding, intracystic echoes can be detected.

The other imaging procedures have less utility in diagnosis compared with ultrasound and are generally not required. CT confirms the presence of one or several round or oval, water-dense lesions, without septation or intracystic formations; dynamic CT shows that the tumors are avascular. In small cysts, recognition of water density may be difficult (the average density of the cyst being obscured by the density of the adjacent liver tissue), and an apparent increase in density may be observed after intravenous injection of contrast medium.

If the patient is living or had been living in an area where hydatid disease is endemic, or if there is any doubt about a possible hydatid cyst, serologic tests for this parasitic infection must be performed (see Ch. 61). Aspiration has been proposed for confirming the diagnosis by showing a clear fluid and by

showing the absence of communication with the biliary tree after intracystic injection of contrast medium (Roemer et al, 1981). It also may be used to rule out the presence of scolices if hydatid disease is suspected.

Course and Complications

In most cases, simple cysts are asymptomatic and remain silent; repeated ultrasound studies usually show no appreciable changes over years. In some patients, the cysts grow slowly. In a few patients, the size of the cysts increases rapidly; such a course, which may be associated with severe pain and discomfort, is observed almost exclusively in women older than 50 years.

Complications are uncommon. Intracystic bleeding is the most frequent (Frisell et al, 1979; Moreaux & Bloch, 1971). It is presumed to result from the erosion of an artery adjacent to the cyst. The clinical manifestations consist of sudden, severe pain and increase in the size of the cyst. The pain resolves in a few days. In a few cases, pain is mild or absent. There is no evidence of anemia, and the biologic liver tests show only a moderate elevation of gamma-glutamyltransferase. On ultrasound, echoic material, corresponding to clots, is present within the cyst; usually this echoic material is mobile, sliding in the inferior part of the cyst. Hemorrhagic cysts also become hyperintense on T1-weighted magnetic resonance imaging (MRI), whereas uncomplicated cysts are hypointense (Fig. 64.2).

Numerous other potential complications have been described, but these are infrequent. Spontaneous rupture may occur into the peritoneal cavity (Akriviadis et al, 1989) or more rarely the pleural cavity or the duodenum (Williamson et al, 1978). In contrast to hydatid cysts, peritoneal perforation of simple cysts is exceptional and self-limited. Severe hemoperitoneum has been described only in patients with polycystic liver disease undergoing dialysis. Bacterial infection, compression of the inferior vena cava (Frisell et al, 1979) that may result in clot formation and pulmonary embolism (Buyse et al, 2004), communication with an intrahepatic duct (Perreau et al, 1965), cholestasis secondary to compression of the bifurcation of the common bile duct (Fig. 64.3) (Cappell, 1988; Clinkscales et al, 1985; Moreaux & Bloch, 1971; Santman et al, 1977), hemobilia, portal hypertension secondary to compression of the portal vein (Lebon et al, 1955), torsion (Soud & Watson, 1974), and carcinoma (Yagi et al, 2004) also have been reported.

Differential Diagnosis

A simple cyst is easily distinguished from liver abscess, necrotic malignant tumor, large hemangioma, and hematoma. The clinical background of these lesions is different. On ultrasound and CT, these lesions rarely appear as purely fluid-filled, sharply defined areas. A few cases of hepatic metastases of neuroendocrine tumors (see Ch. 73b) sometimes can be difficult, however, to distinguish from liver cysts. These malignant tumors can be well tolerated; the necrotic areas may be sharply defined.

The distinction between simple cyst and hydatid disease (see Ch. 61) can be difficult. Several characteristics of simple cysts and hydatid disease (Table 64.1) usually allow a clear distinction between the two diseases. Difficulties may be due to the following: (1) Hydatid disease may have been contracted in an area where this parasitic infection is not endemic; (2) calcifications, septations,

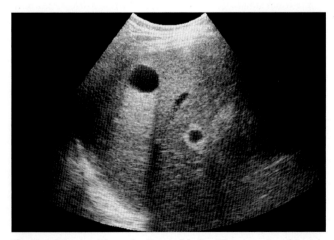

Fig. 64.1. Ultrasound shows simple cyst of the liver. Transverse view of the right lobe of the liver. The cyst corresponds to the round anechoic area. There is accentuation of the echoes beyond the cyst.

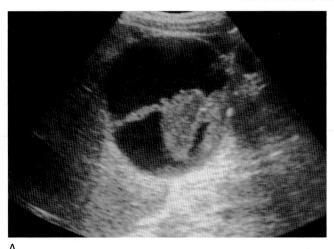

A

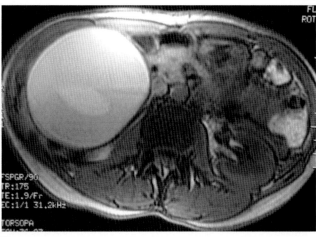

B

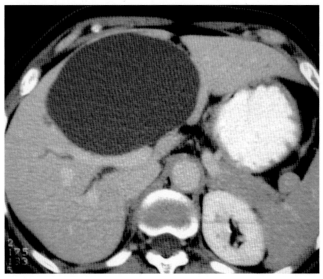

C

Fig. 64.2. Hemorrhagic simple cyst of the liver. **A,** Ultrasound shows echoic material within the cyst corresponding to clots. **B,** On T1-weighted MRI, the cyst is hyperintense in contrast to uncomplicated cysts. **C,** On T2-weighted MRI, the cyst is hyperintense similar to uncomplicated cysts.

and split walls may be absent in hydatid cysts, which become indistinguishable from simple cysts; (3) septations may be mimicked by contiguous simple cysts (Fig. 64.4); (4) serologic tests for hydatid disease may be negative in some patients with hydatid cyst; (5) simple cyst with intracystic clots may resemble hydatid cyst with a split wall or parasitic vesicles or both. In patients in whom the distinction between simple cyst and hydatid cyst cannot be made, microscopic examination of cystic fluid obtained by aspiration can be useful, in particular, when laparoscopic fenestration is considered (Giuliante et al, 2003). Distinction between a hemorrhagic cyst and a cystadenoma may be difficult. The presence of associated typical hepatic cysts is helpful in suggesting the diagnosis of simple cyst (Vuillemin-Bodaghi et al, 1997).

Treatment

Single Cyst

Asymptomatic liver cysts, even when large, need no treatment. When symptoms are present, treatment is indicated only if the symptoms are clearly related to the cyst. One should be cautious before advocating any form of treatment in patients with cysts that are smaller than 8 cm and that do not protrude outside of the liver surface. In case of doubt, it may be helpful to perform

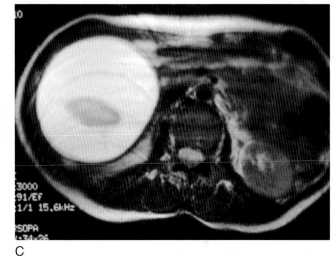

Fig. 64.3. Abdominal CT of a large simple cyst compressing the biliary confluence. Intrahepatic bile ducts of the right liver are enlarged. The portal bifurcation also is compressed.

Table 64.1 Distinctive Characteristics of Simple Cyst and Hydatid Cyst of the Liver

	Simple Cyst	Hydatid Cyst
Septations	Absent	Common
Calcifications	Absent	Common
Split wall	Absent	Possible
Communication with biliary tree	Absent	Possible
Serologic tests for hydatid disease	Negative	Positive*

*In most, but not all, patients with hydatid disease.

an ultrasound-guided aspiration of the cyst as a therapeutic test. If aspiration has no influence on the symptoms, further treatment is not required. After simple aspiration, the cyst inevitably recurs (Saini et al, 1983).

Nonsurgical treatment of hepatic cysts is the injection of a sclerosing agent into the cyst cavity, which aims at the destruction of the epithelial lining. The most frequently used sclerosing agent is ethanol. The amount of ethanol injected is half of the cyst volume, but not exceeding the total amount of 100 mL, and the ethanol is kept in the cyst for 3 to 20 minutes. Complications include severe abdominal pain during intracystic injection (generally caused by extravasation of alcohol into the peritoneal cavity), transient neuropsychic disorders secondary to diffusion of alcohol, hypotension, and inflammatory changes of the cysts (which can make a subsequent partial excision difficult). Minocycline hydrochloride has been used as an alternative to ethanol and seems to be associated with fewer side effects, although it may require multiple injections. Although sclerotherapy has been used for years, few large studies with prolonged follow-up are available (Montorsi et al, 1994; Simonetti et al, 1993; Tanaka et al, 1996; Tikkakoski et al, 1996; Yamada et al, 1994). The success rates range from 65% to 95%. A contraindication

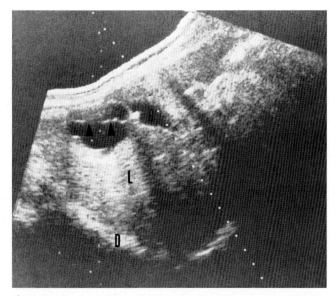

Fig. 64.4. Ultrasound shows simple cyst of the liver. Transverse view of the right upper quadrant of the abdomen. Two contiguous cysts, located in segment V, near the gallbladder, produce a pseudoseptation *(arrowheads)*. L, liver; D, diaphragm.

to this treatment is the presence of bile in the cyst cavity or leakage of contrast media injected in the cyst into the bile duct.

Surgical treatment (see Ch. 65) is by fenestration. The cyst wall protruding outside of the liver is excised to establish a large communication between the cyst and the peritoneal cavity. Fluid continues to be produced by the epithelial lining, but is reabsorbed by the peritoneum. This treatment is extremely simple because symptomatic cysts are virtually always large with a protrusion of part of their wall outside of the liver. There is no need to enter the liver parenchyma. Fenestration is effective, provided that the opening is large enough and the cyst cavity collapses. A small size cyst cavity may persist, especially for cysts located in the upper part of the liver, probably because of adhesions between the opening and the diaphragm; recurrence of symptoms is unusual. When the cyst is very large, fluid secretion may overflow the resorption capacity of the peritoneum, which results in transient ascites.

Fenestration can be performed by open surgery or by laparoscopy (Emmermann et al, 1997; Fabiani et al, 1997; Gigot et al, 1997; Klingler et al, 1997; Martin et al, 1998; Morino et al, 1994). The laparoscopic approach is currently the first choice, although few studies have a follow-up exceeding 3 years. There are, however, two limitations to the laparoscopic approach: (1) When the cyst is located in the upper part of the liver (segment VII or VIII), it is difficult to achieve adequate opening of the cyst; (2) hemorrhage or infection within a liver cyst results in changes that mimic a liver tumor or a parasitic cyst. Open surgery with intraoperative biopsies or complete excision may be required in this setting (Shimada et al, 1998). Finally, laparoscopic fenestration should be performed only if the diagnosis of hydatid disease or cystadenoma has been formally ruled out.

Multiple Large Cysts

Patients with multiple cysts most frequently have one to five large cysts coexisting with a various number of very small cysts. In these patients, symptoms are related only to the large cysts, which should be treated individually as if a single cyst. The small cysts, which are frequently deeply located in the liver, should not be treated. Because of the large surface of exposed epithelium, the risk of transient postoperative ascites is high. Long-term outcome is similar to that in patients with single cysts (Farges & Bismuth, 1995).

CYSTADENOMA AND CYSTADENOCARCINOMA OF THE LIVER

Cystadenoma of the liver is a rare tumor, which has a strong tendency to recur and has malignant potential. Differentiation of this tumor from simple cyst of the liver is important.

Pathology and Pathogenesis

The cystadenoma (see Ch. 70) of the liver is a single, usually large, tumor, measuring 10 to 20 cm in diameter. It has a globular external surface from which cysts of various sizes bulge outward. The cut surface shows multiple loculi of various sizes, limited by thin walls. The loculi usually contain a mucinous fluid (Ishak et al, 1977).

On microscopic examination, the loculi are limited by a single layer of cuboidal or columnar cells resting on a basement membrane. These cells are uniform, with round or oval nuclei;

their cytoplasm is clear or faintly vacuolated; the vacuoles stain positive for mucin. In places, the epithelium forms multiple polypoid or papillary projections. The stroma supporting the epithelium is thick, compact, and cellular, resembling ovarian stroma; it often contains pigmented or foamy macrophages and cholesterol clefts (Ishak et al, 1977).

The pathogenesis of cystadenoma is unknown. A congenital origin from an abnormal intrahepatic bile duct or from misplaced germ cells is possible. The former hypothesis, although generally accepted, does not account for the mucinous epithelium, which borders the loculi. The latter hypothesis would explain the similarity of cystadenoma of the liver and ovarian cyst.

Prevalence and Etiology

Cystadenoma of the liver is a rare tumor. From a review of the literature to 1955, the prevalence of cystadenoma was estimated as 20 times less than that of simple cyst of the liver (Geist, 1955). In our experience, mainly based on the recognition of liver cysts by ultrasound and CT, the prevalence of cystadenoma of the liver seems to be much lower, probably 1000 times less than that of simple cyst of the liver. Cystadenoma of the liver mainly affects women older than 40 (Ishak et al, 1977). Only one case has been reported in a child (Alexander, 1925).

Manifestations and Diagnosis

The presenting symptoms of cystadenoma are abdominal pain, abdominal discomfort, anorexia, nausea, and abdominal swelling. Jaundice is possible, related to the compression of, or the fistulization into, the bile ducts with their obstruction by mucinous material. A large hepatic mass may be palpated. In patients with a small cystadenoma, the disease may be asymptomatic, and clinical examination may be normal. Liver function tests are normal (Cadranel et al, 1994).

Diagnosis of cystadenoma is based mainly on ultrasound and CT. Ultrasound shows a single, large, anechoic, fluid-filled, ovoid or globular area with irregular margins; internal echoes are seen, corresponding to septations delimiting multiple loculi of various sizes and to papillary growths originating from the cystic wall or from the septa (Forrest et al, 1980). CT (Fig. 64.5) shows comparable abnormalities, including a single low-density area, with internal septations and mural nodules. CT is less sensitive than ultrasound for showing internal septations, a characteristic feature of cystadenoma. Thin septations not shown with CT may be visible with ultrasound. The density of the wall of the cyst, septations, and mural nodules is enhanced after intravenous injection of contrast medium (Choi et al, 1989; Frick & Feinberg, 1982; Korobkin et al, 1989). In some patients, the density of the cystic area is higher than the water density (>30 Hounsfield units) (Choi et al, 1989), probably because of the high protein content of the fluid. Calcifications are seen in septations and mural nodules in some patients (Korobkin et al, 1989). On MRI, the tumor is strongly hyperintense on T2-weighted images and usually hypointense on T1-weighted images (Fig. 64.6), although it also may be hyperintense or heterogeneous owing to mucinous or blood content.

Other imaging procedures are of limited interest. Arteriography shows that the intrahepatic arteries are displaced by the tumor. The tumor itself is avascular with multiple clusters of fine vessels

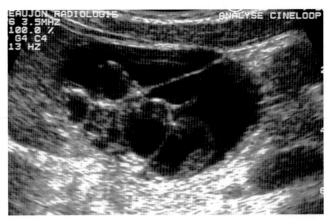

A

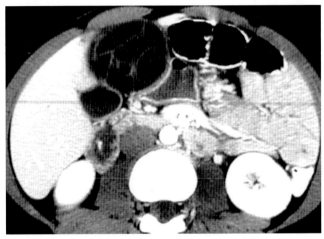

B

Fig. 64.5. Benign cystadenoma of the liver. **A,** Ultrasound shows an anechoic lesion with internal echoes corresponding to septations. **B,** Abdominal CT at the arterial phase. This cystic lesion has a peripheral wall, and the wall and the internal septations are enhanced by the intravenous contrast medium.

in the periphery of the tumor; an accumulation of contrast material in the wall of the cystadenoma, in the septa, and in the papillary growths may be seen in the parenchymal phase (Forrest et al, 1980; Korobkin et al, 1989). Endoscopic retrograde cholangiography shows displacement of the intrahepatic bile ducts by the tumor and no communication between the biliary tree and cystadenoma. Mucinous material may be present in the biliary tree in cases of fistulization.

Serologic tests for hydatid disease must be performed systematically and are negative. Percutaneous aspiration usually provides a mucinous fluid, which is a strong argument in favor of the diagnosis of cystadenoma. If cystadenoma is complicated by cystadenocarcinoma, however, puncture of the cyst theoretically could disseminate malignancy.

Serum CA 19-9 levels may be elevated in patients with cystadenoma. In contrast, a single case of increased CA 19-9 has been reported in a patient with simple cyst. The increased CA 19-9 was attributed to the rupture of the cyst into the systemic circulation (Yamaguchi et al, 1999). In contrast to pancreatic cysts, the various forms of liver cysts (simple cysts, cystadenoma, cystadenocarcinoma) cannot be easily distinguished yet by measuring the values of tumor markers in liver cysts.

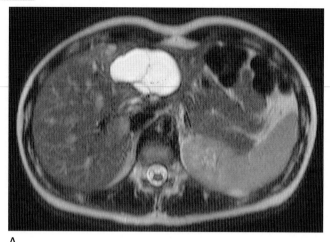 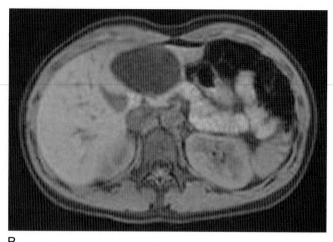

A   B

Fig. 64.6. MRI of a benign cystadenoma. **A,** On T2-weighted images, the lesion is strongly hyperintense and the septations are visible. **B,** On T1-weighted images, the lesion is hypointense.

Cystic fluid CA 19-9 levels are increased in most cystadenomas, but very high levels also may be observed in simple cysts. The accuracy of cystic fluid measurement of ACE, which is frequently increased in cystadenoma, is unknown.

Course and Complications

Cystadenomas grow very slowly. Complications, which may be the first manifestations of the tumor, include cholestasis secondary to compression of the common bile duct (van Roekel et al, 1982) or fistulization into the common bile duct, intracystic hemorrhage, bacterial infection, rupture, recurrence after partial excision, and transformation into cystadenocarcinoma. The risk of transformation of cystadenoma into cystadenocarcinoma is supported by the presence of foci of cystadenocarcinoma within proven cystadenoma (Woods, 1981). Cystadenocarcinoma of the liver develops almost exclusively in a preexisting cystadenoma. Histologically, the malignant epithelium is multilayered, with numerous papillary projections; malignant epithelial cells are dysmorphic and invade the stroma. Malignancy may affect all the epithelium or, more often, only a part of the cystadenoma. Malignant transformation may be suspected by imaging studies when they show large projections protruding in the lumina of the loculi; hemorrhagic content; or septal calcifications (Korobkin et al, 1989; Stanley et al, 1983). Cyst cytology is not accurate in differentiating cystadenoma from cystadenocarcinoma. Malignant tissue can be obtained by biopsy under ultrasound guidance (Iemoto et al, 1983). Cystadenocarcinoma extends progressively into the liver. Obstruction of the biliary tree is due to compression or, more rarely, to obliteration by mucin (Kokubo et al, 1988). Extrahepatic metastases can develop (Iemoto et al, 1983).

Differential Diagnosis

Cystadenoma of the liver must be distinguished from hydatid cyst and simple cyst of the liver. Cystadenoma resembles hydatid cyst in that septations are present in both diseases. The distinctive characteristics of cystadenoma and simple cyst of the liver

are listed in Table 64.2. It can be difficult to make the distinction between cystadenoma and a cluster of contiguous cysts of the liver (the contiguous cysts being interpreted as a single cystadenoma with septations); the distinction between these two diseases is important because their prognosis and treatment are completely different. As emphasized earlier, the presence of additional typical cysts is a strong argument for the diagnosis of simple cysts, whereas cystadenomas are exceptionally multiple.

Treatment

Cystadenoma of the liver, even in an asymptomatic patient, must be treated by complete excision (see Ch. 65). Partial excision exposes the patient to the risk of recurrence and to the risk of cystadenocarcinoma (Lewis et al, 1988). After complete excision, cystadenoma does not recur. Three-year survival after treatment of cystadenocarcinoma is 55% (Barthet et al, 1992).

CILIATED HEPATIC FOREGUT CYSTS

Ciliated cysts have been described in all areas where the foregut extends during the embryonic period, including the sublingual area, esophagus, stomach, ileum, pancreas, and gallbladder.

Table 64.2 Distinctive Characteristics of Cystadenoma and Simple Cyst of the Liver

	Cystadenoma	Simple Cyst
No. cysts	1	≥1
Septations	Present	Absent
Papillary projections	Common	Absent
Cystic fluid	Mucinous	Serous
Recurrence after partial excision	Common	Exceptional
Malignant transformation (cystadenocarcinoma)	Possible	Exceptional

They also may be present within the liver. Although extremely rare, ciliated hepatic cysts warrant special consideration.

Pathology and Pathogenesis

Ciliated hepatic cysts are located within the liver parenchyma, do not communicate with the biliary system, and have a characteristic four-layer border that consists of a pseudostratified ciliated columnar epithelium covering a subepithelial connective tissue, smooth muscle bundles, and an outer fibrous capsule. The lining epithelium may secrete fluids of different composition (from nearly water to viscous or mucous), which explains why its echogenicity may be variable and why calcifications may be present, although exceptionally. The second characteristic of these cysts is that they are subcapsular, usually located on the anterior surface of the liver close to the insertion of the falciform ligament. Two thirds are localized in the left lobe of the liver in segment IV, but right lobe cysts also have been described (Takahiro et al, 2003). The final characteristic of these cysts is that they are classically unilocular and usually less than 4 cm in diameter.

Prevalence and Etiology

Ciliated hepatic cysts, although known since 1857, are exceptional, with fewer than 60 cases reported in the literature, most in the past 20 years of the 20th century. There is no gender predominance, and the age of the patients ranges from 5 to 82 years (mean age 52 years).

Manifestation and Diagnosis

Most ciliated hepatic foregut cysts are asymptomatic and discovered incidentally during abdominal imaging studies or surgical explorations. Abdominal symptoms are rare, probably because of their small size. Two thirds of the cysts are hypoechoic on ultrasound, are hypodense on CT, and do not enhance after injection of contrast material (Fig. 64.7). They are anechoic, as formal biliary cysts, in less than 5% (Horii et al, 2003). Some ciliated cysts also may have an atypical solid tumor appearance on CT and a noncystic appearance on ultrasound (hyperechoic), probably as a result of mucinous material, calcium, and cholesterol crystals within the cyst. In this situation, the differential diagnosis includes cystadenoma or cystadenocarcinoma and may be difficult, especially because CA 19-9 may be expressed by the epithelium of the ciliated cysts, and its serum level may be slightly elevated (Wu et al, 1998). Fine-needle aspiration cytology has been suggested, but its accuracy in this setting is unknown.

Course, Complications, and Treatment

Ciliated hepatic foregut cysts are usually thought to follow a benign course. Compression of adjacent structures is extremely rare, with a single case report of portal compression resulting in portal hypertension (Harty et al, 1998). At least three cases of malignant transformation into squamous cell carcinoma have been reported, however, in recent years (de Lajarte-Thirouard et al, 2002; Furlanetto & Dei Tos, 2002; Vick et al, 1999). Because this transformation has occurred in patients with cysts larger than 10 cm, most authors agree that excision is indicated when the cyst is larger than 4 to 5 cm, enlarges, shows abnormalities in its wall, or is symptomatic, although other authors have broader indications.

POLYCYSTIC LIVER DISEASE

Polycystic liver disease is an autosomal dominant condition responsible for the formation of multiple hepatic cysts that are frequently, but not always, associated with kidney cysts.

Pathology and Pathogenesis

Liver cysts in patients with adult polycystic kidney disease are macroscopically and microscopically similar to simple cysts of

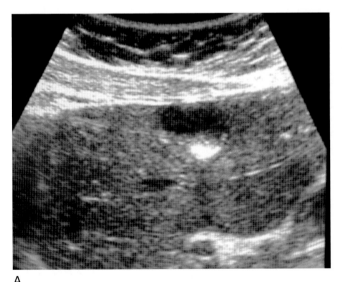

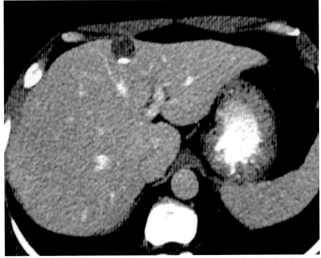

A   B

Fig. 64.7. Ciliated hepatic foregut cyst. **A,** Ultrasound. **B,** CT. The cyst is superficial, small, and not strictly anechoic. A calcification is present at its inferior level.

the liver. The cysts are unilocular, are bordered by a single-layered epithelium, contain a serous fluid, and do not communicate with the biliary tree. The main difference between these two entities concerns the number of the liver cysts. The liver cysts, when present, are multiple in all patients with adult polycystic kidney disease; in contrast, numerous cysts are found only in a few patients with simple cysts of the liver.

In patients with adult polycystic kidney disease, microscopic examination of the liver shows that, in addition to the macroscopic cysts, there are usually numerous microscopic cysts and clusters of multiple bile ductules, designated as von Meyenburg complexes, in the lobules or in the vicinity of the portal spaces. Pathogenesis of the liver cysts associated with adult polycystic kidney disease is similar to that of simple cysts of the liver. The cysts result from dilation of an aberrant bile ductule, probably belonging to a von Meyenburg complex, which has lost its communication with the biliary tree (Melnick, 1975). Despite the large number and the large size of liver cysts, the hepatic parenchymal volume is preserved (Everson et al, 1988), which explains why normal hepatic function and normal intrahepatic circulation is maintained in most of these patients.

Etiology

Polycystic liver disease usually is associated with autosomal dominant polycystic kidney disease, whereas autosomal recessive polycystic renal disease, which is far less frequent, is associated with congenital hepatic fibrosis. Polycystic liver disease associated with autosomal dominant polycystic kidney disease is linked to mutations in either the *PKD1* or *PKD2* gene. *PKD1* (Ward et al, 1996) is located on the short arm of chromosome 16 and expresses polycystin-1; its mutation accounts for 90% of mutations in autosomal dominant polycystic kidney disease families. Most of the remainder are related to a mutation in *PKD2* (Mochizuki et al, 1996), which is located on chromosome 4 and expresses polycystin-2. Polycystic liver disease also may be observed in the absence of renal cystic disease. In this setting it is related to a third mutation, in the *PRKCSH* gene, located on chromosome 19, which encodes hepatocystin (Drenth et al, 2004).

Features of the cysts and their natural history are comparable whatever the mutation, although patients with *PKD2* mutation tend to have later onset of their disease than patients with *PKD1* mutation. Hepatic cysts, similar to simple cysts, are rarely observed before puberty, and their prevalence increases thereafter. Kidney cysts in patients with autosomal dominant polycystic kidney disease always precede the development of hepatic cysts. By the time they reach their 40s, approximately 80% of patients with renal cysts have liver cysts (Table 64.3) (Gabow et al, 1990). The number and size of the liver cysts are greater in women than in men, increase with patient age, and are greater in patients with large renal cysts and severe kidney dysfunction than in patients with small renal cysts and mild renal insufficiency. Similar to simple cysts, men and women have an equal lifetime risk to develop hepatic cysts, but women experience greater numbers and larger sizes of hepatic cysts. Pregnancy and use of female steroid hormones further increase the risk of severe hepatic cystic disease.

Manifestations and Diagnosis

In most patients with adult polycystic kidney disease, the liver cysts are small and sparse and remain clinically silent. In a few patients, numerous larger liver cysts may cause abdominal pain and discomfort; early postprandial fullness, especially when there is severe involvement of the left liver that compresses the stomach; or shortness of breath. At clinical examination of patients with large cysts, the liver is enlarged, sometimes to an enormous size; the cysts may be so tense that they can be confused with solid tumors. There are no signs or symptoms suggesting cholestasis, liver failure, or portal hypertension. Liver tests are usually normal or show only a slight elevation in gamma-glutamyltransferase. Manifestations and complications (and management) are the same whether polycystic liver disease is isolated or associated with polycystic kidney disease (Qian et al, 2003).

Ultrasound and CT show multiple, fluid-filled, round or oval cysts, with sharp margins, in the liver and in the kidneys (Fig. 64.8). Calcification of the cysts has been reported, but is rare (Coffin et al, 1990; Kutcher et al, 1977). Similar to simple cysts, cysts are hyperintense on T2-weighted MRI and hypointense on T1-weighted MRI except when they are complicated by hemorrhage.

Table 64.3   Age and Prevalence of Liver Cysts Shown by Liver Scintiscan* or by Computed Tomography[†] in Patients with Adult Polycystic Kidney Disease

Patient Age (yr)	LIVER SCINTISCAN		COMPUTED TOMOGRAPHY	
	No. Patients Studied	Patients with Liver Cysts (%)	No. Patients Studied	Patients with Liver Cysts (%)
10-19	12	0	0	0
20-29	47	11	1	0
30-39	31	32	15	40
40-49	30	37	17	53
50-59	25	40	20	65
>60	13	77	13	87
Total	*158*	*29*	*66*	*59*

*Milutinovic et al, 1980.
[†]Thomsen & Thaysen, 1988.

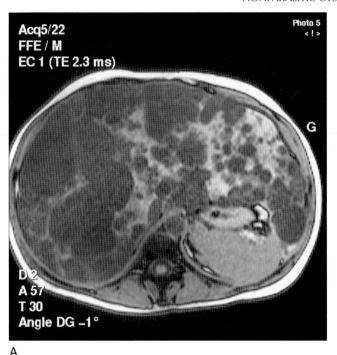

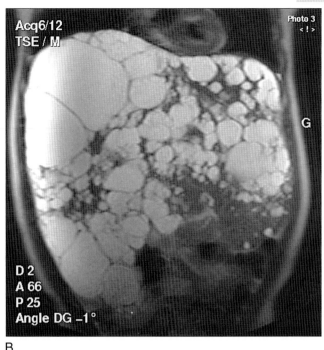

Fig. 64.8. Polycystic liver disease. **A,** Abdominal CT. **B,** T2-weighted MRI. The liver is enlarged and almost completely replaced by multiple cysts. These cysts are large in the right lobe and smaller in the left lobe. The stomach is compressed between the left liver and the spleen.

Course and Complications

Liver cysts grow slowly. In some patients, whose life has been prolonged by hemodialysis or renal transplantation, liver cysts may become enormous. The main complication is bacterial infection of a cyst (Robson & Fenster, 1964; Telenti et al, 1990), which may be facilitated by immunosuppressive drugs administered to renal transplant recipients (Bourgeois et al, 1983). The infected cysts can be recognized by ultrasound and CT, which show echoic material (corresponding to pus) within the cysts (Telenti et al, 1990). Bacterial infection can be severe enough to threaten the patient's life. Another complication, which is relatively common, is intracystic bleeding. Other complications, which are less common, include cholestasis secondary to compression of the bifurcation by large cysts (Ergün et al, 1980; Howard et al, 1976), portal hypertension causing gastrointestinal bleeding (Ratcliffe et al, 1984) or refractory ascites (McGarrity et al, 1986), right atrium compression causing hypotension and leg edema (Lasic et al, 2004), malnutrition owing to compression of the stomach, Budd-Chiari syndrome (Fig. 64.9), and cholangiocellular carcinoma (Levine et al, 1985). Associated conditions include cerebral aneurysm and mitral valve prolapse. Cerebral aneurysms may be linked to the *PKD1* mutation (Rossetti et al, 2003) and have been observed in polycystic liver disease without autosomal dominant polycystic kidney disease. Most of these aneurysms are small and do not seem to be at increased risk of growth or rupture (Gibbs et al, 2004).

Differential Diagnosis

Liver cysts associated with adult polycystic kidney disease must be distinguished from multiple simple cysts of the liver.

First, because adult polycystic kidney disease is transmitted as an autosomal dominant trait, it is usual for one parent or sibling to have been recognized to have the disease. In the case of simple cysts of the liver, which are noninherited malformations, parents and siblings are not affected with the disease. The presentation of adult polycystic kidney disease varies, however, and affected

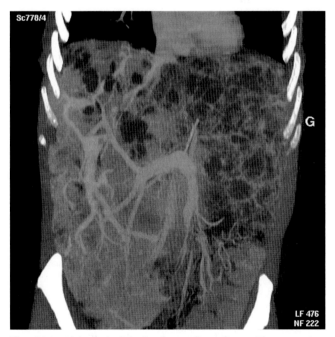

Fig. 64.9. Abdominal CT of polycystic liver disease. Transverse view. The termination of the right and middle hepatic veins is compressed by the cysts, and there is an intrahepatic circulation between the hepatic veins.

individuals may be asymptomatic and unrecognized. Second, multiple renal cysts are associated constantly with liver cysts in adult polycystic kidney disease, whereas renal cysts are absent in multiple simple cysts of the liver. As mentioned earlier, one or a few simple renal cysts may be fortuitously associated with simple cysts of the liver. Patients with this fortuitous association must not be thought to have adult polycystic kidney disease.

Treatment

There are no medical therapies for polycystic liver disease (see Ch. 67). Although secretin triggers secretion by normal intrahepatic bile duct cells, somatostatin analogues have failed to reduce hepatic cyst growth or size (Chauveau et al, 1993). There is no strong evidence that estrogen replacement therapy should be avoided, when indicated. Although there are anecdotal reports of palliation with percutaneous alcohol sclerotherapy or laparoscopic fenestration of the cysts, neither sclerotherapy nor fenestration proves effective in the long-term (Robinson et al, 2004).

Symptoms in polycystic liver disease are related mainly to the volume of the liver, rather than to a specific cyst, and the aim of treatment is to decompress the whole liver or remove as many cysts as possible. These objectives can be achieved, in highly symptomatic patients, by open fenestration, liver resection, or liver transplantation (see Ch. 65). The aim of fenestration is to unroof as many cysts as possible, starting from the superficial cyst and proceeding stepwise to the deeper cysts. The laparoscopic approach does not allow sufficient access and is contraindicated (Kabbej et al, 1996; Morino et al, 1994). The vascular structures that are compressed by the cysts may be inadvertently injured. The volume of fluid aspirated averages 3 L and may be as high as 8 L; postoperative ascites is common and may result in delayed wound healing or in superinfection. Partial liver resection in combination with fenestration of the remnant liver has been proposed (Que et al, 1995; Soravia et al, 1995; Vons et al, 1998) to increase regeneration of the noncystic liver. Liver transplantation should be considered in patients in whom the aforementioned procedures have been unsuccessful, but it has been performed in only a few patients (Jeyarajah et al, 1998; Pirenne et al, 2001; Starzl et al, 1990; Swenson et al, 1998; Washburn et al, 1996).

Consensus is lacking on the indications for treatment procedures. Available data indicate the following: (1) Open fenestration of the maximum number of cysts is associated with significant morbidity, but provides long-term relief of symptoms in patients who do not have diffuse replacement of the liver by cysts (Farges & Bismuth, 1995; Gigot et al, 1997; Vons et al, 1998). (2) Liver resection, which often proves possible owing to an asymmetry in cyst distribution, is a demanding procedure, associated with high morbidity rates, but achieves better results than fenestration alone; long-term sustained reduction in symptoms is observed in more than 90% of patients (Que et al, 1995). (3) Liver transplantation cures patients (Pirenne et al, 2001), but has inherent mortality with a 5-year survival of 69% (U.S. Scientific Registry of Transplant Recipients; available at www.ustransplant.org). Despite its risk, transplantation is the only option in patients with kidney failure resulting from autosomal dominant polycystic kidney disease or malnutrition resulting from massive hepatomegaly.

If liver transplantation (see Ch. 103) is indicated per se, simultaneous renal transplantation should be considered if renal function is impaired. The rationale for a combined liver-kidney transplantation using grafts from the same donor is as follows: (1) Immunosuppression is difficult to manage in patients with renal failure; (2) renal function may deteriorate further after liver transplantation because of the nephrotoxicity of immunosuppressive agents or progression of the kidney disease or both; (3) rejection episodes seem to be fewer in patients receiving both organs from the same donor than from two donors.

Asymptomatic or paucisymptomatic patients should not be operated on. If kidney transplantation is indicated, simultaneous liver transplantation should be anticipated if liver cysts cause incapacitating manifestations. Because immunosuppression after kidney transplantation is similar to that after liver transplantation, the additional risk of simultaneous liver transplantation is related only to surgical complications and not to immunosuppression.

CONGENITAL HEPATIC FIBROSIS

Congenital hepatic fibrosis is a recessive inherited disease that belongs to the family of hepatic ductal plate malformations. It is characterized by large, fibrotic portal spaces containing multiple bile ductules, the main consequence of which is portal hypertension. In contrast to the other conditions presented in this chapter, cysts in congenital hepatic fibrosis remain small. The disease was described as fibrocystic disease of the liver by Grumbach and coworkers in 1954. The name *congenital hepatic fibrosis* was introduced by Kerr and associates in 1961.

Pathology and Pathogenesis

The lesion of congenital hepatic fibrosis consists of portal spaces markedly increased in size because of abundant connective tissue and numerous bile ductules, more or less ectatic, communicating with the biliary tree (Fig. 64.10). Congenital hepatic fibrosis is not simply fibrosis, and bile ductular proliferation is an essential component of the lesion. A few portal spaces remain normal, which explains why congenital hepatic fibrosis may be

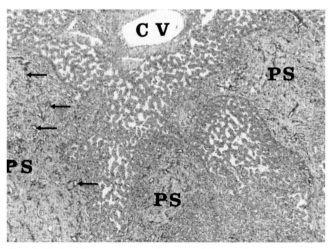

Fig. 64.10. Liver biopsy specimen of congenital hepatic fibrosis. Portal spaces (PS) are markedly increased in size and contain abundant fibrosis and numerous bile ducts *(arrows)*. CV, centrilobular vein.

unrecognized at histologic examination of a small liver biopsy specimen. Some clusters of multiple bile ductules surrounded with fibrosis may be present within the lobules, apart from the portal spaces. Some bile ductules are so markedly dilated that they form microcysts; the microcysts communicate with the biliary tree. Separation between the fibrotic portal spaces and the rest of the liver parenchyma is sharp. The architecture of the liver is normal.

The primary disorder of congenital hepatic fibrosis is likely to be bile ductular proliferation, with fibrosis being secondarily induced by the multiple bile ductules. The initial lesion might be clusters of multiple bile ductules (i.e., von Meyenburg complexes), resembling the initial lesion of the liver cysts associated with adult polycystic kidney disease. In congenital hepatic fibrosis, the abnormal bile ductules maintain their communication with the biliary tree, and as a result, only microcysts are formed. In contrast, in adult polycystic kidney disease, the abnormal bile ductules lose their communication with the biliary tree and dilate markedly and form large cysts.

The mechanism for the development of multiple bile ductules in congenital hepatic fibrosis is unknown. It has been suggested that bile ductular proliferation might result from a disproportionate overgrowth of the biliary epithelium (Nakanuma et al, 1982). A similar disorder affecting the epithelium of the large bile ducts might account for Caroli's disease associated with congenital hepatic fibrosis. A similar mechanism might explain the dilation of the renal collecting tubules and the dilation of pancreatic ducts, two extrahepatic malformations that may be associated with congenital hepatic fibrosis.

Etiology and Prevalence

Congenital hepatic fibrosis is an inherited malformation transmitted as an autosomal recessive trait (Alvarez et al, 1981; De Vos et al, 1988; Kerr et al, 1961; Summerfield et al, 1986). The parents, presumably heterozygous, are phenotypically normal. Men and women are equally affected. Several siblings may be affected. Consanguinity increases the risk of congenital hepatic fibrosis. The prevalence of congenital hepatic fibrosis is not established, but it is probably low and might be similar to another autosomal recessive liver disease, Wilson's disease (i.e., about 1:100,000) (Sheinberg & Sternlieb, 1984). There is no ethnic predominance.

Clinical Manifestations and Diagnosis

The main consequence of congenital hepatic fibrosis is portal hypertension, which is likely to have been present since the patient's birth. In most patients, the disease is recognized at the first episode of gastrointestinal bleeding secondary to ruptured esophageal or gastric varices, which occurs usually between age 5 and 20 years, sometimes later. In a few patients, the disease is recognized before any episode of gastrointestinal bleeding because of blood disorders secondary to hypersplenism, abdominal discomfort secondary to an enlarged spleen, or the presence of abdominal collateral venous circulation. In a few patients with congenital hepatic fibrosis not associated with Caroli's disease, an episode of bacterial cholangitis is the presenting manifestation (De Vos et al, 1988; Erlinger et al, 1969). The disease may

remain completely silent during the lifetime of the patient (Averback, 1977). In other patients, the onset of symptoms may be delayed until the 40s or 50s.

At clinical examination, the liver is often, but not constantly, enlarged. Splenomegaly is present in most patients. An abdominal wall collateral circulation (Cruveilhier syndrome in some patients) is often visible. Ascites is absent. There is no symptom or sign indicating liver failure, in particular, jaundice or spider nevi. Liver tests are normal except for a moderately increased alkaline phosphatase and gamma-glutamyltransferase in a few patients. Endoscopic examination shows esophageal varices. Ultrasound and CT show the liver (and most notably the left lateral segment and caudate lobe) is often enlarged (often hyperechoic because of fibrosis and ductular proliferation), the portal vein is patent (which excludes extrahepatic portal hypertension), the spleen is enlarged, and portacaval anastomoses are present. Associated ductal plate malformations (e.g., biliary hamartoma, Caroli's disease, or choledochal cyst), enlargement of the hepatic artery, and renal abnormalities (polycystic renal disease, parenchymal calcification, or medullary sponge disease) also may be identified on CT (Zeitoun et al, 2004). MRI cholangiography shows an extremely unusual distribution of the biliary tree, with mild and more or less uniform dilation peripherally contrasting with slenderness and poor visibility centrally (Krause et al, 2002). Histologic examination of a hepatic tissue specimen obtained by needle biopsy shows the typical lesion in most patients; however, if the specimen is small, the lesion may be missed because, as mentioned earlier, some of the portal spaces may be normal.

Course and Complications

The course of the disease is dominated by recurrent episodes of gastrointestinal bleeding. These are often well tolerated and usually are not followed by hepatic encephalopathy, ascites, or jaundice. Death is due to massive bleeding, but not to liver dysfunction. The course of congenital hepatic fibrosis resembles that of extrahepatic portal hypertension and differs from that of cirrhosis. Nevertheless, because it is a dynamic disorder with progressive extension of the fibrosis, evolution into secondary biliary cirrhosis is possible (De Ledinghen et al, 1998). Even in the absence of associated Caroli's disease, recurrent episodes of bacterial cholangitis affect a few patients (Alvarez et al, 1981; De Vos et al, 1988; Erlinger et al, 1969). There is a risk of intrahepatic cholangiocarcinoma (Yamato et al, 1998).

Associated Malformations

Congenital hepatic fibrosis is often associated with Caroli's disease, either clinically silent (shown by ultrasound or CT) or causing cholangitis (see later). Congenital hepatic fibrosis likewise often is associated with a renal malformation consisting of ectatic collecting tubules, resembling sponge kidney (Kerr et al, 1962). Dilation affects the medullary and cortical portions of the collecting tubules in congenital hepatic fibrosis, whereas dilation is limited to the medullary portion of the collecting tubules in sponge kidney (Clermont et al, 1967; Fauvert & Benhamou, 1974). This renal malformation is clinically silent except for hematuria or urinary infection or both in a few patients. Dilation of the collecting tubules can be shown by intravenous pyelography revealing enlarged kidneys and coarse streaking of the medulla. These radiologic abnormalities are present in about two thirds of patients (Alvarez et al, 1981; Kerr et al, 1962); their presence is good evidence for, but their absence is not an argument against, the diagnosis of congenital hepatic fibrosis. In some patients with a normal intravenous pyelogram, histologic examination of the kidney may show ectatic collecting tubules (Clermont et al, 1967).

In most patients, dilation of collecting tubules remains stable. In some patients, the ectatic segments lose their communications with the urinary tract and transform into large renal cysts (Dupond et al, 1978); the renal malformation resembles adult polycystic kidney disease. This transformation accounts for the large renal cysts detectable by ultrasound or intravenous pyelography in numerous patients with congenital hepatic fibrosis (Alvarez et al, 1981; Clermont et al, 1967; De Vos et al, 1988; Kerr et al, 1962). This transformation may occur early in infancy or later. In patients with large renal cysts, the renal malformation may cause renal failure or arterial hypertension or both. Other associated malformations are rare and include duplication of the intrahepatic portal vein branches (Alvarez et al, 1981; Odièvre et al, 1977), cystic dysplasia of the pancreas (Kerr et al, 1961), intestinal lymphangiectasia (Chagnon et al, 1982), pulmonary emphysema (Williams et al, 1964), cerebral hemangioma (Wagenvoort et al, 1962), aneurysms of renal and cerebral arteries (Kerr et al, 1961), and cleft palate (Kerr et al, 1961).

Treatment

Active bleeding from ruptured esophageal varices requires blood transfusions, vasopressin (or somatostatin), and endoscopic sclerotherapy. Prevention of recurrent hemorrhage is based on β-blockers or endoscopic sclerotherapy. In the few patients in whom sclerotherapy is unsuccessful, poorly tolerated, or not feasible, surgical portacaval shunt can be considered. Hepatic encephalopathy and liver failure after portosystemic shunt would be less common in patients with congenital hepatic fibrosis than in patients with cirrhosis (Alvarez et al, 1981; De Vos et al, 1988; Kerr et al, 1978). Because of the risk of bacterial infection of the cystic biliary tract, transjugular intrahepatic portacaval shunt has been seldom performed.

CAROLI'S DISEASE

Caroli's disease is a congenital malformation characterized by multifocal dilation of segmental bile ducts, the main consequence of which is recurrent bacterial cholangitis. This malformation was described by Caroli and colleagues in 1958 (Caroli et al, 1958b). This malformation is not a single entity, and, for this reason, the term *Caroli's syndrome* also is used.

Pathology, Classification, and Etiology

Caroli's disease is thought to result from the arrest of or a derangement in the normal embryologic remodeling of ducts. If the large intrahepatic bile ducts are affected, the result is Caroli's disease, whereas abnormal development of the small interlobular bile ducts results in congenital hepatic fibrosis. If all levels of the biliary tree are involved, features of congenital hepatic fibrosis and Caroli's disease are present.

The lesion of Caroli's disease consists of multifocal dilation of the segmental bile ducts. The ectatic portions form cysts of varying size, separated by portions of bile ducts that are normal or regularly dilated. Septa containing portal veins protrude into the lumen of the ectatic bile ducts (dot sign) (Choi et al, 1990). The multifocal dilation may be diffuse, affecting the whole intrahepatic biliary tree (although it may be more marked in a part of the liver), or it may be confined to a part of the liver, often the left lobe or a segment of the left lobe (Caroli et al, 1958a). Cysts are numerous in the diffuse form; in the localized form, there are usually fewer than 10 cysts.

Multifocal dilation of the segmental bile ducts is not a single entity. In about half of the cases, multifocal dilation of the segmental bile ducts is associated with congenital hepatic fibrosis (Fauvert & Benhamou, 1974; Summerfield et al, 1986). In this type of Caroli's disease, the distribution of multifocal dilation is diffuse. As in congenital hepatic fibrosis, the malformation is transmitted as an autosomal recessive trait and may be associated with a renal malformation.

In about half of cases, multifocal dilation of the segmental bile ducts is not associated with congenital hepatic fibrosis (De Vos et al, 1988; Summerfield et al, 1986). In such cases, multifocal dilation may be confined to a part of the liver, usually the left lobe (Caroli et al, 1958a). This type of Caroli's disease is not inherited and usually is not associated with a renal malformation, but it may be associated with other malformations of the biliary tree, in particular, choledochal cyst (Loubeau & Steichen, 1976; Summerfield et al, 1986).

Manifestations and Diagnosis

Caroli's disease, which is likely to be present at birth, remains asymptomatic for the first 5 to 20 years of the patient's life (sometimes longer) and in a few cases during the patient's whole life. Asymptomatic Caroli's disease remains unrecognized except in patients in whom an imaging investigation of the liver is performed for unrelated reasons and in patients in whom congenital hepatic fibrosis has been diagnosed, and multifocal dilation of the segmental bile ducts has been suspected and shown by ultrasound or CT. In most patients, the first episode of bacterial cholangitis occurs in the absence of any apparent precipitating factor. In a few cases, however, bacterial cholangitis is induced by a surgical operation or an invasive investigation on the biliary tree, such as cholecystectomy, choledochotomy, T-tube drainage, intraoperative cholangiography, or endoscopic retrograde cholangiography (Clermont et al, 1967; Grumbach et al, 1954).

The main and often the only symptom of bacterial cholangitis secondary to Caroli's disease is fever without abdominal pain and jaundice. This is in contrast to bacterial cholangitis complicating common bile duct stones, in which fever usually is accompanied by pain or jaundice or both. As a consequence, the first episodes of fever may be not attributed to bacterial cholangitis.

At clinical examination, the liver is usually enlarged. There is no sign or symptom indicating liver dysfunction. In patients with Caroli's disease associated with congenital hepatic fibrosis, manifestations of portal hypertension are present. Liver function tests are normal except for alkaline phosphatase and gamma-glutamyltransferase, which may be moderately increased.

Ultrasound and CT show cysts of various sizes, which are distributed throughout the liver or confined to a part of the liver. The cysts may or may not be associated with tubular dilation of the segmental bile ducts. Ultrasound and CT may show tiny dots within the dilated bile ducts, corresponding to portal branches and hepatic arteries protruding into the lumen of the cysts (Choi et al, 1990).

The main characteristic of these cysts is their communication with the biliary tract. Communication of the cysts with the biliary tree may be obvious (1) because the cysts are in continuity with the large intrahepatic bile ducts, or (2) because the cysts contain biliary stones, or (3) because the cysts contain air. These communications can be shown, when not obvious, by several procedures, including (1) hepatobiliary scintiscan, which shows cold areas in the early phase scans that become hot at the late phase (Stillman et al, 1981); (2) CT after intravenous injection of biliary contrast material, which shows opacification of the cysts; and (3) MRI (Fig. 64.11) (Guy et al, 2002). MRI has replaced direct opacification of the cysts by endoscopic retrograde cholangiography, intraoperative cholangiography, or postoperative cholangiography through a T-tube because of their inherent risk of bacterial cholangitis.

Half of patients with Caroli's disease have a fusiform enlargement of the common bile duct; this may be secondary to the repeat bouts of cholangitis, stone migration, increased bile flow, or associated choledocal cyst. The intrahepatic cysts of Caroli's disease must be distinguished from (1) multiple liver cysts and the liver cysts of adult polycystic kidney disease (these cysts do not communicate with the biliary tract), (2) dilated bile ducts secondary to an obstructed common bile duct, and (3) ectatic bile ducts secondary to primary sclerosing cholangitis (Ludwig et al, 1982, 1986; Theilmann & Stiehl, 1990). The ectactic bile ducts of primary sclerosing cholangitis are usually small; however, they are relatively large in a few cases of sclerosing cholangitis (Ludwig et al, 1982; Theilmann & Stiehl; 1990), in which an erroneous diagnosis of Caroli's disease has been made (Ludwig et al, 1982, 1986).

Course and Complications

The course of Caroli's disease is dominated by recurrent episodes of bacterial cholangitis (see Ch. 58), the frequency of which varies widely. Some patients experience 10 to 20 episodes, whereas others experience only 1 or 2 episodes a year. In patients with frequent episodes of bacterial cholangitis, the prognosis is poor; most die 5 to 10 years after the onset of cholangitis, usually of uncontrolled biliary bacterial infection. Bacterial cholangitis may be complicated by liver abscesses, septicemia, extrahepatic abscesses, and secondary amyloidosis (Fevery et al, 1972).

Caroli's disease often is complicated by intrahepatic stones (Mathias et al, 1978) (see Ch. 40). The bile of patients with Caroli's disease frequently contains cholesterol crystals (Ros et al, 1993). For this reason, most of the stones are pigmented and cholesterol-rich. Such stones are recognized easily by ultrasound, but may be missed by CT when not calcified. These stones can migrate from the cysts into the common bile duct and produce biliary pain, cholestasis, or acute pancreatitis (Sahel et al, 1976). Cholangiocellular carcinoma (see Ch. 52) develops in some patients with Caroli's disease in the monolobar and diffuse forms of the disease (Abdalla et al, 1999; Caroli et al, 1958b; Dayton et al, 1983; Etienne et al, 1987; Summerfield et al, 1986; Totkas & Hohenberger et al, 2000), but because of the rarity of the disease, the frequency with which this occurs is unknown. Reported figures range from 7% to 24% (Bloustein, 1977; Levy et al, 2002). Similar to sclerosing cholangitis, the early diagnosis of malignant transformation is challenging. Hepatocellular carcinoma also has been reported in association with Caroli's disease (Kchir et al, 1990).

Associated Malformations

In patients with Caroli's disease and congenital hepatic fibrosis, the malformations described in association with congenital hepatic

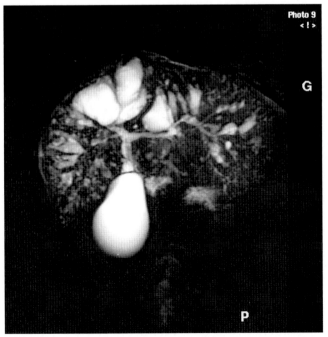

A

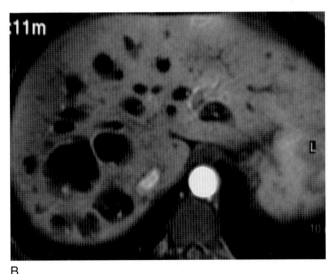

B

Fig. 64.11. MRI of Caroli's disease in its diffuse form, associated with congenital hepatic fibrosis. **A,** MRI reconstruction showing the segmental dilation of the intrahepatic bile ducts. **B,** After injection of contrast medium, tiny dots corresponding to portal branches and hepatic arteries protruding into the lumen of the cysts are visible.

fibrosis may be present. In patients with Caroli's disease with or, more often, without congenital hepatic fibrosis, associated choledochal cyst (see Ch. 63) is relatively common (Loubeau & Steichen, 1976; Summerfield et al, 1986). Exceptionally, Caroli's disease is associated with Laurence-Moon-Biedl-Bardet syndrome (Tsuchiya et al, 1977).

Treatment

Treatment of the episodes of bacterial cholangitis is with appropriate antibiotics. The prevention of recurrent bacterial cholangitis is difficult. Periodic administration of antibiotics is efficacious in some patients, but completely inefficient in others. T-tube drainage is ineffective and may be dangerous in patients with associated congenital hepatic fibrosis; large amounts of water and electrolytes secreted by the multiple bile ductules may be lost through the T-tube, which may result in severe dehydration (Turnberg et al, 1968). Administration of ursodiol is efficient in the prevention of lithiasis and in the treatment of intrahepatic stones (Ros et al, 1993). It is reasonable to administer ursodiol in all patients with Caroli's disease. Transhepatic intubation and drainage of the biliary tree has been used successfully in a few patients (Witlin et al, 1982). Surgical biliary-intestinal anastomoses or endoscopic papillotomy may facilitate the passage of stones from the common bile duct into the intestine; these procedures have long been avoided because they may increase the frequency and severity of the episodes of bacterial cholangitis (Watts et al, 1974). More recent experience suggests, however, that improvement of symptoms can be achieved through complete endoscopic stone clearance in septic patients (Caroli-Bosc et al, 1998).

In the localized form of Caroli's disease, partial hepatectomy is indicated, and excellent results can be expected (Nagasue, 1984; Ramond et al, 1984; Serejo et al, 1988; Thompson et al, 1983). In the diffuse form, if the cysts predominate in a confined part of the liver, partial hepatectomy likewise can be attempted. In such patients, partial hepatectomy may be difficult, however, because of associated congenital hepatic fibrosis and portal hypertension. The long-term results may be compromised because multifocal dilation affecting the remaining liver may be the source of recurrent bacterial cholangitis (Ramond et al, 1984). In the diffuse form without predominance of the cysts in any part of the liver and complicated by severe recurrent bacterial cholangitis, liver transplantation should be considered (Sans et al, 1997; Waechter et al, 2001).

REFERENCES

Abdalla EK, et al, 1999: Monolobar Caroli's disease and cholangiocarcinoma. HPB Surg 11:271-276.

Akriviadis EA, et al, 1989: Spontaneous rupture of nonparasitic cyst of the liver. Gastroenterology 97:213-215.

Alexander RC, 1925: Solitary nonparasitic cysts of the liver. Edinb Med J 32:61-68.

Alvarez F, et al, 1981: Congenital hepatic fibrosis. J Pediatr 99:370-375.

Averback P, 1977: Congenital hepatic fibrosis: asymptomatic adults without renal anomaly. Arch Pathol Lab Med 101:260-261.

Barthet M, et al, 1992: Biliary cystadenocarcinoma: a rare tumor of the liver. Dig Surg 9:285-287.

Bloustein PA, 1977: Association of carcinoma with congenital cystic conditions of the liver and bile ducts. Am J Gastroenterol 67:40-46.

Bourgeois M, et al, 1983: Infection of hepatic cysts following kidney transplantation in polycystic disease. World J Surg 7:629-631.

Buyse S, et al, 2004: Acute pulmonary embolism: a rare complication of a large non-parasitic hepatic cyst. Eur J Gastroenterol Hepatol 16:1241-1244.

Cadranel JF, et al, 1994: Cystadénome du foie: etude clinique, radiologique et anatomopathologique de 5 cas, dont un associé à un cystadénocarcinome. Gastroenterol Clin Biol 18:84-89.

Cappell MS, 1988: Obstructive jaundice from benign, nonparasitic hepatic cysts: identification of risk factors and percutaneous aspiration for diagnosis and treatment. Am J Gastroenterol 83:93-96.

Caremani M, et al, 1993: Echographic epidemiology of non-parasitic hepatic cysts. J Clin Ultrasound 21:115-118.

Caroli J, et al, 1958a: Une affection nouvelle, sans doute congénitale, des voies biliaires: la dilatation kystique unilobaire des canaux hépatiques. Semaine des Hôpitaux de Paris 34:136-143.

Caroli J, et al, 1958b: La dilatation polykystique congénitale des voies biliaires intrahépatiques: essai de classification. Semaine des Hôpitaux de Paris 34:488-495.

Caroli-Bosc FX, et al, 1998: The role of therapeutic endoscopy associated with extracorporeal shock-wave lithotripsy and bile acid treatment in the management of Caroli's disease. Endoscopy 30:559-563.

Carrim ZI, Murchison JT, 2003: The prevalence of simple renal and hepatic cysts detected by spiral computed tomography. Clin Radiol 58:626-629.

Chagnon JP, et al, 1982: Fibrose hépatique congénitale, polykystose rénale et lymphangiectasies intestinales primitive. Gastroenterol Clin Biol 6:326-332.

Chauveau D, et al, 1993: Evaluation of octreotide in massive polycystic liver disease. Presented at the 12th International Congress of Nephrology, Jerusalem, Israel, June 13-18, 1993, 487A.

Choi BI, et al, 1989: Biliary cystademona and cystadenocarcinoma: CT and sonographic findings. Radiology 171:57-61.

Choi BI, et al, 1990: Caroli's disease: central dot sign in CT. Radiology 174:161-163.

Clermont RJ, et al, 1967: Fibrose hépatique congénitale. Can Med Assoc J 97:1272-1278.

Clinkscales NB, et al, 1985: Obstructive jaundice secondary to benign hepatic cyst. Radiology 154:643-644.

Coffin B, et al, 1990: Calcified hepatic and renal cysts in adult dominant polycystic kidney disease. Dig Dis Sci 35:1172-1175.

Dayton MT, et al, 1983: Caroli's disease: a premalignant condition? Am J Surg 145:41-48.

de Lajarte-Thirouard AS, et al, 2002: Squamous cell carcinoma arising in a ciliated hepatic forgut cyst. Pathol Res Pract 198:697-700.

De Ledinghen V, et al, 1998: Case report: secondary biliary cirrhosis possibly related to congenital hepatic fibrosis—evidence of decreased number of portal branch veins and hypertrophic peribiliary vascular plexus. J Gastroenterol Hepatol 13:720-724.

De Vos M, et al, 1988: Congenital hepatic fibrosis. J Hepatol 6:222-228.

Drenth JP, et al, 2004: Molecular characterization of hepatocystin, the protein that is defective in autosomal dominant polycystic liver disease. Gastroenterology 126:1819-1827.

Dupond JL, et al, 1978: Kidney polycystic disease in adult congenital hepatic fibrosis. Ann Intern Med 88:514-515.

Emmermann A, et al, 1997: Laparoscopic treatment of nonparasitic cysts of the liver with omental transposition flap. Surg Endosc 11:734-736.

Ergün H, et al, 1980: Obstructive jaundice caused by polycystic liver disease. Radiology 136:435-436.

Erlinger S, et al, 1969: Les formes angiocholitiques de la fibrose hépatique congénitale. Presse Med 77:1189-1191.

Etienne JC, et al, 1987: Cholangiocarcinome développé sur maladie de Caroli: a propos d'un cas: revue de la littérature. J Chir (Paris) 124:161-164.

Everson GT, et al, 1988: Polycystic liver disease: quantitation of parenchymal and cyst volumes from computed tomography images and clinical correlates of hepatic cysts. Hepatology 8:1627-1634.

Fabiani P, et al, 1997: Laparoscopic fenestration of symptomatic non-parasitic cysts of the liver. Br J Surg (London) 84:321-322.

Farges O, Bismuth H, 1995: Fenestration in the management of polycystic liver disease. World J Surg 19:25-30.

Fauvert R, Benhamou JP, 1974: Congenital hepatic fibrosis. In Schaffner F, et al, (eds): The Liver and Its Diseases. New York, IMS, pp 283-288.

Fevery J, et al, 1972: Congenital dilatation of the intrahepatic bile ducts associated with the development of amyloidosis. Gut 13:604-609.

Flagg RS, Robinson DW, 1967: Solitary non parasitic hepatic cysts: report of oldest known case and review of the literature. Arch Surg 95:964-973.

Forrest ME, et al, 1980: Biliary cystadenomas: sonographic-angiographic-pathologic correlations. AJR Am J Roentgenol 135:723-727.

Frick M, Feinberg SB, 1982: Biliary cystadenoma. AJR Am J Roentgenol 139:393-395.

Frisell J, et al, 1979: Compression of the inferior caval vein: a rare complication of a large non-parasitic liver cyst. Acta Med Scand 205:541-542.

Furlanetto A, Dei Tos AP, 2002: Squamous cell carcinoma arising in a ciliated hepatic foregut cyst. Virchows Arch 441:296-298.

Gabow PA, et al, 1990: Risk factors for the development of hepatic cysts in autosomal dominant polycystic kidney disease. Hepatology 11:1033-1037.

Gaines PA, Sampson MA, 1989: The prevalence and characterization of simple hepatic cysts by ultrasound examination. Br J Radiol 62:335-337.

Geist DC, 1955: Solitary nonparasitic cyst of the liver. Arch Surg 71:867-880.

Gibbs GF, et al, 2004: Follow-up of intracranial aneurysms in autosomal-dominant polycystic kidney disease. Kidney Int 65:1621-1627.

Gigot JF, et al, 1997: Adult polycystic liver disease: is fenestration the most adequate operation for long-term management? Ann Surg 225:286-294.

Giuliante F, et al, 2003: Risk for laparoscopic fenestration of liver cysts. Surg Endosc 17:1735-1738.

Grumbach R, et al, 1954: Maladie fibrokystique du foie avec hypertension portale chez l'enfant: deux observations. Arch Anat Cytol Pathol 30:74-77.

Guy F, et al, 2002: Caroli's disease: magnetic resonance imaging features. Eur Radiol 12:2730-2736.

Harty MP, et al, 1998: Ciliated hepatic foregut cyst causing portal hypertension in an adolescent. AJR Am J Roentgenol 170:688-690.

Horii T, et al, 2003: Ciliated hepatic foregut cyst: a report of one case and a review of the literature. Hepatol Res 26:243-248.

Howard RJ, et al, 1976: Jaundice associated with polycystic liver disease: relief by surgical decompression of the cysts. Arch Surg 111:816-817.

Iemoto Y, et al, 1983: Biliary cystadenocarcinoma diagnosed by liver biopsy performed under ultrasonographic guidance. Gastroenterology 84:399-403.

Ishak KG, et al, 1977: Biliary cystadenoma and cystadenocarcinoma: report of 14 cases and review of the literature. Cancer 39:322-338.

Jeyarajah DR, et al, 1998: Liver and kidney transplantation for polycystic liver disease. Transplantation 66:529-544.

Kabbej M, et al, 1996: Laparoscopic fenestration in polycystic liver disease. Br J Surg 83:1697-1701.

Kchir N, et al, 1990: Maladie de Caroli associée à un hépatocarcinome: a propos d'une observation et revue de la littérature. Semaine des Hôpitaux de Paris 66:1962-1966.

Kerr DNS, et al, 1961: Congenital hepatic fibrosis. QJM 30:91-117.

Kerr DNS, et al, 1962: Lesion resembling medullary sponge kidney in patients with congenital hepatic fibrosis. Clin Radiol 12:85-91.

Kerr DNS, et al, 1978: Congenital hepatic fibrosis: the long term prognosis. Gut 19:514-520.

Klingler PJ, et al, 1997: Treatment of hepatic cysts in the era of laparoscopic surgery. Br J Surg 84:438-444.

Kokubo T, et al, 1988: Mucin-hypersecreting intrahepatic biliary neoplasms. Radiology 168:609-614.

Korobkin M, et al, 1989: Biliary cystadenoma and cystadenocarcinoma: CT and sonographic findings. AJR Am J Roentgenol 153:507-511.

Krause D, et al, 2002: MRI for evaluating congenital bile duct abnormalities. J Comput Assist Tomogr 26:541-552.

Kutcher R, et al, 1977: Calcification in polycystic disease. Radiology 122:77-80.

Larsen KA, 1961: Benign lesions affecting the bile ducts in the postmortem cholangiogram. Acta Pathol Microbiol Immunol Scand 51:47-62.

Lasic LB, et al, 2004: Refractory hypotension and edema caused by right atrial compression in a woman with polycystic kidney disease. Am J Kidney Dis 43:13-17.

Lebon J, et al, 1955: Kyste solitaire du foie. Archives Françaises des Maladies de l'Appareil Digestif 44:1274-1277.

Levine E, et al, 1985: Liver cysts in autosomal-dominant polycystic kidney disease: clinical and computed tomographic study. AJR Am J Roentgenol 145:229-233.

Levy AD, et al, 2002: Caroli's disease: radiologic spectrum with pathologic correlation. AJR Am J Roentgenol 179:1053-1057.

Lewis WD, et al, 1988: Surgical treatment of biliary cystadenoma: a report of 15 cases. Arch Surg 123:563-568.

Loubeau JM, Steichen FM, 1976: Dilatation of intrahepatic bile ducts in choledochal cysts: case report with follow-up and review of the literature. Arch Surg 111:1384-1390.

Ludwig J, et al, 1982: Focal dilatation of intrahepatic bile ducts (Caroli's disease), cholangiocarcinoma, and sclerosis of intrahepatic bile ducts. J Clin Gastroenterol 4:53-57.

Ludwig J, et al, 1986: Intrahepatic cholangiectases and large-duct obliteration in primary sclerosing cholangitis. Hepatology 6:560-568.

Martin IJ, et al, 1998: Tailoring the management of nonparasitic liver cysts. Ann Surg 228:167-172.

Mathias K, et al, 1978: Intrahepatic cystic bile duct dilatations and stone formation: a new case of Caroli's disease. Acta Hepatogastroenterol Belg 25:40-44.

McGarrity TJ, et al, 1986: Refractory ascites associated with polycystic liver disease: treatment with peritoneovenous shunt. Dig Dis Sci 31:217-220.

Melnick PJ, 1975: Polycystic liver: analysis of seventy cases. Arch Pathol Lab Med 59:162-172.

Milutinovic J, et al, 1980: Liver cysts in patients with autosomal dominant polycystic kidney disease. Am J Med 68:741-744.

Mochizuki T, et al, 1996: PKD2, a gene for polycystic kidney disease that encodes an integral membrane protein. Science 272:1339-1342.

Montorsi M, et al, 1994: Percutaneous alcohol sclerotherapy of simple hepatic cysts: results from a multicentre survey in Italy. HPB Surg 8:89-94.

Moreaux J, Bloch P, 1971: Les kystes biliaires solitaires du foie. Archives Françaises des Maladies de l'Appareil Digestif 60:203-224.

Morino M, et al, 1994: Laparoscopic management of symptomatic nonparasitic cysts of the liver: indications and results. Ann Surg 219:157-164.

Nagasue N, 1984: Successful treatment of Caroli's disease by hepatic resection: report of six patients. Ann Surg 200:718-723.

Nakanuma Y, et al, 1982: Caroli's disease in congenital hepatic fibrosis and infantile polycystic disease. Liver 2:346-352.

Odièvre M, et al, 1977: Anomalies of the intrahepatic portal venous system in congenital hepatic fibrosis. Radiology 122:427-430.

Perreau P, et al, 1965: Kyste solitaire non parasitaire du foie: considérations anatomo-cliniques, diagnostiques et thérapeutiques. Archives Françaises des Maladies de l'Appareil Digestif 54:881-888.

Pirenne J, et al, 2001: Liver transplantation for polycystic liver disease. Liver Transplant 7:238-245.

Qian Q, et al, 2003: Clinical profile of autosomal dominant polycystic liver disease. Hepatology 37:164-171.

Que F, et al, 1995: Liver resection and cyst fenestration in the treatment of severe polycystic liver disease. Gastroenterology 108:487-494.

Ramond MJ, et al, 1984: Partial hepatectomy in the treatment of Caroli's disease: report of a case and review of the literature. Dig Dis Sci 29:367-370.

Ratcliffe PJ, et al, 1984: Bleeding oesophageal varices and hepatic dysfunction in adult polycystic kidney disease. BMJ 288:1330-1331.

Robinson TN, et al, 2004: Laparoscopic palliation of polycystic liver disease. Surg Endosc 19:130-132.

Robson GB, Fenster F, 1964: Fatal liver abscess developing in a polycystic liver. Gastroenterology 47:82.

Roemer CE, et al, 1981: Hepatic cysts: diagnosis and therapy by sonographic needle aspiration. AJR Am J Roentgenol 136:1065-1070.

Ros E, et al, 1993: Ursodeoxycholic acid treatment of primary hepatolithiasis in Caroli's syndrome. Lancet 342:404-406.

Rossetti S, et al, 2003: Association of mutation position in polycystic kidney disease 1 (PKD1) gene and development of a vascular phenotype. Lancet 361:2196-2201.

Sahel J, et al, 1976: Maladie de Caroli avec pancréatite aiguë et angiocholite: intérêt diagnostique et thérapeutique de la cholédoco-wirsungographie endoscopique. Nouv Presse Med 5:2067-2069.

Saini S, et al, 1983: Percutaneous aspiration of hepatic cysts does not provide definitive therapy. AJR Am J Roentgenol 141:559-560.

Sans M, et al, 1997: Liver transplantation in patients with Caroli's disease and recurrent cholangitis. Transplant Int 10:241-244.

Santman FW, et al, 1977: Intermittent jaundice: a rare complication of solitary nonparasitic liver cyst. Gastroenterology 72:325-328.

Serejo FF, et al, 1988: Caroli's disease of the left hepatic lobe associated with hepatic fibrosis. J Clin Gastroenterol 10:559-564.

Sheinberg IH, Sternlieb IM, 1984: Wilson's Disease. Philadelphia, Saunders.

Shimada M, et al, 1998: Treatment strategy for patients with cystic lesions mimicking a liver tumor. Arch Surg 133:643-646.

Simonetti G, et al, 1993: Percutaneous treatment of hepatic cysts by aspiration and sclerotherapy. Cardiovasc Interv Radiol 16:81-84.

Soravia C, et al, 1995: Surgery for adult polycystic liver disease. Surgery 117:272-275.

Soud SC, Watson A, 1974: Solitary cyst of the liver presenting as an abdominal emergency. Postgrad Med J 50:48-50.

Spiegel RM, et al, 1978: Ultrasonography of primary cysts of the liver. AJR Am J Roentgenol 131:235-238.

Stanley J, et al, 1983: Evaluation of biliary cystadenoma and cystadenocarcinoma. Gastrointest Radiol 8:245-248.

Starzl TE, et al, 1990: Liver transplantation for polycystic liver disease. Arch Surg 125:575-577.

Stillman A, et al, 1981: Hepatobiliary scanning in diagnosis and management of Caroli disease. Gastroenterology 80:1295 (abstract).

Summerfield JA, et al, 1986: Hepatobiliary fibropolycystic diseases: a clinical and histological review of 51 patients. J Hepatol 2:141-156.

Swenson K, et al, 1998: Liver transplantation for adult polycystic liver disease. Hepatology 28:412-415.

Takahiro H, et al, 2003: Ciliated hepatic foregut cyst: a report of one case and a review of the literature. Hepatol Res 26:243-248.

Tanaka Y, et al, 1996: Examination of percutaneous minocycline hydrochloride injection therapy for hepatic cyst by one-puncture method. Nippon Shokakibyo Gakkai Sasshi 93:828-836.

Telenti A, et al, 1990: Hepatic cyst infection in autosomal dominant polycystic kidney disease. Mayo Clin Proc 65:933-942.

Theilmann L, Stiehl A, 1990: Detection of large intrahepatic cholangiectases in patients with primary sclerosing cholangitis by endoscopic retrograde cholangiography. Endoscopy 22:49-50.

Thompson HH, et al, 1983: Major hepatic resection: a 25-year experience. Ann Surg 197:375-388.

Thomsen HS, Thaysen JH, 1988: Frequency of hepatic cysts in adult polycystic kidney disease. Acta Med Scand 224:381-384.

Tikkakoski T, et al, 1996: Treatment of symptomatic congenital hepatic cysts with single-session percutaneous drainage and ethanol sclerosis: technique and outcome. J Vasc Interv Radiol 7:235-239.

Totkas S, Hohenberger P, 2000: Cholangiocellular carcinoma associated with segmental Caroli's disease. Eur J Surg Oncol 26:520-521.

Tsuchiya R, et al, 1977: Congenital cyst dilatation of the bile ducts associated with Laurence-Moon-Biedl-Bardet syndrome. Arch Surg 112:82-84.

Turnberg LA, et al, 1968: Biliary secretion in a patient with cystic dilatation of the intrahepatic biliary tree. Gastroenterology 54:1155-1161.

van Roekel V, et al, 1982: Cystadenoma of the liver. J Clin Gastroenterol 4:167-172.

Vick DJ, et al, 1999: Squamous cell carcinoma arising in a ciliated hepatic foregut cyst. Arch Pathol Lab Med 123:1115-1117.

Vons C, et al, 1998: Résection hépatique chez les malades atteints de polykystose hépatique. Gastroenterol Clin Biol 22:50-54.

Vuillemin-Bodaghi V, et al, 1997: Imaging of atypical cysts of the liver: study of 26 surgically treated cases. Gastroenterol Clin Biol 21:394-399.

Waechter FL, et al, 2001: The role of liver transplantation in patients with Caroli's disease. Hepatogastroenterology 48:672-674.

Wagenvoort CA, et al, 1962: Subarachnoid hemorrhage due to cerebellar hemangioma associated with congenital hepatic fibrosis and polycystic kidneys: report of a case. Mayo Clin Proc 37:301-306.

Ward CJ, et al, 1996: Polycystin, the polycystic kidney disease 1 protein, is expressed by epithelial cells in fetal, adult, and polycystic kidney. Proc Natl Acad Sci U S A 93:1524-1528.

Washburn WK, et al, 1996: Liver transplantation for adult polycystic liver disease. Liver Transplant Surg 2:17-22.

Watts DR, et al, 1974: Congenital dilatation of the intrahepatic bile ducts. Arch Surg 108:592-598.

Williams R, et al, 1964: Congenital hepatic fibrosis with an unusual pulmonary lesion. J Clin Pathol 17:135-142.

Williamson RCN, et al, 1978: Congenital solitary cysts of the liver and spleen. Br J Surg 65:871-876.

Witlin LT, et al, 1982: Transhepatic decompression of the biliary tree in Caroli's disease. Surgery 91:205-209.

Woods G, 1981: Biliary cystadenocarcinoma: case report of hepatic malignancy originating in benign cystadenoma. Cancer 47:2936-2940.

Wu ML, et al, 1998: Ciliated hepatic foregut cyst mimicking neoplasm. Am J Gastroenterol 93:2212-2214.

Yagi H, et al, 2004: Squamous cell carcinoma of the liver originating from non-parasitic cysts after a 15-year follow-up. Eur J Gastroenterol Hepatol 16:1051-1056.

Yamada N, et al, 1994: Treatment of symptomatic hepatic cysts by percutaneous instillation of minocycline hydrochloride. Dig Dis Sci 39:2503-2509.

Yamaguchi M, et al, 1999: Spontaneous rupture of a nonparasitic liver cyst complicated by intracystic hemorrhage. J Gastroenterol 34:645-648.

Yamato T, et al, 1998: Intrahepatic cholangiocarcinoma arising in congenital hepatic fibrosis: report of an autopsy case. J Hepatol 28:717-722.

Zeitoun D, et al, 2004: Congenital hepatic fibrosis: CT findings in 18 adults. Radiology 231:109-116.

Surgical Management of Cystic Disease of the Liver

65

D. M. NAGORNEY AND J. M. SARMIENTO

Cystic disease of the liver classically is divided into nonparasitic and parasitic cysts (see Chs. 61 and 64). Nonparasitic cysts are more prevalent worldwide, although prevalence may vary significantly by geographic region. Generally, most hepatic cysts, regardless of type, remain asymptomatic. Hepatic function rarely is affected by their presence. When cysts cause symptoms, they are only mildly disruptive of patients' routine lifestyle. Occasionally, cysts are the focus of hemorrhage or infection or produce hepatic dysfunction by bile duct compression or portal hypertension. Liver failure is exceedingly rare. Since the 1990s, the management of cystic disease of the liver has been affected greatly by the evolution of interventional radiographic and laparoscopic techniques. This chapter reviews the major types of cystic diseases of the liver and their clinical management. Although treatment options for symptomatic cysts are presented in a least invasive to most invasive sequence, choice of treatment for any patient must be individualized to the clinical circumstance.

IMAGING

Several imaging modalities, including ultrasonography, computed tomography (CT), and magnetic resonance imaging (MRI), can define cystic disease of the liver accurately. Choice of imaging procedure depends on clinical presentation, patient habitus, specific anatomic definition required, and whether radiographically guided intervention is planned. Generally, ultrasound and CT accurately define the size, location, number, and anatomic relationship of all cysts within the liver. MRI usually is reserved for better definition of the intrahepatic vasculature in polycystic liver disease (PLD). CT is superior to ultrasound in patients with PLD because a global view of the liver is displayed, and superimposition of multiple artifacts seen by ultrasound is eliminated by CT. MRI lacks interventional capabilities currently and should be used only selectively.

Ultrasound (see Ch. 15) is the simplest and least expensive imaging modality used to diagnose hepatic cysts. All cysts are characterized by discrete anechoic or hypoechoic masses. Simple cysts are characterized by acoustic enhancement posterior to the mass. Features of the cyst that aid in the diagnosis of defining cyst type include cyst wall features (thickness and nodularity), cyst number, cyst septa, and cyst density. Simple cysts typically are solitary, thin-walled without focal thickening or nodularity, and anechoic without debris. Simple cysts usually lack septa. The interface of several adjacent cysts may mimic septa, but the lobulated circumference of a cluster of multiple cysts generally permits differentiation from true septa. When septa are present, they usually are seen as transverse lines or planes of variable thickness, which partially traverse the circumference of the cyst. Septa typically are

findings in cystadenomas (Fig. 65.1) and cystadenocarcinomas. Mural or septal nodularity most typically is seen in cystadenocarcinoma (Fig. 65.2). Occasionally, a portion of a vasculobiliary pedicle along the cyst perimeter indents a simple cyst and mimics a septum, but thorough imaging confirms the underlying nature of this pseudoseptum. Hydatid cysts (see Ch. 61) differ from simple cysts and cystadenomas by cyst density, type of septations, and the frequent presence of peripheral calcifications. Hydatid cysts are typically hypoechoic rather than anechoic, contain concentric peripheral daughter cysts within the larger cyst, and may have partial or complete calcification of the cyst wall (Fig. 65.3). Additionally, biliary ductal dilation or intraductal debris, indicating cyst rupture within the biliary tree, may accompany the other features of hydatid disease. Intracystic hemorrhage is recognized by a change in cyst density. A hematocrit sign or layering of blood within the cyst may be seen early after hemorrhage. Diffuse, irregular hyperechogenicity within a cyst is seen several days after hemorrhage and may persist indefinitely. Variable cyst density is common in PLD. Air within cysts occasionally develops with cyst infection, but is a more common residual finding after intervention.

CT (see Ch. 18) features of hepatic cysts are similar to features seen on ultrasound, and cysts are recognized as discrete, hypodense masses. Cyst number, wall thickness and nodularity, septa, and density can be well characterized by CT. CT may reveal septa unrecognized by ultrasound and vice versa. Although CT often identifies small (≤1 cm) intrahepatic masses suspicious for a cyst, ultrasound is more specific for diagnosis of masses this size,

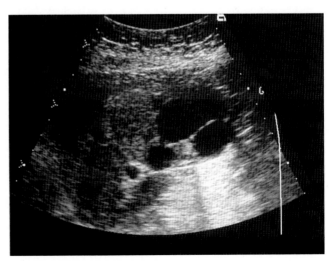

Fig. 65.1. Hepatic ultrasound of cystadenoma. Note various septa across cystadenoma of the left lobe of the liver.

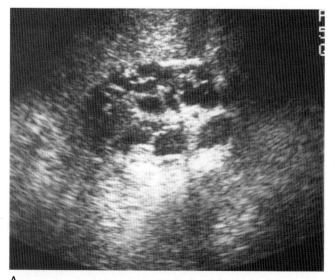

Fig. 65.2. Hepatic ultrasound of cystadenocarcinoma. Note thick, irregular mural nodularity along the periphery and septa of cystadenocarcinoma of the left lobe of liver.

particularly if posterior acoustic enhancement is recognized. Cyst hemorrhage and infection are confirmed by intracystic fluid layering or increased density. Interseptal calcifications may be seen in PLD, but lack the peripheral concentric calcification typically seen in hydatid disease. Both types of calcification can be recognized with CT, however.

Contrast enhancement during CT augments visualization of the portal or hepatic veins, depending on the timing of the imaging acquisition. Early phase imaging defines the portal veins, and later phase imaging defines the hepatic veins. The concurrent presence of ascites and cystic disease of the liver should raise suspicion for hepatic venous outflow obstruction rather than parenchymal dysfunction as a cause. Although all patients with PLD have some component of hepatic venous compression, ascites usually indicates marked compression of all the major hepatic veins and the retrohepatic inferior vena cava. CT often shows large intrahepatic collateral veins in patients with PLD and

hepatic venous outflow obstruction. CT can define the extent of the compression of the major hepatic veins and inferior vena cava and help determine the extent of cyst resection or fenestration required to resolve hepatic venous outflow obstruction. Finally, major vascular enhancement within the cyst wall or mural nodules suggests a cyst-associated malignancy or a cystadenocarcinoma (Fig. 65.4), whereas only various septations occur with cystadenoma (Fig. 65.5).

MRI (see Ch. 19) also can provide accurate imaging of cystic disease of the liver. Because MRI is the most expensive current imaging modality, it should be reserved to address specific issues unresolved by other imaging techniques. MRI findings are similar to CT findings. If CT fails to define hepatic vasculature accurately, MRI can define the vascular anatomy accurately without contrast media, which may be important in patients with PLD and renal failure.

In patients with cystic disease of the liver with jaundice or known hydatid disease and suspected intrabiliary rupture, cholangiography is indicated. Endoscopic retrograde cholangiopancreatography (see Ch. 20) is preferred and documents the site and degree of biliary obstruction or often the site of biliary communication. Endoscopic stenting of the biliary obstruction relieves obstruction and cholangitis, if present. Finally, cholangiography is essential to differentiate bile duct cysts from hepatic cysts with biliary communication. MRI and CT cholangiography also can be employed for definition of the biliary system. Although either of these image reconstructions can define the extrahepatic biliary system accurately, anatomic detail of the intrahepatic ducts is difficult to obtain in PLD, and identification of the origin of biliary fistula is similarly difficult.

Hepatic angiography has little, if any, current role in the diagnosis of cystic disease of the liver. Contrast enhancement on CT and MRI usually provides sufficient anatomic information regarding the hepatic vasculature without angiography. Angiographic access to the major hepatic venous system is useful, however, to measure free and wedge hepatic venous pressures and suprahepatic and infrahepatic inferior vena caval pressures if hepatic venous outflow obstruction is suspected in patients with PLD to

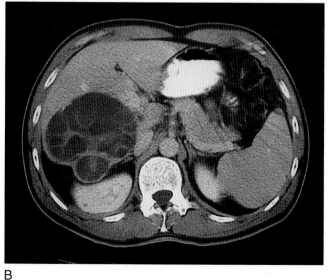

A   B

Fig. 65.3. Hepatic ultrasound **(A)** and CT **(B)** of a hydatid cyst (echinococcal) of the right lobe of the liver. Note multiple daughter cysts along the periphery of the primary cyst cavity (see Ch. 61).

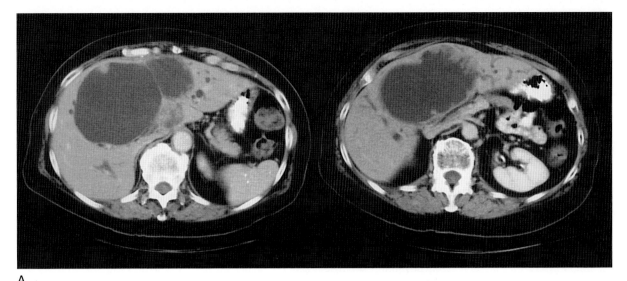

A

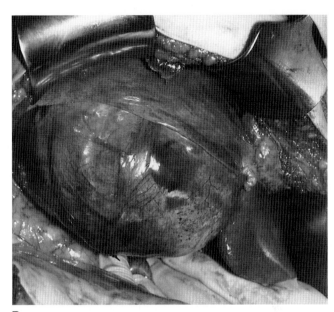

B

Fig. 65.4. A, Abdominal CT of a cystadenocarcinoma of the left lobe of the liver. Note the mural irregularities and papillary projections into the primary cyst *(left)*. An additional CT scan *(right)* of the same cystadenocarcinoma further depicts irregular papillary tumor nodules along the cyst periphery. **B,** Intraoperative photograph of cystadenocarcinoma of the right lobe of the liver.

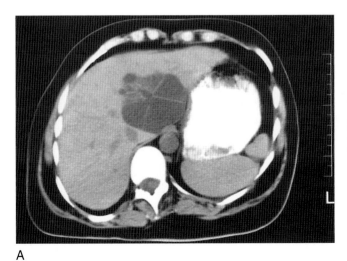

A

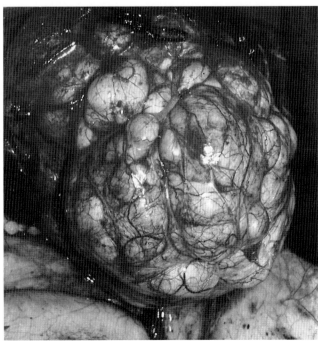

B

Fig. 65.5. A, Abnormal CT of a cystadenoma of the left lobe. Note spoke-wheel septations within the cyst. **B,** Intraoperative photograph of a cystadenoma of the left lobe of the liver. Note the lobulations on the surface of the cystadenoma.

document and quantitate portal hypertension. Angiographic placement of expandable metal stents may be used therapeutically to reduce vascular gradients in nonoperative candidates for relief of ascites.

SIMPLE CYSTS

Simple cysts of the liver are common. Although they were considered rare several decades ago, modern imaging of the liver has confirmed a prevalence of 1% to 5% of the general population. Cyst prevalence based on imaging or autopsy data may underestimate true prevalence, however, given the fact that subcapsular cysts (≤4 mm) are so commonly recognized intraoperatively. Simple cysts are found more frequently in women than in men, and symptomatic cysts are nearly 10 times more frequent in women than men.

Simple cysts may be solitary or multiple, but are usually unilocular. Multilocular cysts usually are formed by the confluence of multiple adjacent cysts. Simple cysts rarely have true septations, but frequently have intrahepatic portal pedicles, which traverse a portion of the cyst periphery, which may mimic septa. The lining of simple cysts is epithelial and secretory, but does not communicate with the biliary tree. The content of simple cysts is usually serous, but can be bile stained, mucoid, bloody, or turbid and thick, presumably from old inspissated hemorrhage. Enlargement of cysts results in compression of adjacent liver parenchyma. The adjacent liver may become atrophic with marked cystic enlargement and compression of the adjacent portal pedicles. The cause of simple cysts is unknown. Disruption and isolation of biliary radicles during embryogenesis is postulated as the most likely etiopathology. Why some simple cysts grow and others remain stable is unknown.

Most patients with simple cysts of the liver are asymptomatic. Symptoms develop insidiously. Usually symptoms include abdominal fullness or pressure, satiety, and mild dyspnea from cyst expansion and compression of adjacent organs. A dull abdominal ache is common in symptomatic cysts, but sharp pain is not, unless intracystic hemorrhage has occurred. Cyst infection usually is associated with fever and rigors. Jaundice may accompany extensive compression of the bile duct confluence or common hepatic duct, but it is rare. Jaundice usually is attributable to concurrent hepatobiliary diseases, rather than to the cyst itself.

Laboratory tests provide no diagnostic aid. Liver function is almost always normal even with diffuse hepatic involvement by PLD. Imaging features of cysts have been discussed previously.

The indications for treatment of simple cysts are symptoms or associated complications. Simple cysts may be complicated by hemorrhage, infection, rupture into the peritoneal cavity or into the biliary tree or adjacent bowel, jaundice, and rarely portal hypertension. Treatment is not indicated for asymptomatic simple cysts, regardless of size. Because symptoms are often vague, an initial image-guided aspiration is warranted to confirm that subsequent definitive treatment would resolve symptoms. If symptoms are unaffected by aspiration, alternative sources of symptoms should be investigated. Aspiration alone should never be used as definitive treatment because cyst recurrence is almost certain.

The treatment of simple cysts of the liver has changed dramatically because of the interventional capacity associated with modern imaging and laparoscopy. Before these advances, open laparotomy for total cyst excision or partial cyst excision (unroofing) was the treatment of choice. Currently, choice of treatment for simple cysts includes aspiration and sclerosis, laparoscopic excision or fenestration, and excision or fenestration at laparotomy. Choice of treatment should be guided by cyst location, number, associated cyst complications, and comorbidity. Generally, because most symptomatic cysts are large, solitary, and uncomplicated, a radiographic-guided approach or laparoscopic approach should be offered initially. Although cyst location itself rarely prevents a radiographic approach, cysts in segments VII and VIII of the liver can pose technical problems if approached laparoscopically. With mobilization of the right lobe, however, access to segments VII and VIII can be achieved. By detaching the cysts in segment VIII from their adherence to the diaphragm, wide laparoscopic fenestration can be performed (Weber et al, 2004). The major problem encountered with unroofing of cysts in segments VII and VIII is the abutment of the rim of the cysts to the diaphragm when the liver returns to its normal position. Frequently, the apposition of cyst rim to diaphragm seals firmly and prevents intraperitoneal drainage of cyst fluid with subsequent cyst recurrence. The hand-assisted technique also is useful in mobilizing the liver and facilitates the fenestration of these cysts. Cysts complicated by

Table 65.1   Aspiration and Sclerosis of Nonparasitic Hepatic Cysts

Reference	Patients (*n*)	Sclerosant	No. Patients with Relief of Symptoms	No. Patients Requiring Repeat Sclerosis	Maximum Duration of Follow-up (mo)
Andersson et al, 1989	9	Alcohol	8	6	54
Furuta et al, 1990	6	Alcohol	6	3	68
Simonetti et al, 1993	30	Alcohol	25	—	36
Montorsi et al, 1994	21	Alcohol	21	—	60
vanSonnenberg et al, 1994	20	Alcohol Tetracycline Doxycycline	17 — —	10 — —	6 — —
Yamada et al, 1994	9	Minocycline	7	3	35
Tikkakoski et al, 1996	25	Alcohol	18	—	—
Larssen et al, 1997	10	Alcohol	8	0	42
Tocchi et al, 2002	6	—	6	—	50
Larssen et al, 2003	7	Alcohol	7	—	47

active hemorrhage or enteric communication are best treated by open laparotomy.

Radiofrequency ablation has been described as useful for definitive treatment of simple cysts. The cystic fluid conducts thermic energy generated by radiofrequency, which ablates epithelia of the cyst. Immediate collapse of the cyst without recurrence after a follow-up of 2 years has been documented. Although preliminary, this experience should prompt further use and assessment of radiofrequency ablation (Rhim et al, 2004).

Percutaneous cyst aspiration and sclerosis under ultrasound or CT guidance has evolved as an effective treatment for uncomplicated hepatic cysts. The patient should be informed that repeat sessions may be required to obtain complete cyst contraction or to treat multiple cysts. Usually after diagnostic aspiration confirms resolution of symptoms and a nonbilious aspirate, repeat radiographic intervention for definitive aspiration and sclerosis is performed. The basic technique for aspiration and sclerosis has been standardized. The cyst is localized by ultrasound or CT and is punctured through the most direct route, carefully avoiding adjacent viscera or lung. A drainage catheter is inserted into the cyst by the Seldinger technique. Cyst contents are aspirated and measured. A cystogram is obtained by injection of water-soluble contrast material to exclude biliary communication or puncture site extravasation into the peritoneal cavity. If exclusion criteria are absent, the contrast material is aspirated and 20 to 100 mL of absolute alcohol is injected, depending on cyst size. While the sclerosant remains in contact with the cyst, the posture of the patient is varied to ensure complete exposure of the sclerosant to the entire cyst wall. The sclerosant is aspirated completely, and the catheter is removed. Some centers repeat sclerosant injection and patient positioning at the same session to ensure complete contact.

Results from current literature are shown in Table 65.1. The reported number of patients treated overall is small, and duration of follow-up has been short. Success, defined as resolution of symptoms and an ablation or reduction of the sclerosed cysts, ranges from 70% to 90%. An example of successful ablation of a single cyst is shown in Fig. 65.6. Repeat aspirations and sclerosant sessions are required frequently. Complications include mild procedure-related pain after injection of alcohol, fever without infection, nausea and vomiting, alcohol intoxication, pleural effusion, peritoneal extravasation, and infection. Rarely, severe prolonged hypotension or death from unintentinal intravascular injection may occur (Gelczer et al, 1998). Overall, morbidity is usually less than 10% (Martin et al, 1998), and mortality has been 0%. Recurrence rates range from 0% to 17%. The frequency of complications and recurrence herein is likely related to evolving techniques and the type and concentration of sclerosing agent, which have varied among reporting centers. A decrease in complications and recurrences and an increase in initial success are likely with further standardization of the technique and sclerosant.

LAPAROSCOPIC CYST EXCISION

Because the treatment of simple cysts does not require complete cyst excision, laparoscopic partial excision or unroofing with intraperitoneal drainage has evolved as effective and preferred treatment (see also Ch. 80). Laparoscopic management has several advantages, including less invasiveness than laparotomy; rapid patient recovery; tissue sampling for histopathology; and cyst wall

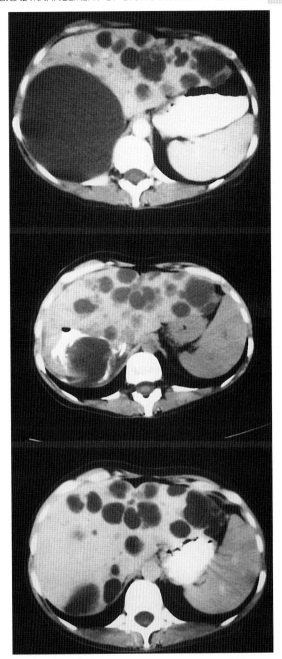

Fig. 65.6. Sequential abdominal CT scans of a large symptomatic right lobe liver cyst in a polycystic liver. *Top panel* shows the dominant cyst before aspiration. *Middle panel* shows contrast material within the cyst (cystogram) after aspiration, but before alcohol injection. *Bottom panel* shows contracted cyst 1 year after alcohol sclerosis.

exposure for inspection, biopsy, or ablation by sclerosant or omentoplasty. Laparoscopic management may be limited by cyst number and intrahepatic location. Generally, if radiologic expertise is unavailable, laparoscopic management should be considered before open laparotomy. Laparoscopic management is indicated in patients with symptomatic superficial cysts located within the anterior liver segments (III, IV, V, and VI) and patients who have not had extensive upper abdominal surgery (Gigot et al, 1996). Most patients with PLD are not candidates for laparoscopic management, unless a large accessible solitary cyst is symptomatic.

Although there are minor technical variations of laparoscopic management, the basic approach has been standardized. After pneumoperitoneum is established, a periumbilical trocar for the camera and two or three subcostal trocars (5 mm or 10 mm) are inserted. The cyst is punctured with a long needle under direct vision if fluid cytology or culture is indicated clinically. Alternatively, the cyst wall is incised with scissors or cautery, and the cyst contents are aspirated. The cyst wall is grasped and excised widely, preferably to its interface with the hepatic parenchyma. Coagulation scissors, Harmonic scalpel (Ethicon Endo-Surgery, Inc, Cincinnati, OH), ultrasonic shears, or Ligasure (Valleylab, Tyco Healthcare Group, Boulder, CO) is used to excise the superficial portion of the cyst wall near the interface of the cyst wall and liver parenchyma. Ultrasonic shears use ultrafast vibration to induce sealing of vessels 3 mm in diameter; the Ligasure induces coagulation in larger vessels (7 mm). Both devices have facilitated safe, expeditious parenchymal transection with minimal risk of hemorrhage.

Endovascular staplers can be used for secure closure of larger vasculobiliary structures recognized intraoperatively at the cyst-parenchymal interface. Histopathology of the excised portion of the cyst is indicated routinely. Often, the liver adjacent to the cyst is attenuated and may contain peripheral bile ducts or vessels. Careful hemostasis is required, and any thickened band along the cyst periphery is clipped or suture ligated. After excision of the superficial cyst wall, the concavity of the residual cyst should be inspected. If irregularities are seen, biopsy is indicated. Simple cysts do not require ablation of the residual cyst lining or omentoplasty. If partial cyst excision has removed more than 50% of the estimated surface area of the cyst, no further therapy other than intraperitoneal drainage of the residual cyst is necessary. If less surface area is excised, or most of the cyst resides within the liver parenchyma, ablation of the cyst lining by direct cautery, argon beam coagulation, topical sclerosant, or omentoplasty may reduce the risk of recurrence. Suction drainage is optional. Laparoscopic ultrasound has been advocated to identify unexpected cysts (deep seated) and to confirm the adequacy of the drainage. One series found that laparoscopic ultrasound changed the surgical plan in one third of the cases (Schachter et al, 2001). It is undetermined whether laparoscopic ultrasound is useful enough for routine use, given the accuracy of CT and MRI for hepatic cyst.

Results of laparoscopic management are shown in Table 65.2. Similar to the experience with percutaneous aspiration and sclerosis, the reported number of patients treated is small, and the duration of follow-up is short. Success, defined as resolution of symptoms without objective cyst recurrence, ranges from 75% to 100%. Conversion to an open laparotomy for treatment in these select patients was required infrequently. Several studies have emphasized the need for careful patient selection, which emphasizes cyst multiplicity and posterior location as contraindications (Emmermann et al, 1997; Gigot et al, 1996; Marks et al, 1998; Martin et al, 1998). Complication rates range from 0% to 15%, and complications include shoulder pain, dyspnea, pleural effusion, ascites, hemorrhage, infection, and subhepatic bile collection. No mortality has been reported. Most series had no morbidity. Recurrence rate was less than 17%. Recurrence after laparoscopic management of simple cysts has been attributed to poor patient selection (Gigot et al, 1996; Martin et al, 1998). Cysts that cannot undergo wide unroofing or cysts that are located within the posterior liver segments are likely to have adjacent diaphragm or retroperitoneum seal in the residual cyst wall and allow for contained secretions and cyst recurrence. Ablation of the residual wall or omentoplasty may reduce recurrence in posteriorly located hepatic cysts treated laparoscopically.

Table 65.2   Laparoscopic Management of Nonparasitic Hepatic Cysts

Reference	Patients (n)	No. Patients Requiring Conversion	No. Patients with Recurrence	Maximum Duration of Follow-up (mo)
Fabiani et al, 1991	4	0	0	15
Morino et al, 1994	4	0	1	22
Albrink et al, 1994	4	0	0	—
Cala et al, 1996	3	0	0	6
Gigot et al, 1996	17	2	3	48
Marks et al, 1998	10	1	0	67
Zacherl et al, 1996	4	0	0	41
Emmermann et al, 1997	18	1	2	43
Koperna et al, 1997	10	1	1	—
Diez et al, 1998	9	0	1	36
Martin et al, 1998	13	0	1	80
Hansman et al, 2001	6	0	0	108
Zacherl et al, 2000	7	—	1	36
Gigot et al, 2001	19	4	2	130
Schachter et al, 2001	10	0	1	30
Tocchi et al, 2002	8	—	2	50
Tagaya et al, 2003	5	—	1	102
Giulante et al, 2003	13	—	—	24
Fiamingo et al, 2003	10	1	1	—

Table 65.3 Laparoscopic Management of Polycystic Liver Disease

Reference	Patients (n)	No. Patients Requiring Conversion	No. Patients with Recurrence	Maximum Duration of Follow-up (mo)
Morino et al, 1994	7	2	3	24
Gigot et al, 1996	9	1	3	17
Kabbej et al, 1996	13	0	8	49
Marks et al, 1998	7	1	4	67
Zacherl et al, 1996	3	0	0	41
Koperna et al, 1997	5	0	0	—
Martin et al, 1998	7	—	5	67
Fiamingo et al, 2003	6	0	2	48

The results of laparoscopic management of PLD are shown in Table 65.3. The reported experience of laparoscopic management of patients with PLD remains anecdotal. Success has been related to type of PLD, which has been arbitrarily classified as follows: type I PLD, numerous large superficial cysts, and type II PLD, innumerable small, diffuse cysts (Morino et al, 1994). More recently, this PLD classification has been modified as follows (Gigot et al, 1996): type I, few large cysts (>7-10 cm); type II, multiple medium cysts (5-7 cm); and type III, diffuse small to medium cysts (<5 cm). Successful laparoscopic management is probable in selected patients with type I PLD, but rare in patients with type II PLD, and exceptional in type III PLD patients (Kabbej et al, 1996). Laparoscopic completion of right or left lobectomies has been described for treatment of PLD, however (Andoh et al, 2004). Although reported mortality is zero, morbidity is significant in patients with PLD. Specifically, ascites and hemorrhage are the major complications (Gigot et al, 1996; Marks et al, 1998; Martin et al, 1998). Thorough cyst fenestration of a massively enlarged polycystic liver is prohibited technically by the gross anatomy. Fenestration refers to the development of windows or openings through adjacent cysts by excision of a portion of the intracystic walls. Generally, wide excision of such walls is only possible peripherally. Central cyst fenestration is precluded because the architectural rigidity of the liver persists through the septa, which contain the hepatic vasculature and bile ducts. Central cysts are inaccessible to decompression because instrument access is prevented by the rigidity of the liver. Any bleeding within the cyst can obscure visual fields quickly and prevent control of hemorrhage.

Laparoscopic management of PLD other than for type I PLD is generally contraindicated.

MANAGEMENT BY LAPAROTOMY

Open laparotomy was the treatment of choice for simple cysts before the evolution of percutaneous radiographic and laparoscopic techniques. The primary surgical approach was wide partial or total cystectomy and occasionally formal hepatic resection. Ablation of residual cyst wall by coagulation or omentoplasty was reported variably. The results of the various open surgical approaches for the treatment of hepatic cysts are shown in Table 65.4. Although the number of reported patients is small, duration of follow-up is longer for open approaches. These data affirm that recurrence after total cystectomy or hepatic resection was zero. Only one postoperative death was reported (Madariaga et al, 1993), and morbidity occurred in less than 10% of patients. In contrast, partial cystectomy was associated with a recurrence rate of 0% to 37%. Recurrence rates have depended on rigor of follow-up and the development of recurrent symptoms. Because simple cysts have no malignant predisposition, most physicians have advised follow-up only for recurrent symptoms. The reported recurrence rate for partial excision (deroofing or fenestration) at open laparotomy is probably underestimated because of expectant follow-up. Caveats related to partial excision at laparoscopy also are applicable at open laparotomy. Wide excision is essential, preferably excising greater than half the cyst to prevent sealing of the cyst remnant by adjacent viscera or diaphragm or residual

Table 65.4 Open Laparotomy for Nonparasitic Hepatic Cysts

Reference	Partial Cystectomy (Recurrence)	Total Cystectomy (Recurrence)	Hepatic Resection (Recurrence)	Maximum Duration of Follow-up (mo)
Sanchez et al, 1991	8 (3)	4 (0)	1 (0)	360
Henne-Bruns et al, 1993	6 (0)	—	—	32
Madariaga et al, 1993	—	—	19 (0)	108
Koperna et al, 1997	29 (0)	—	4 (0)	72
Martin et al, 1998	7 (2)	—	3 (0)	104
Gigot et al, 2001	5 (0)	—	—	130
Hansman et al, 2001	21 (1)	—	1 (0)	108
Tocchi et al, 2002	10 (3)	4 (0)	2 (0)	50

cyst wall contraction and cyst recurrence. If less than half of the cyst is excisable, omentoplasty and ablation of the residual cyst epithelium by coagulation or sclerosant should be performed. Alternatively, hepatic resection prevents recurrence totally.

POLYCYSTIC LIVER DISEASE

In contrast to simple cysts, PLD is inherited as an autosomal recessive trait associated with congenital hepatic fibrosis in infancy or childhood or as an autosomal dominant trait presenting in adulthood. Most autosomal dominant PLD is associated with renal cysts and is linked to mutations in *PKD1* or *PKD2* genes (Everson et al, 2004). Isolated PLD without renal cysts is caused by mutations in the *PRKCSH* gene. Production of *polycystin 1* or *polycystin 2* is altered by mutations of *PKD1* and *PKD2*. Mutations in the *PRKCSH* gene, which encodes for hepatocystin, also cause PLD (Drenth et al, 2004). Investigations have shown that many different mutations in the *PRKCSH* gene exist, likely restricting genetic screening to patients with positive family history or for patients with known disease (Drenth et al, 2004).

PLD progresses insidiously. The number and size of cysts increase with age, female sex, and severity of renal cystic disease and renal dysfunction (Everson et al, 2004). Presentation almost always occurs after puberty. Hepatic failure is rare. Even with marked hepatosplenomegaly and portal hypertension, liver function is well preserved. Ascites usually results from hepatic venous outflow obstruction. PLD in adults also may be associated with multiple cysts of the pancreas, spleen, ovaries, and lungs.

Symptoms also develop insidiously and late in the natural history of PLD. They are caused by increased liver volume and adjacent visceral compression. The most common complaints are increased abdominal girth, chronic dull abdominal pain, satiety, weight loss, dyspnea, physical disability, and descensus. Ascites can be prominent, although other stigmata of chronic liver disease are rare. Physical examination reveals a large nodular liver. Abdominal tenderness over the liver is common, although persistent pain is unusual. Liver function tests are usually normal except for gamma-glutamyltransferase, which often is mildly elevated. Abnormal liver function is usually attributable to concurrent liver disease, usually chronic hepatitis B or C contracted during treatment for chronic renal failure with dialysis. Although diagnosis of PLD is readily confirmed by ultrasound or CT, CT best defines the extent of liver and adjacent organ involvement.

Surgical intervention is reserved for selected patients who exhibit significant impairment of clinical performance status from massive hepatomegaly or from complications of cyst rupture, infection, hemorrhage, or jaundice. Nearly 10% of patients have intracranial aneurysms, and these patients with hypertension are at risk for cerebrovascular hemorrhage. Intracranial aneurysms should be sought in any patient who is a candidate for abdominal surgery. If identified by CT or MRI, aneurysms are treated based on site and size. Choice of treatment for PLD is dictated by size and extent of liver involvement and by complication. For patients with a few dominant cysts, percutaneous cyst aspiration with or without alcohol ablation may provide prolonged symptomatic relief or resolve infection and may be repeated as indicated. For patients with more diffuse PLD, operative management should be considered. Cyst fenestration with intraperitoneal marsupialization and resection have been the mainstays of surgical therapy. Although cyst decompression by fenestration

avoids these risks, decompression is often limited technically by the number and size of cysts and the massive bulk of the liver. Fenestration with intraperitoneal marsupialization has produced temporary symptomatic relief, but long-term reduction of abdominal girth has been documented infrequently. Resection addresses the problem of liver mass, but poses significant risk of biliary ductal injury, vascular compromise, and liver insufficiency because cysts markedly distort the intrahepatic anatomy. In patients who harbor diffuse PLD, orthotopic liver transplantation is effective, but inherently assumes the risks of long-term immunosuppression and rejection.

Treatment approaches should be individualized based on type of PLD. Type I PLD can be approached as a single simple cyst with either percutaneous aspiration and sclerosis or laparoscopic fenestration. Some patients with type II PLD are candidates for laparoscopic management if symptomatic cysts are located in the anterior liver segments (Gigot et al, 1997). Open fenestration or resection should be employed for more diffuse type II PLD. Type III PLD is most problematic (Fig. 65.7). Only extended resection with concurrent fenestration and orthotopic liver transplantation are viable options. Generally, if at least one sector is spared, combined resection/fenestration is preferred. The criteria of sectoral sparing warrant emphasis because vascular viability of the liver depends on the patency of the afferent and efferent venous systems after resection of the cystic liver. If involvement is diffuse without sectoral sparing, orthotopic liver transplantation is preferred.

The results of combined hepatic resection/fenestration and orthotopic liver transplantation for massive PLD are shown in Table 65.5. The number of total patients with PLD treated by either method has been few. Duration of follow-up has been greater for combined hepatic resection/fenestration than for orthotopic liver transplantation. Operative mortality associated with hepatic resection has ranged from 0% to 20%. Morbidity has been significant (>50% of patients). Major complications include perioperative hemorrhage, bile leaks, and ascites. Ascites has been particularly troublesome and likely results from continued cyst secretion from residual fenestrated cysts that exceeds the peritoneal absorptive capacity, disrupted intrahepatic lymphatics, and partial hepatic venous outflow obstruction. Resolution usually occurs with drainage and diuretics. If hepatic venous outflow obstruction is suspected, diagnosis is confirmed by MRI

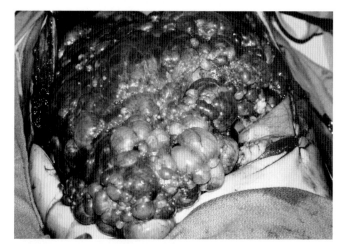

Fig. 65.7. Intraoperative photograph of massive hepatomegaly from adult PLD. Relative sparing of segments VI and VII is not visible.

Table 65.5 Hepatic Resection or Orthotopic Liver Transplantation for Polycystic Liver Disease

Reference	Patients (n)	No. Patients with Relief or Suppression	No. Patients with Recurrence	Maximum Duration of Follow-up (mo)
Resection				
Iwatsuki & Starzl, 1988	6	5	—	65
Sanchez et al, 1991	2	2	0	52
Vauthey et al, 1991	5	5	0	27
Henne-Bruns et al, 1993	8	8	2	48
Madariaga et al, 1993	2	2	2	156
Que et al, 1995	31	29	27	—
Koperna et al, 1997	5	5	0	72
Martin et al, 1998	3	3	0	13
Farges et al, 2003	16	14	2	54
Orthotopic Liver Transplantation				
Starzl et al, 1990	4	3	0	29
Washburn et al, 1996	5	4	0	82
Jeyarajah et al, 1998	6	6	0	67
Swenson et al, 1998	9	8	0	46
Pirenne et al, 2001	16	16	0	120
Ueda et al, 2004	3	3	0	48
Gustafsson et al, 2003	7	7	0	72

documenting hepatic vein or inferior vena cava compression and venous pressure measurements above and below the site of obstruction. Because residual cysts adjacent to the major vasculature are the usual cause, cyst aspiration with sclerosis or reoperation to excise the specific cyst may be indicated (Torres et al, 1994; Udden et al, 1995). Portosystemic shunting or transjugular intrahepatic portosystemic stenting should be avoided. Durability of results has been good, however (Que et al, 1995). Although postoperative cystic degeneration of the residual liver has been postulated, data have shown that cyst progression is usually indolent. Estrogen use postoperatively is contraindicated in women after resection and fenestration.

Hepatic resection with cyst fenestration takes advantage of both operative techniques by removing diffusely cystic liver that cannot be adequately fenestrated and fenestrating cysts in relatively spared liver to preserve liver function. Careful patient selection is required. Candidates for combined resection/fenestration must have at least one anatomic liver sector relatively spared of cystic involvement, near-normal liver function, significant impairment of clinical performance status owing to increased liver mass, and no significant cardiopulmonary compromise. Preoperatively, malnutrition must be corrected enterally or parenterally. Cerebrovascular disease must be excluded. Combined hepatic resection/fenestration is a formidable procedure because of the massively enlarged liver and distortion of the normal distribution of the hepatic vasculature and biliary ductal system by the cysts. The normal vasculature and bile ducts are obscured by the cysts themselves. Consequently, risk of bile duct and vascular injury with potential liver insufficiency is significant. Residual cyst walls retain their secretory capacity and can contribute to troublesome postoperative ascites. At operation, anatomic resection is preceded by lobar vascular isolation. Inflow vascular occlusion is often necessary. The transection plane is developed by sequential cyst fenestration. Intraseptal vessels and bile ducts are suture ligated. Cholecystectomy is performed to eliminate potential confounding diagnostic problems in the future or postoperatively. Perihepatic lymphatics are ligated if divided.

An example of results achieved by combined resection/fenestration as assessed by preoperative and postoperative CT scan is shown in Fig. 65.8. Long-term benefits of combined resection/fenestration will be determined by the rate of progressive cystic degeneration of the spared liver remnant. Current data on the natural history of PLD suggest that progression of cystic disease will be slow, and resection/fenestration will afford the possibility of prolonged benefit. No clinical trials have compared resection/fenestration with liver transplantation for patients with symptomatic polycystic disease.

Orthotopic liver transplantation for PLD is indicated for patients with progressive PLD after resection/fenestration, patients with concurrent liver dysfunction and renal failure, and patients with diffuse PLD without segmental sparing. Operative mortality for orthotopic liver transplantation for PLD is almost 12%. Risk is increased by prior intervention, especially with open abdominal procedures. Orthotopic liver transplantation is particularly challenging in PLD. The massive size of the liver makes the access to the suprahepatic inferior vena cava extremely difficult. Generally, the infrahepatic inferior vena cava is resected en bloc with the liver, and the piggyback technique is avoided (Pirenne et al, 2001). Selective cyst aspiration or fenestration faciliates dissection and exposure of posterior structures. Concurrent renal transplantation has been undertaken in approximately 13% of patients. Although symptomatic relief for the symptoms of hepatomegaly occurred in all surviving patients, long-term follow-up addressing quality of life, hepatorenal function, immunosuppressive complications, and survival is limited. The advent of living donor liver transplantation may affect the strategy for patients with PLD given the incapacitating symptoms but well-preserved liver function. Genetic screening if the potential donor is a relative (see earlier) must be undertaken, however, to obviate subsequent phenotypic PLD in either the recipient or the donor (Ueda et al, 2004).

MISCELLANEOUS CYSTS

Miscellaneous cysts of the liver include traumatic cysts and neoplastic cysts. Traumatic cysts are rare and usually form after incomplete resolution of subcapsular or intrahepatic hematomas or bilomas. They are usually single and have a thick pseudocyst wall and contain thick, bile-stained contents and hematoma.

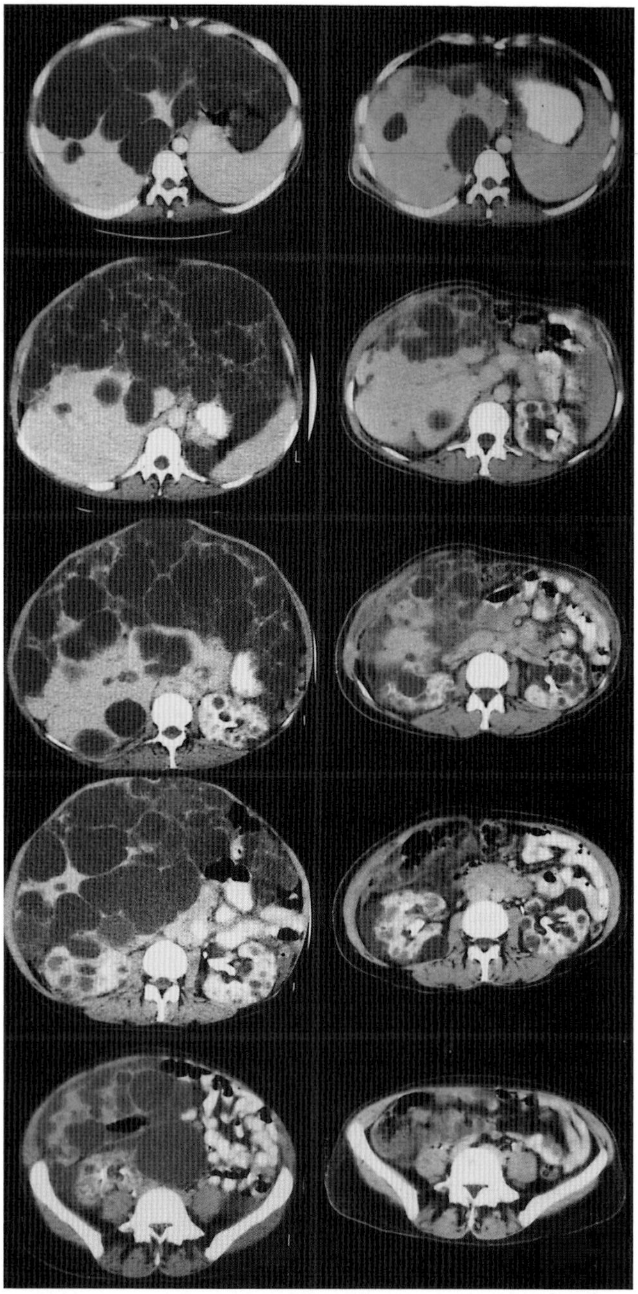

Fig. 65.8. Abdominal CT of a polycystic liver with relative sparing of segments VI and VII before *(left column)* and 5 years after *(right column)* extended left hepatectomy (polysegmentectomy I-V, VIII).

Because traumatic cysts are formed by parenchymal and ductal disruption, they have no epithelial lining. Most traumatic cysts resolve spontaneously. Occasionally, however, an intraparenchymal cyst may persist. If traumatic cysts continue to enlarge, disruption of a major segmental bile duct, which lacks continuity with the extrahepatic duct, must be suspected. If the cyst is symptomatic, complete resection or partial resection with intraperitoneal marsupialization and closure of the ductal defect is effective treatment.

Cystadenomas or cystadenocarcinomas constitute true neoplastic hepatic cysts. As with cystadenomas elsewhere intra-abdominally, they may be serous or mucinous, although the latter is more common. Cystadenomas are more common in

women, and clinical presentation is similar to that of large simple cysts. Preoperative imaging characteristics have been addressed previously. Prominent intraductal septa and focal wall thickening with or without mural nodularity are the hallmarks of cystadenomas on imaging studies. Although the presence of septations or nodular projections within the cyst on imaging classically differentiates cystadenomas from simple cysts, cystadenomas frequently are unilocular. Cyst aspirates may contain elevated levels of CA 19-9 or carcinoembryonic antigen, but, to date, the diagnostic value of these markers is indeterminate, and testing is not routine. If cystadenoma is suspected clinically, complete excision is indicated.

The results for treatment of cystadenomas after excision have been excellent. Partial excision has been associated with a high (>60%) recurrence rate (Davies et al, 1999). Any cyst in which a biopsy has been performed and cystadenoma confirmed requires complete excision. There are two histopathologic subtypes of cystadenomas: (1) simple cystadenoma and (2) cystadenoma with mesenchymal stroma. The latter type of cystadenoma occurs exclusively in women. Although histologically distinct, both subtypes seem to have similar clinical presentation and outcomes (Akwari et al, 1990; Wheeler & Edmonson, 1985).

Mucinous cystadenomas have a malignant potential and require complete excision. Adenocarcinomas may arise from the epithelial lining of a cystadenoma. Cystadenocarcinomas are exceedingly rare, and few have been reported (Ishak et al, 1977). The frequency of liver cysts harboring malignancy is so rare that the possibility of malignancy does not constitute an indication for excision of all cysts. Even symptomatic simple cysts are unusual. If cyst excision is undertaken, any irregularity of the cyst wall requires biopsy to exclude cystadenocarcinoma. If carcinoma is diagnosed, formal hepatic resection is recommended. Hepatic resection may be complicated because of the gross distortion of the intrahepatic ductal anatomy splayed over the cyst wall. Despite this intrahepatic ductal distortion, wide excision with adequate tumor-free margins is required. Consequently, extended lobar resections usually are required. Reported outcomes of hepatic resection for hepatic cystadenocarcinoma are few. Long-term survival has been obtained only after complete excision (Ishak et al, 1977; Wheeler & Edmonson, 1985). Complications associated with excision of cystadenocarcinomas have been similar to that of hepatic resections for intrahepatic malignancies.

Ciliated hepatic foregut cyst is a rare condition with fewer than 60 reported cases worldwide. This cyst likely is related to a developmental anomaly of the anterior foregut, leading to a detached outpouching of the hepatic diverticulum or enteric foregut. The cysts are typically small, solitary, and uniloculated. They contain ciliated pseudostratified columnar epithelium, scattered mucosal cells, loose subepithelial connective tissue, and a fibrous external capsule. They are benign with a low malignant potential (two reported cases). Although typically asymptomatic, resection usually is undertaken because of the inability to distinguish them from neoplastic cysts (Momin et al, 2004).

Hepatic cysts secondary to radiofrequency ablation are seen increasingly. Coagulative necrosis of the tumor and the adjacent hepatic parenchyma causes a radiofrequency ablation cyst (pseudocyst). Necrosis of adjacent bile duct or vessel may affect cyst composition. Resolution is typical, but variable in duration. Infection of radiofrequency ablation cysts is common in the presence of prior biliary drainage procedures or patent sphincterotomy. An infected radiofrequency ablation cyst should be managed as a hepatic abscess.

REFERENCES

Akwari OE, et al, 1990: Hepatobiliary cystadenoma with mesenchymal stroma. Ann Surg 211:18-27.

Albrink MH, et al, 1994: Laparoscopic management of cystic disease of the liver. Am Surg 60:262-266.

Andersson R, et al, 1989: Alcohol sclerotherapy of nonparasitic cysts of the liver. Br J Surg 76:254-255.

Andoh H, et al, 2004: Laparoscopic right hemihepatectomy for a case of polycystic liver disease with right predominance. J Hepatobiliary Pancreat Surg 11:116-118.

Cala Z, et al, 1996: Laparoscopic treatment of nonparasitic cysts of spleen and liver. J Laparoendosc Surg 6:387-391.

Davies W, et al, 1999: Intrahepatic biliary cystadenomas: an institutional experience with 37 cases. HPB Surg 1:141-146.

Diez J, et al, 1998: Laparoscopic treatment of symptomatic cysts of the liver. Br J Surg 85:25-27.

Drenth JP, et al, 2004: Abnormal hepatocystin caused by truncating *PRKCSH* mutations leads to autosomal dominant polycystic liver disease. Hepatology 39:924-931.

Emmermann A, et al, 1997: Laparoscopic treatment of nonparasitic cysts of the liver with omental transposition flap. Surg Endosc 11:734-736.

Everson GT, et al, 2004: Polycystic disease of the liver. Hepatology 40:774-782.

Fabiani P, et al, 1991: Laparoscopic fenestration of biliary cysts. Surg Laparosc Endosc 1:162-165.

Farges O, et al, 2003: Liver resection in the treatment of polycystic liver disease. J Gastrointest Surg 7:280A.

Fiamingo P, et al, 2003: Laparoscopic treatment of simple hepatic cysts and polycystic liver disease. Surg Endosc 17:623-626.

Furuta T, et al, 1990: Treatment of symptomatic non-parasitic liver cysts: surgical treatment versus alcohol injection therapy. HPB Surg 2:269-279.

Gelczer RK, et al, 1998: Complications of percutaneous ethanol ablation. J Ultrasound Med 17:531-533.

Gigot JF, et al, 1996: Laparoscopic treatment of nonparasitic liver cysts: adequate selection of patients and surgical technique. World J Surg 20:556-561.

Gigot JF, et al, 1997: Adult polycystic liver disease: is fenestration the most adequate operation for long-term management? Ann Surg 225:286-294.

Gigot JF, et al, 2001: The surgical management of congenital liver cysts: the need for a tailored approach with appropriate patient selection and proper surgical technique. Surg Endosc 15:357-363.

Giulante F, et al, 2003: Risk for laparoscopic fenestration of liver cysts. Surg Endosc 17:1735-1738.

Gustafsson BI, et al, 2003: Liver transplantation for plycystic liver disease: indications and outcome. Transplant Proc 35:813-814.

Hansman MF, et al, 2001: Management and long-term follow-up of hepatic cysts. Am J Surg 181:404-410.

Henne-Bruns D, et al, 1993: Non-parasitic liver cysts and polycystic liver disease: results of surgical treatment. Hepatogastroenterology 40:1-5.

Ishak KG, et al, 1977: Biliary cystadenoma and cystadenocarcinoma: report of 14 cases and review of the literature. Cancer 39:322-338.

Iwatsuki S, Starzl TE, 1988: Personal experience with 411 hepatic resections. Ann Surg 208:421-434.

Jeyarajah DR, et al, 1998: Liver and kidney transplantation for polycystic disease. Transplantation 66:529-544.

Kabbej M, et al, 1996: Laparoscopic fenestration in polycystic liver disease. Br J Surg 83:1697-2701.

Koperna T, et al, 1997: Nonparasitic cysts of the liver: results and options of surgical treatment. World J Surg 21:850-855.

Larssen TB, et al, 1997: Single-session alcohol scherotherapy in benign symptomatic hepatic cysts. Acta Radiol 38:993-997.

Larssen TB, et al, 2003: Single-session alcohol sclerotherapy in symptomatic benign hepatic cysts performed with a time of exposure to alcohol of 10 min: initial results. Eur Radiol 13:2627-2632.

Madariaga JR, et al, 1993: Hepatic resection for cystic lesions of the liver. Ann Surg 218:610-614.

Marks J, et al, 1998: Laparoscopic liver surgery: a report of 28 patients. Surg Endosc 12:331-334.

Martin IJ, et al, 1998: Tailoring the management of nonparasitic liver cysts. Ann Surg 228:167-172.

Momin TA, et al, 2004: Ciliated hepatic foregut cyst of the left hepatic vein. J Gastrointest Surg 8:601-603.

Montorsi M, et al, 1994: Percutaneous alcohol sclerotherapy of simple hepatic cysts: results from a multicentre survey in Italy. HPB Surg 8:89-94.

Morino M, et al, 1994: Laparoscopic management of symptomatic nonparasitic cysts of the liver: indications and results. Ann Surg 219:157-164.

Pirenne J, et al, 2001: Liver transplantation for polycystic disease. Liver Transplant 7:238-245.

Rhim H, et al, 2004: Radiofrequency thermal ablation of hepatic cyst. J Vasc Interv Radiol 15:95-96.

Que F, et al, 1995: Liver resection and cyst fenestration in the treatment of severe polycystic liver disease. Gastroenterology 108:487-494.

Sanchez H, et al, 1991: Surgical management of nonparasitic cystic liver disease. Am J Surg 161:113-119.

Schachter P, et al, 2001: The role of laparoscopic ultrasound in the minimally invasive management of symptomatic hepatic cysts. Surg Endosc 15:364-367.

Simonetti G, et al, 1993: Percutaneous treatment of hepatic cysts by aspiration and sclerotherapy. Cardiovasc Interv Radiol 16:81-84.

Starzl TE, et al, 1990: Liver transplantation for polycystic liver disease. Arch Surg 125:575-577.

Swenson K, et al, 1998: Liver transplantation for adult polycystic liver disease. Hepatology 28:412-415.

Tagaya N, et al, 2003: Long-term results of laparoscopic unroofing of symptomatic solitary nonparasitic hepatic cysts. Surg Laparosc Endosc 13:76-79.

Tikkakoski T, et al, 1996: Treatment of symptomatic congenital hepatic cysts with single-session percutaneous drainage and ethanol sclerosis: treatment and outcome. J Vasc Interv Radiol 7:235-239.

Tocchi A, et al, 2002: Symptomatic nonparasitic hepatic cysts: options for results of surgical management. Arch Surg 137:154-158.

Torres VE, et al, 1994: Hepatic venous outflow obstruction in autosomal dominant polycystic kidney disease. J Am Soc Nephrol 5:1186-1192.

Udden W, et al, 1995: Hepatic venous outflow obstruction in patients with polycystic liver disease: pathogenesis and treatment. Gut 36:142-145.

Ueda M, et al, 2004: Living-donor liver transplantation for polycystic liver disease. Transplantation 77:480-482.

vanSonnenberg E, et al, 1994: Symptomatic hepatic cysts: percutaneous drainage and sclerosis. Radiology 190:387-392.

Vauthey JN, et al, 1991: Adult polycystic disease of the liver. Br J Surg 78:524-527.

Washburn WK, et al, 1996: Liver transplantation for adult polycystic liver disease. Liver Transplant Surg 2:17-22.

Weber T, et al, 2004: Laparoscopic unroofing of nonparasitic liver cysts within segments VII and VIII: technical considerations. J Laparoendosc Adv Surg Tech 14:37-42.

Wheeler DA, Edmonson HA, 1985: Cystadenoma with mesenchymal stroma (CMS) in the liver and bile ducts: a clinicopathologic study of 17 cases, 4 with malignant change. Cancer 56:1434-1445.

Yamada N, et al, 1994: Treatment of symptomatic hepatic cysts by percutaneous instillation of minocycline hydrochloride. Dig Dis Sci 39:2503-2509.

Zacherl J, et al, 1996: Laparoscopic unroofing of symptomatic congenital liver cysts. Surg Endosc 10:813-815.

Zacherl J, et al, 2000: Long-term results after laparoscopic unroofing of solitary symptomatic congenital liver cysts. Surg Endosc 14:59-62.

Injury and Hemorrhage

Liver, Biliary, and Pancreatic Injury

66a LIVER AND BILE DUCT INJURY

D. DEMETRIADES, A. SALIM, AND T. V. BERNE

ANATOMY

Knowledge of the basic anatomy is essential for optimal operative management of severe liver injuries (see Ch. 1). Some important planes have practical importance in trauma and should be borne in mind. The interlobar plane between the gallbladder anteriorly and the inferior vena cava (IVC) posteriorly runs along the course of the middle hepatic vein. Dissection along the falciform ligament plane should be avoided because of the risk of injury to the portal venous supply to the medial segment of the left lobe (Fig. 66a.1). Good knowledge of the anatomy of the retrohepatic IVC and hepatic veins is crucial in the management of injuries to these structures. The retrohepatic IVC measures about 8 to 10 cm in length. The atriocaval junction is only about 3 cm above the phrenic veins. In about 90% of humans, the IVC is partially encircled by liver parenchyma. In about 7%, the IVC is completely encircled by liver tissue. There are three major hepatic veins and about seven smaller retrohepatic veins. Occasionally, there is a large inferior right hepatic vein. Only about 2 cm of the major hepatic veins course extrahepatically before joining the IVC. In about 85% of humans, the middle hepatic vein fuses with the left hepatic vein before draining into the IVC. A detailed description of the anatomy of the liver is presented in Ch. 1.

EPIDEMIOLOGY

The liver is the most commonly injured intra-abdominal organ after blunt trauma. A review of 825 patients with significant blunt abdominal trauma and an Abbreviated Injury Score (AIS) of 2 or greater admitted to the Los Angeles County–University of Southern California Trauma Center showed liver injuries in 563 (68%) patients and splenic injuries in 493 (60%). The usual mechanisms of injury are anteroposterior compression, deceleration forces with avulsion of the ligaments or the hepatic veins, and direct penetration by a fractured rib.

In penetrating abdominal injuries, the liver is the third most common injured organ after the small bowel and the colon. In 273 patients undergoing laparotomy for gunshot wounds, the small bowel was injured in 38%, the colon in 31%, and the liver in 28%. Low velocity missiles cause localized tissue damage; they are life-threatening only if they transect a major vessel. High velocity missiles cause massive destruction of the liver parenchyma, and they are associated with high mortality.

CLASSIFICATION OF SEVERITY OF HEPATIC INJURIES

Standardized classification of liver injury is important in evaluating and comparing therapeutic interventions. The Organ Injury Scaling Committee of the American Association for the Surgery of Trauma published a classification system that is extensively used now (Table 66a.1) (Moore et al, 1995). The classification is based on operative or computed tomography (CT) scan findings.

CLINICAL PRESENTATION

The clinical presentation of liver injuries depends on the mechanism of injury and the presence or not of significant bleeding and other associated intra-abdominal injuries. Patients with significant blood loss or associated hollow viscus perforation present with hypotension or signs of peritonitis. Most patients with isolated liver injuries are hemodynamically stable on admission and have no signs or minimal signs of peritonitis. In most patients with penetrating trauma, the diagnosis is made intraoperatively,

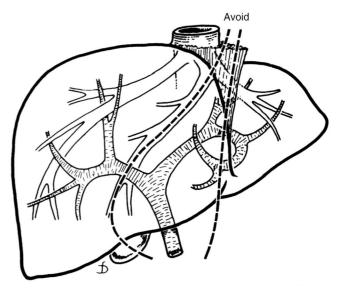

Fig. 66a.1. Dissection along the plane between the gallbladder and IVC may injure the middle hepatic vein. Dissection along the falciform ligament may injure the portal venous supply of the medial segment of the left lobe.

Table 66a.1   Liver Injury Scale*

	Grade[†]	Injury Description	ICD-9	AIS-90
I	Hematoma	Subcapsular, <10% surface area	864.01 864.11	2
	Laceration	Capsular tear, <1 cm parenchymal depth	864.02	2
II	Hematoma	Subcapsular, 10-50% surface area Intraparenchymal, <10 cm in diameter	864.01 864.11	2
	Laceration	1-3 cm parenchymal depth, <10 cm in length		
III	Hematoma	Subcapsular, >50% surface area or expanding; ruptured subcapsular or intraparenchymal hematoma >10 cm or expanding		3
	Laceration	>3 cm parenchymal depth	864.04 864.14	3
IV	Laceration	Parenchymal disruption involving 25-75% of hepatic lobe or 1-3 Couinaud's segments within a single lobe	864.04 864.14	
V	Laceration	Parenchymal disruption involving >75% of hepatic lobe or >3 Couinaud's segments within a single lobe		5
	Vascular	Juxtahepatic venous injuries (i.e., retrohepatic vena cava/ central major hepatic veins)		5
VI	Vascular	Hepatic avulsion		6

*1994 revision.
[†]Advance one grade for multiple injuries, up to grade III.
From Moore EE, et al, 1995: Organ injury scaling: spleen and liver (1994 revision). J Trauma 38:323-324.

whereas in most patients with blunt trauma, the diagnosis is made by CT evaluation.

INVESTIGATIONS

Ultrasound performed by physicians in the emergency department may be helpful in detecting free fluid in the abdomen. Free fluid usually is seen in the space between the liver and the right kidney (Fig. 66a.2). Ultrasound does not provide any information about the source of the free fluid, however, and fluid may be absent in cases with intrahepatic hematomas. A formal ultrasound examination performed by an experienced radiologist may provide reliable information regarding the type and severity of the hepatic injury.

An abdominal CT scan with intravenous contrast administration is the most useful investigation in the evaluation of suspected liver trauma. It provides reliable information about the nature and extent of the injury, the amount of free fluid in the peritoneal cavity, the presence of active bleeding, vascular lesions (false aneurysms or arteriovenous fistulae), and the presence of other associated injuries. CT is a valuable tool in the selection of patients for operation or observation or angiographic embolization (Fig. 66a.3).

Diagnostic peritoneal lavage has largely been replaced by ultrasound and abdominal CT. We perform diagnostic peritoneal aspirate without fluid infusion in rare cases with hemodynamic instability and indeterminate ultrasound results (Fig. 66a.4). The presence of free blood in the peritoneal cavity is not always

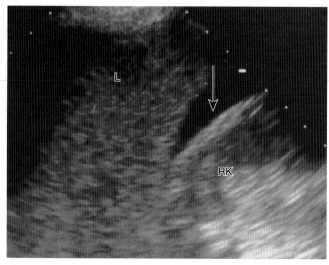

Fig. 66a.2. Ultrasound done as an emergent procedure shows free fluid *(arrow)* between the liver (L) and the right kidney (RK).

an absolute indication for operation. Intraperitoneal fluid infusion for diagnostic peritoneal lavage does not give more information about serious intra-abdominal bleeding than diagnostic peritoneal aspirate, and it interferes with the interpretation of a subsequent CT scan. The high sensitivity of diagnostic peritoneal lavage in detecting small amounts of intraperitoneal blood results in an unacceptably high incidence of nontherapeutic laparotomies.

MANAGEMENT

Nonoperative Management

Selective nonoperative management of blunt liver trauma has become the standard of care. The selection of patients for nonoperative management should be based on the findings of clinical examination and CT evaluation and the presence or not

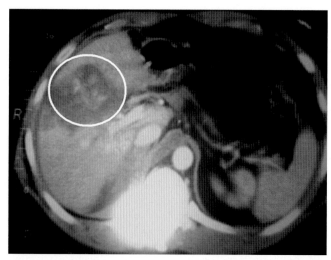

Fig. 66a.3. CT scan with intravenous contrast administration shows a "blush" *(circle)*, which is diagnostic of active bleeding or a false aneurysm. This finding should prompt the surgeon to perform angiographic evaluation in hemodynamically stable patients or a laparotomy in unstable patients.

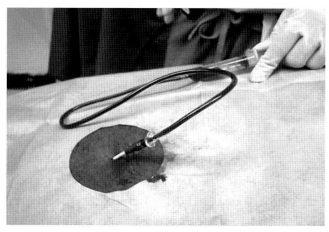

Fig. 66a.4. Diagnostic peritoneal aspirate shows aspiration of gross blood. A standard peritoneal lavage catheter is inserted through a 2-mm incision below the umbilicus and directed toward the pelvis. Aspiration is performed with a syringe. If no blood is aspirated, the procedure is terminated. Diagnostic peritoneal aspirate is indicated in unstable patients with multiple trauma and indeterminate ultrasound results. Stable patients are best investigated by CT scan.

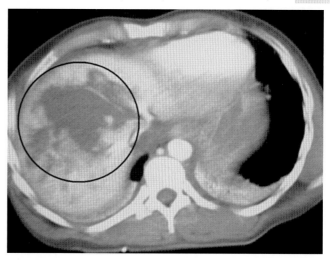

Fig. 66a.5. Grade IV liver injury successfully managed nonoperatively. High-grade injuries do not preclude nonoperative management. Angiographic evaluation should be performed liberally in these cases.

of associated injuries. Hemodynamic stability and no signs of peritonitis are absolute requirements for nonoperative management. Frequent serial clinical evaluations are the cornerstone for successful nonoperative management. Missed associated intra-abdominal injuries are a rare but significant problem associated with nonoperative management. Missed injuries and delayed treatment of injuries may result in significant complications, including death. Such visceral injuries in patients selected for nonoperative management are found in less than 2% to 3% of cases, and the delay in diagnosis is usually only a few hours (Miller et al, 2002; Velmahos et al, 2003). In some cases (e.g., severe head trauma or spinal cord injury), clinical evaluation of the abdomen is difficult, however, and the diagnosis may be delayed several days.

The combination of clinical examination and CT reliably provides a diagnosis or a high index of suspicion in almost all visceral injuries. Important CT findings suggesting intestinal trauma include bowel wall thickening, unexplained free intraperitoneal fluid, free gas, and mesenteric stranding. In suspected cases, a repeat CT scan should be performed a few hours later.

The success rate of nonoperative management of blunt hepatic trauma is high. In some series, the liver injury–specific success rate is 100% (Velmahos et al, 2003). Most treatment failures occur within the first 24 hours of admission. A liver-related failure rarely occurs after the first 24 hours. Identifying independent risk factors of failure of nonoperative management is difficult because of the few patients who experience treatment failure during the observation period. There is some evidence that patients with a high Injury Severity Score, severe liver injuries (grade IV-V), multiple transfusions, or associated chronic liver disease, such as cirrhosis, have an increased risk of failure of nonoperative management. The presence of associated severe head trauma initially was thought to be a relative contraindication for nonoperative management, but subsequent studies failed to confirm this (Keller et al, 1996; Shapiro et al, 2001). Severe head injury often is associated with disseminated intravascular coagulopathy, however, which might increase the risk of bleeding from any injured solid organ. Severity of liver injury is not in itself an absolute contraindication for nonoperative management (Fig. 66a.5). Although some surgeons are reluctant to observe

high-grade liver injuries, many studies have shown that carefully selected high-grade injuries can be managed safely nonoperatively (Goan et al, 1998; Sherman et al, 1995). Angiographic embolization may increase significantly the success rate of nonoperative management of high-grade injuries (Velmahos et al, 2003; Wahl et al, 2002). *The failure rate of nonoperative management in grade IV or V liver injuries is still high.* A retrospective multi-institutional study from 13 level I trauma centers reported nonoperative management in only 14% of grade IV or V injuries (Pachter et al, 1996).

Although nonoperative management of blunt liver trauma has gained widespread acceptance, most penetrating injuries are still treated operatively. There is evidence, however, that selected cases with penetrating trauma can be managed safely nonoperatively. In a South African prospective study of 63 cases with stab wounds to the liver, 33% were managed successfully nonoperatively (Demetriades et al, 1986). Subsequent studies showed that patients with gunshot injuries to the right thoracoabdominal area could be managed nonoperatively (Chmielewski et al, 1995; Renz et al, 1994). In a more recent study from Los Angeles, 21% of isolated gunshot injuries to the liver were managed successfully nonoperatively (Demetriades et al, 1999). Routine CT evaluation of these patients is essential to evaluate the severity of injury and detect active bleeding, pseudoaneurysms, or arteriovenous fistulae (Fig. 66a.6). Selective nonoperative management of gunshot wounds to the abdomen has been used successfully (Demetriades et al, 1997; Velmahos et al, 1997), and a case for nonoperative management of selected cases with gunshot wounds to the liver can be made. This is still a controversial issue, however, and a conservative approach should be used only in trauma centers with experience.

Management of Liver Injuries Selected for Nonoperative Care

Patients with significant liver injuries (grades III-V) selected for nonoperative management should be admitted to the intensive care unit (ICU) for close monitoring of vital signs and hemoglobin and frequent examinations of the abdomen. Patients with high-grade injuries and pooling of contrast material in the hepatic parenchyma ("blush") or significant free blood in the peritoneal

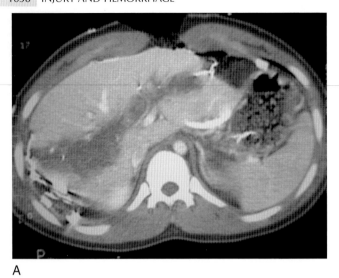 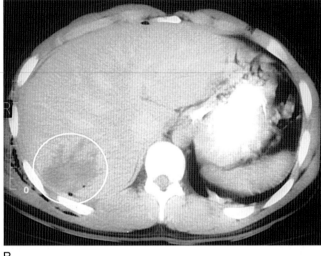

A   B

Fig. 66a.6. A and **B,** Gunshot wounds to the liver managed successfully with nonoperative management. Patients should be hemodynamically stable and have no signs of peritonitis.

cavity should be considered for early angiographic embolization, before hemodynamic instability occurs or blood transfusions are required. Failure of nonoperative management is defined as the development of hemodynamic instability or of "liver-related" multiple transfusions despite angiographic embolization, signs of peritonitis, or abdominal compartment syndrome. These patients require laparotomy and surgical control of the injuries.

Monitoring in an ICU and strict bed rest are required for the first 2 or 3 days. In the absence of other major associated injuries, the patient can be moved to a regular floor with instructions for gradual ambulation. The nature and severity of liver injury should determine how long vigorous physical activities should be avoided. In most cases with liver lacerations, the patient should avoid vigorous physical activities for about 6 to 8 weeks. Experimental evidence indicates that hepatic wounds heal well within 3 weeks, and the bursting strength of the healed area is stronger than the normal liver parenchyma (Dulchavsky et al, 1990). The natural history and prognosis of other liver injuries, such as massive parenchymal damage or large subcapsular or intrahepatic hematomas, are not well known, however. These lesions sometimes enlarge and may rupture after external trauma or cause compression to the surrounding tissues. These patients

may require longer observation before regular activities are resumed. Repeat CT scans are valuable in determining the progress of the lesion and deciding the timing of return to normal activities (Fig. 66a.7). It is strongly recommended that all patients with severe liver injuries be re-evaluated by CT scan before return to vigorous physical activities.

Complications of Nonoperative Management

Nonoperative management of liver injuries is safe; the liver-related complication rate is 2% (Velmahos et al, 2003). Rebleeding from the liver is the most common complication and in most cases occurs within the first few hours or days. Bleeding rarely occurs after the first few days, and it usually is related to a false aneurysm or liver parenchymal necrosis (Gates, 1994). Most patients with recurrent bleeding can be managed safely with angiographic embolization. Other liver-related complications include biloma, abscess, false aneurysm, arteriovenous fistula, hemobilia, intrahepatic biliary strictures, and Budd-Chiari syndrome secondary to compression of the IVC by a liver hematoma (Markert et al, 1997). Most complications can be managed by percutaneous drainage or angiographic embolization, and surgical treatment is rarely necessary.

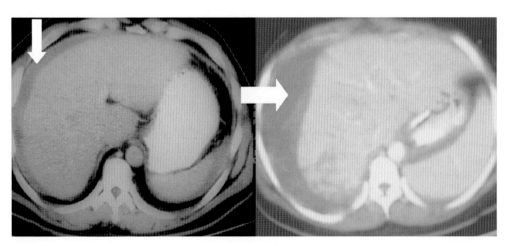

Fig. 66a.7. Small subcapsular hematoma *(left)* and large subcapsular hematoma *(right)* successfully managed nonoperatively. These lesions should be monitored with serial CT scans before return to normal physical activities.

Operative Management of Liver Injuries

Incisions

The abdomen always should be entered through a midline incision because it provides the best exposure for exploration for any intra-abdominal injury. Placement of gauze packs between the liver and the diaphragm displaces the liver downward and improves the exposure. Division of the falciform and coronary ligaments should be performed only if further exposure is required to suture any posterior liver injuries. If the nature of the liver injury precludes suturing, the ligaments should not be divided because they allow more effective perihepatic packing. In complex liver injuries, the exposure may be improved by adding a subcostal incision (Fig. 66a.8A). A median sternotomy should be performed only if an atriocaval shunt is considered (see Fig. 66a.8B). A right thoracotomy is rarely indicated in some cases requiring total liver vascular isolation.

Operative Techniques

In about 80% to 85% of patients undergoing operation, the liver injury can be managed by relatively simple surgical techniques, such as application of local hemostatic agents, electrocoagulation, superficial suturing, or closed drains. The remaining 15% to 20% of cases require more complex surgical techniques. Temporary control of liver bleeding may be achieved by compression of the liver wound. If compression is not effective, cross-clamping of the porta hepatis structures with a vascular clamp (Pringle maneuver) may reduce bleeding.

Deep Liver Lacerations

Bleeding from deep liver lacerations often can be controlled by direct suture ligation of any major bleeders, followed by deep, figure-eight, tension-free sutures (chromic 0 on a large liver needle). The dead space should be obliterated as much as possible to avoid intraparenchymal hematomas. Fears about intrahepatic abscess or hemobilia after deep sutures have been overstated. These complications are relatively rare and can be managed by percutaneous drainage or angiographic embolization. Omental packing of large liver wounds has been a common practice. Although omentum is useful in reducing any dead space, there

is no evidence that it reduces bleeding or bile leak, and in some cases omental ischemic necrosis may occur.

Penetrating Liver Tracts

Severe bleeding from deep bullet or knife tracts in the liver can be a difficult problem. Packing of the tract with hemostatic agents is not effective in controlling significant bleeding. Tractotomy and bleeding control of the bleeders is a commonly used approach. This technique is safe and effective in peripheral injuries. In central tracts, a tractotomy may be associated with severe bleeding from the divided normal parenchyma, however, especially in coagulopathic patients. An alternative to the tractotomy is tamponade using a balloon catheter (Demetriades, 1998; Thomas et al, 1993). The senior author (D.D.) has designed a commercially available sausage-shaped balloon, which results in tamponade along the whole length of the tract (Fig. 66a.9). When the bleeding is controlled, the free end of the catheter is brought out through the skin, and the catheter is occluded. Closed drains are placed near the entry and exit of the tract, and the abdomen is closed. Postoperatively, the patient is observed in the ICU. Indications for angiographic evaluation should be liberal. On day 3 or 4, the balloon is deflated, and the patient is monitored a few hours for any bleeding from the catheter or the closed drains. If no bleeding occurs, the deflated catheter is removed. On the rare occasion when bleeding is observed, the balloon is reinflated for another attempt in a few days. In some cases in which the abdomen is packed, the balloon catheter may be left in the peritoneal cavity until the next planned re-exploration.

Massive Parenchymal Damage

Severe blunt trauma or high velocity gunshot wounds can cause extensive parenchymal damage not amenable to deep suturing (Fig. 66a.10). Nonanatomic resection of the devitalized liver parenchyma may be needed for hemostasis or prevention of subsequent necrosis and sepsis or delayed hemorrhage. The American trauma literature generally does not support anatomic resections because of the associated high mortality rate. It has been postulated that the lack of experience of trauma surgeons with liver resections might be a significant reason for the poor results after partial hepatectomy (Strong et al, 1998). Strong and

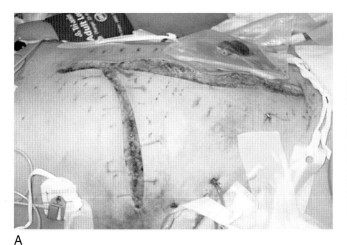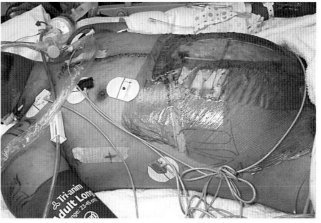

A   B

Fig. 66a.8. A, A midline laparotomy provides good surgical exposure in most liver injuries. In complex injuries, the exposure may be improved by adding a right subcostal incision. **B,** Patient with complex liver injury requiring extension of the laparotomy into a median sternotomy for an atriocaval shunt. This is the strongest indication for a sternotomy. The liver injury was managed with perihepatic packing, and the abdomen was left open to avoid the development of abdominal compartment syndrome.

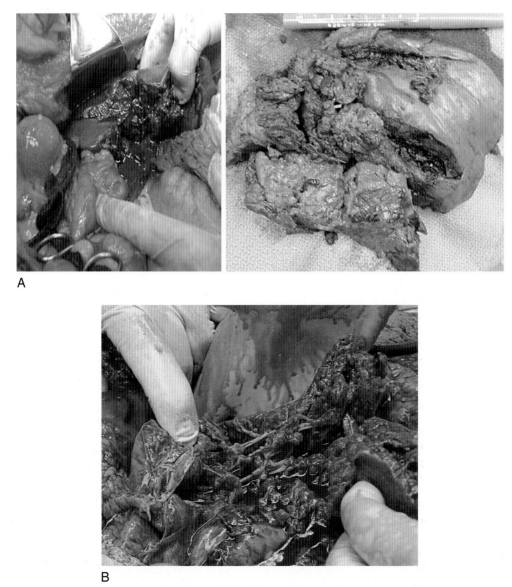

Fig. 66a.9. A and **B,** Custom-made balloon for liver tamponade for controlling bleeding from deep penetrating wounds. The inflated balloon stays in place for 3 to 4 days.

Fig. 66a.10. A, Grade IV liver injury requiring a nonanatomic resection. **B,** Grade V liver injury requiring major nonanatomic resection.

colleagues (1998) reported a low mortality of 8.1% and liver-related morbidity of 19% with anatomic resections. They concluded that anatomic resection for trauma is associated with low morbidity and mortality if performed by experienced hepatobiliary surgeons. Other authors also have reported good results with formal resections (Blumgart et al, 1979; Kasai & Kobayashi, 1993). In practice, major hepatic resections are rarely indicated and should be reserved for destructive parenchymal injuries in which perihepatic packing is not effective in controlling the hemorrhage. Resections should be performed semielectively in selected patients with postoperative liver necrosis. In these cases, the surgeon should not hesitate to use the experience of a hepatobiliary surgeon.

Another suggested alternative method of managing extensive hepatic trauma is wrapping of the liver with absorbable mesh. Despite early enthusiasm and good results (Brunet et al, 1994; Stevens et al, 1991), the technique failed to gain popularity because of its complexity. Perihepatic packing is much simpler and faster than mesh wrapping and is the procedure used by almost all trauma surgeons in cases of complex liver trauma.

Perihepatic packing and damage control is probably the most significant surgical advancement in the management of complex liver injuries. It is effective in controlling life-threatening hemorrhage in most severe liver injuries (Cue et al, 1990; Feliciano et al, 1986; Krige et al, 1992). It often is not effective in many major retrohepatic venous injuries or other major intrahepatic vascular injuries. More recent reports have suggested that even some retrohepatic caval injuries can be managed successfully by packing (Cue et al, 1990). It has been suggested that perihepatic packing should be considered in patients in extremis who have become coagulopathic, hypothermic, and hemodynamically unstable. We firmly believe that packing should be performed much earlier and before complications occur. After rapid evaluation of the severity of the liver injury, the surgeon should make an early decision about management strategy. If the anatomic site and severity of the injury are such that conventional methods are unlikely to be effective in controlling bleeding, perihepatic packing should be instituted.

The technique of packing is important for effective tamponade. The presence of intact hepatic ligaments increases the effectiveness of the tamponade, and they should not routinely be divided. To avoid bleeding from the raw surface of the liver during removal of the laparotomy pads at reoperation, an absorbable mesh is spread over the surface of the liver, before the packing pads or gauze rolls are placed (Fig. 66a.11). The mesh is left in place permanently when the packing is removed 2 or 3 days later. After perihepatic packing, the abdomen is not closed primarily to avoid the development of an abdominal compartment syndrome. Temporary abdominal closure should be performed using one of the described techniques (Brock et al, 1995; Miller et al, 2004). The perihepatic packing should be removed as soon as the patient stabilizes and any coagulopathy and hypothermia are corrected; this is usually possible within 24 to 48 hours. There is evidence that keeping the packing 72 hours does not increase the incidence of local infection, but that prolonged packing (>3 days) is associated with an increased risk of perihepatic infection (Cue et al, 1990).

Selective hepatic artery ligation has been suggested as a useful method of controlling difficult bleeding. Despite earlier enthusiasm (Aaron et al, 1975), it has not gained wide acceptance and is used rarely in trauma. The combination of hepatic artery ligation, parenchymal injury, and hypotension often leads to

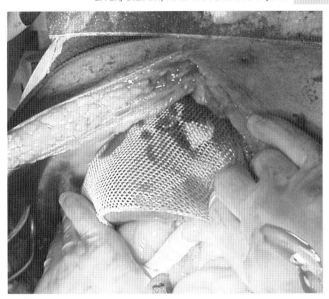

Fig. 66a.11. Application of an absorbable mesh over the surface of the liver before placing the packing pads for perihepatic packing. This technique avoids bleeding from the surface of the liver during removal of the pads at reoperation.

hepatic necrosis. Ligation should be reserved for the rare case of injury to the hepatic artery.

Retrohepatic Vena Cava and Hepatic Vein Injury

Injury to the juxtahepatic major veins is the most lethal form of hepatic trauma. Death usually occurs as a result of massive blood loss or air embolism. The operative findings may include a stable retrohepatic hematoma or severe active bleeding. Stable retrohepatic hematomas should be left undisturbed, and the surgeon should resist the temptation to explore the area because to do this may result in severe hemorrhage and possibly death. Control of severe active bleeding can challenge the skills of even the most experienced trauma surgeon. The bleeding characteristically becomes worse at any attempt to rotate or lift the liver to expose the bleeding site. Good knowledge of the local anatomy is crucial in deciding the operative maneuvers.

Adequate exposure is the cornerstone of the successful management of injury to the retrohepatic veins. Addition of a subcostal incision provides a good exposure to the retrohepatic vessels. Division of the hepatic ligaments and mobilization of the liver may improve the exposure to some extent, but should not be done if perihepatic packing is effective in controlling bleeding. If packing is successful, the abdomen should be closed temporarily and the patient transferred to the ICU. More complex maneuvers should be attempted only if packing is ineffective. In many cases with intrahepatic venous injuries, the bleeding vessel can be exposed directly and ligated through the liver-injured parenchyma. Occasionally, complete division of the liver along the interlobar plane may be necessary for the satisfactory exposure of the vena cava and the confluence of the major hepatic veins (Schrock et al, 1968).

Temporary control of the bleeding can be achieved by using vascular isolation of the liver or intracaval shunts. Vascular isolation is the most commonly used approach and consists of cross-clamping of the aorta below the diaphragm, the suprahepatic and infrahepatic IVC, and the porta hepatis (Fig. 66a.12) (Yellin et al, 1971). Clamping the aorta is essential and should be done

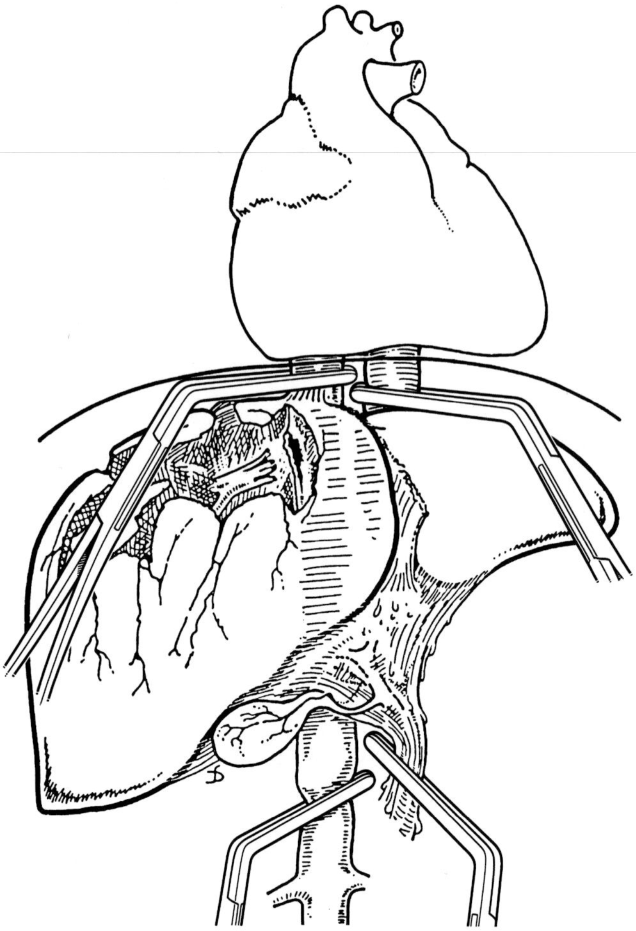

Fig. 66a.12. Vascular isolation of the liver for major retrohepatic venous injuries. The aorta is cross-clamped below the diaphragm. Vascular clamps are applied to the suprahepatic IVC (between the dome of the liver and the right diaphragm), the infrahepatic IVC (above the renal veins), and the porta hepatis (Pringle maneuver).

first to prevent hypovolemic cardiac arrest. Suprahepatic cross-clamping of the IVC can be performed by applying a vascular clamp on the IVC, between the diaphragm and the dome of the liver. The practice of opening the chest to control the intraperi-cardial IVC is not necessary in most patients. Timely and appropriate application of total vascular isolation may yield good results with 70% survival (Miller et al, 2002).

The use of intracaval shunt should be considered in selected complex venous injuries that cannot be managed by other, less aggressive approaches. The laparotomy incision is extended into a median sternotomy, and the pericardium is opened. A tape tourniquet is applied around the intrapericardial IVC. The right atrial appendage is occluded with a vascular clamp, and a 2-0 silk purse-string suture is placed in the appendage. A No. 8 endotracheal tube with a side hole cut at about 8 to 10 cm from the clamped proximal end of the tube is inserted through the purse-string. The tube is guided by the surgeon into the IVC, the balloon is inflated just above the renal veins, and the tape tourniquet around the intrapericardial IVC is tightened (Fig. 66a.13). Alternatively, a No. 36 chest tube might be used as a shunt, keeping in mind that a second tape tourniquet placed around the suprarenal abdominal IVC will be required. Atriocaval shunts reduce the hemorrhage from the injured veins, but they do not achieve complete cessation of the bleeding. The reported

results with atriocaval shunts are generally poor, with a mortality rate of 80% to 90% (Burch et al, 1988; Cogbill et al, 1988). The experience of the surgical team and the timing of the shunt are crucial factors in determining outcome (Khaneja et al, 1997). We have seen a few survivors when the shunt was placed early, before the development of major coagulopathy and severe hypothermia. Other types of shunting that have been used in the management of retrohepatic venous injuries include vena caval balloons inserted through the femoral vein (Pilcher et al, 1977) and extracorporeal venovenous bypass with the use of an interposed pump (Baumgartner et al, 1996; Horwitz et al, 1995). These techniques have been used in only a few case reports.

Other reported techniques for the management of these injuries include hypothermic circulatory arrest (Hartman et al, 1991; Marelli et al, 1995) and emergency liver transplantation (Ginzburg et al, 1998; Jen et al, 1993). Hypothermic circulatory arrest is still an experimental method. Liver transplantation has been performed successfully in many cases, and it should be considered in centers with transplant capabilities.

Liver Hematomas

Many liver hematomas can be managed safely nonoperatively, provided that the patient is hemodynamically stable and has no peritonitis. The discovery of a stable subcapsular or intra-hepatic hematoma during an exploratory laparotomy poses a major dilemma for the surgeon. Exploring these hematomas may precipitate significant bleeding, whereas failure to do so may result in delayed rupture and bleeding. Management is contro-versial; we suggest that deep, stable intraparenchymal hematomas and small or moderate size subcapsular hematomas be left undis-turbed. To rule out bleeding and false aneurysms, postoperative evaluation with contrast CT scan is essential, especially in large intrahepatic hematomas. Large subcapsular hematomas should be explored, and any underlying liver lacerations should be sutured and hemostasis achieved, if necessary, with perihepatic packing.

Other Therapeutic Techniques

Angiographic Embolization (see Chs. 21 and 74)
Interventional radiology has made a significant contribution to the management of bleeding from the liver parenchyma. The threshold for using angiographic evaluation postoperatively in patients with severe liver trauma should be low (Fig. 66a.14). Patients managed with perihepatic packing should be evaluated angiographically liberally and as soon as possible. We transfer these patients directly from the operating room to the angiogra-phy suite. By following this aggressive policy, we have been able to reduce operative mortality in grade IV and V liver injuries (Asensio et al, 2003). We believe that the commonly used prac-tice of observing these patients in the ICU and selecting for angiography only patients who deteriorate has many disadvan-tages. Continued bleeding from the liver may not be diagnosed early, especially in patients with other major associated injuries, and further bleeding may aggravate coagulopathy, hypothermia, and organ failure.

Local Hemostatic Agents
Commercially available fibrin glue products, which can be prepared in the operating room by mixing human fibrinogen and

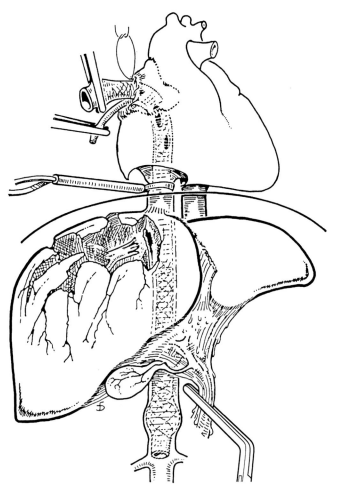

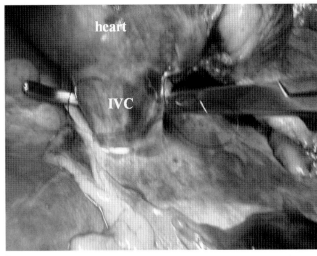

B

Fig. 66a.13. A, Atriocaval shunt for major retrohepatic venous injuries, using a No. 8 endotracheal tube with extra holes through a purse-string in the right atrial appendage. The balloon is inflated above the renal veins, and a tape tourniquet around the intrapericardial IVC is tightened. A Pringle maneuver also is performed. B, Isolation of the suprahepatic IVC inside the pericardium, in preparation for an atriocaval shunt.

A

thrombin, have a useful role in some liver injuries. Experimental work has suggested that fibrin glue controls massive bleeding and eliminates the need for packing in a model of severe liver injury (Cohn et al, 1998). In our experience, fibrin glue is usually effective in minor or moderate slow oozing from the raw subcapsular liver surface or parenchymal lacerations. In the presence of severe hemorrhage, the tissue glue is washed away and is ineffective in controlling bleeding.

Experimental work with dry fibrin sealant dressings has shown impressive results by reducing blood loss, reducing resuscitation volume, and improving survival in hypothermic animals with grade V liver injuries. Control of bleeding was much better than

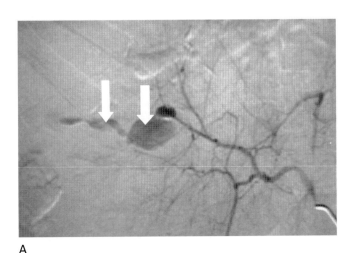

A   B

Fig. 66a.14. Postoperative angiographic evaluation shows a false aneurysm with bleeding (A). Successful embolization was performed (B).

with the use of conventional perihepatic packing (Holcomb et al, 1999). This promising approach has not been tested in clinical studies.

Recombinant Factor VIIa

Intravenous administration of recombinant activated human factor VII (rFVIIa) has been known to be effective in controlling bleeding in hemophiliacs undergoing surgery. Its role in trauma has not been defined clearly. Case reports suggest that rFVIIa may be effective in controlling bleeding in patients with trauma who are coagulopathic (Dutton et al, 2003; Martinowitz et al, 2001b; Sapsford, 2004). Experimental work has shown that early injection of high-dose rFVIIa after severe liver injury decreases bleeding and prolongs survival (Jeronkhimov et al, 2002). Other studies reported no benefit, however, when rFVIIa was administered to noncoagulopathic pigs with grade V liver injuries (Schreiber et al, 2003). In coagulopathic animals with grade V liver injuries, rFVIIa reduced blood loss and restored abnormal coagulation function when used as an adjunct to liver packing (Martinowitz et al, 2001a; Schreiber et al, 2002). In view of the high costs and the lack of strong evidence on the efficacy of rFVIIa, it should be used only in carefully selected coagulopathic patients with severe liver injuries managed with perihepatic packing and as part of an investigative protocol.

POSTOPERATIVE COMPLICATIONS

The incidence of postoperative liver-related complications in surviving patients with severe liver injuries (grades III-V) has been reported to be 50% (Demetriades et al, 2003; Knudson et al, 1994). These complications include early or late hemorrhage, liver necrosis, liver abscess, biloma, biliary fistula, false aneurysm, arteriovenous fistula, hemobilia, and intrahepatic biliary strictures (Demetriades et al, 2003). About 65% of patients with significant liver-related complications are symptomatic and have a clear indication for CT evaluation. The remaining patients have no obvious indication for CT (Demetriades et al, 2003). In a prospective study of asymptomatic patients after operation for severe liver trauma, routine CT evaluation revealed significant liver pathology in 15% (Demetriades et al, 2003).

The timing of clinical presentation of liver-related complications may vary from a few days to many months. Some complications, such as biloma, false aneurysm, or arteriovenous fistula, may remain asymptomatic only to manifest as potentially life-threatening complications at a later stage (Howdieshell et al, 1995; Inoguchi et al, 2001). There is evidence that the presence of bile impairs liver healing by inhibiting the production of granulation tissue and scarring and may predispose to hemobilia (Croce et al, 1994; Sandblom et al, 1976). Early treatment of large bilomas may prevent this complication, infection, or free rupture. In view of these facts, it is recommended that all patients with severe liver injuries undergo routine postoperative CT with intravenous contrast administration.

Recurrent Bleeding

Postoperative bleeding usually occurs during the first few hours after the operation and is usually due to inadequate hemostasis or coagulopathy. Correction of any coagulopathy and hypothermia combined with embolization controls the bleeding in most cases.

If the bleeding is severe and the patient is hemodynamically unstable, however, reoperation and better hemostasis or repacking of the liver should be performed.

Delayed hemorrhage many days or weeks after surgery is usually due to necrotic liver parenchyma or sepsis eroding into an adjacent vessel or due to rupture of a false aneurysm. CT usually reveals the underlying problem and helps with the planning of the appropriate therapeutic intervention. Most cases can be managed successfully by embolization. Subsequent drainage of a liver abscess or surgical débridement of necrotic parenchyma may be required in some cases.

False Aneurysms and Arteriovenous Fistulae

False aneurysms and arteriovenous fistulae are fairly common in severe injuries secondary to penetrating trauma, especially gunshot wounds. Routine postoperative contrast CT can identify the lesions before any complications occur. Unsuspected large false aneurysms may cause compression symptoms from the biliary tree, may rupture into the biliary system and cause hemobilia, or may rupture freely and bleed profusely. Embolization is the therapeutic procedure of choice and is successful in almost all cases (Fig. 66a.15).

Hemobilia

Hemobilia (see Ch. 68) may manifest within days or many weeks after the injury. The classic triad of gastrointestinal hemorrhage, colicky pain in the right upper quadrant, and jaundice is almost never seen in the ICU, where the usual manifestation is an unexplained decrease in hemoglobin and the presence of blood in the nasogastric tube. A history of liver trauma should prompt the surgeon to evaluate for hemobilia by means of contrast CT or angiography. Embolization is the procedure of choice and has a high success rate. Operative intervention is rarely necessary—only in patients with associated necrotic liver parenchyma.

Hepatic Parenchymal Necrosis

Liver parenchymal necrosis is the most common complication of severe liver injury in patients who undergo operation (Demetriades et al, 2003). The combination of parenchymal damage secondary to the injury, deep suturing, prolonged hypotension, and embolization creates the ideal conditions for hepatic necrosis. The typical clinical presentation is unexplained persistent fever and leukocytosis. The diagnosis is confirmed by contrast CT (Fig. 66a.16A). Small areas of necrosis may be managed with observation. Large necrotic areas associated with persistent symptoms may require surgical débridement (see Fig. 66a.16B).

Biliary Fistula

Biliary fistula (see Ch. 43b) after severe liver injury is common and generally has an excellent prognosis. The reported incidence is about 5% (Hollands & Little, 1991; Howdieshell et al, 1995), and incidence increases with the severity of the liver injury.

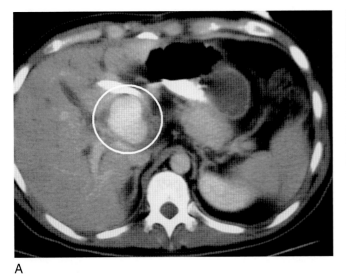

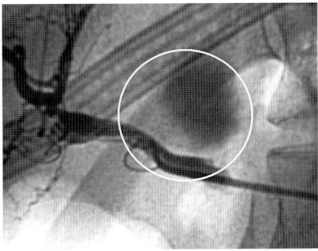

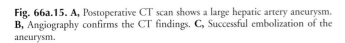

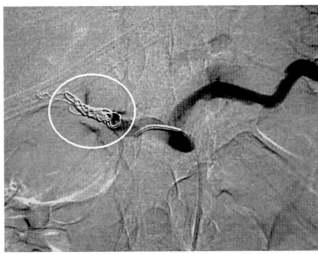

Fig. 66a.15. A, Postoperative CT scan shows a large hepatic artery aneurysm. **B,** Angiography confirms the CT findings. **C,** Successful embolization of the aneurysm.

The definition of biliary fistula as bile drainage of more than 50 mL/day (Cogbill et al, 1988) is useful.

Almost all cases with fistulae originating from the intrahepatic biliary ducts can be managed successfully nonoperatively (see Ch. 43b) (Hollands & Little, 1991; Howdieshell et al, 1995). Most fistulae close spontaneously within a few days, although in some cases it might take several weeks before healing occurs (Hollands & Little, 1991; Howdieshell et al, 1995). It is essential that the surgeon be patient and not contemplate early surgical intervention. Investigations should be considered only after 10 to 14 days of persistent bile leak with no evidence of improvement. Tubography may outline the anatomy of the fistula, but endoscopic retrograde cholangiopancreatography (ERCP) is the most reliable investigation and in addition to its diagnostic value has potential therapeutic applications. Endoscopic sphincterotomy may be considered in cases with prolonged and persistent biliary fistulae (Fig. 66a.17) (Llach et al, 2002; Okan et al, 1999). Endoscopic stenting is reserved mainly for cases with persistent extrahepatic bile duct leaks, although transhepatic stenting may be considered in selected cases with intrahepatic ductal injuries. Operation should be considered in the rare cases when the aforementioned measures fail, such as in fistula secondary to a large necrotic area in the liver.

EXTRAHEPATIC BILIARY TRACT INJURY

Trauma to the extrahepatic biliary tree (see Ch. 43b) is exceedingly rare, occurring in 2% of all abdominal trauma injuries. Of all injuries, 85% are a result of penetrating mechanisms, and of those, 85% involve the gallbladder alone.

Mechanism of Injury

Stab wounds typically result in injuries to the gallbladder, whereas gunshot wounds result in injuries randomly distributed throughout the extrahepatic biliary ductal system. Blunt injuries to the biliary system are much less common and are usually a result of either a crushing force or seatbelt compression or deceleration. The mechanism of gallbladder injury is a blow to the distended organ while the sphincter of Oddi is contracted (Sondenaa et al, 2000). The mechanisms involved in injury to the bile ducts are unclear, but several theories have been postulated, including impingement and compression of the ductal system against the vertebral column (McFadden et al, 1980), blowout injury of the common duct from a sudden increase in intraluminal pressure from rapidly displaced gallbladder bile

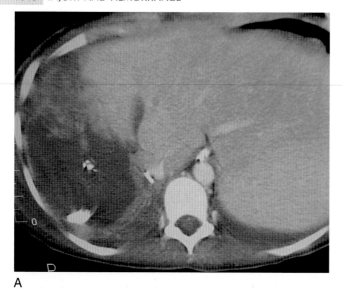

A

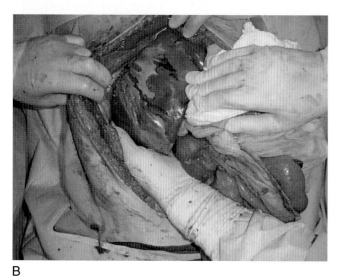

B

Fig. 66a.16. A, CT shows a large area of necrotic liver parenchyma after operation and postoperative embolization. **B,** Because of persistent fever, the patient underwent re-exploration and débridement of the necrotic parenchyma. Note the appearance of the necrotic areas of the liver.

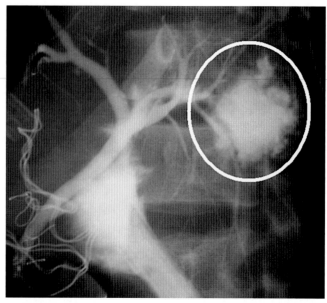

Fig. 66a.17. ERCP after a postoperative persistent biliary leak secondary to a gunshot wound to the liver shows a significant biliary leak. The patient was managed successfully with endoscopic sphincterotomy and observation.

is typically the case for isolated blunt biliary injuries. Patients present days or weeks after the initial trauma with nonspecific symptoms, such as nausea, vomiting, abdominal distention, anorexia, and jaundice. Sterile bile in the peritoneal cavity rarely results in early symptoms. Diagnostic tests, including abdominal ultrasound (see Ch. 15), CT, and technetium 99m hepatobiliary iminodiacetic acid (HIDA) (see Ch. 17) scanning may suggest the presence of an injury. ERCP may prove to be the optimal diagnostic test because of the detailed picture of the biliary tree it provides (Fig. 66a.18). Patients commonly present with abdominal distention, ascites, jaundice, and a remote history of trauma. Biliary injury is suggested when an abdominal paracentesis reveals bilious fluid and subsequently is confirmed by ERCP (see Ch. 20).

Management

The operative management of injuries to the biliary tree varies and usually depends on patient stability, associated injuries, location and extent of the biliary injury, and size of the bile duct (Gerndt et al, 1995). Most injuries to the gallbladder are best treated by cholecystectomy, although cholecystorrhaphy with absorbable sutures has been recommended for simple lacerations (Sharma, 1995).

An attempt should be made to repair the ductal injury if the patient is stable, and if the magnitude of other injuries demanding repair is permissive. Complete duct transections are best managed with a Roux-en-Y biliary-enteric anastomosis. This procedure avoids the high stricture rate, reportedly 55% in some series, associated with primary repair (Howdieshell et al, 1990). Choledochojejunostomy is preferred to choledochoduodenostomy because of the deleterious consequences of a leak from the latter anastomosis. Because the ducts are often less than 1 cm in diameter, a small catheter can be inserted through the jejunal loop to stent the choledochojejunostomy. Incomplete lacerations can be repaired primarily, provided that less than 50% of the

(Kitahama et al, 1982), and shearing force or avulsion at the junction of the fixed portion of the duct within the pancreas and the flexible portion within the hepatoduodenal ligament (Fish & Johnson, 1965). An injury most likely is the result of a combination of these factors. The other structures of the hepatoduodenal ligament, the portal vein and the hepatic artery, are rarely injured in blunt trauma, probably as a result of the increased length, tortuosity, and elasticity of these structures (Kitahama et al, 1982).

Diagnosis

Bile duct injuries usually are diagnosed during laparotomy. A high index of suspicion is necessary because 20% of injuries may go undetected at the initial operation (Michelassi & Ranson, 1985). Patients also may present in a more delayed fashion, which

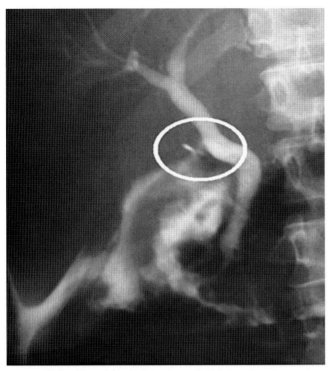

Fig. 66a.18. Cholangiography after a persistent bile leak shows an injury to the common bile duct. The patient was managed successfully with a stent.

duct circumference is injured. Insertion of a T-tube through a separate choledochotomy and repair of the duct injury over the T-tube is preferred. Lacerations involving greater than 50% of the circumference of the duct and lesser injuries where tissue viability is questioned should be treated similar to complete transections. All repairs of the biliary tract must be drained externally by an appropriately placed closed suction drain. If the duct is severed and the patient's condition is so tenuous as to preclude definitive repair, a catheter can be placed into the proximal duct, and an external fistula can be created. The area is drained, and repair is deferred to a later date.

The management of hepatic duct injuries is different from common duct injuries. The lobar and segmental ducts are much smaller, and greater attention to technical detail is necessary. Proximal unilateral hepatic duct injuries can be treated with partial hepatectomy or simple drainage alone perhaps combined with ERCP and stenting to facilitate closure of the leak (Eid et al, 1996). Ligation of the duct is a viable option, even in stable patients, provided that the remainder of the biliary ductal system is intact as shown by an intraoperative cholangiogram (Dawson & Jurkovich, 1991). Bilateral hepatic duct injuries are repaired with biliary-enteric bypass, unless the injury is very proximal; internal drainage with a hepatoportojejunostomy, similar to the Kasai procedure for biliary atresia (Dawson & Jurkovich, 1991) can be performed.

A particularly serious injury is one of the common bile duct in its intrapancreatic course. If the injury is combined with a duodenal or pancreatic injury, a pancreaticoduodenectomy may be warranted. An isolated intrapancreatic complete division of the bile duct should be treated by ligation of the distal duct and reimplantation of the proximal duct into a Roux-en-Y loop of jejunum. Further details on the treatment of biliary injuries are provided in Ch. 43.

Prognosis

The mortality associated with extrahepatic biliary injury is often related to the associated injuries that may be present. Mortality rates range from 13% (Michelassi & Ranson, 1985) to 40% (Kim et al, 1993). Jurkovich and colleagues (1995) found that mortality can be reduced to 11% just by performing biliary-enteric anastomosis for complete transections. Complications include early obstruction owing to hematoma and edema from the injury or repair or both, bile leak, and infection. Late obstruction may occur secondary to stricture, although stricture rates are markedly reduced with a biliary-enteric anastomosis. Patients who return with late stricture formation from primary repair usually have dilated proximal ducts and can be treated with a Roux-en-Y choledochojejunostomy.

REFERENCES

Aaron WS, et al, 1975: Selective ligation of the hepatic artery for trauma of the liver. Surg Gynecol Obstet 141:187-189.

Asensio JA, et al, 2003: Operative management and outcomes in 103 AAST-OIS grades IV and V complex hepatic injuries: trauma surgeons still need to operate, but embolization helps. J Trauma 54:647-653.

Baumgartner F, et al, 1996: Extra-corporal methods of vascular control for difficult IVC procedures. Am Surg 62:246-248.

Blumgart LH, et al, 1979: Hepatic resection for trauma, tumor and biliary obstruction. Br J Surg 66:762-769.

Brock WB, et al, 1995: Temporary closure of open abdominal wounds: the vacuum pack. Am Surg 61:30-35.

Brunet C, et al, 1994: Treatment of hepatic trauma with perihepatic mesh: 35 cases. J Trauma 37:200-204.

Burch JM, et al, 1988: The atriocaval shunt: facts and fiction. Ann Surg 207:555-568.

Chmielewski GW, et al, 1995: Non-operative management of gunshot wounds of the abdomen. Am Surg 61:665-668.

Cogbill TH, et al, 1988: Severe hepatic trauma: a multicenter experience with 1335 liver injuries. J Trauma 28:1433-1438.

Cohn SM, et al, 1998: Fibrin glue terminates massive bleeding after complex hepatic injury. J Trauma 45:662-672.

Croce MA, et al, 1994: Traumatic hepatic artery pseudoaneurysm with hemobilia. Am J Surg 168:235-238.

Cue JI, et al, 1990: Packing and planned re-exploration for hepatic and retroperitoneal hemorrhage: critical refinements of a useful technique. J Trauma 30:1007-1011.

Dawson DL, Jurkovich GJ, 1991: Hepatic duct disruption from blunt abdominal trauma: case report and literature review. J Trauma 31:1698-1702.

Demetriades D, 1998: Balloon tamponade for bleeding control in penetrating liver injuries. J Trauma 44:538-539.

Demetriades D, et al, 1986: Non-operative management of penetrating liver injuries: a prospective study. Br J Surg 73:736-737.

Demetriades D, et al, 1997: Selective non-operative management of gunshot wounds of the anterior abdomen. Arch Surg 132:178-183.

Demetriades D, et al, 1999: Gunshot injuries to the liver: the role of selective non-operative management. J Am Coll Surg 188:343-348.

Demetriades D, et al, 2003: Role of postoperative computed tomography in patients with severe liver injury. Br J Surg 90:1398-1400.

Dulchavsky SA, et al, 1990: Efficacy of liver wound healing by secondary intent. J Trauma 30:44-48.

Dutton RP, et al, 2003: Recombinant factor VIIa for control of hemorrhage: early experience in critical ill trauma patients. J Clin Anesth 15:184-188.

Eid A, et al, 1996: Conservative treatment of a traumatic tear of the left hepatic duct: case report. J Trauma 41:912-913.

Feliciano DV, et al, 1986: Packing for control of hepatic hemorrhage: 58 consecutive patients. J Trauma 26:738-743.

Fish JC, Johnson GL, 1965: Rupture of the duodenum following blunt trauma: a report of a case with avulsion of the papilla of Vater. Ann Surg 162:917-919.

Gates JD, 1994: Delayed hemorrhage with free rupture complicating the non-surgical management of blunt hepatic trauma: a case report and review of the literature. J Trauma 36:572-575.

Gerndt SJ, et al, 1995: Biliary tract injury following blunt abdominal trauma: case reports. J Trauma 39:612-615.

Ginzburg E, et al, 1998: The role of liver transplantation in the subacute trauma patients. Am Surg 64:363-364.

Goan YG, et al, 1998: Non-operative management for extensive hepatic and splenic injuries with significant hemoperitoneum in adults. J Trauma 45:350-364.

Hartman AR, et al, 1991: Profound hypothermic circulatory arrest for the management of a penetrating retrohepatic venous injury: case report. J Trauma 31:1310-1311.

Holcomb JB, et al, 1999: Dry fibrin sealant dressings reduce blood loss, resuscitation volume, and improve survival in hypothermic coagulopathic swine with grade V liver injuries. J Trauma 47:233-240.

Hollands MJ, Little JM, 1991: Post-traumatic bile fistulae. J Trauma 31: 117-120.

Horwitz JR, et al, 1995: Venovenous bypass as an adjunct for the management of a retrohepatic venous injury in a child. J Trauma 39:584-585.

Howdieshell TR, et al, 1990: Management of blunt hepatic duct transection by ligation. South Med J 83: 579-583.

Howdieshell TR, et al, 1995: Biloma and biliary fistula following hepatorrhaphy for liver trauma: incidence, natural history, and management. Am Surg 61:165-168.

Inoguchi H, et al, 2001: Intrahepatic pseudoaneurysm after surgical hemostasis for a delayed hemorrhage due to blunt liver injury: report of case. Surg Today 31:367-370.

Jen LR, et al, 1993: Emergent liver transplantation to salvage a hepatic avulsion injury with a disrupted suprahepatic vena cava. Arch Surg 198:1075-1077.

Jeronkhimov I, et al, 2002: Early injection of high-dose recombinant factor VIIa decreases blood loss and prolongs time from injury to death in experimental liver injury. J Trauma 53:1053-1057.

Jurkovich GJ, et al, 1995: Portal triad injuries. J Trauma 39:426-434.

Kasai T, Kobayashi K, 1993: Searching for the best operative modality for severe hepatic injuries. Surg Gynecol Obstet 177:551-555.

Keller MS, et al, 1996: Associated head injury should not prevent non-operative management of spleen or liver injury in children. J Trauma 41:471-475.

Khaneja SC, et al, 1997: Management of penetrating juxtahepatic inferior vena cava injuries under total vascular occlusion. J Am Coll Surg 184:469-474.

Kim PCW, et al, 1993: Unusual isolated common bile duct injury after blunt trauma. Can J Surg 36:533-536.

Kitahama A, et al, 1982: The extrahepatic biliary tract injury. Ann Surg 196:536-540.

Knudson MM, et al, 1994: Morbidity and mortality following major penetrating liver injuries. Arch Surg 129:256-261.

Krige JE, et al, 1992: Therapeutic perihepatic packing in complex liver trauma. Br J Surg 79:43-46.

Llach J, et al, 2002: Sphincterotomy in the treatment of biliary leakage. Hepatogastroenterology 49:1496-1498.

Marelli D, et al, 1995: Deep hypothermic circulatory arrest for blunt retrohepatic venous injury: a case report. J Trauma 38:609-611.

Markert DJ, et al, 1997: Buddi-Chiari syndrome resulting from intra-hepatic IVC compression secondary to blunt trauma. Clin Radiol 52:384-387.

Martinowitz U, et al, 2001a: Intravenous rFVIIa administered for hemorrhage in hypothermic coagulopathic swine with grade V liver injuries. J Trauma 50:721-729.

Martinowitz U, et al, 2001b: Recombinant activated factor VII for adjunctive hemorrhage control in trauma. J Trauma 51:431-438.

McFadden PM, et al, 1980: Traumatic hepatic duct injury. Am J Surg 139:268-271.

Michelassi F, Ranson JHC, 1985: Bile duct disruption by blunt trauma. J Trauma 25:454-457.

Miller PR, et al, 2002: Associated injuries in blunt solid organ trauma. J Trauma 53:238-242.

Miller PR, et al, 2004: Prospective evaluation of vacuum-assisted fascial closure after open abdomen: planned ventral hernia rate is substantially reduced. Ann Surg 239:608-614.

Moore EE, et al, 1995: Organ injury scaling: spleen and liver (1994 revision). J Trauma 38:323-324.

Okan A, et al, 1999: Endoscopic sphincterotomy in the management of biliary leakage after partial hepatectomy. Hepatogastroenterology 46:790-791.

Pachter HL, et al, 1996: Status of non-operative management of blunt hepatic injuries in 1995: a multicenter experience of 404 patients. J Trauma 40:31-38.

Pilcher DB, et al, 1977: Retrohepatic vena cava balloon shunt introduced via the saphenofemoral junction. J Trauma 17:837-841.

Renz BM, Feliciano DV, 1994: Gunshot wounds to the right thoracoabdomen: a prospective study of non-operative management. J Trauma 37:737-744.

Sandblom P, et al, 1976: The healing of liver wound. Ann Surg 183:679-684.

Sapsford W, 2004: The potential use of recombinant activated factor VII in trauma and surgery. Scand J Surg 93:17-23.

Schreiber MA, et al, 2002: The effect of recombinant factor VIIa on coagulopathic pigs with grade V liver injuries. J Trauma 53:252-257.

Schreiber MA, et al, 2003: The effect of recombinant factor VIIa on non-coagulopathic pigs with grade V liver injuries. J Am Coll Surg 196:691-697.

Schrock T, et al, 1968: Management of blunt trauma to the liver and hepatic veins. Arch Surg 96:698-704.

Shapiro MB, et al, 2001: Non-operative management of solid abdominal organ injuries from blunt trauma: impact of neurological impairment. Am Surg 67:793-796.

Sharma O, 1995: Blunt gallbladder injuries: presentation of twenty-two cases with review of the literature. J Trauma 39:576-580.

Sherman HF, et al, 1995: Non-operative management of adult hepatic injuries. Am J Surg 169:442-454.

Sondenaa K, et al, 2000: Diagnosis of blunt trauma to the gallbladder and bile ducts. Eur J Surg 166:903-907.

Stevens SL, et al, 1991: Total mesh wrapping for parenchymal liver injuries— a combined experimental and clinical study. J Trauma 31:1103-1108.

Strong RW, 1998: Anatomic resections for severe liver trauma. Surgery 123:251-257.

Thomas SV, et al, 1993: Balloon tamponade for liver injuries: case report. J Trauma 34:448-449.

Velmahos GC, et al, 1997: A selective approach to the management of gunshot wounds to the back. Am J Surg 174:342-346.

Velmahos GC, et al, 2003: High success with non-operative management of blunt hepatic trauma. Arch Surg 138:475-480.

Wahl WL, et al, 2002: The need for early angiographic embolization in blunt liver injuries. J Trauma 52:1097-1101.

Yellin AE, et al, 1971: Vascular isolation in treatment of juxtahepatic venous injuries. Arch Surg 102:566-573.

66b PANCREATIC INJURY

D. DEMETRIADES, A. SALIM, AND C. V. R. BROWN

HISTORY

Reports of pancreatic injury date back to the early 19th century. The first reported case was discovered at autopsy by Travers (1827) after an intoxicated woman was struck and killed by a stagecoach. On examination, the pancreas was found to be transversely disrupted. In 1828, Caldwell reported a patient who was stabbed in the abdomen causing the pancreas to protrude through the wound. Having become gangrenous, the protruding pancreas was excised (Caldwell, 1828). Many similar case reports followed, most being found at autopsy or managed with simple ligation and excision of a protruding portion of pancreas. Garre (1904) was the first to operate successfully on a patient with a transected pancreas. This was the first planned surgical procedure for pancreatic injury. Advances over the next century led to improvements in the diagnosis and management of pancreatic wounds. This chapter focuses on the current understanding of the epidemiology, diagnosis, management, and outcomes of pancreatic injuries.

ANATOMY

The retroperitoneal location of the pancreas adds to the complexity in the diagnosis and management of pancreatic injuries. A thorough understanding of pancreatic anatomy and its intimate relationship to surrounding organs is paramount in handling patients with pancreatic trauma appropriately (McClusky et al, 2002a, b, c; Skandalakis et al, 1993). The pancreas is divided into five anatomic regions: head, uncinate process, neck, body, and tail. The head of the pancreas lies within the C-loop of the duodenum, bordered anteriorly by the pylorus and transverse colon and posteriorly by the right kidney, right renal vessels, right gonadal vessels, and IVC. In addition, the common bile duct is intimately related to the head of the pancreas. The common bile duct lies posteriorly, partially or completely embedded within the pancreatic substance (see Ch. 1).

The uncinate process is an extension of the right posterior portion of the head of the pancreas, with great variation in size and shape. The uncinate process usually lies just anterior to the aorta and IVC, but posterior to the superior mesenteric artery and vein. The neck of the pancreas is the 1.5- to 2-cm portion of the pancreas just to the left of the pancreatic head. Similar to the head of the pancreas, the neck is bounded anteriorly by the pylorus, but posteriorly it is closely related to the confluence of the splenic vein and superior mesenteric vein to form the portal vein. Although the area between the neck of the pancreas and the portal vein is usually devoid of venous tributaries, care must be taken when dissecting in this area because several small branches draining the pancreas are occasionally present.

The body of the pancreas usually is defined as the portion of pancreas immediately anterior to the origin of the superior

mesenteric artery and the aorta. The middle colic artery originates from the superior mesenteric artery at the inferior border of the body of the pancreas. Additionally, the body is bordered posteriorly by the left kidney, left renal vessels, left adrenal gland, and splenic vein. Although the splenic vein courses posterior to the body of the pancreas, the splenic artery usually runs along the superior border of the body. Anteriorly, the pancreatic body is covered by the stomach, gastrocolic ligament, and transverse mesocolon. Although defined in an arbitrary fashion, the tail of the pancreas is the most distal portion of pancreatic tissue. The tail is usually quite mobile and reaches the hilum of the spleen, in close approximation with the distal splenic artery and the origin of the splenic vein.

The complex anatomy of the pancreatic ductal system varies widely from patient to patient (see Ch. 1). Originating in the tail of the pancreas, the main pancreatic duct (duct of Wirsung) travels through the tail and body midway between the inferior and superior margins, although more posterior than anterior. During its course through the tail and body, 20 tributaries join the main pancreatic duct. As it reaches the head of the pancreas, the main duct turns caudally and posteriorly. Eventually, the duct turns horizontally to join the surface of the common bile duct before finally entering the wall of the duodenum.

The intricate arterial blood supply and venous drainage of the pancreas play an important role in decision making when managing pancreatic injuries. The pancreas receives its blood supply from the celiac trunk and the superior mesenteric artery. The head of the pancreas is supplied by pancreaticoduodenal arcades, which it shares with the C-loop of the duodenum, preventing pancreatic head resection without duodenal resection. Resection of more than 95% of the pancreas may endanger the blood supply of the duodenum (Fig. 66b.1). The superior pancreaticoduodenal arteries (anterior and posterior branches) are derived from the celiac trunk, which anastomose with the inferior pancreaticoduodenal arcades (anterior and posterior branches) originating from the superior mesenteric artery. Branches originating from the splenic artery (dorsal pancreatic artery, inferior/transverse pancreatic artery, great pancreatic artery, and caudal pancreatic artery), which communicate with collaterals from the pancreaticoduodenal arcades, supply the remainder of the neck, body, and tail. The venous drainage generally parallels the arterial supply, with veins running superficially, and arteries and veins residing posterior to ductal structures. All venous tributaries from the pancreas subsequently drain into the portal vein, splenic vein, and superior and inferior mesenteric veins.

EPIDEMIOLOGY

Although uncommon, the true incidence of pancreatic injury has been difficult to define because it is probably underdiagnosed

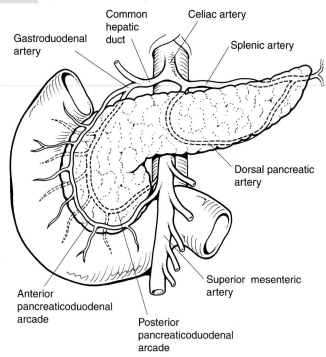

Fig. 66b.1. Blood supply of the head of the pancreas and the C-loop of the duodenum is provided by the anterior and posterior pancreaticoduodenal arcades, preventing pancreatic head resection without resulting in ischemia of the duodenum.

in patients who never undergo laparotomy. The reported incidence varies from 0.2% to 6%, with most injuries (70%) occurring as a result of penetrating trauma. Gunshot wounds (72%) are the most common (Asensio et al, 1999). Over a 10-year period at our institution, 283 of 38,459 (0.7%) patients admitted for trauma sustained a pancreatic injury. Pancreatic injury was more common after penetrating trauma (1.9%) than blunt trauma (0.2%). In addition, penetrating injury occurred in 81% of patients versus blunt trauma in only 19%. The location of pancreatic injury was distributed evenly among the head and neck (37%), body (36%), and tail (26%), with 3% sustaining an injury at multiple sites (Asensio et al, 1999). Because associated injury is the rule, it should be a marker of other intra-abdominal pathology. The most common associated injury is to a hollow viscus (38%), followed by the liver (19%) and spleen (11%). More concerning is the rate of associated major abdominal vascular injury (14%), which is the most common cause of early mortality in patients with pancreatic trauma. Penetrating injuries to the head of the pancreas are associated with a 75% incidence of major vascular injury.

DIAGNOSIS

Organ Injury Grading

Although a variety of organ injury grading systems exist, the most widely accepted is that proposed by the Organ Injury Scaling Committee of the American Association for the Surgery of Trauma in 1990 (Table 66b.1) (Moore et al, 1990). This classification scheme takes into account the type of injury (hematoma or laceration), the presence or absence of duct

Table 66b.1 American Association for the Surgery of Trauma Organ Injury Scale for the Pancreas

Grade	Type of Injury	Description of Injury
I	Hematoma	Minor contusion without duct injury
	Laceration	Superficial laceration without duct injury
II	Hematoma	Major contusion without duct injury or tissue loss
	Laceration	Major laceration without duct injury or tissue loss
III	Laceration	Distal transection or parenchymal injury with duct injury
IV	Laceration	Proximal transection or parenchymal injury
V	Laceration	Massive destruction of pancreatic head

From Moore EE, et al, 1990: Organ injury scaling: II. pancreas, duodenum, small bowel, colon, and rectum. J Trauma 30:1427-1429.

involvement, and the location of pancreatic injury (proximal or distal to superior mesenteric vein). This grading system may be applied to CT, intraoperative, or autopsy findings. Although no absolute decision should be made based solely on the organ injury grade, it can be a useful tool in evaluating and managing patients with pancreatic injury.

Clinical Presentation

Because of its retroperitoneal location and infrequent occurrence, diagnosis of pancreatic injury after blunt trauma can be elusive at best. In addition, clinical presentation is historically unreliable in patients with pancreatic injury. The situation is simplified in patients with peritonitis or hemodynamic instability because they require immediate operation, and the pancreas can be evaluated intraoperatively. Difficulty arises when a patient with suspected blunt pancreatic injury has minimal or no symptoms or cannot be evaluated because of other injuries or intoxication. This diagnostic dilemma requires further evaluation with laboratory tests, radiographic examinations, and serial physical examinations.

Laboratory Investigations

No single laboratory test is sensitive or specific enough to be a stand-alone test in evaluating patients with suspected pancreatic injury. Nevertheless, serum amylase has long been recognized as a marker of pancreatic disease and may assist in diagnosing patients with pancreatic trauma (Elman et al, 1929; Naffziger & McCorkle, 1943). A serum amylase at the time of admission may be particularly unreliable; amylase levels should be followed serially in patients with suspected pancreatic trauma (Takishima et al, 1997). The sensitivity for serum amylase reflecting pancreatic injury ranges from 48% to 89%, and specificity ranges from 64% to 81% (Bouwman et al, 1984; Moretz et al, 1975; Olsen, 1973; Takishima et al, 1997; White & Benfield, 1972). When used as a screening tool after blunt abdominal trauma, a normal serum amylase has a negative predictive value of 93% to 98% (Bouwman et al, 1984; Moretz et al, 1975; Olsen, 1973). Despite the fact that amylase may be released by organs other than the pancreas (salivary glands, bowel), the addition of pancreatic amylase isoenzymes does not seem to improve sensitivity or

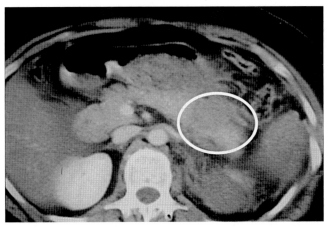

Fig. 66b.2. CT scan with intravenous contrast administration shows a distal pancreatic injury. The admission CT scan may not show the injury. A repeat CT scan several hours after injury is more likely to show the pancreatic injury. Circle shows distal pancreatic resection.

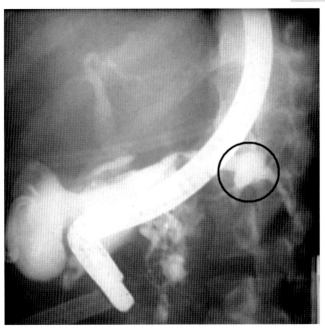

Fig. 66b.3. ERCP shows pancreatic duct leak after blunt trauma (area within circle).

specificity (Bouwman et al, 1984). An isolated elevation of serum amylase does not predict pancreatic injury reliably. Serial amylase determinations are more useful, however, and should be considered in suspected cases.

Radiographic Investigations

Although a wide variety of radiographic tests are used in the evaluation of trauma patients, plain films and ultrasound are of limited value in patients with suspected pancreatic injury. CT with intravenous contrast administration (see Ch. 18) has become the radiologic test of choice to evaluate hemodynamically stable patients with possible pancreatic trauma. Findings on CT specific to the pancreas include pancreatic transection, pancreatic enlargement, hematoma, fluid separating the pancreas and splenic vein, and increased attenuation of fat around the pancreas (Fig. 66b.2). Nonspecific CT scan findings that may represent pancreatic injury are thickening of the anterior renal fascia, fluid in the lesser sac, free fluid (intraperitoneal or extraperitoneal), and associated injuries to local structures. Although these abnormalities may be present with pancreatic injury, CT rarely shows actual pancreatic ductal disruption, making it difficult to comment on the status of the main pancreatic duct by CT alone. Often the admission CT scan is normal; repeat imaging later in the patient's hospital course may be useful. The overall sensitivity for identification of pancreatic injuries by the initial CT scan ranges from 60% to 80% (Ilahi et al, 2002). Although a normal CT scan cannot be relied on to rule out pancreatic injury, an abnormal scan with findings specific for pancreatic injury is invaluable because the positive predictive value ranges from 80% to 100%. Despite its specificity, CT underestimates grade of pancreatic injury in 30% of patients who have injury confirmed at operation (Akhrass et al, 1996).

ERCP may be a useful investigation in selected cases with suspected pancreatic duct disruption and may be used for therapeutic purposes (Canty & Weinman, 2001; Chandler & Waxman, 1996; Hayward et al, 1989; Takishima et al, 2000; Taxier et al, 1980) (Fig. 66b.3). Because ERCP is an invasive

procedure, with its own associated morbidity, a trend in the diagnosis of pancreatic injury has been to use magnetic resonance imaging cholangiopancreatography (MRCP) (see Ch. 19) (Fig. 66b.4). Although the literature regarding MRCP is evolving, the results are encouraging (Fulcher et al, 2000; Nirula et al, 1999). MRCP is diagnostic in 95% to 99% of cases of pancreatic ductal injury, and complete visualization of normal sized pancreatic ducts occurs in 97% of patients. MRCP provides an advantage over CT in that it can assess the ductal status and detail any pancreatic parenchymal injury. As opposed to ERCP, MRCP is noninvasive, but does not permit therapeutic intervention, such as stent placement.

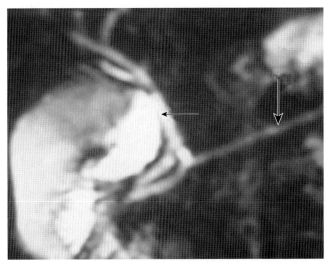

Fig. 66b.4. MRCP shows normal common bile duct (*small arrow*) and pancreatic duct (*large arrow*). MRCP has an advantage over ERCP because it is noninvasive. MRCP does not permit therapeutic interventions, however.

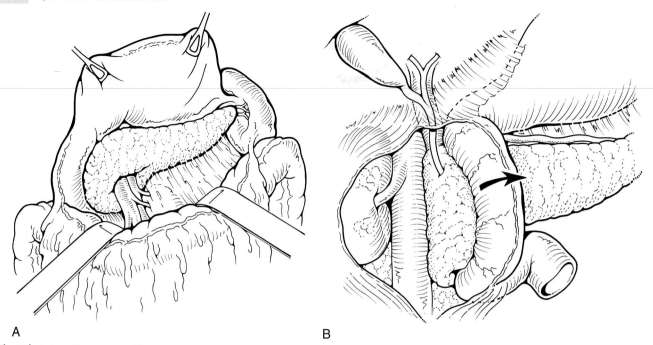

A

B

Fig. 66b.5. A and **B,** Division of the gastrocolic ligament allows exposure and evaluation of the anterior surface of the body and tail of the pancreas. Mobilization of the duodenal loop with the Kocher maneuver allows evaluation of the head of the pancreas.

Intraoperative Investigation

As mentioned previously, many patients with pancreatic injury present with peritonitis or hemodynamic instability, necessitating immediate surgical intervention. In these cases, the pancreas must be evaluated thoroughly at the time of exploration. The first priority is control of hemorrhage; subsequently, the pancreas can be explored in a systematic fashion. Most of the pancreas can be visualized by opening the gastrocolic ligament between the stomach above and the transverse colon below. This maneuver exposes the anterior, inferior, and superior surfaces of the body and tail of the pancreas (Fig. 66b.5A). Occasionally, there may be some attachments between the anterior surface of the pancreas and the posterior stomach; these should be divided. If the tail of the pancreas is not adequately visualized with these maneuvers, the spleen may be mobilized to view the length of the gland adequately.

To explore the head and uncinate process completely, the hepatic flexure of the colon must be completely mobilized. After mobilization of the colon, the duodenum and head of the pancreas are exposed with a generous Kocher maneuver (see Fig. 66b.5B); this allows bimanual palpation of the anterior and posterior surfaces of the head and uncinate process. If access to the posterior portion of the body and tail is necessary, the spleen, splenic flexure, and pancreas must be dissected free from the anterior surface of the left kidney. After sharply freeing the attachments of the spleen and colon, this plane anterior to the kidney usually can be developed with careful blunt dissection. After this thorough mobilization, the pancreas can be inspected from the uncinate process to the tail over its anterior, posterior, inferior, and superior surfaces. If any parenchymal injury is identified, the integrity of the major pancreatic duct must be established.

Most trauma patients have normal sized pancreatic ducts, which can be difficult to visualize. The use of magnifying glasses

and administration of secretin may facilitate visualization of the duct. This brings into question to what lengths one should go to identify a ductal disruption intraoperatively. *We generally do not recommend complex maneuvers to identify a ductal injury that is not readily apparent.* Nevertheless, the surgeon should be familiar with techniques that allow intraoperative study of the pancreatic duct.

Intraoperative pancreatography can be performed in a variety of ways. If the duodenum is already opened, the ampulla of Vater may be cannulated directly. Identification of the ampulla can be difficult, however, especially in the presence of edema or hematoma. Opening the duodenum can lead to complications that probably outweigh the benefit of a pancreatogram. The major duct is cannulated using a pediatric feeding tube, and several milliliters of contrast materials are instilled (Fig. 66b.6). A static or dynamic radiograph is taken to identify contrast extravasation during pancreatography. Amputation of the tail of the pancreas to gain access to the pancreatic duct is mentioned only to condemn.

Although rarely employed at our institution, some centers have advocated the use of intraoperative ERCP to assess the ductal system. This is a time-consuming approach and is rarely used, especially in severe trauma. Finally, visualization of the pancreatic duct may be attempted with intraoperative cholangiopancreatography (Fig. 66b.7). This imaging is performed by injecting contrast material into the gallbladder after clamping of the proximal common bile duct. The administration of morphine to cause contraction of the sphincter of Oddi may aid in visualizing the pancreatic duct. In about 10% of subjects, the common bile duct and pancreatic duct drain separately, and the pancreatic duct is not visualized with this technique. Although we do not favor routine intraoperative cholangiopancreatography in patients with pancreatic trauma, it can be reserved for select situations in which determination of duct integrity is paramount for further management. Most importantly, visualization of the duct

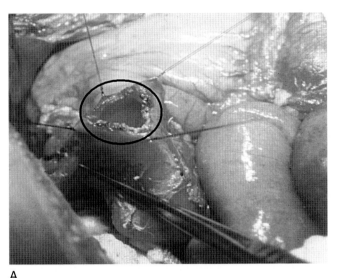 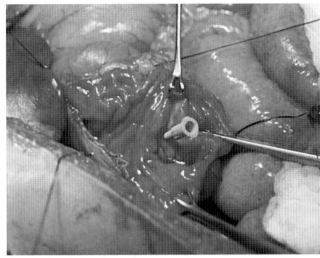

A   B

Fig. 66b.6. A and **B,** Duodenotomy and catheterization of the ampulla of Vater for intraoperative pancreatography. Identification and catheterization of the ampulla may be a difficult task, especially in the presence of hematoma or edema. This approach is rarely indicated.

should be considered only if the surgeon is prepared to act on the findings (e.g., perform a pancreaticoduodenectomy if indicated).

MANAGEMENT

Nonoperative Management

Although standard teaching dictates operative treatment for all pancreatic lesions, nonoperative management may be an option in a select population of patients. Only patients who are hemodynamically stable and have no evidence of peritonitis are

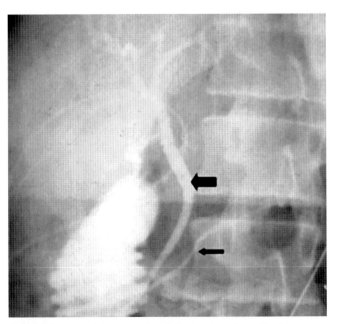

Fig. 66b.7. Normal intraoperative cholangiopancreaticography by contrast injection into the gallbladder. In about 10% of subjects, the common bile duct *(large arrow)* and pancreatic duct *(small arrow)* drain separately, and the pancreatic duct is not visualized with this technique.

potential candidates for nonoperative management. Subsequent decisions for nonoperative management are based on grade of injury. Generally, patients with lower grade injuries (I and II) identified on CT may be considered for nonoperative care, whereas patients with higher grade injuries (III, IV, and V) and duct disruption should undergo laparotomy and repair. This dictum has been challenged, particularly in pediatric patients (Kouchi et al, 1999). In 1997, Keller and associates reviewed all pancreatic injuries in the National Pediatric Trauma Registry. They reported 154 children with pancreatic injury over a 7-year period; 80% sustained grade I and II injuries, and only 20% had higher grade injuries. Although half of patients with higher grade injuries required a pancreatic procedure, only 21% of patients with grade I and II injuries required an operation, with an 80% success rate of nonoperative management. In addition, the frequency of operative management decreased over the last 4 years of the study. It may be difficult to extrapolate these results to adult patients because children rarely (0.12%) have pancreatic duct disruption, whereas adults sustain associated duct injury in 15% of cases. Despite this fact, these results suggest that nonoperative management is safe for lower grade lesions and may be acceptable for select high-grade injuries. The downside to nonoperative management is the development of a pseudocyst or peripancreatic fluid collection (Canty & Weinman, 2001). Pseudocysts are said to occur in 10% to 80% of patients undergoing nonoperative management of pancreatic injury. These complications usually require subsequent percutaneous drainage under CT guidance. ERCP also may be used as an adjunctive tool to stent a pancreatic duct in an attempt at nonoperative treatment.

Operative Management

When faced with operative management of pancreatic trauma, the treatment plan is determined by the overall condition of the patient, the grade of pancreatic injury, the associated injuries, and the experience of the surgeon. Attention to significant associated injuries, in particular, major vascular injury, should take precedence before addressing the pancreatic injury. Most pancreatic injuries (80%) are grade I and II and have no ductal disruption. These injuries are managed best with débridement of nonviable tissue, hemostasis of the pancreatic parenchyma, and wide external drainage with closed suction drains. Although some authors advocate repair of the pancreatic capsule, this may lead to bleeding, further parenchymal damage, or pseudocyst formation. Only the sutures necessary to control bleeding should be adequate. Application of tissue glue on the pancreatic wound may facilitate hemorrhage control and reduce the risk of postoperative leaks. When hemostasis is assured, closed suction drains are placed around the pancreas.

When dealing with higher grade injuries (III, IV, and V) the choice of procedure depends on the location of duct injury. For distal ductal injuries (grade III), a distal pancreatectomy is recommended. If the injury has caused transection of the pancreas, the pancreas is divided at the point of injury, and the distal portion is resected. If a distal ductal injury is identified without complete transection, the pancreas is divided just proximal to the site of injury to preserve as much pancreas as possible. Extensive resection extending to the right of the superior mesenteric vessels may lead to diabetes or exocrine insufficiency. In these cases, the distal pancreas may be preserved and anastomosed to a Roux-en-Y jejunal loop (Fig. 66b.8). The pancreas may be divided sharply between clamps or may be divided with the assistance of a stapling device (Andersen et al, 1980; Sheehan et al, 2002). The distal pancreas usually is resected en

bloc with the spleen, although a spleen-preserving distal pancreatectomy may be considered (Cogbill et al, 1991; Dawson & Scott-Conner, 1986; Pachter et al, 1989; Schein et al, 1991; Warshaw, 1988). Preservation of the spleen may be an option in hemodynamically stable patients without ongoing bleeding who are not hypothermic or acidotic. Spleen-preserving distal pancreatectomy is technically more challenging and may lead to increased blood loss and prolonged operative time. Although not the standard procedure, splenic salvage may be considered in children or other patients in whom splenic preservation is a priority. After the distal pancreas has been resected, attention should be turned to the proximal pancreatic stump. Every effort should be made to identify and ligate individually the main pancreatic duct with nonabsorbable suture, keeping in mind its posterior location within the pancreatic parenchyma. With the main duct ligated, the proximal pancreatic parenchyma should be closed with either mattress sutures or a TA stapling device. Closed suction drains should be placed around the remaining pancreas and the left upper quadrant if the spleen has been removed.

When faced with suspected proximal ductal injuries (grade IV), the surgical options are more varied. In pancreatic head injuries, in the presence of hemodynamic instability or multiple associated injuries or if the surgeon is not experienced in complex pancreatic surgery, no attempt should be made to establish the integrity of the duct or embark on extensive resections. The best therapeutic option is hemostasis and external drainage with closed suction drains. Most patients recover without any significant local complications. Others may develop a fistula or a pancreatic pseudocyst, conditions that can be managed safely nonoperatively. In the presence of a major proximal pancreatic duct injury and associated destructive injury to the duodenum (grade V), a pancreaticoduodenectomy may be necessary (Arsenio et al, 2003). The timing of the procedure should be determined on the basis of the general condition of the patient. The definitive procedure during the first operation should be reserved only for stable patients. In severely compromised patients, damage control with abdominal packing is the procedure of choice during the initial operation. The definitive pancreaticoduodenectomy should be deferred for 24 to 48 hours, after stabilization of the patient. Pancreaticoduodenectomy is rarely indicated, and most surgeons do not perform even one such procedure in their professional lives. Review of 214 pancreatic injuries over 7.5 years at our center showed only 16 (7.4%) pancreaticoduodenectomies. The technique of pancreaticoduodenectomy for trauma is similar to that in elective situations (see Ch. 56). It is strongly recommended that a feeding needle jejunostomy be placed in all cases at risk for postoperative leaks, allowing distal enteral feeding in such cases. Because of the small size of the normal common bile duct, the incidence of late stricture of the choledochojejunostomy is high (Fig. 66b.9).

OUTCOMES

Morbidity

Complications directly related to pancreatic trauma occur in about 25% of patients (Kao et al, 2003). As expected, patients with higher grade injuries (III, IV, and V) have more complications than patients with grade I and II injuries. Most complications can be managed without additional operation, either expectantly or with the assistance of percutaneous techniques.

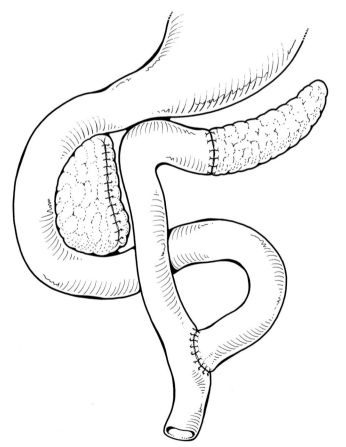

Fig. 66b.8. Anastomosis of the distal pancreatic stump to a Roux-en-Y jejunal loop. Preserving the stump reduces the risk of diabetes or exocrine insufficiency, but increases the risk of perioperative complications because of anastomotic leaks.

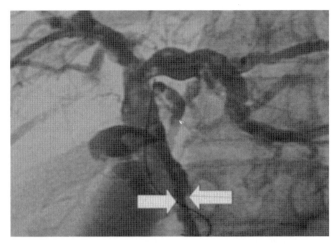

Fig. 66b.9. Percutaneous transhepatic cholangiography shows severe stricture at the choledochojejunostomy site after a pancreaticoduodenectomy for a high velocity gunshot wound of the pancreas and duodenum 5 months earlier.

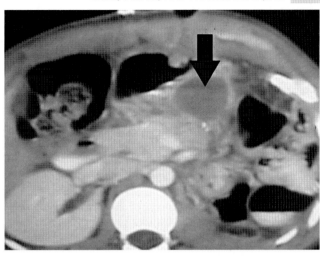

Fig. 66b.10. Small pancreatic pseudocyst after blunt trauma. The patient was managed successfully without any therapeutic intervention.

Persistent Drain Output

After all pancreatic procedures, external drainage with closed suction drains should be used routinely. In some patients, drain output may persist for several days after the operation. A persistent drain output, or pancreatic fistula, is the most common complication after pancreatic trauma and occurs in 10% to 35% of patients (Jurkovich & Bulger, 2004). The fluid should be sampled and sent for an amylase level to confirm a pancreatic source. The prognosis of these fistulae is excellent because almost all close spontaneously within a matter of a few weeks. Administration of a somatostatin analogue may decrease output from drains and may lead to faster resolution of pancreatic leak. Although prophylactic use of a somatostatin analogue has been advocated for elective pancreatic surgery, its prophylactic use in trauma is controversial. Routine parenteral nutrition is not advocated in this group of patients. Many patients tolerate oral feeding without any significant increase in the output of the fistula. Parenteral nutrition should be considered only in patients in whom oral feeding results in an increase of the drainage from the fistula. If drain output persists after a period of conservative management, or there is clinical deterioration, a CT scan should be obtained to rule out an undrained intra-abdominal fluid collection. If this is the case, it can be drained percutaneously. If after several weeks of conservative therapy the drain output continues, MRCP or ERCP is used to evaluate the ductal anatomy and determine the need for stent placement or additional surgical therapy. In our experience, these additional procedures are rarely necessary.

Peripancreatic Fluid Collections

Peripancreatic fluid collections, or pseudocysts if present for several weeks, can complicate traumatic injury of the pancreas. Although the true incidence of peripancreatic fluid collections is unknown, it is likely to become a more common occurrence as a result of the more frequent use of nonoperative treatment of pancreatic injuries. Fluid collections usually are identified incidentally during routine postoperative CT scan or after investigation of upper abdominal symptoms. The natural history of fluid collections depends on the integrity of the main pancreatic duct. If the duct is not injured, most fluid collections should resolve spontaneously without the need for intervention (Fig. 66b-10). If the duct has been injured, the fluid collection may persist and progress to the formation of a pseudocyst. Patients with small fluid collections identified incidentally and who are asymptomatic may be managed expectantly. Repeat imaging may be necessary to confirm resolution. If patients are symptomatic, or the fluid collection is sizable, percutaneous drainage may be necessary (Fig. 66b.11). CT-guided percutaneous drainage suffices in most cases, but if patients have persistent symptoms or drain output, MRCP or ERCP may be necessary to investigate the main pancreatic duct. If MRCP or ERCP identifies a ductal disruption, a stent can be placed, which facilitates the resolution of the fluid collection or persistent drainage. Rarely, patients require reoperation for resection or internal drainage of a pseudocyst.

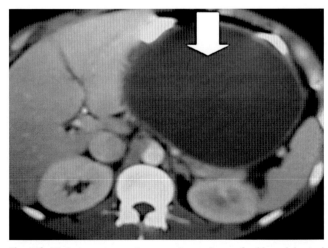

Fig. 66b.11. Large symptomatic pancreatic pseudocyst after blunt abdominal trauma. The patient was managed successfully with percutaneous drainage and ERCP pancreatic duct stenting.

Mortality

Although many patients with pancreatic injury die as a result of associated exsanguinating injuries, overall pancreatic-related mortality ranges from 0.5% to 1%. Some late deaths occur as a result of sepsis and multisystem organ failure, which may or may not be related directly to the pancreatic injury. Although pancreatic complications are not associated directly with mortality, Kao and associates (2003) found a significant correlation between the grade of pancreatic injury and mortality. Patients with grade I and II injury had 7% mortality, whereas patients with higher grade injuries had 29% mortality and an odds ratio for mortality of 2.6. This high percentage most likely represents mortality from more severe associated injuries in patients with higher grade pancreatic injury. Most importantly, patients with pancreatic injuries should have associated injuries and life-threatening hemorrhage addressed first. The pancreatic injury is rarely related to death.

SUMMARY

Pancreatic injuries are uncommon after abdominal trauma and usually are associated with penetrating injury. Most patients who experience pancreatic trauma have significant associated injuries, which are related directly to outcome. In the absence of intraoperative evaluation, the diagnosis of blunt pancreatic injury can be elusive. Because the initial clinical presentation is often unreliable, serial clinical examinations, serial amylase levels, CT scan, and a high index of suspicion are essential. Low-grade pancreatic injuries may be managed nonoperatively in hemodynamically stable patients without peritonitis. When faced with intraoperative evaluation of the pancreas, a systematic and thorough exploration of the pancreas is essential to identify all injuries. Most injuries can be managed with hemostasis and closed suction drainage. Distal ductal injuries are managed best by distal pancreatectomy, with or without splenectomy. Proximal injuries may require extended distal pancreatectomy or simply hemostasis and wide drainage. In pancreatic head injuries, if there is hemodynamic instability or multiple associated injuries, or if the surgeon is not experienced in complex pancreatic surgery, no attempts should be made to establish the integrity of the duct or embark on extensive resections. The safest therapeutic option is hemostasis and external drainage. Pancreaticoduodenectomy is rarely indicated and should be reserved for severe injuries to the head of the pancreas associated with destructive duodenal injuries. Although postoperative complications are common, most pancreas-related complications can be managed safely nonoperatively with observation or radiographic or endoscopic drainage.

REFERENCES

Akhrass R, et al, 1996: Computed tomography: an unreliable indicator of pancreatic trauma. Am Surg 62:647-651.

Andersen DK, et al, 1980: Management of penetrating pancreatic injuries: subtotal pancreatectomy using the autosuture stapler. J Trauma 20:347-349.

Asensio JA, et al, 1999: Management of pancreatic injuries. Curr Probl Surg 36: 325-420.

Asensio JA, et al, 2003: Pancreaticoduodenectomy: a rare procedure for the management of complex pancreaticoduodenal injuries. J Am Coll Surg 197:937-942.

Bouwman DL, et al, 1984: Serum amylase and its isoenzymes: a clarification of their implications in trauma. J Trauma 24:573-578.

Bradley EL, et al, 1998: Diagnosis and management of blunt pancreatic trauma: guidelines from a multiinstitutional review. Ann Surg 227:861-869.

Caldwell DC, 1828: Transylvania J Med 1:116. Quoted by Senn N, 1887: The surgery of the pancreas, as based upon experiments and clinical researches. Am Surg Assoc 4:99-169.

Canty TG, Weinman D, 2001: Management of major pancreatic duct injuries in children. J Trauma 50:1001-1007.

Chandler C, Waxman K, 1996: Demonstration of pancreatic ductal integrity by endoscopic retrograde pancreatography allows conservative surgical management. J Trauma 40:466-468.

Ciesla DJ, Burch JM, 2004: Pancreatic and duodenal injuries. In Cameron JL (ed): Current Surgical Therapy, 8th ed. St Louis, Mosby, pp 959-963.

Cogbill TH, et al, 1991: Distal pancreatectomy for trauma: a multicenter experience. J Trauma 31:1600-1606.

Dawson DL, Scott-Conner CE, 1986: Distal pancreatectomy with splenic preservation: the anatomic basis for a meticulous operation. J Trauma 26:1142-1145.

Elman R, et al, 1929: The volume of blood amylase estimation in the diagnosis of pancreatic disease. Arch Surg 19:943-967.

Fahy BN, et al, 2002: Morbidity, mortality, and technical factors of distal pancreatectomy. Am J Surg 183:237-241.

Fulcher AS, et al, 2000: Magnetic resonance cholangiopancreatography (MRCP) in the assessment of pancreatic duct trauma and its sequelae: preliminary findings. J Trauma 48:1001-1007.

Garre C, 1904: Totaler Querriss des Pankreas durch Naht geheilt. Beit Clin Chir 46:233.

Hayward SR, et al, 1989: Emergent endoscopic retrograde cholangiopancreatography: a highly specific test for acute pancreatic trauma. Arch Surg 124:745-746.

Ilahi O, et al, 2002: Efficacy of computed tomography in the diagnosis of pancreatic injury in adult blunt trauma patients: a single-institutional study. Am Surg 68:704-708.

Jurkovich GJ, Bulger EM, 2004: Duodenum and pancreas. In Moore EE, et al (eds): Trauma, 5th ed. New York, McGraw-Hill, pp 709-734.

Kao LS, et al, 2003: Predictors of morbidity after traumatic pancreatic injury. J Trauma 55:898-905.

Keller MS, et al, 1997: Conservative management of pancreatic trauma in children. J Trauma 42:1097-1100.

Kouchi K, et al, 1999: Nonoperative management of blunt pancreatic injury in childhood. J Pediatr Surg 34:1736-1739.

Lucas CE, 1977: Diagnosis and treatment of pancreatic and duodenal injury. Surg Clin North Am 57:49-65.

McClusky DA, et al, 2002a: Harbinger or hermit? Pancreatic anatomy and surgery through the ages: Part 1. World J Surg 26:1175-1185.

McClusky DA, et al, 2002b: Harbinger or hermit? Pancreatic anatomy and surgery through the ages: Part 2. World J Surg 26:1370-1381.

McClusky DA, et al, 2002c: Harbinger or hermit? Pancreatic anatomy and surgery through the ages: Part 3. World J Surg 26:26:1512-1524.

Moore EE, et al, 1990: Organ injury scaling: II. pancreas, duodenum, small bowel, colon, and rectum. J Trauma 30:1427-1429.

Moretz JA, et al, 1975: Significance of serum amylase level in evaluating pancreatic trauma. Am J Surg 130:739-741.

Naffziger HC, McCorkle HJ, 1943: The recognition and management of acute trauma to the pancreas: with particular reference to the use of the serum amylase test. Ann Surg 118:594-602.

Nirula R, et al, 1999: Magnetic resonance cholangiopancreatography in pancreatic trauma: a new diagnostic modality? J Trauma 47:585-587.

Olsen WR, 1973: The serum amylase in blunt abdominal trauma. J Trauma 12:200-204.

Pachter HL, et al, 1989: Traumatic injuries to the pancreas: the role of distal pancreatectomy with splenic preservation. J Trauma 29:1352-1355.

Schein M, et al, 1991: Splenic conservation in distal pancreatic injury: stay away from the hilum. J Trauma 31:431.

Sheehan MK, et al, 2002: Distal pancreatectomy: does the method of closure influence fistula formation? Am Surg 68:264-268.

Skandalakis LJ, et al, 1993: Surgical embryology and anatomy of the pancreas. Surg Clin North Am 73:661-697.

Takishima T, et al, 1997: Serum amylase level on admission in the diagnosis of blunt injury to the pancreas: its significance and limitations. Ann Surg 226:70-76.

Takishima T, et al, 2000: Pancreatographic classification of pancreatic ductal injuries caused by blunt injury to the pancreas. J Trauma 48:745-752.

Taxier M, et al, 1980: Endoscopic retrograde pancreatography in the evaluation of trauma to the pancreas. Surg Gynecol Obstet 150:65-68.

Travers B, 1827: Rupture of the pancreas. Lancet 12:384.

Warshaw AL, 1988: Conservation of the spleen with distal pancreatectomy. Arch Surg 123:550-553.

White P, Benfield J, 1972: Amylase in the management of pancreatic trauma. Arch Surg 105:158-163.

67

Aneurysm and Arteriovenous Fistula of the Liver and Pancreatic Vasculature

T. DIAMOND AND D. MOLE

The liver is the most frequently injured abdominal organ despite its relatively protected location. Management of liver injuries has changed significantly over the last 2 decades, with significant improvement in outcomes. There is now a broad consensus regarding some areas of management, with development of standard protocols, but in other areas considerable controversy still exists. The general management of liver and pancreatic trauma is outlined in Ch. 66; this chapter specifically addresses trauma to the liver and pancreatic vasculature, aneurysm, and arteriovenous fistula.

INJURIES TO THE HEPATIC PEDICLE AND PANCREATIC VASCULATURE

Injury to the hepatic artery or portal vein in the hepatic pedicle usually occurs in association with liver or pancreatic injuries in blunt trauma. Isolated pedicle injuries may occur in penetrating trauma. In blunt trauma, injury often involves shearing-induced tears or disruption, which tend to occur at the points of maximal fixation—the porta hepatis or the suprapancreatic area where the hepatic pedicle is relatively fixed to the retroperitoneum.

Vascular control may be obtained with a Pringle clamp or sling around the proximal pedicle. Mobilization of the duodenum and head of the pancreas by division of the peritoneum along the lateral border of the duodenum (Kocher maneuver or kocherization) allows better control of bleeding and visualization of the injury, particularly for more inferior pedicle injuries or injuries involving the retropancreatic portion of the portal vein.

When dealing with injuries of the hepatic pedicle, care must be taken to identify the disrupted vessels accurately. Rapid deep placement of large sutures in a hurried attempt to control bleeding should be avoided in view of the risk of injury to the common bile duct. In cases of vascular injury to the pedicle, common bile duct injury also should be suspected, and an operative cholangiogram should be performed to detect this.

Disruption of the right or left hepatic artery may be treated simply by ligation, provided that the ipsilateral portal vein is intact. If the common hepatic artery is bleeding, a simple laceration may be repaired. For more extensive common hepatic artery disruption, if the portal vein is intact, a lot of time should not be spent attempting repair or grafting. If right hepatic artery ligation, common hepatic artery ligation, or cholangiogram is necessary, cholecystectomy should be performed.

Injuries to the portal vein can be difficult to manage. Bleeding from these injuries can be profuse in view of the high flow and the fact that the portal vein, similar to the hepatic veins, cannot contract to reduce bleeding. The portal vein also is relatively inaccessible—in the posterior part of the hepatic pedicle and behind the pancreas. A classification of portal vein injuries describes three types: type A, in which less than 50% of the vein circumference is disrupted; type B, in which more than 50% of the circumference is disrupted, and type C, in which there is complete transection (Coimbra et al, 2004).

If bleeding can be controlled by a soft Pringle clamp or sling, after mobilization of the duodenum and pancreas, the portal vein may be better visualized by division of the peritoneum on the lateral and anterior aspects of the hepatic pedicle, including the prepyloric veins. Further exposure of the area where the vein passes behind the pancreas may be obtained by division of the gastroduodenal artery as in a Whipple procedure. After exposure, careful retraction of the bile duct to the left may allow direct repair of main portal venous tears. Retraction of the lower bile duct and pancreas to the right allows better visualization of a retropancreatic tear. To visualize the retropancreatic portion and the splenoportal junction, the pancreas should be exposed fully by dividing the gastrocolic omentum to allow dissection of the inferior border of the pancreas and the superior mesenteric vein. In most portal vein and splenic vein injuries, disruption of the pancreas also would have occurred, and repair may involve associated pancreatic resection or repair (Henne-Burns et al, 1993). Where bleeding from the retropancreatic portion of the portal vein or splenoportal junction is significant, in a patient in whom the pancreas is intact, division of the neck of the pancreas has been recommended, but this should be avoided if possible because it inflicts further trauma on an already severely injured patient and introduces further potential complications, such as pancreatic leakage and fistula. Use of hemostatic agents and packing, if it achieves hemostasis, is a more logical damage control option in this situation.

Techniques to repair the portal vein include suture repair and vein patch graft for type A and B injuries and end-to-end anastomosis for type C injuries. In type B or C injuries, in which there is major loss of tissue, insertion of a vascular interposition graft, from the superior mesenteric vein to the portal vein at the hilum, may be lifesaving. Emergency portacaval shunt also has been used (Graham et al, 1978; Henne-Burns et al, 1993; Peterson et al, 1979). The theory behind the use of these major surgical procedures was to avoid the splanchnic venous congestion and hemodynamic instability associated with portal vein ligation. Portal vein ligation has been reported with 50% survival, however, and a low incidence of subsequent portal hypertension (Coimbra et al, 2004; Pachter et al, 1979; Stone et al, 1982). Portal vein ligation can be performed only if the hepatic artery is intact or can be repaired. In an unstable patient with coagulopathy, portal vein ligation represents an appropriate damage control option, with avoidance of prolonged surgery in a patient who is unlikely to tolerate it.

HEPATIC ARTERY ANEURYSM

Historical Perspective

Hepatic artery aneurysm was first described by Wilson in 1809 (O'Connor et al, 1995). In 1871, Quincke described a hepatic artery aneurysm in a patient presenting with jaundice, hemobilia, and biliary colic. These symptoms have become known as the classic triad, although they are present in less than 40% of cases (Messina & Shanley, 1997). The first surgical repair was performed in 1903 by Kehr, who ligated the feeding vessel proximal to a common hepatic artery aneurysm (Carr et al, 1996). At the end of the 20th century, endovascular treatment was employed with increasing frequency, and the first successful endovascular stent exclusion of a hepatic artery aneurysm was reported by O'Connor and colleagues in 1995.

Incidence

Hepatic artery aneurysm traditionally was reported to constitute 20% of all splanchnic artery aneurysms, second in incidence to aneurysms affecting the splenic artery (60%) (Feliciano & Pachter, 1999). The true incidence of hepatic artery aneurysms, similar to all splanchnic artery aneurysms, is difficult to ascertain because of selection bias (if the incidence at radiologic examination is used) or observer bias (if the incidence at postmortem examination is used), as shown by two reviews of postmortem findings. When postmortem examination was done in a routine manner, the incidence of all splanchnic artery aneurysms was recorded at 0.01% (Panayiotopoulos et al, 1996), whereas if the postmortem examination was conducted specifically looking for a splanchnic artery aneurysm, the pathologist found one in 10% of cases (Bedford & Lodge, 1960). With these variations in mind, the average incidence is probably 0.2% (Panayiotopoulos et al, 1996).

Although it is unlikely that the incidence of true hepatic artery aneurysm is increasing, the incidental discovery during cross-sectional imaging performed for an unrelated reason is increasing. In addition, the routine use of abdominal computed tomography (CT) in trauma patients has led to the detection of false aneurysms that otherwise might have passed unnoticed (Messina & Shanley, 1997). Likewise, the increasing use of CT in the diagnosis and severity assessment during and after an attack of acute pancreatitis may lead to an increased frequency of diagnosis. Currently, it is estimated that 50% of all hepatic artery aneurysms are false aneurysms (Shanley et al, 1996a), many of which are discovered via circuitous routes, although a definitive study addressing the true variation in incidence of true and false aneurysms has not been performed recently.

Hepatic artery aneurysm has been reported in patients 10 to 93 years old, with presentation most common in the 60s (Abbas et al, 2003). The male-to-female ratio is 2:1, although some authors contend an equal incidence of true aneurysm, with the perceived increase in males being due to an increased association with trauma and alcoholic pancreatitis (Carmeci & McClenathan, 2000; Messina & Shanley, 1997; Miani et al, 1993; Panayiotopoulos et al, 1996; Wagner et al, 1997).

Etiology

The etiology of true hepatic artery aneurysms is unclear. Degeneration of the media is a common histopathologic feature, and atherosclerosis is present in 30% of lesions (Messina & Shanley, 1997). Whether atherosclerosis is causative or occurs as a secondary event during aneurysm formation is contentious. Historically, true aneurysms have been associated with mycotic emboli, although with modern antibiotic usage, this form is becoming restricted to intravenous drug users (Shanley et al, 1996a). Rare causes include polyarteritis nodosa, tuberculosis, inherited diseases of collagen formation, and arteritis (Abbas et al, 2003). False aneurysms account for more than 50% of all hepatic artery aneurysms. This increased incidence is likely to be a result of increased frequency and better survival after major accidental trauma and an increase in iatrogenic trauma, during liver needle biopsy, percutaneous biliary instrumentation, and laparoscopic cholecystectomy (Figs. 67.1 and 67.2) (Bulut et al, 2002; Carr et al, 1996; Duce et al, 2002; Feliciano & Pachter, 1999; Grego et al, 2003; Hossain et al, 2001; Larson et al, 2002). Aneurysms complicating laparoscopic cholecystectomy frequently affect the right hepatic artery, but may be confined to the cystic artery remnant (Tessier et al, 2003). Inflammation, in particular severe acute pancreatitis, can result in lasting damage to the arterial wall and false aneurysm formation (Mallick & Winslet, 2004; Shanley et al, 1996a; Traverso & Kozarek, 1993).

Anatomic Location

Part of the changing pattern of true versus false hepatic artery aneurysms is a shift from an extrahepatic toward an intrahepatic location. In 1970, 80% of all reported aneurysms were extrahepatic, whereas in 1996, this had decreased to 66% (Messina & Shanley, 1997). The Mayo Clinic experience (36 cases during 1980-1998) included an extrahepatic proportion of 80%, but the inclusion of cases dating from 1980 may have influenced this finding (Abbas et al, 2003). In a review of reported cases from the years 1985-1995, Shanley and colleagues (1996a) found the right hepatic artery most commonly affected (47%), followed by the common hepatic artery (22%), the proper hepatic artery (16%), the left hepatic artery (13%), and rarely the cystic artery (1%). Most aneurysms are solitary (83%) (Abbas et al, 2003; Shanley et al, 1996a). Older reviews of combined cases reported a larger proportion in the common and proper hepatic arteries (63%), reflecting the historical preponderance for an extrahepatic location (Feliciano & Pachter, 1999). Hepatic artery aneurysms may be saccular or fusiform, and reports of the maximum transverse diameter range from 1 to 14.5 cm (Abbas et al, 2003). The natural history of these lesions is one of progressive growth, and it is probable that increasing size is associated with an increasing likelihood of rupture, although evidence to support this is lacking. Dissection is rare (Abbas et al, 2003; Carr et al, 1996).

Presentation

The usual mode of presentation of a hepatic artery aneurysm is as an emergency after rupture. The risk of rupture varies. Conservative estimates place the lifetime risk for patients with an aneurysm at less than 20% (Carr et al, 2001), but reporting bias pushes the incidence of rupture toward 60% to 70%

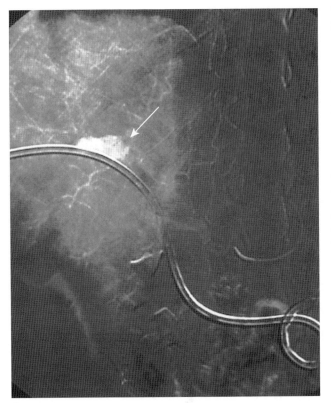

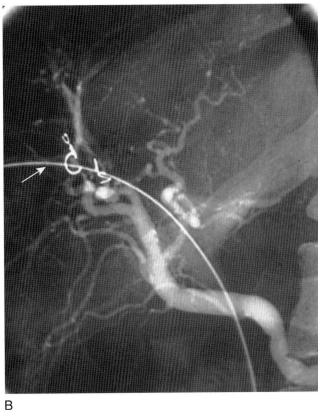

A

B

Fig. 67.1. A and **B,** Hepatic pseudoaneurysm after percutaneous biliary stent insertion (*arrow* in **A**), managed by embolization (*arrow* in **B**).

(Dolapci et al, 2003). Of all hepatic artery aneurysms presenting to one community hospital in the years 1980-1998, 63% were ruptured on presentation (Carmeci & McClenathan, 2000). Rupture occurs into the peritoneal cavity (43%), biliary tree (41%), gastrointestinal tract (11%), or portal vein (5%) (Carr et al, 2001). Of patients who reach the hospital after aneurysm rupture, the mortality ranges from 3% to 40% in larger case series

(Abbas et al, 2003; Shanley et al, 1996a; Tessier et al, 2003). Abdominal pain is present in most patients, usually located in the epigastrium, radiating to the back or right shoulder. Hypovolemic shock is present in 60% of patients with rupture (Carr et al, 1996; Feliciano & Pachter, 1999). Erosion into the biliary tree generates the classic triad of jaundice, hemobilia (see Ch. 68), and biliary colic secondary to intraductal clot or

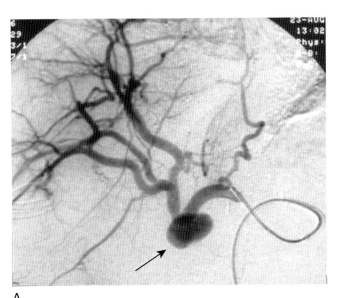

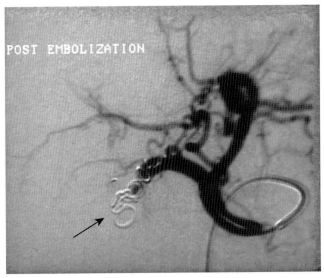

A

B

Fig. 67.2. A and **B,** Pseudoaneurysm of the hepatic artery after laparoscopic cholecystectomy (*arrow* in **A**), managed by embolization (*arrow* in **B**).

external compression of the bile duct in approximately 10% to 50% of patients (Messina & Shanley, 1997; Wagner et al, 1997). Occasionally, a steal phenomenon resulting from transient mesenteric ischemia may lead to postprandial abdominal pain (Rokke et al, 1997). On examination, hepatic artery aneurysms are normally not palpable unless huge, when an expansile mass in the upper abdomen, often with an associated thrill, may be felt or a bruit may be detected on auscultation.

Radiologic Findings

Asymptomatic aneurysms (30-50%) may be detected during radiologic investigations, such as CT, duplex ultrasound, and angiography, performed for other indications. The plain radiographic appearance of an eggshell-like calcification in the right upper quadrant should alert the clinician to the possibility of an undetected aneurysm (Feliciano & Pachter, 1999). If a diagnosis of hepatic artery aneurysm is suspected, contrast-enhanced CT, with computer reconstruction if available, or magnetic resonance angiography, is indicated to delineate the extent of the lesion and relationship to the surrounding anatomy (Howling et al, 1997). Angiography (see Ch. 21) should be used to characterize the hepatic artery blood flow in detail if operative treatment is planned (Messina & Shanley, 1997). Patients chosen for active observation do not require angiography (Athey et al, 1986). Ultrasound has been used to diagnose hepatic artery aneurysms. Because it is more operator and equipment dependent, ultrasound may have a more useful role in the surveillance of small aneurysms in patients who are at high risk of complications after intervention (Athey et al, 1986).

Management

The management of a ruptured hepatic artery aneurysm is emergency volume resuscitation (some centers advocate a degree of permissive hypotension) followed by definitive treatment involving embolization, occlusion, endovascular stenting, or open surgical repair (Carr et al, 2001; Wagner et al, 1997). Occasionally, angiographic techniques may be used to stabilize a hemodynamically compromised patient before open repair. Correction of any coagulation defects is a crucial adjunct to successful surgery.

In the elective setting, an aggressive approach is recommended (Janzen & Simpson, 2000; Kanazawa et al, 1997; Messina & Shanley, 1997). With the exception of the frailest patients, the risk of death after hepatic artery aneurysm rupture outweighs the operative mortality, and most clinicians would advocate active treatment of all but the smallest lesions. The choice of open surgical repair over endovascular treatment (see Figs. 67.1 and 67.2) depends on many factors, including the size and anatomy of the aneurysm, the shape of the sac and its accessibility to endovascular device placement or embolization, the need for restoration of arterial continuity, the general health of the patient, and the previous failure of endovascular repair. One failed angiographic treatment does not preclude further attempts. In their 1985-1995 review, Shanley and colleagues (1996a) recorded angiographic embolization as the most common treatment (37%), followed by open ligation (36%), aneurysmectomy (27%), repair with revascularization (15%), and aneurysmorrhaphy (4%). Only 2% of repairs required liver resection.

Open Repair

Selection of the most appropriate option for repair of a hepatic artery aneurysm depends on the detailed anatomy of the aneurysm and its relationship to neighboring vascular structures, ideally determined preoperatively at angiography. Proximal aneurysms (i.e., aneurysms of the common hepatic artery) may be ligated, with or without removal of the aneurysm sac, without reconstruction (Messina & Shanley, 1997). Collateral circulation through the gastroduodenal and right gastric artery usually is sufficient to prevent ischemic damage to the liver, in the absence of underlying parenchymal disease. If the patient has cirrhosis or is in a state of hemorrhagic shock, the liver substance becomes more sensitive to ischemia, and reconstruction is recommended (Carr et al, 1996; Messina & Shanley, 1997; Shanley et al, 1996a). Ligation of aneurysms of the proper hepatic artery interferes with this collateral circulation and is more likely to induce a degree of ischemic necrosis of the liver. For this reason, arterial reconstruction is recommended for all aneurysms of the proper hepatic artery. Autogenous vein grafts, synthetic grafts, aneurysmorrhaphy with vein patch closure, and direct reimplantation into the aorta all have been used to restore arterial flow. Intrahepatic aneurysms may require liver resection if ligation cannot be performed for technical reasons, such as vessel accessibility. In all situations of repair of hepatic artery aneurysm, control of the feeding and draining vessels may be gained from within the aneurysm itself if surrounding inflammation prevents adequate exposure (Messina & Shanley, 1997).

Outcome

Complications after surgical repair generally relate to ischemic necrosis of the liver distal to the aneurysm, which also may become infected, with abscess formation and sepsis (Abbas et al, 2003; Miani et al, 1993; Rokke et al, 1996, 1997). Endovascular techniques may be complicated by endoleakage around stents, progressive aneurysm enlargement, and failure of complete occlusion of the aneurysm (Sakai et al, 2004; Schick et al, 2004; Stambo et al, 2004; Van den Steen et al, 2003). The outcome of hepatic artery aneurysm repair in the published literature has a clear reporting bias toward a favorable outcome, going against the high mortality associated with rupture. For this reason, an overall survival rate for treated aneurysms cannot be given. There are no reported cases in the literature of surgically repaired hepatic artery aneurysms that have progressed to rupture.

PANCREATICODUODENAL AND GASTRODUODENAL ANEURYSMS

The distinction between true aneurysms of the pancreatic vasculature and pseudoaneurysms, such as pseudoaneurysms related to pancreatitis, is important because they show striking differences in several aspects of diagnosis and management.

True Aneurysms

Ferguson, in 1895, is credited with the first description of a pancreaticoduodenal artery aneurysm (Moore et al, 2004). True aneurysms of the pancreaticoduodenal or gastroduodenal arteries are extremely rare, accounting for 2% and 1.5%, respectively, of all splanchnic artery aneurysms. Moore and colleagues (2004) reviewed all pancreaticoduodenal and gastroduodenal artery aneurysms reported during 1946-2001. The mean age at presentation was 58 years with an approximately equal male and female distribution. Previous series documented a male preponderance, but it is likely that a lack of distinction between true aneurysms and pseudoaneurysms confounded earlier reports (Messina & Shanley, 1997; Moore et al, 2004; Paty et al, 1996; Shanley et al, 1996b).

The pathology of peripancreatic aneurysms is similar to that of hepatic artery aneurysms, with medial degeneration and atherosclerosis evident on histologic examination. Similar to hepatic artery aneurysms, the cause is unclear and probably multifactorial. There is a strong link between celiac occlusion (found in 33% of cases) and peripancreatic aneurysm development, reportedly as a result of hyperdynamic flow through these arteries when they are functioning as collateral vessels (Moore et al, 2004; Paty et al, 1996). In addition, the prevalence of a second aneurysm at remote locations, such as the cerebral vasculature, found in 18% of gastroduodenal artery aneurysms and 24% of pancreaticoduodenal artery aneurysms, suggests a systemic factor contributing to aneurysm formation (Moore et al, 2004).

Presentation follows rupture of the aneurysm in 38% to 62% of patients with pancreaticoduodenal aneurysms and 35% to 56% of patients with gastroduodenal artery aneurysms (Messina & Shanley, 1997; Moore et al, 2004). Abdominal pain is usually present, which may radiate through to the back if the aneurysm has ruptured into the retroperitoneum, as occurs in 50% of pancreaticoduodenal aneurysms (de Perrot et al, 1999b; Wagner et al, 1997). Rupture into the bowel occurs in 18% of pancreaticoduodenal aneurysm ruptures, leading to hematemesis, melena, and other signs of gastrointestinal hemorrhage. Gastroduodenal aneurysms are more likely to erode into the duodenum, with 50% of all reports documenting rupture into the bowel. Rupture also may occur into adjacent vessels and organs, including systemic and portal venous systems, the bile duct, and the pancreatic duct (Panayiotopoulos et al, 1996). Nonruptured aneurysms may present with abdominal pain; gastrointestinal bleeding; a pulsatile mass; and occasionally vomiting, jaundice, and nonspecific bowel disturbance (Shanley et al, 1996b). Of peripancreatic aneurysms, 7% are diagnosed as incidental findings (Moore et al, 2004).

Ruptured peripancreatic artery aneurysms are managed in a similar fashion to ruptured hepatic artery aneurysms, with volume resuscitation and delineation of the anatomy by CT and angiography, including endovascular treatment or angiographic stabilization, if immediate lifesaving laparotomy is not required. Aneurysms that have not ruptured should be treated aggressively in all but the most high-risk patients because the risk of rupture is high and does not seem to be related to size (Carr et al, 2001; Messina & Shanley, 1997; Shanley et al, 1996b; Wagner et al, 1997).

Endovascular treatment is increasingly used in the management of peripancreatic aneurysms, not least because of the poor accessibility and difficult dissection of the retroperitoneum after rupture. In addition, pancreaticoduodenal artery aneurysms often are buried deep within the pancreatic parenchyma and prove challenging to access surgically, and pancreatic resection occasionally is required (de Perrot et al, 1999b). Intraoperative duplex scanning may assist in the diagnosis and delineation of the aneurysm at open operation (Moore et al, 2004). Gastroduodenal artery aneurysms are slightly more accessible after duodenal mobilization, although adherence to the bowel and surrounding inflammation can create difficulties. Revascularization is not required in the absence of celiac axis occlusion (Paty et al, 1996), and some authors advocate that revascularization is not required at all after embolization or ligation of a pancreaticoduodenal or gastroduodenal artery aneurysm (Small et al, 1988). There are reports, however, of severe mesenteric ischemia and death after aneurysm occlusion in the absence of a patent celiac axis. It is probably safer to perform a mesenteric bypass or restore patency to the celiac axis before occlusion of the aneurysm; this may be achieved by open surgery or catheter-based techniques (de Perrot et al, 1999b; Moore et al, 2004; Paty et al, 1996).

Pseudoaneurysms

Most aneurysms affecting the pancreatic and peripancreatic vasculature develop as a complication of pancreatitis (see Ch. 46). Pseudoaneurysms complicate 3% to 10% of cases of acute pancreatitis and 10% to 17% of cases of chronic pancreatitis (de Perrot et al, 1999a; Mallick & Winslet, 2004). In acute pancreatitis, the incidence of pseudoaneurysm increases with disease severity (Flati et al, 2003). Several mechanisms exist by which pancreatic inflammation may lead to pseudoaneurysm formation. Proteolysis, elastolysis, and lipolysis within the pancreatic necrosis and in the retroperitoneum and peripancreatic tissues may damage blood vessels, placing them at a high risk of rupture or pseudoaneurysm formation (Stipa et al, 1994). An expanding pseudocyst may erode into an adjacent vessel, resulting in a pseudoaneurysmal pseudocyst (Flati et al, 2003; Messina & Shanley, 1997; Shanley et al, 1996b). Manipulation of friable tissue during necrosectomy, whether percutaneous, endoscopic transgastric, open, or radiologically guided, may precipitate vascular damage. Infection of pancreatic necrosis with abscess formation may cause further vascular damage, although one series reported a lower incidence of bleeding complications in infected (18%) compared with noninfected (40%) necrosis (Flati et al, 2003).

The temporal relationship of pseudoaneurysm formation with an acute attack of pancreatitis is highly variable and complicated by the fact that the presenting features of abdominal pain, tachycardia, and hypotension are features of pancreatitis itself. The time between onset of pain and presentation to the hospital has been recorded, however, and ranged from 1 to 29 days in one series (de Perrot et al, 1999a). Pseudoaneurysm associated with chronic pancreatitis often is associated with an acute attack or exacerbation. Whether this is the cause of the exacerbation or secondary to a new episode of acute inflammation has not been shown.

The splenic artery is most frequently involved (40%) (Fig. 67.3), followed by the gastroduodenal (30%), pancreaticoduodenal (20%), gastric (5%), and hepatic arteries (2%) (Mallick & Winslet, 2004). Similar to true aneurysms of these arteries, size is not predictive of rupture. Rupture may occur into the retroperitoneum, peritoneal cavity, or any adjacent hollow organ and into neighboring blood vessels (see subsequent section on arteriovenous fistula). Rupture of a pseudoaneurysm during pancreatitis may cause sudden death (7.5% of cases), and bleeding complications have been reported to account for half of all fatalities secondary to acute pancreatitis (Flati et al, 2003). Conservative management of these lesions is associated with a higher overall mortality rate (21-54%) compared with the rate after intervention (18-34%),

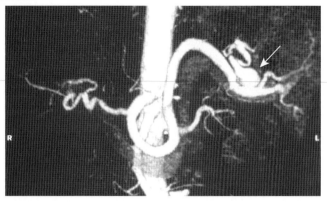

Fig. 67.3. Multislice CT shows a pseudoaneurysm of the splenic artery after necrotizing pancreatitis *(arrow)*.

and definitive treatment is recommended (Flati et al, 2003; Moore et al, 2004; Paty et al, 1996).

The management of pseudoaneurysms associated with pancreatitis is similar to that described previously for true aneurysms, with resuscitation, cross-sectional radiologic imaging, angiography, and endovascular or open surgical definitive therapy. Angiographic techniques are the preferred treatment. If these are not possible or fail in the short-term, open surgery should be performed. A caveat to this recommendation is that open surgery during an attack of acute pancreatitis is hazardous, and timing of surgery is crucial. Delaying surgery until the acute attack of pancreatitis has settled may be beneficial because fewer bleeding complications are seen after delayed rather than early surgery, but conversely, extending the time between diagnosis and intervention increases the chance of rupture of a known pseudoaneurysm. The optimal time for intervention depends on the particulars of each case.

ARTERIOVENOUS FISTULA

Congenital Hepatic Vascular Shunts

Congenital intrahepatic shunts are extremely rare anomalies characterized by abnormal communication between the hepatic arterial system, portal veins, hepatic veins, or systemic veins, owing to disordered embryologic development at around 5 weeks of gestation. Normal development involves anastomosis of the paired vitelline veins as they enter the septum transversum (primitive liver) and intersperse with rapidly proliferating cords of liver cells. Involution of the left vitelline vein with emerging dominance of the right leads to the formation of the terminal portion of the inferior vena cava, the hepatic veins, and the portal veins. The paired umbilical veins, which bring oxygenated blood to the fetus, pass in close proximity to the liver. As the right umbilical vein and a portion of the left umbilical vein become obliterated, a channel forms within the liver called the *ductus venosus* to allow oxygenated blood to bypass the hepatic sinusoids to reach the sinus venosus of the fetal heart. Accidents of development at any of these junctures can result in congenital anomalies (Gallego et al, 2004).

Rare congenital hepatic neoplasms, including infantile hemangioma (hemangioendothelioma), hepatoblastoma, angiosarcoma, and metastatic neuroblastoma, may cause hepatic vascular shunting.

Infantile hemangiomata are benign vascular tumors with a high rate of endothelial cell growth coupled with rapid involution and fibrosis, which frequently exhibit arteriovenous shunting (Horton et al, 1999). Most are symptomatic, presenting with high output congestive heart failure, hepatomegaly, anemia, thrombocytopenia, respiratory distress, and jaundice (Feliciano & Pachter, 1999). They may be associated with other hemangiomata (e.g., of the skin) and hypothyroidism, which worsens heart failure and increases mortality (Keslar et al, 1993). Magnetic resonance imaging (MRI) is the diagnostic modality of choice, showing multiple flow voids within and around lesions, hypointensity on T1-weighted images, and hyperintensity on T2-weighted images (Gallego et al, 2004). The natural history of infantile hemangioma is 6 months of growth followed by 2 to 3 years of involution (Mahboubi et al, 1987). Asymptomatic patients may be closely observed. Symptomatic cases are treated with corticosteroids, with resistant cases receiving interferon alfa. Failure of medical therapy is an indication for angiographic embolization (see Ch. 21) where possible, but the presence of multiple collaterals, which can supply these tumors from the superior mesenteric, renal, phrenic, and intercostal vessels, can jeopardize success. When embolizing tumors with a significant portal venous supply, the portal vein should be embolized before the hepatic arterial component; otherwise, fatal hepatic necrosis may occur. Untreated, the mortality is 85% to 90%. With supportive measures, it is 60%, and with specific treatment, mortality is 30% (Gallego et al, 2004).

True congenital arteriovenous malformations have no growth potential, and they do not regress spontaneously. They usually are localized to one lobe of the liver. Similar to infantile hemangioma, congenital arteriovenous malformations manifest in infancy with congestive heart failure, anemia, and hepatomegaly, but if associated with hereditary telangiectasia, they may pass undetected until late childhood, when heart failure, hepatic ischemia, and portal hypertension ensue (Boon et al, 1996). Duplex ultrasound may show a nest of tortuous vessels with high peak Doppler shifts and venous pulsatility. Contrast-enhanced CT is characterized by homogeneous enhancement in the arterial or early portal venous phase, with rapid washout of contrast material. MRI is useful in distinguishing an arteriovenous malformation from infantile hemangioma: Arteriovenous malformation is more likely if there is delayed uptake of contrast material around the hypertrophic vessels (Gallego et al, 2004). Medical treatment with digoxin and diuretics may help congestive heart failure; otherwise, patients should proceed to embolization or surgical resection. Liver transplantation is indicated in situations of very large or diffuse lesions. The mortality associated with congenital true arteriovenous malformation is reported to be 55% (Knudson & Alden, 1979).

Congenital arterioportal fistulae also present during infancy, but symptoms of portal hypotension predominate, rather than high-output congestive heart failure. These fistulae usually occur in isolation, but may be associated with hereditary hemorrhagic telangiectasia, Ehlers-Danlos syndrome, and biliary atresia (Gallego et al, 2004). Hepatofugal flow in the portal vein precipitates arterialization, followed by splenomegaly, hypersplenism, varix formation, ascites, intestinal malabsorption, and diarrhea (Altuntas et al, 1998). An enlarged hepatic artery and portal vein segment at the site of the fistula may be detectable on duplex ultrasound. Contrast enhancement of the portal vein during the arterial phase on dynamic CT with regional increased arterial flow to compensate for decreased portal perfusion of the area is diagnostic (Gallego et al, 2004). Arteriography and embolization should be performed as soon as possible after diagnosis, to minimize hepatoportal sclerosis and portal radicle fibrosis secondary to portal hypertension (Altuntas et al, 1998). Infants with biliary atresia constitute a special group, however, because liver viability usually depends on arterial inflow. Because embolization of the feeding artery in these children may precipitate fatal liver ischemia, liver transplantation is preferred (Choi et al, 2002).

Congenital portosystemic shunts may be extrahepatic or intrahepatic and are largely a result of accidents during the complex embryologic process of vitelline, umbilical, and hepatoportal venous involution and development described earlier. Extrahepatic portosystemic shunts also are known as Abernethy malformations, from the first reported case in 1793 (Howard & Davenport, 1997). The portal system may empty entirely into the inferior vena cava, with congenital absence of the portal vein, or there may be a side-to-side communication between portal vein and inferior vena cava with a variable degree of shunting. These lesions may occur alone or in combination with other congenital malformations, including biliary atresia, genitourinary tract anomalies, or as part of complex syndromes such as Goldenhar's syndrome (Gallego et al, 2004). Intrahepatic portosystemic shunts may belong to one of four morphologic categories: (1) a single tube connecting the right hepatic vein with the inferior vena cava, (2) multiple small communications confined to a single hepatic segment, (3) multiple communications throughout the liver, and (4) a persistent ductus venosus (Park et al, 1990). Doppler ultrasound is the diagnostic modality of choice (Kudo et al, 1993). The ultrasound findings may be subtle, but the presence of two structures at the liver hilum, the bile duct and an enlarged hepatic artery, rather than three, should prompt a search for an abnormal portosystemic shunt. A pulsatile triphasic or biphasic spectral pattern in the portal and splenic veins should suggest the presence of a portosystemic shunt (Kudo et al, 1993). Portal scintigraphy using rectally administered iodine 123 iodoamphetamine also may be helpful in the diagnosis. If a portosystemic shunt is present, the isotope is detectable in the lungs and liver simultaneously (Gallego et al, 2004). The natural history of portosystemic shunts depends on the shunt ratio and the age of the patient. Intrahepatic shunts in neonates are expected to close in the first 2 years, and active observation is sufficient (Gallego et al, 2004).

Portosystemic venous shunting may result in elevated serum galactose, leading to cataract formation, postprandial hyperglycemia, elevated serum bile acids, and hyperammonemia. Infants are more resistant than adults to hyperammonemia because adults have a more sensitive central nervous system response to ammonia and rapidly develop encephalopathy (Florio et al, 1998). A protein-free diet supplemented with lactulose and branched chain amino acids is a useful adjunct in patients with mild symptoms. The reduced portal inflow in this situation results in a nutritional deficit in hepatocytes, with consequent fatty degeneration and atrophy leading to liver dysfunction. This situation is largely reversible on restoration of normal portal inflow. Shunt ratios greater than 60% nearly always are associated with encephalopathy and should prompt surgical correction (Florio et al, 1998; Gallego et al, 2004; Howard & Davenport, 1997).

Acquired Hepatic Vascular Fistula

Blunt and penetrating trauma (see Ch. 66a), liver cirrhosis, and hepatic neoplasms (see Ch. 71) may result in an acquired fistula between any of the hepatic vessel types. Percutaneous liver biopsy, transhepatic cholangiography, biliary surgery, and gastrectomy also may be complicated by fistula formation, either directly or through an intermediate stage of pseudoaneurysm formation with subsequent rupture into a neighboring vessel (Fig. 67.4) (Choi et al, 2002). Transhepatic chemoembolization of large hepatocellular carcinomas may be followed by fistula formation because a hepatic infarct often occurs. In addition, chemoembolization causes arterioportal shunting for additional reasons not yet elucidated (Bronowicki et al, 1994). Superselective embolization using microcatheters may reduce the incidence of this complication. Acute cholecystitis, liver abscess, cholangitis, and pancreatitis may cause hyperemia of the hepatic artery, with decreased regional portal or hepatic venous flow, encouraging the development of an arterioportal shunt.

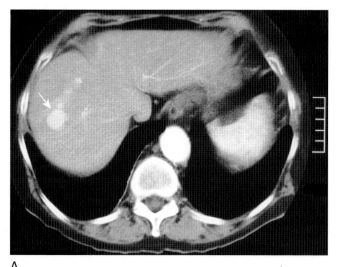
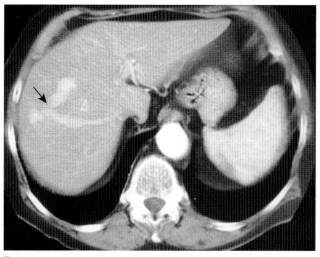

A   B

Fig. 67.4. A and **B,** Contrast-enhanced CT shows an aneurysmal fistula (*arrow* in **A**) between the right portal vein and the right hepatic vein (*arrow* in **B**).

The passage of blood through a fistula may follow one or more anatomic routes (Choi et al, 2002). The transsinusoidal route, where arterial blood passes though the sinusoids and retrogradely into the portal vein owing to high resistance in the hepatic veins, is seen in Budd-Chiari syndrome or liver cirrhosis. A transvasal route is seen in localized portal vein obstruction, such as that caused by tumor thrombus, where flow from the hepatic artery through the vasa vasorum into an unobstructed distal portion of the portal vein occurs. A transplexal route through the peribiliary vascular plexus is seen in complete portal vein obstruction. A transtumoral route may occur when blood may flow though a hypervascular tumor into its draining vein. A direct route along the injury tract may be seen after penetrating trauma. Dynamic CT shows early enhancement of peripheral portal vein branches before the central portal vein and transient hepatic attenuation difference. Transient hepatic attenuation difference is a radiologic sign characterized by transient, peripheral, wedge-shaped hepatic parenchymal enhancement, usually with a straight margin, seen during the hepatic arterial phase of a CT scan (Itai et al, 1995). MRI shows comparable findings, but offers little advantage over CT (Fig. 67.5) (Choi et al, 2002).

Acquired arterioportal fistula follows a progression through three distinct phases (Feliciano & Pachter, 1999). Initial gastrointestinal bleeding secondary to mucosal congestion occurs during the first 6 months after fistula development. Upper gastrointestinal endoscopy shows a friable edematous mucosa, which may bleed. The diagnosis is frequently missed because patients enter a variable quiescent phase as collateral circulation develops 6 months to 5 years after the fistula forms (Feliciano & Pachter, 1999). The resulting portal hypertension, involving most of the splanchnic bed, gives rise to subsequent symptoms of bleeding esophageal varices, ascites, hypersplenism, and splenomegaly. Angiographic localization and treatment of the fistula is the preferred treatment option, but if unsuccessful, owing to technical difficulties or the presence of numerous collateral vessels, open corrective surgery may be performed. The important maneuver is ligation of the arterial feeding vessels, in a similar approach to that for hepatic artery aneurysm. Resection of the fistula proper is not an absolute requisite. Liver resection sometimes may be the only feasible method of treating the lesion (Feliciano &

Pachter, 1999). Long-term follow-up and repeated angiography should be performed because small shunts can slowly open up and symptoms redevelop after the main fistula has been treated, especially in cases of long-standing portal hypertension (Gallego et al, 2004).

Pancreatic Arteriovenous Malformation and Arteriovenous Fistula

Arteriovenous malformations in the pancreas constitute less than 1% of all arteriovenous malformations found in the digestive tract (Chang et al, 2004). Presentation is as frequent in men as in women, usually in the 40s or 50s (Miura et al, 1992). Of cases, 90% are congenital in origin, and one third of these are associated with Osler-Weber-Rendu syndrome (hereditary hemorrhagic telangiectasia) (Chang et al, 2004). Dysregulation of arteriocapillary sphincter function is thought to be etiopathologic (Takiguchi et al, 1995). The vessels most commonly involved in a pancreatic arteriovenous malformation are the splenic artery (42%), gastroduodenal artery (22%), and small pancreatic arteries (22%) (Rezende et al, 2003). Acquired arteriovenous communications within the pancreas are usually the result of trauma, tumor, or inflammation, especially acute and chronic pancreatitis. Arterioportal communications through a pseudocyst have been reported and are associated with a high mortality (75%), even if treated, because they display a significant rebleed rate (30%) (Denys et al, 1998). Rarely, pancreatitis may cause a fistula between the pancreatic duct and portal vein, which is usually thrombosed (Van Steenbergen & Ponette, 1990). In a patient with chronic pancreatitis, signs of subcutaneous fat necrosis, recurrent gram-negative bacteremia, and portal hypertension may suggest a pancreaticoportal fistula (Willis & Brewer, 1989). Conservative management and surgery have been reported as successful. Pancreatic arteriovenous fistula also may occur in a pancreatic allograft after transplantation (Lowell et al, 1996).

The symptom complexes associated with arteriovenous malformations and fistulae may be divided broadly into symptoms of gastrointestinal hemorrhage (seen in 50% of cases) and symptoms of portal hypertension. Of cases, 20% are asymptomatic (Chang et al, 2004). Gastrointestinal bleeding may be caused by rupture of the arteriovenous malformation into the pancreatic duct, with bleeding into the duodenum, bleeding from associated arteriovenous malformations at other sites in the gastrointestinal tract, bleeding esophageal varices, duodenal ulcer secondary to pressure and erosion by the malformation, and hemobilia after bile duct erosion (Aida et al, 2002).

Radiologic diagnosis is traditionally by angiography, but more recent applications of Doppler ultrasound and MRI also are useful (Kurosaki et al, 1993; Tano et al, 1996). Signs at angiography include a racemose network of vessels (from the Latin word *racemus*, meaning "a bunch of grapes"), with dilated tortuous feeding arteries, early venous filling of the portal vein, and early disappearance of the pancreatic stain. A "signal void" area on T1-weighted MRI is demonstrative of rapidly flowing blood in these lesions (Kurosaki et al, 1993).

Arteriovenous malformations of the pancreas grow in size and cause portal hypertension if this is not already present at the time of diagnosis. They should be treated early and aggressively because early treatment can prevent increased portal venous pressure and, more importantly, once portal hypertension is established, treatment of the primary lesion does little to

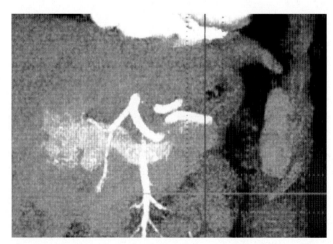

Fig. 67.5. Multislice CT with intravenous contrast administration shows an arterioportal fistula with retrograde filling of the portal vein.

improve symptoms, although it may slow its insidious progression (Sato et al, 2003). Angiographic embolization is a useful first-line therapy for the primary lesion, especially if the feeding artery is single and easily identifiable. Successful embolization frequently is followed by development of collateral vessels and recurrence in 37% of cases (Rezende et al, 2003). Pancreaticoduodenectomy or total pancreatectomy for large lesions or lesions confined to the head of the pancreas is associated with significant procedure-related morbidity and mortality, and an attempt at embolization should be considered before surgery (Iwashita et al, 2002). This combination approach potentially may reduce intraoperative bleeding (Rezende et al, 2003). Distal pancreatectomy for lesions of the body and tail is associated with less operative morbidity and mortality and a more favorable outcome (Miura et al, 1992). Radiation treatment was reported to be successful in one case of a large arteriovenous malformation with previous failed embolization and may be a useful option in patients in whom the risk of complications after major pancreatic surgery is prohibitive (Sato et al, 2003).

REFERENCES

Abbas MA, et al, 2003: Hepatic artery aneurysm: factors that predict complications. J Vasc Surg 38:41-45.

Aida K, et al, 2002: Duodenal ulcer and pancreatitis associated with pancreatic arteriovenous malformation. Eur J Gastroenterol Hepatol 14:551-554.

Altuntas B, et al, 1998: Severe portal hypertension due to congenital hepatoportal arteriovenous fistula associated with intrahepatic portal vein aneurysm. J Clin Ultrasound 26:357-360.

Athey PA, et al, 1986: Sonography in the diagnosis of hepatic artery aneurysms. AJR Am J Roentgenol 147:725-727.

Bedford PD, Lodge B, 1960: Aneurysm of the splenic artery. Gut 1:312-320.

Boon LM, et al, 1996: Hepatic vascular anomalies in infancy: a twenty-seven year experience. J Pediatr 129:346-354.

Bronowicki J, et al, 1994: Transcatheter oily chemoembolisation for hepatocellular carcinoma: a 4-year study of 127 French patients. Cancer 74:16-24.

Bulut T, et al, 2002: False aneurysm of the hepatic artery after laparoscopic cholecystectomy. Acta Chir Belg 102:459-463.

Carmeci C, McClenathan J, 2000: Visceral artery aneurysms as seen in a community hospital. Am J Surg 179:486-489.

Carr SC, et al, 1996: Current management of visceral artery aneurysms. Surgery 120:627-633.

Carr SC, et al, 2001: Visceral artery aneurysm rupture. J Vasc Surg 33:806-811.

Chang S, et al, 2004: Arteriovenous malformation of the pancreas in a patient with gastrointestinal bleeding: helical CT findings. Abdom Imaging 29:259-262.

Choi BI, et al, 2002: Hepatic arterioportal shunts: dynamic CT and MR features. Korean J Radiol 3:1-15.

Coimbra R, et al, 2004: Outcome from traumatic injury of the portal and superior mesenteric veins. Vasc Endovasc Surg 38:249-256.

Denys A, et al, 1998: Arterioportal fistula due to a ruptured pancreatic pseudocyst: diagnosis and endovascular treatment. AJR Am J Roentgenol 170:1205-1206.

de Perrot M, et al, 1999a: Management of bleeding pseudoaneurysms in patients with pancreatitis. Br J Surg 86:29-32.

de Perrot M, et al, 1999b: Management of true aneurysms of the pancreaticoduodenal arteries. Ann Surg 229:416-420.

Dolapci M, et al, 2003: Hepatic artery aneurysm. Ann Vasc Surg 17:214-216.

Duce MN, et al, 2002: Spontaneous thrombosis of a post-traumatic hepatic artery pseudoaneurysm with arterio-biliary fistula in a child: helical CT diagnosis. Pediatr Radiol 32:95.

Feliciano DV, Pachter HL, 1999: Trauma to the liver vasculature, aneurysm and arteriovenous fistula. In Blumgart LH (ed): Surgery of the Liver and Biliary Tract, 3rd ed. Edinburgh, Churchill Livingstone, pp 1301-1318.

Flati G, et al, 2003: Potentially fatal bleeding in acute pancreatitis: pathophysiology, prevention, and treatment. Pancreas 26:8-14.

Florio F, et al, 1998: Congenital intrahepatic portosystemic shunt. Cardiovasc Interv Radiol 21:421-424.

Gallego C, et al, 2004: Congenital hepatic shunts. Radiographics 24:755-772.

Graham JM, et al, 1978: Portal venous system injuries. J Trauma 18:419-422.

Grego FG, et al, 2003: Visceral artery aneurysms: a single center experience. Cardiovasc Surg 11:19-25.

Henne-Burns D, et al, 1993: Injuries of the portal veins in patients with blunt abdominal trauma. HPB Surg 6:163-168.

Horton KM, et al, 1999: CT and MR imaging of benign hepatic and biliary tumours. Radiographics 19:431-451.

Hossain A, et al, 2001: Visceral artery aneurysms: experience in a tertiary-care center. Am Surg 67:432-437.

Howard ER, Davenport M, 1997: Congenital extrahepatic portocaval shunts—the Abernethy malformation. J Pediatr Surg 32:494-497.

Howling SJ, et al, 1997: Hepatic artery aneurysms: evaluation using three-dimensional spiral CT angiography. Clin Radiol 52:227-230.

Itai Y, et al, 1995: Straight border sign of the liver: spectrum of CT appearances and causes. Radiographics 15:1089-1102.

Iwashita Y, et al, 2002: Pancreatic arteriovenous malformation treated by transcatheter embolization. Hepatogastroenterology 49:1722-1723.

Janzen RM, Simpson WT, 2000: Visceral artery aneurysm. Can J Surg 43:301-302.

Kanazawa S, et al, 1997: The diagnosis and management of splanchnic artery aneurysms: report of 8 cases. J Cardiovasc Surg (Torino) 38:479-485.

Keslar PJ, et al, 1993: Infantile haemangioendothelioma of the liver revisited. Radiographics 13:657-670.

Knudson RP, Alden ER, 1979: Symptomatic arteriovenous malformation in infants less than 6 months of age. Pediatrics 64:238-241.

Kudo M, et al, 1993: Intrahepatic portosystemic venous shunt: diagnosis by color Doppler imaging. AJR Am J Roentgenol 88:723-729.

Kurosaki M, et al, 1993: Asymptomatic arteriovenous malformation of the pancreas: demonstration by Doppler ultrasonography and magnetic resonance imaging. Dig Dis Sci 38:1342-1346.

Larson RA, et al, 2002: Stent graft repair of visceral artery aneurysms. J Vasc Surg 36:1260-1263.

Lowell JA, et al, 1996: Mesenteric arteriovenous fistula after vascularized pancreas transplantation resulting in graft dysfunction. Clin Transplant 10:278-281.

Mahboubi S, et al, 1987: Computed tomography, management, and follow-up in infantile haemangioendothelioma of the liver. J Comput Assist Tomogr 11:370-375.

Mallick IH, Winslet MC, 2004: Vascular complications of pancreatitis. JOP 5:328-337.

Messina LM, Shanley CJ, 1997: Visceral artery aneurysms. Surg Clin North Am 77:425-442.

Miani S, et al, 1993: Splanchnic artery aneurysms. J Cardiovasc Surg (Torino) 34:221-228.

Miura Y, et al, 1992: Arteriovenous malformation of the pancreas associated with hepatocellular carcinoma: a case report and review of the literature. Dig Dis Sci 37:1619-1623.

Moore E, et al, 2004: Surgical management of peripancreatic arterial aneurysms. J Vasc Surg 40:247-253.

O'Connor PJ, et al, 1995: The radiological treatment of hepatic artery aneurysms. Clin Radiol 50:792-796.

Pachter HL, et al, 1979: Traumatic injuries of the portal vein: the role of acute ligation. Ann Surg 189:383-385.

Panayiotopoulos YP, et al, 1996: Aneurysms of the visceral and renal arteries. Ann R Coll Surg Engl 78:412-419.

Park JH, et al, 1990: Intrahepatic portosystemic venous shunt. AJR Am J Roentgenol 155:527-528.

Paty PS, et al, 1996: Aneurysms of the pancreaticoduodenal artery. J Vasc Surg 23:710-713.

Peterson SR, et al, 1979: Management of portal vein injuries. J Trauma 19:616-620.

Rezende MB, et al, 2003: Pancreatic arteriovenous malformation. Dig Surg 20:65-69.

Rokke O, et al, 1996: The diagnosis and management of splanchnic artery aneurysms. Scand J Gastroenterol 31:737-743.

Rokke O, et al, 1997: Successful management of eleven splanchnic artery aneurysms. Eur J Surg 163:411-417.

Sakai H, et al, 2004: Successful covering of a hepatic artery aneurysm with a coronary stent graft. Cardiovasc Interv Radiol 27:274-277.

Sato M, et al, 2003: Radiation therapy for a massive arteriovenous malformation of the pancreas. AJR Am J Roentgenol 181:1627-1628.

Schick C, et al, 2004: Hepatic artery aneurysm: treatment options. Eur Radiol 14:157-159.

Shanley CJ, et al, 1996a: Common splanchnic artery aneurysms: splenic, hepatic, and celiac. Ann Vasc Surg 10:315-322.

Shanley CJ, et al, 1996b: Uncommon splanchnic artery aneurysms: pancreaticoduodenal, gastroduodenal, superior mesenteric, inferior mesenteric, and colic. Ann Vasc Surg 10:506-515.

Small DJ, et al, 1988: True aneurysms of the pancreaticoduodenal artery: a rare cause of retroperitoneal bleeding and delayed diagnosis. Br J Surg 75:721.

Stambo GW, et al, 2004: Coil embolization of multiple hepatic artery aneurysms in a patient with undiagnosed polyarteritis nodosa. J Vasc Surg 39:1122-1124.

Stipa F, et al, 1994: Bleeding pseudocyst of the pancreatic head: the role of omentoplasty and local hemostasis. HPB Surg 8:123-128.

Stone HH, et al, 1982: Wounds of the portal venous system. World J Surg 6:335-341.

Takiguchi N, et al, 1995: Pancreatic arteriovenous malformation involving adjacent duodenum in a patient with gastrointestinal bleeding. Am J Gastroenterol 90:1151-1154.

Tano S, et al, 1996: Pancreatic arteriovenous malformation with duodenal ulcer: demonstration by color Doppler ultrasonography. Dig Dis Sci 41:1232-1237.

Tessier DJ, et al, 2003: Iatrogenic hepatic artery pseudoaneurysms: an uncommon complication after hepatic, biliary, and pancreatic procedures. Ann Vasc Surg 17:663-669.

Traverso LW, Kozarek RA, 1993: The Whipple procedure for severe complications of chronic pancreatitis. Arch Surg 128:1047-1050.

Van den Steen G, et al, 2003: Asymptomatic aneurysm of the hepatic artery: management options. Acta Gastroenterol Belg 66:298-302.

Van Steenbergen W, Ponette E, 1990: Pancreaticoportal fistula: a rare complication of chronic pancreatitis. Gastrointest Radiol 15:299-300.

Wagner WH, et al, 1997: Ruptured visceral artery aneurysms. Ann Vasc Surg 11:342-347.

Willis SM, Brewer TG, 1989: Pancreatic duct–portal vein fistula. Gastroenterology 97:1025-1027.

Hemobilia and Bilhemia*

L. H. BLUMGART

DEFINITION

Hemorrhage into the biliary tract occurs when disease or trauma produces an abnormal communication between blood vessels and bile ducts, either within the liver or in the extrahepatic biliary tract. It has been termed *hemobilia* (Sandblom, 1948) from the Greek *haima* ("blood") and the Latin *bilis* ("bile"). *Bilhemia* denotes the rare reverse condition when bile enters the bloodstream (see later).

Hemobilia corresponds to hematuria in urinary tract disease. The two syndromes would be expected to have a close resemblance. Although hematuria is primarily a diagnostic sign of urinary tract disease, hemobilia presents a problem of differential diagnosis with regard to other, more common bleeding sources in the gastrointestinal tract.

Major, profuse hemobilia is rare, but when it occurs, it is not only an essential symptom, but also a dangerous, sometimes life-threatening complication of liver or biliary tract disease or trauma, which may constitute the main reason for treatment. Minor hemobilia is frequent, but rarely of clinical significance. Either the blood remains fluid, flowing unobtrusively into the intestine, or if it coagulates, the clot promptly dissolves through the fibrinolytic activity of the bile. If the clots escape this influence, they remain and may produce symptoms.

Hemorrhage from the pancreas discharging into the pancreatic duct is relatively rare (see later). It may be a cause of bleeding into the biliary tract.

HISTORY

Because of its obscure appearance and apparent rarity, hemobilia was late in becoming an acknowledged entity. It has been discovered repeatedly only to be forgotten again. In 1654, Francis Glisson (Fig. 68.1), in the first detailed description of the anatomy of the liver, discussed the possibility of hemorrhage through the biliary tract: "I believe that if the liver is injured by a contusion, it may lead to blood leaving the body by way of vomit or the stool for there is no doubt that the biliary tract takes unto itself (to the great good of the patient) some of the blood issuing into the liver and leads it down to the intestines. From there it is either impelled upwards through reverse peristalsis or downwards the normal way."

Glisson's observations sank into oblivion, and a century elapsed before the subject of hemorrhage into the biliary tract was brought up again. In Morgagni's epistles (1765), the founder of clinical pathology noted, in the section on the causes of dilation of the biliary tract, that abscesses in the liver and the voiding of sharp gallstones could lead to bleeding through the biliary ducts.

In 1777, Antoine Portal presented a case in which he made the diagnosis before the death of the patient and confirmed it at autopsy. In this early treatise, Portal drew attention to the difficulty of finding the source of hemorrhages in the biliary tract, "when they are slight in quantity and occur but seldom," and to the risk of mistakenly tracing them to a healthy organ, a mistake that has been made repeatedly in the history of hemobilia.

The first case in North America was published by a Boston surgeon, Jackson (1834), who gave a careful clinical and pathologic report of an "aneurysm of the hepatic artery bursting into the hepatic duct," the first direct observation of an abnormal communication between the blood vessels and biliary ducts. In 1871, the German surgeon Quincke gave a masterly account of the course of events in biliary tract hemorrhage and established its three cardinal symptoms—*gastrointestinal hemorrhage, biliary colic,* and *jaundice* (Walt, 1984).

Hemobilia formerly was regarded as a medical curiosity, but it is now being diagnosed with increasing frequency, owing to more

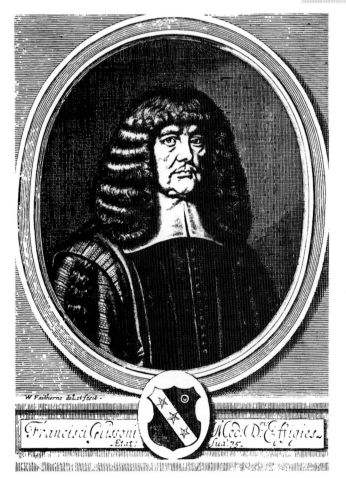

Fig. 68.1. Francis Glisson (1597-1677) gave the first account (1654) of hemorrhage into the biliary tract in his famous treatise *Anatomica Hepatis.*

*Adapted from Chapter 70, by the late J. P. Sandblom, in *Surgery of the Liver and Biliary Tract*, 3rd ed.

widespread knowledge of the syndrome and to improved diagnostic means (Sandblom, 1972). In addition, there is an absolute increase in frequency because of the increase in traffic accidents and especially in iatrogenic trauma through invasive diagnostic and therapeutic procedures, both of which may result in liver injury.

ETIOLOGY

Common causes of the pathologic vascular-biliary communication that gives rise to hemobilia are trauma (either in connection with an accident or caused by medical intervention), gallstones, tumors, inflammatory processes, and vascular disorders. Among miscellaneous causes, many conditions occasionally give rise to hemobilia, including nematodes, blood coagulation defects, choledochal cysts, pancreatitis, and portal hypertension.

The relative frequency is shown in Fig. 68.2A. The proportion noted in the diagrams relates to major hemobilia. A series of more than 500 cases collected from the world literature until 1972 (Sandblom, 1972) is compared with 490 cases from 1988-1998. There is a rapid increase of cases caused by iatrogenic injury (see Fig. 68.2B), and a change of trends is evident: Shock wave lithotripsy is not mentioned after 1992, when laparoscopic cholecystectomy began to be performed. Lithotripsy has been abandoned since the introduction of laparoscopic cholecystectomy. The great difference in numbers of nematodes is probably due to considerable numbers of overlooked cases in the later period (Khurro et al, 1990; Ton That Tung, 1972).

Major hemobilia is uncommon, and most surgeons probably see only a few cases during their career. If cases of minor hemobilia are counted, the number is considerable; gallstone disease and iatrogenic lesions constitute most cases. Biliary tract operations and the passage of gallstones through the biliary tract as a rule are accompanied by minute bleeding from the injured mucosa (Sandblom & Mirkovitch, 1979). Further details of etiologic factors and management are discussed subsequently.

NATURE OF HEMORRHAGE AND CLINICAL MANIFESTATIONS

The course of hemobilia is influenced by the character of the bleeding—whether it is profuse or scanty; prolonged or of short duration; and continuous, a solitary episode, or repeated. Most hemorrhage of consequence is arterial in origin. When only veins are injured, the bleeding is usually slight, but it may be substantial if the portal pressure is elevated. The bleeding in hemobilia may originate in the liver parenchyma or in the intrahepatic or extrahepatic biliary tract, including the gallbladder. The pancreas is a rare source of bleeding (hemosuccus pancreaticus) (see later) (Sandblom, 1970).

The clinical manifestations are due to blood loss and formation of clots in the biliary tract. From its source, the blood passes into the digestive tract and sometimes appears as hematemesis, always as melena. Violent or major hemobilia causes shock and eventually death from exsanguination, unless an emergency intervention is performed. Occult or minor hemobilia (Sandblom & Mirkovich, 1979), if continued, may result in chronic secondary anemia. The author has seen several such cases after chronic blood loss associated with papillary biliary tumors (see Ch. 52)

The blood often coagulates to form a cast of the ducts, especially when trapped above a contracted sphincter of Oddi.

The formation of clots depends on the quality and the quantity of the bleeding, and their fate depends on whether they are dissolved, expelled into the intestine, or retained in the biliary tract. When clots are retained, they act like calculi and cause biliary colic when passing, jaundice when retained, cholecystitis if they lodge in the gallbladder (Cacho et al, 1996; Connihan et al, 1996), and pancreatitis if they obstruct a common channel above the sphincter (Van Os & Petersen, 1996). Only rarely do clots remain long enough to be encrusted and form stones (Luzuy et al, 1987; Olsen, 1982). The fibrinous exudate in cholangitis may form clots of a similar nature (Fig. 68.3F). The great clinical interest of clots is that they often are mistaken for gallstones and are treated inadequately.

PATHOPHYSIOLOGY

The behavior of blood entering the bile stream and the formation and fate of clots in the biliary tract have been studied in model and animal experiments (Sandblom et al, 1977). The profuse bleeding in major hemobilia produces mixed clots of blood and bile, whereas in minor hemobilia, the blood flows immiscibly to the lowest level, where it forms a clot of pure blood, a cast of the lumen with a horizontal surface. There is a notable difference between mixed and pure blood clots. The former have a mushy consistency and dissolve rapidly through the fibrinolytic action of the bile; the latter are solid and tenacious. The mixed ones tend to adhere to the mucosa (see Figs. 68.3E and 68.12). The solid clots float freely in the lumen. When clots are subjected to flowing bile, they eventually are dissolved. Through its fibrinolytic property (King, 1972), the bile plays the same role as does the urine and saliva—to clear the respective ducts of fibrin deposits. A clinical example of the rapidity with which clots are formed and the efficiency of the lytic process is presented in Fig. 68.3B.

When protected from the bile stream, clots may escape this lytic action and remain solid. This situation can occur when the bile flow is diverted through a T-tube above the clot (see Fig. 68.3C) or when it is totally obstructed by the clot itself (Fig. 68.4C). There also may be a persistent clot if the rate of a continuous hemorrhage exceeds the speed of fibrinolysis. These clots often have to be removed actively for relief of the obstructive jaundice.

The clots that are produced by hemobilia have certain characteristics that allow their recognition and differentiation from calculi. They have been studied directly when retrieved at operation (Fig. 68.5) or when observed through the choledochoscope; indirectly, their features may be examined through the defects they cause in cholangiograms. Their form is often ovoid (see Fig. 68.4A), sometimes multilobular (see Figs. 68.3B and 68.8), but rarely round.

Generally, the clots are casts of the lumen where they are produced. When formed in the common duct, they are cylindrical, and on the casts from the lower periampullary duct, one may recognize the impressions of the sphincter; even the pancreatic duct may show (see Fig. 68.4C). When formed in the ampulla, the clots are rounded with one flat surface, which was horizontal at the time of coagulation (see Fig. 68.3D, G, and H). Clotting of blood flowing with the bile stream makes bandlike structures, and clotting in the smaller ducts produces long, branched strings, which often coil up into a ball (see Fig. 68.11B). The color, red at the start, soon becomes dark brown. The consistency varies from mushy and fragile to tenacious and firm (see Fig. 68.5).

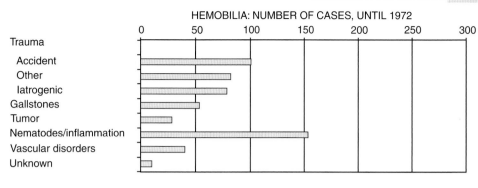

HEMOBILIA: NUMBER OF CASES, UNTIL 1972

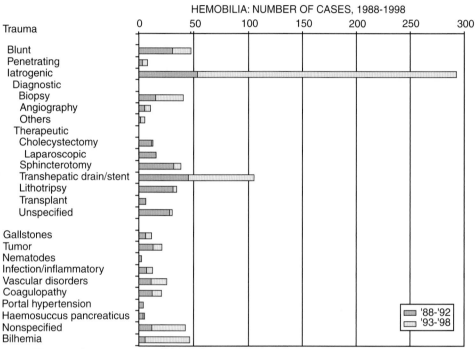

HEMOBILIA: NUMBER OF CASES, 1988-1998

Fig. 68.2. A, Distribution of 545 cases of hemobilia from the world literature until 1972 with respect to cause (Sandblom, 1972), *above,* compared with 490 cases from 1988-1998, *below.* Data are not available, but the proportion of cases associated with iatrogenic trauma undoubtedly has increased. **B,** Iatrogenic trauma, the most common cause of hemobilia, includes transhepatic cholangiography, balloon dilation of an anastomotic stricture, and percutaneous intubations. Note the blood clots in the intrahepatic ducts.

A

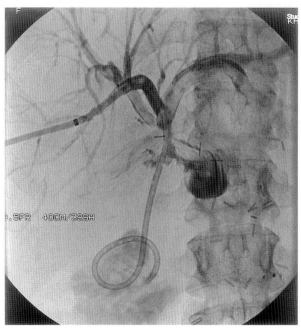

B

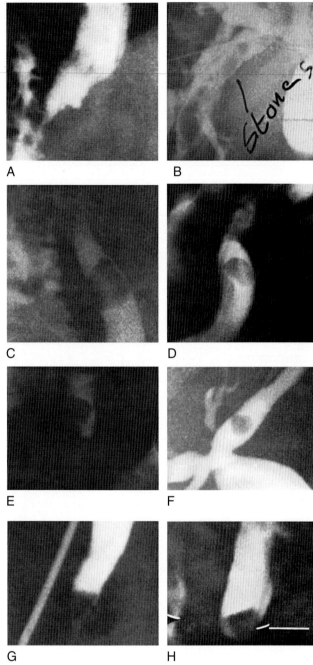

Fig. 68.3. Characteristics of cholangiographic defects caused by clots, which often are misinterpreted as calculi. **A,** This defect with indistinct borders was caused by a blood clot that appeared in connection with choledocholithotomy. The common duct was reopened to ascertain that the defect was not due to a remaining stone. **B,** A fresh multilobar coagulum in an intrahepatic duct immediately after a liver puncture, diagnosed as stones. At operation the next day, only some small fringes remained. **C,** A solid cylindrical clot formed postoperatively, during 3 weeks of total bile drainage after choledocholithotomy. **D,** The remaining resistant fragment of a large, dissolved clot looks like a cast of the ampulla. **E,** A clot resulting from minor hemobilia in an otherwise normal biliary tract during excessive anticoagulant therapy. Note the attachments to the ductal mucosa. **F,** A pure fibrin clot, adhering to the duct wall. **G,** A contrast defect, reported to be caused by a stone, dissolved during 7 days of treatment with saline solution. It looks like, and probably was, a blood clot. **H,** This defect in a postoperative cholangiogram disappeared within 1 week, despite continuous bile drainage. It looks like a cast of the ampulla and was probably due to a clot.

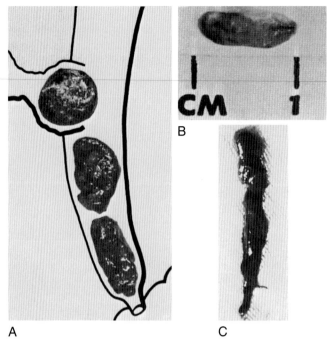

Fig. 68.4. Clots of different aspects. **A,** Drawing of the operative finding with photographs of a stone penetrating into the common duct and two occluding firm clots distally. Their resemblance to stones explains why they often are misinterpreted as such. **B,** A formation removed from a common duct with all the characteristics of clot, but alternately called *debris cluster* and *tissue particle*. **C,** An obstructing blood clot extracted from the common duct in a case of traumatic hemobilia. Note the impression of the sphincter and a cast of the confluence of the pancreatic duct.

The qualities described have induced surgeons who are unaware of hemobilia to give these clots a variety of names, including *inspissated bile, bile plugs,* and *tissue debris* (see Fig. 68.4B). Most of the features that characterize the clots on direct inspection, especially their form, can be recognized in the cholangiogram. A fresh clot, especially when it is mixed with bile, presents an indistinct surface (see Fig. 68.3A). Because of their affinity for

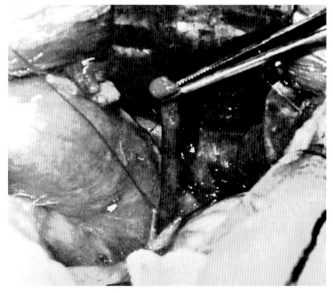

Fig. 68.5. A blood clot, which had caused total obstruction, is extracted from the opened common duct. Its firm consistency is evident.

the mucosa, they often are attached to the wall, sometimes in a stringlike fashion (see Figs. 68.3E and F and 68.12).

These clinical and experimental observations show how important it is for the surgeon to remember that a free body in the biliary tract is not always a stone. If this is the case, the fibrinolytic effect of the bile generally suffices to clear the biliary tract. If a clot continues to cause a total obstruction, which helps it to escape fibrinolysis, it eventually may have to be extracted.

One of the salient features of hemobilia is the tendency for the bleeding to recur repeatedly over months and years. Liver lesions with hemobilia may heal spontaneously (Sandblom, 1972). The cause of this feature is the fact that local liver lesions opening into the biliary tract and exposed to bile heal poorly. In the latter situation, there is a diminished production of fibrinous exudate, granulation tissue, and fibrous scar. As a result, a central cavity becomes lined by easily damaged parenchymal cells rather than by sturdy granulation tissue (Sandblom et al, 1976).

SYMPTOMS

The symptoms of hemobilia include gastrointestinal bleeding, melena in 90% of cases and hematemesis in 60%; biliary colic in 70%; and jaundice in 60%. These events constitute the pathognomonic symptom triad of hemobilia. Gastrointestinal bleeding in connection with biliary symptoms always should arouse suspicion of biliary tract hemorrhage. Hemobilia is known for its periodic appearance (see earlier) and does not often cease spontaneously (Ishaq et al, 2003). Minor hemobilia generally runs an entirely symptomless course, but may show all the signs of solid clot formation.

DIAGNOSIS

The diagnosis of major hemobilia is easy to establish, provided that one is aware of the syndrome. Many cases of hemobilia have been diagnosed too late, at operation (see Fig. 68.5) or at autopsy, or after undue delay when one or more inadequate operations have been performed (Ranniger et al, 1968). When hemorrhage into the biliary tract is suspected, the following diagnostic procedures should be undertaken in turn.

The first investigation should be upper gastrointestinal endoscopy to rule out other bleeding sources and because direct observations of blood flowing from the papilla of Vater are common in hemobilia (Carr-Locke & Westwood, 1980; Czerniak et al, 1988). Endoscopic retrograde cholangiopancreatography (ERCP) sometimes reveals clots in the bile ducts (Ball et al, 1975; Guitron-Cantu et al, 2002; Howdle et al, 1976). A lesion often first appears on ultrasonography (Sandblom & Essinger, 1981) or computed tomography (Krudy et al, 1983); these imaging modalities may show even small traumatic lesions if a hematoma is produced, but not if there is only an arteriobiliary fistula. The ultrasound appearance of intracholecystic blood is described by Laing and colleagues (1997). Clotted blood in the biliary tract produces less distinctive shadows (or defects) than stones, and the shadows often are interpreted as being due to gravel or inspissated bile (see Fig. 68.12). Magnetic resonance imaging (MRI) also can show active bleeding to the biliary tract (Yamamoto et al, 1994), and MRI cholangiopancreatography can improve visualization of the biliary tract and gallbladder (see Ch. 19) (Tseng et al, 2001).

The best way to verify a suspected diagnosis of hemobilia is by selective arteriography of the hepatic artery (see Ch. 21), which reveals the source of a major bleed in most cases (Boijsen et al, 1966; Ranniger et al, 1968) by displacement of the vessels around a liver mass or by filling a true aneurysm (Figs. 68.6 and 68.7). When caught at the right moment, contrast material may be seen traveling down the hepatic duct, proving the existence of a communication with the biliary tract (see Fig. 68.6B) (Kelley et al, 1983). In some cases, the artery also opens into the portal system (Sarr et al, 1984). The arteriographic catheter should not be withdrawn until it has been decided whether embolization of the feeding artery should be considered as treatment. Arteriography is of special value in discovering central liver lesions, which may be difficult or impossible to localize during exploratory laparotomy (see Figs. 68.7 and 68.11).

Cholangiography, postoperatively through a T-tube by means of ERCP or through diagnostic percutaneous liver puncture (Fig. 68.8), may reveal a lesion by contrast filling of a cavity or by demonstration of clots, which appear as defects in the contrast filling (Millbourn, 1951). "In some instances, clots in the biliary tract simulated stone during the investigation, but if their occurrence is borne in mind, no mistakes need to be made" (Arner et al, 1962). Percutaneous transhepatic cholangiography has a complication rate of less than 5% (Redman & Joseph, 1975).

TREATMENT

The treatment of hemobilia depends on the cause of the hemorrhage. Cholecystectomy is done for gallstones, resection for tumors, and embolization or vascular repair for aneurysms. In general, there is a choice between resection of the liver, ligation of the feeding artery (Andreassen & Lindenberg, 1959), or definitive embolization (Asmat & Beckmann, 1983). Refinement of embolization procedures may make this approach the most frequent and first choice.

Liver Resection

Thomeret and coworkers (1957) treated a case of hemobilia from central liver rupture by resecting the right lobe. Since then, numerous successful resections for hemobilia have been reported. Embolization is increasingly preferred, however.

Ligature of the Hepatic Artery

Ligature of the hepatic artery or one of its branches, first done by Kehr (1903) (see Fig. 68.10), nowadays is reserved for cases in which the abdomen has been opened for exploration or repair (see Fig. 68.10) and when embolization is impossible or has been unsuccessful. A condition for ligature of the main artery is free flow through the portal vein, which suffices to nourish the hepatic parenchyma. Ligature often provides only temporary relief (see later).

Arterial Embolization

Arterial embolization (see Ch. 29) (see Fig. 68.6) has become the preferred treatment. Abnormal communications between

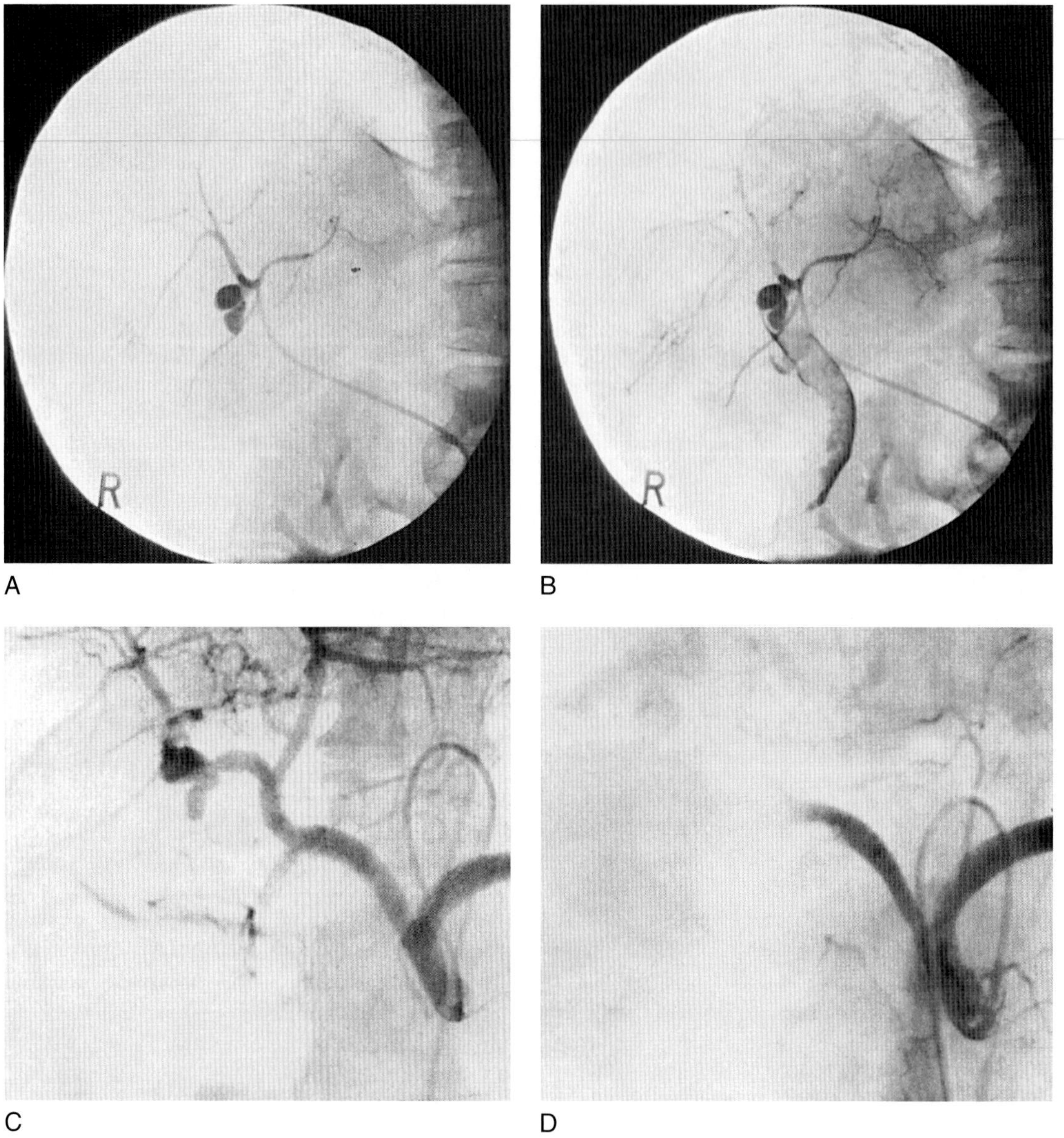

A   B

C   D

Fig. 68.6. After complicated cholecystectomy an iatrogenic pseudoaneurysm developed. It ruptured into the biliary tract and caused exsanguinating hemobilia, diagnosed through duodenal endoscopy and treated successfully with embolization. **A,** Selective arteriogram shows a pseudoaneurysm of the hepatic artery located at the liver hilum. **B,** A few seconds later, the contrast material is seen flowing down the hepatic duct displaying the arteriobiliary fistula. **C and D,** The same aneurysm before and after obliteration of the feeding artery with artificial embolus.
(From Kelley CJ, et al, 1983: Non-surgical management of post-cholecystectomy hemobilia. Br J Surg 70:502 [case of Professor L. H. Blumgart].)

the branches of the hepatic artery and the biliary tract can be selectively occluded by large particulate material of different kinds (Horak et al, 1996). Walter and colleagues (1976) reported the first successful treatment of hemobilia by this method. *Several advantages make embolization preferable to surgery in the treatment of hemobilia.* The risk of hepatic necrosis is minimal because the obstruction can be limited to a segmental branch of the hepatic artery. It is important to perform selective embolization because occlusion of a major hepatic arterial branch not only allows the possibility of rebleeding owing to revascularization, but also makes repeat embolization, which may be necessary, impossible.

Since embolization techniques have been popularized, the overall picture of the therapeutic management of hemobilia patients has changed. Formerly, resection and arterial ligature were performed with equal frequency and with comparable results regarding cure, morbidity, and mortality (Sandblom, 1972). In the 1990s, liver resection decreased to less than 10% of the treated cases, and embolization was used in most cases (Peng et al, 2001), with an overall success rate of about 95% (Curet et al, 1984). No long-term sequelae occurred in patients followed for more than 14 years (Czerniak et al, 1988; Uflacker et al, 1989).

ETIOLOGIC GROUPS

Accidental Trauma

In accidental trauma (see Chs. 66 and 67), there is a great difference in the clinical manifestation of liver lesions that tear the liver capsule and lesions that do not (i.e., subcapsular or central

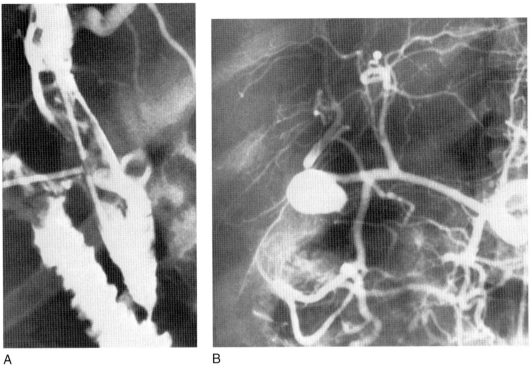

Fig. 68.7. Iatrogenic hemobilia. Operative lesion through forceful instrumental exploration of the bile ducts. **A,** Postoperative cholangiogram after occurrence of profuse hemobilia through the T-tube; the large filling defects represent blood clots. **B,** Hepatic arteriogram revealing the source of the bleeding—a false aneurysm in the right hepatic artery, caused by instrumental lithotomy.

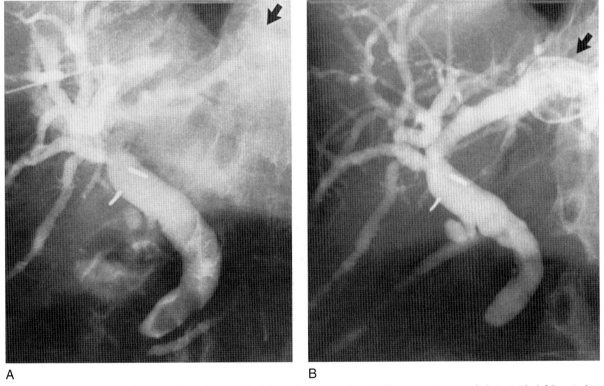

Fig. 68.8. Lesion from transhepatic cholangiography, producing a blood clot in the common duct. **A,** The *arrow* points toward a lesion in the left hepatic duct. Filling defect in the common duct caused by a gelatinous "bile plug," probably a blood clot that disappeared through the sucker. **B,** A postoperative cholangiogram shows the extravasation from the ductal lesion responsible for the hemobilia.

liver ruptures). The former may result in dangerous intra-abdominal hemorrhage and often require an emergency operation. Hemobilia is rare with this lesion because the blood more readily flows into the low pressure intraperitoneal cavity than down through the biliary tract. Traumatic hemobilia is found more often in patients with a central liver rupture causing less acute and more obscure symptoms. If a hepatic vein tears, there is a risk that bile gains access into the circulation, causing jaundice (so-called bilhemia) (see later).

Although the mechanism of penetrating trauma is evident, it is more complicated in blunt trauma. If the liver is compressed, the fragile and inelastic parenchyma tears easily. The disrupting force is greatest in the middle of the organ, which explains the high frequency of central liver rupture. This occurs far more commonly than was recognized before the availability of modern diagnostic measures (Walt, 1984). The central lesion often is combined with smaller superficial rifts caused by the direct force. When the surgeon sees these rifts at emergency exploration, he or she is apt to be satisfied that they represent the major injury and may miss a central rupture that is not grossly visible. The surgeon may create a cavity that predisposes to hemobilia if he or she superficially sutures a deep laceration; hemobilia then may appear later.

Central liver ruptures may be of different sizes, from large cavities to small arteriobiliary fistulae. Occasionally, no or only temporary bleeding occurs, but there may be delayed hemobilia (Rousseau et al, 2004). The course of events in these cavities accounts for the typical clinical history. The rupture tears bile ducts, arteries, and veins, which fill the cavity with bile and blood. If a large artery is torn, exsanguinating gastrointestinal hemorrhage may occur, necessitating emergency surgery to save the patient's life. Usually the cavity fills slowly, however, and the escape of blood and bile is delayed by coagulation in the cavity or in the ducts. Finally, after days, weeks, or months, the pressure in the cavity suddenly forces the clot down the biliary tract into the intestine, followed by a gush of blood and bile.

During these events, the patient first experiences an increasing, dull pain over the liver. Sometimes hepatomegaly can be detected, and there may be signs of obstructive jaundice. Then one day, the patient experiences intense biliary colic, followed by hematemesis and melena. Occasionally, the patient vomits long clots, which are casts of the biliary tract. Relief is usually only temporary; the course of events is repeated over months and years. *The syndrome is characterized by periodicity.* A long interval between trauma and clinically manifest hemobilia may obscure the causal relationship

Although the frequency of major traumatic hemobilia is considerably less than that of minor hemobilia, it is still common enough for every surgeon to be able to diagnose and treat it. The treatment used to be mainly operative, but since it was found that spontaneous healing often occurs, a conservative attitude can be initiated if the hemorrhage has subsided (Hendren et al, 1971). Nonoperative treatment has become the treatment of choice in hemodynamically stable patients and is successful in 50% to 80% of adult cases (Carrillo et al, 1998; Forlee et al, 2004). The rate of complicating hemobilia and bilhemia is about 1% (Yoshida et al, 1987). The healing process must be monitored carefully, and intervention may be necessary later if symptoms recur. At one time, it was thought that packing or drainage was insufficient (Madding & Kennedy, 1971), but in recent years this has been found to be effective (see Ch. 66). If operation is necessary, it should include careful exploration of cavities and precise hemostasis and suture of open bile radicles before packing,

drainage, and closure. If this approach does not suffice, a more radical procedure is necessary (Poulos, et al 1974). In some cases, it may be possible to control bleeding vessels by initial embolization and subsequent drainage should this prove necessary (Carrillo et al, 1999).

Iatrogenic Trauma

To an increasing extent, biliary hemorrhage is reported as a complication of diagnostic and therapeutic procedures on the liver or the bile ducts (see Fig. 68.2B). It is now encountered much more frequently than hemobilia from traffic accidents (see Fig. 68.2) (Sandblom, 1986). Diagnostic liver puncture (see Ch. 22) causes hemobilia in 3% to 7% of cases (Hodgson et al, 2004; Wiechel, 1964). The risk is enhanced if there is portal hypertension or when there is a bleeding tendency. With the common use of percutaneous needle biopsy and percutaneous cannulation of the biliary ducts for cholangiography or drainage, the incidence of patients with hemobilia from iatrogenic trauma has increased threefold (Curet et al, 1984). There may be a three-way communication with a concomitant arterioportal fistula (Sarr et al, 1984; Walter et al, 1976) or bilhemia (Sears et al, 1997). If no hematoma is produced by the lesion, most hemorrhages, even considerable ones, usually stop spontaneously. If intervention becomes necessary, embolization of the feeding artery that supplies the lesion is the procedure of choice (Cacho et al, 1996).

Transhepatic cholangiography (see Ch. 20) was introduced in 1937 (Huard & Do-Xuan-Hop, 1937). It carries an even greater risk of hemobilia than biopsy because of the close relationship between bile ducts and blood vessels (see Fig. 68.3B) (Wiechel, 1964). In a series of 300 cases, 9 developed major hemobilia (Sarr et al, 1984). With adequate control of prothrombin time, however, the risk should be minimal (Hines et al, 1972). The difficulty of finding a bile duct, especially if this is of normal caliber, may require repeated puncture. The production of clots in this form of minor hemobilia often causes diagnostic problems. Because pathologic findings are expected, the clots often are mistaken for stones (see Fig. 68.8).

Endobiliary prostheses now frequently are used for temporary relief of obstructive jaundice secondary to incurable malignancy. In one series of 300 patients, 9 developed profuse hemobilia related to a transhepatic biliary catheter, and 8 were treated successfully with hepatic artery embolotherapy; in 1 patient, the bleeding was ultimately fatal (Sarr et al, 1984). Difficulties in placing the stent caused a fatal bilhemia in one patient (Lunderquist, 1998). Other authors have recorded hemobilia in this setting (Born et al, 2003; Wolters et al, 2003)

Surgery of the biliary tract also may lead to damage to the hepatic artery by suture or by the dissection, which may result in an arteriobiliary fistula or in a false aneurysm leaking or eroding into the extrahepatic bile ducts (Kelley et al, 1983) (see Fig. 68.6). Shock wave lithotripsy with adjuvant endoscopic sphincterotomy had a short-lived international acceptance (see Fig. 68.2A), but has been abandoned because of the high complication rate. In a series of 568 cases, mostly elderly patients, 34 developed hemobilia. A case of hemobilia resulting in death after radiofrequency ablation of a hepatic tumor has been reported (Enne et al, 2004). Hemobilia also may follow placement of a transhepatic portosystemic shunt (Gonzales-Abraldes et al, 2001).

Laparoscopic cholecystectomy has rapidly replaced the open operation in most centers because of reduced hospitalization time despite an equal or greater risk of intraoperative lesions.

Postoperative hemobilia has been reported repeatedly, especially as the result of thermal injuries (Kassasseya et al, 1997) and laser techniques (Genyk et al, 1994). After treating four cases in a year, Stewart and associates (1995) feared that postcholecystectomy hemobilia was enjoying a renaissance in the laparoscopic era, and this has proved to be correct (Journe et al, 2004; Nicholson et al, 1999; Saldinger et al, 2002).

Surgical procedures and instrumental exploration of the intrahepatic ducts often damage their walls with great risk of hemorrhage. Minor bleeding constantly accompanies such procedures, but the hemorrhage generally ceases spontaneously, and the resulting clots promptly dissolve. Even during their ephemeral existence, they may cause diagnostic discussion when they appear on the postexploratory concluding cholangiogram (see Fig. 68.3A).

Forceful instrumental exploration of the biliary tree and extraction of stones can provoke significant hemorrhage (see Fig. 68.7A). Endoscopic sphincterotomy (see Ch. 37) is a common intervention to facilitate passage of stones. When performed with care, it causes only minor, temporary hemorrhage, but several cases of major hemobilia have occurred (Barbier et al, 1996; Mosenkis & Brandt, 1997). Not all surgeons are aware of the vulnerability of the intrahepatic ducts and the dangerous proximity to hepatic arteries. Bleeding from a T-tube occasionally can be caused by local erosion of the mucosa from the inlying tube, but if an arteriogram is done, it frequently exposes another source—a false aneurysm originating from an intraductal lesion, caused by the instrument used (see Fig. 68.7B). As in other kinds of traumatic hemobilia, there is sometimes a considerable interval between trauma and the bleeding episode.

Profuse biliary bleeding rarely complicates elective hepatic resection (see Ch. 80). The author has found minor intraductal bleeding can result in confusing temporary postoperative jaundice. Hemobilia also has been reported after liver transplantation (Tung & Kimmey, 1999).

Inflammation and Nematodes

In cholangitis, clots may appear that consist of pure fibrin from the fibrinous exudate or of blood from the vulnerable, inflamed mucosa or often both concomitantly. Ruptured liver abscess has caused hemobilia in a few cases (Liou et al, 1996). Many cases of hemobilia of an inflammatory nature are caused by nematodes. They have a singular geographic distribution: All originate in Asia or in Africa (e.g., China, Vietnam, and Korea). The causative agent in this category is *Ascaris* (see Ch. 60), a nematode with a tendency to invade the bile ducts, where it frequently produces bleeding (Fig. 68.9). This so-called tropical hemobilia is said to be a common problem in surgical departments in the Far East (Ton That Tung, 1972). In the West, these cases are exceedingly rare (Corr et al, 1997). In India, 500 cases of biliary ascariasis have been reported (Khurro et al, 1990). Suppuration, but no bleeding, is mentioned. Because blood iron levels were low, and no examination for hematochezia was performed, it may be that many cases were overlooked.

Gallstones

In gallstone disease, microscopic hemorrhage is frequent and can be proved in one of four cases with stones in the gallbladder and in one of three with stones in the common duct (Gad, 1962). Macroscopic hemobilia is rare, constituting only about 10% of all major hemobilia cases reported. It generally occurs when large stones erode the cystic artery or penetrate into an adjacent viscus or vessel (see Fig. 68.14) (Ritz et al, 1997). The stones may cause profuse, exsanguinating hemobilia; 11 out of 20 patients in one report bled to death. Hemobilia should be regarded just as seriously, but as a much less frequent complication secondary to neglected gallstones (Joo et al, 2003), as obstructive jaundice, cholecystitis, and pancreatitis.

Tumor

Tumors play an insignificant role as a source of bleeding in the biliary tract, constituting only 6% of all cases of major hemobilia. The malignant tumors outnumber the benign by at least three to one. Liver metastases, which account for the bulk of tumors in the liver, hardly ever cause hemobilia; similarly, hemobilia is not a frequent sequela of primary cancers in the liver (Kitagawa et al, 1999). Hemobilia has been described from metastases in such rare locations as the gallbladder wall (Kubota et al, 2000) or

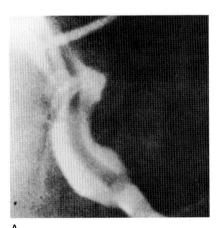
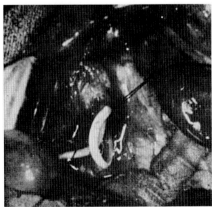
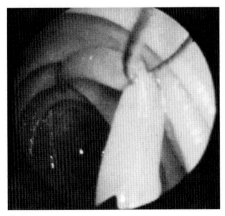

A   B   C

Fig. 68.9. Hemobilia from ascaris. **A,** T-tube cholangiogram visualizes a stringlike filling defect. **B,** Operative extraction of an ascaris through a choledochotomy. **C,** Endoscopic extraction of an ascaris, protruding through the papilla.
(**A,** case of J. Sawyer, Vanderbilt University; **B,** case of G.B. Ong, University of Hong Kong; **C,** courtesy of R. Cavin, Lausanne, Switzerland.)

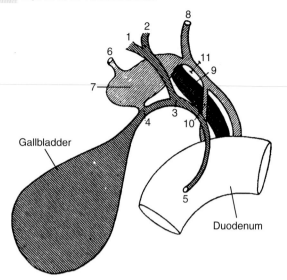

Gallbladder

Duodenum

Fig. 68.10. A case of true aneurysm in the right hepatic artery, rupturing into the gallbladder. This original drawing by Hans Kehr in 1903 shows the pathologic picture in the first case of hemobilia that was treated successfully by operative ligature of the hepatic artery proper.

from melanoma in the ductal mucosa. In cases of hemobilia caused by malignant tumors in the gallbladder (Hernandez-Castillo et al, 2002), the bleeding is most marked if the tumor grows in a polypoid fashion (Strauss, 1929). In the bile ducts, benign adenoma (Teter, 1954), polyps, or polyposis has a protracted course of hemobilia. Papillary tumors of the bile duct also may bleed intermittently (see Chs. 50 and 52). As described earlier, hemobilia may follow radiofrequency ablation of liver tumors (see Ch. 76).

Vascular Disorders

Vascular disease accounts for only 10% of cases of gross hemobilia. The frequency of true aneurysms (Ryan et al, 2002) of the hepatic artery or its branches (Maralcan et al, 2003; Morioka et al, 2004) rupturing into the biliary tract is diminishing with the disappearance of mycotic aneurysms (Fig. 68.10), leaving only aneurysms of atherosclerotic origin or those associated with arteriopathy (e.g., polyarteritis nodosa) (Dutta et al, 2004; Yazici et al, 1997) or trauma. When an aneurysm leaks only, it might give rise to inconspicuous hemobilia (Fig. 68.11), but if it ruptures into the biliary tract, the symptoms are generally stormy with exsanguinating hemorrhage and intense biliary colic. An arterial angiogram should precede an emergency operation or embolization. Most frequently, embolization is the intervention of choice (see Fig. 68.6). Sometimes, vascular lesions associated with arterial hypertension give rise to hemobilia. The structure usually affected is the gallbladder, and the disorder is designated as "apoplexy of the gallbladder." A case of hemobilia from bile duct varices associated with portal hypertension was treated successfully with endoscopic injection sclerotherapy (Ito et al, 1997), and the author has experience of three cases of intraductal varices: one associated with a benign biliary stricture, long-standing biliary tract obstruction, and biliary cirrhosis; one associated with Caroli's disease and portal hypertension; and one associated with alcoholic cirrhosis and accompanying portal hypertension. Chu and associates (2002) reported fatal bleeding from gallbladder varices in a patient with alcoholic cirrhosis.

Coagulation Defects

Hemobilia may result from coagulopathy with or without minimal trauma (Elte et al, 1980), hemophilia, idiopathic thrombocytopenic

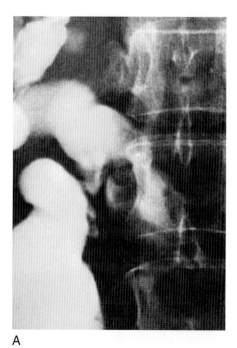

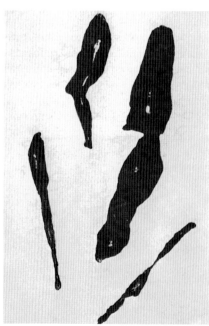

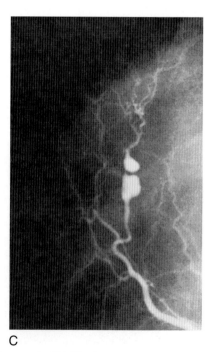

A   B   C

Fig. 68.11. Hemobilia from a source not identified during laparotomy. **A,** Perioperative cholangiogram through the normal gallbladder shows a large oval defect and a couple of bandlike ones below. **B,** Corresponding blood clots, rolled up into a ball, were extracted. **C,** 6 weeks later, the source was identified through arteriography as an aneurysm in the right hepatic artery. Because no further bleeding occurred, a planned embolization was postponed.

purpura (Daidoh et al, 1996), or anticoagulant therapy (see Figs. 68.3E and 68.12). The increasing frequency of the latter probably results in many cases of minor hemobilia with the formation of clots, imitating stones (Fig. 68.12) (Sandblom & Essinger, 1981; Yoshida et al, 1987).

Hemosuccus Pancreaticus

Hemorrhage from the pancreas or from a pancreatic cyst is a rare source of hemobilia (Ross et al, 1991; Sandblom, 1970). Blood from the pancreatic duct, *hemosuccus pancreaticus*, mixes with the bile in the 70% of cases in which the contents of the duct of Wirsung and the common bile duct enter the duodenum through a common channel. This condition also is discussed in Chs. 46 and 48.

The condition is associated most often with chronic pancreatitis. In 50%, pancreatic enzymes produce a pseudoaneurysm in the splenic artery, which ruptures into the pancreatic duct, often through a pseudocyst (Fig. 68.13B) (Yoshida et al, 1987). The author also has encountered this problem arising from aneurysm of the pancreaticoduodenal arcade. In another 30%, pancreatic duct stones eroded an adjacent vessel (see Fig. 68.13A). In only 10% of the cases are the aneursyms congenital or atherosclerotic.

In hemosuccus pancreaticus, the symptom triad is the same as in hemobilia, and there may be increased pancreatic enzymes in the serum. Endoscopy performed during bleeding episodes has often revealed blood extruding from the papilla, and ductography has shown defects caused by clots (see Fig. 68.13A).

The diagnosis should be confirmed by selective angiography of the splenic artery, which often exposes the communication with the duct of Wirsung (see Fig. 68.13B).

Pancreatic pseudocysts are often implicated. Arterial embolization may be unsuitable, and surgical therapy may be necessary. Acute pancreatitis can be associated with hemobilia (Asselah et al, 2001; Machicao et al, 2002).

Bilhemia

Bilhemia denotes the reverse of hemobilia, with bile entering the bloodstream through a communication with the hepatic veins (Clemens & Wittrin, 1975; Sandblom et al, 2000) or with branches of the portal vein (Lagagne et al, 1988). The reversed flow is due to inversion of the pressure gradient (Francois et al, 1994) caused by high intraductal bile pressure, generally resulting from a peripheral obstruction (Fig. 68.14) or low venous pressure. In a large series of cases of obstructive jaundice, the pressure in the bile ducts was invariably higher than in the hepatic veins (Wiechel, 1964). In five instances, gallstones eroded into the portal vein (see Fig. 68.14). The first case was reported in 1559, preceding hemobilia by a century: At the necropsy of Ignatius Loyola, three gallstones were found in the portal vein.

Portal vein bilhemia was recognized relatively recently. The first case (after Loyola), caused by liver biopsy, was described by Brown and Walsh in 1952, and the second, 15 years later by Mehta and Rubenstone (1967). The condition, which was named by Clemens and Wittrin in 1975, is rare but dangerous. Of the 50 cases reported in the literature, 25 were fatal. The cause

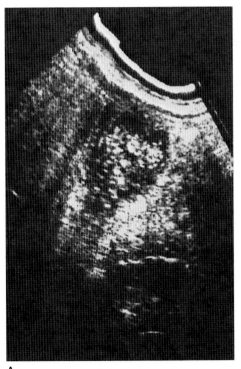

A

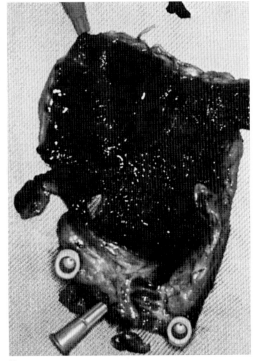

B

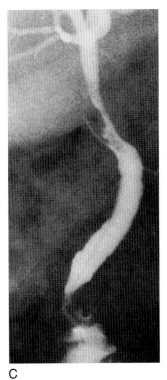

C

Fig. 68.12. Hemobilia caused by clotting defect during anticoagulation therapy. **A,** Sonogram indicating dense material in the gallbladder, interpreted as "microcalculi" or "inspissated bile." **B,** In the gallbladder, there was clotted blood, firmly attached to the wall. **C,** Defects in the perioperative cholangiogram caused by blood clots, the large proximal one attached to the wall and the distal one bandlike.

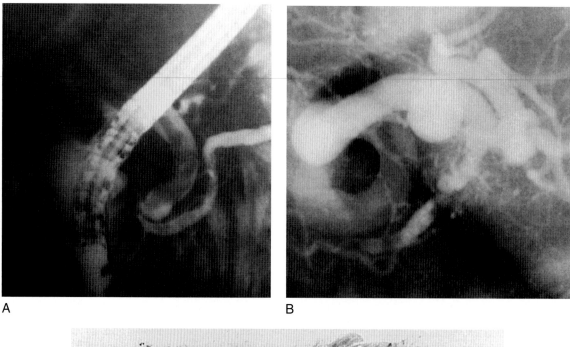

A

B

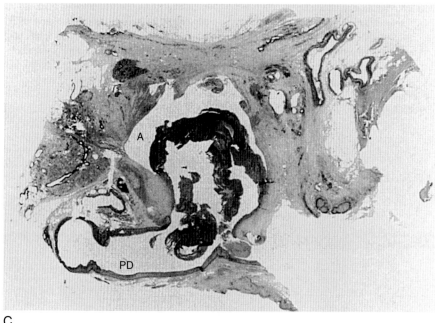

C

Fig. 68.13. Hemosuccus pancreaticus. **A,** ERCP showing wormlike filling defects in the pancreatic and common bile ducts. A stone in the pancreatic duct had eroded into the splenic artery, and esophagogastroduodenoscopy had revealed a blood clot passing through the papilla. **B,** Splenic arteriogram shows an aneurysm with contrast medium flowing into the pancreatic duct. The opening is partly occluded by the clot. The distal pancreas containing the aneurysm was resected. **C,** Histologic section through the communication between the aneurysm (A) containing a thrombus and the pancreatic duct (PD).
(**A,** from Ross C, et al, 1991: Hemosuccus pancreaticus: an unusual cause of upper gastrointestinal hemorrhage. Contemp Surg 38:11. **C,** from Koehler R, et al, 1976: Massive extra-enteric gastrointestinal bleeding: angiographic diagnosis. Diagn Radiol 113:41.)

of the pathologic passage was accidental: blunt trauma in half the cases and iatrogenic injury or manipulation during operation in three cases (Koehler et al, 1978).

The bile flow is often low, with spontaneous closure of the fistula; the condition is apt to be overlooked (Koehler et al, 1978). It acquires clinical significance when a large amount of bile enters the bloodstream. This bile may cause embolization of the lungs (Fig. 68.15) (Brozinsky et al, 1981), which may be fatal (Schmidt-Mutter et al, 2003). Seventeen patients died suddenly

during a difficult placement at percutaneous transhepatic cholangiography of a metallic stent into the common duct. There was evidently a high intraductal pressure and a large amount of bile collected above the obstruction. Great care must be taken in performing invasive procedures in patients with obstructive jaundice.

The symptoms are a *rapidly increasing jaundice with elevated direct bilirubin without increase of liver enzymes*. Septicemia has occurred through bilhemia with infected bile (Morettin &

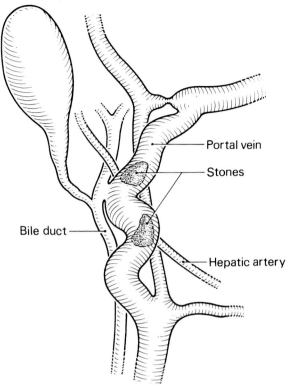

Fig. 68.14. Bilhemia. Gallstones had penetrated into a collateral portal vein. As portal hypertension reversed the pressure gradient between portal circulation and bile flow, bilhemia transformed to hemobilia. (From Sandblom, 1972: Hemobilia, Springfield, IL, Charles C Thomas.)

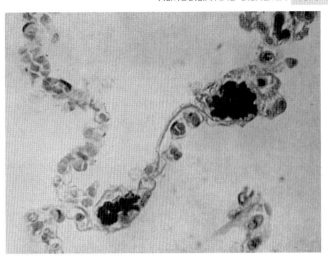

Fig. 68.15. The first case of bilhemia (Brown & Walsh, 1952). The patient died as a result of embolism in connection with percutaneous liver biopsy. Lung with bile present in the capillaries.

Dodd, 1972). Selective arteriography is nondiagnostic in bilhemia, whereas scintigraphy has been useful (Francois et al, 1994). ERCP, in which the contrast material follows the direction of the biliary flow, is the best means to show the fistula (Glaser et al, 1994) (Fig. 68.16).

Treatment aims at release of the ductal obstruction, sometimes through endoscopic sphincterectomy or, with a higher location, through a percutaneous transhepatic drain. This procedure sometimes causes the fistula to close or at least gives temporary relief (Sears et al, 1997). More lasting effect can be obtained with endostenting (Gable et al, 1997). For definitive cure, the affected liver may have to be resected (Clemens & Wittrin, 1975) or the fistula occluded via angiography or ERCP (Struyven et al, 1982).

"The light which experience gives us," says Coleridge, "is a lantern on the stern which shines only on the waves behind us." With a syndrome as comparatively rare as hemobilia, experience has to be replaced by knowledge: a lantern on the bow to enlighten us so that we can recognize the syndrome when we encounter it and know how to handle it.

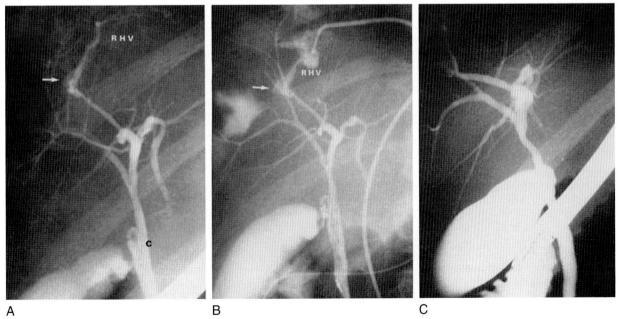

A B C

Fig. 68.16. A, ERCP. Bile ducts injected by catheter (C) positioned in common bile duct. Opacification of fistula *(arrow)* and segmental branch of right hepatic vein (RHV). **B,** Selective opacification of segmental branch of right hepatic vein, fistula *(arrow),* and bile ducts. Balloon catheter positioned as tip to diagnostic catheter. **C,** ERCP 3½ weeks later. Normal biliary pattern.
(From Struyven et al, 1982: Post-traumatic bilhemia: diagnosis and catheter therapy. AJR Am J Roentgenol 138:746.)

REFERENCES

Andreassen M, Lindenberg K, 1959: Late postoperative 'hemobilia' treated with peripheral ligation of the hepatic artery. Surgery 46:870.

Arner O, et al, 1962: Percutaneous transhepatic cholangiography. Surgery 52:561.

Asmat P, Beckmann CF, 1983: Transcatheter embolisation of the liver for control of massive hemobilia in a patient with adenocarcinoma of the gallbladder invading the intrahepatic biliary system. Am J Gastroenterol 78:761.

Asselah T, et al, 2001: Hemobilia causing acute pancreatitis after percutaneous liver biopsy: diagnosis by magnetic resonance cholangiopancreatography. Eur J Gastroenterol Hepatol 13:877.

Ball TJ, et al, 1975: Hemobilia following percutaneous liver biopsy. Gastroenterology 68:1297.

Barbier C, et al, 1996: Aspects radiologiques des complications des sphincterotomies endoscopiques. J Radiol 77:555.

Boijsen E, et al, 1966: Angiographic diagnosis of hepatic rupture. Radiology 86:66.

Born P, et al, 2003: Arterial bleeding as an unusual late complication of percutaneous transhepatic biliary drainage. Endoscopy 35:978.

Brown CY, Walsh GC, 1952: Fatal bile embolism following liver biopsy. Ann Intern Med 36:1529.

Brozinsky S, et al, 1981: Bile emboli: a complication of PTD. J Clin Gastroenterol 3:135.

Cacho G, et al, 1996: Arterioportal fistula and hemobilia with associated acute cholecystitis: a complication of percutaneous liver biopsy. Hepatogastroenterology 43:1020.

Carrillo E, et al, 1998: Non-operative management of blunt hepatic trauma. Br J Surg 85:463.

Carrillo EH, et al, 1999: Interventional techniques are useful adjuncts in nonoperative management of hepatic injuries. J Trauma 46:619.

Carr-Locke DL, Westwood CA, 1980: Endoscopy and endoscopic retrograde cholangiopancreatography finding in traumatic liver injury and hemobilia. Am J Gastroenterol 73:162.

Chu EC, et al, 2002: Fatal spontaneous gallbladder variceal bleeding in a patient with alcoholic cirrhosis. Dig Dis Sci 47:2682.

Clemens M, Wittrin G, 1975: Bilhämie and Hämobilie nach Reitunfall. Taglich Nordw Dtsch Chirurg Vortrag 166.

Connihan T, et al, 1996: Acute cholecystitis resulting from hemobilia after trucut biopsy. Am Surg 65:757.

Corr P, et al, 1997: An unusual cause of haemobilia: biliary ascariasis. Pediatr Radiol 27:348.

Curet O, et al, 1984: Hepatic hemobilia of traumatic or iatrogenic origin: recent advances in diagnosis and therapy, review of the literature from 1976 to 1981. World J Surg 8:1.

Czerniak A, et al, 1988: Hemobilia—a disease in evolution. Arch Surg 123:718.

Daidoh H, et al, 1996: Asymptomatic hemobilia with idiopathic thrombocytopenic purpura. Hepatogastroenterology 43:1470.

Dutta U, et al, 2004: Hemobilia as presenting manifestatin of polyarteritis nodosa. Indian J Gastroenterol 23:71.

Elte P, et al, 1980: Hemobilia after liver biopsy: early detection in a patient with mild hemophilia A. Arch Intern Med 140:839.

Enne M, et al, 2004: Fatal hemobilia after radiofrequency thermal ablation for hepatocellular carcinoma. Surgery 135:460.

Forlee MV, et al, 2004: Haemobilia after penetrating and blunt liver injury: treatment with selective hepatic artery embolisation. Injury 35:23.

Francois D, et al, 1994: Hepatobiliary scintigraphy in a patient with bilhaemia. Eur J Nucl Med 20:1020.

Gable DR, et al, 1997: Endoscopic treatment of posttraumatic 'bilhaemia': case report. J Trauma Injury Infect Crit Care 43:534.

Gad P, 1962: Okkult blodning ved galdesten. Nordisk Medicin 68:1069.

Genyk Y, et al, 1994: Hepatic artery pseudoaneurysm and hemobilia following laser laparoscopic cholecystectomy. Surg Endosc 8:201.

Glaser K, et al, 1994: Traumatic bilhaemia. Surgery 116:24.

Gonzales-Abraldes J, et al, 2001: Selective arterial embolization for life threatening hemobilia after transjugular intrahepatic portosystemic shunt placement. J Hepatol 34:174.

Guitron-Cantu A, et al, 2002: [Endoscopic diagnosis and treatment of nontraumatic bilhemia. A case report]. Rev Gastroenterol Mexico 67:259.

Hendren WH, et al, 1971: Traumatic hemobilia: non-operative management with healing documented by serial angiography. Ann Surg 174:991.

Hernandez-Castillo E, et al, 2002: Haemobilia and gallbladder carcinoma. Dig Liver Dis 34:681.

Hines C, et al, 1972: Percutaneous transhepatic cholangiography. Dig Dis 17:868.

Hodgson RS, et al, 2004: Hematochezia in Crohn's disease caused by late-onset hemobilia following percutaneous liver biopsy. Eur J Gastroenterol Hepatol 16:229.

Horak D, et al, 1996: Poly (2-hydroxyethyl methacrylate) particles for management of hemorrhage of complicated origin: treatment of hemobilia. J Biomed Mater Res 33:193.

Howdle P, et al, 1976: Diagnosis of biliary tract hemorrhage (hemobilia) by endoscopy. Gastrointest Endosc 23:94.

Huard P, Do-Xuan-Hop, 1937: La ponction transhepatique des canaux biliares. Bull Soc Med Chir Indoch 15:1090.

Ishaq M, et al, 2003: Recurrent gastrointestinal bleed. Postgrad Med J 79:243.

Ito T, et al, 1997: Successful endoscopic injection sclerotherapy for bleeding from bile duct varices. J Surg 27:174.

Jackson JBS, 1834: Aneurysm of the hepatic artery bursting into the hepatic duct. Medical Magazine Boston 3:115.

Joo YE, et al, 2003: Hemobilia caused by liver abscess due to intrahepatic duct stones. J Gastroenterol 38:507.

Journe S, et al, 2004: Right hepatic artery pseudoaneurysm and cystic duct leak after laparoscopic cholecystecomy. Surg Endosc 18:554.

Kassasseya A, et al, 1997: Hemobilie apres cholecystectomie laparoscopique. Ann Chir 51:159.

Kehr H, 1903: Der erste Fall von erfolgreicher Unterbindung der Art. Hepatica propria wegen Aneurysm. Med Wochenschr 50:1861.

Kelley CJ, et al, 1983: Non-surgical management of post-cholecystectomy hemobilia. Br J Surg 70:502.

Khurro M, et al, 1990: Hepatobiliary and pancreatic ascariasis in India. Lancet 335:1503.

King JB, 1972: Fibrinolysis by bile. Thromb Diath Haemost 28:279.

Kitagawa K, et al, 1999: Selective transcatheter hepatic arterial chemoembolization for hemobilia from hepatocellular carcinoma: report of three cases. J Vasc Interv Radiol 10:1357.

Koehler LS, et al, 1978: A complication of percutaneous cholangiography resulting in the hypoxia and death of an anesthetized patient. Anesthesiology 49:210.

Koehler R, et al, 1976: Massive extra-enteric gastrointestinal bleeding: angiographic diagnosis. Diagn Radiol 113:41.

Krudy AG, et al, 1983: Hemobilia: computed tomographic diagnosis. Radiology 148:785.

Kubota H, et al, 2000: A patient with undifferentiated carcinoma of gallbladder presenting with hemobilia. J Gastroenterol 35:63.

Lagagne PM, et al, 1988: Bilioportal fistula as a complication of choledochoduodenostomy. Surgery 103:125.

Laing FC, 1997: Hemobilia: sonographic appearances in the gallbladder and biliary tree with emphasis on intracholecystic blood. J Ultrasound Med 16:537.

Liou T-C, et al, 1996: Liver abscess concomitant with hemobilia due to rupture of hepatic artery aneurysm. Hepatogastroenterology 43:241.

Lunderquist A, 1998: Personal communication.

Luzuy F, et al, 1987: Biliary calculi caused by hemobilia. Surgery 102:886.

Machicao VI, et al, 2002: Arterioportal fistula causing acute pancreatitis and hemobilia after liver biopsy. J Clin Gastroenterol 34:481.

Madding GF, Kennedy PA, 1971: Trauma to the Liver, II. Philadelphia, Saunders.

Maralcan G, et al, 2003: Hemobilia in a patient with multiple intrahepatic, hepatic artery aneurysms. Acta Chir Belg 103:113.

Mehta S, Rubenstone AJ, 1967: Pulmonary bile thromboemboli. Am J Clin Pathol 47:490.

Millbourn E, 1951: Cholangiografiskt pånavisade blodkoagel i gallväuagarna i samband med choldochusingrepp. Nord Med 45:103.

Morettin L, Dodd G, 1972: Percutaneous transhepatic cholangiography. Dig Dis 17:831.

Morgagni S, 1765: Liber III. Epist XXXVII:82.

Morioka D, et al, 2004: Hemobilia caused by pseudoaneurysm of the cystic artery. J Gastroenterol Hepatol 19:724.

Mosenkis B, Brandt LJ, 1997: Bleeding causing biliary obstruction after endoscopic sphincterotomy. Am J Gastroenterol 92:708-709.

Nicholson T, et al, 1999: Hepatic artery angiography and embolization for hemobilia following laparoscopic cholecystectomy. Cardiovasc Interv Radiol 22:2.

Olsen WR, 1982: Late complications of central liver injuries. Surgery 92:733.

Peng Z, et al, 2001: Hepatic artery angiography and embolization for hemobilia after hepatobiliary surgery. Chin Med J (Engl) 114:803.

Portal A, 1777: Sur quelques maladies du foie qu'on attribue a? d'autres organes. Histoire de l'Academie Royal Des Sciences 601.

Poulos E, et al, 1974: Traumatic hemobilia treated by massive liver resection. Arch Surg 88:596.

Quincke H, 1871: Ein Fall con Aneurysma der Leberarterise. Berliner Klinische Wochenschrift 8:349.

Ranniger K, et al, 1968: Angiographic diagnosis of an intrahepatic aneurysm as a cause of unexplained bleeding. Radiology 90:507.

Redman H, Joseph R, 1975: Hemobilia and pancreatitis as complications of a percutaneous transhepatic cholangiogram. Dig Dis 20:691.

Ritz J-P, et al, 1997: Hämobile bei cholecystolithiasis als seltene ursache einer massiven oberen gastrointestinalen blutung. Der Chirurg 68:87.

Ross C, et al, 1991: Hemosuccus pancreaticus: an unusual cause of upper gastrointestinal hemorrhage. Contemp Surg 38:11.

Rousseau A, et al, 2004 [Hemobilia after blunt hepatic trauma: a sometimes delayed complication]. Ann Chir 129:41.

Ryan MF, et al, 2002: Hemobilia due to idiopathic hepatic artery aneurysm: case report. Can Assoc Radiol J 53:149.

Saldinger PF, et al, 2002: Cystic artery stump pseudoaneurysm following laparoscopic cholecystectomy. Surgery 131:585.

Sandblom P, 1948: Hemorrhage into the biliary tract following trauma—traumatic hemobilia. Surgery 94:271.

Sandblom P, 1970: Gastrointestinal hemorrhage through the pancreatic duct. Ann Surg 171:61-66.

Sandblom P, 1972: Hemobilia. Springfield, Charles C Thomas.

Sandblom P, 1986: Iatrogenic hemobilia. Am J Surg 151:754.

Sandblom P, Essinger A, 1981: Stones or clots in the biliary tract. Acta Chir Scand 147:673.

Sandblom P, Mirkovitch V, 1979: Minor hemobilia. Ann Surg 190:254.

Sandblom P, et al, 1976: The healing of liver wounds. Ann Surg 184:679.

Sandblom P, et al, 1977: Formation and fate of fibrin clots in the biliary tract. Ann Surg 185:356.

Sandblom P, et al, 2000: Fatal bilhemia. Surgery 127:354.

Sarr MG, et al, 1984: Management of hemobilia associated with transhepatic internal biliary drainage catheters. Surgery 95:603.

Schmidt-Mutter C, et al, 2003: Fatal bile pulmonary embolism after radiofrequency treatment of hepatocellular carcinoma. Surg Endosc 17:2028.

Sears R, et al, 1997: Endoscopic diagnosis and therapy of a case of bilhemia after percutaneous liver biopsy. Gastrointest Endosc 46:276.

Stewart B, et al, 1995: Post-cholecystectomy haemobilia: enjoying a renaissance in the laparoscopic era? Aust N Z J Surg 65:185.

Strauss A, 1929: Über Verblutung aus den Gallenwegen. Monatsschrift der Unfallheil Kunde 36:438.

Struyven J, et al, 1982: Post-traumatic bilhemia: diagnosis and catheter therapy. AJR Am J Roentgenol 138:746.

Teter LF, 1954: Massive hemorrhage from benign adenoma of the biliary duct causing death. J Mich Med Soc 53:62.

Thomeret G, et al, 1957: Rupture traumatique du foie. Mem Acad Chir 83:38.

Ton That Tung, 1972: Les hemobilies tropicales. Chirurgie 98:43.

Tseng JH, et al, 2001: Icteric-type hepatoma: magnetic resonance imaging and magnetic resonance cholangiographic features. Abdom Imaging 26:171.

Tung BY, Kimmey MB, 1999: Biliary complications of orthotopic liver transplantation. Dig Dis 17:133.

Uflacker R, et al, 1989: Hemobilia: transcatheter occlusive therapy and long-term follow-up. Cardiovasc Interv Radiol 12:136.

Van Os E, Petersen BT, 1996: Pancreatitis secondary to percutaneous liver biopsy–associated hemobilia. Am J Gastroenterol 91:577.

Walt A, 1984: Personal communication with P. Sandblom.

Walter JF, et al, 1976: Successful transcatheter embolic control of massive hematobilia secondary to liver biopsy. AJR Am J Roentgenol 127:847-849.

Wiechel KL, 1964: Percutaneous transhepatic cholangiography. Acta Chir Scand Suppl 24:330.

Wolters F, et al, 2003: Delayed massive hemobilia after biliary stenting. Endoscopy 35:976.

Yamamoto F, et al, 1994: A case report of MR imaging of traumatic hemobilia. J Gastroenterol 29:511.

Yazici A, et al, 1997: Polyarteritis nodosa presenting with hemobilia and intestinal hemorrhage. Eur Radiol 7:1059.

Yoshida J, et al, 1987: Hemobilia: review of recent experience with a worldwide problem. Am J Gastroenterol 82:448.

Liver Tumors

Tumors of the Liver—Pathologic Aspects

A. ZIMMERMANN

The main tumors of the liver are derived from the hepatocyte, bile duct epithelium, and endothelial cells. There are other cell systems in the liver, including connective tissue and muscle cells, macrophages, and neuroendocrine cells, but these rarely are regarded as unequivocal origins of tumor. This chapter describes hepatocellular carcinoma (HCC) and other tumors and other aspects that may be relevant to surgical practice.

HEPATOCELLULAR CARCINOMA

HCC (see Ch. 71) is probably the most common tumor that affects men in the world. This tumor is currently the fifth most frequent malignant solid neoplasm worldwide, with greater than 500,000 deaths per year (Parkin et al, 2001). The incidence of HCC has a broad geographic variation owing to the large heterogeneity of risk factors within diverse populations (Bruix et al, 2004; Llovet et al, 2003; Srivatanakul et al, 2004).

Macroscopic Forms

The criteria on which HCCs are grouped macroscopically generally are based on their size and form (Eggel, 1901) or on an assessment of the mode of growth (Nakashima & Kojiro, 1987; Okuda et al, 1984; Peters, 1976). HCCs have been designated in one system as *nodular, massive,* in which a large tumor mass seems to infiltrate surrounding liver parenchyma, or *diffuse,* in which multiple small tumor nodules involve much of the liver (Eggel, 1901). Another system attempts a separation of tumor types according to the apparent pattern of growth and spread (Okuda et al, 1984). In this system, tumors are referred to as *expanding, spreading, multifocal,* or *indeterminate.* Tumors included within the expanding group are characterized by a sharp demarcation between the tumor mass and the compressed and partly atrophic surrounding parenchyma. In support of the concept of the expanding process is the presence of distorted hepatic vessels, including arteries, forming curved structures on the surface of the tumor mass or visible on the cut surface of a tumor (Fig. 69.1). The expanding type sometimes is encapsulated. Capsule formation in a subset of these tumors is considered to begin at a tumor diameter of about 10 mm or greater because no distinct capsule was noted in lesions less than 10 mm (Nakamura et al, 1986). Capsule formation has been suggested to result from defense mechanisms of the host directed against the growth of HCC (Torimura et al, 1991). Other expanding lesions are fibrous, whereas some appear relatively homogeneous, often partly necrotic and hemorrhagic, when large (Fig. 69.2). When there is diffuse fibrosis in an expanding tumor, it is referred to as *sclerosing HCC* (Peters, 1976). Fibrosis may occur

in a septate pattern or focally, with the latter group including fibrolamellar HCC (Berman et al, 1980; Craig et al, 1980).

Lack of demarcation between a tumor and the surrounding tissue characterizes the *spreading* type of HCC, sections of which are composed of dense fibrosis, which extends into and distorts the adjacent nontumor tissue, or of multiple, irregular small tumor nodules varying in size and extending into and interdigitating with surrounding parenchyma. These small cirrhotic-like nodules may involve almost the whole liver. Vessels seem to be incorporated into and not displaced by the tumor mass so that curved arteries do not surround the tumor (Okuda et al, 1977, 1982a, 1982b). The term *diffuse HCC* (Eggel, 1901; Nakashima & Kojiro, 1987) seems to cover the same or a similar subset of tumors. Multicentric origin and intrahepatic spread after portal vein invasion have been discussed as pathogenic mechanisms in this class, and the incidence seems to range from 5.4% to 17%, depending on the sources of material and on differences in interpretation (Nakashima & Kojiro, 1987).

HCC usually not associated with cirrhosis and showing an irregular and indistinct tumor/nontumor boundary has been termed *infiltrative HCCs* (Nakashima & Kojiro, 1987). Large infiltrative HCC seems to correspond to Eggel's massive form. In a larger series, this category accounted for 33% of cases observed (Nakashima & Kojiro, 1987). In a clinically oriented study, this mode of growth has been classified as *invasive tumor* (see later) (Baer et al, 1989).

Some HCCs tend to show a predominantly extrahepatic growth, with much of the tumor mass being visible outside the level of the liver capsule and sometimes with formation of a distinct pedicle. These tumors are called *pedunculated HCC* (Nakashima & Kojiro, 1987). Pedunculated HCCs are divided further into two subtypes: intrahepatic origin (type I) (Nakashima & Kojiro, 1987) and extrahepatic origin (type II) (Miyoshi et al, 1977). In type II lesions it has been demonstrated that an extrahepatic tumor mass was nourished by a branch of the hepatic artery, even though no connection between the HCC and the liver was visualized (Miyoshi et al, 1977). Pedunculated HCCs are included in the category of hanging tumors in the system of Baer and colleagues (1989) (see Ch. 80). The identification of the pedunculated group is significant because even in the case of large tumors limited resection may give excellent results. The awareness that this peculiar growth pattern defines a subset of HCC with probably a different biology and a gross morphology amenable to preoperative diagnosis is underlined by the fact that since its original description (Roux, 1897), more than 30 well-documented cases have been identified, and increasing numbers may be expected in the future as a result of more sophisticated imaging techniques.

The use of the terms *multifocal* and *indeterminate* (Okuda et al, 1984) implies an opinion, rather than a descriptive categorization, but often a consensus may be reached. *Multifocal* reflects the

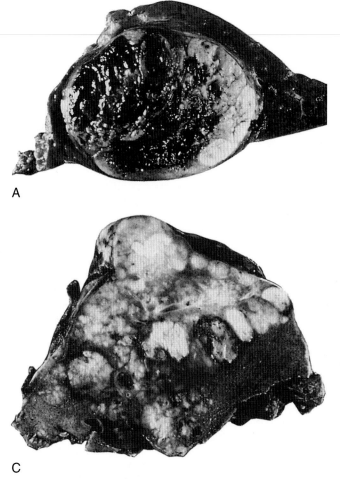

A

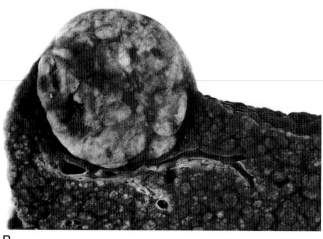

B

C

Fig. 69.1. Modes of growth of HCC. **A,** Pushing tumor grows expansively and compresses the surrounding liver tissue. **B,** Hanging tumor grows with a base adjacent to the free liver edge; note the curved dislocation of a large vein. **C,** Invasive tumor; the tumor border is highly irregular, and no rim of compressed tissue is formed. Resection specimens.

finding of several unconnected small tumors of roughly similar size that do not seem to have developed as metastatic foci arising from a single growth. *Indeterminate* represents tumors that show different features in different parts or are indistinct because of necrosis or hemorrhage (see Fig. 69.2). The difficulties that may arise in gross classification are illustrated by cases of apparently expansive HCC, which on a different section level may show areas of active invasive growth at the periphery (Fig. 69.3).

There are difficulties in achieving reproducible categorization without considerable variation among different workers, and it is evident that terms are employed in different ways in different countries (Liver Cancer Study Group of Japan, 1984; Okuda et al, 1984). The value of using some agreed-on form of categorization, which possibly was regarded as a structured academic exercise in the past, has become more evident with the development of sophisticated new statistical procedures in cancer epidemiology and with the more optimistic approach to therapeutic procedures. A proper and reproducible gross classification of HCC is of particular importance in assessing resectability of large focal liver lesions (i.e., with the exclusion of diffuse forms). It has been shown that, using imaging techniques, a simple morphologic classification can be found for these situations, allowing for a reasonable prediction of resectability (Baer et al, 1989). In the system used by these authors, three different morphologic varieties of tumor have been defined, providing an additional

advantage of this system in that it not only works for HCC, but also for other potentially resectable large tumors occurring in the liver. The first category, *hanging tumors,* is defined as tumors growing with a base adjacent to the free liver edge and hanging in their entirety, or at least their major part, free of

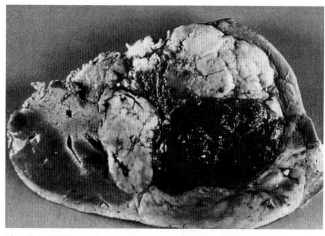

Fig. 69.2. HCC, mostly the pushing (expanding) type. The center of this tumor is involved by massive hemorrhage. Resection specimen.

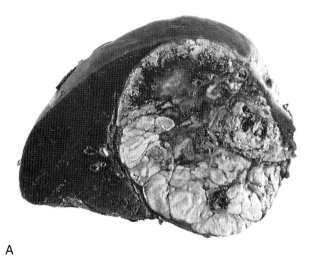

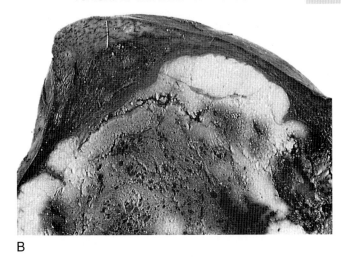

A   B

Fig. 69.3. HCC. **A,** The overall impression of this large tumor is that of a pushing or expanding lesion. **B,** Another section plane discloses several invasive outgrowths visible as white nodular structures clearly different from the necrotic and hemorrhagic central parts of the tumor. Resection specimen.

the rest of the surrounding liver tissue in the abdominal cavity. Tumors in the second category, or *pushing tumors,* grow expansively and compress the surrounding normal liver tissue. The third category comprises *invasive tumors,* which grow without anatomic limits and no clear border so that differentiation of normal from malignant areas of the liver is difficult. Small tumors of less than 5 cm diameter cannot be classified properly within this system because they do not display gross morphologic differences. Examples of these morphologic patterns as occurring in the case of HCC are depicted in Fig. 69.1.

A macroscopic description and classification of HCC may focus on features different from the overall growth pattern. Small HCCs are discussed later. The significance of capsule formation and stromal content has not yet been settled, but there seem to be differences in the incidence of these subgroups in different countries. There is a higher incidence of encapsulated tumors in Japan and a lower incidence of sclerosing tumors in Japan and South Africa (Goodman & Ishak, 1982; Goodman et al, 1985).

Current surgical therapy requires a clear indication of the presence or absence of accompanying cirrhosis (Fig. 69.4). It has been recognized that tumors referred to as *expanding* generally are accompanied by cirrhosis when distinctly encapsulated, but are not accompanied by cirrhosis when there is conspicuous intratumor sclerosis, whether this is focal or diffuse (Figs. 69.5-69.7). Only a few cases of HCC with particularly dense stroma have been reported to be associated with long-term survival, and fibrosis in these instances is accompanied by lymphocytic infiltration (Sonoda et al, 1989). It may be suggested that fibrosis is a result of strong immune and other defense reactions directed against the neoplastic cell population in these situations, and that the biology of disease may depend strongly on complex interactions between epithelial cells and the extracellular matrix in cirrhosis and malignant epithelial tumors. The incidence of hepatocellular tumors with accompanying cirrhosis is generally greater than that of tumors without cirrhosis. Geographic differences may contribute to the type of disease because of unknown factors and because of different diagnostic criteria for cirrhosis (Anthony et al, 1978). It is possible that early deaths from cirrhosis may alter the local incidence of the association between the two conditions. The cause of discrepancies between published accounts of cirrhosis and tumors is unclear, but there are several

possible difficulties. In some series, the liver tumors considered in the reports have included cholangiocarcinomas and HCCs, with a resultant distortion of the incidence of cirrhosis in patients with HCC; another source of error is the poor appreciation of cirrhotic changes so that a category has been suggested, as a safeguard, that groups "cirrhosis or fibrosis or both" (Okuda et al, 1982a) as accompaniments of HCC.

The invasion and formation of tumor emboli in the portal vein is a familiar feature of HCC, supporting the general consensus that intrahepatic spread of HCC mainly occurs via the portal venous system. Portal vein invasion may be associated with

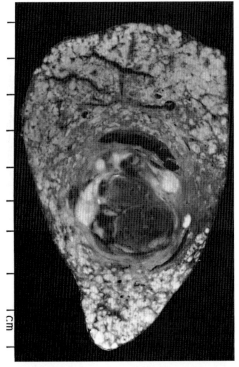

Fig. 69.4. Expanding HCC in a patient with cirrhosis. Note the thin rim of fibrosis surrounding the tumor, the necrosis, and the curved vascular structures distorted by the expanding tumor mass. Resection specimen.

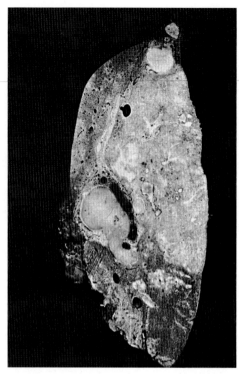

Fig. 69.5. Expanding HCC in noncirrhotic liver. Note the sharp demarcation, the large amount of fibrosis within the tumor, and the invasion of portal vein. Resection specimen.

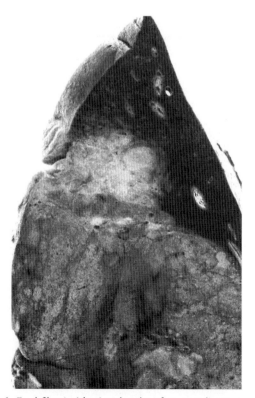

Fig. 69.6. Focal fibrosis *(above)* at the edge of an expanding tumor mass in noncirrhotic liver. Resection specimen.

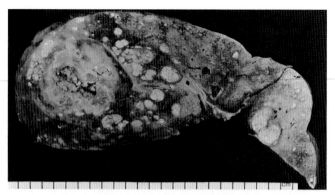

Fig. 69.7. Diffuse spreading HCC. Multiple variably sized tumor foci, some necrotic, in noncirrhotic liver. Resection specimen.

thrombosis of this vessel. Notwithstanding the fact that the developmental steps of the intrahepatic invasion and metastasis cascade are poorly understood (Kondo & Wada 1991), and that the significance of vascular invasion as to outcome has not yet been analyzed sufficiently, the presence or the absence of portal vein involvement should be determined with care at the initial gross examination. In some situations, vascular invasion with formation of tumor plugs is easily detectable, and the probable starting point within a tumor mass and the end of a plug contacting the blood can be reconstructed by careful examination of sequential section planes (Fig. 69.8). Macroscopically, intravascular tumor plugs in some instances may be difficult to distinguish from tumor nodules on section surfaces, but probing with a needle or forceps usually helps to detect the slitlike cleft located between a plug and the vessel wall in cases in which a plug is not completely adherent to the inner surface of a vein.

The morphologic elements that have been determined for a gross description and classification of HCC are an important armamentarium for current and future staging systems of this neoplasm. The issue of staging is discussed in detail elsewhere. Several reviews have addressed this question more recently (Huo et al, 2004; Wildi et al, 2004).

Gross examination of livers or resection specimens harboring tumors may disclose other morphologic changes that are significant in pretreatment diagnostic measures and in understanding the biology of the disease. Peripherally located small and large tumors may exhibit umbilication, which is thought to develop from regression and collapse of a poorly nourished tumor center (Fig. 69.9), the actively growing part of the tumor then forming a mantle zone or a nodular ring around the central depression. Necrosis adjacent to the liver surface may induce secondary inflammatory changes, however, which may produce intriguing changes at imaging. This pattern frequently occurs with liver metastases, but also may be encountered with primary malignant liver tumors. Production of a fibrin-rich exudate on the liver surface at the site of a partly necrotic peripheral tumor mass may be followed by formation of granulation and scar tissue and by adhesion of adjacent tissues (Fig. 69.10; see Fig. 69.9). These lesions may result in localized hypodense areas on computed tomography (CT), indicating apparent extrahepatic invasion by tumor, but histologic examination frequently shows that this is not the case (Weinbren et al, 1987). In some instances, central necrosis associated with inflammatory change and scarring may communicate through a funnel-like structure of variable width with connective tissue, adipose tissue, or even muscle tissue (in the

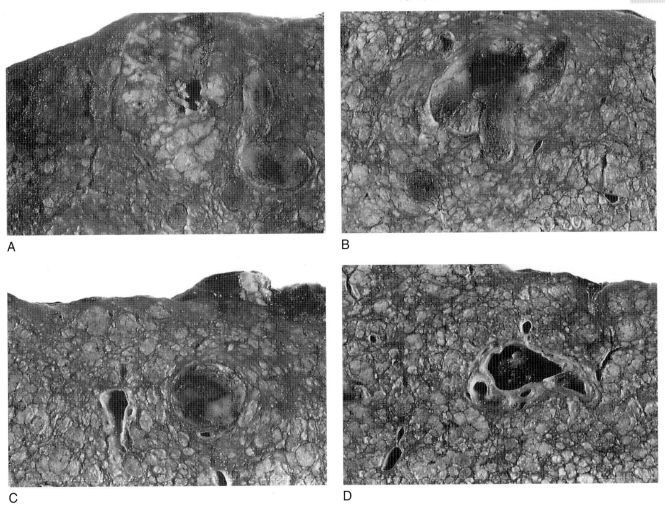

Fig. 69.8. Portal vein invasion by HCC. **A,** Part of the primary tumor is seen, and an adjacent dilated branch of the portal vein is involved by tumor thrombus. **B,** Section plane at about 1 cm from the primary tumor. The tumor thrombus now also involves smaller branches. **C,** The tumor thrombus closely fits the vascular lumen. The lesions may be mistaken as intrahepatic metastasis or a second tumor. **D,** Freely floating end of intravascular tumor thrombus. The liver shows cirrhosis. Resection specimens.

case of a subdiaphragmatic lesion) adherent to the liver capsule (see Fig. 69.10). A similar picture, which is probably visible on CT, may occur when tumor is extending along large intrahepatic preexisting structures, such as a thick tract containing blood vessels and bile ducts (Fig. 69.11).

In some cases, tumor growth can be observed to involve the adipose tissue–containing intrahepatic part of the round ligament (Fig. 69.12). For reasons of comparison with preoperative imaging findings, it may be useful to apply documentation techniques that allow better insight into the internal gross structure of a tumor (e.g., with regard to necrosis, hemorrhage, and angioarchitecture). Production of vascular casts may be informative in some instances, and transillumination of a slice may provide an extremely detailed picture of the internal structure of a tumor (Fig. 69.13).

Small Hepatocellular Carcinomas

A small liver cancer currently is defined as HCC with a maximum diameter of less than 2 cm (Nakashima & Kojiro, 1987), which is important with respect to its biology and treatment (Yamamoto et al, 2004; Zhou et al, 2001). The lack of a widely accepted definition has led to a lot of confusion, and HCCs smaller than 3 to 5 cm have been included in this group, which has mainly gained significance owing to progress in diagnostic imaging techniques. The limit of 2 cm is based on *The General Rules for the Clinical and Pathological Study of Primary Liver Cancer,* issued by the Liver Cancer Study Group of Japan in 1983. A synonymous term used by some authors is *minute HCC.* Small HCCs are found in noncirrhotic and cirrhotic livers, but in autopsy series many small HCCs have been detected in livers that were cirrhotic and highly atrophic (500-800 g) (Nakashima & Kojiro, 1987). Small HCC may remain unchanged in size for a long time, and there have been reports of long survival without specific treatment. In surgical cases, small HCCs usually occur as single lesions; data obtained at necropsy illustrate that single and multiple lesions occur with about the same frequency.

Small HCCs are nodular in shape, are often well differentiated, and display characteristic imaging features (Rapaccini et al, 2004). The last feature may produce considerable diagnostic problems because small HCCs may be difficult to distinguish from large atypical nodules (see later). Lesions less than 2 cm may lack the classic features of HCC, exhibiting a close to normal trabecular architecture and minimal atypia (Kondo et al, 1989). Capsule formation seldom was found in tumors smaller than 1 cm in

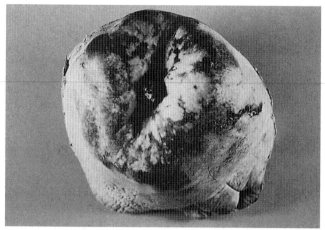

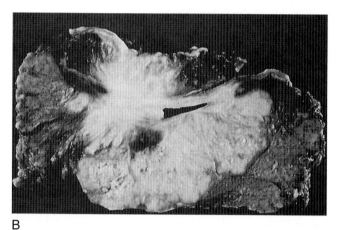

Fig. 69.9. A, Typical umbilication of the tumor as a result of collapse after central necrosis. The central depression of the umbilicated area shows a small tissue mass apparently above the capsular level. **B,** Section plane illustrates that epicapsular masses may not be involved in the tumor. The white core of this exterior lesion consists of connective tissue flanked by diaphragm muscle (dark tissue). The *black triangular structure* is a peritoneal pocket. Resection specimens.

diameter, whereas about 70% of tumors greater than 2 cm in diameter and found in association with cirrhosis had a fibrous capsule (Nakashima & Kojiro, 1987), suggesting that the probability of finding a capsule becomes greater the larger the lesion. Extracapsular growth and portal vein involvement become evident more frequently in tumors reaching or exceeding 3 to 5 cm, but some small HCCs may extend in an invasive fashion even in the early stage (Nakashima & Kojiro, 1987). In one study, detection of invasive growth was the most important parameter influencing tumor recurrence (Hsu et al, 1985), but tumor size as such seems to be a predictive factor for intrahepatic recurrence (Arii et al, 1992) and should be assessed carefully at gross examination of surgical specimens. Similarly, tumor vascularity seems to be significant for prognosis (Toyoda et al, 1997), and the distinct hemodynamic features of these lesions have been studied in detail (Kumada et al, 2004, Wen et al, 2004). More information on the pathology of small HCC is summarized subsequently.

The concept of small HCC could be questioned owing to the argument that, similar to other tumors, any larger HCC would have passed a stage where it was less than 2 or 3 cm in diameter during its evolution. At least a subset of such small and definitely malignant lesions seems to represent a distinct entity, however, with respect to morphology and biology, being different from early HCC. Early HCC has been defined on histologic grounds as a well-differentiated lesion, sometimes still containing Glisson's triads, growing without substantial destruction of the preexisting hepatic framework and seldom showing angioinvasion (Sakamoto et al, 1991). Genomic alterations already can be detected at this early cancer stage (Nagai et al, 1998). Early HCC, when defined as a lesion of 2 cm or less and proposed to represent a stage 0 lesion, seems to have a high rate of surgical cure (Takayama et al, 1998).

Assessment of Radicality: Resection Margin

The aim in performing liver resection is to remove the tumor with a sufficiently large clearance margin from the line of transection (see Ch. 80). What is a sufficient margin? What does a zone of liver tissue free of tumor mean for outcome? How is an

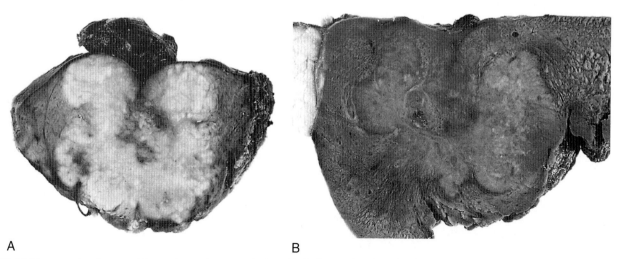

Fig. 69.10. Two examples of tumor with central necrosis communicating with the liver surface through a funnel-like structure. **A,** Very narrow gap and adherent non-neoplastic tissue. **B,** Gap produced by necrosis is larger. It is filled with stroma and granulation tissue. Resection specimens.

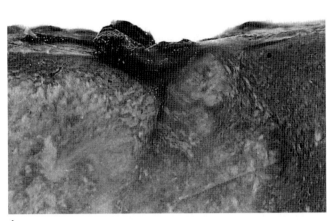
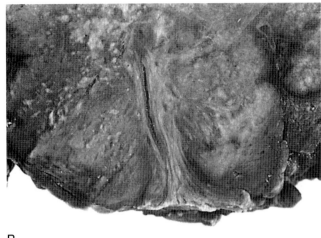

A   B

Fig. 69.11. A, Tumor growth extending to, but not involving, the liver capsule. There is a clear distinction between tumor mass and an adherent non-neoplastic tissue fragment. **B,** Tumor growth along a large preexisting tissue tract containing bile duct and blood vessels. Resection specimens.

"optimal resection margin" assessed? These questions cannot be answered fully at present. Theoretically, intrahepatic spread can occur through portal tracts; systematic wide resection may reduce the recurrence rate. The amount of substance that can be resected is limited, however, by loss of liver function, notwithstanding the fact that the liver has a considerable regenerative power. The question regarding a sufficiently wide clearance margin has been addressed in several studies. In one study, no significant difference between patients with and patients without a disease-free margin of 1 cm from the tumor edge with regard to intrahepatic recurrence was found (Arii et al, 1992). It was suggested that the presence or absence of a 1-cm disease-free margin is an inappropriate factor on which to base a significant differentiation, and that the appropriate distance from the tumor edge to the cut surface should be decided on the basis of the histopathologic properties of the tumor (Arii et al, 1992). Based on the investigation of the incidence of micrometastases, for HCC 3 cm or less, a proximal resection margin and a distal

margin of 1 cm were recommended, whereas for HCC greater than 3 cm, a 1-cm proximal resection margin and 2-cm distal margin were recommended (Shi et al, 2004).

The conjecture of a necessary resection margin was analyzed in a systematic study, and it was found that, among 65 patients with detailed measurement of macroscopic resection margins, a significant reduction of residual histologic disease was observed when a 0.5-cm margin had been established, whereas further extension of the margin had no additional benefit (Lai et al, 1991). Macroscopic assessment of the resection margin within this study was defined by taking the shortest distance measured between the edge of the lesion and the parenchymal transection line, but it also was stressed that gross measurement of a resection margin is an unreliable guide (Lai et al, 1991). A closer look at resection specimens may explain why this is so. A resection surface in most instances is not a flat area, but a complex surface characterized by parenchymal protrusions of variable size, depending on the original state of the tissue and on the resection technique used.

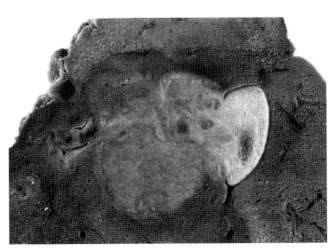

Fig. 69.12. Tumor invasion into the intrahepatic part of the adipose tissue–containing round ligament (to the right of center). Resection specimen.

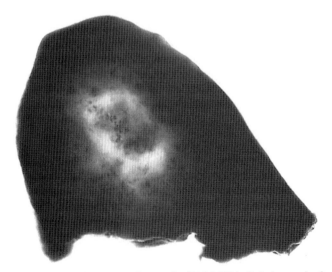

Fig. 69.13. Transillumination photograph of HCC (thick slice). As a result of hemorrhage, this tumor had zones of differing light penetrability. Resection specimen.

Fixation may contribute further to the irregularity of this surface. When performing a measurement, this irregular pattern becomes particularly crucial in situations in which the resected tumor is close to the resection margin because the distance measured (e.g., 0.5 cm) may be in the same range as the size of the protrusions and depressions found on the resection surface; the results strongly depend on the site of measurement.

In principle, the same is true for the geometry of the tumor edge, which may vary from a flat outer surface in the case of an expanding HCC to a highly irregular edge in the case of an invading lesion. Measuring distances on histologic sections to overcome this difficulty is just transposing the problem to another dimension, with an even greater sampling error. Pathologists should cooperate closely with surgeons to arrive at a standardized procedure, including distance categories to be given (realistically in steps of 0.5 cm) and using a protocol that specifies that always the tops of protrusions seen on the resection surface or the depressions found between them are taken as the reference points of measurement.

Microscopic Appearance

Diagnosis of HCC usually is based on the resemblance between tumor cells and normal hepatocytes (Anthony, 1973), and this assessment refers usually to the abundant eosinophilic cytoplasm within a polygonal cell and vesicular nucleus with a recognizable nucleolus (Fig. 69.14). Departures from these cytologic features include cells in which fewer differentiated characteristics are expressed so that primitive, poorly differentiated forms are found or in which cells with marked variations in the appearance

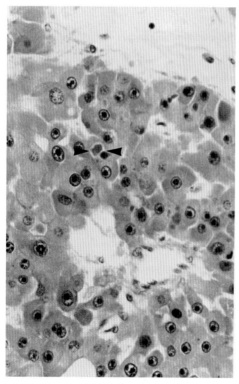

Fig. 69.14. Well-differentiated HCC. Prominent nucleoli, intracanalicular bile pigment inspissates *(arrowheads)*, and noticeable absence of Kupffer cells. (Hematoxylin and eosin stain, ×400.)

of the whole or component parts are observed. In addition, there may be striking variations in the stroma between cells. The arrangement of the cells contributes to the variety of microscopic appearances. On this basis, several types of tumor have been categorized, but it is not yet established fully if these variations reflect differences in behavior and influence prognosis (Berman et al, 1980; Peters, 1976), although some of the histologic features seem to act as prognosticators (Qin & Tang, 2002).

Functional changes in HCC cells also may reflect the degree of differentiation, and the ability to produce and excrete bile sometimes may show a morphologic counterpart in the form of inspissated bile between adjacent cells, probably within canaliculi (see Fig. 69.14). The presence of such inspissated bile implies a higher degree of cellular differentiation (Edmondson & Steiner, 1954; Peters, 1976). Failure to identify bile poses the difficulty of subjective assessment of the extent to which the tumor cells resemble normal liver cells, and although most diagnoses by experienced histopathologists made on this basis are validated, the possibility remains of an occasional tumor of another origin masquerading as HCC. HCC may be categorized as bile producing or consisting of cells resembling hepatocytes or both; the other microscopic variants are recognized on the basis of arrangements of the tumor cells, expression of distinct characteristics within the tumor cells, and production of an abnormal extracellular matrix, for which special procedures may be necessary (Kew, 1983).

Differentiation patterns used for tumor grading at present usually are based on the morphologic characteristics of the tumor cells more than on their arrangement (Hamilton & Aaltonen, 2000). Edmondson and Steiner (1954) divided HCC into grades I through IV, using a previously published classification as the basis (Broders, 1920). A grade I HCC, the most differentiated tumor, consists of a homogeneous cell population strongly resembling hepatocytes, and these cells usually are arranged in a thin trabecular pattern (Fig. 69.15). In most cases, grade I components seem to occur only locally and are associated with a grade II lesion. In grade II HCC, there is still a marked resemblance of the tumor cells to normal hepatocytes, but the nuclei are larger and more hyperchromatic, and the cytoplasm is abundant and often strongly eosinophilic. The nucleus may be laterally displaced as a result of marked development of the endoplasmic reticulum (Fig. 69.16). In grade III HCC, the nuclei are even more hyperchromatic and occupy a greater proportion of the cell; bile formation is noted less frequently, and tumor giant cells are most numerous in this group (Fig. 69.17). Grade IV HCC, which forms the most poorly differentiated group, exhibits large and atypical nuclei located in cells that are often low in cytoplasm. These tumors show a high cellularity, and bile is not easily detected or is not visible at all (Fig. 69.18).

Definition of types and subtypes of HCC is based on the morphology of the neoplastic cell population and the arrangement of these cells within the tumor. This normal hepatocyte plate pattern is recapitulated by many hepatocellular tumors, but hepatocellular plates may become much larger. Between these plates run irregular, thin-walled vascular spaces lined with endothelial cells. These vessels almost always lack Kupffer cells (Peters, 1976), and the presence of hepatic stellate cells is not generally noted (Anthony, 1973; Foster & Berman, 1977). Hepatocellular plates may be only one or two cells thick, in which case tumor cells are difficult to distinguish from normal nonmalignant hepatocytes; in other situations, plates with more than 10 cells occur (macrotrabecular pattern) (Fig. 69.19).

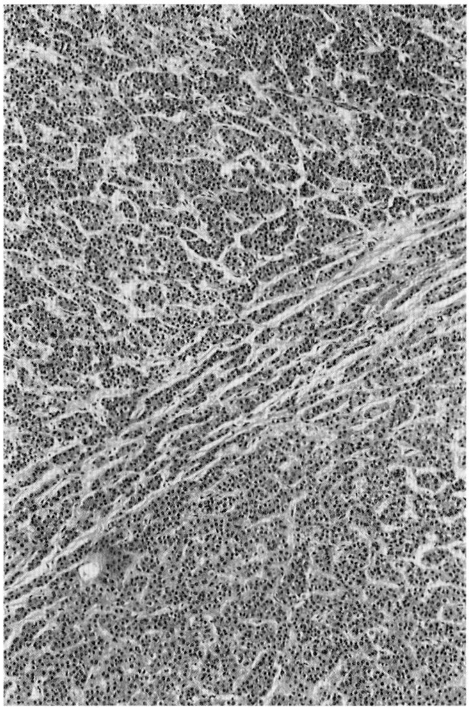

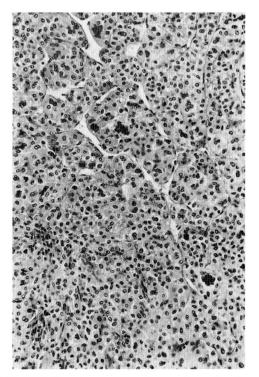

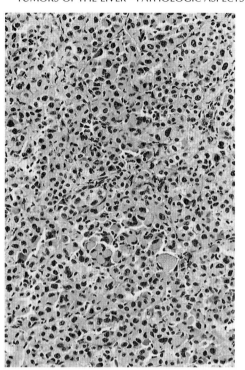

Fig. 69.15. Well-differentiated HCC. The neoplastic cells are arranged in a thin trabecular pattern. (Hematoxylin and eosin stain, ×40.)

Fig. 69.16. HCC grade II according to Edmondson and Steiner (1954). The neoplastic cells still resemble normal hepatocytes, but the nuclei are larger and more hyperchromatic. (Hematoxylin and eosin stain, ×150.)

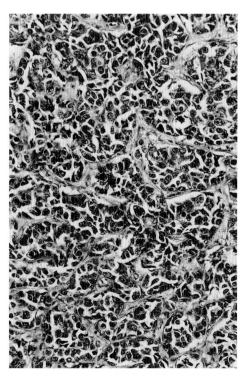

Fig. 69.17. HCC. Note the occurrence of tumor giant cells, a feature most frequently encountered in grade III carcinomas. (Hematoxylin and eosin stain, ×150.)

Fig. 69.18. HCC. This tumor is highly cellular, and its nuclei are more prominent than the cytoplasm (grade IV). (Hematoxylin and eosin stain, ×150.)

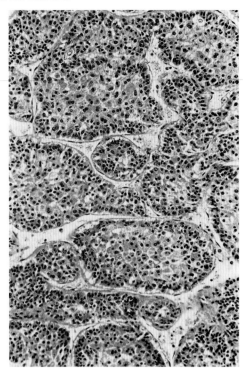

Fig. 69.19. The hepatocellular plates of this HCC are very large and sometimes more than 10 cells thick. This arrangement of cells is termed *a macrotrabecular pattern.* (Hematoxylin and eosin stain, ×40.)

A deviation from the classic trabecular arrangement of hepatocytes is found in instances in which a distinct or enlarged canaliculus forms a central structure surrounded by tumor cells, resulting in some sort of glandular or pseudoglandular pattern (Fig. 69.20). This arrangement is termed an *acinar structure,* and large lumina sometimes are formed. Combinations of these appearances are frequent.

The classification employed by the World Health Organization (Gibson & Sobin, 1978; Hamilton & Aaltonen, 2000) refers to cellular arrangements observed in HCC and defines the following histologic patterns: *trabecular* and *pseudoglandular* or *acinar.* The World Health Organization added two types, which differ from the foregoing: the *compact pattern,* in which a basically trabecular pattern is recognized but the tumor cells grow in apparently solid masses and sinusoids are rendered inconspicuous by compression, and the *scirrhous pattern,* in which areas with abundant fibrous stroma separate cords of tumor cells. The latter pattern is seen mostly after radiation, chemotherapy, and infarction. The morphology of some HCC deviates from the features described so far, and in the following section the histology of these variants is briefly described.

Variants of Hepatocellular Carcinoma

The *clear cell variant* of HCC is a tumor that is predominantly or wholly composed of cells with clear cytoplasm (Fig. 69.21). This variant of HCC may be composed entirely of clear cells or may express these features in a focal pattern only. The pertinent literature was reviewed by Liu and colleagues (2004). In one series, less than 10% of HCC contained a clear cell component, but these cases showed a slightly older mean age of the patients

and a male-to-female ratio of 1.6:1, which is lower than the worldwide ratio of 6.7:1 for other HCC (Buchanan & Huvos, 1974). In a series from East Asia, 12.5% of the cases studied were diffuse clear cell HCC (Lai et al, 1989). The biologic behavior may be similar to (Kishi et al, 1983) or better than (Lai et al, 1989) that of other forms of HCC. In some instances, the clear cell variant is associated with a marked desmoplastic reaction (Buchanan & Huvos, 1974). On an ultrastructural level, substantial quantities of glycogen and lipids can be observed (Wu et al, 1983). Clear cell HCC may be associated with hypoglycemia and hypercholesterolemia (Sasaki et al, 1981), and sudden death from severe hypoglycemia has been reported (Ross & Kurian, 1985).

One group of HCC is characterized by the formation of pleomorphic cells or giant cells or both and is termed the *pleomorphic variant.* HCCs whose giant cells lack the pleomorphism seen in HCC with anaplastic giant cells are termed *hepatic giant cell carcinoma* (Hood et al, 1990) or *HCC with osteoclast-like giant cells* (Kuwano et al, 1984).

Some HCCs contain various cytoplasmic inclusions usually round in shape, which may be periodic acid–Schiff–positive. Another type of inclusion found in some HCC is more dense and more irregularly shaped, is periodic acid–Schiff–negative, and strongly resembles Mallory bodies. Mallory bodies usually are found in neoplastic cells rich in cytoplasm (Fig. 69.22), and tumors harboring numerous Mallory bodies are termed *Mallory body–rich HCCs.* Three distinct patterns of Mallory bodies have been found in human HCC—a clustering type, a diffuse type, and a sparse type (Nakanuma & Ohta, 1986).

Fibrolamellar HCC (fibrolamellar carcinoma) (Fig. 69.23) is a distinct variant of HCC characterized by large polygonal tumor cells embedded in fibrous stroma forming bands or lamellar

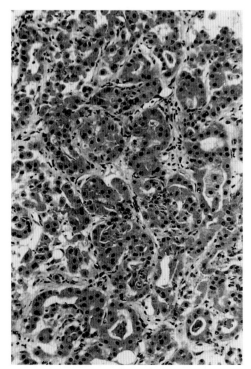

Fig. 69.20. This type of HCC forms lumina lined by neoplastic cells, corresponding to a pseudoglandular or acinar pattern. (Hematoxylin and eosin stain, ×150.)

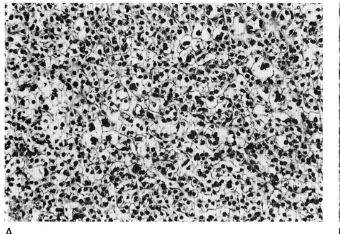
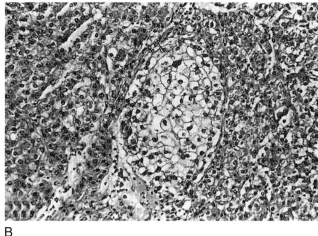

A B

Fig. 69.21. HCC, clear cell variant. **A,** Clear cell change is diffuse. **B,** Clear cell carcinoma nodule is embedded in carcinoma showing the more usual granular cells. (Hematoxylin and eosin stain, ×150.)

structures (Berman et al, 1980; Kaczynski et al, 1996; Saab & Yao, 1996). Similar to ordinary HCC, a clear cell variant has been described (Cheuk & Chan, 2001). In a population-based study of the Surveillance, Epidemiology, and End Results program (1986-1999), fibrolamellar HCC constituted 0.85% of all cases of primary liver cancer and 13.4% of all cases in patients younger than age 40, and the age-adjusted incidence rate for this tumor was 0.02 per 100,000 (El-Serag & Davila, 2004). The marked stromal response is associated with prominent matrix turnover (Schoedel et al, 2003). As in other situations in which distinct fibrosis ensues, fibrogenic cytokines seem to be involved in the excessive stroma formation, in particular, transforming growth factor-β (Orsatti et al, 1997). In contrast to other types of HCC, fibrolamellar HCC seems to express abundantly type 7 cytokeratin and, in some cells, biliary-type cytokeratin 19, which may suggest that the differentiation and origin of this unique tumor are different in some ways from those of other HCCs (Van Eyken et al, 1990a). Fibrolamellar HCC predominates in young adults and was thought to be associated with a more favorable prognosis. A study of 46 patients enrolled in

the Pediatric Intergroup Hepatoma Protocol showed, however, that children with fibrolamellar HCC do not have a favorable prognosis and do not respond any differently to current therapeutic regimens than patients with typical HCC (Katzenstein et al, 2003).

The tumor may be spatially associated with focal nodular hyperplasia (FNH) and sometimes has a morphologic appearance at imaging that is difficult to distinguish from FNH (Saul et al, 1987). Generally, fibrolamellar HCC is larger on first presentation (mean 12 cm) (Berman et al, 1980) than FNH, however,

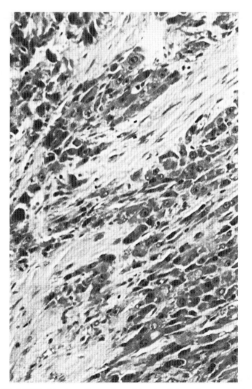

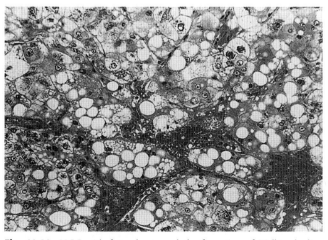

Fig. 69.22. HCC with fatty change and the formation of Mallory bodies. The latter are visualized as distinct, dark inclusions in the cytoplasm of some of the neoplastic cells. (Hematoxylin and eosin stain, ×150.)

Fig. 69.23. HCC, fibrolamellar variant. Islands of large hepatocellular tumor cells between hypocellular mature fibrous tissue.

which is larger than 10 cm in only 3% to 4% of cases (Kerlin et al, 1983). Patients with fibrolamellar HCC are more likely to have abdominal pain (74%) and a palpable abdominal mass (67%) compared with patients with FNH, in whom 80% to 90% of lesions are incidental findings (Saul et al, 1987). A central scarlike lesion may be seen in both tumors, but calcifications indicate fibrolamellar HCC (Friedman et al, 1985). The question of whether fibrolamellar HCC may arise in FNH is not yet resolved. Fibrolamellar HCC has interesting biochemical characteristics that can be used in preoperative evaluation. High serum vitamin B_{12} binding capacity has been proposed as a marker of fibrolamellar HCC (Paradinas et al, 1982), and elevated neurotensin values in serum can be found in patients with fibrolamellar HCC (Collier et al, 1984). Fibrolamellar HCC can express aromatase (Hany et al, 1997), which may result in clinically manifest steroid action, such as gynecomastia (Agarwal et al, 1998).

Some HCCs other than the fibrolamellar variant also may produce large amounts of fibrous stroma and have been described as *sclerosing HCCs*. These tumors usually consist of compressed, sometimes elongated, hepatocytes surrounded by moderately cellular fibrous tissue with some evidence of sinusoidal spaces. In contrast to fibrolamellar HCC, this variety is found in older patients and sometimes is associated with hypercalcemia (Samuelsson & Werner, 1963). Parathyroid hormone–related protein has been detected in this variant (Albar et al, 1996; Kitazawa et al, 1999). It may be confused with cholangiocarcinoma, but does not produce acid mucin. Closely related (or the same) variants, but termed *HCC composed of dense collagenous stroma,* have been found to be associated with long-term survival and may form a distinct morphologic and clinical subset of HCC (Sonoda et al, 1989). In this variant, nodules of cancer cells are separated widely by a dense fibrous stroma containing an abundant lymphocytic infiltration. A high density of lymphocytes also has been observed in a subset of HCC less than 3 cm (Wada et al, 1998), indicating that several and eventually clinically relevant subtypes of HCC may have this distinct feature.

A few (about 4%) HCCs consist of cytokeratin-expressing and vimentin-expressing spindle cells and multinucleated cells. Without immunohistochemistry, these tumors are difficult to identify as epithelial in origin and are known as *HCC with sarcomatous change* or *sarcomatoid HCC* (Haratake & Horie, 1991; Kakizoe et al, 1987). They lack α-fetoprotein (AFP) in serum or show low AFP levels only and are characterized by a high incidence of extrahepatic metastases.

Fat (triglyceride) droplets are observed in many HCCs, but fatty change in some instances represents a dominant morphologic feature. These tumors appear yellow on gross examination and may be termed *fatty HCC* (Yoshikawa et al, 1988) or lipid-rich clear cell HCC (Orikasa et al, 2001). Histologic examination discloses numerous macrovesicular structures in the cytoplasm of the tumor cells; these structures have been shown to contain neutral fat when examined in frozen sections (Fig. 69.24). HCCs with extensive fatty metamorphosis are usually well-differentiated, sometimes large tumors that may contain considerable amounts of bile. Features seen on imaging (Yoshikawa et al, 1988) have to be distinguished from other nodular lesions known to accumulate fat, such as fatty macroregenerative nodules in nonsteatotic liver cirrhosis (Terada et al, 1989a). Similar to other groups of epithelial tumors, HCC may consist of small cells, which is termed *small cell carcinoma of the liver* (Zanconati et al, 1996). In cases in which a high density of dilated sinusoid-like vessels is

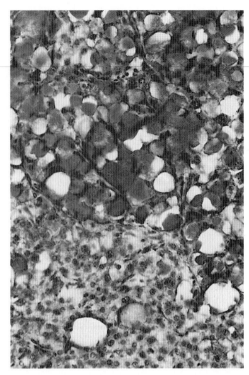

Fig. 69.24. HCC with strong fatty change (so-called fatty HCC). In this frozen section, droplets of dark-staining neutral fat are visible in tumor cells. Large vacuoles represent gaps formerly occupied by lipid droplets.

a hallmark of the tumor, the term *pelioid HCC* has been proposed (Peters, 1976).

Mixed/Combined Hepatocellular Carcinoma–Cholangiocarcinoma

Mixed/combined HCC-cholangiocarcinoma (HCC-CC) represents an uncommon group of primary hepatic carcinomas presenting features of hepatocelullar and cholangiocellular epithelial differentiation. Previously, some of these lesions were regarded as *collision tumors* (Goodman et al, 1985). In the more recent literature, *combined HCC-CC* is more commonly used, but a stringent definition of this tumor group is still needed. In particular, the relationship of combined HCC-CC to either HCC or CC is still controversial. The variability in interpretation and classification has caused divergent results when analyzing clinical features and outcomes. It has been reported that the demographic and clinical features of patients with combined tumors were most similar to those of patients with cholangiocarcinoma (Jarnagin et al, 2002). It has been proposed that combined HCC-CC might be a variant of HCC with cholangiocellular features (Yano et al, 2003). In regard to gender distribution, combined HCC-CC seems to be intermediate between HCC and cholangiocarcinoma (Jarnagin et al, 2002). In one study of 21 patients from South Asia, increased serum AFP was present in 61.5%, and histologic evidence of cirrhosis or chronic hepatitis was present in 77.8% (Ng et al, 1998). In a group of patients from Korea, the prevalence of cirrhosis in combined HCC-CC patients was intermediate between HCC and cholangiocarcinoma (Koh et al, 2005). In contrast, an investigation with a small population of Asian heritage patients showed that combined tumors were not associated with chronic liver disease (Jarnagin et al, 2002). The overall survival times were short, suggesting that the clinical features of combined HCC-CC are more akin to HCC than to cholangiocarcinoma (Ng et al, 1998). Another study found overall survival rates for combined HCC-CC to be shorter than for HCC, however (Yano et al, 2003). There was a trend of cholangiocellular differentiation to worsen prognosis (Jarnagin et al, 2002).

These tumors have been subclassified further according to their main growth patterns. A single nodular variant has been separated from a multinodular variant. The single nodular type shows a pattern of infiltration similar to HCC, whereas the multinodular type resembles intrahepatic cholangiocarcinoma (Sasaki et al, 2001). Based on CT, three enhancement patterns reflecting three types of masses have been described (Sanada et al, 2005). More detailed investigations of histology, immuno-histochemistry, and RNA expression have added considerably to better understanding of these tumors and their features of biphenotypic differentiation. It has been shown that combined HCC-CC contains areas morphologically intermediate between HCC and cholangiocarcinoma (transitional-type tumors), and that more than 90% exhibit mRNA signals for albumin also in cholangiocarcinoma-like areas (Tickoo et al, 2002).

Pathogenetically, a derivation of the mixed cell lineages from bipotential hepatic progenitor cells may be assumed (Kim et al, 2004). This view may be supported by the finding of rare hepatic tumors in adults that have features of hepatic progenitor cell origin (*hepatic stem cell malignancies*) (Theise et al, 2003). A detailed study of the allelic status of several chromosomes in combined HCC-CC revealed a highest frequency of loss of heterozygosity (LOH) on 4q and 17p, followed by 8p and 16q. The genetic patterns observed were allocated to three possible pathways of origin: (1) collision tumor, in which two independent neoplastic clones develop in close proximity; (2) single clonal tumor with homogeneous genetic background in both components, but divergent differentiation; and (3) single clonal process in which genetic heterogeneity in the process of clonal evolution parallels histologic diversity (Fujii et al, 2000). In regard to cell differentiation in combined tumors, a role of the hepatocyte growth factor/c-met tyrosine receptor kinase system has been discussed (Varnholt et al, 2002).

Other Morphologic Features of Hepatocellular Carcinoma

It is well known that HCCs arising in hemochromatosis fail to show accumulation of stainable iron (Hirota et al, 1982), with a few intriguing exceptions. A similar phenomenon has been observed during experimental carcinogenesis in rodents over-loaded with iron (Williams & Yamamoto, 1972). A lack of capa-bility of liver cells to produce hemosiderin may represent a diagnostic marker, and iron-negative foci in siderotic macroregen-erative nodules in human cirrhotic livers have been suggested to be a marker for incipient neoplastic lesions (Terada & Nakanuma, 1989).

Some HCCs accumulate copper, which can be detected using histochemical methods, and it has been reported that the serum copper concentration is sometimes higher in patients with HCC than in patients with liver cirrhosis not associated with HCC (Miatto et al, 1985). Accumulation of large amounts of copper and copper-binding protein (orcein-positive) has been found

chiefly in the fibrolamellar variant of HCC (Lefkowitch et al, 1983), but metallothionein and copper and zinc levels generally are associated with tumor differentiation in HCC (Tashiro-Itoh et al, 1997). Prominent copper accumulation also has been shown in some small or minute HCCs (Haratake et al, 1986). Some neoplastic liver cells may develop a disorder of the handling of copper or of copper-binding proteins, which is expressed in an early stage of tumor evolution.

There are some unusual instances in which HCC produces substances that occur in some rare metabolic disorders (e.g., *black HCC* occurred in a patient without Dubin-Johnson syndrome, but the tumor contained pigment strongly resembling the pigment found in the latter disorder) (Roth et al, 1982). A sarcoid-like reaction sometimes may be encountered within HCC, the granulomas being characterized by epithelioid cells, Langerhans-type giant cells, and varying numbers of lympho-cytes (Fig. 69.25) (Nakashima & Kojiro, 1987). This reaction may represent a mechanism of immunosurveillance or anti-tumor immune reaction, but nonspecific, fortuitous phenomena cannot be excluded (e.g., a foreign body–type response to some disintegration products of the tumor).

Morphology of Small Hepatocellular Carcinoma

Small HCCs (see earlier) are of interest in light of their natural history and their clinical significance (Belli et al, 1989; Ebara et al, 1986), and it is necessary to analyze whether their morphol-ogy differs from that of larger HCC, or whether they represent only a smaller histologic window of the overall histology well known for other lesions. Several studies have addressed this question in the past. It generally is agreed that many small HCCs (i.e., lesions <2 cm in diameter) have a well-differentiated

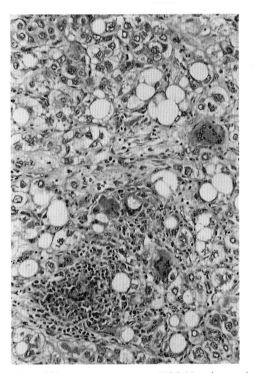

Fig. 69.25. Sarcoid-like reaction occurring in a HCC. Note the granuloma and several giant cells of the Langhans type. (Hematoxylin and eosin stain, ×150.)

appearance and are difficult to diagnose (Kojiro, 1989; Kondo et al, 1990). In a systematic study, 60% of tumors had cells arranged in trabecules of almost normal thickness (normotrabecular pattern). Such a pattern may lead to considerable problems for the pathologist in the case of small samples. Additional alterations, such as nuclear crowding (similar to dysplastic nodules; see later) (Terasaki et al, 1998), occasional microacinar formation, and an increase in cytoplasmic basophilia, may be of some diagnostic help (Kondo et al, 1987). Other potentially useful criteria include fatty change, the presence of Mallory bodies, storage of excessive copper, accumulation of bile and glycogen, clear cell clusters, and the formation of a fibrous capsule (Haratake et al, 1986; Kojiro, 1989; Kondo et al, 1990; Motohashi et al, 1992; Nakanuma & Ohta, 1984; Nakanuma et al, 1981; Terada et al, 1989b).

Notwithstanding the possibility that all these criteria in some instances may combine and facilitate a clear diagnosis, many cases remain where the histologic diagnosis of small HCC is difficult or impossible, and where its distinction from large, but reactive nodules cannot be made. To circumvent these difficulties, more sophisticated and mainly morphometric methods have been worked out and applied to this type of lesion (Motohashi et al, 1990, 1992). In studies of this type, the use of morphometric parameters, such as the nuclear shape factor, has allowed HCC to be differentiated correctly from conditions such as HCC-like lesions, but further work is needed to develop reliable strategies suitable for situations in which most of the diagnosis depends on histologic assessment. What is relevant with regard to the evolution of small lesions is also largely unknown. Minute HCCs seem to undergo no appreciable change for many years (Yoshida et al, 1982), whereas others have a more rapid evolution. Theoretically, capsule formation may act as some sort of barrier, at least in a mechanistic sense, and fibrous capsules have been found in small HCCs less than 3 cm in diameter (Nakashima, 1989). No relationship between the thickness of the capsule and the degree of tumor differentiation has been found, however (Ohno, 1985). Conversely, connective tissues (as components of capsules) are structures of considerable biologic plasticity and have the capability of turnover so that the mere presence of a capsule may not have much effect on limiting the size of a tumor that has started to grow invasively. The demonstration of invasiveness may be significant in the evaluation of small or early HCC, particularly portal tract invasion (Nakano et al, 1981).

Special Examinations of Hepatocellular Carcinoma

Special examinations of HCC include ultrastructural, immunohistochemical, and, more recently, molecular biologic examinations, such as in situ hybridization, polymerase chain reaction, and other analyses performed with extracted tumor DNA. Transmission electron microscopy shows well-differentiated HCC cells containing abundant mitochondria, which may not be so evident in cells that appear to be poorly differentiated on examination by light microscopy (Ma & Biempica, 1971), and so electron microscopy does not always provide valuable confirmatory evidence in the diagnosis of HCC. In contrast, immunohistochemical methods for diagnosing liver tumors have evolved rapidly in recent years, and the antigens detectable by this approach include those of typical hepatocyte export proteins, components of the cytoskeleton (in particular, intermediate filament proteins), membrane glycoproteins and receptors,

hormone and growth factor receptors, and components of the extracellular matrix. Although a broad array of cellular and extracellular components has been tested so far, relatively few have gained an established position in the diagnosis of HCC (Varma & Cohen, 2004).

Among the export proteins produced and secreted by hepatocytes and their neoplastic offspring, *AFP* is probably the most important. Immunoreactive AFP is found as a granular reaction product in the cytoplasm of some, but not all, HCC (Fig. 69.26) (Kojiro et al, 1981), and its distribution has been analyzed in several studies (Ganjei et al, 1988; Hirohashi et al, 1983; Otsuru et al, 1988). AFP immunohistochemistry may be used to separate acinar-type HCC from cholangiocarcinoma, which is clearly AFP negative, even though visible expression of AFP in HCC may be found in less than 20% of cases (Ganjei et al, 1988). Other export proteins known to occur in HCC are α_1-antitrypsin and ferritin (Fig. 69.27) (Ganjei et al, 1988).

HCC cells express a typical pattern of cytoskeletal intermediate filaments. Normal human hepatocytes contain only cytokeratins 8 and 18 of the catalogue of Moll, whereas bile duct cells express cytokeratins 7, 8, 18, and 19. In most instances, the cytokeratin pattern of normal hepatocytes is preserved in their neoplastic offspring (Johnson et al, 1988; Lai et al, 1989; Van Eyken

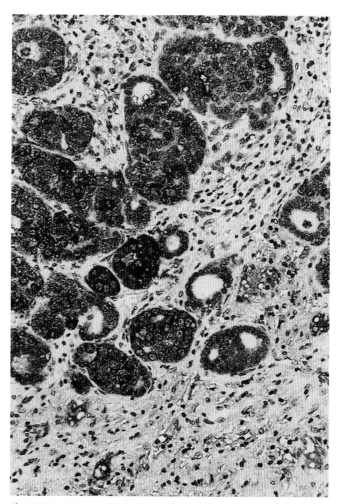

Fig. 69.26. Expression of α-fetoprotein in a mixed trabecular and acinar HCC. Expression is visible in the form of a dark reaction product within the tumor cells. (Immunoperoxidase stain.)

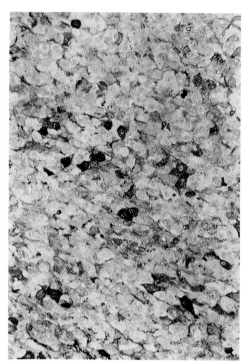

Fig. 69.27. Expression of ferritin in HCC. A few of the neoplastic cells are shown to have a dark-staining reaction product in the cytoplasm. (Immunoperoxidase stain.)

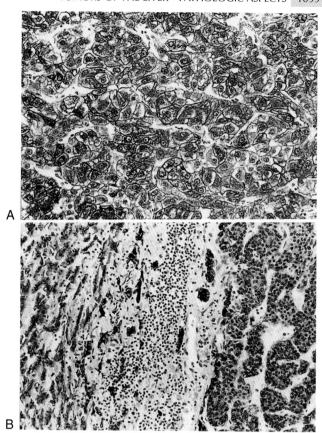

Fig. 69.28. Cytokeratin expression in HCC. **A,** Expression of cytokeratins typical of hepatocytes (CAM 5.2, an antibody system directed against cytokeratins 8 and 18). The cell periphery is strongly stained. **B,** Expression of the biliary-type cytokeratin 19 at the border of HCC. The cells of non-neoplastic ductules are strongly positive, whereas neither the HCC nor the normal hepatocytes show staining. (Immunoperoxidase stain.)

et al, 1988), the situation in fibrolamellar HCC being a notable exception (Van Eyken et al, 1990a). In a larger series, 17 of 34 cases of HCC showed reactivity only with monoclonal anti-cytokeratins 8 and 18, but an aberrant expression of the biliary-type cytokeratin 19 also may be noted (Terada et al, 1995; Van Eyken et al, 1988), indicating that, at least at the cytoskeletal level, some sort of bidirectional differentiation may occur (Fig. 69.28). In addition to the above-listed components, hepatocyte-specific antigens have been tested with the goal to identify HCC more easily (Minervini et al, 1997).

HCC may express receptors for signal substances, growth factors, and hormones. These include the transferrin receptor, of which an intense expression has been noted in HCC (Sciot et al, 1988), in contrast to benign liver cell tumors (Sciot et al, 1990), but the significance of this finding has not yet been clarified. It generally is accepted that the liver is one of the target organs for estrogens, and a possible correlation of estrogens with the development of liver tumors has been suggested by many reports of oral contraceptive–associated liver cell adenoma and HCC (see later). As in some geographic regions, most HCCs occur in men with cirrhosis; elevated estrogen and decreased testosterone levels in serum also have been suggested to play a role in hepatocarcinogenesis.

Estrogen receptors can be shown in cell populations by immunohistochemical and biochemical methods, but the results obtained so far for HCC do not allow final conclusions to be drawn. Some authors have found estrogen receptors to be decreased in the HCC compared with the surrounding tissue (Francavilla et al, 1991), whereas others have found that some, but not all, specimens of HCC show elevated levels of either estrogen or androgen receptors (Eagon et al, 1991). These conflicting results may be due at least in part to the biologic

fragility of steroid hormone receptors or to the low amounts of receptors present in hepatic tissue. To overcome the difficulties posed by some methods, including immunohistochemistry, new techniques are increasingly being developed to detect small amounts of crucial substances (e.g., measuring receptor mRNA using Northern blot analysis and the polymerase chain reaction). Using these methods, androgen receptor mRNA has been shown in human HCC (Nakagama et al, 1991). Refined methods also are needed to understand better the production, turnover, and biologic significance of other compounds and receptors found in HCC, such as epidermal growth factor, fibroblast growth factor, and insulin-like growth factor II (Lamas et al, 1991; Motoo et al, 1991).

Extracellular Matrix of Hepatocellular Carcinoma

The extracellular matrix of the liver, consisting of cells and their specific products, plays an important role in mediating the normal development and maintenance of the normal architecture of this organ. In particular, the maintenance of hepatocyte shape, polarity, and position may be strongly influenced by the extracellular matrix, as are at least some of the liver cell functions (Gleiberman et al, 1989). Theoretically, it may be anticipated that the interaction between epithelial cells and the extracellular matrix may be disturbed in the case of neoplastic growth, and that such changes may be amenable to morphologic examination.

The cellular products that form a large part of the extracellular matrix consist of members of the collagen family of proteins (Van der Rest & Garrone, 1991), collagen-associated fibrillar proteins, elastin, mucopolysaccharides, and basement membranes, the last being composed of a whole array of proteins (e.g., collagen type IV, laminin, nidogen, entactin). Normal and neoplastic cells are capable of producing or interacting with these components; interaction usually is mediated by distinct types of receptors, such as integrins, nonintegrin proteins, sulfated polysaccharides, and glycolipids (Mecham, 1991). It is currently thought that these interactions play a crucial role in the pathogenesis of neoplastic cell spread and tissue remodeling.

Laminin, a large glycoprotein with several subunits (A, B1, B2, S, and M), is an integral basement membrane protein (Beck et al, 1990), which in the normal liver is distributed in the basement membranes of blood vessels, the epithelial basement membranes of the bile ducts, and under the capsular mesothelium. Most authors agree that laminin is not, or only sparsely, deposited in the perisinusoidal space, which is in keeping with the fact that no continuous basement membrane is seen in the extracellular matrix in this area. Under normal conditions, laminin synthesis does not seem to be a function of hepatocytes, but rather of mesenchymal, endothelial, and bile duct epithelial cells (Milani et al, 1989); however, some laminin chains may be expressed by fetal hepatocytes and hepatocytes in culture (Rescan et al, 1990). Immunohistochemical studies on HCC have shown that laminin is deposited in these tumors in a peritrabecular or periacinar pattern (Fig. 69.29) (Donato et al, 1989; Grigioni et al, 1987, 1991; Liétard et al, 1998), indicating that HCC can produce basement membrane glycoproteins.

Similarly, HCC may express other known components of basement membranes and of the extracellular matrix as a whole, such as fibronectin (see Fig. 69.29) (Donato et al, 1989), with an alternative splicing pattern of its mRNA (Matsui et al, 1997), collagens type III and IV (Donato et al, 1989; Grigioni et al, 1991; Gulubova, 1997), heparan sulfate proteoglycan (Roskams et al, 1998), and tenascin (Yamada et al, 1992; Zhao et al, 1996). The potential biologic significance of these findings is emphasized by the observations that basement membrane or laminin phenotypic expression may be influenced by the degree of tumor differentiation (Grigioni et al, 1987, 1991), and that the production of these extracellular matrix components may modify tumor cell adhesion, locomotion, and invasion (Zimmermann & Keller, 1987). Synthesis of extracellular matrix components also may represent a significant mechanism of capsule formation around HCC (Torimura et al, 1991), with extracellular matrix production probably mediated by myofibroblast-like cells (Ooi et al, 1997), which generally seem to play a pivotal role in stroma formation in liver tumors (Terada et al, 1996; Tran Van Nhieu et al, 1998).

Another extracellular matrix molecule that appears to be located mainly at the crucial epitheliomesenchymal interface is tenascin (Anbazhagan et al, 1990; Jones et al, 1989). In HCC, tenascin expression was found at the sites of invasion (i.e., where remodeling of the extracellular matrix is thought to occur) (Yamada et al, 1992), which is of particular interest because tenascin has been shown to stimulate tumor cell proliferation and to decrease cellular adhesiveness (Chiquet-Ehrismann et al, 1986, 1988). The mechanisms regulating the turnover of extracellular matrix proteins in liver tumors are only partially known, but fibrogenic cytokines, including transforming growth factor-β1 and its isoforms and receptors (Orsatti et al, 1997), and extracellular matrix–degrading enzymes, such as metalloproteinases and their inhibitors (Harada et al, 1998; Musso et al, 1997), play a significant role.

Growth of Hepatocellular Carcinoma

Overall growth characteristics of HCC may be estimated in vivo by assessing tumor doubling times based on sequential imaging of the lesions and, in the future, by performing solid organ volumetry using Cavalieri's method on CT scans (Pache et al, 1992). The assessment of the growth fractions depends on appropriate tissue samples. Growth rates so far have been estimated mainly in small or minute HCC, and it has been found that doubling times vary considerably, also with respect to the patient population studied. An increase in diameter of 1 cm may take a few months to several years. Longer time periods probably are related to the observation that small HCCs may enter phases

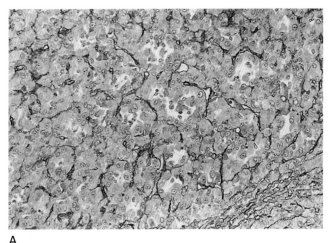

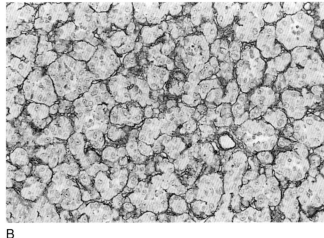

A   B

Fig. 69.29. Expression of extracellular matrix proteins in HCC. **A,** Laminin is deposited in these tumors in a peritrabecular fashion. **B,** A similar pattern is found with fibronectin. (Immunoperoxidase stain.)

of very slow or even undetectable growth (Cottone et al, 1989; Ebara et al, 1986; Oka et al, 1990; Okazaki et al, 1989; Sheu et al, 1985; Yoshida et al, 1982).

Growth of tumors is the result of two mechanisms counteracting each other:(1) increase of mass via proliferation of tumor cells and production of stroma, vessels, and other tissue components and (2) loss of mass through cell decay (necrosis and apoptosis) and cell emigration. With respect to increase in tumor cell number, several methods are now available for analyzing the nuclear DNA content of HCC cells and for estimating the proliferation pattern of the cells involved. Proliferating cells can be assessed by use of DNA labeling of cells brought into culture or employing immunohistochemistry (antibodies directed against Ki-67, proliferating cell nuclear antigen, DNA polymerase) (Seki et al, 1992; Terada & Nakanuma, 1992). Using the bromodeoxyuridine technique in vivo, a wide variation in the labeling indices of HCC has been found, with a tendency of less differentaited tumors to show a higher proliferation fraction (Tarao et al, 1989). In principle, similar findings have been obtained by estimating proliferating cell nuclear antigen, which is correlated with Ki-67 labeling (Hall et al, 1990) and flow cytometric data (Garcia et al, 1989). Ki-67 labeling seems to be related to tumor differentiation (Ng et al, 1995), and HCC with elevated proliferation showed a shorter survival (Soini et al, 1996). In a more recent study, however, neither Ki-67 nor proliferating cell nuclear antigen was an independent prognostic parameter, whereas high fractions of proliferating cells were predictive of early relapse (Nolte et al, 1998).

The assessment of proliferative activity and DNA ploidy patterns (Fujimoto et al, 1991; Kuo et al, 1987; Nagasue et al, 1992) is also of significance when estimating the transition from precursor lesions to fully established cancer and the disease progression. Proliferating cell nuclear antigen labeling has been performed in nodule-in-nodule lesions (see later), and it was found that the labeling index was high in the inner components, intermediate in the outer part of the nodules, and low in the surrounding parenchyma (Matsuno et al, 1990). Similar to proliferating cell nuclear antigen, a higher labeling of HCC compared with the adjacent liver tissue has been noted when analyzing the Ki-67 antigen (Grigioni et al, 1989). Generally, hepatocyte proliferation seems to be a powerful parameter for predicting HCC development in liver cirrhosis (Borzio et al, 1998), and further progression of established tumors is associated with variable proliferation, but also changes in nuclear DNA ploidy (Oriyama et al, 1998).

Although loss of tissue through necrosis is well known for HCC, the complex phenomenon of tumor cell apoptosis (also termed *programmed cell death*) counteracting an increase in cellularity brought about by proliferation has been studied in more detail, specifically in relation to future therapies of HCC, only more recently (Schuchmann & Galle, 2004). Apoptosis occurs in HCC (Hino et al, 1996), and it seems to be associated with the expression of a factor modulating apoptosis (i.e., *p53*) (Zhao & Zimmermann, 1997). The role of one of the most important mediators of programmed cell death, Fas, is still controversial in HCC, however (Higaki et al, 1996; Jiang et al, 1999; Kubo et al, 1998; Watson, 1999). Expression of an apoptosis protector, *bcl*-2, has been observed in HCC (Zhao et al, 1994a), and data regarding expression by HCC of numerous known factors regulating apoptosis are rapidly increasing (Fields et al, 2004; Park et al, 2004; Persad et al, 2004; Watanabe et al, 2004). The biologic significance of apoptosis is underlined by

the observation that a low degree of apoptosis and necrosis is associated with shortened survival in HCC (Soini et al, 1996), probably as a result of the phenomenon that reduced cell loss in these situations is overcompensated by proliferative activity.

Several factors that have been shown to exert a regulatory influence on cell proliferation and differentiation in other tissues also have been shown to play a role in HCC. These factors include basic fibroblast growth factor (Kin et al, 1997), transforming growth factor-α (Nalesnik et al, 1998), transforming growth factor-β (Bedossa et al, 1995; Ito et al, 1991), insulin-like growth factor-II (Sohda et al, 1997), and hepatocyte growth factor and the receptor c-met (Noguchi et al, 1996; Ogasawara et al, 1998; Zhao & Zimmermann, 1998). The links between genetic changes occurring in HCC and the expression of such factors and of members of signaling pathways are currently being studied.

Invasion and Spread of Hepatocellular Carcinoma

The question of whether a second tumor mass in the liver represents a metastatic deposit or an independent tumor, including nodular precursor lesions, has been discussed in detail (Peters, 1976), and the distinction is sometimes unclear, particularly in the case of small tumors detected in a cirrhotic liver (Kishi et al, 1983). The evidence of intrahepatic spread of HCC is persuasive (Willis, 1948), however, and is easily documented in instances in which several small tumor foci are grouped around a large tumor. These foci frequently are supported by the presence of grossly or microscopically visible angioinvasion, including invasion of the portal vein. The latter seems to be of considerable clinical significance because only three factors (performance status, tumor thrombus in the main portal vein trunk, and age) were shown to have independent prognostic value (Okada et al, 1992). Tumor vascularization and angioarchitecure are ratelimiting factors not only for tumor growth, but also for spread. Invasion, which is a complex sequence of events starting with loss of intercellular adhesion, differential adhesion on the matrix (Masumoto et al, 1999), and tumor cell locomotion and continuing with adhesion (via specific receptors) on vessel wall structures and traffic through the vessel wall itself, crucially depends on the interface between invading cells and lymph or blood vessels.

The angioarchitecture of HCC has been studied using selective celiac angiography (Bierman et al, 1951), percutaneous catheterization (Seldinger, 1958), and contrast medium injection at autopsy (Nakashima & Kojiro, 1986). In arteriograms, HCCs are generally hypervascular, whereas, in comparison, cholangiocellular carcinomas appear hypovascular, which could be due to different balances between angiogenesis and antiangiogenesis involving an intricate network of factors, including vascular endothelial growth factor (VEGF) and its receptors, angiopoietins 1 and 2, thrombospondin-1, and endostatin (Kawahara et al, 1998; Poon et al, 2004; Sun & Tang, 2004; Torimura et al, 2004; Zhao et al, 2003). The sinusoidal vascular pattern seen in many HCCs may facilitate spread because the invasion interface is large, and the traveling distances for migrating cells are shorter. It has been shown, however, that with progressive tumor dedifferentiation, endothelial cells forming the vascular channels in HCC lose the phenotype of sinusoidal endothelial cells (Nakamura et al, 1997). The contact surface between tumor cells and vascular channels can be augmented secondarily by the formation of cavernous channels found in portal tracts in the vicinity of portal vein branches obstructed by tumor (Terada et al, 1989c).

With respect to pathogenic mechanisms involved in intra-tumorous and peritumorous vessel formation, progress has been made regarding angiogenic and antiangiogenic factors (Imura et al, 2004; Rundell, 1998; Sheibani & Frazier, 1999). Studies on HCC performed so far emphasize the significance of factors inducing the formation of endothelial cells and of vascular channels, in particular, VEGF. VEGF is overexpressed in HCC (El-Assal et al, 1998; Torimura et al, 1998), and the expression of VEGF seems to be related to disease progression (Chow et al, 1997) and to tumor grade (Yamaguchi et al, 1998). In contrast, another vascular growth factor, platelet-derived endothelial growth factor, has not been shown to play a significant role in HCC (Yamamoto et al, 1998), suggesting that a differential expression of angiogenic factors may determine the distinct angioarchitecture seen in HCC. VEGF also affects hepatocellu-lar junctions and by this may exert a direct influence on invasion mechanisms (Schmitt et al, 2004). Angiogenesis in HCC also is related to maxtrix turnover involved in invasion and spread, through the action of metalloproteinase networks (Ishii et al, 2003).

Of particular interest is the switch from a liver-specific type of vascularity to an angioarchitecture typical for pathways leading to liver cell cancer. Not much is known about these phenomena, but expression of one marker, CD34, is lacking in liver cirrhosis, is focally present in nodular precursor lesions, and is clearly detectable in HCC, suggesting a progressive change in the vascularity pattern as a function of progressive transformation (Kimura et al, 1998). Because tumor spread seems to depend crucially on angioarchitecture, a more detailed study of angio-genesis and vasculogenesis and of antiangiogenesis may become an important field for future treatment strategies. Of similar importance are the pathogenic mechanisms involved in intrava-sation of tumor cells. On migration in the extracellular space, mediated by basic fibroblast growth factor in HCC (Kin et al, 1997), neoplastic cells come into receptor-mediated contact with vessels and afterward may be able to invade vascular channels.

As in other tumors, invasion of tissue in HCC needs the action of enzymes degrading the matrix, in particular, metallo-proteinases (Yamamoto et al, 1997). On transmigration through vessel walls, the intravasation process starts, which leads to distribution of cancer cells within the streaming blood. Several mechanisms are involved in this complex process. It has been shown that, apart from matrix metalloproteinases, the urokinase plasminogen activator receptor and, by implication, the uro-kinase plasminogen activator play significant roles. The urokinase plasminogen activator/plasmin system seems to have a dual role in the intravasation process—the activation of proteinases (chiefly prometalloproteinase MMP9) and the facilitation of invasion across the endothelium itself or the promotion of the release of tumor cells into the blood after intravasation has been accom-plished (Quigley & Armstrong, 1998). Intravascular spread is modulated by several factors. Tumor pressure increases with capsule formation, and the pressure gradient between the tumor and the portal vein may be a causal factor in the dispersal of tumor cells into the portal vein (Tanaka et al, 1997). With respect to the take of dislodged tumor cells and their subsequent growth to form a metastasis, only few data are available so far. It has been shown that an integral membrane protein belonging to the TM4 family, KAI1, exerts a crucial action as a metastasis suppressor in HCC (Guo et al, 1998).

Regarding the histomorphology of intrahepatic metastatic lesions, the criteria for their identification include growth pattern, shape, and similarity to the suggested primary tumor (Kondo & Wada, 1991; Nakanuma et al, 1986). Although careful histologic examination in many instances may suffice to identify a second focus as being due to spread, more refined techniques need to be employed to study this important field (e.g., by comparing the clonal features of putative primary and secondary lesions). HCC sometimes may present unusual patterns of growth and spread. Neoplastic growth within bile ducts may occur, followed by obstructive jaundice and what has been termed *icteric hepatoma* (Lin, 1976). These situations, which may be confused with other causes of obstruction, seem to be associated with direct invasion from the primary tumor or from adjacent tumor thrombus in the portal vein (Nakashima & Kojiro, 1986). Intraductal invasion by HCC rarely may produce tumor fragments in the common hepatic duct, causing obstructive jaundice (Kiev et al, 1990). Another particular growth pattern is presented by HCC with prominent intra-atrial tumor growth; this situation is associated with frequent and marked edema of the lower extremities and marked venous dilation in the abdominal wall (Kojiro et al, 1984).

Other Epithelial Tumors

Several other discrete masses may need to be distinguished from HCC. The resemblance varies from superficial and macroscopic to profound and requiring more refined analysis. At the macro-scopic level, most solid masses may simulate HCC. When associ-ated with cirrhosis, the neoplasm is usually larger than hyperplastic nodules, is softer, retains less iron (Williams & Yamamoto, 1972), and provides little difficulty in diagnosis. The main problems relate to masses without accompanying cirrhosis. Masses that most resemble HCC are cholangiocarcinoma, metastatic tumor, FNH, hepatocellular adenoma, and some large nodular hyper-plasias (Knowles & Wolff, 1976; Phillips et al, 1973).

HEPATOCELLULAR ADENOMA

Hepatocellular adenoma (see Ch. 70) consists of thick liver plates of regular, larger than normal, and usually glycogen-rich tumor cells with regular nuclei and not particularly prominent nucleoli and usually without mitotic figures (Fig. 69.30) (Ishak, 1979). Focal necroses and hemorrhages are commonly present in adenomas associated with contraceptive steroid administra-tion, but not in adenomas lacking such an association. Rarely, formation of bone marrow (Ranaldi et al, 1993) or of myxoid tissue (Galassi et al, 1995) can occur. Mitosis, variability in nuclear size, and deviations of cell arrangement from trabecular to other structures may occur in some (usually large) adenomas. Such alterations may pose considerable difficulties for diagnosis, but are regarded as significant and generally indicate the possi-bility of malignant change (Tesluk & Lawrie, 1981). Morphologic examination may not allow in every instance a clear decision to be made as to whether such lesions are still benign or are already malignant. So far, new methods, such as immunohistochemistry, do not contribute more to differential diagnosis than the strict application of histologic criteria in these situations (Koelma et al, 1986). Similarly, it is still difficult to identify early adenomatous lesions. A more recent study has led

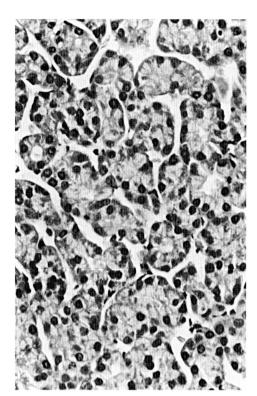

Fig. 69.30. Regular pale cells of hepatic adenoma. No mitoses or nuclear variability. Resection specimen. (Hematoxylin and eosin stain, ×400.)

to the concept of hepatic micronodules suggested to represent adenoma precursors (Lepreux et al, 2003a). The cells of origin of hepatocellular adenoma are not yet known, although hepatic progenitor cells have been identified in hepatocellular adenoma (Libbrecht et al, 2001a).

Steroid hormones play a role in the etiology of at least a large fraction of hepatocellular adenomas. There is a marked increase in the relative risk of hepatocellular adenoma with duration of oral contraceptive use of more than 60 months with an estimated annual incidence of 0.3 to 0.4 cases of hepatocellular adenoma per 100,000 women per year. Continuation of oral contraceptive use may result in the development of other hepatocellular adenoma, and hepatocellular adenoma may progress during pregnancy (Athanassion & Craigo, 1998) and postpartum (Rooks et al, 1979), sometimes with liver adenomatosis (see later) (Le Bail et al, 1992). Although activation of the Wnt signaling pathway seems to be important in a subset of hepatic adenomas, this activation does not seem to be directly linked to hormonal receptor status (Torbenson et al, 2002). Hepatocellular adenoma also can be induced by androgens (Soe et al, 1992), and receptors for estrogens and androgens have been detected in these tumors (Cohen et al, 1998), but also in HCC and cell lines derived thereof (Villa et al, 1995; Yu L et al, 1997).

Hepatocellular adenomas may or may not regress after discontinuation of oral contraceptive use (Buehler et al, 1982, Marks et al, 1988), but resolution after discontinuation of therapy may be associated with subsequent evolution into HCC (Gordon et al, 1986). The question as to which group of hepatocellular adenomas bears the highest risk of transformation into a malignant phenotype has not yet been answered fully (Ferrell, 1993; Foster & Berman, 1994; Gyorffy et al, 1989; Ito et al, 2003; Scott et al, 1996; Tao, 1991, 1992). Some types of

hepatocellular adenoma deviate from the classic presentation of this tumor and may lead to differential diagnostic problems. Occasionally, hepatocellular adenoma may show heavy iron deposition (Abdulkader et al, 2004a). Giant hepatocellular adenomas are associated with a particularly high incidence of rupture (Ramakrishna et al, 1996).

Liver cell adenoma occurs in combination with FNH (Friedman et al, 1984; Grange et al, 1987; Laurent et al, 2003) (e.g., after danazol therapy) (Bartley et al, 2004) and may manifest as multiple discrete lesions, particularly in association with glycogenosis type Ia (Coire et al, 1987; Howell et al, 1976; Poe & Snover, 1988; Volmar et al, 2003). In the latter situation, transformation into HCC may occur (Grossman et al, 1981). Apart from glycogenosis type Ia, hepatocellular adenoma also has been found in association with glycogenosis type IV (Alshak et al, 1994). Childhood hepatocellular adenoma can occur in familial adenomatous polyposis (Bala et al, 1997), in hirsutism with elevated levels of cortisol and corticotropin (Khoo et al, 1994), and in tyrosinemia. Situations with more than three lesions are termed *liver adenomatosis,* which occurs in patients with no history of steroid use (Arsenault et al, 1996; Chiche et al, 2000; Flejou et al, 1985; Gokhale & Whitington, 1996; Ribeiro et al, 1998; Skarupa et al, 2004), but is rarely associated with hereditary hemochromatosis (Radhi & Loewy, 2000). Liver adenomatosis can present as multiple calcified masses (Khan et al, 1992) and has been observed in glycogenosis type Ia (Karasawa et al, 1998). Familial occurrence of liver cell adenoma in association with diabetes mellitus has been reported (Foster et al, 1978). A familial form of liver adenomatosis has been shown to be associated with hepatocyte nuclear factor 1α inactivation (Bacq et al, 2003). Several reports have shown the association of liver cell adenoma with amyloidosis (Fievet et al, 1990; Poe & Snover, 1988; Zangeneh et al, 1969).

In recent years, molecular methods have been employed to characterize further the origin and biology of liver cell adenomas. In most adenomas analyzed so far, LOH at chromosome 12q was the only recurrent genetic alteration, a region including the *TCF1* gene encoding hepatocyte nuclear factor 1 (HNF-1). Biallelic inactivation of *TCF1* was detected in most adenomas, suggesting that this is an important event in the occurence of adenoma (Bluteau et al, 2002). Heterozygous germline mutations of HNF-1α are associated with maturity-onset diabetes of the young type 3. HNF-1α gene inactivation has been found to indicate cosegregation between liver adenomatosis and maturity-onset diabetes of the young type 3 (Reznik et al, 2004). Liver adenomas show alterations of the Wnt/β-catenin pathway. Part of the adenomas show interestitial deletions of the β-catenin gene resulting in truncated forms of the protein, suggesting that Wnt signaling anomalies play a role in the formation of these lesions (Chen et al, 2002). Mutation of the adenomatous polyposis coli (APC) gene encoding a protein of the Wnt signaling pathway has been found in liver cell adenoma (Blaker et al, 2004). Cell cycle deregulation in liver cell adenoma also may be related to changes in INK4a-ARF on chromosome 9p21 encoding two tumor suppressor genes, *p16* (INK4a) and *p14* (ARF) (Tannapfel et al, 2002).

Bile Duct Adenoma

The bile duct adenoma, usually a small (1-3 cm), well-demarcated, dense white mass found in a subcapsular position, consists of irregular intertwined small ductlike structures, with well-formed lumina and basement membranes and separated by abundant fibrous connective tissue, often containing lymphocytes. These foci are not encapsulated, but are clearly distinguished from surrounding hepatocyte cords, although sometimes abutting or fusing with a portal tract. The benign appearance of the ducts enmeshed in fibrous tissue is characteristic, and this is unlikely to be confused on microscopy with HCC (Edmondson, 1976). Atypical bile duct adenoma has been reported to have a clear cell phenotype (Albores-Saavedra et al, 2001).

Focal Nodular Hyperplasia

FNH (see Ch. 70) possesses the macroscopic characteristics of a discrete pale to beige mass, with a superficial resemblance to HCC; the differences include a thin, but defined fibrous capsule; a variegated and in part nodular cut surface; and frequently a central stellate scar that also is visualized at imaging (Wanless et al, 1985). Histology shows an arrangement of normal or thick hepatocyte plates coursed by variably sized fibrous bands containing abundant small bile ducts (which are lacking in liver cell adenoma), but lacking interlobular bile ducts; abnormal blood vessels; and an infiltrate of lymphocytes (Fig. 69.31). Most hepatocyte nuclei are uniform, small, and probably diploid, in contradistinction to the nuclei of normal adult liver, which usually contains several ploidy classes of nuclei. Although regarded as a hallmark of FNH, the scarlike lesions are not a constant finding. In a study of 305 lesions, only 49% of the FNH lesions had one to three macroscopic scars (Nguyen et al, 1999). The field of FNH currently is rapidly evolving, and diagnostic criteria will have, at least in part, to be revised (Bioulac-Sage et al, 2001). In particular, the diagnosis of FNH in needle biopsy specimens is difficult. In the case of

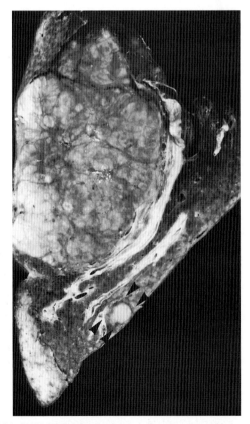

Fig. 69.31. FNH. Well-defined pale mass of moderately uniform parenchyma traversed by fine fibrous tissue and separated from noncirrhotic parenchyma. A second smaller lesion is present *(arrow)*. Resection specimen.

a typical imaging presentation, biopsy of the liver may not be required, but a study of 30 patients revealed that the diagnosis of FNH on biopsy was reached in 58.3% in patients with two or fewer imaging criteria (Fabre et al, 2002).

FNH has been proposed to be subclassified into several variants—a classic group and a nonclassic group, with the latter consisting of the telangiectatic form, a mixed hyperplastic and adenomatous form, and a form with atypia of large cell type (Nguyen et al, 1999). In the telangiectatic variant of FNH, dilated sinusoidal areas surrounding compact areas are a distinct feature. This variant differs from typical FNH at imaging by the frequent lack of a central scar, lesion heterogeneity, a different magnetic resonance imaging pattern, and persistent contrast enhancement on delayed contrast-enhanced CT (Attal et al, 2003). Multiple lesions are associated with vascular anomalies in the adjacent non-nodular liver substance, supporting the concept that multiple telangiectatic FNH lesions are a reaction to focal ischemia induced by various mechanisms (Lepreux et al, 2003c). Based on the finding that telangiectatic FNH shares some features with liver cell adenoma, this variant of FNH has been analyzed by use of molecular techniques. The clonal features and the angiopoietin expression profile were compatible with the view that telangiectatic FNH is a variant of hepatocellular adenoma (*teleangiectatic hepatocellular adenoma*) (Paradis et al, 2004).

In conjunction with typical FNH, additional small nodules detectable by modern imaging techniques can be found, which are sometimes difficult to identify as FNH. Lepreux and associates (2003b) have presented the criteria to diagnose such FNH-like nodules reliably as possible precursor lesions of FNH. These nodules also are significant in the context of FNH lacking key morphologic features (Lepreux et al, 2002) and of FNH-like areas that can arise in liver cirrhosis (Quaglia et al, 2003).

FNH and FNH-like nodules are now well known to develop in hepatic venous outflow obstruction, including Budd-Chiari syndrome (Ibarrola et al, 2004; Maetani et al, 2002) and in other circulatory disorders of the liver, including portal vein thrombosis (Buresu et al, 2004). FNH itself harbors vascular and in part diagnostic anomalies (specifically, thick-walled abnormal vessels of intermediate phenotype in the portal tract–like spaces). In addition, the perisinusoidal spaces in FNH exhibit an aberrant extracellular matrix associated with abnormal fibrillin-1 expression (Lepreux et al, 2004). For FNH and other hyperplastic disorders, pathogenic mechanisms involved in these situations have been discussed (Kondo 2001; Kondo et al, 2004).

Similar to liver cell adenoma, FNH has been observed in association with the use of oral contraceptive steroids (Scott et al, 1984) and may occur together with adenoma (Friedman et al, 1984; Grange et al, 1987). FNH has been found to be associated with several types of malformation (including malformations of the liver, e.g., arteriovenous malformations at the liver hilum), hemangiomata of the liver, and several other tumors (e.g., in siblings with glioblastoma). The significance of these associations is unclear. The pathogenic significance of circulatory and vascular factors in FNH has been supported by the observation of an increased expression of the angiopoietin-1–to–angiopoietin-2 ratio and of the presence of functional Tie-2 receptor in FNH (Paradis et al, 2003). A further study showed that the phenotype of endothelial cells lining the vascular channels in FNH differ from those in the remaining liver, associated with a downregulation of angiotensin I converting enzyme/CD143 (Gräntzdörffer et al, 2004).

ETIOLOGY AND PATHOGENESIS OF HEPATOCELLULAR CARCINOMA (see also Ch. 71)

Many epidemiologic studies show that risk factors and causes of HCC include hepatitis viruses, alcohol, chemicals, hormones, cirrhosis, and metabolic diseases, in particular, hemochromatosis (Colombo, 1992; Johnson, 1996). Hepatotropic viruses (hepatitis B virus [HBV] and hepatitis C virus [HCV]) play a significant role in the etiology of HCC. The most detailed knowledge regarding the etiology and pathogenesis of HCC has been gained by studying chronic viral infection of the liver (Anzola, 2004; Arbuthnot & Kew, 2001; Block et al, 2003; Bruix & Llovet, 2003; Szabo et al, 2004; Van Dekken et al, 2003). There exists a synergy of viral hepatitis and alcohol on the risk of HCC (Yuan et al, 2004). HBV is likely to be one of the most frequent causes of HCC; this is based on population studies, the detection of HBV antigens or genomic components or both in cells, and animal models (Arthur et al, 1984; Beasley, 1988; Bréchot et al, 1985; Hann et al, 2004; Kuang et al, 2004; MacNab et al, 1976; Marion et al, 1980; Ohbayashi, 1976; Pollicino et al, 2004; Summers et al, 1978; Vogel et al, 1970; Wang et al, 2004a; You et al, 2004).

The pathogenic mechanisms involved in HBV-induced HCC, in particular the role of the HBx antigen in affecting signal pathways, have been discussed in detail. Integrated parts of the HBV genome are observed in many HCCs arising in chronic HBV infection (Wang et al, 2004b), but integration may be nonselective. It has been shown that the *HBx* gene induces liver cancer in transgenic mice (Kim et al, 1991). *HBx* also interacts in a complex way with several regions of the human genome, including the *p53* region involved in the regulation of cell proliferation and apoptosis (Hsu et al, 1991; Koike, 1995; Truant et al, 1995), and *HBx* is essential for the activation of Wnt/β-catenin signaling known to be involved in carcinogenesis (Cha et al, 2004). Numerous studies support the evidence that HCV infection also is connected with HCC (Kasahara et al, 1998; Naoumov et al, 1997; Okuda et al, 1987; Tanaka et al, 2004). A high prevalence of anti-HCV antibodies has been found in patients with HCC (Yu et al, 1990), and HCV RNA sequences can be isolated from tumor tissue (Herr et al, 1993; Saito K et al, 1997). HCC in HCV infection can develop in noncirrhotic livers.

Among exogenous toxic agents, alcohol seems to be a major cause of HCC, particularly in the West (Nalpas et al, 1995; Popper et al, 1981). In almost every instance, there is accompanying cirrhosis, but it is unknown whether this is the most important pathogenic factor (Bréchot et al, 1982; Lieber 1975). Although there is no evidence that ethanol is a direct-acting carcinogen (Mills et al, 1981), it might affect DNA metabolism via the formation of acetaldehyde. The role of ethanol is complicated by the fact that alcohol-induced liver disease shows an increased prevalence of HCV infection (Pares et al, 1990) and iron overload.

In certain parts of the world, aflatoxin is believed to be involved in hepatocarcinogenesis (Krishnamarchari et al, 1975; Omer et al, 2004; Onyemelukwe et al, 1980; Wogan, 1976). Putative mechanisms of pathogenesis have been studied in individuals infected by HBV (Kew, 2003; Yu et al, 1997), and the gene for aflatoxin B1–aldehyde reductase is located in a region of chromosome 1 that frequently is mutated in human tumors, including liver tumors (Praml et al, 1998). Steroidal sex hormones are other exogenous agents that may induce HCC (Davis et al, 1975; Henderson et al, 1983; Klatskin, 1977; Mays & Christopherson, 1984; Neuberger et al, 1980; Sweeney & Evans, 1976; Tesluk & Lawrie, 1981).

Cirrhosis has been reported to be a major cause of HCC, regardless of the etiology (Kew & Popper, 1984; Nzeako et al, 1996; Popper et al, 1981). Apart from the effect of continuously increased cell turnover (Preat et al, 1984), direct metabolic effects occurring in a subset of cirrhosis may play a role (Greene, 1982; Powell & Kerr, 1975; Weinberg & Finegold, 1983; Weinberg et al, 1977). This role is particularly obvious in cases of iron overload states, especially hemochromatosis (Hsing et al, 1995; Kowdley et al, 1995). Among genetic hemochromatosis patients, the risk of developing HCC may be about 200-fold compared with a normal population (Bradbear et al, 1985; Finch & Finch, 1955; Niederau et al, 1985). Other metabolic disorders sometimes complicated by HCC include α_1-antitrypsin deficiency (Eriksson & Hagerstrand, 1974; Liebermann et al, 1975; Propst et al, 1994; Rawlings et al, 1974; Zhou & Fischer, 1998), Wilson's disease (Cheng et al, 1992; Guan et al, 1985; Polio et al, 1989; Wilkinson et al, 1983), porphyrias (Andant et al, 1997), tyrosinemia, and glycogenoses. Some of these disorders may lead to cholestasis, and chronic and severe cholestasis may play a pathogenic role, such as in biliary atresia, neonatal giant cell hepatitis, and Byler's disease (Deoras & Dicus, 1973; Roth & Duncan, 1951; Ugarte & Gonzales-Crussi 1981) and, in adults, primary biliary cirrhosis (Gluskin et al, 1985; Krasner et al, 1979; Melia et al, 1984; Nakanuma et al, 1990a) (perhaps via formation of macroregenerative nodules) (Nakanuma et al, 1990b; Terada et al, 1989d) and primary sclerosing cholangitis (Snook et al, 1989; Wee et al, 1985).

Obesity and the spectrum of fatty liver disease have been shown to play an increasing role in the pathogenesis of primary liver tumors. Nonalcoholic fatty liver disease (NAFLD) is characterized by hepatic macrovesicular steatosis (macrosteatosis) in the absence of a history of significant alcohol consumption or other known liver disease. The histologic spectrum of NAFLD ranges from nonalcoholic fatty liver alone to nonalcoholic steatohepatitis, which is the most relevant form of NAFLD in regard to the development of chronic liver disease (Brunt & Tiniakos, 2005; Brunt et al, 2004; Sass et al, 2005; Zafrani, 2004). A histologic scoring system for NAFLD has been designed and validated (Kleiner et al, 2005). Nonalcoholic steatohepatitis has a distinct natural history and is a progressive disease in a significant proportion of patients, in which liver fibrosis or cirrhosis occurs in 20% of patients over a 10-year period, whereas nonalcoholic fatty liver alone seems to confer progression to fibrosis or cirrhosis in about 3% of the patients (McCullough, 2004). The pathogenic pathways involved in NAFLD and its spectrum of lesions seem to involve the differential expression of several genes and gene products (Younossi et al, 2005).

It was noted previously that obesity confers an elevated risk for HCC in cirrhosis, but that this higher risk was confined to alcoholic liver disease (Nair et al, 2002). Evidence now suggests, however, that chronic liver disease caused by nonalcoholic fatty liver disease, including nonalcoholic steatohepatitis, is an important risk factor for HCC that rivals that of carcinogenesis in HCV-related cirrhosis, particularly in older men (Bugianesi et al, 2002; Caldwell et al, 2004; Cotrim et al, 2000; Cuadrado et al, 2005; McCullough, 2004; Qian & Fan, 2005). So far, most HCCs developing in the context of nonalcoholic fatty liver disease have been observed in patients with liver cirrhosis (Shimada et al, 2002). The pathogenesis of HCC developing in NAFLD has not yet been clarified. Similar to other situations of chronic liver disease, fibrosis or cirrhosis may play a significant role. Distinct genes potentially altered in NAFLD may be involved, however, in hepatic carcinogenic pathways. The novel tumor suppressor gene, *PTEN,* mapping to chromosome 10q23.3 and encoding a dual specificity phosphatase, is impaired, deleted, or weakly expressed in HCC and HCC cell lines (Dong-Dong et al, 2003; Zhang et al, 2004). Liver-specific deletion of Pten in mice results in fatty liver and insulin hypersensitivity (Stiles et al, 2004) and in steatohepatitis and HCC (Horie et al, 2004), suggesting a possible pathogenic link.

A strong association is reported with vena cava obstruction and chronic Budd-Chiari syndrome (see Ch. 100) attributed to congenital malformations, such as membranes and webs (Nakamura et al, 1986; Okuda et al, 1982a, 1982b; Simson, 1982). Budd-Chiari syndrome can be associated with nodular hepatic hyperplasia, indicating increased growth and cell turnover. A close association between inferior vena cava obstruction and HCC in Africa is seen mainly in areas where additional causative factors may play a role (Kew & Popper, 1984; Kew et al, 1989).

Over the years, numerous molecular events likely to be involved in hepatic carcinogenesis have been identified, including altered expression of oncogenes, tumor suppressor genes, and growth factors and their receptors; changes in signaling proteins; and deviations in the expression of proteins regulating checkpoints and progression of the cell cycle. Further discussion of these mechanisms is beyond the scope of this chapter, and the reader is referred to pertinent reviews (Coleman, 2003; Feitelson et al, 2004; Locker, 2004; Nishida et al, 2003; Suriawinata & Xu, 2004; Thorgeirsson & Grisham, 2002; Voorhoeve & Agami, 2004).

PRECURSOR LESIONS OF HEPATOCELLULAR CARCINOMA

Based on typical patterns observed in experimental hepatic carcinogenesis, numerous investigations have focused on potential precursors of human HCC associated with distinct morphologic and molecular patterns (Hytiroglou, 2004; Schwartz, 1998). The lesions identified so far mainly comprise liver cell dysplasia (LCD) and a broad spectrum of more or less atypical nodular lesions associated or not associated with liver cirrhosis. After a phase of confusing terminology, the picture is now becoming clearer (Hytiroglou, 2004; Kojiro, 2004; Roncalli, 2004), and some of the major aspects are summarized in this section.

LCD, which denotes a situation in which morphologically atypical hepatocytes in a structurally normal liver or within cirrhotic nodules are found, originally was observed and described in hepatitis B surface antigen–positive livers of Ugandan patients and emphasized as a preneoplastic change (Anthony, 1976). Subsequently, other studies arrived at controversial interpretations regarding the precancerous nature of LCD (Schwartz, 1998). In Western countries, the etiology of liver cirrhosis has not been shown conclusively to be of relevance for the presence of LCD (Theise et al, 1992), but LCD is observed relatively frequently in HCV infection (Ferrel et al, 1992). The question regarding the preneoplastic significance of LCD is complicated by the facts that (1) LCD and the subtypes of it are not yet clearly defined, and (2) cellular atypias similar to LCD occur in large liver nodules grossly and microscopically deviating from usual cirrhotic or regenerative nodules (see later) and thought to be nodular precursors of HCC.

Morphologically, LCD usually is classified as being of the small cell (Watanabe et al, 1983) or large cell type, with the latter being broken down further into variants with hyperchromatic or hypochromatic nuclei. The hypothesis that LCD, the pathogenesis of which is largely unknown, may represent a precancerous state is based on several observations. Some LCD cells show a marked increase in DNA content allowing their distinction from normal hepatocytes and regenerating hepatocytes by use of karyometry, and the karyometric features of the large cell variant of LCD are closest to those of well-differentiated HCC, whereas the features of small cell LCD closely reflect those of poorly differentiated HCC (Zhao et al, 1994b). The degree of DNA aneuploidy increases from low-degree to high-degree dysplasia (Thomas et al, 1992), and numerical chromosome aberrations have been observed in large cell LCD (Terris et al, 1997), even though, based on studies of patients with cirrhosis and HCC, large cell LCD did not seem to represent a direct malignant precursor (Lee et al, 1997) or was found to be an independent risk factor for liver cancer (Libbrecht et al, 2001b).

With respect to proliferative activity, LCD cells may be similar to HCC (Adachi et al, 1993, Zhao et al, 1994b), particularly with regard to the small cell variant. An abnormal growth pattern of LCD cells is associated with alterations in the extracellular matrix and of regulatory proteins. Similar to atypical liver cell nodules, small cell LCD is characterized by an abnormal tenascin and type IV collagen expression, reflecting the defective matrix pattern seen in HCC (Zhao et al, 1996). In contrast to malignant hepatocellular tumors, transforming growth factor-β1, which regulates cell proliferation and fibrogenesis, was not detectable in LCD (Zhao & Zimmermann, 1998). Among oncogene proteins, the hepatocyte growth factor receptor, c-met protein, is expressed in small cell LCD (Zhao & Zimmermann, 1998), and LCD cells are reactive for the tumor suppressor, p53 protein, the latter phenomenon being associated with an increased level of apoptosis of the cells involved (Zhao & Zimmermann, 1997). It seems that LCD represents a liver cell population that clearly deviates from normal or regenerating hepatocytes not only with regard to morphology, but also with regard to several biologic parameters. Further studies are needed to clarify the preneoplastic significance of LCD (Hytiroglou, 2004; Le Bail et al, 1997).

Atypical nodular lesions chiefly encountered in cirrhotic livers have been described under a host of different terms, including *macroregenerative nodules, large nodules, atypical nodules, adenomatous hyperplasia* (with or without atypia), *borderline nodules,* and *dysplastic nodules* (Hytiroglou, 2004; Hytiroglou et al, 1995; Kondo et al, 1987; Matsui et al, 1989; Nakanuma et al, 1990b, 1998; Ohta & Nakanuma, 1987; Okuda, 1992; Pompili et al, 1991; Sakamoto et al, 1991; Schwartz, 1998; Sugihara et al, 1987; Sugitani et al, 1998; Takayama et al, 1990; Terada et al, 1989d; Theise, 1995; Wada et al, 1988). Modern imaging modalities detect these small (i.e., usually 1-2 cm) lesions of the liver. They differ from HCC particularly because they usually show no enhancement on angiography. These nodular lesions also are easily detectable on cut surfaces of liver resection specimens, explants, and autopsy livers owing to their size, color, and, frequently, bulging features; sometimes they are located within other nodular structures (nodule-in-nodule lesions). Histologically, atypical nodules are identifiable by an aberrant trabecular structure, particularly well seen with reticulin stains (Bergman et al, 1997), and eventually by the presence of dysplastic cells.

An International Working Party (1995) proposed a new classification of atypical hepatocellular lesions, mainly placing emphasis on the dysplastic focus and the dysplastic nodule and suggesting that former terms, such as *adenomatous hyperplasia*, should be abandoned. According to the terminology proposed, a *dysplastic focus* is a cluster of hepatocytes less than 1 mm in diameter with dysplasia, but without definite histologic criteria of malignancy. These lesions usually occur in cirrhosis, and large and small cell LCD may be found together. A *dysplastic nodule*, this term replacing previously used names for larger nodular lesions, is a nodular region of hepatocytes at least 1 mm in diameter with dysplasia, but without definite histologic criteria of malignancy. These nodules are usually, but not always, found in cirrhotic livers; they can protrude from the liver, and a nodule-in-nodule pattern may be observed. Dysplastic nodules are subdivided further into low grade or high grade (with respect to the degree of dysplasia), with the term *high-grade dysplastic nodule* corresponding to the former term *borderline nodule*. As dysplastic nodules enlarge, new vessels composed of nontriadal arteries become dominant, indicating abnormal angiogenesis. For the high-grade variant, a further subdivision has been proposed, comprising nodules with diffuse small cell change or pseudogland formation; nodules with nodule-in-nodule–type lesions with small cell dysplasia, clear cell change, or Mallory body clustering; and nodules with microfoci of HCC (Park et al, 1998).

What is the evidence that dysplastic foci or nodules may represent bona fide precursors of HCC? Clinical observations indicate that dysplastic nodules can evolve into liver cancer (Borzio et al, 2003; Efremidis & Hytiroglou, 2002; Kim et al, 2000; Seki et al, 2000). Several features of dysplastic nodules make it likely that these lesions are positioned in a pathway potentially leading to malignancy. Immunohistochemically, these nodules deviate from ordinary cirrhotic nodules (Hytiroglou, 2004; Terada et al, 1995), and particularly nodules with a nodule-in-nodule pattern show increased proliferative activity (Theise et al, 1996). Nodules with increasing degrees of dysplasia may show overexpression of *p53* (similar to non-nodular dysplasia; see earlier), in that neither *p53* overexpression nor mutation was found in low-grade dysplastic nodules, but *p53* overexpression or mutation was found in more than 40% of high-grade lesions (Kang et al, 1998). Telomerase activation is an early event in the development of such nodules (Hytiroglou et al, 1998). By testing LOH, it has been shown that dysplastic nodules may be monoclonal lesions (Aihara et al, 1996; Theise, 1996), even though polyclonality also has been observed in large nodules (Piao et al, 1997). Taken together, there is increasing evidence that, similar to other organs, a morphologic and genetic/molecular base is present to induce a dysplasia-carcinoma sequence also in the liver (Taguchi et al, 2002; Van Dekken et al, 2003).

The clonal expansion of dysplastic nodules is supported further by the observation that these nodules undergo a reduction of activated stellate cells (Park et al, 1997). Abnormal angiogenesis, which is well known for HCC, seems to ensue early in the development of putative precursor nodules and gradually proceeds during the nodule-to-HCC sequence (Terada & Nakanuma, 1995). Notwithstanding an increasing amount of information suggesting the precancerous nature of dysplastic nodular lesions, many of the findings outlined earlier require specific and sometimes time-consuming methods, and one would like to have an approach allowing for the rapid identification of features predicting malignant transformation, particularly in daily routine. Several easily detectable features of dysplastic nodules have been worked out and shown to have significant predictive value. These characteristics include an increased ratio of nuclear density, clear cell change, small cell dysplasia, and fatty change, all of which are associated with a high risk for evolution to HCC (Terasaki et al, 1998).

VASCULAR TUMORS

Tumors arising from endothelial cells and mainly in adults include the most common primary tumor of the liver, cavernous hemangioma, which is a benign tumor with an incidence in hospital autopsies of approximately three times that of HCC (an underestimate because small lesions probably are not always recorded); angiosarcoma, which is an aggressively malignant vascular tumor with an incidence of 1:30 to 1:80 that of HCC (Pollard & Millward-Sadler, 1974); and epithelioid hemangioendothelioma, which is a rare, more indolent variety (Ishak et al, 1984). Important histogenetic aspects of the spectrum of endothelial cell tumors have been reviewed (Bell, 2003).

Cavernous Hemangioma

Cavernous hemangioma (see Ch. 70) consists of multiple vascular channels, supported by collagenous walls lined by a single layer of endothelial cells (Fig. 69.32). These tumors are sharply demarcated from surrounding liver tissue; have a spongy, dark red appearance; and are frequently partly necrotic, sometimes completely fibrosed, and rarely calcified (Fig. 69.33). The tumors vary in size, and tumors larger than 4 cm are referred to

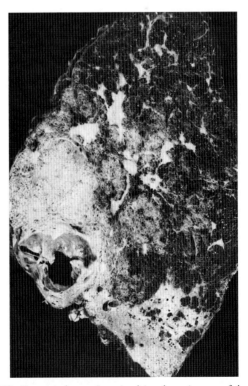

Fig. 69.32. Cavernous hemangioma involving the major part of the resected right lobe of the liver. There are many minute foci of hemangiomata on the lower side near the resection margin.

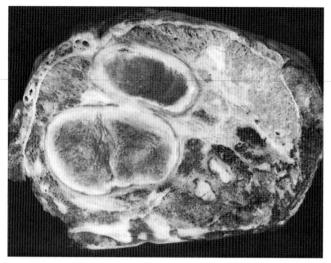

Fig. 69.33. Cavernous hemangioma with necrotic foci. Resected specimen.

as *giant hemangiomata* by some authors (Behar et al, 1963). Hemangiomata seen at surgery seem to show a higher incidence of pedunculated forms (15-20%) (Shumacker, 1942) compared with very few pedunculated tumors at autopsy (Oschner & Halpert, 1958). This difference may be due to the fact that larger tumors become pedunculated because of their size and for the same reason may become symptomatic (Dehner & Ishak, 1971), eventually via arterioportal shunting (Srivastava et al, 1998). Thrombi in the process of organization are frequently present, and there are many foci of fibrosis. These may replace vascular channels in part or all of the tumor; in the case of fibrosis, only a sclerosed mass representing the vascular lesion may remain. Giant hemangiomata can undergo inflammatory changes and become symptomatic (Pol et al, 1998).

Although cavernous hemangioma can be diagnosed on biopsy material, percutaneous biopsies should not be performed. With needle biopsy, there is the risk of provoking massive and uncontrollable hemorrhage, and results can be unreliable, with a significant false negative rate in large lesions that may prove to be malignant. Among 40 needle biopsies reported in a series, there was one false positive diagnosis of hemangioma, which subsequently was proved to be HCC (Schwartz, 1987).

Some large or giant hemangiomata show a particular relationship to the adjacent liver tissue, and this makes them amenable to surgical enucleation (Baer et al, 1989; Zimmermann & Baer, 1996) (see Ch. 80). When histologically analyzing the interfaces between the periphery of the hemangioma and the hepatic tissue, four major patterns of interface morphology can be defined. The first pattern, which may be termed *fibrolamellar interface,* is characterized by a capsule-like fibrous lamella of variable thickness. It contains small blood vessels (arteries and veins), which seem to traverse the fibrous border or may follow the contour of the periphery of the tumor in a more or less parallel fashion. Hepatic tissue outside this lamella may be atrophic, and portal tracts with bile ductule proliferations are sometimes seen. The second pattern, *interdigitating interface,* reveals that peripheral components of the hemangioma are interdigitating with hepatic parenchyma without the formation of a fibrous lamella. Islands of lobular or nodular liver tissue may be deeply situated within tumor septa. In the third pattern, *compression interface,* the

periphery of the tumor is in direct contact with hepatic tissue, forming a curvilinear border without major intercalation. Adjacent parenchyma shows zonal atrophy. Large blood channels may be seen in this area, corresponding to dilated portal vein branches or to hemangioma-like foci (microhemangiomata). The fourth pattern, *irregular or spongy interface,* is characterized by a highly irregular border of the hemangioma, with numerous foci of liver parenchyma interspersed between dilated blood channels. Within this spongy structure, the outer border of the tumor can barely be delineated (Fig. 69.34).

Some liver hemangiomata deviate from the standard morphology. Liver hemangiomata tend to develop regressive changes characterized by an increase of fibrous matrix. There are also lesions with a distinct fibrous phenotype and abnormal thick-walled blood vessels, termed *sclerosed hemangiomata* (Makhlouf & Ishak, 2002).

Hemangiomata of the liver can be accompanied by hemangiomata of other organs (Willis, 1948) and may be multiple. Occasionally, a large hemangioma is accompanied by many small lesions. Large tumors may produce symptoms as a result of pressure or rupture (Shumacker, 1942) or effects on coagulation, which mainly have the features of a consumptive coagulopathy (Martinez et al, 1973). There is a significant association between liver hemangiomata and FNH (Vilgrain et al, 2003).

The cause of cavernous hemangioma is unknown, but the action of steroid hormones may be involved (Takahashi et al, 1998), in particular, female sex steroids (Glinkova et al, 2004). Familial hepatic hemangioma is known, indicating genetic factors (Moser et al, 1998). Cavernous hemangioma occurs with greater frequency in adults than in children, although figures in children sometimes are confused by the inclusion of hemangioendothelioma (Ishak, 1976); these are usually distinguished, however, and the incidence in children is agreed to be lower than in adults (Landing, 1976) and lower than the incidence of capillary hemangioma (Dehner & Ishak, 1971). There is a higher incidence in women, ranging from 1.3 to 6 times that in men (Edmondson, 1958). Sex hormones may contribute to the enlargement and to symptoms (Morley et al, 1974), but it is not postulated that sex hormones cause hemangiomata.

Cavernous hemangioma is usually characteristic on macroscopic and microscopic examination, but at times resemblances have been remarked between this tumor and other conditions. These conditions include peliosis hepatis, hemorrhagic teleangiectasia (Osler-Rendu-Weber), infantile hemangioendothelioma, malignant vascular tumors, and metastases of several vascular malignant tumors. Hepatic infantile angiomata may be confounded with vascular malformations of the liver; these lesions may be distinguished by endothelial reactivity for an endothelial marker, GLUT1, which, in contrast to malformations, is positive in the hemangioma group (Mo et al, 2004).

Peliosis hepatis consists of distended vascular spaces with variable survival of endothelium, but without the thin fibrous walls characteristic of hemangioma. Hemorrhagic telangiectasia consists essentially of anastomosing veins and capillaries, enmeshed in fibrous tissue and generally involving the portal tract regions of the liver of a patient with cutaneous vascular lesions (Martini, 1959). Hemangioendothelioma is a distinctive capillary angioma without fibrous walls and containing distorted vessels and ducts with isolated islands of hepatocytes. Vascular HCC, sometimes referred to as the *pelioid variety of HCC* (Peters, 1976), is dominated by the epithelial elements.

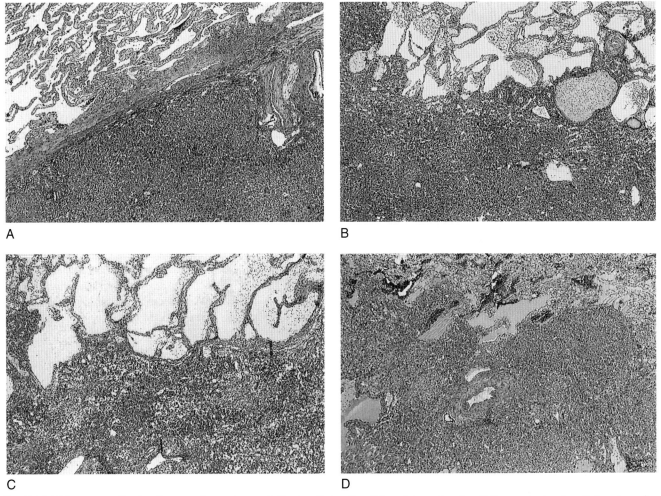

Fig. 69.34. Different types of border of cavernous hemangiomata. **A,** Fibrolamellar interface. **B,** Interdigitating interface. **C,** Compression interface. **D,** Irregular surface.

Vascular metastatic tumors, such as deposits of Kaposi's sarcoma, are essentially distinguished by their particular type of cell.

Angiosarcoma

Similar to other malignant mesenchymal tumors of the liver, hepatic angiosarcoma is rare (<1% of primary hepatic malignancies), but it represents the most frequent sarcoma of the liver, amounting to about one third of these lesions (Molina & Hernandez, 2003). The essential nature of this tumor is that of proliferating variably differentiated endothelial cells with associated fibriosis, sometimes solid, sometimes hemorrhagic, but usually recognizable microscopically (Weinbren, 1976). Multiple tumors are found more frequently than single masses; they vary in size and sometimes contain blood-filled cavities. They are not associated with cirrhosis, but depending on the cause, there may be extensive fibrosis involving portal and perisinusoidal regions (Weinbren, 1976). The tumor cells closely resemble endothelial cells and are seen for the most part flanking surviving hepatocyte plates and separated from them by a layer of fibrous tissue. This sinusoidal pattern is most frequent. Sometimes tumor cells have a cuboidal shape, and papillary formations may develop in which tumor cells surround single hepatocytes enclosed in fibrous tissue. More solid foci resembling spindle cell sarcoma occur in some areas, and poorly differentiated giant cell forms are noted (Weinbren, 1976). Mitotic activity varies. Extramedullary hematopoiesis is often present, but phagocytic activity is rare. Ultrastructurally, angiosarcoma cells are seen to infiltrate the parenchyma, to dissect the hepatocyte cords, to infiltrate sinusoids, and to have a close association with red blood cells (Phillips et al, 1987). The basement membranes are discontinuous and frequently are absent, and Weibel-Palade bodies are not seen.

Remote from the main tumor masses, there are often less obvious changes, which are otherwise difficult to evaluate. These changes involve an enlargement and an increase in the number of endothelial cells, sometimes with the formation of distorted nuclei. These endothelial tumor cells are generally well differentiated, always line vascular spaces, and may be difficult to distinguish from normal or reactive endothelial cells. A further category of tumor pattern has been delineated, and this involves the formation of blood-filled spaces often surrounded by thick fibrous walls, which seem to be lined by the tumor cells. This cavernous type is the microscopic counterpart of the macroscopic blood-filled cavities characteristic of this tumor (Figs. 69.35-69.37).

There are changes in other elements, in tumor-bearing regions and in parts of the liver that appear to be tumor-free.

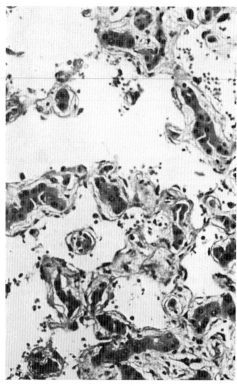

Fig. 69.35. Angiosarcoma showing characteristic endothelial cells attached by scaffolding-like fibrous tissue to liver plates. Necropsy specimen. (Hematoxylin and eosin stain, ×200.)

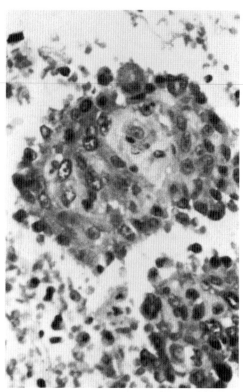

Fig. 69.36. Angiosarcoma showing surviving hepatocyte, surrounding fibrosis, and papillary-like tumor of endothelial tumor cells. Necropsy specimen. (Hematoxylin and eosin stain, ×400.)

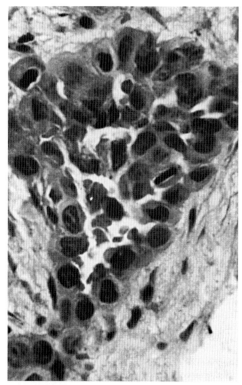

Fig. 69.37. Epithelioid region of angiosarcoma with plump tumor cells lining the vascular space. Necropsy specimen. (Hematoxylin and eosin stain, ×600.)

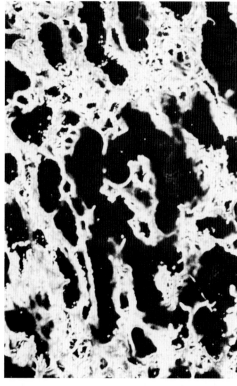

Fig. 69.38. Gross sinusoidal reticulin fibrosis regarded as a precancerous lesion and portent for angiosarcoma. (Gordon and Sweet reticulin and dark ground illumination stain, ×600.)

Perisinusoidal reticulin fibers are prominent between tumor-bearing sinusoids and hepatocyte plates, and the increased collagen apparently lies in the perisinusoidal space of Disse (Fig. 69.38). This collagenization varies from a minor inconspicuous increase in reticulin fibers to a marked increase in fibers that obstruct the lumen and that are associated with trapping or loss of hepatocytes.

The cause of angiosarcoma of the liver cannot always be established, but there is compelling evidence from population studies that exposure to certain chemical agents is operative in the development of this tumor (Lee et al, 1996). These include chronic exposure to arsenic (Centeno et al, 2002) (e.g., in vineyard workers) (Roth, 1957) and arsenical medication for psoriasis, thorium dioxide (Lipshutz et al, 2002; Srinivasan & Dean, 1997; Visfeldt & Poulsen, 1972) and, more importantly, vinyl chloride (Bosetti et al, 2003; Lewis & Rempala, 2003). The elevated incidence of angiosarcoma of the liver owing to exposure to vinyl chloride monomer is still of interest, although the number of cases is decreasing (Lee, 1982). Approximately 100 cases have been reported, mostly in the United States, Germany, and France (Lee, 1982), but safety measures to protect workers cleaning autoclaves (removing solid polymer polyvinyl chloride) are now efficient, and a screening program has been set up. This is important because surveillance must continue as the latent period may extend to more than 20 years. It has been estimated that 200 to 1200 cases may be expected to occur in Western Europe and 350 in the United States over the next 20 to 30 years, and that we are at about the halfway stage in the appearance of vinyl chloride monomer–related hemangiosarcoma (Forman et al, 1985). The pathogenic role of vinyl chloride is not clear, but the substance has been shown to induce connexin 37 mutations in a rat model of angiosarcoma (Saito T et al, 1997). The role of the tumor suppressor gene, *p53*, has been studied (Barbin et al, 1997; Smith et al, 1998). A probably significant effect of oncogenes is emphasized by the observation that sporadic and thorotrast-induced hepatic angiosarcomas manifest frequent and multiple point mutations in K-*ras*-2 (Przegodzki et al, 1997).

Rare causes of angiosarcoma include androgenic and anabolic steroids (Falk et al, 1979), diethylstilbestrol (Ham et al, 1980), oral contraceptive steroids (Monroe et al, 1981), phenelzine (Daneshmend et al, 1979), and von Recklinghausen's disease (Andreu et al, 1997). More recently, molecular abnormalities in angiosarcomas have been identified, including vinyl chloride–induced mutations of K-*ras*-2 (Weihrauch et al, 2002a), changes of the ARF-*p53* pathway (Weihrauch et al, 2002b), and alteration of p16INK4A (Tannapfel et al, 2001).

Diagnostic difficulties arise in situations of early or incipient hemangiosarcoma of the liver, as in other primary sites. Lesions may be discrete, but foci of dilated sinusoid-like structures may occur, associated with focal hypercellularity (visible even at low magnification), owing to increased numbers of endothelial, Kupffer, and Ito cells, which become increasingly abnormal. Within these clusters of cells, atypical endothelial cells may be recognized using factor VIII–associated antigen immunohistochemistry, which has been shown to give positive staining in some cases of angiosarcoma of the liver (Schmid & Beham, 1987). Excess collagen and reticulin fibers are deposited in the atypical areas, mainly in and around the sinusoids. The differential diagnosis of angiosarcoma includes metastatic vascular tumors, metastatic sarcomas, embryonic sarcoma (Vermess et al, 1984), and an unusual form of vascular tumor, epithelioid hemangioendothelioma (see later) (Ishak et al, 1984).

Rare Vascular Tumors

Epithelioid Hemangioendothelioma of the Liver

Epithelioid hemangioendothelioma of the liver is an unusual vascular tumor, the forerunner of which originally was found in the lung, considered epithelial in origin, and termed *intravascular bronchioloalveolar tumor*. Ishak and colleagues (1984) defined this lesion for cases occurring in the liver and used the term *epithelioid hemangioendothelioma*. A primitive, reticuloendothelial cell has been proposed as forming a relevant cell lineage, the tumor being a neoplastic analogue of wound healing (Demetris et al, 1997).

Most of the reports on this tumor have been reviewed more recently (Pokharna et al, 1997). The tumor rarely can mimic Budd-Chiari syndrome (Walsh et al, 1998) and may extensively calcify (Den Bakker et al, 1998). Grossly, the tumors are often multiple and involve both liver lobes. The lesions are generally white and firm to hard. Microscopically, two types of neoplastic cells (dendritic and epithelioid) are found to infiltrate sinusoids and intrahepatic veins of all sizes. The endothelial nature of the epithelioid cell type had formerly been acknowledged, owing to detection of pinocytotic activity of the cells and the expression of Weibel-Palade bodies, leading to the term now generally used (Weiss & Enzinger, 1982). Dendritic cells exhibit a marked variety of shapes and sizes, whereas epithelioid cells do not show surface projections and have a more abundant cytoplasm (Fig. 69.39). An immunohistochemical study showed that neoplastic cells express factor VIII–related antigen, but no reactivity for epithelial markers (Scoazec et al, 1989). The biologic behavior of this tumor is complex. It can be regarded as a neoplasm of intermediate malignancy, progressive, and with unpredictable outcome. Although the prognosis seems to be much more favorable than that for angiosarcoma, extrahepatic metastases occurred in 28% in the series reported by Ishak and colleagues (1984). There are reports of patients who have been treated with orthotopic liver transplantation, with a prospective 5-year actuarial survival rate more than 70% (Kelleher et al, 1989).

Infantile Hemangioendothelioma

Although rare, this lesion is the most common mesenchymal tumor of the liver in childhood (see Ch. 72), and most cases are

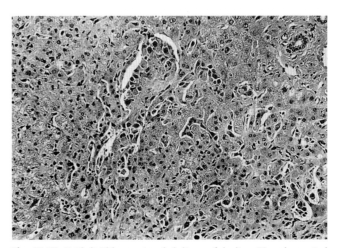

Fig. 69.39. Epithelioid hemangioendothelioma of the liver. Note the atypical cells with abundant cytoplasm invading the sinusoidal spaces. (Hematoxylin and eosin stain, ×150.)

encountered within the first few months of life (Dehner & Ishak, 1971; Ishak, 1976). Most tumors are solitary, but 40% are multicentric throughout the liver. Although many tumors are benign, large tumor size, increased growth rate, and type 2 histology may indicate aggressive behavior. Clinical presentation is dominated by hepatomegaly, but cardiac failure owing to intratumorous arteriovenous shunting and consumptive coagulopathies also may occur. Type 1 lesions show vascular channels lined by plump endothelial cells without atypia. Type 2 lesions have an atypical morphology with irregularly branched channels lined by pleomorphic endothelial cells, with papillary structures (Kanai et al, 1998, Klosowski et al, 1998). Thrombosis and infarction are frequent, as are foci of extramedullary hematopoiesis.

Hepatic Hemangioblastoma

Capillary hemangioblastomas are benign vascular tumors that occur in association with the phakomatosis von Hippel–Lindau disease. Visceral involvement in von Hippel–Lindau disease is well known, including that in the liver, but it usually manifests with simple cysts or adenomas. Hemangioblastoma in this disorder is primarily a tumor of the central nervous system, particularly in the posterior cranial fossa. This vascular tumor also may arise in the liver, however, forming nodules replacing large areas of hepatic parenchyma (Hayasaka et al, 1999; Rojiani et al, 1991) and grossly mimicking in some way the lesion pattern seen in infantile hemangioendothelioma. The histology and immunohistochemical appearance are identical to those of the corresponding cerebellar tumor.

Hepatic Angiomyolipoma

Angiomyolipoma is a tumor that develops in several organs, including the liver, but is particularly well known in the kidneys, where it can occur in the form of multiple nodules. In the liver, angiomyolipomas occur as solitary or multiple lesions, usually in the right lobe; they may reach more than 30 cm in size (Ng et al, 2003; Ren et al, 2003). Hepatic and renal lesions can develop together. About 5% to 10% of hepatic angiomyolipomas are associated with renal angiomyolipoma and tuberous sclerosis. In the latter situation, hepatic angiomyolipomas can be associated with pulmonary lymphangioleiomyomatosis, a further lesion typically related to tuberous sclerosis (Kim et al, 2003). Besides mature-looking adipocytes, this benign tumor contains spindle and polygonal cells expressing smooth muscle actin and desmin, and the distinct cell type found in angiomyolipomas is related to the system of perivascular epithelioid cells or PEC (Hoffman et al, 1997; Linton et al, 1991; Messiaen et al, 1996).

RARE HEPATIC TUMORS

As is the case with most viscera, in addition to its specialized elements, the liver is composed of a large variety of other tissues, and tumors may arise from any of these. Various forms of connective tissue, neuroendocrine tissue, and lymphoreticular tissue tumors have been observed, and usually these resemble similar tumors arising in other organs and tissues. In general, they occur with a much lower incidence than the tumors already referred to, although several are reported as occurring more frequently in children (Edmondson, 1958; Landing, 1976). Although consideration of rare tumors usually is not part of the preoperative assessment, and little has been contributed so far to pathogenetic

or epidemiologic studies from their subsequent accurate microscopical definition, several intrahepatic tumors that have attracted some attention are discussed here.

Benign Nonepithelial Tumors

Leiomyomatous tumors of the liver (benign and malignant) usually are interpreted as primary only with the exclusion of similar lesions in other organs (Burdette, 1975). Hepatic leiomyomas are rare lesions (Demel, 1926; Hawkins et al, 1980; Rios-Dalenz, 1965), and they have been observed mainly in immunodeficient or transplanted patients with or without Epstein-Barr virus infection (Bail et al, 1996; Cheuk et al, 2002; Wachsberg et al, 1994). Hepatic leiomyomas sometimes are of the myxoid variant (Yoon et al, 1998).

Fibromas are rarely encountered in the liver, but may grow to a considerable size (Edmondson, 1958; Formiggini, 1953). A pedunculated variant has been reported, which may enter the differential diagnosis of other, better known tumors with a pedunculated growth (Formiggini, 1953). One subset of benign liver nodules is characterized by a high lipid content. These lesions, which may be termed *fatty tumors* (or *fatty nodules*) of the liver, are important in a clinical setting, particularly when one has to sort out reactive or benign from malignant neoplastic cell populations. The diagnosis of fatty focal lesions or tumors of the liver is often possible using ultrasound or CT. Fatty lesions may consist of hepatocytes or represent the nodular progeny of nonhepatocyte liver tissue (Ishak, 1976).

Although diffuse fatty change of the liver is an extremely common change, lesions with a nonuniform (focal or nodular) pattern of lipid deposition are less frequently observed. In some situations, hepatocytes show a focal fatty change, usually in the context of well-known steatogenic conditions (Brawer et al, 1980). A nodular aspect of focal fatty change results only in situations in which fatty change ensues in preexisting nodular parenchyma. Fatty macroregenerative nodules in nonsteatotic liver cirrhosis have been described (Terada et al, 1989a). A marked accumulation of lipid can be found in liver cell adenomas and, rarely, in HCC (fatty HCC) (Yoshikawa et al, 1988).

Lipid-rich tumors of nonhepatocyte origin include lipoma (Ishak, 1976; Ramchand et al, 1970), myelolipoma (Rubin et al, 1984), and angiomyolipoma (see earlier) (Pounder, 1982). All of these lesions are situated within the liver and should not be confused with the common hepatic pseudolipomas or coelomic fat ectopia, which are always found on the surface of the liver (Karhunen, 1985).

Mature Teratomas

Relatively few cases of hepatic teratoma have been reported, and most have occurred in children, although adults also have been affected (Robinson & Nelson, 1986). Most of the hepatic teratomas described so far have been tridermal (i.e., composed of elements of mesoderm, ectoderm, and endoderm). Grossly, they are partially cystic and multilobular and may contain a thick, yellow to white fluid. Teratoma mixed with hepatoblastoma has been reported (Misugi & Reiner, 1965). A mature hepatic teratoma in an anencephalic fetus had some similarity to neuromuscular hamartoma or so-called benign Triton tumor (Robinson & Nelson, 1986). Mature teratoma of the liver may be associated with chromosomal anomalies (e.g., trisomy 13) (Dische & Gardner, 1978).

Malignant Nonepithelial Tumors

Apart from malignant vascular tumors, which were discussed earlier, sarcomas and other malignant nonepithelial tumors of the liver are uncommon findings.

Undifferentiated Embryonal Sarcoma (Embryonal Sarcoma)

Undifferentiated embryonal sarcoma of the liver appears on imaging as a cystic tumor, usually regarded preoperatively as a benign cystic tumor (Chowdhary et al, 2004), sometimes mimicking hydatid cysts, or as a necrotic metastasis (Barnes et al, 1981; Wooten et al, 1978). Undifferentiated embryonal sarcoma is a highly aggressive tumor that generally manifests in children (Bisogno et al, 2002; Kim et al, 2002; Stocker & Ishak, 1978), but also has been reported in adults (Stocker & Ishak, 1978; Vermess et al, 1984). It has been estimated that undifferentiated embryonal sarcoma constitutes 13% of all hepatic tumors in children (Weinberg & Finegold, 1983). The tumor can occur in conjunction with mesenchymal hamartoma of the liver (see later) (Begueret et al, 2001; De Chadarevian et al, 1994; Lauwers et al, 1997; O'Sullivan et al, 2001). Formerly, this tumor was termed *embryonal sarcoma, malignant mesenchymoma, embryonal rhabdomyosarcoma, fibromyxosarcoma, embryonal hepatoma,* or simply *sarcoma of the liver.* In a review of 31 patients, 51.6% were 6 to 10 years old, and there was no sex preponderance (Stocker & Ishak, 1978). The right lobe of the liver was involved more frequently. Serum AFP was normal in two cases. Eighteen patients (58%) died of the disease.

The essential features consist of pleomorphic spindle cells, often with multinucleated, irregularly shaped cells in a loose and frequently myxoid connective tissue, and containing eosinophilic intracytoplasmic globules staining for periodic acid–Schiff. Immunohistochemistry has shown that part of the spindled cells exhibit a smooth muscle differentiation (Nishio et al, 2003). There is usually substantial necrosis in which hemorrhage may occur. Differentiated elements usually are not encountered, although undifferentiated embryonal sarcoma may be confused with angiosarcoma, leiomyosarcoma, and fibrosarcoma (hence, the host of terms formerly used).

The origin of this tumor is still unknown, but it has been suggested that it may derive from a multipotent precursor cell able to differentiate along stromal and epithelial lines (Walker et al, 1992). Immunohistochemical studies indicated that this tumor shows phenotypic diversity comparable with that of malignant fibrous histiocytoma with or without additional rhabdomyosarcomatous or leiomyosarcomatous differentiation (Aoyama et al, 1991). Cells expressing cytokeratins also can be found (Leuschner et al, 1990), and coexpression of vimentin and cytokeratin has been observed (Lack et al, 1991). Cytogenetic analyses have shown that this tumor has near-triploid and near-hexaploid clones with several chromosomal rearrangements, similar to other sarcomas (Ilisko et al, 1998). Comparative genomic hybridization has revealed multiple chromosomal amplifications and deletions in undifferentiated embryonal sarcoma (Sowery et al, 2001).

Leiomyosarcoma of the Liver

Primary leiomyosarcoma of the liver can occur (Fong & Ruebner, 1974), but should be sorted out carefully from metastatic lesions, which may develop with considerable delay (17 years in one report) (Hanada et al, 1985). Of the little more than 15 hepatic leiomyosarcomas reported so far (Chen, 1983), 2 were vascular leiomyosarcomas related to hepatic veins (MacMahon & Ball, 1971), and 1 was a primary hepatic vascular leiomyosarcoma of probable portal vein origin (Sundaresan et al, 1990).

Malignant Mesenchymal Hepatic Tumors of Uncertain Origin

Malignant rhabdoid tumor (see also the paragraph on pediatric liver tumors), a clinically aggressive tumor most commonly arising in the kidney during childhood, but also observed in adults, has rarely been seen in the liver (Gonzales-Crussi et al, 1982b; Parham et al, 1988). This neoplasm, also termed *primary hepatic malignant tumor with rhabdoid features,* is morphologically characterized by sheets of cells that have peculiar eosinophilic cytoplasmic inclusions, which are composed of intermediate cytoskeletal filaments. There is still controversy regarding the cell of origin and lineage of differentiation of malignant rhabdoid tumor, although immunohistochemical investigations have shown that cells of this rapidly fatal tumor may express cytokeratins, in addition to vimentin (Parham et al, 1988; Scheimberg et al, 1996).

Among apparently primary hepatic tumors, the group classifed as *malignant hepatic mixed tumor* or *hepatoblastoma* in adults is among the least common. These lesions comprise epithelial and mesenchymal elements, but are different from teratomas. Since its first description (Walter, 1896), little more than 20 cases have been reported, with an age range of 19 to 78 years (average 51.1 years) (Kawarada et al, 1985). Malignant hepatic mixed tumors may develop into single or multinodular, sometimes very large, lesions, but correct diagnosis has been established only at autopsy in 87.5% of the cases reported so far (Kawarada et al, 1985). In addition to epithelial components, which resemble those occurring in hepatoblastomas in children, mesenchymal elements, including cartilage, osteoid, and bone, are seen. Most of the epithelial cells seem to be derived from hepatocytes, although signs of keratinocyte differentiation have been observed (Kawarada et al, 1985). It has been proposed that malignant hepatic mixed tumors should be differentiated into hepatocytic and nonhepatocytic malignant mixed tumors (Kawarada et al, 1985). Giant cell tumors resembling osteoclastomas of the bone have been reported as occurring in extraosseous sites, including the liver (Munoz et al, 1980).

Malignant Non-Hodgkin Lymphoma of the Liver

The involvement of the liver in non-Hodgkin lymphoma (NHL) is relatively common, particularly in advanced disease (Jaffe, 1987). In contrast, primary NHL of the liver is a rare disorder (Lei, 1998; Santos et al, 2003). Because the cells forming the malignant cell population of NHL can circulate and recirculate in the body (at least in some types of NHL), it may be difficult to assess where a malignant lymphoproliferative disorder has taken its origin, and this holds true for the situations in which the apparent initial manifestation of NHL was the liver. Nevertheless, the occurrence of primary NHL of the liver has been documented (Lei, 1998; Zafrani & Gaulard, 1993). Most cases have had a poor prognosis (Miller et al, 1983; Osborne et al, 1985).

Among B cell NHL, the liver can be involved by large B cell lymphoma, which predominates in some studies, but also by rarer types of NHL, such as mucosa-associated lymphoid tissue–type lymphomas (primary hepatic low-grade B cell NHL of mucosa-associated lymphoid tissue) (Isaacson et al, 1995), sometimes associated with primary biliary cirrhosis (Prabhu et al, 1998). Primary extramedullary plasmacytoma of the liver is extremely rare (Weichhold et al, 1995). A distinct hepato-tropic type of NHL is hepatosplenic γδ T cell lymphoma. There seems to be a male preponderance, and the median age at diagnosis is about 20 years. Liver sinusoids are markedly expanded by neoplastic T cells, with sparing of portal tracts, in contrast to CLL. Polymerase chain reaction analysis exhibits T cell receptor–γ gene rearrangement (Belhadj et al, 2003; Chang & Arber, 1998; Cooke et al, 1996; Gaulard et al, 2003). In addition to the γδ T cell variant, some hepatic T cell NHLs exhibit an αβ cell lineage (hepatosplenic αβ T cell lymphomas) (Macon et al, 2001).

There is increasing evidence that chronic HCV infection is associated with NHL (mainly of the B cell lineage), even in the absence of essential mixed cryoglobulinemia. An increased HCV prevalence among NHL patients has been found chiefly by studies in Italy, Japan, and France, suggesting a strong regional variation (Bronowicki et al, 2003; Mizorogi et al, 2000; Talamini et al, 2004). Aspects of an association between HCV infection and lymphomagenesis have been reviewed in detail (Negri et al, 2004).

A particular type of lymphocyte expansion is Epstein-Barr virus–associated post-transplant lymphoproliferative disorder. This is a frequently fatal complication that develops mainly after bone marrow grafting from unrelated donors, but it also can localize to liver allografts and may have a donor origin (Lones et al, 1997; Pham et al, 1998; Rizkalla et al, 1997). In biopsy specimens, post-transplant lymphoproliferative disorder may be difficult to distinguish from acute liver rejection.

NHL can develop in association with HCV infection (Pozzato et al, 1994) and may occur together with HCV-associated liver tumors. The more specific question of NHL occurring in acquired immunodeficiency syndrome (AIDS) is addressed subsequently.

Primary Hepatic Carcinoid Tumors and Other Liver Tumors with Neuroendocrine Features

Although carcinoid tumors (see Ch. 73b) are seen commonly in the gastrointestinal tract, they are extremely rare in the liver, and some of the primary carcinoid tumors reported to be found in the liver have been described as *cholangiocarcinomas* or *HCC with a carcinoid component* (Barsky et al, 1984). The diagnosis of primary neuroendocrine tumors of the liver can be difficult because this organ is the most frequently encountered site for metastatic carcinoid tumors from other organs. Primary carci-noid tumors of the liver are thought to derive from neuro-endocrine cells located in the biliary tract lining. Argyrophil cells and somatostatin-containing cells are physiologically present in the intrahepatic biliary tree. Of 20 livers analyzed, 65% had argyrophil cells, 50% had somatostatin-containing cells, 2 had

argentaffin cells, 2 had serotonin-containing cells, and 1 had pancreatic polypeptide–containing cells (Kurumaya et al, 1989). In light of these findings, one theoretically would expect more primary hepatic tumors with neuroendocrine features.

Of the few primary hepatic carcinoid tumors studied so far, some showed the typical features known for other carcinoids on light microscopy, electron microscopy, and immunohisto-chemistry (Andreola et al, 1990; Sioutos et al, 1991). At the ultrastructural level, cytoplasmic dense granules can be found, sometimes admixed with intermediate filaments and other organelles (Sioutos et al, 1991). Epithelial differentiation is emphasized by the finding of cytokeratin expression (Sautner et al, 1988). In a few cases, production of one polypeptide may predominate. A pancreatic polypeptide–producing apudoma of the liver has been reported (Warner et al, 1980) and a malignant apudoma of the liver was associated with symptomatic intractable hypoglycemia (Ali et al, 1978).

More intriguing are situations where cells with electron microscopy or immunohistochemistry neuroendocrine features are seen in primary hepatic tumors not showing the morphology of carcinoid tumors or apudomas. Electron microscopic exami-nation of fibrolamellar HCC of the liver revealed the presence of neurosecretory granules, which were sparse in some cells and abundant in others (Payne et al, 1986), and cells with neuroen-docrine differentiation have been observed in hepatoblastoma (Ruck et al, 1990). HCC may express carcinoid features (Barsky et al, 1984) or can be associated with the carcinoid syndrome (Primack et al, 1971). Using a set of antibodies directed against general neuroendocrine markers and the Grimelius method, it has been shown that neuroendocrine differentiation may occur in several primary neoplasms of the liver, including HCC, biliary carcinoma, and hemangioendothelioma (Wang et al, 1991). These observations warrant further investigation because they may change our view with regard to the definition of neuro-endocrine cells and shed more light on the modulation of cell functions and the differentiation capabilities of hepatic tumor cells. Neuroendocrine substances may be generally used by the liver as signal agents in autocrine or paracrine regulatory circuits and may be expressed in the programming of neoplastic cell growth or in remodeling processes (e.g., in ductular reaction), where expression of neuroendocrine markers and of neural cell adhesion molecule has been observed (Roskams et al, 1990).

Hepatic Tumors and Tumor-like Lesions in Acquired Immunodeficiency Syndrome

The reason why hepatic tumors in AIDS are discussed under the heading, "rare hepatic tumors," is based on the fact that the neoplastic processes and lesions mimicking them occurring in the setting of AIDS are rare in immunocompetent hosts. Visceral Kaposi's sarcoma is rare in individuals with an intact immune system. One third of patients with AIDS who have cutaneous involvement with Kaposi's sarcoma also may have hepatic Kaposi's sarcoma (Schneiderman et al, 1987). Visceral manifestations of Kaposi's sarcoma may be macroscopic or microscopic and are likely to remain undetected ante mortem in many cases, although internal Kaposi's sarcoma may be present even when no manifestation is seen on the skin (Gottlieb et al, 1983; Guarda et al, 1984). Liver involvement is macroscopically visible in the form of multiple dark or purplish lesions, typically situated in subcapsular and hilar regions (Glasgow et al, 1985;

Herndier & Friedman, 1992). Histologically, nodules consisting of spindle cells and atypical vascular channels are seen, mainly within portal tracts (Friedman, 1988; Glasgow et al, 1985). Widespread visceral Kaposi's sarcoma may worsen the prognosis. A striking decrease in survival at 24 months was found in patients with endoscopic evidence of Kaposi's sarcoma (11%) compared with patients without evidence of visceral disease (88%) (Friedman SL et al, 1985).

Atypical vascular structures occurring in hepatic Kaposi's sarcoma should be distinguished from other, but clearly reactive, vascular anomalies known to occur in the liver of patients with AIDS. Peliosis hepatis may develop in AIDS (Czapar et al, 1986; Scoazec et al, 1988). Neoplastic vascular processes have to be separated from bacillary angiomatosis, which can produce a disseminated disease in immunocompromised hosts, and which is known to occur in the liver (LeBoit, 1990). Several cases of bacillary angiomatosis associated with peliosis hepatis have been reported (Perkocha et al, 1990). Typically, one notes clusters of blood-filled spaces with a fibromyxoid stroma, cellular infiltrates, and, sometimes, deposition of a granular material that may correspond to bacilli (Perkocha et al, 1990). Within the lesion, intact bacilli can be shown using the Warthin-Starry, Brown-Hopps, Brown-Brenn, or Steiner's silver stains or by using electron microscopy. A gram-negative agent was identified bearing phylogenetic similarities to rickettsia-like organisms (Relman et al, 1990).

In patients with AIDS, the hepatobiliary system can be involved by NHL, and hepatic involvement is particularly common, having been seen in one series in one third of NHL patients with any gastrointestinal tract involvement (Ziegler et al, 1984). Liver manifestation may be macroscopic or microscopic and may be present in the absence of lymphadenopathy (Lisker-Melman et al, 1989). When large, the lesions can be solid or even cystic, with fluid accumulation (Nyberg et al, 1986). Involvement of the gallbladder (Ziegler et al, 1982) and the common bile duct (Kaplan et al, 1989) has been described. Diagnostic criteria for hepatobiliary NHL in AIDS have been reviewed (Herndier & Friedman, 1992). Hodgkin's disease involving the liver has been reported to occur in human immunodeficiency virus (HIV)–infected patients, and it may be more aggressive than in HIV-negative individuals (Knowles et al, 1988).

Tumor-like Lesions

Rarely, nodular neoplastic growths of the liver are mimicked by lesions of reactive or inflammatory character. These alterations are termed *inflammatory pseudotumor of the liver,* of which about 30 cases have been reported (Horiuchi et al, 1990; Pokorny et al, 1991). Notwithstanding this low reported frequency, inflammatory pseudotumors may become increasingly recognized as a result of the more frequent use of imaging methods. The etiology and pathogenesis of these lesions are still unknown. Initial symptoms are abdominal pain, fever, and weight loss; jaundice is uncommon. Most cases are solitary and located in the right liver lobe (Horiuchi et al, 1990). Male patients predominate, and the highest incidence occurs in infants and young adults. Angiography usually shows hypovascularity or even an apparently avascular lesion, and CT reveals a mass of low density. The histologic picture is dominated by infiltrates consisting of lymphocytes, plasma cells and foamy macrophages, lymphoid follicles, granuloma formation, foreign body giant cells, marked

fibrosis, and occasionally occlusive phlebitis of relatively large portal vein branches (Horiuchi et al, 1990; Pokorny et al, 1991). In young children, solitary lesions may involve the porta hepatis (Stamatakis et al, 1979). Most lesions reported so far have been resected. In a review, only 4 of 29 patients did not undergo resection, but 2 of these patients were alive and well 4 and 5 years after diagnosis (Horiuchi et al, 1990). *Inflammatory pseudotumor of the liver* should not be confused with a similar term used to denote regenerating hyperplastic nodules in cirrhosis—*hepatocellular pseudotumor in the cirrhotic liver* (Nagasue et al, 1984).

Another solitary lesion that may mimic neoplastic liver disease on ultrasound is the so-called solitary necrotic nodule of the liver (Shepherd & Lee, 1983). These lesions are usually benign, and an origin in hemangiomata is confirmed for most alterations of this type studied so far (Sundaresan et al, 1991).

LIVER TUMORS IN INFANCY

The discussion of pathologic aspects of hepatic tumors has been directed mainly toward lesions in patients outside the pediatric age group and has dealt with most of the tumors for which surgery might be contemplated. It is appropriate, however, to refer to some tumors in infancy and childhood that may be encountered in surgical practice (see Ch. 72).

Hepatoblastoma

Hepatoblastoma is a rare solid embryonic hepatic neoplasm of childhood apparently recapitulating several developmental phases of the liver (Ishak & Glunz, 1967; Keeling, 1971). Although hepatoblastoma is the most common malignant liver tumor in childhood (Perilongo et al, 2002), with an expected annual incidence of 1 case per 1 million children younger than 15 years old, it represents only 0.8% to 1% of all childhood malignant tumors. The male-to-female ratio is about 2.2:1 (Darbari et al, 2003). Most cases are detected in children younger than 5 years old, and few cases are seen in the neonatal period. A total of 65% to 70% are diagnosed in children younger than 2 years old. AFP is elevated in most (90-95%) patients. Hepatoblastoma rarely may occur in adults (Carter, 1969). The etiology and pathogenesis have not been clarified so far.

Low birth weight (<1000 g) may represent a risk factor in that this group of children is overrepresented in patients having hepatoblastoma (Ikeda et al, 1998). Findings of the Surveillance, Epidemiology and End Results program of the United States suggest that an increased incidence of hepatoblastoma coincides with the improved survival of children with low birth weight (Ross & Gurney, 1998). One study suggested that hepatoblastoma with unfavorable biologic behavior develops in children who are extremely premature at birth (Ikeda et al, 1998). Apart from very low birth weight, AFP levels may represent an important prognosticator (Von Schweinitz et al, 1997). Although most cases of hepatoblastoma are sporadic, familial occurrence is known (Sotelo-Avila et al, 1975), and an association with hereditary disorders (i.e., Beckwith-Wiedemann syndrome and familial APC syndrome) has been noted (Kingston et al, 1983). Some cases of hepatoblastoma are considered as extracolic manifestations of APC because long-term survivors of hepatoblastoma (chiefly boys) and relatives of children with hepatoblastoma can develop APC (Giardiello et al, 1996). Hepatoblastoma patients later developing APC also may show retinal pigment epithelium hypertrophy as in Gardner's syndrome. Hepatoblastoma has been encountered in association with precocious puberty; these patients have elevated levels of human chorionic gonadotropin in the serum and focal intracellular human chorionic gonadotropin positivity in tumor cells (Arshad et al, 1982). Fetal components of hepatoblastoma are usually diploid, whereas embryonal parts are aneuploid (Rugge et al, 1998).

Cytogenetically, patients with hepatoblastoma may exhibit trisomy of chromosome 20 (as in some APC families), of chromosome 8, and of the q arm of chromosome 2. Additional anomalies comprise double minute chromosomes, unbalanced translocations involving chromosomes 1 and 4, breakpoints in chromosome 1, and deletions of the short arm of chromosome 1 (Kraus et al, 1996; Rodriguez et al, 1991; Sainati et al, 1998). The significance of these changes is unknown. Molecular genetic analyses also have shown an allelic loss of the region 11p15.5, a region frequently altered in Beckwith-Wiedemann syndrome and harboring, among others, the gene of the autocrine growth factor insulin-like growth factor II (Albrecht et al, 1994).

Macroscopically, the right liver lobe is involved in 60% to 70% of cases, and most tumors manifest with a smooth or lobulated contour (Fig. 69.40). Multifocality or diffuse infiltration is uncommon. Most hepatoblastomas weigh 400 to 500 g at time of diagnosis and measure 5 to 20 cm in diameter. The TNM staging system employed for the pretreatment assessment of disease is not optimal for hepatoblastoma. The Childhood Liver Tumors Study Group of the International Society of Pediatric Oncology devised a new system called *PRETEXT* (Pre Treatment Extent of Disease) (MacKinlay & Pritchard, 1992), which is not synonymous with other staging systems (Conran et al, 1992; Von Schweinitz et al, 1997). Gross examination of resection specimens reveals solid and cystic structures, a nodular architecture, and sometimes a mucoid appearance. Greenish nodules (deposition of bile), calcifications (especially post-treatment), hemorrhage, and necrosis also may be encountered. Gross blood vessel invasion is unusual, but it may be impressive when it occurs (see Fig. 69.40).

Originally, two basic histologic types were identified: an epithelial type, with a fetal or an embryonal pattern or a combination of both, and a mixed type, which consists of primitive mesenchymal cells in addition to the epithelial components. Later, a third distinctive pattern was added, the anaplastic pattern (Kasai & Watanabe, 1970). A fourth pattern (macrotrabecular) subsequently was described (Gonzales-Crussi et al, 1982a). The criteria for histologic classification of hepatoblastomas have been reviewed (Rowland, 2002). A variant of the mixed type of hepatoblastoma contains elements of all three germ layers and has been named *teratoid hepatoblastoma* (Manivel et al, 1986). A histologic classification based on epithelial and mesenchymal components has been proposed (Conran et al, 1992). The classification currently employed by the Childhood Liver Tumors Study Group of the International Society of Pediatric Oncology is as follows:

Hepatoblastoma, wholly epithelial type
    Fetal subtype
    Embryonal subtype
    Macrotrabecular subtype
    Small cell undifferentiated subtype (formerly anaplastic subtype)
Hepatoblastoma, mixed epithelial and mesenchymal type
    Without teratoid features
    With teratoid features
Hepatoblastoma, not otherwise specified

The fetal subtype refers to a tumor where any part is composed of small, round, uniform cells with abundant cytoplasm and distinct cytoplasmic membranes. Thin trabeculae are formed (two to three cells thick). The embryonal subtype shows cells arranged in sheets of irregular, angulated cells with a high nucleo-cytoplasmic ratio, increased nuclear chromatin, and indistinct cytoplasmic membranes. The macrotrabecular subtype refers to a tumor in which trabeculae more than 10 cells thick are present in a repetitive pattern. The large trabeculae contain fetal- or embryonal-type cells, or a third, larger, hepatocyte-like cell type, or a combination of all three cell types; the macrotrabecular phenotype refers to a growth pattern rather than a distinct subtype. Small cell undifferentiated hepatoblastoma (originally

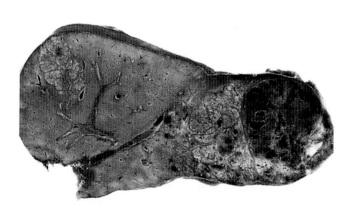

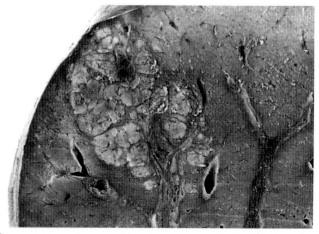

A   B

Fig. 69.40. Hepatoblastoma. **A,** The primary tumor can be seen on the *right-hand side of the figure*; it shows hemorrhage and necrosis. The neoplasm has invaded an intrahepatic portal vein branch *(center of figure)* and has spread to form an intrahepatic metastasis *(left-hand upper corner)*. **B,** Metastasis at higher magnification. Note the numerous nodular outgrowths centered around the vascular tree. Resection specimen.

designated *anaplastic*) consists of a diffuse population of small cells with scant cytoplasm and indistinct cell membranes, resembling neuroblastoma cells. The mixed pattern shows a combination of fetal or embryonal patterns intermixed with primitive spindled mesenchymal cells. Osteoid-like material is a common feature. The mixed pattern with teratoid features contains the aforementioned epithelial and mesenchymal elements and various combinations of foci of mature cartilage, skeletal muscle, intestinal-type and keratinized squamous epithelium, and melanin pigment (Conran et al, 1992). The prognostic significance of these patterns has been analyzed (Haas et al, 1989, Conran et al, 1992). Immunohistochemistry has shown that AFP may be expressed in cells of the fetal and embryonal types, but not in the small cell pattern (Abenoza et al, 1987). Neuroendocrine differentiation in hepatoblastomas has been shown, indicating the multidirectional differentiation of this tumor (Ruck et al, 1990).

There is evidence that histologic subtypes of hepatoblastoma are associated with tumor biology. The small cell undifferentiated phenotype generally is regarded as a high-risk morphology (Haas et al, 1989; Lack et al, 1982; Ortega et al, 2000). It has been shown that a focal (partial or predominant) expression of a small cell phenotype in completely resected hepatoblastomas has an unfavorable effect on outcome (Haas et al, 2001). The macrotrabecular subtype is suggested to be unfavorable as well, but the data are still sparse. Only two systematic studies performed so far have referred to this morphology; one uncovered an unfavorable effect, whereas the other found no prognostic effect. In contrast to these two morphotypes, a purely fetal pattern of hepatoblastoma has a favorable effect on outcome.

Within the frame of large pathology reviews, other phenotypes of hepatoblastoma and related tumors have emerged. A subset of hepatoblastomas exhibits ductlike profiles consisting of cholangiocyte-like cells, a tumor variant proposed to be termed *hepatoblastoma with cholangioblastic features* or *cholangioblastic hepatoblastoma* (Zimmermann, 2002). A bile duct cell component also is evident in rare tumors in some way mimicking an abnormal ductal plate (*ductal plate tumors*) (Gornicka et al, 2001; Zimmermann, 2002). A novel liver cell tumor developing in older children and young adolescents expressing a hepatocyte-like phenotype, but being different from HCC, has been described under the term *transitional liver cell tumor,* "transitional" meaning that the cells involved theoretically hold a position intermediate between hepatoblasts and mature hepatocytes (Prokurat et al, 2002). Transitional liver cell tumor is a highly aggressive lesion that usually manifests as large tumors associated with high or very high serum AFP levels. The issue of emerging phenotypes in the hepatoblastoma family of tumors has been reviewed (Zimmermann, 2005).

More recent investigations have aimed at better understanding of the cells involved in the development of hepatoblastoma and their growth regulation. One cell lineage dominating hepatoblastoma is the hepatocyte and the precursors thereof. That a hepatocyte differentiation pathway seems to start early in hepatoblastoma carcinogenesis is underlined by the observation that a typical marker for the parenchymal cell, Hep Par 1, is expressed in all hepatoblastomas (Fasano et al, 1998), apart from lineage-specific cytokeratins (Van Eyken et al, 1990b). Of particular interest is the question as to whether hepatoblastoma takes its origin from hepatic precursor cells. Ductal plate and bile duct cells in developing human liver express, in association with certain cytokeratins, hematopoietic stem cell markers,

such as c-kit and CD 34 (Lemmer et al, 1998), and the role of such cells, which may reappear as oval cells in the regenerating liver or as tumor cells, is currently being analyzed. The identification of so-called small epithelial cells corresponding to oval cells of the rat in human hepatoblastoma supports the hypothesis that hepatoblastoma may derive from a pluripotent stem cell (Ruck et al, 1996). The finding that antigens associated with oval cells can be observed in hepatoblastoma supports this hypothesis (Ruck et al, 1997).

The clonal expansion of putative precursor cells, their modes of proliferation and differentiation, and the regulation thereof are only partially known. Apart from intracellular regulators of growth involved in hepatoblastoma, such as igf2 and h19 (Li et al, 1998), cell-to-cell and cell-to-matrix contacts mediated by adhesion molecules play a role (Von Schweinitz et al, 1996). The proliferative activity of embryonal components seems to be higher than that of fetal components (Rugge et al, 1998), but the growth characteristics of small undifferentiated cells has not been clarified. Transforming growth factor-α, a potent stimulator of hepatic cell proliferation, is expressed in better differentiated hepatoblastoma, whereas less differentiated components do not depend on growth stimulation by this cytokine (Kiss et al, 1998). Alterations in the cyclin-dependent kinase inhibitor A gene family do not seem to play a significant role for the growth of hepatoblastoma, whereas changes in the cell division cycle regulators, cyclins D, seem to be involved (Iolascon et al, 1998). A further gene that is altered in hepatoblastoma is the *PLK1* oncogene, encoding an execution protein of cytokinesis, Polo-like kinase-1. This gene is highly expressed in hepatoblastomas and indicates a poor prognosis (Yamada et al, 2004). A few putative tumor suppressor genes also may be altered in hepatoblastoma (e.g., the paternally imprinted polyspecific transporter gene *BWR1A* (Beckwith-Wiedemann–related gene 1A) assigned to 11p15.5, a region implicated in Beckwith-Wiedemann syndrome (Albrecht et al, 2004).

Investigations have shown that complex alterations in signal transduction pathways occur in hepatoblastomas, in particular changes in the Wnt/beta-catenin signaling pathway (Buendia, 2002). Beta-catenin is central to the converging Wnt, beta-catenin, and cadherin pathways, where it forms a signaling complex with axin, the APC tumor suppressor protein, glycogen synthase kinase 3β, and other proteins (Nelson & Nusse, 2004). Mutations in the beta-catenin gene represent the most frequent molecular alteration in sporadic hepatoblastoma detected so far (Buendia, 2002). Mutations of the degradation targeting box of the beta-catenin gene favor the bypassing of the proteasomal degradation of beta-catenin and a preferential shift of the protein into the cell nucleus, where it can be detected by immunohistochemistry. Nuclear localization of beta-catenin related to the respective gene mutations is a prognosticator in hepatoblastoma (Park et al, 2001), and beta-catenin mutations are associated with poorly differentiated histology in these tumors (Takayasu et al, 2001).

Hepatocellular Carcinoma

The morphologic features of HCC (see Ch. 72) in childhood are similar to the features of its adult counterpart except in the lack of underlying liver cirrhosis in many pediatric cases (Schmidt et al, 1985; Weinberg & Finegold, 1983). HCC is uncommon in children younger than 5 years old, but may occur in infants. A distinct variant, fibrolamellar HCC, occurs in the noncirrhotic livers of older children and young adults (see earlier). Associations of HCC and its possible causes and liver cell adenoma in children already have been discussed.

Mesenchymal Hamartoma

Mesenchymal hamartoma (see Ch. 72), a rare tumor, is characterized macroscopically by a lobulated, multicystic, or solid nonencapsulated mass or a pedunculated lesion, usually occurring in children younger than age 2 years and located in the right liver lobe in 75% to 80% of cases (Arfa et al, 2003; Stocker & Ishak 1983). It is the third most common hepatic tumor in infants, after hepatoblastoma and hemangioendothelioma. A progressively enlarging liver mass, usually without other clinical manifestations, is the most frequent presentation in a child younger than 2 years old. The median age at diagnosis is about 10 months, but the lesion has been observed prenatally, in the neonatal period, as late as 10 years old (Alwaidh et al, 1997; Bejvan et al, 1997; Tovbin et al, 1997), and in adults (Drachenberg et al, 1991). Clinicopathologic differences between pediatric and adult cases were identified by Cook and coworkers (2003).

Mesenchymal hamartoma of the liver may be associated with an unexpected elevation of serum AFP and may mimic hepatoblastoma, particularly in cases where cysts are lacking (Boman et al, 2004). Histologically, the predominant component is a fibrous or loose myxoid stroma containing epithelial-lined structures resembling bile ducts. A variable contribution of a cholangiocyte lineage also is documented by use of immunohistochemistry (Abdulkader et al, 2004b). Lymphangioma-like structures may be encountered. At DNA cytometric analysis, most mesenchymal hamartomas are diploid, but a subset is aneuploid (Otal et al, 1994). Distinct chromosomal aberrations have been described in part of the lesions, including a recurrent translocation involving chromosome band 19q13.4 (Bove et al, 1998; Rakheja et al, 2004), suggesting that at least a subset of the hamartomas may be true neoplasms. The lesion is benign and resectable without much difficulty in most patients. There also is evidence that mesenchymal hamartoma (even very large lesions) may spontaneously regress and calcify (Narasimhan et al, 2004). An intriguing question is whether undifferentiated embryonal sarcoma might arise in mesenchymal hamartoma of the liver. Support for a relationship between undifferentiated embryonal sarcoma and mesenchymal hamartoma is based on a few reports only (however, in part with the demonstration of shared genetic anomalies), and the association remains tenuous (Begueret et al, 2001; De Chadarevian et al, 1994; Lauwers et al, 1997; O'Sullivan et al, 2001).

A novel, smooth muscle tissue–containing variant of a hepatic hamartomatous lesion has been described under the term *myoid hamartoma of the liver* (Gornicka et al, 2004). Undifferentiated embryonal sarcoma of the liver and infantile hemangioendothelioma have been discussed together with other mesenchymal tumors of the liver earlier.

Malignant Rhabdoid Tumor of the Liver

Malignant rhabdoid tumor, a highly malignant neoplasm, is particularly well known as a renal tumor (Beckwith & Palmer, 1978), but extrarenal malignant rhabdoid tumor is established for several organs, including the liver. About 18 cases of hepatic malignant rhabdoid tumor have been reported so far (Yuri et al, 2004). Malignant rhabdoid tumor has a characteristic histology, with medium-sized to large, so-called rhabdoid cells frequently showing a paranuclear eosinophilic inclusion body ultrastructurally consisting of cytoskeletal filaments and immunoreactive for cytokeratins and vimentin (Haas et al, 1981; Yuri et al, 2004). The presence of rhabdoid cells is a feature occurring in several tumors, including carcinomas, but is a particularly distinct hallmark of malignant rhabdoid tumor. Rhabdoid cells resemble rhabdomyoblasts, but do not belong to a myoid cell lineage. The origin of the rhabdoid cell is still unknown. When detected in a tumor, the cells generally indicate a highly aggressive phenotype. It has been shown that mutated codons of the cytokeratin 8 gene in malignant rhabdoid tumor are located in the important region involved in the conformational change of intermediate filaments (Shiratsuchi et al, 2002).

Atypical teratoid rhabdoid intracranial tumors and some extrarenal malignant rhabdoid tumors exhibit mutations of the *hSNF5/INI1* gene (Biegel et al, 2002). The tumor suppressor *hSNF5 (integrase interactor)/INI1* is a component of the adenosine triphosphate–dependent chromatin remodeling *hSWI/SNF* complex. It induces cell cycle arrest (Reincke et al, 2003) and modulates cell growth via control of the G_1-S checkpoint (Versteege et al, 2002), repression of cyclin D1 transcription (Zhang et al, 2002), and actin cytoskeleton organization (Medjkane et al, 2004).

Hepatobiliary Rhabdomyosarcoma

Rhabdomyosarcoma of the biliary tract is a very rare, but clinically characteristic lesion in children. It is a highly aggressive tumor. At diagnosis, 75% of children are younger than 5 years old. Pediatric hepatobiliary rhabdomyosarcoma accounts for only 0.8% of all rhabdomyosarcomas and 1.3% of all liver tumors (Aggarwal et al, 2004; Kebudi et al, 2003). Growth of hepatobiliary rhabdomyosarcoma closely follows the walls of the intrahepatic or extrahepatic bile ducts or both, sometimes with intraluminal growth resulting in the typical botryoid (grapelike) features, associated with prestenotic dilation of the ducts involved. Hepatobiliary rhabdomyosarcoma is usually of the embryonal type, and the histology reflects the patterns known for other situations in which embryonal rhabdomyosarcoma develops in association with a mucosal surface.

Pediatric Hepatic Tumors Related to Perivascular Epithelioid Cells

Hepatic angiomyolipoma that is related to the perivascular epithelioid cell system has been discussed in the section on vascular tumors. Unusual and sometimes huge neoplasms occurring in the hepatic ligaments of children and apparently derived from perivascular epithelioid cells have been reported. These novel types of clear cell PEComas, not related to tuberous sclerosis and originating from the falciform or round ligaments of children and young adults, are termed *clear cell epithelioid tumors* (Tanaka et al, 2000) or *clear cell myomelanocytic tumors* (Folpe et al, 2000) of hepatic ligaments.

ACKNOWLEDGMENT

The excellent secretarial help of Erna H. Kramel is greatfully acknowledged.

REFERENCES

Abdulkader I, et al, 2004a: Liver-cell adenomas with heavy iron deposition. Int J Surg Pathol 12:245-250.

Abdulkader I, et al, 2004b: Mesenchymal hamartoma of the liver: clinico-pathological, immunohistochemical and flow cytometric study of two cases. Hepatol Res 28:216-219.

Abenoza P, et al, 1987: Hepatoblastoma: an immunohistochemical and ultra-structural study. Hum Pathol 18:1025-1035.

Adachi E, et al, 1993: Proliferating cell nuclear antigen in hepatocellular carcinoma and small cell liver dysplasia. Cancer 72:2902-2909.

Agarwal VR, et al, 1998: Molecular basis of severe gynecomastia associated with aromatase expression in a fibrolamellar hepatocellular carcinoma. J Clin Endocrinol Metab 83:1797-1800.

Aggarwal K, et al, 2004: Botryoid rhabdomyosarcoma of common bile duct. Ind J Pediatr 71:363-364.

Aihara T, et al, 1996: Clonal analysis of precancerous lesion of hepatocellular carcinoma. Gastroenterology 111:455-461.

Albar JP, et al, 1996: Immunohistochemical detection of parathyroid hormone-related protein in a rare variant of hepatic neoplasm (sclerosing hepatic carcinoma). Hum Pathol 27:728-731.

Albores-Saavedra J, et al, 2001: Atypical bile duct adenoma, clear cell type: a previously undescribed tumor of the liver. Am J Surg Pathol 25:956-960.

Albrecht S, et al, 1994: Loss of maternal alleles on chromosome arm 11p in hepatoblastoma. Cancer Res 54:5041-5044.

Albrecht S, et al, 2004: Allelic loss but absence of mutations on the polyspecific transporter gene BWR1A on 11p15.5 in hepatoblastoma. Int J Cancer 111:627-632.

Ali M, et al, 1978: Malignant APUDoma of the liver with symptomatic intractable hypoglycemia. Cancer 42:686-692.

Alshak NS, et al, 1994: Hepatocellular adenoma in glycogen storage disease type IV. Arch Pathol Lab Med 118:88-91.

Alwaidh MH, et al, 1997: Mesenchymal hamartoma of the liver: a case report. Pediatr Radiol 27:247-249.

Anbazhagan R, et al, 1990: The distribution of immunoreactive tenascin in the epithelial-mesenchymal junctional areas of benign and malignant squamous epithelia. Virchows Arch B 59:59-63.

Andant C, et al, 1997: Occurrence of hepatocellular carcinoma in a case of hereditary coproporphyria. Am J Gastroenterol 92:1389-1390.

Andreola S, et al, 1990: A clinico-pathologic study of primary hepatic carcinoid tumors. Cancer 65:1211-1218.

Andreu V, et al, 1997: Plexiform neurofibromatosis and angiosarcoma of the liver in von Recklinghausen disease. Am J Gastroenterol 92:1229-1230.

Anthony PP, 1973: Primary carcinoma of the liver: a study of 282 cases in Ugandan Africans. J Pathol 110:37-48.

Anthony PP, 1976: Precursor lesions for liver cancer in humans. Cancer Res 36:2579-2583.

Anthony PP, et al, 1978: The morphology of cirrhosis. J Clin Pathol 31:395-414.

Anzola M, 2004: Hepatocellular carcinoma: role of hepatitis B and hepatitis C viruses proteins in hepatocarcinogenesis. J Viral Hepat 11:383-393.

Aoyama C, et al, 1991: Undifferentiated (embryonal) sarcoma of the liver: a tumour of uncertain histogenesis showing divergent differentiation. Am J Surg Pathol 15:615-624.

Arbuthnot P, Kew M, 2001: Hepatitis B virus and hepatocellular carcinoma. Int J Exp Pathol 82:77-100.

Arfa MN, et al, 2003: Cystic mesenchymal hamartoma of the liver: report of a case and review of the literature. Hepatogastroenterology 50(suppl 2): ccxlix-ccli.

Arii S, et al, 1992: Predictive factors for intrahepatic recurrence of hepatocellular carcinoma after partial hepatectomy. Cancer 69:913-919.

Arsenault TM, et al, 1996: Hepatic adenomatosis. Mayo Clin Proc 71:478-480.

Arshad RR, et al, 1982: Virilizing hepatoblastoma: precocious sexual development and partial response of pulmonary metastases to cis-platinum. CA Cancer J Clin 32:293-295.

Arthur MJP, et al, 1984: Hepatitis B, hepatocellular carcinoma, and strategies for prevention. Lancet 1:607-610.

Athanassion AM, Craigo SD, 1998: Liver masses in pregnancy. Semin Perinatol 22:166-177.

Attal P, et al, 2003: Telangiectatic focal nodular hyperplasia: US, CT, and MR imaging findings with histopathologic correlation in 13 cases. Radiology 228:465-472.

Bacq Y, et al, 2003: Familial liver adenomatosis associated with hepatocyte nuclear factor 1alpha inactivation. Gastroenterology 125:1470-1475.

Baer HU, et al, 1989: Resectability of larger focal liver lesions. Br J Surg 76:1042-1045.

Bail B, et al, 1996: Cystic smooth-muscle tumor of the liver and spleen associated with Epstein-Barr virus after renal transplantation. Am J Surg Pathol 20: 1418-1425.

Bala S, et al, 1997: Childhood hepatocellular adenoma in familial adenomatous polyposis: mutations in adenomatous polyposis coli gene and p53. Gastroenterology 112:919-922.

Barbin A, et al, 1997: p53 gene mutation pattern in rat liver tumors induced by vinyl chloride. Cancer Res 57:1695-1698.

Barnes PA, et al, 1981: Pitfalls in the diagnosis of hepatic cysts by computed tomography. Radiology 141:129-133.

Barsky SH, et al, 1984: Hepatocellular carcinoma with carcinoid features. Hum Pathol 15:892-894.

Bartley J, et al, 2004: Hepatocellular adenoma and focal nodular hyperplasia after long-term use of danazol for endometriosis: a case report. Arch Gynecol Obstet 269:290-293.

Beasley RP, 1988: Hepatitis B virus: the major etiology of hepatocellular carcinoma. In Fortner JC, Rhoads JE (eds): Accomplishment in Cancer Research 1987. Philadelphia, Lippincott.

Beck K, et al, 1990: Structure and function of laminin: anatomy of a multidomain glycoprotein. FASEB J 4:148-152.

Beckwith JB, Palmer NF, 1978: Histopathology and prognosis of Wilms tumor: results from the First National Wilms' Tumor Study. Cancer 41:1937-1948.

Bedossa P, et al, 1995: Transforming growth factor-beta1 (TGF-beta 1) and TGF-beta 1 receptors in normal, cirrhotic and neoplastic human livers. Hepatology 21:760-766.

Begueret H, et al, 2001: Hepatic undifferentiated embryonal sarcoma: malignant evolution of mesenchymal hamartoma? Study of one case with immunohistochemical and flow cytometric emphasis. J Hepatol 34:178-179.

Behar A, et al, 1963: Acquired hypofibrinogenemia associated with a giant cavernous hemangioma of the liver. Am J Clin Pathol 40:78-82.

Bejvan SM, et al, 1997: Prenatal evaluation of mesenchymal hamartoma of the liver: gray scale and power Doppler sonographic imaging. J Ultrasound Med 16:227-229.

Belhadj K, et al, 2003: Hepatosplenic γδ T-cell lymphoma is a rare clinicopathologic entity with poor outcome: report on a series of 21 patients. Blood 102:4261-4269.

Bell CD, 2003: Endothelial cell tumors. Microsc Res Tech 60:165-170.

Belli L, et al, 1989: Reappraisal of surgical treatment of small hepatocellular carcinomas in cirrhosis: clinicopathological study of resection or transplantation. Dig Dis Sci 34:1571-1575.

Bergman S, et al, 1997: The usefulness of the reticulin stain in the differential diagnosis of liver nodules on fine-needle aspiration biopsy cell block preparations. Mod Pathol 10:1258-1264.

Berman MM, et al, 1980: Hepatocellular carcinoma: polygonal cell type with fibrous stroma—an atypical variant with a favorable prognosis. Cancer 46: 1448-1455.

Biegel JA, et al, 2002: The role of INI1 and the SWI/SNF complex in the development of rhabdoid tumors: meeting summary from the workshop on childhood atypical teratoid/rhabdoid tumors. Cancer Res 62:323-328.

Bierman HR, et al, 1951: Studies of blood supply of tumors in man: vascular pattern of the liver by hepatic arteriography in vivo. J Natl Cancer Inst 12:107-131.

Bioulac-Sage P, et al, 2001: Diagnosis of focal nodular hyperplasia: not so easy. Am J Surg Pathol 25:1322-1325.

Bisogno G, et al, 2002: Undifferentiated sarcoma of the liver in childhood: a curable disease. Cancer 94:252-257.

Blaker H, et al, 2004: Analysis of somatic APC mutations in rare extracolonic tumors of patients with familial adenomatous polyposis coli. Genes Chromosomes Cancer 41:93-98.

Block TM, et al, 2003: Molecular viral oncology of hepatocellular carcinoma. Oncogene 22:5093-5107.

Bluteau O, et al, 2002: Bi-allelic inactivation of TCF1 in hepatic adenomas. Nat Genet 32:312-315.

Boman F, et al, 2004: Mesenchymal hamartomas of the liver may be associated with increased serum alpha foetoprotein concentrations and mimic hepatoblastomas. Eur J Pediatr Surg 14:63-66.

Borzio M, et al, 1998: Hepatocyte proliferation rate is a powerful parameter for predicting hepatocellular carcinoma development in liver cirrhosis. J Clin Pathol Mol Pathol 51:96-101.

Borzio M, et al, 2003: Impact of large regenerative, low grade and high grade dysplastic nodules in hepatocellular carcinoma development. J Hepatol 39:208-214.

Bosetti C, et al, 2003: Occupational exposure to vinyl chloride and cancer risk: a review of the epidemiologic literature. Eur J Cancer Prev 12:427-430.

Bove KE, et al, 1998: Third report of t(19q)(13.4) in mesenchymal hamartoma of liver with comments on link to embryonal sarcoma. Pediatr Dev Pathol 1:438-442.

Bradbear RA, et al, 1985: Cohort study of internal malignancy in genetic hemochromatosis and other chronic nonalcoholic liver disease. J Natl Cancer Inst 75:81-84.

Brawer MK, et al, 1980: Focal fatty change of the liver, a hitherto poorly recognized entity. Gastroenterology 78:247-252.

Bréchot C, et al, 1982: Evidence that hepatitis B virus has a role in liver cell carcinoma in alcoholic liver disease. N Engl J Med 306:1384-1387.

Bréchot C, et al, 1985: Hepatitis B virus DNA in patients with chronic liver disease and negative tests for hepatitis B surface antigen. N Engl J Med 312:270-276.

Broders AC, 1920: Squamous-cell epithelioma of the lip, a study of five hundred thirty seven cases. JAMA 74:656-664.

Bronowicki JP, et al, 2003: Primary lymphoma of the liver: clinico-pathological features and relationship with HCV infection in French patients. Hepatology 37:781-787.

Bruix J, Llovet JM, 2003: Hepatitis B virus and hepatocellular carcinoma. J Hepatol 39(suppl 1):S59-S63.

Bruix J, et al, 2004: Focus on hepatocellular carcinoma. Cancer Cell 5:215-219.

Brunt EM, Tiniakos DG, 2005: Pathological features of NASH. Front Biosci 10:1475-1484.

Brunt EM, et al, 2004: Nonalcoholic steatohepatitis: histologic features and clinical correlations with 30 blinded biopsy specimens. Hum Pathol 35:1070-1082.

Buchanan TF, Huvos AG, 1974: Clear-cell carcinoma of the liver: a clinico-pathological study of 13 patients. Am J Clin Pathol 61:529-539.

Buehler H, et al, 1982: Regression of liver cell adenoma: a follow-up study of three consecutive patients after discontinuation of oral contraceptive use. Gastroenterology 82:775-782.

Buendia MA, 2002: Genetic alterations in hepatoblastoma and hepatocellular carcinoma: common and distinctive aspects. Med Pediatr Oncol 39:530-535.

Bugianesi E, et al, 2002: Expanding the natural history of nonalcoholic steato-hepatitis: from cryptogenic cirrhosis to hepatocellular carcinoma. Gastroenterology 123:134-140.

Burdette WJ, 1975: Neoplasms of the liver. In Schiff L (ed): Diseases of the Liver, 4th ed. Philadelphia, Lippincott, p 1070.

Buresu C, et al, 2004: Liver nodules resembling focal nodular hyperplasia after portal vein thrombosis. J Hepatol 41:499-500.

Caldwell SH, et al, 2004: Obesity and hepatocellular carcinoma. Gastroenterology 127(suppl 1):S97-S103.

Carter R, 1969: Hepatoblastoma in the adult. Cancer 23:191-197.

Centeno JA, et al, 2002: Pathology related to chronic arsenic exposure. Environ Health Perspect 110(suppl 5):883-886.

Cha C, et al, 2004: Surgical therapy for hepatocellular carcinoma. Adv Surg 38:363-376.

Chang KL, Arber DA, 1998: Hepatosplenic γδ T-cell lymphoma—not just an alphabet soup. Adv Anat Pathol 5:21-29.

Chen KTK, 1983: Hepatic leiomyosarcoma. J Surg Oncol 24:325-328.

Chen YW, et al, 2002: P53 and Wnt signaling in benign neoplasms: beta-catenin mutations in hepatic adenoma but not in focal nodular hyperplasia. Hepatology 36:927-935.

Cheng WSC, et al, 1992: Hepatocellular carcinoma in a case of Wilson's disease. Liver 12:42-45.

Cheuk W, Chan JK, 2001: Clear cell variant of fibrolamellar carcinoma of the liver. Arch Pathol Lab Med 125:1235-1238.

Cheuk W, et al, 2002: Epstein-Barr virus–associated smooth muscle tumour: a distinctive mesenchymal tumour of immunocompromised individuals. Pathology 34:245-249.

Chiche L, et al, 2000: Liver adenomatosis: reappraisal, diagnosis, and surgical management: eight new cases and review of the literature. Ann Surg 231:74-81.

Chiquet-Ehrismann R, et al, 1986: Tenascin: an extracellular matrix protein involved in tissue interactions during fetal development and oncogenesis. Cell 47:131-139.

Chiquet-Ehrismann R, et al, 1988: Tenascin interferes with fibronectin action. Cell 53:383-390.

Chow NH, et al, 1997: Expression of vascular endothelial growth factor in normal liver and hepatocellular carcinoma: an immunohistochemical study. Hum Pathol 28:698-703.

Chowdhary SK, et al, 2004: Undifferentiated embryonal sarcoma in children: beware of the solitary liver cyst. J Pediatr Surg 39:E9-E12.

Cohen C, et al, 1998: Sex and androgenic steroid receptor expression in hepatic adenomas. Hum Pathol 29:1428-1432.

Coire CI, et al, 1987: Hepatic adenomata in type Ia glycogen storage disease. Arch Pathol Lab Med 111:166-169.

Coleman WB, 2003: Mechanisms of human hepatocarcinogenesis. Curr Mol Med 3:573-588.

Collier NR, et al, 1984: Neurotensin secretion by fibrolamellar carcinoma of the liver. Lancet 1:538-540.

Colombo M, 1992: Hepatocellular carcinoma. J Hepatol 15:225-236.

Conran RM, et al, 1992: Hepatoblastoma: the prognostic significance of histologic type. Pediatr Pathol 12:167-183.

Cook JR, et al, 2003: Mesenchymal hamartoma of the liver in the adult: association with distinct clinical features and histological changes. Hum Pathol 33:893-898.

Cooke CB, et al, 1996: Hepatosplenic T-cell lymphoma: a distinct clinicopathologic entity of cytotoxic γδ T-cell origin. Blood 88:4265-4274.

Cotrim HP, et al, 2000: Nonalcoholic steatohepatitis and hepatocellular carcinoma: natural history? Am J Gastroenterol 95:3018-3019.

Cottone M, et al, 1989: Asymptomatic hepatocellular carcinoma in Child's A cirrhosis. Gastroenterology 96:1566-1571.

Craig JR, et al, 1980: Fibrolamellar carcinoma of the liver: a tumor of adolescents and young adults with distinctive clinicopathologic features. Cancer 46:372-379.

Cuadrado A, et al, 2005: Non-alcoholic steatohepatitis (NASH) and hepatocellular carcinoma. Obes Surg 15:442-446.

Czapar CA, et al, 1986: Peliosis hepatis in the acquired immunodeficiency syndrome. Arch Pathol Lab Med 110:611-613.

Daneshmend TK, et al, 1979: Angiosarcoma of liver associated with phenelzine. BMJ 2:1679.

Darbari A, et al, 2003: Epidemiology of primary hepatic malignancies in U.S. children. Hepatology 38:560-566.

Davis M, et al, 1975: Histological evidence of carcinoma in a hepatic tumour associated with oral contraceptives. BMJ 4:496-498.

De Chadarevian JP, et al, 1994: Undifferentiated (embryonal) sarcoma arising in conjunction with mesenchymal hamartoma of the liver. Mod Pathol 7:490-493.

Dehner LP, Ishak KG, 1971: Vascular tumors of the liver in infants and children: a study of 30 cases and review of the literature. Arch Pathol 92:101-111.

Demel P, 1926: Ein operierter Fall von Lebermyom. Virchows Arch 261:881-884.

Demetris AJ, et al, 1997: Hepatic epithelioid hemangioendothelioma: biological questions based on pattern of recurrence in an allograft and tumor immunophenotype. Am J Surg Pathol 21:263-270.

Den Bakker MA, et al, 1998: Subtotal liver calcification due to epithelioid hemangioendothelioma. Pathol Res Pract 194:189-194.

Deoras MP, Dicus W, 1973: Hepatocarcinoma associated with biliary cirrhosis. Arch Pathol 86:338-341.

Dische MR, Gardner HA, 1978: Mixed teratoid tumor of the liver and neck in trisomy 13. Am J Clin Pathol 69:631-637.

Donato MF, et al, 1989: Distribution of basement membrane components in human hepatocellular carcinoma. Cancer 63:272-279.

Dong-Dong L, et al, 2003: Expression and significance of new tumor suppressor gene PTEN in primary liver cancer. J Cell Mol Med 7:67-71.

Drachenberg CB, et al, 1991: Adult mesenchymal hamartoma of the liver: report of a case with light microscopic, FNA cytology, immunohistochemistry, and ultrastructural studies and review of the literature. Mod Pathol 4:392-395.

Eagon PK, et al, 1991: Quantitation of estrogen and androgen receptors in hepatocellular carcinoma and adjacent normal human liver. Dig Dis Sci 36:1303-1308.

Ebara M, et al, 1986: Natural history of minute hepatocellular carcinoma smaller than three centimeters complicating cirrhosis. Gastroenterology 90:289-298.

Edmondson HA, 1958: Tumors of the liver and intrahepatic bile duct. In: Atlas of Tumor Pathology, section 7, part 25. Armed Forces Institute of Pathology.

Edmondson HA, 1976: Benign epithelial tumors and tumorlike lesions of the liver. In Okuda M, Peters RL (eds): Hepatocellular Carcinoma. New York, Wiley, pp 309-330.

Edmondson HA, Steiner PE, 1954: Primary carcinoma of the liver: a study of 100 cases among 48,900 necropsies. Cancer 7:462-503.

Efremidis SC, Hytiroglou P, 2002: The multistep process of hepatocarcinogenesis in cirrhosis with imaging correlation. Eur Radiol 12:753-764.

Eggel H, 1901: Ueber das primäre Carcinom der Leber. Beiträge zur Pathologischen Anatomie und Allgemeinen Pathologie 30:506-604.

El-Assal ON, et al, 1998: Clinical significance of microvessel density and vascular endothelial growth factor expression in hepatocellular carcinoma and surrounding liver: possible involvement of vascular endothelial growth factor in the angiogenesis of cirrhotic liver. Hepatology 27:1554-1562.

El-Serag HB, Davila JA, 2004: Is fibrolamellar carcinoma different from hepatocellular carcinoma? A US population-based study. Hepatology 39: 798-803.

Eriksson S, Hagerstrand I, 1974: Cirrhosis and malignant hepatoma in alpha-1-AT deficiency. Acta Med Scand 195:451-458.

Fabre A, et al, 2002: Histologic scoring of liver biopsy in focal nodular hyperplasia with atypical presentation. Hepatology 35:414-420.

Falk H, et al, 1979: Hepatic angiosarcoma associated with androgenic-anabolic steroids. Lancet 2:1120-1123.

Fasano M, et al, 1998: Immunohistochemical evaluation of hepatoblastomas with use of the hepatocyte-specific marker, hepatocyte paraffin 1, and the polyclonal anti-carcinoembryonic antigen. Mod Pathol 11:934-938.

Feitelson MA, et al, 2004: Early molecular and genetic determinants of primary liver malignancy. Surg Clin North Am 84:339-354.

Ferrel L, et al, 1992: Incidence and diagnostic features of macroregenerative nodules vs. small hepatocellular carcinoma in cirrhotic livers. Hepatology 16:1372-1381.

Ferrell LD, 1993: Hepatocellular carcinoma arising in a focus of multilobular adenoma: a case report. Am J Surg Pathol 17:525-529.

Fields AC, et al, 2004: Survivin expression in hepatocellular carcinoma: correlation with proliferation, prognostic parameters, and outcome. Mod Pathol 17: 1378-1385.

Fievet P, et al, 1990: Systemic AA amyloidosis induced by liver cell adenoma. Gut 31:361-363.

Finch SC, Finch CA, 1955: Idiopathic hemochromatosis, and iron storage disease: A. iron metabolism in hemochromatosis. Medicine 34:381-430.

Flejou JF, et al, 1985: Liver adenomatosis: an entity distinct from liver adenoma? Gastroenterology 89:1132-1138.

Folpe AL, et al, 2000: Clear cell myomelanocytic tumor of the falciform ligament/ligamentum teres: a novel member of the perivascular epithelioid clear cell family of tumors with a predilection for children and young adults. Am J Surg Pathol 24:1239-1246.

Fong JA, Ruebner BH, 1974: Primary leiomyosarcoma of the liver. Hum Pathol 5:115-119.

Forman D, et al, 1985: Exposure to vinyl chloride and angiosarcoma of the liver: a report of the register of cases. Br J Indust Med 42:750-753.

Formiggini B, 1953: Osservazioni sopra un caso di fibroma peduncolato del fegato presubilmente congenito. Clin Pediatr 35:295-298.

Foster JH, Berman MM, 1977: Solid Liver Tumors. Philadelphia, Saunders.

Foster JH, Berman MM, 1994: The malignant transformation of liver cell adenomas. Arch Surg 129:712-717.

Foster JH, et al, 1978: Familial liver-cell adenoma and diabetes mellitus. N Engl J Med 299:239-241.

Francavilla A, et al, 1991: Role of estrogens and epidermal growth factor in hepatocellular carcinoma (HCC). Dig Dis Sci 36:1299-1302.

Friedman AC, et al, 1985: Fibrolamellar hepatocellular carcinoma. Radiology 157:583-587.

Friedman SL, 1988: Gastrointestinal and hepatobiliary neoplasms in AIDS. Gastroenterol Clin North Am 17:465-486.

Friedman SL, et al, 1984: Simultaneous occurrence of hepatic adenoma and focal nodular hyperplasia: report of a case and review of the literature. Hepatology 4:536-540.

Friedman SL, et al, 1985: Gastrointestinal Kaposi's sarcoma in patients with acquired immunodeficiency syndrome: endoscopic and autopsy findings. Gastroenterology 89:102-108.

Fujii H, et al, 2000: Genetic classification of combined hepatocellular-cholangiocarcinoma. Hum Pathol 31:1011-1017.

Fujimoto J, et al, 1991: Flow cytometric DNA analysis of hepatocellular carcinoma. Cancer 67:939-944.

Galassi A, et al, 1995: Benign myxoid hepatocellular tumor: a variant of liver cell adenoma. Liver 15:233-235.

Ganjei P, et al, 1988: Histologic markers in primary and metastatic tumors of the liver. Cancer 62:1994-1998.

Garcia RL, et al, 1989: Analysis of proliferative grade using anti-PCNA/cyclin monoclonal antibodies in fixed, embedded tissues: comparison with flow cytometric analysis. Am J Pathol 134:733-739.

Gaulard P, et al, 2003: γδ T-cell lymphomas. Semin Hematol 40:233-243.

Giardiello FM, et al, 1996: Hepatoblastoma and APC gene mutation in familial adenomatous polyposis. Gut 39:867-869.

Gibson JB, Sobin LH, 1978: International Histological Classification of Tumours 20: Histological Typing of Tumours of the Liver, Biliary Tract and Pancreas. Geneva, World Health Organization.

Glasgow BJ, et al, 1985: Clinical and pathologic findings of the liver in the acquired immune deficiency syndrome (AIDS). Am J Clin Pathol 85:582-588.

Gleiberman AS, et al, 1989: Synthesis of alpha-fetoprotein in hepatocytes is co-ordinately regulated with cell-cell and cell-matrix interactions. Mol Biol Med 6:95-107.

Glinkova V, et al, 2004: Hepatic haemangiomas: possible association with female sex hormones. Gut 53:1352-1355.

Gluskin LE, et al, 1985: Hepatocellular carcinoma in a patient with precirrhotic primary biliary cirrhosis. J Clin Gastroenterol 7:441-444.

Gokhale R, Whitington PF, 1996: Hepatic adenomatosis in an adolescent. J Pediatr Gastroenterol Nutr 23:482-486.

Gonzales-Crussi F, et al, 1982a: Hepatoblastoma: attempt at characterization of histologic subtypes. Am J Surg Pathol 6:599-612.

Gonzales-Crussi F, et al, 1982b: Infantile sarcoma with intracytoplasmic filamentous inclusions: distinctive tumor of possible histiocytic origin. Cancer 49:2365-2375.

Goodman ZD, Ishak GI, 1982: Hepatocellular carcinoma in woman—probable lack of etiologic association with oral contraceptive steroids. Hepatology 2:440-444.

Goodman ZD, et al, 1985: Combined hepatocellular cholangiocarcinoma: a histologic and immunohistochemical study. Cancer 55:124-135.

Gordon SC, et al, 1986: Resolution of a contraceptive-steroid-induced hepatic adenoma with subsequent evolution into hepatocellular carcinoma. Ann Intern Med 105:547-549.

Gornicka B, et al, 2001: Immature hepatic tumor of bimodal differentiation in a young adult patient: a novel lesion expressing beta-catenin and mimicking a distinct phase of hepatogenesis. J Hepatol 34:955-961.

Gornicka B, et al, 2004: Myoid hamartoma of the liver—a novel variant of hamartoma developing in the hilar region and imitating a malignant liver tumor. Med Sci Monit 10:CS23-CS26.

Gottlieb MS, et al, 1983: The acquired immunodeficiency syndrome. Ann Intern Med 99:208-220.

Grange JD, et al, 1987: Liver adenoma and focal nodular hyperplasia in a man with high endogeneous sex steroids. Gastroenterology 93:1409-1413.

Gräntzdörffer I, et al, 2004: Angiotensin I-converting enzyme (CD 143) is down-regulated in focal nodular hyperplasia of the liver. Am J Surg Pathol 28:84-88.

Greene HL, 1982: Glycogen storage diseases. Semin Liver Dis 2:291-301.

Grigioni WF, et al, 1987: Hepatocellular carcinoma: expression of basement membrane glycoproteins: an immunohistochemical approach. J Pathol 152: 325-332.

Grigioni WF, et al, 1989: Primary liver neoplasms: evaluation of proliferation index using MoAb Ki67. J Pathol 158:23-29.

Grigioni WF, et al, 1991: Evaluation of hepatocellular carcinoma aggressiveness by a panel of extracellular matrix antigens. Am J Pathol 138:647-654.

Grossman H, et al, 1981: Hepatic ultrasonography in type I glycogen storage disease (Von Gierke disease): detection of hepatic adenoma and carcinoma. Radiology 141:753-756.

Guan R, et al, 1985: Primary hepatocellular carcinoma associated with Wilson's disease in a young woman. Postgrad Med J 61:357-359.

Guarda LA, et al, 1984: Acquired immunodeficiency syndrome: postmortem findings. Am J Clin Pathol 81:549-557.

Gulubova MV, 1997: Collagen type III and type IV detection in and around human hepatocellular carcinoma. Gen Diagn Pathol 142:155-163.

Guo XZ, et al, 1998: KAI1, a new metastasis suppressor gene, is reduced in metastatic hepatocellular carcinoma. Hepatology 28:1481-1488.

Gyorffy EJ, et al, 1989: Transformation of hepatic cell adenoma to hepatocellular carcinoma due to oral contraceptive use. Ann Intern Med 110:489-490.

Haas JE, et al, 1981: Ultrastructure of malignant rhabdoid tumor of the kidney: a distinct renal tumor of children. Hum Pathol 12:646-657.

Haas JE, et al, 1989: Histopathology and prognosis in childhood hepatoblastoma and hepatocarcinoma. Cancer 64:1082-1095.

Haas JE, et al, 2001: Small cell undifferentiated histology in hepatoblastoma may be unfavorable. Cancer 15:3130-3134.

Hall PA, et al, 1990: Proliferating cell nuclear antigen (PCNA) immunolocalization in paraffin sections: an index of cell proliferation with evidence of deregulated expression in some neoplasms. J Pathol 162:285-294.

Ham JM, et al, 1980: Haemangioendothelial sarcoma of the liver associated with long-term estrogen therapy in a man. Dig Dis Sci 25: 879-883.

Hamilton SR, Aaltonen LA (eds), 2000: Tumours of the Digestive System: Pathology and Genetics. World Health Organization Classification of Tumours. Lyon, IARC Press.

Hanada M, et al, 1985: Hepatic metastasis 17 years following resection of low-grade leiomyosarcoma of the rectum. Acta Pathol Jpn 35:243-249.

Hann HW, et al, 2004: Preneoplastic markers of hepatitis B virus–associated hepatocellular carcinoma. Cancer Res 64:7329-7335.

Hany MA, et al, 1997: A childhood fibrolamellar hepatocellular carcinoma with increased aromatase activity and a near triploid karyotype. Med Pediatr Oncol 28:136-138.

Harada T, et al, 1998: Membrane-type matrix metalloproteinase-1 (MT1-MMP) gene is overexpressed in highly invasive hepatocellular carcinoma. J Hepatol 28:231-239.

Haratake J, Horie A, 1991: An immunohistochemical study of sarcomatoid liver carcinoma. Cancer 68:93-97.

Haratake J, et al, 1986: Minute hepatoma with excessive copper accumulation. Arch Pathol Lab Med 110:192-194.

Hawkins EP, et al, 1980: Primary leiomyoma of the liver. Am J Surg 4:301-303.

Hayasaka K, et al, 1999: Hepatic hemangioblastoma: an unusual presentation of von Hippel–Lindau disease. J Comput Assist Tomogr 23:565-566.

Henderson BE, et al, 1983: Hepatocellular carcinoma associated with the use of oral contraceptives. Br J Cancer 48:437-440.

Herndier BG, Friedman SL, 1992: Neoplasms of the gastrointestinal tract and hepatobiliary system in acquired immundeficiency syndrome. Semin Liver Dis 12:128-141.

Herr W, et al, 1993: Hepatitis C virus-associated primary hepatocellular carcinoma in a noncirrhotic liver. Clin Invest 71:49-53.

Higaki K, et al, 1996: Fas antigen expression and its relationship with apoptosis in human hepatocellular carcinoma and noncancerous tissues. Am J Pathol 149:429-437.

Hino N, et al, 1996: Apoptosis and proliferation of human hepatocellular carcinoma. Liver 16:123-129.

Hirohashi S, et al, 1983: Distribution of alphafetoprotein and immunoreactive carcinoembryonic antigen in human hepatocellular carcinoma and hepatoblastoma. Jpn J Clin Oncol 13:37-44.

Hirota N, et al, 1982: Resistance to iron accumulation and presence of hepatitis B surface antigen in preneoplastic and neoplastic lesions in human hemochromatotic livers. Hepatogastroenterology 29:49-51.

Hoffman AL, et al, 1997: Hepatic angiomyolipoma: two case reports of caudate-based lesions and review of the literature. Liver Transpl Surg 3:46-53.

Hood DL, et al, 1990: Hepatic giant cell carcinoma: an ultrastructural and immunohistochemical study. Am J Clin Pathol 93:111-116.

Horie Y, et al, 2004: Hepatocyte-specific Pten deficiency results in steatohepatitis and hepatocellular carcinomas. J Clin Invest 113:1774-1783.

Horiuchi R, et al, 1990: Inflammatory pseudotumor of the liver: clinicopathologic study and review of the literature. Cancer 65:1583-1590.

Howell RR, et al, 1976: Hepatic adenomata with type I glycogen storage disease. JAMA 236:1481-1484.

Hsing AW, et al, 1995: Cancer risk following primary hemochromatosis: a population-based cohort study in Denmark. Int J Cancer 60:160-162.

Hsu HC, et al, 1985: Prognostic histologic features of resected small hepatocellular carcinoma (HCC) in Taiwan: a comparison with resected large HCC. Cancer 56:672-680.

Hsu IC, et al, 1991: Mutational hotspot in the p53 gene in human hepatocellular carcinoma. Nature 350:427-428.

Huo TI, et al, 2004: Staging for hepatocellular carcinoma: look for a perfect classification system. J Hepatol 40:1041-1042.

Hytiroglou P, 2004: Morphological changes of early human hepatocarcinogenesis. Semin Liver Dis 2:65-75.

Hytiroglou P, et al, 1995: Macroregenerative nodules in a series of adult cirrhotic liver explants: issues of classification and nomenclature. Hepatology 21:703-708.

Hytiroglou P, et al, 1998: Telomerase activity in precancerous hepatic nodules. Cancer 82:1831-1838.

Ibarrola C, et al, 2004: Focal nodular hepatocellular nodules in hepatic venous outflow obstruction: a clinicopathological study of four patients and 24 nodules. Histopathology 44:172-179.

Ikeda H, et al, 1998: Development of unfavorable hepatoblastoma in children of very low birth weight: results of a surgical and pathologic review. Cancer 82:1789-1796.

Ilisko M, et al, 1998: Cytogenetic findings in an embryonal sarcoma of the liver. Cancer Genet Cytogenet 102:142-144.

Imura S, et al, 2004: Correlation of vascular endothelial cell proliferation with microvessel density and expression of vascular endothelial growth factor and basic fibroblast growth factor in hepatocellular carcinoma. J Med Invest 5:202-209.

International Working Party, 1995: Terminology of nodular hepatocellular lesions. Hepatology 22:983-993.

Iolascon A, et al, 1998: Analysis of CDKN2A, CDKN2B, CDKN2C, and cyclin Ds gene status in hepatoblastoma. Hepatology 27:989-995.

Isaacson PG, et al, 1995: Primary low-grade hepatic B-cell lymphoma of mucosa-associated lymphoid tissue (MALT) type. Am J Surg Pathol 19:571-575.

Ishak KG, 1976: Mesenchymal tumors of the liver. In Okuda K, Peters RL (eds): Hepatocellular Carcinoma. New York, Wiley, pp 247-307.

Ishak KG, 1979: Hepatic neoplasms associated with contraceptive and anabolic steroids. Recent Results Cancer Res 66:73-128.

Ishak KG, Glunz PR, 1967: Hepatoblastoma and hepatocarcinoma in infancy and childhood: report of 47 cases. Cancer 20:396-422.

Ishak KG, et al, 1984: Epithelioid haemangioendothelioma of the liver: a clinicopathologic and follow-up study of 32 cases. Hum Pathol 15:839-852.

Ishii Y, et al, 2003: A study on angiogenesis-realted matrix metalloproteinase networks in primary hepatocellular carcinoma. J Exp Cancer Res 22:461-470.

Ito M, et al, 2003: Liver cell adenoma with malignant transformation: a case report. World J Gastroenterol 9:2379-2381.

Ito N, et al, 1991: Elevated levels of transforming growth factor beta messenger RNA and its polypeptide in human hepatocellular carcinoma. Cancer Res 51:4080-4083.

Jaffe E, 1987: Malignant lymphomas: pathology of hepatic involvement. Semin Liver Dis 17:257-268.

Jarnagin WR, et al, 2002: Combined hepatocellular and cholangiocarcinoma: demographic, clinical, and prognostic factors. Cancer 94:2040-2046.

Jiang S, et al, 1999: Apoptosis in human hepatoma cell lines by chemotherapeutic drugs via Fas-dependent and Fas-independent pathways. Hepatology 29:101-110.

Johnson DE, et al, 1988: The diagnostic utility of the keratin profiles of hepatocellular carcinoma and cholangiocarcinoma. J Surg Pathol 12:187-197.

Johnson PJ, 1996: The epidemiology of hepatocellular carcinoma. Eur J Gastroenterol Hepatol 8:845-849.

Jones FS, et al, 1989: A cDNA clone for cytotactin contains sequences similar to epidermal growth factor-like repeats and segments of fibronectin and fibrinogen. Proc Natl Acad Sci U S A 85:2186-2190.

Kaczynski J, et al, 1996: Fibrolamellar hepatocellular carcinoma in an area with a low incidence of primary liver cancer: a retrospective study. Eur J Surg 162:367-371.

Kakizoe S, et al, 1987: Hepatocellular carcinoma with sarcomatous change: clinicopathologic and immunohistochemical studies of 14 autopsy cases. Cancer 59:310-316.

Kanai N, et al, 1998: Infantile hemangioendothelioma of the liver associated with anomalous dilated and tortuous vessels on the placental surface. Pediatr Surg Int 13:175-176.

Kang YK, et al, 1998: p53 mutation and overexpression in hepatocellular carcinoma and dysplastic nodules in the liver. Virchows Arch 432:27-32.

Kaplan LD, et al, 1989: Primary bile duct lymphoma in the acquired immunodeficiency syndrome. Ann Intern Med 110:161-162.

Karasawa Y, et al, 1998: A case of glycogen storage disease type Ia with multiple hepatic adenomas and G727T mutation in the glucose-6-phosphatase gene, and a comparison with other mutations previously reported. Am J Gastroenterol 93:1550-1553.

Karhunen PJ, 1985: Hepatic pseudolipoma. J Clin Pathol 38:877-879.

Kasahara A, et al, 1998: Risk factors for hepatocellular carcinoma and its incidence after interferon treatment in patients with chronic hepatitis C. Osaka Liver Disease Study Group. Hepatology 27:1394-1402.

Kasai M, Watanabe I, 1970: Histologic classification of liver-cell carcinoma in infancy and childhood and its clinical evaluation: a study of 70 cases in Japan. Cancer 25:551-563.

Katzenstein HM, et al, 2003: Fibrolamellar hepatocellular carcinoma in children and adolescents. Cancer 97:2006-2012.

Kawahara N, et al, 1998: Enhanced expression of thrombospondin-1 and hypovascularity in human cholangiocarcinoma. Hepatology 28:1512-1517.

Kawarada Y, et al, 1985: Nonhepatocytic malignant mixed tumor primary in the liver: report of two cases. Cancer 55:1790-1798.

Kebudi R, et al, 2003: Rhabdomyosarcoma of the biliary tree. Pediatr Int 45:469-471.

Keeling JW, 1971: Liver tumours in infancy and childhood. J Pathol 103:69-85.

Kelleher MB, et al, 1989: Epithelioid hemangioendothelioma of liver: clinicopathological correlation of 10 cases treated by orthotopic liver transplantation. Am J Surg Pathol 13:999-1008.

Kerlin P, et al, 1983: Hepatic adenomas and focal nodular hyperplasia. Gastroenterology 84:994-1002.

Kew MC, 1983: Hepatocellular carcinoma. Postgrad Med J 59:78-87.

Kew MC, 2003: Synergistic interaction between aflatoxin B1 and hepatitis B virus in hepatocarcinogenesis. Liver Int 23:405-409.

Kew MC, Popper H, 1984: Relationship between hepatocellular carcinoma and cirrhosis. Semin Liver Dis 4:136-146.

Kew MC, et al, 1989: The role of membranous obstruction of the inferior vena cava in the etiology of hepatocellular carcinoma in Southern African blacks. Hepatology 9:121-125.

Khan SS, et al, 1992: Case report: liver adenomatosis presenting as multiple calcified masses. Clin Radiol 45:206-207.

Khoo US, et al, 1994: Cholestatic liver cell adenoma in a child with hirsutism and elevated serum levels of cortisol and ACTH. Histopathology 25:586-588.

Kiev J, et al, 1990: Obstructive jaundice caused by hepatoma fragments in the common hepatic duct. J Clin Gastroenterol 12:207-213.

Kim CM, et al, 1991: HBx gene of hepatitis B virus induced liver cancer in transgenic mice. Nature 351:317-320.

Kim DY, et al, 2002: Undifferentiated (embryonal) sarcoma of the liver: combination treatment by surgery and chemotherapy. J Pediatr Surg 37:1419-1423.

Kim H, et al, 2004: Primary liver carcinoma of intermediate (hepatocyte-cholangiocyte) phenotype. J Hepatol 40:298-304.

Kim NR, et al, 2003: Pulmonary lymphangioleiomyomatosis and multiple hepatic angiomyolipomas in a man. Pathol Int 53:231-235.

Kim SR, et al, 2000: Hepatocellular carcinoma transforming from dysplastic nodule with background of non-B non-C chronic persistent hepatitis. J Hepatol 33:857-858.

Kimura H, et al, 1998: Angiogenesis in hepatocellular carcinoma as evaluated by CD34 immunohistochemistry. Liver 18:14-19.

Kin M, et al, 1997: Basic fibroblast growth factor regulates proliferation and motility of human hepatoma cells by an autocrine mechanism. J Hepatol 27:677-687.

Kingston JE, et al, 1983: Association between hepatoblastoma and polyposis coli. Arch Dis Child 58:959-962.

Kishi K, et al, 1983: Hepatocellular carcinoma: a clinical and pathologic analysis of 57 hepatectomy cases. Cancer 51:542-548.

Kiss A, et al, 1998: Expression of transforming growth factor-alpha in hepatoblastoma. Cancer 83:670-677.

Kitazawa R, et al, 1999: In situ demonstration of parathyroid hormone–related protein mRNA in sclerosing hepatic carcinoma. Virchows Arch 435:137-142.

Klatskin G, 1977: Hepatic tumours: possible relationship to use of oral contraceptives. Gastroenterology 73:386-394.

Kleiner DE, et al, 2005: Design and validation of a histological scoring system for nonalcoholic fatty liver disease. Hepatology 41:1313-1321.

Klosowski S, et al, 1998: Extreme hyperbilirubinemia in a neonate with hepatic haemangio-endothelioma. Eur J Pediatr 157:521-522 (letter).

Knowles DM, Wolff M, 1976: Focal nodular hyperplasia of the liver: a clinico-pathologic study and review of the literature. Hum Pathol 7:533-545.

Knowles DM, et al, 1988: Lymphoid neoplasia associated with the acquired immunodeficiency syndrome (AIDS). Ann Intern Med 108:744-753.

Koelma IA, et al, 1986: Hepatocellular carcinoma, adenoma, and focal nodular hyperplasia: comparative histopathologic study with immunohistochemical parameters. Arch Pathol Lab Med 110:1035-1040.

Koh KC, et al, 2005: Clinicopathologic features and prognosis of combined hepatocellular and cholangiocarcinoma. Am J Surg 189:120-125.

Koike K, 1995: Hepatitis B virus HBx gene and hepatocarcinogenesis. Intervirol 38:134-142.

Kojiro M, 1989: Pathologic characteristics of early hepatocellular carcinoma. Kan Tan Sui 18:835-839.

Kojiro M, 2004: Focus on dysplastic nodules and early hepatocellular carcinoma: an Eastern point of view. Liver Transplant 10(2 suppl 1):S3-S8.

Kojiro M, et al, 1981: Distribution of albumin- and/or α-fetoprotein–positive cells in hepatocellular carcinoma. Lab Invest 44:221-226.

Kojiro M, et al, 1984: Hepatocellular carcinoma with intraatrial tumor growth: a clinicopathologic study of 18 autopsy cases. Arch Pathol Lab Med 108:989-992.

Kondo F, 2001: Benign nodular hepatocellular lesions caused by abnormal hepatic circulation: etiological analysis and introduction of a new concept. J Gastroenterol Hepatol 16:1319-1328.

Kondo F, et al, 1987: Morphological clues for the diagnosis of small hepatocellular carcinoma. Virchows Arch 411:15-21.

Kondo F, et al, 1989: Biopsy diagnosis of well-differentiated hepatocellular carcinoma based on new morphologic criteria. Hepatology 9:751-755.

Kondo F, et al, 1990: Biopsy diagnosis of well differentiated hepatocellular carcinoma based on new morphologic markers of hepatocellular carcinoma. Cancer 65:84-87.

Kondo F, et al, 2004: Nodular lesions associated with abnormal liver circulation. Intervirology 47:277-287.

Kondo Y, Wada K, 1991: Intrahepatic metastasis of hepatocellular carcinoma: a histopathologic study. Hum Pathol 22:125-130.

Kowdley KV, et al, 1995: Primary liver cancer and survival in patients undergoing liver transplantation for hemochromatosis. Liver Transpl Surg 1:237-241.

Krasner N, et al, 1979: Hepatocellular carcinoma in primary biliary cirrhosis: report of four cases. Gut 20:255-258.

Kraus JA, et al, 1996: Loss of heterozygosity on chromosome 1 in human hepatoblastoma. Int J Cancer 67:467-471.

Krishnamarchari KAVR, et al, 1975: Hepatitis due to aflatoxicosis. Lancet 2:1061-1063.

Kuang SY, et al, 2004: Specific mutations of hepatitis B virus in plasma predict liver cancer development. Proc Natl Acad Sci U S A 101:3575-3580.

Kubo K, 1998: The Fas system is not significantly involved in apoptosis in human hepatocellular carcinoma. Liver 18:117-123.

Kumada T, et al, 2004: Assessment of tumor hemodynamics in small hepatocellular carcinoma: comparison of Doppler ultrasonography, angiography-assisted computed tomography, and pathological findings. Liver Int 24:425-431.

Kuo SH, et al, 1987: Cytophotometric measurements of nuclear DNA content in hepatocellular carcinoma. Hepatology 7:330-332.

Kurumaya H, et al, 1989: Endocrine cells in the intrahepatic biliary tree in normal livers and hepatolithiasis. Arch Pathol Lab Med 113:143-147.

Kuwano H, et al, 1984: Hepatocellular carcinoma with osteoclast-like giant cells. Cancer 54:837-842.

Lack EE, et al, 1982: Hepatoblastoma: a clinical and pathologic study of 54 cases. Am J Surg Pathol 6:693-705.

Lack EE, et al, 1991: Undifferentiated (embryonal) sarcoma of the liver: clinical and pathologic study of 16 cases with emphasis on immunohistochemical features. Am J Surg Pathol 15:1-16.

Lai ECS, et al, 1991: Hepatectomy for larger hepatocellular carcinoma: the optimal resection margin. World J Surg 15:141-145.

Lai YS, et al, 1989: Expression of cytokeratins in normal and diseased livers and in primary liver carcinomas. Arch Pathol Lab Med 113:134-138.

Lamas E, et al, 1991: Localization of insulin-like growth factor II and hepatitis B virus mRNAs and proteins in human hepatocellular carcinoma. Lab Invest 64:98-104.

Landing BH, 1976: Tumors of the liver in childhood In Okuda M, Peters RL (eds): Hepatocellular Carcinoma. New York, Wiley, pp 205-226.

Laurent C, et al, 2003: Association of adenoma and focal nodular hyperplasia: experience of a single French academic center. Comp Hepatol 2:6.

Lauwers GY, et al, 1997: Hepatic undifferentiated (embryonal) sarcoma arising in mesenchymal hamartoma. Am J Surg Pathol 21:1248-1254.

Le Bail B, et al, 1992: Liver adenomatosis with granulomas in two patients on long-term oral contraceptives. Am J Surg Pathol 16:982-987.

Le Bail B, et al, 1997: Prevalence of liver cell dysplasia and association with HCC in a series of 100 cirrhotic liver explants. J Hepatol 27:835-842.

LeBoit PE, 1990: The expanding spectrum of a new discase, bacillary angiomatosis. Arch Dermatol 126:808-811.

Lee FI, 1982: Vinyl chloride–induced liver disease. J R Coll Physicians 16:226-230.

Lee FI, et al, 1996: Occupationally related angiosarcoma of the liver in the United Kingdom 1972-1994. Gut 39:312-318.

Lee RG, et al, 1997: Large cell change (liver cell dysplasia) and hepatocellular carcinoma in cirrhosis: matched case-control study, pathological analysis, and pathogenetic hypothesis. Hepatology 26:1415-1422.

Lefkowitch JH, et al, 1983: Copper and copper-binding protein in fibrolamellar liver cell carcinoma. Cancer 51:97-100.

Lei KIK, 1998: Primary non-Hodgkin's lymphoma of the liver. Leuk Lymphoma 29:293-299.

Lemmer ER, et al, 1998: Isolation from human fetal liver of cells co-expressing CD 34 haematopoietic stem cell and CAM 5.22 pancytokeratin markers. J Hepatol 29:450-454.

Lepreux S, et al, 2002: Focal nodular hyperplasia lacking some key histopathological features making the diagnosis difficult. Virchows Arch 440:445-446.

Lepreux S, et al, 2003a: The identification of small nodules in liver adenomatosis. J Hepatol 39:77-85.

Lepreux S, et al, 2003b: FNH-like nodules: possible precursor lesions in patients with focal nodular hyperplasia. Comp Hepatol 26:7.

Lepreux S, et al, 2003c: Multiple telangiectatic focal nodular hyperplasia: vascular abnormalities. Virchows Arch 442:226-230.

Lepreux S, et al, 2004: Expression of fibrillin-1 in focal nodular hyperplasia of the liver: a role in microcirculation adaptability. Comp Hepatol 3(suppl 1):S57.

Leuschner I, et al, 1990: Undifferentiated sarcoma of the liver in childhood: morphology, flow cytometry, and literature review. Hum Pathol 21:68-76.

Lewis R, Rempala G, 2003: A case-cohort study of angiosarcoma of the liver and brain cancer at a polymer production plant. J Occup Environ Med 45:538-545.

Li X, et al, 1998: Promoter-specific methylation and expression alterations of *igf2* and *h19* are involved in human hepatoblastoma. Int J Cancer 75:176-180.

Libbrecht L, et al, 2001a: Hepatic progenitor cells in hepatocellular adenoma. Am J Surg Pathol 25:1388-1396.

Libbrecht L, et al, 2001b: Predictive value of liver cell dysplasia for development of hepatocellular carcinoma in patients with non-cirrhotic and cirrhotic chronic viral hepatitis. Histopathology 39:66-73.

Lieber CS, 1975: Liver disease and alcohol: fatty liver, alcoholic hepatitis, cirrhosis and their interrelationships. Ann N Y Acad Sci 252:63-84.

Liebermann J, et al, 1975: Hepatocellular carcinoma and intermediate alpha-1-antitrypsin deficiency (MZ phenotype). Am J Clin Pathol 64:304-310.

Liétard J, et al, 1998: Laminin isoforms in non-tumoral and tumoral human livers: expression of alpha1, beta1, beta2 and gamma1 chain mRNA and an alpha chain homologous to the alpha2 chain. J Hepatol 28:691-699.

Lin TY, 1976: Tumors of the liver. In Bockus HL (ed): Gastroenterology. Philadelphia, Saunders, pp 522-533.

Linton PL, et al, 1991: Angiomyolipoma of the liver: immunohistochemical study of a case. Liver 11:158-161.

Lipshutz GS, et al, 2002: Thorotrast-induced liver neoplasia: a collective review. J Am Coll Surg 195:713-718.

Lisker-Melman M, et al, 1989: Primary lymphoma of the liver in a patient with acquired immunodeficiency syndrome and chronic hepatitis B. Am J Gastroenterol 84:1445-1448.

Liu JH, et al, 2004: Clear cell and non-clear cell hepatocellular carcinoma: a case report and literature review. Kaohsiung 20:78-82.

Liver Cancer Study Group of Japan, 1983: The General Rules for the Clinical and Pathological Study of Primary Liver Cancer. Tokyo, Kanehara.

Liver Cancer Study Group of Japan, 1984: Primary liver cancer in Japan. Cancer 54:1747-1755.

Llovet JM, et al, 2003: Hepatocellular carcinoma. Lancet 362:1907-1917.

Locker J, 2004: A new way to look at liver cancer. Hepatology 40:521-523.

Lones MA, et al, 1997: Donor origin of posttransplant lymphoproliferative disorder localized to a liver allograft: demonstration by fluorescence in situ hybridization. Arch Pathol Lab Med 121:701-706.

Ma MH, Biempica L, 1971: Normal human liver cell: cytochemical and ultra-structural studies. Am J Pathol 62:353-390.

MacKinlay GA, Pritchard J, 1992: A common language for childhood liver tumours. Pediatr Surg 7:325-326.

MacMahon HE, Ball HG, 1971: Leiomyosarcomas of the hepatic vein and the Budd-Chiari syndrome. Gastroenterology 61:239-243.

MacNab GM, et al, 1976: Hepatitis B surface antigen produced by a human hepatoma cell line. Br J Cancer 34:509-515.

Macon WR, et al, 2001: Hepatosplenic αβ T-cell lymphomas: a report of 14 cases and comparison with hepatosplenic γδ T-cell lymphomas. Am J Surg Pathol 25:285-296.

Maetani Y, et al, 2002: Benign hepatic nodules in Budd-Chiari syndrome: radiologic-pathologic correlation with emphasis on the central scar. AJR Am J Roentgenol 178:869-875.

Makhlouf HR, Ishak KG, 2002: Sclerosed hemangioma and sclerosing carvernous hemangioma of the liver: a comparative clinicopathologic and immunohistochemical study with emphasis on the role of mast cells in their histogenesis. Liver 22:70-78.

Manivel C, et al, 1986: Teratoid hepatoblastoma: the nosologic dilemma of solid embryonic neoplasms of childhood. Cancer 57:2168-2174.

Marion PL, et al, 1980: State of hepatitis B viral DNA in a human hepatoma cell line. J Virol 33:795-806.

Marks WH, et al, 1988: Failure of hepatic adenomas to regress after discontinuation of oral contraception: an association with focal nodular hyperplasia and uterine leiomyoma. Ann Surg 208:190-195.

Martinez J, et al, 1973: Hypofibrinogenemia associated with hemangioma of the liver. Am J Clin Pathol 59:192-197.

Martini GA, 1959: Cirrhosis of the Liver in Hereditary Hemorrhagic Telangiectasia. Proceedings of the First World Congress on Gastroenterology, vol 2. Baltimore, Williams & Wilkins, pp 857-858.

Masumoto A, et al, 1999: Role of beta1 integrins in adhesion and invasion of hepatocellular carcinoma. Hepatology 29:68-74.

Matsui O, et al, 1989: Adenomatous hyperplastic nodules in the cirrhotic liver: differentiation from hepatocellular carcinoma with MR imaging. Radiology 173:123-126.

Matsui S, et al, 1997: Expression, localization and alternative splicing pattern of fibronectin messenger RNA in fibrotic human liver and hepatocellular carcinoma. J Hepatol 27:843-853.

Matsuno Y, et al, 1990: Heterogeneity of proliferative activity in nodule-in-nodule lesions of small hepatocellular carcinoma. Jpn J Cancer Res 81:1137-1140.

Mays ET, Christopherson W, 1984: Hepatic tumors induced by sex steroids. Semin Liver Dis 4:147-157.

McCullough AJ, 2004: The clinical features, diagnosis and natural history of nonalcoholic fatty liver disease. Clin Liver Dis 8:521-533.

Mecham RP, 1991: Receptors for laminin on mammalian cells. FASEB J 5:2538-2546.

Medjkane S, et al, 2004: The tumor suppressor hSNF5/INI1 modulates cell growth and actin cytoskeleton organization. Cancer Res 64:3406-3413.

Melia WM, et al, 1984: Hepatocellular carcinoma in primary biliary cirrhosis: detection by alpha-fetoprotein. Gastroenterology 87:660-663.

Messiaen T, et al, 1996: Hepatic angiomyo(myelo)lipoma: difficulties in radiological diagnosis and interest of fine needle aspiration biopsy. Liver 16:338-341.

Miatto O, et al, 1985: Diagnostic and prognostic value of serum copper and plasma fibrinogen in hepatic carcinoma. Cancer 55:774-778.

Milani S, et al, 1989: Cellular localization of laminin gene transcripts in normal and fibrotic human liver. Am J Pathol 134:1175-1182.

Miller ST, et al, 1983: Primary hepatic or hepatosplenic non-Hodgkin's lymphoma in children. Cancer 52:2285-2288.

Mills PR, et al, 1981: Evidence of previous hepatitis B virus infection in alcoholic cirrhosis. BMJ 282:437-438.

Minervini MI, et al, 1997: Utilization of hepatocyte-specific antibody in the immunocytochemical evaluation of liver tumors. Mod Pathol 10:686-692.

Misugi K, Reiner CB, 1965: A malignant true teratoma of liver in childhood. Arch Pathol 80:409-412.

Miyoshi M, et al, 1977: A case of pedunculated hepatoma with spontaneous rupture. Acta Hepatol Jpn 18:765-772.

Mizorogi F, et al, 2000: Hepatitis C virus infection in patients with B-cell non-Hodgkin's lymphoma. Intern Med 39:112-117.

Mo JQ, et al, 2004: GLUT1 endothelial reactivity distinguishes hepatic infantile hemangioma from congenital hepatic vascular malformation with associated capillary proliferation. Hum Pathol 35:200-209.

Molina E, Hernandez A, 2003: Clinical manifestations of primary hepatic angiosarcoma. Dig Dis Sci 48:677-682.

Monroe PS, et al, 1981: Hepatic angiosarcoma: possible relationship to long-term oral contraceptive ingestion. JAMA 246:64-65.

Morley JE, et al, 1974: Enlargement of cavernous haemangioma associated with exogenous administration of oestrogens. South Afr Med J 1:695-697.

Moser C, et al, 1998: [Familial giant hemangiomas of the liver: study of a family and review of the literature]. Schweiz Rundsch Med Prax (Switzerland) 87:461-468 (in German).

Motohashi I, et al, 1990: Micromorphometric investigation of hepatocellular carcinoma (HCC) and HCC-like lesions with particular emphasis on nuclear and cellular pleomorphism. Acta Hepatol Jpn 31:1274-1281.

Motohashi I, et al, 1992: Morphological differences between hepatocellular carcinoma and hepatocellular carcinoma-like lesions. Hepatology 16:118-126.

Motoo Y, et al, 1991: Expression of epidermal growth factor and fibroblast growth factor in human hepatocellular carcinoma: an immunohistochemical study. Liver 11:272-277.

Munoz PA, et al, 1980: Osteoclastoma-like giant cell tumor of the liver. Cancer 46:771-779.

Musso O, et al, 1997: In situ detection of matrix metalloproteinase-2 (MMP2) and the metalloproteinase inhibitor TIMP2 transcripts in human primary hepatocellular carcinoma and in liver metastasis. J Hepatol 26:593-605.

Nagai H, et al, 1998: Genomic alterations in early stage human hepatocellular carcinomas. Cancer 82:454-461.

Nagasue N, et al, 1984: Hepatocellular pseudotumor in the cirrhotic liver: report of three cases. Cancer 54:2487-2494.

Nagasue N, et al, 1992: Comparison between diploid and aneuploid hepatocellular carcinomas: a flow cytometric study. Br J Surg 79:667-670.

Nair S, et al, 2002: Is obesity an independent risk factor for hepatocellular carcinoma in cirrhosis? Hepatology 3:150-155.

Nakagama H, et al, 1991: Expression of androgen receptor mRNA in human hepatocellular carcinomas and hepatoma cell lines. Hepatology 14:99-102.

Nakamura S, et al, 1997: Immunohistochemical studies on endothelial cell phenotype in hepatocellular carcinoma. Hepatology 26:407-415.

Nakamura T, et al, 1986: Obstruction of the inferior vena cava in the hepatic portion and the hepatic veins. Angiology 19:479-498.

Nakano M, et al, 1981: A histopathological study of early hepatocellular carcinoma (HCC): portal tract invasion and progression to advanced HCC. Acta Hepatol Jpn 22:266-272.

Nakanuma Y, Ohta G, 1984: Small hepatocellular carcinoma containing many Mallory bodies. Liver 4:128-133.

Nakanuma Y, Ohta G, 1986: Expression of Mallory bodies in hepatocellular carcinoma in man and its significance. Cancer 57:81-86.

Nakanuma Y, et al, 1981: Cytoplasmic expression in hepatocellular carcinoma. Acta Hepatol Jpn 22:266-272.

Nakanuma Y, et al, 1986: Incidental solitary hepatocellular carcinoma smaller than 1 cm in size found at autopsy: a morphometric study. Hepatology 6: 631-635.

Nakanuma Y, et al, 1990a: Hepatocellular carcinoma in primary biliary cirrhosis: an autopsy study. Hepatology 11:1010-1016.

Nakanuma Y, et al, 1990b: "Atypical adenomatous hyperplasia" in liver cirrhosis: low-grade hepatocellular carcinoma or borderline lesion? Histopathology 17:27-35.

Nakanuma Y, et al, 1998: Analytical histopathological diagnosis of small hepatocellular nodules in chronic liver disease. Histol Histopathol 13:1077-1087.

Nakashima O, 1989: Pathomorphological study on early hepatocellular carcinoma: a study on capsule and septum formation. Acta Hepatol Jpn 30:28-34.

Nakashima T, Kojiro M, 1986: Pathologic characteristics of hepatocellular carcinoma. Semin Liver Dis 6:259-266.

Nakashima T, Kojiro K, 1987: Hepatocellular Carcinoma: An Atlas of Its Pathology. Tokyo, Springer-Verlag.

Nalesnik MA, et al, 1998: Transforming growth factor alpha (TGFalpha) in hepatocellular carcinomas and adjacent hepatic parenchyma. Hum Pathol 29:228-234.

Nalpas B, et al, 1995: Hepatocellular carcinoma in alcoholics. Alcohol 12:117-120.

Naoumov NV, et al, 1997: Hepatitis C virus infection in the development of hepatocellular carcinoma in cirrhosis. J Hepatol 27:331-336.

Narasimhan KL, et al, 2004: Conservative management of giant hepatic mesenchymal hamartoma. Indian J Gastroenterol 23:26.

Negri E, et al, 2004: B-cell non-Hodgkin's lymphoma and hepatitis C virus infection: a systematic review. Int J Cancer 111:1-8.

Nelson WJ, Nusse R, 2004: Convergence of Wnt, beta-catenin, and cadherin pathways. Science 303:1483-1487.

Neuberger J, et al, 1980: Oral-contraceptive-associated liver tumours: occurrence of malignancy and difficulties in diagnosis. Lancet 1:273-276.

Ng IOL, et al, 1995: Ki-67 antigen expression in hepatocellular carcinoma using monoclonal antibody MIB1: a comparison with proliferating cell nuclear antigen. Am J Clin Pathol 104:313-318.

Ng IO, et al, 1998: Combined hepatocellular-cholangiocarcinoma: a clinicopathologic study. J Gastroenterol Hepatol 13:34-40.

Ng KK, et al, 2003: Hepatic angiomyolipoma. Surgery 133:594-595.

Nguyen BN, et al, 1999: Focal nodular hyperplasia of the liver: a comprehensive pathologic study of 305 lesions and recognition of new histologic forms. Am J Surg Pathol 23:1441-1454.

Niederau C, et al, 1985: Survival and causes of death in cirrhosis and in noncirrhotic patients with primary hemochromatosis. N Engl J Med 313:1256-1266.

Nishida N, et al, 2003: Chromosomal instability and human hepatocarcinogenesis. Histol Histopathol 18:897-909.

Nishio J, et al, 2003: Undifferentiated (embryonal) sarcoma of the liver in middle-aged adults: smooth muscle differentiation determined by immunohistochemistry and electron microscopy. Hum Pathol 34:246-252.

Noguchi O, et al, 1996: Gene expressions of c-met and hepatocyte growth factor in chronic liver disease and hepatocellular carcinoma. J Hepatol 24:286-292.

Nolte M, et al, 1998: Expression of proliferation associated antigens and detection of numerical chromosome aberrations in primary human liver tumours: relevance to tumour characteristics and prognosis. J Clin Pathol 51:47-51.

Nyberg DA, et al, 1986: AIDS-related lymphomas: evaluation by abdominal CT. Radiology 159:59-63.

Nzeako UC, et al, 1996: Hepatocellular carcinoma in cirrhotic and noncirrhotic livers: a clinico-histopathologic study of 804 North American patients. Am J Clin Pathol 105:65-75.

Ogasawara H, et al, 1998: Hepatocyte growth factor stimulates DNA synthesis in rat preneoplastic hepatocytes but not in liver carcinoma cells. Gastroenterology 114:775-781.

Ohbayashi A, 1976: Genetic and familial aspects of liver cirrhosis and hepatocellular carcinoma. In Okuda K, Peters RL (eds): Hepatocellular Carcinoma. New York, Wiley, pp 43-51.

Ohno H, 1985: Pathological studies on fibrous capsule of so-called encapsulated hepatocellular carcinomas. Acta Hepatol Jpn 26:727-738.

Ohta G, Nakanuma Y, 1987: Comparative study of the three nodular lesions in cirrhosis: adenomatoid hyperplasia, adenomatoid hyperplasia with intermediate lesions, and small hepatocollular carcinoma. In Okuda K, Ishak KG (eds): Neoplasms of the Liver. Berlin, Springer-Verlag, pp 177-187.

Oka H, et al, 1990: Prospective study of early detection of hepatocellular carcinoma in patients with cirrhosis. Hepatology 12:680-687.

Okada S, et al, 1992: Prognostic factors in patients with hepatocellular carcinoma receiving systemic chemotherapy. Hepatology 16:112-117.

Okazaki N, et al, 1989: Evaluation of the prognosis for small hepatocellular carcinoma based on tumor volume doubling time. Cancer 63:2207-2210.

Okuda K, 1992: Hepatocellular carcinoma: recent progress. Hepatology 15: 948-963.

Okuda K, et al, 1977: Clinicopathological features of encapsulated hepatocellular carcinoma: a study of 26 cases. Cancer 40:1240-1245.

Okuda K, et al, 1982a: Hepatocellular carcinoma arising in non cirrhotic and highly cirrhotic livers: a comparative study of histopathology and frequency of hepatitis B markers. Cancer 49:450-455.

Okuda K, et al, 1982b: A clinical and pathological study of diffuse type hepatocellular carcinoma. Liver 2:176-192.

Okuda K, et al, 1984: Gross anatomic features of hepatocellular carcinoma from three disparate geographic areas: proposal of a new classification. Cancer 54:2165-2173.

Okuda K, et al, 1987: Changing incidence of hepatocellular carcinoma in Japan. Cancer Res 47:4967-4972.

Omer RE, et al, 2004: Population-attributable risk of dietary aflatoxins and hepatitis B virus infection with respect to hepatocellular carcinoma. Nutr Cancer 48:15-21.

Onyemelukwe OG, et al, 1980: Aflatoxin B1 in hepatocellular carcinoma. Trop Geogr Med 32:237-240.

Ooi LPJ, et al, 1997: Evidence that "myofibroblast-like" cells are the cellular source of capsular collagen in hepatocellular carcinoma. J Hepatol 26: 798-807.

Orikasa H, et al, 2001: Lipid-rich clear-cell hepatocellular carcinoma arising in non-alcoholic steatohepatitis in a patient with diabetes mellitus. J Submicrosc Cytol Pathol 33:195-200.

Oriyama T, et al, 1998: Progression of hepatocellular carcinoma as reflected by nuclear DNA ploidy and cellular differentiation. J Hepatol 28:142-149.

Orsatti G, et al 1997: Lamellar fibrosis in the fibrolamellar variant of hepatocellular carcinoma: a role for transforming growth factor beta. Liver 17: 152-156.

Ortega JA, et al, 2000: Randomized comparison of cisplatin/vincristine/fluorouracil and cisplatin/continuous infusion doxorubicin for treatment of pediatric hepatoblastoma: a report from the Children's Cancer Group and the Pediatric Oncology Group. J Clin Oncol 18:2665-2675.

Osborne MB, et al, 1985: Primary lymphoma of the liver: ten cases and a review of the literature. Cancer 56:2902-2910.

Oschner JL, Halpert B, 1958: Cavernous hemangioma of the liver. Surgery 43:577-582.

O'Sullivan MJ, et al, 2001: Undifferentiated embryonal sarcoma with unusual features arising within mesenchymal hamartoma of the liver: report of a case and review of the literature. Pediatr Dev Pathol 4:482-489.

Otal TM, et al, 1994: Mesenchymal hamartoma of the liver: DNA flow cytometric analysis of eight cases. Cancer 74:1237-1242.

Otsuru A, et al, 1988: Analysis of alpha-fetoprotein gene expression in hepatocellular carcinoma and liver cirrhosis by in situ hybridisation. Cancer 62: 1108-1112.

Pache JC, et al, 1992: Vertical light microscopy (LM) sections and parallel computed tomography (CT) scans for the stereology of human lung and other organs. International Congress of Pathology, Madrid (abstract).

Paradinas FJ, et al, 1982: High serum vitamin B_{12} binding capacity as a marker of the fibrolamellar variant of hepatocellular carcinoma. BMJ 285: 840-842.

Paradis V, et al, 2003: A quantitative gene expression study suggests a role for angiopoietins in focal nodular hyperplasia. Gastroenterology 124: 651-659.

Paradis V, et al, 2004: Telangiectatic focal nodular hyperplasia: a variant of hepatocellular adenoma. Gastroenterology 126:1323-1329.

Pares A, et al, 1990: Hepatitis C virus antibodies in chronic alcoholic patients: association with severity of liver injury. Hepatology 12:1295-1299.

Parham DM, et al, 1988: Malignant rhabdoid tumor of the liver: evidence for epithelial differentiation. Arch Pathol Lab Med 112:61-64.

Park SS, et al, 2004: Involvement of c-Src kinase in the regulation of TGF-beta1-induced apoptosis. Oncogene 23:6272-6281.

Park WS, et al, 2001: Nuclear localization of beta-catenin is an important prognostic factor in hepatoblastoma. J Pathol 193:483-490.

Park YN, et al, 1997: Hepatic stellate cell activation in dysplastic nodules: evidence for an alternate hypothesis concerning human hepatocarcinogenesis. Liver 17:271-274.

Park YN, et al, 1998: Neoangiogenesis and sinusoidal "capillarization" in dysplastic nodules of the liver. Am J Surg Pathol 22:656-662.

Parkin DM, et al, 2001: Estimating the world cancer burden: GLOBOCAN 2000. Int J Cancer 94:153-156.

Payne CM, et al, 1986: Fibrolamellar carcinoma of the liver: a primary, malignant oncocytic carcinoid? Ultrastruct Pathol 10:539-552.

Perilongo G, et al, 2002: Hepatic tumours. In Souhami RL, et al (eds): Oxford Textbook of Oncology, vol 2, 2nd ed. Oxford, Oxford University Press, pp 2657-2668.

Perkocha LA, et al, 1990: Clinical and pathological features of bacilliary peliosis hepatis in association with human immunodeficiency virus infection. N Engl J Med 323:1581-1586.

Persad R, et al, 2004: Overexpression of caspase-3 in hepatocellular carcinomas. Mod Pathol 17:861-867.

Peters RL, 1976: Pathology of hepatocellular carcinoma. In Okuda M, Peters RL (eds): Hepatocellular Carcinoma. New York, John Wiley & Sons, pp 107-168.

Pham H, et al, 1998: Occurrence of gammopathies and lymphoproliferative disorders in liver transplant recipients randomized to tacrolimus (FK 506)- or cyclosporine-based immunosuppression. Liver Transpl Surg 4:146-151.

Phillips MJ, et al, 1973: Benign liver tumours: classification and ultrastructural pathology. Cancer 32:463-470.

Phillips MJ, et al, 1987: The Liver: An Atlas and Text of Ultrastructural Pathology. New York, Raven Press.

Piao Z, et al, 1997: Clonality of large regenerative nodules in liver cirrhosis. Liver 17:251-256.

Poe R, Snover DC, 1988: Adenomas in glycogen storage disease type I: two cases with unusual histologic features. Am J Surg Pathol 12:477-483.

Pokharna RK, et al, 1997: Primary epithelioid haemangioendothelioma of the liver: case report and review of the literature. J Clin Pathol 50:1029-1031.

Pokorny CS, et al, 1991: Inflammatory pseudotumor of the liver causing biliary obstruction: treatment by biliary stenting with 5-years follow-up. J Clin Gastroenterol 13:338-341.

Pol B, et al, 1998: Inflammatory process complicating giant hemangioma of the liver: report of three cases. Liver Transpl Surg 4:204-207.

Polio J, et al, 1989: Hepatocellular carcinoma in Wilson's disease. J Clin Gastroenterol 11:220-224.

Pollard SM, Millward-Sadler GH, 1974: Malignant haemangioendothelioma involving the liver. J Clin Pathol 27:214-221.

Pollicino T, et al, 2004: Hepatitis B virus maintains its pro-oncogenic properties in the case of occult HBV infection. Gastroenterology 126:102-110.

Pompili M, et al, 1991: Review of adenomatous hyperplastic nodules in liver cirrhosis: pathological features, imaging diagnosis and prognostic significance. Gastroenterol Int 4:120-124.

Poon RT, et al, 2004: Prognostic significance of serum vascular endothelial growth factor and endostatin in patients with hepatocellular carcinoma. Br J Surg 91:1354-1360.

Popper H, et al, 1981: Pathology of alcoholic liver diseases. Semin Liver Dis 1:203-216.

Pounder DJ, 1982: Hepatic angiomyolipoma. Am J Surg Pathol 6:677-681.

Powell LW, Kerr JFR, 1975: The pathology of the liver in hemochromatosis. Pathobiol Annu 5:317-337.

Pozzato G, et al, 1994: Low-grade malignant lymphoma, hepatitis C virus infection, and mixed cryoglobulinemia. Blood 84:3047-3053.

Prabhu RM, et al, 1998: Primary hepatic low-grade B-cell lymphoma of mucosa-associated lymphoid tissue (MALT) associated with primary biliary cirrhosis. Mod Pathol 11:404-410.

Praml C, et al, 1998: Cloning of the human aflatoxin B1-aldehyde reductase gene at 1p35-1p36.1 in a region frequently altered in human tumor cells. Cancer Res 58:5014-5018.

Preat V, et al, 1984: Promoting effect of portocaval anastomosis in rat hepatocarcinogenesis. Carcinogenesis 5:1151-1154.

Primack A, et al, 1971: Hepatocellular carcinoma with the carcinoid syndrome. Cancer 27:1182-1189.

Prokurat A, et al, 2002: Transitional liver cell tumors (TLCT) in older children and adolescents: a novel group of aggressive tumors expressing beta-catenin. Med Pediatr Oncol 39:510-518.

Propst T, et al, 1994: Prevalence of hepatocellular carcinoma in alpha-1-antitrypsin deficiency. J Hepatol 21:1006-1011.

Przegodzki RM, et al, 1997: Sporadic and Thorotrast-induced angiosarcomas of the liver manifest frequent and multiple point mutations in K-ras-2. Lab Invest 76:153-159.

Qian Y, Fan JG, 2005: Obesity, fatty liver and liver cancer. Hepatobiliary Pancreat Dis Int 4:173-177.

Qin LX, Tang ZY, 2002: The prognostic significance of clinical and pathological features in hepatocellular carcinoma. World J Gastroenterol 8:193-199.

Quaglia A, et al, 2003: Focal nodular hyperplasia-like areas in cirrhosis. Histopathology 42:14-21.

Quigley JP, Armstrong PB, 1998: Tumor cell intravasation Alu-cidated: the chick embryo opens the window. Cell 94:281-284.

Radhi JM, Loewy J, 2000: Hepatocellular adenomatosis associated with hereditary hemochromatosis. Postgrad Med J 76:100-102.

Rakheja D, et al, 2004: Hepatic mesenchymal hamartoma with translocation involving chromosome band 19q13.4: a recurrent abnormality. Cancer Genet Cytogenet 153:60-63.

Ramakrishna B, et al, 1996: Large encapsulated hepatocellular adenoma in a male. Liver 16:235-236.

Ramchand S, et al, 1970: Lipoma of the liver. Arch Pathol 90:331-333.

Ranaldi R, et al, 1993: Hepatocellular adenoma with areas of bone marrow: report of a case. Am J Surg Pathol 17:952-953.

Rapaccini GL, et al, 2004: Hepatocellular carcinoma < 2 cm in diameter complicating cirrhosis: ultrasound and clinical features in 153 consecutive patients. Liver Int 24:124-130.

Rawlings W, et al, 1974: Hepatocellular carcinoma and partial deficiency of alpha-1-antitrypsin (MZ). Ann Intern Med 81:771-773.

Reincke BS, et al, 2003: INI1 expression induces cell cycle arrest and markers of senescence in malignant rhabdoid tumor cells. J Cell Physiol 194:303-313.

Relman DA, et al, 1990: The agent of bacillary angiomatosis: an approach to the identification of uncultured pathogens. N Engl J Med 323:1573-1580.

Ren N, et al, 2003: Diagnosis and treatment of hepatic angiomyolipoma in 26 cases. World J Gastroenterol 9:1856-1858.

Rescan PY, et al, 1990: Differential expression of laminin chains and receptor (LBP-32) in fetal and neoplastic hepatocytes compared to normal adult hepatocytes in vivo and in culture. Am J Pathol 137:701-709.

Reznik Y, et al, 2004: Hepatocyte nuclear factor-1 alpha inactivation: cosegregation between liver adenomatosis and diabetes phenotypes in two maturity-onset diabetes of the young (MODY) 3 families. J Clin Endocrinol Metab 89:1476-1480.

Ribeiro A, et al, 1998: Management of liver adenomatosis: results with a conservative surgical approach. Liver Transpl Surg 4:388-398.

Rios-Dalenz JD, 1965: Leiomyoma of the liver. Arch Pathol Lab Med 79:54-59.

Rizkalla KS, et al, 1997: Key features distinguishing post-transplantation lymphoproliferative disorders and acute liver rejection. Mod Pathol 10: 708-715.

Robinson RA, Nelson L, 1986: Hepatic teratoma in an anencephalic fetus. Arch Pathol Lab Med 110:655-657.

Rodriguez E, et al, 1991: Abnormalities of 2q: a common genetic link between rhabdomyosarcoma and hepatoblastoma? Genes Chromosomes Cancer 3:122-127.

Rojiani AM, et al, 1991: Hepatic hemangioblastoma: an unusual presentation in a patient with von Hippel–Lindau disease. Am J Surg Pathol 15:81-86.

Roncalli M, 2004: Hepatocellular nodules in cirrhosis: focus on diagnostic criteria on liver biopsy: a Western experience. Liver Transplant 10:S9-S15.

Rooks JB, et al, 1979: Epidemiology of hepatocellular adenoma: the role of oral contraceptive use. JAMA 242:644-648.

Roskams T, et al, 1990: Neuroendocrine features of reactive bile ductules in cholestatic liver disease. Am J Pathol 137:1019-1025.

Roskams T, et al, 1998: Heparan sulphate proteoglycan expression in human primary liver tumors. J Pathol 185:290-297.

Ross JA, Gurney A, 1998: Hepatoblastoma incidence in the United States from 1973 to 1992. Med Paediat Oncol 30:141-142.

Ross JS, Kurian S, 1985: Clear cell hepatocellular carcinoma: sudden death from severe hypoglycemia. Am J Gastroenterol 80:188-194.

Roth D, Duncan P, 1951: Primary carcinoma of the liver after giant cell hepatitis in infancy. Cancer 8:986-991.

Roth F, 1957: Arsen und Lebertumoren (Hämangioendotheliom). Zeitschrift für Krebsforschung 61:468-503.

Roth JA, et al, 1982: A black hepatocellular carcinoma with Dubin-Johnson-like pigment and Mallory bodies: a histochemical and ultrastructural study. Am J Surg Pathol 6:375-382.

Roux J, 1897: Un cas de cancer primitif du foie avec pericholécystite calculeuse et perforation intestinale. Revue Medicale de la Suisse Romande 17:114-119.

Rowland JM, 2002: Hepatoblastoma: assessment of criteria for histologic classification. Med Pediatr Oncol 39:478-483.

Rubin E, et al, 1984: Myelolipoma of the liver. Cancer 54:2043-2046.

Ruck P, et al, 1990: Neuroendocrine differentiation in hepatoblastoma: an immunohistochemical investigation. Am J Surg Pathol 14:847-855.

Ruck P, et al, 1996: Small epithelial cells and the histogenesis of hepatoblastoma: electron microscopic, immunoelectron microscopic, and immunohistochemical findings. Am J Pathol 148:321-329.

Ruck P, et al, 1997: Hepatic stem-like cells in hepatoblastoma: expression of cytokeratin 7, albumin and oval cell associated antigens detected by OV-1 and OV-6. Histopathology 31:324-329.

Rugge M, et al, 1998: Hepatoblastoma: DNA nuclear content, proliferative indices, and pathology. Liver 18:128-133.

Rundell K, 1998: The basic science underlying antiangiogenesis therapies: meeting report. Biochem Biophys Acta 1378:R27-R31.

Saab S, Yao F, 1996: Fibrolamellar hepatocellular carcinoma: case reports and review of the literature. Dig Dis Sci 41:1981-1985.

Sainati L, et al, 1998: Cytogenetic analysis of hepatoblastoma: hypothesis of cytogenetic evolution in such tumors and results of a multicentric study. Cancer Genet Cytogenet 104:39-44.

Saito K, et al, 1997: Detection of hepatitis C virus RNA sequences in hepatocellular carcinoma and its precursors by microdissection polymerase chain reaction. Arch Pathol Lab Med 121:400-403.

Saito T, et al, 1997: Connexin 37 mutations in rat hepatic angiosarcomas induced by vinyl chloride. Cancer Res 57:375-377.

Sakamoto M, et al, 1991: Early stages of multistep hepatocarcinogenesis: adenomatous hyperplasia and early hepatocellular carcinoma. Hum Pathol 22:172-178.

Samuelsson S, Werner I, 1963: Hepatic carcinoma simulating hyperparathyroidism. Acta Med Scand 73:539-547.

Sanada Y, et al, 2005: A clinical study of 11 cases of combined hepatocellular-cholangiocarcinoma: assessment of enhancement patterns on dynamic computed tomography before resection. Hepatol Res 32:185-195.

Santos ES, et al, 2003: Primary hepatic non-Hodgkin's lymphomas: case report and review of the literature. Am J Gastroenterol 98:2789-2793.

Sasaki A, et al, 2001: Clinicopathologic study of mixed hepatocellular and cholangiocellular carcinoma: modes of spreading and choice of surgical treatment by reference to macroscopic type. J Surg Oncol 76:37-46.

Sasaki K, et al, 1981: Hepatic clear cell carcinoma associated with hypoglycemia and hypercholesterolemia. Cancer 47:820-822.

Sass DA, et al, 2005: Nonalcoholic fatty liver disease: a clinical review. Dig Dis Sci 50:171-180.

Saul SH, et al, 1987: The fibrolamellar variant of hepatocellular carcinoma: its association with focal nodular hyperplasia. Cancer 60:3049-3055.

Sautner D, et al, 1988: Autoptisch gesichertes primäres Leberkarzinoid. Pathologe 9:115-118.

Scheimberg I, et al, 1996: Primary hepatic malignant tumor with rhabdoid features: a histological, immunocytochemical, and electron microscopic study of four cases and a review of the literature. Am J Surg Pathol 20:1394-1400.

Schmid C, Beham A, 1987: Angiosarkom der Leber und Nierenzellkarzinom mit Panmyelopathie nach Thorotrastapplikation vor 40 bzw. 41 Jahren. Fallberichte mit immunhistochemischen Untersuchungen. Pathologe 8:177-182.

Schmidt D, et al, 1985: Primary malignant hepatic tumors in childhood. Virchows Arch 407:387-405.

Schmitt M, et al, 2004: Disruption of hepatocellular tight junctions by vascular endothelial growth factor (VEGF): a novel mechanism for tumor invasion. J Hepatol 41:274-283.

Schneiderman DJ, et al, 1987: Hepatic disease in patients with the acquired immunodeficiency (AIDS). Hepatology 7:925-930.

Schoedel KE, et al, 2003: HGF, MET, and matrix-related proteases in hepatocellular carcinoma, fibrolamellar variant, cirrhotic and normal liver. Mod Pathol 16:14-21.

Schuchmann M, Galle PR, 2004: Sensitizing to apoptosis—sharpening the medical sword. J Hepatol 40:335-336.

Schwartz MR, 1998: Liver cell dysplasia and other atypical lesions: new insights and applications. Adv Anat Pathol 5:99-105.

Schwartz SI, 1987: Cavernous hemangioma of the liver: a single institution report of 16 resections. Ann Surg 205:456-465.

Sciot R, et al, 1988: Transferrin receptor expression in human hepatocellular carcinoma: an immunohistochemical study of 34 cases. Histopathology 12:53-63.

Sciot R, et al, 1990: Transferrin receptor expression in benign tumours and in hepatoblastoma of the liver. Histopathology 16:59-62.

Scoazec JY, et al, 1988: Peliosis hepatis and sinusoidal dilatation during infection by the human immunodeficiency virus (HIV): an ultrastructural study. Am J Pathol 131:38-47.

Scoazec JY, et al, 1989: Epithelioid hemangioendothelioma of the liver: an ultrastructural study. Hum Pathol 20:673-681.

Scott DL, et al, 1984: Oral contraceptives, pregnancy, and focal nodular hyperplasia of the liver. JAMA 251:1461-1463.

Scott FR, et al, 1996: Hepatocellular carcinoma arising in an adenoma: value of Qbend 10 immunostaining in diagnosis of liver cell carcinoma. Histopathology 28:472-474.

Seki S, et al, 1992: An analysis of proliferating cells in biopsy specimens from patients with small hepatocellular carcinoma. Cancer 69:2433-2439.

Seki S, et al, 2000: Outcomes of dysplastic nodules in human cirrhotic liver: a clinicopathological study. Clin Cancer Res 6:3469-3473.

Seldinger SI, 1958: Catheter-replacement of the needle in percutaneous arteriography: a new technique. Acta Radiol 39:368-376.

Sheibani N, Frazier WA, 1999: Thrombospondin-1, PECAM-1, and regulation of angiogenesis. Histol Histopathol 14:285-294.

Shepherd NA, Lee G, 1983: Solitary necrotic nodules of the liver simulating hepatic metastases. J Clin Pathol 36:1181-1183.

Sheu JC, et al, 1985: Growth rate of asymptomatic hepatocellular carcinoma and its clinical implications. Gastroenterology 89:259-266.

Shi M, et al, 2004: Micrometastases of solitary hepatocellular carcinoma and appropriate resection margin. World J Surg 28:376-381.

Shimada M, et al, 2002: Hepatocellular carcinoma in patients with non-alcoholic steatohepatitis. J Hepatol 37:154-160.

Shiratsuchi H, et al, 2002: Mutation analysis of human cytokeratin 8 gene in malignant rhabdoid tumor: a possible association with intracytoplasmic inclusion body formation. Mod Pathol 15:146-153.

Shumacker HB, 1942: Hemangioma of the liver: discussion of symptomatology and report of patients treated by operation. Surgery 11:209-222.

Simson IW, 1982: Membranous obstruction of the inferior vena cava and hepatocellular carcinoma in South Africa. Gastroenterology 82:171-178.

Sioutos N, et al, 1991: Primary hepatic carcinoid tumor: an electron microscopic and immunohistochemical study. Am J Clin Pathol 95:172-175.

Skarupa DJ, et al, 2004: Hepatocellular adenomatosis is a rare entity that may mimic other hepatocellular lesions. Ann Diagn Pathol 8:43-49.

Smith SJ, et al, 1998: Molecular epidemiology of p53 protein mutations in workers exposed to vinyl chloride. Am J Epidemiol 147:302-308.

Snook JA, et al, 1989: Fibrolamellar hepatocellular carcinoma complicating ulcerative colitis with primary sclerosing cholangitis. Gut 30:243-245.

Soe KL, et al, 1992: Liver pathology associated with the use of anabolic-androgenic steroids. Liver 12:73-79.

Sohda T, et al, 1997: Co-localisation of insulin-like growth factor II and the proliferation marker MIB1 in hepatocellular carcinoma cells. J Clin Pathol 50:135-137.

Soini Y, et al, 1996: Hepatocellular carcinomas with a high proliferation index and a low degree of apoptosis and necrosis are associated with a shortened survival. Br J Cancer 73:1025-1030.

Sonoda T, et al, 1989: Long-term surviving patients with hepatocellular carcinoma comprised of dense collagenous stroma. Am J Gastroenterol 84:1087-1091.

Sotelo-Avila C, et al, 1975: Neoplasms associated with Beckwith's syndrome. Am J Pathol 78:41a.

Sowery RD, et al, 2001: Comparative genomic hybridization detects multiple chromosomal amplifications and deletions in undifferentiated embryonal sarcoma of the liver. Cancer Genet Cytogenet 126:128-133.

Srinivasan R, Dean HA, 1997: Thorotrast and the liver-revisited. J Toxicol Clin Toxicol 35:199-202.

Srivastava DN, et al, 1998: Pedunculated hepatic haemangioma with arterio-portal shunt: treated with angioembolization and surgery. Australas Radiol 42:151-153.

Srivatanakul P, et al, 2004: Epidemiology of liver cancer : an overview. Asian Pacific J Cancer Prev 5:118-125.

Stamatakis JD, et al, 1979: Benign inflammatory tumor of the common bile duct. Br J Surg 66:257-258.

Stiles B, et al, 2004: Liver-specific deletion of negative regulator Pten results in fatty liver and insulin hypersensitivity. Proc Natl Acad Sci U S A 101:2082-2087.

Stocker JT, Ishak KG, 1978: Undifferentiated (embryonal) sarcoma of the liver: report of 31 cases. Cancer 42:336-348.

Stocker JT, Ishak KG, 1983: Mesenchymal hamartoma of the liver: report of 30 cases and review of the literature. Pediatr Pathol 1:245-247.

Sugihara S, et al, 1987: A resected case of hepatocellular carcinoma associated with adenomatous hyperplasia of the liver. Jpn J Gastroenterol 84:1320-1324.

Sugitani S, et al, 1998: Hyperplastic foci reflect the risk of multicentric development of human hepatocellular carcinoma. J Hepatol 28:1045-1053.

Summers J, et al, 1978: A virus similar to human hepatitis B virus associated with hepatitis and hepatoma in woodchucks. Proc Natl Acad Sci U S A 75:4533-4537.

Sun HC, Tang ZY, 2004: Angiogenesis in hepatocellular carcinoma: the retrospectives and perspectives. J Cancer Res Clin Oncol 130:307-319.

Sundaresan M, et al, 1990: Primary hepatic vascular leiomyosarcoma of probable portal vein origin. J Clin Pathol 43:1036.

Sundaresan M, et al, 1991: "Solitary" necrotic nodules of the liver: an aetiology reaffirmed. Gut 32:1378-1380.

Suriawinata A, Xu R, 2004: An update on the molecular genetics of hepatocellular carcinoma. Semin Liver Dis 24:77-88.

Sweeney EC, Evans DJ, 1976: Hepatic lesions in patients treated with synthetic anabolic steroids. J Clin Pathol 29:626-633.

Szabo E, et al, 2004: Similarities and differences in hepatitis B and C virus–induced hepatocarcinogenesis. Pathol Oncol Res 10:5-11.

Taguchi K, et al, 2002: Morphologic approach to hepatocellular carcinoma development in man: de novo or the so-called "dysplastic nodule-carcinoma" sequence? Oncol Rep 9:737-743.

Takahashi T, et al, 1998: Multiple liver hemangiomas enlargement during long-term steroid therapy for myasthenia gravis. Dig Dis Sci 43:1553-1561.

Takayama T, et al, 1990: Malignant transformation of adenomatous hyperplasia to hepatocellular carcinoma. Lancet 336:1150-1153.

Takayama T, et al, 1998: Early hepatocellular carcinoma as an entity with a high rate of surgical cure. Hepatology 28:1241-1246.

Takayasu H, et al, 2001: Frequent deletions and mutations of the beta-catenin gene are associated with overexpression of cyclin D1 and fibronectin and poorly differentiated histology in childhood hepatoblastoma. Clin Cancer Res 7:901-908.

Talamini R, et al, 2004: Non-Hodgkin's lymphoma and hepatitis C virus: a case-control study from northern and southern Italy. Int J Cancer 1:380-385.

Tanaka H, et al, 2004: Prospective study on the risk of hepatocellular carcinoma among hepatitis C virus–positive blood donors focusing on demographic factors, alanine aminotransferase level at donation and interaction with hepatitis B virus. Int J Cancer 112:1075-1080.

Tanaka T, 1997: Factors regulating tumor pressure in hepatocellular carcinoma and implications for tumor spread. Hepatology 26:283-287.

Tanaka Y, et al, 2000: HMB-45/melan-A and smooth muscle actin-positive clear cell epithelioid tumor arising in the ligamentum teres hepatis: additional example of clear "sugar" tumors. Am J Surg Pathol 24:1295-1299.

Tannapfel A, et al, 2001: p16INK4A-alterations in primary angiosarcoma of the liver. J Hepatol 35:62-67.

Tannapfel A, et al, 2002: INK4a-ARF alterations in liver cell adenoma. Gut 51:253-258.

Tao LC, 1991: Oral contraceptive–associated liver cell adenoma and hepatocellular carcinoma: cytomorphology and mechanism of malignant transformation. Cancer 68:341-347.

Tao LC, 1992: Are oral contraceptive–associated liver cell adenomas premalignant? Acta Cytol 36:338-344.

Tarao K, et al, 1989: Difference in the in vitro uptake of bromodeoxyuridine between liver cirrhosis with and without hepatocellular carcinoma. Cancer 64:104-109.

Tashiro-Itoh T, et al, 1997: Metallothionein expression and concentrations of copper and zinc are associated with tumor differentiation in hepatocellular carcinoma. Liver 17:300-306.

Terada T, Nakanuma Y, 1989: Iron-negative foci in siderotic macroregenerative nodules in human cirrhotic liver: a marker of incipient neoplastic lesions. Arch Pathol Lab Med 113:916-920.

Terada T, Nakanuma Y, 1992: Cell proliferative activity in adenomatous hyperplasia of the liver and small hepatocellular carcinoma. Cancer 70:591-598.

Terada T, Nakanuma Y, 1995: Multiple occurrence of borderline hepatocellular nodules in human cirrhotic livers: possible multicentric origin of hepatocellular carcinoma. Virchows Arch 427:379-383.

Terada T, et al, 1989a: Fatty macroregenerative nodule in non-steatotic liver cirrhosis: a morphologic study. Virchows Arch A 415:131-136.

Terada T, et al, 1989b: Mallory body clustering in adenomatous hyperplasia in human cirrhotic livers. Hum Pathol 20:886-890.

Terada T, et al, 1989c: Development of cavernous vasculatures in livers with hepatocellular carcinoma: an autopsy study. Liver 9:172-178.

Terada T, et al, 1989d: Macroregenerative nodules of the liver in primary biliary cirrhosis: report of two autopsy cases. Am J Gastroenterol 84:418-421.

Terada T, et al, 1995: Distribution of cytokeratin 19–positive biliary cells in cirrhotic nodules, hepatic borderline nodules (atypical adenomatous hyperplasia) and small hepatocellular carcinomas. Mod Pathol 8:371-379.

Terada T, et al, 1996: Alpha-smooth muscle actin–positive stromal cells in cholangiocarcinomas, hepatocellular carcinomas and metastatic liver carcinomas. J Hepatol 24:706-712.

Terasaki S, et al, 1998: Histological features predicting malignant transformation of nonmalignant hepatocellular nodules: a prospective study. Gastroenterology 115:1216-1222.

Terris B, et al, 1997: Interphase cytogenetic analysis reveals numerical chromosome aberrations in large liver cell dysplasia. J Hepatol 27:313-319.

Tesluk H, Lawrie J, 1981: Hepatocellular adenoma—its transformation of carcinoma in a user of oral contraceptives. Arch Pathol Lab Med 105:296-299.

Theise ND, 1995: Macroregenerative (dysplastic) nodules and hepatocarcinogenesis: theoretical and clinical considerations. Semin Liver Dis 15:360-371.

Theise ND, 1996: Cirrhosis and hepatocellular neoplasia: more like cousins than like parent and child. Gastroenterology 111:526-528 (editorial).

Theise ND, et al, 1992: Macroregenerative nodules and hepatocellular carcinoma in forty-four sequential adult liver explants with cirrhosis. Hepatology 16:949-955.

Theise ND, et al, 1996: Low proliferative activity in macroregenerative nodules: evidence for an alternate hypothesis concerning human hepatocarcinogenesis. Liver 16:134-139.

Theise ND, et al, 2003: Hepatic "stem cell" malignancies in adults: four cases. Histopathology 43:263-271.

Thomas RM, et al, 1992: Liver cell dysplasia: a DNA aneuploid lesion with distinct morphologic features. Hum Pathol 23:496-503.

Thorgeirsson SS, Grisham JW, 2002: Molecular pathogenesis of human hepatocellular carcinoma. Nat Genet 31:339-346.

Tickoo SK, et al, 2002: Combined hepatocellular-cholangiocarcinoma: a histopathologic, immunohistochemical, and in situ hybridization study. Am J Surg Pathol 26:989-997.

Torbenson M, et al, 2002: Hepatic adenomas: analysis of sex steroid receptor status and the Wnt signaling pathway. Mod Pathol 1:189-196.

Torimura T, et al, 1991: Mechanism of fibrous capsule formation surrounding hepatocellular carcinoma. Arch Pathol Lab Med 115:365-371.

Torimura T, et al, 1998: Increased expression of vascular endothelial growth factor is associated with tumor progression in hepatocellular carcinoma. Hum Pathol 29:986-991.

Torimura T, et al, 2004: Overexpression of angiopoietin-1 and angiopoietin-2 in hepatocellular carcinoma. J Hepatol 40:799-807.

Tovbin J, et al, 1997: Hepatic mesenchymal hamartoma: a pediatric tumor that may be diagnosed prenatally. Ultrasound Obstet Gynecol 10:63-65.

Toyoda H, et al, 1997: Significance of tumor vascularity as a predictor of long-term prognosis in patients with small hepatocellular carcinoma treated by percutaneous ethanol injection therapy. J Hepatol 26:1055-1962.

Tran Van Nhieu J, et al, 1998: Myofibroblasts and hepatocellular carcinoma: an in vivo and in vitro study. J Hepatol 29:120-128.

Truant R, et al, 1995: Direct interaction of the hepatitis B virus HBx protein with p53 leads to inhibition by HBx of p53 response element-directed transactivation. J Virol 69:1851-1859.

Ugarte N, Gonzales-Crussi F, 1981: Hepatoma in siblings with progressive familial cholestatic cirrhosis of childhood. Am J Pathol 76:172-177.

Van Dekken H, et al, 2003: Genetic evaluation of the dysplasia-carcinoma sequence in chronic viral liver disease: a detailed analysis of two cases and review of the literature. Acta Histochem 105:29-41.

Van der Rest M, Garrone R, 1991: Collagen family of proteins. FASEB J 5:2814-2823.

Van Eyken P, et al, 1988: Cytokeratin expression in hepatocellular carcinoma: an immunohistochemical study. Hum Pathol 19:562-568.

Van Eyken P, et al, 1990a: Abundant expression of cytokeratin 7 in fibrolamellar carcinoma of the liver. Histopathology 17:101-107.

Van Eyken P, et al, 1990b: A cytokeratin-immunohistochemical study of hepatoblastoma. Hum Pathol 2:302-308.

Varma V, Cohen C, 2004: Immuohistochemical and molecular markers in the diagnosis of hepatocellular carcinoma. Adv Anat Pathol 11:239-249.

Varnholt H, et al, 2002: C-met and hepatocyte growth factor expression in combined hepatocellular and cholangiocarcinoma. Oncol Rep 9:35-41.

Vermess M, et al, 1984: Misleading appearance of a rare malignant liver tumour on computed tomography: report of a case of primary undifferentiated (embryonal) sarcoma of the liver. Br J Radiol 57:262-265.

Versteege I, et al, 2002: A key role of the hSNF5/INI1 tumour suppressor in the control of the G1-S transition of the cell cycle. Oncogene 21:6403-6412.

Vilgrain V, et al, 2003: Prevalence of hepatic hemangioma in patients with focal nodular hyperplasia: MR imaging analysis. Radiology 229:75-79.

Villa E, et al, 1995: Variant estrogen receptor messenger RNA species detected in human primary hepatocellular carcinoma. Cancer Res 55:498-500.

Visfeldt J, Poulsen H, 1972: On the histopathology of liver and liver tumours in thorium-dioxide patients. Acta Pathol Microbiol Scand A Pathol 80:97-108.

Vogel CL, et al, 1970: Hepatitis-associated antigen in Ugandan patients with hepatocellular carcinoma. Lancet 2:621-624.

Volmar KE, et al, 2003: Hepatic adenomatosis in glycogen storage disease type Ia: report of a case with unusual histology. Arch Pathol Lab Med 127:e402-e405.

Von Schweinitz D, et al, 1996: Expression of cell adhesion molecules and common acute lymphoblastic leukemia antigen in hepatoblastoma. Virchows Arch 429:235-241.

Von Schweinitz D, et al, 1997: Prognostic factors and staging systems in childhood hepatoblastoma. Int J Cancer 74:595-599.

Voorhoeve PM, Agami R, 2004: Unraveling human tumor suppressor pathways: a tale of the INK4A locus. Cell Cycle 3:616-620.

Wachsberg RH, et al, 1994: Two leiomyomas of the liver in an adult patient with AIDS: CT and MR appearance. J Comput Assist Tomogr 18:156-157.

Wada K, et al, 1988: Large regenerative nodules and dysplastic nodules in cirrhotic livers: a histopathologic study. Hepatology 8:1684-1688.

Wada Y, et al, 1998: Clinicopathological study on hepatocellular carcinoma with lymphocytic infiltration. Hepatology 27:407-414.

Walker NI, et al, 1992: Undifferentiated (embryonal) sarcoma of the liver: pathologic findings and long-term survival after complete surgical resection. Cancer 69:52-59.

Walsh MM, et al, 1998: Epithelioid hemangioendothelioma of the liver mimicking Budd-Chiari syndrome. Arch Pathol Lab Med 122: 846-848.

Walter M, 1896: Ueber das multiple Auftreten primärer, bösartiger Neoplasmen. Archiv für Klinik und Chirurgie 53:1-58.

Wang J, et al, 1991: "Neuroendocrine" differentiation in primary neoplasms of the liver. J Pathol 163:61-67.

Wang Y, et al, 2004a: Characterization of HBV integrants in 14 hepatocellular carcinomas: association of truncated X gene and hepatocellular carcinogenesis. Oncogene 8:142-148.

Wang Y, et al, 2004b: HBsAg and HBx knocked into the p21 locus causes hepatocellular carcinoma in mice. Hepatology 39:318-324.

Wanless IR, et al, 1985: On the pathogenesis of focal nodular hyperplasia of the liver. Hepatology 5:1194-1200.

Warner TFCS, et al, 1980: Pancreatic-polypeptide-producing apudoma of the liver. Cancer 46:1146-1151.

Watanabe J, et al, 2004: Prognostic significance of Bcl-xL in human hepatocellular carcinoma. Surgery 135:604-612.

Watanabe S, et al, 1983: Morphologic studies of the liver cell dysplasia. Cancer 51:2197-2205.

Watson A, 1999: The role of Fas in apoptosis induced by anticancer drugs. Hepatology 29:280-281 (editorial).

Wee A, et al, 1985: Hepatobiliary carcinoma associated with primary sclerosing cholangitis and chronic ulcerative colitis. Hum Pathol 16: 719-726.

Weichhold W, et al, 1995: Primary extramedullary plasmacytoma of the liver. Am J Surg Pathol 19:1197-1202.

Weihrauch M, et al, 2002a: Mutation analysis of K-ras-2 in liver angiosarcoma and adjacent nonneoplastic liver tissue from patients occupationally exposed to vinyl chloride. Environ Mol Mutagen 40:36-40.

Weihrauch M, et al, 2002b: Abnormalities of the ARF-p53 pathway in primary angiosarcomas of the liver. Hum Pathol 3:884-892.

Weinberg AG, Finegold MJ, 1983: Primary hepatic tumors of childhood. Hum Pathol 14:512-537.

Weinberg AG, et al, 1977: The occurrence of hepatoma in the chronic form of hereditary tyrosinemia. J Pediatr 88:434-438.

Weinbren K, 1976: Histopathology of liver lesions assosiated with exposure to vinyl chloride monomer. Proc R Soc Med 69:299-303.

Weinbren K, et al, 1987: Apparent extra-hepatic invasion by metastatic tumours in the liver. Clin Radiol 38:357-362.

Weiss SW, Enzinger FM, 1982: Epithelioid hemangioendothelioma: a vascular tumour often mistaken for a carcinoma. Cancer 50:970-981.

Wen YL, et al, 2004: Detection of intratumoral vascularity in small hepatocellular carcinoma by coded phase inversion harmonics. Intervirology 47:169-178.

Wildi S, et al, 2004: Critical evaluation of the different staging systems for hepatocellular carcinoma. Br J Surg 91:400-408.

Wilkinson ML, et al, 1983: Wilson's disease and hepatocellular carcinoma: possible protective role of copper. Gut 24:767-771.

Williams GM, Yamamoto RS, 1972: Absence of stainable iron from preneoplastic lesions in rat liver with 8-hydroxyquinoline-induced siderosis. J Natl Cancer Inst 49:685-692.

Willis RA, 1948: Pathology of Tumours. London, Butterworth.

Wogan GN, 1976: Aflatoxins and their relationship to hepatocellular carcinoma. In Okuda K, Peters RL (eds): Hepatocellular Carcinoma. New York, Wiley, pp 25-41.

Wooten WB, et al, 1978: Computed tomography of necrotic hepatic metastases. AJR Am J Roentgenol 131:839-842.

Wu PC, et al, 1983: Clear cell carcinoma of liver: an ultrastructural study. Cancer 52:504-507.

Yamada S, et al, 1992: Tenascin expression in human chronic liver disease and in hepatocellular carcinoma. Liver 12:10-16.

Yamada S, et al, 2004: Expression profiling and differential screening between hepatoblastomas and the corresponding normal livers: identification of high expression of the PLK1 oncogene as a poor-prognostic indicator of hepatoblastomas. Oncogene 23:5901-5911.

Yamaguchi R, et al, 1998: Expression of vascular endothelial growth factor in human hepatocellular carcinoma. Hepatology 28:68-77.

Yamamoto A, et al, 1998: Thymidine phosphorylase (platelet-derived endothelial cell growth factor), microvessel density and clinical outcome in hepatocellular carcinoma. J Hepatol 29:290-299.

Yamamoto H, et al, 1997: Relation of enhanced secretion of active matrix metalloproteinases with tumor spread in human hepatocellular carcinoma. Gastroenterology 112:1290-1296.

Yamamoto M, et al, 2004: Favorable surgical outcomes in patients with early hepatocellular carcinoma. Ann Surg 239:395-399.

Yano Y, et al, 2003: Combined hepatocellular and cholangiocarcinoma: a clinicopathologic study of 26 resected cases. Jpn J Clin Oncol 33:283-287.

Yoon GS, et al, 1998: Primary myxoid leiomyoma of the liver. Arch Pathol Lab Med 122:1112-1115.

Yoshida T, et al, 1982: Minute hepatocellular carcinoma without appreciable change in size for seven years: a case report. Cancer 49:1491-1495.

Yoshikawa J, et al, 1988: Fatty metamorphosis in hepatocellular carcinoma: radiologic features in 10 cases. Am J Radiol 151:717-720.

You SL, et al, 2004: Seropositivity of hepatitis B e antigen and hepatocellular carcinoma. Ann Med 36:215-224.

Younossi ZM, et al, 2005: A genomic and proteomic study of the spectrum of nonalcoholic fatty liver disease. Hepatology 42:665-674.

Yu L, et al, 1997: Heterogeneity in androgen receptor levels and growth response to dihydrotestosterone in sublines derived from human hepatocellular carcinoma line (KYN-1). Liver 17:35-40.

Yu MC, et al, 1990: Prevalence of hepatitis B and C viral markers in black and white patients with hepatocellular carcinoma in the United States. J Natl Cancer Inst 82:1038-1041.

Yu M-W, et al, 1997: Effect of aflatoxin metabolism and DNA adduct formation on hepatocellular carcinoma among chronic hepatitis B carriers in Taiwan. J Hepatol 27:320-330.

Yuan JM, et al, 2004: Synergism of alcohol, diabetes, and viral hepatitis on the risk of hepatocellular carcinoma in blacks and whites in the U.S. Cancer 101:1009-1017.

Yuri T, et al, 2004: Malignant rhabdoid tumor of the liver: case report and literature rview. Pathol Int 54:623-629.

Zafrani ES, 2004: Non-alcoholic fatty liver disease: an emerging pathological spectrum. Virchows Arch 444:3-12.

Zafrani ES, Gaulard P, 1993: Primary lymphoma of the liver. Liver 13:57-61.

Zanconati F, et al, 1996: Small cell carcinoma of the liver: a hitherto unreported variant of hepatocellular carcinoma. Histopathology 29:449-453.

Zangeneh F, et al, 1969: Hepatorenal glycogenosis (type I glycogenosis) and carcinoma of the liver. J Pediatr 74:73-83.

Zhang L, et al, 2004: Study of the PTEN gene expression and FAK phosphorylation in human hepatocarcinoma tissues and cell lines. Mol Cell Biochem 262:25-33.

Zhang ZK, et al, 2002: Cell cycle arrest and repression of cyclin D1 transcription by INI1/hSNF5. Mol Cell Biol 22:5975-5988.

Zhao M, Zimmermann A, 1997: Apoptosis in human hepatocellular carcinoma and in liver cell dysplasia is correlated with p53 protein immunoreactivity. J Clin Pathol 50:394-400.

Zhao M, Zimmermann A, 1998: Liver cell dysplasia: reactivities for c-met protein, Rb protein, E-cadherin and transforming growth factor-beta1 in comparison with hepatocellular carcinoma. Histol Histopathol 13: 657-670.

Zhao M, et al, 1994a: Immunohistochemical detection of bcl-2 protein in liver lesions: bcl-2 protein is expressed in hepatocellular carcinomas but not in liver cell dysplasia. Histopathology 25:237-245.

Zhao M, et al, 1994b: Three types of liver cell dysplasia (LCD) in small cirrhotic nodules are distinguishable by karyometry and PCNA labelling, and their features resemble distinct grades of hepatocellular carcinoma. Histol Histopathol 9:73-83.

Zhao M, et al, 1996: Tenascin and collagen type IV expression in liver cell dysplasia and in hepatocellular carcinoma. Histol Histopathol 11: 323-333.

Zhao ZC, et al, 2003: The molecular mechanism underlying angiogenesis in hepatocellular carcinoma: the imbalance activation of signaling pathways. Hepatobiliary Pancreat Dis Int 2:529-536.

Zhou H, Fischer H-P, 1998: Liver carcinoma in PiZ alpha-1-antitrypsin deficiency. Am J Surg Pathol 22:742-748.

Zhou XD, et al, 2001: Experience of 1000 patients who underwent hepatectomy for small hepatocellular carcinoma. Cancer 91:1479-1486.

Ziegler JL, et al, 1982: Outbreak of Burkitt's-like lymphoma in homosexual men. Lancet 2:631-633.

Ziegler JL, et al, 1984: Non-Hodgkin's lymphoma in 90 homosexual men: relation to generalized lymphadenopathy and the acquired immunodeficiency syndrome. N Engl J Med 311:565-570.

Zimmermann A, 2002: Hepatoblastoma with cholangioblastic features ("cholangioblastic hepatoblastoma") and other liver tumors with a bimodal differentiation in young patients. Med Pediatr Oncol 39:487-491.

Zimmermann A, 2005: The emerging family of hepatoblastoma tumours: from ontogenesis to oncogenesis. Eur J Cancer 41:1503-1514.

Zimmermann A, Baer HU, 1996: Fibrous tumor-liver interface in large hepatic neoplasms: its siginificance for tumor resection and enucleation. Liver Transpl Surg 2:192-199.

Zimmermann A, Keller HU, 1987: Locomotion of tumor cells as an element of invasion and metastasis. Biomed Pharmacother 41:337-344.

Benign Liver Lesions

J. BELGHITI, V. VILGRAIN, AND V. PARADIS

A consequence of extensive use of liver ultrasonography is the detection of asymptomatic tumors. In the absence of underlying chronic liver disease, most of these lesions correspond to benign liver tumors, including cystic and solid lesions. Cystic tumors are discussed in Chs. 64 and 65. Solid benign lesions include a broad spectrum of regenerative and true neoplastic processes (Table 70.1). Based on the cell of origin, most frequent solid benign tumors can be classified into two groups according to epithelial or mesenchymal origins. Epithelial lesions include hepatocellular (focal nodular hyperplasia [FNH] and adenoma) and cholangiocellular (bile duct adenoma) tumors. Mesenchymal tumors originating from blood vessels include hemangioma, tumors originating from adipose tissue include angiolipoma, and tumors originating from muscle tissue include leiomyoma. Mesenchymal hamartomas originate from mixed epithelial and mesenchymal tissues. Most solid benign liver lesions, including hemangioma, FNH, and regenerative processes, remain asymptomatic, do not increase in volume, and do not require any treatment or follow-up. By contrast, hepatic adenoma may be associated with serious complications, indicating surgical resection.

Understanding of the clinical, biologic, radiologic, and pathologic characteristics of each tumor is important for accurate diagnosis and appropriate management. Advances in imaging studies allow an accurate diagnosis in most cases, reducing the use of percutaneous biopsy to a few patients and limiting resections for final diagnosis to exceptional cases. The most frequent benign liver cell lesions include hemangioma, FNH, and hepatocellular adenoma. Because radiologic imaging is crucial in diagnosis and management, considerable emphasis is placed on the role of radiologic study (see Chs. 15, 18, and 19).

CAVERNOUS HEMANGIOMA

Hepatic hemangiomata are probably the most common of all liver tumors. These tumors occur at all ages. Because of the difference in histologic structure between the adult and the infantile forms and the different clinical presentation, however, they are regarded as separate entities (Hobbs, 1990). Only hemangioma of the liver in adults is discussed in this chapter.

Pathogenesis and Pathology

The prevalence of hemangioma in the general population ranges from 1% to 20% (Semelka & Sofka, 1997) with a large predominance in women with a 5:1 female-to-male ratio (Biecker et al, 2003; Mergo & Ros, 1998; Trotter & Everson, 2001). In adults, hemangiomata usually are found in patients with a mean age of 50 years, equally in the left and right lobes of the liver, and most are less than 5 cm in diameter. Hemangiomata measuring 10 cm or more are referred to as *giant hemangiomata* (Fig. 70.1). The pathogenesis of hemangiomata is not well understood. Some of these

tumors have estrogen receptors, and accelerated growth has been observed with high estrogen states, such as associated with puberty, pregnancy, oral contraceptive use, and androgen treatment. These findings suggest that hormonal effect may be a pathogenic mechanism (Biecker et al, 2003; Cobey & Salem, 2004; Trotter & Everson, 2001). Macroscopic examination shows well-delineated, flat, red-blue lesions that may collapse partially on sectioning. Some degree of fibrosis, calcification, and thrombosis may be observed, most commonly on the largest lesions. Microscopically, hemangiomata are composed of cavernous vascular spaces lined by flattened endothelium underlying fibrous septa of various widths (Fig. 70.2). Small hemangiomata may become entirely fibrous, appearing as a "solitary fibrous nodule."

Clinical and Biologic Data

Most hemangiomata are less than 5 cm and found incidentally during ultrasound or computed tomography (CT) examination of the abdomen for unrelated reasons (Trotter & Everson, 2001). They remain stable in size (Takayasu et al, 1990) or show minimal increase in diameter over time (Nghiem et al, 1997). Few observations of significant enlargement of a hemangioma have been reported (Nghiem et al, 1997; Takayasu et al, 1990). Pain related to an uncomplicated hemangioma probably is due to associated disorders, such as gallbladder disease, liver cysts, gastroduodenal ulcers, or hiatal hernia (Farges et al, 1995). Large hemangiomata can be asymptomatic or may manifest as an abdominal mass or pain. Large lesions located in the left lobe of the liver may cause pressure effects on adjacent structures with resulting symptoms.

Liver function tests, including alkaline phosphatase and gamma-glutamyltransferase, are normal. Standard laboratory tests associated with a large hepatic tumor with mild symptoms could be helpful in the diagnosis of hemangioma. Complications are observed mostly in large hemangiomata and include (1) alterations of internal architecture, such as inflammation; (2) alteration in coagulation, which could lead to systemic disorders; (3) hemorrhage, which can cause hemoperitoneum; and (4) compression of adjacent structures.

Some cases of inflammatory processes complicating giant hemangioma have been reported (Takayasu et al, 1990). The prevalence is probably underestimated. Signs and symptoms of an inflammatory process include low-grade fever, weight loss, abdominal pain, accelerated erythrocyte sedimentation rate, anemia, thrombocytosis, and increased fibrinogen level. The imaging features are those of giant hemangioma. Clinical and laboratory abnormalities disappear after surgical excision of the hemangioma (Bornman et al, 1987; Pateron et al, 1991; Pol et al, 1998).

Kasabach-Merritt syndrome is a rare complication of hepatic hemangioma in adults. It is a coagulopathy consisting of intravascular coagulation, clotting, and fibrinolysis within the hemangioma (About et al, 1994). The initially localized coagulopathy may progress to secondary increased systemic fibrinolysis and

Table 70.1   Histologic Classification of Benign Liver Lesions and Main Clinical Data

Epithelial Lesions

Hepatocytes	Liver cell adenoma	Very rare Associated with oral contraceptives High rate of complications (bleeding, malignant transformation)
	Focal nodular hyperplasia	Rare Female predominance No risk of complication
	Nodular regenerative hyperplasia	Very rare Associated with systemic diseases and drugs Portal hypertension a complication
	Focal fatty change	Common Associated with diabetes, obesity, hepatitis C virus, and malnutrition No risk of complication
Biliary cells	Bile duct adenoma	Rare No risk of complication
	Biliary hamartoma (Von Meyenburg complex)	Very rare Development anomaly No risk of complication

Nonepithelial Lesions

Mesenchymal	Hemangioma	Common Female predominance Very low risk of complication
	Angiomyolipoma	Rare Associated with tuberous sclerosis No risk of complication
	Lipoma, myelolipoma	Exceptional No risk of complication
Heterotopia	Adrenal, pancreatic, or splenic tissues	Exceptional Very low risk of complication
Others	Peliosis hepatis	Exceptional Associated with androgens, oral contraceptives, drugs, malignancies, tuberculosis No risk of complication
	Inflammatory pseudotumor	Very rare Associated with general syndromes No risk of complication

thrombocytopenia (Maceyko & Camisa, 1991), leading to a fatal outcome in 20% to 30% of patients.

Intratumoral hemorrhage is rarely encountered in hepatic hemangioma. It can occur spontaneously or after anticoagulation therapy. The symptoms consist of acute-onset vomiting and epigastric pain (Graham et al, 1993). The bleeding is suggested by intratumoral high attenuation on nonenhanced CT scans and high signal intensity on T1-weighted magnetic resonance imaging (MRI). Spontaneous rupture of a hemangioma is exceptional; a PubMed Medline search identified only 32 cases of spontaneous rupture (Corigliano et al, 2003). Taking into account the high prevalence of these tumors, this extremely rare complication should not have an impact on the therapeutic indication or on the specific advice to patients, who often are worried by the presence of a liver tumor.

Imaging

Most hemangiomata can be diagnosed accurately by imaging studies alone because there are usually characteristic imaging features. On ultrasonography (see Ch. 15), the classic appearance of hemangioma is that of an echogenic mass of uniform density, less than 3 cm in diameter, with acoustic enhancement and sharp margins (Fig. 70.3). No vascular pattern is identified on color Doppler ultrasound. The potential of contrast-enhanced harmonic ultrasound to characterize liver lesions has been highlighted. In hemangiomata, the absence of intratumoral vessels in

the arterial phase and peripheral nodular enhancement in the portal phase are the most typical patterns and are observed in 76% and 88%, respectively (Isozaki et al, 2003). Peripheral globular enhancement in the portal phase and isoechoic pattern on late phase also are observed in most atypical hemangiomata larger than 3 cm (Quaia et al, 2002).

Strict criteria for the diagnosis of hemangioma on CT (see Ch. 18) were described previously. These criteria were (1) low attenuation on noncontrast CT; (2) peripheral enhancement of the lesion followed by a central enhancement on contrast CT; and (3) contrast enhancement of the lesion on delayed scans (Freeny & Marks, 1986). These criteria have been updated with the helical multiphasic CT technique. The presence of peripheral puddles at the arterial phase has a sensitivity of 67%, a specificity of 99%, and a positive predictive value of 86% for hemangioma (Nino-Murcia et al, 2000). A hallmark of liver hemangioma is isoattenuation with the arterial system (Fig. 70.4) (Van Leeuwen et al, 1996). Hemangiomata that are the most difficult to characterize are lesions smaller than 3 cm because they may not show nodular enhancement, but often enhance homogeneously during the hepatic arterial or portal venous phase (Kim et al, 2001).

The role of MRI in the characterization of liver hemangiomata was established in 1985 (Itai et al, 1985; Starck et al, 1985). The classic appearance of a liver hemangioma is a hypointense lesion on T1-weighted sequences and a strongly hyperintense lesion on heavily T2-weighted sequences with a "lightbulb" pattern. Gadolinium chelate administration and dynamic serial postcontrast MRI is performed in all cases. Hemangiomata identified

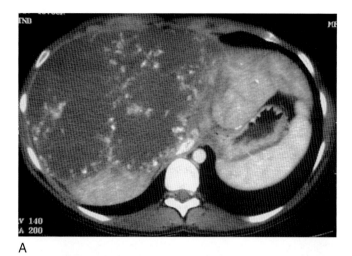

A

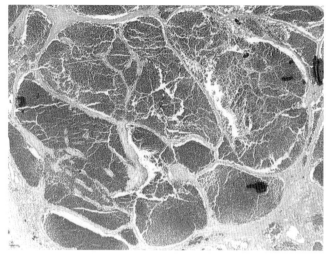

Fig. 70.2. Hemangioma is composed of cavernous vascular spaces lined by flattened endothelium underlying fibrous septa of various widths. The vascular spaces are filled with red blood cells.

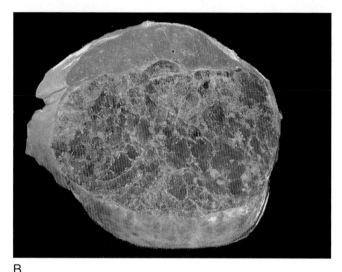

B

Fig. 70.1. Giant hemangioma. **A,** Portal-venous phase helical CT and centripetal contrast enhancement. **B,** Macroscopic view of hemangioma shows a well-delineated, flat lesion, consisting of large vascular spaces filled with blood cells.

Usually typical early, peripheral, globular enhancement is observed, however, with typical hyperintensity on T2-weighted MRI at the periphery. The progressive centripetal enhancement of the lesion, although present, does not lead to complete filling.

Rapidly filling hemangiomata are infrequent (16% of all hemangiomata) and seem to occur significantly more often in small lesions (42% of hemangiomata <1 cm in diameter) (Hanafusa et al, 1995). CT and MRI show immediate homogeneous enhancement at arterial phase, which makes differentiation from other hypervascular tumors difficult. T2-weighted images may be helpful, but hypervascular tumors, such as islet cell metastases, also are hyperintense on such images. Accurate diagnosis is made with delayed phase CT or MRI because hemangiomata remain hyperattenuating or hyperintense, whereas hypervascular metastases do not.

Another important finding in diagnosis of hemangioma is attenuation equivalent to that of the aorta during all phases of CT.

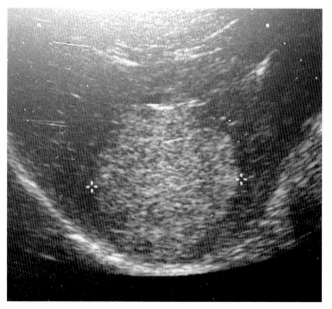

Fig. 70.3. Ultrasound of a typical hemangioma. The lesion is echoic, is homogeneous, and has sharp margins.

with this technique have the following features: (1) peripheral hyperintense nodules with a nonintact ring immediately after contrast administration, (2) progressive centripetal enhancement that is most intense at 90 seconds, (3) undulating nodular contour of the inner ring margin, and (4) persistent homogeneous enhancement without heterogeneous or peripheral washout (Fig. 70.5) (Semelka et al, 1994). Technetium 99m pertechnetate–labeled red blood cell single-photon emission CT also is quite specific, but comparison with MRI showed that MRI had a higher sensitivity and specificity than single-photon emission CT, especially for lesions less than 2 cm in diameter (Birnbaum et al, 1990).

Two types of hemangiomata have an atypical imaging pattern. One type can be diagnosed if the clinician is aware of large hemangiomata, rapidly filling or very slow filling hemangiomata, and hemangiomata with arterial-portal venous shunt. The second type of hemangiomata cannot be diagnosed with imaging and require biopsy. Large hemangiomata are often heterogeneous (Coumbaras et al, 2002; Danet et al, 2003) and are termed *giant hemangiomata* when they exceed 6 to 12 cm in diameter. At imaging, large hemangiomata often appear heterogeneous with marked central areas corresponding to thrombosis, extensive hyalinization, and fibrosis.

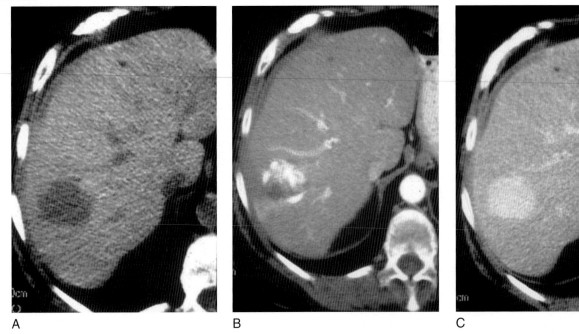

A   B   C

Fig. 70.4. Multiphasic helical CT of a typical hemangioma. **A,** On precontrast CT, the lesion is hypodense. After contrast medium injection, the lesion enhances with peripheral puddling (**B**) and becomes homogeneously hyperdense on delayed phase imaging (**C**).

Very slow filling hemangiomata appear as hypoattenuating lesions on multiphasic examination, or they have tiny enhancing dots that do not progress to the classic globular enhancement. They are estimated to account for 8% to 16% of the cases. These hemangiomata are problematic in patients with malignancy.

Arterial-portal venous shunts are associated mainly with hepatic malignancy, but also can be seen in benign liver masses (Kim et al, 2001), in particular, hemangiomata. They consist of early parenchymal enhancement associated with early filling of the portal vein. They are not related to the size of the lesion, but they are seen more frequently in hemangiomata with rapid enhancement. Other atypical hemangiomata are calcified hemangiomata, hyalinized hemangiomata, cystic hemangiomata, pedunculated hemangiomata, and hemangiomata with fluid-fluid level.

Hemangiomata developing in abnormal liver are difficult to diagnose. Hemangiomata in fatty liver usually appear hypoechoic at ultrasound and hyperattenuating at nonenhanced CT (Marsh et al, 1989). MRI is more helpful than CT. With progressive cirrhosis, hemangiomata are likely to decrease in size and become more fibrotic and difficult to diagnose radiologically (Brancatelli et al, 2001). Association of hepatic hemangioma and FNH is frequent (25% of cases) and not fortuitous (Mathieu et al, 1989; Vilgrain et al, 2003). FNH is considered to be a hyperplastic response caused by focal increased arterial flow in the hepatic parenchyma and, similar to hemangioma, is thought to have a vascular origin. When the tumors have typical imaging features, diagnosis can be made with confidence.

Liver hemangioma has been considered a contraindication to needle biopsy for many years because of the high risk of hemorrhage. Several series of percutaneous biopsy in liver hemangiomata have been reported, however, and the contraindications should be reconsidered. No serious complications were observed in two large series: one in 47 biopsy specimens obtained using a core-needle biopsy (Heilo & Stenwig, 1997) and one in 114 patients having fine-needle aspiration biopsy (Caldironi et al, 1998).

In the latter series, two minor accidents were observed, resulting in profuse bleeding of a giant hemangioma, and resolved with medical care. As in other tumors, a cuff of normal hepatic parenchyma should be interposed between the capsule and the margin of the hemangioma. Indications for percutaneous biopsy should be restricted to atypical cases despite a combination of imaging modalities. Sensitivity and overall accuracy are reported in more than 90% (Caldironi et al, 1998; Nakaizumi et al, 1990).

Management

Whatever the size, there is no treatment for *asymptomatic hemangioma*. When the diagnosis is established, it is not necessary to adopt therapeutic or specific measures. The patient should be reassured about the rare occurrence of growth and the extremely low risk of complication. There is no argument for interrupting oral contraceptive use or avoiding pregnancy, and follow-up is not justified. In our experience of hundreds of patients with hemangioma, the main complication of hemangioma has been surgical operation. Although in specialized centers liver resection mortality has declined dramatically to less than 1%, there is a risk of intraoperative bleeding and postoperative biliary fistula, which should be considered unacceptable considering the benign nature of these lesions.

Indications for treatment include severe symptoms, complications, and inability to exclude malignancy (Yoon et al, 2003). Surgical resection is the definitive treatment; other, less effective options include hepatic artery ligation and radiation therapy. Radiation therapy can reduce the size of the lesion (Gaspar et al, 1993). Long-term effects of radiation therapy on the liver and adjacent structures can be deleterious, however, and the relief of symptoms is not well documented. Arterial embolization, which may be considered for the temporary control of hemorrhage, has limited success and occasionally is associated with morbidity

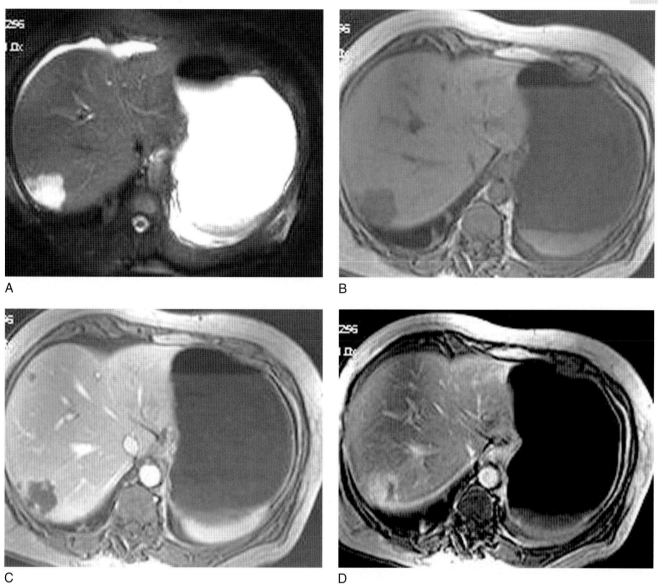

Fig. 70.5. MRI of a typical hemangioma. **A,** The lesion is strongly hyperintense on T2-weighted image. **B,** The lesion is strongly hypointense on T1-weighted image. **C** and **D,** Postgadolinium T1-weighted MRI sequences. Progressive and globular enhancement is noted at the periphery followed by central and delayed enhancement.

(Reading et al, 1988). Arterial ligation may be considered during surgical procedures, allowing manual decompression of large hemangiomata and facilitating their manipulation and enucleation (see Ch. 80) (Yoon et al, 2003).

When indicated, the only treatment to be considered is resection (Herman et al, 2005). When performed in specialized units, a variety of techniques can be used, including enucleation, hepatic resection, and laparoscopic techniques. The choice of excision requires consideration of the size and anatomic location of the lesion. Studies comparing enucleation with anatomic resection showed that enucleation is associated with fewer intra-abdominal complications and especially lower rate of biliary fistula (Gedaly et al, 1999; Kuo et al, 1994). One explanation might be that vital structures are compressed by the hemangioma, and enucleation within the fibrous space spares bile ducts and major vessels from damage (Kuo et al, 1994). After identification and ligation of the main feeding arteries to the lesion, enucleation allows the preservation of a maximal amount of functional liver. The use of

the Cavitron ultrasonic surgical aspiration system with concomitant control of the inflow vessels facilitates the dissection of the plane between the lesion and the liver. In some cases, it may be safer to perform a formal anatomic liver resection, however. Laparoscopic resection of liver hemangioma has been reported (Karahasanoglu et al, 2001). Liver transplantation also has been used successfully to treat symptomatic patients with technically unresectable complicated giant hemangiomata (Browers et al, 1997; Ferraz et al, 2004; Tapetes et al, 1995).

FOCAL NODULAR HYPERPLASIA

Pathogenesis and Pathology

FNH is the second most common benign liver process, after hemangioma. It is a benign, tumor-like condition predominantly diagnosed in women 30 to 50 years old; FNH is not influenced by oral contraceptives (International Working Party, 1995; Ishak, 1979). FNH is considered a hyperplastic reaction resulting from arterial malformation (Wanless et al, 1985). This hypothesis, suggesting that increased arterial flow hyperperfuses the local liver parenchyma leading to secondary hepatocellular hyperplasia, has been reinforced by molecular data showing that FNH is a polyclonal regenerative process (Gaffey et al, 1996; Paradis et al, 1997). This regenerative process induced in a specific vascular territory could explain the absence of size changes. Such lesions display a typical pathologic pattern for radiologists and pathologists. Grossly, FNH is a well-circumscribed, unencapsulated, usually solitary mass, characterized by a central fibrous scar that radiates into the liver parenchyma (Fig. 70.6). Histologically, FNH is composed of benign-appearing hepatocytes arranged in nodules that are delineated by fibrous septa originating from the central scar. In the fibrous septa, large and dystrophic vessels, ductular proliferation, and inflammatory cells are observed. The hepatocytes are hyperplastic, arranged in liver plates of normal or slightly increased thickness (see Fig. 70.6B and C). Hepatocytes may be hydropic related to cholestatic changes. Inside the lesion, steatosis may be observed.

Besides this classic form of FNH, several variant lesions are being described with increased frequency and commonly are classified as "nontypical FNH" by radiologists. This group is heterogeneous, including FNH without central fibrous scar, lesions displaying telangiectatic changes, and lesions with adenomatous features (Nguyen et al, 1999). On histologic examination, FNH without macroscopic central fibrous scar exhibits all the pathologic elementary features of classic FNH (Fig. 70.7). Molecular studies showed, however, that in this group of atypical FNH, lesions displaying telangiectatic changes, so-called telangiectatic form of FNH, are clonal processes and should be regarded as a variant form of liver cell adenoma, rather than FNH (Bioulac-Sage et al, 2005; Paradis et al, 2004). Histologic diagnosis of these atypical lesions is difficult on fine-needle biopsy and in most cases may be achieved only on surgical resection specimens (Fabre et al, 2002). Pathologic features of this entity are described in Ch. 60.

Clinical and Biologic Data

Most FNH lesions are asymptomatic and are discovered incidentally during liver ultrasound examination. In few patients with large tumors, FNH may be discovered because of abdominal pain or discomfort. Large lesions located in the left lobe of the liver may cause pressure effects on adjacent structures with

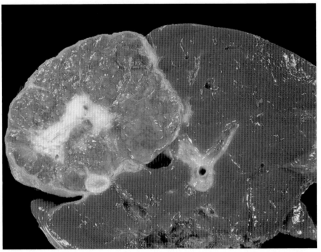

A

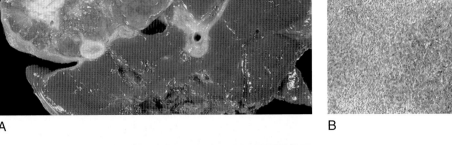

B

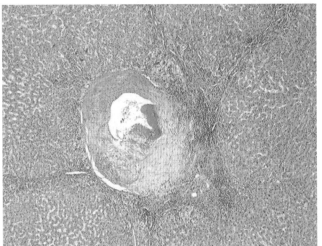

C

Fig. 70.6. A, Macroscopic view of FNH, which is well circumscribed, displays a central fibrous scar that radiates and delineates liver parenchyma nodules. Adjacent liver is normal. **B,** On trichrome staining, fibrous bands spread across the FNH, delineating hepatocellular nodules. Vascular spaces are observed inside the fibrous tissue. **C,** On hematoxylin and eosin staining, in the fibrous bands, large and dystrophic vessels and inflammatory cells are observed (the corresponding image is seen in Fig. 70-10).

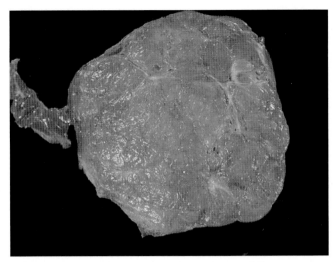

Fig. 70.7. Pedunculated FNH, without macroscopic central fibrous scar.

resulting symptoms. The lesion may be felt when it is pedunculated, and it can be responsible for acute episodes of pain secondary to torsion of the pedicle. It has been proposed that some FNH developing below Glisson's capsule could cause pain (Buetow et al, 1996). In most cases, pain related to FNH is probably due to associated disorders. Complications of FNH, such as rupture or bleeding, are exceptional and usually are related to atypical forms of FNH with specific imaging and biologic features, such as so-called telangiectatic FNH, which should be classified as an adenoma (see later). No malignant transformation of FNH has been reported.

Liver function tests are normal in nearly 80% of cases (Belghiti et al, 1993). Abnormalities include mild elevation of gamma-glutamyltransferase and alkaline phosphatase in patients with large FNH causing extrinsic compression of intrahepatic biliary ducts. Slight elevation of serum transaminase levels could be due to the presence of associated steatosis in the underlying liver parenchyma. Results reflecting the presence of an inflammatory process, including accelerated erythrocyte sedimentation rate and increased fibrinogen level, should lead one to consider the occurrence of the telangiectatic form of FNH.

Imaging

FNH is usually slightly hypoechoic or isoechoic at ultrasound. Some lesions are detected only because they displace the surrounding vessels. Lobulated contours and hypoechoic halo are often observed. The central scar is slightly hyperechoic, but is often difficult to visualize at ultrasound (20% of cases) (Shamsi et al, 1993). Color and power Doppler improve the detection of this lesion. Typical findings on color Doppler include the presence of a central feeding artery with a stellate or spoke-wheel pattern corresponding to the artery running from the central scar to fibrous septa (Fig. 70.8). Doppler spectral analysis shows in most cases an intralesional pulsatile waveform with high diastolic flow and low resistive index (Uggowitzer et al, 1997). Large draining vessels may be identified in the periphery at the tumor margins.

Ultrasound contrast agents and nonlinear continuous imaging modes at low mechanical index seem to be promising tools to characterize FNH better at ultrasound. Most lesions enhance at the very arterial phase (85% and 96%) (Dietrich et al, 2005; Kim et al, 2004), with a central vascular supply and centrifugal filling to the periphery (Fig. 70.9). The lesion becomes homogeneously hyperechoic in the late arterial phase and is slightly hyperechoic or isoechoic in the late portal and sinusoidal phases in most cases (77%) (Kim et al, 2004). The scar appears hypoechoic on arterial and portal phases.

CT examination includes the acquisition of nonenhanced and enhanced images, with the latter performed during the arterial, portal, and delayed phases after administration of intravenous iodinated contrast material injected with a high flow rate. On precontrast CT scans, FNH is shown as a focal hypodense or isodense mass. A central hypodense scar is depicted in only one third of the cases (Shamsi et al, 1993). Calcifications within the central scar are rare and observed in only about 1% of the cases (Caseiro-Alves et al, 1996).

Because of the prominent arterial supply to FNH, the lesion enhances rapidly at the arterial phase of contrast-enhanced CT in most cases (89-100%) (Brancatelli et al, 2001), and the lesion-to-liver contrast is high. Lesion contour is well demarcated and may be lobulated. At that time, the central scar is hypodense and appears more evident than on unenhanced CT scans (60%). Central arteries are detected on multidetector-row helical CT in

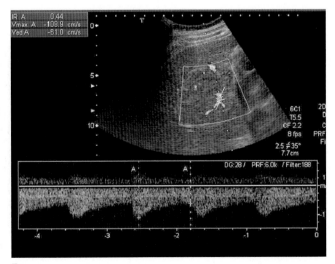

A   B

Fig. 70.8. Ultrasound of a typical FNH. **A,** The lesion is homogeneous and nonencapsulated. **B,** Doppler ultrasound shows central signals of arterial flow.

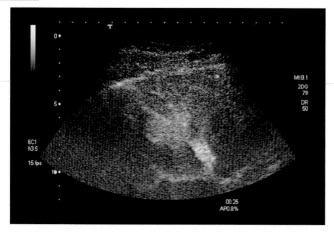

Fig. 70.9. Contrast sonography in FNH shows a rapid and homogeneous enhancement, which slightly persists on delayed phase.

relatively hypoattenuating central scar (Buetow et al, 1996). On delayed images of the liver, FNH is isodense relative to normal liver, and in most cases, central scars appear isoattenuating or hyperattenuating (Carlson et al, 2000). A central scar is observed more often in large lesions than in small lesions. Multiphasic helical CT highlights that mean attenuation values of FNH in the arterial phase are significantly higher than in hepatocellular adenoma (Ruppert-Kohlmayr et al, 2001).

Precontrast MRI sequences include T1-weighted gradient recalled echo (with in-phase and opposed phase images) and T2-weighted fast spin echo or turbo spin echo (TSE) sequences. Postcontrast sequences are performed in the arterial, portal, and delayed phases. Typical FNH is isointense or hypointense on T1-weighted images (94-100%) and isointense or slightly hyperintense on T2-weighted images (94-100%) (Vilgrain et al, 1992). The minimal difference in signal intensity between FNH and the normal liver parenchyma on precontrast MRI sequences is a key finding and is related to the normal hepatocytes within FNH, which are rearranged. The central scar is hypointense on T1-weighted images and strongly hyperintense on T2-weighted images (78-84%) (Mortelé et al, 2000). Another key finding is the lesion homogeneity (96%) apart from the central scar. After administration of gadolinium chelates, the enhancement is similar to that observed on contrast-enhanced

most cases (Choi & Freeny, 1998). At the portal phase of contrast-enhanced CT, lesion enhancement decreases, and the lesion may be isodense or slightly hyperdense relative to normal liver (Fig. 70.10). Small-sized FNH may be barely visible, whereas large FNH is visualized because of deformity in the liver contour, displacement of adjacent vessels, or depiction of a

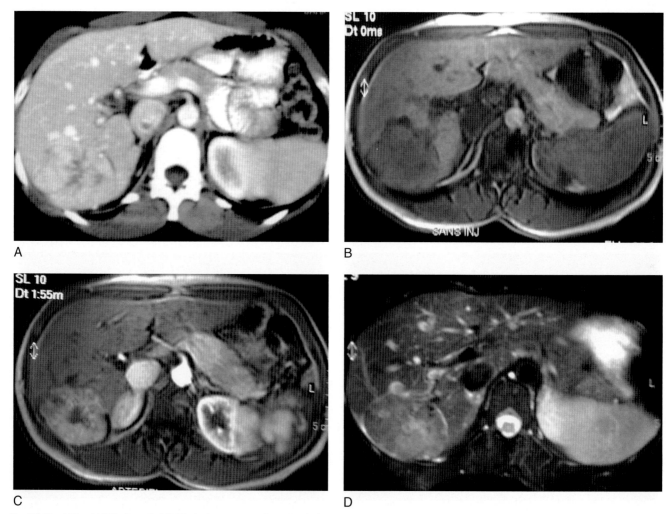

Fig. 70.10. CT and MRI of a typical FNH. **A,** On contrast-enhanced CT, the lesion enhances homogeneously at the arterial phase. **B** and **C,** Pre- and postcontrast gadolinium T1-weighted MRI sequences. MRI shows a homogeneous lesion that enhances strongly after contrast administration. Note that the central scar does not enhance at the arterial phase (**C**). **D,** T2-weighted MRI sequence. The lesion is isointense and contains a hyperintense scar (see corresponding pathologic view in Fig. 70.6).

CT: dramatic enhancement in the arterial phase, followed by isointensity of the lesion during the portal venous phase. On delayed phase imaging, the central scar shows high signal intensity because of the accumulation of contrast material in the fibrous tissue. Images obtained 10 minutes after contrast administration are usually more helpful than images obtained at the equilibrium phase (3-5 minutes postcontrast). Specific contrast media, such as paramagnetic iron oxide–based, manganese-based, or gadolinium-based contrast agents, with hepatobiliary elimination are targeted at the Kupffer cells and the hepatocytes and can be used to highlight the hepatocellular origin of the lesions (Ba-Ssalamah et al, 2002; Grazioli et al, 2005).

Atypical forms of FNH maybe difficult to diagnose. Some FNH may have no scar even at pathology, especially FNH measuring less than 3 cm in diameter (Fig. 70.11). Rarely, scars remain hypodense or isodense on delayed scans or are hypointense on T2-weighted images. Other atypical findings include lesion heterogeneity or hyperintensity on T1-weighted images, which may be caused by various pathologic changes, including fat deposition (mostly in patients with steatosis) (Stanley et al, 2002). Although FNH is a nonencapsulated lesion, capsule-like enhancement may be observed on portal vein and on delayed phase scans or MRI (Choi & Freeny, 1998). This enhancement corresponds to dilated vessels and sinusoids around FNH. Rarely, large FNHs

are responsible for portal vein or hepatic vein compression, and transient alterations in the enhancement of normal liver may be detected. In the latter case, nonvisualization of hepatic veins and development of aberrant small veins may mimic Budd-Chiari syndrome (Rangheard et al, 2002).

Telangiectatic FNH, as described by Wanless and colleagues (1989), differs from classic FNH because arteries have hypertrophied muscular media, but no intimal proliferation, and these abnormal vessels drain directly into the adjacent sinusoids. At imaging, telangiectatic FNH also differs from classic FNH because of the following: heterogeneous pattern, hyperintensity on T1-weighted images, strong hyperintensity on T2-weighted images, absence of central scar in most cases, and persistent lesion enhancement on delayed phase images (Fig. 70.12) (Attal et al, 2003). Molecular studies have shown, however, that telangiectatic FNHs display a molecular pattern closer to that of hepatocellular adenomas than to FNH (Paradis et al, 2004).

Although FNH is mainly a solitary lesion, multiple lesions are observed in 20% to 30% of cases. FNH is associated with hepatic hemangiomata, and in two studies, 20% to 23% of the FNH patients had associated hepatic hemangiomata (Mathieu et al, 1989; Vilgrain et al, 2003). The simultaneous occurrence of FNH and hepatocellular adenoma has been infrequently documented (3.6%). This association could be coincidental

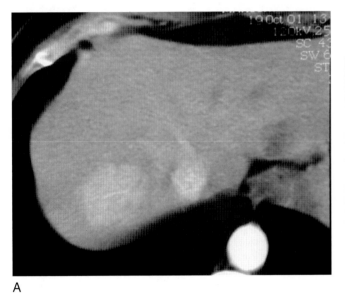

A

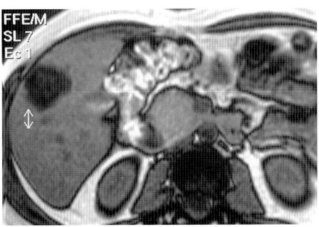

B

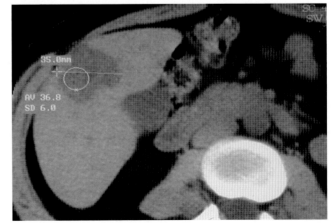

C

Fig. 70.11. Presence of two atypical FNHs in the same patient. **A,** The first lesion at the dome does not contain any scar. **B,** The second lesion adjacent to the gallbladder contains fat well shown by the decrease in signal intensity on opposed phase T1-weighted MRI. **C,** Fat also is evident on precontrast CT.

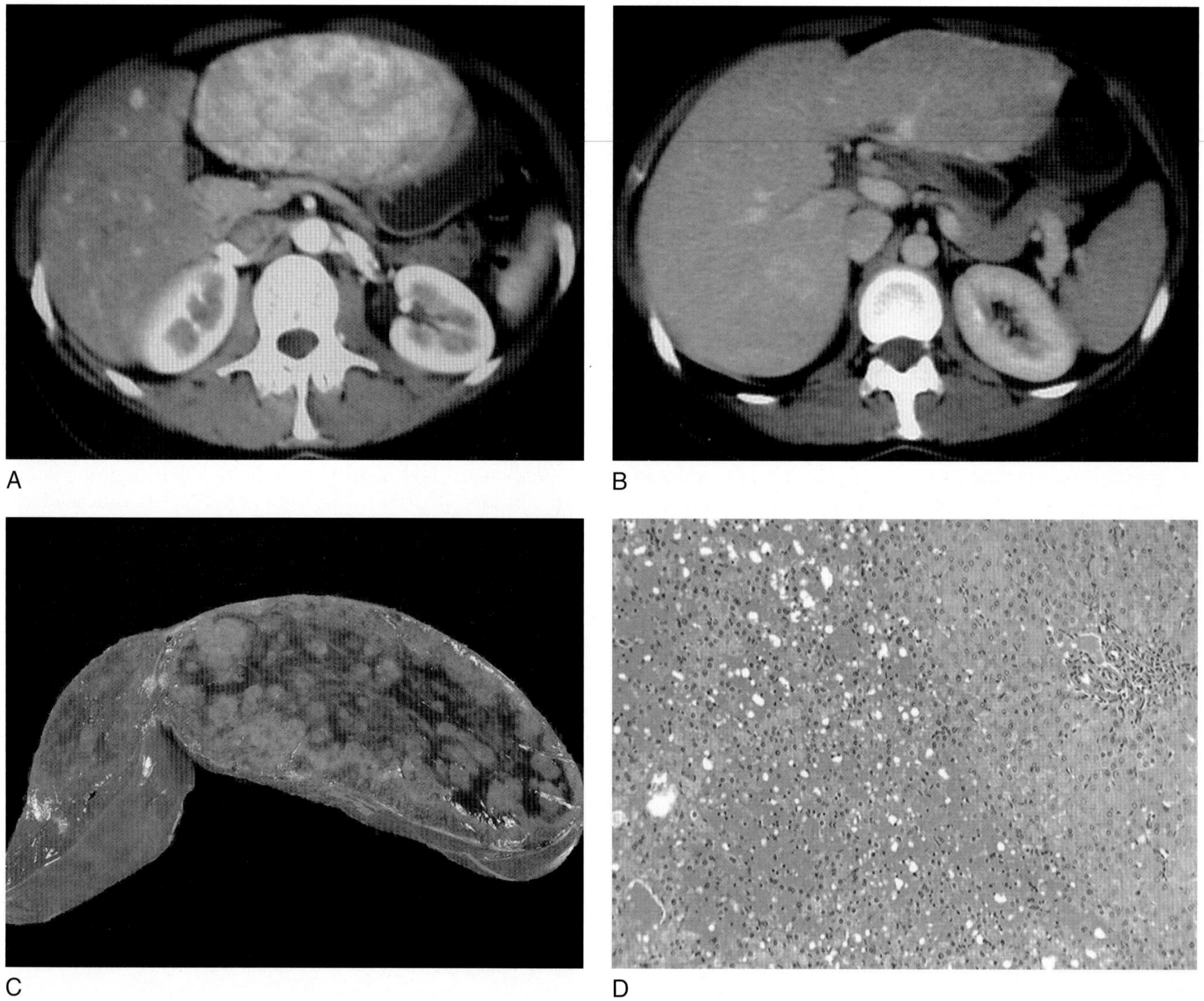

Fig. 70.12. Telangiectatic FNH. **A** and **B,** CT shows a pedunculated lesion with heterogeneous enhancement at the arterial phase **(A),** with absence of washout on delayed phase **(B). C,** Macroscopically, the lesion is well delineated, of heterogeneous color with extensive areas of telangiectasis, giving a pattern of nodularity. No fibrous changes were present. **D,** Histologically, the lesion is composed of liver cells arranged in a trabecular pattern. A few, short fibrous septa containing several small vessels without evident ductular proliferation are observed.

or favored by angiogenic abnormalities, tumor-induced growth factors, or thrombosis and local arteriovenous shunting (Laurent et al, 2003). Association of FNH with fibrolamellar hepatocellular carcinoma is controversial. Some authors consider fibrolamellar carcinoma to be the malignant counterpart of FNH (Vecchio et al, 1984); however, no malignant transformation has been observed. Also, FNH may be associated with other extrahepatic vascular abnormalities (Wanless et al, 1989).

Most studies show that MRI has higher sensitivity (70%) and specificity (98%) for FNH than ultrasound and CT. Accuracy of contrast-enhanced ultrasound cannot be established firmly. The higher sensitivity and specificity of MRI probably is related to the combination of soft tissue characteristics and the vascularity of the lesions. FNH mainly occurs in young adults in whom avoidance of radiation is crucial.

Two points must be stressed: First, the prevalence of typical features of FNH ranges from 22% to 70% and may be explained by variations in the stringency of the criteria used to diagnose FNH and recruitment bias. Second, the diagnosis of FNH is based on a combination of features, and none of them are specific to FNH.

There is a role for liver biopsy in FNH when imaging cannot establish the diagnosis firmly. The contribution of cytology to the diagnosis is poor, in contrast to histology, seen on a biopsy specimen, which may be obtained percutaneously, laparoscopically, or by laparotomy. We have shown that in the absence of radiologic diagnostic criteria in FNH, a histologic diagnosis could be made in most cases (Fabre et al, 2002). Most atypical tumors on imaging were nonclassic forms of FNH at pathology, but using a scoring system incorporating major and minor diagnostic features and concomitant analysis of noninvolved parenchyma, FNH can be recognized on biopsy (Fabre et al, 2002).

Management

Whatever the size and the number of lesions, there is no treatment for asymptomatic FNH when the diagnosis is firmly established. This lesion should be considered as a regenerative procedure rather than a tumor. The occurrence of this lesion in men should not modify the indication of conservative treatment. FNH has no risk of malignant potential, and there is no risk of complication. The patient should be reassured about the absence of complications and the natural history of this lesion, which remains stable in most cases or even could decrease and disappear after 50. Although it has been recommended to discontinue oral contraceptives, it has been shown that neither the size nor the number of FNH lesions is influenced by oral contraceptive use (Mathieu et al, 2000). There is no argument to support interrupting oral contraceptive use or avoiding pregnancy, and follow-up is not justified.

Surgical resection is indicated in doubtful cases or in symptomatic patients. Symptomatic patients with confirmed FNH should be investigated thoroughly to exclude other pathology before attributing symptoms to the liver lesion. In some symptomatic patients with large FNH located in the right liver or in segment I, transarterial embolization has been advocated to determine the relationship between the lesion and symptoms (De Rave & Hussain, 2002; Kehagias et al, 2001). Resection should be considered if it can be performed in specialist hepatobiliary units with no mortality and acceptable morbidity (Belghiti et al, 1993; Landen et al, 1993; Nagorney, 1995; Weimann et al, 1997). The development of a laparoscopic liver approach has increased the number of FNHs resected, without convincing arguments in favor of resection (Cherqui, 2003; Descottes et al, 2003). Resection is indicated in patients with large symptomatic FNH located in the left liver and in patients with pedunculated lesions. Liver resection with a surgical margin may be a safer resection procedure than enucleation because FNH is often surrounded by large veins.

HEPATOCELLULAR ADENOMA

Pathogenesis and Pathology

Hepatocellular adenoma is a rare, benign liver neoplasm that is strongly associated with oral contraceptive use and androgen steroid therapy (Coombes et al, 1978; Nime et al, 1979). Its incidence is estimated to be 0.1 per year per 100,000 in non–oral contraceptive users and 3 to 4 per 100,000 in long-tem oral contraceptive users (Wittekind, 1995). The risk for developing adenoma increases with the duration of oral contraceptive use and with the estrogen content of the oral contraceptive used (Rosenberg, 1991). Hepatocellular adenoma also can occur spontaneously or be associated with underlying metabolic diseases, including type I glycogen storage disease, iron overload related to β-thalassemia, and diabetes mellitus (Barthelemes & Tait, 2005).

Hepatocellular adenoma is usually solitary, sometimes pedunculated, with a diameter that can reach 30 cm. Large subcapsular vessels commonly are found on macroscopic examination. On cut sections, the tumor is well delineated, sometimes encapsulated, with a fleshy appearance ranging in color from white to brown (Fig. 70.13). Adenoma frequently displays heterogeneous areas of necrosis or hemorrhage or both. Histologically, hepatocellular adenoma consists of a proliferation of benign hepatocytes arranged in a trabecular pattern. The normal liver architecture organization is absent. Small thin vessels usually are found throughout the tumor (Fig. 70.14). Hepatocytes may have intracellular fat or increased glycogen. A certain degree of cellular atypia can be detected, especially in patients who have taken steroids for many years. In that context, differential diagnosis with hepatocellular carcinoma may be difficult. Malignant transformation can occur, but is rare (see later) (Gyorffy et al, 1989). After withdrawal of the oral contraceptive, the tumor may regress or rarely enlarge.

Some atypical forms of FNH (i.e., telangiectatic and mixed hyperplastic and adenomatous FNH) should be included in the group regarded as hepatocellular adenomas. More recent studies showed that such lesions are clonal processes and display molecular changes similar to the changes observed in adenomas (Paradis et al, 2004). Macroscopically, telangiectatic FNH is well delineated and unencapsulated and shows significant areas of vascular changes, without any fibrous scar (see Fig. 70.12). They initially were described by Wanless and colleagues (1989) as multiple nodules and were labeled *multiple FNH syndrome*. Similar to adenomas, they occur in women taking oral contraceptives. Microscopic examination of these lesions shows transitional morphologic features between adenoma and FNH. In all cases, there is no central fibrous scar. Few and short fibrous septa containing several small vessels without evident ductular proliferation are observed throughout the telangiectatic form of FNH, which

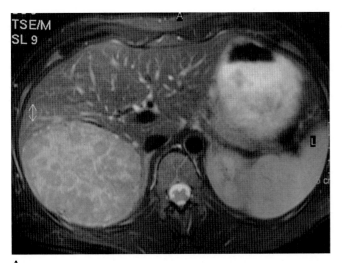

A

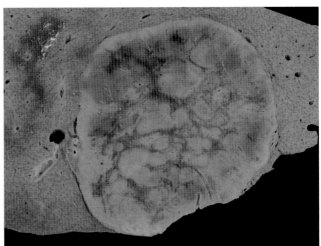

B

Fig. 70.13. Hepatocellular adenoma. **A,** T2-weighted MRI shows a large, heterogeneous lesion in the right liver with strong hyperintensity. **B,** Macroscopically, the lesion is well delineated, unencapsulated, and tan to yellow with some vascular changes.

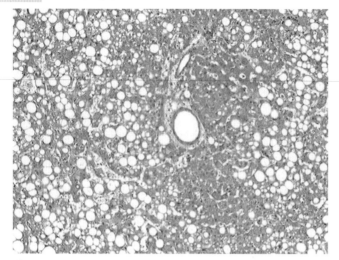

Fig. 70.14. Histologic aspect of adenoma shows a cellular proliferation of well-differentiated hepatocytes with steatotic changes. Throughout the lesion, small isolated arteries with thin walls are observed.

display significant vascular changes of telangiectatic type (Wanless et al, 1989). The hyperplastic and adenomatous form of FNH is characterized histologically by two alternating aspects: one resembling telangiectatic type, the other simulating adenoma. Taken together, these forms represent less than 20% of atypical FNH in large surgical series (Nguyen et al, 1999). Both lesions are now recognized as variant forms of hepatocellular adenomas and may be managed as adenomas. Based on more recent molecular studies, it seems that an upgraded classification of benign liver epithelial cells is required for pathologists, radiologists, and clinicians to enable correct management of such lesions.

Clinical and Biologic Data

Although patients with adenoma are more likely to present with symptoms, most patients, especially if they have small tumors, are asymptomatic (Trotter & Everson, 2001; Weimann et al, 2000). Tumors are discovered during diagnostic workup of elevated liver enzymes and during liver ultrasound monitoring of pregnancy or for other reasons. Large adenomas may cause a sensation of right upper quadrant fullness or discomfort. Adenoma is clinically important because of its tendency to bleed spontaneously, resulting in hemorrhage and infarction in the tumor. A review of series of adenomas shows that the risk of spontaneous bleeding is 20% to 40% (Barthelemes & Tait, 2005). The risk of bleeding is increased in women taking oral contraceptives, during pregnancy, and when tumors are greater than 5 cm in diameter (Terkivatan et al, 2000, 2001b). About 10% of patients present acutely with severe abdominal pain secondary to intraperitoneal rupture and hemoperitoneum, which may be associated with hypovolemic shock. Hemorrhage results in acute pain and discomfort accompanied by anorexia, nausea, vomiting, and fever. Although tumor rupture with hemoperitoneum is an alarming manifestation, hemodynamic instability is rare except in patients treated with anticoagulation (Marini et al, 2002). The risk of malignant transformation of adenoma is 10% (Barthelemes & Tait, 2005). This risk is higher in men and in patients with large adenoma. Most cases of hepatocellular carcinoma develop at the site of liver cell adenoma, and malignancy is discovered on the analysis of the surgical specimen (Barthelemes & Tait, 2005).

Liver function tests are normal in patients with small adenomas, whereas in patients with large tumors, gamma-glutamyltransferase and alkaline phosphatase levels usually are elevated (Belghiti et al, 1993). In the absence of malignancy, serum α-fetoprotein is normal.

Imaging

At ultrasound, hepatocellular adenoma usually is seen as a well-delineated heterogeneous hepatic mass. The hyperechogenicity of hepatocellular adenoma is attributed to the presence of fat and glycogen. Anechoic or hypoechoic areas correspond to hemorrhagic foci and necrosis. Doppler studies show no intratumoral signal in half of cases, mainly owing to massive fat deposit or hemorrhagic or necrotic changes. In the other cases, various patterns of Doppler signals may be observed located at the center or at the periphery of the lesions (Golli et al, 1994). Ultrasound contrast media show in noncomplicated adenomas intense enhancement during the arterial phase, whereas the lesion becomes isoechoic or slightly hypoechoic during the portal and delayed phases. On nonenhanced CT, hepatocellular adenomas are predominantly isodense, but may appear hypodense or heterogeneous (especially in lesions >4 cm). In rare instances, areas of hyperdensities are seen and are due to intratumoral hemorrhage (Fig. 70.15). On contrast-enhanced CT scans, the lesions are mostly hypervascular and heterogeneous on the arterial phase and become isodense or hypodense on the portal phase as a result of arteriovenous shunting. Distinctive findings between FNH and hepatocellular adenoma are the smooth surface (95%), the presence of necrosis or hemorrhage (25%), and the tumor capsule (25%) (Ichikawa et al, 2000).

Because of its higher sensitivity for fat and hemorrhage, MRI is one of the best methods for characterization of hepatocellular adenoma. On MRI, hepatocellular adenoma appears hyperintense or isointense on T1-weighted images and mildly hyperintense on T2-weighted images (see Fig. 70.13). Hyperintensity on T1-weighted images (present in >50% of cases) can be attributed to the fatty content of the lesion, hemorrhagic necrosis, and frequent marked sinusoidal dilation or peliosis. The presence of a fatty component can be assessed by fat-suppressed or in-phase and opposed phase imaging (Fig. 70.16). Heterogeneity of signal intensity has been considered one of the most constant features of hepatocellular adenoma as a result of the wide range of pathologic changes that can occur within the lesion, observed in more than 50% of the MRI series. Hepatocellular adenoma also shows variable features in regard to vascularity on dynamic gadolinium-enhanced MRI, but is in most cases hypervascular in the arterial phase. Tumor heterogeneity, peripheral capsule, or hyperintensity on T1-weighted images was shown in 90% of patients and in 88% of hepatic adenomas (Arrivé et al, 1994). Using these criteria, definite differentiation between hepatocellular adenoma and FNH is possible in most patients, whereas it is less evident with hepatocellular carcinoma.

Treatment

Prevention of bleeding or malignant transformation or both is guaranteed with surgical resection. Small lesions (<3 cm in diameter) that have a low risk of complication initially could be observed after cessation of oral contraceptive use and avoidance

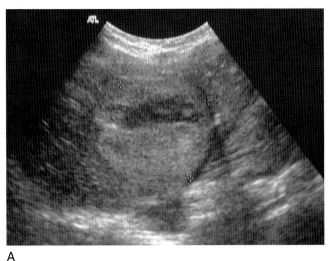

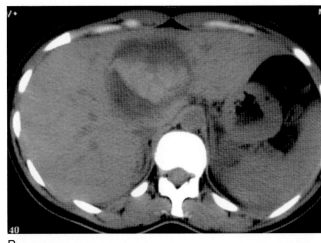

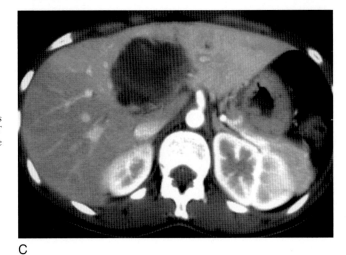

Fig. 70.15. Hemorrhagic hepatocellular adenoma. **A** and **B,** The lesion is heterogeneous on ultrasound (**A**) and precontrast CT (**B**). **C,** Arterial phase CT shows lack of lesion hypervascularity, which is related to the hemmorhage. The hyperdensity on precontrast CT reflects the hemorrhage.

of pregnancy (Terkivatan et al, 2001a). Many studies have shown regression and complete resolution of adenomas after cessation of oral contraceptive use (Andersen & Packer, 1976; Aseni et al, 2001; Bühler et al, 1982; Steinbrecher et al, 1981). Other authors have not noted any changes, however, after discontinuation of oral contraceptive use (Marks et al, 1988). *In patients with adenomas greater than 4 cm in diameter, surgical resection is indicated.* The operative approach should be tailored to the location and the size of the tumor. In most cases, anatomic or segmental resection is the best option (Nagorney, 1995; Weimann et al, 1997). Although there is a risk of malignancy within the tumor, there is no need for a large resection margin, allowing complete resection through a laparoscopic approach (Descottes et al, 2003).

Many authors consider ruptured adenoma a life-threatening situation justifying emergency resection (Flowers et al, 1990; Iwatsuki et al, 1990). This strategy resulted in a mortality of 8%, however (Rooks et al, 1979; Shortell & Schwartz, 1991). The extent of resection and operative risk can be reduced by delaying surgery for several months (Marini et al, 2002; Terkivatan et al, 2001b). After stabilization of the patient and selective hepatic artery embolization, the tumor size decreases. The absorption of the hematoma surrounding the tumor allows an easier elective resection with a low risk of transfusion (Marini et al, 2002). The risk of malignancy in the area of the tumor leads us to consider liver resection even if the tumor is not visible on imaging.

This conservative management includes stopping oral contraceptive use. Although recurrence of solitary adenoma has not been reported after resection, discontinuation of oral contraceptive use is still recommended to the patient (Barthelemes & Tait, 2005). Pregnancy should be followed by sequential ultrasound liver examination.

Multiple Adenomas and Adenomatosis

Review of the literature on patients with multiple adenomas, including adenomatosis, does not support an arbitrary classification based on clinical and imaging characteristics (Fig. 70.17) (Barthelemes & Tait, 2005; Jovine et al, 2004; Ribeiro et al, 1998). Patients with multiple adenomas are predominantly women, and oral contraceptive use was present in more than 80% of cases (Barthelemes & Tait, 2005). Patients with glycogen storage disease type I are at risk of developing multiple adenomas (see Fig. 70.17) (Labrune et al, 1997). The risk of bleeding, which is similar to that in patients with solitary adenoma, is present only in tumors larger than 4 cm in diameter (Barthelemes & Tait, 2005; Ribeiro et al, 1998). The risk of malignant transformation is approximately 10%, similar to that in patients with solitary adenoma (Barthelemes & Tait, 2005). Although the risk of malignant transformation is particularly high in large tumors,

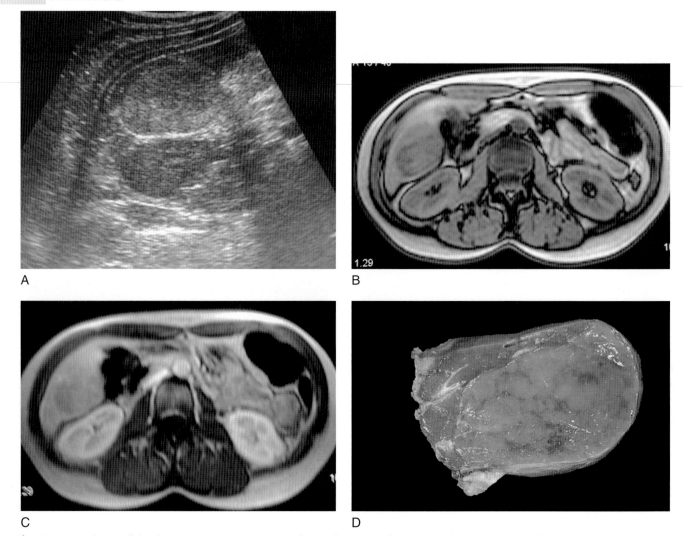

Fig. 70.16. Fatty hepatocellular adenoma. **A,** Hyperechogenicity on ultrasound. **B,** Opposed phase T1-weighted MRI sequence shows a strong hypointensity and a drop in signal intensity compared with in phase imaging. **D,** Macroscopically, the lesion is yellow with shiny and hemorrhagic areas. No necrosis is noted.

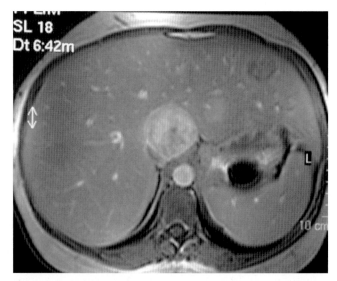

Fig. 70.17. Multiple adenomas. Postgadolinium T1-weighted MRI shows three lesions on the same slice (one in the caudate lobe and two in the left lobe) with different signal intensity and enhancement.

there are some observations of multiple degenerated tumors in the same patient (Chiche et al, 2000).

Except for the number of lesions, no difference is observed between imaging features of adenomatosis and solitary adenomas. We have shown that there are three different MRI patterns of liver adenomatosis that correlate to three different pathologic forms: the steatotic form, the peliotic form (Fig. 70.18), and the mixed form (Lewin et al, 2005). Whether these different types could be associated with specific genetic profiles needs to be shown. The search for genetic alterations in hepatocellular adenomas is promising. A high risk of malignancy potentially associated with β-catenin activation and the absence of hepatocyte nuclear factor 1 (HNF 1) and β-catenin mutations associated with a high risk of bleeding could be suggested. Currently, the management of patients with multiple adenomas is based on the size and number of tumors.

Taking into account the risk of bleeding and malignant transformation, the management of these patients, in whom surgical excision of all the tumors is often impossible, is challenging. Because the risk of complication (including malignancy) is related to the tumor size, resection of all adenomas (≥5 cm) should be performed. In some patients with large bilobar tumors, resection could be performed in two steps. Tumors located in one lobe are

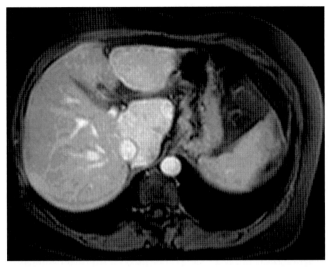

Fig. 70.18. Presence of two peliotic forms of adenoma (caudate and left lobes).

resected during a first procedure followed some weeks later by a second procedure resecting tumors located in the remnant liver. There is no need to resect small tumors. After resection of large tumors, patients should be observed with a close imaging follow-up and serum α-fetoprotein measurement to document the volume and number stability of remaining small adenomas (Ribeiro et al, 1998). With this conservative approach and long-term follow-up of small lesions, we showed that the rate of tumor growth was less than 10%, whereas tumors decreased in size or disappeared in approximately 5% of cases (Belghiti et al, 2005). Although some of our patients with remaining small adenomas experienced pregnancy without changes in tumor size, discontinuation of oral contraceptive use is recommended.

Liver transplantation is not indicated to prevent bleeding or cancer and is unwarranted in benign conditions given the good outcome with surgical resection of large tumors (Ribeiro et al, 1998). In patients with malignancy located in only one tumor, resection is a safe and efficient option, whereas in patients with multiple and disseminated malignancies, liver transplantation is followed by rapid recurrence (Belghiti et al, 2005). A specific and aggressive treatment, including liver transplantation, is not justified in patients with multiple adenomas.

OTHER LESIONS

Fatty Lesions of the Liver

Angiomyolipoma

Hepatic angiomyolipoma is a rare fatty tumor, composed of varying portions of fat, epithelioid and spindled smooth cells, and thick-walled blood vessels. It occurs frequently in the kidney and rarely in the liver. This rare tumor may occur as a solitary mass or as an associated finding with tuberous sclerosis (Hooper et al, 1994). These lesions predominantly affect women at any age, are often larger than 5 cm in diameter, and are well circumscribed and red to yellow (Hoffman et al, 1997). No malignant transformation has been reported. Patients usually have no symptoms, and most of these tumors are found incidentally on routine ultrasound studies. Liver tests are normal. The accuracy of preoperative diagnosis is low as a result of variable imaging appearances

owing to the varying content of the three components and the rarity of the lesion. The fat component of angiomyolipoma varies from 10% to 90% (Hooper et al, 1994).

Typically, angiomyolipoma appears hyperechoic, hypodense on unenhanced CT scans, and markedly enhanced on the arterial phase with central vascular opacification (Fig. 70.19). The presence of large central vessels within the lesions (so-called macroaneurysms) is characteristic of angiomyolipoma. MRI also is an important diagnostic technique that allows fat suppression and multiphase dynamic contrast-enhanced scanning. MRI generally shows a marked hypersignal in T1-weighted images suppressible in fat-saturated sequences. The lesions have various imaging characteristics because of the different proportions of smooth muscle, fat, and vessels (Yan et al, 2002). The amount of fat may be too small to be detected, and some angiomyolipomas may mimic hepatocellular lesions (Arblade et al, 1996). The accuracy of needle biopsy can be reinforced by using HMB-45 reactivity, which labels the epithelioid cell component (Arblade et al, 1996). When the diagnosis is established, careful observation with serial follow-up is recommended in asymptomatic patients (Hoffman et al, 1997; Sawai et al, 1998).

Lipoma

Hepatic lipomas are rarer than angiomyolipomas and can occur sporadically. They are homogeneous and circumscribed, show fat attenuation on CT, and do not enhance after intravenous administration of contrast material. On MRI, lipomas are hyperintense on T1-weighted images and moderately hyperintense on T2-weighted images. The key finding is the decrease in signal intensity on fat-suppressed or opposed phase MRI sequences (Horton et al, 1999). Microscopic analysis shows well-differentiated adipose tissue without any significant changes. There is no need to resect lipoma.

Bile Duct Adenoma

Bile duct adenoma, also called *benign cholangioma,* is a benign, asymptomatic mass that typically is discovered incidentally at imaging studies, surgery, or autopsy. This rare benign lesion of the liver is usually a well-circumscribed, subcapsular nodule

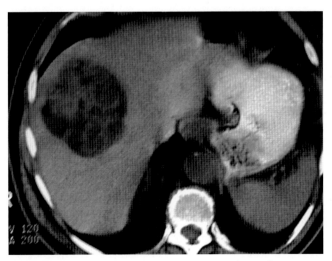

Fig. 70.19. Typical angiomyolipoma. Precontrast CT shows a heterogeneous lesion that contains fat.

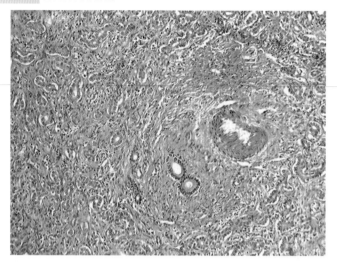

Fig. 70.20. Bile duct adenoma is a proliferation of noncystic biliary structures, lined by a cuboidal epithelium, within a dense fibrous stroma. A portal tract is included in the lesion.

with a diameter of less than 1 cm consisting of the proliferation of noncystic biliary structures within a dense fibrous stroma (Fig. 70.20) (Allaire et al, 1988). No relationship between this tumor and cholangiocarcinoma has been shown. Its only clinical significance lies in the possible confusion with biliary hamartoma.

Biliary Hamartoma

Biliary hamartoma, also known as the Von Meyenburg complex, is a developmental anomaly of small intrahepatic bile ducts and composed of bile ductules, inflammatory cells, and fibrosis (Fig. 70.21; see Table 70.1) (Neri et al, 2004). The main practical problem raised by this tumor is for the pathologist because its possible discovery during surgery for carcinoma of another abdominal organ leads the surgeon to perform a biopsy for frozen-section diagnosis. A pathologist who is unaware of this

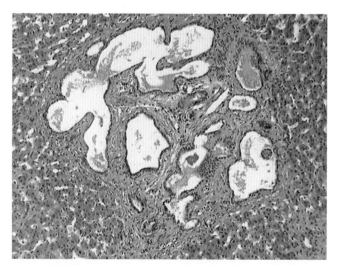

Fig. 70.21. Biliary hamartoma (Von Meyenburg complex) comprises bile ductules of various size and shape having dilated lumina, surrounded by fibrous tissue and some inflammatory cells.

rare entity may be puzzled and tempted to call the lesion metastatic carcinoma. Treatment is not required.

Inflammatory Pseudotumors

Inflammatory pseudotumor is a rare benign tumor commonly found in the lung that can mimic a malignant tumor in the liver. Inflammatory pseudotumors of the liver (IPL) also are referred to as inflammatory myofibroblastic tumors. They are three times more common in men than in women, are more frequently seen in the non-European population, and have an average age of presentation of 35 years (Koea et al, 2003). Most of these lesions are located near the gallbladder or related to the biliary tree, sometimes mimicking a malignant biliary stricture (Koea et al, 2003; Locke et al, 2005). Patients with IPL typically present with vague constitutional symptoms, such as fever, abdominal pain, and weight loss (Zamir et al, 1998). The predominantly inflammatory pattern of pathology and the associated systemic reaction suggest an underlying infectious agent (Koea et al, 2003). Hematologic tests are generally normal or show an acute-phase response with elevated white blood cell count, usually neutrophilia, and elevated platelet count. Liver function tests are abnormal, with elevations in alkaline phosphatase and gamma-glutamyltransferase being the most commonly seen abnormalities. Imaging studies often show large tumors that are diffuse and infiltrative. Two different patterns are described: (1) a well-limited pattern appearing as a hypodense nonenhancing lesion on CT and hyperintense on T2-weighted images, surrounded by a thick capsule and resembling a solitary necrotic tumor of the liver and (2) a more aggressive pattern with an ill-demarcated lesion mimicking cholangiocarcinoma (Fig. 70.22) (Chirica et al, 2005). Portal vein occlusion within the lesion has been reported. A biopsy is often necessary to differentiate IPL from other tumors.

On gross sections, IPL is tan and usually unencapsulated and may show indistinct borders with the surrounding parenchyma. Histologic examination reveals myofibroblasts, polyclonal plasma cells, and fibrous tissue. The pathogenesis of this lesion is still debated. In the tumoral hypothesis, authors suggest that some IPL may be of follicular dendritic cell origin (Shek et al, 1998). Differentiating IPL from malignant liver tumors has assumed greater importance since the 1990s because hepatic surgery has become safer, and a more aggressive approach toward hepatic resection has been adopted. This change has resulted in some investigators advocating hepatic resection for IPL because of the possible destructive nature of IPL or its malignant potential (Li et al, 1989). IPL are benign lesions, however, with no malignant potential, and numerous reports suggest that the natural history of these lesions is complete resolution (Koea et al, 2003). It also has been suggested that steroid administration accelerates resolution of IPL (Maze et al, 1999). IPL can be managed safely nonoperatively.

Peliosis

Peliosis is characterized by multiple blood-filled pools of various sizes in liver parenchyma without lobular systematization. Secondary changes, including fibrosis, may occur secondarily. Peliosis is observed mostly in users of androgenic-anabolic steroids or other drugs and in association with several pathologic diseases, such as severe tuberculosis and malignancies. Imaging findings often mimic true tumors because they are well limited and

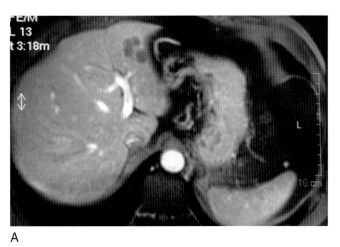

A

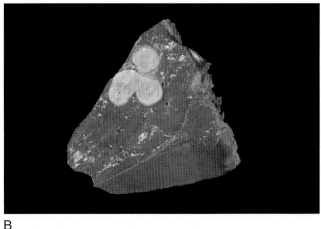

B

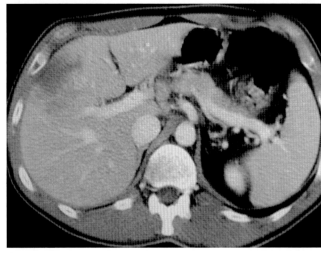

C

Fig. 70.22. Inflammatory pseudotumor of the liver. **A,** Solid and necrotic appearance on postgadolinium T1-weighted MRI sequence. **B,** Macroscopic analysis shows a subcapsular, well-limited, trefoil-shaped, white lesion corresponding to necrosis. A thin fibrous capsule is observed at the border of the lesion. **C,** Aggressive pattern mimicking cholangiocarcinoma on CT.

strongly hyperintense on T2-weighted MRI and enhance at the arterial phase on CT or MRI. The persistent contrast uptake within the lesion is due to the blood-pooled condition (Verswijvel et al, 2003). Treatment should include withdrawal of the possible causative agents and specific treatment (e.g., antibiotics) in patients with either primary or secondary infections.

Focal Fatty Changes

Hepatic steatosis is generally a diffuse process. An uneven and focal distribution of fat is quite common in the liver and may manifest as fatty sparing and focal fatty change (Wanless, 2002). Although the pathogenesis is not well understood, regional hypoxia of hepatic tissue is thought to play a role (Zeppa et al, 2002). Most patients have underlying disease, such as diabetes, obesity, hepatitis C, or malnutrition. Lesions often are discovered incidentally on imaging studies. Characteristically, focal fatty sparing is seen in the posterior aspect of segment IV, appearing hypoechoic relative to the fatty liver, hyperdense on precontrast and postcontrast CT, and hypointense on T1-weighted MRI. Conversely, focal fatty changes are predominantly seen adjacent to the falciform ligament (Itai & Saida, 2002). Imaging findings are related to their fatty content: hyperechoic, hypodense on CT and hyperintense on T1-weighted MRI. Rarely, focal fatty changes

are multiple, so-called pseudotumoral steatosis. Showing the fatty component by MRI is crucial; however, some of these tumor-like lesions may be mistaken for other hepatic tumors, and liver biopsy may be required for definitive diagnosis (Zeppa et al, 2002).

Heterotopic Tissue

The presence of heterotopic tissue within the liver has been described occasionally, and diagnosis usually is established after surgical excision. Adrenal rest tumors usually are located subcapsularly and may be difficult to distinguish histologically from liver cell adenoma (Edmonson, 1958). Pancreatic heterotopia has been reported, and a metaplastic origin of the pancreatic tissue from the intrahepatic biliary epithelium has been suggested (Suzuki et al, 1999). Splenic ectopia should be considered in the differential diagnosis of hepatic lesions detected postsplenectomy (Davidson & Reid, 1997). Splenosis is the autotransplantation of splenic tissue, most commonly seen after traumatic splenic rupture and splenectomy. Splenosis is a rare asymptomatic lesion, indistinguishable from a liver tumor by standard preoperative evaluation, and could be misinterpreted as hepatocellular carcinoma or breast metastatic disease (D'Angelica et al, 1998; Foroudi et al, 1999). Nuclear medicine is highly specific for the diagnosis of splenosis.

REGENERATIVE PROCESS

Nodular Regenerative Hyperplasia

Nodular regenerative hyperplasia (NRH) is a relatively rare, benign diffuse micronodular transformation of the liver that has been referred to by many names in the literature, including *nodular transformation, noncirrhotic nodulation,* and *partial nodular transformation.* It is a distinct disease entity characterized by diffuse involvement of the liver with nodules composed of hyperplastic hepatocytes. NRH should not be confused with the regenerative nodules of cirrhosis or FNH (Federle & Brancatelli, 2001).

NRH is often an incidental finding at laparotomy and is found in approximately 3% of livers at autopsy (Craig et al, 1989; Wanless, 1990). It appears as pale, bulging nodules, mostly less than 1.5 cm in diameter (Trotter & Everson, 2001). Histologic examination reveals the regeneration of hepatocytes with multinucleated hepatocytes and thickened regenerating hepatocytes with centrilobular atrophy. These regenerating nodules also compress the central veins curvilinearly, and there is a lack of fibrotic reaction. NRH and hepatocellular adenoma share a similar benign process and histologic elements and are difficult to distinguish from each other based on a single-needle biopsy. Multiple biopsy specimens are often helpful because NRH is a diffuse or multinodular process, whereas hepatic adenoma is a solitary process in which the remainder of the liver is normal (Mortelé & Ros, 2002).

The pathogenesis of NRH is not well known. One proposed theory hypothesizes that a primary vascular process leads to obliteration of portal vein, which induces ischemia, atrophy of hepatocytes in the central zone, and proliferation of hepatocytes (Al-Mukhaizeem et al, 2004). The other theory proposes that a preneoplastic process leads to NRH based on the reported high prevalence of hepatocyte dysplasia (20-42%) and hepatocellular carcinoma formed in livers of patients with NRH (Dogan et al, 2003). The prevalence of NRH was reported to be around 2% (Biecker et al, 2003). NRH mostly affects patients older than age 50 years, and the gender distribution of NRH varies. A wide spectrum of systemic diseases and drugs also is associated with NRH. Examples include myeloproliferative disorders, lymphoproliferative disorders, chronic vascular disorders, rheumatologic and collagen vascular diseases (rheumatoid arthritis, Felty's syndrome, polyarteritis nodosa, amyloidosis, and primary biliary cirrhosis), solid organ transplantation (renal and liver transplantation), and use of steroids or chemotherapeutic agents (Mortelé & Ros, 2002). This disease also often is associated with hepatoportal sclerosis.

Clinically, NRH usually causes no symptoms and is discovered incidentally during imaging studies or surgery. Some patients present mainly with symptoms of portal hypertension, such as hepatomegaly, splenomegaly, ascites, or esophageal varices, owing to the compression of the main portal vein at the hepatic hilum. Other cholestatic symptoms also can occur (Arvanitaki & Adler, 2001). Mild and nonspecific elevated liver function tests may be seen. Rarely, hepatic failure, rupture of the liver, or malignant transformation can occur (Dogan et al, 2003). Because of these clinical features, the diagnosis of NRH should be considered in patients with clinical signs of portal hypertension and normal or mildly abnormal liver function tests, in whom other causes of portal hypertension have been excluded.

Imaging findings are nonspecific, and histologic examination is often warranted. In most cases, imaging shows normal hepatic parenchyma. In rare cases, NRH has a pseudotumoral appearance as well-delineated hypoechoic or isoechoic nodules at ultrasound, hypoattenuating nodules on CT with variable enhancement, hyperintense lesions on T1-weighted MRI, and isointense or hypointense to normal liver on T2-weighted MRI (Casillas et al, 1997; Clouet et al, 1999; Horita et al, 2002; Mortelé & Ros, 2002). Accurate diagnosis should be confirmed with histologic examination before treatment. In highly suspicious cases, open biopsy is indicated to obtain an adequate sample of hepatic tissue because percutaneous needle biopsies may give false negative results (Biecker et al, 2003). Management depends on the clinical symptoms. In asymptomatic patients, no treatment is recommended except for periodic follow-up to monitor for development of hepatocellular carcinoma, although this is rare. In patients with complications of portal hypertension, appropriate management, including drug therapy, endoscopic therapy, or portacaval shunt, is necessary (Biecker et al, 2003). Rarely, patients may progress to liver failure and finally require liver transplantation (Trotter & Everson, 2001).

Focal Nodular Hyperplasia–Like Lesions

FNH-like lesions are lesions that histopathologically resemble FNH, but are seen in patients with liver disease or liver vessel abnormalities. The most common causes of liver diseases responsible for FNH-like lesion development are Budd-Chiari syndrome, hereditary hemorrhagic telangiectasia, and congenital hepatic fibrosis (Buscarini et al, 2004; Vilgrain et al, 1999; Zeitoun et al, 2004). All of these diseases induce severe liver flow alterations with decreased portal vein blood flow and markedly increased hepatic artery blood flow. FNH-like lesions may be a hepatic response to increased arterial inflow. Similarly, FNH-like lesions have been reported in patients with portal vein thrombosis (Bureau et al, 2004); imaging findings of FNH-like lesions are similar to FNHs arising in normal liver, and they may contain a central scar. Because the liver signal is abnormal in Budd-Chiari syndrome the FNH-like lesions are mostly hyperintense on T1-weighted MRI and hypointense on T2-weighted MRI. However, they still enhance strongly at the arterial phase. In contrast to FNH, FNH-like lesions may become more numerous and grow over time.

REFERENCES

About I, et al, 1994: Hémangiome hépatique géant non résécable et syndrome de Kasabach-Merritt. Rev Med Interne 15:846-850.

Allaire GS, et al, 1988: Bile duct adenoma: a study of 152 cases. Am J Surg Pathol 12:708-715.

Al-Mukhaizeem KA, et al, 2004: Nodular regenerative hyperplasia of the liver: an under-recognized cause of portal hypertension in hematological disorders. Am J Hematol 75:225-230.

Andersen PH, Packer JT, 1976: Hepatic adenoma—observations after estrogen withdrawal. Arch Surg 111:898-900.

Arblade S, et al, 1996: Angiomyolipome hépatique simulant une tumeur hépatocytaire. Gastroenterol Clin Biol 20:1022-1026.

Arrivé L, et al, 1994: Hepatic adenoma: MR findings in 51 pathologically proved lesions. Radiology 193:507-512.

Arvanitaki M, Adler M, 2001: Nodular regenerative hyperplasia of the liver: a review of 14 cases. Hepatogastroenterology 48:1425-1429.

Aseni P, et al, 2001: Rapid disappearance of hepatic adenoma after contraceptive withdrawal. J Clin Gastroenterol 33:234-236.

Attal P, et al, 2003: Telangiectatic focal nodular hyperplasia: US, CT, and MR imaging findings with histopathologic correlation in 13 cases. Radiology 228:465-472.

Barthelemes L, Tait IS, 2005: Liver cell adenomas and liver cell adenomatosis. HPB Surg 7:186-196.

Ba-Ssalamah A, et al, 2002: Atypical focal nodular hyperplasia of the liver: imaging features of nonspecific and liver-specific MR contrast agents. AJR Am J Roentgenol 179:1447-1456.

Belghiti J, et al, 1993: Resection of presumed benign liver tumours. Br J Surg 80:380-383.

Belghiti J, et al, 2005: Specific management for multiple liver cell adenoma: is it justified? Hepatology 42(suppl 1):296A.

Biecker E, et al, 2003: Benign hepatic tumours. Z Gastroenterol 41:191-200.

Bioulac-Sage P, et al, 2005: Clinical morphologic, and molecular features defining so-called telangiectatic focal nodular hyperplasias of the liver. Gastroenterology 128:1211-1218.

Birnbaum BA, et al, 1990: Definitive diagnosis of hepatic hemangiomas: MR vs Tc-99m labeled red blood cell SPECT. Radiology 176:95-105.

Bornman PC, et al, 1987: Giant hepatic hemangiomas: diagnostic and therapeutic dilemmas. Surgery 101:445-449.

Brancatelli G, et al, 2001: Focal nodular hyperplasia: CT findings with emphasis on multiphasic helical CT in 78 patients. Radiology 219:61-68.

Browers MAM, et al, 1997: Surgical treatment of giant haemangioma of the liver. Br J Surg 84:314-316.

Buetow PC, et al, 1996: Focal nodular hyperplasia of the liver: radiologic-pathologic correlation. Radiographics 16:369-388.

Bühler H, et al, 1982: Regression of liver cell adenoma: a follow up study of three consecutive patients after discontinuation of oral contraceptive use. Gastroenterology 82:775-782.

Bureau C, et al, 2004: Liver nodules ressembling focal nodular hyperplasia after portal vein thrombosis. J Hepatology 41:499-500.

Buscarini E, et al, 2004: High prevalence of hepatic focal nodular hyperplasia in subjects with hereditary hemorrhagic telangiectasia. Ultrasound Med Biol 30:1089-1097.

Caldironi MW, et al, 1998: Echo-guided fine-needle biopsy for the diagnosis of hepatic angioma: a report on 114 cases. Minerva Chir 53:505-509.

Carlson SK, et al, 2000: CT of focal nodular hyperplasia of the liver. AJR Am J Roentgenol 174:705-712.

Caseiro-Alves F, et al, 1996: Calcification in focal nodular hyperplasia: a new problem for differentiation from fibrolamellar hepatocellular carcinoma. Radiology 198:889-892.

Casillas C, et al, 1997: Pseudotumoral presentation of nodular regenerative hyperplasia of the liver: imaging in five patients including MR imaging. Eur Radiol 7:654-658.

Cherqui D, 2003: Laparoscopic liver resection. Br J Surg 90:644-646.

Chiche L, et al, 2000: Liver adenomatosis: reappraisal, diagnosis and surgical management: eight new cases and review of the literature. Ann Surg 231:74-81.

Chirica M, et al, 2005: Major hepatectomy for peripheral papillary cholangiocarcinoma with hilar extension in a patient with situs ambiguous. Gastroenterol Clin Biol 29:456-460.

Choi CS, Freeny PC, 1998: Triphasic helical CT of hepatic focal nodular hyperplasia: incidence of atypical findings. AJR Am J Roentgenol 170:391-395.

Clouet M, et al, 1999: Imaging features of nodular regenerative hyperplasia of the liver mimicking hepatic metastases. Abdom Imaging 24:258-261.

Cobey FC, Salem RR, 2004: A review of liver masses in pregnancy and a proposed algorithm for their diagnosis and management. Am J Surg 187:181-191.

Coombes GB, et al, 1978: An androgen-associated hepatic adenoma in a trans-sexual. Br J Surg 65:869-870.

Corigliano N, et al, 2003: Hemoperitoneum from a spontaneous rupture of a giant hemangioma of the liver: report of a case. Surg Today 33:459-463.

Coumbaras M, et al, 2002: CT and MR imaging features of pathologically proven atypical giant hemangioma of the liver. AJR Am J Roentgenol 179:1457-1463.

Craig JR, et al, 1989: Tumors of the liver and intrahepatic bile ducts. In Atlas of Tumor Pathology, Second Series Fascicle 26. Washington, DC, Armed Forces Institute of Pathology.

Danet IM, et al, 2003: Giant hemangioma of the liver: MR imaging characteristics in 24 patients. Magn Reson Imaging 21:95-101.

D'Angelica M, et al, 1998: Isolated hepatic splenosis: first reported case. HPB Surg 11:39-42.

Davidson LA, Reid IN, 1997: Intrahepatic splenic tissue. J Clin Pathol 50:532-533.

De Rave S, Hussain SM, 2002: A liver tumour as an incidental finding: differential diagnosis and treatment. Scand J Gastroenterol Suppl 236:81-86.

Descottes B, et al, 2003: Laparoscopic liver resection of benign liver tumors. Surg Endosc 17:23-30.

Dietrich CF, et al, 2005: Contrast-enhanced endoscopic ultrasound with low mechanical index: a new technique. Z Gastroenterol 43:1219-1223.

Dogan E, et al, 2003: Nodular regenerative hyperplasia of the liver: a case report. Turk J Gastroenterol 14:64-67.

Edmonson HA, 1958: Tumors of the Liver and Intrahepatic Bile Ducts. Atlas of Tumor Pathology, Section 7, Fascicle 25. Washington, DC, Armed Forces Institute of Pathology.

Fabre A, et al, 2002: Histological scoring of liver biosy in focal nodular hyperplasia with atypical presentation. Hepatology 35:414-420.

Farges O, et al, 1995: Cavernous hemangiomas of the liver: are there any indications for resection? World J Surg 19:19-24.

Federle MP, Brancatelli G, 2001: Imaging of benign hepatic masses. Semin Liver Dis 21:237-249.

Ferraz AA, et al, 2004: Liver transplant for the treatment of giant hepatic hemangioma. Liver Transpl 10:1436-1437.

Flowers BF, et al, 1990: Ruptured hepatic adenoma: a spectrum of presentation and treatment. Am Surg 56:380-383.

Foroudi F, et al, 1999: Splenosis mimicking metastases from breast carcinoma. Clin Oncol (R Coll Radiol) 11:190-192.

Freeny PC, Marks WM, 1986: Hepatic hemangioma: dynamic bolus CT. AJR Am J Roentgenol 147:711-719

Gaffey MJ, et al, 1996: Clonal analysis of focal nodular hyperplasia of the liver. Am J Pathol 148:1089-1096.

Gaspar L, et al, 1993: Radiation therapy in the unresectable cavernous hemangioma of the liver. Radiother Oncol 29:45-50.

Gedaly R, et al, 1999: Cavernous hemangioma of the liver: anatomic resection vs. enucleation. Arch Surg 134:407-411.

Golli M, et al, 1994: Hepatocellular adenoma: color Doppler US and pathologic correlations. Radiology 190:741-744.

Graham E, et al, 1993: Symptomatic liver hemangioma with intra-tumor haemorrhage treated by angiography and embolization during pregnancy. Obstet Gynecol 81:813-816.

Grazioli L, et al, 2005: Accurate differentiation of focal nodular hyperplasia from hepatic adenoma at gadobenate dimeglumine-enhanced MR imaging: prospective study. Radiology 236:166-177.

Gyorffy EJ, et al, 1989: Transformation of hepatic cell adenoma to hepatocellular carcinoma due to oral contraceptive use. Ann Intern Med 110:489-490.

Hanafusa K, et al, 1995: Hepatic hemangioma: findings with two-phase CT. Radiology 196:465-469.

Heilo A, Stenwig AE, 1997: Liver hemangioma: US-guided 18-gauge core-needle biopsy. Radiology 204:719-722.

Herman P, et al, 2005: Management of hepatic hemangiomas: a 14-year experience. J Gastrointest Surg 9:853-859.

Hobbs KE, 1990: Hepatic hemangiomas. World J Surg 14:468-471.

Hoffman A, et al, 1997: Hepatic angiomyolipoma: two cases reports of caudate-based lesions and review of the literature. Liver Transplant Surg 3:46-53.

Hooper LD, et al, 1994: Multiple hepatorenal angiomyolipomas: diagnosis with fat suppression, gadolinium-enhanced MRI. Abdom Imaging 19:549-551.

Horita T, et al, 2002: Significance of magnetic resonance imaging in the diagnosis of nodular regenerative hyperplasia of the liver complicated with systemic lupus erythematosus: a case report and review of the literature. Lupus 11:193-196.

Horton KM, et al, 1999: CT and MR imaging of benign hepatic and biliary tumors. Radiographics 19:431-451.

Ichikawa T, et al, 2000: Hepatocellular adenoma: multiphasic CT and histopathologic finding in 25 patients. Radiology 214:861-868.

International Working Party, 1995: Terminology of nodular hepatocellular lesions. Hepatology 22:983-993.

Ishak KG, 1979: Hepatic neoplasms associated with contraceptive and anabolic steroids: carcinogenesis hormones. In Lingerman CH (ed): Recent Results in Cancer Research. New York, Springer-Verlag, pp 72-128.

Isozaki T, et al, 2003: Differential diagnosis of hepatic tumors by using contrast enhancement patterns at US. Radiology 229:798-805.

Itai Y, Saida Y, 2002: Pitfalls in liver imaging. Eur Radiol 12:1162-1174.

Itai Y, et al, 1985: Noninvasive diagnosis of small cavernous hemangioma of the liver: advantage of MRI. AJR Am J Roentgenol 145:1195-1199.

Iwatsuki S, et al, 1990: Excisional therapy for benign hepatic lesions. Surg Gynecol Obstet 171:240-246.

Jovine E, et al, 2004: Intrahepatic rupture of a caudate lobe adenoma in liver adenomatosis. J Hepatobiliary Pancreat Surg 11:324-329.

Karahasanoglu T, et al, 2001: Laparoscopic enucleation of giant liver hemangioma. Surg Endosc 15:1489.

Kehagias D, et al, 2001: Focal nodular hyperplasia: imaging findings. Eur Radiol 11:202-212.

Kim MJ, et al, 2004: Evaluation of hepatic focal nodular hyperplasia with contrast-enhanced gray scale harmonic sonography: initial experience. J Ultrasound Med 23:297-305.

Kim T, et al, 2001: Discrimination of small hepatic hemangiomas from hypervascular malignant tumors smaller than 3 cm with three-phase helical CT. Radiology 219:699-706.

Koea JB, et al, 2003: Inflammatory pseudotumor of the liver: demographics, diagnosis, and the case for nonoperative management. J Am Coll Surg 196:226-235.

Kuo YT, et al, 1994: Imaging diagnosis of cavernous hemangioma of the rib—one case report and review of the literature.Gaoxiong Yi Xue Ke Xue Za Zhi 10:469-473.

Labrune P, et al, 1997: Hepatocellular adenomas in glycogen storage disease type I and III: a series of 43 patients and review of the literature. J Pediatr Gastroenterol Nutr 24:276-279.

Landen S, et al, 1993: Focal nodular hyperplasia of the liver: a retrospective review of 20 patients managed surgically. Acta Chir Belg 93:94-97.

Laurent C, et al, 2003: Association of adenoma and focal nodular hyperplasia: experience of a single French academic center. Comp Hepatol 2:6.

Lewin M, et al, 2006: MR imaging of liver adenomatosis: classification of a heterogeneous entity with a pathological correlation. Radiology, in press.

Li GH, et al, 1989: Inflammatory pseudotumor of the liver. J Surg Oncol 42:244-248.

Locke JE, et al, 2005: Inflammatory pesudotumor of the liver. J Hepatobiliary Pancreat Surg 12:314-316.

Maceyko RF, Camisa C, 1991: Kasabach-Merritt syndrome. Pediatr Dermatol 8:113-136.

Marini P, et al, 2002: Management of spontaneous rupture of liver tumours. Dig Surg 19:109-113.

Marks WH, et al, 1988: Failure of hepatic adenomas (HCA) to regress after discontinuance of oral contraceptives—an association with focal nodular hyperplasia (FNH) and uterine leiomyoma. Ann Surg 208:190-195.

Marsh JI, et al, 1989: Hepatic hemangioma in the presence of fatty infiltration: an atypical sonographic appearance. Gastrointest Radiol 14:262-264.

Mathieu D, et al, 1989: Association of focal nodular hyperplasia and hepatic hemangioma. Gastroenterology 97:154-157.

Mathieu D, et al, 2000: Oral contraceptive use and focal nodular hyperplasia of the liver. Gastroenterology 118:560-564.

Maze GL, et al, 1999: Inflammatory pseudotumor of the liver and pregnancy. Am J Gastroenterol 94:529-530.

Mergo PJ, Ros PR, 1998: Benign lesions of the liver. Radiol Clin North Am 36:319-331.

Mortelé KJ, Ros PR, 2002: Benign liver neoplasms. Clin Liver Dis 6:119-145.

Mortelé KJ, et al, 2000: CT and MR imaging findings in focal nodular hyperplasia of the liver: radiologic-pathologic correlation. AJR Am J Roentgenol 175:687-692.

Nagorney DM, 1995: Benign hepatic tumors: focal nodular hyperplasia and hepatocellular adenoma. World J Surg 19:13-18.

Nakaizumi A, et al, 1990: Diagnosis of hepatic cavernous hemangioma by fine-needle aspiration biopsy under ultrasonic guidance. Gastrointest Radiol 15:39-42.

Neri S, et al, 2004: Biliary hamartomas (Von Meyenburg complex): magnetic resonance imaging in a case report. Intern Med J 34:71-72.

Nghiem HV, et al, 1997: Cavernous hemangiomas of the liver: enlargement over time. AJR Am J Roentgenol 169:137-140.

Nguyen BN, et al, 1999: Focal nodular hyperplasia of the liver: a comprehensive pathologic study of 305 lesions and recognition of new histologic forms. Am J Surg Pathol 23:1441-1454.

Nime F, et al, 1979: The histology of liver tumors in oral contraceptive users observed during a national survey by the American College of Surgeons Commission on Cancer. Cancer 44:1481-1489.

Nino-Murcia M, et al, 2000: Focal liver lesions: pattern-based classification scheme for enhancement at arterial phase CT. Radiology 215:746-751.

Paradis V, et al, 1997: Evidence for the polyclonal nature of focal nodular hyperplasia of the liver by the study of X chromosome inactivation. Hepatology 26:891-895.

Paradis V, et al, 2004: Telangiectatic focal nodular hyperplasia: a variant of hepatocellular adenoma. Gastroenterology 126:1323-1329.

Pateron D, et al, 1991: Giant hemangioma of the liver with pain, fever, and abnormal liver tests: report of two cases. Dig Dis Sci 36:524-527.

Pol B, et al, 1998: Inflammatory process complicating giant hemangioma of the liver: a report of three cases. Liver Transplant Surg 4:204-207.

Quaia E, et al, 2002: Characterization of liver hemangiomas with pulse inversion harmonic imaging. Eur Radiol 12:537-544.

Rangheard AS, et al, 2002: Focal nodular hyperplasia inducing hepatic vein obstruction. AJR Am J Roentgenol 179:759-762.

Reading NG, et al, 1988: Hepatic haemangioma: a critical review of diagnosis and management. QJM 67:431-445.

Ribeiro A, et al, 1998: Management of liver adenomatosis: results with a conservative surgical approach. Liver Transplant Surg 4:388-398.

Rooks JB, et al, 1979: Epidemiology of hepatocellular adenoma—the role of oral contraceptive use. JAMA 242:644-648.

Rosenberg L, 1991: The risk of liver neoplasia in relation to combined oral contraceptive use. Contraception 43:643-652.

Ruppert-Kohlmayr AJ, et al, 2001: Focal nodular hyperplasia and hepatocellular adenoma of the liver: differentiation with multiphasic helical CT. AJR Am J Roentgenol 176:1493-1498.

Sawai J, et al, 1998: Angiomyolipoma of the liver: case report and collective review of cases diagnosed from fine needle aspiration biopsy specimens. J Hepatobiliary Pancreat Surg 5:333-338.

Semelka RC, Sofka CM, 1997: Hepatic hemangiomas. Magn Reson Imaging Clin N Am 5:241-253.

Semelka RC, et al, 1994: Hepatic hemangiomas: a multi-institutional study of appearance on T2-weighted and serial gadolinium-enhanced gradient-echo MR images. Radiology 192:401-406.

Shamsi K, et al, 1993: Focal nodular hyperplasia of the liver: radiologic findings. Abdom Imaging 18:32-38.

Shek TWH, et al, 1998: Intra-abdominal follicular dentritic cell tumour: a rare tumour in need of recognition. Histopathology 33:465.

Shortell CK, Schwartz SI, 1991: Hepatic adenoma and focal nodular hyperplasia. Surg Gynecol Obstet 173:426-431.

Stanley G, et al, 2002: CT findings ans histopathology of intratumoral steatosis in focal nodular hyperplasia: case report and review of the literature. J Comput Assist Tomogr 26:815-817.

Starck DD, et al, 1985: Magnetic resonance imaging of cavernous hemangioma of the liver: tissue-specific characterization. AJR Am J Roentgenol 145:213-222.

Steinbrecher UP, et al, 1981: Complete regression of hepatocellular adenoma after withdrawal of oral contraceptives. Dig Dis Sci 26:1045-1050.

Suzuki K, et al, 1999: Heterotopic pancreatic tissue associated with intra- and extrahepatic choledochal cyst. Pathol Int 49:759-762.

Takayasu K, et al, 1990: Computed tomography of a rapidly growing hepatic hemangioma. J Comput Assist Tomogr 14:143-145.

Tapetes K, et al, 1995: Orthotopic liver transplantation for benign hepatic neoplasms. Arch Surg 130:153-156.

Terkivatan T, et al, 2000: Management of hepatocellular adenoma during pregnancy. Liver 20:186-187.

Terkivatan T, et al, 2001a: Indications and long-term outcome of treatment for benign hepatic tumors: a critical appraisal. Arch Surg 136:1033-1038.

Terkivatan T, et al, 2001b: Treatment of ruptured hepatocellular adenoma. Br J Surg 88:207-209.

Trotter JF, Everson GT, 2001: Benign focal lesions of the liver. Clin Liver Dis 5:17-42.

Uggowitzer M, et al, 1997: Power Doppler imaging and evaluation of the resistive index in focal nodular hyperplasia of the liver. Abdom Imaging 22:268-273.

Van Leeuwen MS, et al, 1996: Focal liver lesions: characterization with triphasic spiral CT. Radiology 201:327-336.

Vecchio FM, et al, 1984: Fibrolamellar carcinoma of the liver: the malignant counterpart of focal nodular hyperplasia with oncocytic change. Am J Clin Pathol 81:521-526.

Verswijvel G, et al, 2003: Peliosis hepatis presenting as a multifocal hepatic pseudotumor: MR findings in two cases. Eur Radiol 13:40-44.

Vilgrain V, et al, 1992: Focal nodular hyperplasia of the liver: MR imaging and pathologic correlation in 37 patients. Radiology 184:699-703.

Vilgrain V, et al, 1999: Hepatic nodules in Budd-Chiari syndrome: imaging features. Radiology 210:443-450.

Vilgrain V, et al, 2003: Prevalence of hepatic hemangioma in patients with focal nodular hyperplasia: MR imaging analysis. Radiology 229:75-79.

Wanless IR, 1990: Micronodular transformation (nodular regenerative hyperplasia) of the liver: a report of 64 cases among 2,500 autopsies and a new classification of benign hepatocellular nodules.Hepatology 11:787-797.

Wanless IR, 2002: Benign liver tumors. Clin Liver Dis 6:513-552.

Wanless IR, et al, 1985: On the pathogenesis of focal nodular hyperplasia. Hepatology 5:1194-1120.

Wanless IR, et al, 1989: Multiple focal nodular hyperplasia of the liver associated with vascular malformations of various organs and neoplasia of the brain. Mod Pathol 2:456-462.

Weimann A, et al, 1997: Benign liver tumors: differential diagnosis and indications for surgery. World J Surg 21:983-990.

Weimann A, et al, 2000: Critical issues in the diagnosis and treatment of hepatocellular adenoma. HPB Surg 2:25-32.

Wittekind C, 1995: Hepatocellular carcinoma and cholangiocarcinoma. In Hermanek P, Gospodarowicz MK, Henson DE, et al (eds): Prognostic Factors in Cancer. Berlin, Springer, pp 88-93.

Yan F, et al, 2002: Hepatic angiomyolipoma: various appearances on two-phase contrast scanning of spiral CT. Eur J Radiol 41:12-18.

Yoon SS, et al, 2003: Diagnosis, management and outcomes of 115 patients with hepatic hemangioma. J Am Coll Surg 197:392-402.

Zamir D, et al, 1998: Inflammatory pseudotumor of the liver—a rare entity and a diagnostic challenge. Am J Gastroenterol 93:1538-1540.

Zeitoun D, et al, 2004: Congenital hepatic fibrosis: CT findings in 18 adults. Radiology 231:109-116.

Zeppa P, et al, 2002: Fine needle aspiration biopsy of hepatic focal fatty change: a report of two cases. Acta Cytol 46:567-570.

Hepatocellular Carcinoma

71

J. BRUIX, M. SALA, AND J. M. LLOVET

Hepatocellular carcinoma (HCC) is the most frequent primary liver tumor. It currently represents the fifth most common cancer worldwide and is the third major case of cancer death. Its incidence presents a marked geographic difference (Table 71.1) (Bosch et al, 2004; Parkin et al, 2001). Asia and sub-Saharan Africa constitute high-risk areas with yearly rates exceeding 20 per 100,000 population. Southern Europe and Japan have intermediate rates, and rates are low in Northern Europe and North America (Bosch et al, 2004; Parkin et al, 2001). Several registries have shown that the incidence figures have changed slightly during the past several years. Vaccination plans against hepatitis B virus (HBV) and improvement in health standards have decreased the incidence in some high-risk areas, such as Taiwan (Chang et al, 1997). The incidence is decreasing in some European countries, where the risk of HCC is linked significantly to chronic infection with hepatitis C virus (HCV) that was acquired decades ago when health care was less concerned by blood-borne viral disease. By contrast, HCC incidence is increasing in the United States (El Serag & Mason, 1999) and in Northern Europe (Bosch et al, 2004), probably reflecting the different timing in the appearance of risk factors, mostly HCV infection (Tanaka et al, 2002). Finally, a major risk factor for HCC is alcohol intake, and this also varies widely in different countries. Aflatoxin B1 uptake (Chen et al, 1996), cigarette smoking, and heavy alcohol consumption are independent risk factors and may have synergistic effects (Jee et al, 2004; Kuper et al, 2000).

In all areas of the world, cirrhosis underlies HCC in almost 90% of the cases (Bruix et al, 2004a; Fattovich et al, 2004). Cirrhosis is related to chronic HBV and HCV, which contribute to HCC development in 80% of cases. Alcohol consumption is a frequent cofactor, and surveys indicate that a significant proportion of HCC in cryptogenic cirrhosis is due to nonalcoholic fatty liver disease (Calle et al, 2003; El Serag et al, 2001; Regimbeau et al, 2004), a condition associated with diabetes or obesity (Day, 2002). Because of the obesity epidemic, this currently infrequent cause may gain relevance in the near future. Follow-up studies have disclosed that HCC development is now the most frequent cause of death in patients with cirrhosis (Benvegnu et al, 2004; Degos et al, 2000; Sangiovanni et al, 2004). Prevention, diagnosis, and treatment of this neoplasm are major areas of clinical and research activity.

The mean annual incidence of HCC in cirrhotic patients in the West is 3% to 4%, and this figure increases in parallel to liver function impairment (Benvegnu et al, 2004; Bolondi et al, 2001; Degos et al, 2000; Ikeda et al, 1993; Sangiovanni et al, 2004). Some specific characteristics have been associated with a higher risk. The most consistent are male sex, advanced age (this being a surrogate for the duration of the underlying liver disease), and increased α-fetoprotein (AFP) concentration (Bruix & Sherman, 2005; Bruix et al, 2001). HBV and HCV coinfection imply a higher risk (Fattovich et al, 2004), whereas coinfection with human immunodeficiency virus has been associated with a more aggressive phenotype and lack of therapeutic benefit (Puoti et al, 2004). Irregular regeneration, high proliferative stage, and presence of dysplastic foci in biopsy samples also have been correlated with higher HCC incidence during follow-up, but the need of tissue sampling has prevented their robust validation and wide clinical acceptance (Bruix et al, 2004a).

RISK FACTORS AND PREVENTION

All types of cancer are the consequence of genetic changes that accumulate through time, ultimately conferring a survival advantage to cells with an abnormal phenotype. The relationship between chronic hepatitis and long-lasting liver damage with HCC development suggests that persistent inflammation is a key factor leading to cancer. Maintained injury and repair with high proliferation rate increase the risk for DNA mutation (Arbuthnot & Kew, 2001). In addition to genetic damage secondary to inflammation, HBV itself may have direct genetic or epigenetic effects, being able to integrate into the host genome (Brechot, 2004). This integration into the host genome is accompanied by rearrangement and increased mutagenesis that may affect crucial target genes (Ferber et al, 2003; Ryu, 2003). HCV is an RNA virus and does not integrate into host DNA.

The most effective prevention of HCC is based on the avoidance of the acquisition of viral infection or of toxin intake. There is effective vaccination for HBV, and the vaccination plans in Taiwan have shown the efficacy of this action in diminishing cancer rates in children and adults (Chang et al, 1997). Proper controls in health care settings prevent HCV dissemination through blood transmission. Alcohol intake should be the target of health campaigns in the community, and aflatoxin contamination of food can be prevented by avoiding grain storage in humid conditions. The epidemic of obesity with associated nonalcoholic steatohepatitis leading to HCC has to be controlled by health education.

If viral infection is already present, it has been shown that a decrease in viral replication and subsequently of chronic hepatic damage could result in a reduced incidence of HCC in the long-term (Liaw et al, 2004; Yoshida et al, 1999). Effective therapy is available for HCV and HBV, and secondary prevention may be feasible for both agents. If chronic liver disease already has caused cirrhosis, however, it is unclear if antiviral therapy has any preventive capacity because cell damage and transformation already may be present (Baffis et al, 1999; Camma et al, 1999; Heathcote, 2004; Lok, 2004). In patients with HBV infection, the genetic damage may occur in the absence of major liver insult, and this would explain the appearance of HCC in an otherwise healthy liver. This circumstance is more frequent in areas where viral transmission occurs early after birth or in childhood, stressing the benefits of HBV vaccination. Secondary prevention in patients with chronic liver disease requires the prior recognition of the affected individuals, but currently there is no proof of the cost-effectiveness of population screening for viral liver disease, and this is not recommended (Chou et al, 2004).

Table 71.1 Incidence of Hepatocellular Carcinoma According to Geographic Area and Distribution of Risk Factors

Geographic Area	Age-Adjusted Incidence Rate Male/Female	RISK FACTORS HCV	HBV	Alcohol	Other
Europe		60-70%	10-15%	20%	10%
Western Europe	5.8/1.6				
Southern	9.8/3.4				
Northern	2.6/1.3				
North America		50-60%	20%	20%	—
Northern	4.1/1.6				
Southern	4.8/3.6				
Asia and Africa		20%	70%	10%	Aflatoxin
(Japan)		70%	10-20%	10%	10%
Eastern Asia	35.4/12.6				
Southeast Asia	18.3/5.7				
Middle Africa	24.2/12.9				
World	14.9/5.5				

Modified from Llovet JM, et al, 2003: Hepatocellular carcinoma. Lancet 362:1907-1917.

SCREENING AND RECALL OF HIGH-RISK INDIVIDUALS

Randomized controlled trials comparing screening versus no screening are lacking, and the establishment of surveillance for HCC in patients with cirrhosis is based on expert opinion (Bolondi, 2003). The aim of screening is to detect HCC at an early stage, when the tumor could be cured (Bruix et al, 2001). Success of screening depends on several factors, including adequate ultrasound performance, accurate diagnostic and staging criteria, and timely availability of curative treatments. If these requirements are not met, screening will never result in an increase of life expectancy. Even when accounting for the potential lead-time bias (i.e., patients apparently surviving longer simply because their tumors were diagnosed earlier) and length-time bias (i.e., the interval between screenings misses the more aggressive tumors that will be detected when symptoms appear), it is assumed that screening results in more frequent detection of early stage HCC with more common application of effective treatment and improved outcome. Effective treatment and long-term cure are feasible with early detection, and diagnosis at the symptomatic stage reflects an advanced evolutionary stage and lack of effective treatment. Based on these arguments, the European Association for the Study of the Liver (EASL) panel of experts suggested 6-monthly abdominal ultrasound scanning and AFP measurements for patients with liver cirrhosis who would be treated if diagnosed with HCC (Bruix et al, 2001). This recommendation excludes patients with severe associated conditions and patients with advanced liver disease who are already candidates for transplantation. If this is not an option, screening for HCC aiming to detect early tumor will never be followed by treatment, and it makes no clinical sense.

AFP is known to have a reduced sensitivity for diagnosis (Trevisani et al, 2001). Performance of AFP is even poorer for early detection (Sherman, 2001), and its main usefulness is to identify high-risk individuals. Accordingly, screening is based mostly on regular ultrasound scanning. On detection of an abnormal finding, patients have to be evaluated. Fig. 71.1 depicts

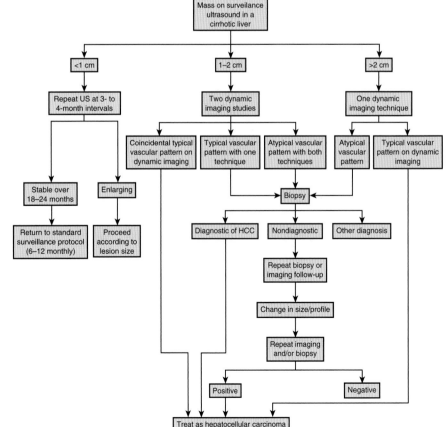

Fig. 71.1. Screening strategy as proposed in the AASLD Practice Guidelines. (From Bruix J, Sherman M, 2005: Management of hepatocellular carcinoma. Hepatology 42:1208-1236.)

Table 71.2   Diagnostic Criteria for Hepatocellular Carcinoma

Cytohistologic criteria

Noninvasive criteria (cirrhotic patients)
    Focal lesion 1-2 cm: two imaging techniques* with arterial
        hypervascularization and venous washout
    Focal lesion >2 cm: one imaging technique with arterial
        hypervascularization and venous washout

*Techniques to be considered: contrast ultrasound, dynamic CT, and MRI.
From Bruix J, Sherman M, 2005: Management of hepatocellular carcinoma. Hepatology 42:1208-1236.

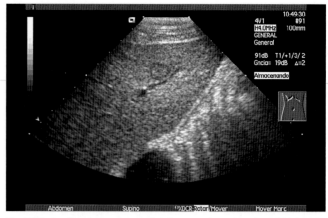

Fig. 71.3. Small nodule measuring less than 2 cm located in the right lobe. The nodule is heterogeneous and appears as a thin hypoechoic capsule. Fine-needle aspiration biopsy established the diagnosis of HCC. Early detection of this small tumor allows effective therapy to be initiated. (Courtesy of Dr. Bianchi.)

the recall strategy proposed by American Association for the Study of Liver Diseases (AASLD) panel, and Table 71.2 summarizes proposed diagnostic criteria (Bruix & Sherman, 2005). Nodules measuring less than 1 cm in a cirrhotic liver may not correspond to a malignant focus in 50% of cases (Fracanzani et al, 2001); even so, their confident diagnosis is almost not feasible with current diagnostic tools. Close follow-up to detect any increase in size is recommended (Bruix & Sherman, 2005). Nodules in a cirrhotic liver that are larger than 1 cm can be diagnosed as HCC if the vascular profile on imaging techniques is characteristic of this neoplasm, that is, intense contrast uptake in the arterial phase followed by contrast washout in the delayed venous phase (Bruix & Sherman, 2005). In a tumor larger than 2 cm in diameter, a single dynamic imaging technique suffices to establish the diagnosis. By contrast, in tumors between 1 and 2 cm, it is necessary to base the diagnosis on the coincidental findings of two imaging techniques, choosing among contrast ultrasound, dynamic CT, and MRI (Fig. 71.2). If the characteristic dynamic profile is not recognized by imaging techniques, it is recommended that the diagnosis be based on fine needle biopsy (Fig. 71.3). This is so even in the presence of increased AFP values because cholangiocarcinoma and hepatic metastases may produce AFP (Bruix & Sherman, 2005). It has to be stressed that biopsy does not have 100% sensitivity and, hence, a negative result does not exclude HCC.

Tumor staging is done through ultrasound, spiral CT, and MRI; the last-mentioned is the most sensitive to detect nodules smaller than 2 cm (Burrel et al, 2003). The technical advances in these techniques have made angiography unnecessary for diagnosis and staging. Other tumor markers, such as protein induced by vitamin K absence (PIVKA) (Marrero et al, 2003; Tanaka et al, 1999), glypican-3 (Capurro et al, 2003; Sung et al, 2003), and AFP fractions (Hayashi et al, 1999), have been proposed to be used alone or in combination with AFP, but their usefulness in routine clinical practice is not established.

STAGING AND PROGNOSTIC EVALUATION

Staging systems are crucial tools to stratify patients into different subgroups according to prognosis. Ideally, they should establish a link with treatment and predict outcome after therapy. A well-validated and internationally accepted staging system is

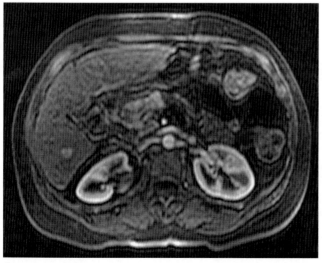

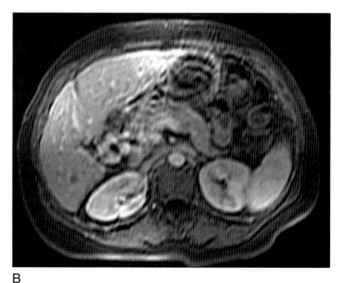

A   B

Fig. 71.2. A, MRI depicts a small nodule with arterial enhancement after contrast administration. **B,** The nodule exhibits washout of the contrast material in the venous phase. This is the characteristic pattern of HCC. (Courtesy of Dr. Ayuso.)

lacking in HCC. In most tumors, the prognosis is related mainly to tumor stage at the time of diagnosis. The presence of underlying liver disease makes prognostic evaluation of patients with HCC more complex because liver disease influences outcome and the possibility of treatment.

This need to take into account tumor stage and liver function explains why one-dimensional systems taking into account one of the two aspects have no power to predict outcome or to establish the best treatment. This is the case for the TNM system (AJCC, 2002) or the Child-Pugh classification (Pugh et al, 1973). Despite several modifications over time, the TNM system is still not valid because it relies predominantly on pathologic findings. Combination with a rough assessment of the underlying liver status (cirrhosis versus no cirrhosis) (Vauthey et al, 2002) offers some advantages, but still lacks accuracy to predict prognosis in nonsurgical cases. The Okuda classification is based on rough assessment of tumor burden (on imaging or surgery) and liver function. It stratifies patients into three groups with different outcomes (Okuda et al, 1985), but its main capacity is to identify end-stage patients. Several additional scoring systems have been proposed in Uganda (Primack et al, 1975), the United States (Stuart et al, 1996), Barcelona (Calvet et al, 1990), France (Chevret, et al 1999), Italy (Cancer of the Liver Italian Program [CLIP] investigators, 1998), Austria (Schoniger-Hekele et al, 2000), Hong Kong (Leung et al, 2002) and Japan (Kudo et al, 2003; Omagari et al, 2004) (Table 71.3). The relevant prognostic parameters are not the same in all systems, and despite their capacity to stratify subjects, none of them has shown transportability: Strata of patients do not have the same survival in different settings. The major usefulness of these systems is the identification of end-stage patients with a poor prognosis, but none of these systems provides any link to treatment indication. This lack of reproducibility indicates major heterogeneity among the different studies, and currently there is no widely accepted universal scoring and staging system.

The Barcelona Clinic Liver Cancer staging strategy avoids the use of a single scoring system for all patients. Instead, it divides patients into four major groups (early, intermediate, advanced, and end stage) and develops a prognostic model within each group taking into account the impact of treatment (Fig. 71.4) (Bruix et al, 2004a; Llovet et al, 1999a). This model was constructed based on the results obtained in the setting of several cohort studies and randomized controlled trials. The proposal constitutes a regularly updated staging classification derived from the combination of the data of several independent prognostic studies in different disease stages and treatments. Because it links staging with treatment indication, it has become a widely used clinical tool for treatment decision making. It considers variables related to tumor stage, liver functional status, physical status, and cancer-related symptoms. Patients at an early stage present with solitary tumors (usually <5 cm) or two or three nodules (none >3 cm). Depending on the degree of liver function impairment, patients may benefit from curative therapies, such as resection, transplantation, or percutaneous ablation. The 5-year survival ranges from 50% to 70%. The intermediate stage comprises patients with large or multifocal tumors with preserved liver function and no cancer-related symptoms or vascular invasion. They may benefit from transarterial chemoembolization and achieve a 50% survival at 3 years. Patients at advanced stage have cancer-related symptoms or vascular invasion or extrahepatic spread, and their median survival is less than 1 year. There is no effective treatment for these patients, and the optimal policy is to recruit them in research trials. Finally, end-stage patients are patients with major impairment of liver function or major cancer-related symptoms with severe deterioration of physical condition as reflected by a performance status greater than 2. Their short-term prognosis is poor, and they should receive palliative care (Bruix et al, 2004a).

TREATMENT STRATEGY

The selection of the best treatment in patients with HCC is the result of the evaluation of several factors, among which the most relevant are the status of the underlying liver and the tumor stage (see Chs. 2 and 88). Accurate definition of the status of the

Table 71.3 Prognostic Scores Proposed for Stratification of Hepatocellular Carcinoma Patients According to Expected Outcome

Reference	N	Treated Patients	Tumor	Liver Function	General Health
Calvet et al, 1990	206	28%	Tumor size, metastases	Bilirubin, ascites, GGT, renal function	Constitutional syndrome, age
Stuart et al, 1996	314	None	Portal thrombosis, AFP	Albumin	—
CLIP, 1998	435	42%	Portal thrombosis, tumor burden, AFP	Child-Pugh	—
Chevret et al, 1999	761	53%	Portal thrombosis, AFP	Child-Pugh, alkaline phosphatase	Karnofsky
Llovet et al, 1999a	102	100%	Portal thrombosis, extrahepatic spread	—	PST, constitutional syndrome
Villa, 2000	96	100%	Estrogen receptors	Bilirubin	—
CUPI, 2002	926	58%	TNM, AFP	Bilirubin, ascites, alkaline phosphatase	Symptoms
Kudo et al, 2003	722	?	TNM Japan	Child-Pugh	—
Omagari et al, 2004	177	8%	TNM Japan, PIVKA	Child-Pugh, ICG 15	—

PST, performance status test.

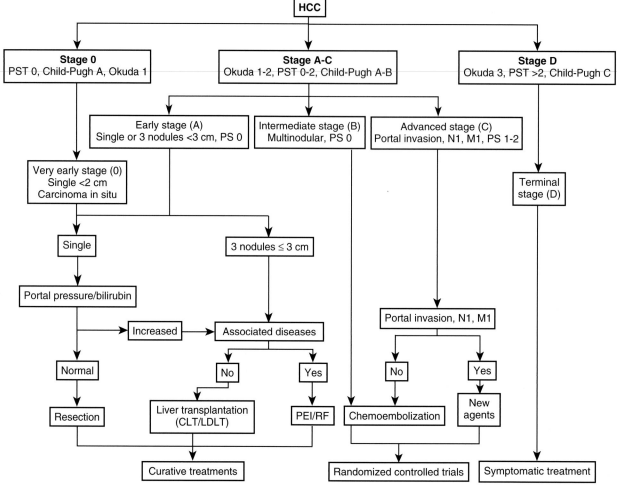

Fig. 71.4. Staging system and treatment strategy according to the Barcelona Clinic Liver Cancer criteria. Patients are stratified according to clinical, tumor, and biochemical characteristics into four major groups: early, intermediate, advanced, and terminal. Treatment selection is decided according to stage allocation. CLT, cadaveric liver transplantation; LDLT, live donor liver transplantation; PEI, percutaneous ethanol injection; PST, performance status test; RF, radiofrequency. (Modified from Llovet JM, et al, 2003: Hepatocellular carcinoma. Lancet 362:1907-1917.)

nontumor liver is crucial. The few patients in whom HCC appears in a noncirrhotic liver are good candidates for liver resection. Major lobectomies are well tolerated, and resection is the first-line option (Regimbeau et al, 1999). By contrast, in most patients, cirrhosis underlies HCC, and the degree of functional impairment may preclude safe surgery (see Chs. 80 and 82). In these patients, the first-line treatment should be liver transplantation (see Chs. 103 and 106), and if this is not feasible, they should be considered for percutaneous ablation through any of the available techniques (ethanol injection, radiofrequency, cryotherapy, microwave) (see Ch. 76). These options are thought to offer potential long-term cure. The sole palliative approach that has been shown to have a positive impact in survival is transarterial chemoembolization (Llovet et al, 2003). All these approaches are discussed in other chapters; we briefly discuss the Barcelona strategy to select the best option for each patient (see Fig. 71.4).

The liver function is assessed initially through the Child-Pugh classification, and this is combined with a detailed evaluation of tumor extent (Bruix et al, 2004a). This assessment has to search for the presence of daughter nodules, vascular invasion, extrahepatic disease, and portal vein thrombosis. Extrahepatic disease

is ruled out by chest CT scan and bone scintigraphy. The general condition of the patient not only includes consideration of comorbid conditions that may increase perioperative or intervention-related morbidity and mortality, but also the assessment of cancer-related symptoms as reflected by their performance status score (Sorensen et al, 1993). This provides an evaluation similar to the Karnofsky index, although simpler. Heavily affected (performance status 3-4) patients belong to terminal disease stage and should receive palliative treatment.

Liver resection (see Chs. 80, 82, and 83) is the first-line treatment in patients with solitary tumors who do not present with underlying cirrhosis and in patients with HCC in well-compensated cirrhosis (Belghiti et al, 2002; Bruix et al, 2004a). This status cannot be assessed through the Child-Pugh classification. Only patients with normal bilirubin concentration and absence of clinically relevant portal hypertension should be considered optimal candidates for resection (Llovet et al, 1999b). They tolerate the intervention without risk of hepatic decompensation, and survival at 5 years is approximately 70%. Hepatic vein catheterization is the most accurate tool to measure portal pressure, and a hepatic pressure gradient less than 10 mm Hg is the best cutoff value. Patients with portal hypertension are at high risk of liver decompensation and death after surgery, and their survival at 5 years is less than 50%.

Liver transplantation (see Chs. 103 and 106) is offered to patients who do not fit the optimal profile for resection and present with solitary tumors less than 5 cm or with two or three nodules, each less than 3 cm. Vascular invasion and extrahepatic dissemination should be ruled out, and patients should not have general contraindications for liver transplantation. Percutaneous treatment is proposed if expected waiting time exceeds 6 months, and all patients also are proposed to enter the live donor program (Sala et al, 2004b).

If patients are not candidates for surgery, they are offered *percutaneous ablation* (Gaiani et al, 2003). Radiofrequency is the main technique, with ethanol injection being used in the presence of contraindications for radiofrequency (i.e., subcapsular location, vicinity of gallbladder or heart). The best results of ablation are achieved in solitary tumors smaller than 2 cm. These achieve 100% necrosis in 90% of the cases, and recurrence rate is similar to resection (Sala et al, 2004a).

Patients with more advanced disease (large or multifocal HCC) without portal vein invasion are candidates for *transarterial chemoembolization* (see Ch. 74) if liver function is preserved and they are still free of cancer-related symptoms. Response to this locoregional approach is associated with improved survival, and it is the sole palliative therapy that has a statistically significant impact on outcome (Bruix et al, 2004b; Lo et al, 2002; Llovet & Bruix, 2003). If chemoembolization is not feasible, but patients still present with preserved liver function (Child-Pugh A-B) without major cancer-related symptoms, they are considered for research therapeutic trials. If patients are diagnosed at a terminal stage identified by severe liver function deterioration (Child-Pugh C), and the extent of the tumor prevents transplantation and has induced severe cancer-related symptoms (performance status >2), patients are offered palliative care (Bruix et al, 2004a).

FUTURE PROSPECTS

Major research in recent years has been devoted to allowing an earlier diagnosis of HCC and more accurate staging at the time of diagnosis. The improvements in treatment have had a minor impact because most patients still are diagnosed at an advanced stage when there is no option for long-term cure. The effective treatments available today should be considered invasive, and it is hoped that active laboratory research should translate into new instruments to predict the biology of the tumor and identify new treatment targets. This development already has occurred in breast cancer (Perou et al, 2000; Somiari et al, 2003; Van de Vijver et al, 2002), prostate cancer (Dhanasekaran et al, 2001; Grubb et al, 2003), lung cancer (Yanagisawa et al, 2003), non-Hodgkin B lymphoma (Alizadeh et al, 2000), and melanoma (Bittner et al, 2000). Molecular profiling is evolving using gene or protein profiling (Golub et al, 1999; Khan et al, 2001; Rosenblatt et al, 2004), and it is expected to affect diagnosis, evaluation, and treatment of patients with liver cancer.

SUMMARY

The incidence of HCC has a marked geographic heterogeneity. Although years ago HCC was considered an infrequent neoplasm in Europe and North America, more recent epidemiologic surveys have shown that its incidence in these areas has increased significantly. HCC is associated with chronic liver diseases, usually related to viral infection or toxic agents, such as alcohol. Despite major advances in detection, diagnosis, and treatment, only a few patients currently are diagnosed at early stages and become candidates for treatments offering potential long-term cure (resection, transplantation, and percutaneous ablation). Most patients with this malignancy still are diagnosed at an intermediate or advanced stage. At this evolutionary stage, the only therapy that has been shown to offer a significant survival benefit is transarterial chemoembolization, but this can be applied in only a few cases. There is an urgent need to develop better detection and diagnostic strategies aimed at increasing the proportion of patients diagnosed at an early stage who could receive effective therapy. In addition, active translational research should help to develop new therapeutic tools that could result in a significant improvement of the long-term survival of patients diagnosed at advanced stage.

REFERENCES

American Joint Committee on Cancer, 2002: Cancer Staging Handbook, New York, Springer.

Alizadeh AA, et al, 2000: Distinct types of diffuse large B-cell lymphoma identified by gene expression profiling. Nature 403:503-511.

Arbuthnot P, Kew M, 2001: Hepatitis B virus and hepatocellular carcinoma. Int J Exp Pathol 82:77-100.

Baffis V, et al, 1999: Use of interferon for prevention of hepatocellular carcinoma in cirrhotic patients with hepatitis B or hepatitis C virus infection. Ann Intern Med 131:696-701.

Belghiti J, et al, 2002: Resection of hepatocellular carcinoma: a European experience of 328 cases. Hepatogastroenterology 49:41-46.

Benvegnu L, et al, 2004: Natural history of compensated viral cirrhosis: a prospective study on the incidence and hierarchy of major complications. Gut 53:744-749.

Bittner M, et al, 2000: Molecular classification of cutaneous malignant melanoma by gene expression profiling. Nature 406:536-540.

Bolondi L, 2003: Screening for hepatocellular carcinoma in cirrhosis. J Hepatol 39:1076-1084.

Bolondi L, et al, 2001: Surveillance programme of cirrhotic patients for early diagnosis and treatment of hepatocellular carcinoma: a cost-effectiveness analysis. Gut 48:251-259.

Bosch FX, et al, 2004: Primary liver cancer: worldwide incidence and trends. Gastroenterology 127(5 suppl 1):S5-S16.

Brechot C, 2004: Pathogenesis of hepatitis B virus–related hepatocellular carcinoma: old and new paradigms. Gastroenterology 127(5 suppl 1):S56-S61.

Bruix J, et al, 2001: Clinical management of hepatocellular carcinoma: conclusions of the Barcelona-2000 EASL Conference. J Hepatol 35:421-430.

Bruix J, et al, 2004a: Focus on hepatocellular carcinoma. Cancer Cell 5:215-219.

Bruix J, et al, 2004b: Chemoembolization for hepatocellular carcinoma. Gastroenterology 127(5 suppl 1):S179-S188.

Burrel M, et al, 2003: MRI angiography is superior to helical CT for detection of HCC prior to liver transplantation: an explant correlation. Hepatology 38:1034-1042.

Calle EE, et al, 2003: Overweight, obesity, and mortality from cancer in a prospectively studied cohort of U.S. adults. N Engl J Med 348:1625-1638.

Calvet X, et al, 1990: Prognostic factors of hepatocellular carcinoma in the west: a multivariate analysis in 206 patients. Hepatology 12:753-760.

Camma C, et al, 1999: Chronic hepatitis C and interferon alpha: conventional and cumulative meta-analyses of randomized controlled trials. Am J Gastroenterol 94:581-595.

Cancer of the Liver Italian Program (CLIP) Investigators, 1998: A new prognostic system for hepatocellular carcinoma: a retrospective study of 435 patients. Hepatology 28:751-755.

Capurro M, et al, 2003: Glypican-3: a novel serum and histochemical marker for hepatocellular carcinoma. Gastroenterology 125:89-97.

Chang MH, et al, 1997: Universal hepatitis B vaccination in Taiwan and the incidence of hepatocellular carcinoma in children. N Engl J Med 336:1855-1859.

Chen CJ, et al, 1996: Elevated aflatoxin exposure and increased risk of hepatocellular carcinoma. Hepatology 24:38-42.

Chevret S, et al, 1999: A new prognostic classification for predicting survival in patients with hepatocellular carcinoma. Groupe d'Etude et de Traitement du Carcinome Hepatocellulaire. J Hepatol 31:133-141.

Chou R, et al, 2004: Screening for hepatitis C virus infection: a review of the evidence for the U.S. Preventive Services Task Force. Ann Intern Med 140:465-479.

Day CP, 2002: Non-alcoholic steatohepatitis (NASH): where are we now and where are we going? Gut 50:585-588.

Degos F, et al, 2000: Hepatitis C virus–related cirrhosis: time to occurrence of hepatocellular carcinoma and death. Gut 47:131-136.

Dhanasekaran SM, et al, 2001: Delineation of prognostic biomarkers in prostate cancer. Nature 412:822-826.

El Serag HB, Mason AC, 1999: Rising incidence of hepatocellular carcinoma in the United States. N Engl J Med 340:745-750.

El Serag HB, et al, 2001: The role of diabetes in hepatocellular carcinoma: a case-control study among United States Veterans. Am J Gastroenterol 96:2462-2467.

Fattovich G, et al, 2004: Hepatocellular carcinoma in cirrhosis: incidence and risk factors. Gastroenterology 127(5 suppl 1):S35-S50.

Ferber MJ, et al, 2003: Integrations of the hepatitis B virus (HBV) and human papillomavirus (HPV) into the human telomerase reverse transcriptase (hTERT) gene in liver and cervical cancers. Oncogene 22:3813-3820.

Fracanzani AL, et al, 2001: Contrast-enhanced Doppler ultrasonography in the diagnosis of hepatocellular carcinoma and premalignant lesions in patients with cirrhosis. Hepatology 34:1109-1112.

Gaiani S, et al, 2003: Review article: percutaneous treatment of hepatocellular carcinoma. Aliment Pharmacol Ther 17(suppl 2):103-110.

Golub TR, et al, 1999: Molecular classification of cancer: class discovery and class prediction by gene expression monitoring. Science 286:531-537.

Grubb RL, et al, 2003: Signal pathway profiling of prostate cancer using reverse phase protein arrays. Proteomics 3:2142-2146.

Hayashi K, et al, 1999: Usefulness of measurement of *Lens culinaris* agglutinin-reactive fraction of alpha-fetoprotein as a marker of prognosis and recurrence of small hepatocellular carcinoma. Am J Gastroenterol 94:3028-3033.

Heathcote EJ, 2004: Prevention of hepatitis C virus–related hepatocellular carcinoma. Gastroenterology 127:S294-S302.

Ikeda K, et al, 1993: A multivariate analysis of risk factors for hepatocellular carcinogenesis: a prospective observation of 795 patients with viral and alcoholic cirrhosis. Hepatology 18:47-53.

Jee SH, et al, 2004: Cigarette smoking, alcohol drinking, hepatitis B, and risk for hepatocellular carcinoma in Korea. J Natl Cancer Inst 96:1851-1856.

Khan J, et al, 2001: Classification and diagnostic prediction of cancers using gene expression profiling and artificial neural networks. Nat Med 7:673-679.

Kudo M, et al, 2003: Prognostic staging system for hepatocellular carcinoma (CLIP score): its value and limitations, and a proposal for a new staging system, the Japan Integrated Staging Score (JIS score). J Gastroenterol 38:207-215.

Kuper H, et al, 2000: Tobacco smoking, alcohol consumption and their interaction in the causation of hepatocellular carcinoma. Int J Cancer 85:498-502.

Leung TW, et al, 2002: Construction of the Chinese University Prognostic Index for hepatocellular carcinoma and comparison with the TNM staging system, the Okuda staging system, and the Cancer of the Liver Italian Program staging system: a study based on 926 patients. Cancer 94:1760-1769.

Liaw YF, et al, 2004: Lamivudine for patients with chronic hepatitis B and advanced liver disease. N Engl J Med 351:1521-1531.

Llovet JM, Bruix J, 2003: Systematic review of randomized trials for unresectable hepatocellular carcinoma: chemoembolization improves survival. Hepatology 37:429-442.

Llovet JM, et al, 1999a: Prognosis of hepatocellular carcinoma: the BCLC staging classification. Semin Liver Dis 19:329-338.

Llovet JM, et al, 1999b: Intention-to-treat analysis of surgical treatment for early hepatocellular carcinoma: resection versus transplantation. Hepatology 30:1434-1440.

Lo CM, et al, 2002: Randomized controlled trial of transarterial lipiodol chemoembolization for unresectable hepatocellular carcinoma. Hepatology 35:1164-1171.

Lok AS, 2004: Prevention of hepatitis B virus–related hepatocellular carcinoma. Gastroenterology 127(5 suppl 1):S303-S309.

Marrero JA, et al, 2003: Des-gamma carboxyprothrombin can differentiate hepatocellular carcinoma from nonmalignant chronic liver disease in American patients. Hepatology 37:1114-1121.

Okuda K, et al, 1985: Natural history of hepatocellular carcinoma and prognosis in relation to treatment: study of 850 patients. Cancer 56:918-928.

Omagari K, et al, 2004: Preliminary analysis of a newly proposed prognostic scoring system (SLiDe score) for hepatocellular carcinoma. J Gastroenterol Hepatol 19:805-811.

Parkin DM, et al, 2001: Estimating the world cancer burden: Globocan 2000. Int J Cancer 94:153-156.

Perou CM, et al, 2000: Molecular portraits of human breast tumours. Nature 406:747-752.

Primack A, et al, 1975: A staging system for hepatocellular carcinoma: prognostic factors in Ugandan patients. Cancer 35:1357-1364.

Pugh RN, et al, 1973: Transection of the oesophagus for bleeding oesophageal varices. Br J Surg 60:646-649.

Puoti M, et al, 2004: Hepatocellular carcinoma in HIV-infected patients: epidemiological features, clinical presentation and outcome. AIDS 18:2285-2293.

Regimbeau JM, et al, 1999: Is surgery for large hepatocellular carcinoma justified? J Hepatol 31:1062-1068.

Regimbeau JM, et al, 2004: Obesity and diabetes as a risk factor for hepatocellular carcinoma. Liver Transpl 10(2 suppl 1):S69-73.

Rosenblatt KP, et al, 2004: Serum proteomics in cancer diagnosis and management. Annu Rev Med 55:97-112.

Ryu WS, 2003: Molecular aspects of hepatitis B viral infection and the viral carcinogenesis. J Biochem Mol Biol 36:138-143.

Sala M, et al, 2004a: Initial response to percutaneous ablation predicts survival in patients with hepatocellular carcinoma. Hepatology 40:1352-1360.

Sala M, et al, 2004b: Selection of candidates with HCC for transplantation in the MELD era. Liver Transpl 10(10 suppl 2):S4-S9.

Sangiovanni A, et al, 2004: Increased survival of cirrhotic patients with a hepatocellular carcinoma detected during surveillance. Gastroenterology 126:1005-1014.

Schoniger-Hekele M, et al, 2000: Hepatocellular carcinoma in Austria: aetiological and clinical characteristics at presentation. Eur J Gastroenterol Hepatol 12:941-948.

Sherman M, 2001: Alphafetoprotein: an obituary. J Hepatol 34:603-605.

Somiari RI, et al, 2003: High-throughput proteomic analysis of human infiltrating ductal carcinoma of the breast. Proteomics 3:1863-1873.

Sorensen JB, et al, 1993: Performance status assessment in cancer patients: an inter-observer variability study. Br J Cancer 67:773-775.

Stuart KE, et al, 1996: Hepatocellular carcinoma in the United States: prognostic features, treatment outcome, and survival. Cancer 77:2217-2222.

Sung YK, et al, 2003: Glypican-3 is overexpressed in human hepatocellular carcinoma. Cancer Sci 94:259-262.

Tanaka Y, et al, 1999: Sensitive measurement of serum abnormal prothrombin (PIVKA-II) as a marker of hepatocellular carcinoma. Hepatogastroenterology 46:2464-2468.

Tanaka Y, et al, 2002: A comparison of the molecular clock of hepatitis C virus in the United States and Japan predicts that hepatocellular carcinoma incidence in the United States will increase over the next two decades. Proc Natl Acad Sci U S A 99:15584-15589.

Trevisani F, et al, 2001: Serum alpha-fetoprotein for diagnosis of hepatocellular carcinoma in patients with chronic liver disease: influence of HBsAg and anti-HCV status. J Hepatol 34:570-575.

Van de Vijver MJ, et al, 2002: A gene-expression signature as a predictor of survival in breast cancer. N Engl J Med 347:1999-2009.

Vauthey JN, et al, 2002: Simplified staging for hepatocellular carcinoma. J Clin Oncol 20:1527-1536.

Villa E, et al, 2000: Natural history of inoperable hepatocellular carcinoma: estrogen receptors' status in the tumor is the strongest prognostic factor for survival. Hepatology 32:233-238.

Yanagisawa K, et al, 2003: Proteomic patterns of tumour subsets in non-small-cell lung cancer. Lancet 362:433-439.

Yoshida H, et al, 1999: Interferon therapy reduces the risk for hepatocellular carcinoma: national surveillance program of cirrhotic and noncirrhotic patients with chronic hepatitis C in Japan. IHIT Study Group. Inhibition of Hepatocarcinogenesis by Interferon Therapy. Ann Intern Med 131:174-181.

Hepatic Tumors in Childhood

72

M. P. LA QUAGLIA

An appreciation of hepatic segmental anatomy (see Ch. 1) has led to major advances in hepatic surgery, especially for tumors. In addition, the irresistible but still mysterious stimulus to hepatic regeneration has allowed larger and more extensive resections. Eighty-five percent of the liver can be removed safely in small infants, greatly increasing the scope for cure. There also have been advances in understanding tumor biology and clinical behavior. This chapter addresses benign and malignant tumors of the liver and biliary tract encountered in infancy, childhood, and adolescence.

HISTORY

Between 310 and 280 B.C., Herophilus and Erasistratus first presented a description of hepatic anatomy. In the late 1880s, hepatic resection was attempted, but advances in anesthesia and antisepsis would be required before a successful outcome could be realized. Wendel used avascular anatomic planes in the liver to perform a hepatic resection in 1910 (McClusky et al, 1997). Progress in hepatic surgery has been based on an appreciation of hepatic segmental anatomy as described by Couinaud (Bismuth, 1982; Couinaud, 1986, 1992) (see "Historical Perspective" at the beginning of this book). The distribution of the portal and hepatic veins delimits each hepatic segment, which has a unique portal vein and hepatic artery branch and bile duct. Knowledge of this anatomy allows control of the vascular structures before division of the hepatic parenchyma making major hepatic resections feasible (see Ch. 1). Bloodless hepatic dissection is crucial in infants and small children, who may have a total blood volume of less than 1 L. In the pediatric literature, Martin and Woodman (1969) reported that hepatoblastomas could be treated by hepatic lobectomy, and modern hepatic resection is soundly based on principles of segmental hepatic anatomy.

A second important historical finding was the sensitivity of some tumors, especially hepatoblastoma, to systemic chemotherapy (Fegiz et al, 1977). Chemotherapy caused significant reductions in tumor volume, and previously unresectable hepatoblastomas became resectable (Filler et al, 1991; Reynolds, 1995). Presently, the standard of practice is to administer neoadjuvant systemic chemotherapy to patients with hepatoblastoma, unless the tumor is clearly resectable at diagnosis.

In addition, there has been a greater appreciation of the biology of hepatic epithelial malignancies, especially the differences between hepatoblastoma and hepatocellular carcinoma (HCC). These differences include the relatively good prognosis of hepatoblastoma compared with HCC in childhood, the importance of complete surgical resection of the primary hepatic tumor, and the association of hepatoblastoma with certain clinical syndromes (Exelby et al, 1975; Koishi et al, 1996; Schneid et al, 1997; Simms et al, 1995; Tsai et al, 1996; Vaughan et al, 1995). Finally, the first application of hepatic transplantation to a childhood liver tumor was reported by Heimann and colleagues in 1987.

A series of pediatric liver tumor patients treated by hepatic transplantation was reported in 1992 (Tagge et al, 1992). There is continued interest in using this modality for unresectable hepatic malignancies in childhood and adolescence (Pichlmayr et al, 1995; Pinna et al, 1997; Superina & Bilik, 1996).

MALIGNANT TUMORS

The distribution of the most common malignant hepatic tumors is depicted in Fig. 72.1. Hepatoblastoma is the most common and is a success story in pediatric oncology.

Hepatoblastoma

Incidence

Primary malignant liver tumors constitute approximately 1.1% of childhood malignancies in Western nations. The overall incidence of primary liver cancer published by the Surveillance Epidemiology and End Results program (SEER) is 5 cases/1 million children in the 0- to 4-year age group, and 1 case/1 million in the 5- to 9-year, 10- to 14-year, and 14- to 19-year groups (National Cancer Institute, 1995). Liver cancers constitute 0.5% to 2% of all pediatric solid tumors and about 5% of abdominal tumors in childhood (Weinberg & Finegold, 1983). Hepatoblastomas are the most common primary hepatic tumors of childhood, constituting 43% to 64% of all hepatic neoplasms in one large series (Mann et al, 1990; Stocker, 1994; Weinberg & Finegold, 1983). Hepatoblastoma accounts for 91% of primary hepatic tumors in children younger than 5 years old (Darbari et al, 2003). Hepatoblastoma constitutes less than 1% of hepatic malignancies when adult age groups are included (Kaczynski et al, 1996). The Liver Cancer Study Group of Japan (1987)

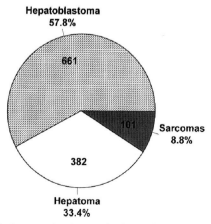

Fig. 72.1. The frequency distribution of malignant hepatic tumors in childhood as compiled from reported large series (Exelby et al, 1975; Weinberg & Finegold, 1983).

identified 30 hepatoblastomas (0.6%) in a cohort of 4658 patients of all ages diagnosed over a 2-year period. Hepatoblastoma affects 1 child younger than 15 years old in 1 million per year (Finegold, 1994). There are approximately 50 to 70 new cases per year in the United States with a male-to-female ratio of 1.7:1 (Lampkin et al, 1985). Although there are sporadic reports of hepatoblastoma in adults (Bortolasi et al, 1996; Harada et al, 1995; Inoue et al, 1995; Kacker et al, 1995; Parada et al, 1997), the median age at diagnosis is about 18 months, and most cases occur before age 2½ to 3 years (Exelby et al, 1975). In one study of more than 17,000 autopsies performed on newborns, only one small hepatic adenoma was identified (Werb et al, 1992). There are case reports, however, of congenital hepatoblastoma (Endo et al, 1996). Finally, the incidence of hepatoblastoma may be increasing (Blair & Birch, 1994). The incidence of hepatoblastoma was 0.6 per 1 million in the years 1973-1977 and increased to 1.2 per 1 million in 1993-1997 (Darbari et al, 2003).

Hepatoblastoma may occur in siblings (Fraumeni et al, 1969; Ito et al, 1987; Napoli & Campbell, 1977; Surendran et al, 1989). It is most strongly associated with familial polyposis (Giardiello et al, 1996; Iwama & Mishima, 1994), Gardner's syndrome (Hartley et al, 1990), and Beckwith-Wiedemann syndrome (Koishi et al, 1996; Tsai et al, 1996). In familial polyposis, there seems to be an increased incidence of hepatoblastoma in first-degree relatives of the patients with polyposis. Beckwith-Wiedemann syndrome is associated with Wilms' tumor, rhabdomyosarcoma, adrenocortical carcinoma, and hepatoblastoma. There also may be an association between hepatoblastoma and trisomy 18 (Bove et al, 1996).

Hepatoblastoma also is associated with low birth weight (Ikeda et al, 1997; Reynolds et al, 2004). It is unknown whether developmental abnormalities associated with prematurity or interventions, such as early total parenteral nutrition, are the causative agent. These tumors also are reported in patients with congenital anomalies, such as cleft palate, cardiovascular and renal anomalies including multicystic kidney, and absence of the right adrenal gland (Rao et al, 1989). There also are at least two reports of hepatoblastoma occurring in patients with biliary atresia (Taat et al, 2004). There is no evidence associating hepatoblastoma with hepatitis B or C infection or any other chronic viral hepatitis. These patients usually do not have cirrhosis or inborn errors of metabolism.

Pathology

The five histologic subtypes observed in hepatoblastoma are fetal, embryonal, mixed mesenchymal, macrotubular, and anaplastic or small cell. These subtypes are differentiated based on the findings with light microscopy. All tumor cells appear smaller than nonneoplastic hepatocytes. Extramedullary hematopoiesis is notably present and may be related to constitutive cytokine production by the tumor cells (von Schweinitz et al, 1995a). The fetal type grows in trabeculae and resembles fetal hepatic cells. Embryonic hepatoblastoma cells grow in noncohesive sheets and resemble embryonic cells. Some hepatoblastomas contain mesenchymal tissue along with the epithelial component. Calcification also may appear in these tumors, and there is one report of a patient with osteosarcomatous elements in the hepatoblastoma and associated pulmonary metastases (Alcantar, 1985).

Another subtype consists of small round blue cells that are reminiscent of neuroblastoma cells. This anaplastic or small cell variant is rare, but particularly virulent with a strong metastatic

potential (Dehner & Manivel, 1988). The importance of subtyping in hepatoblastoma is the association between prognostic risk and subtype illustrated in Fig. 72.2 (Gonzalez-Crussi et al, 1982; Lack et al, 1982). Some studies have indicated that the fetal histologic subtype has a better prognosis. In contrast, patients with the rare anaplastic variant usually do poorly (Dehner & Manivel, 1988).

Basic Biology

Few cellular models of hepatoblastoma exist, and immortalized cell lines have been difficult to establish. In one cell line, isolated from a human hepatoblastoma, growth factors that were required for maximal growth included 10% fetal bovine serum, insulin, transferrin, hydrocortisone, and epidermal growth factor (Manchester et al, 1995). This cell line clearly expressed the oncogenes c-myc and Ha-ras and epidermal growth factor receptor. Antibodies that blocked the epidermal growth factor receptor inhibited cell growth, but the significance of oncogene expression remains to be determined. In another study, elevated hepatocyte growth factor levels were found in the serum of 10 of 22 (45%) patients with hepatoblastoma. The hepatocyte growth factor receptor, c-met, was identified on the surface of the epithelial component of these tumors (von Schweinitz et al, 1997a). Addition of hepatocyte growth factor causes proliferation in hepatoblastoma-derived cell lines.

In more recent studies, small epithelial cells characteristic of hepatic stem cells have been observed in human hepatoblastomas of various subtypes (Ruck & Xiao, 2002). Also, chromosome 8q amplification is associated with a worsened prognosis and has been correlated with overexpression of the transcription factor, PLAG1, which transactivates the insulin-like growth factor (IGF)2-p3 promoter (Zatkova et al, 2004). Significantly, the demethylation of IGF2-p3 is associated with increased expression of IGF2 in nude mouse xenografts of the hepatoblastoma cell line, Hep T1 (Eriksson et al, 2001). Finally, telomerase and its regulatory protein (human telomerase reverse transcriptase) expression levels have been correlated with poor outcome in human hepatoblastoma (Hiyama et al, 2004). Tamoxifen may inhibit hepatoblastoma cells by reducing telomerase levels (Brandt et al, 2005).

The well-known thrombocytosis associated with untreated hepatoblastoma and the presence of extramedullary hematopoiesis in these tumors is fascinating. It was shown that hepatoblastoma

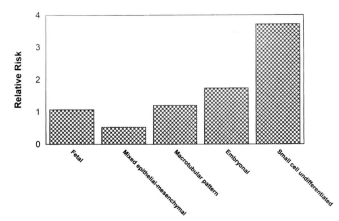

Fig. 72.2. Graph depicts the risk of death for patients with fetal histology hepatoblastoma adjusted for age, sex, and stage and compared with other histopathologic subtypes.

cells secrete interleukin-1β, and that this causes secretion of interleukin-6 from surrounding fibroblasts and endothelial cells (von Schweinitz et al, 1993). Other factors, such as erythropoietin and stem cell factor, have been localized to the cytoplasm of hepatoblastoma cells. Thrombopoietin has been identified in hepatoblastoma tissue and serum from a patient, but its correlation with the thrombocytosis associated with this neoplasm is unclear (Komura et al, 1998).

Loss of heterozygosity on chromosome 11p15.5 and 1p36 has been described in hepatoblastoma (Albrecht et al, 1994; Kraus et al, 1996). Investigations into both of these regions suggest that each may contain a tumor suppressor gene, but this has not been proved. Trisomy 20 and trisomy of all or part of chromosome 2 also have been reported (Swarts et al, 1996). The abnormality of the long arm of the second chromosome (2q) may provide a common genetic link between hepatoblastoma and rhabdomyosarcoma (Rodriguez et al, 1991). In another study that used comparative genomic hybridization to analyze 18 tumors from Europe and Japan, the most frequent genetic losses included regions 13q21-q22 (28%) and 9p22-pter (22%) (Gray et al, 2000). The most frequent gains of genetic material were on chromosomes 2q23-q23 (33%) and 1q24-q25 (28%).

Perhaps the most exciting new insight is the association between hepatoblastoma and familial adenomatous polyposis syndrome (Bala et al, 1997; Cetta et al, 1997). In one study of 13 hepatoblastomas obtained from non–familial adenomatous polyposis patients, 69% had mutations in the adenomatous polyposis coli (*APC*) gene (Oda et al, 1996). Li and coworkers (1987) suggested that hepatoblastoma is an associated feature of familial polyposis coli. In one case of siblings with hepatoblastoma, a shared *APC* gene mutation was identified (Thomas et al, 2003).

Clinical Findings

The most common presenting sign of hepatoblastoma is an asymptomatic abdominal mass. The child is often in good health, and the tumor usually is discovered incidentally when an attentive parent, grandparent, or clinician discovers the mass on a routine examination or while bathing the child (Fabre et al, 2004). Patients with the anaplastic variant of hepatoblastoma, who often have distant metastases at diagnosis, are more frequently symptomatic. Accompanying symptoms, such as pain, irritability, minor gastrointestinal disturbances, fever, and pallor, occur in smaller numbers of patients. Significant weight loss is unusual, although patients may fail to thrive. In most series of hepatoblastomas and HCCs, a few patients present acutely with tumor rupture and intraperitoneal hemorrhage (Brown et al, 1993). Rarely, hepatoblastoma manifests with sexual precocity (Muraji et al, 1985). There is one report of a hepatoblastoma patient presenting with a biliary fistula (Daniel & Kifle, 1989). Finally, hepatoblastoma may present as a cardiac tumor (Wang et al, 2003).

A mild anemia associated with a markedly elevated platelet count is observed in most patients at diagnosis. The platelet count can range into the millions. As noted previously, the cause is probably secondary to abnormal cytokine release.

Measurement of serum α-fetoprotein (AFP) is well established as an initial tumor marker in the diagnosis of hepatoblastoma and a means of monitoring the therapeutic response (Van Tornout et al, 1993). The normal level in most laboratories is less than 20 ng/mL, whereas the AFP level at diagnosis in hepatoblastoma patients can range from normal to 7.7×10^6 ng/mL. It is estimated that the AFP is elevated in 84% to 91% of patients with hepatoblastoma (Lack et al, 1982). One study reported a mean AFP level in hepatoblastoma of 3 million ng/mL. In comparison, the mean in pediatric patients with HCC was about 200,000 ng/mL (Ortega et al, 1991). In infants younger than 1 year of age, the AFP is normally elevated; it is highest at birth (Fig. 72.3).

Some authors suggest that subfractionation more reliably indicates whether the increased AFP is secondary to a hepatoblastoma or HCC, an endodermal sinus tumor, or benign liver disease (Tsuchida et al, 1997). The half-life of AFP is about 6 days, and in one study 24 of 31 (77%) patients had levels decline by at least 1 log before second-look surgery (Walhof et al, 1988). Sixteen of these 32 patients eventually had AFP levels decline to normal at the end of therapy and had no clinical or radiographic evidence of hepatoblastoma at this point. Finally, 15 of 16 (94%) patients who attained a complete response also showed a decline in AFP levels of 2 logs or more before second-look surgery (Van Tornout et al, 1997). A large early decline in AFP levels was an independent predictor of survival in multivariate analysis. It has been stated that a low initial AFP level is associated with worse

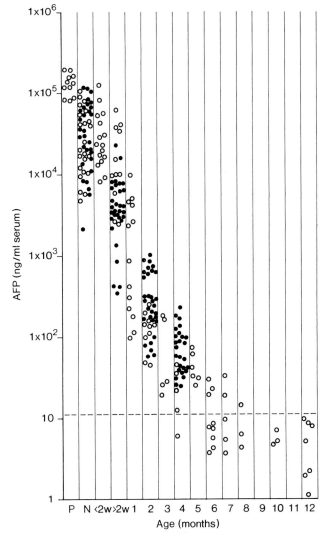

Fig. 72.3. Graph shows the time decay of AFP levels in normal infants during the first year of life.
Data from Wu JT, et al, 1981: Serum alpha fetoprotein (AFP) levels in normal infants. Pediatr Res 15:50-52.

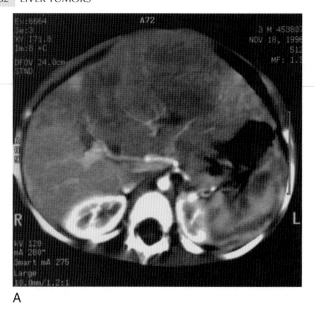
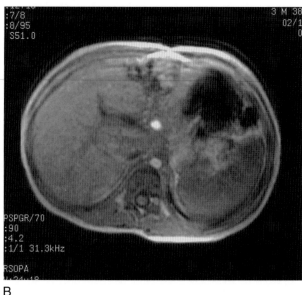

Fig. 72.4. A, CT of a patient with hepatoblastoma before induction chemotherapy. **B,** MRI of the same patient after four courses of vincristine, cisplatin, and 5-fluorouracil.

survival (von Schweinitz et al, 1995b), but this has not been confirmed in multivariate analysis (von Schweinitz et al, 1994a). Anaplastic hepatoblastomas may be associated with lower AFP levels, however (Tsunoda et al, 1996).

When interpreting the AFP level, it is important to realize that normal AFP levels are very high at birth and decrease over the first 6 months of life. Premature newborns may have AFP levels in the range of 100,000 ng/mL. Term newborns also can have relatively high levels (10^4-10^5 ng/mL). By age 2 months, most infants have levels ranging from 100 to 1000 ng/mL, and by age 6 months, levels should be less than 100 ng/mL. Usually, levels decrease to normal (<20 ng/mL) after 6 to 7 months, but may remain elevated for 1 year after birth (Ohama et al, 1997).

Imaging

The first imaging study is usually an abdominal ultrasound (see Ch. 15). If duplex technique is employed, tumor vascularity can be gauged, and the hepatic veins can be assessed (Bates et al, 1990). The ultrasonographer also should search for anomalies of the genitourinary system and rule out tumor thrombus in either the vena cava or the hepatic veins. Computed tomography (CT) (see Ch. 18) is useful to identify pulmonary metastases, identify diffuse hepatic involvement, and determine resectability. Oral and intravenous contrast material is used (Fig. 72.4A). CT scans can be performed quickly and completed in less than 2 minutes in helical scanners; this greatly shortens the required period of sedation for infants or small children. It has the added advantage of being a quick and reliable screening method for pulmonary metastases. CT angiography (CT portography) uses CT with fine cuts and an increased amount of intravenous contrast material to image hepatic tumors and the hepatic venous anatomy. CT portography may provide as much information as magnetic resonance imaging (MRI).

MRI (see Ch. 19) is useful for evaluating hepatic lesions and their relationship to vascular structures (see Fig. 72.4B). MRI can show the hepatic veins, the vena cava, and bile ducts (Ohnuma et al, 1991). MRI of a hepatoblastoma patient after neoadjuvant chemotherapy is shown in Fig. 72.4B.

Positron emission tomography has been used to identify hepatoblastoma recurrence and to search for sites of metastatic disease, but may not be reliable for lesions smaller than 6 to 10 mm (Wong et al, 2004).

Staging

Most studies to date have used the clinical grouping defined by the Children's Cancer Group and the Pediatric Oncology Group (Table 72.1). The impact of clinical group on relative risk of death from disease is shown in Fig. 72.5. More recently, the TNM classification has been used (Table 72.2) (Brower et al, 1998). A pretreatment extent of disease staging system has been used extensively by the International Society of Pediatric Oncology liver group, SIOPEL (Fig. 72.6) (Aronson et al, 2005). This PRETEXT system was compared with pathologic findings in 110 patients and was correct in 51%, overstaged in 37%, and understaged in 12%. The authors compared this system with the Children's Cancer Group/Pediatric Oncology Group and TNM schemes and claimed a better correlation with risk status. This finding may be debatable, but to allow closer comparison of results between SIOPEL and the Children's Oncology Group, all liver tumor patients in future Children's Oncology Group studies will undergo PRETEXT staging.

Table 72.1 Intergroup Liver Tumor Clinical Groups for Pediatric Epithelial Hepatic Malignancies

Clinical Group	Criteria
I	Complete resection as initial treatment
IIA	Complete resection after chemotherapy or irradiation
IIB	Residual disease confined to one lobe
III	Disease involving both lobes
IIIB	Regional nodes involved
IV	Distant parenchymal metastases (extent of primary tumor irrelevant)

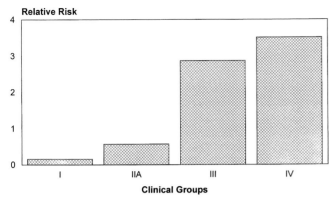

Relative Risk

Fig. 72.5. The relative risk of death for hepatoblastoma patients for each clinical group.

Treatment

Multiple studies support the effectiveness of systemic chemotherapy combined with complete surgical resection of the primary hepatic tumor (Gauthier et al, 1986; von Schweinitz et al, 1994a, 1994b, 1995b). Survival depends on removal of the primary liver tumor in most cases. Historically, the combination of doxorubicin and cisplatin was used with great success. Other regimens include vincristine, 5-fluorouracil, and cisplatin (Douglass et al, 1993) and ifosfamide, cisplatin, and doxorubicin (von Schweinitz et al, 1997b). The combination of cisplatin plus doxorubicin was compared with cisplatin plus 5-fluorouracil plus vincristine in a combined Children's Cancer Group/Pediatric Oncology Group (intergroup) study (Ortega et al, 2000). The efficacy was thought to be similar, but there were more complications with the doxorubicin-containing regimen accounting for equivalent event-free survivals. A more detailed review of the analysis suggested, however, that the doxorubicin-containing arm had an improved disease-specific survival. This finding implied that with better management of toxicity, patient outcome might be better with a doxorubicin-containing regimen. In addition, a clinical trial that used a combination of cisplatin and carboplatin had to be terminated because of poor tumor response, suggesting that platinum-based monotherapy as proposed by SIOPEL was not as effective as combination chemotherapy. At present, the

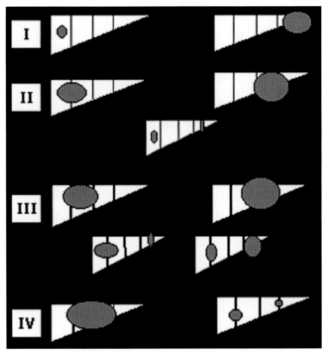

Fig. 72.6. The PRETEXT staging system as used by SIOPEL.
From Aronson DC, et al, 2005: Predictive value of the pretreatment extent of disease system in hepatoblastoma: results from the International Society of Pediatric Oncology Liver Tumor Study Group SIOPEL-1 study. J Clin Oncol 23:1245-1252.

recommendation for initial treatment of hepatoblastomas is with cisplatin, 5-fluorouracil, and vincristine. Doxorubicin frequently is added in high-risk patients. Clinical trials in the Children's Oncology Group and SIOPEL are planned to evaluate the use of doxorubicin, irinotecan, and other agents, especially in high-risk patients.

The first clinical decision is whether to initiate neoadjuvant chemotherapy or proceed with resection. Extensive tumors usually shrink with chemotherapy, facilitating resection, whereas chemotherapy might be lessened or avoided in some patients by resection at diagnosis. In one study, the rate of shrinkage was high after initiation of chemotherapy, but declined after two cycles had been administered (Fig. 72.7) (Medary et al, 1996). Exquisite clinical judgment and good communication between members of the multidisciplinary team are crucial. About 46% of hepatic malignancies are resectable at diagnosis (Ortega et al, 1991). Often, resection is not feasible if tumors are large and involve both hepatic lobes. Preoperative (neoadjuvant) chemotherapy results in tumor shrinkage and makes subsequent resection easier (Reynolds, 1995). To confirm the diagnosis, an initial biopsy is required. For unresectable tumors, the initial surgical procedure should include a diagnostic biopsy and placement of a vascular access device for chemotherapy. A second laparotomy is performed after four cycles of chemotherapy if imaging studies show a good response and the tumor appears resectable. Complete resection of the primary tumor is necessary for survival and may require extended hepatic lobectomies or complex biliary reconstructions. The patient should receive several cycles of chemotherapy after definitive resection. In hepatoblastoma, reports have suggested that gross total resection of the primary lesion may be adequate for cure in chemoresponsive tumors (Dicken et al, 2004; Schnater et al, 2002).

Table 72.2 TNM Staging for Hepatic Malignancies

Primary Tumor (T)

TX	Primary tumor cannot be assessed
T0	No evidence of primary tumor
T1	Solitary tumor without vascular invasion
T2	Solitary tumor with vascular invasion or multiple tumors none more than 5 cm
T3	Multiple tumors more than 5 cm or tumor involving a major branch of the portal or hepatic vein(s)
T4	Tumor(s) with direct invasion of adjacent organs other than the gallbladder or with perforation of visceral peritoneum

Stage Grouping

Stage I	T1	N0	M0
Stage II	T2	N0	M0
Stage IIIA	T3	N0	M0
IIIB	T4	N0	M0
IIIC	Any T	N1	M0
Stage IV	Any T	Any N	M1

From American Joint Committee on Cancer, 2002: AJCC Cancer Staging Manual, 6th ed.

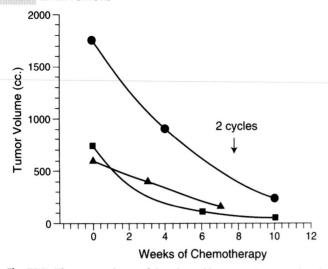

Fig. 72.7. The tumor volumes of three hepatoblastoma patients are plotted versus time from initiation of chemotherapy. There is a significant reduction in tumor volume that is most rapid during the first two cycles of induction chemotherapy.
(Data from Medary I, et al, 1996: Kinetics of primary tumor regression with chemotherapy: implications for the timing of surgery. Ann Surg Oncol 3:521-525.)

In one study, the 1-year survival for patients presenting with metastases was no different from patients with localized tumors (Van Tornout et al, 1997). In another study by SIOPEL, the 5-year overall and event-free survivals for children with hepatoblastoma who presented with pulmonary metastases were 57% and 28%, respectively (Perilongo et al, 2000). This study suggested that 25% to 30% of patients with synchronous pulmonary metastases are curable. It is still necessary to resect the primary liver tumor, and pulmonary metastasectomy should be done only if the primary site is controlled (Schnater et al, 2002). Many pulmonary metastases resolve with chemotherapy, but thoracotomy and resection sometimes are required for larger or persistent metastatic lesions (Passmore et al, 1995). Some radiation oncologists have treated pulmonary metastases with external-beam radiotherapy in an approach similar to that used for Wilms' tumors, but with 18 to 20 Gy administered (Habrand et al, 1992). Pulmonary radiation may be associated with significant pulmonary toxicity.

Outcome

Overall survival of 60% to 70% is achievable with non–stage IV hepatoblastoma except for the very aggressive small cell (anaplastic) variant. As noted earlier, approximately 50% of patients who present with pulmonary metastases are curable. If gross disease remains in the primary site, survival falls to zero. Some patients with microscopic residual tumor are curable with continued chemotherapy and may benefit from external-beam radiotherapy to the primary hepatic site. In multivariate analysis, factors that have been independent predictors of worsened prognosis include a high TNM stage, unresectable tumor, bilobar involvement and multifocality, AFP less than 100 ng/mL or greater than 10^5 ng/mL, distant metastases, embryonal versus fetal histology, and vascular invasion (von Schweinitz et al, 1997c). Resection of many hepatoblastomas may be easier after chemotherapy, and complete resection of the primary hepatic tumor is necessary for survival.

Future Directions

Advances in hepatic anatomy have allowed more extensive resections so that even very large and bilobar tumors can be removed

successfully. Segmental resection also is feasible and may allow resection of multifocal lesions. Hepatic transplantation for unresectable primary lesions can be effective for tumors confined to the liver (Achilleos et al, 1996; Superina & Bilik, 1996; Tagge et al, 1992). Table 72.3 summarizes reported series that used hepatic transplantation in the treatment of hepatoblastoma. Liver transplantation for hepatoblastoma has the best outcome when done as the primary procedure, rather than as a salvage procedure. Accurate preoperative assessment of resectability is mandatory. Cases with extensive extrahepatic extension or vascular invasion have had poor outcomes with total hepatectomy and hepatic transplantation.

Chemoembolization, which involves arteriographic injection of occluding thrombogenic materials (Angiostat collagen) combined with chemotherapeutic agents, such as cisplatin or doxorubicin, into the arterial circulation to the tumor (Malogolowkin et al, 1993), had shown initial promise, but is rarely used in clinical practice in children at present. Using this technique, the concentration of chemotherapeutic agents can be increased 50-fold to 100-fold in the embolized tumor. The average decrease in tumor size was 84% in one study (Clouse et al, 1994), and unresectable hepatoblastomas may become resectable with this intervention (Berthold et al, 1986). In a variation of this approach, some researchers have used superselective intra-arterial radiometabolic therapy for malignant hepatic tumors (Maini et al, 1996; Order et al, 1996). Other new approaches include treatment with anti-AFP antibodies, interleukin-2, and viral transfection vectors to attack malignant hepatic cells (Geiger, 1996; Huber & Richards, 1996; Ji & St, 1997; Ramani et al, 1997). Finally, a prospective study of patients with fetal histology tumors might refine further the role of adjuvant chemotherapy in this subtype.

Hepatocellular Carcinoma (Hepatoma)

Epidemiology

HCC (see Ch. 71) accounts for 23% of pediatric liver tumors, but is rare in infancy (Finegold, 1994). Approximately 1.4 cases per 1 million children exist in the United States (Ni et al, 1997). The Liver Cancer Study Group of Japan (1987) reported no cases in children age 4 years or younger in a series of 2286 patients with histologically reviewed tumors. Historical series without pathologic review may report a higher rate of infantile HCC owing to misdiagnosis of some early hepatoblastomas (Exelby et al, 1975). We have had personal experience of infants with well-documented HCC, however. HCC affects about 0.5 children younger than age 15 years per 1 million per year. SEER data indicate that HCC accounts for 87% of primary hepatic malignancies in the 15- to 19-year age group (Darbari et al, 2003). The incidence is bimodal with an early peak that is lower than that of hepatoblastoma. Most of these early cases occur before 5 years of age. A second peak occurs between 13 and 15 years of age. The median age at presentation of fibrolamellar carcinoma, a variant of HCC, is 20 years, and it is rarely observed before age 10 years. There is a male predominance (1.3-3.2:1) for HCC. In areas endemic for hepatitis B, the male-to-female ratio may be reversed at 0.2:1. Approximately 35 to 40 new HCCs are diagnosed per year in the pediatric age group in the United States. The incidence in the years 1973-1977 versus 1993-1997 decreased from 0.45 to 0.29 cases per 1 million (Darbari et al, 2003).

Hepatitis B and C infection correlates with the incidence of HCC. In Asia, 85% of these patients (adult and pediatric) are

Table 72.3 Reports of Hepatic Transplantation in the Treatment of Hepatoblastoma*

Reference	No. Transplanted	Overall Survival	Comment
Tiao et al, 2005	8—5 primary, 2 for gross residual after resection, 1 for liver failure after resection and chemotherapy	7	1 patient died 7 yr after liver transplant from post-transplant–related lymphoma
Urata et al, 2004	1 (living related)	1 (alive at 38 mo)	Transplant necessitated by complete portal vein obstruction
Otte et al, 2004	12 transplanted in SIOPEL—7 primary transplant, 5 rescue transplant	85% of primary at 10 yr; 40% of rescue at 10 yr	—
Otte et al, 2004 (literature review)	142 transplanted—106 primary transplant; 41 rescue transplant	82% of primary at 6 yr; 30% of rescue at 6 yr	—
Cillo et al, 2003	7 transplanted	56% at 5 yr	2 patients died of recurrent disease
Srinivasan et al, 2002	13 transplanted—12 primary transplant; 1 rescue transplant	All primary alive at mean of 33 mo (range 1-108 mo); 1 rescue died of respiratory failure 3 wk after transplant (NED)	—
Molmenti et al, 2002	9 transplanted	3 deaths, 1 recurrence	—
Reyes et al, 2002	12 transplanted	83% at 5 yr	—
Al-Qabandi et al, 1999	8 transplanted	5 NED at median 22 mo (range 2-78 mo); 2 died from recurrence, 1 from sepsis	3 whole, 5 reduced grafts
Lockwood et al, 1993	1 transplanted	NED at 36 mo	Carboplatin used
Tagge et al, 1992	6 transplanted	5 survivors	—
Koneru et al, 1991	12 transplanted	6 survivors; 3 died from tumor recurrence, and 3 died from other causes	Vascular invasion and anaplastic histology were adverse prognostic factors
Barton & Keller, 1989	1 transplanted	NED at 18 mo	Patient with Goldenhar's syndrome

*Transplantation can be effective in the treatment of hepatoblastoma when used in conjunction with multiagent chemotherapy. Salvage or secondary transplants are associated with a worse prognosis, suggesting that a rigorous assessment of resectability should be done before exploration.
NED, no evidence of disease.

hepatitis B surface antigen positive, whereas this is found in only 10% to 25% of patients in the United States. The relative risk for the development of HCC is 250:1 for patients with chronic active hepatitis compared with patients without hepatitis surface antigen positivity (Brower et al, 1998). Hepatitis C antibodies are found in 20% of patients with HCC. In one report, an infant with a history of neonatal hepatitis developed HCC (Moore L et al, 1997).

Other conditions associated with the development of HCC include cirrhosis, α_1-antitrypsin deficiency, tyrosinemia, aflatoxin ingestion, hemochromatosis, hepatic venous obstruction, androgen and estrogen exposure, Alagille syndrome (arteriohepatic dysplasia), and thorotrast administration (Wegmann et al, 1996). There is also a report of childhood HCC developing in a patient with neurofibromatosis (Ettinger & Freeman, 1979). A universal vaccination program against hepatitis B has reduced the incidence of HCC in Taiwan. The average annual incidence of HCC in children 6 to 14 years old declined from 0.70 per 100,000 children during 1981-1986 to 0.36 during 1990-1994 ($P<.01$) coincident with widespread administration of the hepatitis B vaccine (Chang et al, 1997). The mortality rate also decreased during this period. Antiviral therapy with lamivudine reduced the risk of development of HCC in patients with chronic hepatitis B infection and cirrhosis or fibrosis (Liaw et al, 2004).

In one comparative study of pediatric HCC and hepatoblastoma, numerous discriminating features were reported (Chan et al, 2002). The mean age at presentation was 18 months for hepatoblastoma versus 10 years for HCC. The initial resectability of HCC was 45% and did not improve with chemotherapy, whereas 91% of hepatoblastomas could be completely resected before or after chemotherapy. Tumor rupture occurred in 36% of hepatoblastomas versus 9% of HCCs. Most importantly, the survival of patients with HCC was much worse.

Pathology (see Ch. 69)
HCCs are highly invasive and often multicentric at diagnosis with frequent hemorrhage and necrosis. Nuclear pleomorphism, nucleolar prominence, and the absence of extramedullary hematopoiesis are observed, and the cells are larger than normal hepatocytes. Low-grade HCCs may look similar to normal hepatocytes, especially if a limited amount of tissue is sampled. Invasiveness, especially vascular invasion, is a hallmark of these tumors. Extrahepatic dissemination to portal lymph nodes, lungs, and bones is frequent at diagnosis and strongly affects survival. HCCs naturally progress from capsular invasion followed by extracapsular extension, then vascular invasion, and finally intrahepatic metastases (Toyosaka et al, 1996). There is a strong correlation between intrahepatic metastases and portal vein thrombosis; this suggests that efferent tumor vessels anastomose to the portal rather than the hepatic veins, allowing intrahepatic spread and explaining the multicentricity that is a hallmark of HCC. Fibrolamellar HCC is a histologic variant seen in older children and young adults. It has been thought that this variant was associated with a better prognosis (Greenberg & Filler, 1989). Studies indicate, however, that when stage is controlled for, the

survival is similar between standard HCC and its fibrolamellar variant.

Biology and Molecular Biology

Most investigations into the basic biology of HCC involve study of hepatitis B and its relationship to carcinogenesis (Scaglioni et al, 1996). In one in vivo model in which rats developed HCC after prolonged feeding with glyceryl trinitrate, K-*ras* point mutations were identified in 8 of 18 animals developing tumors (Tamano et al, 1996). There were no *p53* mutations. Cytogenetic data indicate that chromosomal abnormalities are complex, but no consistent patterns have been established (Terris et al, 1997).

Clinical Findings

Children and adolescents with HCC frequently present with palpable abdominal masses (40%), but many are symptomatic at diagnosis (Ni et al, 1997). Pain is frequent (38%) and may occur in the absence of an obvious mass. Constitutional disturbances, such as anorexia, malaise, nausea and vomiting, and significant weight loss, occur with greater frequency. Jaundice is an uncommon feature of either disease. AFP is elevated in approximately 85% of patients, with most levels greater than 1000 ng/mL (Brower et al, 1998). Although elevated, these levels are usually lower than levels measured in hepatoblastoma patients; 10% may present with tumor rupture and a hemoperitoneum (Brower et al, 1998).

Staging

The staging schemes listed for hepatoblastoma also are used for HCC in childhood.

Treatment

Long-term survival is impossible without complete resection. Because of a high incidence of multifocality within the liver, extra-hepatic extension to regional lymph nodes, vascular invasion, and distant metastases, complete resection is often impossible. Infiltration with thrombosis of portal and hepatic venous branches is common, and even the vena cava may be involved. Historically, the same chemotherapy protocols that were used for hepatoblastoma also were applied to HCCs in childhood. Cisplatin, in particular, has had activity against HCC (Bower et al, 1996). Because of

the poor survival of patients with HCC, present thinking is to apply new and innovative approaches to these cancers.

Unresectable HCCs can be palliated with embolization with or without added chemotherapeutic agents or radioisotopes (Maini et al, 1996). Percutaneous intralesional injection of ethanol also has been of palliative benefit when lesions are small (Ryu et al, 1997). Radiofrequency ablation of these tumors, percutaneously or at laparoscopy/laparotomy, has been associated with tumor resolution and prolonged survival (Inamori et al, 2004; Koda et al, 2004; Raut et al, 2005; Santambrogio et al, 2003). Lin and coworkers (2004) reported that radiofrequency ablation was superior to ethanol injection in HCCs that were 4 cm or less in diameter (see Ch. 76).

Outcome

The overall survival from HCC in childhood approaches zero, and it remains a therapeutic problem (Table 72.4). Occasionally, resection of localized lesions results in long-term survival. The trend is to separate HCC from hepatoblastoma in clinical studies because of its greatly differing biologic behavior.

Future Directions

Gene therapy with viral vectors that attack dividing cells is being investigated. Hepatocytes rarely divide unless stimulated by liver resection. Viruses, such as herpes, attack dividing cells and can be molecularly manipulated to contain cytotoxic genes. Modified herpesvirus can be transfected efficiently into hepatoma cells (Carew et al, 1998; Tung et al, 1996). One group has used an adenovirus vector to deliver murine endostatin to tumors in nude mice injected with HCC cells with a resultant reduction in tumor growth (Li et al, 2004).

Rhabdomyosarcoma of the Extrahepatic Bile Ducts

Incidence

Embryonal rhabdomyosarcoma of the extrahepatic bile ducts is rare. Ten cases were reported in the Intergroup Rhabdomyosarcoma Studies I and II, constituting 0.8% of confirmed tumors in those studies (Ruymann et al, 1985).

Table 72.4   Comparison of Resectability and Survival for Hepatoblastoma and Hepatocellular Carcinoma in Childhood

Reference	HEPATOBLASTOMA Resectability (%)	Survival (%)	HEPATOCELLULAR CARCINOMA Resectability (%)	Survival (%)
Exelby et al, 1975	60	35 overall; 60 in complete resection	34	13 overall; 35 in complete resection
Ehrlich et al, 1997	77	87	—	—
Stringer et al, 1995	90	67	—	—
Ni et al, 1997	—	—	9.8	10 (1 yr)
Hata, 1990	—	42	—	—
Ortega et al, 1991	48	67	13	21
Douglass et al, 1993	77 (group III)	90% groups I, II; 67% group III	—	—
von Schweinitz et al, 1995b	89	73	—	—
Moore SW, et al, 1997	—	—	33	16.6 (at 5 yr)
Weitman et al, 1997	—	0 progression-free survival at 2 yr	—	—
Lee & Ko, 1998	—	47% at 5 yr	—	17% at 5 yr
Chan et al, 2002	91	—	45	—
Ho et al, 2004	—	55% at 3 yr	—	0 at 3 yr

Pathology

Most tumors are of the embryonal histopathologic subtype. They often show botryoid characteristics similar to other rhabdomyosarcomas that arise in a hollow viscus. About 40% of patients develop distant metastases, but mortality is most often due to the effects of local invasion (Lack et al, 1981). Rhabdomyosarcoma of the liver, but not involving the bile ducts, also has been reported, but is very rare (Horowitz et al, 1987).

Presentation

Patients range in age from 1 to 9 years at diagnosis. The typical presentation includes intermittent jaundice and may include loss of appetite and episodes of cholangitis (Charcot's triad) (Perisic et al, 1991). Hepatomegaly and a palpable abdominal mass are usual (Lack et al, 1981; Nagaraj et al, 1977). The diagnosis may be confused with hepatitis with resultant delay in specific therapy. It also can be mistaken for a choledochal cyst (Sanz et al, 1997).

Imaging

Ultrasonography shows a hilar or intrahepatic mass that may be confused with a choledochal cyst (Friedburg et al, 1984; Geoffray et al, 1987). Although CT or MRI may provide information about extension and metastases (Ng et al, 1997), they do not establish the diagnosis. Imaging may be more accurate for extrahepatic ductal involvement (Roebuck et al, 1998).

Treatment

Surgical exploration and biopsy are necessary to establish the diagnosis in most cases. Often a hilar lymph node provides diagnostic material, but carefully sampling the primary tumor may be necessary. A core needle biopsy or aspiration cytology may be adequate for diagnosis. Entry into the bile ducts themselves should be avoided if possible. Intraoperative ultrasound (see Ch. 23) is helpful in identifying the course of biliary structures. Initial complete resection before chemotherapy may be difficult or impossible because of the extensive nature of these tumors. Also, microscopic submucosal extension is common, and resection margins are often microscopically positive despite the normal appearance of the intrahepatic bile ducts.

It is probably better to establish the diagnosis with a biopsy and begin systemic chemotherapy. Chemotherapy reduces the tumor size and allows a cleaner resection at second-look surgery. During the initial biopsy, hilar and left gastric lymph node sampling is performed to determine whether these nodal echelons require added radiotherapy. In the series reported from the Intergroup Rhabdomyosarcoma Study, 6 of the 10 patients underwent initial resection, but all had microscopic or minimal gross disease left behind (Ruymann et al, 1985). The only four survivors were in this group, however. None of the four patients in whom resection was not attempted survived. In another report of three consecutive cases from a single institution, all patients presented with jaundice, cachexia, and abdominal mass (Martinez-F et al, 1982). The tumor arose in the common hepatic duct in two children and the left hepatic duct in the third. The technical difficulty of prechemotherapy resection is illustrated by the fact that intrahepatic extension was noted in all, making complete resection impossible. Two of these patients are alive and disease-free at 9 months and 14 years, whereas the third died as a result of progressive disease at 33 months. All received radiotherapy in addition to multiagent chemotherapy. Jaundice was not a late problem.

The need for aggressive surgical resection of biliary rhabdomyosarcomas was challenged in a report by Spunt and associates (2000). They reported 25 patients with this diagnosis from Intergroup Rhabdomyosarcoma studies I through IV and noted that although only 29% of these patients underwent a gross total resection before or after multiagent chemotherapy, the overall 5-year survival rate was 78%. They concluded that surgery was important for diagnosis and staging, but was not necessary for long-term survival with present chemotherapeutic agents. They also noted that the use of biliary drains in patients undergoing aggressive surgery was associated with a high rate of serious infections.

The surgical approach is a bile duct resection, and a Roux-en-Y jejunostomy is the favored reconstruction. Intraoperative cholangiography is recommended to ensure adequate bile drainage. The 4 of these 10 patients who survived were alive and disease-free 6 months to 6 1/2 years from diagnosis.

Future Directions

Presently, the need for radiation or even surgical resection has been questioned. In the future, some of these patients may be treated by chemotherapy alone after establishment of the diagnosis. If a complete radiologic response is documented after neoadjuvant chemotherapy, no further intervention except observation may be needed. This requires further study. Embryonal rhabdomyosarcoma of the extrahepatic bile ducts is rare, is locally invasive, and requires multidisciplinary treatment. Initial biopsy followed by chemotherapy and resection at a second-look procedure is the standard course.

Embryonal Sarcoma

Incidence

Embryonal sarcoma (malignant mesenchymoma or undifferentiated sarcoma in the older literature) is a rare primary hepatic neoplasm that occurs in older children. In one study, there were 2 cases out of 1102 (0.2%) primary liver tumors analyzed (Flemming et al, 1995). The age at diagnosis ranges from 5 to 16 years (Newman et al, 1989; Vetter et al, 1989). Embryonal sarcoma constitutes 14% of malignant liver tumors occurring in children 6 to 10 years old (Yedibela et al, 2000).

Pathology

Microscopically, these tumors appear as a pleomorphic or undifferentiated sarcoma. There may be areas of entrapped liver. Primitive mesenchymal cells with occasional small cysts and ducts lined with benign-appearing epithelium are sometimes present at the periphery (Gallivan et al, 1983). Some reports have suggested that embryonal sarcoma of the liver may represent malignant degeneration of a mesenchymal hamartoma (Begueret et al, 2001; O'Sullivan et al, 2001).

Clinical Presentation

A right upper quadrant abdominal mass and pain are significant presenting symptoms. Fever also may be prominent. Spontaneous rupture was reported in a woman (Yedibela et al, 2000).

Imaging

These malignancies often appear hypodense (dark) on CT and have a bright peripheral fibrous pseudocapsule. A case is shown in Fig. 72.8. They can be very bulky tumors and sometimes are confused with cystic liver disease (Orozco et al, 1991; Tozzi et al, 1992). These tumors may have the appearance of a solitary liver

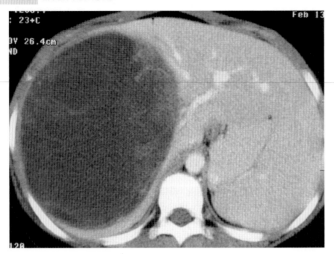

Fig. 72.8. CT showing the radiologic characteristics of malignant mesenchymoma.

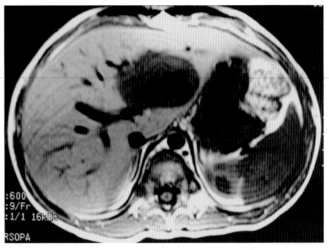

Fig. 72.9. Leiomyosarcoma of the liver in a patient with acquired immuno-deficiency syndrome (CT scan).

cyst in childhood (Chowdhary et al, 2004) or mimic a hydatid cyst (Aggarwal et al, 2001).

Treatment and Outcome

Embryonal sarcomas of the liver are treated with resection and adjuvant chemotherapy (Kadomatsu et al, 1992). Cisplatin, doxorubicin, cyclophosphamide, dacarbazine, actinomycin, and other agents have been used in combination with radiotherapy (Newman et al, 1989; Vetter et al, 1989). Complete surgical resection should be attempted and usually requires a hepatic lobectomy for tumor clearance. Although past reports have cited a poor prognosis, we have seen long-term survival with a combination of modern multiagent chemotherapy and complete resection.

Leiomyosarcoma

Patients with human immunodeficiency virus (HIV) infection are experiencing an increasing incidence of smooth muscle tumors (Norton et al, 1997; Ross et al, 1992). Leiomyosarcoma of the liver has been reported in more than 20 patients; the youngest was 9 years old. Adjuvant therapy is ineffective, and these tumors must be resected for control. They tend to be low grade or have an indeterminate malignant potential. Supportive and antiretroviral therapy is given through the perioperative period. A case of HIV-associated leiomyosarcoma is shown in Fig. 72.9.

Primary Hepatic Rhabdoid Tumor

Incidence

Rhabdoid tumors are very rare, highly malignant, sarcoma-like neoplasms that usually involve the kidney or central nervous system (Vujanic et al, 1996). It can be primary in extrarenal sites, including extremity, paraspinal, and cervical soft tissues and the liver (Honda et al, 1996; Jimenez-Heffernan et al, 1998; Kelly et al, 1998).

Pathology

Histopathologic examination shows a high-grade round cell neoplasm with abundant cytoplasm and containing cells with cytoplasmic filamentous inclusions (White et al, 1999). The cells are frequently positive for vimentin and epithelial antigens. Cytogenetic abnormalities on chromosome 22 are nonrandom and may have significance.

Imaging

There are no distinct radiologic features.

Clinical Presentation

The diagnosis may be suspected if widespread metastases, including central nervous system dissemination, are found with a hepatic mass. One case with spontaneous rupture has been reported (Kelly et al, 1998).

Treatment

These tumors are highly resistant to treatment. Disease confined to the liver should be resected if possible. Treatment with dose-intense, antisarcoma-type chemotherapy is warranted.

Outcome

Although an initial period of control is feasible, these tumors are likely to recur and metastasize.

Angiosarcoma

Some authors describe angiosarcoma as the malignant form of hemangioendothelioma in children (Falk et al, 1981; Noronha & Gonzalez-Crussi, 1984). Arsenic exposure has been associated with malignant progression from hemangioendothelioma to hemangiosarcoma (Falk et al, 1981). In one report of 10 cases of hepatic angiosarcoma in childhood, 6 patients were female and 4 were male (Selby et al, 1992). The median age at diagnosis was 3.7 years (range 1.5-7 years). Histologically, hypercellular whorls of spindled sarcoma cells are observed interspersed with bile ducts, blood vessels, and collagen. Intracellular periodic acid–Schiff–positive globules are present in most cases, and focal factor VIII staining may be seen. Six of seven patients with follow-up died from disease with a mean follow-up of 10 months. Complete resection is required for cure, but there is a high rate of recurrence, and consideration should be given to adjuvant chemotherapy.

Malignant Germ Cell Tumors

Primary malignant germ cell tumors of the liver are very rare and may present as teratomas, choriocarcinomas, or yolk sac tumors (Theegarten et al, 1998). In childhood, these may respond well to neoadjuvant chemotherapy followed by resection. Usually, a regimen containing cisplatin, ifosfamide, and bleomycin is employed.

Primary Hepatic Non-Hodgkin Lymphoma

Primary non-Hodgkin lymphoma of the liver occurs in childhood and may compose 5% of primary hepatic malignancies in this age group (Gururangan et al, 1992). Burkitt's and other types of small cell noncleaved lymphoma have been reported (Huang et al, 1997; Mills 1988). The primary treatment of lymphoma in childhood is chemotherapy, which usually results in complete resolution of the hepatic mass. Resection is rarely, if ever, indicated.

Hepatic Metastases

The liver is a relatively frequent site of metastatic disease in childhood. Non-Hodgkin lymphoma, neuroblastoma, rhabdomyosarcoma, rhabdoid tumors, Wilms' tumor, desmoplastic small round cell tumor, adrenal cortical carcinoma, osteogenic sarcomas, and a host of other malignancies may metastasize to the liver. There are few data to determine the correct surgical approach to these lesions. Criteria for surgical removal of hepatic metastases include control of the primary site, a solitary or limited number of metastases, good performance status, and a reasonable expectation of prolonged survival or cure. A helpful finding is some response of the metastatic lesions to adjuvant chemotherapy. MRI is helpful in the diagnosis and evaluation of hepatic metastases. We have had experience with 11 patients (age range 4.3-21 years) who underwent hepatic metastasectomy. The overall survival in this group was 20%, but local hepatic control was greater than 85%.

Neuroblastoma
Hepatic metastases from neuroblastoma are relatively uncommon except in newborns and infants with stage 4S disease. In this situation, the liver involvement is a hallmark of the disease (Komuro et al, 1998). In stage 4S, hepatic tumors generally resolve, although they may increase alarmingly in size before this happens. The increase in size usually causes pulmonary and vena caval impairment and may require relief by placement of an abdominal silo similar to that used for congenital abdominal wall defects.

Wilms' Tumor
Wilms' tumor metastasizes to the liver in about 12% of cases (Cohen & Siddiqui, 1982), and this usually is associated with unfavorable histology (Breslow et al, 1986; Thomas et al, 1991). Resection of localized residual disease may be beneficial in well-selected cases. In one report, four cases of Wilms' tumor with metastases to the liver underwent hepatic resection with 80% 2-year survival. Two patients survived 14 and 17 years (Morrow et al, 1982). This experience also is noted in other reports of Wilms' tumor (Hagiwara et al, 1982).

Osteogenic Sarcoma
Calcified hepatic metastases sometimes are observed in patients with osteogenic sarcoma (Shapiro et al, 1988). There are no reports defining the role of liver resection when this is encountered.

Desmoplastic Small Round Cell Tumor
Hepatic involvement with desmoplastic small round cell tumor is frequent and usually associated with a fatal outcome (Kushner et al, 1996; Mazuryk et al, 1998; Ordonez, 1998). The pattern of metastases is diffuse leaving no spared segments that would allow resection. Complete resection is associated with a significant survival advantage in this disease (Schwarz et al, 1998). Future strategies include chemoembolization and arterial infusion therapy. Hepatic radiation to a level of 3000 cGy is ineffective.

Rhabdomyosarcoma
The liver follows regional lung, lymph nodes, and bone as a site of rhabdomyosarcoma metastases (Shimada et al, 1987). Resection of liver metastases is usually not feasible because of diffuse hepatic involvement and the presence of metastases in other sites.

Colon Cancer
Colon cancer can occur in childhood (LaQuaglia et al, 1992). About 50% of these patients have signet ring tumors. The pattern of spread is over peritoneal surfaces, rather than through the portal system, and hepatic metastases usually occur late despite massive peritoneal disease.

Malignant Peripheral Nerve Cell Tumor
Malignant peripheral nerve cell tumors are likely to metastasize to the liver in childhood and adolescence. The pattern of metastases is usually miliary, and the tumors do not respond well to chemotherapy (Probst-Cousin et al, 1997).

Adrenocortical Carcinoma
Adrenocortical carcinoma also may metastasize to the liver, although concomitant pulmonary and retroperitoneal metastases are usually present as well (Arico et al, 1992). Treatment is usually platinum-based chemotherapy, and surgery is rarely done.

Rhabdoid Tumor
Rhabdoid tumor most commonly originates from the kidney and can metastasize to liver (White et al, 1999). It also may be primary to the liver, but this is rare. The pattern for hepatic metastases is usually diffuse and not amenable to surgical resection. Chemotherapy protocols suitable for sarcoma are usually employed (Vujanic et al, 1996).

Hepatic Evaluation and Resection

Surgical Anatomy
The schema of hepatic anatomy most useful for the surgeon is based on the work of Couinaud; this is described in other chapters. The principles of hepatic resection in small children and infants are the same as those for adults (see Ch. 80).

Hepatic Regeneration
The liver in a child is able to regenerate quickly, even after massive resections (see Ch. 4) and administration of systemic

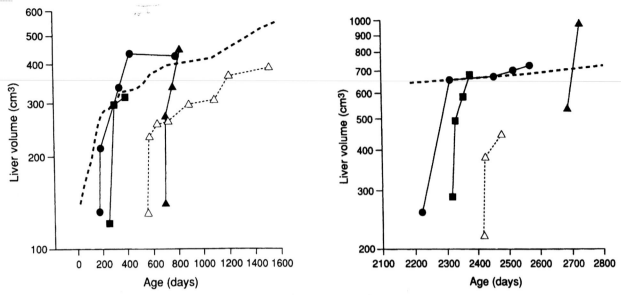

Fig. 72.10. Graphs show the rapid recovery of hepatic volume to normal levels for age after major resections in childhood. The graphs show regeneration in two different age groups.
(Data from Wheatley JM, et al, 1996: Liver regeneration in children after major hepatectomy for malignancy—evaluation using a computer-aided technique of volume measurement. J Surg Res 61:183-189.)

chemotherapy (Shamberger et al, 1996; Wheatley et al, 1996). In most patients, there is a rapid recovery to the normal volume for age (Fig. 72.10).

EVALUATION OF A CHILD WITH A HEPATIC MASS

Patients presenting with a suspected hepatic mass first undergo a history and physical examination. Blood work should include a complete blood count, liver function tests, coagulation studies, and tumor markers. Tumor markers include a serum AFP and β-human chorionic gonadotropin. Doppler ultrasound is done to determine whether a mass is cystic or solid, determine the patency of the portal and hepatic veins and vena cava, and identify satellite lesions. At present, MRI provides the greatest amount of information concerning the lesion and surrounding veins and bile ducts. CT portography has been shown to give anatomic information equal to MRI. If a malignant tumor is suspected, thoracic CT is done to identify metastases. A tissue diagnosis is mandatory if malignancy is suspected after the workup. Percutaneous needle core or aspiration biopsy is useful for hepatoblastomas, but may not be definitive in the case of HCC. Open or laparoscopic biopsy is acceptable if necessary. The surgeon must do a thorough diagnostic workup and determine resectability before exploration. Often a team approach with a pediatric surgeon and an experienced hepatobiliary surgeon is helpful.

BENIGN HEPATIC TUMORS

Benign hepatic tumors (see Ch. 70) accounted for less than 35% of 1250 pediatric liver tumors in one study (Finegold, 1994). Benign tumors of the liver that occur in childhood include hemangiomata or vascular malformations, hepatocytic adenomas, focal nodular hyperplasia, mesenchymal hamartomas, and various types of cysts or cystic disease. The distribution of common benign hepatic tumors of childhood is illustrated in Fig. 72.11.

Hemangiomata or Vascular Malformations

Hemangiomata are lesions characterized by endothelial-lined vascular spaces that vary in size and extent (Ehren et al, 1983; Ishak, 1976). They sometimes are classified as hamartomas and are the most common skin lesions observed in childhood. Hemangioendotheliomas are highly proliferative cellular lesions of variable malignant potential. In contrast, venous malformations and cavernous hemangiomata are distinguished by a lack of cellularity and large vascular spaces. Arteriovenous malformations are the rarest pathologic subtype and are distinguished by abnormal anastomoses between arteries and veins. Venous malformations, cavernous hemangiomata, and arteriovenous malformations may be associated with significant shunting that results in congestive heart failure.

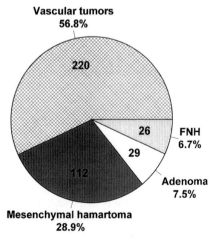

Fig. 72.11. The frequency distribution of benign hepatic tumors in childhood (Exelby et al, 1975; Weinberg & Finegold, 1983). This graph is based on surgical or pathologic series of patients. With modern imaging techniques, the frequency of asymptomatic vascular tumors that are discovered incidentally is undoubtedly much higher (Flemming et al, 1995). FNH, focal nodular hyperplasia.

Incidence

The overall incidence of endothelial-lined vascular tumors of the liver in childhood is probably unknown because many are asymptomatic. Vascular lesions taken together represent 13% to 18% of symptomatic hepatic tumors in childhood (Exelby et al, 1975; Finegold, 1994). Hepatic hemangiomata are more common in girls by 2:1 (Mulliken, 1988).

Presentation and Diagnosis

An abdominal mass is probably the most frequent sign of a vascular tumor of the liver. Multiple hemispheric cutaneous hemangiomata may be present and warn the physician of possible visceral lesions. A systolic bruit sometimes can be heard over the enlarged liver. Infants with large, actively perfused vascular lesions may present with congestive heart failure. Rarely, jaundice, disseminated intravascular coagulation, or hemorrhagic shock from intraperitoneal rupture may be present. Rupture can be precipitated by percutaneous needle biopsy (Hobbs, 1990). Imaging studies are usually all that is required to confirm the diagnosis. Tumor extent and tissue characterization are assessed using MRI with standard spin echo T1-weighted and T2-weighted imaging (Powers et al, 1994). Intravenous administration of gadopentetate dimeglumine (gadolinium) can produce greater resolution. Vascular lesions can be seen as intensely white on T2-weighted images, and this study is often accurate enough to be definitive. Arteriography rarely is indicated given the detail and accuracy of modern imaging techniques. Open biopsy can result in massive hemorrhage.

Treatment

Asymptomatic lesions do not require treatment, and many hepatic hemangiomata regress after the first year of life. Patients with congestive heart failure are admitted to the intensive care unit and treated with digitalis and furosemide. If the heart failure remains refractory to these maneuvers, hepatic artery embolization or direct surgical ligation may be necessary (de Lorimier et al, 1967; Herlin et al, 1988). Hepatic arterial embolization may be successful in controlling symptoms, but rapid development of collateral vessels can make subsequent resection or embolization difficult. Transfusion of blood and platelets may be required for disseminated intravascular coagulation. Interferon alfa therapy for symptomatic angiomatosis and hemangioendothelioma is being used with success in individual patients (Le Luyer et al, 2000).

Patients who present with rupture of a vascular tumor and hemorrhagic shock usually require hepatic resection. Initial hepatic arterial embolization may control bleeding temporarily and allow stabilization and safer surgery (Takvorian et al, 1988). Hepatic resection also may be required in some cases associated with congestive heart failure. Blood loss in these complicated procedures may be reduced using hemodilution techniques (Kitahara et al, 1995; Schaller et al, 1984).

Outcome

The overall prognosis for benign hepatic vascular lesions is good. Most patients do not require operative intervention, and most cellular lesions start to regress after the first year of life. Angiosarcomatous degeneration of benign hemangioendotheliomas has been reported in five patients from one institution (Weinberg & Finegold, 1983). Three of the five were treated with radiotherapy to the benign hemangioendotheliomas before the development of angiosarcoma. This and other reports from the literature have correlated radiotherapy of benign vascular tumors

with subsequent malignant degeneration, usually to angiosarcoma (Costello & Seywright, 1990).

Hemangioendothelioma

In one report of 16 infants and children, 15 presented with hepatomegaly, 7 with congestive heart failure, and 4 with associated cutaneous lesions (Holcomb et al, 1988). The Kasabach-Merrit syndrome, a platelet-trapping coagulopathy, also has been observed (von Schweinitz et al, 1995c). These lesions may appear very cellular, but do not metastasize. If a primary lesion produces symptoms, resection is indicated for relief.

Hemangioblastoma

Hemangioblastoma of the liver usually is associated with von Hippel–Lindau disease (Rojiani et al, 1991). In infancy and childhood, these lesions appear very cellular, but distant metastases are uncommon. Complete resection should be performed and is usually curative. Hemangioblastomas of the central nervous system and retina have been treated with interferon alfa-2a, but without striking resolution, although two retinal lesions showed shrinkage (Niemela et al, 2001).

Mesenchymal Hamartoma

Mesenchymal hamartomas are usually solitary hepatic masses occurring in infants. They are usually multicystic, and the cysts are lined with flattened biliary epithelium or endothelium. There is abundant and actively growing mesenchyme associated with distended lymphatics. It is postulated that mesenchymal hamartomas arise in areas of focal intrahepatic biliary atresia; this results in distal bile duct obstruction and hepatocellular necrosis (Cooper et al, 1989). Others have hypothesized that these lesions arise in conjunction with anomalies of vascular development. This explains the occurrence of small hemangiomata that are observed in close proximity to mesenchymal hamartomas (Srouji et al, 1978). Cytogenetic analysis has only rarely been performed on these tumors, but a consistent 19q13.4 breakpoint has been identified (Mascarello & Krous, 1992).

Epidemiology

Mesenchymal hamartomas account for 6% of primary liver tumors in childhood, and there is a male predominance. In one study, 4 of 134 patients with space-occupying liver lesions had mesenchymal hamartomas (Yen et al, 2003). Two thirds of these tumors are diagnosed in infants younger than 1 year of age, although presentation in the teenage years has been described. In one study of 18 such tumors, the mean age at diagnosis was 16 months (DeMaioribus et al, 1990).

Presentation and Diagnosis

Most mesenchymal hamartomas present as an enlarging abdominal mass or hepatomegaly and are usually not otherwise symptomatic (Srouji et al, 1978). They can grow to great size causing respiratory distress or evidence of caval obstruction. Ultrasound, CT, and MRI are the most useful diagnostic studies. Fig. 72.12 shows MRI of a huge mesenchymal hamartoma. Often an open biopsy is necessary to make the diagnosis. Giant hepatic cysts

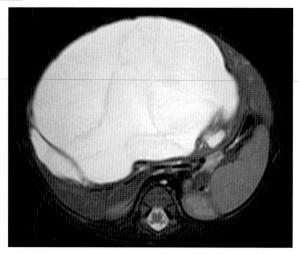

Fig. 72.12. T2-weighted MRI of a massive mesenchymal hamartoma.

in fetuses also have been diagnosed on ultrasound (Tsao et al, 2002).

Treatment

Anatomic resection (hepatic lobectomy) is effective treatment, especially for large lesions. Because of the mesenchymal component, these lesions have a definite capsule that facilitates enucleation of large central mesenchymal hamartomas that are not amenable to lobectomy. Enucleation was done in the case illustrated in Fig. 72.12. Occasionally, it is necessary to marsupialize a large cystic lesion, but only if it is not feasible to remove this lesion completely. This approach may not be successful (Meinders et al, 1998). One report using sequential CT scans documented initial expansion followed by involution of a mesenchymal hamartoma (Barnhart et al, 1997). It has been postulated that in utero decompression of giant hepatic cysts would improve the outcome in these patients (Tsao et al, 2002).

Outcome

These patients do well with all forms of therapy. In one study of 18 patients, 13 who were available for follow-up were alive and well 1 month to 24 years after treatment (mean 5 years) (DeMaioribus et al, 1990).

Focal Nodular Hyperplasia and Hepatocellular Adenoma

Focal nodular hyperplasia and hepatocytic adenomas are benign hepatocellular proliferations that are more common in adults than in children (see Ch. 70). Hepatic adenomas are expected with type I glycogen storage disease after the first decade of life and may be multiple (Saito et al, 1984). Focal nodular hyperplasia also has been described in a patient with type I glycogen storage disease (Sakatoku et al, 1996). Hepatic adenomas also have grown in patients undergoing androgen therapy for hematologic disorders, after danazol use, and in woman on oral contraceptives (Fermand et al, 1990). Both tumors have been correlated with a high estrogen environment (Sakatoku et al, 1996). There is also a report of focal nodular hyperplasia developing in children treated for other solid malignancies (Bouyn et al, 2003). These authors postulated that a vascular injury secondary to chemotherapy or radiation was the causal factor. Focal nodular

hyperplasia is distinguished from adenoma by the presence of fibrous septa that contain bile ducts and an inflammatory infiltrate. In one report, 5 of 39 unresected hepatic adenomas developed HCC (Foster & Berman, 1994).

Epidemiology

Less than 2% of hepatic tumors in childhood are focal nodular hyperplasia or hepatocellular adenomas (Weinberg & Finegold, 1983). Both lesions have been described in infants and teenagers. Most patients are younger than 5 years of age at presentation, and there is a female predominance (Nagorney, 1995). There is an association with contraceptive use in adults, but no defined association between exogenous hormone administration in childhood and adolescence. Focal nodular hyperplasia has been reported in an infant antenatally exposed to corticosteroids (Prasad et al, 1995). In one report of 48 benign liver tumors in childhood, there were three cases (6%) of focal nodular hyperplasia and two cases of hepatocellular adenoma (4%) (Ehren et al, 1983).

Presentation and Diagnosis

These patients usually present with an asymptomatic abdominal mass. Hepatocellular adenomas are more likely to be symptomatic and may present with rupture and resultant hemorrhage causing an acute abdomen. Both lesions are well encapsulated on imaging studies. Because focal nodular hyperplasia is associated with fibrous septa, abdominal ultrasound and CT may show a distinctive central "scar." Hepatic adenomas may show encapsulation on imaging studies, but histologic sections may be difficult to distinguish from HCC. In childhood, these tumors may attain great size, contributing to symptoms. In one report of six cases in childhood, the average tumor size was 7.5 cm (range 2.5-10 cm) (Lack & Ornvold, 1986). The tumor was localized to the right lobe in four of the six and was bilobar in the remaining two. Superparamagnetic oxide–enhanced MRI may discriminate between hepatic adenoma and focal nodular hyperplasia (Beets-Tan et al, 1998).

Treatment

It is best to remove adenomas because of the difficulty of differentiating them from low-grade HCCs, uncertainty about future malignant degeneration, and the possibility of rupture and hemorrhage (Westaby et al, 1983). Resection also results in relief of preoperative symptoms (Hutton et al, 1993). An anatomic liver resection usually is required, and we have employed extended left hepatectomy successfully in children to treat this lesion (Glick et al, 2000). Laparoscopic resection of these lesions also has been done (Marks et al, 1998; Samama et al, 1998). Embolization of unresectable lesions is an option if they are large or symptomatic. Unresectable and asymptomatic cases of focal nodular hyperplasia are observed using serial abdominal ultrasound, MRI, and clinical examination.

Outcome

Most patients do well after hepatic resection. In one study of six patients with focal nodular hyperplasia and two with an adenoma, there were six long-term survivors (Lack & Ornvold, 1986). Three patients with focal nodular hyperplasia were alive 4 to 17 years after hepatic lobectomy. Two other patients were followed with observation alone and were alive and well 13 and 15 years later. The one death in this group was from leukemia with an incidental finding of focal nodular hyperplasia. One of the two patients with an adenoma survived for 10.5 years after lobectomy, whereas the second died as a result of postoperative hemorrhage. In general, anatomic resection is preferable.

Cysts and Cystic Disease

Solitary Cysts

There are multiple case reports of solitary, congenital, nonparasitic liver cysts in childhood (Hernandez-Siverio et al, 1988; Pul & Pul, 1995). They are extremely rare, but have been increasingly noted as incidental findings on ultrasound or CT performed for other reasons. Cysts are simple and not multilocular, they often have a bluish appearance at laparotomy, and the wall usually has three layers. The lining is generally cuboidal or columnar, although mucinous or squamous epithelium is reported. The middle layer comprises vascular elements, and the outer layer comprises compressed hepatocytes, collagen, muscle fibers, and bile ducts (Jones, 1994). The central contents are straw-colored and clear and are not under high pressure, as is the case with parasitic cysts. Most of these cysts are located in the right, anteroinferior hepatic lobe (segment V), and occasionally they are pedunculated.

Most solitary cysts are asymptomatic and do not require therapy. Older patients sometimes complain of abdominal pain or sensation of fullness. Rarely, a large cyst ruptures, and torsion of a pedunculated cyst has been reported. Nine percent of solitary cysts may be associated with extrahepatic biliary obstruction and jaundice secondary to external bile duct compression by the cyst. These cysts do not affect longevity, and malignant degeneration has not been reported. This must be considered when planning therapy. Solitary, asymptomatic cysts do not require therapy. If the cyst is symptomatic, simple percutaneous aspiration usually is followed by recurrence, but aspiration followed by ethanol injection (sclerotherapy) may be an effective treatment. More commonly, operative intervention is required. Preoperative MRI or Doppler ultrasound is necessary to determine proximity to the portal and hepatic veins. Cysts that are neither adherent nor in proximity to these vascular structures are excised. Hepatic lobectomy may be necessary for symptomatic cysts that adhere to major veins. Occasionally, marsupialization is a viable alternative. Injection of contrast media into the cyst can rule out a rare communication with the biliary tract. Cysts discovered incidentally at laparotomy should be left alone if less than 5 cm in diameter. Aspiration of cysts that are between 5 cm and 10 cm in diameter should be performed to confirm the diagnosis. Aspiration is followed by excision of the cyst wall. For large cysts, especially if there has been previous inflammation or the cyst wall is near major venous or biliary branches, an anatomic liver resection is indicated (Iwatsuki et al, 1990). This resection avoids unnecessary bleeding and the risk of postoperative biliary fistula.

Adult-type polycystic disease involving the liver has been reported with right lobar replacement and sparing of the left hepatic lobe (Marcellini et al, 1986). This was effectively treated by right hepatic lobectomy. Embryonal sarcoma of the liver sometimes can be confused with a solitary cyst (Chowdhary et al, 2004). Percutaneous needle aspiration and biopsy may be required to establish the diagnosis.

REFERENCES

Achilleos OA, et al, 1996: Unresectable hepatic tumors in childhood and the role of liver transplantation. J Pediatr Surg 31:1563-1567.

Aggarwal S, et al, 2001: Embryonal sarcoma of the liver mimicking a hydatid cyst in an adult. Trop Gastroenterol 22:141-142.

Albrecht S, et al, 1994: Loss of maternal alleles on chromosome arm 11p in hepatoblastoma. Cancer Res 54:5041-5044.

Alcantar VC, 1985: Hepatoblastoma associated with osteosarcoma. Rev Mex Pediatr 52:389-392.

Al-Qabandi W, et al, 1999: Orthotopic liver transplantation for unresectable hepatoblastoma: a single center's experience. J Pediatr Surg 34:1261-1264.

Arico M, et al, 1992: Partial response after intensive chemotherapy for adrenal cortical carcinoma in a child. Med Pediatr Oncol 20:246-248.

Aronson DC, et al, 2005: Predictive value of the pretreatment extent of disease system in hepatoblastoma: Results from the International Society of Pediatric Oncology Liver Tumor Study Group SIOPEL-1 study. J Clin Oncol 23:1245-1252.

Bala S, et al, 1997: Childhood hepatocellular adenoma in familial adenomatous polyposis: mutations in adenomatous polyposis coli gene and p53. Gastroenterology 112:919-922.

Barnhart DC, et al, 1997: Conservative management of mesenchymal hamartoma of the liver. J Pediatr Surg 32:1495-1498.

Barton JW, Keller MS, 1989: Liver transplantation for hepatoblastoma in a child with congenital absence of the portal vein. Pediatr Radiol 20:113-114.

Bates SM, et al, 1990: Hepatoblastoma: detection of tumor vascularity with duplex Doppler US. Radiology 176:505-507.

Beets-Tan RG, et al, 1998: Hepatic adenoma and focal nodular hyperplasia: MR findings with superparamagnetic iron oxide-enhanced MRI. Clin Imaging 22:211-215.

Begueret H, et al, 2001: Hepatic undifferentiated embryonal sarcoma: malignant evolution of mesenchymal hamartoma? Study of one case with immunohistochemical and flow cytometric emphasis. J Hepatol 34:178-179.

Berthold F, et al, 1986: Combination chemotherapy and chemoembolization in the treatment of primary inoperable hepatoblastoma. Klin Padiatr 198:257-261.

Bismuth H, 1982: Surgical anatomy and anatomical surgery of the liver. World J Surg 6:3-9.

Blair V, Birch JM, 1994: Patterns and temporal trends in the incidence of malignant disease in children: II. Solid tumours of childhood. Eur J Cancer 30A:1498-1511.

Bortolasi L, et al, 1996: Hepatoblastoma in adult age: a report of two cases. Hepatogastroenterology 43:1073-1078.

Bouyn CI, et al, 2003: Hepatic focal nodular hyperplasia in children previously treated for a solid tumor: incidence, risk factors, and outcome. Cancer 97:3107-3113.

Bove KE, et al, 1996: Hepatoblastoma in a child with trisomy 18: cytogenetics, liver anomalies, and literature review. Pediatr Pathol Lab Med 16:253-262.

Bower M, et al, 1996: Fibrolamellar hepatocellular carcinoma responsive to platinum-based combination chemotherapy. Clin Oncol (R Coll Radiol) 8:331-333.

Brandt S, et al, 2005: The tamoxifen-induced suppression of telomerase activity in the human hepatoblastoma cell line hepG2: a result of post-translational regulation. J Cancer Res Clin Oncol 131:120-128.

Breslow NE, et al, 1986: Clinicopathologic features and prognosis for Wilms' tumor patients with metastases at diagnosis. Cancer 58:2501-2511.

Brower ST, et al, 1998: Pancreatic cancer, hepatobiliary cancer, and neuroendocrine cancers of the GI tract. In Pazdur R, et al (eds): Cancer Management: A Multidisciplinary Approach. Huntington, NY, Published Research & Representation, Inc., pp 113-148.

Brown BF, et al, 1993: Hepatoblastoma: a rare pediatric neoplasm. Mil Med 158:51-55.

Carew JF, et al, 1998: Efficient gene transfer to human squamous cell carcinomas by the herpes simplex virus type 1 amplicon vector. Am J Surg 176:404-408.

Cetta F, et al, 1997: Hepatoblastoma and APC gene mutation in familial adenomatous polyposis. Gut 41:417.

Chan KL, et al, 2002: Paediatric hepatoblastoma and hepatocellular carcinoma: retrospective study. Hong Kong Med J 8:13-17.

Chang MH, et al, 1997: Universal hepatitis B vaccination in Taiwan and the incidence of hepatocellular carcinoma in children. Taiwan Childhood Hepatoma Study Group. N Engl J Med 336:1855-1859.

Chowdhary SK, et al, 2004: Undifferentiated embryonal sarcoma in children: beware of the solitary liver cyst. J Pediatr Surg 39:E9-E12.

Cillo U, et al, 2003: Liver transplantation for the management of hepatoblastoma. Transplant Proc 35:2983-2985.

Clouse ME, et al, 1994: Hepatic arterial chemoembolization for metastatic neuroendocrine tumors. Digestion 55:92-97.

Cohen MD, Siddiqui A, 1982: Liver metastases in Wilms' tumour. Clin Radiol 33:539-540.

Cooper K, et al, 1989: Mesenchymal hamartoma of the liver: a report of 5 cases. S Afr Med J 75:295-298.

Costello SA, Seywright M, 1990: Post-irradiation malignant transformation in benign haemangioma. Eur J Surg Oncol 16:517-519.

Couinaud C, 1986: Surgical anatomy of the liver: several new aspects. Chirurgie 112:337-342.

Couinaud C, 1992: The anatomy of the liver. Ann Ital Chir 63:693-697.

Daniel E, Kifle A, 1989: An unusual presentation of hepatoblastoma. Ethiop Med J 27:231-234.

Darbari A, et al, 2003: Epidemiology of primary hepatic malignancies in U.S. children. Hepatology 38:560-566.

Dehner LP, Manivel JC, 1988: Hepatoblastoma: an analysis of the relationship between morphologic subtypes and prognosis. Am J Pediatr Hematol Oncol 10:301-307.

de Lorimier AA, et al, 1967: Hepatic-artery ligation for hepatic hemangiomatosis. N Engl J Med 277:333-337.

DeMaioribus CA, et al, 1990: Mesenchymal hamartoma of the liver: a 35-year review. Arch Surg 125:598-600.

Dicken BJ, et al, 2004: Association between surgical margins and long-term outcome in advanced hepatoblastoma. J Pediatr Surg 39:721-725.

Douglass EC, et al, 1993: Cisplatin, vincristine, and fluorouracil therapy for hepatoblastoma: a Pediatric Oncology Group study. J Clin Oncol 11:96-99.

Ehren H, et al, 1983: Benign liver tumors in infancy and childhood: report of 48 cases. Am J Surg 145:325-329.

Ehrlich PF, et al, 1997: Improved long-term survival with preoperative chemotherapy for hepatoblastoma. J Pediatr Surg 32:999-1002.

Endo EG, et al, 1996: Neonatal hepatoblastoma metastatic to the choroid and iris. Arch Ophthalmol 114:757-761.

Eriksson T, et al, 2001: Methylation changes in the human IGF2 p3 promoter parallel IGF2 expression in the primary tumor, established cell line, and xenograft of a human hepatoblastoma. Exp Cell Res 270:88-95.

Ettinger LJ, Freeman AI, 1979: Hepatoma in a child with neurofibromatosis. Am J Dis Child 133:528-531.

Exelby PR, et al, 1975: Liver tumors in children in the particular reference to hepatoblastoma and hepatocellular carcinoma: American Academy of Pediatrics Surgical Section Survey 1974. J Pediatr Surg 10:329-337.

Fabre M, et al, 2004: Hepatic tumors in childhood: experience on 245 tumors and review of literature. Ann Pathol 24:536-555.

Falk H, et al, 1981: Review of four cases of childhood hepatic angiosarcoma—elevated environmental arsenic exposure in one case. Cancer 47:382-391.

Fegiz G, et al, 1977: A case report of hepatoblastoma treated by chemotherapy and hepatic lobectomy. World J Surg 1:407-414.

Fermand JP, et al, 1990: Danazol-induced hepatocellular adenoma. Am J Med 88:529-530.

Filler RM, et al, 1991: Preoperative chemotherapy in hepatoblastoma. Surgery 110:591-556.

Finegold MJ, 1994: Tumors of the liver. Semin Liver Dis 14:270-281.

Flemming P, et al, 1995: Mesenchymal tumors of the liver: their frequency and histopathological diagnostic problems in surgical investigations. Verh Dtsch Ges Pathol 79:116-119.

Foster JH, Berman MM, 1994: The malignant transformation of liver cell adenomas. Arch Surg 129:712-717.

Fraumeni JF Jr, et al, 1969: Hepatoblastoma in infant sisters. Cancer 24:1086-1090.

Friedburg H, et al, 1984: Sonographic and computed tomographic features of embryonal rhabdomyosarcoma of the biliary tract. Pediatr Radiol 14:436-438.

Gallivan MV, et al, 1983: Undifferentiated ("embryonal") sarcoma of the liver: ultrastructure of a case presenting as a primary intracardiac tumor. Pediatr Pathol 1:291-300.

Gauthier F, et al, 1986: Hepatoblastoma and hepatocarcinoma in children: analysis of a series of 29 cases. J Pediatr Surg 21:424-429.

Geiger JD, 1996: Surgery for hepatoblastoma in children. Curr Opin Pediatr 8:276-282.

Geoffray A, et al, 1987: Ultrasonography and computed tomography for diagnosis and follow-up of biliary duct rhabdomyosarcomas in children. Pediatr Radiol 17:127-131.

Giardiello FM, et al, 1996: Hepatoblastoma and APC gene mutation in familial adenomatous polyposis. Gut 39:867-869.

Glick RD, et al, 2000: Extended left hepatectomy (left hepatic trisegmentectomy) in childhood. J Pediatr Surg 35:303-307.

Gonzalez-Crussi F, et al, 1982: Hepatoblastoma: attempt at characterization of histologic subtypes. Am J Surg Pathol 6:599-612.

Gray SG, et al, 2000: Comparative genomic hybridization reveals population-based genetic alterations in hepatoblastomas. Br J Cancer 83:1020-1025.

Greenberg M, Filler RM, 1989: Hepatic tumors. In Pizzo PA, Poplack DG (eds): Principles and Practice of Pediatric Oncology. Philadelphia, Lippincott, pp 697-711.

Gururangan S, et al, 1992: Primary hepatic tumours in children: a 26-year review. J Surg Oncol 50:30-36.

Habrand JL, et al, 1992: Is there a place for radiation therapy in the management of hepatoblastomas and hepatocellular carcinomas in children? Int J Radiat Oncol Biol Phys 23:525-531.

Hagiwara M, et al, 1982: Multimodal treatment of advanced adult Wilms tumor. J Urol 127:535-538.

Harada T, et al, 1995: Adult hepatoblastoma: case report and review of the literature. Aust N Z J Surg 65:686-688.

Hartley AL, et al, 1990: Epidemiological and familial aspects of hepatoblastoma. Med Pediatr Oncol 18:103-109.

Hata Y, 1990: The clinical features and prognosis of hepatoblastoma: follow-up studies done on pediatric tumors enrolled in the Japanese Pediatric Tumor Registry between 1971 and 1980. Part I. Committee of Malignant Tumors, Japanese Society of Pediatric Surgeons. Jpn J Surg 20:498-502.

Heimann A, et al, 1987: Hepatoblastoma presenting as isosexual precocity: the clinical importance of histologic and serologic parameters. J Clin Gastroenterol 9:105-110.

Herlin T, et al, 1988: Treatment of unresectable hepatoblastoma with cisplatin, vincristine and 5-fluorouracil. Eur J Pediatr 147:514-515.

Hernandez-Siverio N, et al, 1988: Solitary, non-parasitic hepatic cyst in childhood. An Esp Pediatr 28:269-270.

Hiyama E, et al, 2004: High expression of telomerase is an independent prognostic indicator of poor outcome in hepatoblastoma. Br J Cancer 91:972-979.

Ho SY, et al, 2004: Hepatic angiosarcoma presenting as hepatic rupture in a patient with long-term ingestion of arsenic. J Formos Med Assoc 103:374-379.

Hobbs KE, 1990: Hepatic hemangiomas. World J Surg 14:468-471.

Holcomb GW, et al, 1988: Experience with hepatic hemangioendothelioma in infancy and childhood. J Pediatr Surg 23:661-666.

Honda M, et al, 1996: Case report: intrahepatic cholangiocarcinoma with rhabdoid transformation. J Gastroenterol Hepatol 11:771-774.

Horowitz ME, et al, 1987: Hepatic undifferentiated (embryonal) sarcoma and rhabdomyosarcoma in children: results of therapy. Cancer 59:396-402.

Huang CB, et al, 1997: Primary Burkitt's lymphoma of the liver: report of a case with long-term survival after surgical resection and combination chemotherapy. J Pediatr Hematol Oncol 19:135-138.

Huber BE, Richards CA, 1996: Regulated expression of artificial chimeric genes contained in retroviral vectors: implications for virus-directed enzyme prodrug therapy (VDEPT) and other gene therapy applications. J Drug Target 3:349-356.

Hutton KA, et al, 1993: Focal nodular hyperplasia of the liver in childhood. Eur J Pediatr Surg 3:370-372.

Ikeda H, et al, 1997: Association between hepatoblastoma and very low birth weight: a trend or a chance? J Pediatr 130:557-560.

Inamori H, et al, 2004: Laparoscopic radiofrequency ablation of hepatocellular carcinoma in the caudate lobe by using a new laparoscopic US probe with a forward-viewing convex-array transducer. Gastrointest Endosc 60:628-631.

Inoue S, et al, 1995: Successful resection of a large hepatoblastoma in a young adult: report of a case. Surg Today 25:974-977.

Ishak KG, 1976: Primary hepatic tumors in childhood. Prog Liver Dis 5:636-667.

Ito E, et al, 1987: Type Ia glycogen storage disease with hepatoblastoma in siblings [published erratum appears in Cancer 1987;60:723] Cancer 59:1776-1780.

Iwama T, Mishima Y, 1994: Mortality in young first-degree relatives of patients with familial adenomatous polyposis. Cancer 73:2065-2068.

Iwatsuki S, et al, 1990: Excisional therapy for benign hepatic lesions. Surg Gynecol Obstet 171:240-246.

Ji W, St CW, 1997: Inhibition of hepatitis B virus by retroviral vectors expressing antisense RNA. J Viral Hepat 4:167-173.

Jimenez-Heffernan JA, et al, 1998: Pathological case of the month: primary hepatic malignant tumor with rhabdoid features. Arch Pediatr Adolesc Med 152:509-510.

Jones RS, 1994: Surgical management of non-parasitic liver cysts. In Blumgart LH (ed): Surgery of the Liver and Biliary Tract. London, Churchill Livingstone, pp 1211-1218.

Kacker LK, et al, 1995: Hepatoblastoma in an adult with biliary obstruction and associated portal venous thrombosis. HPB Surg 9:47-49.

Kaczynski J, et al, 1996: Incidence of primary liver cancer and aetiological aspects: a study of a defined population from a low-endemicity area. Br J Cancer 73:128-132.

Kadomatsu K, et al, 1992: Undifferentiated (embryonal) sarcoma of the liver: report of three cases. Surg Today 22:451-455.

Kelly DM, et al, 1998: Spontaneous rupture of a malignant rhabdoid tumour of the liver. Pediatr Surg Int 14:111-112.

Kitahara S, et al, 1995: Successful left trisegmentectomy for ruptured hepatoblastoma using intraoperative transarterial embolization. J Pediatr Surg 30:1709-1712.

Koda M, et al, 2004: Percutaneous sonographically guided radiofrequency ablation with artificial pleural effusion for hepatocellular carcinoma located under the diaphragm. AJR Am J Roentgenol 183:583-588.

Koishi S, et al, 1996: Myelodysplasia in a child with Beckwith-Wiedemann syndrome previously treated for hepatoblastoma with multi-agent chemotherapy. J Pediatr Hematol Oncol 18:419-420 (letter).

Komura E, et al, 1998: Thrombopoietin in patients with hepatoblastoma. Stem Cells 16:329-333.

Komuro H, et al, 1998: Congenital mediastinal dumbbell neuroblastoma with spontaneous regression of liver metastases. Pediatr Surg Int 14:86-88.

Koneru B, et al, 1991: Liver transplantation for hepatoblastoma: the American experience. Ann Surg 213:118-121.

Kraus JA, et al, 1996: Loss of heterozygosity on chromosome 1 in human hepatoblastoma. Int J Cancer 67:467-471.

Kushner BH, et al, 1996: Desmoplastic small round-cell tumor: prolonged progression-free survival with aggressive multimodality therapy. J Clin Oncol 14:1526-1531.

Lack EE, Ornvold K, 1986: Focal nodular hyperplasia and hepatic adenoma: a review of eight cases in the pediatric age group. J Surg Oncol 33:129-135.

Lack EE, et al, 1981: Botryoid rhabdomyosarcoma of the biliary tract. Am J Surg Pathol 5:643-652.

Lack EE, et al, 1982: Hepatoblastoma: a clinical and pathologic study of 54 cases. Am J Surg Pathol 6:693-705.

Lampkin BC, et al, 1985: Solid malignancies in children and adolescents. Surg Clin North Am 65:1351-1386.

LaQuaglia MP, et al, 1992: Prognostic factors and outcome in patients 21 years and under with colorectal carcinoma. J Pediatr Surg 27:1085-1089.

Lee CL, Ko YC, 1998: Survival and distribution pattern of childhood liver cancer in Taiwan. Eur J Cancer 34:2064-2067.

Le Luyer B, et al, 2000: Use of interferon in a case of hepatic hemangioma. Arch Pediatr 7:1201-1204.

Li FP, et al, 1987: Hepatoblastoma in families with polyposis coli. JAMA 257:2475-2477.

Li GC, et al, 2004: Treatment of hepatocellular carcinoma with a novel gene-viral therapeutic system CNHK300-murine endostatin. Zhonghua Yi Xue Za Zhi 84:943-948.

Liaw YF, et al, 2004: Lamivudine for patients with chronic hepatitis B and advanced liver disease. N Engl J Med 351:1521-1531.

Lin SM, et al, 2004: Radiofrequency ablation improves prognosis compared with ethanol injection for hepatocellular carcinoma < or = 4 cm. Gastroenterology 127:1714-1723.

Liver Cancer Study Group of Japan, 1987: Primary liver cancer in Japan: sixth report. Cancer 60:1400-1411.

Lockwood L, et al, 1993: Cisplatin-resistant metastatic hepatoblastoma: complete response to carboplatin, etoposide, and liver transplantation. Med Pediatr Oncol 21:517-520.

Maini CL, et al, 1996: Superselective intra-arterial radiometabolic therapy with I-131 lipiodol in hepatocellular carcinoma. Clin Nucl Med 21:221-226.

Malogolowkin MH, et al, 1993: Chemoembolization (CE) for progressive hepatoblastoma (HB) in children. Proc Annu Meet Am Soc Clin Oncol 12:A1450 (meeting abstract).

Manchester KM, et al, 1995: Establishment and characterization of a novel hepatoblastoma-derived cell line. J Pediatr Surg 30:553-558.

Mann JR, et al, 1990: Malignant hepatic tumours in children: incidence, clinical features and aetiology. Paediatr Perinat Epidemiol 4:276-289.

Marcellini M, et al, 1986: Adult polycystic liver disease in childhood: a case report. Ital J Surg Sci 16:217-221.

Marks J, et al, 1998: Laparoscopic liver surgery: a report on 28 patients. Surg Endosc 12:331-334.

Martin LW, Woodman KS, 1969: Hepatic lobectomy for hepatoblastoma in infants and children. Arch Surg 98:1-7.

Martinez-F, et al, 1982: Rhabdomyosarcoma of the biliary tree: the case for aggressive surgery. J Pediatr Surg 17:508-511.

Mascarello JT, Krous HF, 1992: Second report of a translocation involving 19q13.4 in a mesenchymal hamartoma of the liver. Cancer Genet Cytogenet 58:141-142.

Mazuryk M, et al, 1998: Benefit of aggressive multimodality therapy with autologous stem cell support for intra-abdominal desmoplastic small round cell tumor. Bone Marrow Transplant 21:961-963.

McClusky DA 3rd, et al, 1997: Hepatic surgery and hepatic surgical anatomy: historical partners in progress. World J Surg 21:330-342.

Medary I, et al, 1996: Kinetics of primary tumor regression with chemotherapy: implications for the timing of surgery. Ann Surg Oncol 3:521-525.

Meinders AJ, et al, 1998: Mesenchymal hamartoma of the liver: Failed management by marsupialization. J Pediatr Gastroenterol Nutr 26:353-355.

Mills AE, 1988: Undifferentiated primary hepatic non-Hodgkin's lymphoma in childhood. Am J Surg Pathol 12:721-726.

Molmenti EP, et al, 2002: Treatment of unresectable hepatoblastoma with liver transplantation in the pediatric population. Am J Transplant 2:535-538.

Moore L, et al, 1997: Hepatocellular carcinoma following neonatal hepatitis. Pediatr Pathol Lab Med 17:601-610.

Moore SW, et al, 1997: Hepatocellular carcinoma in children. Pediatr Surg Int 12:266-270.

Morrow CE, et al, 1982: Hepatic resection for secondary neoplasms. Surgery 92:610-614.

Mulliken JB, 1988: Diagnosis and natural history of hemangiomas. In Mulliken JB, Young AE (eds): Vascular Birthmarks: Hemangiomas and Malformations. Philadelphia, Saunders, pp 41-62.

Muraji T, et al, 1985: The prognostic implication of hypercholesterolemia in infants and children with hepatoblastoma. J Pediatr Surg 20:228-230.

Nagaraj HS, et al, 1977: Rhabdomyosarcoma of the bile ducts. J Pediatr Surg 12:1071-1074.

Nagorney DM, 1995: Benign hepatic tumors: focal nodular hyperplasia and hepatocellular adenoma. World J Surg 19:13-18.

Napoli VM, Campbell WG Jr, 1977: Hepatoblastoma in infant sister and brother. Cancer 39:2647-2650.

National Cancer Institute, 1995: SEER Cancer Statistics Review, 1973-1992: Tables and Graphs, National Cancer Institute. NIH Publication No. 96-2789. Bethesda, MD, National Institutes of Health.

Newman KD, et al, 1989: Malignant mesenchymoma of the liver in children. J Pediatr Surg 24:781-783.

Ng KK, et al, 1997: Three-dimensional magnetic resonance cholangiopancreatography for evaluation of obstructive jaundice. J Formos Med Assoc 96:586-592.

Ni YH, et al, 1997: Hepatocellular carcinoma in childhood: clinical manifestations and prognosis. Cancer 68:1737-1741.

Niemela M, et al, 2001: Interferon alpha-2a therapy in 18 hemangioblastomas. Clin Cancer Res 7:510-516.

Noronha R, Gonzalez-Crussi F, 1984: Hepatic angiosarcoma in childhood: a case report and review of the literature. Am J Surg Pathol 8:863-871.

Norton KI, et al, 1997: Leiomyosarcoma of the kidney in an HIV-infected child. Pediatr Radiol 27:557-558.

Oda H, et al, 1996: Somatic mutations of the APC gene in sporadic hepatoblastomas. Cancer Res 56:3320-3323.

Ohama K, et al, 1997: Alpha-fetoprotein (AFP) levels in normal children. Eur J Pediatr Surg 7:267-269.

Ohnuma N, et al, 1991: The role of magnetic resonance imaging for treatment in children with malignant solid tumor. Nippon Geka Gakkai Zasshi 92:1143-1146.

Order SE, et al, 1996: Preliminary experience of infusional brachytherapy using colloidal 32P. Ann Acad Med Singapore 25:347-351.

Ordonez NG, 1998: Desmoplastic small round cell tumor: I. A histopathologic study of 39 cases with emphasis on unusual histological patterns. Am J Surg Pathol 22:1303-1313.

Orozco H, et al, 1991: Undifferentiated (embryonal) sarcoma of the liver: report of a case. Rev Invest Clin 43:255-258.

Ortega JA, et al, 1991: Effective treatment of unresectable or metastatic hepatoblastoma with cisplatin and continuous infusion doxorubicin chemotherapy: a report from the Children's Cancer Study Group. J Clin Oncol 9:2167-2176.

Ortega JA, et al, 2000: Randomized comparison of cisplatin/vincristine/fluorouracil and cisplatin/continuous infusion doxorubicin for treatment of pediatric hepatoblastoma: a report from the Children's Cancer Group and the Pediatric Oncology Group. J Clin Oncol 18:2665-2675.

O'Sullivan MJ, et al, 2001: Undifferentiated embryonal sarcoma with unusual features arising within mesenchymal hamartoma of the liver: report of a case and review of the literature. Pediatr Dev Pathol 4:482-489.

Otte JB, et al, 2004: Liver transplantation for hepatoblastoma: results from the International Society of Pediatric Oncology (SIOP) study SIOPEL-1 and review of the world experience. Pediatr Blood Cancer 42:74-83.

Parada LA, et al, 1997: Cytogenetic abnormalities and clonal evolution in an adult hepatoblastoma. Am J Surg Pathol 21:1381-1386.

Passmore SJ, et al, 1995: Prolonged survival following multiple thoracotomies for metastatic hepatoblastoma. Med Pediatr Oncol 24:58-60.

Perilongo G, et al, 2000: Hepatoblastoma presenting with lung metastases: treatment results of the first cooperative, prospective study of the International Society of Paediatric Oncology on childhood liver tumors. Cancer 89:1845-1853.

Perisic VN, et al, 1991: Cholestasis caused by biliary botryoid sarcoma. Eur J Pediatr Surg 1:242-243.

Pichlmayr R, et al, 1995: Role of liver transplantation in the treatment of unresectable liver cancer. World J Surg 19:807-813.

Pinna AD, et al, 1997: Treatment of fibrolamellar hepatoma with subtotal hepatectomy or transplantation. Hepatology 26:877-883.

Powers C, et al, 1994: Primary liver neoplasms: MR imaging with pathologic correlation. Radiographics 14:459-482.

Prasad VK, et al, 1995: Hepatic focal nodular hyperplasia in infant antenatally exposed to steroids. Lancet 346:371 (letter).

Probst-Cousin S, et al, 1997: Malignant peripheral nerve sheath tumor with extensive miliary metastases: a case report. Gen Diagn Pathol 142:357-360.

Pul N, Pul M, 1995. Congenital solitary nonparasitic cyst of the liver in infancy and childhood. J Pediatr Gastroenterol Nutr 21:461-462.

Ramani K, et al, 1997: Novel gene delivery to liver cells using engineered virosomes. FEBS Lett 404:164-168.

Rao PS, et al, 1989: Multicystic kidney in association with hepatoblastoma—a case report. Jpn J Surg 19:583-585.

Raut CP, et al, 2005: Significant long-term survival after radiofrequency ablation of unresectable hepatocellular carcinoma in patients with cirrhosis. Ann Surg Oncol 12:616-628.

Reyes JD, et al, 2000: Liver transplantation and chemotherapy for hepatoblastoma and hepatocellular cancer in childhood and adolescence. J Pediatr 136:795-804.

Reynolds M, 1995: Conversion of unresectable to resectable hepatoblastoma and long-term follow-up study. World J Surg 19:814-816.

Reynolds P, et al, 2004: Birth characteristics and hepatoblastoma risk in young children. Cancer 100:1070-1076.

Rodriguez E, et al, 1991: Abnormalities of 2q: a common genetic link between rhabdomyosarcoma and hepatoblastoma. Genes Chromosomes Cancer 3:122-127.

Roebuck DJ, et al, 1998: Hepatobiliary rhabdomyosarcoma in children: diagnostic radiology. Pediatr Radiol 28:101-108.

Rojiani AM, et al, 1991: Hepatic hemangioblastoma: an unusual presentation in a patient with von Hippel-Lindau disease. Am J Surg Pathol 15:81-86.

Ross JS, et al, 1992: Primary hepatic leiomyosarcoma in a child with the acquired immunodeficiency syndrome. Hum Pathol 23:69-72.

Ruck P, Xiao JC, 2002: Stem-like cells in hepatoblastoma. Med Pediatr Oncol 39:504-507.

Ruymann FB, et al, 1985: Rhabdomyosarcoma of the biliary tree in childhood: a report from the Intergroup Rhabdomyosarcoma Study. Cancer 56:575-581.

Ryu M, et al, 1997: Therapeutic results of resection, transcatheter arterial embolization and percutaneous transhepatic ethanol injection in 3225 patients with hepatocellular carcinoma: a retrospective multicenter study. Jpn J Clin Oncol 27:251-257.

Saito Y, et al, 1984: Anesthetic management and metabolic control of a patient with von Gierke's disease (glycogen storage disease type I) associated with hepatic adenoma. Masui 33:1395-1399.

Sakatoku H, et al, 1996: Focal nodular hyperplasia in an adolescent with glycogen storage disease type I with mesocaval shunt operation in childhood: a case report and review of the literature. Acta Paediatr Jpn 38:172-175.

Samama G, et al, 1998: Laparoscopic anatomical hepatic resection: report of four left lobectomies for solid tumors. Surg Endosc 12:76-78.

Santambrogio R, et al, 2003: Safety and efficacy of laparoscopic radiofrequency ablation of hepatocellular carcinoma in patients with liver cirrhosis. Surg Endosc 17:1826-1832.

Sanz N, et al, 1997: Rhabdomyosarcoma of the biliary tree. Pediatr Surg Int 12:200-201.

Scaglioni PP, et al, 1996: Recent advances in the molecular biology of hepatitis B virus. Baillieres Clin Gastroenterol 10:207-225.

Schaller RT Jr, et al, 1984: The advantages of hemodilution anesthesia for major liver resection in children. J Pediatr Surg 19:705-710.

Schnater JM, et al, 2002: Surgical view of the treatment of patients with hepatoblastoma: results from the first prospective trial of the International Society of Pediatric Oncology Liver Tumor Study Group. Cancer 94:1111-1120.

Schneid H, et al, 1997: The Beckwith-Wiedemann syndrome phenotype and the risk of cancer. Med Pediatr Oncol 28:411-415.

Schwarz RE, et al, 1998: Desmoplastic small round cell tumors: prognostic indicators and results of surgical management. Ann Surg Oncol 5:416-422.

Selby DM, et al, 1992: Angiosarcoma of the liver in childhood: a clinicopathologic and follow-up study of 10 cases. Pediatr Pathol 12:485-498.

Shamberger RC, et al, 1996: Long-term hepatic regeneration and function in infants and children following liver resection. J Am Coll Surg 182:515-519.

Shapiro RS, et al, 1988: Case report: calcified liver metastases from osteosarcoma. J Comput Assist Tomogr 12:196-198.

Shimada H, et al, 1987: Pathology of fatal rhabdomyosarcoma: report from Intergroup Rhabdomyosarcoma Study (IRS-I and IRS-II). Cancer 59:459-465.

Simms LA, et al, 1995: Genetic mosaicism at the insulin locus in liver associated with childhood hepatoblastoma. Genes Chromosomes Cancer 13:72-73.

Spunt SL, et al, 2000: Aggressive surgery is unwarranted for biliary tract rhabdomyosarcoma. J Pediatr Surg 35:309-316.

Srinivasan P, et al, 2002: Orthotopic liver transplantation for unresectable hepatoblastoma. Transplantation 74:652-655.

Srouji MN, et al, 1978: Mesenchymal hamartoma of the liver in infants. Cancer 42:2483-2489.

Stocker JT, 1994: Hepatoblastoma. Semin Diagn Pathol 11:136-143.

Stringer MD, et al, 1995: Improved outcome for children with hepatoblastoma. Br J Surg 82:386-391.

Superina R, Bilik R, 1996: Results of liver transplantation in children with unresectable liver tumors. J Pediatr Surg 31:835-839.

Surendran N, et al, 1989: Hepatoblastoma in siblings. J Pediatr Surg 24:1169-1171.

Swarts S, et al, 1996: Significance of extra copies of chromosome 20 and the long arm of chromosome 2 in hepatoblastoma. Cancer Genet Cytogenet 91:65-67.

Taat F, et al, 2004: Hepatoblastoma in a girl with biliary atresia: coincidence or co-incidence. Pediatr Blood Cancer 43:603-605.

Tagge EP, et al, 1992: Resection, including transplantation, for hepatoblastoma and hepatocellular carcinoma: impact on survival. J Pediatr Surg 27:292-296.

Takvorian P, et al, 1988: Hepatic rupture after puncture biopsy: value of embolization. Apropos of a case with hepatoblastoma. Pediatrie (Bucur) 43:531-533.

Tamano S, et al, 1996: Histogenesis and the role of p53 and k-*ras* mutations in hepatocarcinogenesis by glyceryl trinitrate (nitroglycerin) in male F344 rats. Carcinogenesis 17:2477-2486.

Terris B, et al, 1997: Interphase cytogenetic analysis reveals numerical chromosome aberrations in large liver cell dysplasia. J Hepatol 27:313-319.

Theegarten D, et al, 1998: Mixed malignant germ cell tumour of the liver. Virchows Arch 433:93-96.

Thomas D, et al, 2003: Familial hepatoblastoma and APC gene mutations: renewed call for molecular research. Eur J Cancer 39:2200-2204.

Thomas PR, et al, 1991: Prognostic implications of hepatic adhesion, invasion, and metastases at diagnosis of Wilms' tumor. The National Wilms' Tumor Study Group. Cancer 68:2486-2488.

Tiao GM, et al, 2005: The current management of hepatoblastoma: a combination of chemotherapy, conventional resection, and liver transplantation. J Pediatr 146:204-211.

Toyosaka A, et al, 1996: Pathologic and radiographic studies of intrahepatic metastasis in hepatocellular carcinoma: the role of efferent vessels. HPB Surg 10:97-103.

Tozzi MC, et al, 1992: The hepatic malignant mesenchymoma: a case report. Eur J Pediatr 151:488-491.

Tsai SY, et al, 1996: Hepatoblastoma in an infant with Beckwith-Wiedemann syndrome. J Formos Med Assoc 95:180-183.

Tsao K, et al, 2002: Fetal therapy for giant hepatic cysts. J Pediatr Surg 37:E31.

Tsuchida Y, et al, 1997: The role of subfractionation of alpha-fetoprotein in the treatment of pediatric surgical patients. J Pediatr Surg 32:514-517.

Tsunoda Y, et al, 1996: Non-alpha-fetoprotein-producing anaplastic hepatoblastoma cell line. In Vitro Cell Dev Biol Anim 32:194-196 (letter).

Tung C, et al, 1996: Rapid production of interleukin-2–secreting tumor cells by herpes simplex virus–mediated gene transfer: implications for autologous vaccine production. Hum Gene Ther 7:2217-2224.

Urata H, et al, 2004: Strategy for the treatment of unresectable hepatoblastoma: neoadjuvant chemotherapy followed by delayed primary operation or liver transplantation. Int Surg 89:95-99.

Van Tornout JM, et al, 1993: Rate and magnitude of decline in alphafetoprotein (AFP) levels in treated children with unresectable or metastatic hepatoblastoma (HB) are indicators of outcome: a report from the Children's Cancer Group. Proc Annu Meet Am Soc Clin Oncol 12:A1408 (meeting abstract).

Van Tornout JM, et al, 1997: Timing and magnitude of decline in alpha-fetoprotein levels in treated children with unresectable or metastatic hepatoblastoma are predictors of outcome: a report from the Children's Cancer Group. J Clin Oncol 15:1190-1197.

Vaughan WG, et al, 1995: Favorable outcome in children with Beckwith-Wiedemann syndrome and intraabdominal malignant tumors. J Pediatr Surg 30:1042-1044.

Vetter D, et al, 1989: Hepatic undifferentiated (or embryonal) sarcoma: diagnostic and therapeutic problems apropos of botryoid rhabdomyosarcoma. Gastroenterol Clin Biol 13:98-103.

von Schweinitz D, et al, 1993: Production of interleukin-1 beta and interleukin-6 in hepatoblastoma. Int J Cancer 53:728-734.

von Schweinitz D, et al, 1994a: Clinico-pathological criteria with prognostic relevance in hepatoblastoma. Eur J Cancer 30A:1052-1058.

von Schweinitz D, et al, 1994b: Results of the HB-89 study in treatment of malignant epithelial liver tumors in childhood and concept of a new HB-94 protocol. Klin Paediatr 206:282-288.

von Schweinitz D, et al, 1995a: Extramedullary hematopoiesis and intratumoral production of cytokines in childhood hepatoblastoma. Pediatr Res 38:555-563.

von Schweinitz D, et al, 1995b: Complete resection before development of drug resistance is essential for survival from advanced hepatoblastoma—a report from the German Cooperative Pediatric Liver Tumor Study HB-89. J Pediatr Surg 30:845-852.

von Schweinitz D, et al, 1995c: Liver tumors in neonates and very young infants: diagnostic pitfalls and therapeutic problems. Eur J Pediatr Surg 5:72-76.

von Schweinitz D, et al, 1997a: Hepatocyte growth factor in pediatric hepato-blastoma. Langenbecks Arch Chir Suppl Kongressbd 114:37-40.

von Schweinitz D, et al, 1997b: Efficiency and toxicity of ifosfamide, cisplatin and doxorubicin in the treatment of childhood hepatoblastoma: study committee of the Cooperative Paediatric Liver Tumour Study HB89 of the German Society for Paediatric Oncology and Haematology. Eur J Cancer 33:1243-1249.

von Schweinitz D, et al, 1997c: Prognostic factors and staging systems in child-hood hepatoblastoma. Int J Cancer 74:593-599.

Vujanic GM, et al, 1996: Rhabdoid tumour of the kidney: a clinicopathological study of 22 patients from the International Society of Paediatric Oncology (SIOP) nephroblastoma file. Histopathology 28:333-340.

Walhof CM, et al, 1988: Half-life of alpha-fetoprotein in patients with a teratoma, endodermal sinus tumor, or hepatoblastoma. Pediatr Hematol Oncol 5:217-227.

Wang JN, et al, 2003: Cardiac tumors in infants and children. Acta Paediatr Taiwan 44:215-219.

Wegmann W, et al, 1996: [Liver cell carcinoma as a late complication of Alagille syndrome (arterio-hepatic dysplasia)]. Leber Magen Darm 26:157-158, 161-163.

Weinberg AG, Finegold MJ, 1983: Primary hepatic tumors of childhood. Hum Pathol 14:512-537.

Weitman S, et al, 1997: Pediatric phase II cancer chemotherapy trials: a Pediatric Oncology Group study. J Pediatr Hematol Oncol 19:187-191.

Werb P, et al, 1992: Survey of congenital tumors in perinatal necropsies. Pathology 24:247-253.

Westaby D, et al, 1983: Androgen-related primary hepatic tumors in non-Fanconi patients. Cancer 51:1947-1952.

Wheatley JM, et al, 1996: Liver regeneration in children after major hepatec-tomy for malignancy—evaluation using a computer-aided technique of volume measurement. J Surg Res 61:183-189.

White FV, et al, 1999: Congenital disseminated malignant rhabdoid tumor: a distinct clinicopathologic entity demonstrating abnormalities of chromo-some 22q11. Am J Surg Pathol 23:249-256.

Wong KK, et al, 2004: The use of positron emission tomography in detecting hepatoblastoma recurrence—a cautionary tale. J Pediatr Surg 39:1779-1781.

Yedibela S, et al, 2000: Undifferentiated, embryonal sarcoma as a rare cause of spontaneous liver rupture in adults. Chirurg 71:101-105.

Yen JB, et al, 2003: Hepatic mesenchymal hamartoma. J Paediatr Child Health 39:632-634.

Zatkova A, et al, 2004: Amplification and overexpression of the IGF2 regulator PLAG1 in hepatoblastoma. Genes Chromosomes Cancer 39:126-137.

73a SURGICAL TREATMENT OF HEPATIC METASTASES FROM COLORECTAL CANCER

R. TAYLOR AND Y. FONG

The liver is the most common site for hematogenous metastasis from colorectal cancers. A quarter of patients with primary colorectal carcinoma are found to have synchronous hepatic metastasis (Bengmark & Hafstrom, 1969). Nearly half of patients who undergo resection of the colorectal primary eventually develop metachronous liver metastasis (Bozzetti et al, 1987; Ekberg et al, 1987). In patients with isolated hepatic metastases, the extent of liver disease is the prime determinant of survival, and when left untreated, the survival is measured in months (Bengmark & Hafstrom, 1969; Bengtsson et al, 1981; Klein et al, 1992; Oxley & Ellis, 1969; Wood et al, 1976). Despite improvements in regional therapies, systemic chemotherapies, and biologic agents, survival is rarely longer than 3 years (Baker et al, 1976; Buroker et al, 1978; Cunningham et al, 2004; Doroshow et al, 1990; Erlichman et al, 1988; Grage et al, 1979; Hurwitz et al, 2004; Kemeny et al, 1990; Macdonald et al, 1976; Nordic Gastrointestinal Tumor Adjuvant Therapy Group, 1989; Petrelli et al, 1987; Saltz et al, 2000).

Over the last 3 decades, surgery has been shown to be safe and potentially curative in the treatment of colorectal metastases to the liver. The current 5-year survival after a margin-negative hepatic resection is 40%; 10-year survival approaches 20%. Although no prospective randomized trials comparing liver resection with systemic, regional, or other local therapies have been performed, the outcome for patients after liver resection for metastatic colorectal cancer is sufficiently favorable that surgery is now considered a standard therapy in this disease (Wagner et al, 1984; Wilson & Adson, 1976).

This chapter reviews the data supporting the use of liver resection for the treatment for metastatic colorectal carcinoma. More recent results of hepatic resection, including operative morbidity, mortality, and long-term survival; the most significant developments, including new staging systems to stratify this diverse group of patients; and the role of new imaging techniques for preoperative evaluation are reviewed. Numerous systemic chemotherapies and biologic therapies have been approved for use in colorectal cancer, and the current use of these agents to prevent recurrence after resection or to downstage unresectable disease is reviewed in an attempt to put into clinical context the choice of agents as adjuvant and neoadjuvant therapies.

NATURAL HISTORY OF METASTASES FROM COLORECTAL CANCER

The outcome of untreated metastatic colorectal cancer has been well studied. The median survival is 5 to 10 months, 2-year survival is unusual, and 5-year survival is extremely rare. Jaffe and colleagues (1968) reported a median survival of 5 months with no 5-year survivors. Similar results have been reported by Bengmark and Hafstrom (1969), Goslin and associates (1982), Bengtsson and coworkers (1981), Finan and colleagues (1985), and De Brauw and colleagues (1987) (Table 73a.1).

Most studies indicate that prognosis is most closely related to the extent of liver replacement by tumor (Arnaud et al, 1984; Bengmark et al, 1982; Bengmark & Hafstrom, 1969; Bengtsson et al, 1981; Pettavel & Morgenthaler, 1978; Wagner et al, 1984; Wood et al, 1976). In a retrospective study of 113 patients from the Glasgow Royal Infirmary, Wood and associates (1976) reported a 1-year survival rate of 5.7% for patients with widespread liver disease, 27% for patients with metastases localized to a single segment or lobe of liver, and 60% for patients with a solitary metastasis. Patients with solitary metastases had a mean survival of 25 months. Similarly, Wagner and coworkers (1984) showed that 20% of patients who had an unresected solitary liver lesion lived 3 years.

In both of the aforementioned reports (Wagner et al, 1984; Wood et al, 1976), the authors attempted to distinguish potentially resectable from unresectable disease. In the study by Wood and associates (1976), 13 patients were thought retrospectively to have potentially resectable disease, and for this subgroup, the 1-year, 3-year, and 5-year survival for untreated disease was 77%, 23%, and 8% (compared with 15%, 0%, and 0% for the unresectable group) (1 case). Similarly, Wagner and coworkers (1984) reported the 3-year and 5-year survival for untreated resectable disease to be 14% and 2% (compared with 4% and 0% for unresectable disease). Even though solitary lesions or unilobar disease seem to have better prognoses, the 5-year survival is still consistently less than 3%.

To rule out patient selection as the sole reason for the improved survival after resection (Silen, 1989), many case controlled studies have been undertaken. Wilson and Adson (1976) studied the survival of 60 patients treated with hepatic resection compared with 60 patients with a comparable number of lesions and extent of disease not subjected to surgery. Hepatic resection was associated with a 5-year and 10-year survival of 25% and 19%, whereas no patient in the unresected group survived to 5 years. In a similar study, the 5-year survival for 116 patients treated by liver resection was 25% compared with 2% for the 70 patients with potentially resectable metastases who did not undergo liver resection (Wagner et al, 1984). Scheele and colleagues (1991) compared 183 patients with resected tumor with 62 resectable patients who were not subjected to surgery and 920 patients with unresectable disease. The median survival was 30 months, 14.2 months, and 6.9 months. Although the patients with limited

Table 73a.1 Natural History of Liver Metastasis from Colorectal Cancer

Reference	N	No. Liver Metastases	Median Mean (mo)	SURVIVAL 1 Yr (%)	3 Yr (%)	5 Yr (%)
Bengmark & Hafstrom, 1969	173	40 (24.5%)	—*	5.7	0	0
Cady et al, 1970	269	—	13	—	—	—
Oxley & Ellis, 1969	640	112 (18%)	—	27	4	1
Wood et al, 1976	113	—	6.6	15	3	1
Bengtsson et al, 1981	155	25 (16%)	—	—	—	—
Wagner et al, 1984	252	—	—	49	7	2
Scheele et al, 1990	921	6.9	—	—	—	0
Stangl et al, 1994	484	—	7.5	—	—	1
Rougier et al, 1995	318	—	5.7	—	—	—

*— indicates data not specified.

unresected disease lived longer than patients with unresectable disease, no patient in either group survived 5 years.

These uniformly poor results in untreated stage IV colon cancer, even in the presence of a single isolated hepatic metastasis, provided the rationale for increasingly aggressive hepatectomies in the treatment of this disease. Hepatectomy represents the only currently established chance for cure or prolonged disease-free survival and is now accepted as the standard of care for patients with resectable liver metastases from a colorectal primary.

MEDICAL TREATMENT OF METASTATIC COLORECTAL DISEASE TO THE LIVER (see Ch. 77)

Since the 1970s, the most widely employed agent in the treatment of metastatic colorectal cancer has been 5-fluorouracil (5-FU), used alone or in combination with other chemotherapies. The response rate of hepatic metastases to 5-FU alone is consistently less than 30% (Baker et al, 1976; Buroker et al, 1978; Grage et al, 1979; Macdonald et al, 1976). The most widely employed regimens over the last 3 decades have used this agent alone or in combination with others (Baker et al, 1976; Buroker et al, 1978; Doroshow et al, 1990; Erlichman et al, 1988; Grage et al, 1979; Kemeny et al, 1990; Macdonald et al, 1976; Petrelli et al, 1987). A complete response is rare, and the median survival is 1 year or less.

In the 1990s, the most common first-line regimen for metastatic colorectal cancer was the combination of 5-FU and leucovorin. Tumor response occurs in approximately one third of patients (Advanced Colorectal Cancer Meta-Analysis Project, 1992; de Gramont et al, 1997). In 2000, two studies compared systemic therapy with irinotecan (CPT-11) in combination with 5-FU/leucovorin versus 5-FU/leucovorin alone in previously untreated patients with stage IV colorectal cancer. Saltz and colleagues (2000) showed that treatment with the irinotecan-containing regimen resulted in a longer progression-free survival (7 versus 4.3 months), a higher response rate (39% versus 21%), and longer survival (median 14.8 months versus 12.6 months). Douillard and coworkers (2000) reported similar results. Irinotecan with 5-FU/leucovorin became the standard treatment for nonresectable stage IV colorectal cancer. Subsequently, oxaliplatin plus 5-FU/leucovorin was accepted as another reasonable first-line regimen based on a significantly improved response rate of 40% to 60% (de Gramont et al, 2000; Goldberg et al,

2004) and median survival of 19.5 months (compared with 15 months with 5-FU/leucovorin alone) (Goldberg et al, 2004). Two novel targeted biologic agents effective against colorectal cancer have been introduced. Cetuximab, an epidermal growth factor receptor antagonist, now is accepted as an effective agent against unresectable colorectal metastases (Cunningham et al, 2004). Bevacizumab (Avastin), a monoclonal antibody against vascular endothelial growth factor, also has been approved. In a study comparing the use of bevacizumab plus irinotecan and 5-FU/leucovorin with 5-FU/leucovorin alone, the bevacizumab-containing regimen was associated with a longer overall survival (median 20.3 months versus 15.6 months) and a higher response rate (44.8% versus 34.8%) (Hurwitz et al, 2004). Currently, a patient without prior systemic therapy has an almost 50% chance of responding to modern systemic therapy and can be expected to have a median survival of approximately 18 to 20 months without resection. Nevertheless, unresected patients still rarely live beyond 3 years.

These encouraging results are for first-line therapy. If a patient fails first-line therapy, the results are less encouraging. Response rates of 20% or less can be expected whether the patient receives an oxaliplatin (Bensmaine et al, 2001; Comella et al, 2002), irinotecan (Cunningham et al, 1998), or biologic regimen (Cunningham et al, 2004).

RESULTS OF RESECTION FOR COLORECTAL LIVER METASTASES

Over the last 3 decades, an increasingly aggressive surgical approach has resulted in abundant data to support hepatectomy as a potentially curative approach for metastatic colorectal cancer. The rationale for a regional approach to what normally would be thought of as a systemic process is based on the concept that tumor cells from gastrointestinal malignancies, especially colorectal cancer, spread hematogenously via the portal circulation, making the liver the first site of metastasis in most patients (Weiss et al, 1986). This stepwise spread of cancer from primary site to liver and from there to other organs provides an opportunity to prevent dissemination of tumor to other sites by direct treatment of hepatic metastases. In this way, metastatic colorectal cancer differs from most other metastatic malignancies. In addition, the remarkable ability of the liver to regenerate after hepatic resection (see Ch. 4) has enabled aggressive surgical options for hepatic metastases. In patients with normal hepatic reserve, removal of 80% of the liver is possible, with regeneration largely occurring in the first few weeks.

Long-Term Results

In 1978, Foster provided the first multi-institutional data encouraging liver resection for metastatic colorectal cancer. In this collected series from 99 institutions, liver resections were associated with a 20% 5-year survival, clearly superior to the 0% 5-year survival associated with any other therapy available at the time (Foster, 1978). Since then, many large single-institution and multi-center reports have shown that liver resection is effective and can be potentially curative in the treatment of this disease (Table 73a.2) (Doci et al, 1991; Iwatsuki et al, 1986; Logan et al, 1982; Morrow et al, 1982; Vogt et al, 1991; Younes et al, 1991). Three of these studies are particularly worthy of mention. In 1986, Hughes and associates published a multicenter survey study involving 859 patients treated by potentially curative liver resection; they reported the actuarial 5-year patient survival to be 33%. More recently, Nordlinger and colleagues (1996) reported an analysis from a multicenter series of more than 1500 patients subjected to liver resection for hepatic colorectal metastases with 2-year and 5-year survival rates of 64% and 28%. Fong and coworkers (1999) analyzed data from 1001 patients from a single institution and showed even more favorable results. In this study, surgical resection resulted in a 5-year survival for nearly 40% of patients and a median survival of longer than 40 months (Fong et al, 1999).

Liver resection has become the standard treatment for metastatic lesions from colorectal primaries. With many series reporting long-term survival for these patients, even before the era of modern chemotherapy, 5-year, 10-year, and 20-year survivals with hepatic resection can be expected to reach 40%, 25%, and 20% (Butler et al, 1986; Nordlinger et al, 1987; Scheele et al, 1991). There is no doubt that surgery alone can cure a subset of patients. Because these long-term results with surgery are significantly better than the results in untreated patients or patients treated with systemic chemotherapy, it would be impossible, on ethical grounds, to set up a randomized study to compare the two therapeutic modalities. The safety and efficacy of surgical resection compare favorably with alternative treatments.

Outcome and Surgical Volume

Numerous studies have correlated perioperative outcome with hospital volume for hepatectomy. Choti and colleagues (1998) and Glasgow and associates (1999), using the state registries in Maryland and in California, found that hepatectomies performed at a high volume center improved outcome as measured by perioperative mortality, length of hospital stay, and cost. A study by Fong and coworkers (2005) also found that long-term survival was significantly improved for patients treated by hepatectomy at a high volume center. Using data from the National Medicare Database, the authors showed that perioperative outcome correlated with surgical expertise, and notably the survival advantage

Table 73a.2   Results of Hepatic Resection for Metastatic Colorectal Cancer

Reference	N	Operative Mortality	1-Yr Survival (%)	3-Yr Survival (%)	5-Yr Survival (%)	10-Yr Survival (%)	Median (mo)
Foster, 1978	78	5	—*	—	22	—	—
Thompson et al, 1983	22	11	80	37	31	—	18
Adson et al, 1984	141	3	80	42	25	—	—
Fortner et al, 1984	75	7	89	57	35	—	—
Butler et al, 1986	62	10	—	50	34	21	—
Iwatsuki et al, 1986	60	0	95	53	45	—	—
Hughes et al, 1986	607	—	—	—	33	—	—
Nordlinger et al, 1987	80	5	75	41	25	18	—
Cobourn et al, 1987	56	0	—	—	25	—	—
Schlag et al, 1990	122	4	85	40	30	—	32
Doci et al, 1991	100	5	—	28	—	28	—
Younes et al, 1991	133	—	91	—	—	—	—
Rosen et al, 1992	280	4	84	47	25	—	—
Scheele et al, 1995	434	4	85	45	33	20	40
Jamison et al, 1997	280	4	84	—	27	20	33
Fong et al, 1999	1001	2.8	89	57	36	22	42
Minagawa et al, 2000	235	0.85	—	51	38	26	—
Choti et al, 2002	226	1	93	57	40	26	46
Belli et al, 2002	181	—	91.2	55.3	39.8	—	—
Kato et al, 2003	585	0†	—	—	33	—	—
Mutsaerts et al, 2005	102	3	—	—	29	—	—

*— indicates data not specified.
†Patients who died perioperatively were excluded from study.

was not lost after the perioperative period. These data lend support to the concept of regionalization of hepatectomies to high volume centers.

PROGNOSTIC VARIABLES AND STAGING SYSTEMS

All patients with colorectal metastases by definition are grouped as stage IV in the TNM staging system, but considerable diversity exists within this group. The prognosis of a patient with a solitary liver metastasis found years after resection of a node-negative right colon cancer is different from the prognosis of a patient with synchronously discovered diffuse bilateral liver metastases at the time of operation for a perforated node-positive colon cancer. A classification system that can discriminate between these patients and provide meaningful prognostic information is essential. This classification system must enable the comparison of patients from diverse publications and facilitate patient selection for adjuvant therapy or clinical trials.

To define a new classification system, clinical and pathologic variables that predict survival in this population must be defined. In the population of patients with isolated hepatic metastases from colorectal cancer, clinical and pathologic variables can be classified broadly into three categories: (1) clinical and pathologic variables associated with the primary tumor, (2) clinical variables associated with the presentation of the liver metastases, and (3) pathologic characteristics of the liver metastases (Table 73a.3). The disparate results between studies are due to the relatively small sample sizes in most early studies because of the difficulty in performing a reliable multivariate analysis on small numbers of patients. These studies are nevertheless important in providing the preliminary data that have guided more recent large cohort studies.

Characteristics of the Patient and Primary Tumor

Although age has not been found consistently to be a significant prognostic variable for long-term survival (Ballantyne & Quin, 1993; Cady et al, 1992; Hughes et al, 1988), this is likely due to patient selection. Most clinicians are reluctant to perform liver resections in elderly patients, particularly those with comorbidities. The data on the effect of gender on prognosis are conflicting, but some reports have shown better outcomes in women than in men (Adson, 1987; Holm et al, 1989). The location of primary cancer does not seem to affect outcome, with no significant differences in survival for patients with rectal versus colon cancers (Adson, 1987; Doci et al, 1991). The stage of the primary is a major prognostic factor for outcome, however (Doci et al, 1991; Hughes et al, 1986). Regional nodal involvement by tumor predicts a poorer overall survival (Hughes et al, 1989). Liver metastases found synchronously with the colorectal primary tumor also predict a poor outcome (Ballantyne & Quin, 1993). The cellular differentiation of primary cancer has not been shown to influence outcome independently (Doci et al, 1991).

Clinical Characteristics of Liver Metastases

The clinical presentation of hepatic metastases most often correlated with poor outcome is a short disease-free interval between presentation of the primary cancer and the development of liver metastases (Hughes et al, 1986; Rosen et al, 1992; Scheele et al, 1991). Multiple tumors (Hughes et al, 1986; Rosen et al, 1992), bilateral tumors (Pass et al, 1985), large tumor size (Hughes et al, 1986; Stephenson et al, 1988), and markedly elevated preoperative carcinoembryonic antigen (CEA) (Hughes et al, 1986; Nordlinger et al, 1996) are additional predictors

Table 73a.3 Predictors of Recurrence after Hepatic Resection for Metastatic Colorectal Cancer

Reference	Patient Age	Primary Stage	METASTASES Synchronous	Size	No.	Bilobar	Satellite	Chemotherapy	Surgical Margin	CEA
Foster, 1978	—	N	N	Y	Y	—	—	—	—	—
Adson et al, 1984	—	Y	N	N	N	N	—	—	—	—
Fortner et al, 1984	N	Y	—	N	N	—	—	N	—	N
Butler et al, 1986	N	Y	N	N	N	—	—	N	N	—
Iwatsuki et al, 1986	N	Y	N	Y	Y	—	—	Y	—	—
Cobourn et al, 1987	—	N	N	—	Y	—	N	—	—	—
Nordlinger et al, 1987	—	—	—	N	N	—	—	—	—	—
Hughes et al, 1988	—	Y	Y	Y	Y	Y	—	Y	Y	Y
Schlag et al, 1990	—	—	Y	—	—	—	—	—	—	—
Doci et al, 1991	N	Y	N	N	N	N	—	—	—	N
Scheele et al, 1991	N	Y	Y	N	N	N	Y	—	Y	—
Younes et al, 1991	—	N	N	Y	Y	—	—	—	—	Y
Cady et al, 1992	N	N	N	N	Y	—	—	—	Y	Y
Rosen et al, 1992	—	N	N	N	N	—	Y	—	N	—
Scheele et al, 1995	N	Y	Y	Y	N	N	Y	—	Y	Y
Nordlinger et al, 1996	Y	Y	Y	Y	Y	N	—	—	Y	Y
Fong et al, 1997	N	Y	Y	Y	Y	Y	—	Y	Y	Y
Fong et al, 1999	N	Y	Y	Y	Y	Y	—	—	Y	Y

of recurrence and death from disease. The prognosis is better for fewer than four tumors; however, even when more than four tumors are found, complete resection of the metastases is still better than systemic therapy alone (Cady et al, 1992; Fortner et al, 1984; Hughes et al, 1986). A tumor size greater than 5 cm diameter also is associated with a poorer outcome. A CEA level greater than 200 ng/mL is associated with early recurrence and death from disease, whereas a CEA of less than 5 ng/mL has been associated with a greater than 50% 5-year disease-free survival (Cady et al, 1992; Hughes et al, 1988).

Operative and Pathologic Characteristics of Liver Metastases

Anatomic resections are associated with a significantly lower rate of positive margins, and patients subjected to anatomic resection had a better outcome than patients subjected to wedge resections (DeMatteo et al, 2000) (see Ch. 83). The reason for this is technical-anatomic resections allow definition of resection planes along major hepatic veins and prevent inadvertent incision into the tumor. Wedge resections usually are guided by palpation and may be plagued by difficulties in exposure and retraction. The attendant problems of poor visibility and impaired tactile sense at the depth of the resection often lead to tearing of the specimen along the hard tumor–soft liver interface, resulting in a positive margin (see Ch. 80). Higher operative blood loss and transfusion requirements have been found to be associated with an increased number of perioperative complications and mortality, but not with a worse long-term survival (Kooby et al, 2003b). The most important operative finding associated with adverse long-term survival to date is extrahepatic disease (Adson et al, 1984; Cady & McDermott, 1985; Ekberg et al, 1987; Fortner et al, 1984; Hughes et al, 1986; Rosen et al, 1992). Aside from limited, resectable pulmonary metastases, particularly in patients showing response to systemic chemotherapy (DeMatteo et al, 1999; Smith et al, 1992), the existence of extrahepatic disease should be considered a contraindication for hepatectomy. Other unmistakable predictors of recurrence are involvement of the resection margin by tumor (Cady & McDermott, 1985; Hughes et al, 1986) and hepatic satellite lesions (Gayowski et al, 1994; Scheele et al, 1995).

A pathologic feature that frequently has been overlooked is intrabiliary invasion and intraluminal growth of metastatic liver tumors. Okano and associates (1999), in a clinicopathologic review of 355 colorectal liver metastases, observed histologic bile duct invasion in 42% and macroscopic invasion in 12%. Two thirds of tumors with macroscopic invasion were well-differentiated with less vascular involvement, and correspondingly the 5-year survivals were significantly better in these tumors (80% versus 57%). The same group later showed that the histology of the primary tumor was well-differentiated adenocarcinoma in 100% of patients with intrahepatic biliary invasion of metastases (Kubo et al, 2002). By contrast, when intrabiliary extension is significant enough to cause jaundice or to be detected as an intrabiliary filling defect on preoperative imaging, the tumors are rarely resectable with a 5-year survival of 0% in unresected patients (Povoski et al, 2000). These preoperative findings are relatively infrequent, and intraoperative recognition is more common than clinical and radiographic recognition. A diligent examination of the resected liver tissue may identify unsuspected bile duct involvement, which could have implications for a negative margin status and for long-term prognosis.

Clinical Risk Score

Two large studies have allowed for robust multivariate analyses of prognostic variables. Nordlinger and colleagues (1996) reported on a multicenter series of more than 1500 patients. Fong and colleagues (1999) reported on a single-institution series of 1001 patients with similar results in both studies. In the latter series, the seven parameters that were found to be independent predictors of prognosis were (1) the presence of extrahepatic disease, (2) a positive resection margin, (3) nodal metastases from primary cancer, (4) a short disease-free interval, (5) largest tumor greater than 5 cm, (6) more than one liver metastasis, and (7) CEA greater than 200 ng/mL. The first two parameters are data that are determined intraoperatively only because preoperative evidence of extrahepatic disease and inability to obtain negative margins would be relative contraindications to surgery. There is no role for surgical debulking in this setting. Using the last five criteria, a preoperative clinical risk score (CRS) system was created (Table 73a.4) with each positive criterion counting as 1 point. This CRS is a simple, easily remembered staging system for classifying patients with liver-exclusive metastatic colorectal cancer (Fig. 73a.1).

The presence of any one of these characteristics still was associated with a 5-year survival of 24% to 34%, and no single criterion can be considered a contraindication to resection. The total score out of 5 is highly predictive of outcome. A score of 2 or less places a patient in a good prognostic group, for whom resection is ideal. For scores of 3 or 4, outcome is less favorable, and patients should be considered for aggressive trials of adjuvant therapy. For a score of 5, long-term disease-free survivors rarely are encountered, and resections in this high-risk group should be accompanied by trials of adjuvant therapy.

Current Use of Clinical Risk Score

This prognostic scoring system has been verified by independent investigators from Norway (Mala et al, 2002), indicating that it is applicable in a variety of populations outside of a large tertiary U.S. center. This CRS also has proved useful in selection of patients for neoadjuvant therapy and ablative therapies and in stratification of patients enrolled in clinical trials (Table 73a.5). This CRS also now is being used to help select the extent and sophistication of preoperative assessment. A high CRS has been associated with sufficiently high incidence of occult metastatic disease that fluorodeoxyglucose positron emission tomography (FDG PET) can be justified as a preoperative test (Schussler-Fiorenza et al, 2004). The multitude of tests available for preoperative staging and the relatively high cost of newer imaging modalities necessitate a risk stratification tool to identify patients who are most and least likely to have their management altered by the results of the test.

Table 73a.4   Prognostic Scoring System for Hepatic Colorectal Metastases*

Node-positive primary tumor
Disease-free interval <12 mo between colon resection and appearance of metastases
Size of largest lesion >5 cm
>1 tumor
CEA >200 ng/dL

*Sum of points with 1 point assigned for each positive criterion.

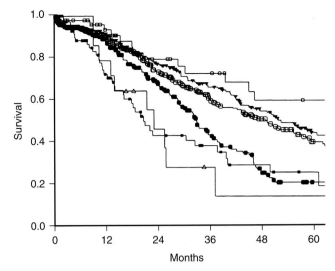

Fig. 73a.1. Survival after hepatic resection as related to CRS. *Open box*, score = 0 (*n* = 52); *filled triangle*, score = 1 (*n* = 262); *open circle*, score = 2 (*n* = 350); *filled circle*, score = 3 (*n* = 243); *filled box*, score = 4 (*n* = 80); *open triangle*, score = 5 (*n* = 14). *P* = .00001.
(From Fong Y, et al, 1999: Clinical score for predicting recurrence after hepatic resection for metastatic colorectal cancer: analysis of 1001 consecutive cases. Ann Surg 230:314. Copyright © 1999 Lippincott Williams & Wilkins.)

The yield from laparoscopy (Jarnagin et al, 2001) in the preoperative staging of patients with hepatic colorectal metastases also has been correlated with the CRS. For patients with a high CRS, a laparoscopy can save patients with disseminated disease from having a laparotomy, minimizing morbidity and hospital stay, whereas patients with a low CRS can avoid the added anesthesia and operating room time associated with a negative laparoscopy.

Molecular Determinants of Outcome

Molecular characteristics of the tumors constitute an evolving area that is likely to become important in postoperative stratification of risk of recurrence and cancer outcome. There are reports that molecular characteristics that predict response to

chemotherapy, such as tumor thymidylate synthase levels or levels of the transcription factor E2F-1, are important in outcome (Banerjee et al, 2000). It is likely that these and other molecular determinants will be incorporated into postoperative prognostic scales in the future.

PREOPERATIVE INVESTIGATIONS

The selection of patients for hepatic metastasectomy depends on patient operability and tumor resectability. The criteria for patient operability are similar to the criteria considered for any major laparotomy. A history of cardiac and pulmonary disease must be investigated because these patients are at significant risk for perioperative complications. Pulmonary compromise secondary to the long upper abdominal incision and the development of a right sympathetic pleural effusion may predispose to pneumonia. This risk can be reduced by avoiding a subcostal incision and using an upper midline incision with a rightward extension above the umbilicus. In addition, dramatic intravascular fluid shifts and electrolyte imbalances, which may occur perioperatively, can precipitate cardiac ischemia and arrhythmia. Finally, any previous liver disease that might have impaired hepatic function should be evaluated because this determines the volume of liver than can be resected safely.

Preoperative investigations before resection of metastatic colon cancer are directed at (1) establishing the diagnosis, (2) anatomically defining the liver lesion for diagnosis and surgical planning, and (3) staging to rule out extrahepatic disease. A confirmatory biopsy of hepatic lesions is indicated to confirm the diagnosis only when the clinical picture is unclear. Metastatic tumors and benign hepatic lesions usually can be differentiated by imaging modalities, including ultrasound, magnetic resonance imaging (MRI), and PET, as discussed further on. The risk of tract seeding from percutaneous fine-needle aspiration seems to be quite small with only a few case reports in the literature. The workup to determine the extent of disease includes imaging (see later) and recent colonoscopy (within 6 months). Because a detailed discussion of each imaging modality is beyond the scope of this chapter, the following discussion focuses on the practical aspects of imaging for preoperative workup of patients with hepatic colorectal metastases.

Role of Preoperative Imaging

Computed Tomography

Computed tomography (CT) (see Ch. 18) has become indispensable in the staging of patients with metastatic colorectal cancer. CT scans of the chest, abdomen, and pelvis are obtained routinely, although the yield from a CT scan of the chest in identifying metastatic tumors is small (Kronawitter et al, 1999). The most important images in the evaluation of the liver are obtained in the portal venous phase. The arterial phase images in a typical triphasic scan are not useful in identifying metastatic colorectal lesions because these lesions are not very vascular. Arterial phase images are used mainly to identify benign vascular lesions, such as hemangiomata, that are common and can be mistaken for colorectal metastases. In addition, arterial phase images can be used to define the arterial anatomy of the liver to aid in placement of hepatic arterial infusion (HAI) pumps (see Ch. 79). Standard CT scanning in this disease consists of a triphasic scan

Table 73a.5 Clinical Risk Score and Survival in Patients Undergoing Liver Resection for Metastatic Colorectal Cancer*

| Score | FONG ET AL | | MALA ET AL | |
	5-Yr Survival (%)	Median Survival (mo)	5-Yr Survival (%)	Median Survival (mo)
0	60	74	42	40
1	44	51		39
2	40	47		30
3	20	33	12	20
4	25	20		37
5	14	22	—†	—†

*Data from two studies (Fong et al, 1999; Mala et al, 2002).
†In Mala et al, there were no patients classified with a clinical risk score of 5.

with 5- to 7-mm-thick slices. When scans are intended for reconstruction of the hepatic arterial anatomy, 1.5-mm-thick overlapping slices are obtained.

Metastatic lesions from colorectal primaries tend to respect the liver capsule and intersegmental planes and push structures away, rather than invade directly into them (Baer et al, 1989; Scheele, 1989). Even very large lesions that appear to involve the inferior vena cava on CT often do not, and such appearances should not preclude exploration. Similarly, diaphragmatic invasion is rare, and approximation of the diaphragm by a large tumor should not deter the surgeon from exploration (Weinbren & Blumgart, 1986).

Magnetic Resonance Imaging

MRI (see Ch. 19) is most useful in diagnosing equivocal hepatic lesions and in defining the relationship of tumors to the hepatic vasculature and the biliary tree with MRI cholangiopancreatography. In particular, MRI is superb in diagnosing benign lesions, such as hemangiomata, adenomas, and fibronodular hyperplasia, and in delineating metastases in a fatty liver, where CT may not show small lesions clearly. MRI should be performed if lesions are equivocal or in patients with fatty liver from obesity, diabetes, prior chemotherapy, or other metabolic causes. MRI is most beneficial in the scenario where a patient has a fatty liver, a high CEA, and no detectable lesions by CT. MRI is much more expensive than CT and should not be used routinely.

Ultrasonography

Ultrasonography (see Ch. 15) is a relatively inexpensive test that may provide detailed information about the number, extent, and anatomic relationship of the hepatic tumor, but it is highly operator dependent. In expert hands, this examination is highly sensitive in finding small metastatic lesions within the liver. Ultrasound gives information regarding the size of the tumor and extent of liver involvement. It is the least expensive method for diagnosing cystic lesions of the liver. Duplex ultrasound can define the proximity of the tumor to vascular hilar structures, hepatic veins, and the inferior vena cava and in many cases may obviate the need for angiography (Gibson et al, 1986; Hann et al, 1996).

Hepatic Angiography and Computed Tomography Portography

Direct hepatic angiography (see Ch. 21) has largely been replaced by the less invasive CT angiography and MRI angiography. The main indication for direct angiography at present is for CT portography. This is a technique whereby contrast material is administered directly into the splanchnic bed by injection into the superior mesenteric artery. CT images acquired after a suitable delay provide portal phase pictures of the liver that are highly sensitive for even small metastatic tumors (Sica et al, 2000). The invasive nature of the test and the relatively high false positive rate resulting from perfusion defects limit the utility of this test. Nevertheless, it may be useful for patients with multiple small tumors or to rule out other smaller tumors not identified by other cross-section imaging modalities and may provide valuable information for patients with very high CEA levels and negative results on other imaging modalities.

Inferior Vena Cavography

There is virtually no role for inferior vena cavography in the evaluation of patients with metastatic colorectal cancer. MRI and duplex ultrasound usually yield sufficient details for surgical planning.

Positron Emission Tomography

An exciting innovation in imaging for patients with metastatic colorectal cancer is the advent of whole body PET (see Ch. 17). The most common tracer used in PET scanning is FDG, a glucose analogue that cannot proceed down the glycolytic pathway and accumulates within glucose-avid cancer cells, such as colorectal metastases. The FDG can be imaged to localize the distribution of metastases (Fig. 73a.2). Strasberg and coworkers (2001) examined the utility of this imaging modality in guiding surgical therapy for patients determined by CT to have resectable disease. Of 43 patients, they found 6 additional cases of unresectable disease by FDG PET (14%). In addition, of the 37 patients explored for resection, 35 underwent resection (95%) with a 77% 3-year survival (Strasberg et al, 2001). These are highly encouraging data for use of FDG PET in this patient population because they indicate that FDG PET not only alters surgical therapy by improving staging, but also improves long-term outcome by enhancing patient selection. In the United States, the use of FDG PET for staging, diagnosis, and restaging for colorectal cancer was approved by Medicare in 2001 (Kelloff et al, 2005).

Role of Laparoscopic Staging

Laparoscopy (see Ch. 23) has been shown to be a useful tool for staging patients with hepatic malignancies (Babineau et al, 1994; Jarnagin et al, 2000; John et al, 1994). This minimally invasive technique is particularly good at identifying peritoneal disease or

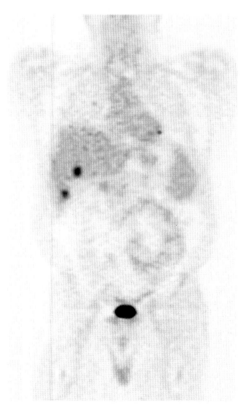

Fig. 73a.2. A patient with two potentially resectable hepatic metastases in the right lobe of the liver. FDG PET identified abnormal uptake in the left lingula of the lung; a biopsy was performed, and this was found to represent an extrahepatic colorectal cancer metastasis.

the involvement of periportal lymph nodes not apparent on preoperative imaging. When laparoscopy is employed, laparotomy can be avoided in 78% of patients with unresectable disease (Potter et al, 2000). In these patients, laparoscopy can decrease the morbidity of operation, shorten hospital stay, decrease cost, and shorten the delay to systemic therapy (Jarnagin et al, 2001).

In cases in which laparoscopy yields no additional findings, this diagnostic procedure lengthens anesthetic time and increases cost. Its use should be limited to patients who have a significant risk of having unresectable disease. Laparoscopy is indicated in cases in which the results of imaging studies are suspicious, but not diagnostic for extrahepatic tumor, such as suspicious peritoneal nodules or enlarged lymph nodes. Jarnagin and colleagues (2001) also have shown that the CRS predicts yield of laparoscopy. In patients with a CRS greater than 2, the likelihood of occult metastatic disease identified at laparoscopy was 42% compared with 12% in patients with a CRS of 2 or less. Laparoscopy should be routine in patients with a CRS greater than 2.

Synchronous Metastases and Timing of Resection

The timing of hepatic resection in patients presenting with liver metastases during workup for the primary tumor is controversial. Some suggest that synchronous diagnosis of metastases portends a worse prognosis (Scheele et al, 1995), perhaps as a result of a failure to detect micrometastatic foci in the liver. Delaying hepatic resection may increase survival in the surgically resected group by selecting out the patients with aggressive tumor biology who would be unlikely to derive a survival benefit from resection. Although delayed resection does not seem to impair survival, it does increase the volume of resected liver, a factor that is predictive of postoperative complications (Lambert et al, 2000). Simultaneous resection does have the advantage, however, of avoiding the morbidity of a second laparotomy. In many studies, a one-stage procedure has been shown to be safe with no differences in overall survival between immediate versus delayed liver resection (Vogt et al, 1991). In one study, age greater than 70 years and poorly differentiated histology of the primary predicted decreased overall survival (Tanaka et al, 2004). If simultaneous resection can be performed without changing the overall operative mortality, it is a reasonable approach, whereas if the liver and colon resections are extensive or if the patient is frail, a staged approach is often preferable.

Preoperative Algorithm

The preoperative preparation and planning before hepatic resection of colorectal metastases must be meticulous to avoid unexpected findings or obstacles at the time of laparotomy. A systematic approach to a colorectal cancer patient who is referred for consideration of hepatic resection can facilitate a thorough patient workup and minimize unnecessary investigations.

OPERATIVE TECHNIQUE (see Chs. 80-83)

The principles of hepatic resection are no different for colorectal metastases than for any other hepatic surgery. The immediate preoperative preparation includes a single dose of prophylactic antibiotics and placement of sequential compression devices to prevent the development of deep vein thromboses. The choice of incision includes a subcostal, long midline, or a short midline with a rightward extension approximately 3 cm above the umbilicus. The latter is used most frequently at our institution because it provides excellent exposure, while minimizing the length of incision in the upper abdomen, potentially reducing postoperative pulmonary compromise. The maintenance of a low central venous pressure (<5 mm Hg) can reduce operative blood loss by decreasing bleeding from the hepatic venous radicles during dissection (see Chs. 25 and 80). Maintenance of low central venous pressure can be facilitated by performing the dissection with the patient in 15 degrees of Trendelenburg, which increases the venous return to the heart and improves cardiac output.

Intraoperative Staging and Role of Intraoperative Ultrasound

As with any laparotomy for cancer, the abdomen must be explored thoroughly for evidence of extrahepatic metastases. In particular, the celiac axis and portocaval and hilar lymph nodes must be palpated, and any suspicious nodes should be removed and examined by frozen section. Most surgeons routinely use intraoperative ultrasound after mobilization of the liver. With experience, this practice may detect 5% to 10% of lesions missed on noninvasive imaging with CT, MRI, and transabdominal ultrasound (Boldrini et al, 1987; Machi et al, 1987, 1991; Olsen, 1990; Stone et al, 1994). In addition, intraoperative ultrasound can delineate better the interior anatomy of the liver, including intrahepatic vessels, and hepatic resection can be performed more safely and in a more anatomically oriented fashion. In addition to the initial planning, the operation can be monitored by the repeated use of intraoperative ultrasound because the resection line is displayed in relation to the lesion and blood vessels. Several reports, from the pre–FDG PET scan era, have shown that surgical management of hepatic tumors has been changed by the use of intraoperative ultrasound in 30% to 50% of operations (Castaing et al, 1986; Rifkin et al, 1987). The extent of resection depends on the number and location of metastases relative to the portal triads and hepatic veins. As previously mentioned, anatomic resections, which are facilitated by intraoperative ultrasound, are preferred to wedge resections. Anatomic resections permit excision of parenchymal areas distal to the index tumor, where vascular micrometastases tend to occur, and, most importantly they are less likely to have positive margins (2% versus 16%) (Weber et al, 2000).

POSTOPERATIVE MANAGEMENT (see Chs. 24-26)

Immediate Postoperative Care

Metabolic derangements are common in the postoperative period after liver resection and are due to hepatic insufficiency and hepatic regeneration. Hypoproteinemia and hypoglycemia may indicate early hepatic insufficiency, but they are usually transient. Hypokalemia and hypophosphatemia occur on postoperative day 2 as the liver begins to consume these electrolytes for regeneration. These metabolic conditions should be treated supportively with an intravenous infusion of 5% dextrose and half normal saline and 15 to 30 mEq/L of potassium phosphate.

Alkaline phosphatase and transaminase elevations are common, and hyperbilirubinemia may occur. Abnormalities in coagulation or platelets also may occur and should be treated if the international normalized ratio is greater than 1.5 or the platelets are less than 50,000/μL. Hepatic regeneration occurs rapidly. DNA synthesis is initiated in hepatocytes 10 to 12 hours after surgery, and most of the hepatic mass has returned within 1 week. Subsequent architectural arrangement continues over the next few weeks, but in most cases this is complete in 6 weeks.

Perioperative Mortality and Morbidity

For a surgical approach to be widely accepted, it must be not only efficacious, but also safe and feasible. Major liver resection can be performed with acceptable mortality and morbidity. Using proper patient selection, preoperative staging, and surgical expertise, metastatic hepatectomies can result in prolonged disease-free survival and cure.

Mortality

The mortality associated with an elective liver resection for colorectal metastases has decreased significantly over the last 3 decades, and since the 1990s it has been uniformly less than 10% in all major series (Butler et al, 1986; Cobourn et al, 1987; Hughes et al, 1986; Nordlinger et al, 1987; Pagana, 1986; Rosen et al, 1992; Scheele et al, 1991; Schlag et al, 1990; Younes et al, 1991). Advances in understanding of liver anatomy, resection techniques, and anesthetic care have translated into favorable survival rates after even the most extensive resections. Results from the best centers have reached a plateau at an operative mortality of 3% to 5% (see Table 73a.2). Most deaths

occur from perioperative hemorrhage or liver failure. Mortality is unlikely to improve further because although technical advances have improved safety, surgeons have taken an increasingly aggressive approach to hepatic resections. Most patients and surgeons are willing to accept a 3% to 5% mortality for a surgical resection because it represents the only potentially curative approach to an aggressive cancer.

Morbidity

Removing a significant portion of the liver produces significant metabolic and immunologic derangements, and this is the major contributor to the relatively high complication rate associated with hepatectomy. The reported complication rate in most series is greater than 20% (Table 73a.6), but this is likely an underestimate resulting from the retrospective nature of most reports. Other nonspecific morbidities include cardiac, pulmonary, and infectious complications. The incidence of myocardial complications is relatively low (approximately 1%) (Doci et al, 1991; Fortner et al, 1984; Nordlinger et al, 1987; Scheele et al, 1991) and reflects the careful selection of patients for liver resection. Pulmonary complications are more frequent and are due to the large upper abdominal incision and the postsurgical sympathetic pleural effusions. Symptomatic pleural effusions that may require tube thoracostomy occur in 5% to 10% of cases (Coppa et al, 1985; Nordlinger et al, 1987). Pneumonia occurs in 5% to 22% of cases (Doci et al, 1991; Schlag et al, 1990), and pulmonary embolism occurs in 1% of cases (Cunningham et al, 1994; Scheele et al, 1991).

Of liver-specific complications, the most ominous is liver failure, which occurs after 3% to 8% of all major hepatic resections (Cunningham et al, 1994; Doci et al, 1991; Scheele et al, 1991; Schlag et al, 1990). Bile leak and biliary fistula occur in

Table 73a.6 Complications of Liver Resection*

	Scheele et al, 1992	Schlag et al, 1990	Doci et al, 1991	Fortner et al, 1984	Nordlinger et al, 1987	Coelho et al, 2004	Mala et al, 2002	Jarnagin et al, 2002	Cady et al, 1998
Total resections	219	122	100	75	80	83	146	1803	244
Liver-related complications									
Hemorrhage	7 (3)	—†	3	1 (1)	1 (1)	—	4‡ (3)	18	1
Bile fistula	8 (4)	5 (4)	4	—	—	11	2 (1)	—	2
Perihepatic abscess	4 (2)	11 (9)	5	5 (7)	2 (3)	—	—	110	1
Liver failure	17 (8)	—	3	3 (4)	1 (1)	6	—	99	1
Renal failure	3 (1)	—	1	—	—	—	—	—	—
Portal vein thrombosis	—	—	—	1 (1)	—	1	1 (<1)	9	—
Infections									
Wound	—	7 (6)	—	1 (1)	—	2	—	94	2
Sepsis	—	3 (2)	2	—	4 (5)	—	3 (2)	39	2
General complications									
GI bleed	—	—	—	—	—	5	—	21	0
DVT	2 (1)	—	—	1 (1)	—	—	—	24	<1
Pulmonary embolism	4 (2)	—	—	1 (1)	1 (1)	—	—	—	<1
Cardiac/MI	2 (1)	6 (5)	1	1 (1)	1 (1)	1	1 (<1)	21	3
Pneumonia	—	10 (8)	22	3 (4)	—	7	13 (9)	54	1
Pleural effusion	—	—	—	6 (8)	3 (4)	11	—	154	2

*Number (%).
†— indicates data not specified.
‡One patient was operated on twice for hemorrhage.
DVT, deep vein thrombosis; GI, gastrointestinal; MI, myocardial infarction.

approximately 4% (Scheele et al, 1991; Schlag et al, 1990). Perihepatic abscess occurs in 2% to 10% (Doci et al, 1991; Fortner et al, 1984; Nordlinger et al, 1987; Scheele et al, 1991; Schlag et al, 1990). Significant hemorrhage is rare (1-3%), but is a major cause of perioperative mortality. The high incidence of complications does not always translate into prolonged hospital stay, and if treated appropriately and rapidly, most complications do not result in poor outcome. For major liver resections, the reported median hospital stay from centers experienced in liver surgery is less than 2 weeks. In a study of more than 1800 liver resections performed in a single center, including 544 trisegmentectomies, the median hospital stay was 8 days, and intensive care unit admission was required for only 112 patients (Jarnagin et al, 2002).

FOLLOW-UP AFTER RESECTION

There is no consensus regarding the extent and frequency of follow-up after surgery for primary colorectal cancer because it has not been shown conclusively to improve survival (Kjeldsen et al, 1997; Makela et al, 1995; Ohlsson et al, 1995; Schoemaker et al, 1998). Similarly, no conclusive data show improved survival with close follow-up after hepatic resection for colorectal cancer metastases. Nevertheless, patients who have undergone hepatic resection usually are monitored in an attempt to identify early recurrence that may be amenable to further resection for cure. Currently, most patients undergo serial physical examination, serum CEA level, annual chest x-ray, and CT of the abdomen and pelvis every 3 to 4 months for the first 2 years and then every 6 months for the next 5 years.

ROLE OF ADJUVANT THERAPY

Patterns of Recurrence

Most patients surviving after liver resection die of recurrent disease (Bozzetti et al, 1987; Ekberg et al, 1987; Maeda et al, 1992), indicating that disease undetected at the time of surgery is responsible for failures. The most common sites for failure are the liver or lung (Table 73a.7). In 45% to 75% of cases, the liver is involved as a site of recurrence after liver resection (Bozzetti et al, 1987; Hohenberger et al, 1990; Maeda et al, 1992;

Nordlinger et al, 1987); this explains the number of studies that have examined the use of hepatically directed adjuvant therapy.

Adjuvant Systemic Chemotherapy

No prospective study examining the utility of adjuvant systemic chemotherapy after complete hepatic resection of colon cancer has been completed to date. Results from four retrospective studies using systemic 5-FU–based chemotherapy are equivocal. Two respective studies from the Memorial Sloan-Kettering Cancer Center (MSKCC) reported by Butler and colleagues (1986) and Fortner and associates (1984) found no improvement in survival with adjuvant chemotherapy. In a small study from the University of Pittsburgh, Iwatsuki and coworkers (1986) reported that 22 patients who received chemotherapy had a significantly better survival than 38 patients who did not receive chemotherapy ($P<.05$). Hughes and coworkers (1986), in a report of collected series from 24 institutions, found that patients who received postoperative chemotherapy had a better overall survival, but the reported differences were small. Insufficient details were given to allow rigorous comparison of the groups studied. At present, there are no conclusive data on use of newer regimens, such as oxaliplatin, irinotecan, and bevacizumab, as adjuvant chemotherapy after liver resection for colorectal metastases. Although the use of oxaliplatin-based or irinotecan-based chemotherapies in this setting is commonplace, there are no clear data from comparative studies supporting such practice.

Adjuvant Hepatic Arterial Infusion Chemotherapy
(see Ch. 79)

Because the liver is the most common site for tumor recurrence after liver resection and is the sole site of recurrence in 40% of patients (Nordlinger et al, 1987), regional chemotherapy, via the hepatic artery, is a theoretically attractive mode of adjuvant therapy. The rationale for HAI of chemotherapy is based on the concept that most metastatic liver tumors preferentially derive their blood supply from the hepatic artery, whereas normal hepatic tissue relies on the portal venous blood supply. In addition, the ability of the hepatic parenchyma to extract and metabolize chemotherapy drugs to nontoxic metabolites offers a unique opportunity to administer highly toxic drug levels to tumor

Table 73a.7 Sites of Initial Recurrence After Liver Resection for Colorectal Metastasis*

Reference	N	Recurrences	Median Follow-Up (mo)	Liver	Liver and Other	Lung	Lung and Other	Colon/Rectum	Other
Hughes et al, 1986	607	424	—†	149 (35)	42 (10)	73 (17)	—	33 (8)	61 (14)
Schlag et al, 1990	122	80	—	17 (14)	55 (45)	—	—	—	8 (7)
Butler et al, 1986	62	30	—	10 (33)	10 (33)	—	—	—	10
Ekberg et al, 1987	68	53	20	19 (28)	25 (47)	3 (6)	12 (23)	8 (15)	—
Bozzetti et al, 1987	45	28	18	11 (39)	5 (18)	5 (17)	—	—	—
Nordlinger et al, 1987	80	51	—	21 (42)	13 (26)	11 (22)	—	11 (22)	—
Fortner, 1988	69	45	—	8 (12)	—	16 (23)	—	—	—
Suzuki et al, 1997	64	45	—	31 (48)	—	16 (25)	—	—	16 (25)

*Number (%).
†— indicates data not specified.

cells, while minimizing systemic toxicity. The ideal agent should have a steep dose-response curve to maximize local antitumour activity, a high extraction rate to minimize systemic toxicity, and rapid total body clearance when infusion is discontinued. The most extensively studied agent is 5-fluorouracil-2-deoxyuridine (FUDR), an analogue of 5-FU that can be concentrated 100-fold to 400-fold in the liver because of a 95% hepatic extraction ratio (Ensminger et al, 1978). For a more detailed discussion of the technical aspects of regional chemotherapy, see Ch. 79.

Hepatic Arterial Infusion as Palliative Therapy

Most of the data on regional hepatic chemotherapy is derived from studies of patients with unresectable disease (see Ch. 79). Randomized trials have shown that HAI is a safe treatment for colorectal metastasis to the liver that produces a significantly higher response rate than systemic chemotherapy (48-62% and 0-21%, respectively) (Chang et al, 1987; Hohn et al, 1989; Kemeny et al, 1987; Martin et al, 1990; Rougier et al, 1992). This increase in response rate has translated to an improved survival in only one study (Chang et al, 1987) in a subset analysis. In this study from the National Cancer Institute (Chang et al, 1987), if patients with portal lymph nodes positive for metastatic cancer were excluded from the analysis, the 2-year survival for intra-arterial chemotherapy was 47%, significantly better than the 13% survival with systemic chemotherapy ($P = .03$). There are several potential reasons why the superior response rates with HAI in the individual trials did not translate into greater survival benefit. First, because patients were randomized preoperatively, technical problems with pump placement and unexpectedly high rates of extrahepatic disease discovered at laparotomy led to a substantial number of patients, assigned to HAI arms, who never received regional therapy (range 0-34%). This may have led to an underestimation of benefit when using an intention-to-treat analysis. Second, lack of experience in certain centers and the absence of a strict, predetermined dose-reduction scheme in several trials may have led to greater toxicities and fewer cycles of therapy, which may have offset any survival benefit. Finally, three trials (conducted by MSKCC [Kemeny et al, 1987], the Northern California Oncology Group [Hohn et al, 1989], and the City of Hope [Wagman et al, 1990]) allowed crossover to HAI therapy for patients who progressed on systemic chemotherapy, further diluting any survival benefit based on intention to treat. In the study by Kemeny and associates (1987), 60% of patients randomized to systemic chemotherapy eventually crossed over to HAI, and in that group of patients the median survival was 18 months, whereas patients who could not cross over because of technical reasons had a median survival of 8 months.

The Cancer and Leukemia Group B is the most recently completed trial comparing systemic 5-FU/leucovorin with HAI of FUDR, leucovorin, and dexamethasone (Kemeny et al, 2003b). No crossover was permitted. Only 135 patients, out of an accrual goal of 340, were randomized, in part because of delays caused by a temporary halt in production of FUDR and implantable pumps by their respective manufacturers. The response rate (48% versus 25%; $P = .009$) was higher in the HAI group, with time to hepatic progression better in the HAI arm (9.8 months versus 7.3 months; $P = .017$) and time to extrahepatic progression better in the systemic arm (7.8 months versus 23.3 months; $P = .0007$). The median overall survival time was significantly better in the HAI arm (22.7 months versus 19.8 months; $P = .027$) (Kemeny et al, 2003b). The extrahepatic toxicities also were greater in the systemic group, with neutropenia in 45%, stomatitis in 24%, and diarrhea in 16% compared with 2%, 0%, and 5% in the FUDR group. Quality of life also was improved in the HAI group with better physical functioning (Rand-36, $P = .038$) and fewer symptoms (Memorial Symptom Assessment Scale [MSAS] $P = .017$) at 3 months.

Hepatic Arterial Infusion as Adjuvant Therapy (see Ch. 79)

Four reasonably sized, randomized trials of adjuvant regional chemotherapy have been completed, with three positive trials (Kemeny MM et al, 2002; Kemeny N et al, 1999; Lygidakis et al, 2001) and one negative trial (Lorenz et al, 1998). The negative trial, reported by Lorenz and coworkers (1998), found no difference in outcome for patients treated with resection alone versus patients treated with resection and regional 5-FU chemotherapy when analyzed on an intention-to-treat basis. This study had a high operative mortality rate in patients randomized to regional therapy (8%) and used 5-FU, which has a much lower regional extraction rate than FUDR and a higher incidence of dose-limiting systemic toxicity. In addition, the investigators used implanted ports, rather than a pump, with the result that technical complication prevented the use of chemotherapy in a significant number of patients randomized to regional therapy. Consequently, only 74% of patients assigned to HAI started this treatment, and only 30% completed it, emphasizing the importance of technical expertise when delivering regional chemotherapy (Lorenz et al, 1998).

Two large U.S. studies showed efficacy of regional adjuvant therapy. In an Intergroup study (Eastern Cooperative Oncology Group/South West Oncology Group) of 109 patients randomized to surgery alone or surgery plus HAI-FUDR, the 4-year hepatic disease–free survival was significantly better in the HAI group (67% versus 43%; $P = .03$) (Kemeny et al, 2002). In a larger single institution study from MSKCC, 156 patients were randomized to resection plus systemic 5-FU or resection plus combined systemic 5-FU and HAI-FUDR. The patients who were treated with regional therapy had a significantly better 2-year survival (86% versus 72%; $P = .03$) and markedly improved liver disease control. The 10-year follow-up to this study showed a significantly improved disease-free survival for patients treated with regional therapy (31.3 months versus 17.2 months) (Fig. 73a.3) (Kemeny & Gonen, 2005).

Current and future studies will explore regimens that combine HAI chemotherapy with FUDR and with systemic chemotherapy with newer agents such as irinotecan (CPT-11), oxaliplatin, bevacizumab, and cetuximab (Erbitux). This strategy would employ the most effective systemic therapy combined with the use of the most effective regional therapy for potential synergistic action against the metastases.

Phase I and II studies combining systemic CPT-11 with HAI-FUDR or combining systemic oxaliplatin with HAI-FUDR are being undertaken at many centers. In the palliative setting, the response rate of nonresectable hepatic colorectal metastases to CPT-11/HAI-FUDR as second-line therapy is 74% (Kemeny et al, 2001). This compares favorably to the 20% response rate expected for treatment with any systemic regimen as second-line therapy. A phase I/II study of adjuvant HAI with floxuridine and dexamethasone with intravenous irinotecan after resection of hepatic metastases from colon cancer showed the safety and feasibility of this regimen (Kemeny et al, 2003a). With a median follow-up of 40 months, the 2-year survival rate was 89%. Results from studies examining systemic oxaliplatin and HAI-FUDR are equally promising, with response rates of greater than

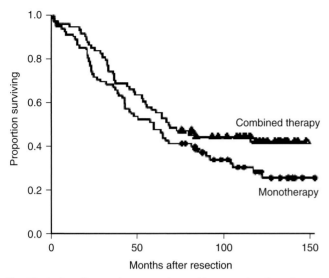

Fig. 73a.3. Overall survival among patients with metastatic colorectal cancer who were treated with HAI plus systemic chemotherapy (combined therapy) or with systemic chemotherapy alone (monotherapy).
(From Kemeny N, Gonen M, 2005: Hepatic arterial infusion after liver resection. N Engl J Med 352:734. Copyright © 2005 Massachusetts Medical Society.)

80% (Kemeny & Gonen, 2005) in the palliative setting. In a MSKCC phase I study, 36 patients (89% previously treated) with unresectable hepatic metastases received HAI of FUDR/dexamethasone plus either systemic oxaliplatin/5-FU/leucovorin or systemic oxaliplatin and irinotecan (Kemeny et al, 2005). Both regimens were well tolerated, and response rates were 90% and 87% with median survival times of 36 months and 22 months. Active investigation is now directed at determining whether combined systemic and regional chemotherapy is efficacious as an adjuvant therapy after liver resection. The American College of Surgical Oncology group presently is enrolling for a study of HAI with FUDR and dexamethasone in combination with intravenous oxaliplatin and 5-FU and leucovorin as adjuvant treatment in patients with resectable hepatic metastases from colorectal cancer (Alberts et al, 2004). While awaiting the results of ongoing trials, regional FUDR should be considered for adjuvant chemotherapy in patients at high risk for liver recurrence, particularly if the patient had failed systemic therapy previously.

NEOADJUVANT CHEMOTHERAPY FOR DOWNSTAGING OF UNRESECTABLE DISEASE

Improved response rates with new chemotherapeutic agents have the potential to render formerly unresectable patients resectable. In addition, neoadjuvant chemotherapy has the theoretical advantage of treating micrometastatic disease early and functioning as an in vivo test of chemoresponsiveness to a particular agent. Bismuth and colleagues (1996) were the first to publish this observation in a report examining 330 consecutive patients presenting to their institution with unresectable disease. They found that a combination of folinic acid, leucovorin, and oxaliplatin converted 53 of these patients to resectable disease. The long-term outcome of these patients after resection was similar to patients at their institution who were found initially to have resectable disease (Bismuth et al, 1996). Since then, numerous trials have shown the ability of neoadjuvant systemic chemotherapy

to render 3% to 41% of patients resectable (Adam et al, 2001; Alberts et al, 2003; De La Cámara et al, 2004; Delaunoit et al, 2004; Falcone et al, 2004; Giacchetti et al, 1999; Pozzo et al, 2004; Quenet et al, 2004; Wein et al, 2001). Patients who undergo complete resection have a median survival of 30 to 60 months (Alberts et al, 2003; Giacchetti et al, 1999). In the largest prospective study, 95 of 701 patients (14%) were rendered resectable with neoadjuvant 5-FU/leucovorin and either irinotecan or oxaliplatin. The factors associated with resectability and 5-year survival were large and critically located lesions, as opposed to multinodular disease and extrahepatic metastases (Adam et al, 2004a). Patients with tumor progression during preoperative chemotherapy have a significantly worse outcome, with a 5-year survival of 8% versus 37% and 30% for patients with objective tumor response or tumor stabilization (Adam et al, 2004b). Patients with tumor progression still had a poor prognosis even when a potentially curative hepatic resection was performed.

Data suggest that regional chemotherapy also may convert patients with unresectable liver metastases to resectable. Clavien and associates (2002), using HAI-FUDR with or without leucovorin, induced resectability in 6 (26%) of 23 previously treated patients (including 20 patients previously treated with irinotecan). The actuarial survival rates at 3 years were 84% for responders to neoadjuvant therapy compared with 40% for nonresponders. At MSKCC, 44 pretreated patients with extensive liver metastases received HAI-FUDR and dexamethasone plus oxaliplatin-based systemic chemotherapy as part of two phase I trials (Leonard et al, 2004). The study population in this trial had a high preoperative CRS (Fong et al, 1999) with many patients with more than four metastases, metastases greater than 5 cm in size, more than 25% liver involvement with tumor, a CEA level greater than 10 ng/dL, and previous chemotherapy exposure. Despite this high CRS, the objective response rate was 82%, resulting in complete gross resection of tumor in 9 (20%) of the 44 patients and a median survival for all patients of 26 months.

Neoadjuvant chemotherapy with newer agents, including oxaliplatin and irinotecan, has been associated with hepatic sinusoidal obstruction (Rubbia-Brandt et al, 2004) and hepatic steatosis (Kooby et al, 2003a; Parikh et al, 2003). More importantly, severe steatohepatitis has been reported with the administration of neoadjuvant chemotherapy, particularly in obese patients (Fernandez et al, 2005). In these patients, consideration should be given to preoperative liver biopsy to evaluate the histology of the liver parenchyma. In patients in whom liver function is compromised, preoperative portal vein embolization may be advisable to induce hypertrophy of the liver uninvolved with tumor. This finding provides an additional argument to proceed with surgery in resectable patients, particularly if they are obese, and undertake chemotherapy postoperatively when the liver has regenerated.

Steatohepatitis is not the only peril of neoadjuvant chemotherapy for the liver surgeon. A preoperatively treated liver is more fibrotic, often with perivascular adhesions. The planes of resection are difficult to dissect, making the procedure more challenging overall. Despite the operative complexity, the perioperative morbidity and mortality in the trials of resection after neoadjuvant chemotherapy do not seem to be higher than series of de novo hepatic resection (Adam et al, 2001, 2004b; De La Cámara et al, 2004; Pozzo et al, 2004; Quenet et al, 2004).

One last controversial issue is the treatment of a patient with a complete clinical response to neoadjuvant chemotherapy.

When there is no visible tumor left to resect, should a blind resection, based on the site of previous metastasis, be undertaken? No series to date have followed a cohort of patients with this clinical response to determine the outcomes and patterns of recurrence. Our current practice is to use intraoperative ultrasound to attempt to identify the lesion, and if this is not possible, we perform a hepatic resection of the area previously involved with tumor. This is not, however, a universally accepted practice.

Although the studies showing a high rate of R0 resection after preoperative chemotherapy are encouraging, they should not be used as justification to treat every patient with neoadjuvant chemotherapy. Neoadjuvant chemotherapy can be costly, with a regimen containing 5-FU, leucovorin, oxaliplatin, and bevacizumab costing more than $20,000 per month. As previously mentioned, these regimens can bring about steatosis, which has been shown to complicate subsequent liver surgery, and progression on neoadjuvant chemotherapy can portend a very poor prognosis. Currently, there are no recommended selection criteria, chemotherapy regimen, or duration of therapy for neoadjuvant treatment. Patients who present with liver lesions that are potentially resectable for cure should be offered a surgical resection because there are no definite data supporting a neoadjuvant chemotherapeutic approach.

REPEAT RESECTION FOR RECURRENCE AFTER RESECTION

As previously mentioned, the most common site for recurrence after resection of hepatic colorectal metastases is the liver, and it is the sole site of recurrence in 15% to 40% of cases

(Table 73a.8). In the absence of extrahepatic disease and in a patient with a good performance status and adequate hepatic reserve, a repeat hepatectomy may be considered, and approximately one third of recurrence is amenable to further resection (Bozzetti et al, 1992; Fortner, 1988). The presence of adhesions and the altered anatomy of the liver, particularly the position of the vasculature and biliary system, make this a technically challenging surgery. Nonetheless, many reports have shown the safety and the utility of repeat resection for recurrent hepatic-only disease (see Table 73a.8) (Bozzetti et al, 1992; Butler et al, 1986; Fortner, 1988; Griffith et al, 1990; Hohenberger et al, 1990; Lange et al, 1989; Nordlinger et al, 1987; Vaillant et al, 1993) with an operative mortality of less than 3% and morbidity similar to initial resections (Bozzetti et al, 1992; Lange et al, 1989). Reported complications include biliary fistula, hepatic duct stenosis, hemorrhage, hepatic failure, and subphrenic abscess. More importantly the 5-year overall survival ranged from 31% to 41% with a median survival of 30 to 46 months.

The largest series published to date is a combined series of 126 patients who underwent repeat resection from MSKCC and the University of Frankfurt Medical Center (Petrowsky et al, 2002). The operative procedures included 90 minor resections and 36 resections of a lobe or more. The 1-year, 3-year, and 5-year survivals were 86%, 51%, and 34%; there are 19 actual 5-year survivors to date. By multivariate regression analysis (proportional hazard model), number of lesions greater than 1 ($P = .01$) and tumor size greater than 5 cm ($P = .04$) were independent prognostic indicators of reduced survival. In contrast to the results of previous smaller studies (Adam et al, 1997; Bozzetti et al, 1992), the interval between the first and second liver resection did not seem to be predictive of outcome. In selected patients,

Table 73a.8   Results of Past Studies on Repeat Hepatic Resections

Reference	All Liver	Liver Only Recurrence	Resected	Mortality	Median 2-Yr Survival	5-Yr Survivors	Survivors NED	Follow-Up Patients (Mo)
Butler et al, 1986	62	10	2	0/2	—*	0	0	6, 17
Nordlinger et al, 1987	80	21	6	0/6	—	1	0	2, 12
Fortner, 1988	380	8	3	0/3	—	1	0	5
Lange et al, 1989	82	—	9	0/9	15	3	0	1, 3, 23, 35
Griffith et al, 1990	106	—	9	1/9	23	3	1	17, 42, 40, 6, 17
Hohenberger et al, 1990	105	12	6	0/6	23	1	0	—
Stone et al, 1990	95	27	10	0/10	25	5	0	31, 15, 43
Bozzetti et al, 1992	120	34	10	1/11	23	3	0	15, 17, 24, 42
Vaillant et al, 1993	189	60	16	1/16	33	9	2	26, 33, 38, 93
Elias et al, 1993	279	—	28	1/28	30	—	—	—
Que & Nagorney, 1994	—	—	21	1/21	40.8	—	1	—
Fong et al, 1994	499	—	25	0/25	30.2	—	0	8, 10, 24, 26, 29, 30, 59
Adam et al, 1997	—	—	—	—	—	—	—	—
Tuttle et al, 1997	—	—	23	0/23	—	7	—	—
Yamamoto et al, 1999	—	—	75	0/75	—	23	—	—
Muratore et al, 2001	—	—	29	1/29	—	—	—	—
Suzuki et al, 2001	—	—	26	0/26	—	8	—	—
Petrowsky et al, 2002	—	—	126	2/126	—	43	—	—

*— indicates data not specified.
NED, no evidence of disease.

with a low tumor burden, further resection of the liver is safe and can translate into prolonged survival after recurrence of colorectal liver metastases. In the absence of medical contraindications to major surgery, repeat resection should be considered the standard of care. There is a higher likelihood of further recurrence, however, and the study of adjuvant therapy should be encouraged in these patients.

CONCLUSION

Partial hepatectomy for metastases from colorectal cancer is the standard of care for patients with resectable, isolated hepatic disease. It can be performed with an acceptable morbidity and mortality, results in prolonged survival, and offers the only potential for cure. The advent of new and more efficacious regional and systemic chemotherapies will increase the therapeutic options for patients, including adjuvant and neoadjuvant chemotherapy. This multimodal treatment may improve further the cure rate for what was thought of as a terminal disease only a few decades ago.

REFERENCES

Adam R, et al, 1997: Repeat hepatectomy for colorectal liver metastases. Ann Surg 225:51-62.

Adam R, et al, 2001: Five-year survival following hepatic resection after neoadjuvant therapy for nonresectable colorectal (liver) metastases. Ann Surg Oncol 8:347-353.

Adam R, et al, 2004a: Rescue surgery for unresectable colorectal liver metastases downstaged by chemotherapy: a model to predict long-term survival. Ann Surg 240:644-657.

Adam R, et al, 2004b: Tumor progression while on chemotherapy: a contraindication to liver resection for multiple colorectal metastases? Ann Surg 240:1052-1061.

Adson MA, 1987: Resection of liver metastases: when is it worthwhile? World J Surg 11:511-520.

Adson MA, et al, 1984: Resection of hepatic metastases from colorectal cancer. Arch Surg 119:647-651.

Advanced Colorectal Cancer Meta-Analysis Project, 1992: Modulation of fluorouracil by leucovorin in patients with advanced colorectal cancer: evidence in terms of response rate. J Clin Oncol 10:896-903.

Alberts SR, et al, 2003: Liver resection after 5-fluorouracil, leucovorin and oxaliplatin for patients with metastatic colorectal cancer (MCRC) limited to the liver: a North Central Cancer Treatment Group (NCCTG) phase II study. 2003 ASCO annual meeting. Proc Am Soc Clin Oncol 22:263 (abstract 1053).

Alberts SR, et al, 2004: Safety of systemic capecitabine and oxaliplatin administered with hepatic arterial infusion (HAI) of floxuridine (FUDR) following resection of colorectal metastases (M-CRC) confined to the liver: A North Central Cancer Treatment Group (NCCTG) phase II intergroup trial. 2004 ASCO Gastrointestinal Cancers Symposium. Proc Am Soc Clin Oncol 2004 ASCO Gastrointestinal Cancers Symposium (abstract 205). www.asco.org/portal/site/ASCO/menuitem.

Arnaud JP, et al, 1984: Natural history of colorectal carcinoma with untreated liver metastases. Surg Gastroenterol 3:37-42.

Babineau TJ, et al, 1994: Role of staging laparoscopy in the treatment of hepatic malignancy. Am J Surg 167:151-155.

Baer HU, et al, 1989: Resectability of large focal liver lesions. Br J Surg 76:1042-1044.

Baker LH, et al, 1976: Phase III comparison of the treatment of advanced gastrointestinal cancer with bolus weekly 5-FU vs. methyl-CCNU plus bolus weekly 5-FU. Cancer 38:1-7.

Ballantyne GH, Quin J, 1993: Surgical treatment of liver metastases in patients with colorectal cancer. Cancer 71:4252-4266.

Banerjee D, et al, 2000: Levels of E2F-1 expression are higher in lung metastasis of colon cancer as compared with hepatic metastasis and correlate with levels of thymidylate synthase. Cancer Res 60:2365-2367.

Belli G, et al, 2002: Liver resection for hepatic metastases: 15 years of experience. J Hepatobiliary Pancreat Surg 9:607-613.

Bengmark S, Hafstrom L, 1969: The natural history of primary and secondary malignant tumors of the liver. Cancer 23:198-202.

Bengmark S, et al, 1982: Metastatic disease in the liver from colorectal cancer: an appraisal of liver surgery. World J Surg 6:61-65.

Bengtsson G, et al, 1981: Natural history of patients with untreated liver metastases from colorectal cancer. Am J Surg 141:586-589.

Bensmaine MA, et al, 2001: Factors predicting efficacy of oxaliplatin in combination with 5-fluorouracil (5-FU) +/− folinic acid in a compassionate-use cohort of 481 5-FU-resistant advanced colorectal cancer patients. Br J Cancer 85:509-517.

Bismuth H, et al, 1996: Resection of nonresectable liver metastases from colorectal cancer after neoadjuvant chemotherapy. Ann Surg 224:509-520.

Boldrini G, et al, 1987: The systematic use of operative ultrasound for detection of liver metastases during colorectal surgery. World J Surg 11:622-627.

Bozzetti F, et al, 1987: Patterns of failure following surgical resection of colorectal cancer liver metastases. Ann Surg 205:264-270.

Bozzetti F, et al, 1992: Repeated hepatic resection for recurrent metastases from colorectal cancer. Br J Surg 79:146-148.

Buroker T, et al, 1978: 5-FU infusion with mitomycin-C versus 5-FU infusion with methyl-CCNU in the treatment of advanced colon cancer. Cancer 42:1228-1233.

Butler J, et al, 1986: Hepatic resection for metastases of the colon and rectum. Surg Gynecol Obstet 162:109-113.

Cady B, McDermott WV, 1985: Major hepatic resection for metachronous metastases from colon cancer. Ann Surg 201:204-209.

Cady B, et al, 1970: Survival of patients after colonic resection for carcinoma with simultaneous liver metastases. Surg Gynecol Obstet 131:697-700.

Cady B, et al, 1992: Technical and biological factors in disease-free survival after hepatic resection for colorectal cancer metastases. Arch Surg 127:561-569.

Cady B, et al, 1998: Surgical margin in hepatic resection for colorectal metastasis: a critical and improvable determinant of outcome. Ann Surg 227:566-571.

Castaing D, et al, 1986: Utility of operative ultrasound in the surgical management of liver tumors. Ann Surg 204:600-605.

Chang AE, et al, 1987: A prospective randomized trial of regional versus systemic continuous 5-fluorodeoxyuridine chemotherapy in the treatment of colorectal liver metastases. Ann Surg 206:685-693.

Choti MA, et al, 1998: Should hepatic resections be performed at high-volume referral centers? J Gastrointest Surg 2:11-20.

Choti MA, et al, 2002: Trends in long-term survival following liver resection for hepatic colorectal metastases. Ann Surg 235:759-766.

Clavien PA, et al, 2002: Downstaging of hepatocellular carcinoma and liver metastases from colorectal cancer by selective intra-arterial chemotherapy. Surgery 131:433-442.

Cobourn CS, et al, 1987: Examination of patient selection and outcome for hepatic resection for metastatic disease. Surg Gynecol Obstet 165:239-246.

Coelho JC, et al, 2004: Liver resection: 10-year experience from a single institution. Arq Gastroenterol 41:229-233.

Comella P, et al, 2002: Oxaliplatin plus raltitrexed and leucovorin-modulated 5-fluorouracil i.v. bolus: a salvage regimen for colorectal cancer patients. Br J Cancer 86:1871-1875.

Coppa GF, et al, 1985: Hepatic resection for metastatic colon and rectal cancer: an evaluation of preoperative and postoperative factors. Ann Surg 202:203-208.

Cunningham D, et al, 1998: Randomised trial of irinotecan plus supportive care versus supportive care alone after fluorouracil failure for patients with metastatic colorectal cancer. Lancet 352:1413-1418.

Cunningham D, et al, 2004: Cetuximab monotherapy and cetuximab plus irinotecan in irinotecan-refractory metastatic colorectal cancer. N Engl J Med 351:337-345.

Cunningham JD, et al, 1994: One hundred consecutive hepatic resections: blood loss, transfusion and operative technique. Arch Surg 129:1050-1056.

De Brauw LM, et al, 1987: Diagnostic evaluation and survival analysis of colorectal cancer patients with liver metastases. J Surg Oncol 34:81-86.

de Gramont A, et al, 1997: Randomized trial comparing monthly low-dose leucovorin and fluorouracil bolus with bimonthly high-dose leucovorin and fluorouracil bolus plus continuous infusion for advanced colorectal cancer: a French intergroup study. J Clin Oncol 15:808-815.

de Gramont A, et al, 2000: Leucovorin and fluorouracil with or without oxaliplatin as first-line treatment in advanced colorectal cancer. J Clin Oncol 18:2938-2947.

De La Cámara J, et al, 2004: Triplet therapy with oxaliplatin, irinotecan, 5-fluorouracil and folinic acid within combined modality approach in patients with liver metastases from colorectal cancer. 2004 ASCO Annual Meeting. J Clin Oncol 22:3593.

Delaunoit TP, et al, 2004: Chemotherapy-allowed resection of metastatic colorectal cancer: a cooperative group experience. Proc Am Soc Clin Oncol

2004 ASCO Gastrointestinal Cancers Symposium (abstract 196). www.asco.org/portal/site/ASCO/menuitem.

DeMatteo RP, et al, 1999: Outcome after resection of both liver and lung metastases in patients with colorectal cancer. 1999 ASCO annual meeting. Proc Am Soc Clin Oncol 18:249a (abstract 958).

DeMatteo RP, et al, 2000: Anatomic segmental hepatic resection is superior to wedge resection as an oncologic operation for colorectal liver metastases. J Gastrointest Surg 4:178-184.

Doci R, et al, 1991: One hundred patients with hepatic metastases from colorectal cancer treated by resection: analysis of prognostic determinants. Br J Surg 78:797-801.

Doroshow JH, et al, 1990: Prospective randomized comparison of fluorouracil versus fluorouracil and high-dose continuous infusion leucovorin calcium for the treatment of advanced measurable colorectal cancer in patients previously unexposed to chemotherapy. J Clin Oncol 8:491-501.

Douillard JY, et al, 2000: Irinotecan combined with fluorouracil compared with fluorouracil alone as first-line treatment for metastatic colorectal cancer: a multicentre randomised trial. Lancet 355:1041-1047.

Ekberg H, et al, 1987: Pattern of recurrence in liver resection for colorectal secondaries. World J Surg 11:541-547.

Elias D, et al, 1993: Repeat hepatectomy for cancer. Br J Surg 80:1557-1562.

Ensminger WD, et al, 1978: A clinical pharmacological evaluation of hepatic arterial infusions of 5-fluoro-2-deoxyuridine and 5-fluorouracil. Cancer Res 38:3784-3792.

Erlichman C, et al, 1988: A randomized trial of fluorouracil and folinic acid in patients with metastatic colorectal carcinoma. J Clin Oncol 6:469-475.

Falcone A, et al, 2004: Surgical resection of metastases (mts) after biweekly chemotherapy with irinotecan, oxaliplatin and 5-fluorouracil/leucovorin (FOLFOXIRI) in initially unresectable metastatic colorectal cancer (MCRC). 2004 ASCO Annual Meeting Proceedings. J Clin Oncol 22:3553.

Fernandez FG, et al, 2005: Effect of steatohepatitis associated with irinotecan or oxaliplatin pretreatment on resectability of hepatic colorectal metastases. J Am Coll Surg 200:845-853.

Finan PJ, et al, 1985: Factors affecting survival in patients presenting with synchronous hepatic metastases from colorectal cancer: a clinical and computer analysis. Br J Surg 72:373-377.

Fong Y, et al, 1994: Repeat hepatic resections for metastatic colorectal cancer. Ann Surg 220:657-662.

Fong Y, et al, 1997: Liver resection for colorectal metastases. J Clin Oncol 15:938-946.

Fong Y, et al, 1999: Clinical score for predicting recurrence after hepatic resection for metastatic colorectal cancer: analysis of 1001 consecutive cases. Ann Surg 230:309-318.

Fong Y, et al, 2005: Long-term survival is superior after resection for cancer in high-volume centers. Ann Surg 242:540-544.

Fortner JG, 1988: Recurrence of colorectal cancer after hepatic resection. Am J Surg 155:378-382.

Fortner JG, et al, 1984: Multivariate analysis of a personal series of 247 consecutive patients with liver metastases from colorectal cancer. Ann Surg 199:306-316.

Foster JH, 1978: Survival after liver resection for secondary tumors. Am J Surg 135:389-394.

Gayowski TJ, et al, 1994: Experience in hepatic resection for metastatic colorectal cancer: analysis of clinical and pathological risk factors. Surgery 116:703-711.

Giacchetti S, et al, 1999: Long-term survival of patients with unresectable colorectal cancer liver metastases following infusional chemotherapy with 5-fluorouracil, leucovorin, oxaliplatin and surgery. Ann Oncol 10:663-669.

Gibson RN, et al, 1986: Bile duct obstruction: radiologic evaluation of level, cause and tumor resectablitiy. Radiology 160:43-47.

Glasgow RE, et al, 1999: The relationship between hospital volume and outcomes of hepatic resection for hepatocellular carcinoma. Arch Surg 134:30-35.

Goldberg RM, et al, 2004: A randomized controlled trial of fluorouracil plus leucovorin, irinotecan, and oxaliplatin combinations in patients with previously untreated metastatic colorectal cancer. J Clin Oncol 22:23-30.

Goslin R, et al, 1982: Factors influencing survival in patients with hepatic metastases from adenocarcinoma of the colon and rectum. Dis Colon Rectum 25:749-754.

Grage TB, et al, 1979: Results of a prospective randomized study of hepatic artery infusion with 5-fluorouracil versus intravenous 5-fluorouracil in patients with hepatic metastases from colorectal cancer: a Central Oncology Group study. Surgery 86:550-555.

Griffith KD, et al, 1990: Repeat hepatic resections for colorectal metastases. Br J Surg 77:230-233.

Hann LE, et al, 1996: Malignant hepatic hilar tumors: can ultrasonography be used as an alternative to angiography with CT arterial portography for determination of resectability? J Ultrasound Med 15:37-45.

Hohenberger P, et al, 1990: Tumor recurrence and options for further treatment after resection of liver metastases in patients with colorectal cancer. J Surg Oncol 44:245-251.

Hohn DC, et al, 1989: A randomized trial of continuous intravenous versus hepatic intraarterial floxuridine in patients with colorectal cancer metastatic to the liver: the Northern California Oncology Group trial. J Clin Oncol 7:1646-1654.

Holm A, et al, 1989: Hepatic resection of metastasis from colorectal-carcinoma—morbidity, mortality, and pattern of recurrence. Ann Surg 209:428-434.

Hughes KS, et al, 1986: Resection of the liver for colorectal carcinoma metastases: a multi-institutional study of patterns of recurrence. Surgery 100:278-284.

Hughes KS, et al, 1988: Resection of the liver for colorectal carcinoma metastases: a multi-institutional study of long-term survivors. Dis Colon Rectum 31:1-4.

Hughes K, et al, 1989: Surgery for colorectal cancer metastatic to the liver. Surg Clin North Am 69:339-359.

Hurwitz H, et al, 2004: Bevacizumab plus irinotecan, fluorouracil, and leucovorin for metastatic colorectal cancer. N Engl J Med 350:2335-2342.

Iwatsuki S, et al, 1986: Liver resection for metastatic colorectal cancer. Surgery 100:804-810.

Jaffe BM, et al, 1968: Factors influencing survival in patients with untreated hepatic metastases. Surg Gynecol Obstet 127:1-11.

Jamison RL, et al, 1997: Hepatic resection for metastatic colorectal cancer results in cure for some patients. Arch Surg 132:505-511.

Jarnagin WR, et al, 2000: A prospective analysis of staging laparoscopy in patients with primary and secondary hepatobiliary malignancies. J Gastrointest Surg 4:34-43.

Jarnagin WR, et al, 2001: A clinical scoring system predicts the yield of diagnostic laparoscopy in patients with potentially resectable hepatic colorectal metastases. Cancer 91:1121-1128.

Jarnagin WR, et al, 2002: Improvement in perioperative outcome after hepatic resection: analysis of 1,803 consecutive cases over the past decade. Ann Surg 236:397-406.

John TG, et al, 1994: Superior staging of liver tumors with laparoscopy and laparoscopic ultrasound. Ann Surg 220:711-719.

Kato T, et al, 2003: Therapeutic results for hepatic metastasis of colorectal cancer with special reference to effectiveness of hepatectomy: analysis of prognostic factors for 763 cases recorded at 18 institutions. Dis Colon Rectum 46: S22-S31.

Kelloff GJ, et al, 2005: Progress and promise of FDG-PET imaging for cancer patient management and oncologic drug development. Clin Cancer Res 11:2785-2808.

Kemeny MM, et al, 2002: Combined-modality treatment for resectable metastatic colorectal carcinoma to the liver: surgical resection of hepatic metastases in combination with continuous infusion of chemotherapy—an intergroup study. J Clin Oncol 20:1499-1505.

Kemeny N, Gonen M, 2005: Hepatic arterial infusion after liver resection. N Engl J Med 352:734-735.

Kemeny N, et al, 1987: Intrahepatic or systemic infusion of fluorodeoxyuridine in patients with liver metastases from colorectal carcinoma. Ann Intern Med 107:459-465.

Kemeny N, et al, 1990: Interferon alpha-2a and 5-fluorouracil for advanced colorectal carcinoma. Cancer 66:2470-2475.

Kemeny N, et al, 1999: Hepatic arterial infusion of chemotherapy after resection of hepatic metastases from colorectal cancer. N Engl J Med 341: 2039-2048.

Kemeny N, et al, 2001: Phase I study of hepatic arterial infusion of floxuridine and dexamethasone with systemic irinotecan for unresectable hepatic metastases from colorectal cancer. J Clin Oncol 19:2687-2695.

Kemeny N, et al, 2003a: Phase I/II study of hepatic arterial therapy with floxuridine and dexamethasone in combination with intravenous irinotecan as adjuvant treatment after resection of hepatic metastases from colorectal cancer. J Clin Oncol 21:3303-3309.

Kemeny NE, et al, 2003b: Hepatic arterial infusion (HAI) versus systemic therapy for hepatic metastases from colorectal cancer: a CALGB randomized trial of efficacy, quality of life (QOL), cost effectiveness, and molecular markers. Proc Am Soc Clin Oncol (abstract 1010). 2003 ASCO annual meeting. www.asco.org/portal/site/ASCO/menuitem.

Kemeny N, et al, 2005: Phase I trial of systemic oxaliplatin combination chemotherapy with hepatic arterial infusion in patients with unresectable liver metastases from colorectal cancer. J Clin Oncol 23:4888-4896.

Kjeldsen BJ, et al, 1997: A prospective randomized study of follow-up after radical surgery for colorectal cancer. Br J Surg 84:666-669.

Klein B, et al, 1992: Inhibiting IL-6 in human multiple myeloma. Curr Top Microbiol Immunol 182:237-244.

Kooby DA, et al, 2003a: Impact of steatosis on perioperative outcome following hepatic resection. J Gastrointest Surg 7:1034-1044.

Kooby DA, et al, 2003b: Influence of transfusions on perioperative and long-term outcome in patients following hepatic resection for colorectal metastases. Ann Surg 237:860-869.

Kronawitter U, et al, 1999: Evaluation of chest computed tomography in the staging of patients with potentially resectable liver metastases from colorectal carcinoma. Cancer 86:229-235.

Kubo M, et al, 2002: Less aggressive features of colorectal cancer with liver metastases showing macroscopic intrabiliary extension. Pathol Int 52:514-518.

Lambert LA, et al, 2000: Interval hepatic resection of colorectal metastases improves patient selection. Arch Surg 135:473-479.

Lange JF, et al, 1989: Repeat hepatectomy for recurrent malignant tumors of the liver. Surg Gynecol Obstet 169:119-126.

Leonard GD, et al, 2004: Liver resection after hepatic arterial infusion (HAI) plus systemic oxaliplatin (Oxal) combinations in pretreated patients with extensive unresectable colorectal liver metastases. 2004 ASCO Annual Meeting Proceedings. J Clin Oncol 22:3542.

Logan SE, et al, 1982: Hepatic resection of metastatic colorectal carcinoma. Arch Surg 117:25-28.

Lorenz M, et al, 1998: Randomized trial of surgery versus surgery followed by adjuvant hepatic arterial infusion with 5-fluorouracil and folinic acid for liver metastases of colorectal cancer. Ann Surg 228:756-762.

Lygidakis NJ, et al, 2001: Metastatic liver disease of colorectal origin: the value of locoregional immunochemotherapy combined with systemic chemotherapy following liver resection. Results of a prospective randomized study. Hepatogastroenterology 48:1685-1691.

Macdonald JS, et al, 1976: 5-fluorouracil (5-FU), methyl-CCNU, and vincristine in the treatment of advanced colorectal cancer: phase II study utilizing weekly 5-FU. Cancer Treat Rep 60:1597-1600.

Machi J, et al, 1987: Intraoperative ultrasonography in screening for liver metastases from colorectal cancer: comparative accuracy with traditional procedures. Surgery 101:678-684.

Machi J, et al, 1991: Accuracy of intraoperative ultrasonography in diagnosing liver metastasis from colorectal cancer: evaluation with postoperative follow-up results. World J Surg 15:551-557.

Maeda T, et al, 1992: Trial of percutaneous hepatic cryotherapy: preliminary report. Nippon Geka Gakkai Zasshi 93:666.

Makela JT, et al, 1995: Five-year follow-up after radical surgery for colorectal cancer: results of a prospective randomized trial. Arch Surg 130:1062-1067.

Mala T, et al, 2002: Hepatic resection for colorectal metastases: can preoperative scoring predict patient outcome? World J Surg 26:1348-1353.

Martin JK, et al, 1990: Intra-arterial floxuridine vs systemic fluorouracil for hepatic metastases from colorectal cancer. Arch Surg 125:1022-1027.

Minagawa M, et al, 2000: Extension of the frontiers of surgical indications in the treatment of liver metastases from colorectal cancer: long-term results. Ann Surg 231:487-499.

Morrow CE, et al, 1982: Hepatic resection for secondary neoplasms. Surgery 92:610-614.

Muratore A, et al, 2001: Repeat hepatectomy for colorectal liver metastases: a worthwhile operation? J Surg Oncol 76:127-132.

Mutsaerts EL, et al, 2005: Prognostic factors and evaluation of surgical management of hepatic metastases from colorectal origin: a 10-year single-institute experience. J Gastrointest Surg 9:178-186.

Nordic Gastrointestinal Tumor Adjuvant Therapy Group, 1989: Superiority of sequential methotrexate, fluorouracil, and leucovorin to fluorouracil alone in advanced symptomatic colorectal carcinoma: a randomized trial. J Clin Oncol 7:1437-1446.

Nordlinger B, et al, 1987: Hepatic resection for colorectal liver metastases. Ann Surg 205:256-263.

Nordlinger B, et al, 1996: Surgical resection of colorectal carcinoma metastases to the liver: a prognostic scoring system to improve case selection, based on 1568 patients. Association Francaise de Chirurgie. Cancer 77:1254-1262.

Ohlsson B, et al, 1995: Follow-up after curative surgery for colorectal carcinoma: randomized comparison with no follow-up. Dis Colon Rectum 38:619-626.

Okano K, et al, 1999: Macroscopic intrabiliary growth of liver metastases from colorectal cancer. Surgery 126:829-834.

Olsen AK, 1990: Intraoperative ultrasonography and the detection of liver metastases in patients with colorectal cancer. Br J Surg 77:998-999.

Oxley EM, Ellis H, 1969: Prognosis of carcinoma of the large bowel in the presence of liver metastases. Br J Surg 56:149-152.

Pagana TJ, 1986: A new technique for hepatic infusional chemotherapy. Semin Surg Oncol 2:99-102.

Parikh AA, et al, 2003: Perioperative complications in patients undergoing major liver resection with or without neoadjuvant chemotherapy. J Gastrointest Surg 7:1082-1088.

Pass H, et al, 1985: Detection of pulmonary metastases in patients with osteogenic and soft-tissue sarcomas: the superiority of CT-scans compared with conventional linear tomograms using dynamic anlysis. J Clin Oncol 3:1261-1265.

Petrelli N, et al, 1987: A propective randomized trial of 5-fluorouracil versus 5-fluorouracil and high-dose leucovorin versus 5-fluorouracil and methotrexate in previously untreated patients with advanced colorectal carcinoma. J Clin Oncol 5:1559-1565.

Petrowsky H, et al, 2002: Second liver resections are safe and effective treatment for recurrent hepatic metastases from colorectal cancer: a bi-institutional analysis. Ann Surg 235:863-871.

Pettavel J, Morgenthaler F, 1978: Protracted arterial chemotherpy of liver tumors: an experience of 107 cases over a 12-year period. Prog Clin Cancer 7:217-233.

Potter MW, et al, 2000: A critical appraisal of laparoscopic staging in hepatobiliary and pancreatic malignancy. Surg Oncol 9:103-110.

Povoski SP, et al, 2000: Recognition of intrabiliary hepatic metastases from colorectal adenocarcinoma. HPB Surg 11:383-390.

Pozzo C, et al, 2004: Neoadjuvant treatment of unresectable liver disease with irinotecan and 5-fluorouracil plus folinic acid in colorectal cancer patients. Ann Oncol 15:933-939.

Que FG, Nagorney DM, 1994: Resection of 'recurrent' colorectal metastases to the liver. Br J Surg 81:255-258.

Quenet F, et al, 2004: Resection of previously unresectable liver metastases from colorectal cancer (LMCRC) after chemotherapy (CT) with CPT-11/L-OHP/LV5FU (Folfirinox): a prospective phase II trial. 2004 ASCO Annual Meeting Proceedings. J Clin Oncol 22:3613.

Rifkin M, et al, 1987: Intraoperative ultrasound of the liver: an important adjunctive tool for decision making in the operating room. Ann Surg 205:465.

Rosen CB, et al, 1992: Perioperative blood transfusion and determinants of survival after liver resection for metastatic colorectal carcinoma. Ann Surg 216:492-505.

Rougier P, et al, 1992: Hepatic arterial infusion of floxuridine in patients with liver metastases from colorectal carcinoma: long-term results of a prospective randomized trial. J Clin Oncol 10:1112-1118.

Rougier P, et al, 1995: Prospective study of prognostic factors in patients with unresected hepatic metastases from colorectal cancer. Fondation Francaise de Cancerologie Digestive. Br J Surg 82:1397-1400.

Rubbia-Brandt L, et al, 2004: Severe hepatic sinusoidal obstruction associated with oxaliplatin-based chemotherapy in patients with metastatic colorectal cancer. Ann Oncol 15:460-466.

Saltz LB, et al, 2000: Irinotecan plus fluorouracil and leucovorin for metastatic colorectal cancer. Irinotecan Study Group. N Engl J Med 343:905-914.

Scheele J, 1989: Segment oriented resection of the liver: rationale and technique in hepato-biliary and pancreatic malignancies. In Lygidakis NJ, Tytgat GNJ (eds): Hepatobiliary and Pancreatic Malignancies. New York, Thieme, pp 219-247.

Scheele J, et al, 1990: Hepatic metastases from colorectal carcinoma: impact of surgical resection on natural history. Br J Surg 77:1241-1246.

Scheele J, et al, 1991: Indicators of prognosis after hepatic resection for colorectal secondaries. Surgery 110:13-29.

Scheele J, et al, 1995: Resection of colorectal liver metastases. World J Surg 19:59-71.

Schlag P, et al, 1990: Resection of liver metastases in colorectal cancer—competitive analysis of treatment results in synchronous versus metachronous metastases. Eur J Surg Oncol 16:360-365.

Schoemaker D, et al, 1998: Yearly colonoscopy, liver CT, and chest radiography do not influence 5-year survival of colorectal cancer patients. Gastroenterology 114:7-14.

Schussler-Fiorenza CM, et al, 2004: Clinical risk score correlates with yield of PET scan in patients with colorectal hepatic metastases. J Gastrointest Surg 8:150-157.

Sica GT, et al, 2000: CT and MR imaging of hepatic metastases. AJR Am J Roentgenol 174:691-698.

Silen W, 1989: Hepatic resection for metastases from colorectal carcinoma is of dubious value. Arch Surg 124:1021-1024.

Smith JW, et al, 1992: Resection of hepatic and pulmonary metastases from colorectal cancer. Surg Oncol 1:399-404.

Stangl R, et al, 1994: Factors influencing the natural history of colorectal liver metastases. Lancet 343:1405-1410.

Stephenson KR, et al, 1988: Perioperative blood transfusions are associated with decreased time to recurrence and decreased survival after resection of colorectal liver metastases. Ann Surg 208:679-687.

Stone MD, et al, 1990: Surgical therapy for recurrent liver metastases from colorectal cancer. Arch Surg 125:718-721.

Stone MD, et al, 1994: Intraoperative ultrasound imaging of the liver at the time of colorectal cancer resection. Arch Surg 129:431-435.

Strasberg SM, et al, 2001: Survival of patients evaluated by FDG-PET before hepatic resection for metastatic colorectal carcinoma: a prospective database study. Ann Surg 233:293-299.

Suzuki S, et al, 1997: Surgical management of recurrence after resection of colorectal liver metastases. J Hepatobiliary Pancreat Surg 4:103-112.

Suzuki S, et al, 2001: Impact of repeat hepatectomy on recurrent colorectal liver metastases. Surgery 129:421-428.

Tanaka K, et al, 2004: Outcome after simultaneous colorectal and hepatic resection for colorectal cancer with synchronous metastases. Surgery 136:650-659.

Thompson HH, et al, 1983: Major hepatic resection: a 25 year experience. Ann Surg 197:375.

Tuttle TM, et al, 1997: Repeat hepatic resection as effective treatment for recurrent colorectal liver metastases. Ann Surg Oncol 4:125-130.

Vaillant JC, et al, 1993: Repeat liver resection for recurrent colorectal metastases. Br J Surg 80:340-344.

Vogt P, et al, 1991: Resection of synchronous liver metastases from colorectal cancer. World J Surg 15:62-67.

Wagman LD, et al, 1990: A prospective, randomized evaluation of the treatment of colorectal cancer metastatic to the liver. J Clin Oncol 8:1885-1893.

Wagner JS, et al, 1984: The natural history of hepatic metastases from colorectal cancer: a comparison with resective treatment. Ann Surg 199:502-508.

Weber SM, et al, 2000: Survival after resection of multiple hepatic colorectal metastases. Ann Surg Oncol 7:643-650.

Wein A, et al, 2001: Impact of surgery on survival in palliative patients with metastatic colorectal cancer after first line treatment with weekly 24-hour infusion of high-dose 5-fluorouracil and folinic acid. Ann Oncol 12:1721-1727.

Weinbren HK, Blumgart LH, 1986: Pathological changes in the liver and computed tomography. Recent Results Cancer Res 100:58-67.

Weiss L, et al, 1986: Haematogenous metastatic patterns in colonic carcinoma: an analysis of 1541 necropsies. J Pathol 150:195-203.

Wilson SM, Adson MA, 1976: Surgical treatment of hepatic metastases from colorectal cancers. Arch Surg 111:330-334.

Wood CB, et al, 1976: A retrospective study of the natural history of patients with liver metastases from colorectal cancer. Clin Oncol 2:285-288.

Yamamoto J, et al, 1999: Repeat liver resection for recurrent colorectal liver metastases. Am J Surg 178:275-281.

Younes RN, et al, 1991: The influence of intraoperative hypotension and perioperative blood transfusion on disease-free survival in patients with complete resection of colorectal liver metastases. Ann Surg 214:107-113.

73b HEPATIC METASTASES FROM PRIMARY NEUROENDOCRINE TUMORS

D. M. NAGORNEY, T. D. ATWELL, AND F. G. QUE

The liver remains second only to regional lymph nodes as the dominant site of metastases from all gastrointestinal tract malignancies. Because progression of hepatic metastases is the predominant cause of death in patients with gastrointestinal cancers, these metastases have been the focus of multiple therapeutic approaches. Progress has been significant for medical and surgical approaches. Most importantly, the accumulated experience documenting the survival potential of hepatic resection for selected patients with colorectal metastases (see Ch. 73a) has prompted evaluation of this approach for essentially any other malignancy metastatic to the liver. It is unclear whether similar approaches would be effective for noncolorectal metastases.

Interest in hepatic resection for gastrointestinal neuroendocrine cancers (NECs) has increased. Resection of metastatic NECs to the liver is appealing because these cancers have a route of metastatic origin through the portal venous system similar to colorectal cancers, and their typical natural history is strikingly prolonged compared with other gastrointestinal tract cancers and other solid tumors. Initial experience with hepatic resection for neuroendocrine metastases (Foster & Berman, 1977) suggested that patients might benefit in terms of survival and symptom relief from clinical endocrinopathies in an era when antihormonal and antineoplastic therapies for such cancers were unavailable. Although neuroendocrine metastases are encountered infrequently, the attractiveness of hepatic resection for these metastases has grown because of several clinical observations: (1) the protracted natural history of NECs compared with other gastrointestinal tract cancers, (2) the often prolonged duration of intrahepatic disease before evidence of extrahepatic progression, (3) the clinical impression that the severity of clinical endocrinopathies correlates with the intrahepatic volume of metastatic disease, (4) the frequent resectability of the primary and regional neuroendocrine tumors despite metastatic disease, and (5) the rarity of underlying concomitant hepatic disease (fibrosis or cirrhosis). As a result of these observations, hepatic resection and, less commonly, hepatic transplantation for metastatic NEC have been undertaken with increasing frequency. This chapter (1) details the evidence supporting the premises for hepatic resection of neuroendocrine metastases; (2) presents the current outcomes for hepatic resection, hepatic transplantation, and ablative therapy for metastatic neuroendocrine tumors; and (3) presents an algorithm for long-term management of patients with neuroendocrine tumors metastatic to the liver.

CLASSIFICATION OF GASTROENTEROPANCREATIC NEUROENDOCRINE TUMORS

Most neuroendocrine metastases to the liver are of gastrointestinal or pancreatic origin (see Ch. 57), or so-called gastroenteropancreatic (GEP) tumors (Rindi et al, 1998). GEP neuroendocrine tumors historically are divided into two broad types: carcinoid and noncarcinoid. Either type may or may not be associated with hormone production causing a clinical endocrinopathy (functional or nonfunctional). Traditionally, gastrointestinal carcinoids have been classified by their site of origin—foregut (lung, thymus, stomach, duodenum, pancreas, bile duct, gallbladder, and liver), midgut (small intestine, appendix, and proximal colon), and hindgut (distal colon and rectum)—because of the various biologic and biochemical features shown within these groups. In contrast, pancreatic neuroendocrine tumors have been classified by whether they are functional or not.

Regardless of origin, neuroendocrine tumors are similar histopathologically. Many histologic and morphologic features may be shared by benign and malignant tumors. Histologically, neuroendocrine tumors typically are well differentiated, and atypia and mitoses are rare. Neuroendocrine tumors stain positive for chromogranin A, neuron-specific enolase, and synaptophysin, which confirms neuroendocrine cell origin. In addition to neural markers, neuroendocrine tumors also stain positively for one or more endocrine hormones immunohistochemically. Even nonfunctioning neuroendocrine tumors may stain positively for one or more hormonal markers. Morphologically, neuroendocrine tumors can be solitary or multiple and solid or cystic. Tumor size alone is not a reliable indicator of malignancy. Neuroendocrine tumors greater than 2 cm throughout the GEP tract have a greater probability of malignant behavior, however, than tumors less than 2 cm. Gross or microscopic vascular invasion may occur for any GEP neuroendocrine tumors, although major vascular invasion is most typical of pancreatic NECs. Only the confirmed presence of metastases confers an unequivocal diagnosis of malignancy.

A spectrum of clinical behavior for NECs has long been observed ranging from an indolent, benign course to an aggressive clinical course with rapid cancer progression and death. To distinguish the clinical behavior of neuroendocrine tumors, several histopathologic classifications have been proposed. For GEP neuroendocrine tumors, two schemes have been employed. The initial classification stratified GEP neuroendocrine tumors as benign, low-grade malignancy, and high-grade malignancy (Capella et al, 1995). Subsequently, the World Health Organization (WHO) on the basis of a consensus conference of pathologists proposed four subtypes: benign, uncertain, low-grade malignancy, and high-grade malignancy (Solcia et al, 2000). The WHO classification was proposed primarily for neuroendocrine tumors of pancreatic origin, but is applicable to all GEP neuroendocrine tumors. Each histopathologic subtype can be subclassified further as functioning or nonfunctioning. Such histopathologic typing of GEP neuroendocrine tumors distinguishing clinical behavior is likely to influence interpretation of outcomes after surgical management. Regardless of classification system, clinically surgeons addressing NEC metastatic to the liver encounter only low-grade or high-grade malignancy.

Gastrointestinal carcinoid cancers produce a variety of proteins and peptide hormones (Onaitis et al, 2000; Schnirer et al, 2003). The most common is serotonin. Foregut tumors have low serotonin content. Occasionally, 5-hydroxy-L-tryptophan, growth hormone, and corticotropin are secreted. Midgut carcinoids have high serotonin content and frequently cause the classic carcinoid syndrome. Midgut carcinoids frequently secrete kinins and prostaglandins, which have synergistic interactions with 5-hydroxy-L-tryptophan metabolites, although midgut carcinoids may produce any gut hormone. The absence of endocrine syndromes also may be related to the presence of biologically inactive peptides. Hindgut carcinoids rarely contain serotonin. Almost all NECs are positive for the neuroendocrine markers chromogranin A and neuron-specific enolase, but serum levels have correlated poorly with prognosis (Tomassetti et al, 2001).

Peptides produced by neuroendocrine tumors of the pancreas in decreasing order of frequency are pancreatic polypeptide, glucagon, insulin-proinsulin, somatostatin, gastrin, vasoactive intestinal polypeptide, and parathormone-like polypeptide (Gumbs et al, 2002; Mansour & Chen, 2004). Some tumors occasionally produce multiple peptides of which more than one can be active and result in overlapping clinical syndromes. The eight major functioning endocrinopathies associated with pancreatic neuroendocrine tumors and their frequency of malignancy are insulinoma (10%), gastrinoma (50%), glucagonoma (70%), somatostatinoma (80%), GRFoma (30%), VIPoma (40%), ACTHoma or CRHoma (100%), and PTHoma (100%) (Gumbs et al, 2002; Mansour & Chen, 2004). Nonfunctional neuroendocrine tumors of the pancreas imply the production of an inactive peptide, subclinical hormone production, or no peptide production at all. Reviews for the specific endocrinopathies from pancreatic neuroendocrine tumors are cited for reference to recognize their implications in clinical management (Gumbs et al, 2002; Mansour & Chen, 2004).

EPIDEMIOLOGY

A brief overview of the most commonly encountered primary GEP neuroendocrine tumors is presented because combined resection of the primary and regional extent of disease and hepatic metastases is frequently undertaken. Various technical aspects of resection of the most common primary GEP NECs are addressed because the principles in the management of these cancers can be extrapolated to other GEP NECs.

Gastrointestinal carcinoids typically are diagnosed in individuals around 60 years of age. There is a female predominance (60%) and a racial prevalence of African Americans. Gastrointestinal carcinoids constitute nearly 75% of all carcinoids, with the remainder primarily of bronchopulmonary origin. The distribution of gastrointestinal carcinoids is as follows: small intestine (35%), rectum (23%), appendix (19%), colon (12%), stomach (6%), duodenum (4%), and hepatobiliary-pancreatic (2%) (Modlin et al, 2003). The relative incidence of gastric and rectal carcinoids has increased over the last 3 decades, but carcinoids have decreased in the appendix. Gastrointestinal carcinoids frequently are associated with noncarcinoid tumors: small intestine (29%), stomach (21%), and appendix (18%). Overall, localized disease characterizes the presentation of rectal (80%) and gastric (70%) carcinoids, and nonlocalized disease characterizes colonic (80%) and small intestine (67%) carcinoids. Although gastrointestinal carcinoids generally are believed to behave benignly, 13% of patients have metastatic disease at presentation, and overall 5-year survival for gastrointestinal carcinoid is only 67% (Kulke & Mayer, 1999).

Nonfunctional NECs of the pancreas are distributed equally between sexes (Hochwald et al, 2001). NEC of the pancreas occurs in 0.5 to 1 person per 100,000 population. Nonfunctional NEC accounts for approximately 50% of pancreatic NEC in most series. Wide variations in incidence among types of NEC likely are related to the definition of *nonfunctional*. Nonfunctional NECs grow slowly, and there is a slight predominance in the distal pancreas. They are usually larger than pancreatic ductal cancers. Abdominal and back pain, anorexia, weight loss, and fatigue are the most common symptoms. Jaundice is less frequent than in pancreatic ductal cancers. Steatorrhea is rare. Multicentricity is frequent (15%). Rarely, patients may present with gastrointestinal hemorrhage from tumor erosion into the adjacent gastrointestinal tract or from sinistral portal hypertension secondary to splenic vein obstruction. Duration of symptoms is often prolonged (median 10 months). Symptom duration is significantly longer for functional than nonfunctional NECs. The epidemiology of functional pancreatic neuroendocrine tumors varies widely with or without multiple endocrine neoplasia syndrome and is beyond the scope of this chapter (references are provided).

Small Intestine Carcinoids

Small intestine carcinoids are the most common gastrointestinal carcinoid (Kulke & Mayer, 1999; Modlin et al, 2003). Patients usually present with abdominal pain, obstructive symptoms, diarrhea, and gastrointestinal bleeding. Small intestine carcinoids account for 90% of patients with carcinoid syndrome. Approximately 20% of patients with carcinoid syndrome have clinically evident carcinoid heart disease (resulting in tricuspid or other valve insufficiency), and an even larger proportion have occult heart disease detectable by echocardiography. Small intestine carcinoids often are associated with dense mesenteric fibrosis, intestinal obstruction, and intestinal ischemia secondary to vessel compression by metastatic regional lymph nodes and local release of vasoactive hormones (mesenteric angiopathy) (Eckhauser et al, 1981). Nearly 30% of patients have multiple gastrointestinal carcinoids, and more than a third of patients have concurrent noncarcinoid cancers. Besides regional lymph node metastases, these carcinoids frequently metastasize to the liver, peritoneum, retroperitoneal nodes, and ovaries.

Resection is the only potentially curative treatment for small intestine carcinoids (Hellman et al, 2002b; Loftus & van Heerden, 1995; Soreide et al, 1992; Woodside et al, 2004). Because of the frequency of the associated syndrome, careful preoperative evaluation and preparation is necessary. When suspected clinically, baseline urinary 5-hydroxyindoleacetic acid levels should be obtained. The extent and site of the primary small intestine carcinoid can be defined by barium contrast gastrointestinal series or by small bowel enteroclysis. Further imaging of the abdomen and chest for metastatic disease is best defined by contrast-enhanced CT. CT often identifies mesenteric adenopathy and stranding characteristic of regionally advanced small bowel carcinoids even without identification of the site of the primary carcinoid on small bowel studies. Assessment of the relationship of the regional lymphatic metastases to the vessels of the small bowel is important in planning resection of the primary and regional extent of disease. Despite the often desmoplastic reaction adjacent to the involved regional lymph nodes, resection is feasible, unless there is extensive invasion of the third portion of the duodenum and the uncinate process of the pancreas or circumferential arterial and venous encasement without patent proximal arterial collaterals or distal mesenteric arteries large enough for reconstruction (Öhvrall et al, 2000). Although not anatomically useful in planning operations, somatostatin receptor scintigraphy or scanning with Octreoscan is useful in evaluating the overall disease extent and the site of the primary when not recognized by other studies and when modifying treatment strategies (Slooter et al, 2001). The role of MRI is increasing primarily in assessing the extent of hepatic metastases. MRI is particularly sensitive in detecting small metastases within the liver and often detects disease not seen by other imaging techniques, including CT. MRI has limited applicability for defining the site of the primary carcinoid, however.

The recognition of carcinoid heart disease demands a thorough cardiac evaluation (Fox & Khattar, 2004). The major implication of carcinoid heart disease is the presence of right heart failure and the consequently elevated systemic venous pressures that can cause a pulsatile liver (implying hepatic vein pressures of >25 mm Hg) and precludes hepatic resection if present. The presence of clinically significant carcinoid heart disease dictates medical treatment and occasionally valve replacement before resection of the primary small intestine carcinoid and the hepatic metastases. Survival after surgical repair of carcinoid heart disease is improved compared with medical treatment, even without surgical treatment of hepatic metastases (Connolly et al, 1995). Some patients may be candidates for hepatic resection after repair of carcinoid heart disease depending on objective decreases in systemic venous hypertension and the degree of functional cardiac improvement (Connolly et al, 2002; McDonald et al, 1999).

Any patient with the carcinoid syndrome requires preoperative and intraoperative somatostatin analogue therapy to prevent a carcinoid crisis (Oberg et al, 2004). Carcinoid crisis refers to a clinical syndrome of life-threatening intraoperative hypotension or hypertension and severe flushing with or without concurrent bronchospasm or arrhythmias. The frequency and factors predictive of this perianesthetic complication are unknown. Prevention is essential, and appropriate treatment should be prescribed in all patients undergoing intervention for metastatic carcinoid tumors (Kinny et al, 2001). Short-acting analogues are preferred even if the patient has received the long-acting analogue within 30 days. Management should consist of subcutaneous short-acting somatostatin analogue on call to operation and intravenous infusion of the analogue throughout the operation and in recovery. Additional intraoperative increases in infusion rates are appropriate for unexplained intraoperative hemodynamic instability.

Resection of small intestine carcinoids should encompass the primary tumor, any multicentric tumors (which may require intraoperative small intestine enteroscopy to be recognized), and the regional lymph nodes. When intestinal ischemia is present, bowel resection is indicated. Resection of the regional lymph nodes is often possible by keeping the dissection immediately adjacent to the nodes and retracting the visceral vessels away from the involved nodes (Hellman et al, 2002b). Preservation of the blood supply to the gastrointestinal tract is essential in preventing a short bowel syndrome. As mentioned previously, preoperative CT with intravenous contrast administration defines which patients have resectable nodal disease, which is very difficult to assess intraoperatively. Resection of hepatic metastases generally is indicated only if complete resection of the primary

and regional disease is feasible. Resection of hepatic metastases should be performed concurrently if all gross metastases can be excised. If more than 90% of the hepatic disease can be resected (or ablated), cytoreductive resection should be considered because survival and symptom-free quality of life may be improved (Knox et al, 2004; Sarmiento et al, 2003). Staged resections can be performed with similar expectations in outcomes. Overall 5-year survival for small intestine carcinoid ranges from 50% to 67%.

Pancreatic Neuroendocrine Cancers (see Ch. 57)

An aggressive operative approach generally is warranted for NECs of the pancreas (Chen et al, 1998; Hochwald et al, 2001; Matthews et al, 2002; Phan et al, 1998; Solorzano et al, 2001). Resection remains the treatment of choice for patients with localized NEC of the pancreas and many patients with hepatic metastases. Resection of the primary NEC and the regional lymph nodes is generally possible despite their often large size. The site of the primary NEC dictates the extent and type of pancreatectomy: pancreaticoduodenectomy for head NEC and distal pancreatectomy/splenectomy for body-tail NEC. Pancreatic NECs are often large and tend to displace adjacent arteries, rather than invade or encase them, which increases the resectability of these pancreatic NECs compared with ductal variants. In contrast, venous invasion is common, and frequently a tumor thrombus is recognized on preoperative imaging or during operation. Resection is generally possible after proximal and distal control of the major portal venous tributaries because the thrombus usually is not fixed to the endothelium. These thrombi may be fragile, however, so compression should be minimized to prevent fracture and migration into the intrahepatic portal venous system. Bulky nodal metastases should not preclude resection as is the case for pancreatic ductal cancers. All gross nodal disease should be excised during resection. Whether formal lymphadenectomies should be performed routinely is controversial, but it is noteworthy that regional lymph nodes are a predominant site of late recurrence, which suggests that a more thorough lymphadenectomy may be valuable for maintenance of quality of life, particularly in patients with functioning NECs. Enucleation should be reserved for patients with small superficial neuroendocrine tumors (<2 cm) without overt regional lymph node metastases or patients with significant comorbidity and highly symptomatic endocrinopathies. The definitive role of enucleation for uncertain neuroendocrine tumors (WHO classification) or alternatively spleen-sparing distal pancreatectomy is unknown. For patients with NECs locally invasive to adjacent structures or the gastrointestinal tract, en bloc resection should be done. Laparoscopic techniques are applicable if a similar extent of pancreatectomy is as feasible as that by open techniques (Fernandez-Cruz et al, 2002). Concurrent resection of primary pancreatic NEC and hepatic metastases can be performed safely, although staged resections may be preferable, particularly in patients with involvement of the head of the pancreas (Sarmiento et al, 2002). Overall actuarial 5-year survival for NECs of the pancreas ranges from 45% to 63% with a median survival of 4 years.

Because of the indolent and unpredictable course of NECs of the pancreas, palliative resection of the primary tumor may be warranted even in the presence of extensive distant disease. Resection of the primary NEC is indicated when the patient presents with overt gastrointestinal bleeding or large symptomatic ulcers from malignant invasion of the stomach or duodenum. For patients with obstructive jaundice, operative biliary bypass should be strongly considered in contrast to biliary endoprostheses owing to the expectedly prolonged natural history. Similarly, duodenal bypass should be considered for large unresectable pancreatic head NECs because of the potential long-term survival.

NATURAL HISTORY

Regardless of whether NECs are classified as carcinoid or noncarcinoid, the natural history of patients with unresected or unresectable hepatic metastases generally has been similar. Overall, patients with unresected hepatic metastases from NEC have an approximately 30% 5-year survival (Proye, 2001). Several factors may affect the natural history of carcinoid and noncarcinoid cancers. The presence of liver metastases alone is the most significant factor adversely affecting outcome (Chu et al, 2002; Moertel, 1987). Five-year survival with and without liver metastases from NECs is approximately 30% to 40% and 90% to 100%. Poorly differentiated NEC and progressive neuroendocrine metastases in the liver (>25% volume increase on two CT scans within 3 months) further adversely affect survival in patients with hepatic metastases (Madeira et al, 1998). Progression in size or number of hepatic neuroendocrine metastases can be expected in 90% after a median follow-up of 11.5 months (Skinazi et al, 1996). Carcinoid heart disease, which occurs only in the presence of metastatic carcinoid tumor to the liver, independently predicts poor survival. The survival of patients with clinically severe carcinoid heart disease is approximately 1.6 years with only a 31% survival rate at 3 years, unless cardiac surgery is undertaken successfully (Connolly et al, 1995; Fox & Khattar, 2004). Although uncontrolled endocrinopathies from functioning metastatic NECs may cause life-threatening conditions (e.g., severe hypoglycemia from insulinoma, gastrointestinal perforation from gastrinoma), documentation that the overall frequency of such events has affected the natural history of these patients is lacking. Conversely, it is likely that clinical control of endocrinopathies can affect the natural history of NEC, although specific studies documenting clinical control of endocrinopathies by antihormonal therapy with objective tumor responses have not been well documented (except for gastrinoma before and after the use of H_2 blockers or proton-pump inhibitors) (Norton et al, 2003a).

Similar to carcinoid tumors, the 5-year survival of patients with pancreatic NECs ranges from 30% to 40% with a median survival of approximately 40 months (Chen et al, 1998; Thompson et al, 1985). It is unclear whether the presence or absence of clinical endocrinopathies affects the natural history of patients with metastatic NEC from the pancreas. The specific NEC likely affects overall natural history, however. In a series of 35 patients with hepatic metastases, of which 60% were from gastrinomas, the 5-year survival was approximately 70%. The frequency of patients with hepatic metastases at presentation is greater for nonfunctioning than functioning NECs. The prognosis also is affected by the extent of metastatic NEC in the liver (Chamberlain et al, 2000; Phan et al, 1998). Five-year survival was 24% with greater than 75% tumor replacement of the liver, whereas 5-year survival approached 80% for less than 50% tumor replacement. High-grade malignancy frequently is associated with nonfunctional pancreatic NEC and adversely affects natural history.

HEPATIC RESECTION FOR NEUROENDOCRINE METASTASES

The current mainstay of treatment for gastrointestinal NECs metastatic to the liver is resection. Although hepatic resection of malignancy is employed most often with curative intent, the tumor biology of these typically indolent and slow growing cancers renders them less responsive to more commonly employed palliative therapies, such as chemotherapy and radiation; surgical resection with palliative intent (cytoreduction) may afford patients a real and significant advantage in palliation and prolong survival (Sutcliffe et al, 2004). The focus on palliation and extension of life, rather than on complete remission, is conceptually a paradigm shift because most hepatic resections are undertaken for cure in patients with metastatic solid cancers.

The treatment of hepatic metastases from NECs is aimed at reduction of the mass of malignant tissue (cytoreduction) chiefly for two reasons. First, metastatic gastrointestinal neuroendocrine tumors are usually indolent and slow growing because most are low-grade malignancies (WHO classification) (Solcia et al, 2000). Chemotherapeutic and radiotherapeutic regimens targeted at rapidly dividing cells are relatively ineffective, targeting only a paucity of the total population of malignant cells. Second, symptoms secondary to expression and secretion of biologically active peptides by these tumors are directly related to overall mass of tumor, although production of peptides may be heterogeneous among individual metastases. Similarly, pain and debilitating decrease in performance status may have a negative impact on quality of life for nonfunctional NECs metastatic to the liver. Cytoreduction of the tumor is the most direct and immediately effective method to provide symptomatic relief. These reasons, coupled with improved safety for hepatic resection, have prompted hepatic resection as a primary therapeutic option for patients with functional and nonfunctional metastatic GEP NECs. Based on these premises, hepatic cytoreduction, whether by hepatic resection or transplantation, should address clinical endocrinopathies and improve survival, and as a corollary, the duration of response should be proportional to the extent of the debulking or cytoreduction of the metastatic NEC.

Currently, hepatic resection of metastatic NEC is recommended if the primary tumor and regional disease are resectable or resected, and greater than 90% of hepatic metastases are resectable or ablatable. Our initial results showed that debulking hepatic resection could be performed safely, and overall survival was approximately 75% at 4 years (Que et al, 1995). There was no significant difference in survival between patients undergoing complete or incomplete resection. Mean duration of symptom response was nearly 2 years. Subsequently, our findings in 170 patients undergoing hepatic resections showed that symptoms resolve in 98% of patients. Median time to symptom recurrence was 45 months, and 59% of patients experienced recurrent symptoms at 5 years. Overall survival was 61% and 35% at 5 and 10 years, and perioperative mortality was 1.2%. Recurrence was 84% at 5 years, however, and 94% at 10 years (Fig. 73b.1) (Sarmiento et al, 2003). Examples of results obtained from cytoreductive hepatic resection for NECs are shown in Fig. 73b.2.

Table 73b.1 summarizes the current literature for hepatic resection of neuroendocrine metastases. The cumulative findings for these reports support an aggressive operative approach for metastatic NEC. Overall 5-year survival ranges from 47% to 92%, with a median of 74%. Only four perioperative deaths have occurred among the reported total of 384 patients.

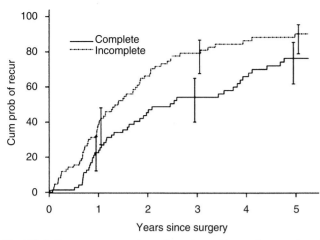

Fig. 73b.1. Recurrence rate was lower for patients with complete resection of the tumor (complete versus incomplete resection, 76% versus 91% at 5 years, median time to recurrence 30 months versus 16 months; $P=.0004$ by the log-rank test). Cum Prob of Recur, cumulative probability of recurrence.
(From Sarmiento JM, et al, 2003: Surgical treatment of neuroendocrine metastases to the liver: a plea for resection to increase survival. J Am Coll Surg 197:29-37. With permission from American College of Surgeons.)

Resolution of endocrine symptoms exceeded 90% of patients when reported. Duration of response was not abstractable for this review. Although most patients reported to date have had metastatic carcinoid tumor to the liver, survival has not differed appreciably among patients with carcinoid and noncarcinoid (primarily islet cell cancers) cancers, which is not unexpected given that all GEP NECs are histopathologically analogous, albeit immunohistochemically different. Our findings do not support the postulate that functional status affects outcome. Although complete resection of hepatic metastases has been undertaken more frequently, survival has not been significantly different between patients with complete or incomplete hepatic resection of NEC metastases if the latter cytoreduction exceeds 90% of the estimated tumor volume (Que et al, 1995). Significant improvement in quality of life and survival has been confirmed for patients undergoing hepatic resection of greater than 90% of metastatic tumor volume (Knox et al, 2004). These data suggest that hepatic resection of metastases is safe and clinically effective, and overall operative survival is nearly double compared with survival in patients with unresected metastases. Complete resection remains the goal of cytoreductive hepatic resection because progression rate and median time to clinical recurrence are significantly reduced by incomplete resection. Few other factors related to the primary NEC, metastatic disease, or the patient have been correlated with survival.

The frequency of reported recurrence to date has been high (>80% at 5 years). Because the recurrence clearly implies intrahepatic progression of residual metastases from debulking resections (R2) or occult hepatic metastases, these findings dictate that a subsequent plan for treatment for hepatic metastases is necessary. Although cure of patients with metastatic NECs is infrequent, prolonged palliation is probable. Patterns of intrahepatic recurrence have not been well studied. Intrahepatic recurrence is typically multicentric in our experience. The extent and distribution of the hepatic recurrence dictate the choice of therapy. For solitary recurrences, either resection or ablation is appropriate. Given that serial imaging usually identifies small recurrences, percutaneous ablative approaches often are preferable.

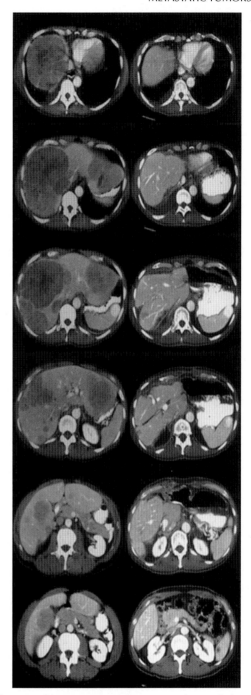

Fig. 73b.2. CT of a patient with metastatic carcinoid tumor before *(left)* and 18 months after *(right)* cytoreductive hepatic resection. Intrahepatic recurrences were ablated by percutaneous radiofrequency ablation.

Repeat hepatic resection is advised for lesions in sites that preclude safe radiofrequency ablation (RFA) (i.e., surface metastases adjacent to bowel, near bile ducts, or near diaphragm). Sequential ablation or resection is undertaken as recurrence is recognized until precluded by extent of recurrence within the liver. Extensive recurrent intrahepatic metastases are treated by embolization or chemoembolization with or without systemic chemotherapy in the absence of extrahepatic disease and chemotherapy in the presence of extrahepatic disease. A scheme for management of neuroendocrine metastases to the liver is outlined in Fig. 73b.3.

Table 73b.1   Hepatic Resection for Metastatic Neuroendocrine Cancer

Reference	No. Patients	Perioperative Mortality (No.)	Postoperative Symptom Control (%)	5-Yr Survival (%)
Chen et al, 1998	15	0	—	73
Chamberlain et al, 2000	34	2	90	76
Grazi et al, 2000	19	0	95	92
Nave et al, 2001	31	0	—	47
Yao et al, 2001	16	0	100	70
Jaeck et al, 2001	13	0	100	68
Ringe et al, 2001	31	0	—	47
El Rassi et al, 2002	11*	0	100	91
	15†	0	100	50
Norton et al, 2003a	16	0	100	82
Sarmiento et al, 2003	170	2	96	61
Knox et al, 2004	13	—	100	85

*Curative.
†Cytoreductive.

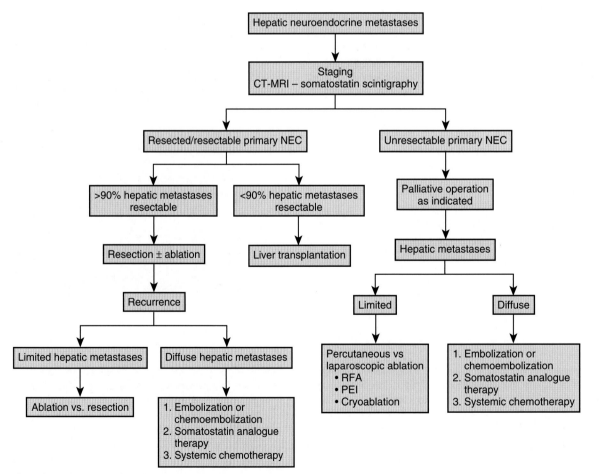

Fig. 73b.3. Management algorithm for patients with neuroendocrine liver metastases.

Hepatic Transplantation for Neuroendocrine Metastases

Orthotopic liver transplantation (OLT) has been employed increasingly to treat metastatic NEC. Given the protracted natural history of NEC, it was postulated that metastases from NEC may be limited to the liver for protracted periods. The liver itself may foster such growth by a variety of mechanisms, which may not be present extrahepatically. Regardless of the mechanisms, OLT during the period of intrahepatic disease may be curative or at least significantly palliative. In contrast to debulking or cytoreductive partial hepatectomy, OLT addresses all hepatic disease. The attractiveness of complete hepatic resection and the high recurrence rate of NEC after partial hepatectomy have warranted ongoing investigation of OLT for metastatic NEC.

Table 73b.2 summarizes the current literature of OLT for NEC. As with partial hepatectomy, OLT is indicated if the primary and regional NEC has been resected, and distal metastases have been excluded by octreotide scintigraphy and dynamic CT or MRI. Outcomes have been reported for 185 patients. Results and selection criteria have varied, and actual duration of follow-up has been limited. One-year survival has ranged from 50% to 100% (mean 82%) and 5-year survival from 36% to 89% (mean 57%) with a mean follow-up of 36 months. Only 12 patients have been reported as actual disease-free 5-year survivors. Symptomatic relief from clinical endocrinopathies, when present, has been uniformly complete, but duration of symptomatic relief after OLT has not been clearly documented. The high rate of recurrence after transplantation may be due to poor patient selection. Several studies have attempted to identify prognostic indicators. Factors examined include age, anatomic location of the primary tumor, extent of primary operation, extent of liver disease, Ki67 index, E-cadherin expression, genetic instability ($p53$), and histologic features. Age younger than 50 years, limited liver disease, low Ki67 index, regular E-cadherin staining, and complete local-regional primary cancer control for more than 1 year correlated with prolonged survival (Fernández et al, 2003). These limited data preclude routine use as selection criteria until confirmed further.

The role of OLT for NEC based on current evidence remains undefined (Fernández et al, 2003). OLT should be considered as an investigative treatment alternative in specialty centers. Referral probably should be considered in patients with resected primary NEC after a period of disease stability with exclusion of any extrahepatic disease. It is unclear whether other biologic or genetic markers would improve the reliability for selection.

Radiofrequency Ablation of Neuroendocrine Hepatic Metastases

Multiple minimally invasive ablative modalities exist for the treatment of liver tumors, including cryotherapy; percutaneous ethanol injection; and thermal techniques, such as RFA, microwave ablation, and interstitial laser thermotherapy. Currently, RFA is likely the most widely used ablative technique because of its effectiveness in treating larger tumors, versatility, ease of use, and relatively low risk of complications (Bleicher et al, 2003; Giovannini & Seitz, 1994; Livraghi et al, 2003; Pearson et al, 1999; Wong et al, 2001).

The application of RFA for metastatic NEC arose after its efficacy was established in the treatment of hepatocellular carcinoma and metastatic colorectal cancer (Curley et al, 1999; Pawlik et al, 2003; Solbiati et al, 2001a; Wood et al, 2000). Local tumor control is achieved in 82% to 98% of treated metastases, although duration of follow-up varies (Bleicher et al, 2003; Bowles et al, 2001; Curley et al, 2000; de Baere et al, 2000; Pawlik et al, 2003; Pearson et al, 1999; Rhim & Dodd, 1999; Solbiati et al, 2001a). Local recurrence rates were greater in patients with colorectal metastases and less in patients with neuroendocrine hepatic metastases (Bleicher et al, 2003; Solbiati et al, 2001b), which may relate to different morphologic characteristics of these tumors. Successful ablation typically occurred in the treatment of small metastases (<3 cm) (de Baere et al, 2000; Kettenbach et al, 2003; Solbiati et al, 2001b; Wood et al, 2000). Only 50% of large tumors (>5 cm) were ablated completely, even with repeated ablation (Goldberg & Ahmed, 2002).

Published experience with RFA for neuroendocrine hepatic metastases has been limited. RFA has been employed primarily and as an adjunct to resection. Objective tumor destruction has been well documented and has been shown to be highly effective in local tumor control, with local recurrence in 3% to 5%

Table 73b.2 Hepatic Transplantation for Metastatic Neuroendocrine Cancer

Reference	No. Patients	Median Follow-Up (mo)	1-Yr Survival (%)	5-Yr Survival (%)	Actual 5-Yr Disease-Free
Frilling et al, 1998	4	54	50	50	0
Lehnert, 1998	103	—	70	47	7*
Lang et al, 1999	10	33	100	—	1
Pascher et al, 2000	4	42	100	50	1
Coppa et al, 2001	9	39	100	70	—
Ringe et al, 2001	9	24	67	—	0
Olausson et al, 2002	9	22	89	—	0
El Rassi et al, 2002	5	52	80	40	0
Cahlin et al, 2003	7	36	100	0	0
Rosenau et al, 2002	19	38	89	80	3
Florman et al, 2004	11	30	73	36	1
Fenwick et al, 2004	2	70	100	50	1

*Actual duration of follow-up and current disease status of these patients is undefined.

of treated metastases (Berber et al, 2002; Hellman et al, 2002a). Duration of follow-up is insufficient to determine actual durability of local control given the protracted natural history of NEC. Progression of hepatic metastases has occurred in approximately 30% of patients within 2 years (Berber et al, 2002; Hellman et al, 2002a). Specific factors of the hepatic metastases, such as site, degree of necrosis or fibrosis, and hormonal markers, have not yet been correlated to RFA response.

RFA has been effective in relieving clinical endocrinopathies related to neuroendocrine hepatic metastases. Nearly 90% of patients have experienced some degree of symptom relief after ablation (Berber et al, 2002; Hellman et al, 2002a; Henn et al, 2003; Siperstein & Berber, 2001; Siperstein et al, 1997). Duration of relief from symptoms usually has extended for 10 months or longer (Berber et al, 2002; Henn et al, 2003). These findings parallel the findings reported after hepatic resection of metastatic NEC (Chamberlain et al, 2000; Sarmiento et al, 2003). For limited hepatic metastases, RFA can achieve similar results percutaneously. In the setting of extrahepatic disease, isolated hepatic ablation has a limited effect on symptoms (Henn et al, 2003). Clinical efficacy depends on the volume and site of extrahepatic tumor and the specific hormone expression.

Serum and urine neuroendocrine tumor markers are generally proportional to tumor burden (Moertel, 1987). The response of such markers to RFA has varied. In a study of 34 patients treated with intraoperative RFA, only 65% of patients had a decrease in serum tumor markers after ablation (Berber et al, 2002). Persistently elevated tumor markers after RFA likely reflect patient selection, completeness of ablation, and occult or overt NEC within the abdomen or elsewhere. A favorable response in reduction of serum tumor markers after ablation may predict the durability of symptomatic response and be associated with improved survival and decreased incidence of disease progression (Berber et al, 2002).

Ethanol Ablation of Hepatic Neuroendocrine Metastases

Ethanol ablation also has been incorporated into the treatment of primary and secondary hepatic neoplasms, including metastases from neuroendocrine malignancies in selected patients (Castells et al, 1993; Giovannini, 2002; Giovannini & Seitz, 1994; Lencioni et al, 1995; Livraghi et al, 1995, 1999; Shiina et al, 1993). Several studies have documented a complete intrahepatic response in patients with hepatic neuroendocrine metastases treated with percutaneous ethanol injection (Livraghi et al, 1991). Percutaneous ethanol injection permits ablation of metastases located adjacent to structures at risk of damage by RFA.

Highly selective ethanol ablation can be performed on metastases located adjacent to vital structures (e.g., the hepatic flexure of the colon); metastases adjacent to large vessels vulnerable to the heat-sink effect; and metastases adjacent to central bile ducts, where subsequent biliary stricture may occur (Fig. 73b.4). Metastases of very small size also can be ablated successfully with ethanol, with limited collateral injury to adjacent liver.

Cryoablation of Hepatic Neuroendocrine Metastases

Intraoperative cryoablation is effective in the treatment of primary and secondary tumors of the liver (Finlay et al, 2000; Mahvi & Lee, 1999; Neeleman et al, 2001; Seifert et al, 1998a; Sheen et al, 2002; Zhou & Tang, 1998). Based on a collective

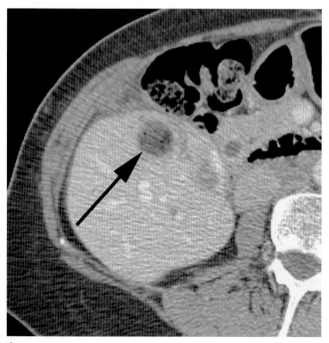

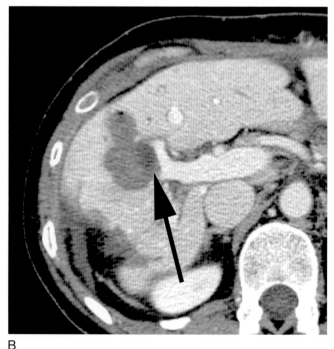

A   B

Fig. 73b.4. Ethanol ablation of critically located neuroendocrine hepatic metastases. **A,** CT with intravenous contrast administration shows nonenhancing, low-density, post–ethanol ablation changes within treated 2-cm carcinoid hepatic metastasis *(arrow),* located near the hepatic flexure of the colon. RFA was deferred because of risk of thermal injury to colon. **B,** CT with intravenous contrast administration shows combined RFA and ethanol ablation changes in a carcinoid metastasis located adjacent to the right anterior portal vein. *Arrow* indicates subtle low-density ethanol changes medially in the treated tumor. Ethanol was used selectively owing to the relative cooling of the ablation zone by adjacent blood flow, which could result in inadequate ablation ("heat-sink effect").

review of circa 1990s literature, local recurrence develops in about 30% of cryoablated tumors (Seifert et al, 1998a). In a direct comparison of cryoablation and RFA in the treatment of primary and secondary hepatic tumors, RFA was shown to be more effective in local control (2% versus 14% local recurrence) with fewer complications (3% versus 41% complication rate) (Chung et al, 2001; Pearson et al, 1999).

Current experience with cryoablation for hepatic neuroendocrine metastases reflects ablations performed intraoperatively (Bilchik et al, 1997; Cozzi et al, 1995; Goering et al, 2002; Seifert et al, 1998b). Most often, intraoperative cryoablation is performed in conjunction with resection of the primary tumor and hepatic metastases (Cozzi et al, 1995; Seifert et al, 1998b). Local control of neuroendocrine hepatic metastases has occurred in 95% of treated tumors (Chung et al, 2001; Cozzi et al, 1995; Seifert et al, 1998b), which is similar to other ablative techniques. Some relief of symptoms has been shown in all patients, even with recognized subtotal ablative debulking (Bilchik et al, 1997; Cozzi et al, 1995; Seifert et al, 1998a). Postoperative ablative adjuvant therapy with long-acting somatostatin analogue can prolong symptom-free survival (Chung et al, 2001).

Guidelines for Ablation

General guidelines in the ablation of liver metastases are analogous to the treatment of hepatocellular carcinoma and colorectal metastases. Recognizing the prolonged survival and clinical endocrinopathies of metastatic NEC, broader application of ablation as a component of multimodal treatment is warranted. Because reports of surgical experience have shown that cytoreduction of NEC can improve patient survival and symptoms considerably, the corollary of an aggressive ablation of progressive hepatic neuroendocrine metastases should provide similar patient benefit. There are three clinical scenarios for ablation of neuroendocrine hepatic metastases: (1) adjunct to concurrent surgical resection of hepatic metastases, (2) treatment of limited hepatic metastases in patients unfit for operation, and (3) primary hepatic therapy when clinical expertise or intraoperative circumstances preclude safe resection. Palliation of symptoms is an inherent aim for all patients with functional neuroendocrine symptoms.

RFA complements intraoperative resection of hepatic neuroendocrine metastases. Given the extensive hepatic tumor burden typically encountered, ablation affords selective treatment of metastases located deep in the liver or in sites not further resectable after partial hepatectomy. Adjunctive RFA optimizes debulking of hepatic metastases, reduces the extent of resection, and increases overall candidacy for surgical treatment.

Resection is precluded in many patients with neuroendocrine metastases to the liver because of the extent of tumor burden, comorbid disease, or prior hepatic resection. In such patients, percutaneous ablation allows less invasive tumor debulking. In contrast to non-neuroendocrine metastases, there is justification based on surgical experience for subtotal debulking of significant hepatic tumor by the ablation of multiple metastases (Fig. 73b.5). Generally, if the metastasis is visible with imaging, it can be treated in some manner with percutaneous ablation using either RFA or ethanol ablation, provided that there is sufficient preserved liver parenchyma to prevent hepatic decompensation.

This large volume ablation contrasts with the ablation of limited disease. Such a patient might have one or two very small hepatic metastases such that surgical resection might be considered

overly aggressive given the effectiveness of percutaneous RFA in treating such tumors (Fig. 73b.6). Percutaneous treatment typically is performed on an outpatient basis and obviates the longer hospitalization after resection. Given the inevitable recurrence of metastases after surgical resection (Sarmiento et al, 2003), percutaneous ablation is well suited for a patient who has undergone prior liver surgery. In contrast to surgical resection, ablation can be performed easily on multiple occasions based on occurrence of new metastases.

RFA of neuroendocrine hepatic metastases allows a relatively noninvasive mechanism to treat patient symptoms, similar to the role of hepatic resection. In our experience, less than 5% of patients are treated solely for tumor-related symptoms. Such ablative treatment is usually twofold with debulking of the hepatic tumor and secondary symptom management (Fig. 73b.7).

MEDICAL TREATMENT OF HEPATIC NEUROENDOCRINE METASTASES

Approaches for the medical treatment of metastatic NECs include somatostatin analogues, chemotherapy, immunotherapy, embolization or chemoembolization, and internal irradiation with iodine 131 conjugates (de Vries et al, 2002; Sutcliffe et al, 2004).

Somatostatin Analogues

Octreotide is a synthetic somatostatin analogue with a significantly longer half-life and duration of action than native somatostatin (Lamberts et al, 1996). It is primarily cytostatic, but also can be cytotoxic. The effect of somatostatin analogues is mediated through type 2 and 5 somatostatin receptors, inhibiting the cellular release of hormone. Response may correlate to somatostatin receptor scintigraphy (Janson et al, 1994). The analogues also can affect cell cycle arrest in G_1 phase, induce apoptosis, and inhibit angiogenesis. Lanreotide is currently the longest acting slow-release analogue. Octreotide dose is 100 to 500 μg three times daily, and lanreotide dose is 60 to 120 mg every 4 weeks.

Somatostatin analogues have been associated with a biochemical response in approximately 70% of patients and symptomatic relief in 60% to 90% of patients (Oberg et al, 2004). Objective reduction in tumor size (>50% of largest diameter) has occurred in less than 10% of patients. Stabilization of NECs has been observed in 36% to 70% of patients for a median duration of 12 months (Oberg et al, 2004). As expected, symptomatic response has been correlated with improved quality of life. Response to somatostatin analogue therapy varies by type of NEC. As noted previously, short-acting somatostatin analogue therapy is used to prevent or to treat the carcinoid crisis periprocedurally for any intervention, including resection, transplantation, ablation, or embolization. Somatostatin analogue treatment generally is well tolerated. Steatorrhea, diarrhea, abdominal discomfort, and biliary sludge or gallstones can develop, but rarely preclude continued use (Kaltsas et al, 2004; Kvols et al, 1987; Trendle et al, 1997).

Chemotherapy

Systemic chemotherapy generally is reserved for patients with advanced or progressive disease in whom other treatment efforts have failed (Brentjens & Saltz, 2001; Kaltsas et al, 2001; Oberg,

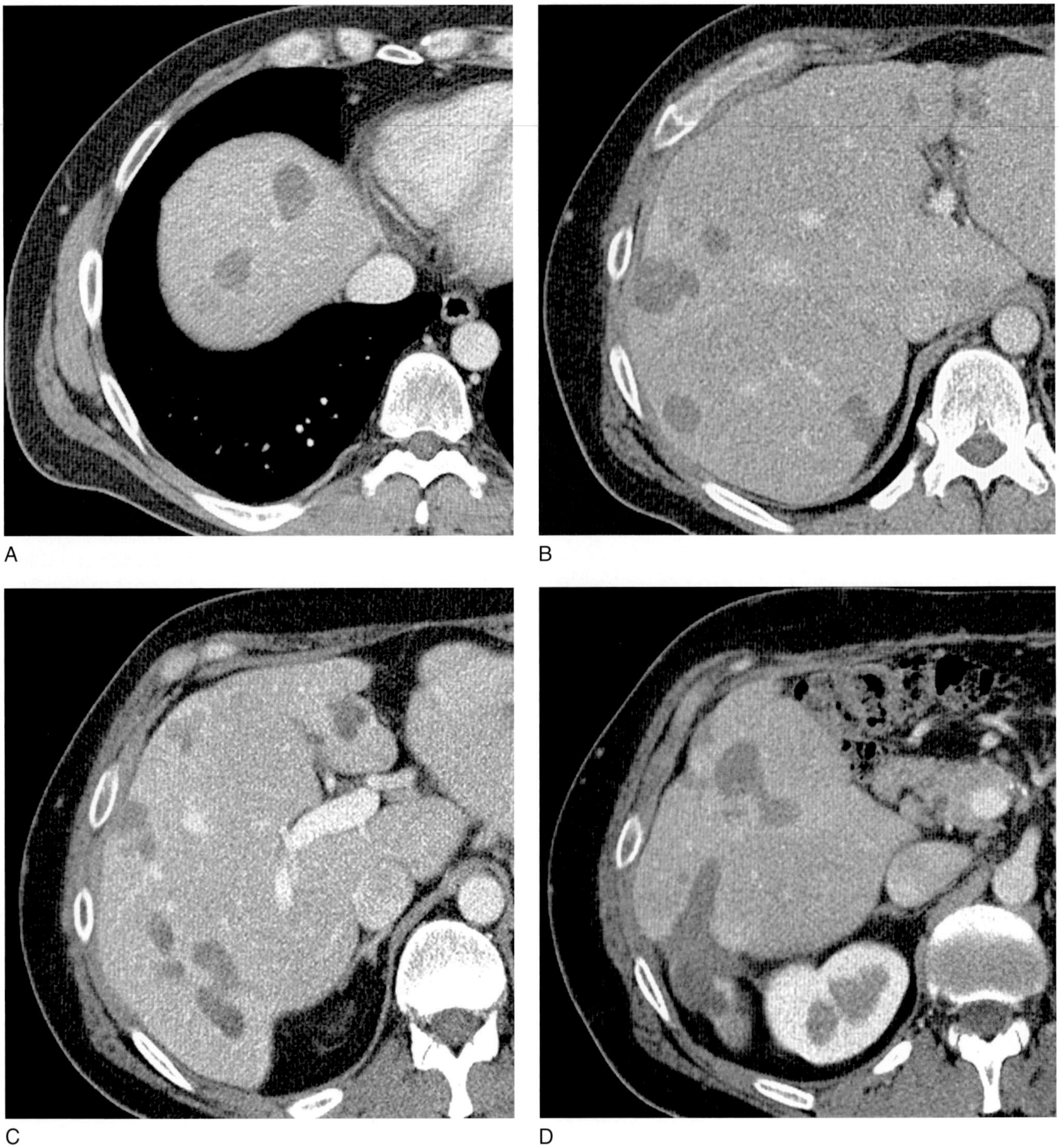

Fig. 73b.5. RFA of multiple neuroendocrine hepatic metastases. This patient with metastatic islet cell carcinoma has undergone four RFA procedures with the treatment of 50 metastases, including the treatment of 19 metastases in a single percutaneous ablation session. **A-D**, CT after intravenous contrast administration shows extensive nonenhancing ablation defects throughout the liver.

2003; Rivera & Ajani, 1998). Patients with pancreatic NECs have been more responsive to chemotherapy than patients with carcinoid tumors (Rivera & Ajani, 1998). Streptozocin-based combinations with 5-FU and doxorubicin have resulted in objective responses in 45% to 69% of patients (Kaltsas et al, 2001; Moertel et al, 1992; Oberg, 2001). Median duration of response for high-grade NEC is approximately 8 to 9 months. Carcinoid tumors may be less sensitive to cytotoxic agents because of the preponderance of low-grade malignant (well-differentiated) histology and low proliferation index (Bajetta et al, 2002). Dacarbazine, 5-FU, and epirubicin combination therapy has achieved objective tumor response in approximately 30% of patients with carcinoid tumors (Bajetta et al, 2002; Oberg, 2003). Median duration of response for carcinoid tumors is approximately 6 months.

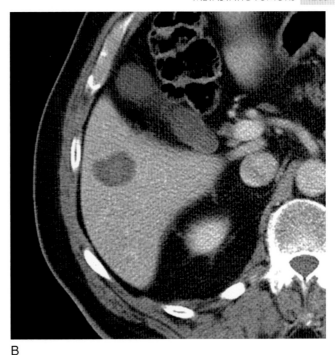

A   B

Fig. 73b.6. Percutaneous RFA of metastatic carcinoid in nonsurgical patient. **A**, CT with intravenous contrast administration shows subtle hyperenhancing solitary 2.3-cm metastasis in the right lobe of the liver *(arrow)*. Given limited disease and surgical risk in this 115-kg patient, the metastasis was treated with RFA. **B**, CT obtained 3 months after ablation shows no recurrent tumor.

Interferon Alfa

Systemic interferon alfa may be used to treat advanced NEC. The mechanism of interferon alfa is mediated through direct inhibitors of the cell cycle (G_1/S phase) and of protein and hormone production, through antiangiogenesis, and indirectly through increased immune stimulation (Oberg et al, 2004). Although an objective tumor response is seen in only 10% to 15%, symptomatic and biochemical responses have been observed in approximately 40% to 60% of patients (Biesma et al, 1992; Fjallskog et al, 2002; Jacobsen et al, 1995; Moertel et al, 1989; Oberg et al, 1986, 2004). Disease stabilization has occurred in 40% to 60% of patients. Adverse reactions to interferon alfa are common and may dictate discontinuation. Chronic fatigue and hematologic cytopenias are the most common side effects.

Embolization of Hepatic Neuroendocrine Metastases

Neuroendocrine metastases are intensely hypervascular. Embolization of the hepatic arteries results in ischemia of the metastases and causes variable degrees of tumor necrosis, which can alleviate symptoms or endocrinopathies (Perry et al, 1994). Embolization alone or in combination with intra-arterial chemotherapy (chemoembolization) has been employed for relief of symptoms. Repeated embolization is possible depending on the interventional vascular technique employed (selective or nonselective). Objective tumor responses to embolization alone ranged from 30% to 70% with similar symptomatic response rates (Brown et al, 1999; Oberg et al, 2004). Intermittent or temporary dearterialization with the use of an implantable hepatic artery occluder provides similar symptomatic relief for 6 to 12 months (Bengmark et al, 1982). Duration of response has

ranged from 15 to 30 months. Chemotherapy after embolization has prolonged duration of response (Moertel et al, 1994). These findings, coupled with the theoretical advantages of high intrahepatic concentration afforded by arterial infusion of chemotherapeutic agents, prompted evaluation of chemoembolization. Although chemoembolization has been employed for metastatic NEC, range and duration of response have been similar to embolization alone (Fiorentini et al, 2004; Yao et al, 2001). To date, no randomized trial comparing embolization with and without chemotherapy has confirmed a significant difference in outcomes or response.

Complications are generally tolerable, although significant. Postembolization syndrome, consisting of nausea, right upper quadrant abdominal pain, fever, and elevation of serum transaminases usually lasting for 3 to 7 days, is common. Parenteral analgesics, intravenous hydration, and antipyretics are often necessary. Antibiotic prophylaxis is recommended for embolization. Other side effects include gallbladder necrosis, hepatic abscess, and renal failure. Patients with large (>5-10 cm) metastases and patients with greater than 50% to 70% hepatic replacement are at greater risk of complications. Sequential lobar embolization may reduce the severity of the postembolization syndrome and risk of complications. Mortality after embolization has ranged from 2% to 7%.

PRIMARY HEPATIC NEUROENDOCRINE TUMORS

Albeit rare, NECs may arise primarily within the liver. Hepatobiliary NECs accounted for only 2% of all gastrointestinal carcinoids in the Surveillance Epidemiology and End Results database over a 30-year period, and primary hepatic carcinoids accounted for less than half of these tumors (Modlin et al, 2003).

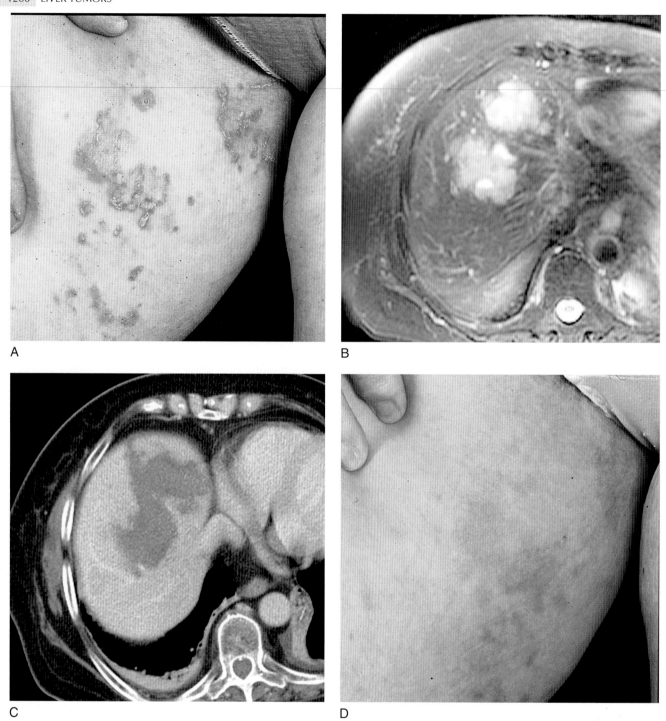

A

B

C

D

Fig. 73b.7. Percutaneous RFA for relief of symptoms secondary to metastatic glucagonoma (serum glucagon 16,000 pg/mL). **A,** Symptomatic necrolytic migratory erythema, days before ablation session. **B,** MRI shows multiple hyperintense hepatic metastases. **C,** CT performed hours after RFA shows large corresponding non-enhancing ablation defect in the liver parenchyma. The patient's rash resolved within days of the RFA. **D,** At 2-month follow-up, the patient was asymptomatic with healed rash and serum glucagon 3700 pg/mL.
(From Atwell TD, et al: Radiofrequency ablation of neuroendocrine metastases. In vanSonnenberg E, et al [eds], 2005: Tumor Ablation: Principles and Practice. New York, Springer Business and Science Media, pp 332-340).

Most reports of primary hepatic carcinoids are single case experiences, and case series are usually limited to fewer than six patients (Knox et al, 2003; Soga, 2002). Primary hepatic carcinoids have similar histopathologic and immunohistochemical findings as extrahepatic carcinoids. Most primary hepatic carcinoids are nonfunctional and rarely are associated with the carcinoid syndrome. Because they can be functional and can be associated with a specific endocrinopathy and not limited only to the carcinoid syndrome, however, they probably should be termed primary *hepatic neuroendocrine tumors* and not hepatic carcinoids.

The diagnosis presumes a thorough search and exclusion of an extrahepatic NEC. The cell of origin is unknown. Pancreatic heterotopia has been postulated as a source of these tumors.

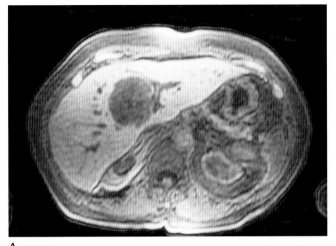
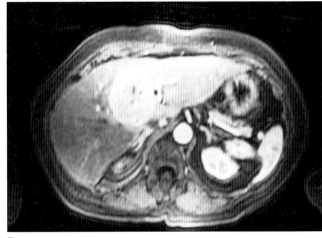

A   B

Fig. 73b.8. A and **B**, MRI (T1 [**B**] and T2 [**A**]) of a primary hepatic NEC depicting the expected features of a discrete hypervascular solitary mass residing centrally within the liver.

Some tumors may arise from intrahepatic biliary tract radicles because carcinoids of the extrahepatic biliary tract are more common. Most primary hepatic neuroendocrine tumors arise centrally or perihilarly within the liver. Finally, some primary hepatic neuroendocrine tumors may be metastases from an occult primary NEC or a primary NEC that had spontaneously regressed. A history of prior GEP resections warrants careful pathologic review of the resected specimen to exclude a missed primary NEC. Conversely, the absence of an identifiable extrahepatic site of NEC after resection is posited as evidence supporting the liver as a primary site.

There is a female predominance (65%), and mean age at presentation is 50 years. Typical symptoms and signs at presentation include abdominal pain, jaundice, weight loss, and, rarely, a specific endocrinopathy. The imaging features are similar to other neuroendocrine tumors (Fig. 73b.8). The criteria for resectability of primary hepatic NEC are similar to other hepatic malignancies. Because of the central location within the liver, extended lobar hepatic resections frequently are required for resection of these tumors. Hepatic transplantation also has been employed.

A review of the literature estimates overall 5-year and 10-year survivals of 78% and 59% (Knox et al, 2003). Among the 44 patients reported to have had hepatic resections for treatment, 5-year and 10-year survivals were 80% and 68% (Knox et al, 2003). Predictors of long-term survival have been few, and analysis of such factors is limited by the low prevalence of primary hepatic NEC. Hepatic multicentricity and bilaterality, extrahepatic metastases at the time of resection, advanced age, and gender have not correlated adversely with survival. Recurrence within the liver is common, and repeat resections have been reported and associated with further prolongation of survival. Hepatic transplantation also has proved effective for primary hepatic NEC deemed unresectable otherwise by standard techniques (Fenwick et al, 2004). The overall and disease-free survival after hepatic transplantation is similar to that of standard resection, albeit limited in duration of follow-up and number of patients reported. Current data preclude assessment of antihormonal therapy and chemotherapy, although anecdotal reports suggest that responses are similar to the responses in patients with extrahepatic NEC.

REFERENCES

Bajetta E, et al, 2002: Efficacy of a chemotherapy combination for the treatment of metastatic neuroendocrine tumours. Ann Oncol 13:614-621.

Bengmark S, et al, 1982: Temporary liver dearterialization in patients with metastatic carcinoid disease. World J Surg 6:46-53.

Berber E, et al, 2002: Laparoscopic radiofrequency ablation of neuroendocrine liver metastases. World J Surg 26:985-990.

Biesma B, et al, 1992: Recombinant interferon alpha-2b in patients with metastatic apudomas: effect on tumours and tumour markers. Br J Cancer 66:850-855.

Bilchik AJ, et al, 1997: Cryosurgical palliation of metastatic neuroendocrine tumors resistant to conventional therapy. Surgery 122:1040-1047.

Bleicher RJ, et al, 2003: Radiofrequency ablation in 447 complex unresectable liver tumors: lessons learned. Ann Surg Oncol 10:52-58.

Bowles BJ, et al, 2001: Safety and efficacy of radiofrequency thermal ablation in advanced liver tumors. Arch Surg 136:864-869.

Brentijens R, Saltz L, 2001: Islet cell tumors of the pancreas: the medical oncologist's perspective. Surg Clin North Am 81:527-542.

Brown KT, et al, 1999: Particle embolization of hepatic neuroendocrine metastases for control of pain and hormonal symptoms. J Vasc Interv Radiol 10:397-403.

Cahlin C, et al, 2003: Liver transplantation for metastatic neuroendocrine tumor disease. Transplant Proc 35:809-810.

Capella C, et al, 1995: Revised cassification of neuroendocrine tumours of the lung, pancreas, and gut. Virch Arch 425:547-560.

Castells A, et al, 1993: Treatment of small hepatocellular carcinoma in cirrhotic patients: a cohort study comparing surgical resection and percutaneous ethanol injection. Hepatology 18:1121-1126.

Chamberlain RS, et al, 2000: Hepatic neuroendocrine metastases: does intervention alter outcomes? J Am Coll Surg 190:432-445.

Chen H, et al, 1998: Isolated liver metastases from neuroendocrine tumors: does resection prolong survival? J Am Coll Surg 187:88-93.

Chu QD, et al, 2002: Predictive factors associated with long-term survival in patients with neuroendocrine tumors of the pancreas. Ann Surg Oncol 9:855-862.

Chung MH, et al, 2001: Hepatic cytoreduction followed by a novel long-acting somatostatin analog: a paradigm for intractable neuroendocrine tumors metastatic to the liver. Surgery 130:954-962.

Connolly HM, et al, 1995: Outcome of cardiac surgery of carcinoid heart disease. J Am Coll Cardiol 25:410-416.

Connolly HM, et al, 2002: Carcinoid heart disease: impact of pulmonary valve replacement on right ventricular function and remodeling. Circulation 106:151-156.

Coppa J, et al, 2001: Resection versus transplantation for liver metastases from neuroendocrine tumors. Transplant Proc 33:1537-1539.

Cozzi PJ, et al, 1995: Cryotherapy treatment of patients with hepatic metastases from neuroendocrine tumors. Cancer 76:501-509.

Curley SA, et al, 1999: Radiofrequency ablation of unresectable primary and metastatic hepatic malignancies: results in 123 patients. Ann Surg 230:1-8.

Curley SA, et al, 2000: Radiofrequency ablation of hepatocellular cancer in 110 patients with cirrhosis. Ann Surg 232:381-391.

de Baere T, et al, 2000: Radiofrequency ablation of 100 hepatic metastases with a mean follow-up of more than 1 year. AJR Am J Roentgenol 175:1619-1625.

de Vries H, et al, 2002: Diagnostic, surgical, and medical aspect of the midgut carcinoid. Cancer Treat Rev 28:11-25.

Eckhauser FE, et al, 1981: Mesenteric angiopathy, intestinal gangrene, and midgut carcinoids. Surgery 90:720-728.

El Rassi ZS, et al, 2002: Primary and secondary liver endocrine tumors: clinical presentation, surgical approach and outcome. Hepatogastroenterology 49:1340-1346.

Fenwick SW, 2004: Hepatic resection and transplantation for primary carcinoid tumors of the liver. Ann Surg 239:210-219.

Fernández JA, et al, 2003: Role of liver transplantation in the management of metastatic neuroendocrine tumors. Transplant Proc 35:1832-1833.

Fernandez-Cruz L, et al, 2002: Outcome of laparoscopic pancreatic surgery: endocrine and nonendocrine tumors. World J Surg 26:1057-1065.

Finlay IG, et al, 2000: Resection with cryotherapy of colorectal hepatic metastases has the same survival as hepatic resection alone. Eur J Surg Oncol 26:199-202.

Fiorentini G, et al, 2004: Intra-arterial hepatic chemoembolization in liver metastases from neuroendocrine tumors: a phase II study. J Chemother 16:293-297.

Fjallskog ML, et al, 2002: Treatment of malignant endocrine pancreatic tumors with a combination of alpha-interferon and somatostatin analogs. Med Oncol 19:35-42.

Florman S, et al, 2004: Liver transplantation for neuroendocrine tumors. J Gastrointest Surg 8:208-212.

Foster JH, Berman MM (eds), 1977: Solid Liver Tumors. Philadelphia, Saunders.

Fox DJ, Khattar RS, 2004: Carcinoid heart disease: presentation, diagnosis, and management. Heart 90:1224-1228.

Frilling A, et al, 1998: Liver transplantation in patients with liver metastases of neuroendocrine tumors. Transplant Proc 30:3298-3300.

Giovannini M, 2002: Percutaneous alcohol ablation for liver metastasis. Semin Oncol 29:192-195.

Giovannini M, Seitz JF, 1994: Ultrasound-guided percutaneous alcohol injection of small liver metastases: results in 40 patients. Cancer 73:294-297.

Goering JD, et al, 2002: Cryoablation and liver resection for noncolorectal liver metastases. Am J Surg 183:384-389.

Goldberg SN, Ahmed M, 2002: Minimally invasive image-guided therapies for hepatocellular carcinoma. J Clin Gastroenterol 35:S115-S129.

Grazi GL, et al, 2000: Highly aggressive policy of hepatic resections for neuroendocrine liver metastases. Hepatogastroenterology 47:481-486.

Gumbs AA, et al, 2002: Review of the clinical, histological, and molecular aspects of pancreatic endocrine neoplasms. J Surg Oncol 81:45-53.

Hellman P, et al, 2002a: Radiofrequency tissue ablation using cooled tip for liver metastasis of neuroendocrine tumors. World J Surg 26:1052-1056.

Hellman P, et al, 2002b: Effect of surgery on the outcome of midgut carcinoid disease with lymph node and liver metastases. World J Surg 26:991-997.

Henn AR, et al, 2003: Percutaneous radiofrequency ablation of hepatic metastases for symptomatic relief of neuroendocrine syndromes. AJR Am J Roentgenol 181:1005-1010.

Hochwald SN, et al, 2001: Nonfunctional pancreatic islet cell tumors. In Doherty G, Skogseid B (eds): Surgical Endocrinology. Philadelphia, Lippincott Williams & Wilkins, pp 361-373.

Jacobsen MB, et al, 1995: Interferon-alpha 2b, with or without prior hepatic artery embolization: clinical response and survival in mid-gut carcinoid patients. The Norwegian Carcinoid Study. Scand J Gastroenterol 30:789-796.

Jaeck D, et al, 2001: Hepatic metastases of gastroenteropancreatic neuroendocrine tumors: safe hepatic surgery. World J Surg 25:689S-692S.

Janson ET, et al, 1994: [111In-DTPA-D-Phe1] octreotide scintigraphy in patients with carcinoid tumours: the predictive value for somatostatin analogue treatment. Eur J Endocrinol 131:577-581.

Kaltsas G, et al, 2001: The role of chemotherapy in the nonsurgical management of malignant neuroendocrine tumours. Clin Endocrinol 55:575-587.

Kaltsas GA, et al, 2004: The diagnosis and medical management of advanced neuroendocrine tumors. Endocr Rev 25:458-511.

Kettenbach J, et al, 2003: Percutaneous saline-enhanced radiofrequency ablation of unresectable hepatic tumors: initial experience in 26 patients. AJR Am J Roentgenol 180:1537-1545.

Kinny MAO, et al, 2001: Perianaesthetic risks and outcomes of abdominal surgery for metastatic carcinoid tumours. Br J Anaesth 87:447-452.

Knox CD, et al, 2003: Long-term survival after resection for primary hepatic carcinoid tumor. Ann Surg Oncol 10:1171-1175.

Knox CD, et al, 2004: Survival and functional quality of life after resection of hepatic carcinoid metastasis. J Gastrointest Surg 8:653-659.

Kulke MH, Mayer RJ, 1999: Carcinoid tumors. N Engl J Med 340:858-868.

Kvols LK, et al, 1987: Treatment of metastatic islet cell carcinoma with a somatostatin analogue (SMS 201-995). Ann Intern Med 107:162-168.

Lamberts SWJ, et al, 1996: Octreotide. N Engl J Med 334:246-254.

Lang H, et al, 1999: Total hepatectomy and liver transplantation for metastatic neuroendocrine tumors of the pancreas—a single center experience with ten patients. Lang Arch Surg 384:370-377.

Lehnert T, 1998: Liver transplantation for metastatic neuroendocrine carcinoma. Transplantation 66:1307-1312.

Lencioni R, et al, 1995: Treatment of small hepatocellular carcinoma with percutaneous ethanol injection: analysis of prognostic factors in 105 Western patients. Cancer 76:1737-1746.

Livraghi T, et al, 1991: Liver metastases: results of percutaneous ethanol injection in 14 patients. Radiology 179:709-712.

Livraghi T, et al, 1995: Hepatocellular carcinoma and cirrhosis in 746 patients: long-term results of percutaneous ethanol injection. Radiology 197:101-108.

Livraghi T, et al, 1999: Small hepatocellular carcinoma: treatment with radio-frequency ablation versus ethanol injection. Radiology 210:655-661.

Livraghi T, et al, 2003: Treatment of focal liver tumors with percutaneous radio-frequency ablation: complications encountered in a multicenter study. Radiology 226:441-451.

Loftus JP, van Heerden JA, 1995: Surgical management of gastrointestinal carcinoid tumors. Adv Surg 28:317-336.

Madeira I, et al, 1998: Prognostic factors in patients with endocrine tumours of the duodenopancreatic area. Gut 43:422-427.

Mahvi DM, Lee FT Jr, 1999: Radiofrequency ablation of hepatic malignancies: is heat better than cold? Ann Surg 230:9-11.

Mansour JC, Chen H, 2004: Pancreatic endocrine tumors. J Surg Res 120:139-161.

Matthews BD, et al, 2002: Surgical experience with functioning pancreatic neuroendocrine tumors. Am Surg 68:660-665.

McDonald ML, et al, 1999: Carcinoid heart disease and carcinoid syndrome: successful surgical treatment. Ann Thorac Surg 67:537-539.

Modlin IM, et al, 2003: A 5-decade analysis of 13,715 carcinoid tumors. Cancer 97:934-959.

Moertel CG, 1987: Karnofsky memorial lecture: an odyssey in the land of small tumors. J Clin Oncol 5:1502-1522.

Moertel CG, et al, 1989: Therapy of metastatic carcinoid tumor and the malignant carcinoid syndrome with recombinant leukocyte A interferon. J Clin Oncol 7:865-868.

Moertel CG, et al, 1992: Streptozocin-doxorubicin, streptozocin-fluorouracil or chlorozotocin in the treatment of advanced islet-cell carcinoma. N Engl J Med 326:519-523.

Moertel CG, et al, 1994: The management of patients with advanced carcinoid tumors and islet cell carcinomas. Ann Intern Med 120:302-309.

Nave H, et al, 2001: Surgery as primary treatment in patients with liver metastases from carcinoid tumors: a retrospective, unicentric study over 13 years. Surgery 129:170-175.

Neeleman N, et al, 2001: Cryosurgery as treatment modality for colorectal liver metastases. Hepatogastroenterology 48:325-329.

Norton JA, et al, 2003a: Morbidity and mortality of aggressive resection in patients with advanced neuroendocrine tumors. Arch Surg 138:859-866.

Norton JA, et al, 2003b: Aggressive surgery for metastatic liver neuroendocrine tumors. Surgery 134:1057-1065.

Oberg K, 2001: Chemotherapy and biotherapy in the treatment of neuroendocrine tumours. Ann Oncol 12(suppl 2):S111-S114.

Oberg K, 2003: Diagnosis and treatment of carcinoid tumors. Expert Rev Anticancer Ther 3:863-877.

Oberg K, et al, 1986: Treatment of malignant carcinoid tumors with human leukocyte interferon: long-term results. Cancer Treat Rep 70:1297-1304.

Oberg K, et al, 2004: Guidelines for the management of gastroenteropancreatic neuroendocrine tumours (including bronchopulmonary and thymic neoplasms). Acta Oncol 43:617-625.

Öhvrall U, et al, 2000: Method for dissection of mesenteric metastases in mid-gut carcinoid tumors. World J Surg 24:1402-1408.

Olausson M, et al, 2002: Indication and results of liver transplantation in patients with neuroendocrine tumours. World J Surg 26:998-1004.

Onaitis MW, et al, 2000: Gastrointestinal carcinoids: characterization by site of origin and hormone production. Ann Surg 232:549-556.

Pascher A, et al, 2000: Primary and secondary hepatic manifestation of neuroendocrine tumors. Lang Arch Surg 385:265-270.

Pawlik TM, et al, 2003: Combined resection and radiofrequency ablation for advanced hepatic malignancies: results in 172 patients. Ann Surg Oncol 10:1059-1069.

Pearson AS, et al, 1999: Intraoperative radiofrequency ablation or cryoablation for hepatic malignancies. Am J Surg 178:592-599.

Perry LJ, et al, 1994: Hepatic arterial embolization for metastatic neuroendocrine tumors. Surg 116:1111-1116.

Phan GQ, et al, 1998: Surgical experience with pancreatic and peripancreatic neuroendocrine tumors: review of 125 patients. J Gastrointest Surg 2:472-482.

Proye C, 2001: Natural history of liver metastases of gastroenteropancreatic neuroendocrine tumors: place for chemoembolization. World J Surg 25:685-688.

Que FG, et al, 1995: Hepatic resection for neuroendocrine carcinomas. Am J Surg 169:36-42.

Rhim H, Dodd GD 3rd, 1999: Radiofrequency thermal ablation of liver tumors. J Clin Ultrasound 27:221-229.

Rindi G, et al, 1998: Cell biology, clinicopathological profile, and classification of gastro-enteropancreatic endocrine tumors. J Mol Med 76:413-420.

Ringe B, et al, 2001: Treatment of hepatic metastases from gastroenteropancreatic neuroendocrine tumors: role of liver transplantation. World J Surg 25:697-699.

Rivera E, Ajani JA, 1998: Doxorubicin, streptozocin, and 5-fluorouracil chemotherapy for patients with metastatic islet-cell carcinoma. Am J Clin Oncol 21:36-38.

Rosenau J, et al, 2002: Ki67, E-cadherin, and p53 as prognostic indicators of long-term outcome after liver transplantation for metastatic neuroendocrine tumors. Transplantation 73:386-394.

Sarmiento JM, et al, 2002: Concurrent resections of pancreatic islet cell cancers with synchronous hepatic metastases: outcomes of an aggressive approach. Surgery 132:976-983.

Sarmiento JM, et al, 2003: Surgical treatment of neuroendocrine metastases to the liver: a plea for resection to increase survival. J Am Coll Surg 197:29-37.

Schnirer II, et al, 2003: Carcinoid: comprehensive review. Acta Oncol 42:672-692.

Seifert JK, et al, 1998a: A collective review of the world literature on hepatic cryotherapy. J R Coll Surg Edinb 43:141-154.

Seifert JK, et al, 1998b: Cryotherapy for neuroendocrine liver metastases. Semin Surg Oncol 14:175-183.

Sheen AJ, et al, 2002: Cryotherapeutic ablation of liver tumours. Br J Surg 89:1396-1401.

Shiina S, et al, 1993: Percutaneous ethanol injection therapy for hepatocellular carcinoma: results in 146 patients. AJR Am J Roentgenol 160:1023-1028.

Siperstein AE, Berber E, 2001: Cryoablation, percutaneous alcohol injection, and radiofrequency ablation for treatment of neuroendocrine liver metastases. World J Surg 25:693-696.

Siperstein AE, et al, 1997: Laparoscopic thermal ablation of hepatic neuroendocrine tumor metastases. Surgery 122:1147-1154.

Skinazi F, et al, 1996: Liver metastases of digestive endocrine tumours: natural history and response to medical treatment. Eur J Gastroenterol Hepatol 8:673-678.

Slooter GD, et al, 2001: Somatostatin receptor imaging, therapy and new strategies in patients with neuroendocrine tumours. Br J Surg 88:31-40.

Soga J, 2002: Primary hepatic endocrinomas (carcinoids and variant neoplasms): a statistical evaluation of 126 reported cases. J Exp Clin Cancer Res 21:457-468.

Solbiati L, et al, 2001a: Percutaneous radio-frequency ablation of hepatic metastases from colorectal cancer: long-term results in 117 patients. Radiology 221:159-166.

Solbiati L, et al, 2001b: Radiofrequency thermal ablation of hepatic metastases. Eur J Ultrasound 13:149-158.

Solcia E, et al, 2000: Histological Typing of Neuroendocrine Tumors. World Health Organization Classification of Tumor. New York. Springer.

Solorzano CC, et al, 2001: Nonfunctioning islet cell carcinoma of the pancreas: survival results in a contemporary series of 163 patients. Surgery 130:1078-1085.

Soreide O, et al, 1992: Surgical treatment is a principle in patients with advanced abdominal carcinoid tumors. Surgery 111:48-54.

Sutcliffe R, et al, 2004: Management of neuroendocrine liver metastases. Am J Surg 187:39-46.

Thompson GB, et al, 1985: Carcinoid tumors of gastrointestinal tract: presentation, management and prognosis. Surgery 98:1054.

Tomassetti P, et al, 2001: Diagnostic value of plasma chromogranin in neuroendocrine tumours. Eur J Gastroenterol Hepatol 13:55-58.

Trendle MC, et al, 1997: Incidence and morbidity of cholelithiasis in patients receiving chronic octreotide for metastatic carcinoid and malignant islet cell tumors. Cancer 79:830-834.

Wong SL, et al, 2001: Radiofrequency ablation for unresectable hepatic tumors. Am J Surg 182:552-557.

Wood TF, et al, 2000: Radiofrequency ablation of 231 unresectable hepatic tumors: indications, limitations, and complications. Ann Surg Oncol 7:593-600.

Woodside KJ, et al, 2004: Current management of gastrointestinal carcinoid tumors. J Gastrointest Surg 8:742-756.

Yao KA, et al, 2001: Indications and results of liver resection and hepatic chemoembolization for metastatic gastrointestinal neuroendocrine tumors. Surgery 130:677-685.

Zhou XD, Tang ZY, 1998: Cryotherapy for primary liver cancer. Semin Surg Oncol 14:171-174.

73c NONCOLORECTAL NON-NEUROENDOCRINE METASTASES

J. WEITZ AND R. P. DEMATTEO

Hepatic resection is a well-established therapy for patients with liver metastases from colorectal or neuroendocrine carcinoma. Surgical resection of liver metastases from colorectal cancer results in a 3-year survival rate of 30% to 61% and a 5-year survival rate of 16% to 51%, depending on patient selection (Fong et al, 1997, 1999; Scheele et al, 1995; Schlag et al, 1990). In patients with hepatic neuroendocrine metastases, 5-year survival rates of 76% have been achieved with surgical resection, and some surgeons occasionally employ liver transplantation (Chamberlain et al, 2000; Lehnert, 1998). In contrast, the role of hepatectomy in patients with liver metastases from noncolorectal, non-neuroendocrine (NCNN) tumors is not well defined, but the number of reports on this topic is increasing.

SERIES SUMMARIZING MULTIPLE PRIMARY TUMOR TYPES

Most current reports regarding hepatectomy for metastases of NCNN tumors combine multiple primary tumor types to have a large enough number of patients to analyze. Despite this approach, most series still are limited by a small number of patients or inclusion of patients with neuroendocrine metastases (Benevento et al, 2000; Buell et al, 2000; Elias et al, 1998; Goering et al, 2002; Hamy et al, 2000; Hemming et al, 2000; Karavias et al, 2002; Laurent et al, 2001; Schwartz, 1995; Takada et al, 2001; van Ruth et al, 2001; Yamada et al, 2001).

Goering and colleagues (2002) reported the outcome of 48 patients who had undergone liver resection or ablation for liver metastases from noncolorectal tumors. With a median follow-up of 48 months, the 5-year survival rate was 39%, and the median overall survival was 45 months. There was no difference in survival between patients treated with liver resection versus cryotherapy. The 3-year survival for patients with primary neuroendocrine ($n = 13$), genitourinary ($n = 16$), and soft tissue tumors ($n = 15$) was 91%, 52%, and 34% ($P = .26$).

Elias and colleagues (1998) performed hepatectomy in 147 patients with liver metastases from a noncolorectal primary. Operative mortality was 2%. The overall 5-year survival rate was 36% with the following results for different primary tumors: breast cancer ($n = 35$) 20%, neuroendocrine tumor ($n = 27$) 74%, testicular cancer ($n = 20$) 46%, sarcoma ($n = 13$) 18%, and gastric cancer ($n = 11$) 20%. The authors pointed out that the overall survival was similar to their results obtained in 270 patients undergoing liver resection for metastases of colorectal cancer.

Hemming and associates (2000) performed liver resections in 37 patients with NCNN primaries. After a median follow-up of 22 months, the overall 5-year survival rate was 45%. Curative resection and primary tumor type were independent prognostic markers of overall survival in this series. In the subgroup with nongastrointestinal primaries ($n = 30$), the overall 5-year survival rate was 60% compared with 0% for patients with gastrointestinal primaries ($n = 7$; $P = .01$).

Laurent and coworkers (2001) analyzed the outcome of 39 patients undergoing potentially curative resection of NCNN liver metastases. Patients had primary gastrointestinal ($n = 15$), genitourinary ($n = 12$), or miscellaneous ($n = 12$) tumors. The 5-year survival for the entire group was 35%. Notably, 5-year survival was 100% for patients with a disease-free interval from removal of the primary that exceeded 24 months versus 10% otherwise ($P < .01$). No other prognostic parameters were identified.

The MSKCC experience of patients who underwent hepatic resection for metastases from NCNN carcinoma was analyzed by Weitz and associates (2004). The objectives of this study were to define perioperative and long-term outcome and to define prognostic factors for survival in 141 patients who underwent resection for liver metastases from NCNN carcinoma during the period April 1981–April 2002. Table 73c.1 depicts the primary tumor types. The median operative time was 238 minutes (interquartile range 180-321 minutes), and the median blood loss was 600 mL (interquartile range 250-1420 mL). The median length of hospital stay was 9 days (interquartile range 7-12 days). Of 141 (33%) patients, 46 developed postoperative complications, but the 30-day mortality was 0%. The median follow-up was 26 months, with a median follow-up of 35 months for survivors. The actuarial 3-year relapse-free survival rate was 30% (median 17 months). The actuarial 3-year cancer-specific survival rate was 57% (median 42 months). Primary tumor type and length of disease-free interval from the primary tumor were significant independent prognostic factors for relapse-free and cancer-specific survival (Figs. 73c.1-73c.3, Table 73c.2). Margin status was significant for cancer-specific survival and showed a strong trend in relapse-free survival. Patients with a primary reproductive tract tumor who underwent R0 resection had the best outcome, with an actuarial 3-year cancer-specific survival of 78%. In the group of patients with primary non–reproductive tract tumors, survival after R0 resection was influenced largely by the length of the disease-free interval. Patients with a disease-free interval of 24 months or less achieved an actuarial 3-year survival of 36%, but only 5% were free of relapse after 3 years. Patients with a non–reproductive tract primary and a disease-free interval of more than 24 months had an actuarial 3-year cancer-specific survival of 72% and an actuarial 3-year relapse-free survival of 30%. There were 14 actual 5-year survivors in this group. Laparoscopy might be a reasonable staging tool for these patients. D'Angelica and coworkers (2002) examined 30 patients with potentially resectable liver metastases of NCNN tumors. Nine of these patients had unresectable disease, six of whom were identified by laparoscopy.

Table 73c.1 Primary Tumor Type of Patients Undergoing Liver Resection for Metastatic Noncolorectal, Non-neuroendocrine Tumors

Primary Tumor	No. (%)
Breast	29 (20)
Melanoma	17 (12)
Reproductive tract	39 (28)
Testicular	20 (14)
Gynecologic	19 (14)
Ovarian	12
Endometrium	4
Cervix	2
Fallopian tube	1
Adrenocortical	15 (11)
Renal	11 (8)
Gastrointestinal	12 (9)
Stomach	3
Duodenum	1
Pancreas	5
Ampulla	2
Anal	1
Other	13 (9)
Lung	4
Salivary gland	3
Nasopharynx	2
Glottis	1
Tonsil	1
Thyroid	1
Sweat gland	1
Unknown	5 (3)

Data from Weitz J, et al, 2004: Partial hepatectomy for metastases from non-colorectal, non-neuroendocrine carcinoma. Ann Surg 241:269-276.

SERIES FOCUSING ON ONE PRIMARY TUMOR TYPE

Sarcoma

The largest surgical series of patients with sarcoma metastatic to the liver comprises 56 patients who underwent liver resection (DeMatteo et al, 2001). These patients were selected from 331 patients with liver metastases from sarcomas who had been admitted to MSKCC during the years 1982-2000. Gastrointestinal stromal tumors and leiomyosarcomas were the most common histology (Fig. 73c.4). There were no perioperative deaths in patients undergoing complete resection of the tumor. The 5-year overall survival rate was 30% with a median of 39 months in completely resected patients. Patients who did not undergo complete resection had a 5-year survival of only 4% (Fig. 73c.5). A disease-free interval of less than 24 months was a significant adverse prognostic parameter for survival on univariate and multivariate analysis (Fig. 73c.6).

The treatment strategy for patients with liver metastases from gastrointestinal stromal tumors has changed since the development of the targeted agent imatinib mesylate, which achieves dramatic tumor response rates (Corless et al, 2004; DeMatteo, 2002). Imatinib is now the first-line treatment. Resection is considered for patients when they reach the maximal response to imatinib if all gross tumor can be removed and for patients who have immediate or limited acquired resistance to the drug (Antonescu et al, 2005).

Breast Cancer

In a small proportion (4-5%) of patients with breast cancer, liver metastases are the only sign of disseminated disease (Fig. 73c.7) (Elias et al, 2003). Although it has not been formally proven that liver resection prolongs survival for selected patients with liver metastases of breast cancer, actuarial 5-year survival was 34% to 61% in more recently published series (Elias et al, 2003; Vlastos et al, 2004). Patients with liver metastases of breast cancer receiving chemotherapy only rarely, if ever, survive 5 years (Wyld et al, 2003). Even with aggressive systemic chemotherapy, the median survival for patients with isolated liver metastases of breast cancer was only 23 to 27 months, with time to progression of 8 to 10 months in two more recent trials (Atalay et al, 2003). Resection for liver metastases of breast cancer may prolong survival for a subset of highly selected patients (Singletary et al, 2003).

Table 73c.3 summarizes the published studies of liver resection for metastatic breast cancer. Meaningful comparisons between

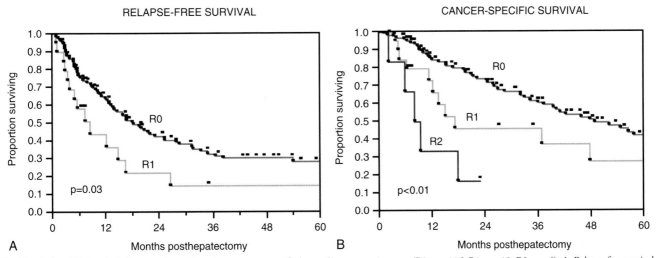

Fig. 73c.1. A and **B,** Survival after resection of hepatic metastases stratified according to margin status (R0, *n* = 116; R1, *n* = 19; R2, *n* = 6). **A,** Relapse-free survival. **B,** Cancer-specific survival.
(From Weitz J, et al, 2004: Partial hepatectomy for metastases from non-colorectal, non-neuroendocrine carcinoma. Ann Surg 241:269-276.)

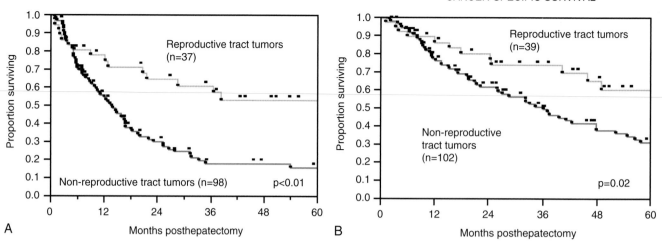

Fig. 73c.2. A and **B,** Survival after resection of hepatic metastases stratified according to primary tumor type (reproductive tract versus non–reproductive tract tumors) (patients with R2 resection were excluded for relapse-free survival). **A,** Relapse-free survival. **B,** Cancer-specific survival.
(From Weitz J, et al, 2004: Partial hepatectomy for metastases from non-colorectal, non-neuroendocrine carcinoma. Ann Surg 241:269-276.)

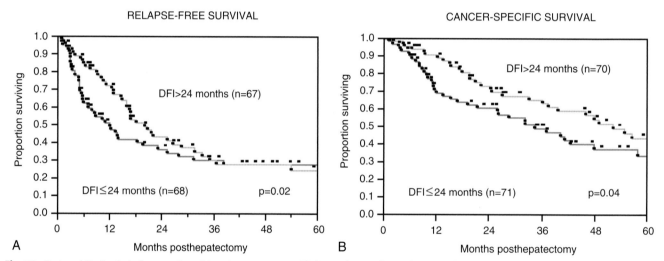

Fig. 73c.3. A and **B,** Survival after resection of hepatic metastases stratified according to disease-free interval (DFI) (patients with R2 resection were excluded for relapse-free survival) **A,** Relapse-free survival. **B,** Cancer-specific survival.
(From Weitz J, et al, 2004: Partial hepatectomy for metastases from non-colorectal, non-neuroendocrine carcinoma. Ann Surg 241:269-276.)

Table 73c.2   Multivariate Analysis of Prognostic Factors of Patients Undergoing Liver Resection for Metastatic Noncolorectal, Non-neuroendocrine Carcinoma

		RELAPSE-FREE SURVIVAL		**CANCER-SPECIFIC SURVIVAL**	
		Hazard Ratio (95% CI)	**P Value**	**Hazard Ratio (95% CI)**	**P Value**
Disease-free interval	≤24 mo	1.4 (1.1-1.8)	.02	1.4 (1.0-1.8)	.03
	>24 mo	Reference		Reference	
Primary tumor	Adrenocortical	0.9 (0.5-1.6)	<.01	0.7 (0.4-1.3)	.02
	Breast	0.9 (0.6-1.5)		1.0 (0.6-1.7)	
	Gastrointestinal	0.6 (0.3-1.1)		0.8 (0.3-1.5)	
	Reproductive tract	0.4 (0.2-0.6)		0.4 (0.2-0.7)	
	Melanoma	1.0 (0.5-1.9)		1.5 (0.7-2.7)	
	Renal	1.1 (0.5-2.2)		0.7 (0.3-1.3)	
	Other	1.6 (0.8-2.9)		1.7 (0.3-1.3)	
	Unknown	Reference		Reference	
Margin status	R0	Reference	.08	Reference	<.01
	R1	1.8 (0.9-3.2)		2.1 (1.1-4.1)	
	R2	ND*		2.7 (0.8-7.9)	

*ND, not determined (relapse-free survival patients with incomplete macroscopic resection [*n* = 6] were not included in the analysis).
CI, confidence interval.
Data from Weitz J, et al, 2004: Partial hepatectomy for metastases from non-colorectal, non-neuroendocrine carcinoma. Ann Surg 241:269-276.

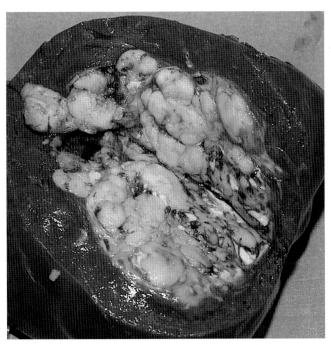

Fig. 73c.4. Right hepatectomy for a liver metastasis from gastrointestinal stromal tumor.

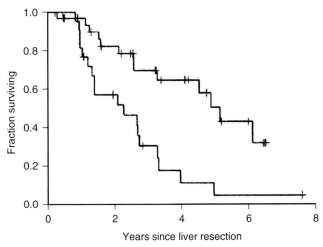

Fig. 73c.6. Disease-specific survival of patients after complete resection of liver metastases from sarcoma with a disease-free interval of more than 2 years (*upper line, n* = 32) versus less than 2 years (*lower line, n* = 24; *P* = .002). (From DeMatteo RP, et al, 2001: Results of hepatic resection for sarcoma metastatic to the liver. Ann Surg 234:540-548.)

these studies cannot be made because they are heterogeneous studies reporting small patient numbers with different inclusion criteria and treatment strategies. Valid criteria for selecting patients who might benefit from hepatic resection for metastases of breast cancer cannot be defined at this time. A common recommendation is that patients with extrahepatic disease should not undergo liver resection, even though some studies did not find a worse prognosis for such patients. Some authors also suggest that patients first should undergo systemic chemotherapy, and that only patients who do not progress should undergo liver resection. Formal randomized trials confirming this strategy have not been performed.

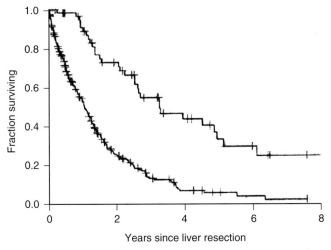

Fig. 73c.5. Disease-specific survival of patients with liver metastases from sarcoma who underwent complete resection (*upper line, n* = 56) versus other treatment (*lower line, n* = 275; *P* = .0001). (From DeMatteo RP, et al, 2001: Results of hepatic resection for sarcoma metastatic to the liver. Ann Surg 234:540-548.)

Melanoma

Melanoma recurs after potentially curative resection in approximately one third of patients, with almost every organ being at risk (Allen & Coit, 2002). Hepatic metastases are diagnosed in about 10% to 20% of patients with stage IV melanoma, even though it is well documented that most patients have liver metastases on postmortem examination. Patients with liver metastases of melanoma as the initial site of metastatic disease have a very poor prognosis with a median survival of 4.4 months (Rose et al, 2001). Most patients with liver metastases of melanoma have unresectable disease owing to extrahepatic disease or disseminated hepatic metastases. This is shown by a study from the John Wayne Cancer Institute and the Sydney Melanoma Unit (Rose et al, 2001). During the years 1971-1999, 26,204 patients with melanoma were seen in these institutions, and 1750 patients (6.7%) had liver metastases. Only 34 patients underwent surgical exploration for attempted liver resection, and hepatectomy was performed in 24 patients. Of these 24 patients, 12 had synchronous extrahepatic disease. Eighteen patients could be rendered disease-free surgically. The 10 patients who underwent only exploration had a median survival of 4 months. The overall survival of all patients with liver metastases treated nonoperatively was 6 months. Overall survival in the patients who underwent complete resection was 28 months with a median disease-free survival of 12 months. One patient is still alive more than 10 years postoperatively. The actuarial 5-year overall survival was 29%. Complete gross resection and histologically negative margins were associated with an improved disease-free survival, and complete gross resection showed a trend for improved overall survival (*P* = .06).

From this experience, one might conclude that extrahepatic disease per se is not a contraindication for resection as long as all disease is resectable. Selection of patients is crucial, which is well documented in this study. Only 1.4% of all patients with liver metastases underwent hepatic resection, and these patients had a median disease-free interval of 58 months before presenting with hepatic metastases. Several other small series in the literature mostly contain less than 10 patients undergoing liver resection for metastatic melanoma, with median survival times of 10 to

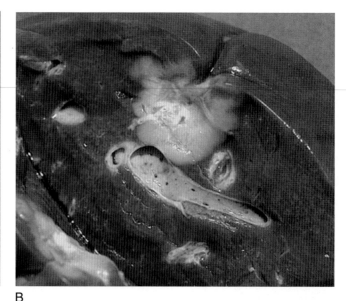

Fig. 73c.7. Liver metastasis of breast cancer. **A,** CT scan shows the lesion *(arrow)* to have early peripheral contrast enhancement. **B,** The patient underwent resection of segments II and III; a gross photograph of the sectioned specimen is shown.

51 months (Rose et al, 2001). Repeat hepatic resection might be beneficial for some patients who can be rendered disease-free surgically (Mondragon-Sanches et al, 1999).

Uveal melanoma is a distinct entity that seems to have a different tumor biology, and it commonly spreads to the liver. About 50% to 80% of patients with uveal melanoma who develop distant metastases have liver involvement. Hsueh and colleagues (2004) reported 112 patients with metastatic uveal melanoma, with 78 patients having liver metastases. A total of 24 patients underwent surgical resection for metastases (5 with liver metastases). A multivariate analysis showed surgical resection, but not site of metastasis, to be a significant predictor of survival.

The median survival for patients undergoing resection was 38 months in this series, with a 5-year survival of 39%. Aoyama and coworkers (2000) presented a series of 12 patients with metastatic uveal melanoma (9 with liver metastases). Median recurrence-free survival after complete resection was 19 months, with a median overall survival exceeding 27 months, emphasizing that selected patients with metastatic melanoma may benefit from surgical resection. Most patients with liver metastases from uveal melanoma are not candidates for surgical resection, however. For these patients, regional chemotherapy might offer increased response rates and probably increased overall survival compared with other treatment options (Feldman et al, 2004).

Table 73c.3 Results of Liver Resection for Metastatic Breast Cancer*

Reference	No. Patients	Median Survival (mo)†	Adverse Prognostic Factors	Comments
Vlastos et al, 2004	31	63	None	Inclusion criteria: no extrahepatic disease
Elias et al, 2003	54	34	Negative receptor status (OR 3.5)	Inclusion criteria: no extrahepatic disease; no disease progression on chemotherapy
Carlini et al, 2002	17	53	None	Inclusion criteria: no extrahepatic disease
Pocard et al, 2000	49	42	Short disease-free interval; node-positive primary	Inclusion criteria: good performance status; objective response on chemotherapy; 1-3 liver metastases
Selzner et al, 2000	17	27	Short disease-free interval	6041 patients with breast cancer were treated during the study interval at the authors' institution.
Yoshimoto et al, 2000	25	34	None	67% of patients developed recurrence in the liver
Seifert et al, 1999	15	57	None	Inclusion criteria: no extrahepatic disease
Raab et al, 1998	34	41.5‡	R1 resection; local recurrence of primary tumor	59% of patients with isolated metastasis

*Only series including >10 patients are presented.
†Overall survival.
‡For patients undergoing R0 resection.
OR, odds ratio.

Gastric and Pancreatic Cancer

Most reports on liver resection for NCNN metastases of gastrointestinal origin are based on patients with gastric cancer. Patients undergoing hepatic resection for metastatic gastric cancer are highly selected, as apparent in the report of Ochiai and colleagues (1994), who treated 6540 patients with gastric cancer. Liver resection for metastases was performed in only 30 of these patients (0.46%). Table 73c.4 summarizes more recently published data. There have been a few long-term survivors.

Only a handful of long-term survivors have been reported after the resection of liver metastases from pancreatic ductal adenocarcinoma (Detry et al, 2003). Consequently, surgery cannot be recommended for these patients. For other primary malignant tumors of the pancreas that show a less aggressive tumor biology, such as solid pseudopapillary tumor of the pancreas, resection of liver metastases might be justified (Martin et al, 2002).

Renal Carcinoma

About 10% of patients with renal tumors develop liver metastases, and they have a dismal prognosis with less than 10% of the patients surviving beyond 1 year. About 2% to 4% of patients develop hepatic disease that is amenable to complete surgical resection. Several series in the literature report fewer than 10 patients undergoing liver resection for metastatic renal tumors, with survival exceeding 5 years in about 13% of patients (Alves et al, 2003). In one series, 14 patients with liver metastases of renal tumors underwent hepatic resection (Alves et al, 2003). Median survival was 26 months with a 3-year survival of 26%. Patients with a disease-free interval less than 24 months and patients with a diameter of the metastases exceeding 5 cm showed a worse prognosis. In patients with recurrence after hepatic resection, survival was better for patients who could undergo a repeat hepatectomy. In patients with hepatic metastases of renal tumors in whom a complete resection seems possible, surgical exploration may be justified.

Reproductive Tract Tumors

Effective chemotherapeutic regimens are available for most reproductive tumors. Surgical resection is only one component of a multimodal approach to the treatment of liver metastases from these tumors. The development of liver metastases is a well-defined adverse prognostic factor for patients with germ cell tumors (Gholam et al, 2003). Rivoire and associates (2001) attempted to define guidelines for the resection of liver metastases from germ cell tumors. They examined 37 patients who had undergone liver resection for metastatic germ cell tumors. All patients had received cisplatin-based chemotherapy before surgery. Median survival was 54 months with an overall 5-year survival rate of 62%. The authors defined three prognostic factors associated with a worse outcome: pure embryonal carcinoma in the primary tumor, liver metastasis greater than 3 cm, and presence of viable residual disease after chemotherapy. Because no patients with liver tumors of less than 1 cm had viable disease, the authors recommended a nonsurgical approach for these patients. Male patients with liver tumors greater than 3 cm in diameter represented a high-risk group that may not benefit from surgical resection. Hepatic resection was recommended for the other subgroups.

Hahn and coworkers (1999) presented data regarding 57 patients undergoing liver resection for metastatic testicular cancer after systemic chemotherapy. In 48 patients, concomitant cytoreductive procedures for extrahepatic disease were performed. The overall 2-year survival rate was 97.1%. Pathologic analysis of resected specimens showed either a benign lesion or only necrotic tumor in 58% of specimens. Three of five patients with active disease with persistently elevated serum markers died during follow-up, underlining the importance of response to chemotherapy as a predictor of outcome.

Patients with metastatic ovarian or fallopian tube carcinoma usually do not present with isolated liver metastases because recurrence is usually diffuse. Cytoreductive surgery that reduces disease to less than 1 cm when combined with chemotherapy is an accepted treatment approach. For these diseases, liver resection may be necessary because of true liver metastases or secondary liver involvement by peritoneal disease. A median overall survival of 62 months after hepatic resection has been described with this approach in 24 patients, with 18 patients having extrahepatic disease at the time of hepatectomy (Yoon et al, 2003). In this study, complete resection of all gross disease was possible in 21 patients, whereas in 3 patients tumor debulking to less than 1 cm was performed. Merideth and coworkers (2003) reported 26 patients undergoing liver resection for metachronous metastases

Table 73c.4 Results of Liver Resection for Metastatic Gastric Cancer*

Reference	No. Patients	Median Survival[†]	Adverse Prognostic Factors	Comments
Sakamoto et al, 2003	22	21.4 mo	>1 liver metastasis	Inclusion criteria: no extrahepatic disease
Shirabe et al, 2003	36	3-yr survival 26%	Lymphatic invasion[‡]; venous invasion[‡]; >3 liver metastases	4 actual 5-yr survivors; 61% of patients developed liver recurrence
Okano et al, 2002	19	3-yr survival 34%	Synchronous metastases; >1 liver metastasis; no fibrous pseudocapsule of metastasis	4 actual 5-yr survivors; 63% of patients developed liver recurrence
Ambiru et al, 2001	40	2-yr survival 27%	Synchronous metastases	6 actual 5-yr survivors; 72% of patients developed liver recurrence
Fujii et al, 2001	12	16.3 mo	Disease-free interval <12 mo; metastases >5 cm	—

*Only series including >10 patients are presented.
[†]Overall survival.
[‡]Primary tumor.

from ovarian carcinoma; cytoreduction was suboptimal (residual tumor >1 cm) in 5 patients. Overall median disease-related survival was 26.3 months, and a disease-free interval exceeding 12 months and optimal cytoreduction were associated with improved outcome. Other reports also justify hepatic resection in metastatic ovarian carcinoma (Bristow et al, 1999; Chi et al, 1997).

Liver resection for metastases from cervical and endometrial cancer have been reported in the literature with an overall survival of 7 to 50 months (Tangjitgamol et al, 2004). Selected patients may benefit from hepatectomy. Because of the small number of published cases, however, no general conclusions can be drawn from the available data.

Other Primary Tumors

Resection of liver metastases of lung cancer has been reported, and in selected patients long-term survival has been achieved. Di Carlo and associates (2003) summarized the available data from the literature. Liver resection was performed in 14 patients with liver metastases from lung cancer, and 2 patients lived longer than 5 years.

Patients presenting with liver metastases from an unknown primary tumor are a challenge to manage because median overall survival is approximately 5 months. Liver resection or ablative therapy might be appropriate for some patients in whom all disease can be destroyed or removed, but a median disease-free survival of only 6.5 months was reported in a recent study (Hawksworth et al, 2004).

CRITICAL EVALUATION OF LIVER RESECTION FOR METASTATIC NONCOLORECTAL NON-NEUROENDOCRINE TUMORS

Before discussing the rationale of liver resection for metastatic NCNN tumors, one should try to analyze the reason for the relative success of liver resection for metastatic colorectal cancer. As a result of the favorable long-term outcome after resection and the improved safety of liver resection, the treatment strategy of patients with liver metastases arising from primary colorectal cancers has changed in the last 2 decades. Liver metastases from colorectal cancer no longer are viewed as indicators of untreatable, widespread, systemic disease, and cure is still possible with surgery in some patients.

Two different concepts explain the relatively favorable outcome of patients undergoing hepatectomy for liver metastases from colorectal cancer. First, the tumor biology of metastatic colorectal cancer may be different from that of other solid tumors. Tumor cell dissemination of colorectal cancer via the bloodstream may be inefficient and could lead to death of most of the tumor cells shed into the bloodstream before the development of clinically significant metastases. Implantation of circulating colorectal tumor cells in the liver may be particularly effective owing to the expression of particular adhesion molecules (Mizuno et al, 1998; Sugarbaker, 1993; Weiss, 1990). The second reason may be the venous drainage of the large intestine via the portal vein to the liver. Tumor cells reaching the liver through the portal vein may be effectively entrapped by the liver, preventing systemic spread. If this concept is correct, tumor cells must overcome hepatic filtration to reach the systemic circulation and cause distant metastases (Sugarbaker, 1993).

Both notions are substantiated by clinical and experimental findings. It could be shown that the liver is an effective filter for colorectal cancer cells because these cells can be found more frequently in blood samples obtained from the portal vein compared with blood samples from the vena cava (Koch et al, 2001). Tumor biology also is important, however, because the most relevant prognostic factors after resection of colorectal liver metastases, such as length of disease-free interval and nodal status of primary tumor, are at least in part surrogates for tumor biology (Fong et al, 1999).

These concepts are crucial when trying to define the value of surgical resection of noncolorectal liver metastases. Except for gastrointestinal primaries, the liver is not the primary filter for venous blood from the organs being discussed in this chapter. Liver metastases from nongastrointestinal cancers indicate systemic tumor spread; this makes selection of patients with good tumor biology a crucial factor to offer hepatic resection to patients who may benefit the most. Tumor biology depends mainly on the primary tumor type, which is shown by the fact that relapse-free and cancer-specific survival for patients with reproductive tract primary tumors is significantly longer compared with that of patients with non–reproductive tract primary tumors in most studies. When selecting patients for liver resection, it also is important to select patients with more favorable tumor biology within a particular histology. Disease-free interval between the treatment of the primary tumor and the development of liver metastasis may be a valid surrogate marker in this respect, with a longer disease-free interval being associated with less aggressive tumor biology. Most studies support this concept because patients with a longer disease-free interval show a longer relapse-free and cancer-specific survival after hepatectomy. The biologic behavior of liver metastases also is most likely linked to the behavior of the primary tumor because in some studies positive lymph node status or venous invasion of the primary tumor predicts worse outcome after hepatectomy for liver metastases. Tumor biology also determines whether a patient would respond to systemic chemotherapy. Chemotherapy might be an important component when managing these patients, as shown for hepatic metastases of reproductive tract primary tumors.

Another important point that should be considered when contemplating hepatic resection for a patient with NCNN metastases is the likelihood of achieving a microscopically complete tumor resection. In most studies, long-term survival can be achieved only if the tumor can be removed completely, which depends on tumor-related factors and surgical expertise. When summarizing the published data, primary tumor type, length of disease-free interval, and pathologic features of the primary tumor may be valid criteria to assess the potential outcome after a planned hepatic resection for patients with metastatic NCNN tumors. By applying these criteria, long-term survival after potentially curative resection of liver metastases can be achieved. The use of systemic chemotherapy to assess the biologic behavior of the tumor also should be considered, although randomized trials validating this approach are lacking.

CONCLUSION

Hepatic resection for metastatic NCNN tumors is safe and is associated with a favorable outcome in highly selected patients. Primary tumor type and disease-free interval seem to be valid selection parameters. Because hepatic resection is often the only modality offering a potential cure, it should be considered in some patients with metastases from NCNN tumors.

REFERENCES

Allen P, Coit DG, 2002: The surgical management of metastatic melanoma. Ann Surg Oncol 9:762-770.

Alves A, et al, 2003: Hepatic resection for metastatic renal tumors: is it worthwhile? Ann Surg Oncol 10:705-710.

Ambiru S, et al, 2001: Benefits and limits of hepatic resection for gastric metastases. Am J Surg 181:279-283.

Antonescu CR, et al, 2005: Acquired resistance to imatinib in gastrointestinal stromal tumor occurs through secondary gene mutation. Clin Cancer Res 11:4182-4190.

Aoyama T, et al, 2000: Protracted survival after resection of metastatic uveal melanoma. Cancer 89:1561-1568.

Atalay G, et al, 2003: Clinical outcome of breast cancer patients with liver metastases alone in the anthracycline-taxane era: a retrospective analysis of two prospective, randomised metastatic breast cancer trials. Eur J Cancer 39:2439-2449.

Benevento A, et al, 2000: Results of liver resection as treatment for metastases from noncolorectal cancer. J Surg Oncol 74:24-29.

Bristow RE, et al, 1999: Survival impact of surgical cytoreduction in stage IV epithelial ovarian cancer. Gynecol Oncol 72:278-287.

Buell JF, et al, 2000: Hepatic resection: effective treatment for primary and secondary tumors. Surgery 128:686-693.

Carlini M, et al, 2002: Liver metastases from breast cancer: results of surgical resection. Hepatogastroenterology 49:1597-1601.

Chamberlain RS, et al, 2000: Hepatic neuroendocrine metastases: does intervention alter outcomes? J Am Coll Surg 190:432-445.

Chi DS, et al, 1997: Hepatic resection for metastatic gynecologic carcinomas. Gynecol Oncol 66:45-51.

Corless CL, et al, 2004: Biology of gastrointestinal stromal tumors. J Clin Oncol 22:3813-3825.

D'Angelica M, et al, 2002: Staging laparoscopy for potentially resectable noncolorectal, nonneuroendocrine liver metastases. Ann Surg Oncol 9:204-209.

DeMatteo RP, 2002: The GIST of targeted cancer therapy: a tumor (gastrointestinal stromal tumor), a mutated gene (c-kit), and a molecular inhibitor (STI571). Ann Surg Oncol 9:831-839.

DeMatteo RP, et al, 2001: Results of hepatic resection for sarcoma metastatic to the liver. Ann Surg 234:540-548.

Detry O, et al, 2003: Liver resection for noncolorectal, nonneuroendocrine metastases. Acta Chir Belg 103:458-462.

Di Carlo I, et al, 2003: Liver metastases from lung cancer: is surgical resection justified? Ann Thorac Surg 76:291-293.

Elias D, et al, 1998: Resection of liver metastases from a noncolorectal primary: indications and results based on 147 monocentric patients. J Am Coll Surg 187:493.

Elias D, et al, 2003: An attempt to clarify indications for hepatectomy for liver metastases from breast cancer. Am J Surg 185:158-164.

Feldman ED, et al, 2004: Regional treatment options for patients with ocular melanoma metastatic to the liver. Ann Surg Oncol 11:290-297.

Fong Y, et al, 1997: Liver resection for colorectal metastases. J Clin Oncol 15:938-946.

Fong Y, et al, 1999: Clinical score for predicting recurrence after hepatic resection for metastatic colorectal cancer: analysis of 1001 consecutive cases. Ann Surg 230:309-318.

Fujii K, et al, 2001: Resection of liver metastasis from gastric adenocarcinoma. Hepatogastroenterology 45:368-371.

Gholam D, et al, 2003: Advanced seminoma—treatment results and prognostic factors for survival after first-line, cisplatin-based chemotherapy and for patients with recurrent disease: a single-institution experience in 145 patients. Cancer 98:745-752.

Goering JD, et al, 2002: Cryoablation and liver resection for noncolorectal liver metastases. Am J Surg 183:384-389.

Hahn TL, et al, 1999: Hepatic resection of metastatic testicular carcinoma: a further update. Ann Surg Oncol 6:640-644.

Hamy AP, et al, 2000: Hepatic resections for non-colorectal metastases: forty resections in 35 patients. Hepatogastroenterology 47:1090-1094.

Hawksworth J, et al, 2004: Surgical and ablative treatment for metastatic adenocarcinoma to the liver from unknown primary tumor. Am Surg 70:512-517.

Hemming AW, et al, 2000: Hepatic resection of noncolorectal nonneuroendocrine metastases. Liver Transpl 6:97-101.

Hsueh EC, et al, 2004: Prolonged survival after complete resection of metastases from intraocular melanoma. Cancer 100:122-129.

Karavias DD, et al, 2002: Liver resection for metastatic non-colorectal non-neuroendocrine hepatic neoplasms. Eur J Surg Oncol 28:135-139.

Koch M, et al, 2001: Comparative analysis of tumor cell dissemination in mesenteric, central and peripheral venous blood in patients with colorectal cancer. Arch Surg 136:85-89.

Laurent C, et al, 2001: Resection of noncolorectal and nonneuroendocrine liver metastases: late metastases are the only chance of cure. World J Surg 25:1532-1536.

Lehnert T, 1998: Liver transplantation for metastatic neuroendocrine carcinoma: an analysis of 103 patients. Transplantation 66:1307-1312.

Martin R, et al, 2002: Solid-pseudopapillary tumor of the pancreas: a surgical enigma? Ann Surg Oncol 9:35-40.

Merideth MA, et al, 2003: Hepatic resection for metachronous metastases from ovarian carcinoma. Gynecol Oncol 89:16-21.

Mizuno N, et al, 1998: Importance of hepatic first-pass removal in metastasis of colon carcinoma cells. J Hepatol 28:865-877.

Mondragon-Sanches R, et al, 1999: Repeat hepatic resection for recurrent metastatic melanoma. Hepatogastroenterology 46:459-461.

Ochiai T, et al, 1994: Hepatic resection for metastatic tumours from gastric cancer: analysis of prognostic factors. Br J Surg 81:1175-1178.

Okano K, et al, 2002: Hepatic resection for metastatic tumors from gastric cancer. Ann Surg 235:86-91.

Pocard M, et al, 2000: Hepatic resection in metastatic breast cancer: results and prognostic factors. Eur J Surg Oncol 26:155-159.

Raab R, et al, 1998: Liver metastases of breast cancer: results of liver resection. Anticancer Res 18:2231-2233.

Rivoire M, et al, 2001: Multimodality treatment of patients with liver metastases from germ cell tumors. Cancer 92:578-587.

Rose DM, et al, 2001: Surgical resection for metastatic melanoma to the liver: the John Wayne Cancer Institute and Sydney Melanoma Unit Experience. Arch Surg 136:950-955.

Sakamoto Y, et al, 2003: Surgical resection of liver metastases of gastric cancer: an analysis of a 17-year experience with 22 patients. Surgery 133:507-511.

Scheele J, et al, 1995: Resection of colorectal liver metastases. World J Surg 19:59-71.

Schlag P, et al, 1990: Resection of liver metastases in colorectal cancer: competitive analysis of treatment results in synchronous versus metachronous metastases. Eur J Surg Oncol 16:360-365.

Schwartz SI, 1995: Hepatic resection for noncolorectal nonneuroendocrine metastases. World J Surg 19:72-75.

Seifert JK, et al, 1999: Liver resection for breast cancer metastases. Hepatogastroenterology 46:2935-2940.

Selzner M, et al, 2000: Liver metastases from breast cancer: long-term survival after curative resection. Surgery 127:383-389.

Shirabe K, et al, 2003: Analysis of the prognostic factors of liver metastasis of gastric cancer after hepatic resection: a multi-institutional study of the indications for resection. Hepatogastroenterology 50:1560-1563.

Singletary E, et al, 2003: A role of curative surgery in the treatment of selected patients with metastatic breast cancer. Oncologist 8:241-251.

Sugarbaker PH, 1993: Metastatic inefficiency: the scientific basis for resection of liver metastases from colorectal cancer. J Surg Oncol 3(suppl):158-160.

Takada Y, et al, 2001: Hepatic resection for metastatic tumors from noncolorectal carcinoma. Hepatogastroenterology 48:83-86.

Tangjitgamol S, et al, 2004: Role of surgical resection for lung, liver, and central nervous system metastases in patients with gynecological cancer: a literature review. Int J Gynecol Cancer 14:399-422.

van Ruth S, et al, 2001: Metastasectomy for liver metastases of non-colorectal primaries. Eur J Surg Oncol 27:662-667.

Vlastos G, et al, 2004: Long-term survival after an aggressive surgical approach in patients with breast cancer hepatic metastases. Ann Surg Oncol 11:869-874.

Weiss L, 1990: Metastatic inefficiency. Adv Cancer Res 54:159-211.

Weitz J, et al, 2004: Partial hepatectomy for metastases from non-colorectal, non-neuroendocrine carcinoma. Ann Surg 241:269-276.

Wyld L, et al, 2003: Prognostic factors for patients with hepatic metastases from breast cancer. Br J Cancer 89:284-290.

Yamada H, et al, 2001: Hepatectomy for metastases from non-colorectal and non-neuroendocrine tumor. Anticancer Res 21:4159-4162.

Yoon SS, et al, 2003: Resection of recurrent ovarian or fallopian tube carcinoma involving the liver. Gynecol Oncol 91:383-388.

Yoshimoto M, et al, 2000: Surgical treatment of hepatic metastases from breast cancer. Br Cancer Res Treat 59:177-184.

Embolization of Liver Tumors

74

C. J. YOON AND J. W. CHUNG

Primary and secondary cancers of the liver present a challenging problem in clinical oncology. They cause tremendous morbidity and mortality. Hepatocellular carcinoma (HCC) (see Ch. 71) is the fifth most common cancer and the third most common cause of cancer-related death in the world (Montalto et al, 2002; Parkin et al, 2001). In addition to its greatest incidence in Asia and sub-Saharan Africa, where hepatitis B is endemic, the incidence of HCC has been increasing steadily in the United States and Western Europe, owing to the high prevalence of chronic hepatitis C (El-Serag et al, 2003; Tanaka et al, 2002). Surgery has been considered only potentially curative (Bismuth & Majno, 2000; Mor et al, 1998). Less than a third of patients are candidates for hepatic resection because of extreme tumor extension, multiplicity of tumor foci, and associated advanced liver cirrhosis at the time of diagnosis (Llovet et al, 2003). In addition, surgery has been plagued by high recurrence rates. The cumulative recurrence rate reaches 70% at 5 years after surgery, including true recurrence and de novo tumors (Bismuth & Majno, 2000). Currently, orthotopic or living donor liver transplantation is considered the treatment of choice in selected patients with HCC. A critical impediment of this treatment is limited availability of donors (Jonas et al, 2001; Yao FY et al, 2001).

Liver metastasis from colorectal cancer (see Ch. 73a) is the most common hepatic malignancy. Only 25% of patients are candidates for surgery, and about 60% of patients who undergo curative surgery for colorectal cancer ultimately develop regional or distant recurrence (Chiappa et al, 1999; Liu et al, 2003). Despite frequent extrahepatic spread, about half of deaths of patients with colorectal cancers are attributable to liver metastases (Fong et al, 1999; Geoghegan & Scheele, 1999).

To date, systemic chemotherapy has shown limited therapeutic effects for primary and secondary hepatic malignancies. Tumor response rates to various chemotherapeutic regimens are less than 30%. Most investigative efforts have converged on developing and testing methods of local control of these tumors. The transcatheter hepatic arterial approach has been outstanding among these methods over past 2 decades.

Transcatheter arterial chemoembolization (TACE) for liver tumors was first reported by Doyon and colleagues (1974), and chemoembolization using absorbable gelatin sponge (Gelfoam) and anticancer drugs was reported by Yamada and associates (1983). In the early 1980s, iodized oil (Lipiodol; Andre Guerbet, Aulnay-sous-Bois, France), a lymphangiographic dye, was found to remain selectively in the neovasculature and extravascular spaces of liver tumors when it was injected into the hepatic artery (Konno et al, 1983; Nakamura et al, 1983). Thereafter, TACE with iodized oil mixed with different anticancer agents or, more often, with the emulsion of iodized oil and anticancer drugs followed by Gelfoam embolization has been increasingly used as an effective means of palliation for unresectable or postoperatively recurrent tumors and as an alternative to surgery even for resectable tumors.

BASIC PRINCIPLES IN EMBOLIZATION OF LIVER TUMORS

Blood Supply of Liver Tumors

The normal liver receives a dual blood supply from the hepatic artery and the portal vein. Approximately one third of the normal hepatic blood flow comes from the hepatic artery, and the other two thirds comes from the portal vein. About half of the oxygen requirement of the liver is supplied by the portal vein. Primary and secondary liver tumors derive 90% of their blood supply from the hepatic artery with a smaller (10%) contribution from the portal vein (Ackerman, 1974; Kan et al, 1983). Hepatocarcinogenesis is a multistep process involving parenchymal arterialization, sinusoidal capillarization, and development of unpaired arteries (neoangiogenesis), causing gradual change in blood supply from portal to arterial (Park et al, 1998). These hemodynamic changes have been evidenced on imaging modalities, including Doppler ultrasound (Suzuki et al, 2003), computed tomography (CT) (Tajima et al, 2002b), and magnetic resonance imaging (MRI) (Levy, 2002). It is logical to use intra-arterial treatment for targeting HCC while normal liver is spared. In an experimental study, 10 times higher intratumoral concentration of chemotherapeutic agent was observed when it was given through the hepatic artery rather than through the portal vein (Sigurdson et al, 1987).

In reality, the blood supply of liver tumors varies according to their developmental stage and growth pattern. Although encapsulated nodular HCC is totally supplied by the hepatic artery, well-differentiated or early HCC, small nodular tumors such as daughter nodules and intrahepatic metastases, and extracapsular infiltrating edge of advanced HCC are supplied by the portal vein and the hepatic artery (Goseki et al, 1995; Wakasa et al, 1990). Similar observations have been made in metastatic liver tumors. Micrometastases less than 200 μm seem to be supplied mainly by sinusoidal blood. With continuing growth, tumor vessels develop, and the arterial supply dominates in the advanced tumors (Ackerman, 1974; Strohmeyer et al, 1987). Even in the advanced stage, most liver metastases have a distinct portal blood supply to the tumor periphery (Strohmeyer et al, 1987; Taniguchi et al, 1993). These liver tumors with portal blood supply can be resistant to intra-arterial embolotherapy. To treat the tumor fraction partly supplied by the portal vein, Nakao and colleagues (1986) simultaneously embolized the hepatic artery and portal vein and showed a better rate of necrosis.

Not only hepatic arteries, but also extrahepatic collateral arteries can supply liver tumors (Charnsangavej et al, 1982; Tanabe et al, 1998). It was shown that extrahepatic collaterals commonly supply large HCC without proximal hepatic artery occlusion at their initial presentation (Chung et al, 1998; Kim et al, 2005). The anatomic location of the tumor adjacent to the bare area and suspensory ligaments of the liver or direct invasion or adhesion to the adjacent organ seems to be the primary cause of the development of extrahepatic collaterals (Fig. 74.1). Attenuation or occlusion of the hepatic artery may exaggerate the degree of collateral circulation.

Hepatic Artery Embolization

In the past, hepatic artery ligation was tried to induce ischemic necrosis of the tumor (Mori et al, 1966). Its effect of tumor regression and symptomatic improvement was temporary because proximal occlusion of the hepatic artery induces rapid development of collateral circulation to the peripheral hepatic arteries (Fig. 74.2). Peripheral hepatic artery occlusion by transcatheter arterial embolization (TAE) should be done to minimize the development of collateral circulation and induce selective ischemic necrosis of HCC. For this purpose, it is important to select the proper size of particulate embolic materials. The optimal size of particulate embolic materials should be bigger than the size of arteriovenous shunt in liver tumors and peribiliary plexus to avoid the risk of pulmonary embolization and bile duct necrosis. It has not been determined, however, what kind and size of embolic material are ideal for effective treatment of liver tumors while sparing normal parenchyma. In general, smaller embolic materials penetrate more peripheral arteries than larger ones and can induce more effective embolization of tumor vasculature, while the risk of normal parenchyma injury increases simultaneously (Cay et al, 1996; Doppman et al, 1978; Nishioka et al, 1994).

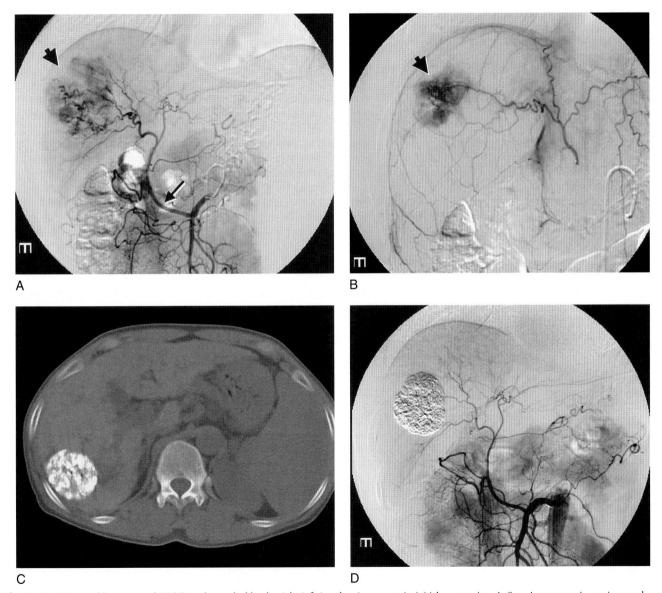

Fig. 74.1. A 56-year-old woman with HCC partly supplied by the right inferior phrenic artery at its initial presentation. **A,** Superior mesenteric arteriogram shows the origin of the common hepatic artery from the superior mesenteric artery *(long arrow)* and a hypervascular mass with a lobulating contour. Defective margin at the superior lateral aspect of the mass *(short arrow)* suggests the possibility of an extrahepatic collateral arterial supply. **B,** Right inferior phrenic arteriogram reveals tumor stain at that site *(arrow)*. **C,** TACE was performed with a mixture of 10 mL of iodized oil and 50 mg of doxorubicin hydrochloride followed by Gelfoam (soaked with mitomycin C) embolization. Two weeks later, iodized oil CT shows even uptake of iodized oil throughout the tumor. **D,** Four months later, follow-up angiogram shows disappearance of tumor vascularity and shrunken tumor mass with compact iodized oil uptake.

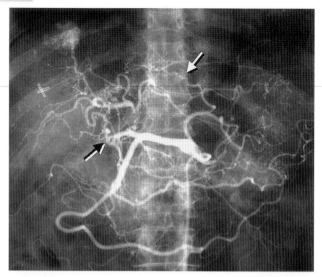

Fig. 74.2. Development of collateral circulation after hepatic artery ligation in a 67-year-old woman with HCC. Hepatic arteriogram shows occluded proper hepatic artery owing to surgical ligation and development of multiple collateral channels along the hepatoduodenal ligament (*black arrow*) and lesser omentum (*white arrow*).

To date, many embolic materials have been used for TAE, such as gelatin sponge particle microspheres (Nishioka et al, 1994), autologous blood clot (Gunji et al, 2002), polyvinyl alcohol particle (Ramsey et al, 2002), cyanoacrylate (Winkelbauer et al, 1995), and absolute ethanol (Matsui et al, 1993). In current clinical practice, absorbable gelatin sponge particles are the most frequently used embolic material in TAE. Gelatin sponge particles of 500 to 1000 µm do not cause serious hepatic damage in experimental animals and humans with good hepatic functional reserve (Cho et al, 1976; Kan et al, 1993; Sonomura et al, 1997). With the introduction of subsegmental embolization at tumor feeding arteries using microcatheters, TAE using smaller sized microspheres is under clinical investigation. Several experimental and clinical trials using various sizes of microspheres showed that particles smaller than 40 µm preferentially (6-12 times) accumulates in tumor vasculature, but may pass through sinusoids and tumor-related arteriovenous shunt into the systemic circulation and can cause serious embolic complications (Bastian et al, 1998; Brown, 2004).

For safe and effective TAE, it is important to recognize tumor-related arteriovenous shunt before the procedure. In patients with HCC, angiographic incidence has been reported in 31.2%: shunting into the portal vein in 28.8% and hepatic vein in 2.4% (Ngan & Peh, 1997). The more liver parenchyma that is occupied by the tumor, the more arteriovenous shunts exist (Fig. 74.3). The arteriovenous shunt is associated with poor prognosis (Granov et al, 1992) and is frequently problematic in TAE of liver tumors (Sugano et al, 1994; Walser et al, 1996). Severe arterioportal shunt can cause hepatofugal portal flow, ascites, and variceal bleeding. In patients with prominent arteriovenous shunt, it is recommended first to embolize the shunt with gelatin sponge particles, coils, and ethanol before TAE (Furuse et al, 1997; Huang et al, 2004). After embolization for massive arterioportal shunt, hepatofugal portal flow may convert to hepatopetal, and performance status and ascites may be improved (Furuse et al, 1997; Morse et al, 1985).

Transcatheter Arterial Chemoembolization

TACE is a targeted therapy that combines intra-arterial chemotherapy and arterial embolization. This combination may induce highly concentrated chemotherapy and ischemic damage on the tumor, which is likely to be synergistic in producing tumor necrosis (Ramsey et al, 2002; Yu & Keeffe, 2003). Hepatic arterial embolization induces not only ischemic necrosis of tumor, but also failure of transmembrane pumps in tumor cells, resulting in greater absorption of chemotherapeutic agents by the tumor cells (Kruskal et al, 1993). In addition, because of reduced arterial flow after embolization, the chemotherapeutic agents can remain within tumor tissue for prolonged periods. It has been reported that the tissue concentration of chemotherapeutic agents within tumor is more than 40 times higher than surrounding normal liver several months after TACE (Konno, 1990; Sasaki et al, 1987; Sawada, 1989).

An iodized oil has been used successfully not only as an embolic material, but also as a carrier of chemotherapeutic agents (Raoul et al, 1992). When injected into the hepatic artery, an iodized oil persists selectively in the tumor for a few weeks or months because of the hemodynamic difference between hypervascular hepatic tumors and the liver parenchyma and presumably the absence of Kupffer cells in the tumor (Bhattacharya et al, 1994; Kan et al, 1994). Nakajo and coworkers (1998) reported that iodine 131 iodized oil accumulated in vascular tumors 7.5 to 21 times more than in adjacent normal parenchyma. If a stable mixture of an iodized oil and chemotherapeutic agents is infused into the hepatic artery, the chemotherapeutic agent can be delivered locally to HCC together with the iodized oil as a carrier. The chemotherapeutic agent was released slowly from the mixture in patients who underwent hepatectomy (Nakamura et al, 1989). In contrast, in the normal liver parenchyma, the iodized oil injected into the hepatic artery usually does not occlude the hepatic artery and accumulates in the peripheral portal vein through multiple arterioportal communications and subsequently passes through the sinusoids into the systemic circulation (Chung et al, 1993).

In preparing a mixture of an iodized oil and chemotherapeutic agents, the chemotherapeutic drugs usually are dissolved in a water-soluble contrast agent and emulsified in iodized oil with a pumping method (Fig. 74.4). An anticancer drug–iodized oil solution or suspension can be made depending on the physical characteristics of anticancer drugs. Many centers use a single chemotherapeutic agent, such as doxorubicin, whereas others use combinations of different drugs, such as cisplatin, mitomycin, or 5-fluorouracil. Japanese investigators have used styrene maleic acid neocarzinostatin (SMANCS). It is highly lipophilic and is expected to be a more stable agent when mixed with iodized oil (Abe et al, 2000; Okusaka et al, 2002). No data show clear superiority for any cytotoxic agent. Cisplatin may confer a slightly better survival, when used as a cisplatin–iodized oil suspension, based on nonrandomized data (Kamada et al, 2001; Ueno et al, 2000). If a sufficient amount of a mixture of an iodized oil and anticancer drug is injected to fill in the peripheral portal vein around the tumor and followed by hepatic artery embolization, TACE has the effect of combined arterial and portal blockage, which may work to treat the tumor fraction partly supplied by the portal vein (Figs. 74.5 and 74.6).

Regarding antitumor effect, TACE with anticancer drug–iodized oil mixture followed by embolization showed greater tumor necrosis and better survival of patients than TACE with

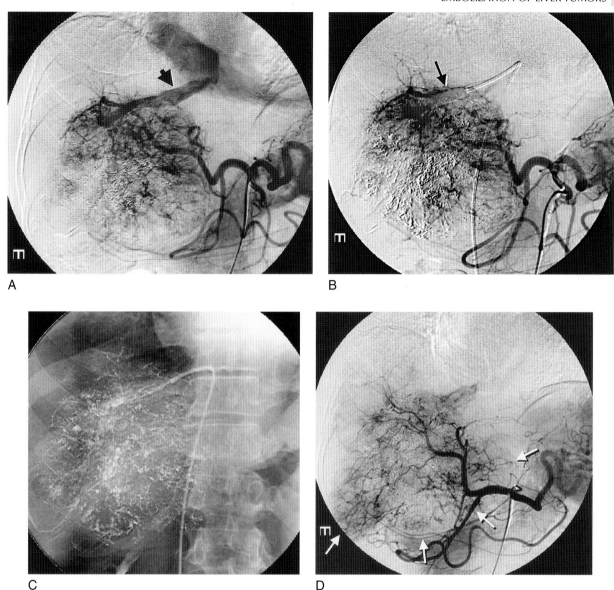

Fig. 74.3. Severe arteriovenous shunt into the middle hepatic vein managed by TACE after balloon occlusion of the middle hepatic vein in a 66-year-old man with HCC. **A,** Celiac arteriogram shows huge hypervascular mass with severe arteriovenous shunt into the middle hepatic vein *(arrow)*. **B,** After balloon occlusion of the middle hepatic vein *(arrow)*, celiac arteriography was repeated and confirmed the disappearance of the shunt. With the balloon inflated, TACE was performed with a mixture of 10 mL of iodized oil and 50 mg of doxorubicin hydrochloride followed by Gelfoam embolization. **C,** Completion radiograph with the balloon deflated shows successful accumulation of iodized oil in the mass without untoward pulmonary embolization. **D,** Three months later, follow-up angiogram shows remarkably decreased arteriovenous shunt and the tumor fraction supplied by the hepatic arteries. There is an overgrowth of the tumor fraction supplied by omental arteries *(arrows).*

anticancer drug–iodized oil mixture alone (Ikeda et al, 2004; Maeda et al, 2002; Suzuki et al, 1997; Takayasu et al, 1987). In a prospective study by Nakamura and colleagues (1994), the long-term survival rate improved in patients treated with doxorubicin–iodized oil emulsion and gelatin sponge embolization compared with patients treated with doxorubicin and gelatin sponge embolization. Concerning the effect of chemotherapeutic agents in TACE, a few clinical studies showed that anticancer drugs have additional therapeutic effect in TACE when they are used in emulsion with iodized oil (Chang et al, 1994). Kawai and associates (1992) compared the therapeutic effects of TACE in the presence versus the absence of doxorubicin

for treatment of HCC. Although there was no survival benefit, tumor marker decreased to a significantly greater extent in the group that received the doxorubicin–iodized oil mixture. These results suggest that therapeutic effect of TACE is caused by the synergy of an iodized oil, anticancer drugs, and arterial embolization.

In patients with compromised liver function, preserving liver function is sometimes more important than inducing complete necrosis of tumors. Greater antitumor effect of a chemoembolic regimen is associated with greater normal parenchyma damage. When the more potent regimen is used, it should be delivered more selectively to the tumor-feeding arteries.

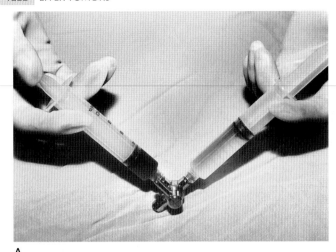

A

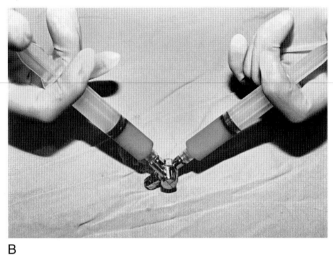

B

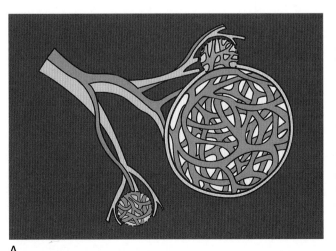

C

Fig. 74.4. Preparation of a mixture of iodized oil and doxorubicin hydrochloride. **A** and **B,** Every 10 mg of doxorubicin hydrochloride was dissolved in 0.5 mL of the water-soluble contrast medium; iodized oil and dissolved doxorubicin hydrochloride were drawn separately into syringes interconnected with a three-way stopcock (**A**) and emulsified by means of vigorous pushing of each syringe in alternation (**B**). **C,** Light photomicrograph shows the formation of oil in water in oil–type emulsion with variable sized (10-50 µm) water droplets containing doxorubicin hydrochloride in the oil base.

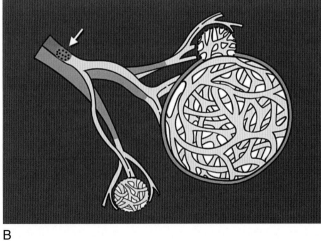

A

B

Fig. 74.5. Diagram for the concept of subsegmental or segmental TACE using iodized oil. **A,** The diagram illustrates the exclusive arterial supply for encapsulated nodular HCC and mixed arterial and portal venous supply for the portion of extracapsular invasion and small HCC without capsule formation. **B,** If a sufficient amount of a mixture of iodized oil and anticancer drug is injected through a tumor feeding artery, not only the tumor neovasculature, but also the peripheral portal veins around the tumor are filled with the emulsion. Subsequent hepatic artery embolization *(arrow)* may result in the effect of combined arterial and portal blockage, and tumor fraction with mixed arterial and portal venous supply can be treated effectively by the combined effect of high-dose chemotherapy and ischemia.

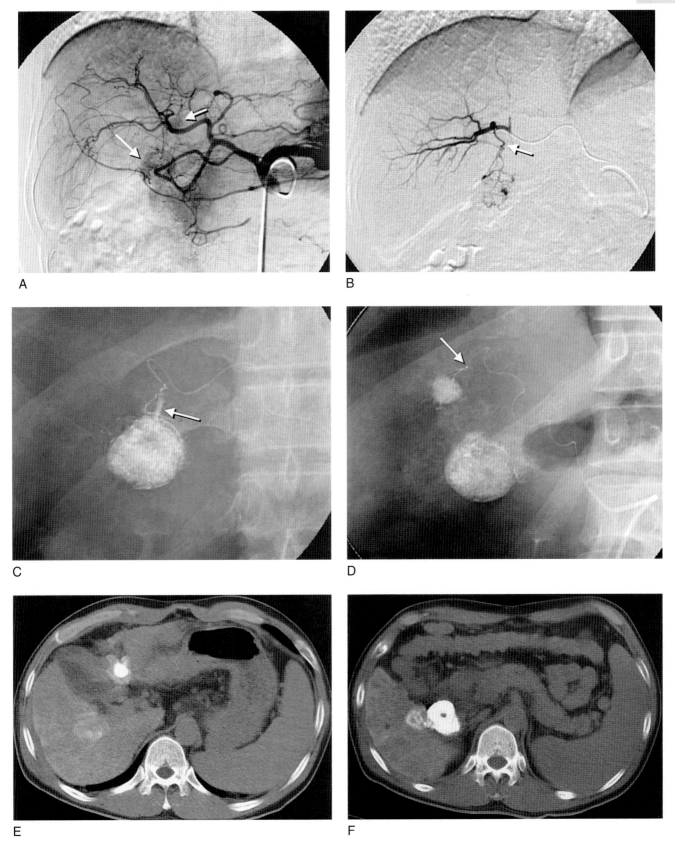

Fig. 74.6. Subsegmental TACE in a 43-year-old man with multinodular HCC. **A,** Celiac arteriogram shows two hypervascular tumor nodules *(arrows)* in the liver. **B,** The larger mass is supplied by a feeding artery *(arrow)* from the right posterior segmental branch. **C,** Subsegmental chemoembolization was performed by selective catheterization of the tumor-feeding artery and injection of an emulsion of 5 mL of iodized oil and 30 mg of doxorubicin hydrochloride. Gelfoam embolization was not performed because sufficient stagnation of blood flow was achieved after injecting the emulsion. Note the filling with iodized oil of the peripheral portal branch *(arrow)* accompanying the tumor-feeding artery. **D,** Subsegmental chemoembolization also was performed for the tumor located in hepatic segment IV by selective catheterization of the tumor-feeding artery *(arrow)*. **E** and **F,** Iodized oil CT reveals compact retention of iodized oil in the nodules.

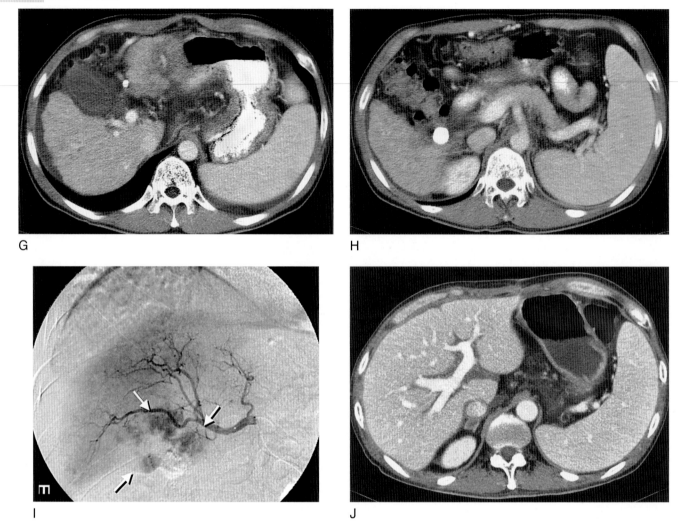

Fig. 74.6, cont'd. G and **H,** Follow-up CT scan 2 years later shows shrunken tumors without evidence of viable portion. **I,** Five years later, celiac arteriogram shows local recurrence around the original tumor *(arrows).* **J,** With the progression of liver cirrhosis and local tumor recurrence, the patient finally underwent liver transplantation.

PATIENT SELECTION

Patients should have liver tumors that are known to respond to chemoembolization and show hypervascularity on hepatic arteriography. Tumors that frequently have these features include HCC; cholangiocarcinoma; and metastases from colorectal or gastric cancer, ocular melanoma, islet cell tumors, carcinoid, and sarcoma. In general, hepatic arterial embolization is indicated in patients with the tumor confined to the liver. Embolization may be indicated with an extrahepatic tumor, however, when intrahepatic tumor is the main source of morbidity and mortality. Benign liver tumors, such as giant hemangioma, hepatic adenoma, and symptomatic epithelioid hemangioendothelioma, also can be treated with TAE or TACE (Fok et al, 1996; Giavroglou et al, 2003).

Another important consideration in patient selection is liver function, especially in patients with HCC. In contrast to other malignancies, the prognosis of HCC patients is related not only to the extent of tumor growth, but also to liver function because most patients with HCC have underlying liver disease. Methods to assess the functional status of the liver and prognosis of HCC

include the Child-Pugh classification, Okuda staging, and the Cancer of the Liver Italian Program (CLIP) score. These staging systems do not indicate, however, which patients would benefit from TACE (CLIP Investigators, 2000; Farinati et al, 2000; Ueno et al, 2001). The Barcelona Clinic Liver Cancer staging system was developed to allow for the indication of the best therapy for each stage of HCC (Llovet et al, 1999). In this staging system, TACE was recommended for intermediate stage (Okuda staging 1-2, performance score 0, and large or multinodular HCC) and some advanced stage (Okuda 1-2, performance score 1, no extrahepatic HCC) HCC. These general guidelines are not always applicable in clinical situations, however.

Spontaneous rupture of HCC has been an emergent indication for TACE regardless of underlying liver function. Even in patients with advanced liver cirrhosis, nodular HCC showing exophytic growth can be managed safely by superselective TACE to prevent tumor rupture without deteriorating liver function. TACE also is indicated for symptom relief in patients with liver tumors that are resistant to conservative management. These symptoms include intractable abdominal pain (Young et al, 1993) and hypercalcemia (Suzuki et al, 1998).

The patency of the portal venous system should be evaluated carefully because portal vein invasion is a well-known major prognostic factor in any kind of treatment for liver tumors. Portal vein occlusion increases the risk of hepatic insufficiency and hepatic infarction after TACE (Chung et al, 1996). TACE can be performed safely and effectively in patients with a limited parenchymal tumor and adequate liver function, however (Chung et al, 1995). Even in patients with HCC invading and occluding the main portal vein, occlusion can be treated safely if hepatopetal collateral flow is present (Fig. 74.7) (Fan et al, 2001; Lee et al, 1997; Tazawa et al, 2001). TACE should be performed carefully with a reduced amount of chemoembolic agents and selective administration of them into tumor-feeding arteries.

Although there are no absolute contraindications to TACE, the combination of two or three major bad prognostic indicators (massive or diffuse tumor involvement, presence of hepatic insufficiency or failure, and portal vein invasion) is considered as a contraindication to TACE because of its ineffectiveness and the risk of complications, including hepatic insufficiency. In addition, patients with contraindications to chemotherapy (severe thrombocytopenia or leukopenia, cardiac or renal insufficiency) and anaphylactoid reactions to the contrast media should not be treated.

PROCEDURE

Underlying hepatic functional reserve should be evaluated first with laboratory tests and assessment for the presence or absence of ascites and hepatic encephalopathy. The baseline serum level of tumor markers (e.g., α-fetoprotein and PIVKA-II [*P*roteins *i*nduced by *V*itamin *K* *A*ntagonism or *A*bsence] in HCC) should be measured before treatment to monitor changes after treatment. By means of cross-sectional imaging studies, the size and extent of the tumor, the tumor growth pattern (expansile versus replacing or infiltrating), and macroscopic angioinvasion into the hepatic and portal veins are evaluated. For successful segmental embolization, accurate segmental localization of the tumor is crucial, and cross-sectional images are useful for that purpose. In addition, imaging studies of the chest, abdomen, and pelvis are recommended to assess comorbid disease and ensure the presence or absence of metastatic disease.

Before undergoing TACE, patients fast overnight and are hydrated at a rate of 200 mL/hr. After infiltration of local anesthetic, the Seldinger technique is used to gain access to the common femoral artery. Initial diagnostic visceral arteriography is performed to determine arterial anatomy to the liver and patency of the portal vein. For complete angiography, all hepatic arteries should be adequately opacified, and all feeding arteries of the tumor should be identified. Anatomic variations of celiac trunk and hepatic arteries commonly are encountered (see Fig. 74.2). With the introduction of multidetector row helical CT, these anatomic variations can be predicted before the procedure by careful review of the arterial phase scan. Among hepatic artery variations, the right hepatic artery commonly arises from the superior mesenteric artery, and the left hepatic artery commonly arises from the left gastric artery. Celiac and superior mesenteric arteriography should be routinely performed. Frequently, additional views in different angles and magnifications and superselective injection with use of microcatheters are necessary to identify small feeding arteries. To avoid nontargeted embolization, it is important to recognize the origin of the cystic artery and the right gastric artery and the existence of the long falciform artery and the accessory left gastric artery originating from the left hepatic artery.

The treatment protocol should be individualized according to the hepatic functional reserve, tumor extent, and major portal vein invasion. Every effort should be made to preserve nontumorous liver parenchyma from chemoembolization. The best way to maximize the treatment effect and to minimize procedure-related complications is to perform superselective chemoembolization of all tumor feeders. Patients with focal lesions should undergo selective (segmental or subsegmental) embolization, in which a catheter or microcatheter is placed more selectively into the feeding artery in closer proximity to the tumor (see Fig. 74.6). Many investigators use a helical CT scan combined with an angiography system for identifying the tumor-feeding subsegmental artery and for immediate postprocedural assessment (Iwamoto et al, 2003).

After the catheter is positioned in the appropriate artery, the mixture of iodized oil and chemotherapeutic agent is injected. The dose of iodized oil and chemotherapeutic agent depends on the size and vascularity of the tumor. The generally accepted upper limit of iodized oil is 15 mL. For a small tumor, enough iodized oil to saturate the entire tumor neovasculature could be administered. The end point for the mixture administration is stasis in tumor-feeding arteries or appearance of iodized oil in portal vein branches. If there is persistent flow in the tumor-feeding arteries after infusion of chemotherapeutic mixture, hepatic artery embolization is performed. Gelatin sponge particles are the embolic agents most frequently used because they degrade in a few weeks, allowing repeat treatment (Fig. 74.8). Polyvinyl alcohol particle is another commonly used embolic agent; it causes a more permanent arterial occlusion (Ramsey et al, 2002). In the presence of prominent arterioportal arteriovenous shunting, it is recommended first to embolize the shunt. After adequate blockage of the shunt, chemoembolization can be performed in the usual fashion (see Fig. 74.3).

Development of extrahepatic collaterals supplying liver tumors prohibits effective control of the tumor by hepatic artery chemoembolization. Extrahepatic collaterals include inferior phrenic artery, omental artery, internal mammary artery, colic branch of superior mesenteric artery, adrenal artery, intercostal artery, renal capsular artery, and gastric arteries (Chung et al, 1998; Kim HC et al, 2005; Kim JH et al, 1995; Miyayama et al, 2001; Nakai et al, 2001; Park et al, 2003; Won et al, 2003). When the hepatic artery and extrahepatic collaterals supply the tumor, additional chemoembolization of the extrahepatic collaterals can be tried to increase the therapeutic efficacy of TACE (Fig. 74.9; see Figs. 74.1 and 74.8). These extrahepatic collaterals can be used to continue chemoembolization for patients with hepatic artery occlusion.

Intra-arterial lidocaine and intravenous narcotic analgesics are given before the procedure to relieve pain during and after TACE (Lee et al, 2001). After the procedure, antiemetics and oral narcotics are continued for 3 to 7 days, if needed. Routine administration of prophylactic antibiotics is not recommended (Geschwind et al, 2002; Ong et al, 2004; Song et al, 2001).

Laboratory studies of liver function and serum level of tumor markers should be repeated in 2 to 4 weeks. Iodized oil CT can be checked 1 to 2 weeks after TACE to assess the pattern of iodized oil uptake by the tumor. Multiphase helical CT may be repeated 4 to 8 weeks after TACE to determine local or remote site tumor recurrence. If there is any evidence of viable tumor on imaging studies or serum level of tumor markers or both, patients return for a second session of TACE in 4 to 16 weeks.

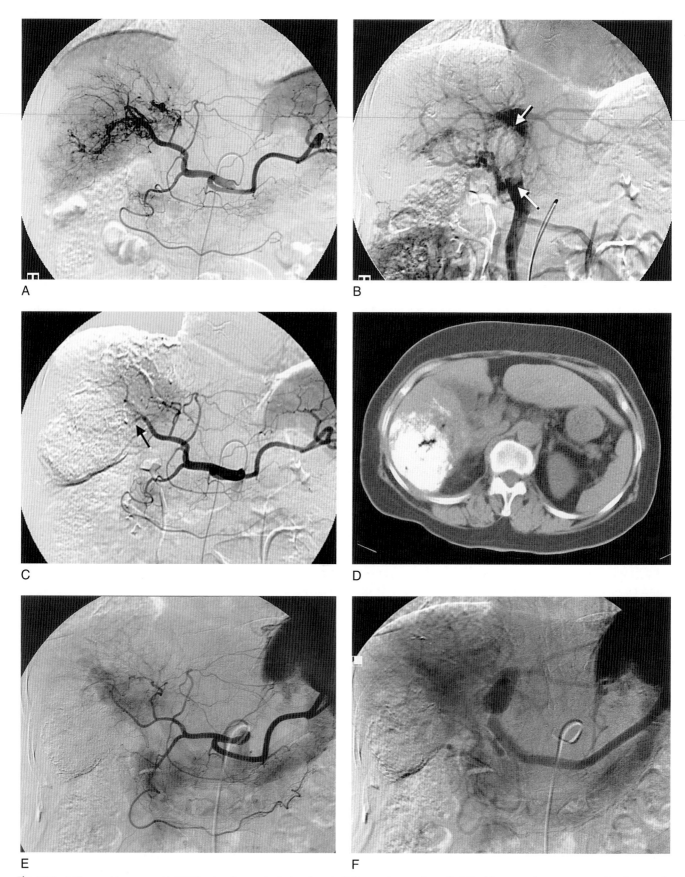

Fig. 74.7. A 69-year-old woman with HCC and main portal vein invasion. **A,** Celiac arteriogram shows ill-defined hypervascular tumor occupying the posterior segment of the right hepatic lobe. **B,** Portogram shows near-total occlusion of the main portal vein by a protruding tumor thrombus from the right portal vein *(arrows)*. **C,** TACE was performed with a mixture of 10 mL of iodized oil and 50 mg of doxorubicin hydrochloride followed by Gelfoam embolization, especially at the posterior segmental branch of the right hepatic artery. Postembolization celiac arteriogram shows complete cessation of blood flow through the embolized posterior segmental branch *(arrow)*. **D,** Iodized oil CT taken 2 weeks later shows retention of iodized oil in the primary tumor and surrounding liver parenchyma with air bubble formation. **E** and **F,** Follow-up celiac arteriogram 4 months later shows markedly decreased tumor vascularity and recanalized main portal vein.

Continued

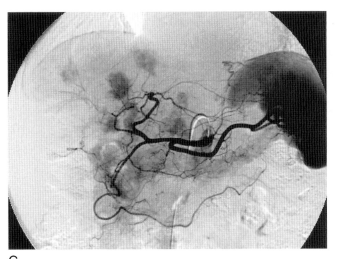

G

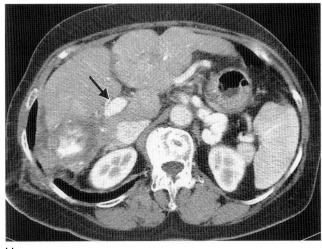

H

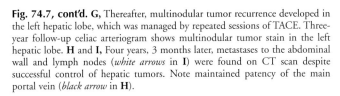

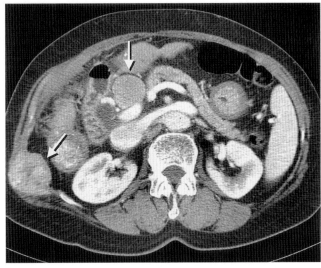

I

Fig. 74.7, cont'd. G, Thereafter, multinodular tumor recurrence developed in the left hepatic lobe, which was managed by repeated sessions of TACE. Three-year follow-up celiac arteriogram shows multinodular tumor stain in the left hepatic lobe. **H** and **I,** Four years, 3 months later, metastases to the abdominal wall and lymph nodes (*white arrows* in **I**) were found on CT scan despite successful control of hepatic tumors. Note maintained patency of the main portal vein (*black arrow* in **H**).

Based on a retrospective comparison, survival rates and tolerability of TACE seemed to be higher when treatment was repeated only when progression of HCC was noted radiographically (Ernst et al, 1999).

THERAPEUTIC EFFICACY OF TRANSCATHETER ARTERIAL CHEMOEMBOLIZATION

Hepatocellular Carcinoma

CT is the most valuable modality to assess the therapeutic effect of TACE (Takayasu et al, 2000). The portion of the tumor that retains iodized oil can be considered necrotic, particularly when a sufficiently long interval exists between TACE and the CT scan (Lim & Han, 2002; Okusaka et al, 2000). Homogeneous, complete retention of iodized oil in the tumor and surrounding liver means better therapeutic effect than defective, inhomogeneous retention (Choi et al, 1992; Nishimine et al, 1994). When the serum level of α-fetoprotein or PIVKA-II is elevated because of HCC, it can be a good indicator of treatment response (see Fig. 74.8L). Because local or remote site recurrence

may occur without elevation of the serum level of those tumor markers, however, imaging studies using ultrasound and helical CT should be done at regular intervals.

Numerous studies have shown that TACE induces partial or complete tumor necrosis (Fig. 74.9). The extent of tumor necrosis after TACE has been reported to range from 50% to 100% (Itsubo et al, 2002; Matsui et al, 1994; Veltri et al, 1998). Matsui and colleagues (1993) reported complete necrosis in about 70% of 100 small hypervascular HCCs less than 4 cm in diameter treated by subsegmental TACE. The 1-year and 4-year local recurrence rates after a single treatment session were 18% and 33%. The 1-year and 4-year survival rates in patients with Child class A or B disease were 100% and 67%. Several studies have suggested predictors of favorable tumor response, including small, encapsulated, expansive, hypervascular tumors and long-term retention of iodized oil on CT (Itsubo et al, 2002; Kuroda et al, 1991; Matsuo et al, 1997; Nakamura et al, 1993). TACE seems markedly less effective in patients with large or diffuse, replacing-type tumors and presence of extranodular growth. Pathologically, trabecular-type HCC showed more prominent necrosis than scirrhous, compact, or well-differentiated HCC (Jinno et al, 1992). Yamada and coworkers (1995) performed a

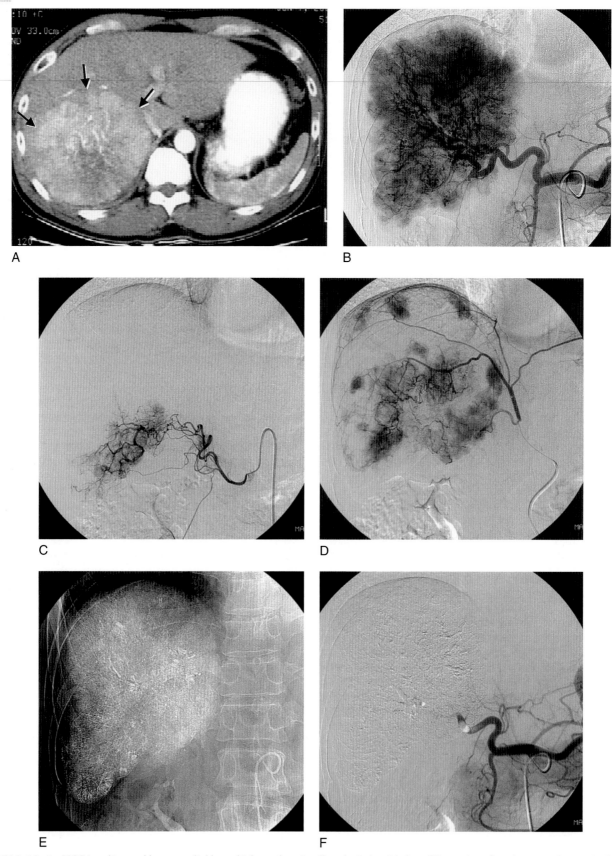

Fig. 74.8. Massive HCC in a 43-year-old man supplied by multiple extrahepatic collaterals. **A,** Arterial phase CT scan shows huge hypervascular mass in the right hepatic lobe. **B,** Celiac arteriogram shows a well-demarcated hypervascular mass with multinodular confluent appearance. **C** and **D,** Selective angiograms of the renal capsular artery (**C**) and the right inferior phrenic artery (**D**) also show multifocal tumor stain. TACE was performed with a mixture of 20 mL of iodized oil and 100 mg of doxorubicin hydrochloride followed by Gelfoam embolization at the right hepatic artery and extrahepatic collaterals. **E** and **F,** Postembolization plain radiograph (**E**) and celiac arteriogram (**F**) show diffuse uptake of iodized oil in the tumor and complete occlusion of the right hepatic artery.

Continued

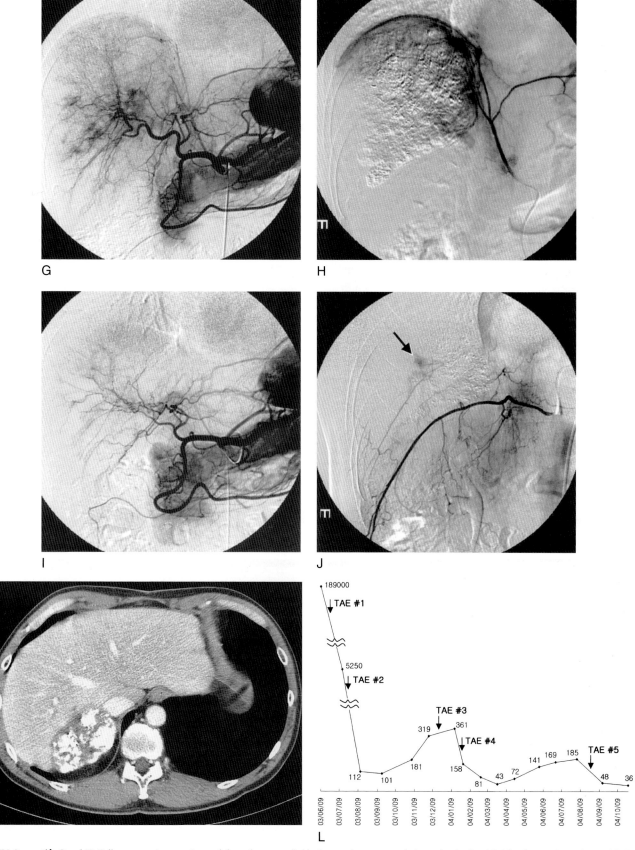

Fig. 74.8, cont'd. G and **H,** Follow-up angiograms 1 month later show remarkably decreased tumor vascularity and stain. **I** and **J,** After four sessions of repeat TACE over 1 year, 4 months, there is no evidence of tumor stain on celiac arteriogram (**I**). Arteriogram of the 11th intercostals shows small tumor stain from its diaphragmatic branch (*arrow* in **J**). TACE was performed via the diaphragmatic branch using a microcatheter. **K,** Follow-up CT scan shows markedly shrunken primary tumor with a thick capsule, persistent iodized oil retention, and well-preserved nontumorous hepatic parenchyma. **L,** Sequential changes in the serum level of α-fetoprotein (ng/mL) during repeat TACE procedures.

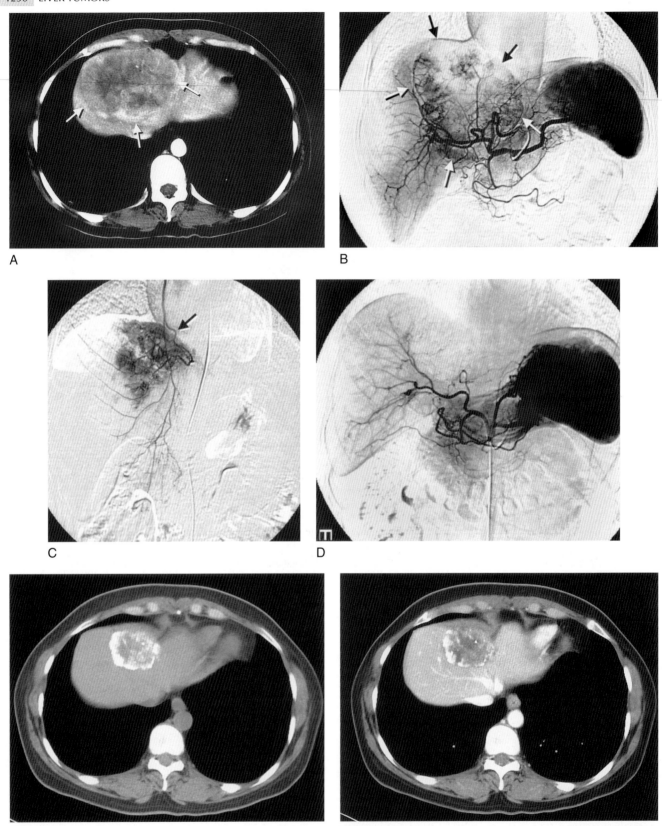

Fig. 74.9. HCC supplied by the right internal mammary artery as an extrahepatic collateral at its initial presentation in a 34-year-old woman. **A,** Initial CT scan shows a large tumor abutting the anterosuperior aspect of the diaphragm *(arrows).* **B,** Celiac arteriogram shows large hypervascular mass occupying the medial segment of the left hepatic lobe and extending to the adjacent segments *(white arrows).* There is a defect in tumor stain at the superior aspect of the tumor *(black arrows)* suggesting the presence of extrahepatic collateral supply. **C,** Right internal mammary arteriogram shows tumor stain at the area exactly matched with the defect in tumor stain on celiac arteriogram. TACE was performed with a mixture of 15 mL of iodized oil and 50 mg of doxorubicin hydrochloride followed by Gelfoam embolization at the right hepatic artery and the diaphragmatic branch of the right internal mammary artery *(arrow).* **D,** Follow-up celiac arteriogram 39 months later shows no evidence of residual tumor. **E and F,** Nine-year follow-up CT scans show markedly shrunken tumor without evidence of enhancing viable tumor.

retrospective study including 1310 patients with unresectable HCC and reported better survival rates in patients with tumors smaller than 5 cm compared with patients with larger tumors. One-year, 2-year, and 3-year survival rates were 72%, 55%, and 47% versus 51%, 28%, and 13%.

Dozens of case-control and retrospective studies have shown that there is a survival benefit in patients treated with TACE compared with untreated patients (Aoyama et al, 1992; Bronowicki et al, 1994; Rose et al, 1998; Sangro et al, 1998). A retrospective study reported that 1-year, 3-year, and 5-year survival rates were 55%, 26%, and 13% in the TACE group compared with 13%, 3%, and 0% in the nontreated group (Sangro et al, 1998). Bronowicki and associates (1994) performed a case-control study, stratifying 254 patients according to Child-Pugh classification and Okuda staging. The survival rates in treated patients were significantly higher (64%, 38%, 27%, and 27% at 1, 2, 3, and 4 years) than in nontreated patients (18%, 6%, and 5% at 1, 2, and 3 years).

Early randomized studies were unable to show a significant difference in patient survival between patients who underwent TACE and patients who were treated conservatively (Groupe d'Etude et de Traitement du Carcinome Hépatocellulaire, 1995; Pelletier et al, 1990, 1998). These studies had limitations, however, because they included heterogeneous techniques and protocols of TACE (different chemotherapeutic or embolic agents, various treatment interval, and presence or absence of iodized oil). The first randomized trial by Pelletier and coworkers (1990) compared patients treated by TACE using doxorubicin and gelatin sponge powder with a nontreated group. The survival rate was not significantly different between the two groups and even lower in the treated group. This trial has an important defect, however, in that gelatin sponge powder may cause more deterioration of liver function than gelatin sponge particles (Kan et al, 1993). In a relatively large study (96 patients) performed by a French cooperative group (Groupe d'Etude et de Traitement du Carcinome Hépatocellulaire, 1995), TACE was performed using cisplatin mixed with iodized oil and gelatin sponge particles. Although the survival rate was more favorable in treated patients (63% versus 44% at 1 year and 38% versus 26% at 2 years), the difference was not statistically significant. This study was later criticized because most patients underwent TACE every 2 months, and causes of deaths were unrelated to tumor growth (Stuart, 2003).

A few more recent randomized studies showed a survival benefit of TACE (Bruix et al, 1998; Llovet et al, 2002; Lo et al, 2002). Llovet and colleagues (2002) divided 112 patients into the three groups: control group, embolization alone group, and TACE using iodized oil and doxorubicin group. This trial showed a statistically significant benefit of TACE on survival compared with the control group (mean survival 28.7% versus 17.9%; 2-year survival 63% versus 27%; P=.009). Similarly, in a randomized study including 80 patients with unresectable HCC, the 2-year survival rate was significantly better in the TACE group (31% versus 11%; P=.002) (Lo et al, 2002). Camma and coworkers (2002) performed a meta-analysis of 18 randomized controlled trials and concluded that TACE significantly reduced the overall 2-year mortality rate (odds ratio 0.54). Lee and coworkers (2002) performed a prospective study to evaluate therapeutic efficacy of TACE compared with hepatic resection for operable HCC. TACE was as effective as hepatic resection in the subpopulations with the International Union against Cancer (UICC) tumor stage of T3N0M0 and adequate liver

function and even with UICC T1-2N0M0 HCC when an iodized oil was compactly retained in the tumor.

There is a controversy about the role of TACE in potential candidates of hepatic resection. TACE has been performed before hepatic resection, mainly in patients with large tumors to reduce tumor volume. Majno and associates (1997) showed that downstaging (42%) or complete necrosis (50%) was achieved in 49 patients and was associated with improved disease-free survival rate. Other workers have reported that tumor-free survival rate and cumulative survival rate were improved by preoperative TACE in small (DiCarlo et al, 1998) and large (Lu et al, 1999; Zhang et al, 2000) HCC. In another randomized trial of 52 patients with resectable large HCC, TACE seemed to increase operative difficulties and lead to worse survival (Wu et al, 1995).

Liver transplantation has been shown to be the best treatment for early stage HCC. Twenty-five percent of patients waiting for transplantation develop contraindications owing to tumor progression within 6 months (Goldberg et al, 2000). TACE has been used as bridge therapy to inhibit tumor growth while waiting for transplantation (see Fig. 74.6). A few nonrandomized studies were performed, but results were contradictory. Some investigators reported that TACE could increase survival or decrease postoperative tumor recurrence (Harnois et al, 1999; Martin et al, 1996; Troisi et al, 1998). Other studies postulated that TACE produced no survival benefit (Mazzaferro et al, 1996). Further study is needed for accurate evaluation of efficacy of TACE in downstaging and inhibiting tumor progression before liver resection and transplantation. In this indication, TACE competes with thermal ablation and limited resection to control tumor progression.

Although surgical resection is the treatment of choice in management of HCC, high postoperative recurrence remains an unresolved problem. In a prospective study, Cha and colleagues (2003) reported a recurrence rate of 55% at a median follow-up of 26 months. Of recurrent tumors, 83% were detected in liver; the liver was the only site of disease in 74%. Several risk factors for early postoperative recurrence have been verified, including incomplete encapsulation, tumor size greater than 5 cm, and vascular invasion (Cha et al, 2003; Ren et al, 2004; Tanaka et al, 1999; Yamanaka et al, 2000).

Minimal intrahepatic metastasis has been regarded as the main cause of early postoperative recurrence (Ouchi et al, 2000). Treatment of minimal intrahepatic metastasis is essential for prevention of postoperative recurrence of HCC. Intra-arterial injection of the mixture of iodized oil and anticancer drug (chemolipiodolization) has been used as adjuvant therapy for preventing postoperative recurrence of HCC (Schwartz et al, 2002; Shimoda et al, 2001). Several investigators showed that adjuvant chemolipiodolization significantly improved local recurrence rate and survival in patients with risk factors. A randomized study showed adjuvant chemoembolization was associated with frequent extrahepatic recurrences, however, and a worse outcome in patients without risk factors (Lai et al, 1998). Postoperative adjuvant TACE is limited to patients with high risk of early recurrence.

Because most recurrent HCC after curative resection manifests in multiple or diffuse patterns involving both lobes of remnant liver, TACE has been used as primary treatment in these patients (Fig. 74.10) (Nagasue et al, 1990; Takayasu et al, 1992). The survival benefit provided by TACE in patients with recurrent HCC after resection has been verified in many studies (Nakoa et al, 1991; Park et al, 1993; Takayasu et al, 1992). The survival

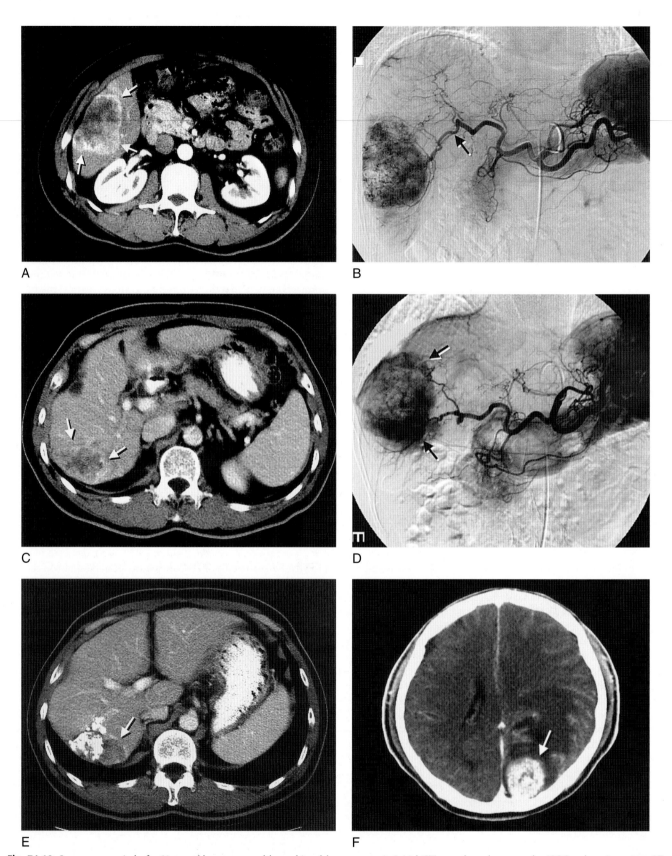

Fig. 74.10. Long-term survival of a 53-year-old man managed by multimodal treatments. **A,** Initial CT scan shows hypervascular HCC at hepatic segment VI *(arrows)*. **B,** Celiac arteriogram shows a nodular hypervascular mass supplied by a hypertrophied segmental hepatic artery *(arrow)*. After TACE, the patient underwent tumorectomy. **C** and **D,** One year, 6 months later, the tumor recurred at the right hepatic lobe *(arrows)*. Extrahepatic collateral supply from the right inferior phrenic artery also was found (not seen). TACE was performed via the right hepatic artery and inferior phrenic artery. **E,** Follow-up CT scan after three sessions of TACE shows persistent viable tumor at the medial aspect of the mass *(arrow)*. At that time, pulmonary metastasis was found in the lung. The patient underwent hepatic tumorectomy, metastasectomy of the lung, and systemic chemotherapy. **F,** Ten months after reoperation, brain MRI revealed an enhancing brain metastasis *(arrow)*. The patient underwent radiotherapy for the metastasis, and follow-up MRI revealed markedly decreased size of the metastatic tumor (not seen). Pulmonary metastasis slowly progressed with continued systemic chemotherapy.

Continued

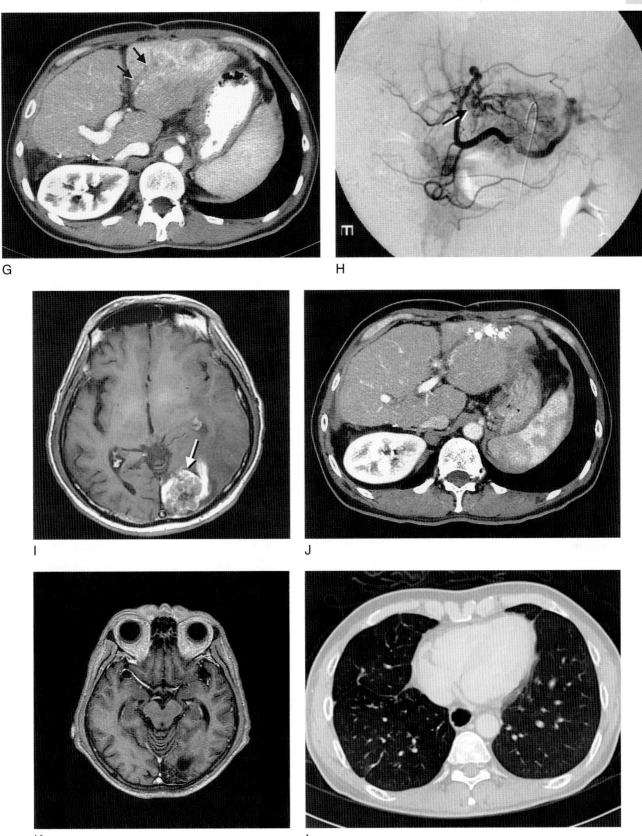

Fig. 74.10, cont'd. G and **H,** One year, 6 months after reoperation, CT scan **(G)** and celiac arteriogram **(H)** show tumor recurrence at hepatic segment III with segmental portal vein invasion *(arrows)*. Segmental TACE was performed. **I,** One year, 6 months after initial radiotherapy for the brain metastasis, follow-up brain MRI revealed regrowth of the enhancing metastatic mass *(arrow)*. Radiotherapy for the brain metastasis was performed again. **J,** Follow-up liver CT after TACE shows shrunken tumor with no evidence of viable portion. Systemic chemotherapy continued, and pulmonary metastasis responded to it. **K** and **L,** Brain MRI **(K)** and chest CT scan **(L)** 6 years after initial presentation show no evidence of disease.

rates in patients who underwent TACE were 64% to 88% at 1 year, 24% to 57% at 2 years, and 5% to 45% at 3 years, which were better than the survival rates of patients who were treated conservatively (Nakoa et al, 1991; Takayasu et al, 1989, 1992).

Spontaneous rupture of HCC is a life-threatening condition with a poor prognosis. Emergency embolization in this clinical setting is an effective treatment (Fig. 74.11). On angiography, only vascular tumors are identified, and extravasation of the contrast medium is uncommon (<20%). Immediate control of bleeding is possible in most patients (Okazaki et al, 1991; Zhu et al, 1996). Ngan and colleagues (1998) reported the results of embolization in 33 patients with HCC rupture. Bleeding was stopped in 32 patients, and median survival of patients with hyperbilirubinemia was significantly worse than survival of patients without hyperbilirubinemia (1 week versus 15 weeks). Because of high operative mortality, the treatment of choice in hemodynamically unstable patients with ruptured HCC is embolization (Dewar et al, 1991; Zhu et al, 1996).

Colorectal Metastases

Colorectal cancers are the most important causes of liver metastases (see Ch. 73a). Liver metastases develop in 60% of patients with colorectal cancer, and these patients frequently die as a result of hepatic failure. In contrast to other common malignancies, such as lung or breast, colorectal cancer frequently metastasizes to the liver as the only site. Surgical resection is the treatment of choice and is potentially curative therapy. Surgical resection is not indicated, however, in two thirds of patients because of number or location of the lesions, hepatic function, or comorbid illnesses (Fusai & Davidson, 2003; Meyers et al, 2003; Penna & Nordlinger, 2002).

Intra-arterial chemotherapy has been used successfully as primary or adjuvant therapy after resection for colorectal liver metastases (Kemeny et al, 2002; Kohnoe et al, 2002; Riel et al, 2000; Tono et al, 2000). Colorectal tumors are not as hypervascular as HCC, limiting the ability to deliver adequate chemotherapy and embolic agent (Shankar et al, 1996; Yamaguchi et al, 2000). TACE has been investigated mainly as a second-line therapy after systemic chemotherapy has failed. As expected, tumor response rates are not as high as the response rates in HCC. Several studies reported response rates of approximately 25% (Lang & Brown, 1993; Martinelli et al, 1994). In a randomized study, partial remission of the tumor was achieved in 20.8%, and mean survival in patients with liver-only metastases was 15 months (Salman et al, 2002). Although any benefit on survival has not been proved, TACE increased the response rate compared with systemic chemotherapy (Martinelli et al, 1994; Salman et al, 2002; Sanz-Altamira et al, 1997).

Neuroendocrine Metastasis

Neuroendocrine tumors (see Ch. 73b), such as pancreatic islet cell and gastrointestinal carcinoid tumors, frequently metastasize to the liver by the time of diagnosis. These tumors have been a common indication for TACE because they are generally hypervascular and often confined to liver (Fig. 74.12). To date, many studies have reported high response rates (70-90%) (Kim et al, 1999; Kirchkoff et al, 2000; Nakaoka et al, 2000; Roche et al, 2003; Venook, 1999; Yao et al, 2001). In a retrospective study by Yao and colleagues (2001), 90% of the patients (17 of 20) showed

significant radiographic (7 patients) or clinical (10 patients) response, and median survival was 32 months. Dominguez and associates (2000) reported that TACE using streptozotocin as a chemotherapeutic agent produced comparable results to other series using doxorubicin or 5-fluorouracil. Sequential and periodic TACE is required for effective palliation. A phase II clinical study was performed by Diamandidou and coworkers (1998) attempting TACE with microencapsulated cisplatin particles; this study showed a clinical response in 67% and objective decrease in the tumor in 77% of patients. Although most studies have reported excellent survival rates after TACE (median survival at least 2 years), it is unclear whether TACE significantly improves survival because prolonged survival may occur even in advanced disease.

Because these tumors are not associated with liver cirrhosis, morbidity after TACE is lower than with tumors of HCC. Until the introduction of somatostatin analogues, exacerbation of the symptoms of carcinoid or carcinoid crisis was common after TACE. Since somatostatin analogues have been used routinely during and after TACE, this complication occurs in only a small percentage of patients.

Other Diseases

Gastrointestinal stromal tumors represent a subset of mesenchymal tumors that involve stomach (60%), the small bowel (30%), and other parts of the gastrointestinal tract. A small bowel gastrointestinal stromal tumor has a high tendency for malignant behavior, and the liver is the most common site of metastasis. Surgical resection is the treatment of choice for single metastasis, but more than half of patients with malignant gastrointestinal stromal tumors have unresectable disease. Because this tumor is frequently hypervascular, TACE may be a good alternative treatment for unresectable liver metastases (Fig. 74.13). Mavligit and coworkers (1995) reported that TACE produced a major (>50% regression) tumor response in 70% of patients, lasting 8 to 31 months. More recent studies have shown a high level of efficacy of imatinib mesylate, a tyrosine kinase inhibitor, with more than 70% complete and partial responses in an unresectable gastrointestinal stromal tumor (Demetri et al, 2002). TACE is recommended for unresectable liver metastasis that does not respond to imatinib mesylate.

Liver metastasis develops in two thirds of patients with ocular melanoma. This metastatic tumor rapidly advances (median survival 2-6 months). A few reports have shown that TACE is effective palliation for this tumor (Feldman et al, 2004; Mavligit et al, 1988). A retrospective study of 201 patients compared cisplatin-based TACE with systemic chemotherapy and reported that TACE produced an acceptable response rate (36%) (Bedikian et al, 1995). Because most patients die of systemic disease, locoregional therapy such as TACE is unlikely to improve survival of patients with these tumors.

Combined Therapy with Other Treatment

There are many treatment options (see Chs. 76, 77, and 79) for liver tumors, including surgery, transcatheter arterial treatments, percutaneous ablation therapy, systemic therapy, and radiotherapy. All of these treatments have advantages and disadvantages. The best patient outcomes can be achieved by adopting a multimodality approach (see Fig. 74.10).

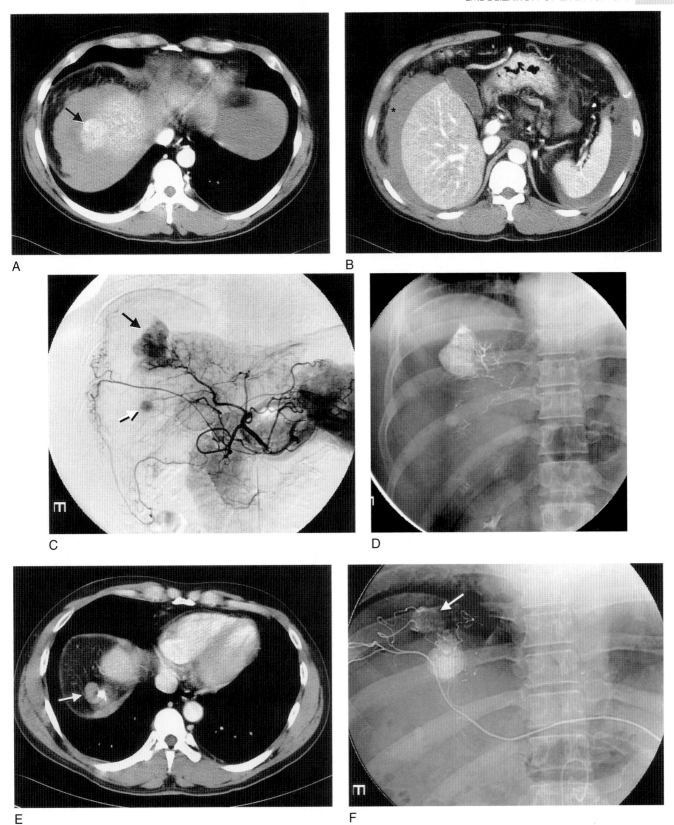

Fig. 74.11. Ruptured HCC in a 36-year-old man with development of collateral supply from omental arteries. **A** and **B,** Enhanced liver CT scans shows a tumor with exophytic growth at the dome of the right hepatic lobe *(arrow)* and large amount of hemoperitoneum (*). **C,** Celiac arteriogram shows exophytic hypervascular mass *(black arrow)* without active extravasation of contrast material. There is another small nodular tumor in the right hepatic lobe *(white arrow)*. **D,** TACE was performed with a mixture of 5 mL of iodized oil and 30 mg of doxorubicin hydrochloride followed by Gelfoam embolization. Completion plain radiograph shows compact iodized oil uptake in the tumor nodules. **E,** Four months later, CT scan revealed recurrent viable tumor at the peripheral aspect of the exophytic mass *(arrow)*. **F,** The tumor was supplied by an omental artery *(arrow)* arising from the splenic artery.

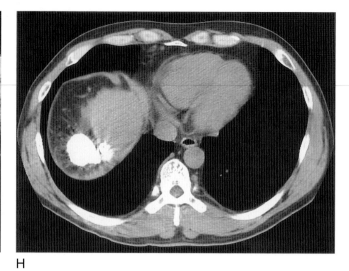

G

H

Fig. 74.11, cont'd. G, Two years later, celiac arteriogram shows marginal tumor recurrence supplied by a different omental artery arising from the right gastroepi-ploic artery *(arrow)*. **H,** Iodized oil CT after TACE via the omental artery shows dense accumulation of iodized oil in the recurrent tumor and surrounding omental edema.

TACE has been proposed before percutaneous treatment of HCC, such as percutaneous ethanol injection (PEI), and radio-frequency ablation. The purpose of TACE is to reduce the size of large tumors for application of percutaneous treatments or to obtain a synergistic effect on tumor necrosis by combining both procedures (Tanaka et al, 1991). TACE enhances the diffusion of ethanol within tumor tissue, causing more extensive tumor necrosis during PEI procedures (Lencioni et al, 1994; Veltri et al, 1998). Several trials have shown that combined TACE-PEI therapy significantly improves initial therapeutic response rate and reduces local recurrence rate in small and large HCC (Bartolozzi et al, 1995; Kamada et al, 2002; Koda et al, 2001). Koda and colleagues (2001) compared the combined therapy

with PEI alone in 52 patients with small HCC. In their study, the combined therapy improved local recurrence rates (8.7% and 19.3% versus 26.9% and 80.1% at 1 year and 3 years) and survival rates in small (<2 cm) HCC. Kamada and associates (2002) compared the therapeutic effect of this combined therapy and TACE alone in 69 patients with small (<3 cm) HCC. The 5-year survival rates were better in the combined therapy group than in the TACE alone group (50% versus 22%). The survival rates of these studies were comparable to the survival rates with surgical resection. In addition, this combined therapy prolongs survival in patients with large HCC (Yamamoto et al, 1997). In a prospective comparative study of 132 patients with unresectable HCC, median survival time was better in the TACE-PEI group

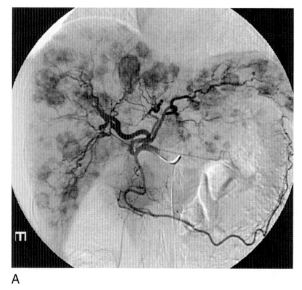

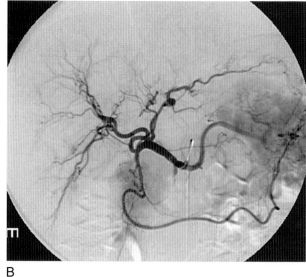

A

B

Fig. 74.12. Liver metastasis of rectal carcinoid in a 36-year-old woman. **A,** Celiac arteriogram shows numerous metastatic nodules scattered in the both hepatic lobes. Initial TACE was performed with a mixture of 7 mL of iodized oil and 40 mg of doxorubicin hydrochloride followed by Gelfoam embolization. **B,** Follow-up celiac arteriogram 2 years later after eight sessions of repeat TACE shows markedly improved metastatic lesions.

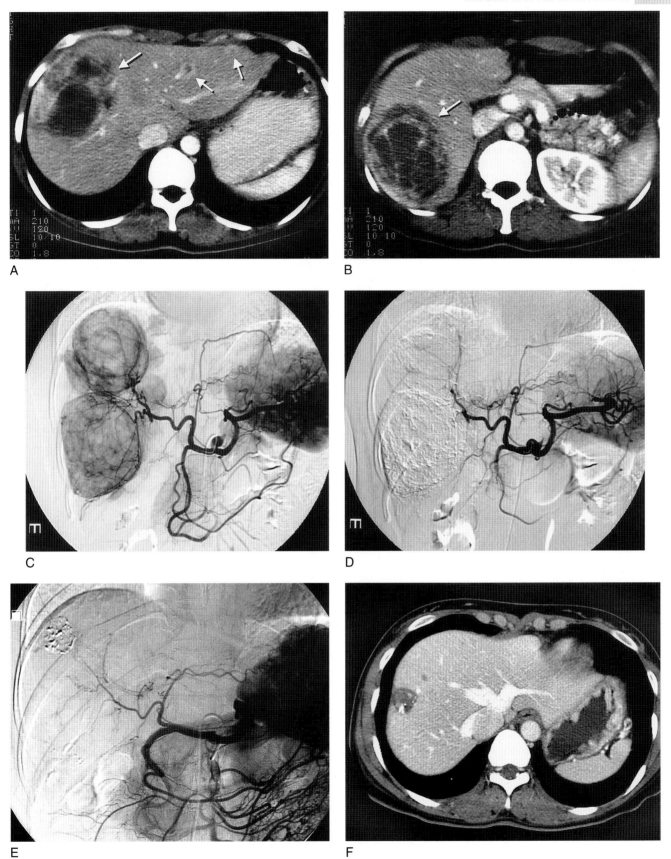

Fig. 74.13. Liver metastasis of gastrointestinal stromal tumor of the stomach in a 34-year-old woman. **A** and **B,** CT scans of the liver show multiple metastatic tumors in the both hepatic lobes *(arrows).* **C,** Celiac arteriogram shows variable sized multiple hypervascular tumors in the liver. **D,** Initial TACE was performed with a mixture of 10 mL of iodized oil and 50 mg of doxorubicin hydrochloride followed by Gelfoam embolization. Completion arteriogram shows successful devascularization of the tumor. **E,** After three sessions of repeat TACE, there is no evidence of hypervascular mass in the liver on celiac arteriogram. **F,** Eight-year follow-up CT scan shows no evidence of viable tumor in the liver.

(25 months) compared with the PEI group (18 months), TACE group (8 months), and conservatively treated group (2 months) (Allgaier et al, 1998).

Another combined approach has aimed for synergy effect of flow reduction and thermal injury (Goldberg et al, 2000). Rossi and associates (2000) performed radiofrequency ablation after hepatic arterial embolization in 62 patients with HCC (3.5-8.5 cm) and observed a 1-year survival rate of 87% and recurrence rate of 19%. The survival benefit conferred by this combined therapy also has been verified in patients with metastatic colorectal cancer (Bloomston et al, 2002). Combined therapy using laser thermal ablation and TACE also has been tried. Pacella and coworkers (2001) achieved complete necrosis in 90% (27 of 30), with a local recurrence rate of 7% at 3 years.

COMPLICATIONS

TACE is associated with diverse complications. Procedure-related mortality is less than 5% (Berger et al, 1995; Ernst et al, 1999; Sakamoto et al, 1998). The incidence of major complications has been reported to be less than 5%, including liver abscess, parenchymal infarction, intrahepatic aneurysm, pulmonary embolism, ischemic cholecystitis or gallbladder infarction, pseudocirrhosis, hepatorenal syndrome, carcinoid crisis, liver rupture, and gastric or duodenal ulcerations (De Baere et al, 1996; Kim et al, 2001; Song et al, 2001). Patients with procedure-related complications usually have predisposing factors (Chung et al, 1996). Important predisposing factors are major portal vein obstruction, compromised hepatic functional reserve, biliary obstruction, previous biliary surgery, excessive amount of iodized oil, hepatic arterial occlusion after repeat TACE, and nonselective embolization (Chung et al, 1996; Song et al, 2001). Recognition of predisposing factors before the procedure and selective embolization with an adequate amount of chemoembolic material and careful postprocedure monitoring of patients can prevent major complications in most patients.

Postembolization Syndrome

Postembolization syndrome is a self-limited condition; nevertheless, it is an important complication of TACE that prolongs hospitalization and postpones additional treatment. It manifests as fever, nausea, vomiting, and dull right upper quadrant pain (Okuda et al, 1985; Venook et al, 1990). Possible causes of the pain are acute ischemia of liver parenchyma, distention of the liver capsule, and gallbladder ischemia secondary to inadvertent embolization of the cystic artery. Leung and colleagues (2001) reported that gallbladder embolization and dose administered are associated with this syndrome. Intra-arterial administration of lidocaine before and during TACE can be helpful to prevent or reduce pain (Lee et al, 2001; Romano et al, 2003). Fever after TACE usually is considered to be the result of tumor necrosis. Paye and coworkers (1999) suggested, however, that fever and cytolysis after TACE are caused by injury of nontumorous parenchyma, rather than by tumor necrosis. Pulmonary embolism of iodized oil also causes a febrile reaction (Chung et al, 1993). These symptoms can be controlled by antiemetics, analgesics, antipyretics, and hydrocortisone.

Liver Failure

The most serious complication of TACE is hepatic insufficiency. In a prospective study including 197 sessions of TACE, acute liver failure developed in 20% of patients, and 3% of cases were irreversible. Hyperbilirubinemia, prolonged prothrombin time, higher dose of anticancer drug, and advanced cirrhosis were associated with irreversible failure (Chan et al, 2002). TACE does not induce significant liver dysfunction in patients with Child classification A or B cirrhosis despite embolization of relatively proximal (proper or right/left main) hepatic arteries (Caturelli et al, 2000). Most cases of liver dysfunction that require hospitalization develop in patients with Child C disease (Shah et al, 1998).

Liver Infarction

Although the iodized oil is selectively retained in tumor neovasculature, TACE also adversely affects nontumorous liver parenchyma. The normal liver of experimental animals tolerates even a large amount of iodized oil (0.5-2 mL/kg) well (Kan et al, 1993). Treatment with iodized oil alone also is ineffective in hepatic tumors. The addition of anticancer drugs to the iodized oil increases the therapeutic effect on malignant tumors with some hepatic damage, which includes small areas of hepatic infarction. Hepatic artery embolization with the combination of iodized oil and gelatin sponge particles has the effect of combined arterial and portal blockage. Consequently, with better therapeutic effects, hepatic artery embolization with the combination has a higher risk of hepatic necrosis and atrophy of nontumorous liver parenchyma than does embolization with iodized oil or gelatin sponge particles alone.

Portal vein obstruction is a well-known risk factor for hepatic failure and infarction after hepatic artery embolization. In patients with major portal vein obstruction, TACE should be performed with a reduced amount of chemoembolic agents and selective administration of the agents into tumor-feeding arteries. Especially when there is preexisting hepatic insufficiency, TACE seems to be contraindicated because of the risk of acute hepatic failure.

Cirrhosis and chronic hepatitis frequently compromise the liver with HCC. A safe dose of iodized oil to the compromised liver has not been determined yet. It generally is recommended that, in patients with Child-Pugh class B or C, the amount of iodized oil used should be limited to less than 5 to 10 mL according to the severity of hepatic decompensation. The iodized oil should be injected to tumor-feeding arteries as selectively as possible.

In an experimental study, the liver with biliary obstruction was susceptible to hepatic infarction, which can be explained by means of the decreased portal venous inflow that accompanies biliary obstruction. Acute hepatic failure and sepsis can develop after TACE for HCC with biliary obstruction (Chung et al, 1996). Usually patients with biliary obstruction have extensive parenchymal tumor. In that case, adequate decompression of the biliary system should be performed first before trying TACE. The amounts of embolic agents used during TACE should be reduced to prevent bile duct injury (Kim HK et al, 2001). A few patients with HCC and biliary obstruction have localized parenchymal tumor, however, and their biliary obstruction is caused by the ingrowth of tumor from the peripheral bile duct. In these circumstances, TACE can be tried first before biliary drainage procedure with great caution and careful postprocedure monitoring of patients.

Septicemia

TACE or hepatic arterial embolization has been reported to induce septicemia. Chen and colleagues (1999) reported that 7 of 176 TACE procedures (4%) were associated with symptomatic bacterial infection, including sepsis, liver abscess, and infected biloma. In a retrospective study by Chung and associates (1996), 10 (1.1%) of 942 TACE procedures were associated with septicemia. Fatal sepsis is rare, however, and mostly develops in patients with predisposing factors, such as portal vein or biliary obstruction, ascites, and biliary-enteric anastomosis. Routine administration of prophylactic antibiotics is not recommended.

Liver Abscess

Liver abscess develops after 0.5% to 2% of TACE procedures (Kim W et al, 2001). Song and coworkers (2001) conducted a retrospective study to determine predisposing factors to liver abscess based on 6202 TACE procedures in 2190 patients with hepatic tumors. Liver abscess developed in 14 patients (0.6%): 3 of 263 (1.1%) patients with portal vein obstruction, 3 of 54 (5.6%) patients with metastatic hepatic tumors, and 5 of 36 (13.9%) patients with biliary abnormalities. Among all of the potential predisposing factors, prior biliary-enteric bypass surgery has been reported as the most important predisposing factor for intrahepatic abscess after TACE (Kim W et al, 2001; Ong et al, 2004; Song et al, 2001). Aggressive prophylactic antibiotic administration with bowel preparation before TACE is recommended to prevent abscess formation in these patients (Geschwind et al, 2002). Liver abscess may result in a fatal outcome if it is detected too late or managed inappropriately. It can be managed successfully with percutaneous drainage and parenteral antibiotics (Fig. 74.14) (Song et al, 2001). The benefit-to-risk ratio should be evaluated carefully in patients with biliary-enteric anastomosis and indications for TACE.

Bile Duct Injury

In contrast to normal liver parenchyma, intrahepatic bile ducts are supplied by peribiliary capillary plexus from hepatic artery. Ischemic injury of the bile ducts can develop after TACE. The incidence of this complication has been reported as 2% to 12.5%, including intrahepatic biloma, focal stricture of common duct, and diffuse dilation of intrahepatic bile duct (Kim HK et al, 2001; Kobayashi et al, 1993). The intrahepatic bile duct injury may cause obliteration of the adjacent portal vein and liver parenchyma atrophy (Yu et al, 2001). Intrahepatic biloma is a major complication, which can result in biliary stasis with cholangitis, abscess formation, and sepsis. A large study by Sakamoto and colleagues (2003) reported that the incidence of biloma is higher in patients with metastatic liver tumor than in patients with HCC. It seems to develop more easily in noncirrhotic livers and when selective embolization of distal arterial branches is performed, rather than proximal occlusion (Yu et al, 2002). Most patients with this complication are asymptomatic, but when

there are signs of infection, percutaneous drainage is required (Sakamoto et al, 2003).

Extrahepatic Nontargeted Embolization

Another major category of complications of TACE is unintentional extrahepatic embolization. When the cystic artery is occluded during the procedure, gallbladder infarction occurs in 75% to 90% of patients. Although most cases of gallbladder infarction show a self-limited clinical course, more serious conditions have been reported, such as gallbladder perforation and gangrenous or emphysematous cholecystitis, which necessitate surgery or percutaneous cholecystostomy (Kuroda et al, 1983; Tarazov et al, 2000). It is recommended to infuse chemoembolic agents into the tumor-feeding artery distal to the origin of the cystic artery.

Splenic infarction is caused by reflux of embolic materials into the splenic artery during embolization or arteriography after embolization. It frequently is symptomatic, producing a dull pain in the left upper quadrant, but self-limited (Takayasu et al, 1984). With celiac artery stenosis or splenomegaly secondary to portal hypertension, the flow direction of the common hepatic artery can be reversed, and the risk of splenic artery embolization increases (Sakamoto et al, 1998).

Acute pancreatitis can complicate nonselective TAE of HCC with an incidence ranging from 1.7% (acute clinical pancreatitis) to 40% (biologic pancreatitis) (Khan et al, 1993). This complication probably is caused by embolic materials regurgitated into the pancreaticoduodenal artery and occluded peripheral portion of the pancreatic vascular bed, leading to ischemia of the pancreas (Kishimoto et al, 1989). Superselective embolization with a microcatheter prevents this complication.

Skin complications can develop after TACE of extrahepatic collateral vessels, such as internal mammary artery and intercostal artery (Arora et al, 1999). Painful induration and discoloration are observed, but transmural necrosis that requires skin graft is uncommon. A supraumbilical skin rash can develop if the emulsion of iodized oil and anticancer drug flows into the falciform artery. When a dilated falciform artery arising from the left hepatic artery is identified, embolization of the falciform artery with coils before TACE of the left hepatic artery is needed to prevent this complication (Baysal et al, 1998; Ueno et al, 1995).

In TACE, at least some proportion of iodized oil injected into the hepatic artery must leave the liver through normal hepatic vasculature or an arteriovenous hepatic shunt, which causes embolization of the pulmonary vascular network in all patients who undergo TACE. The amount of the iodized oil injected is the most important factor in the production of symptomatic pulmonary oil embolism (Chung et al, 1993). To prevent pulmonary oil embolism, it is recommended to use no more than 15 mL of iodized oil, administer it superselectively, and observe arteriovenous hepatic shunts carefully on initial arteriograms and during the procedure. TACE of the inferior phrenic artery frequently results in pulmonary complications, including iodized oil accumulation in the lung field, consolidation, and pleural effusion (Tajima et al, 2002a). Early recognition and embolization of arteriovenous shunt is necessary to prevent these complications. When a large amount of iodized oil accumulates in lung parenchyma, respiratory symptoms of cough, hemoptysis, and dyspnea develop 2 to 5 days after TACE. The chest radiograph shows diffuse bilateral pulmonary parenchymal infiltration.

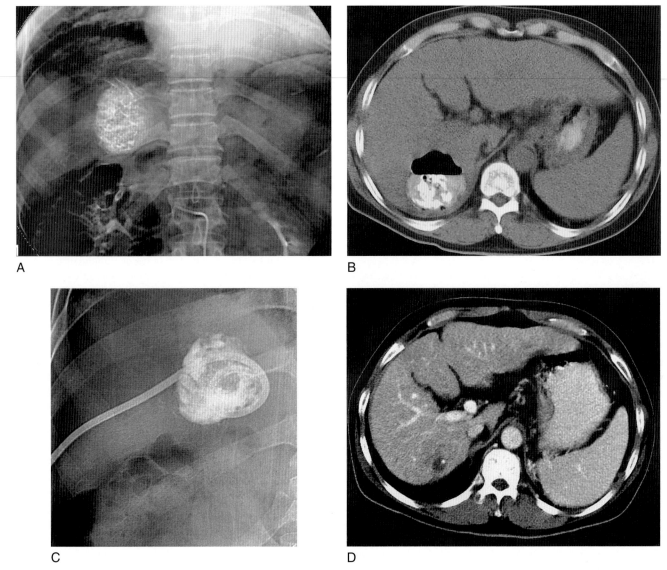

Fig. 74.14. Liver abscess formation after chemoembolization and treatment with percutaneous drainage procedure in a 55-year-old man. **A,** Plain radiograph obtained after chemoembolization shows selective iodized oil accumulation in the tumor. **B,** Noncontrast CT scan 2 weeks later shows air-fluid level in the tumor. **C,** Percutaneous drainge catheter was inserted into the abscess cavity. **D,** Follow-up CT scan 1 month later shows remarkable shrinkage of the tumor without evidence of viable tumor.

The symptoms, arterial hypoxemia, and radiographic abnormality clear 10 to 28 days after TACE in most cases (Chung et al, 1993).

Gastrointestinal Bleeding

Hematemesis or melena may occur after TACE in 8.5% to 15% of cases (Lin et al, 1996; Wu et al, 2002). The causes of this complication are gastroesophageal varices, acute gastric mucosal lesion, acute ulcer, and rarely Mallory-Weiss syndrome. Variceal bleeding may develop after angiography and TACE (Lin et al, 1996). Nonvariceal bleeding, which is usually milder than variceal bleeding, is probably due to inadvertent embolization of the accessory left gastric arteries that arise from the left hepatic artery and the right gastric artery that arises from the proper hepatic artery (Hirakawa et al, 1988). If these gastric branches are

not recognized before the procedure, and appropriate protective measures are not taken, gastric complications are unavoidable. Embolization of gastric branches with coil or balloon occlusion of proper hepatic artery can redirect the blood flow.

Coagulation and Fibrinolysis

Disseminated intravascular coagulopathy after TACE has been reported (Katsushima et al, 1990; Sakon et al, 1991). In patients with this complication, laboratory findings indicate coagulation and fibrinolysis are activated. There is a marked reduction of platelet count and fibrinogen level, which precede symptoms of disseminated intravascular coagulopathy. There should be an awareness of this rare condition for early detection and proper management.

Iatrogenic Vascular Injury

During the TACE procedure, iatrogenic arterial injury, such as dissection, may occur in the visceral arteries. The two most common sites of dissection are the celiac artery and the proper hepatic artery. Although iatrogenic dissection of the arteries heals spontaneously in most patients, and subsequent TACE is possible via the dissected arteries, it may result in complete obstruction or pseudoaneurysm formation (So et al, 2003; Yoon et al, 1995). Skillful angiographic technique can prevent unexpected hepatic artery injury with the tip of catheters or guidewires. Proximal hepatic artery injury makes it impossible to perform complete and selective chemoembolization.

CONCLUSION

Advances in catheter technology and chemoembolic materials and accumulation of knowledge about the procedure and tumor blood supply may improve the effectiveness of the treatment and reduce procedure-related complications in chemoembolization of hepatic tumors. The treatment protocol or procedure optimally should be tailored for each patient, considering his or her hepatic function, the status of the portal vein, and the extent of the tumor.

REFERENCES

Abe S, et al, 2000: Focal therapeutic efficacy of transcatheter arterial infusion of styrene maleic acid neocarzinostatin for hepatocellular carcinoma. J Gastroenterol 35:28-33.

Ackerman NB, 1974: The blood supply of experimental liver metastases: IV. changes in vascularity with increasing tumor growth. Surgery 75:589-596.

Allgaier HP, et al, 1998: Survival benefit of patients with inoperable hepatocellular carcinoma treated by a combination of transarterial chemoembolization and percutaneous ethanol injection—a single-center analysis including 132 patients. Int J Cancer 79:601-605.

Aoyama K, et al, 1992: Evaluation of transcatheter arterial embolization with epirubicin-lipiodol emulsion for hepatocellular carcinoma. Cancer Chemother Pharmacol 31:S55-S59.

Arora R, et al, 1999: Cutaneous complications of hepatic chemoembolization via extrahepatic collaterals. J Vasc Interv Radiol 10:1351-1356.

Bartolozzi C, et al, 1995: Treatment of large HCC: transcatheter arterial chemoembolization combined with percutaneous ethanol injection versus repeated transcatheter arterial chemoembolization. Radiology 197: 812-818.

Bastian P, et al, 1998: Chemo-embolization of experimental liver metastases: Part I. distribution of biodegradable microspheres of different sizes in an animal model for the locoregional therapy. Eur J Pharm Biopharm 46:243-254.

Baysal T, et al, 1998: Supraumbilical dermal sclerosis and fat necrosis from chemoembolization of hepatocellular carcinoma. J Vasc Interv Radiol 9: 645-647.

Bedikian AY, et al, 1995: Treatment of uveal melanoma metastatic to the liver: a review of the M. D. Anderson Cancer Center experience and prognostic factors. Cancer 76:1665-1670.

Berger DH, et al, 1995: Hepatic artery chemoembolization or embolization for primary and metastatic liver tumors: post-treatment management and complications. J Surg Oncol 60:116-121.

Bhattacharya S, et al, 1994: Iodized oil in the treatment of hepatocellular carcinoma. Br J Surg 81:1563-1571.

Bismuth H, Majno P, 2000: Hepatobiliary surgery. J Hepatol 32:208-224.

Bloomston M, et al, 2002: Transcatheter arterial chemoembolization with or without radiofrequency ablation in the management of patients with advanced hepatic malignancy. Am Surg 68:827-831.

Bronowicki JP, et al, 1994: Transcatheter oily chemoembolization for hepatocellular carcinoma: a 4-year study of 127 French patients. Cancer 74:16-24.

Brown KT, 2004: Fatal pulmonary complications after arterial embolization with 40-120-μm tris-acryl gelatin microspheres. J Vasc Interv Radiol 15: 197-200.

Bruix J, et al, 1998: Transarterial embolization versus symptomatic treatment in patients with advanced hepatocellular carcinoma: results of a randomized, controlled trial in a single institution. Hepatology 27:1578-1583.

Camma C, et al, 2002: Transarterial chemoembolization for unresectable hepatocellular carcinoma: meta-analysis of randomized controlled trials. Radiology 224:47-54.

Caturelli E, et al, 2000: Transcatheter arterial chemoembolization for hepatocellular carcinoma in patients with cirrhosis: evaluation of damage to nontumorous liver tissue—long-term prospective study. Radiology 215:123-128.

Cay O, et al, 1996: Targeting of different ethiodized oil–doxorubicin mixtures to hypovascular hepatic metastases with intraarterial and intraportal injections. J Vasc Interv Radiol 7:409-417.

Cha C, et al, 2003: Predictors and patterns of recurrence after resection of hepatocellular carcinoma. J Am Coll Surg 197:753-758.

Chan AO, et al, 2002: A prospective study regarding the complications of transcatheter intraarterial lipiodol chemoembolization in patients with hepatocellular carcinoma. Cancer 94:1747-1752.

Chang JM, et al, 1994: Transcatheter arterial embolization with or without cisplatin treatment of hepatocellular carcinoma: a randomized controlled study. Cancer 74:2449-2453.

Charnsangavej C, et al, 1982: Angiographic classification of hepatic arterial collaterals. Radiology 144:485-494.

Chen C, et al, 1999: Bacterial infections associated with hepatic arteriography and transarterial embolization for hepatocellular carcinoma: a prospective study. Clin Infect Dis 29:161-166.

Chiappa A, et al, 1999: Survival after repeat hepatic resection for recurrent colorectal metastases. Hepatogastroenterology 46:1065-1070.

Cho KJ, et al, 1976: Effects of experimental hepatic artery embolization on hepatic function. AJR Am J Roentgenol 127:563-567.

Choi BI, et al, 1992: Therapeutic effect of transcatheter oily chemoembolization therapy for encapsulated nodular hepatocellular carcinoma: CT and pathologic findings. Radiology 182:709-713.

Chung JW, et al, 1993: Pulmonary oil embolism after transcatheter oily chemoembolization of hepatocellular carcinoma. Radiology 187:689-693.

Chung JW, et al, 1995: Hepatocellular carcinoma and portal vein invasion: results of treatment with transcatheter oily chemoembolization. AJR Am J Roentgenol 165:315-321.

Chung JW, et al, 1996: Hepatic tumors: predisposing factors for complications of transcatheter oily chemoembolization. Radiology 198:33-40.

Chung JW, et al, 1998: Transcatheter oily chemoembolization of the inferior phrenic artery in hepatocellular carcinoma: the safety and potential therapeutic role. J Vasc Interv Radiol 9:495-500.

CLIP (Cancer of the Liver Italian Program) Investigators, 2000: Prospective validation of the CLIP score: a new prognostic system for patients with cirrhosis and hepatocellular carcinoma. Hepatology 31:840-845.

De Baere T, et al, 1996: Liver abscess formation after local treatment of liver tumors. Hepatology 23:1436-1440.

Demetri GD, et al, 2002: Efficacy and safety of imatinib mesylate in advanced gastrointestinal stromal tumors. N Engl J Med 347:472-480.

Dewar GA, et al, 1991: Management of bleeding liver tumours in Hong Kong. Br J Surg 78:463-466.

Diamandidou E, et al, 1998: Two-phase study of hepatic artery vascular occlusion with microencapsulated cisplatin in patients with liver metastases from neuroendocrine tumors. AJR Am J Roentgenol 170:339-344.

DiCarlo V, et al, 1998: Preoperative chemoembolization of hepatocellular carcinoma in cirrhotic patients. Hepatogastroenterology 45:1950-1954.

Dominguez S, et al, 2000: Hepatic arterial chemoembolization with streptozotocin in patients with metastatic digestive endocrine tumours. Eur J Gastroenterol Hepatol 12:151-157.

Doppman JL, et al, 1978: Proximal versus peripheral hepatic artery embolization experimental study in monkeys. Radiology 128:577-588.

Doyon D, et al, 1974: L'embolisation artérielle hépatique dans les tumeurs malignes du foie. Ann Radiol 17:593-603.

El-Serag HB, et al, 2003: The continuing increase in the incidence of hepatocellular carcinoma in the United States: an update. Ann Intern Med 139: 817-823.

Ernst O, et al, 1999: Treatment of hepatocellular carcinoma by transcatheter arterial chemoembolization: comparison of planned periodic chemoembolization and chemoembolization based on tumor response. AJR Am J Roentgenol 172:159-164.

Fan J, et al, 2001: Multimodality treatment in hepatocellular carcinoma patients with tumor thrombi in portal vein. World J Gastroenterol 7:28-32.

Farinati F, et al, 2000: How should patients with hepatocellular carcinoma be staged? Validation of a new prognostic system. Cancer 89:2266-2273.

Feldman ED, et al, 2004: Regional treatment options for patients with ocular melanoma metastatic to the liver. Ann Surg Oncol 11:290-297.

Fok TF, et al, 1996: Hepatic haemangioendothelioma presenting with early heart failure in a newborn: treatment with hepatic artery embolization and interferon. Acta Paediatr 85:1373-1375.

Fong Y, et al, 1999: Clinical score for predicting recurrence after hepatic resection for metastatic colorectal cancer: analysis of 1001 consecutive cases. Ann Surg 230:309-318.

Furuse J, et al, 1997: Hepatocellular carcinoma with portal vein tumor thrombus: embolization of arterioportal shunts. Radiology 204:787-790.

Fusai G, Davidson BR, 2003: Management of colorectal liver metastases. Colorectal Dis 5:2-23.

Geoghegan JG, Scheele J, 1999: Treatment of colorectal liver metastases. Br J Surg 86:158-169.

Geschwind JF, et al, 2002: Influence of a new prophylactic antibiotic therapy on the incidence of liver abscesses after chemoembolization treatment of liver tumors. J Vasc Interv Radiol 13:1163-1166.

Giavroglou C, et al, 2003: Arterial embolization of giant hepatic hemangiomas. Cardiovasc Interv Radiol 26:92-96.

Goldberg SN, et al, 2000: Thermal ablation therapy for focal malignancy: a unified approach to underlying principles, techniques, and diagnostic imaging guidance. AJR Am J Roentgenol 174:323-331.

Goseki N, et al, 1995: Nourishment of hepatocellular carcinoma cells through the portal blood flow with and without transcatheter arterial embolization. Cancer 76:736-742.

Granov AM, et al, 1992: Arterioportal fistulas (APF) in liver tumors: prognosis in relation to treatment. HPB Surg 5:87-94.

Groupe d'Etude et de Traitement du Carcinome Hépatocellulaire, 1995: A comparison of lipiodol chemoembolization and conservative treatment for unresectable hepatocellular carcinoma. N Engl J Med 332:1256-1261.

Gunji T, et al, 2002: Long-term outcomes of transcatheter arterial chemoembolization with autologous blood clot for unresectable hepatocellular carcinoma. Int J Oncol 21:427-432.

Harnois DM, et al, 1999: Preoperative hepatic artery chemoembolization followed by orthotopic liver transplantation for hepatocellular carcinoma. Liver Transpl Surg 5:192-199.

Hirakawa M, et al, 1988: Gastroduodenal lesions after transcatheter arterial chemo-embolization in patients with hepatocellular carcinoma. Am J Gastroenterol 83:837-840.

Huang MS, et al, 2004: Comparison of long-term effects between intra-arterially delivered ethanol and Gelfoam for the treatment of severe arterioportal shunt in patients with hepatocellular carcinoma. World J Gastroenterol 10:825-829.

Ikeda M, et al, 2004: Transcatheter arterial chemotherapy with and without embolization in patients with hepatocellular carcinoma. Oncology 66:24-31.

Itsubo M, et al, 2002: Subsegmental transcatheter arterial embolization for small hepatocellular carcinoma. Hepatogastroenterology 49:735-739.

Iwamoto S, et al, 2003: Angiographic subsegmentectomy for the treatment of patients with small hepatocellular carcinoma. Cancer 97:1051-1056.

Jinno K, et al, 1992: Clinicopathological study on combination therapy consisting of arterial infusion of lipiodol-dissolved SMANCS and transcatheter arterial embolization for hepatocellular carcinoma. Cancer Chemother Pharmacol 31:S7-S12.

Jonas S, et al, 2001: Vascular invasion and histopathologic grading determine outcome after liver transplantation for hepatocellular carcinoma in cirrhosis. Hepatology 33:1080-1086.

Kamada K, et al, 2001: Long-term prognosis of patients undergoing transcatheter arterial chemoembolization for unresectable hepatocellular carcinoma: comparison of cisplatin lipiodol suspension and doxorubicin hydrochloride emulsion. J Vasc Interv Radiol 12:847-854.

Kamada K, et al, 2002: Combination of transcatheter arterial chemoembolization using cisplatin-lipiodol suspension and percutaneous ethanol injection for treatment of advanced small hepatocellular carcinoma. Am J Surg 184:284-290.

Kan Z, et al, 1983: In vivo microscopy of hepatic tumors in animal models: a dynamic investigation of blood supply to hepatic metastases. Radiology 187:621-626.

Kan Z, et al, 1993: Distribution and effect of iodized poppyseed oil in the liver after hepatic artery embolization: experimental study in several animal species. Radiology 186:261-266.

Kan Z, et al, 1994: Role of Kupffer cells in iodized oil embolization. Invest Radiol 29:990-993.

Katsushima S, et al, 1990: Hepatic neoplasms: effects of transcatheter arterial embolization on coagulation and fibrinolysis. Radiology 174:747-750.

Kawai S, et al, 1992: Prospective and randomized clinical trial for the treatment of hepatocellular carcinoma: a comparison of lipiodol-transcatheter arterial embolization with and without adriamycin (first cooperative study).

The Cooperative Study Group for Liver Cancer Treatment of Japan. Cancer Chemother Pharmacol 31:S1-S6.

Kemeny MM, et al, 2002: Combined-modality treatment for resectable metastatic colorectal carcinoma to the liver: surgical resection of hepatic metastases in combination with continuous infusion of chemotherapy—an intergroup study. J Clin Oncol 20:1499-1505.

Khan KN, et al, 1993: Pancreatic tissue damage by transcatheter arterial embolization for hepatoma. Dig Dis Sci 38:65-70.

Kim HC, et al, 2005: Recognizing extrahepatic collateral vessels that supply hepatocellular carcinoma to avoid complications of transcatheter arterial chemoembolization. Radiographics 25:S25-S39.

Kim HK, et al, 2001: Ischemic bile duct injury as a serious complication after transarterial chemoembolization in patients with hepatocellular carcinoma. J Clin Gastroenterol 32:423-427.

Kim JH, et al, 1995: Transcatheter arterial embolization of the internal mammary artery in hepatocellular carcinoma. J Vasc Interv Radiol 6:71-74.

Kim W, et al, 2001: Risk factors for liver abscess formation following hepatic chemoembolization. J Vasc Interv Radiol 12:965-968.

Kim YH, et al, 1999: Selective hepatic arterial chemoembolization for liver metastases in patients with carcinoid tumor or islet cell carcinoma. Cancer Invest 17:474-478.

Kirchkoff T, et al, 2000: Chemoembolization of hepatic metastases from intestinal neuroendocrine tumours. Eur J Gastroenterol Hepatol 12:141-143.

Kishimoto W, et al, 1989: Acute pancreatitis after transcatheter arterial embolization (TAE) for hepatocellular carcinoma. Am J Gastroenterol 84:1396-1399.

Kobayashi S, et al, 1993: Postmortem survey of bile duct necrosis and biloma in hepatocellular carcinoma after transcatheter arterial chemoembolization therapy: relevance to microvascular damages of peribiliary capillary plexus. Am J Gastroenterol 88:1410-1415.

Koda M, et al, 2001: Combination therapy with transcatheter arterial chemoembolization and percutaneous ethanol injection compared with percutaneous ethanol injection alone for patients with small hepatocellular carcinoma: a randomized control study. Cancer 92:1516-1524.

Kohnoe S, et al, 2002: Protracted hepatic arterial infusion with low-dose cisplatin plus 5-fluorouracil for unresectable liver metastases from colorectal cancer. Surgery 131:S128-S134.

Konno T, 1990: Targeting cancer chemotherapeutic agents by use of lipiodol contrast medium. Cancer 66:1897-1903.

Konno T, et al, 1983: Effect of arterial administration of high-molecular-weight anticancer agent SMANCS with lipid lymphographic agent on hepatoma. Eur J Cancer Clin Oncol 19:1053-1065.

Kruskal JB, et al, 1993: In vivo and in vitro analysis of the effectiveness of doxorubicin combined with temporary arterial occlusion in liver tumors. J Vasc Interv Radiol 4:741-748.

Kuroda C, et al, 1983: Gallbladder infarction following hepatic transcatheter arterial embolization: angiographic study. Radiology 149:85-89.

Kuroda C, et al, 1991: Limitation of transcatheter arterial chemoembolization using iodized oil for small hepatocellular carcinoma: a study in resected cases. Cancer 67:81-86.

Lai EC, et al, 1998: Postoperative adjuvant chemotherapy after curative resection of hepatocellular carcinoma: a randomized controlled trial. Arch Surg 133:183-188.

Lang EK, Brown CL Jr, 1993: Colorectal metastases to the liver: selective chemoembolization. Radiology 189:417-422.

Lee HS, et al, 1997: The safety and efficacy of transcatheter arterial chemoembolization in the treatment of patients with hepatocellular carcinoma and main portal vein obstruction. Cancer 79:2087-2094.

Lee HS, et al, 2001: Intraarterial lidocaine administration for relief of pain resulting from transarterial chemoembolization of hepatocellular carcinoma: its effectiveness and optimal timing of administration. Cardiovasc Interv Radiol 24:368-371.

Lee HS, et al, 2002: Therapeutic efficacy of transcatheter arterial chemoembolization as compared with hepatic resection in hepatocellular carcinoma patients with compensated liver function in a hepatitis B virus–endemic area: a prospective cohort study. J Clin Oncol 20:4459-4465.

Lencioni R, et al, 1994: Transcatheter arterial embolization followed by percutaneous ethanol injection in the treatment of hepatocellular carcinoma. Cardiovasc Interv Radiol 17:70-75.

Leung DA, et al, 2001: Determinants of postembolization syndrome after hepatic chemoembolization. J Vasc Interv Radiol 12:321-326.

Levy AD, 2002: Malignant liver tumors. Clin Liver Dis 6:147-164.

Lim HK, Han JK, 2002: Hepatocellular carcinoma: evaluation of therapeutic response to interventional procedures. Abdom Imaging 27:168-179.

Lin DY, et al, 1996: Gastrointestinal bleeding after hepatic transcatheter arterial embolization in patients with hepatocellular carcinoma. Gastrointest Endosc 43:132-137.

Liu L, et al, 2003: Current treatment for liver metastases from colorectal cancer. World J Gastroenterol 9:193-200.

Llovet JM, et al, 1999: Prognosis of hepatocellular carcinoma: the BCLC staging classification. Semin Liver Dis 19:329-338.

Llovet JM, et al, 2002: Arterial embolisation or chemoembolisation versus symptomatic treatment in patients with unresectable hepatocellular carcinoma: a randomized controlled trial. Lancet 359:1734-1739.

Llovet JM, et al, 2003: Hepatocellular carcinoma. Lancet 362:1907-1917.

Lo CM, et al, 2002: Randomized controlled trial of transarterial lipiodol chemoembolization for unresectable hepatocellular carcinoma. Hepatology 35:1164-1171.

Lu CD, et al, 1999: Preoperative transcatheter arterial chemoembolization and prognosis of patients with hepatocellular carcinomas: retrospective analysis of 120 cases. World J Surg 23:293-300.

Maeda S, et al, 2002: Survival and local recurrence rates of hepatocellular carcinoma patients treated by transarterial chemolipiodolization with and without embolization. Hepatol Res 23:202-210.

Majno PE, et al, 1997: Influence of preoperative transarterial lipiodol chemoembolization on resection and transplantation for hepatocellular carcinoma in patients with cirrhosis. Ann Surg 226:688-701.

Martin M, et al, 1996: Intrahepatic arterial chemoembolization for hepatocellular carcinoma and metastatic neuroendocrine tumors in the era of liver transplantation. Am Surg 62:724-732.

Martinelli DJ, et al, 1994: Utility of embolization or chemoembolization as second-line treatment in patients with advanced or recurrent colorectal carcinoma. Cancer 74:1706-1712.

Matsui O, et al, 1993: Small hepatocellular carcinoma: treatment with subsegmental transcatheter arterial embolization. Radiology 188:79-83.

Matsui O, et al, 1994: Subsegmental transcatheter arterial embolization for small hepatocellular carcinomas: local therapeutic effect and 5-year survival rate. Cancer Chemother Pharmacol 33:84-88.

Matsuo N, et al, 1997: Optimal lipiodol volume in transcatheter arterial chemoembolotherapy for hepatocellular carcinoma: study based on lipiodol accumulation patterns and histopathologic findings. Semin Oncol 24: S6-61-S6-70.

Mavligit GM, et al, 1988: Regression of ocular melanoma metastatic to the liver after hepatic arterial chemoembolization with cisplatin and polyvinyl sponge. JAMA 260:974-976.

Mavligit GM, et al, 1995: Gastrointestinal leiomyosarcoma metastatic to the liver: durable tumor regression by hepatic chemoembolization infusion with cisplatin and vinblastine. Cancer 75:2083-2088.

Mazzaferro V, et al, 1996: Liver transplantation for the treatment of small hepatocellular carcinomas in patients with cirrhosis. N Engl J Med 334: 693-699.

Meyers MO, et al, 2003: Locoregional strategies for colorectal hepatic metastases. Clin Colorectal Cancer 3:34-44.

Miyayama S, et al, 2001: Hepatocellular carcinoma with blood supply from omental branches: treatment with transcatheter arterial embolization. J Vasc Interv Radiol 12:1285-1290.

Montalto G, et al, 2002: Epidemiology, risk factors, and natural history of hepatocellular carcinoma. Ann N Y Acad Sci 963:13-20.

Mor E, et al, 1998: Treatment of hepatocellular carcinoma associated with cirrhosis in the era of liver transplantation. Ann Intern Med 129:643-653.

Mori W, et al, 1966: Hepatic artery ligation and tumor necrosis in the liver. Surgery 59:359-363.

Morse SS, et al, 1985: Hepatoma, arterioportal shunting, and hyperkinetic portal hypertension: therapeutic embolization. Radiology 155:77-82.

Nagasue N, et al, 1990: Assessment of pattern and treatment of intrahepatic recurrence after resection of hepatocellular carcinoma. Surg Gynecol Obstet 171:217-222.

Nakai M, et al, 2001: Hepatocellular carcinoma: involvement of the internal mammary artery. Radiology 219:147-152.

Nakajo M, et al, 1998: Biodistribution and in vivo kinetics of iodine-131 lipiodol infused via the hepatic artery of patients with hepatic cancer. J Nucl Med 29:1066-1077.

Nakamura H, et al, 1983: Transcatheter embolization of hepatocellular carcinoma: assessment of efficacy in case of resection following embolization. Radiology 147:401-405.

Nakamura H, et al, 1989: Transcatheter oily chemoembolization of hepatocellular carcinoma. Radiology 170:783-786.

Nakamura H, et al, 1993: Response to transcatheter oily chemoembolization in hepatocellular carcinoma 3 cm or less: a study in 50 patients who underwent surgery. Hepatogastroenterology 40:6-9.

Nakamura H, et al, 1994: Five-year survival after transcatheter chemoembolization for hepatocellular carcinoma. Cancer Chemother Pharmacol 33: S89-S92.

Nakao N, et al, 1986: Hepatocellular carcinoma: combined hepatic, arterial, and portal venous embolization. Radiology 161:303-307.

Nakaoka R, et al, 2000: Repeated hepatic arterial chemoembolization therapy for management of a patient with metastatic carcinoid tumors of the liver. Am J Gastroenterol 95:1842-1843.

Nakoa N, et al, 1991: Recurrent hepatocellular carcinoma after partial hepatectomy: value of treatment with transcatheter arterial chemoembolization. AJR Am J Roentgenol 156:1177-1179.

Ngan H, Peh WC, 1997: Arteriovenous shunting in hepatocellular carcinoma: its prevalence and clinical significance. Clin Radiol 52:36-40.

Ngan H, et al, 1998: The role of hepatic arterial embolization in the treatment of spontaneous rupture of hepatocellular carcinoma. Clin Radiol 53: 338-341.

Nishimine K, et al, 1994: Segmental transarterial chemoembolization with Lipiodol mixed with anticancer drugs for nonresectable hepatocellular carcinoma: follow-up CT and therapeutic results. Cancer Chemother Pharmacol 33:S60-S68.

Nishioka Y, et al, 1994: A study of embolizing materials for chemo-embolization therapy of hepatocellular carcinoma: effects of particle size and dose on chitin-containing cis-diamminedichloroplatinum (II) albumin microsphere antitumor activity in VX2 hepatic tumor model rabbits. Biol Pharm Bull 17:1251-1255.

Okazaki M, et al, 1991: Intraperitoneal hemorrhage from hepatocellular carcinoma: emergency chemoembolization or embolization. Radiology 180: 647-651.

Okuda K, et al, 1985: Natural history of hepatocellular carcinoma and prognosis in relation to treatment: study of 850 patients. Cancer 56:918-928.

Okusaka T, et al, 2000: Evaluation of the therapeutic effect of transcatheter arterial embolization for hepatocellular carcinoma. Oncology 58:293-299.

Okusaka T, et al, 2002: Transcatheter arterial embolization with zinostatin stimalamer for hepatocellular carcinoma. Oncology 62:228-233.

Ong GY, et al, 2004: Liver abscess complicating transcatheter arterial embolization: a rare but serious complication: a retrospective study after 3878 procedures. Eur J Gastroenterol Hepatol 16:737-742.

Ouchi K, et al, 2000: Prediction of recurrence and extratumor spread of hepatocellular carcinoma following resection. J Surg Oncol 75:241-245.

Pacella CM, et al, 2001: Hepatocellular carcinoma: long-term results of combined treatment with laser thermal ablation and transcatheter arterial chemoembolization. Radiology 219:669-678.

Park JH, et al, 1993: Postoperative recurrence of hepatocellular carcinoma: results of transcatheter arterial chemoembolization. Cardiovasc Interv Radiol 16:21-24.

Park SI, et al, 2003: Extrahepatic collateral supply of hepatocellular carcinoma by the intercostal arteries. J Vasc Interv Radiol 14:461-468.

Park YN, et al, 1998: Neoangiogenesis and sinusoidal "capillarization" in dysplastic nodules of the liver. Am J Surg Pathol 22:656-662.

Parkin DM, et al, 2001: Estimating the world cancer burden: GLOBOCAN 2000. Int J Cancer 94:153-156.

Paye F, et al, 1999: Cytolysis following chemoembolization for hepatocellular carcinoma. Br J Surg 86:176-180.

Pelletier G, et al, 1990: A randomized trial of hepatic arterial chemoembolization in patients with unresectable hepatocellular carcinoma. J Hepatol 11: 181-184.

Pelletier G, et al, 1998: Treatment of unresectable hepatocellular carcinoma with lipiodol chemoembolization: a multicenter randomized trial. J Hepatol 29:129-134.

Penna C, Nordlinger B, 2002: Colorectal metastasis (liver and lung). Surg Clin North Am 82:1075-1090.

Ramsey DE, et al, 2002: Chemoembolization of hepatocellular carcinoma. J Vasc Interv Radiol 13:S211-S221.

Raoul JL, et al, 1992: Chemoembolization of hepatocellular carcinomas: a study of the biodistribution and pharmacokinetics of doxorubicin. Cancer 70: 585-590.

Ren ZG, et al, 2004: Postoperative adjuvant arterial chemoembolization improves survival of hepatocellular carcinoma patients with risk factors for residual tumor: a retrospective control study. World J Gastroenterol 10: 2791-2794.

Riel JM, et al, 2000: Hepatic arterial 5-fluorouracil in patients with liver metastases of colorectal cancer: single-centre experience in 145 patients. Ann Oncol 11: 1563-1570.

Roche A, et al, 2003: Trans-catheter arterial chemoembolization as first-line treatment for hepatic metastases from endocrine tumors. Eur Radiol 13: 136-140.

Romano M, et al, 2003: Chemoembolization for hepatocellular carcinoma: effect of intraarterial lidocaine in peri- and post-procedural pain and hospitalization. Radiol Med (Torino) 105:350-355.

Rose AT, et al, 1998: Hepatocellular carcinoma outcomes based on indicated treatment strategy. Am Surg 64:1128-1135.

Rossi S, et al, 2000: Percutaneous radio-frequency thermal ablation of nonresectable hepatocellular carcinoma after occlusion of tumor blood supply. Radiology 217:119-126.

Sakamoto I, et al, 1998: Complications associated with transcatheter arterial embolization for hepatic tumors. Radiographics 18:605-619.

Sakamoto I, et al, 2003: Intrahepatic biloma formation (bile duct necrosis) after transcatheter arterial chemoembolization. AJR Am J Roentgenol 181:79-87.

Sakon M, et al, 1991: Effects of transcatheter hepatic arterial embolization on coagulation and fibrinolysis in patients with hepatocellular carcinoma. Am J Gastroenterol 86:1800-1803.

Salman HS, et al, 2002: Randomized phase II trial of embolization therapy versus chemoembolization therapy in previously treated patients with colorectal carcinoma metastatic to the liver. Clin Colorectal Cancer 2:173-179.

Sangro B, et al, 1998: Prognosis of hepatocellular carcinoma in relation to treatment: a multivariate analysis of 178 patients from a single European institution. Surgery 124:575-583.

Sanz-Altamira PM, et al, 1997: Selective chemoembolization in the management of hepatic metastases in refractory colorectal carcinoma: a phase II trial. Dis Colon Rectum 40:770-775.

Sasaki Y, et al, 1987: A new approach to chemoembolization therapy for hepatoma using ethiodized oil, cisplatin, and gelatin sponge. Cancer 60:1194-1203.

Sawada S, 1989: Transcatheter oily chemoembolization of hepatocellular carcinoma. Radiology 170:783-786.

Schwartz JD, et al, 2002: Neoadjuvant and adjuvant therapy for resectable hepatocellular carcinoma: review of the randomized clinical trials. Lancet Oncol 3:593-603.

Shah SR, et al, 1998: Tumor ablation and hepatic decompensation rates in multi-agent chemoembolization of hepatocellular carcinoma. QJM 91:821-828.

Shankar A, et al, 1996: The vascularity of colorectal liver metastases. Eur J Surg Oncol 22:389-396.

Shimoda M, et al, 2001: Prophylactic chemolipiodolization for postoperative hepatoma patients. Hepatogastroenterology 48:493-497.

Sigurdson ER, et al, 1987: Tumor and liver drug uptake following hepatic artery and portal vein infusion. J Clin Oncol 5:1836-1840.

So YH, et al, 2003: Balloon fenestration of iatrogenic celiac artery dissection. J Vasc Interv Radiol 14:493-496.

Song SY, et al, 2001: Liver abscess after transcatheter oily chemoembolization for hepatic tumors: incidence, predisposing factors, and clinical outcome. J Vasc Interv Radiol 12:313-320.

Sonomura T, et al, 1997: Dependency of tissue necrosis on gelatin sponge particle size after canine hepatic artery embolization. Cardiovasc Interv Radiol 20:50-53.

Strohmeyer T, et al, 1987: Angioarchitecture and blood supply of micro- and macrometastases in human livers: an anatomic-pathological investigation using injection-techniques. J Hepatol 4:181-189.

Stuart K, 2003: Chemoembolization in the management of liver tumors. Oncologist 8:425-437.

Sugano S, et al, 1994: Intrahepatic arteriovenous shunting due to hepatocellular carcinoma and cirrhosis, and its change by transcatheter arterial embolization. Am J Gastroenterol 89:184-188.

Suzuki K, et al, 1998: Transcatheter arterial chemo-embolization for humoral hypercalcemia of hepatocellular carcinoma. Gastroenterol Jpn 23:29-36.

Suzuki M, et al, 1997: Indication of chemoembolization therapy without gelatin sponge for hepatocellular carcinoma. Semin Oncol 24:S6-110-S6-115.

Suzuki Y, et al, 2003: Clinical utility of sequential imaging of hepatocellular carcinoma by contrast-enhanced power Doppler ultrasonography. Eur J Radiol 48:214-219.

Tajima T, et al, 2002a: Pulmonary complications after hepatic artery chemoembolization or infusion via the inferior phrenic artery for primary liver cancer. J Vasc Interv Radiol 13:893-900.

Tajima T, et al, 2002b: Sequential hemodynamic change in hepatocellular carcinoma and dysplastic nodules: CT angiography and pathologic correlation. AJR Am J Roentgenol 178:885-897.

Takayasu K, et al, 1984: Splenic infarction, a complication of transcatheter hepatic arterial embolization for liver malignancies. Radiology 151:371-375.

Takayasu K, et al, 1987: Hepatocellular carcinoma: treatment with intraarterial iodized oil with and without chemotherapeutic agents. Radiology 163:345-351.

Takayasu K, et al, 1989: Clinical and radiologic assessments of the results of hepatectomy for small hepatocellular carcinoma and therapeutic arterial embolization for postoperative recurrence. Cancer 64:1848-1852.

Takayasu K, et al, 1992: Postresection recurrence of hepatocellular carcinoma treated by arterial embolization: analysis of prognostic factors. Hepatology 16:906-911.

Takayasu K, et al, 2000: Comparison of CT findings with resected specimens after chemoembolization with iodized oil for hepatocellular carcinoma. AJR Am J Roentgenol 175:699-704.

Tanabe N, et al, 1998: Hepatocellular carcinomas supplied by inferior phrenic arteries. Acta Radiol 39:443-446.

Tanaka K, et al, 1991: Hepatocellular carcinoma: treatment with a combination therapy of transcatheter arterial embolization and percutaneous ethanol injection. Radiology 179:713-717.

Tanaka K, et al, 1999: Use of transcatheter arterial infusion of anticancer agents with lipiodol to prevent recurrence of hepatocellular carcinoma after hepatic resection. Hepatogastroenterology 46:1083-1088.

Tanaka Y, et al, 2002: A comparison of the molecular clock of hepatitis C virus in the United States and Japan predicts that hepatocellular carcinoma incidence in the United States will increase over the next two decades. Proc Natl Acad Sci U S A 99:1584-1589.

Taniguchi H, et al, 1993: Blood supply and drug delivery to primary and secondary human liver cancers studied with in vivo bromodeoxyuridine labeling. Cancer 71:50-55.

Tarazov PG, et al, 2000: Ischemic complications of transcatheter arterial chemoembolization in liver malignancies. Acta Radiol 41:156-160.

Tazawa J, et al, 2001: Radiation therapy in combination with transcatheter arterial chemoembolization for hepatocellular carcinoma with extensive portal vein involvement. J Gastroenterol Hepatol 16:660-665.

Tono T, et al, 2000: Limited but definite efficacy of prophylactic hepatic arterial infusion chemotherapy after curative resection of colorectal liver metastases: a randomized study. Cancer 88:1549-1556.

Troisi R, et al, 1998: Multimodal treatment for hepatocellular carcinoma on cirrhosis: the role of chemoembolization and alcoholization before liver transplantation. Clin Transplant 12:313-319.

Ueno K, et al, 1995: Embolization of the hepatic falciform artery to prevent supraumbilical skin rash during transcatheter arterial chemoembolization for hepatocellular carcinoma. Cardiovasc Interv Radiol 18:183-185.

Ueno K, et al, 2000: Transcatheter arterial chemoembolization therapy using iodized oil for patients with unresectable hepatocellular carcinoma: evaluation of three kinds of regimens and analysis of prognostic factors. Cancer 88:1574-1581.

Ueno S, et al, 2001: Discrimination value of the new Western prognostic system (CLIP score) for hepatocellular carcinoma in 662 Japanese patients. Hepatology 34:529-534.

Veltri A, et al, 1998: Effect of preoperative radiological treatment of hepatocellular carcinoma before liver transplantation: a retrospective study. Cardiovasc Interv Radiol 21:393-398.

Venook AP, 1999: Embolization and chemoembolization therapy for neuroendocrine tumors. Curr Opin Oncol 11:38-41.

Venook AP, et al, 1990: Chemoembolization for hepatocellular carcinoma. J Clin Oncol 8:1108-1114.

Wakasa K, et al, 1990: Effect of transcatheter arterial embolization on the boundary architecture of hepatocellular carcinoma. Cancer 65:913-919.

Walser RH, et al, 1996: Diagnostic angioscintigraphic evaluation of malignant hepatic tumors before catheter embolization: determination of shunt, flow distribution, and reflux. Cardiovasc Interv Radiol 19:77-81.

Winkelbauer FW, et al, 1995: Hepatic artery embolotherapy of hepatic metastases from carcinoid tumors: value of using a mixture of cyanoacrylate and ethiodized oil. AJR Am J Roentgenol 165:323-327.

Won JY, et al, 2003: Supplemental transcatheter arterial chemoembolization through a collateral omental artery: treatment for hepatocellular carcinoma. Cardiovasc Interv Radiol 26:136-140.

Wu CC, et al, 1995: Preoperative transcatheter arterial chemoembolization for resectable large hepatocellular carcinoma: a reappraisal. Br J Surg 82:122-126.

Wu JX, et al, 2002: Factors related to acute upper gastrointestinal bleeding after transcatheter arterial chemoembolization in patients with hepatocellular carcinoma. Ai Zheng 21:881-884.

Yamada R, et al, 1983: Hepatic artery embolization in 120 patients with nonresectable HCC. Radiology 148:397-401.

Yamada R, et al, 1995: Transcatheter arterial chemoembolization (TACE) in the treatment of unresectable liver cancer. World J Surg 19:795-800.

Yamaguchi A, et al, 2000: Correlation between angiographically assessed vascularity and blood flow in hepatic metastases in patients with colorectal carcinoma. Cancer 89:1236-1244.

Yamamoto K, et al, 1997: Evaluation of combined therapy with chemoembolization and ethanol injection for advanced hepatocellular carcinoma. Semin Oncol 24:S6-50-S6-55.

Yamanaka J, et al, 2000: Clinicopathologic analysis of stage II-III hepatocellular carcinoma showing early massive recurrence after liver resection. J Gastroenterol Hepatol 15:1192-1198.

Yao FY, et al, 2001: Liver transplantation for hepatocellular carcinoma: expansion of the tumor size limits does not adversely impact survival. Hepatology 33:1394-1403.

Yao KA, et al, 2001: Indications and results of liver resection and hepatic chemoembolization for metastatic gastrointestinal neuroendocrine tumors. Surgery 130:677-682.

Yoon DY, et al, 1995: Iatrogenic dissection of the celiac artery and its branches during transcatheter arterial embolization for hepatocellular carcinoma: outcome in 40 patients. Cardiovasc Interv Radiol 18:16-19.

Young N, et al, 1993: Symptom relief and survival after chemo-embolization with adriamycin, lipiodol and gelfoam for hepatocellular carcinoma. Australas Radiol 37:173-176.

Yu AS, Keeffe EB, 2003: Management of hepatocellular carcinoma. Rev Gastroenterol Disord 3:8-24.

Yu JS, et al, 2001: Bile duct injuries leading to portal vein obliteration after transcatheter arterial chemoembolization in the liver: CT findings and initial observations. Radiology 221:429-436.

Yu JS, et al, 2002: Predisposing factors of bile duct injury after transcatheter arterial chemoembolization (TACE) for hepatic malignancy. Cardiovasc Interv Radiol 25:270-274.

Zhang Z, et al, 2000: The effect of preoperative transcatheter hepatic arterial chemoembolization on disease-free survival after hepatectomy for hepatocellular carcinoma. Cancer 89:2606-2612.

Zhu LX, et al, 1996: Spontaneous rupture of hepatocellular carcinoma. Br J Surg 83:602-607.

Radiotherapy of Liver Tumors

75a SELECTIVE INTERNAL RADIATION THERAPY FOR LIVER TUMORS

R. S. STUBBS AND M. M. CORREIA

The most common primary cancer occurring worldwide is hepatocellular carcinoma (HCC) (see Ch. 71), which without effective treatment carries a prognosis of only 3 to 6 months. Most other common cancers spread to the liver before the patient dies, and generally liver metastases are the most important determinant of the time of death. In a few cancers, notably colorectal cancer (CRC), the liver may be the only macroscopic site of disease at the time of death (see Ch. 73a). This fact makes regional approaches to liver tumors attractive as a means of occasionally curing patients, but more often extending the life of such patients.

Regional approaches to liver tumors include resection, ablation, radiation therapy, and regional chemotherapy. Such approaches are particularly attractive for tumors for which systemic therapy is currently of limited or short-lived benefit. The number, size, or site of liver tumors most often precludes the option of resection or ablation. Until more recently, the use of radiation therapy has been severely limited because of the poor tolerance of normal liver parenchyma to radiation and the propensity for the development of fatal radiation hepatitis if whole liver doses greater than 30 to 35 Gy are delivered (Ingold et al, 1965).

The technique of selective internal radiation therapy (SIRT) has been developed to provide a therapeutic option for tumors localized to the liver, almost regardless of site, size, or number (Fig. 75a.1). The opportunity exists for use of SIRT as a stand-alone modality or in conjunction with regional chemotherapy or systemic chemotherapy.

SIRT relies on the knowledge that liver tumors, regardless of vascularity and type, derive most of their blood supply from the hepatic artery, whereas the normal liver substance derives most of its blood supply from the portal vein (Matsui et al, 1991; Taylor et al, 1979). For this reason, if suitable radiation sources are delivered into the liver via the hepatic artery, and in a form that binds to or is trapped within liver tumors, a degree of selective uptake is achieved. This selective uptake may permit tumoricidal doses of radiation to be delivered where otherwise they could not. In theoretical terms, selective uptake might be achieved by linking a radiation source to (1) microspheres, which become trapped in capillary beds; (2) antibodies, which bind to tumor-specific antigens; or (3) substances such as lipiodol, which are known to bind to particular liver tumors. In practical terms, clinical experience to date has been limited largely to the use of yttrium 90 (^{90}Y) bound to glass or resin microspheres or iodine 131 (^{131}I) incorporated into lipiodol.

RADIATION SOURCES

Iodine 131 Lipiodol

Lipiodol is a poppy seed oil known to be cleared more slowly from HCC cells than from normal liver cells, which means it is retained by HCC cells after hepatic arterial injection for a longer period than by normal hepatocytes (Raoul et al, 1988). Because lipiodol is naturally iodinated, it can be imaged on plain x-rays and computed tomography (CT) scans and be readily iodinated with ^{131}I to become a therapeutic agent as a source of radiation. This property has been exploited in the technique of lipiodol CT (Nakayama et al, 2001; Ngan 1990; Yumoto et al, 1985), which can be helpful in imaging small multifocal HCC in the setting of cirrhosis (Okayasu et al, 1988; Yumoto et al, 1985). Similarly, ^{131}I-lipiodol has been widely used alone as a medium for SIRT or mixed with a variety of chemotherapeutic agents in the technique of transarterial chemoembolization (TACE) (Brans et al, 2003; Ho et al, 1998; Raoul et al, 1994, 1997; Rindani et al, 2002).

^{131}I is a relatively low energy, mixed γ and β emitter with a half-life of 8 days. It has maximum penetration in human tissue of 1 to 2 mm. Because of γ emissions, stringent radiation protection measures are required during and after administration for the safety of the patient, visitors, and staff. The half-life of 8 days means these measures must be maintained for 1 to 2 weeks after delivery, necessitating hospitalization and isolation for 10 to 14 days depending on the dose given. Collection and special disposal of all human waste is required throughout this period after ^{131}I-lipiodol administration.

^{131}I-Lipiodol usually is delivered into the hepatic artery over a few minutes, under fluoroscopic control, via a catheter placed by Seldinger technique. Anomalous hepatic arterial vessels may preclude the treatment or dictate the need for embolization of one or more aberrant vessels before ^{131}I-lipiodol injection. Doses of 500 to 2000 MBq are used per treatment, with three to five repeat treatments being given at 3-month intervals. Doses given generally are determined by issues of radiation exposure to health professionals and the required duration of patient isolation, which can be 10 to 14 days after a single dose. ^{131}I-lipiodol is most suited to the treatment of HCC, but some other tumors, including some neuroendocrine tumors, have been shown to be lipiodol-avid and for that reason may be suitable for this

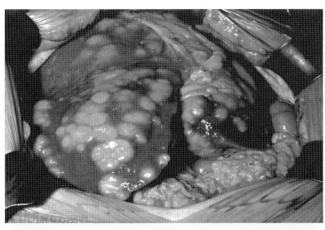

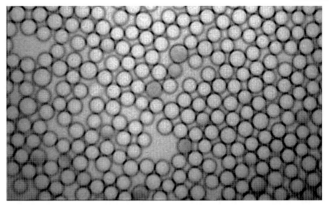

Fig. 75a.2. Photomicrograph of ⁹⁰Y microspheres (SIR-spheres) used for SIRT.

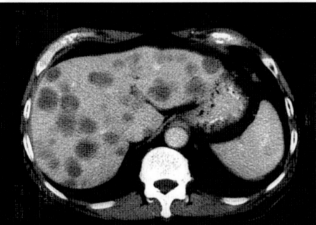

Fig. 75a.1. Extensive colorectal liver metastases suitable for SIRT. Such extensive disease is not suitable for any other locally ablative therapy.

approach (Hewitt et al, 1998). The requirements for special radiation protection measures to be taken for 10 to 14 days starting with the dispensing and administration of ¹³¹I-lipiodol make it a much less convenient source of radiation for clinical use than ⁹⁰Y, which is a pure β emitter.

Yttrium 90 Microspheres

⁹⁰Y is a high energy pure β emitter with a half-life of 64 hours that can be linked to microspheres. These characteristics make it particularly suitable for clinical use. Its relatively high energy emissions give it maximum penetration in human tissue of around 11 mm, arguably rendering it more appropriate than ¹³¹I-lipiodol for use in a large solid organ such as the liver. Issues of radiation protection for patients, visitors, and staff are minimal and easily addressed. Outpatient treatment or 1- to 2-day hospitalization is the norm. Because there is effectively no passage of ⁹⁰Y into body fluids after hepatic arterial injection of the labeled microspheres, the management of patients undergoing SIRT with ⁹⁰Y is generally straightforward.

Two varieties of ⁹⁰Y microspheres are currently commercially available. The Therasphere (MDS Nordion) is a glass microsphere containing ⁹⁰Y, and SIR-spheres (Sirtex Medical Ltd, Lake Forest, IL) are resin microspheres coated with ⁹⁰Y (Fig. 75a.2). Both are approximately 25 to 35 mm in diameter and become trapped in the capillary bed of liver tumors after hepatic artery administration.

From this position, they set up a zone of radiation around each microsphere. Average doses of around 2 GBq are given by the administration of approximately 4 to 8 million Theraspheres or 20 to 40 million SIR-spheres. Neither the Therasphere dose nor the SIR-spheres dose is sufficient to create significant devascularization. Any therapeutic benefit is related to the radiation delivered. Delivery of either type of microsphere achieves a high degree of selective uptake within liver tumors resulting in a high dose of radiation to the tumor with little or no risk of serious radiation hepatitis. This approach is potentially applicable to a wide variety of primary and secondary liver tumors. Estimates of average absorbed doses of radiation to tumors after a single dose are in the vicinity of 150 to 250 Gy, with average doses to normal liver parenchyma being in the vicinity of 15 to 25 Gy (Lau et al, 1998). Although these doses are average doses rather than uniform doses, based on point source radiation, they compare favorably with normal tumoricidal doses of 50 to 60 Gy given by external-beam radiation in other contexts. Although a single treatment is the norm, repeat treatments can be given with good effect, if a good response to the initial treatment was obtained (Lau et al, 1998; Stubbs & Wickremesekera, 2004a, 2004b).

The concept of using ⁹⁰Y microspheres for SIRT is not new, and studies date back to the 1960s, when ⁹⁰Y ceramic microspheres were administered percutaneously into the hepatic artery via an angiographic catheter (Ariel, 1965; Ariel & Pack, 1967). Interest in this approach declined for a time because of complications, such as bone marrow depression related to dissociation or leaching of ⁹⁰Y from the microspheres, radiation gastritis and ulceration resulting from inadvertent delivery of microspheres into the small vessels of the stomach and duodenum, and radiation hepatitis and pulmonary fibrosis (Grady, 1979; Mantravadi et al, 1982). The problem of leaching was overcome by the development of Theraspheres and SIR-spheres in the 1980s and 1990s, and this together with a better understanding of the issues related to safe administration has led to renewed interest in and development of SIRT for liver tumors.

POTENTIAL HAZARDS

Leaching of ⁹⁰Y from microspheres is not seen with the current commercially available products, but if it were to occur, the principal clinical effect would be bone marrow depression because of uptake of the free ⁹⁰Y into bone. Radiation hepatitis is a theoretical concern with the delivery of large doses of

^{90}Y to the liver, but in practical terms, this seldom becomes clinically manifest using currently employed dosing schedules. Radiation pneumonitis is another theoretical concern, which would result if sufficient microspheres passed via arteriovenous shunts from the liver to the pulmonary vasculature. Potential for this complication can be determined by performing a nuclear medicine scan after administration of a small, harmless dose of technetium 99m macroaggregated albumin (^{99m}Tc-MAA) into the hepatic artery before the performance of SIRT (Fig. 75a.3). Because the particle size of the MAA is similar to that of the microspheres, the distribution of the former approximately indicates the distribution of the latter. Provided that less than 13% of the ^{99m}Tc-MAA passes to the lungs (liver-lung shunt), it is considered safe to administer standard doses of ^{90}Y microspheres, and radiation pneumonitis is not seen (Leung et al, 1995). A shunt of greater than 13% is almost never seen in patients with CRC liver metastases, but is seen frequently in patients with cirrhosis or HCC or both. The final and most troublesome of the potential risks is radiation injury to foregut structures, resulting from the passage of some of the ^{90}Y microspheres to these structures from vessels arising from the hepatic artery. In this respect, the gastroduodenal artery, right gastric artery, and pancreaticoduodenal branches are the most worrying. Gastric or duodenal ulceration with associated pain, nausea, and vomiting are a major problem for patients when they occur. The injury is slow to heal, and the symptoms respond poorly to medication. Although ^{99m}Tc-MAA scanning (see Fig. 75a.3) is also capable of identifying many patients at risk of major damage to the gastroduodenum from inadvertent perfusion of these structures, it is not totally reliable in this respect. The key to preventing these complications lies with the method and manner of ^{90}Y microsphere administration into the hepatic artery.

TECHNICAL CONSIDERATIONS

Hepatic Arterial Delivery

Safe and effective delivery of ^{90}Y microspheres requires administration into the liver via the hepatic artery with minimal or no misperfusion through small branches into other foregut structures (i.e., stomach, duodenum, and pancreas). In most situations, the goal is treatment of the whole liver, but occasionally tumor may be confined to one side of the liver, making unilateral or selective treatment an option. In our experience, whole liver treatment is best accomplished at a single treatment session, but some prefer to treat one side of the liver by selective percutaneous catheterization followed by the other side, some time later. Although this latter approach may have advantages in terms of protection against inadvertent misperfusion of the foregut, it has major cost implications and carries with it a significant risk of incomplete treatment. This situation may occur because of patient or physician unwillingness to proceed to the other side, owing to changes in the patient's status in the interim.

Hepatic arterial delivery may be by percutaneous catheter using the Seldinger technique (Lau et al, 1998) or via a surgically implanted hepatic artery port (Stubbs et al, 2001). For whole liver delivery, the latter is inherently safer and more reliable because complete isolation of the hepatic arterial supply from that of the foregut can be achieved at the time of surgery. Anomalous hepatic arterial supply can be dealt with more easily by vessel ligation, ensuring treatment of the whole liver. The technique of port placement must be meticulous (see Ch. 79) and can be assisted by the use of either methylene blue, which we prefer, or fluorescein and a Wood's lamp to ensure isolation of the liver from other foregut structures (Wickremesekera et al, 2000). The use of a surgically implanted port has the added advantage of permitting delivery of hepatic arterial chemotherapy after SIRT, which may be of additional benefit to patients with liver-only CRC metastases. The internal diameter of the port catheter should be at least 0.8 mm to avoid the risk of occlusion with microspheres during delivery and the possibility of catheter "blowout" when such an occlusion is being cleared by forceful injection. Delivery through a percutaneous catheter is appealing, but calls for particular safeguards. One must be prepared for having to embolize anomalous arteries and small branches passing to the foregut. The gastroduodenal artery is usually dealt with easily, but the right gastric artery when it arises from the left hepatic artery is more problematic. This situation is easily missed and can result in serious radiation gastritis and perforation after SIRT. Ideally, the catheter should be

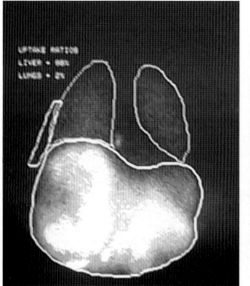

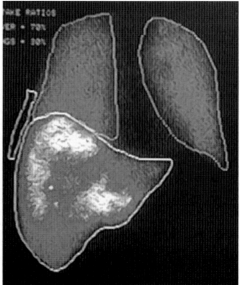

Fig. 75a.3. MAA scan before SIRT shows a liver-lung shunt of 2% in a patient with metastatic CRC (**A**) and 30% in a patient with metastatic leiomyosarcoma (**B**), which was not suitable for SIRT.

A   B

5-Fr or larger to overcome the potential for catheter blockage during microsphere administration, but often only a 3-Fr Tracker catheter can be placed. Selective catheterization may be appropriate for unilateral tumors or if treatment is planned for two sessions. This approach diminishes considerably the risk of radiation damage to foregut structures associated with a percutaneous technique. The option of repositioning the catheter or placing a second selective catheter at the one session does exist, but currently is not commonly exercised.

Yttrium 90 Microsphere Administration

SIRT is usually administered as a single treatment under mild sedation and intravenous analgesia. This can be accomplished as an outpatient procedure with the patient going home within 24 hours, as is commonly the case in the United States. In our practice, SIRT is ordinarily timed for the same admission as placement of a hepatic artery port or percutaneous catheter placement, and the patient remains in the hospital for 48 hours after SIRT. We and other authors administer a small dose of angiotensin II (50 µg) or phenylephrine (0.5 mg) into the hepatic artery immediately before administration of ^{90}Y microspheres to enhance tumor uptake. This enhancement occurs because of the relatively greater vasoconstriction achieved by these agents in normal liver arterioles compared with tumor arterioles (Burton et al, 1988). SIRT with ^{90}Y microspheres is accomplished in 5 to 10 minutes using a specially constructed acrylic delivery system (Fig. 75a.4) that allows for pulsed delivery of the microspheres in a total volume of approximately 40 to 60 mL. No special isolation of the patient or handling of body fluids is required because the ^{90}Y microspheres are trapped within capillary beds, are nondegradable, and are a source of pure β radiation, which is almost totally shielded by the abdominal/chest wall.

Dosing with ^{90}Y microspheres generally has been crudely tailored to the percentage of liver replacement by tumor. Much of

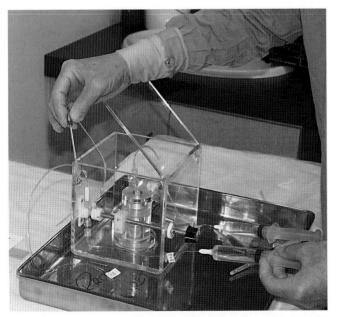

Fig. 75a.4. Acrylic apparatus for delivery of SIR-spheres. The 5-mm-thick acrylic box would provide a partial shield from any spilled SIR-spheres. The SIR-spheres themselves are contained within a glass vial held within a 10-mm-thick acrylic case, which is positioned in the center of the apparatus.

the published experience has employed whole liver doses of 2 GBq for 25% liver replacement, 2.5 GBq for 25% to 50% liver replacement, and 3 GBq for more than 50% liver replacement (Gray et al, 2000; Stubbs et al, 2001). These doses are adjusted by approximately 60% and 40% for selective right and left liver administration, respectively. It is doubtful that doses of 3 GBq are necessary, and we now generally give either 2 GBq or 2.5 GBq depending on less than or greater than 50% liver replacement. Although with external-beam radiation, doses are described as absorbed doses (in Gy), it is not possible to do this with SIRT because delivery is nonuniform, being based on a point source of radiation. Although it is possible to calculate average absorbed doses achieved by SIRT, to do so entails numerous assumptions based on estimates of tumor-to-normal liver uptake and of tumor volume versus liver volume. For this reason, doses administered normally are described in terms of actual radiation dose in Ci or Bq. Delivery of the above-mentioned doses can be calculated to result in average absorbed doses to liver tumor of 200 to 300 Gy (Lau et al, 1998).

After hepatic arterial administration, the distribution of microspheres is nonuniform within normal liver and liver tumor and varies according to the arterial blood supply with a marked tendency to distribute to the peripheral edges of the tumors (Campbell et al, 2000; Kennedy AS et al, 2004). Although supralethal doses of radiation generally are delivered to liver tumors by SIRT techniques, the nonhomogeneous distribution of microspheres achieved together with the point source of the radiation means that some of the cells within any tumor mass probably receive sublethal doses of radiation and survive. The treatment should not be regarded as potentially curative, although on rare occasions it may be.

ASSOCIATED OR ADJUVANT TREATMENT

It follows that if SIRT cannot be regarded as curative, it is desirable that additional therapy be given at some stage, if this option exists. This additional therapy may take the form of regional chemotherapy, which has been shown to have efficacy in CRC liver metastases (Meta-Analysis Group in Cancer, 1996), or it may entail systemic therapy. Sometimes all other therapeutic options have been exhausted, in which case the SIRT must be considered stand-alone therapy and be recognized as palliative.

Much of the published experience in CRC comes from groups that have chosen to follow SIRT with ongoing regional 5-fluorouracil (Stubbs et al, 2001) or fluorodeoxyuridine (Gray et al, 2000). Such an approach makes good sense for patients with disease confined to the liver, leaving as it does systemic chemotherapy options for patients who subsequently fail regional treatment or develop sites of extrahepatic involvement. In other circumstances, the preference may be to follow SIRT with systemic chemotherapy. It might be argued that in the context of isolated CRC liver metastases, such an approach simply deprives the patient of the advantages regional treatment can offer at that stage of their disease in terms of minimizing treatment side effects. That SIRT confers additional benefit to regional chemotherapy has been established by a randomized study in which treatment with SIR-spheres plus regional fluorodeoxyuridine was compared with regional fluorodeoxyuridine alone. The combined treatment produced a higher response rate (72% versus 44%) and superior 2-year survival rates (39% versus 29%) than the regional chemotherapy alone (Gray et al, 2001). It is our policy in patients with isolated CRC liver metastases to follow SIRT with 12 months of regional chemotherapy, giving 4 days of continuous 5-fluorouracil each month (Stubbs et al, 2001). We prefer 5-fluorouracil to fluorodeoxyuridine because of the complete absence of hepatobiliary toxicity with 5-fluorouracil, which eliminates the need for regular dosage adjustments based on close monitoring of liver function tests after regional chemotherapy.

CLINICAL INDICATIONS AND PATIENT SELECTION

The tumors for which the most experience has been gained to date are HCC (Lau et al, 1998) and CRC liver metastases (Gray et al, 2000; Stubbs et al, 2001). The doses of radiation delivered are such that there is reason to consider the option whenever liver-only tumor or liver-predominant tumor is identified. This section describes the tumors for which, in our experience, benefit can be expected.

Hepatocellular Carcinoma

Liver resection and transplantation are the best options for patients with HCC and are almost the only options that can achieve cure. Few patients with HCC meet the criteria for transplantation, however, and only a small proportion are suitable for surgical excision, either because of size or location within the liver or because of poor underlying liver reserve related to the underlying liver disease. TACE is used in many centers as the principal option for nonresectable HCC. SIRT is another candidate treatment in this situation and has many potential advantages over TACE. In particular, SIRT is not associated with the same morbidity as TACE when given to patients with underlying liver disease, is more often required only as a single treatment, and does not entail the same period of hospitalization. SIRT with ^{90}Y microspheres is generally well tolerated even in Child's class C patients and may be considered in the setting of portal venous thrombosis (Salem et al, 2004). SIRT with ^{131}I-lipiodol is safe in patients with portal venous thrombosis (Raoul et al, 1994), which is not the case for chemoembolization techniques. It is considered advisable, however, to reduce the dose of ^{90}Y microspheres in the presence of poor liver function in patients with cirrhosis. In situations in which the tumor is unilateral, risk of liver damage can be reduced by selective administration of microspheres to that side alone.

No direct comparisons between the outcomes after SIRT with ^{90}Y microspheres and ^{131}I-lipiodol in HCC have been made. ^{90}Y has numerous potential advantages over ^{131}I as a radiation source, including ease of administration, shorter half-life (and hospital stay), and higher energy (and tumor penetration). Although clinical experience with SIR-spheres shows no obvious loss of efficacy in large lesions, treatment with ^{131}I-lipiodol indicates that large lesions are less likely to respond than smaller ones (Ho et al, 1998). SIRT with ^{131}I-lipiodol has been shown to be at least as effective as chemoembolization in patients with HCC, with strikingly better patient tolerance and a correspondingly reduced risk (Raoul et al, 1997).

Colorectal Metastases

CRC (see Ch. 73a) liver metastases are particularly suitable for regional treatment because of their propensity to be confined to

the liver for an extended period, even up to the time of death (Weiss et al, 1986). Considerable experience with the use of SIRT has been gained in numerous centers, and consistently high response rates have been observed after this treatment. Most published experience in liver-only CRC metastases has followed SIRT with hepatic artery chemotherapy in patients who generally have not been subjected to modern systemic chemotherapy regimens involving irinotecan and oxaliplatin. Excellent responses to SIRT can be expected whether it is used as first-line therapy for liver metastases or subsequently. No agreement currently exists, however, in regard to how SIRT techniques are best employed in patients with CRC. Our view, based on personal experience, proposes SIRT with subsequent regional chemotherapy as first-line treatment for patients with extensive liver-only metastases, and systemic therapy is reserved for progressive liver-only disease or for when extrahepatic disease develops. SIRT, with or without regional chemotherapy, still should be considered, however, after failure of systemic chemotherapy when and if the disease remains confined to the liver. Even patients who are symptomatic and whose prognosis may be measured only in weeks can benefit from the treatment and occasionally can be returned to an asymptomatic state for extended periods. In some instances, nonresectable disease is rendered resectable (Fig. 75a.5) or multiple deposits are reduced to a few, which at a later date may be amenable to other ablative techniques, further extending survival.

Other Metastases

To date, experience with non-CRC metastases is limited to small numbers of patients, largely because liver-only metastases are relatively uncommon for non-CRC. Theoretical considerations regarding the dose of radiation administered by SIRT do suggest, however, that SIRT with ^{90}Y microspheres is probably worth considering whenever nonresectable liver-only metastases are found. We and others have limited experience with SIRT in neuroendocrine tumors (especially carcinoids), melanoma, cholangiocarcinoma, renal cell carcinoma, breast cancer, pancreatic cancer, gastric cancer, and cervical cancer. We now use it as our preferred treatment for carcinoid tumor and continue to use it for most other primary sites except melanoma, provided that the disease is confined to the liver.

ASSESSMENT OF RESPONSE

The parameters most often employed for judging efficacy of a cancer treatment are response rate, time to progression, and survival time. Although extension of survival time is the goal of all new treatments, it is becoming increasingly difficult to prove because of the propensity of patients to move to another treatment option when one has failed. This means greater reliance must be placed on response rates and time to progression. Conventionally, response rates have been based on changes of the sum of the products of perpendicular diameters of index lesions, usually measured by CT scan 2 to 3 months after start of treatment (Miller et al, 1981). Although this method is well validated for the assessment of responses to chemotherapy, this is not the case for ablative techniques, such as cryotherapy, radiofrequency ablation, and SIRT, in which complete or partial responses may be achieved despite initial size increases (Yang & Johnson, 1999). Assessments of the response based on size changes 2 to 3 months

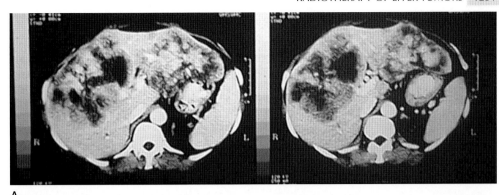

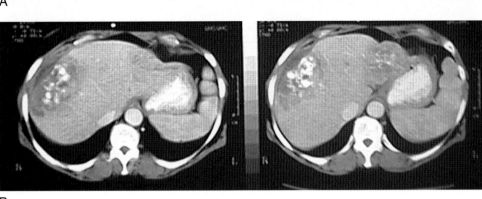

Fig. 75a.5. CT scan showing CRC liver metastases before SIRT (**A**) and 6 months after SIRT (**B**). In this case, the nonresectable disease was rendered resectable.

A

B

after SIRT may well grossly underestimate efficacy and lead to premature changes of therapy (Stubbs et al, 2002).

Groups with appreciable experience with SIRT all have noted marked discrepancies between response rates based on size criteria and based on tumor marker data (Gray et al, 2000; Lau et al, 1998; Stubbs et al, 2001), and we have come to consider that tumor marker changes in the 2 to 3 months after SIRT, where a suitable tumor marker exists, are the most reliable indicator of response to treatment, with the proviso that no major increase in size of any previously seen lesion is observed. We have documented that in CRC patients undergoing SIRT, maximum reduction in size and even complete disappearance of index

lesions can take 21 months (median 12 months) (Fig. 75a.6) (Stubbs et al, 2002). Many groups can give examples of complete histologic response revealed only after surgical excision of residual mass lesions (Fig. 75a.7) (Lau et al, 1998). At times, lesions not revealed by CT before SIRT may become apparent after SIRT and subsequently regress, indicating a response to SIRT rather than progression. It is important to be mindful of these issues when assessing responses to SIRT.

Corroboration is provided by the only currently published report of an evaluation of response to SIRT in CRC liver metastases comparing fluorodeoxyglucose positron emission tomography (PET), CT, magnetic resonance imaging (MRI),

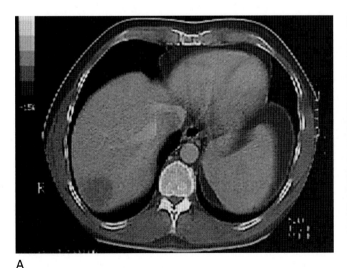

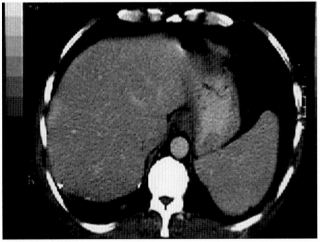

A

B

Fig. 75a.6. CT scan showing one CRC liver metastasis (**A**) and complete disappearance of this index lesion 12 months after SIRT (**B**).

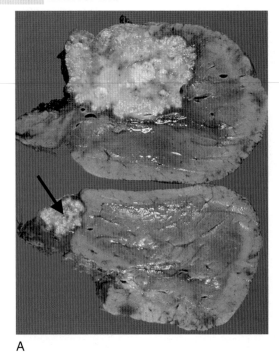

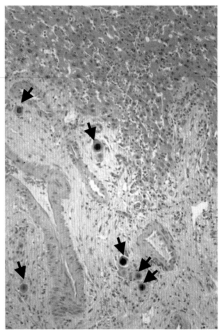

Fig. 75a.7. A, Resected specimen of residual mass 6 months after SIRT for two large CRC liver metastases. **B,** Photomicrograph of one of the lesions shows no residual tumor. The other showed some residual tumor. Several microspheres are evident in each of the sections *(arrows).*

A

B

and carcinoembryonic antigen (CEA). Thirteen lobes in eight consecutive patients with CRC liver metastases treated with ^{90}Y glass microspheres were studied. A metabolic response assessed by PET was noted in a significantly higher proportion of the lobes than was a size reduction evaluated by CT or MRI (12 lobes versus 2 lobes; $P < .0002$). After treatment, serum CEA decreased significantly and correlated better with PET responses than with either CT or MRI size changes. PET seems to be an accurate indicator of treatment response (Wong et al, 2002). A similar conclusion was reached in a multicenter U.S. experience of 190 patients treated with SIRT. Objective responses at 2 months were noted by CT in 35%, by CEA in 70%, and by PET in 90% of patients treated (Kennedy A et al, 2004).

CLINICAL RESULTS

Iodine 131 Lipiodol

The first account of treating nonresectable HCC with ^{131}I-lipiodol was in 1986 (Park et al, 1986), and since that time many small series have been reported. All series attest to the safety of the technique and the occurrence of dramatic tumor responses in more than 50% of patients, whether judged clinically, by tumor marker, or by imaging techniques. Complete tumor destruction is seen sometimes, based on histologic examination of subsequently resected "residual tumor." Response rates are usually highest for small tumors (<4 cm) and reduce with increasing tumor size (Yoo et al, 1991). Currently, the most commonly advocated and used treatment for nonresectable localized HCC is TACE, which has been used throughout the world with modest survival advantage being confirmed by meta-analysis (Llovet & Bruix, 2003). The risk of liver failure is high in patients with compromised liver function, however. In the largest published experience of ^{131}I-lipiodol, this treatment was compared with TACE in a prospective randomized trial involving 142 patients

with Okuda stage I or II HCC. No difference in survival was observed, but a complete absence of life-threatening complications or procedure-related mortality in the ^{131}I-lipiodol–treated group compared favorably with a 27% incidence of life-threatening complications and 9.4% mortality in the TACE-treated group (Raoul et al, 1997). No studies have been undertaken making a direct comparison between SIRT and ^{131}I-lipiodol or SIRT and TACE. At our institution, SIRT is the preferred treatment for nonresectable HCC based on the high expected response rate, its relative safety, and its ease of delivery.

The concept of using ^{131}I-lipiodol in an adjuvant setting after hepatic resection for HCC to address potential residual disease or microscopic multifocal disease was introduced by Lau and colleagues (1999) from the Chinese University in Hong Kong. They reported a small randomized controlled trial of 43 patients in which they examined the benefits of postoperative ^{131}I-lipiodol after curative resection of HCC. Twenty-one patients were treated with a single dose of 1850 MBq of ^{131}I-lipiodol 6 weeks after surgery without significant treatment-related toxicity. The median disease-free survival was improved from 13.6 months (2.1-68.3 months) in the control group to 57.2 months (0.4-69.7 months) in the ^{131}I-lipiodol-treated group ($P = .037$), and overall 3-year survival was improved from 46.3% to 86.4% ($P = .039$). They concluded that adjuvant postoperative ^{131}I-lipiodol significantly improves prognosis after curative resection of HCC (Lau et al, 1999).

In a similar vein, Partensky and associates (2000) from Lyon reported a phase II study in which 28 patients were treated with adjuvant ^{131}I-lipiodol 2 to 3 months after potentially curative hepatectomy for HCC. A repeat dose was given to 16 of the patients 2 years after the first treatment. No clinically significant adverse effects were noted, and the investigators recorded a median time to recurrence of 28 months (12-62 months) with overall survival time of 86% at 3 years and 65% at 5 years. They commented that this compares favorably with the expected results of resection alone in this group of patients (Partensky et al, 2000);

this study provides some corroboration for the conclusion reached by Lau and colleagues (1999).

Yttrium 90 Microspheres

Two different types of ^{90}Y microspheres are currently available for clinical use: Therasphere and SIR-spheres. The principal difference between the two relates to their specific gravity and specific activity. Both are of similar size. The Therasphere is a glass microsphere, which makes it heavier than the resin-based SIR-spheres. Although a similar dose of radiation (2-3 GBq) usually is administered regardless of the type of microspheres employed, the number of Theraspheres required to achieve this dose is around 20% of the number of SIR-spheres required. Although comparable results have been reported for the two products, there are theoretical reasons to consider that the flow characteristics and distribution of the lighter SIR-spheres might be better, and the consequence of any Theraspheres reaching nontarget sites might be greater in terms of associated toxicity because of the the the higher specific activity. In the absence of direct comparative clinical studies, however, these differences remain theoretical.

Hepatocellular Carcinoma

Many clinical reports appeared in the literature during the early 1990s related to the use of glass microspheres in patients with inoperable HCC. These reports comprised relatively small numbers of patients, but each reported encouraging responses in most patients, with probable survival advantage in many. Toxicity related to peptic ulceration and major upper gastrointestinal bleeding was a problem, however (Shepherd et al, 1992; Tian et al, 1996; Yan et al, 1993).

The largest experience in the world of treating nonresectable HCC with SIR-spheres comes from the Chinese University of Hong Kong, where more than 300 patients have been treated since 1990. In 1998, the investigators reported an experience of 71 patients in whom the treatment was well tolerated with no life-threatening toxicity, no liver failure, and no major gastrointestinal bleeding (Lau et al, 1998). Responses were assessed by serial tumor marker data and CT. α-Fetoprotein levels were increased in 46 patients before treatment, and in 41 of these patients (89%), there was a greater than 50% decrease after a single treatment with SIRT, with normalization of α-fetoprotein levels being achieved in 10 of these. Although no complete responses were seen on CT, a partial response with 51% to 87% reduction in tumor volume was observed in 19 patients (26%) 4 to 10 months after the first treatment. Only six patients (8.5%) showed progressive disease immediately after SIRT, as indicated by the appearance of new hepatic lesions or distant metastases. SIRT was repeated in 15 patients with up to five treatments being given. Median survival from diagnosis for all patients was 9.4 months (range 1.8-46.4 months) with actuarial survival at 12 and 24 months of 45% and 18%. Lau and colleagues (1998) regarded these results as encouraging, although they observed that the treatment group represented only 10% of their patients and had to be regarded as a select group. They concluded that a prospective randomized trial would be necessary to confirm the efficacy of the treatment. Such a trial has not yet been undertaken.

In 2004, the same group reported a series of 49 patients with unresectable HCC treated with systemic chemotherapy or SIRT or both in an effort to downstage the disease to the point

that hepatic resection might become possible. The chemotherapy employed was either single agent doxorubicin or cisplatin, interferon alfa, doxorubicin, and 5-fluorouracil. Thirty-two patients (65.3%) had combination chemotherapy alone, 8 patients (16.3%) had single agent chemotherapy alone, 4 patients (8.2%) received SIRT alone, and 5 patients (10.2%) received chemotherapy and SIRT sequentially. Major hepatic resection was achieved in 28 (57.1%) patients, and in 13 of these patients complete tumor destruction was noted in the resected specimens. The 1-year, 3-year, and 5-year survival rates were 98%, 64%, and 57%; median survival was 85.9 months. The investigators concluded that downstaging of unresectable HCC was possible with aggressive use of SIRT or systemic chemotherapy or both with good long-term control being achieved in a small proportion of patients (Lau et al, 2004).

In 2000, Dancey and coworkers from Toronto reported treating 22 HCC patients with Theraspheres with encouraging results, but appreciable, mainly self-limiting, toxicity. They reported responses in 20% of patients, stable disease in another 55%, and median survival of 54 weeks. Carr (2004) published a significant experience of 65 unresectable HCC patients treated with Theraspheres. Forty-six patients received only one treatment, and 19 received repeat treatments (generally two). The median dose delivered was 134 Gy, typically as either 5 or 10 GBq. Clinical toxicities included nine episodes of abdominal pain and two episodes of acute cholecystitis requiring cholecystectomy. Bilirubin increased by more than 200% in 25 patients (30.5%) during 6 months of therapy, although 18 of these patients had only transient elevation. Forty-two patients (64.6%) had a substantial decrease in tumor vascularity in response to therapy, and 25 patients (38.4%) showed a partial response by CT. Median survival for 42 Okuda stage I patients was 649 days (historical comparison 244 days) and for 23 Okuda stage II patients was 302 days (historical comparison 64 days). Ultimately of 42 deaths, 21 were due to liver failure, 6 to tumor progression, and 3 to metastases. Carr (2004) concluded that Therasphere seems to be a relatively safe and effective therapy for advanced stage unresectable HCC (Fig. 75a.8).

The safety of SIRT in the setting of portal vein thrombosis until more recently has been unclear. Carr's patients (see previously) included some patients with portal vein thrombosis, without obvious consequence. Salem and colleagues (2004) reported on the use of Theraspheres in 15 patients with unresectable HCC and portal vein thrombosis, but no evidence of cavernous transformation. The aim of the study was to evaluate hepatic toxicity using serum total bilirubin. They concluded that SIRT was well tolerated and safe in patients with compromised portal venous flow in one or both first-order divisions of the portal vein (Salem et al, 2004).

Colorectal Liver Metastases

Early clinical reports using ^{90}Y microspheres to treat CRC liver metastases also entailed use of glass microspheres and first appeared in the late 1980s (Herba et al, 1988). This experience and that of others reported in the early 1990s (Anderson et al, 1992; Andrews et al, 1994) was similar to that for HCC in that encouraging response rates were seen, but significant problems occurred with gastroduodenal ulceration and sometimes with major life-threatening bleeding. The additional problem for patients with CRC liver metastases was the common development of extrahepatic disease, which occasionally diminished the value of a good response within the liver. The problems of

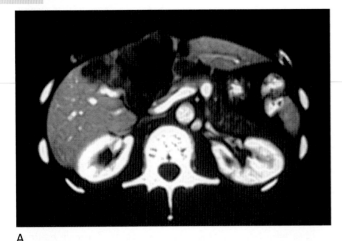

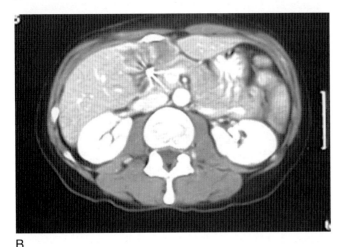

Fig. 75a.8. CT showing nonresectable HCC in a noncirrhotic liver (**A**) and the same liver about 9 months later, showing an excellent response (**B**).

comparing treatment with SIRT plus hepatic arterial chemotherapy with chemotherapy alone using the same regimen. In this trial, SIRT plus hepatic arterial fluorodeoxyuridine was compared with hepatic arterial fluorodeoxyuridine alone in 74 patients. The patients treated with SIRT showed a significant advantage in terms of tumor responses and progression-free survival (Gray et al, 2001).

In our experience, SIRT is well tolerated and relatively easily administered with an average hospital stay of 2 days. Response rates are high, but vary according to the method of assessment. Based on reduction of CEA, about 90% show a response to treatment, with the lowest CEA generally being seen after 2 months (Fig. 75a.9) (Stubbs et al, 2001). In our first 100 patients treated with SIRT for CRC metastases, we observed a reduction in tumor size on CT in 68%, stable disease in 21% (Fig. 75a.10), and progressive liver disease in 11% of patients. Survival seems to be improved based on comparison with historical untreated controls. Expected survival in untreated patients with multiple widespread liver metastases or numerous large, nonresectable metastases is 6 to 12 months from diagnosis and less from treatment (Finan et al, 1985; Stangl et al, 1994). Median survival for the 100 patients undergoing SIRT was 16.2 months from diagnosis and 11 months from treatment. For a subgroup of 41% of the patients, who did not develop extrahepatic disease within 6 months of SIRT, survival was significantly greater, with a median survival of 21.6 months from SIRT. Fig. 75a.11 shows the Kaplan-Meier survival curve for our first 100 patients. Most of these patients were being treated at a time before irinotecan and oxaliplatin were available.

A Canadian experience of Theraspheres in 37 patients treated predominantly for metastatic CRC liver metastases in the years 1986-1994 was reported in 2002. Although no major procedural, hematologic, or pulmonary complications occurred, late gastroduodenal ulceration did occur 6 to 8 weeks after treatment in three patients. Beneficial effects were noted on repeat scanning in the 15 patients with identifiable marker lesions. These changes varied from decreased CT attenuation and sharper tumor-liver interface to ultrasound evidence of liquefaction necrosis and reduction in size (Herba & Thirlwell, 2002).

Other Liver Metastases

At this time, there are no meaningful published data regarding the efficacy of SIRT in non-CRC liver metastases, largely because

gastroduodenal ulceration seemed to decrease after the development of resin microspheres, which have a lower specific gravity than glass microspheres and for that reason may distribute more appropriately after hepatic arterial infusion. A group from Perth, Western Australia, first presented their clinical experience of the resin microsphere (later named SIR-sphere) in 1992 (Gray et al, 1992). There was minimal major morbidity and a high rate of response or stable disease. These investigators initiated the practice of following SIRT in patients with CRC liver metastases with hepatic artery chemotherapy in an effort to prolong the response time within the liver.

The experience of Gray's group, which began in the mid-1980s, totals approximately 300 patients, most of whom had CRC. Our own experience began in 1997, and since that time we have acquired an experience of more than 200 procedures in approximately 180 patients; 132 of our patients have had CRC metastases. The experience of both groups is similar as revealed in published reports (Gray et al, 2000; Stubbs et al, 2001). Most patients who have received SIRT with SIR-spheres for CRC liver metastases also have received ongoing hepatic arterial chemotherapy with fluorodeoxyuridine (Gray et al, 2000) or 5-fluorouracil (Stubbs et al, 2001) after SIRT. Although assessments of survival and responses are confounded by this ongoing chemotherapy, some clarification of the issues is provided by a randomized trial

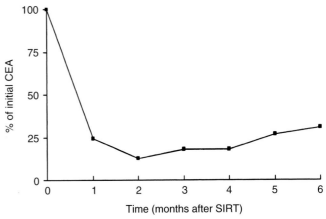

Fig. 75a.9. Graph showing median CEA levels (expressed as a percentage of pretreatment value) after SIRT in 100 patients with CRC liver metastases.

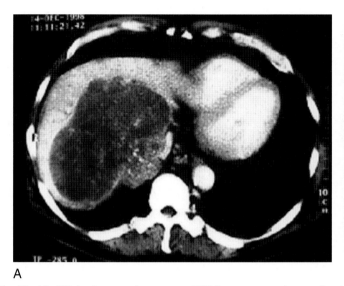 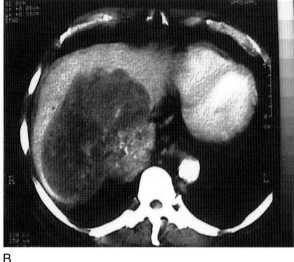

Fig. 75a.10. CT showing extensive recurrent CRC liver metastases 4 years after right hepatectomy (**A**) and 10 months after SIRT (**B**); the tumor showed no increase in size.

of the relatively less frequent occurrence of liver-only metastatic disease for non-CRC primaries. Most units that have developed an experience with SIRT have used it in the treatment of a variety of other tumors, however, where other treatment options have been exhausted or are of limited value. These include neuroendocrine cancer (especially carcinoid tumor), peripheral cholangiocarcinoma, renal cell carcinoma, esophagogastric cancer, pancreatic cancer, cervical cancer, adenocarcinoma of unknown origin, and melanoma. Of these tumors, SIRT is particularly valuable in the setting of carcinoid tumor, where we have come to expect very good responses, including resolution of carcinoid syndrome, in 75% of patients (Fig. 75a.12). We have been discouraged by poor efficacy in patients with metastatic melanoma in the liver and are no longer inclined to offer it in this setting.

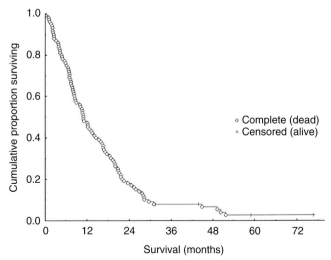

Fig. 75a.11. Kaplan-Meier survival curve showing actuarial survival of 100 patients with CRC liver metastases treated with SIRT.

Safety, Complications, and Adverse Effects

SIRT generally is very well tolerated even when administered to the whole liver. Many patients experience self-limiting pain and nausea for 48 hours. Lethargy and anorexia are to be expected and can be profound for 6 weeks after treatment. The principal and most dangerous complications of SIRT relate to radiation hepatitis, radiation pneumonitis, and peptic ulceration caused by inadvertent exposure of the gastroduodenum to ^{90}Y microspheres. Classically, radiation hepatitis manifests with deteriorating liver function and portal hypertension resulting from a veno-occlusive-type problem. Radiation pneumonitis manifests as increasing shortness of breath with parenchymal fibrosis. Both entities present weeks after the delivery of radiation and are frequently fatal.

In practical terms, clinical manifestations of radiation hepatitis are rarely seen with the doses of ^{90}Y microspheres currently recommended for delivery. If seen, the most likely scenarios involve deterioration of liver function in the context of preexisting liver disease (i.e., cirrhosis) or jaundice associated with progressive liver failure and death weeks after SIRT in a patient with no underlying liver disease. The risk of this latter occurrence is probably around 0.5% to 1%, based on experience to date. Subclinical evidence of radiation hepatitis is, however, more common. In our experience, a rising alkaline phosphatase and gamma-glutamyltransferase for 6 months or so in the face of good tumor response occurs in approximately 25% of patients and presumably indicates a degree of radiation hepatitis. We also have noted the development of mild portal hypertension with evidence of splenic enlargement on follow-up scans in a significant proportion of patients after SIRT. Moroz and coworkers (2001) documented many changes 12 months after SIRT that are likely to be indicative of subclinical radiation hepatitis, including a reduction in the volume of normal hepatic parenchyma by an average of 17%, an increase in portal vein diameter by an average of 9%, and an average increase in splenic volume of 48%. Neither they nor we have seen complications related to portal hypertension arising after SIRT, although it makes surgery a little more difficult. Liver resection after SIRT is, however,

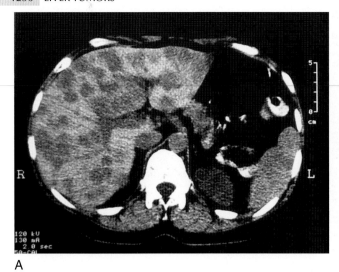
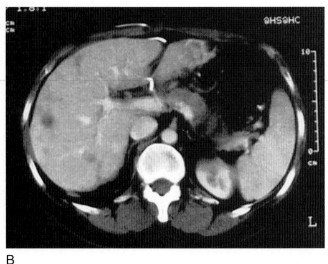

A   B

Fig. 75a.12. CT scan showing extensive carcinoid metastases causing carcinoid syndrome **(A)** and the same liver 3 months after SIRT with SIR-spheres **(B).** All symptoms had disappeared.

possible without major or obvious impairment of liver regeneration. Macroscopically, the liver is abnormally soft and appears finely nodular (similar to the chemotherapy-affected liver), but on light microscopy there is no major abnormality (Fig. 75a.13).

It is said that radiation pneumonitis should not occur after SIRT if a liver-lung shunt of less than 13% is revealed by the pre-SIRT MAA scan (Leung et al, 1995), although we have seen one probable case of nonfatal radiation pneumonitis after SIRT for HCC when the shunt was measured at 11% (Fig. 75a.14). Unreported fatalities are known to have occurred when this advice has not been heeded. A shunt of 13% is rare in patients with CRC liver metastases, but may be seen in 20% of patients with HCC.

The major source of morbidity after SIRT is inadvertent delivery of microspheres to foregut structures (Fig. 75a.15) resulting in peptic ulceration in the stomach, duodenum, or occasionally esophagus. This ulceration can be troublesome for many months and responds poorly to medical treatment. In our hands, the safest approach has been by delivery through a surgically implanted port. In 180 procedures, we have seen major morbidity (principally peptic ulceration) in 11 of 128 (8.6%) patients treated via a port and 13 of 52 (25%) patients treated via a percutaneous arterial catheter ($P < .05$, χ^2). We have seen one death from gastric perforation secondary to severe radiation gastritis 30 days after SIRT via a femoral catheter and another from sepsis complicating acute pancreatitis $2\frac{1}{2}$ months after receiving SIRT via a port.

In an experience of 180 procedures, we have seen 24 (13.3%) important complications after SIRT. The nature of these complications is detailed in Table 75a.1. Thirteen patients (7.2%) developed peptic ulceration within 2 months of SIRT, of whom two experienced acute upper gastrointestinal bleeding, and in one of these, emergency surgery was required followed by an uneventful recovery. In this experience, four deaths (2.2%) occurred that were directly attributable to the SIRT (see Table 75a.1), and another four deaths occurred in patients with advanced disease and deteriorating condition, in whom the SIRT was poorly tolerated and would have contributed to the timing of death.

Repeat Treatment

Although SIRT generally is planned as a single treatment, under some circumstances it is appropriate to repeat the treatment. We would consider doing so, provided that a good response had been obtained from the initial treatment, and provided that the major problem remains largely confined to the liver. Many groups have adopted this approach and employed repeat treatments with good outcomes. We have given repeat treatment to 19 patients, including 15 with CRC metastases (Fig. 75a.16), 1 with carcinoid metastases, 1 with HCC, 1 with renal cell carcinoma, and 1 with melanoma. The median time between first and second treatments was 15 months, and the median repeat dose was 2 GBq. Although all patients who received a repeat dose had shown a good response to the initial treatment, 44% did so again on the second occasion with stable disease being

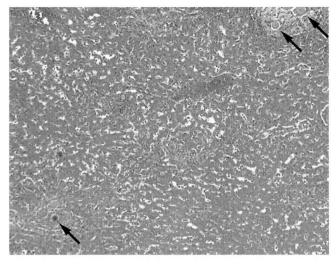

Fig. 75a.13. Photomicrograph of liver parenchyma after SIRT with SIR-spheres *(arrows)* showing normal architecture.

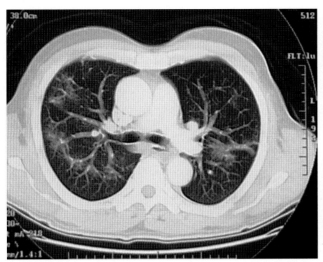
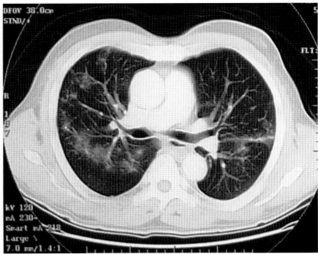

Fig. 75a.14. CT scan of a patient who developed radiation pneumonitis 6 to 8 weeks after receiving SIRT with SIR-spheres for nonresectable HCC. The MAA shunt had been 11% before SIRT.

achieved for a time in another 44%. One patient died as a direct result of the treatment in fulminant liver failure from hepatic necrosis 4 days after SIRT. Another, who was in poor condition before SIRT died after 6 weeks and may have had his death advanced by the repeat treatment. The median survival for patients who received repeat SIRT was 20 months from the first treatment, which compares favorably with a median survival of 11 months for the whole group. The median survival after the second SIRT was 9.21 months.

CONCLUSION

Radiation therapy has long been known to be an effective treatment for cancer. Use of this modality for liver tumors has been limited, however, because of poor tolerance by normal hepatic parenchyma that has limited the dose of radiation able to be given. Selective internal radiation therapy using either ^{90}Y microspheres or ^{131}I-lipiodol delivered directly into the hepatic artery allows for tumoricidal doses of radiotherapy to be administered with little indication of serious liver damage. Although this approach has not yet been used widely for the regional treatment of nonresectable liver tumors, its use in numerous centers around the world for HCC and CRC liver metastases establishes it as a potentially valuable modality worthy of further use and investigation. SIRT is particularly valuable for liver tumors without other good treatment options at present (e.g., HCC, neuroendocrine metastases). Its role in the treatment of CRC liver metastases is not so clear because it comes at a time when systemic chemotherapy is undergoing such change and improvement. The best results to date have been achieved with patients in whom SIRT has been used as first-line therapy for liver-only metastases followed by regional chemotherapy. Good results with SIRT also have been seen in second-line situations, although its use in patients with poor performance status (Karnofsky score <70) is probably unwise.

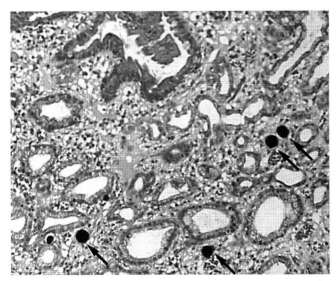

Fig. 75a.15. Photomicrograph showing SIR-spheres in the duodenum after SIRT *(arrows)*. The patient presented with an acute bleed 4 weeks after SIRT for CRC liver metastases from a duodenal ulcer, which required surgical management.

Table 75a.1 Significant Complications Occurring After 180 Selective Internal Radiation Therapy Procedures with SIR-Spheres

Complication	No.	Deaths
Peptic ulceration	13	1
Deterioration of liver function	3	
Cardiac arrest	1	
Myocardial infarction	1	
Radiation hepatitis	2	2
Radiation pneumonitis	1	
Biliary stricture	1	
Acute pancreatitis	1	1
Liver abscess	1	

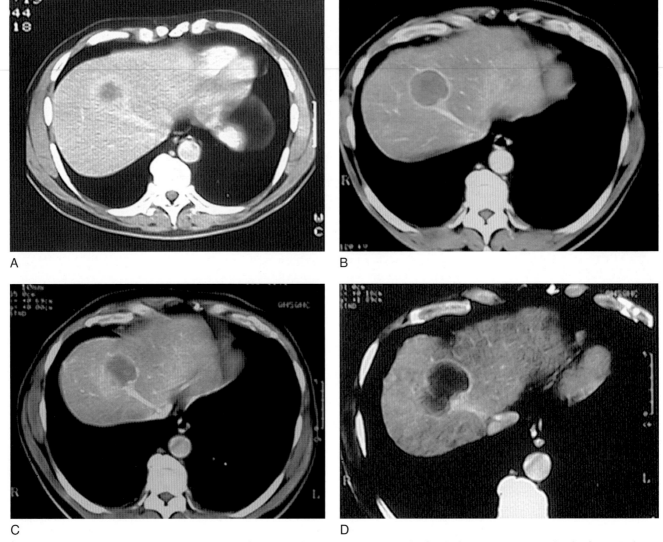

Fig. 75a.16. CT scan of renal carcinoma liver metastasis before SIRT with SIR-spheres **(A),** 9 months after the first SIRT **(B),** 15 months after first SIRT showing tumor recurrence at the margin **(C),** and 3 months after repeat SIRT with SIR-spheres **(D).**

Further use and investigation is likely to define the place of SIRT better in the management of CRC liver metastases specifically and liver tumors in general.

REFERENCES

Anderson JH, et al, 1992: Glass yttium-90 microspheres for patients with colorectal liver metastases. Radiother Oncol 25:137-139.

Andrews JC, et al, 1994: Hepatic radioembolization with yttrium-90 containing glass microspheres: preliminary results and clinical follow-up. J Nucl Med 35:1637-1644.

Ariel IM, 1965: Treatment of inoperable primary pancreatic and liver cancer by the intra-arterial administration of radioactive isotopes (Y⁹⁰ radiating microspheres). Ann Surg 162:267-278.

Ariel IM, Pack GT, 1967: Treatment of inoperable cancer of the liver by intra-arterial radioactive isotopes and chemotherapy. Cancer 20: 793-804.

Brans B, et al, 2003: Intra-arterial radionuclide therapy for liver tumors: effect of selectivity of catheterization and 131I-Lipiodol delivery on tumour uptake and response. Nucl Med Commun 24:391-396.

Burton MA, et al, 1988: Effect of angiotensin II on blood flow in the transplanted sheep squamous cell carcinoma. Eur J Cancer Clin Oncol 24:1373-1376.

Campbell AM, et al, 2000: Analysis of the distribution of intra-arterial microspheres in human liver following hepatic yttrium-90 microsphere therapy. Phys Med Biol 45:1023-1033.

Carr BI, 2004: Hepatic arterial ⁹⁰Yttrium glass microspheres (Therasphere) for unresectable hepatocellular carcinoma: interim safety and survival data on 65 patients. Liver Transpl 10:S107-S110.

Dancey JE, et al, 2000: Treatment of nonresectable hepatocellular carcinoma with intrahepatic ⁹⁰Y-microspheres. J Nucl Med 41:1673-1681.

Finan PJ, et al, 1985: Factors affecting survival in patients presenting with synchronous hepatic metastases from colorectal cancer: a clinical computer analysis. Br J Surg 72:373-377.

Grady ED, 1979: Internal radiation therapy of hepatic cancer. Dis Colon Rectum 22:371-375.

Gray B, et al, 2000: Treatment of colorectal liver metastases with SIR-spheres plus chemotherapy. Gastrointest Cancer 3:249-257.

Gray B, et al, 2001: Randomised trial of SIR-Spheres plus chemotherapy versus chemotherapy alone for treating patients with liver metastases from primary large bowel cancer. Ann Oncol 12:1711-1720.

Gray BN, et al, 1992: Regression of liver metastases following treatment with Yttrium-90 microspheres. Aust N Z J Surg 62:105-110.

Herba MJ, Thirlwell MP, 2002: Radioembolization for hepatic metastases. Semin Oncol 29:152-159.

Herba MJ, et al, 1988: Hepatic malignancies: improved treatment with intraarterial Y-90. Radiology 169:311-314.

Hewitt PM, et al, 1998: Lipiodol avidity of neuroendocrine liver metastases. Eur J Surg Oncol 24:558-561.

Ho S, et al, 1998: Internal radiation therapy for patients with primary or metastatic hepatic cancer. Cancer 83:1894-1907.

Ingold JA, et al, 1965: Radiation hepatitis. Am J Roentgenol Radium Ther Nucl Med 93:200-208.

Kennedy A, et al, 2004: 90Y microspheres in the treatment of colorectal liver metastases: USA experience. International Congress on Anti-Cancer Treatment-15th International Congress, Paris.

Kennedy AS, et al, 2004: Pathologic response and microdosimetry of 90Y microspheres in man: review of four explanted whole livers. Int J Radiat Oncol Biol Phys 60:1552-1563.

Lau WY, et al, 1998: Selective internal radiation therapy for nonresectable hepatocellular carcinoma with intraarterial infusion of 90Yttrium microspheres. Int J Radiat Oncol Biol Phys 40:583-592.

Lau WY, et al, 1999: Adjuvant intra-arterial iodine-131-labelled lipiodol for resectable hepatocellular carcinoma: a prospective randomised trial. Lancet 353:797-801.

Lau WY, et al, 2004: Salvage surgery following downstaging of unresectable hepatocellular carcinoma. Ann Surg 240:299-305.

Leung TW, et al, 1995: Radiation pneumonitis after selective internal radiation treatment with intraarterial 90Yttrium-microspheres for inoperable hepatic tumours. Int J Radiat Oncol Biol Phys 33:919-924.

Llovet J, Bruix J, 2003: Systematic review of randomized trials for unresectable hepatocellular carcinoma: chemoembolization improves survival. Hepatology 37:429-442.

Mantravadi RV, et al, 1982: Intraarterial Yttrium 90 in the treatment of hepatic malignancy. Radiology 142:783-786.

Matsui O, et al, 1991: Benign and malignant nodules in cirrhotic livers: distinction based on blood supply. Radiology 178:493-497.

Meta-Analysis Group in Cancer, 1996: Reappraisal of hepatic arterial infusion in the treatment of nonresectable liver metastases from colorectal cancer. J Natl Cancer Inst 88:252-258.

Miller AB, et al, 1981: Reporting results of cancer treatment. Cancer 47:207-214.

Moroz P, et al, 2001: Effect of selective internal radiation therapy and hepatic arterial chemotherapy on normal liver volume and spleen volume. J Surg Oncol 78:248-252.

Nakayama A, et al, 2001: Value of lipiodol computed tomography and digital subtraction angiography in the era of helical biphasic computed tomography as preoperative assessment of hepatocellular carcinoma. Ann Surg 234:56-62.

Ngan H, 1990: Lipiodol computerized tomography: how sensitive and specific is the technique in the diagnosis of hepatocellular carcinoma? Br J Radiol 63:771-775.

Okayasu I, et al, 1988: Selective and persistent deposition and gradual drainage of iodized oil, lipiodol in hepatocellular carcinoma after injection into the feeding artery. Am J Clin Pathol 90:536-544.

Park CH, et al, 1986: Evaluation of intrahepatic I-131 ethiodol on a patient with hepatocellular carcinoma: therapeutic feasibility study. Clin Nucl Med 11:514-517.

Partensky C, et al, 2000: Intra-arterial iodine 131-labeled lipiodol as adjuvant therapy after curative liver resection for hepatocellular carcinoma: a phase 2 clinical study. Arch Surg 135:1298-1300.

Raoul JL, et al, 1988: Hepatic artery injection of I-131-labeled lipiodol: Part I. biodistribution study results in patients with hepatocellular carcinoma and liver metastases. Radiology 168:541-545.

Raoul JL, et al, 1994: Randomized controlled trial for hepatocellular carcinoma with portal vein thrombosis: intra-arterial iodine-131-iodized oil versus medical support. J Nucl Med 35:1782-1787.

Raoul JL, et al, 1997: Prospective randomized trial of chemoembolization versus intra-arterial injection of 131I-labeled-iodized oil in the treatment of hepatocellular carcinoma. Hepatology 26:1156-1161.

Rindani RB, et al, 2002: 131I lipiodol therapy for unresectable hepatocellular carcinoma. Aust N Z J Surg 72:210-214.

Salem R, et al, 2004: Use of Yttrium-90 glass microspheres (Therasphere) for the treatment of unresectable hepatocellular carcinoma in patients with portal vein thrombosis. J Vasc Interv Radiol 15:335-345.

Shepherd FA, et al, 1992: A phase I dose escalation trial of Yttrium-90 microspheres in the treatment of primary hepatocellular carcinoma. Cancer 70:2250-2254.

Stangl R, et al, 1994: Factors influencing the natural history of colorectal liver metastases. Lancet 343:1405-1410.

Stubbs RS, Wickremesekera SK, 2004a: Selective internal radiation therapy (SIRT): a new modality for treating patients with colorectal liver metastases. HPB Surg 6:133-139.

Stubbs RS, Wickremesekera SK, 2004b: Experience with repeat selective internal radiation therapy (SIRT) with SIR-spheres for non-resectable liver tumors. HPB Surg 6(suppl 1):108.

Stubbs RS, et al, 2001: Selective internal radiation therapy with 90Yttrium microspheres for extensive colorectal liver metastases. J Gastrointest Surg 5:294-302.

Stubbs RS, et al, 2002: Assessment of response to selective internal radiation therapy (SIRT) in patients with colorectal liver metastases. HPB Surg 9:76.

Taylor I, et al, 1979: The blood supply of colorectal liver metastases. Br J Cancer 39:749-756.

Tian JH, et al, 1996: Ultrasound-guided internal radiotherapy using Yttrium-90-glass microspheres for liver malignancies. J Nucl Med 37:958-963.

Weiss L, et al, 1986: Haematogenous metastatic patterns in colonic carcinoma: an analysis of 1541 necropsies. J Pathol 150:195-203.

Wickremesekera J, et al, 2000: Hepatic artery access ports: recognising and avoiding the problems. Aust N Z J Surg 70:496-502.

Wong CY, et al, 2002: Evaluating 90Y-glass microsphere treatment response of unresectable colorectal liver metastases by [18F]FDG PET: a comparison with CT or MRI. Eur J Nucl Med 29:815-820.

Yan ZP, et al, 1993: An experimental study and clinical pilot trials on Yttrium-90 glass microspheres through the hepatic artery for treatment of primary liver cancer. Cancer 72:3210-3215.

Yang WT, Johnson PJ, 1999: Monitoring response to treatment in liver tumours. Baillieres Best Pract Res Clin Gastroenterol 13:637-654.

Yoo HS, et al, 1991: Nodular hepatocellular carcinoma: treatment with subsegmental intraarterial injection of iodine-131-labeled iodized oil. Cancer 68:1878-1884.

Yumoto Y, et al, 1985: Hepatocellular carcinoma detected by iodized oil. Radiology 154:19-24.

75b EXTERNAL-BEAM RADIATION THERAPY FOR PRIMARY HEPATOCELLULAR CARCINOMA AND BILIARY DISEASE

R. WAGMAN

Historically, the use of radiation therapy for liver tumors has been reserved for large, unresectable lesions. Early studies, before the era of CT-guided treatment, including randomized reports from Hong Kong and the United States (Friedman et al, 1988; Lai et al, 1986), noted high rates of liver dysfunction and low tumor response after radiation therapy to the whole liver (Ingold et al, 1954; Nerenstone et al, 1988). These findings are not surprising because the ability of radiation therapy to control tumors generally is related to the size of the lesion and the total dose given, whereas the risk of significant liver damage increases with increased dose and volume of liver irradiated (Emami et al, 1991; Hall & Cox, 1994).

Improvements in imaging and localizing techniques have allowed for increasingly accurate targeting of radiation to part of the liver as opposed to the whole organ. This is a crucial advance because many reports have shown that a part of the liver can tolerate a higher radiation level than the whole liver (Dawson et al, 2000; Emami et al, 1991; Lawrence et al, 1992). Higher doses of radiation have been found to improve tumor control probability for HCC (Dawson et al, 2000; Park et al, 2002; Seong et al, 2003).

Radiation therapy has been used increasingly since the 1990s for primary treatment of unresectable liver tumors. The role of radiation for intrahepatic malignancies is evolving as radiation evolves. New abilities to target therapy to minimize normal tissue damage, in conjunction with improved understanding of the biology of these tumors and their responses to therapy, are likely to redefine the use of this modality.

TECHNICAL INNOVATIONS IN RADIATION THERAPY PLANNING AND DELIVERY

A potentially major innovation in portal approaches is CT-assisted three-dimensional conformal radiation therapy (3D-CRT). 3D-CRT is based on the simple observation that improvements in tumor definition and dosage delivery should enhance the ability of radiation therapy to improve control of many tumor types. True 3D-CRT uses diagnostic CT or MRI to define normal and target structures over 20 to 30 slices and reconstructs these structures from the standpoint of each potential treatment beam (Figs. 75b.1 and 75b.2). These plans often use four to six fields or more, and, importantly, it is possible to visualize the dose distributions in three planes, allowing accurate assessment of dose to critical structures. By virtue of its accurate representation of target and critical tissues, treatment theoretically can be delivered with increasingly tight margins. Although there is an increased risk of geographic miss, especially with a moving target, such as the liver, there is the potential for reduced normal tissue complications at the same dose level (Cho et al, 1999).

In the United States, the University of Michigan has pioneered the use of high-dose, partial-liver irradiation. The investigators described their results on use of conformal therapy in conjunction with intra-arterial chemotherapy in 43 patients with unresectable hepatobiliary disease (27 with HCC) (Dawson et al, 2000). Doses ranged from 28.5 to 90 Gy and were based on the amount of normal liver that could be effectively excluded from the fields using three-dimensional treatment planning, multiple conformal portals, and immobilization. Initially, patients received whole liver irradiation, a practice later abandoned because of toxicity and ineffectiveness. Of 25 assessable patients in whom partial liver was treated for local disease, there was a 68% overall response rate (one complete response). Nine patients failed in the treated site; the median potential follow-up is 26.5 months. In this series, there was one case of radiation hepatitis and six cases of significant gastrointestinal toxicity when tumors and fields were near the stomach and duodenum. The median survival was 16 months overall and 11 months for patients with local but unresectable HCC. For patients treated with 70 Gy or more, the median survival had not yet been reached at the time of publication of these results (>16.4 months compared with 11.6 months for patients treated with lower doses; $P = .003$). Further data from China, Taiwan, and Thailand confirm that 3D-CRT is effective and feasible for nonoperable HCC, with significant tumor response in most patients and 3-year overall survivals of 79% to 97% for patients with small primaries and 35% for patients with advanced primaries. Prognostic variables for survival on multivariate analysis, in addition to dose of radiation, were number of tumors, size of tumor, and mean hepatic dose (Chen & Guan, 2003a, 2003b; Cheng et al, 2002; Pattaranutaporn et al, 2001; Wu & Chen, 2003a, 2003b).

A further technical innovation in radiation therapy has been the development of intensity-modulated radiation therapy (IMRT). IMRT, in contrast to conventional radiation, does not use a single, large, fixed source beam of radiation; rather, thousands of tiny, thin beams of varying intensity are delivered to the body from many different angles (Fig. 75b.3); the result is that the tumor can be targeted more accurately by a beam that exactly matches the shape of the tumor, while theoretically minimizing damage to the surrounding normal tissue by exposing it to only extremely low intensity radiation (Boyer et al, 2001; Oncology Net Guide, 2004). Cheng and coworkers (2002) analyzed 12 of their patients treated with 3D-CRT for HCC who developed radiation-induced liver dysfunction; these patients were replanned using IMRT. With comparable target coverage between 3D-CRT and IMRT, IMRT was able to obtain a large reduction in normal tissue complication probabilities for the liver, kidneys, stomach, and spinal cord. The mean dose to the entire liver did increase with IMRT, however; further study is needed

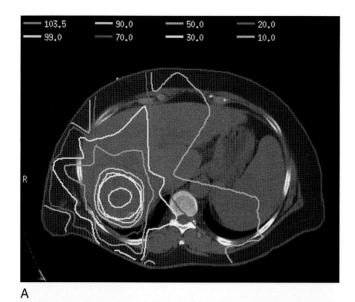

A

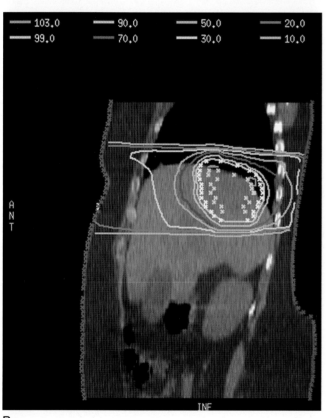

B

Fig. 75b.1. 3D-CRT.

to determine the true risk-to-benefit ratio of IMRT for treatment of liver tumors (Cheng et al, 2002).

As noted earlier, 3D-CRT and IMRT offer the ability to tighten the margin around the target volume. A barrier to the implementation of these techniques in the abdomen has been the movement and deformation of intra-abdominal organs with respiration. Some series have found that the liver moves 1 to 8 cm in the superior-inferior direction with respiration, whereas smaller shifts are found from anterior to posterior and from side to side. Because a typical radiation treatment takes 5 to 10 minutes,

there is significant movement of liver and intrahepatic target over the course of the treatment. With significant improvements in conformal techniques, methods to account for this movement are becoming increasingly important to ensure that the tumor does not move out of (and that normal tissue does not move into) the radiation field during treatment (Gierga et al, 2004; Rosu et al, 2003). Use of gating of respiration, whereby the delivery of dose is synchronized with patient respiration, has been proposed as one method to overcome the challenges posed by moving organs and has been shown to allow for sparing of normal tissues and for dose escalation (Fig. 75b.4) (Ten Haken et al, 1996; Wagman et al, 2003; Wong et al, 1999).

ALTERED FRACTIONATION SCHEDULES

The primary alternative fractionation scheme used in the United States is hyperfractionation; twice-daily treatments were used in the University of Michigan series (Dawson et al, 2000; Lawrence et al, 1992). The basic rationale for hyperfractionation is that the use of small dose fractions allows higher total doses to be administered within the tolerance of late-responding normal tissues; hyperfractionation also allows for increasing radiosensitization of tumor cells through cell cycle redistribution and lesser dependence on oxygenation. The rapid doubling time of HCC tumors (estimated at 41 days) suggests that this type of tumor would respond favorably to hyperfractionation (Ang, 1998). In a nonrandomized study by the Radiation Therapy Oncology Group (RTOG) (Stillwagon et al, 1989), 194 patients with advanced HCC (70-80% had metastases or had failed prior treatment) received treatment to the whole liver. Conventional fractionation (3 Gy four times per week to 21 Gy) was used in 135 patients; 59 received 24 Gy in 1.2-Gy fractions twice daily. Concurrent doxorubicin and 5-fluorouracil were given intravenously every other day to both groups. The response rate for both fractionation schemes was only approximately 20%. Acute toxicity, including esophagitis and thrombocytopenia, occurred significantly more often in the group that received twice-daily radiation.

Another RTOG study on patients with hepatic metastases found that 33 Gy given at 1.5 Gy twice daily resulted in an unacceptably high rate of liver injury; doses of 27 Gy and 30 Gy did not carry the same risk (Russell et al, 1993). The role of twice-daily treatments in the work of Robertson and colleagues (1997) cannot be elucidated at this time because of the preliminary nature of their results. Given the persuasive theoretical rationale for hyperfractionation and the need to decrease long-term morbidity, further studies seem worthwhile.

Others investigators have suggested that, with exceedingly conformal treatments and effective immobilization, use of high dose-per-fraction (hypofractionated) radiation therapy can overcome the effect of sublethal damage repair seen with low dose-per-fraction treatment. Sublethal damage repair is the reason that, with multiple small fractions, a larger total dose is required to achieve the same biologic effect as for a single dose regimen. Herfarth and colleagues (2001) reported the results of a phase I/II trial evaluating 60 liver tumors (4 primary HCC, 56 metastases) in 37 patients. Patients were treated on a dose escalation protocol with single fractions ranging from 14 to 26 Gy; median tumor size was 10 cm³. Actuarial local control was 81% at 18 months after therapy, and no major side effects were observed. Similarly, Blomgren and associates (1998) reported their results

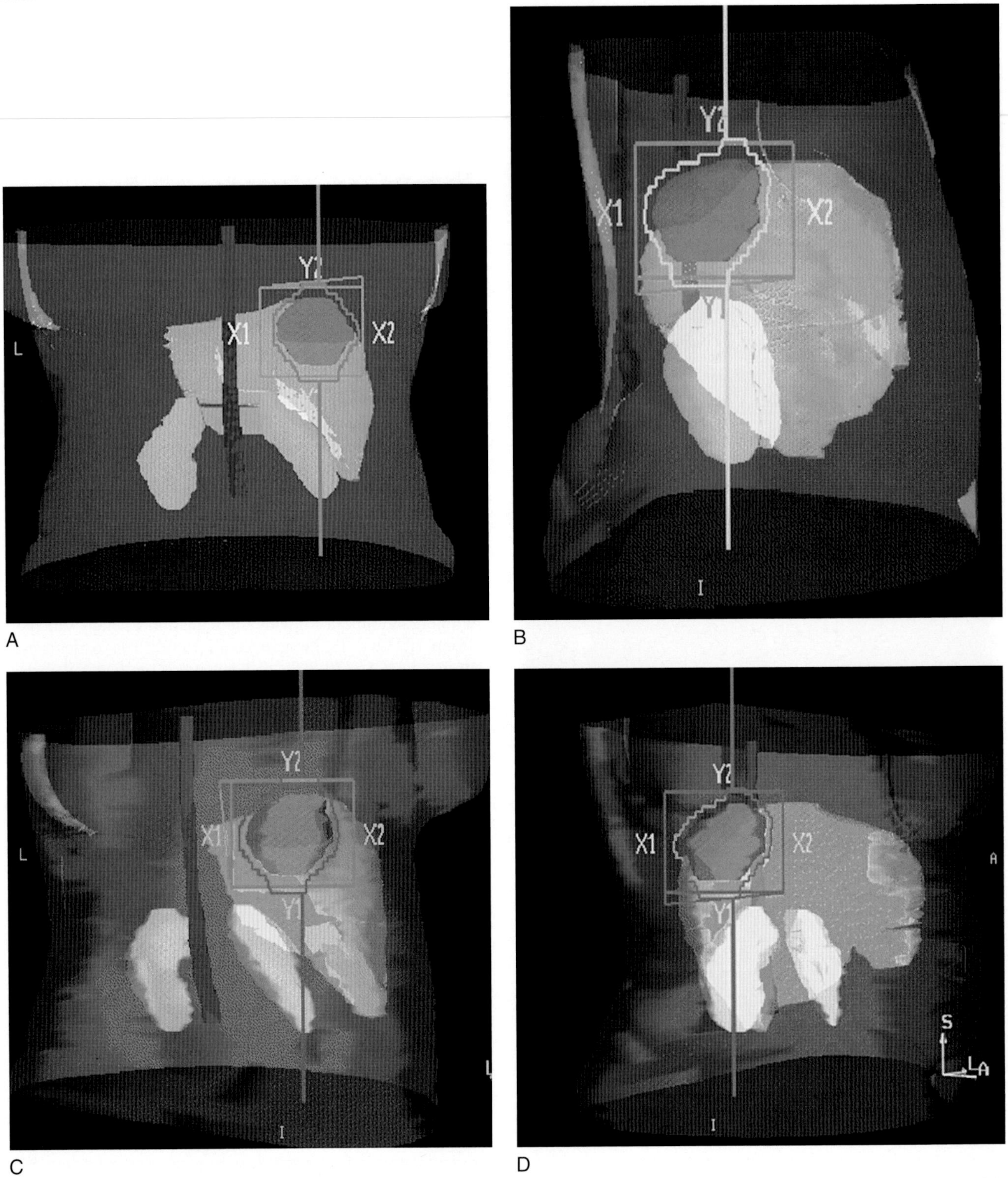

Fig. 75b.2. A, Beam's eye view, posterior field. **B,** Beam's eye view, right anterior oblique field #1. **C,** Beam's eye view, right posterior oblique field. **D,** Beam's eye view, right anterior oblique #2.

on 27 patients (11 patients with primary HCC) treated with 15 to 45 Gy delivered in one to three fractions. Local tumor control was achieved in all primary liver tumors treated with 20 Gy or more, at a mean follow-up of 12 months (range 1.5-38 months); average survival was 13.4 months (range 1.5-39 months). The predominant cause of death was progressive liver cirrhosis and progression of extrahepatic disease (9 of 11 patients) (Blomgren et al, 1998; Fuss & Thomas, 2004). Wulf and coworkers (2001) also reported actuarial local control of 76% at 1 year and 61% at two years in 24 hepatic lesions treated with three 10-Gy fractions of irradiation. Lastly, Wada and coworkers (2004) treated 34 patients with 42 lesions (11 liver patients, with 6 patients

Fig. 75b.3. IMRT plan.

having primary liver cancers) with 3D-CRT given as three fractions of 15 Gy each. They observed a 2-year tumor control probability of 83.6%, with a significant increase in tumor control probability for tumors less than 3 cm in diameter (2-year tumor control probability of 95% versus 58.3% for tumors <3 cm versus ≥3 cm; $P = .0022$) (Wada et al, 2004). Ongoing studies are being conducted at the University of Colorado (Schefter et al, 2003), the Technical University of Munich, Germany (Wulf et al, 2001), and the University of Texas Health Science Center (Fuss et al, 2003).

PROTON BEAM THERAPY

Although conventional external-beam irradiation employs photons, which deposit dose almost exponentially, considerable interest has been directed to development of particles that deposit less dose distal to the target. Proton beams have such a characteristic depth-dose pattern; known as the *Bragg peak*, this characteristic pattern, when applied to a modulated beam, provides constant dose deposition with depth until near the end of the range, where the dose peaks out to a high value followed by

Fig. 75b.4. Variant real-time position management (RPM) respiratory gating system.
(From Yorke E, Lovelock DM: Advanced treatment techniques I. In A Practical Guide to Intensity Modulated Radiation Therapy. Madison, WI, Medical Physics Publishing.)

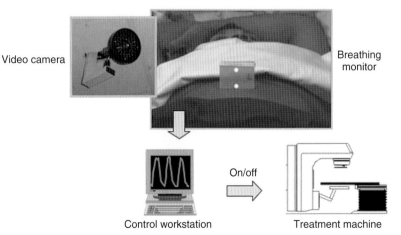

Video camera

Breathing monitor

Control workstation

On/off

Treatment machine

a rapid falloff to zero (Suit, 2002). The Bragg peak is of particular theoretical benefit for patients with HCC, who often have significant underlying liver dysfunction and may be more susceptible to damage even from low doses of irradiation.

The largest reported experience with proton beam therapy for HCC is from Tsukuba University in Japan. Tokuuye and colleagues (2003) reported on 163 patients with medically or technically unresectable HCC treated with proton therapy with or without transarterial embolization or percutaneous ethanol injection or both. A median dose of 72 Gy in 16 fractions over 3.2 weeks was given to part of the liver, with 5-year local control and survival rates of 83.2% and 24.7%. Eighty-five percent of all patients developed additional tumors within the remaining hepatic parenchyma (Tokuuye et al, 2003). These authors also reported that significant hypertrophy can be seen of the remaining liver tissue, and, as in surgical treatment, this seems to be closely related to the preserved functional capacity of the untreated liver volume (Ohara et al, 1997). These newer modalities may be able to minimize normal tissue effects via precise dose localization and should be investigated further.

BRACHYTHERAPY

Much work has been done with various radioisotopes; a full discussion of this modality is the subject of another chapter. In brief, ^{131}I-lipiodol has considerable theoretical appeal given its avid uptake by HCC cells, and numerous small studies have shown it to be associated with a short-lived decrease in tumor size and α-fetoprotein values (Kemeny & Schneider, 1989). A prospective randomized trial found significant improvement in local control, disease-free survival and overall survival for patients who underwent curative resection followed by a single dose of intra-arterial ^{131}I-lipiodol compared with postresection observation. With a median follow-up of 34.6 months, the recurrence rate for the adjuvant treatment group was 28.5% versus 59% for the control group ($P=.04$). Three-year overall survival in the treatment and control groups was 86.4% and 46.3% ($P=.039$) (Lau et al, 1999).

Several institutions also plan to investigate ^{90}Y-labeled lipiodol because of its advantages as a β emitter. Another agent of interest is ferritin, which is found in relatively high levels around HCC cells. ^{131}I-antiferritin and ^{125}I-antiferritin have been used alone or in combination with external-beam radiation, chemotherapy, mixed bacterial vaccines, and hepatic artery ligation. A study from China of 41 patients treated with hepatic artery ligation and intra-arterial antibody showed an increased resectability rate and higher 3-year overall survival rate compared with control subjects (25% versus 7%) (Fan et al, 1992). A randomized RTOG trial (Order et al, 1991) comparing intravenous chemotherapy with ^{131}I-antiferritin confirmed a comparable response rate (25%); in this series, a small but definable group of patients became surgically resectable after radiation therapy. In this series, all patients received "induction" whole liver irradiation (21 Gy in seven fractions) and intravenous doxorubicin/5-fluorouracil chemotherapy 4 to 6 weeks before randomization. Also, radiolabeled monoclonal antibody work shows early promise. Zeng and coworkers (1993) treated 23 unresectable patients with hepatic artery ligation and ^{131}I-Hepama-1, an anti-HCC monoclonal antibody. They found a 75% partial response rate as measured by tumor size and α-fetoprotein level and achieved a 48% resection rate. Direct injection of radioisotopes (high dose rate iridium 192

or ^{90}Y microspheres) into liver tumors also has been evaluated, with response ranging from complete pathologic response to stable disease, and seems to be well tolerated (Ho et al, 1998; Ii et al, 2001; Ricke et al, 2004).

MULTIMODALITY THERAPY

Data suggests that the use of combined radiation therapy and embolization may give promising results. Median survivals with this approach range from 14 to 23.5 months, with reported local control rates of greater than 70% and 3-year overall survival rates of 22% to 40%, even though most patients included in these studies had advanced disease (Table 75b.1) (Cheng et al, 2000; Guo et al, 2003; Li B et al, 2003; Seong et al, 1999, 2000; Yamada et al, 2003). Similarly, combinations of chemotherapy, whether delivered intra-arterially or intravenously concurrently with radiation therapy, may enhance the efficacy of radiation (Figs. 75b.5 and 75b.6).

BILE DUCT CANCERS

Bile duct cancers (see Ch. 52) are rare tumors, representing only a small fraction of all gastrointestinal cancers. Only a few tertiary centers to date have had meaningful experience with them. Similar to HCC, complete resection is the most effective and only potentially curative treatment. Although proximal location within the biliary tree historically has been associated with a worse outcome compared with distal locations, studies have found that it is actually the ability to undergo complete resection that most dictates prognosis (Jarnagin, 2000). Even after complete resection, however, local-regional recurrences are exceedingly common (>50%) (Boerma, 1990; Heron et al, 2003). In their review of a decade of experience at Memorial Sloan-Kettering Cancer Center, of 76 patients with hilar cholangiocarcinoma, 52 patients (68%) had disease recurrence; 38 (65%) were isolated local-regional recurrences (Jarnagin et al, 2003). The tumor-related cause of death in most patients is local persistence of disease and resultant biliary obstruction, liver failure, or intestinal obstruction (Gunderson et al, 1999; Jarnagin et al, 2003).

Adjuvant radiation therapy has been used, but given the rarity of these tumors, data are largely retrospective. Similar to HCC, poor results with irradiation of bile duct cancers have led to the belief that they are intrinsically radioresistant. There is no evidence, however, that bile duct tumor cells have an inherent radioresistance, but rather, as with HCC, that the doses of radiation generally administered have been limited by the surrounding structures. As for HCC, some more recent reports indicate that radiation limited to relatively small fields but reaching higher dose levels, combined with more modern surgical approaches and techniques, may have a positive effect on outcome (Gerhards et al, 2003; Jarnagin, 2000).

Gerhards and colleagues (2003) described a significant increase in median survival with the use of postoperative radiation therapy, external beam (42.3 ± 4.9 Gy, given as 1.1 Gy three times daily) with or without intraluminal brachytherapy (average dose 10.4 ± 1.7 Gy); in their series, median survival was 24 months with radiation therapy (41 patients) versus 8 months without radiation therapy (20 patients). Todoroki and coworkers (2000) described their experience with 63 patients treated with resection followed by intraoperative radiation therapy (21 ± 0.6 Gy)

Table 75b.1   Results of Multimodality Therapy

Reference	N	Stage	Treatment	Response Rate (%)	Local Control	Overall Survival	Median Survival
Yasuda, 1999	102	unresectable	TAE + PEI → EBRT (36-70 Gy) in 44 patients with largest tumors	NR	53% versus 32.7% (RT versus no RT)	81% versus 55% (3 yr)	NR
Seong et al, 2000	27	AJCC III—17; IVA—10	All failed previous TACE; EBRT (51.8 ± 7.9 Gy)	66.7	NR	33.2% (3 yr)	14 mo
Seong et al, 1999	30	AJCC III—10; IVA—20	TACE + Gelfoam embolization → EBRT (44 ± 0.3 Gy)	63.3	NR	22.2% (3 yr)	17 mo
Cheng et al, 2000	25	Okuda I—6; II—18; III—1	Lipiodol/Gelfoam embolization pre or post EBRT (16), PEI (1), EBRT (46.9 ± 5.9 Gy)	NR	78% (2 yr)	41% (2 yr)	19.2 mo
Li et al, 2003	45	AJCC IIIA—27; IIIB—18	TACE → 3D-CRT (50.4 Gy) → TACE	NR	73% (3 yr—crude)	22.6% (3 yr)	23.5 mo
Guo et al, 2003	76	Okuda I—29; II—46; III—1	TACE → EBRT (30-50 Gy) (compared with 89 patients treated with TACE alone)	47 versus 28.1 (RT versus no RT)	NR	28.6% 9.5% (3 yr); 19.3% versus 7.2% (5 yr)	19 mo (versus 10 mo)

EBRT, external beam radiation; NR, not reported; PEI, percutaneous ethanol injection; RT, radiation therapy; TACE, transarterial chemoembolization; TAE, transarterial embolization; 3D-CRT, 3-dimensional conformal radiation therapy.

followed by postoperative external-beam radiation therapy (43.6 Gy; range 27-61.2 Gy). Of 47 patients with microscopic residual disease, 28 received radiation therapy. Local control and 5-year survival rates were significantly higher in the adjuvant radiation therapy group than in the no radiation group (79.2% and 33.9% versus 31.2% and 13.5%) (Todoroki et al, 2000). Similarly, Heron and associates (2003) reported a survival benefit for proximal and distal bile duct cancers treated with adjuvant radiation therapy (36 patients) versus surgery alone (22 patients) (average external beam dose 46 Gy [range 27-60 Gy]; average brachytherapy dose 25 Gy [range 9-33 Gy]). Schoenthaler and coworkers (1992) reported that the median survival for patients with microscopic residual was 21.5 months when treated with adjuvant photon irradiation and 11 months when radiation therapy was not used (P=.0109) (61 months with charged particles; P=.0005). In contrast, although Gonzalez Gonzalez and colleagues (1999) reported that the total radiation dose was of prognostic significance with regard to margin status, patients receiving a total dose greater than 55 Gy had a shorter survival than patients treated with a lower dose; late complications included duodenal stenosis, upper digestive tract bleeding, and cholangitis. A large French study of 552 patients at 55 centers has been cited as showing no radiation effect, but only 5% of these patients received any form of radiation therapy (Reding et al, 1991). Overall, it seems from the bulk of the data that there is a small but definite subset of patients with unfavorable

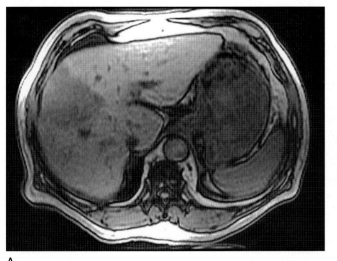
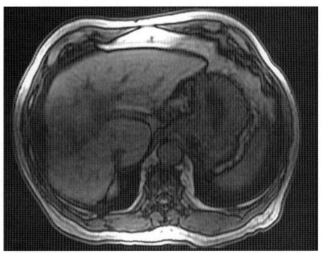

A   B

Fig. 75b.5. A, Patient 1, HCC before radiotherapy (axial, T1 weighted). **B,** Patient 1, HCC 1 year after radiotherapy (axial, T1 weighted).

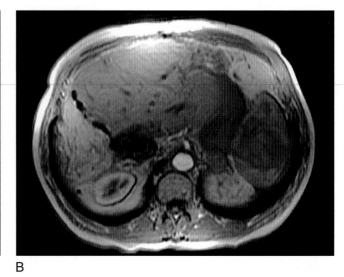

A   B

Fig. 75b.6. A, Patient 2, MRI before radiotherapy (T1 after gadolinium administration). **B,** Patient 2, MRI 10 months after radiotherapy (T1 after gadolinium administration).

disease who benefit from aggressive local therapy, but that toxicity can be high.

For unresectable bile duct cancers, combinations of external-beam radiation therapy and brachytherapy have been found to achieve reasonable local control and improvement in quality of life. Takamura and colleagues (2003) treated 93 patients with unresectable bile duct cancers with external-beam radiation (50 Gy in 25 fractions) followed by low-dose brachytherapy with iridium 192 (27-50 Gy; mean 39.2 Gy) delivered into an expandable metallic endoprosthesis placed into the duct. Median survival in this population was 12 months, with 1-year, 3-year, and 5-year actuarial survivals of 50%, 10%, and 4% (Takamura et al, 2003). Similarly, Shin and coworkers (2003) found a prolongation of the median time to tumor recurrence in patients treated with external-beam radiation in combination with high-dose brachytherapy compared with external-beam radiation alone (9 months versus 5 months) and a significant improvement in 2-year actuarial survival (21% versus 0%; $P=.015$). Data from Memorial Sloan-Kettering Cancer Center and Thomas Jefferson University hospital also support the use of concurrent chemotherapy with external-beam radiation and brachytherapy, with reports of median survivals of 12 to 24 months with this approach (Alden & Mohiuddin, 1994; Minsky et al, 1991). Crane and associates (2002) reported a trend for improved local control with higher doses of radiation therapy in their series of 52 patients treated with radiation therapy and, in 38 patients, concurrent chemotherapy. Radiation therapy also has been noted to be effective for the palliation of obstructive jaundice (Dvorak et al, 2002; Mayer et al, 2003).

Techniques to minimize toxicity and maximize local tumor control are similar to the techniques used for HCC and include 3D-CRT, brachytherapy/intraoperative radiation therapy, and charged particles. The earliest reports on 3D-CRT are from the University of Michigan. In a phase I study, Robertson and colleagues (1997) treated 16 patients with bile duct cancers with concurrent hepatic arterial bromodeoxyuridine and conformal radiation (1.5 Gy per fraction twice daily to dose range 24-66 Gy, depending on fractional volume of normal liver excluded from the high-dose volume). Acute toxicity included thrombocytopenia and leukopenia, and subacute or late complications included duodenal ulcers (two patients) and hemorrhagic gastritis (one patient); these complications occurred in patients treated to 66 Gy using treatment fields that extended inferiorly to the duodenum (Robertson et al, 1997). Wu and coworkers (2003a) used 3D-CRT for 21 patients with unresectable hilar cholangiocarcinoma, with a median overall survival rate of 16.5 months. The role of chemotherapy in combination with external-beam radiation is unclear; however, extrapolation from data on pancreatic, stomach, and colorectal carcinoma suggests a possible benefit to combining systemic therapy with aggressive local therapy. Shimizu and associates (2000) applied high-speed MRI to help delineate the target volume of bile duct and liver tumors and noted that integration of this technology has the potential to determine the target more precisely than conventional CT.

As noted previously, intraoperative radiation therapy and intraluminal brachytherapy are frequently used for bile duct cancers. Overall, there seems to be a small trend toward improved survival with the use of a boost, whether intraoperative radiation therapy or brachytherapy (Jarnagin, 2000). The potential advantages are clear: First, the area is reasonably accessible via stents placed during surgery or by the interventional radiologist; second, a high dose can be limited to a few surrounding centimeters. The risk of serious short-term toxicity is low, although most series report rates of cholangitis of 30% to 50%. Long-term complications secondary to the high doses and use of stents are common and include stricture, bowel obstruction, and bleeding. In addition, the rapid dose falloff means that some of the high-risk area may lie outside the high-dose area, so brachytherapy should be used only in conjunction with external-beam radiation therapy. No study has shown that brachytherapy alone has anything but the briefest of palliative effects. Reports of high-dose brachytherapy are beginning to appear in the literature (Kurisu et al, 1991; Lu et al, 2002). Lu and associates (2002) found improvements in response and median survival with increasing dose of high-dose boost in a phase I/II trial (median survivals of 9 months, 12.2 months, and 20.3 months with 52 Gy, 59 Gy, and 66 Gy total dose); all patients had received external-beam therapy first (total dose 45 Gy).

The use of charged particles has been reported by Lawrence Berkeley Laboratory, where 22 patients were treated with curative intent from 1977-1987 with helium or neon or both (Schoenthaler et al, 1994). The median survival times were 6.5 months, 11 months, and 14 months for patients treated with surgery alone, conventional adjuvant photon irradiation, and adjuvant irradiation with charged particles. Multivariate analysis showed that the extent of residual disease predicted outcome, and that patients with microscopic residual disease had increased median survival times with radiation therapy, especially when charged particles were used. Zurlo and coworkers (2000) analyzed many rival plans for patients with pancreatic and biliary tumors, and found that use of 3D-CRT or IMRT plans would entail a risk close to 5% for serious complications to the kidneys, liver, or bowel. In contrast, proton fields obtained better dose conformation and allowed for a boost to be delivered to all patients without excessive risk of morbidity.

TREATMENT COMPLICATIONS

Short-term toxicity associated with standard external-beam radiation therapy to the upper abdomen includes nausea, vomiting, malaise, fatigue, and weight loss; many patients with indwelling catheters have intermittent fevers. Long-term post–radiation therapy complications, particularly duodenal, have been reported in the literature at rates that seem to vary with survival times. Other dose-limiting structures include the kidneys and liver, as noted previously. Radiation-induced liver dysfunction characteristically appears 2 to 6 weeks after completion of radiation therapy to the liver. The severity of symptoms and physical findings vary widely, but most commonly patients report rapid weight gain and increase in abdominal girth. On physical examination, a markedly enlarged liver and ascites are often noted. On laboratory evaluation, liver function tests and, in particular, alkaline phosphatase are elevated. Pathologically, the acute changes of radiation-induced liver dysfunction involve the centrilobular region and include severe sinusoidal congestion, hyperemia or hemorrhage, and atrophy of the central hepatic cells. Late changes include atrophy of the centrilobular hepatic cords, minimal sinusoidal distention by red blood cells, and thickening of the central vein wall. Treatment ranges from observation to aggressive salt restriction, diuretic therapy, and paracentesis. The place of steroids is unclear (Ingold et al, 1954).

As described earlier, efforts to minimize dose to nearby radiosensitive structures and to minimize complications are ongoing. Further development of systemic therapies designed to enhance the radiation sensitivity and promote control of micrometastases is required (Chenoufi et al, 1998). Preliminary reports on gene therapy for these malignancies are intriguing (Chung et al, 2002; Kawashita et al, 1999; Li XJ et al, 2003).

SUMMARY

HCC and bile duct cancers, although historically thought to be radioresistant, have been found to show responsiveness to radiation therapy in a dose-dependent manner. As progress in the ability to target radiation therapy is made, whether by technical advances in external-beam delivery, brachytherapy, or charged particle therapy or the use of combined treatments (e.g., chemotherapy, arterial embolization, gene therapy), the therapeutic ratio in these diseases is likely to improve.

REFERENCES

Alden ME, Mohiuddin M, 1994: The impact of radiation dose in combined external beam and intraluminal Ir-192 brachytherapy for bile duct cancer. Int J Radiat Oncol Biol Phys 28:945-951.

Ang KK, 1998: Fractionation effects in clinical practice. In Leibel SA, Phillips TL (eds): Textbook of Radiation Oncology. Philadelphia, Saunders.

Blomgren H, et al, 1998: Radiosurgery for tumors in the body: clinical experience using a new method. J Radiosurg 1:63-74.

Boerma E, 1990: Research in the results of resection of the hilar bile duct cancer. Surgery 108:572-580.

Boyer AL, et al, 2001: Intensity-modulated radiotherapy: current status and issues of interest. Int J Radiat Oncol Biol Phys 51:880-914.

Chen LH, Guan J, 2003a: Evaluation of three-dimensional conformal radiation therapy for small primary hepatocellular carcinoma. Di Yi Jun Yi Da Xue Xue Bao 23:260-261.

Chen LH, Guan J, 2003b: Value of conformal radiotherapy for middle stage or advanced primary hepatocellular carcinoma. Di Yi Jun Yi Da Xue Xue Bao 23:55-57.

Cheng JC, et al, 2000: Local radiotherapy with or without transcatheter arterial chemoembolization for patients with unresectable hepatocellular carcinoma. Int J Radiat Oncol Biol Phys 47:435-442.

Cheng JC, et al, 2002: Radiation-induced liver disease after three-dimensional conformal radiotherapy for patients with hepatocellular carcinoma: dosimetric analysis and implication. Int J Radiat Oncol Biol Phys 54:156-162.

Chenoufi N, et al, 1998: In vitro demonstration of synergy between radionuclide and chemotherapy. J Nucl Med 39:900-903.

Cho KH, et al, 1999: Cost-benefit analysis of three dimensional conformal radiation therapy. Acta Oncol 38:603-611.

Chung SM, et al, 2002: The use of a genetically engineered herpes simplex virus (R7020) with ionizing radiation for experimental hepatoma. Gene Ther 9:75-80.

Crane CH, et al, 2002: Limitations of conventional doses of chemoradiation for unresectable biliary cancer. Int J Radiat Oncol Biol Phys 53:969-974.

Dawson LA, et al, 2000: Escalated focal liver radiation and concurrent hepatic artery fluorodeoxyuridine for unresectable intrahepatic malignancies. J Clin Oncol 18:220-221.

Dvorak J, et al, 2002: Intraluminal high dose rate brachytherapy in the treatment of bile duct and gallbladder carcinomas. Hepatogastroenterology 49:916-917.

Emami B, et al, 1991: Tolerance of normal tissue to therapeutic irradiation. Int J Radiat Oncol Biol Phys 21:109-122.

Fan Z, et al, 1992: Radioiodinated anti-hepatocellular carcinoma (anti-HCC) ferritin: targeting therapy, tumor imaging and anti-antibody response in HCC patients with hepatic arterial infusion. J Cancer Res Clin Oncol 118:371-376.

Friedman MA, et al, 1988: Phase III trial of irradiation plus chemotherapy for patients with hepatic metastases and hepatoma: experience of the Northern California Oncology Group. NCI Monogr 6:259-264.

Fuss M, Thomas CR, 2004: Stereotactic body radiation therapy: an ablative treatment option for primary and secondary liver tumors. Ann Surg Oncol 11:1380-1381.

Fuss M, et al, 2003: Daily stereotactic ultrasound targeting for intensity-modulated radiotherapy (IMRT) of abdominal malignancies. Proc ASCO 322:346.

Gerhards MR, et al, 2003: Results of postoperative radiotherapy for resectable hilar cholangiocarcinoma. World J Surg 27:173-179.

Gierga DP, et al, 2004: Quantification of respiration-induced abdominal tumor motion and its impact on IMRT dose distributions. Int J Radiat Oncol Biol Phys 58:1584-1595.

Gonzalez Gonzalez D, et al, 1999: Role of radiotherapy, in particular intraluminal brachytherapy, in the treatment of proximal bile duct carcinoma. Ann Oncol 10(suppl 4):215-220.

Gunderson LL, et al, 1999: Conformal irradiation for hepatobiliary malignancies. Ann Oncol 10(suppl 4):S221-S225.

Guo W, et al, 2003: Comparison between chemoembolization combined with radiotherapy and chemoembolization alone for large hepatocellular carcinoma. World J Gastroenterol 9:1697-1701.

Hall EJ, Cox JD, 1994: Physical and biologic basis of radiation therapy. In Cox JD (ed): Moss' Radiation Oncology, 7th ed. Philadelphia, Mosby, pp 33-35.

Herfarth KK, et al, 2001: Stereotactic single-dose radiation therapy of liver tumors: results of a phase I/II trial. J Clin Oncol 19:164-170.

Heron DE, et al, 2003: Cholangiocarcinoma: the impact of tumor location and treatment strategy on outcome. Am J Clin Oncol 26:422-428.

Ho S, et al, 1998: Internal radiation therapy for patients with primary or metastatic hepatic cancer. Cancer 83:1894-1907.

Ii N, et al, 2001: Advanced hepatocellular carcinoma—feasibility and clinical impact of high-dose-rate brachytherapy on the treatment of lesions growing into biliary trees, portal veins and the vena cava. Gan To Kagaku Ryoho 28:1498-1500.

Ingold J, et al, 1954: Radiation hepatitis. AJR Am J Roentgenol 93:200-208.

Jarnagin WR, 2000: Cholangiocarcinoma of the extrahepatic bile ducts. Semin Surg Oncol 19:156-176.

Jarnagin WR, et al, 2003: Patterns of initial disease recurrence after resection of gallbladder carcinoma and hilar cholangiocarcinoma: implications for adjuvant therapeutic strategies. Cancer 98:1659-1700.

Kawashita J, et al, 1999: Regression of hepatocellular carcinoma in vitro and in vivo by radiosensitizing suicide gene therapy under the inducible and spatial control of radiation. Hum Gene Ther 19:1509-1519.

Kemeny N, Schneider A, 1989: Regional treatment of hepatic metastases and hepatocellular carcinoma. Curr Prob Cancer 13:197-283.

Kurisu K, et al, 1991: High dose-rate intraluminal brachytherapy for bile duct carcinoma after surgery. Radiother Oncol 21:65-66.

Lai E, et al, 1986: Treatment of unresectable hepatocellular carcinoma: results of a randomized controlled trial. World J Surg 10:501-509.

Lau W, et al, 1999: Adjuvant intra-arterial iodine-131 labeled lipiodol for resectable hepatocellular carcinoma: a prospective randomized trial. Lancet 353:797-801.

Lawrence TS, et al, 1992: The use of 3-D dose volume analysis to predict radiation hepatitis. Int J Radiat Oncol Biol Phys 23:781-788.

Li B, et al, 2003: Study of local three-dimensional conformal radiotherapy combined with transcatheter arterial chemoembolization for patients with stage III hepatocellular carcinoma. Am J Clin Oncol 26:e92-e99.

Li XJ, et al, 2003: Ionizing radiation-regulated killing of human hepatoma cells by liposome-mediated CdglyTK gene delivery. Shen Wu Hua Xue Yu Sheng Wu Wu Li Xue Bao 35:64-70.

Lu JJ, et al, 2002: High-dose-rate remote afterloading intracavitary brachytherapy for the treatment of extrahepatic biliary duct carcinoma. Cancer J 8:74-78.

Mayer R, et al, 2003: Palliative treatment of unresectable bile duct tumors. Acta Med Aust 30:1-10.

Minsky BD, et al, 1991: Extrahepatic biliary system cancer: an update of a combined modality approach. Am J Clin Oncol 14:433-437.

Nerenstone SR, et al, 1988: Clinical trials in primary hepatocellular carcinoma: current status and future directions. Cancer Treat Rev 15:1-31.

Ohara K, et al, 1997: Radiation tolerance of cirrhotic livers in relation to the preserved functional capacity: analysis of patients with hepatocellular carcinoma treated by focused proton beam radiotherapy. Int J Radiat Oncol Biol Phys 38:367-372.

Oncology Net Guide, 2004: Beyond radiotherapy: intensity modulated radiation therapy. 5:52-54.

Order S, et al, 1991: A randomized prospective trial comparing full dose chemotherapy to 131I-antiferritin: an RTOG study. Int J Radiat Oncol Biol Phys 20:953-963.

Park HC, et al, 2002: Dose-response relationship in local radiotherapy for hepatocellular carcinoma. Int J Radiat Oncol Biol Phys 54:150-155.

Pattaranutaporn P, et al, 2001: Three-dimensional conformal radiation therapy and periodic irradiation with the deep inspiration breath-hold technique for hepatocellular carcinoma. J Med Assoc Thai 84:1692-1700.

Reding R, et al, 1991: Surgical management of 552 carcinomas of the extrahepatic bile ducts (gallbladder and periampullary tumors excluded). Ann Surg 213:236-241.

Ricke J, et al, 2004: CT-guided interstitial brachytherapy of liver malignancies alone or in combination with thermal ablation: phase I-II results of a novel technique. Int J Radiat Oncol Biol Phys 58:1496-1505.

Robertson J, et al, 1997: Long-term results of hepatic artery fluorodeoxyuridine and conformal radiation therapy for primary hepatobiliary cancers. Int J Radiat Oncol Biol Phys 37:325-330.

Rosu M, et al, 2003: Alterations in normal liver doses due to organ motion. Int J Radiat Oncol Biol Phys 57:1472-1479.

Russell AH, et al, 1993: Accelerated hyperfractionated hepatic irradiation in the management of patients with liver metastases: results of the RTOG dose-escalating protocol. Int J Radiat Oncol Biol Phys 27:117-123.

Schefter T, et al, 2003: Hypofractionated extracranial stereotactic radiotherapy for liver tumors. Int J Radiat Oncol Biol Phys 57(suppl):S282.

Schoenthaler R, et al, 1992: Definitive postoperative irradiation of bile duct carcinoma with charged particles and/or photons. Int J Radiat Oncol Biol Phys 27:75.

Schoenthaler R, et al, 1994: Carcinoma of the extrahepatic bile ducts: the University of California at San Francisco experience. Ann Surg 219:267-274.

Seong J, et al, 1999: Combined transcatheter arterial chemoembolization and local radiotherapy of unresectable hepatocellular carcinoma. Int J Radiat Oncol Biol Phys 43:393-397.

Seong J, et al, 2000: Local radiotherapy for unresectable hepatocellular carcinoma patients who failed with transcatheter arterial chemoembolization. Int J Radiat Oncol Biol Phys 47:1331-1335.

Seong J, et al, 2003: Clinical results and prognostic factors in radiotherapy for unresectable hepatocellular carcinoma: a retrospective study of 158 patients. Int J Radiat Oncol Biol Phys 55:329-336.

Shimizu S, et al, 2000: High-speed magnetic resonance imaging for four-dimensional treatment planning of conformal radiotherapy of moving body tumors. Int J Radiat Oncol Biol Phys 48:471-474.

Shin HS, et al, 2003: Combination of external beam irradiation and high-dose-rate intraluminal brachytherapy for inoperable carcinoma of the extrahepatic bile ducts. Int J Radiat Oncol Biol Phys 57:105-112.

Stillwagon G, et al, 1989: 194 hepatocellular cancers treated by radiation and chemotherapy combinations: toxicity and response: a RTOG study. Int J Radiat Oncol Biol Phys 17:1223.

Suit H, 2002: The Gray Lecture 2001: coming technical advances in radiation oncology. Int J Radiat Oncol Biol Phys 53:798-809.

Takamura A, et al, 2003: Intraluminal low-dose-rate 192-Ir brachytherapy combined with external beam radiotherapy and biliary stenting for unresectable extrahepatic bile duct carcinoma. Int J Radiat Oncol Biol Phys 57:1357-1365.

Ten Haken R, et al, 1996: Potential benefits of eliminating planning target volume expansions for patient breathing in the treatment of liver tumors. Int J Radiat Oncol Biol Phys 36:167-174.

Todoroki T, et al, 2000: Benefits of adjuvant radiotherapy after radical resection of locally advanced main hepatic duct carcinoma. Int J Radiat Oncol Biol Phys 46:581-587.

Tokuuye K, et al, 2003: Clinical results of proton radiotherapy for hepatocellular carcinoma. Int J Radiat Oncol Biol Phys 57(suppl):S383.

Wada H, et al, 2004: Univariate analysis of factors correlated with tumor control probability of three-dimensional conformal hypofractionated high-dose radiotherapy for small pulmonary or hepatic tumors. Int J Radiat Oncol Biol Phys 58:1114-1120.

Wagman R, et al, 2003: Respiratory gating for liver tumors: use in dose escalation. Int J Radiat Oncol Biol Phys 55:659-668.

Wong JW, et al, 1999: The use of active breathing control (ABC) to reduce margin for breathing motion. Int J Radiat Oncol Biol Phys 44:911-919.

Wu DH, Chen LH, 2003a: Therapeutic effect of three-dimensional conformal radiotherapy on hilar cholangiocarcinoma. Di Yi Jun Yi Da Xue Xue Bao 23:1217-1218.

Wu DH, Chen LH, 2003b: Therapeutic effects of 3-dimensional conformal radiotherapy for small hepatocellular cancers and multi-factor analysis of the prognosis. Di Yi Jun Yi Da Xue Xue Bao 23:1056-1058.

Wulf J, et al, 2001: Stereotactic radiotherapy of targets in the lung and liver. Strahlenther Onkol 177:645-655.

Yamada K, et al, 2003: Prospective trial of combined transcatheter arterial chemoembolization and three-dimensional conformal radiotherapy for portal vein tumor thrombus in patients with unresectable hepatocellular carcinoma. Int J Radiat Oncol Biol Phys 57:113-119.

Yasuda S, et al, 1999: Radiotherapy for large hepatocellular carcinoma combined with transcatheter arterial embolization and percutaneous ethanol injection therapy. Int J Oncol 15:467-473.

Zeng Z, et al, 1993: Radioimmunotherapy for unresectable hepatocellular carcinoma using 131I-Hepama-1 mAb: preliminiary results. J Cancer Res Clin Oncol 119:257-259.

Zurlo A, et al, 2000: The role of proton therapy in the treatment of large irradiation volumes: a comparative planning study of pancreatic and biliary tumors. Int J Radiat Oncol Biol Phys 48:277-288.

76

Ablation of Liver Tumors

76a PERCUTANEOUS METHODS FOR ABLATION OF HEPATIC NEOPLASMS

R. LENCIONI AND D. CIONI

Hepatocellular carcinoma (HCC) (see Ch. 71) is the fifth most common cancer, and its incidence is increasing worldwide because of the dissemination of hepatitis B virus and hepatitis C virus infections. Patients with cirrhosis are at the highest risk of developing HCC and should undergo surveillance programs to detect the tumor at an early, asymptomatic stage (Bruix et al, 2001). Patients with early stage HCC—as defined by the Barcelona Clinic Liver Cancer staging classification (Bruix & Llovet, 2002)—should be considered first for surgical treatment options, which may achieve 60% to 70% 5-year survival in well-selected patients (Llovet et al, 2003). Hepatic resection is best indicated for patients with a single tumor and well-preserved liver function, who have neither abnormal bilirubin nor clinically relevant portal hypertension. Less than 5% of cirrhotic patients with HCC fit these criteria, however (Llovet et al, 1999). Liver transplantation benefits patients who have decompensated cirrhosis and one tumor smaller than 5 cm or three or fewer nodules smaller than 3 cm each, but donor shortage greatly limits its applicability. This difficulty may be overcome in part by living donation, which requires a highly skilled surgical team (Belghiti & Kianmanesh, 2003; Schwartz, 2004).

Advances in surgical techniques during the 1980s and 1990s have led to effective treatment for selected patients with hepatic metastases. Surgical resection of colorectal cancer metastatic to the liver results in a 5-year survival rate of 40% (see Ch. 73a), and liver metastases from other primary tumors, such as neuroendocrine carcinoma and genitourinary tumors, are treated effectively with liver resection (Bentrem et al, 2005; Weitz et al, 2005) (see Ch. 73c). Only 10% to 25% of patients with metastases isolated to the liver are eligible for resection, however, because of extent and location of the disease or concurrent medical conditions (Lencioni et al, 2004a). Treatment of nonoperable or nonresectable patients with systemic or intra-arterial chemotherapy is not entirely satisfactory in terms of survival outcomes (Jonker et al, 2000).

Image-guided techniques for local tumor treatment have emerged as viable therapeutic options for patients with limited hepatic malignant disease who are not surgical candidates. Several methods for chemical ablation or thermal tumor destruction through localized heating or freezing have been developed and clinically tested (Table 76a.1). Although chemical and hyperthermic ablation techniques have been widely performed via a percutaneous approach, most experience with cryotherapy has involved an open or laparoscopic approach. This subchapter focuses on the percutaneous use of chemical and hyperthermic ablation in the treatment of HCC and hepatic metastases.

ELIGIBILITY CRITERIA

To evaluate eligibility for percutaneous ablation, a careful clinical, laboratory, and imaging assessment has to be performed in each patient by a multidisciplinary team. Laboratory tests should include measurement of serum tumor markers, such as α-fetoprotein (AFP) for HCC and carcinoembryonic antigen (CEA) for colorectal metastases, and a full evaluation of the patient's coagulation status. A prothrombin time ratio (normal time to patient's time) greater than 50% and a platelet count greater than $50,000/\mu L$ are required to keep the risk of bleeding at an acceptable low level. The tumor staging protocol must be tailored to the kind of malignancy present. In patients with HCC, staging should include abdominal ultrasound and spiral computed tomography (CT) or dynamic magnetic resonance imaging (MRI), although in selected cases chest CT and bone scintigraphy may be needed to exclude extrahepatic tumor spread. Whole body CT and positron emission tomography may be required to stage patients with hepatic metastases properly.

Percutaneous treatment is accepted as the best therapeutic choice for patients with early stage HCC who are not surgical candidates (Bruix et al, 2001; Lencioni et al, 2004b). Patients are required to have a single tumor smaller than 5 cm or three or fewer nodules smaller than 3 cm each, no evidence of vascular invasion or extrahepatic spread, performance status test of 0, and liver cirrhosis in Child-Pugh class A or B. In the setting of metastatic disease, percutaneous ablation generally is indicated for patients with colorectal cancer oligometastases isolated to the liver who are not eligible for surgery (Gillams & Lees, 2005; Lencioni et al, 2004a). Selected patients with limited hepatic and pulmonary colorectal metastatic disease may qualify for percutaneous treatment (Berber et al, 2005; Lencioni et al, 2004c). In patients with hepatic metastases from other primary cancers, promising initial results have been reported in the treatment of breast and endocrine tumors (Abe et al, 2005; Liang et al, 2003). The number of lesions should not be considered an absolute contraindication to percutaneous ablation if successful treatment of all metastatic deposits can be accomplished. Nevertheless, most centers preferentially treat patients with four or fewer lesions. Tumor size is crucial to predict the outcome of percutaneous ablation. Imaging studies underestimate the size of metastatic deposits. The target tumor should not exceed 3 to 4 cm in longest axis to ensure complete ablation with most of the currently available devices.

Pretreatment imaging must define the location of each lesion carefully with respect to surrounding structures. Lesions located

Table 76a.1   Percutaneous Methods for Ablation of Hepatic Neoplasms

Chemical Ablation

Ethanol injection
Acetic acid injection

Thermal Ablation

Radiofrequency ablation
Microwave ablation
Laser ablation
Cryoablation

along the surface of the liver can be considered for percutaneous ablation, although their treatment requires adequate expertise and may be associated with a higher risk of complications. Thermal ablation of superficial lesions that are adjacent to any part of the gastrointestinal tract must be avoided because of the risk of thermal injury of the gastric or bowel wall (Rhim et al, 2004). The colon seems to be at greater risk than the stomach or small bowel for thermally mediated perforation. Gastric complications are rare, likely owing to the relatively greater wall thickness of the stomach or the rarity of surgical adhesions along the gastrohepatic ligament. The mobility of the small bowel also may provide the bowel with greater protection compared with the relatively fixed colon. A laparoscopic approach or the use of special techniques, such as intraperitoneal injection of dextrose to displace the bowel, can be considered in such instances. Treatment of lesions adjacent to the gallbladder or to the hepatic hilum risks thermal injury to the biliary tract. In experienced hands, thermal ablation of tumors located in the vicinity of the gallbladder was shown to be feasible, although it was associated in most cases with self-limited iatrogenic cholecystitis (Chopra et al, 2003). In contrast, thermal ablation of lesions adjacent to hepatic vessels is possible because flowing blood usually protects the vascular wall from thermal injury. In these cases, the risk of incomplete treatment of the neoplastic tissue close to the vessel may increase because of the heat loss by convection. The potential risk of thermal damage to critical structures should be weighed against benefits on a case-by-case basis.

CHEMICAL ABLATION

The seminal technique used for local ablation of hepatic tumors is percutaneous ethanol injection (PEI). Ethanol induces coagulation necrosis of the lesion as a result of cellular dehydration, protein denaturation, and chemical occlusion of small tumor vessels. PEI is a well-established technique for the treatment of nodular-type HCC. HCC nodules have a soft consistency and are surrounded by a firm cirrhotic liver. Consequently, injected ethanol diffuses within them easily and selectively, leading to complete necrosis of about 70% of small lesions (Shiina et al, 1991). An alternate method for chemical ablation is acetic acid injection. Although acetic acid injection has been reported to increase the success rate of PEI, this technique has been used by very few investigators worldwide. PEI and other methods of chemical ablation are ineffective in the treatment of metastatic lesions. As opposed to HCC, ethanol diffusion within hepatic metastases is uneven, resulting in largely incomplete ablation

with necrotic areas and viable tissue irregularly mixed (Livraghi et al, 1991).

Ethanol Injection

PEI is best administered by using ultrasound guidance because ultrasound allows for continuous real-time monitoring of the injection. This monitoring is crucial to realize the pattern of tumor perfusion and to avoid excessive ethanol leakage outside the lesion. Fine noncutting needles, with either a single end hole or multiple side holes, are commonly used for PEI. PEI usually is performed under local anesthesia and does not require patient hospitalization. The treatment schedule includes four to six sessions performed once or twice weekly. The number of treatment sessions and the amount of injected ethanol per session may vary greatly according to the size of the lesion, the pattern of tumor perfusion, and the compliance of the patient.

Although there have not been any prospective randomized trials comparing PEI and best supportive care or PEI and surgical resection, several retrospective studies have provided indirect evidence that PEI improves the natural history of HCC. The long-term outcomes of patients with small tumors who were treated with PEI were similar to the outcomes reported in surgical series, with 5-year survival rates ranging from 41% to 53% in Child A patients (Table 76a.2). Two cohort studies and one retrospective case-control study comparing surgical resection and PEI failed to identify any difference in survival, despite the finding that patients in PEI groups had poorer liver function (Table 76a.3). These data show that PEI is a useful treatment for patients with early stage HCC and suggest that surgical resection may achieve better results only after strict candidate selection.

Table 76a.2   Studies Reporting Long-Term Survival Outcomes of Patients with Early Stage Hepatocellular Carcinoma Who Underwent Percutaneous Ethanol Injection

Reference	No. Patients	SURVIVAL RATES (%)		
		1-yr	3-yr	5-yr
Shiina et al, 1993	98	85	62	52
Lencioni et al, 1995	105	96	68	32
Livraghi et al, 1995				
Child A, single HCC <5 cm	293	98	79	47
Child B, single HCC <5 cm	149	93	63	29
Ryu et al, 1997				
Stage I, 1-3 HCC <3 cm*	110	98	84	54
Stage II, 1-3 HCC <3 cm*	140	91	65	45
Lencioni et al, 1997				
Child A, 1 HCC <5 cm or 3 HCC <3 cm	127	98	79	53
Child B, 1 HCC <5 cm or 3 HCC <3 cm	57	88	50	28
Pompili et al, 2001				
Child A, 1-2 HCC <5 cm	111	94	62	41
Teratani et al, 2002				
Age <70 yr	516	90	65	40
Age >70 yr	137	83	52	27

*Clinical stage according to the Liver Cancer Study Group of Japan.

Table 76a.3   Studies Comparing Surgical Resection and Percutaneous Ethanol Injection in Treatment of Early Stage Hepatocellular Carcinoma

Reference	No. Patients	SURVIVAL RATES (%)			P
		1-yr	3-yr	5-yr	
Castells et al, 1993*					NS
Surgical resection	33	81	44	NA	
PEI	30	83	55	NA	
Yamamoto et al, 2001*					NS
Surgical resection	58	97	84	61	
PEI	39	100	82	59	
Daniele et al, 2003†					NS
Surgical resection	17	82	63	NA	
PEI	65	91	65	NA	

*Cohort study.
†Retrospective case-control study.
NA, not available; NS, not significant.

Although PEI is a low-risk procedure, severe complications have been reported. In a multicenter survey including 1066 patients, 1 death (0.1%) and 34 complications (3.2%), including 7 cases of tumor seeding (0.7%), were reported (Di Stasi et al, 1997). The major limitation of PEI is the high local recurrence rate, which may reach 33% in lesions smaller than 3 cm and 43% in lesions exceeding 3 cm (Khan et al, 2000; Koda et al, 2000). The injected ethanol does not always accomplish complete tumor necrosis because of its inhomogeneous distribution within the lesion, especially in the presence of intratumoral septa, and the limited effect on extracapsular cancerous spread. PEI is unable to create a safety margin of ablation in the liver parenchyma surrounding the nodule and may not destroy tiny satellite lesions that—even in small tumors—may be located in close proximity of the main nodule.

Injection of large volumes of ethanol in a single session performed under general anesthesia has been reported to enable successful PEI treatment of large or infiltrating HCC (Livraghi et al, 1998). Results of single-session PEI are based on uncontrolled investigations. When critically compared with data about the natural history and prognosis of untreated nonsurgical HCC patients, the benefits of the procedure are not evident.

Acetic Acid Injection

Acetic acid injection has been proposed as a viable alternative to PEI for the treatment of HCC. Two studies compared acetic acid injection and PEI. In the first study, 60 patients with small HCC lesions were entered into a randomized trial. The 1-year and 2-year survival rates were 100% and 92% in the acetic acid injection group and 83% and 63% in the PEI group. A multivariate analysis of prognostic factors showed that treatment was an independent predictor of survival (Ohnishi et al, 1998). In contrast, in a prospective comparative study including 63 patients treated by acetic acid injection and 62 patients treated by PEI, no significant survival differences were observed between the two treatment groups (Huo et al, 2003). This alternate option for chemical ablation had limited diffusion and was not tested in large series of patients. The reported survival outcomes are not better than the outcomes obtained by several authors with PEI.

THERMAL ABLATION

Application of localized heating or freezing enables in situ destruction of malignant liver tumors, preserving normal liver parenchyma. The thermal ablative therapies involved in clinical practice can be classified as hepatic hyperthermic treatments—including radiofrequency ablation (RFA) (see Ch. 76c), microwave ablation, and laser ablation—or hepatic cryotherapy. Hepatic hyperthermic treatments are performed mostly via a percutaneous approach, whereas an open or laparoscopic approach has been widely adopted for hepatic cryotherapy (see Ch. 76b). This discussion focuses on percutaneous hyperthermic ablation in the treatment of HCC and hepatic metastases.

The thermal damage caused by heating depends on the tissue temperature achieved and the duration of heating. Heating of tissue at 50°C to 55°C for 4 to 6 minutes produces irreversible cellular damage. At temperatures between 60°C and 100°C, almost immediate coagulation of tissue is induced, with irreversible damage to mitochondrial and cytosolic enzymes of the cells. At temperatures greater than 100°C, tissue vaporizes and carbonizes (Goldberg et al, 2000). For adequate destruction of tumor tissue, the entire target volume must be subjected to cytotoxic temperatures. Different physical mechanisms are involved in hepatic hyperthermic treatments to generate a lethal temperature. RFA is based on the interaction of an alternating electric current with living tissue. At a high-frequency setting (460-480 kHz), the current causes agitation of ions in the adjacent tissue, which generate frictional heat that extends into the tissue by conduction. Microwave ablation relies on high-frequency electromagnetic radiation that is generated to heat the intracellular water molecules of the surrounding tissue. The resulting heat energy leads to irreversible cellular damage. Laser ablation consists of a coherent, monochromatic, and highly collimated beam of light. Focusing such light energy into the liver tumor results in heat production and coagulation.

An important factor that affects the success of thermal ablation is the ability to ablate all viable tumor tissue and an adequate tumor-free margin. To achieve rates of local tumor recurrence with thermal ablation that are comparable to rates obtained with hepatic resection, a 360-degree, 1-cm-thick, tumor-free margin should be produced around each tumor (Goldberg et al, 2000). This cuff is necessary to ensure that all microscopic invasions around the periphery of a tumor have been eradicated. The target diameter of an ablation ideally should be 2 cm larger than the diameter of the tumor that undergoes treatment (Fig. 76a.1).

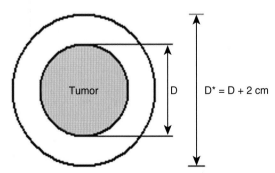

Fig. 76a.1. Schematic model of a thermal ablation. The target diameter of the ablation zone (D*) ideally should be 2 cm larger than the diameter of the tumor that undergoes treatment (D).

A 5-cm ablation device can be used to treat a 3-cm diameter tumor. Otherwise, multiple overlapping ablations have to be performed (Dodd et al, 2001).

Thermal ablation usually is performed under conscious sedation or general anesthesia with standard cardiac, pressure, and oxygen monitoring. Targeting of the lesion can be performed with ultrasound, CT, or MRI. The guidance system is chosen largely on the basis of operator preference and local availability of dedicated equipment, such as CT fluoroscopy or open MRI systems. A percutaneously inserted metallic coil can be placed during the proper phase of contrast enhancement as a target to facilitate ablation of tumors poorly seen on CT or ultrasound (Adam et al, 2004). During the procedure, important aspects to be monitored include how well the tumor is being covered, and whether any adjacent normal structures are being affected at the same time. Although the transient hyperechoic zone that is seen at ultrasound within and surrounding a tumor during and immediately after RFA can be used as a rough guide to the extent of tumor destruction, MRI currently is the only imaging modality with validated techniques for real-time temperature monitoring. To control an image-guided ablation procedure, the operator can use the image-based information obtained during monitoring or an automated system that terminates the ablation at a critical point in the procedure. At the end of the procedure, most systems allow one to ablate the needle tract, which is aimed at preventing any tumor cell dissemination.

Contrast-enhanced ultrasound performed after the end of the procedure may allow an initial evaluation of treatment effects. Contrast-enhanced CT and MRI are recognized as the standard modalities to assess treatment outcome, although promising initial results have been reported using positron emission tomography. CT and MRI performed after treatment show successful ablation as a nonenhancing area with or without a peripheral enhancing rim (Figs. 76a.2 and 76a.3). The enhancing rim that may be observed along the periphery of the ablation zone appears as a relatively concentric, symmetric, and uniform process in an area with smooth inner margins. This is a transient finding that represents a benign physiologic response to thermal injury (initially, reactive hyperemia; subsequently, fibrosis and giant cell reaction).

Benign periablational enhancement needs to be differentiated from irregular peripheral enhancement owing to residual tumor that occurs at the treatment margin. In contrast to benign periablational enhancement, residual unablated tumor often grows in scattered, nodular, or eccentric patterns (Goldberg et al, 2003). Later follow-up imaging studies should be aimed at detecting the recurrence of the treated lesion (i.e., local tumor progression), the development of new hepatic lesions, or the emergence of extrahepatic disease.

Radiofrequency Ablation (see Ch. 76c)

The goal of RFA is to induce thermal injury to the tissue through electromagnetic energy deposition. The patient is part of a closed-loop circuit that includes a radiofrequency generator, an electrode needle, and a large dispersive electrode (ground pads). An alternating electric field is created within the tissue of the patient. Because of the relatively high electrical resistance of tissue compared with the metal electrodes, there is marked agitation of the ions present in the target tissue that surrounds the electrode, as the tissue ions attempt to follow the changes in direction of alternating electric current. The agitation results in frictional heat around the electrode. The discrepancy between the small surface area of the needle electrode and the large area of the ground pads causes the generated heat to be focused and concentrated around the needle electrode.

In the initial experience with RFA, a major limitation of the technique was the small volume of ablation created by conventional monopolar electrodes. These devices were capable of producing cylindrical ablation zones not greater than 1.6 cm in the short axis. Multiple electrode insertions were necessary to treat all but the smallest lesions. Subsequently, several strategies for increasing the ablation zone achieved with RFA have been used. Major progress occurred with the introduction of modified electrodes, including internally cooled electrodes and multitined expandable electrodes (Goldberg et al, 2003). Internally cooled electrodes consist of dual lumen electrodes with an exposed active tip of variable length. Internal cooling is obtained

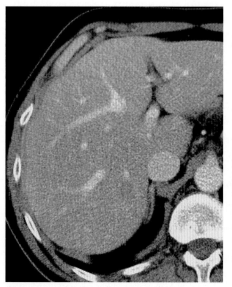
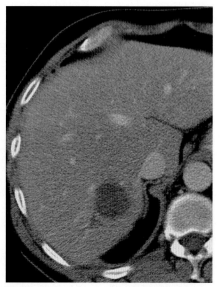

A   B

Fig. 76a.2. CT assessment of the outcome of radiofrequency thermal ablation of hepatic metastasis. **A,** Pretreatment contrast-enhanced CT scan shows the lesion as a small hypoattenuating nodule in segment VII. **B,** Contrast-enhanced CT scan obtained 1 month after the procedure shows a nonenhancing ablation zone encompassing the treated lesion and a cuff of surrounding tissue. The findings are consistent with complete tumor ablation.

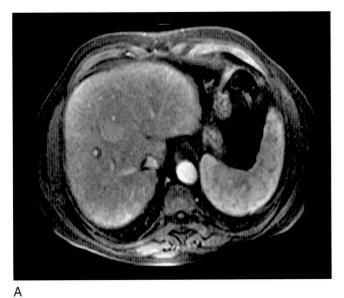 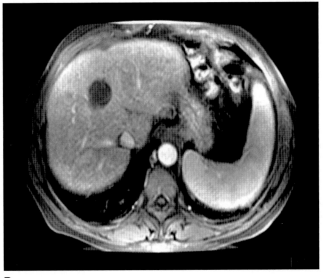

A   B

Fig. 76a.3. MRI of the outcome of radiofrequency thermal ablation of HCC. **A,** Pretreatment MRI obtained in the arterial phase of the dynamic study shows the lesion as a small hyperintense nodule in segment VIII. **B,** At MRI obtained 1 month after the procedure, the lesion is replaced by a nonenhancing ablation zone. The findings are consistent with complete tumor ablation.

by continuous perfusion with chilled saline and is aimed at preventing overheating of tissues nearest to the electrode to minimize carbonization and gas formation around the tip. Multitined expandable electrodes have an active surface that can be increased substantially by prongs deployed from the tip. In application, the tip of the needle is advanced to the target lesion, and the curved electrodes are deployed into the tumor according to the desired volume of ablation.

Most early clinical research with RFA was conducted in the framework of feasibility studies, aimed at showing the local effect and the safety of the procedure (Curley et al, 1999; Lencioni et al, 1998; Solbiati et al, 1997; Wood et al, 2000). More recently, the clinical efficacy of RFA has been evaluated in the treatment of HCC and colorectal hepatic metastases.

Treatment of Hepatocellular Carcinoma

RFA has been the most widely assessed alternative to PEI for local ablation of HCC (see Ch. 71). Histologic data from explanted liver specimens in patients who underwent RFA showed that tumor size and presence of large (≥3 mm) abutting vessels significantly affect local treatment effect. Complete tumor necrosis was shown by pathology in 83% of tumors less than 3 cm and 88% of tumors in a nonperivascular location (Lu et al, 2005). In two comparative studies, the rates of complete tumor response as shown by post-treatment CT were higher in patients who underwent RFA compared with patients who underwent PEI (Ikeda et al, 2001; Livraghi et al, 1999).

Two randomized studies compared RFA versus PEI for the treatment of early stage HCC (Table 76a.4). In the first trial, Child A or B patients with either uninodular tumor less than 5 cm or three or fewer tumors less than 3 cm each were randomly assigned to receive RFA or PEI (Lencioni et al, 2003). The overall survival rates at 1 and 2 years were 100% and 98% in the radiofrequency group and 96% and 88% in the PEI group. Despite the tendency favoring RFA, the observed difference did not reach statistical significance, likely because of the short follow-up period. One-year and 2-year recurrence-free survival

rates were significantly higher in RFA-treated patients than in PEI-treated patients, however, and RFA was confirmed as an independent prognostic factor for local recurrence-free survival by a multivariate analysis (Lencioni et al, 2003). In the second study, patients with HCCs 4 cm or less were randomly assigned to three groups (conventional PEI group, higher dose PEI group, and RFA group) (Lin et al, 2004). The overall and the cancer-free survival rates were highest in the RFA group, and multivariate analysis determined that tumor size, tumor differentiation, and method of treatment (RFA versus both methods of PEI) were significant factors in relation to local tumor progression, overall survival, and cancer-free survival.

Two studies reported the long-term survival outcomes of RFA-treated patients (Table 76a.5). In the first study, 206 patients with early stage HCC who were not candidates for resection or transplantation were enrolled in a prospective, intention-to-treat clinical trial (Lencioni et al, 2005a). RFA was considered as the

Table 76a.4 Randomized Studies Comparing Radiofrequency Ablation and Percutaneous Ethanol Injection in Treatment of Early Stage Hepatocellular Carcinoma

Reference	No. Patients	SURVIVAL RATES (%)			P
		1-yr	3-yr	5-yr	
Lencioni et al, 2003					NS
Radiofrequency ablation	52	100	98	NA	
PEI	50	96	88	NA	
Lin et al, 2004					<.05*
RFA	50	90	82	74	
Conventional PEI	46	85	61	50	
Higher dose PEI	50	88	63	55	

*RFA versus conventional PEI, *P*=.014; radiofrequency ablation versus higher dose PEI, *P*=.023.
NA, not available; NS, not significant.

Table 76a.5 Studies Reporting Long-Term Survival Outcomes of Patients with Early Stage Hepatocellular Carcinoma Who Underwent Percutaneous Radiofrequency Ablation

Reference	No. Patients	SURVIVAL RATES (%)		
		1-yr	3-yr	5-yr
Lencioni et al, 2005a				
Child A, 1 HCC <5 cm or 3 HCC <3 cm	144	100	76	51
Child B, 1 HCC <5 cm or 3 HCC <3 cm	43	89	46	31
Tateishi et al, 2005				
Naive patients*	319	95	78	54
Non-naive patients†	345	92	62	38

*Patients who received RFA as primary treatment.
†Patients who received RFA for recurrent tumor after previous treatment including resection, ethanol injection, microwave ablation, and transarterial embolization.

Table 76a.6 Studies Reporting Long-Term Survival Outcomes of Patients with Colorectal Hepatic Metastases Who Underwent Percutaneous Radiofrequency Ablation

Reference	No. Patients	SURVIVAL RATES (%)		
		1-yr	3-yr	5-yr
Solbiati et al, 2001	117	93	46	NA
Lencioni et al, 2004a	423	86	47	24
Gillams et al, 2004	73	99	58	30

NA, not available.

first-line nonsurgical treatment and was performed in 187 (91%) of 206 patients; 19 (9%) of 206 patients had to be excluded from RFA because of the unfavorable location of the tumor. In patients who underwent RFA, survival depended on the severity of the underlying cirrhosis and the tumor multiplicity. Patients in Child class A had 3-year and 5-year survival rates of 76% and 51%, whereas patients in Child class B had 3-year and 5-year survival rates of 46% and 31%. In the second study, 319 patients received RFA as primary treatment (naive patients), and 345 patients received RFA for recurrent tumor after previous treatment, including resection, PEI, microwave ablation, and transarterial embolization (Tateishi et al, 2005). The cumulative survival rates at 3 and 5 years were 78% and 54% for naive patients and 62% and 38% for non-naive patients. In a comparative study of RFA versus surgical resection in patients with a Child-Pugh score of 5 and a single HCC less than 4 cm in diameter, no differences in overall survival rates and cumulative recurrence-free survival rates were observed, despite a higher rate of local recurrence in the RFA group (Hong et al, 2005).

Despite the many published reports, some questions are still unanswered. Some authors have reported that RFA may be a safe and effective bridge to liver transplantation (Fontana et al, 2002; Wong et al, 2004). Randomized studies are needed, however, to determine advantages and disadvantages of RFA with respect to transcatheter arterial chemoembolization for HCC patients awaiting transplantation. Studies have reported encouraging initial results in the treatment of large HCC lesions with a combination of RFA and balloon catheter occlusion of the tumor arterial supply or prior transcatheter arterial chemoembolization (Kitamoto et al, 2003; Lencioni et al, 2005b; Yamasaki et al, 2002). Further clinical trials are warranted, however, to determine the impact of this approach on survival.

Treatment of Hepatic Metastases

Many studies have investigated the use of RFA in the treatment of limited hepatic metastatic disease in patients who were excluded from surgery (see Ch. 73). Two early studies reported rates of complete response that did not exceed 60% to 70% (Lencioni et al, 1998; Solbiati et al, 1997). Subsequently, owing to the advances in radiofrequency technique, reported rates of successful local tumor control after RFA substantially increased. In two series, RFA allowed eradication of 91% of 100 metastases and 97% of

74 metastases (De Baere et al, 2000; Helmberger et al, 2001). Data on long-term survival of patients with hepatic colorectal metastases who were not eligible for surgery and who underwent RFA have been reported (Table 76a.6). In particular, in two series including patients with five or fewer lesions, each 5 cm or less in diameter, the 5-year survival rate was 24% to 30% (Gillams & Lees, 2004; Lencioni et al, 2004a). These figures are substantially higher than those obtained with any chemotherapy regimens and provide indirect evidence that RFA improves survival in patients with limited hepatic metastatic disease.

Studies analyzed the role of RFA with respect to surgical resection. In one study, 418 patients with colorectal metastases isolated to the liver were treated with hepatic resection, RFA plus resection, RFA only, or chemotherapy only. Overall survival for patients treated with RFA plus resection or RFA only was greater than for patients who received chemotherapy only. Overall survival was highest after resection, however: 4-year survival rates after resection, RFA plus resection, and RFA only were 65%, 36%, and 22% (Abdalla et al, 2004). In another study, the outcome of patients with solitary colorectal liver metastasis treated by surgery or by RFA did not differ. The survival rate at 3 years was 55% for patients treated with surgery and 52% for patients who underwent RFA (Oshowo et al, 2003). Other authors used RFA instead of repeated resection for the treatment of liver tumor recurrence after partial hepatectomy (Elias et al, 2002). The potential role of performing RFA during the interval between diagnosis and resection as part of a "test-of-time" management approach was investigated (Livraghi et al, 2003a). Eighty-eight consecutive patients with colorectal liver metastases who were potential candidates for surgery were treated with RFA. Among the 53 patients in whom complete tumor ablation was achieved after RFA, 98% were spared surgical resection because they remained disease-free or because they developed additional metastases leading to unresectability. No patient in whom RFA did not achieve complete tumor ablation became unresectable as a result of the growth of the treated metastases.

Complications

Three separate multicenter surveys reported acceptable morbidity and mortality rates for a minimally invasive technique. The mortality rate ranged from 0.1% to 0.5%, the major complication rate ranged from 2.2% to 3.1%, and the minor complication rate ranged from 5% to 8.9% (Rhim, 2005). The most common causes of death were sepsis, hepatic failure, colon perforation, and portal vein thrombosis; the most common complications were intraperitoneal bleeding, hepatic abscess, bile duct injury, hepatic decompensation, and grounding pad burns (Bleicher et al, 2003;

De Baere et al, 2003; Livraghi et al, 2003b). Minor complications and side effects were usually transient and self-limiting. An uncommon late complication of RFA can be tumor seeding along the needle tract. In patients with HCC, tumor seeding occurred in 8 (0.5%) of 1610 cases in a multicenter survey (Livraghi et al, 2003b) and in 1 (0.5%) of 187 cases in a single institution series (Lencioni et al, 2005a). Lesions with subcapsular location and an invasive tumoral pattern, as shown by a poor differentiation degree, seem to be at higher risk for such a complication (Llovet et al, 2001). Although these data indicate that RFA is a relatively safe procedure, a careful assessment of the risks and benefits associated with the treatment has to be made in each patient by a multidisciplinary team.

Microwave Ablation

Microwave ablation is the term used for all electromagnetic methods of inducing tumor destruction by using devices with frequencies greater than or equal to 900 kHz. The passage of microwaves into cells or other materials containing water results in the rotation of individual molecules. This rapid molecular rotation generates and uniformly distributes heat, which is instantaneous and continuous until the radiation is stopped. Microwave irradiation creates an ablation area around the needle in a column or round shape, depending on the type of needle used and the generating power (Lu et al, 2001).

Most clinical studies of microwave ablation investigated the usefulness of the technique in the treatment of HCC. The local effect of treatment was assessed in explanted livers by examining the histologic changes of the tumor after microwave ablation. In one study, 89% of 18 small tumors were ablated completely (Yamashiki et al, 2003). Coagulative necrosis with faded nuclei and eosinophilic cytoplasm were the predominant findings in the ablated areas. There also were areas in which the tumors maintained their native morphologic features as if the area were fixed, but their cellular activity was destroyed as shown by succinic dehydrogenase stain. One study compared microwave ablation and PEI in a retrospective evaluation of 90 patients with small HCC (Seki et al, 1999). The overall 5-year survival rates for patients with well-differentiated HCC treated with microwave ablation and PEI were not significantly different. Among the patients with moderately or poorly differentiated HCC, overall survival with microwave ablation was significantly better than with PEI. In a large series including 234 patients, the 3-year and 5-year survival rates were 73% and 57% (Dong et al, 2003). At a multivariate analysis, tumor size, number of nodules, and Child-Pugh classification had a significant effect on survival (Liang et al, 2005). Only one randomized trial compared the effectiveness of microwave ablation with that of RFA (Shibata et al, 2002). Seventy-two patients with 94 HCC nodules were randomly assigned to RFA and microwave ablation groups. In this study, the data were analyzed with respect to lesions and not to patients. Although no statistically significant differences were observed with respect to the efficacy of the two procedures, a tendency favoring RFA was recognized with respect to local recurrences and complication rates.

Limited data have been reported so far concerning the use of microwave ablation in the treatment of hepatic metastases. In one study, 30 patients with multiple metastatic colorectal tumors in the liver who were potentially amenable to hepatic resection were randomly assigned to treatment with microwave

coagulation (14 patients) or hepatectomy (16 patients). One-year and 3-year survival rates and mean survival times were 71%, 14%, and 27 months in the microwave group and 69%, 23%, and 25 months in the hepatectomy group (Shibata et al, 2000). The difference between these two groups was not statistically significant. Other authors have reported initial promising results in the treatment of hepatic metastases from other primary sites (Abe et al, 2005; Liang et al, 2003).

Laser Ablation

The term *laser ablation* should be used for ablation with light energy applied via fibers directly inserted into the tissue. A variety of laser sources and wavelengths are available. In addition, different types of laser fibers, modified tips, and single or multiple laser applicators can be used. From a single, bare 400-μm laser fiber, a spherical volume of coagulative necrosis 2 cm in diameter can be produced. Use of higher power results in charring and vaporization around the fiber tip. Two methods have been developed for producing larger volumes of necrosis. The first consists of firing multiple bare fibers arrayed at 2-cm spacing throughout a target lesion, whereas the second uses cooled-tip diffuser fibers that can deposit 30 W over a large surface area, diminishing local overheating (Vogl et al, 1995).

To date, few data are available concerning the clinical efficacy of laser ablation. No randomized trials to compare laser ablation with any other treatment have been published so far. In one study including 74 patients with early stage HCC, overall survival rates were 68% at 3 years and 15% at 5 years (Pacella et al, 2001). Two single institution series of patients with liver metastases from colorectal cancer who underwent laser ablation reported 5-year survival rates ranging from 4% to 37%, likely reflecting differences in equipment and inclusion criteria (Christophi et al, 2004; Vogl et al, 2004). Laser ablation seems to be relatively safe, with a major complication rate less than 2% (Vogl et al, 2002). The major drawback of current laser technology seems to be the small volume of ablation that can be created with a single probe insertion. Insertion of multiple fibers is technically cumbersome and may not be feasible in lesions that are not conveniently located. New devices could overcome this limitation.

CONCLUSION

Several percutaneous techniques have been developed to treat patients with liver malignancies who are not candidates for surgery. These minimally invasive procedures can achieve effective and reproducible tumor destruction with acceptable morbidity. Percutaneous ablation is accepted as the best therapeutic choice for patients with early stage HCC when resection and transplantation are precluded. PEI is the seminal technique for local ablation of HCC and may achieve a 5-year survival rate of 50% in selected Child A patients. RFA constitutes the most assessed alternative technique. On the basis of the identified evidence, RFA seems to reach higher cumulative survival and recurrence-free survival rates compared with PEI. RFA also has become a viable treatment method for patients with limited hepatic metastatic disease from colorectal cancer who are not eligible for surgical resection. Further trials are needed to establish the clinical efficacy of the other percutaneous treatments. Percutaneous ablation techniques can be used appropriately only when the therapeutic strategy is decided by a multidisciplinary team and is tailored to the individual patient and to the features of the disease.

REFERENCES

Abdalla EK, et al, 2004: Recurrence and outcomes following hepatic resection, radiofrequency ablation, and combined resection/ablation for colorectal liver metastases. Ann Surg 239:818-825.

Abe H, et al, 2005: Open-configuration MR-guided microwave thermocoagulation therapy for metastatic liver tumors from breast cancer. Breast Cancer 12:26-31.

Adam A, et al, 2004: Percutaneous coil placement prior to radiofrequency ablation of poorly visible hepatic tumors. Eur Radiol 14:1688-1691.

Belghiti J, Kianmanesh R, 2003: Surgical techniques used in adult living donor liver transplantation. Liver Transpl 9(10 suppl 2):S29-S34.

Bentrem DJ, et al, 2005: Surgical therapy for metastatic disease to the liver. Annu Rev Med 56:139-156.

Berber E, et al, 2005: Predictors of survival after radiofrequency thermal ablation of colorectal cancer metastases to the liver: a prospective study. J Clin Oncol 23:1358-1364.

Bleicher RJ, et al, 2003: Radiofrequency ablation in 447 complex unresectable liver tumors: lessons learned. Ann Surg Oncol 10:52-58.

Bruix J, Llovet JM, 2002: Prognostic prediction and treatment strategy in hepatocellular carcinoma. Hepatology 35:519-524.

Bruix J, et al, 2001: Clinical management of hepatocellular carcinoma: conclusions of the Barcelona-2000 EASL conference. European Association for the Study of the Liver. EASL Panel of Experts on HCC. J Hepatol 35:421-430.

Castells A, et al, 1993: Treatment of small hepatocellular carcinoma in cirrhotic patients: a cohort study comparing surgical resection and percutaneous ethanol injection. Hepatology 18:1121-1126.

Chopra S, et al, 2003: Radiofrequency ablation of hepatic tumors adjacent to the gallbladder: feasibility and safety. AJR Am J Roentgenol 180:697-701.

Christophi C, et al, 2004: Long-term survival of patients with unresectable colorectal liver metastases treated by percutaneous interstitial laser thermotherapy. World J Surg 28:987-994.

Curley SA, et al, 1999: Radiofrequency ablation of unresectable primary and metastatic malignancies: results in 123 patients. Ann Surg 230:1-8.

Daniele B, et al, 2003: Hepatic resection and percutaneous ethanol injection as treatments of small hepatocellular carcinoma: a Cancer of the Liver Italian Program (CLIP 08) retrospective case-control study. CLIP Investigators. J Clin Gastroenterol 36:63-67.

De Baere T, et al, 2000: Radiofrequency ablation of 100 hepatic metastases with a mean follow-up of more than 1 year. AJR Am J Roentgenol 175:1619-1625.

De Baere T, et al, 2003: Adverse events during radiofrequency treatment of 582 hepatic tumors. AJR Am J Roentgenol 181:695-700.

Di Stasi M, et al, 1997: Percutaneous ethanol injection in the treatment of hepatocellular carcinoma: a multicenter survey of evaluation practices and complication rates. Scand J Gastroenterol 32:1168-1173.

Dodd GD 3rd, et al, 2001: Radiofrequency thermal ablation: computer analysis of the size of the thermal injury created by overlapping ablations. AJR Am J Roentgenol 177:777-782.

Dong B, et al, 2003: Percutaneous sonographically guided microwave coagulation therapy for hepatocellular carcinoma: results in 234 patients. AJR Am J Roentgenol 180:1547-1555.

Elias D, et al, 2002: Percutaneous radiofrequency thermoablation as an alternative to surgery for treatment of liver tumour recurrence after hepatectomy. Br J Surg 89:752-756.

Fontana RJ, et al, 2002: Percutaneous radiofrequency thermal ablation of hepatocellular carcinoma: a safe and effective bridge to liver transplantation. Liver Transpl 8:1165-1174.

Gillams AR, Lees WR, 2004: Radio-frequency ablation of colorectal liver metastases in 167 patients. Eur Radiol 14:2261-2267.

Gillams AR, Lees WR, 2005: Radiofrequency ablation of colorectal liver metastases. Abdom Imaging 30:419-426.

Goldberg SN, et al, 2000: Thermal ablation therapy for focal malignancies: a unified approach to underlyng principles, techniques, and diagnostic imaging guidance. AJR Am J Roentgenol 174:323-331.

Goldberg SN, et al, 2003: Image-guided tumor ablation: proposal for standardization of terms and reporting criteria. International Working Group on Image-Guided Tumor Ablation. Radiology 228:335-345.

Helmberger T, et al, 2001: Radiofrequency ablation of liver metastases: technique and initial results. Radiology 41:69-76.

Hong SN, et al, 2005: Comparing the outcomes of radiofrequency ablation and surgery in patients with a single small hepatocellular carcinoma and well-preserved hepatic function. J Clin Gastroenterol 39:247-252.

Huo TI, et al, 2003: Comparison of percutaneous acetic acid injection and percutaneous ethanol injection for hepatocellular carcinoma in cirrhotic patients: a prospective study. Scand J Gastroenterol 38:770-778.

Ikeda M, et al, 2001: Radiofrequency ablation and percutaneous ethanol injection in patients with small hepatocellular carcinoma: a comparative study. Jpn J Clin Oncol 31:322-326.

Jonker DJ, et al, 2000: Survival benefit of chemotherapy in metastatic colorectal cancer: a meta-analysis of randomized controlled trials. Br J Cancer 82:1789-1794.

Khan KN, et al, 2000: Prospective analysis of risk factors for early intrahepatic recurrence of hepatocellular carcinoma following ethanol injection. J Hepatol 32:269-278.

Kitamoto M, et al, 2003: Radiofrequency ablation in the treatment of small hepatocellular carcinomas: comparison of the radiofrequency effect with and without chemoembolization. AJR Am J Roentgenol 181:997-1003.

Koda M, et al, 2000: Predictive factors for intrahepatic recurrence after percutaneous ethanol injection therapy for small hepatocellular carcinoma. Cancer 88:529-537.

Lencioni R, et al, 1995: Treatment of small hepatocellular carcinoma with percutaneous ethanol injection: analysis of prognostic factors in 105 Western patients. Cancer 76:1737-1746.

Lencioni R, et al, 1997: Long-term results of percutaneous ethanol injection therapy for hepatocellular carcinoma in cirrhosis: a European experience. Eur Radiol 7:514-519.

Lencioni R, et al, 1998: Radio-frequency thermal ablation of liver metastases with a cooled-tip electrode needle: results of a pilot clinical trial. Eur Radiol 8:1205-1211.

Lencioni R, et al, 2003: Small hepatocellular carcinoma in cirrhosis: randomized comparison of radiofrequency thermal ablation versus percutaneous ethanol injection. Radiology 228:235-240.

Lencioni R, et al, 2004a: Percutaneous radiofrequency ablation of hepatic colorectal metastases: technique, indications, results, and new promises. Invest Radiol 39:689-697.

Lencioni R, et al, 2004b: Percutaneous ablation of hepatocellular carcinoma: state-of-the-art. Liver Transpl 10(2 Suppl 1):S91-S97.

Lencioni R, et al, 2004c: Radiofrequency ablation of lung malignancies: where do we stand? Cardiovasc Interv Radiol 27:581-590.

Lencioni R, et al, 2005a: Early-stage hepatocellular carcinoma in cirrhosis: long-term results of percutaneous image-guided radiofrequency ablation. Radiology 234:961-967.

Lencioni R, et al, 2005b: Percutaneous image-guided radiofrequency ablation in the therapeutic management of hepatocellular carcinoma. Abdom Imaging 30:401-408.

Liang P, et al, 2003: Prognostic factors for percutaneous microwave coagulation therapy of hepatic metastases. AJR Am J Roentgenol 181:1319-1325.

Liang P, et al, 2005: Prognostic factors for survival in patients with hepatocellular carcinoma after percutaneous microwave ablation. Radiology 235:299-307.

Lin SM, et al, 2004: Radiofrequency ablation improves prognosis compared with ethanol injection for hepatocellular carcinoma < or = 4 cm. Gastroenterology 127:1714-1723.

Livraghi T, et al, 1991: Liver metastases: results of percutaneous ethanol injection in 14 patients. Radiology 179:709-712.

Livraghi T, et al, 1995: Hepatocellular carcinoma and cirrhosis in 746 patients: long-term results of percutaneous ethanol injection. Radiology 197:101-108.

Livraghi T, et al, 1998: Long-term results of single-session percutaneous ethanol injection in patients with large hepatocellular carcinoma. Cancer 83:48-57.

Livraghi T, et al, 1999: Small hepatocellular carcinoma: treatment with radiofrequency ablation versus ethanol injection. Radiology 210:655-661.

Livraghi T, et al, 2003a: Percutaneous radiofrequency ablation of liver metastases in potential candidates for resection: the "test-of-time approach." Cancer 97:3027-3035.

Livraghi T, et al, 2003b: Treatment of focal liver tumors with percutaneous radio-frequency ablation: complications encountered in a multicenter study. Radiology 226:441-451.

Llovet JM, et al, 1999: Intention-to-treat analysis of surgical treatment for early hepatocellular carcinoma: resection versus transplantation. Hepatology 30:1434-1440.

Llovet JM, et al, 2001: Increased risk of tumor seeding after percutaneous radiofrequency ablation for single hepatocellular carcinoma. Barcelona Clinic Liver Cancer (BCLC) Group. Hepatology 33:1124-1129.

Llovet JM, et al, 2003: Hepatocellular carcinoma. Lancet 362:1907-1917.

Lu DS, et al, 2005: Radiofrequency ablation of hepatocellular carcinoma: treatment success as defined by histologic examination of the explanted liver. Radiology 234:954-960.

Lu MD, et al, 2001: Hepatocellular carcinoma: US-guided percutaneous microwave coagulation therapy. Radiology 221:167-172.

Ohnishi K, et al, 1998: Prospective randomized controlled trial comparing percutaneous acetic acid injection and percutaneous ethanol injection for small hepatocellular carcinoma. Hepatology 27:67-72.

Oshowo A, et al, 2003: Comparison of resection and radiofrequency ablation for treatment of solitary colorectal liver metastases. Br J Surg 90:1240-1243.

Pacella CM, et al, 2001: Laser thermal ablation in the treatment of small hepatocellular carcinoma: results in 74 patients. Radiology 221:712-720.

Pompili M, et al, 2001: Prognostic factors for survival in patients with compensated cirrhosis and small hepatocellular carcinoma after percutaneous ethanol injection therapy. Cancer 92:126-135.

Rhim H, 2005: Complications of radiofrequency ablation in hepatocellular carcinoma. Abdom Imaging 30:409-418.

Rhim H, et al, 2004: Radiofrequency thermal ablation of abdominal tumors: lessons learned from complications. Radiographics 24:41-52.

Ryu M, et al, 1997: Therapeutic results of resection, transcatheter arterial embolization and percutaneous transhepatic ethanol injection in 3225 patients with hepatocellular carcinoma: a retrospective multicenter study. Jpn J Clin Oncol 27:251-257.

Schwartz M, 2004: Liver transplantation for hepatocellular carcinoma. Gastroenterology 127(5 suppl 1):S268-S276.

Seki T, et al, 1999: Percutaneous microwave coagulation therapy for patients with small hepatocellular carcinoma: comparison with percutaneous ethanol injection therapy. Cancer 85:1694-1702.

Shibata T, et al, 2000: Microwave coagulation therapy for multiple hepatic metastases from colorectal carcinoma. Cancer 89:276-284.

Shibata T, et al, 2002: Small hepatocellular carcinoma: comparison of radiofrequency ablation and percutaneous microwave coagulation therapy. Radiology 223:331-337.

Shiina S, et al, 1991: Percutaneous ethanol injection therapy for hepatocellular carcinoma: a histopathologic study. Cancer 68:1524-1530.

Shiina S, et al, 1993: Percutaneous ethanol injection therapy for hepatocellular carcinoma: results in 146 patients. AJR Am J Roentgenol 160:1023-1028.

Solbiati L, et al, 1997: Hepatic metastases: percutaneous radio-frequency ablation with cooled-tip electrodes. Radiology 205:367-373.

Solbiati L, et al, 2001: Percutaneous radio-frequency ablation of hepatic metastases from colorectal cancer: long-term results in 117 patients. Radiology 221:159-166.

Tateishi R, et al, 2005: Percutaneous radiofrequency ablation for hepatocellular carcinoma. Cancer 103:1201-1209.

Teratani T, et al, 2002: Hepatocellular carcinoma in elderly patients: beneficial therapeutic efficacy using percutaneous ethanol injection therapy. Cancer 95:816-823.

Vogl TJ, et al, 1995: Malignant liver tumors treated with MR imaging-guided laser-induced thermotherapy: technique and prospective results. Radiology 196:257-265.

Vogl TJ, et al, 2002: Malignant liver tumors treated with MR imaging-guided laser-induced thermotherapy: experience with complications in 899 patients (2,520 lesions). Radiology 225:367-377.

Vogl TJ, et al, 2004: Colorectal carcinoma metastases in liver: laser-induced interstitial thermotherapy—local tumor control rate and survival data. Radiology 230:450-458.

Weitz J, et al, 2005: Partial hepatectomy for metastases from noncolorectal, nonneuroendocrine carcinoma. Ann Surg 241:269-276.

Wong LL, et al, 2004: Pre-transplant treatment of hepatocellular carcinoma: assessment of tumor necrosis in explanted livers. Clin Transplant 18:227-234.

Wood TF, et al, 2000: Radiofrequency ablation of 231 unresectable hepatic tumors: indications, limitations, and complications. Ann Surg Oncol 7:593-600.

Yamamoto J, et al, 2001: Treatment strategy for small hepatocellular carcinoma: comparison of long-term results after percutaneous ethanol injection therapy and surgical resection. Hepatology 34:707-713.

Yamasaki T, et al, 2002: Percutaneous radiofrequency ablation therapy for patients with hepatocellular carcinoma during occlusion of hepatic blood flow: comparison with standard percutaneous radiofrequency ablation therapy. Cancer 95:2353-2360.

Yamashiki N, et al, 2003: Histopathological changes after microwave coagulation therapy for patients with hepatocellular carcinoma: review of 15 explanted livers. Am J Gastroenterol 98:2052-2059.

76b CRYOTHERAPY FOR LIVER TUMORS*

M. D'ANGELICA

Hepatic resection is the standard of care for resectable primary and metastatic liver tumors confined to the liver (Cha et al, 2002; Fong et al, 1999; Scheele et al, 1995). Most patients with malignant liver tumors are not amenable to potentially curative resection, however, because of anatomic, functional, or prognostic factors. Local control of hepatic malignancy, even when considered unresectable, may change the natural history of these diseases. Several prospective and retrospective analyses have shown liver failure to be a common cause of death in patients with unresected liver tumors (Nagorney & Gigot, 1996; Wagner et al, 1984). Ablative techniques offer an alternative treatment strategy that, by decreasing hepatic tumor load (and possibly eliminating it), may prolong survival and change the cause of death in patients with unresectable liver tumors. These concepts led to the development of ablative therapies for unresectable hepatic tumors. Cryotherapy has been and remains one of the most important ablative techniques used for liver tumors.

PATIENT POPULATION

Hepatocellular Carcinoma

HCC is one of the most common malignancies in the world with more than 1 million cases occurring each year worldwide (see Ch. 71) (Okuda et al, 1993). It is well known that HCC is the most common malignancy in Southeast Asia and in sub-Saharan Africa owing to endemic viral hepatitis, but since the 1990s its incidence has increased significantly in the United States and other Western countries (El-Serag & Mason, 1999). In the United States, the mortality for HCC remains greater than 90%. Of patients presenting with HCC, only 15% to 25% are operable, and fewer are resectable with curative intent (Farmer et al, 1994). Most patients with unresectable disease have tumor confined to the liver, however. At a regional referral center for liver cancer, 79% of patients had disease localized to the liver, whereas only 24% were candidates for resection (Adam et al, 1997). More than half of patients presenting with primary liver cancer are potential candidates for hepatic regional therapy, of which a significant number may be amenable to ablative techniques.

Metastatic Disease

The liver is one of the most common sites of metastatic spread, particularly from gastrointestinal malignancies (see Ch. 73). Most malignancies that recur in the liver do so in combination with extrahepatic metastases, making resectional or ablative regional therapies unsuitable management strategies. In contrast, recurrences from colorectal primary tumors are localized to the liver in approximately one third of patients allowing use of potentially curative regional interventions. Only a small proportion of patients with metastases confined to the liver are operable, and an even smaller fraction are resectable owing to technical and prognostic factors. By evaluating all patients with hepatic colorectal metastases at a single center, Scheele and colleagues (1995) found 21% of patients with synchronous disease and 51% of patients with metachronous disease to be potentially resectable. Most patients with metastatic disease confined to the liver are not candidates for resectional therapies, but are potentially eligible for regional ablative treatments. Systemic and regional chemotherapy for metastatic colorectal cancer has improved dramatically with median survivals of greater than 20 months now commonly reported. Additionally, response rates for systemic chemotherapy are generally greater than 50% and combined with regional chemotherapy approach 90%. Resectional and ablative therapies now must be interpreted in the context of effective chemotherapy, opening the door for downstaging of unresectable tumors and adjuvant therapy for borderline resectable tumors.

GENERAL INDICATIONS FOR NONRESECTIONAL THERAPY OF LIVER TUMORS

Numerous patient-related and tumor-related factors conspire to make liver tumors "inoperable" or "unresectable." General and hepatic-related comorbidities are common contraindications to hepatic resection and are often independent of the extent of disease or proposed operation. Elderly patients with significant cardiac or pulmonary disease are often considered inoperable because of prohibitive perioperative risk. Most patients with HCC have limited hepatic reserve secondary to cirrhosis or portal hypertension or both, which often preclude a safe liver resection. Many technical factors make hepatic malignancy unresectable. Insufficient future liver remnant, involvement of all three hepatic veins, and involvement of portal inflow to both lobes of the liver are examples of such technical issues. Many techniques to deal with technically unresectable tumors have been developed, such as portal vein embolization, parenchymal-sparing segmental-based resections, and two-stage operations. Nonetheless, most liver tumors are still unresectable. Another important reason patients have been considered inoperable relates to the biology and potential curability of the liver disease. Often factors such as size, number of tumors, and other biologic factors make the risk of an operation greater than the potential benefit—even if the patient is technically resectable.

Cryotherapy has been used to treat many primary and metastatic liver tumors; however, extensive experience exists only for hepatic metastases from colorectal and neuroendocrine primary tumors and for primary liver cancer. Cryotherapy should be

*Adapted from Ch. 80 "Cryotherapy for Liver Tumors" in *Surgery of the Liver and Biliary Tract*, 3rd ed, 2000.

considered a second-line alternative to liver resection in patients with resectable disease. In the situations enumerated previously in which resection is not possible or safe, however, cryotherapy can provide a relatively effective alternative therapy with less morbidity than open hepatic resection. The most pronounced benefits of cryotherapy in these situations are that it can be applied without a large incision, it can preserve maximal parenchyma, and it can minimize the overall surgical insult to the patient. Absolute indications and contraindications for cryoablation are undefined. Cryotherapy often is employed in combination with resection to treat contralateral tumors in a small remnant. Cryotherapy also can treat close or involved margins effectively to prevent local recurrence without compromising large amounts of additional normal liver parenchyma.

PATHOPHYSIOLOGY OF CRYOABLATION

The methods by which subzero temperatures destroy tumors are not tissue specific. Normal and neoplastic tissues are sensitive to extreme cold. Cryotherapy causes cell death by a variety of physical and chemical mechanisms depending on the rate of cooling, absolute depth of hypothermia, rate of thawing, number of freeze-thaw cycles used, and delayed effects of post-thaw ischemia.

When a cryoprobe is inserted into the liver, three overlapping zones of injury develop within the iceball. Rapid tissue freezing occurs closest to the cryoprobe. The rate of freezing decreases in proportion to the distance from the probe, creating zones of intermediate and slow cooling. Similarly, a gradient of temperature develops in the iceball, decreasing $3°C/mm$ to $10°C/mm$ from $-170°C$ near the probe to just below $0°C$ at the periphery of the cryolesion. The dynamics of the freezing process cause different mechanisms of injury in these three idealized zones (Gage & Baust, 1998; Mascarenhas & Ravikumar, 1998).

Cooling Rate

The rate at which tissue cools affects the proportion of cells killed by a single freeze cycle. Maximal cell death is achieved at slow and rapid cooling rates (although from different mechanisms), whereas greatest cell survival is seen with intermediate cooling rates. Cellular dehydration causes lethal injury at slow cooling rates, whereas rapidly cooled cells are destroyed by the mechanical action of ice crystallization and expansion.

Slow Cooling Rates

Intracellular and extracellular fluids are complex solutions containing varying amounts of protein, macromolecules, and electrolytes. The presence of solutes in water depresses its freezing point and allows it to supercool rather than crystallize below $0°C$. Because the composition of the intracellular and extracellular compartments differ markedly, the extracellular fluid freezes before the intracellular fluid. As ice forms in the extracellular space, solutes are excluded, making the remaining fluid hyperosmolar. Cellular dehydration occurs as the unfrozen intracellular water flows out of the cell along the osmotic gradient. At a critical level of dehydration, no further fluid can be extracted from the cell because the intracellular macromolecules become concentrated enough to equalize the osmotic gradient across the cell membrane.

The ion concentration across the membrane becomes deranged, however, allowing ions to flow into the cell from the hypertonic extracellular fluid to re-establish the Gibbs-Donnon equilibrium. As a consequence of cellular dehydration, the intracellular pH and ion concentrations are altered, proteins denature, and membranes and membrane-bound enzyme systems are disrupted. Some cells die as a direct result of dehydration, whereas others require the added insult provided during isotonic rehydration, which occurs during the thaw cycle. When the cryolesion thaws, the extracellular fluid melts first, briefly creating a relatively hypotonic environment. Water flows into the hyperosmolar and hypertonic cells causing them to swell, burst, or die. This type of injury predominates in the slowly cooled zone at the periphery of the cryolesion.

Intermediate Cooling Rates

With intermediate cooling rates ($1-10°C/min$), the cells dehydrate as the extracellular fluid turns to ice. The temperature falls fast enough, however, to freeze the intracellular water before cellular dehydration reaches the critical level to produce irreversible cell injury. Intracellular ice formation excludes solutes, increasing the intracellular osmotic concentrations, equalizing the osmotic gradient across the cell membrane, and stopping further cellular dehydration. As a result, the critical level of dehydration allowing influx of solutes is not reached, protecting the cell from the lethal injury caused by water influx secondary to isotonic rehydration during the thaw cycle. Cells in the zone of intermediate cooling do not suffer the consequences of the cellular dehydration, and their survival is improved.

Rapid Cooling Rates

Rapidly frozen tissue is destroyed by an altogether different mechanism. Cooling rates on the order of $50°C/min$, found only in close proximity to the cryoprobe, cause intracellular fluid to freeze before cellular dehydration occurs. Intracellular ice is particularly lethal. Small ice crystals coalesce, causing a physical grinding action that disrupts organelles and cellular membranes leading to reproducible and certain cell death.

Depth of Hypothermia

Independent of the cooling rate, extensive tissue injury occurs at temperatures less than $-20°C$, and temperatures less than $-40°C$ are lethal for almost all tumor cells. The mechanism of cell injury at these temperatures is the formation of intracellular ice. At higher temperatures, the rate of cooling influences the rate of ice formation and the mechanism of cell death; however, when the temperature is less than $-40°C$, almost all of the water within the cell is frozen, ensuring complete tissue ablation. For cryotherapy to be reliable, all targeted tissue must reach these levels of hypothermia to achieve reproducible and certain cell death. This is the theoretical goal of cryotherapy. This level of hypothermia is not consistently reached at the periphery of the iceball, where temperatures may be $0°C$.

The sensitivity of different tissues to hypothermia varies considerably. Most normal hepatocytes die at $-15°C$ to $-20°C$, whereas at $-10°C$ most hepatocytes survive. Bile ducts, connective tissue, and vascular structures tolerate slightly lower temperatures than hepatocytes. In contrast, liver tumors tend to require deeper hypothermia to $-40°C$ for complete and reliable cell death. As a general rule, the $-40°C$ isotherm is located approximately three quarters the distance from the probe to the edge of the iceball as seen at intraoperative sonography. To reach this level of hypothermia and obtain reliable ablation at the tumor margin, the iceball is extended 1 cm beyond the peripheral edge of the tumor.

Thawing Process

Further damage to tissue occurs during the thawing process and varies according to the rate of the thaw. Rapid thawing of frozen tissue tends to increase cell survival, whereas slow thawing is more destructive than either rapid or slow cooling. In slowly thawed tissue, the extracellular ice melts before the intracellular ice, briefly making the extracellular fluid relatively hypo-osmolar compared with the intracellular fluid. Free water flows down this osmotic gradient into the cells, causing them to swell and ultimately burst. Simultaneously, the ice within the cell undergoes recrystallization, especially in the temperature range of −20°C to −25°C. Recrystallization is a process during which the ice crystals reform, coalesce, and enlarge, mechanically disrupting the cellular membranes. The effects of thawing are potentiated by allowing the entire lesion to reach ambient temperature slowly and passively.

Repeated Freeze-Thaw Cycles

Repeated freeze-thaw cycles in animal models have been shown to move the margin of reliable complete cell kill outwardly by producing larger iceballs more rapidly (Poppendiek et al, 1967). This movement is due to increased thermoconductivity of the previously frozen liver. Tissue near the cryoprobe is ablated adequately with one freeze-thaw cycle because low enough temperatures are achieved to ensure complete cellular destruction. The added benefit of multiple cycles occurs in the periphery of the tumor where the depth of hypothermia is unpredictable and the cell kill is unreliable. Early histologic signs of cellular damage in lesions undergoing multiple freeze-thaw cycles are more dramatic, confirming the added benefit of multiple freeze-thaw cycles.

Microvascular Effects

In addition to the acute physicochemical and structural damage to the cell and its environment, the lethal effects of cryoablation are potentiated by disruption of vascular structures, which causes delayed hypoxia and necrosis (Rubinsky et al, 1990). The vascular effects are acute and chronic. Freezing at slow cooling rates causes the radius of the sinusoids to increase by a factor of 2, which is equivalent to increasing the volume in the intravascular space by a factor of 4. The expansion of the vascular space tears the endothelium, exposing and disrupting the underlying basement membrane. Platelet thrombi develop, and permeability increases, leading to swelling and microcirculatory failure. The tissues supplied by these damaged vessels become ischemic and necrotic. This mechanism of injury is more important in the intermediate and slow cooling zones, where direct cellular injury by intracellular ice formation or dehydration is not reliable.

For maximal benefit, cryosurgery should be performed so that there is rapid freeze, slow thaw, and repeated freeze-thaw cycles. Experimental evidence has shown, however, that high flow venules at the periphery of an iceball are crucial in shutting down the microcirculation of the tumor, and repeated cycles do not seem to improve this effect (Richter et al, 2005). It also has been shown in experimental models that the serine protease inhibitor aprotinin decreases platelet trapping and improves tissue destruction in cryolesions (Kollmar et al, 2004). The effects of cryosurgery on tissues are a result of direct cellular damage secondary to physicochemical effects and indirect cell damage secondary to loss of cellular integrity and destruction of vascular channels.

Morphologic and Histologic Changes After Cryotherapy

Immediately after thawing, the area of liver treated with cryoablative techniques appears dark red, swollen, and usually well demarcated. Histologic examination reveals congestion of the hepatic sinusoids associated with hemorrhage. There are decreased levels of cellular glycogen and an absolute reduction in the number of mitochondria. With time, the lesion takes on a light gray color and slowly resorbs over the ensuing weeks. Microscopically, this period correlates with polymorphonuclear cell and macrophage infiltration of the tissue. The cryolesion is progressively replaced with fibrous tissue. There is usually a persistent area of necrosis and fibrosis, but occasionally the lesion is completely resorbed.

Immunologic Effects of Cryoablation

In early studies of cryotherapy, anecdotal reports of regression of untreated tumor sites suggested a generalized tumor-specific immunologic response to the cryoablated lesion (Faraci et al, 1975). These effects have not been substantiated in animal or human models. It is unlikely that an antitumor immune response enhances the effect of cryotherapy.

OPERATIVE TECHNIQUE

Hepatic cryotherapy can be performed via a variety of approaches, including percutaneous, laparoscopic, and open methods. The open approach allows the most flexibility and accuracy. Cryotherapy at laparotomy also is less anatomically limiting than minimally invasive approaches and permits treatment of lesions in areas that are difficult to access by the other methods. The difficulty with the open approach is the morbidity that accompanies a major abdominal incision. Minimally invasive cryotherapy techniques have been developed and are increasingly popular. The technology of laparoscopic instrumentation and percutaneous localization continues to improve, and the role of these techniques continues to increase.

Preoperative Preparation

The extent, location, and proximity of the liver tumor to the hepatic vascular and biliary structures should be defined by careful review of preoperative imaging studies. Patients with more than 40% of the liver replaced with tumor are not candidates for cryoablative techniques because it is difficult to ablate this volume of tumor, and the perioperative morbidity is prohibitive. In general, the same preoperative preparations are required before cryosurgery as for liver resection because a small percentage of patients may be converted to resection owing to unexpected resectability or intraoperative complications. Two devastating complications associated with hepatic cryotherapy are the cryoshock syndrome, a complex of coagulopathy and renal and pulmonary failure, and intraoperative hypothermia (Seifert et al, 1998). Preoperative hydration is important to decrease the incidence of renal dysfunction (Bagia et al, 1998). Hypothermia is another significant complication that can be alleviated using heated fluid and airway circuits and a Bair Hugger (Arizant Healthcare, Eden Prairie, MN) warming system (Onik, 1993). Blood and blood products should be made available for the infrequent cases of intraoperative bleeding.

Cryotherapy at Laparotomy (Open Cryotherapy)

The abdomen is approached through a right subcostal or bilateral subcostal incision with vertical extension in the midline. The peritoneal cavity is explored thoroughly to detect extrahepatic metastatic disease. Enlarged lymph nodes, particularly those in the porta hepatis, are evaluated by frozen section. The liver is mobilized from its ligamentous attachments and examined bimanually. Using a 5-mHz intraoperative ultrasound transducer, each Couinaud segment of the liver is systematically scanned to determine the extent of disease and its relationship to the hepatic vascular and biliary structures. Suspicious lesions undergo ultrasound-directed core biopsies for histologic confirmation. All lesions seen on preoperative studies should be confirmed by intraoperative ultrasound or biopsy or both.

When an operative strategy is defined, the porta hepatis is encircled for the possibility of needing Pringle's maneuver during the procedure. The cryoprobe is introduced into the center of each lesion under ultrasound guidance. The placement is confirmed sonographically by viewing the probe in two or three

perpendicular planes. In general, it is preferable to introduce the cryoprobe through the anterior surface of the liver while monitoring the introduction of the probe and formation of the iceball with the ultrasound transducer placed on the posterior side of the liver. Intraoperative ultrasound allows safe placement of the probe, avoiding injury to major intrahepatic vascular and biliary structures. To minimize tumor spillage and to avoid "cracking" the surface of the tumor, the cryoprobe is optimally inserted through normal liver before entering the tumor.

Depending on the depth of the lesion, direct introduction of the probe into the tumor or wire-guided, Seldinger-style localization may be used. The Seldinger technique is best used for deep intraparenchymal and nonpalpable tumors. First, the tumor is identified by intraoperative ultrasound. An echogenic needle is passed into the center of the lesion under ultrasound guidance and subsequently is exchanged for a J wire (Fig. 76b.1A). When the J wire is in place, the tract of the wire is dilated with a coaxial dilator and peel-away sheath. The dilator is withdrawn, and the cryoprobe is inserted through the sheath into the center of the tumor. The position of the cryoprobe is evaluated again using ultrasound in two or three different axes. The probe must be placed through the center of the tumor with the tip near the opposite margin to encompass the tumor completely within the cryolesion.

It is crucial to tailor the type of cryoprobe and freezing technique to the size and location of the tumor. The temperature gradient within the iceball significantly affects the efficacy of the procedure. The temperature near the probe approximates that of liquid nitrogen, whereas at the periphery of the iceball, the tissue may be only a few degrees below 0°C. In addition, the rate of cooling is determined by the size of the probe, the flux of refrigerant, and the thermoconductivity of the uninsulated portion of the probe. To achieve maximum tumor ablation, the operator must understand the physical properties of the cryotherapy system.

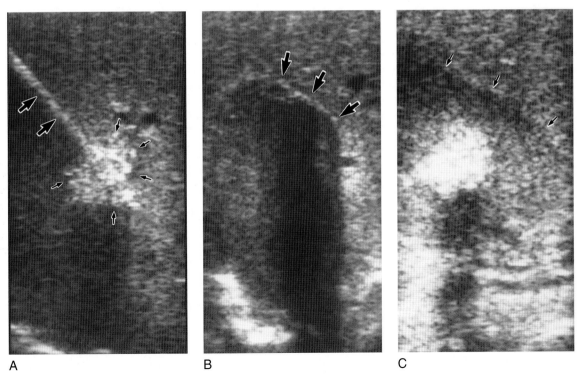

A   B   C

Fig. 76b.1. A, Ultrasound of an echogenic wire–guided localization of an intraparenchymal hepatic metastasis. *Large arrows* indicate the J wire. *Small arrows* indicate the margins of the tumor. **B,** Intraoperative ultrasound of the iceball. *Arrows* indicate the limits of the freeze front. **C,** Ultrasound of the thawed iceball showing the halo appearance caused by edema around the ablated tumor. *Arrows* indicate margins of edema.

The system we use employs vacuum insulated probes and supercooled liquid nitrogen refrigerant. It permits the use of four simultaneous and completely independent probe placements. Two probes are available with this system, accommodating different size tumors. The 3-mm blunted probe creates a cryolesion 4 cm in diameter, whereas the 8-mm trocar point probe creates a freeze-zone 6 cm. Two 8-mm probes, used in tandom, create a 10-cm cryolesion (Ravikumar et al, 1991b). Other systems have flat-faced probes that can be applied to a flat surface creating a hemispheric shaped cryolesion of 3 to 4 cm, which can be helpful to treat close margins (Gruenberger et al, 2001).

When the trajectory is chosen, and appropriate placement of the probes is accomplished, the liver is insulated from surrounding tissues using laparotomy pads, towels, or rubber mats. After the probe is placed, and the surrounding tissue is protected, the freezing process is started. At −100°C, the probe sticks to the tissue allowing placement of additional probes safely without dislodging the first probe. Two or three probes can be placed in the liver at the same time. We do not recommend treating more than three lesions simultaneously because it is difficult to monitor concurrent cryoablations adequately, and there is a higher incidence of intraoperative hypothermia.

Maximal cooling is started, and real-time ultrasound monitoring of the freeze process is carried out. The freeze front is seen as a hyperechoic rim with posterior acoustic shadowing (see Fig. 76b.1B). Cooling continues until the freeze front extends 1 cm beyond the ultrasound margin of the tumor. Typically, the freezing process takes 8 to 15 minutes to complete depending on the efficiency of the cryotherapy system and the size of the tumor. The freeze zone shown by intraoperative ultrasound closely approximates the pathologic and histologic volume of cryonecrosis.

After completion of the first freeze cycle, the tissue is allowed to thaw passively. Active rewarming is unnecessary and may adversely influence results. Complete thawing of the tumor may take 20 to 30 minutes, extending the overall operative time. Because cryotherapy failure usually occurs at the periphery of the iceball, it is necessary only to thaw the most peripheral centimeter of the iceball before initiating the second freeze cycle; this reduces operative time without compromising clinical efficacy. The second freeze-thaw cycle is accomplished in a similar fashion.

After completion of the second freeze-thaw cycle, the probe is actively rewarmed, allowing it to disengage before the tumor completely thaws. The probe tract is packed with absorbable knitted fabric such as Surgicel or another hemostatic material, and gentle pressure is applied to the liver, preventing delayed hemorrhage from the probe tract. Rough handling of the thawing iceball may cause a cleavage plane to develop at the interface of the iceball and the normal liver parenchyma, which can cause massive bleeding. Generally, the probe insertion tract stops bleeding promptly as the coagulation cascade activates at body temperature. After the two freeze-thaw cycles, the treated volume usually remains hyperechoic on ultrasound, whereas the surrounding normal liver becomes hypoechoic owing to edema. This gives the treated tumor a "halo" appearance on imaging studies (see Fig. 76b.1C).

POSTOPERATIVE CARE

Drains are not used, and the abdomen is closed in the routine fashion. Postoperative care is usually unremarkable. Fluid shifts tend to be minimal, and patients usually can be fed on postoperative day 2. There is usually a transient elevation of the liver enzymes, leukocytosis, decrease in platelet count, and fairly high fevers in the early postoperative period. The increase in the liver transaminases is related directly to the volume of liver treated and usually resolves within 1 week. The platelet count falls for the first few days, then stabilizes, only to return to normal or supranormal levels in 7 to 10 days. Less commonly, the coagulation profile deteriorates with increased partial thromboplastin and prothrombin times and elevation of serum levels of fibrin split products and D dimer. Clinically significant disseminated intravascular coagulopathy is rare. Pleural effusions are common, as a result of liver mobilization and treatment of areas adjacent to the diaphragm. Most of the early consequences of the surgery resolve spontaneously. The hospital stay is generally less than 6 days.

LAPAROSCOPIC CRYOTHERAPY

The introduction of videolaparoscopy and refinement of cryoprobe and ultrasound technology have allowed the development of laparoscopic cryoablative therapy. The laparoscopic cryoprobes are 40 cm long and can pass through a 5-mm port. Because the probes are not malleable, expertise in laparoscopic hepatic ultrasound and accurate placement of the working trocars are essential. Patients with lesions in segments VI and VII can be placed in the right-side up position to maximize exposure. The wire-guided Seldinger technique described earlier has been adapted to facilitate accurate placement of the laparoscopic cryoprobe. The dilators have been modified to make them stiffer than the dilators used in the open procedure. The probe is passed into the sheath, and the sheath is retracted to the liver edge during the freeze-thaw cycles. The cryoablation is completed under laparoscopic vision and ultrasound monitoring. A split screen image allows simultaneous viewing of the probe and the ultrasound image of the developing iceball.

The reported experience with laparoscopic cryotherapy is scant, and the patients are highly selected. With the expansion of RFA and its laparoscopic application, laparoscopic cryoablation has become less popular, and further publications have not been forthcoming. Reports have been limited to small case series (generally <10 patients), but the technique seems to be safe and effective in these highly selected patients (Seifert & Junginger, 2004). Despite current technologic limitations, the advantages of the laparoscopic approach are that it is minimally invasive, it eliminates the morbidity associated with a laparotomy incision, and it decreases the length of hospitalization and overall recovery.

PERCUTANEOUS CRYOTHERAPY APPROACHES

Percutaneous approaches for cryotherapy are established, although they have been relatively slow to develop; this is likely related to the explosion in popularity of percutaneous RFA. This approach originally was limited by the large diameter of current cryoprobes, location of the tumors, and accurate radiologic localization. Despite these problems, several moderate sized series have been published, which confirm the feasiblity and safety of this approach. Guidance most typically was performed with CT or with ultrasound, but more recently, techniques using MRI have been developed (Huang et al, 2002; Silverman et al, 2004).

FOLLOW-UP OF PATIENTS TREATED BY CRYOTHERAPY

Although cryotherapy is an accepted procedure for HCC and liver metastases, prospective and comparative data supporting its efficacy are limited. It is important that a reasonably standardized follow-up of patients with careful documentation of recurrence patterns and disease-specific outcome be collected on all patients. Follow-up of patients after cryotherapy comprises history and physical examination, contrast-enhanced CT scans, and tumor markers. The patient should undergo clinical evaluation, serial liver tests, and tumor marker determinations every 3 to 4 months for 2 years and then every 6 months. CEA and AFP levels usually reach their nadir at 4 to 8 weeks after ablation (Steele et al, 1990).

CT scans of the liver should be obtained at least every 6 months for the first 2 years. It is important to obtain an early CT scan within a few weeks after treatment to be used as a baseline. Successfully treated tumors initially appear larger than the original lesion because of swelling and the additionally treated margin of normal tissue (Fig. 76b.2). Subsequently, the lesion decreases in size and may disappear completely. Gas bubbles may be seen within the necrotic tumor and may be a result of the packed probe tract. These bubbles rarely indicate hepatic abscess and should not be acted on unless there are other signs of sepsis. In 3 to 6 months, the lesions shrink leaving a persistent area of fibrosis and architectural distortion.

TECHNICAL CONSIDERATIONS

Inflow Occlusion

The flow of warm blood through vessels adjacent to the tumor may act as cold sinks and change the conformation of the iceball and alter tumor ablation near the vessel. Some groups have used inflow occlusion with Pringle's maneuver to diminish these effects. Experimental studies have not confirmed these assertions in the porcine model, in which clamping the hepatoduodenal ligament did not alter the size of the iceball formed, the amount of liver necrosis, or the incidence of large vessel infarction (Kahlenberg et al, 1998). The relative contraindication to cryoablation near vessels may be only theoretical. Further evaluation of this problem is necessary.

Monitoring the Iceball

Most investigators use ultrasound to monitor the iceball because the pathologic size of liver necrosis closely correlates with the ultrasound size of the iceball. Others have used thermocouples to monitor the temperature at the margin of the iceball; however, this is an unnecessarily invasive procedure that provides no important additional information. Electrical impedance through the cryolesion is not as accurate as ultrasound in defining adequate ablation. MRI is a promising technology because it can accurately evaluate temperature gradients within the iceball in real time. Spectroscopic information obtained by MRI also may provide accurate information on cellular necrosis. MRI is generally unavailable in most operating and interventional radiology suites and remains an investigational tool.

Bile Duct Warming

To protect the major bile ducts from the adverse effects of cryotherapy, some surgeons cannulated the bile ducts to circulate warmed fluids during the cryoablation. At present, there is not enough evidence to support this invasive procedure.

COMPLICATIONS OF CRYOTHERAPY

The complications of hepatic cryotherapy can be broadly classified into operative, technical, and late problems. The operative complications include complications that are not specific to cryotherapy, whereas the technical and late complications are directly related to the procedure (Table 76b.1). The overall morbidity rate ranges from 10% to 40%, and the mortality rate ranges from 0% to 5% (Seifert & Junginger, 2004).

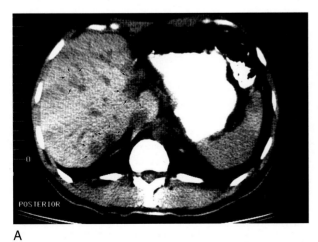
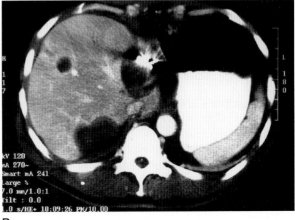

A   B

Fig. 76b.2. A, Pretreatment CT scan shows multiple liver metastases *(arrows)* in a patient who previously had undergone resection of segments II and III for metastatic disease. **B,** CT scan 7 days after cryotherapy of five metastatic tumors. The area of necrosis is larger than the original lesions.

Table 76b.1   Complications After Hepatic Cryotherapy: Summary of 869 Patients in 20 Series

Complication	Incidence (%)	Range (%)
Cracking of iceball	19*	1-25
Hemorrhage	3.7	0-13
Coagulopathy	3.8	0-8
Acute renal failure	1.4	0-17
Bile fistula/biloma	2.9	0-10
Intra-abdominal abscess	1.7	0-9
Pleural effusion	6.3	4-18
Death	1.6	0-8

*Reported in only 5 of 20 studies.
Adapted from Seifert JK, et al, 1998: A collective review of the world literature on hepatic cryotherapy. J R Coll Surg Edinb 43:141-154.

Generalized Hypothermia

Generalized hypothermia, a potentially serious adverse event, is generally rare, but depends on the number of lesions treated and their proximity to blood vessels, especially the vena cava and hepatic veins. The consequences of intraoperative hypothermia are multiple and include cardiac depression, arrhythmias, and coagulopathy. These effects can be ameliorated by warming parenteral fluid and using closed circulation body warmers and heating blankets. Perhaps most importantly, treatment of multiple large lesions simultaneously should be avoided.

Hemorrhage

After removal of the cryoprobe, hemorrhage through the probe tract is common. The blood does not clot because the activity of the enzymes that activate the coagulation factors is depressed by the localized hypothermia. Pressure and hemostatic materials usually control the probe tract bleeding. More significantly, the tumor can crack at the interface with the normal uncryoablated tissue. Massive hemorrhage can ensue, requiring transfusion, packing, or even conversion to resection. Careful handling of the frozen tissue and gentle extraction of the cryoprobe can minimize this complication, which has been reported in 0% to 25% of treated patients. Diligent use of intraoperative ultrasound to avoid moderate sized vessels during probe placement minimizes this problem.

Bile Fistula and Bile Collections

Bile collections are reported after cryotherapy, affecting approximately 3% of patients in collected series (Seifert et al, 1998). Bile collections and fistulae are most common when superficial lesions are treated. Late strictures of the major bile ducts owing to injury during the freezing process may occur and predispose patients to cholangitis. The risk is increased for cryoablated tumors located near the hepatic hilum or the bifurcation of the major biliary ducts. No long-term studies have confirmed this risk of bile duct injury and late stricture.

Cryoshock

Cryoshock is a complex of multisystem organ failure, renal failure, and disseminated intravascular coagulopathy after cryotherapy and is potentially lethal. The cause of this symptom complex is unknown, but it is responsible for 18% of deaths after hepatic cryotherapy. In a survey of all groups using cryotherapy, cryoshock was reported in only 21 of 2173 patients undergoing hepatic cryotherapy for tumor (Seifert & Morris, 1999). The cause of this phenomenon is likely related to systemic release of proinflammatory cytokines, such as tumor necrosis factor, interleukin-1, interleukin-2, and interleukin-6. Experimental studies have correlated the risk of this syndrome with larger ablations and with higher systemic levels of these cytokines (Ng et al, 2004; Seifert et al, 2002).

Mortality

The overall early mortality for cryotherapy is low, 1.5% (range 0-8%) (Seifert & Junginger, 2004). In expert hands, the operative mortality for major hepatic resection is similar. The most common causes of death after hepatic cryotherapy are not specific to the cryotherapy, but rather to cardiac and pulmonary comorbidities. The more common treatment-specific causes of death include cryoshock, liver failure, and hemorrhage.

LONG-TERM RESULTS OF CRYOABLATION

Hepatocellular Carcinoma

Cryoablation of primary liver cancer has been reported in more than 200 patients. The outcome of these reported series is difficult to interpret, however, because many patients were treated with cryotherapy in combination with resection, chemotherapy, or hepatic artery ligation. There is about a 60% (range 40-82%) reduction in AFP levels after cryotherapy in patients in whom AFP was elevated preoperatively. Reduction of AFP serum levels after cryotherapy does not clearly translate into a survival benefit.

For primary liver cancer patients treated with cryotherapy alone, the 5-year actuarial survival is approximately 30%. As expected, survival correlates well with the biologic characteristics of the tumor, of which size seems to be the most important. Zhou and colleagues (1996) showed that 5-year actuarial survival was 48% for tumors less than 5 cm, whereas it was only 25% for larger tumors. The pattern of recurrence is predominately in the liver after cryotherapy; however, the reports typically do not describe whether the cryotherapy was complete or what the intended margin was. Additionally, it is often not reported whether the tumor recurred in the treated area, or whether these recurrences were separate intrahepatic distant tumor resulting from intrahepatic metastases or new primaries. Few studies contain longitudinal survival information, and these results must be corroborated by larger multicenter studies controlling for tumor size, number of lesions treated, and adequacy of treatment.

It is difficult to compare the results of resection (see Chs. 71 and 80) or PEI (see Ch. 76a) with cryotherapy because the reported series generally are not comparable in terms of tumor characteristics. The operative mortality for resection of HCC historically has been 6% to 8% in most series, but now with better selection criteria and improved techniques mortality is generally less than 5%. The median survival is approximately 30 months with 5-year actuarial survivals of 30% to 40%. Similar survivals are reported in selected patients who undergo PEI; however, these are performed in highly selected patients. Livraghi and coworkers (1995) reported a multicenter trial of PEI for HCC that included 746 patients. Survival was related to the size of the lesion, number of tumors, and Child stage of the associated cirrhosis. For unifocal tumors less than 5 cm, the 5-year actuarial survival rates were 47%, 29%, and 0% for Child A, B, and C. Even in the presence of multifocal disease, 36% of patients with Child A cirrhosis survived 5 years after PEI. Similar results have been reported by Castells and associates (1993), in a comparative study of resection and PEI for HCC less than 4 cm. At 4 years, survival was equivalent for the two modalities.

Hepatic artery infusion chemotherapy, hepatic artery ligation, and systemic chemotherapy all have 25% response rates for HCC. These responses have not led to improved survival, however. These approaches remain investigational at present.

Survival after cryoablation is comparable to other modalities with a lower mortality than most resection series. Because of patient selection and the combination of therapies used with cryotherapy, comparisons with other modalities are, for the most part, meaningless. For now it is likely that cryotherapy will complement resection and PEI, but not replace them at present as first-line treatment for primary liver cancer. The rapid development of RFA is also a major competitor for the treatment of HCC. Future directions may include hepatic artery infusional chemotherapy after ablative therapies for unresectable tumors.

Liver Metastases

Liver metastases arising from colorectal, lung, pancreas, and stomach primary tumors constitute the most common malignant tumors of the liver (see Ch. 73). Most cancers that metastasize to the liver do so in combination with extrahepatic dissemination. The natural history and pattern of recurrence for *colorectal cancer* is different. Of the approximately 160,000 new cases each year, half develop liver metastases within 5 years of diagnosis. Approximately 20% of these patients (16,000 patients) develop metastatic disease confined to the liver. Only a quarter (4000-5000 patients) are amenable to hepatic resection with curative intent. The remaining 12,000 patients with liver-only colorectal metastases are candidates for regional therapies to the liver. The number of patients being considered for liver resection is now increasing because of improved resectional techniques and the dramatic improvements in adjuvant chemotherapy.

The ultimate goal of regional treatment of liver metastases is increased survival. Long-term follow-up of patients after cryotherapy for liver metastases is currently inadequate. Most published studies do not have follow-up exceeding 2 years, and fewer groups have treated enough patients to draw valid conclusions regarding the efficacy of cryotherapy in this setting. In recent years, series with adequate follow-up to report 3-year and 5-year survival have been published, albeit with relatively small numbers. In addition, cryotherapy has been used primarily as a salvage procedure or in combination with other treatment modalities, including resection or hepatic artery ligation or infusion, which obscures the results for cryotherapy alone. The value of cryotherapy used as a sole modality is difficult, if not impossible, to assess and compare with other modalities.

Ravikumar and associates (1991a) reported overall and disease-free actuarial survivals of 78% and 39% at 5 years for 18 patients undergoing complete cryoablation of liver metastases. These encouraging results have not been duplicated in more recent studies probably because of less stringent selection criteria. Most series (Table 76b.2) report median overall survival of 2 years after cryoablation of liver metastases. In 24 patients treated with cryotherapy, regardless of whether the ablation was complete or not, Ravikumar and associates (1991b) reported disease-free and overall survival rates of 24% and 63%. Similarly, Weaver and colleagues (1995) found that 11% of patients were disease-free at a mean follow-up of 30 months, and 62% of treated patients were alive at 24 months after cryoablation. Seifert and Morris (1998), in a series of 116 patients with colorectal metastases, showed a median survival of 26 months, and 13% of patients were alive at 5 years. More recent publications have reported 4-year and 5-year actuarial survival ranging from 22% to 36% (Kerkar et al, 2004; Rivoire et al, 2002; Seifert et al, 2004). Despite the wide variation in outcome with cryotherapy, some patients in each of the series achieved durable survival with this treatment. Actual follow-up is greater than 5 years for individual patients suggesting that cryotherapy can be curative in some cases. Based on the worldwide data, it seems that durable local control is achieved in about 20% of patients treated with cryotherapy.

Because the series reporting survival are generally small and include patients treated with cryotherapy in combination with resection for control of inadequate margins, and patients receiving hepatic artery infusion chemotherapy, the results cannot be combined for a proper meta-analysis. Because there are no randomized trials of cryotherapy, Tandan and coworkers (1997) undertook a critical comparative review of resection and cryoablation of colorectal liver metastases. This analysis reviewed 178 studies published from 1973 to 1995. Only studies with survival data exceeding 2 years and for liver resection if the series included more than 60 patients, were included. Four cryotherapy and nine resection studies met these minimum inclusion criteria. The median follow-up times for the two procedures were 12 to 28.8 months for cryotherapy and 21 to 69 months for liver resection. The data on liver resection were found to be more valid and consistent, but this review supported a role for cryotherapy in the management of liver metastases. Based on this evaluation, the authors concluded that cryosurgery offers potential advantages in the treatment of liver metastases, cryotherapy should not be used in cases of resectable disease outside of a clinical trial, and randomized trials comparing the two modalities are needed.

Survival seems to be related to the size of the lesions, the volume of liver replaced by tumor, a low pretreatment serum CEA level, absence of extrahepatic metastases, and whether the lesion underwent complete ablation. Normalization of an elevated precryotherapy CEA has been a favorable prognostic factor. Failure to achieve this normalization of CEA probably results from residual unrecognized micrometastatic disease.

Complete response at the treated site ranges from 60% to 90%, and most recurrences are at sites away from the cryolesion. The pattern of recurrence in these patients is primarily in the liver, with or without synchronous extrahepatic disease. This finding underscores the need for additional therapy to reduce further the incidence of hepatic recurrence. With the improvements in regional and systemic chemotherapy, the utility of cryotherapy combined with chemotherapy has been shown, even in grossly unresectable patients (Kemeny et al, 2001). An additional use for cryoablation is in the treatment of close or inadequate margins.

Table 76b.2   Survival After Cryotherapy: Review of Published Series

Author	Type of Tumor	No. Patients	Type of Treatment	Median Survival (mo)	Median Disease-Free Survival	Overall Actuarial Survival
Zhou et al, 1996	HCC	167	C; C+H; C+R	—	—	32% (5 yr)
Haddad et al, 1998	CRM, PLC, other	31	C; C+R	18	~7	—
Seifert & Morris, 1998	CRM	116	C; C+R; C+H	26	—	13% (5 yr)
Yeh et al, 1997	CRM	24	C; C+R	31	~20	85% (3 yr)
Adam et al, 1997	HCC, CRM	34	C; C+R	NR @ 16	—	52% (2 yr)
Korpan, 1997	CRM	63	C; C+R	—	—	44% (5 yr)
Shafir et al, 1996	CRM, HCC, other	39	C	NR @ 14	—	65% (3 yr)
Crews et al, 1997	CRM, HCC, other	40	C	—	—	30% (5 yr)
Weaver et al, 1995	CRM, other	140	C; C+R	22	11% @ 30	62% (2 yr)
Wrens et al, 1997	HCC	12	C	19	—	—
Ravikumar et al, 1991b	CRM, HCC	32	C; C+R	—	—	63%
Onik et al, 1991	CRM	18	C; C+R	33% @ 29	—	—
Lam et al, 1998	HCC	4	C; C+R	1 NED, 3 AWD @ 12-23	—	—
Lezoche et al, 1998	CRM, other	18	C	78% NED @ 11	—	—
McKinnon et al, 1996	CRM, PLC	11	C; C+R	73% @ 18	—	—
Heniford et al, 1998	CRM, other	12	C	83% @ 11	—	—
Dale et al, 1998	CRM	6	C; C+R	100% @ 17	—	—
Sheen et al, 2002	CRM, other	57	C; C+R	22	12	—
Rivoire et al, 2002	CRM	57	C; C+R	—	—	36% (4 yr)
Seifert et al, 2004	CRM	55	C; C+R	—	—	26% (5 yr)
Kerkar et al, 2004	HCC, CRM, other	98	C	33	—	22% (5 yr)

AWD, alive with disease; C, cryotherapy; CRM, colorectal metastases; H, hepatic artery ligation/infusion; NED, no evidence of disease; NR, not reached; PLC, primary liver cancer; R, resection.

Edge cryotherapy in these situations has resulted in good local tumor control (Gruenberger et al, 2001). Survival after hepatic resection of liver metastases (20-58%) is substantially better than after cryotherapy, but the patient populations are not comparable. Cryotherapy generally has been reserved for patients who are unable to undergo resection and might have a poorer prognosis.

SUMMARY

Because most patients who present with hepatic tumors are unresectable, cryotherapy has a role in the treatment of primary and metastatic liver tumors. With improving chemotherapy for metastases, cryotherapy and other ablative techniques may play a larger role in the management of bilobar tumors and technically unresectable tumors. Its availability expands the possible treatments for unresectable disease and allows resection in combination with ablation for more marginal candidates. It is unclear whether cryotherapy improves outcome for primary or metastatic disease, but preliminary data suggest that it is as good as, if not better than, other nonresectional treatment options. Cryotherapy can be performed safely in patients with significant comorbidity.

The problem of recurrence in the untreated liver after ablative techniques suggests that cryotherapy, similar to hepatic resection and other regional therapies, is not the final answer to hepatic tumors. Innovative approaches combining systemic or regional chemotherapy or both are needed to control micrometastatic disease. For now, cryotherapy expands the possible treatments of these diseases and may alter the natural history of the tumor recurrence, while having an impact on survival.

Cryoassisted hepatic resection is also possible, and the technique for performing this procedure is detailed in Ch. 80.

REFERENCES

Adam R, et al, 1997: Place of cryotherapy in the treatment of malignant liver tumors. Ann Surg 225:39-50.

Bagia JS, et al, 1998: Renal impairment in hepatic cryotherapy. Cryobiology 36:263-267.

Castells A, et al, 1993: Treatment of small hepatocellular carcinoma in cirrhotic patients: a cohort study comparing resection and percutaneous ethanol injection. Hepatology 18:1121-1126.

Cha C, et al, 2002: Surgery and ablative therapy for hepatocellular carcinoma. J Clin Gastroenterol 35(suppl 2):S130-S137.

Crews KA, et al, 1997: Cryosurgical ablation of hepatic tumors. Am J Surg 174:614-618.

Dale PS, et al, 1998: Cryosurgical ablation of unresectable hepatic metastases. J Surg Oncol 68:242-245.

El-Serag HB, Mason AC, 1999: Rising incidence of hepatocellular carcinoma in the United States. N Engl J Med 340:745-750.

Faraci RP, et al, 1975: The effect of curative cryotherapy on tumor-specific immune response of C57 mice. Cryobiology 12:175-179.

Farmer DG, et al, 1994: Current treatment modalities for hepatocellular carcinoma. Ann Surg 219:236-247.

Fong Y, et al, 1999: Clinical score for predicting recurrence after hepatic resection for metastatic colorectal cancer: analysis of 1001 consecutive cases. Ann Surg 230:309-318.

Gage AA, Baust J, 1998: Mechanism of tissue injury in cryosurgery. Cryobiology 37:171-186.

Gruenberger T, et al, 2001: Reduction in recurrence risk for involved or inadequate margins with edge cryotherapy after liver resection for colorectal metastases. Arch Surg 136:1154-1157.

Haddad FF, et al, 1998: Clinical experience with cryotherapy for advanced hepatobiliary tumors. J Surg Res 75:103-108.

Heniford BT, et al, 1998: Laparoscopic cryoablation of hepatic metastases. Semin Surg Oncol 15:194-201.

Huang A, et al, 2002: Phase I study of percutaneous cryotherapy for colorectal liver metastasis. Br J Surg 89:303-310.

Kahlenberg MS, et al, 1998: Clinicopathologic effects of cryotherapy on hepatic vessels and bile ducts in a porcine model. Ann Surg Oncol 5:713-718.

Kemeny N, et al, 2001: Phase I study of hepatic arterial infusion of floxuridine and dexamethasone with systemic irinotecan for unresectable hepatic metastases from colorectal cancer. J Clin Oncol 19:2687-2695.

Kerkar S, et al, 2004: Long term follow up and prognostic factors for cryotherapy of malignant liver tumors. Surgery 136:770-779.

Kollmar O, et al, 2004: Aprotinin inhibits local platelet trapping and improves tissue destruction in hepatic cryosurgery. Surgery 136:624-632.

Korpan NN, 1997: Hepatic cryosurgery for liver metastases. Ann Surg 225:193-201.

Lam C, et al, 1998: Hepatic cryotherapy for recurrent hepatocellular carcinoma after hepatectomy. J Surg Oncol 68:104-106.

Lezoche E, et al, 1998: Ultrasound guided laparoscopic cryoablation of hepatic tumors: preliminary report. World J Surg 22:829-836.

Livraghi T, et al, 1995: Hepatocellular carcinoma in 746 patients: long-term results of percutaneous ethanol injection. Radiology 197:101-108.

Mascarenhas BA, Ravikumar TS, 1998: Experimental basis for hepatic cryotherapy. Semin Surg Oncol 14:110-115.

McKinnon JG, et al, 1996: Cryosurgery for malignant tumours of the liver. Can J Surg 39:401-406.

Nagorney DM, Gigot JF, 1996: Primary epithelial hepatic malignancies: etiology, epidemiology and outcome after subtotal and total hepatic resection. Surg Oncol Clin N Am 5:283-300.

Ng KK, et al, 2004: Comparison of systemic responses of radiofrequency ablation, cryotherapy and surgical resection in a porcine liver model. Ann Surg Oncol 11:650-657.

Okuda K, et al, 1993: Neoplasms of the liver. In Schiff L, Schiff R (eds): Diseases of the Liver. Philadelphia, Lippincott, pp 1236-1296.

Onik G, 1993: Hepatic cryotherapy with and without the Bair-Hugger. J Surg Oncol 52:185-187.

Onik G, et al, 1991: Ultrasound guided hepatic cryosurgery in the treatment of metastatic colon carcinoma. Cancer 67:901-907.

Poppendiek DE, et al, 1967: Thermal conductivity measurements and predictions for biological fluids and tissues. Cryobiology 4:318-327.

Ravikumar TS, et al, 1991a: Experimental and clinical observations on hepatic cryotherapy for colorectal metastases. Cancer Res 51:6323-6327.

Ravikumar TS, et al, 1991b: A 5-year study of cryotherapy in the treatment of liver tumors. Arch Surg 126:1520-1524.

Richter S, et al, 2005: Arteriolovenular shunting critically determines shutdown of microcirculation upon cryotherapy in tumor-bearing rat liver. Ann Surg Oncol 12:303-312.

Rivoire M, et al, 2002: Combination of neoadjuvant chemotherapy with cryotherapy and surgical resection for the treatment of unresectable liver metastases from colorectal carcinoma. Cancer 95:2283-2292.

Rubinsky B, et al, 1990: The process of freezing and the mechanism of damage during hepatic cryosurgery. Cryobiology 27:85-97.

Scheele J, et al, 1995: Resection of colorectal liver metastases. World J Surg 19:59-71.

Seifert JK, Junginger T, 2004: Cryotherapy for liver tumors: current status, perspectives, clinical results and review of literature. Technol Cancer Res Treat 3:151-163.

Seifert JK, Morris DL, 1998: Prognostic factors after cryotherapy for hepatic metastases from colorectal cancer. Ann Surg 228:201-208.

Seifert JK, Morris DL, 1999: World survey on the complications of hepatic and prostate cryotherapy. World J Surg 23:109-114.

Seifert JK, et al, 1998: A collective review of the world literature on hepatic cryotherapy. J R Coll Surg Edinb 43:141-154.

Seifert JK, et al, 2002: Large volume hepatic freezing: association with significant release of the cytokines interleukin-6 and tumor necrosis factor alpha in a rat model. World J Surg 26:1333-1341.

Shafir M, et al, 1996: Cryoablation of unresectable malignant liver tumors. Am J Surg 171:27-31.

Sheen AJ, et al, 2002: Cryotherapeutic ablation of liver tumors. Br J Surg 89:1396-1402.

Silverman SG, et al, 2004: Three-dimensional assessment of MRI-guided percutaneous cryotherapy of liver metastases. AJR Am J Roentgenol 183:707-712.

Steele G, et al, 1990: New surgical treatments for recurrent colorectal cancer. Cancer 65:723-730.

Tandan VR, et al, 1997: Long-term survival after hepatic cryotherapy versus surgical resection for metastatic colorectal carcinoma: a critical review of the literature. Can J Surg 40:175-181.

Wagner TS, et al, 1984: The natural history of hepatic metastases from colorectal cancer: a comparison with resective treatment. Ann Surg 199:502-508.

Weaver ML, et al, 1995: Hepatic cryosurgery in treating colorectal metastases. Cancer 76:210-214.

Wrens SM, et al, 1997: Is cryosurgical ablation appropriate for treating hepatocellular carcinoma? Arch Surg 132:599-604.

Yeh KA, et al, 1997: Cryosurgical ablation of hepatic metastases from colorectal carcinomas. Am Surg 63:63-68.

Zhou X, et al, 1996: Ablative approach for primary liver cancer. Surg Oncol Clin N Am 5:379-390.

76c RADIOFREQUENCY THERMAL ABLATION OF LIVER TUMORS

T. G. ZOGAKIS AND A. J. BILCHIK

Surgical treatment is the "gold standard" for patients with liver metastases or primary liver tumors. Cure rates of 30% to 50% can follow the resection of liver metastases from colorectal cancer (Fong et al, 1997) (see Ch. 73a). Resection is possible in only about 20% of patients (Cady et al, 1998); most hepatic malignancies are surgically inaccessible or associated with a large tumor burden or inadequate hepatic reserve. Patients with unresectable disease may be candidates for systemic therapy (see Ch. 77), local ablative techniques (see Ch. 76) (PEI, microwave tumor coagulation, interstitial laser photocoagulation, cryosurgical ablation, or RFA), or hepatic-directed therapy (hepatic artery ligation, chemoembolization, or hepatic artery perfusion).

Multiple clinical trials have evaluated RFA for the treatment of primary liver tumors and liver metastases. Animal experiments in the early 1990s determined the size and shape of ablations that could be achieved in the liver (Rossi et al, 1990). Rossi and colleagues (1996) subsequently showed the effectiveness of RFA for the treatment of HCC in humans. Other trials have proved that RFA can control primary and metastatic liver lesions with few associated complications. The U.S. Food and Drug Administration approved RFA for generic tissue ablation in 1996 and for ablation of unresectable hepatic metastases in 2000.

RFA destroys tumor by generating heat within a lesion. During RFA, a high-frequency alternating current changes the direction of ions around an alternating electrode charge; this creates frictional energy and heat conduction. As tissue temperature increases to greater than 45°C, loss of cellular structure and protein denaturing result in tumor cell death. RFA can be performed in the operating room via celiotomy or laparoscopy or in the radiology suite by a percutaneous approach. It can be used with other modes of liver-directed therapy, such as resection and hepatic artery perfusion, and it can be used in conjunction with systemic therapy for other sites of metastatic disease. RFA continues to evolve with the introduction of new technology that increases the field of ablation and simplifies the technique.

RADIOFREQUENCY ABLATION TECHNOLOGY

RFA destroys tissue by generating enough heat to denature cell protein and cause cell death (Fig. 76c.1). Cell death can occur instantaneously at 60°C, a temperature achieved by all RFA devices. During RFA, an electrical generator produces a current that alternates directions rapidly. Charged molecules in the tissue follow the direction of the changing current; this results in friction, which produces heat. The current around the ablation electrode creates a relatively uniform zone of conductive heat that radiates out from the electrode. If tissue impedance is low, an expanding spherical zone of ablated tissue is created. As the temperature increases, tissue charring and desiccation occur.

Also, nitrogen gas forms, which can be seen on ultrasound as air bubbles in the tissue. Both of these events raise tissue impedance and inhibit heat conduction, inhibiting further tissue ablation. The spherical size of the ablated tissue is proportional to the square of the radiofrequency current (radiofrequency power density). It also depends on the size of the electrode and the duration of the applied energy. The radiofrequency power density decreases in proportion to the square of the distance from the electrode, resulting in a rapid decrease in tissue temperature with increasing distance from the electrode (Strasberg & Linehan, 2003). Changing technology strives to improve ablation zones by limiting impedance and increasing the radiofrequency power density.

Early RFA electrodes were unipolar. Because they produced a 1.5- to 2-cm cylindrical zone of ablated tissue, only tumors less than 2 cm in diameter could be ablated. These electrodes eventually were replaced by single electrodes that deployed multiarray tines (multiarray electrodes) to create a larger, more spherical zone of ablation. The current multiarray electrodes described subsequently can ablate fields of 4 to 5 cm in diameter. Technologic developments to reduce tissue impedance and increase the ablation zone would allow progressively larger tumors to be treated with single ablations.

Three different companies are producing radiofrequency electrodes and generators for commercial use in the United States. RITA Medical Systems (Fremont, CA) and Boston Scientific (Natick, MA) use multiarray electrodes (Fig. 76c.2). The RITA system has a single electrode through which multiple tines are deployed. The ablation is performed at sequential steps of electrode deployment. Thermoprobes measure temperature in the ablation zone, and an automated adjustment is made to maintain a steady temperature during the ablation. The electrode/generator system measures temperature and time as end points of ablation. This system was modified by the addition of saline perfusion to reduce impedance and increase the diameter of the ablation field to 7 cm. The Boston Scientific system automatically adjusts current according to tissue impedance; temperature is not measured. The multiarray umbrella-shaped electrode can ablate fields of about 4 cm. Radionics (Burlington, MA) uses a three-pronged electrode; each electrode is internally perfused with cold saline. The current is sent in pulses, and the system measures impedance and temperature. Ablation zones can reach 5 cm in diameter.

At least two other companies produce radiofrequency electrodes for use in Europe. Celon (Teltow, Germany) has a bipolar electrode that eliminates the need for a neutral electrode and can ablate an area 5 to 6 cm in diameter. Berchtold (Tuttlingen, Germany) has a monopolar electrode that contains small holes for saline perfusion; perfusion reduces tissue impedance and allows larger zones of ablation. This system also uses an impedance-controlled radiofrequency generator.

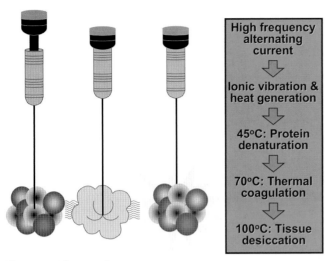

Fig. 76c.1. Schematic of RFA.

TECHNICAL ASPECTS OF RADIOFREQUENCY ABLATION

Patients who present with primary or metastatic liver tumors should be evaluated for curative resection. Patients whose performance status or disease location or distribution prohibits resection may be candidates for RFA. Before RFA, all patients should undergo CT, MRI, or fluorodeoxyglucose positron emission tomography. If these whole body imaging techniques reveal extrahepatic sites of metastatic disease, systemic therapy may be considered a better option than resection or RFA in some cases. Neuroendocrine tumors are an exception in that patients may benefit from debulking. Extrahepatic disease often does not exclude a patient with neuroendocrine tumor from RFA. Baseline hepatic function should be assessed through laboratory indicators of synthetic function and Child-Pugh classification of liver dysfunction. A thorough history and physical examination are essential to determine patient performance and prior treatment history.

If a surgical approach is undertaken, laparoscopy can reveal extrahepatic disease, and intraoperative ultrasound can identify intrahepatic disease. A 30-degree angled laparoscope can be used to examine all parietal and visceral peritoneal surfaces, the lesser sac, omentum, and viscera. If extrahepatic disease is found, RFA should not be done, and systemic treatment should be considered. A flexible 7.5-MHz ultrasound probe is used to evaluate the liver and determine the proximity of liver lesions to major vascular and biliary structures. The exact location of hepatic metastases affects the technical approach for RFA.

If extrahepatic and extensive intrahepatic disease has been ruled out, ablation can take place. Ultrasound during surgical or percutaneous RFA or CT during percutaneous RFA is used to guide the probe into the lesion, and the ablation is monitored by real-time ultrasound imaging of an expanding hyperechogenic zone (Fig. 76c.3). Depending on the maximal ablation size achievable by the probe, multiple overlapping ablations may be needed to destroy a tumor and produce a surrounding rim of necrosis. This situation can be technically challenging. Ultrasound cannot reliably distinguish between ablated and normal tissue, so ablation should begin at the most posterior portion of the tumor. The probe can be withdrawn in approximately 2-cm increments to create sequential overlapping zones of ablated tissue. If target temperatures are not reached, as may be the case for lesions near major vascular structures (heat-sink), the tines are withdrawn slightly or rotated approximately 45 degrees to increase the temperature in the region of ablation. Each ablation should create a 1-cm margin of treated normal parenchyma to ensure complete tumor destruction and reduce the risk of local recurrence. After ablation, the probe tract is cauterized as the RFA needle is withdrawn, to prevent hemorrhage and tumor seeding of the needle tract.

RFA can be performed by celiotomy (open), laparoscopy, or a percutaneous approach. The choice of technique depends on the patient's condition, the number and location of liver tumors, and the skill of the physician performing the ablation. Each approach offers certain advantages and disadvantages that must be weighed to determine the best approach for the individual patient.

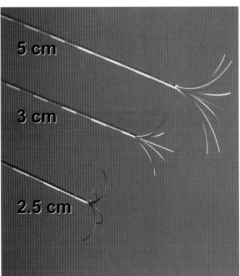

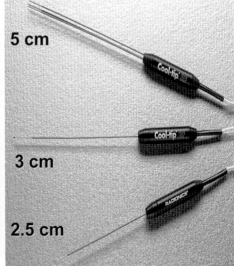

Fig. 76c.2. RITA *(left)* and Radionics *(right)* probes used for RFA.

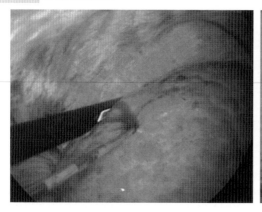 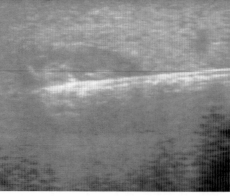

Fig. 76c.3. Ultrasound-guided RFA.

Percutaneous Radiofrequency Ablation

A skilled interventional radiologist typically performs percutaneous RFA as an outpatient procedure under ultrasound or CT guidance. The patient is sedated or given a local anesthetic. Some liver lesions are inaccessible by a percutaneous approach, but can be accessed by a surgical approach. Other lesions can be approached percutaneously, but are problematic. Ablation of lesions at the dome of the liver might result in thermal injury to the diaphragm. Introduction of an air pocket to separate the diaphragm and liver can avoid diaphragmatic thermal injury (Ramin et al, 2004), but requires skill and may result in complications such as diaphragmatic injury or pneumothorax. Tumors near the periphery of the liver may be problematic because of the risk of thermal injury to other visceral structures, such as the small bowel, stomach, or transverse colon; with an open technique, these structures can be retracted away from the liver. Finally, a percutaneous approach through the chest cavity introduces the risk of pneumothorax and possible intrathoracic tumor seeding. A percutaneous approach is less invasive than a surgical approach and may be preferable in patients with comorbid conditions or poor medical status.

Open or Laparoscopic Radiofrequency Ablation

RFA via celiotomy or laparoscopy is performed in the operating room by a surgeon, while the patient is under general anesthesia. In contrast to the percutaneous approach, a surgical approach allows visual inspection of the intra-abdominal cavity for extrahepatic disease. Intraoperative ultrasound is used to evaluate the liver for intrahepatic lesions not seen on preoperative imaging. In a study of 308 patients undergoing laparoscopic RFA with intraoperative hepatic ultrasound, preoperative imaging failed to identify extrahepatic disease in 12% of patients and additional hepatic lesions in 33% of patients (Bilchik et al, 2000). Similarly, Siperstein and coworkers (2000) found that 30% of patients who underwent laparoscopic ultrasound of the liver before RFA had additional metastatic nodules not apparent on preoperative CT scan. Larger liver lesions (>5 cm) are more easily treated with an operative approach than percutaneously. These lesions may require multiple overlapping ablations. Intraoperative occlusion of the portal triad can increase the ablation zone by decreasing the heat-sink effect created by nearby vessels. A surgical approach is sometimes necessary when other treatments are used in combination with RFA. A surgical approach is ideal for patients who

have bilobar liver metastases and may benefit from concomitant liver resection. Larger liver lesions may be resected, whereas smaller lesions in the opposite lobe may be treated by RFA.

Laparoscopy is less invasive than celiotomy and patients often require slightly shorter hospital stays. In some cases, a celiotomy is needed because of decreased access to the liver and limited position of the ultrasound and RFA probes under laparoscopy. Laparoscopy may not be possible if there are multiple adhesions in the abdomen from prior operations or if the tumor cannot be approached safely. In this case, a celiotomy is warranted.

Monitoring and Follow-Up

After laparoscopic RFA or percutaneous RFA, patients usually are admitted to the hospital for 24 hours or discharged home the same day; after open RFA (celiotomy), patients usually are hospitalized for 3 to 5 days. In all cases, red blood cell count, leukocyte counts, liver function tests, and temperature are closely monitored. RFA typically causes mild transient elevations of liver function tests, core temperature, and leukocyte count. These should normalize within about 3 days. Continued elevation, especially 5 days or more after RFA, may indicate a potential complication and should prompt further clinical investigation. Tumor markers, such as CEA for colorectal cancer metastasis and AFP for HCC, also can be used to monitor patients as appropriate. Immediate evaluation for pneumothorax may be necessary after percutaneous RFA.

Contrast-enhanced CT scans obtained within 3 months after RFA should be compared with preprocedure CT scans. Liver necrosis from RFA can be seen as a nonenhancing dark region. When complete necrosis of the tumor is achieved, the resulting necrotic zone exceeds the original tumor size. Postprocedure CT scans are important to determine the success of RFA and to monitor the liver for evidence of recurrence.

CURRENT PRACTICE

RFA has been used mainly for unresectable HCC or metastatic disease confined to the liver. Tumors may be deemed unresectable based on size, number, location, or doubling time. Selection of patients is based initially on a thorough preoperative workup that includes imaging to evaluate for other sites of disease, prior response to other therapies, and the nature of the disease. Occasionally, patients with hepatic and nonhepatic sites of metastasis respond to chemotherapy; if systemic therapy eliminates all nonhepatic metastases, and if its effects prove durable over several months, RFA of hepatic metastases may be considered, but this represents a small subset of unique patients. Some patients have resectable disease, but limited hepatic reserve. A patient with cirrhosis and HCC might not have enough hepatic reserve for tumor resection, but would tolerate RFA. In other patients, resection of larger lesions and RFA of smaller lesions can treat liver disease completely, while maintaining hepatic reserve. Finally, patients who have multiple comorbid factors may not be good candidates for an operation and may be best treated by a less invasive approach such as RFA.

Radiofrequency Ablation of Hepatic Metastases

Many patients with colorectal cancer have metastases confined to the liver, and most of these patients have unresectable disease at presentation. In these patients, RFA can be used to treat liver metastases with good success and low morbidity. Solbiati and coworkers (2001) used percutaneous RFA to treat 179 colorectal metastases in 117 patients. About 11% of the patients had extrahepatic disease at the time of treatment, and 89% received chemotherapy before and/or after RFA. There was one major complication, one minor complication, and no deaths. The estimated median survival was 36 months. At 18 months postablation, 44% of the patients had developed local recurrence. Time of onset and frequency of local recurrence were related to lesion size.

Although this study supports the fact that RFA can treat colorectal liver metastasis successfully, it does not support RFA as a replacement for resection. The 3-year survival rate of 46% after RFA in this study was lower than that reported after resection of colorectal metastases (57%) (Fong et al, 1999). No randomized prospective trial has compared RFA versus resection of colorectal liver metastases. One retrospective study (Abdalla et al, 2004) reported a higher rate of 3-year survival with resection (73%) compared with RFA (37%). Resection should remain the first treatment option for liver metastases from colorectal cancer.

Radiofrequency Ablation of Hepatocellular Carcinoma

In the past, unresectable HCC was often treated with PEI, chemoembolization, or cryosurgery. RFA is used more frequently now for the treatment of HCC and can serve as a bridge to transplantation. RFA offers many advantages over PEI and cryoablation. In general, PEI requires multiple treatments and needle insertions to treat a single lesion, whereas RFA can treat the entire tumor with one or two probe insertions. Compared with cryoablation, RFA is associated with less blood loss, less thrombocytopenia, and a shorter hospital stay (Bilchik et al, 2000). Cryoablation also carries the risk of a systemic inflammatory response that can result in renal insufficiency, coagulopathy, hypotension, and death. This type of systemic response has not been reported with RFA.

Clinical trials of RFA for HCC have shown promising results. Lencioni and colleagues (1998) showed a higher rate of complete necrosis (91% versus 85%) and a lower rate of local recurrence (4% versus 17%) for RFA than PEI. In a study of patients with HCC less than 3 cm in size, complete response rate was 90% with RFA and 80% with PEI (Livraghi et al, 1999). The same group reported a complete response rate of 47.6% in patients who underwent percutaneous RFA of HCC larger than 3 cm (Livraghi et al, 2000). In contrast, Poon and coworkers (2004a) achieved a complete response rate of 91% for RFA of large (>3 cm) HCC. Rates of local recurrence, distant intrahepatic recurrence, and extrahepatic metastasis were independent of tumor size. The difference in these two studies may reflect the latter's use of a cool-tip cluster electrode, usually with a surgical approach. This approach would allow a larger ablation and possibly better positioning of the RFA probe.

Although RFA can achieve local control with little morbidity or mortality, there is still debate concerning whether it can replace resection for HCC. In a comparison of resection and percutaneous RFA, Vivarelli and associates (2004) reported longer rates of disease-free survival and 3-year overall survival after resection (50% and 65%) versus RFA (20% and 33%). These differences might have reflected the RFA group's higher rates of Child B cirrhosis and multinodular tumors. In contrast, two studies from Korea (Cho et al, 2005; Hong et al, 2005) reported no difference in 3-year overall survival in patients who underwent percutaneous RFA versus surgical resection for Child A or noncirrhotic HCC. In both studies, patients had one to three hepatic tumors no larger than 4 to 5 cm and no extrahepatic disease. Local recurrence rate (at the site of the previous resection or ablation) was higher in the RFA group than the resection group in both studies. These studies indicate that RFA may be similar to hepatic resection in certain patients with HCC. Further studies with longer follow-up are necessary to define this subgroup better.

Radiofrequency Ablation of Hepatic Recurrence

Patients who develop a series of hepatic recurrences after resection, RFA, or other therapy may be candidates for sequential RFA. An illustrative case is a patient who underwent complete cryosurgical ablation of 15 liver metastases from colorectal cancer (Fig. 76c.4). About 6 months later, the patient developed an isolated liver metastasis, which was treated successfully with RFA. Over the next several years, liver disease recurred about every 6 months; each time the recurrent lesions were treated completely with RFA. The patient's overall condition remained stable until 7 years after initial diagnosis of liver metastases, when brain metastasis and rib metastasis were identified. At that time, however, his liver was free of disease. In this patient, sequential RFA was a successful long-term management strategy that prolonged life and preserved hepatic function. RFA may be the treatment of choice for carefully selected patients with recurrent hepatic disease.

TUMOR RESPONSE AND RECURRENCE

CT or MRI typically is used to evaluate response rates; ultrasound does not accurately predict the extent of necrosis after RFA and should not be used to determine response (Solbiati et al, 1997). CT with contrast enhancement reveals a hypovascular ablated field with a rim of hypervascular inflammatory tissue. The rim enhancement area should disappear over several months as inflammation resolves. The treatment area should encompass the tumor and at least a 1-cm rim of normal tissue. Comparing preoperative imaging with postoperative imaging is important to determine that the tumor was treated adequately. Patients should

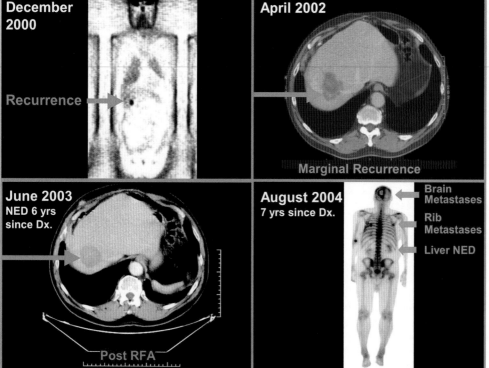

Fig. 76c.4. Patient with metastatic colorectal carcinoma to the liver was treated with multiple RFA treatment for recurrences in the liver. He ultimately developed rib and brain metastases 7 years after his first liver-directed therapy.

receive serial CT scans after RFA to identify recurrences. Recurrences appear as irregular nonenhancing areas on contrast CT (Fig. 76c.5).

Complete and Incomplete Response Rates to Radiofrequency Ablation

Response rates vary from 48% to 98% across studies (Table 76c.1), in part because of differences in the size of treated lesions. Livraghi and colleagues (1999, 2000) evaluated percutaneous RFA in patients with HCC. The rate of complete response was 48% for tumors larger than 3 cm (Livraghi et al, 2000), but increased to 90% for smaller tumors (Livraghi et al, 1999). The success rate was lower for infiltrating versus noninfiltrating HCC. Similarly, Lencioni and coworkers (1998) found a statistically significant difference in response rates to percutaneous RFA for metastatic liver lesions greater than 3 cm (53%) versus less than 3 cm (87%). Larger lesions typically require overlapping ablations. Areas of treated tumor may obscure ultrasound imaging of untreated tumor resulting in higher treatment failures and recurrences.

The approach to RFA also influences response rates. Curley and associates (2000) reported that 6 of 76 patients who underwent percutaneous RFA had an incomplete response, whereas all 34 patients who underwent laparoscopic or open RFA had a complete response. This difference might be explained by better hepatic imaging with intraoperative ultrasound during laparoscopy or celiotomy than with transabdominal ultrasound during percutaneous RFA. Another possibility is that intraoperative probe positioning may be more accurate than percutaneous placement of the probe.

Tumor location adjacent to large vessels also influences response rates. Blood flow from large vessels creates a heat-sink effect that

cools surrounding tissue and increases the temperature necessary for complete ablation. Large vessels are resistant to high temperatures that can damage surrounding tissue. Lu and colleagues (2002) found that porcine vessels smaller than 3 mm thrombosed or necrosed during RFA; vessels larger than 5 mm were not affected. In a porcine model, vascular occlusion during RFA increased the volume of necrosis and prolonged the exposure of tissue to high temperatures (Chinn et al, 2001). De Baere and coworkers (2002) evaluated vascular inflow occlusion in patients undergoing RFA of tumors that were large (>35 mm) or near large blood vessels. Balloon inflow occlusion significantly increased the area of ablation. These studies support the use of Pringle's maneuver to ablate tumors near major blood vessels more effectively and improve response rates. Pringle's maneuver must

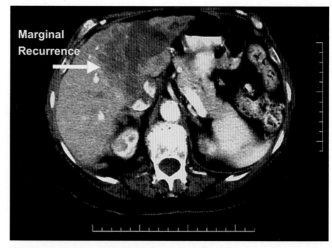

Fig. 76c.5. Recurrence after RFA as seen on CT scan.

Table 76c.1 Response Rates to Radiofrequency Ablation

Reference	Tumor Type (No. Patients)	RFA Approach	Complete Response Rate per Lesion
Solbiati et al, 1997	Metastases	Percutaneous	18/31 (58%)
Rossi et al, 1998	HCC (23), metastases (14)	Percutaneous	44/45 (98%)
Lencioni et al, 1998	Metastases	Percutaneous	41/53 (77%)
Livraghi et al, 1999	HCC ≤3 cm	Percutaneous	47/52(90%)
Siperstein et al, 2000	HCC (11), metastases (170)	Laparoscopic	178/181 (98%)
Livraghi et al, 2000	HCC >3 cm	Percutaneous	60/126 (48%)
Curley et al, 2000	HCC	Percutaneous, laparoscopic, open	104/110 (95%) per patient
Llovet et al, 2001	HCC ≤5 cm	Percutaneous	21/32 (65%)
Livraghi et al, 2001	Metastases from breast cancer	Percutaneous	59/64 (92%)
Solbiati et al, 2001	Metastases from colorectal cancer	Percutaneous	176/179 (98%)
Livraghi et al, 2003a	Metastases from colorectal cancer	Percutaneous	85/134 (63%)
Total			*729/897 (81%)*

be used with caution, however, in cirrhotic patients because it may increase the likelihood of portal vein thrombosis (DeBaere et al, 2003).

Rates of Recurrence at Radiofrequency Ablation Site

Recurrence rates are difficult to interpret across studies. Some authors report recurrences after complete ablation as determined by early postoperative CT or MRI, whereas others do not confirm complete response by postoperative imaging and report recurrences based on follow-up imaging. Investigators may report recurrence rates within the whole liver rather than recurrence rates at the site of ablation. The length of follow-up also affects the recurrence rate. Table 76c.2 summarizes the recurrence rates reported in various studies. Bowles and associates (2001) evaluated 76 patients undergoing RFA of 328 tumors. Sixteen patients underwent repeated ablation for recurrences or new lesions. There were 30 recurrences at the site of a prior ablation. Patients with large tumors, tumor vascular invasion, and hepatic dysfunction had a statistically higher recurrence rate. Solbiati and coworkers (2001) evaluated 117 patients undergoing percutaneous RFA of colorectal metastases; time to local recurrence and frequency of recurrences were influenced by lesion size. Similarly, we found that tumor size significantly influenced local recurrence of metastatic disease, independent of RFA technique

Table 76c.2 Local Recurrence After Radiofrequency Ablation of Hepatic Tumors

Reference	Follow-up (mo)	Tumor Type (No. Patients)	RFA Approach	No. Recurrences per Lesion Ablated
Rossi et al, 1996	Mean 22.6	HCC	Percutaneous	2/54 (4%)
Solbiati et al, 1997	Mean 18.1	Metastases	Percutaneous	9/27 (33%)
Rossi et al, 1998	Mean 10	HCC	Percutaneous	1/24 (4%)
Rossi et al, 1998	Mean 12	Metastases	Percutaneous	1/16 (6%)
Lencioni et al, 1998	Mean 6.5	Metastases	Percutaneous	5/41 (12%)
Bilchik et al, 1999	Median 6	HCC (7), metastases (43)	Percutaneous, laparoscopic, open	3/132 (2%)
Curley et al, 1999	Median 15	HCC (11), metastases (75)	Percutaneous, open	3/169 (1.8%)
Siperstein et al, 2000	Mean 13.9	HCC (11), metastases (170)	Laparoscopic	22/181 (12%)
Curley et al, 2000	Median 19	HCC	Percutaneous, laparoscopic, open	4/149 (2.7%)
De Baere et al, 2000	Mean 13.7	Metastases	Percutanous, open	9/100 (9%)
Llovet et al, 2001	Median 10	HCC ≤5 cm	Percutaneous	2/32 (6%)
Livraghi et al, 2001	Median 19	Metastases from breast cancer	Percutaneous	5/64 (8%)
Bowles et al, 2001	Mean 15	HCC, metastases	Percutaneous, laparoscopic, open	30/328 (9%)
Solbiati et al, 2001	Range 6-52	Metastases from colorectal cancer	Percutaneous	70/179 (39%)
Berber et al, 2002	Mean 1.6	Metastases from neuroendocrine tumors	Laparoscopic	6/227 (3%)
Bleicher et al, 2003	Mean 11	Metastases	Percutaneous, laparoscopic, open	52/447 (12%)
Total				*224/2170 (10%)*

(Bleicher et al, 2003; Wood et al, 2000). No study has shown that differences in technique influence the rate of recurrence after a complete response.

SURVIVAL AFTER RADIOFREQUENCY ABLATION

Few studies to date report survival rates after RFA (Table 76c.3). Studies that report survival data differ in patient selection, follow-up time, tumor type, and RFA approach, which make them difficult to compare. Four studies have evaluated survival after RFA for HCC, and 1-year survival rates range from 78% to 94%. Three-year survival rates vary from 33% (Vivarelli et al, 2004) to 68% (Rossi et al, 1996) and may be related to the type of probe used and amount of disease per patient treated. Rossi and coworkers (1996) treated tumors that were 3 cm in diameter or smaller using a monopolar or bipolar RFA method. Vivarelli and colleagues (2004) used a RITA probe to treat tumors with a mean diameter of 4 cm. About half of the patients in Vivarelli's study had more than one tumor nodule treated, whereas only two patients in Rossi's study had more than one tumor nodule treated. These differences influence outcome and when evaluating studies related to survival need to be taken into account.

The 3-year survival after RFA for colorectal cancer ranges from 37% to 46% (Abdalla et al, 2004; Solbiati et al, 2001). In both studies, more than 50% of the patients had only one tumor ablated. Solbiati and colleagues (2001) ablated liver lesions in 13 patients who had extrahepatic metastases, whereas Abdalla and associates (2004) ablated liver lesions of patients with localized hepatic disease only. These two studies also differ in the method of RFA; Solbiati and colleagues (2001) performed a percutaneous approach and Abdalla and associates (2004) performed an open approach. Some patients in the Abdalla study had a hepatic arterial infusion pump placed, which may have resulted in a slightly better outcome for this group. More studies need to be done to evaluate outcome further with longer follow-up times.

COMPLICATIONS OF RADIOFREQUENCY ABLATION

Reported morbidity and mortality rates associated with RFA (Table 76c.4) can be difficult to interpret, in part because technical approaches vary. Some investigators combine RFA with other treatments, such as cryoablation or liver resection; addition of a second procedure may increase the complication rate.

Ablation of multiple tumors also increases the risk of complications such as bleeding or bile leak. Early studies often used multiple sequential RFAs for treatment of a single hepatic tumor because the monopolar electrode gave a smaller thermal ablation field than the current cluster electrodes. The multiple ablations required to destroy larger tumors increased the potential for complications.

The reporting of morbidities is not standardized. Some authors regard low-grade fevers, transient liver function test elevations, small pleural effusions, and right upper quadrant pain as minor complications, whereas others believe these are expected events that should not be reported. As expected, studies undertaken at institutions with skilled interventionalists or surgeons report fewer complications. Variations in patient selection and disease type also confound interpretation of results. Patients with HCC have different comorbid factors than patients with colorectal metastases. Their preprocedural state may influence the outcome of RFA.

Direct complications of RFA include biloma, biliary fistula, ascites, hepatic insufficiency, arteriovenous fistula, symptomatic pleural effusion, abscess, pain, hemorrhage, hydropneumothorax, pneumothorax, and thermal injury to surrounding structures. Burns related to grounding pads also have been reported; these can be avoided by proper positioning of the pads, by using more pads for longer ablations, and by following manufacturer's directions carefully. Other potential complications are those related to an operative procedure, such as myocardial infarction, cardiac arrhythmias, and pneumonia.

As illustrated by the following two cases, RFA should be undertaken only by skilled physicians able to identify and manage its complications and only at centers equipped with appropriate staff and equipment for acute care. Fig. 76c.6 shows a bile duct injury caused by RFA of a colorectal cancer metastasis near the porta hepatis. The injury was treated with endoscopic retrograde cholangiopancreatography and biliary stenting. Fig. 76c.7 shows a hepatic artery pseudoaneurysm attributed to RFA of liver metastases. This pseudoaneurysm was treated successfully with embolization by a skilled interventionalist.

The best way to avoid potential complications of percutaneous RFA is to understand its technical limitations. A large multicenter study reported morbidity and mortality rates of 0.3% and 2.2% (Livraghi et al, 2003b). In this study, about 33% of all mortalities and 10% of morbidities were associated with gastrointestinal thermal injury and perforation. Patients with prior abdominal surgeries resulting in adhesions and patients with peripheral liver tumors had an increased risk for gastrointestinal injury during percutaneous ablation. The authors recommended consideration

Table 76c.3   Survival Data for Radiofrequency Ablation of Various Tumor Types

Reference	Follow-up (mo)	Tumor Type (No. Patients)	RFA Approach	SURVIVAL (%) 1-yr	2-yr	3-yr	4-yr
Rossi et al, 1996	Mean 22.6	HCC (39)	Percutaneous	94	86	68	40
Solbiati et al, 2001	Range 6-52	Metastases from colorectal cancer (117)	Percutaneous	93	69	46	—
Llovet et al, 2001	Median 10	HCC (32)	Percutaneous	85	—	—	—
Elias et al, 2002	Mean 14.4	HCC (5), metastases (42)	Percutaneous	88	55	—	—
Abdalla et al, 2004	Mean 21	Metastases from colorectal cancer (57)	Open	—	—	37	22
Vivarelli et al, 2004	Mean 15.6	HCC (79)	Percutaneous	78	—	33	—
Poon et al, 2004b	Median 13	HCC (80)	Percutaneous, laparoscopic, open	84	—	—	—

Table 76c.4 Morbidity and Mortality Rates of Radiofrequency Ablation

Reference	Tumor Type (No. Patients)	RFA Approach	Morbidity	Mortality
Rossi et al, 1996	HCC (39), metastases (11)	Percutaneous	0/48 (0%)	0/48 (0%)
Solbiati et al, 1997	Metastases	Percutaneous	1/16 (6%)	0/16 (0%)
Rossi et al, 1998	HCC (23), metastases (14)	Percutaneous	0/37 (0%)	0/37 (0%)
Lencioni et al, 1998	Metastases	Percutaneous	0/29 (0%)	0/29 (0%)
Curley et al, 1999	HCC (11), metastases (75)	Percutaneous, open	3/123 (2%)	0/123 (0%)
Livraghi et al, 1999	HCC ≤3 cm	Percutaneous	5/42 (12%)	0/42 (0%)
Bilchik et al, 1999	HCC (7), metastases (43)	Percutaneous, laparoscopic, open	0/50 (0%)	2/50 (4%)
Curley et al, 2000	HCC	Percutaneous, laparoscopic, open	14/110 (13%)	0/110 (0%)
De Baere et al, 2000	Metastases	Percutaneous, open	5/54 (9%)	0/54 (0%)
Livraghi et al, 2000	HCC >3 cm	Percutaneous	7/114 (6%)	1/114 (0.8%)
Wood et al, 2000	Metastases	Percutaneous, laparoscopic, open	7/84 (8%)	3/84 (4%)
Livraghi et al, 2001	Metastases from breast cancer	Percutaneous	2/24 (8%)	0/24 (0%)
Llovet et al, 2001	HCC ≤5 cm	Percutaneous	8/32 (25%)	0/32 (0%)
Wong et al, 2001	HCC, metastases	Open, percutaneous (1)	8/40 (20%)	0/40 (0%)
Bowles et al, 2001	HCC, metastases	Percutaneous, laparoscopic, open	7/76 major and 17/76 minor	1/76 (1%)
Solbiati et al, 2001	Metastases from colorectal cancer	Percutaneous	2/117 (2%)	0/117 (0%)
Zagoria et al, 2002	Metastases	Percutaneous, open	5/38 (13%)	1/38 (2%)
Berber et al, 2002	Metastases from neuroendocrine cancer	Laparoscopic	2/34 (6%)	0/34 (0%)
De Baere et al, 2003	HCC, metastases	Percutaneous, open	Not reported per patient	5/312 (2%)
Livraghi et al, 2003a	Metastases from colorectal cancer	Percutaneous	3/88 (3%)	0/88 (0%)
Bleicher et al, 2003	Metastases	Percutaneous, laparoscopic, open	3/153 (2%)	18/153 (12%)
Livraghi et al, 2003b	HCC, metastases	Percutaneous	50/2320 (2%)	6/2320 (0.3%)
Curley et al, 2004	HCC, metastases	Percutaneous, laparoscopic	58/608 (9%)	3/608 (0.5%)
Total			*183/4161 (4%)*	*28/4549 (0.6%)*

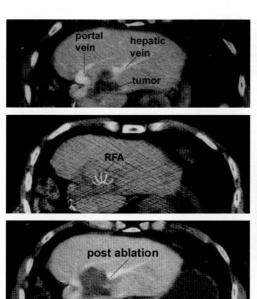

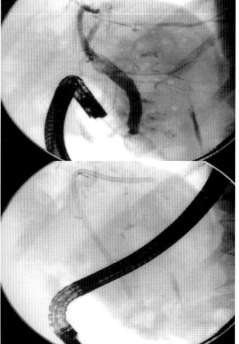

Fig. 76c.6. Biliary injury after RFA treated with stent placement.

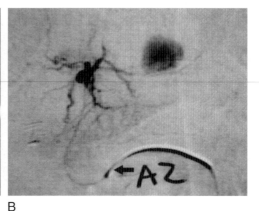

A   B

Fig. 76c.7. Hepatic artery pseudo-aneurysm after RFA.

of open or laparoscopic RFA instead of percutaneous RFA for tumors within 1 cm of the liver edge or gallbladder.

Injury to the diaphragm also is a potential complication during percutaneous RFA, especially when tumors at the dome of the liver are treated. In an animal model, carbon monoxide was introduced into the peritoneal cavity to separate the diaphragm and the liver; although this reduced severe diaphragmatic injury during superficial hepatic RFA (Ramin et al, 2004), the technique needs further clinical testing. Hepatic dome tumors should be treated by an open or laparoscopic approach.

Abscess, one of the most frequent complications of RFA, typically occurs 1 week after ablation and requires percutaneous or surgical drainage (De Baere et al, 2003; Wood et al, 2000). Patients with biliary-enteric anastomosis or biliary stenting seem to have a higher rate of abscess formation. All patients undergoing RFA should receive periprocedural antibiotics that cover coliforms and skin flora. Temperature and leukocyte counts should be followed after the procedure. Any continued elevation should prompt CT imaging for possible hepatic abscess.

Reports of tumor seeding vary from 0.5% to 12% (De Baere et al, 2003; De Sio et al, 2001; Llovet et al, 2001), possibly reflecting differences in follow-up. Llovet and colleagues (2001) found that tumor seeding during RFA was related to subcapsular tumor location and poor tumor differentiation. Recent tumor biopsy, multiple needle insertions, and tumor hemorrhage during treatment also may increase the risk of needle tract seeding. This complication can be avoided by limiting the number of needle insertions, angling the needle to traverse normal hepatic parenchyma before entering the tumor, and cauterizing the tract on withdrawal of the needle. Nicoli and coworkers (2003) reported rapid diffusion of neoplastic cells after the creation of an arteriovenous fistula following RFA. The authors attributed seeding of tumor cells to the pressure gradient between the high-pressure tumor arteries and the low-pressure portal system. This is the only report of this complication in several thousand RFAs to date.

Injury to bile ducts during RFA can result in stenosis and proximal biliary dilation. Most physicians agree that tumors within 15 to 20 mm of a major bile duct should not be treated by RFA (Mulier et al, 2002). Elias and coworkers (2001) introduced intraductal cooling to prevent RFA-associated biliary stenosis. They infused cooled (4°C) Ringer's lactate through a catheter after choledochotomy. Intraductal cooling was undertaken in 13 patients undergoing RFA of tumors within 6 mm of a central bile duct; one patient had a local recurrence, and one developed biliary stenosis (Elias et al, 2004). Biliary stenting also

can avoid biliary injury during ablation of tumors near the bile ducts (Wood et al, 2000).

RADIOFREQUENCY ABLATION VERSUS RESECTION

There is no prospective, randomized controlled trial of RFA versus resection for the treatment of primary liver carcinoma or hepatic metastases. One retrospective study of 358 patients with colorectal liver metastases compared resection, RFA plus resection, RFA alone, and laparotomy with biopsy (Abdalla et al, 2004). RFA was used for cure when complete resection was not possible. All patient-related and tumor-related factors known to influence outcome were similar among the groups. The rate of recurrence was 84% after RFA alone, 63% after RFA plus resection, and 52% after resection alone. Local recurrence (in the area treated) was more common after RFA plus resection (9%) than RFA alone (5%) or resection alone (2%). The 3-year rate of overall survival was 73% after resection, 43% after RFA plus resection, and 37% after RFA alone. Patients who underwent RFA had a survival advantage over patients who underwent biopsy with or without chemotherapy.

Another study by Vivarelli and colleagues (2004) evaluated surgical resection versus percutaneous RFA for the treatment of HCC. This study was performed at two different centers; RFA was performed at one center and resection at the other. Overall and disease-free survivals were significantly better after resection. Patients treated with RFA had more liver lesions and a higher Child classification, however, both of which may have influenced outcome. Matched treatment groups are needed to compare RFA with resection. Currently, we do not advocate RFA in patients who are candidates for resection.

CONCLUSION

RFA can treat primary or metastatic liver tumors with success rates of 90% and little morbidity or mortality. It can be applied via an operative or percutaneous approach. An operative approach allows accurate assessment for the presence of extrahepatic disease and a better evaluation of intrahepatic disease. An operative approach also can isolate the liver from adjacent organs that could be injured during ablation, and it allows placement of the RFA probe in lesions that could not be reached by a percutaneous approach. Operative RFA should be considered instead of percutaneous RFA for patients who are medically fit to undergo an operation, but have unresectable disease.

A randomized prospective study is necessary to determine survival and recurrence rates after RFA versus resection. For now, resection remains the initial choice for patients whose disease is confined to the liver. RFA may be an alternative for patients unable to undergo resection because of limited hepatic reserve, bilobar disease, or poor medical status; in these cases, RFA can be very successful, and its results may be durable. Although RFA provides local control of liver disease, its impact on survival is unclear. Systemic therapy should be used to treat or prevent other sites of metastatic disease.

As the field of RFA has evolved, improvements in bipolar and multipolar probe technology have allowed for larger zones of ablation and higher rates of complete response. Newer probes are now able to treat larger lesions with a single focused ablation. This new technology has reduced limitations of tumor size on adequate response and recurrence rates. Meanwhile, more surgeons are becoming skilled in the technique of RFA. The future application of RFA for liver-directed therapy seems promising.

REFERENCES

Abdalla EK, et al, 2004: Recurrence and outcomes following hepatic resection, radiofrequency ablation, and combined resection/ablation for colorectal liver metastases. Ann Surg 239:818-827.

Berber E, et al, 2002: Laparoscopic radiofrequency ablation of neuroendocrine liver metastases. World J Surg 26:985-990.

Bilchik AJ, et al, 1999: Radiofrequency ablation: a minimally invasive technique with multiple applications. Cancer J Sci Am 5:356-361.

Bilchik AJ, et al, 2000: Cryosurgical ablation and radiofrequency ablation for unresectable hepatic malignant neoplasms. Arch Surg 135:657-664.

Bleicher RJ, et al, 2003: Radiofrequency ablation in 447 complex unresectable liver tumors: lessons learned. Ann Surg Oncol 10:52-58.

Bowles BJ, et al, 2001: Safety and efficacy of radiofrequency thermal ablation in advanced liver tumors. Arch Surg 136:864-869.

Cady B, et al, 1998: Surgical margin in hepatic resection for colorectal metastasis: a critical and improvable determinant of outcome. Ann Surg 227:556-571.

Chinn SB, et al, 2001: Effect of vascular occlusion on radiofrquency ablation of the liver: Results in a porcine model. AJR Am J Roentgenol 176:789-795.

Cho CM, et al, 2005: Radiofrequency ablation versus surgical resection in the treatment of hepatocellular carcinoma; retrospective comparative study. Korean J Hepatol 11:59-71.

Curley SA, et al, 1999: Radiofrequency ablation of unresectable primary and metastatic hepatic malignancies: results in 123 patients. Ann Surg 230:1-8.

Curley SA, et al, 2000: Radiofrequency ablation of hepatocellular cancer in 110 patients with cirrhosis. Ann Surg 232:381-391.

Curley SA, et al, 2004: Early and late complications after radiofrequency ablation of malignant liver tumors in 608 patients. Ann Surg 239:450-458.

De Baere T, et al, 2000: Radiofrequency ablation of 100 hepatic metastases with a mean follow-up of more than 1 year. Am J Radiol 175:1619-1625.

De Baere T, et al, 2002: Percutaneous radiofrequency ablation of hepatic tumors during temporary venous occlusion. AJR Am J Roentgenol 178:53-59.

De Baere T, et al, 2003: Adverse events during radiofrequency treatment of 582 hepatic tumors. Am J Radiol 181:695-700.

De Sio I, et al, 2001: Tumor dissemination after radiofrequency ablation of hepatocellular carcinoma. Hepatology 34:609-610.

Elias D, et al, 2001: Intraductal cooling of the main bile duct during intraoperative radiofrequency ablation. J Surg Oncol 76:297-300.

Elias D, et al, 2002: Percutaneous radiofrequency thermoablation as an alternative to surgery for treatment of liver tumour recurrence after hepatectomy. Br J Surg 89:752-756.

Elias D, et al, 2004: Intraductal cooling of the main bile ducts during radiofrequency ablation prevents biliary stenosis. J Am Coll Surg 198:717-721.

Fong Y, et al, 1997: Liver resection for colorectal metastases. J Clin Oncol 15:938-946.

Fong Y, et al, 1999: Clinical score for predicting recurrence after hepatic resection for metastatic colorectal cancer: analysis of 1001 consecutive cases. Ann Surg 230:309-318.

Hong SN, et al, 2005: Comparing the outcomes of radiofrequency ablation and surgery in patients with a single small hepatocellular carcinoma and well-preserved hepatic function. J Clin Gastroenterol 39:247-252.

Lencioni R, et al, 1998: Radio-frequency thermal ablation of liver metastases with a cooled-tip electrode needle: results of a pilot clinical trial. Eur Radiol 8:1205-1211.

Livraghi T, et al, 1999: Small hepatocellular carcinoma: treatment with radio-frequency ablation versus ethanol injection. Radiology 210:655-661.

Livraghi T, et al, 2000: Hepatocellular carcinoma: radio-frequency ablation of medium and large lesions. Radiology 214:761-768.

Livraghi T, et al, 2001: Percutaneous radio-frequency ablation of liver metastases from breast cancer: initial experience in 24 patients. Radiology 220:146-149.

Livraghi T, et al, 2003a: Percutaneous radiofrequency ablation of liver metastases in potential candidates for resection: the "test of time approach." Cancer 97:3027-3035.

Livraghi T, et al, 2003b: Treatment of focal liver tumors with percutaneous radio-frequency ablation: complications encountered in a multicenter study. Radiology 226:441-451.

Llovet JM, et al, 2001: Increased risk of tumor seeding after percutaneous radiofrequency ablation for single hepatocellular carcinoma. Hepatology 33:1124-1129.

Lu DS, et al, 2002: Effect of vessel size on creation of hepatic radiofrequency lesions in pigs: assessment of the "heatsink" effect. AJR Am J Roentgenol 178:47-51.

Mulier S, et al, 2002: Complications of radiofrequency coagulation of liver tumours. Br J Surg 89:1206-1222.

Nicoli N, et al, 2003: A case of rapid intrahepatic dissemination of hepatocellular carcinoma after radiofrequency thermal ablation. Am J Surg 188:165-167.

Poon RT, et al, 2004a: Effectiveness of radiofrequency ablation for hepatocellular carcinomas larger than 3 cm in diameter. Arch Surg 139:281-287.

Poon RT, et al, 2004b: Radiofrequency ablation for subcapsular hepatocellular carcinoma. Ann Surg 11:281-289.

Ramin SS, et al, 2004: Minimizing diaphragmatic injury during radiofrequency ablation: efficacy of intraabdominal carbon dioxide insufflation. Am J Radiol 183:197-200.

Rossi S, et al, 1990: Thermal lesions induced by 480 khz localized current field in guinea pig and pig liver. Tumori 76:54-57.

Rossi S, et al, 1996: Percutaneous RF interstitial thermal ablation in the treatment of hepatic cancer. AJR Am J Roentgenol 167:759-768.

Rossi S, et al, 1998: Percutaneous treatment of small hepatic tumors by an expandable RF needle electrode. AJR Am J Roentgenol 170:1015-1022.

Siperstein A, et al, 2000: Local recurrence after laparoscopic radiofrequency thermal ablation of hepatic tumors. Ann Surg Oncol 7:106-113.

Solbiati L, et al, 1997: Percutaneous US-guided RF tissue ablation of liver metastases: results of treatment and follow-up in 16 patients. Radiology 202:195-203.

Solbiati L, et al, 2001: Percutaneous radio-frequency ablation of hepatic metastases from colorectal cancer: long-term results in 117 patients. Radiology 221:159-166.

Strasberg SM, Linehan D, 2003: Radiofrequency ablation of liver tumors. Curr Prob Surg 40:451-498.

Wong SL, et al, 2001: Radiofrequency ablation for unresectable hepatic tumors. Am J Surg 182:552-557.

Wood TF, et al, 2000: Radiofrequency ablation of 231 unresectable hepatic tumors: indications, limitations, and complications. Ann Surg Oncol 7:593-600.

Vivarelli M, et al, 2004: Surgical resection versus percutaneous radiofrequency ablation in the treatment of hepatocellular carcinoma on cirrhotic liver. Ann Surg 240:102-107.

Zagoria RJ, et al, 2002: Complications of radiofrequency ablation of liver metastases. Am Surg 68:204-209.

Chemotherapy of Liver Tumors

77a SYSTEMIC THERAPY FOR HEPATOCELLULAR CARCINOMA

G. K. ABOU-ALFA AND L. B. SALTZ

Hepatocellular carcinoma (HCC) (see Ch. 71) is one of the most common solid tumor malignancies worldwide. Its incidence mirrors that of chronic liver injury, which is most commonly due to viral hepatitis infection. Other causes of chronic liver injury and cirrhosis include alcohol, metabolic diseases, and environmental exposures. Western Africa and China have the highest incidence per capita of HCC (McGlynn et al, 2001). There is also a concerning rising incidence of HCC in North America (El-Serag & Mason, 1999). A threefold increase in the age-adjusted rates for HCC associated with hepatitis C, from 2.3 per 100,000 in 1993-1995 to 7 per 100,000 in 1996-1998, has been observed. This increase is most likely explained primarily by the increased incidence of hepatitis C that has been seen in North America during this time.

Most of the etiologic agents that cause HCC lead initially to cirrhosis. Although this is not universally the case, especially in hepatitis B–related HCC, it still would seem prudent for any therapeutic or preventive strategies to address both of these major risk factors to the patient's health and survival: the malignancy itself and the underlying cirrhosis.

Many chemotherapeutic agents have been shown to produce responses in some patients with HCC. With the lack of any clear impact on survival reported so far, however, there is still no widely accepted standard chemotherapy for this disease. HCC is considered to be a relatively chemotherapy-resistant malignancy. By the same token, the role of neoadjuvant and adjuvant therapy remains questionable in this disease, despite some promising preliminary data. A better understanding of the mechanisms of resistance and the biology of the disease would be likely to be helpful in developing more effective therapies.

HEPATOCELLULAR CARCINOMA AND CIRRHOSIS—TWO DISEASES IN ONE

Cirrhosis is as likely to have an impact on a patient's overall survival outcome as is the tumor itself. The need to evaluate the cirrhosis status of patients with liver cancer has long been recognized. A scoring system originally developed by Child (1964) consisted of three parameters: jaundice (bilirubin), ascites, and encephalopathy. Pugh and colleagues (1973) later updated this scoring system; they added an assessment of hepatic synthetic function by evaluating serum albumin levels and prothrombin time (Table 77a.1). This combined score is now known as the Child-Pugh score (see Chs. 2, 80, 82, and 88). It is the most commonly used scoring system for liver cirrhosis. The pitfall from the oncologist's perspective of the Child-Pugh score is that it does not incorporate any parameters that relate to the cancer itself. This score was not developed for oncologic purposes. Still, the Child-Pugh score can serve as a useful predictor of outcome

and can serve as a guide for when the probability of mortality from the cirrhosis is excessive enough to make the risks of anticancer therapy hard to justify. The synthetic hepatic function may be so significantly impaired and the prognosis may be so limited for a patient with a Child-Pugh C score that, for safety purposes, the decision not to treat such a patient with cytotoxic therapy may be warranted. A patient with an unresected HCC in a cirrhotic liver and Child-Pugh C score has a predicted median survival of only approximately 3 months, regardless of the presence or absence of cancer. There is no evidence that anticancer chemotherapy would have an impact on survival at any Child-Pugh stage (Ebara et al, 1998). In such situations, the use of chemotherapeutic agents is far more likely to lead to detrimental toxicity rather than to clinical benefit.

Okuda and coworkers (1985) recognized the need for an HCC staging system that incorporated factors related to the cirrhosis and the tumor itself and developed the Okuda staging system. Believing that a simple and practical system was essential, Okuda and coworkers (1985) limited the scoring system to four variables: albumin, bilirubin, ascites, and tumor size as a percentage function to the size of the liver (>50% or <50%).

The Okuda staging system (see Ch. 2) served as a platform for more advanced and sophisticated prospective scoring systems that used the Cox proportional hazard regression model. The Cancer of the Liver Italian Program (CLIP) investigators (1998, 2000) developed a scoring system that found the independent prognostic variables for patients with HCC to be the Child-Pugh score plus three additional variables that relate to the tumor itself: tumor morphology (as assessed by the number of lesions and extent in the liver), presence or absence of portal vein thrombosis, and α-fetoprotein level (Table 77a.2). Patients with high score of

Table 77a.1 Child-Pugh Scoring System

Parameter	POINTS		
	1	**2**	**3**
Albumin (g/dL)	>3.5	2.8-3.5	<2.8
Bilirubin (mg/dL)	<2	2-3	>3
Ascites	Absent	Slight	Moderate
Encephalopathy	None	I-II	III-IV
PT (INR)	<1.7	1.8-2.3	>2.3
Score	**Points**		
A	5-6		
B	7-9		
C	10-15		

Table 77a.2 Cancer of the Liver Italian Program Scoring System

Parameter	SCORE		
	0	**1**	**2**
Child-Pugh score	A	B	C
Tumor morphology	Uninodular and extension ≤50%	Multinodular and extension ≤50%	Massive or extension >50%
Portal vein thrombosis	No	Yes	—
AFP (ng/dL)	<400	≥400	—
Score	0 1 2 3	4-6	

AFP, α-fetoprotein.

4 to 6 were shown to have a median survival of only 3.2 months. The CLIP score was tested mainly in patients with hepatitis C.

In contrast to the CLIP score, the Chinese University Prognostic Index (CUPI), another scoring system that is based on multivariate analysis, was developed mainly in patients with hepatitis B–associated HCC (Leung et al, 2002a). This prognostic index identified bilirubin, alkaline phosphatase, presence or absence of ascites, tumor stage based on TNM staging, and α-fetoprotein levels as the most important predictors of outcome. In addition, and for the first time, a clinical assessment parameter of the presence or absence of symptoms at presentation was incorporated (Table 77a.3). An important aspect of the CUPI index is the different weights attributed to the different parameters. The median survival of the highest risk group was close to 1 month.

The aforementioned scoring and staging systems have shown success in identifying patients with advanced stage HCC and cirrhosis, for whom supportive care is likely to be the most appropriate therapeutic approach. In contrast, another scoring system, the Barcelona Clinic Liver Cancer Group (BCLC) (Llovet et al, 1999), was developed with the aim of fine-tuning the differences between patients with early stage disease, something the Okuda staging system fails to do. By the same token, the BCLC staging system had limited permutations for patients with advanced disease

Table 77a.3 Chinese University Prognostic Index (CUPI) Scoring System

Parameter	Weight (CUPI Score)					
Bilirubin (mg/dL)	<1.9	0	1.9-2.8	3	≥2.9	4
Ascites	Present	3				
Alkaline phosphatase	≥200 IU/L	3				
TNM stage	I and II	−3	IIIa and IIIb	−1	IVa and IVb	0
AFP (ng/mL)	≥500	2				
Disease symptoms on presentation	None	−4				

Risk Group	Score
Low	−7-1
Intermediate	2-7
High	8-12

AFP, α-fetoprotein.

and regrouped patients with unresectable disease, with Okuda stage I or II, or with Child-Pugh A or B in the same category of advanced disease. As such, the ability of the BCLC to provide prognostic information for more advanced patients is limited.

Each of these scoring or staging systems has limitations. It is important to incorporate one of these staging systems in a patient's assessment before considering therapy. In the case of hepatitis B etiology, the CUPI scoring index seems to be the most appropriate choice. The CLIP system is likely to be more applicable to hepatitis C–related cases. For other, nonviral etiologies, the Child-Pugh system may be most appropriately used.

Platelet levels have not been shown to be of any prognostic significance for patients with cirrhosis and HCC; however, they do play a major role in regard to the decision to treat or not treat a patient with systemic chemotherapy. With advancing cirrhosis and increased platelet pooling into an enlarging spleen, platelet levels can decrease to less than 75,000/μL, potentially compromising the ability to deliver chemotherapy safely.

ROLE OF CHEMOTHERAPY IN HEPATOCELLULAR CARCINOMA

Doxorubicin

Almost all classes of chemotherapy have been assessed in HCC (Nerenstone et al, 1988). Doxorubicin is one of the most studied drugs in this disease; this is partly due to what so far has been an irreproducible reported response rate of 79%, originally reported by Olweny and associates (1975). This early report from the mid-1970s did not use computed tomography (CT) or magnetic resonance imaging (MRI), which are available and used routinely today. Most "responses" were determined on the basis of physical examinations of the liver or using a colloidal gold liver scan. Neither of these measuring techniques would be acceptable as evidence of a response on clinical trials by current standards. Many subsequent attempts to try to reproduce this high response rate have been made, but to no avail. At least 12 additional trials of doxorubicin, as a single agent (Barbare et al, 1984; Chlebowski et al, 1984; Ihde et al, 1977; Johnson et al, 1978; Sciarrino, 1985; Vogel et al, 1977; Williams & Melia, 1980) and in combination (Choi et al, 1984; Falkson et al, 1978, 1987; Melia et al, 1983; Olweny et al, 1980), failed to show such a high response rate or any survival benefit over supportive care (two of these trials also included patients with cholangiocarcinoma) (Falkson et al, 1987).

For the most part, little attention was paid in the many doxorubicin trials to stratification of patients based on their liver function, and only four studies reported some form of scoring regarding the accompanying cirrhosis. Most importantly, none of these studies used well-defined radiologic criteria for response (e.g., CT scan), and many response assessments were done via the crude measure of using clinical examination. Further attempts to explain the response rate initially reported by Olweny and colleagues (1975) based on disease etiology, hepatitis B, or ethnicity (African population) also failed to support or confirm the initial positive result. As discussed subsequently, a recently completed randomized study, which is the only trial that treated a large, homogeneous population of HCC patients with single-agent doxorubicin and used contemporary imaging methods and response criteria, found a confirmed objective response rate of 12% (Yeo et al, 2004).

Table 77a.4   Response Rates to Single Chemotherapeutic Agents in Hepatocellular Carcinoma

Drug	No. Patients	Objective Response (%)	Reference
Cisplatin	35	17	Falkson et al, 1987
Etoposide	24	18	Melia et al, 1983
Mitoxantrone	35	0	Falkson et al, 1987
Vinblastine	25	8	Damrongsak et al, 1973
Capecitabine	37	13	Lozano et al, 2000
Gemcitabine	20	5	Kubicka et al, 2001
Irinotecan	14	7	O'Reilly et al, 2001
Paclitaxel	20	0	Chao et al, 1998

Other Chemotherapeutic Agents

Other older and newer chemotherapeutic agents also have been studied in HCC (Table 77a.4). Many agents, such as cisplatin (Falkson et al, 1987) and etoposide (Melia et al, 1983), have shown similar response rates to the rates reported using doxorubicin—in the 15% to 20% range. Other agents were not as effective: Mitoxantrone had 0% response rate (Falkson et al, 1987), and vinblastine had 8% response rate (Damrongsak et al, 1973), both in small series of 25 to 35 patients. Newer agents have not shown consistently higher responses and sometimes have seemed to have less activity than older agents. In small series of 15 to 37 patients, capecitabine showed a 13% response rate (Lozano et al, 2000); gemcitabine, 5% (Kubicka et al, 2001); irinotecan, 7% (O'Reilly et al, 2001); and paclitaxel, 0% (Chao et al, 1998). This study may represent a lesser degree of activity; however, it is also possible that this may represent different standards used in declaring responses in current versus older investigations.

Combination Chemotherapy

Combination chemotherapy seemed to improve the response rates, but with no clear impact on survival (Table 77a.5). In a phase II trial comprising 25 patients, 5-fluorouracil plus leucovorin showed a response rate of 28% (Porta et al, 1995); 5-fluorouracil

Table 77a.5   Response Rates to Combination Chemotherapeutic Agents in Hepatocellular Carcinoma

Drugs	No. Patients	Objective Response (%)	Reference
5-Fluorouracil, leucovorin	25	28	Porta et al, 1995
5-Fluorouracil, doxorubicin	38	13	Baker et al, 1977
Epirubicin, etoposide	36	39	Bobbio-Pallavicini et al, 1997
5-Fluorouracil, interferon alfa-2b	28	18	Patt et al, 1993
Cisplatin, interferon alfa-2b	30	13.3	Ji et al, 1996

plus doxorubicin, 13% (38 patients) (Baker et al, 1977); and epirubicin plus etoposide, 39% (36 patients) (Bobbio-Pallavicini et al, 1997). Perhaps the most interesting additions to chemotherapy are interferon alfa and interferon beta. Interferon is normally produced in response to a hepatitis viral infection. In addition to its immunomodulatory activity, however, interferon was found to have a potential role as an antiproliferative agent directed against tumor cells. As a single agent, interferon alfa-2b showed only a limited response rate of 7% in a Gastrointestinal Tumor Study Group trial (1990). This disappointing low response, in addition to increased toxicity owing to the use of high doses of interferon, led to testing lower doses in combination with chemotherapy. Adding interferon to 5-fluorouracil (Patt et al, 1993) or cisplatin (Ji et al, 1996) showed response rates of 31% and 13% in individual trials. Results have been inconsistent, however, and favorable activity has not been seen in other trials that have incorporated interferon into 5-fluorouracil–based (Stuart et al, 1996) or doxorubicin-based (Kardinal et al, 1993) regimens.

The preliminary indication of some activity for interferon set the stage for a more intense combination for cisplatin, interferon, doxorubicin, and 5-fluorouracil, which became commonly known as PIAF (Patt et al, 1998). PIAF subsequently was modified and tested in the outpatient setting (Leung et al, 2002b). This phase II trial of 50 patients showed a response rate of 26%. More importantly, 18% (nine patients) had their tumor resected after therapy; of these resected patients, four had a pathologic complete response noted in the resected tumor. There was considerable hematologic toxicity, and two treatment-related deaths were reported owing to neutropenic fever in this 50-patient cohort.

These data led to a randomized phase III trial of doxorubicin versus a PIAF combination (Yeo et al, 2004). This trial showed the same 26% response rate for PIAF versus 12% for single-agent doxorubicin. The study failed, however, to show any survival advantage in favor of the PIAF combination (8.6 months versus 6.8 months; $P = .83$). Despite this trial having a negative outcome of its primary end point, it did provide several important and useful pieces of information. First, as noted earlier, it identified what can be realistically considered the true response rate, by current standards of response definition and determination, of doxorubicin in HCC, and that response rate is 12%. This is the number clinicians realistically must go by, considering that it emanates from a well-conducted current phase III study that required pathologic confirmation and modern radiologic modalities to assess response. Although the study failed to provide support for use of PIAF as a routine palliative therapy for advanced disease, one might consider it in the neoadjuvant setting in a select number of patients with potentially resectable tumors.

RESISTANCE OF HEPATOCELLULAR CARCINOMA TO CHEMOTHERAPY

HCC cells are relatively well differentiated and carry several mechanisms of drug resistance. HCC comprises highly resistant clones of cancer cells (DeVita & Abou-Alfa, 2000); this has been shown not only through clinical experience, but also in experimental work, such as the rat hepatocyte model studied by Farber and others (Farber & Rubin, 1991; Solt et al, 1977). The HCC cells carry a high *genetic mutational load*, which makes them less amenable to the destructive actions of chemotherapy. HCC cells usually contain a high level of dihydropyrimidine dehydrogenase, which potentially makes them relatively resistant to 5-fluorouracil (Jiang et al, 1997). HCC cells also overexpress the multidrug resistance gene *MDR1* (Chenivesse et al, 1993) and the gene product P-glycoprotein (Soini et al, 1996). This overexpression may help explain the resistance of HCC to paclitaxel (O'Reilly et al, 2001) and the relatively low true response rate to doxorubicin (Leung et al, 1999). T138067-sodium, a novel antimicrotubule agent, in contrast to the taxanes and the vinca alkaloids, was shown to be active in preclinical models against multidrug resistance variants of different malignant cell lines (Shan et al, 1999). In a phase II study in patients with HCC, overcoming the multidrug resistance effect was minimal, with a 10% partial response rate reported (Leung et al, 2002b).

As discussed earlier, cirrhosis is often a key clinical factor present in patients with HCC. Many trials, especially older trials, have failed to stratify or select for adequate hepatic function. This failure can lead to excessive toxicity and inadequate assessment of the agent being investigated because of an excessive need for dose attenuations. Although it is clear that there are no highly active agents in this disease, the possibility that a higher degree of activity for some agents might be identified in a trial of patients with good hepatic function cannot be excluded. Nevertheless, currently available agents offer inadequate treatment options to patients with HCC, and the identification of new agents and novel treatment strategies is sorely needed.

INVESTIGATIONAL CYTOTOXIC AGENTS

Newer cytotoxic agents that have embedded properties that may help overcome some mechanisms of resistance in HCC are being evaluated, but have not yet proved useful. Nolatrexed dihydrochloride is a nonclassic lipophilic inhibitor of thymidylate synthase that is not catabolized by dihydropyrimidine dehydrogenase. It lacks a glutamate side chain and has reduced potential transport-associated resistance (Webber et al, 1993). Nolatrexed has been studied in two different clinical trials. It has shown disappointing results, however, with an 8% response rate in a phase II North American study (Stuart et al, 1999) and no responses in a randomized phase II study in Hong Kong (Mok et al, 1999). Nevertheless, a phase III trial is pending completion.

T138067 is an antimicrotubular non–P-glycoprotein substrate that, in contrast to paclitaxel, which showed no activity, has shown a modest 9% response in chemotherapy-naive patients (Leung et al, 2002b). A randomized phase III trial of T138067 versus doxorubicin in patients with advanced HCC has been initiated and is pending completion. Given the limited degree of activity seen with these newer agents in phase II trials, it is difficult to be enthusiastic about the prospects for the phase III outcomes of trials for these agents to improve greatly the outlook for HCC patients.

NOVEL BIOLOGIC THERAPIES IN HEPATOCELLULAR CARCINOMA

The advent of novel targeted therapeutics, and the continued lack of a standard of care for advanced HCC, led to a fast-growing interest in identifying and evaluating relevant targets in HCC along the signal transduction pathways (Fig. 77a.1) (Abou-Alfa & Morse, 2004). At the cell surface, ligands bind to different cell receptors that initiate a cascade of signals that lead

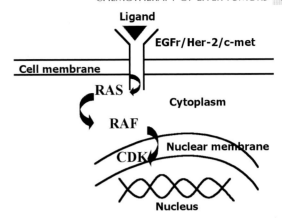

Fig. 77a.1. Potential targets for HCC therapy along the signal transduction pathway.

to cell duplication. This phenomenon can go unchecked despite multiple feedback mechanisms, leading to continued cell replication and oncogenesis. The epidermal growth factor receptor is one of the most well-studied therapeutic targets. Several authors reported no difference in expression of epidermal growth factor receptor between HCC and noncancerous diseased liver tissues (Hamazaki et al, 1997; Harada et al, 1999), whereas others reported overexpression in 17% of HCC cases (Kiss et al, 1997). OSI-774 (erlotinib), an epidermal growth factor receptor–specific receptor tyrosine kinase inhibitor, was tested in HCC as part of a phase II trial (Philip et al, 2004). For unclear reasons, only 20 of 35 patients who initiated therapy were considered evaluable in that study. Three of the 20 evaluable patients had a partial radiologic response, and 7 were progression-free at 6 months. Although the drug was well tolerated, it still leaves the role of epidermal growth factor receptor in HCC in question. Other anti–epidermal growth factor receptor new targeted therapies, particularly the monoclonal antibodies that so far have shown more activity in colorectal cancer, still may warrant investigation.

Another receptor, Her-2/neu, also has been found to be relatively rarely expressed in human HCC tissues (Hsu et al, 2002), leaving the role of trastuzumab in HCC still in question. A more promising target is the hepatocyte growth factor and its receptor c-met, which were found to be overexpressed in 33% and 20% of human HCC (Kiss et al, 1997). An effective targeted therapy against cytokine hepatocyte growth factor or its epithelial receptor, c-met, is under development and would warrant clinical investigation in HCC.

Downstream of surface receptors, and on the cytoplasmic side of the cellular membrane, is the anchoring protein Ras, which is mutated in many cancers. Its relevance in HCC has been debated, however. Conflicting reports showed no pathogenic correlation between Ras and HCC (Tada et al, 1990), whereas others showed a 15% expression in patients with HCC of different etiologies, such as hepatitis B, hepatitis C, and alcoholic cirrhosis (Weihrauch et al, 2001). A higher percentage (42%) was found among patients with HCC who had previous vinyl chloride exposure averaging 9942 ppm-years. The rate-limiting step of Ras processing and anchoring to the cell membrane is a post-translational farnesylation of a cytosine residue located at its carboxyl terminal (Kato et al, 1992). Several farnesylation inhibitors have been studied, including simvastatin (Mazume et al, 1999) and pravastatin (Kawata et al, 1994, 2001). Other potential modalities to block Ras activity include CAAX box peptidomimetic farnesyltransferase inhibitors and geranylgeranyltransferase inhibitors. To date, none have been tested formally in HCC.

Downstream from Ras, the Raf/MEK/ERK signaling pathway plays a key role in the neoplastic transformation of hepatocytes at the level of Raf kinase. Preclinical studies have shown the activation of MEK1/2 and its downstream target mitogen-activated protein kinase in HCC tumors (Huynh et al, 2003). In hepatitis C virus infection, the virus core proteins result in high basal activity of Raf-1, which itself leads to a sustained response to epidermal growth factor by hepatocytes, resulting in an increased possibility of neoplastic transformation (Giambartolomei et al, 2001). Sorafenib (BAY 43-9006) is a novel signal transduction Raf-1 kinase inhibitor (Wilhelm et al, 2004). A phase II study assessing antitumor activity of BAY 43-9006 in patients with advanced inoperable HCC showed a modest 5.1% partial response rate, but a 55% stable disease as best response (Abou-Alfa et al, 2004). Two other aspects of sorafenib are discussed later.

At the nuclear membrane, the cell cycle transitional points are under control of the cyclin-dependent kinases. Flavopiridol, a cyclin-dependent kinase 1, 2, and 4 inhibitor (Carlson et al, 1996; Losiewicz et al, 1994), already has been tested extensively in several studies and in combination with irinotecan in a broad array of solid tumor malignancies as part of a phase I trial (Shah et al, 2003). In this phase I trial, two patients with metastatic HCC had prolonged stable disease with this drug combination. Single-agent irinotecan showed minimal activity in a phase II trial (Kubicka et al, 2001). This concept is being assessed further in a phase II study of flavopiridol and irinotecan in HCC, currently under way.

Despite some initial disappointments, angiogenesis is an appealing target for novel therapeutics, especially with the positive data reported on the antiangiogenic agent bevacizumab in colorectal cancer (Hurwitz et al, 2004). In that report, patients with advanced colorectal cancer were randomized to irinotecan, 5-fluorouracil, and leucovorin (the standard care at that time) plus placebo versus irinotecan, 5-fluorouracil, and leucovorin plus bevacizumab. Patients on the bevacizumab-containing arm showed an increased response rate of 45% versus 35% and a statistically significant improvement in survival (20.3 months versus 15.6 months). These positive findings in colorectal cancer raise optimism that this approach may have some merit in HCC as well. Investigations into this area are beginning.

A preliminary report of an ongoing study of single-agent bevacizumab in patients with advanced HCC (Schwartz et al, 1985) noted one partial response, and 8 patients with stable disease were reported among 10 evaluable patients in a still accruing study. Bevacizumab as a single agent has minimal activity in colorectal cancer (Mitchell et al, 2005). As in colorectal cancer, it may be that the optimal benefit from an antiangiogenic agent would be realized when it is combined with an active cytotoxic regimen.

Another putatively antiangiogenic agent that has been evaluated in HCC is thalidomide. In a phase II trial evaluating thalidomide in patients with advanced HCC, 1 of 32 evaluable patients showed a partial response, and 31% had stable disease (Patt et al, 2005). The neurotoxicity encountered was formidable, however, and the authors did not recommend thalidomide at the doses studied. As with bevacizumab, the possibility that a combination of thalidomide and cytotoxic chemotherapy could have more significant activity does exist; however, this hypothesis has not been explored yet, and a lower dose of thalidomide presumably would have to be tested.

Based on newer data regarding the mechanisms of action of sorafenib, we can now add this agent to the list of antiangiogenic agents. Sorafenib, a small-molecule tyrosine kinase inhibitor of Raf kinase, also has been found to have inhibitory activity against the tyrosine kinases of vascular endothelial growth factor receptors 2 and 3 and platelet-derived growth factor receptor (Wilhelm et al, 2004). As noted earlier, this agent, which had only modest single-agent activity, now is being investigated in a randomized phase II trial in combination with doxorubicin versus doxorubicin alone.

ASSESSMENT OF RADIOLOGIC RESPONSE IN HEPATOCELLULAR CARCINOMA

In contrast to early clinical trials conducted in the 1970s, in which assessment of response depended mainly on clinical evaluation, the advent of radiologic technologies, including contrast-enhanced CT, triphasic CT, and MRI, has helped improve clinicians' ability to assess disease extent and tumor response to therapy in a more objective manner. Despite these improved imaging modalities, HCC remains one of the most difficult tumors to evaluate radiologically. This difficulty is due in part to the infiltrative nature of these tumors, their poor margination, and their hypervascularity, all of which make it hard to define their exact margins. In addition, there is growing recognition that response also can be assessed through dynamic measures, such as necrosis and blood flow to the tumor. In a completed phase II trial of the antiangiogenic and Raf kinase inhibitor sorafenib in HCC (Abou-Alfa et al, 2004), we observed tumor necrosis, but not actual tumor regression, associated with declines in α-fetoprotein in several patients. These patients experienced an actual increase in tumor volume, albeit with MRI evidence of substantial central necrosis, raising the question of a possible overall antitumor benefit from the investigational drug despite objective progression as measured by conventional radiologic techniques. The implications of this observation are unclear. The correlation of this observed necrosis with other parameters of clinical benefit is the subject of ongoing investigation.

New approaches to assess response to therapy are being investigated. Dynamic contrast-enhanced MRI has been shown to be useful in studying the pathophysiology of tumors (Taylor et al, 1999; Yuh, 1999) and possibly response (Morgan et al, 2003). In view of the antiangiogenic activity of drugs such as sorafenib, this technology could be helpful in assessing parameters of interest, such as microvascular density, vascular permeability, and the extravascular extracellular space (Knopp et al, 1999). Dynamic contrast-enhanced MRI also is being investigated as an early indicator of response or failure of an agent. Several studies have shown that successful therapies result in early changes (within 48 hours) in dynamic contrast-enhancement MRI parameters, which may prove to be more accurate as an early indication of response (Barentsz et al, 1998; Brasch et al, 1997; Pham et al, 1998). Studies evaluating novel therapeutics in HCC would be most valuable if they incorporated correlative radiologic studies such as the ones described herein.

NEOADJUVANT CHEMOTHERAPY

In some instances, surgical resection of a localized large primary HCC tumor might be feasible if disease regression is achieved. Neoadjuvant therapy as a concept may render some unresectable tumors surgically approachable and may contribute to better outcome by possibly eradicating microscopic local and systemic disease. Different modalities have been studied in the context of neoadjuvant therapy for HCC, but none so far has been shown to add any survival benefit over surgery alone.

Transarterial chemoembolization (TACE) (see Ch. 74) has been evaluated in multiple randomized studies. A randomized trial of one to five TACE applications before surgery (24 patients) versus surgery alone (28 patients) did not offer a benefit as neoadjuvant therapy (Wu et al, 1995). TACE had no effect on 33% of the patients who had the intervention; these patients remained with stable disease or had progression. No difference was found between the two groups in operative morbidity or mortality rates and pathologic staging. The disease-free survival rate in the two groups was similar, but the incidence of extrahepatic cancer recurrence was higher in the neoadjuvant group (57% versus 23%; $P = .03$), and 5-year survival also was significantly worse in the TACE group (30% versus 60%; $P = .01$).

The experience with transarterial embolization (without chemotherapy) has not been any different. One study randomized 97 patients to transarterial embolization plus surgery versus surgery alone. Despite an increased rate of necrosis in the transarterial embolization group, disease-free survival rate did not differ between the two groups (39% versus 31.1%) (Yamasaki et al, 1996).

Experience with immunoembolization (Lygidakis & Tsiliakos, 1996), radiation (Tang et al, 1995), chemoradiation (Sitzmann & Abrams, 1993), and transarterial yttrium 90 microspheres (Lau et al, 1998) is limited. None of these techniques so far have been shown to confer a survival advantage, however, when administered in the neoadjuvant setting.

Chemotherapy-based clinical trials in the neoadjuvant setting have lagged in view of the discouraging response rates seen in the advanced disease setting. This situation has changed with the advent of the more intense chemoimmunotherapy PIAF combination (Patt et al, 1998). As discussed earlier, this study showed a 26% partial response rate in patients with HCC. Of 13 patients who achieved a partial response, 9 (18%) underwent surgical resection, and 4 had a pathologic complete response (i.e., no viable tumor at surgery). The results of a randomized phase III trial (Yeo et al, 2004) of doxorubicin versus PIAF did not show a survival benefit for the combination, although the trial was not designed to answer a neoadjuvant question. This combination carries substantial treatment-related morbidity and mortality. Most of these excellent performance status patients had grade 3 or higher hematologic toxicity, and two deaths occurred secondary to neutropenic sepsis. The role of PIAF may be worthy of investigation specifically in a neoadjuvant trial, but the routine use of this combination in this setting should be regarded as investigational at this time.

With the lack of any systemic chemotherapy conferring either a significant disease-free or overall survival advantage, HCC still lacks a standard of care neoadjuvant approach. If newer combinations can show more substantial response rates, clinical trials of novel therapeutics most likely will proceed next to evaluation in that setting.

ADJUVANT THERAPY

Regardless of the surgical techniques that have improved in the last decade, numerous patients with resected HCC have recurrence of their disease (Ziparo et al, 2002). In two large series,

the recurrence rate after surgical resection was about 80% over a cumulative 5-year experience (Chen et al, 1994), with almost half of the resected patients experiencing recurrence in the liver (Poon et al, 1999). The experience with liver transplantation has been better, with lower recurrence rates; however, this is a nonrandomized comparison, and transplant patients are selected more carefully and in general have a lower extent of disease (Mazzaferro et al, 1996). Although liver transplantation eliminates the cirrhotic fertile ground for recurrence (Nissen et al, 2004), it cannot answer the need of every patient with HCC because of the limited supply of organs, and because of its limited efficacy in other than small tumors. The question of adjuvant therapy to reduce the risk of recurrence after surgical resection remains an important and pressing one.

With the lack of a standard active systemic chemotherapy for advanced disease, chemotherapy has never been considered seriously in the adjuvant setting. One small randomized study investigated oral carmofur (1-hexylcarbamoyl-5-fluorouracil) versus no therapy (Yamamoto et al, 1996). The study randomized and stratified 67 patients based on Liver Cancer Study Group of Japan (1994) staging. The regimen was poorly tolerated and offered no survival advantage for stage I or II disease. Disease-free survival for stage I patients showed a tangible advantage of 60% versus 30% at 3 years and 50% versus 20% at 5 years ($P = .04$). Disease-free survival is not the meaningful end point in an adjuvant trial, however, and this trial was suspended prematurely owing to 56% of the treated patients having unacceptable side effects.

Hepatic arterial chemotherapy (see Ch. 79), with or without systemic chemotherapy, also has been used in the adjuvant setting in HCC. A randomized study combining hepatic arterial epirubicin and systemic epirubicin and carmofur versus no further therapy (Ono et al, 1997) showed no survival or disease-free survival benefit. Side effects led to the discontinuation of therapy in 21% of randomized patients. In addition, a randomized trial of hepatic artery epirubicin versus the same therapy plus oral tegafur showed no difference in survival or rate of recurrence between the two groups (Kohno et al, 1996). There was no description of any difference in side effects between the two arms of this study.

Another attempt at improving the efficacy of adjuvant therapy was through the use of chemoembolization with or without systemic chemotherapy. An improvement in disease-free survival was reported in a randomized study of a bolus hepatic arterial infusion of lipiodol containing doxorubicin and mitomycin C versus no adjuvant therapy after surgical resection (32% versus 12% at 3 years; $P = .02$) (Izumi et al, 1994). No survival advantage was reported, however. Another trial randomized patients to hepatic artery emulsion of iodized oil and cisplatin and intravenous epirubicin (Lai et al, 1998). This trial showed a worse disease-free survival in the treatment group at 3 years (18% versus 48%; $P = .04$). A third study of transarterial chemoembolization versus no further therapy after surgical resection showed a survival advantage in patients defined at risk for residual tumor and recurrence (Ren et al, 2004). These risk factors included tumor diameter greater than 5 cm, multiple nodules, and vascular invasion. Five-year survival was 44.36% in the adjuvant TACE group versus 37.40% in the control group ($P = .0216$).

In an attempt to improve the outcome of adjuvant therapy, Lau and colleagues (1999) randomized patients to transarterial iodine-133–lipiodol versus no adjuvant therapy after surgical resection. Lipiodol contains 38% iodine by weight. The Lau group converted the inert iodine through an atom-to-atom exchange into radioactive therapy. The results were encouraging, showing not only an improvement in disease-free-survival in favor of the adjuvant therapy arm of 74% versus 36% (P=.037), but also a statistically significant improvement in 3-year overall survival of 85% in the treatment group versus 46% in the control group (P=.039). This remains the only positive adjuvant therapy study with a survival benefit in HCC. It is a small exploratory trial, however, that requires confirmation in a larger setting. Currently, iodine-133–lipiodol is not available in the United States.

Immune modulators also have been tested in the adjuvant setting. These studies included an attempt at infusing autologous lymphocytes that were cultured with interleukin-2 and antibodies to CD-3 versus no therapy (Takayama et al, 2000), hepatic arterial infusion of doxorubicin and interleukin-2 plus an infusion of lymphokine-activated killer cells versus hepatic arterial doxorubicin (Kawata et al, 1995), oral acyclic retinoids versus placebo (Muto et al, 1996), and interferon alfa versus no therapy (Kubo et al, 2001). None of these studies reported a survival advantage, with the exception of the retinoid study, which showed a survival advantage on further follow-up 2 years after the study was originally reported (Muto et al, 1999). Six-year survival was 74% in the acyclic retinoid group versus 46% in the placebo group (P=.04).

Active immunization also has been evaluated in the adjuvant setting for HCC. An HCC vaccine consisting of autologous formalin-fixed tumor tissue fragments, biodegradable microparticles containing human granulocyte-macrophage colony-stimulating factor and human interleukin-2, and tuberculin was tested in a small randomized trial (Kuang et al, 2004). Nineteen patients received three intradermal vaccinations at 2-week intervals beginning 4 to 6 weeks after hepatic resection, whereas 22 patients received no further therapy after surgical resection. In a median follow-up of 15 months, the risk of recurrence in the vaccinated patients was reduced by 81% (P=.003). Vaccination significantly prolonged overall survival by 89% (P=.01). The vaccine was most effective in preventing recurrence in patients with small tumors. Twelve vaccinated patients showed a positive delayed-type hypersensitivity response, and 92% of those patients were recurrence-free at the end of the trial. Adverse effects were limited to grade 1 or 2 skin toxicities, such as erythema, dry desquamation, and pruritus. This is a very small trial that is intriguing, but larger confirmatory data are required before we can assess the merits of this approach fully.

A more aggressive approach was attempted in a small pilot study comprising five patients who, after receiving an orthotopic liver transplant for HCC, received a nonmyeloablative preparative regimen of fludarabine combined with total body irradiation or cyclophosphamide followed by allogeneic peripheral stem cell transplant, which was performed 16 to 135 days after orthotopic liver transplantation with human leukocyte antigen–matched donors (Soderdahl et al, 2003). The aim of the study was to see if a stable mixed donor chimerism could be sustained; this was observed in one of two patients with HCC. Chimerism analysis 36 days after peripheral stem cell transplant showed 100% donor T cells and 90% donor myeloid cells in peripheral blood. This patient was reportedly doing well, albeit with only 10 months follow-up after orthotopic liver transplantation. Investigators have used almost every therapeutic modality to attempt to reduce the risk of recurrence of HCC after surgical resection or transplantation. Although there have been some rare positive outcomes reported, most of those were part of very

small series or lacked the statistical power to show true evidence of a survival advantage.

For immunization strategies, it is still unclear if the necessary goal is to eradicate the underlying etiologic virus that was the culprit for the development of HCC or to kill any remaining tumor cells using cytotoxic therapies. Both explanations may be at work, as illustrated by Kawata and associates (Kawata et al, 1995) and Soderdahl and coworkers (Soderdahl et al, 2003). These concepts warrant further elucidation and assessment in larger randomized trials. Until these questions and many others, such as the molecular predictors of recurrence, are answered or identified, there is no standard adjuvant therapy for resected HCC, and adjuvant treatment outside of a clinical trial cannot be supported by available data at this time.

CONCLUSION

The incidence of HCC is increasing, especially in developed countries, mainly as a result of an increased incidence of hepatitis C. Trying to treat HCC means that the underlying cirrhosis and the cancer itself need to be addressed. A good and thorough understanding of the cirrhosis is imperative as part of understanding the status of the disease and to help identify the appropriate therapies that a physician might recommend. Helpful scores include the Child-Pugh, CLIP, and CUPI scores.

In the case of advanced HCC, systemic chemotherapies have yielded low response rates and no overall survival benefit, and no particular agent or regimen can be considered an appropriate standard of care. The best recommendation in appropriate patients still may be to join a clinical trial where feasible. Finding a better therapy for advanced HCC not only means developing better therapeutics, but also having a better way of assessing the disease. The infiltrative nature of HCC, the poor margination, and hypervascularity limit the use and benefit of standard radiologic techniques such as CT and MRI. Newer modalities that evaluate the dynamic aspects of the cancer are in development and parallel the investigation of novel biologics in the treatment of HCC. So far, neoadjuvant and adjuvant therapies have failed to be proven effective in HCC, and their routine use cannot be recommended. HCC remains one of the most prevalent cancers worldwide and one of the most challenging to treat. Only with a better understanding of the biology of the tumor, the advent of new therapeutic and diagnostic concepts, and increased research efforts, can we realistically expect that significant progress in treating this disease will be made.

REFERENCES

Abou-Alfa GK, Morse M, 2004: Novel therapies targeted at signal transduction in liver tumors. In Clavien PA (ed): Malignant Liver Tumors: Current and Emerging Therapies, 2nd ed. Sudbury, Mass, Jones & Bartlett, p 307.

Abou-Alfa GK, et al, 2004: Phase II study of BAY 43-9006, a novel Raf kinase and VEGFR inhibitor, in patients with advanced hepatocellular carcinoma (HCC). Fourth International Meeting on Hepatocellular Carcinoma: Eastern and Western Experiences, Hong Kong. Asian J Surg 28:S80.

Baker LH, et al, 1977: Adriamycin and 5-fluorouracil in the treatment of advanced hepatoma: a Southwest Oncology Group study. Cancer Treat Reports 61:1595-1597.

Barbare JC, et al, 1984: Carcinome hépatocellulaire sur cirrhose: traitement par la Doxorubicine. Essai phase II. Bull Cancer 71:442-445.

Barentsz JO, et al, 1998: Evaluation of chemotherapy in advanced urinary bladder cancer with fast dynamic contrast-enhanced MR imaging. Radiology 207: 791-797.

Bobbio-Pallavicini E, et al, 1997: Epirubicin and etoposide combination chemotherapy to treat hepatocellular carcinoma patients: a phase II study. Eur J Cancer 33:1784-1788.

Brasch R, et al, 1997: Assessing tumor angiogenesis using macromolecular MR imaging contrast media. J Magn Reson Imaging 7:68-74.

Carlson BA, et al, 1996: Flavopiridol induces G1 arrest with inhibition of cyclin-dependent kinase (CDK) 2 and CDK4 in human breast carcinoma cells. Cancer Res 56:2973-2978.

Chao Y, et al, 1998: Phase II and pharmacokinetic study of paclitaxel therapy for unresectable hepatocellular carcinoma patients. Br J Cancer 78:34-39.

Chen MF, et al, 1994: Postoperative recurrence of hepatocellular carcinoma: two hundred five consecutive patients who underwent hepatic resection in 15 years. Arch Surg 129:738-742.

Chenivesse X, et al, 1993: MDR1 (multidrug resistance) gene expression in human primary liver cancer and cirrhosis. J Hepatol 18:168-172.

Child CG, 1964: The Liver and Portal Hypertension. Philadelphia, Saunders.

Chlebowski RT, et al, 1984: Doxorubicin (75 mg/m²) for hepatocellular carcinoma: clinical and pharmacokinetic results. Cancer Treat Reports 68:487-491.

Choi TK, et al, 1984: Chemotherapy for advanced hepatocellular carcinoma: Adriamycin versus quadruple chemotherapy. Cancer 53:401-405.

CLIP investigators, 1998: A new prognostic system for hepatocellular carcinoma: a retrospective study of 435 patients. The Cancer of the Liver Italian Program (CLIP) investigators. Hepatology 28:751-755.

CLIP investigators, 2000: Prospective validation of the CLIP score: a new prognostic system for patients with cirrhosis and hepatocellular carcinoma. The Cancer of the Liver Italian Program (CLIP) investigators. Hepatology 31:840-845.

Damrongsak C, et al, 1973: Vinblastine in the treatment of carcinoma of liver. J Med Assoc Thailand 56:370-372.

DeVita VT Jr, Abou-Alfa GK, 2000: Therapeutic implications of the new biology. Cancer J 6(suppl 2):S113.

Ebara M, et al, 1998: Natural course of small hepatocellular carcinoma with underlying cirrhosis: a study of 30 patients. Hepatogastroenterology 45(suppl 3):1214-1220.

El-Serag HB, Mason AC, 1999: Rising incidence of hepatocellular carcinoma in the United States. N Engl J Med 340:745-750.

Falkson G, et al, 1978: Chemotherapy studies in primary liver cancer: a prospective randomized clinical trial. Cancer 42:2149-2156.

Falkson G, et al, 1984: Primary liver cancer: an Eastern Cooperative Oncology Group Trial. Cancer 54:970-977.

Falkson G, et al, 1987: A random phase II study of mitoxantrone and cisplatin in patients with hepatocellular carcinoma: an ECOG study. Cancer 60:2141-2145.

Farber E, Rubin H, 1991: Cellular adaptation in the origin and development of cancer. Cancer Res 51:2751-2761.

Gastrointestinal Tumor Study Group, 1990: A prospective trial of recombinant human interferon alpha 2B in previously untreated patients with hepatocellular carcinoma. The Gastrointestinal Tumor Study Group. Cancer 66:135-139.

Giambartolomei S, et al, 2001: Sustained activation of the Raf/MEK/Erk pathway in response to EGF in stable cell lines expressing the hepatitis C virus (HCV) core protein. Oncogene 20:2606-2610.

Hamazaki K, et al, 1997: Epidermal growth factor receptor in human hepatocellular carcinoma. Cancer Detect Prev 21:355-360.

Harada K, et al, 1999: Transforming growth factor-alpha and epidermal growth factor receptor in chronic liver disease and hepatocellular carcinoma. Liver 19:318-325.

Hsu C, et al, 2002: HER-2/neu overexpression is rare in hepatocellular carcinoma and not predictive of anti-HER-2/neu regulation of cell growth and chemosensitivity. Cancer 94:415-420.

Hurwitz H, et al, 2004: Bevacizumab plus irinotecan, fluorouracil, and leucovorin for metastatic colorectal cancer. N Engl J Med 350:2335-2342.

Huynh H, et al, 2003: Over-expression of the mitogen-activated protein kinase (MAPK) kinase (MEK)-MAPK in hepatocellular carcinoma: its role in tumor progression and apoptosis. BMC Gastroenterol 3:19.

Ihde DC, et al, 1977: Adriamycin therapy in American patients with hepatocellular carcinoma. Cancer Treat Reports 61:1385-1387.

Izumi R, et al, 1994: Postoperative adjuvant hepatic arterial infusion of Lipiodol containing anticancer drugs in patients with hepatocellular carcinoma. Hepatology 20:295-301.

Ji SK, et al, 1996: Combined cis-platinum and alpha interferon therapy of advanced hepatocellular carcinoma. Korean J Intern Med 11:58-68.

Jiang W, et al, 1997: Dihydropyrimidine dehydrogenase activity in hepatocellular carcinoma: implication in 5-fluorouracil-based chemotherapy. Clin Cancer Res 3:395-399.

Johnson PJ, et al, 1978: Induction of remission in hepatocellular carcinoma with doxorubicin. Lancet 1:1006-1009.

Kardinal CG, et al, 1993: Combined doxorubicin and alpha-interferon therapy of advanced hepatocellular carcinoma. Cancer 71:2187-2190.

Kato K, et al, 1992: Isoprenoid addition to Ras protein is the critical modification for its membrane association and transforming activity. Proc Natl Acad Sci U S A 89:6403-6407.

Kawata A, et al, 1995: Adjuvant chemoimmunotherapy for hepatocellular carcinoma patients: Adriamycin, interleukin-2, and lymphokine-activated killer cells versus Adriamycin alone. Am J Clin Oncol 18:257-262.

Kawata S, et al, 1994: Modulation of the mevalonate pathway and cell growth by pravastatin and d-limonene in a human hepatoma cell line (Hep G2). Br J Cancer 69:1015-1020.

Kawata S, et al, 2001: Effect of pravastatin on survival in patients with advanced hepatocellular carcinoma: a randomized controlled trial. Br J Cancer 84:886-891.

Kiss A, et al, 1997: Analysis of transforming growth factor (TGF)-alpha/epidermal growth factor receptor, hepatocyte growth factor/c-met, TGF-beta receptor type II, and p53 expression in human hepatocellular carcinomas. Clin Cancer Res 3:1059-1066.

Knopp MV, et al, 1999: Pathophysiologic basis of contrast enhancement in breast tumors. J Magn Reson Imaging 10:260-266.

Kohno H, et al, 1996: Postoperative adjuvant chemotherapy after radical hepatic resection for hepatocellular carcinoma (HCC). Hepatogastroenterology 43:1405-1409.

Kuang M, et al, 2004: Phase II randomized trial of autologous formalin-fixed tumor vaccine for postsurgical recurrence of hepatocellular carcinoma. Clin Cancer Res 10:1574-1579.

Kubicka S, et al, 2001: Phase II study of systemic gemcitabine chemotherapy for advanced unresectable hepatobiliary carcinomas. Hepatogastroenterology 48:783-789.

Kubo S, et al, 2001: Effects of long-term postoperative interferon-alpha therapy on intrahepatic recurrence after resection of hepatitis C virus-related hepatocellular carcinoma: a randomized, controlled trial. Ann Intern Med 134:963-967.

Lai EC, et al, 1998: Postoperative adjuvant chemotherapy after curative resection of hepatocellular carcinoma: a randomized controlled trial. Arch Surg 133:183-188.

Lau WY, et al, 1998: Selective internal radiation therapy for nonresectable hepatocellular carcinoma with intraarterial infusion of 90 yttrium microspheres. Int J Radiat Oncol Biol Phys 40:583-592.

Lau WY, et al, 1999: Adjuvant intra-arterial iodine-131-labelled lipiodol for resectable hepatocellular carcinoma: a prospective randomised trial. Lancet 353:797-801.

Leung TW, et al, 1999: Complete pathological remission is possible with systemic combination chemotherapy for inoperable hepatocellular carcinoma. Clin Cancer Res 5:1676-1681.

Leung TW, et al, 2002a: Construction of the Chinese University Prognostic Index for hepatocellular carcinoma and comparison with the TNM staging system, the Okuda staging system, and the Cancer of the Liver Italian Program staging system: a study based on 926 patients. Cancer 94:1760-1769.

Leung TW, et al, 2002b: A phase II study of T138067-sodium in patients (pts) with unresectable hepatocellular carcinoma (HCC). Proc Am Soc Clin Oncol 21:S572.

Liver Cancer Study Group of Japan, 1994: Predictive factors for long term prognosis after partial hepatectomy for patients with hepatocellular carcinoma in Japan. The Liver Cancer Study Group of Japan. Cancer 74:2772-2780.

Llovet JM, et al, 1999: Prognosis of hepatocellular carcinoma: the BCLC staging classification. Semin Liver Dis 19:329-338.

Losiewicz MD, et al, 1994: Potent inhibition of CDC2 kinase activity by the flavonoid L86-8275. Biochem Biophys Res Commun 201:589-595.

Lozano R, et al, 2000: Oral capecitabine (Xeloda) for the treatment of hepatobiliary cancers (hepatocellular carcinoma, cholangiocarcinoma, and gallbladder cancer). Proc Am Soc Clin Oncol 19:S1025.

Lygidakis NJ, Tsiliakos S, 1996: Multidisciplinary management of hepatocellular carcinoma. Hepatogastroenterology 43:1611-1619.

Mazume H, et al, 1999: Effect of simvastatin, a 3-hydroxy-3-methylglutaryl coenzyme A reductase inhibitor, on alpha-fetoprotein gene expression through interaction with the ras-mediated pathway. J Hepatol 30:904-910.

Mazzaferro V, et al, 1996: Liver transplantation for the treatment of small hepatocellular carcinomas in patients with cirrhosis. N Engl J Med 334:693-699.

McGlynn KA, et al, 2001: International trends and patterns of primary liver cancer. Int J Cancer 94:290-296.

Melia WM, et al, 1983: Induction of remission in hepatocellular carcinoma: a comparison of VP 16 with adriamycin. Cancer 51:206-210.

Mitchell EP, et al, 2005: High-dose bevacizumab in combination with FOLFOX4 improves survival in patients with previously treated advanced colorectal cancer: results from the Eastern Cooperative Oncology Group (ECOG) study E3200. American Society of Clinical Oncology Gastrointestinal Cancers Symposium, May 14-17, 2005, Orlando, Florida, Programs/Proceedings abstract 169a, p 168.

Mok TS, et al, 1999: A multi-centre randomized phase II study of nolatrexed versus doxorubicin in treatment of Chinese patients with advanced hepatocellular carcinoma. Cancer Chemother Pharmacol 44:307-311.

Morgan B, et al, 2003: Dynamic contrast-enhanced magnetic resonance imaging as a biomarker for the pharmacological response of PTK787/ZK 222584, an inhibitor of the vascular endothelial growth factor receptor tyrosine kinases, in patients with advanced colorectal cancer and liver metastases: results from two phase I studies. J Clin Oncol 21:3955-3964.

Muto Y, et al, 1996: Prevention of second primary tumors by an acyclic retinoid, polyprenoic acid, in patients with hepatocellular carcinoma. Hepatoma Prevention Study Group. N Engl J Med 334:1561-1567.

Muto Y, et al, 1999: Prevention of second primary tumors by an acyclic retinoid in patients with hepatocellular carcinoma. N Engl J Med 340:1046-1047.

Nerenstone SR, et al, 1988: Clinical trials in primary hepatocellular carcinoma: current status and future directions. Cancer Treat Rev 15:1-31.

Nissen NN, et al, 2004: Emerging role of transplantation for primary liver cancers. Cancer J 10:88-96.

Okuda K, et al, 1985: Natural history of hepatocellular carcinoma and prognosis in relation to treatment: study of 850 patients. Cancer 56:918-928.

Olweny CL, et al, 1975: Treatment of hepatocellular carcinoma with adriamycin: preliminary communication. Cancer 36:1250-1257.

Olweny CL, et al, 1980: Further experience in treating patients with hepatocellular carcinoma in Uganda. Cancer 46:2717-2722.

Ono T, et al, 1997: Adjuvant chemotherapy with epirubicin and carmofur after radical resection of hepatocellular carcinoma: a prospective randomized study. Semin Oncol 24:S6-18-S6-25.

O'Reilly EM, et al, 2001: A phase II study of irinotecan in patients with advanced hepatocellular carcinoma. Cancer 91:101-105.

Patt YZ, et al, 1993: Low serum alpha-fetoprotein level in patients with hepatocellular carcinoma as a predictor of response to 5-FU and interferon-alpha-2b. Cancer 72:2574-2582.

Patt YZ, et al, 1998: Systemic therapy with platinol, interferon α 2b, doxorubicin and 5-fluorouracil (PIAF) for treatment of non-resectable hepatocellular carcinoma. Proc Am Soc Clin Oncol 17:S1159.

Patt YZ, et al, 2005: Thalidomide in the treatment of patients with hepatocellular carcinoma. Cancer 103:749-755.

Pham CD, et al, 1998: Magnetic resonance imaging detects suppression of tumor vascular permeability after administration of antibody to vascular endothelial growth factor. Cancer Invest 16:225-230.

Philip PA, et al, 2004: Phase II trial of erlotinib (OSI-774) in patients with hepatocellular or biliary cancer. 2004 ASCO Annual Meeting Proceedings (Post-Meeting Edition). J Clin Oncol 22:4025.

Poon RT, et al, 1999: Intrahepatic recurrence after curative resection of hepatocellular carcinoma: long-term results of treatment and prognostic factors. Ann Surg 229:216-222.

Porta C, et al, 1995: 5-Fluorouracil and d,l-leucovorin calcium are active to treat unresectable hepatocellular carcinoma patients: preliminary results of a phase II study. Oncology 52:487-491.

Pugh RN, et al, 1973: Transection of the oesophagus for bleeding oesophageal varices. Br J Surg 60:646-649.

Ren ZG, et al, 2004: Postoperative adjuvant arterial chemoembolization improves survival of hepatocellular carcinoma patients with risk factors for residual tumor: a retrospective control study. World J Gastroenterol 10:2791-2794.

Schwartz JD, 2005: Bevacizumab in hepatocellular carcinoma (HCC) for patients without metastasis and without invasion of the portal vein. Proc Am Soc Oncol 23:338s (abstract 4122).

Sciarrino E, et al, 1985: Adriamycin treatment for hepatocellular carcinoma: experience with 109 patients. Cancer 56:2751-2755.

Shah MA, et al, 2003: Mature results of a phase I study of irinotecan and flavopiridol: a clinically and biologically active regimen. Proc Am Soc Clin Oncol 22:S1051.

Shan B, et al, 1999: Selective, covalent modification of beta-tubulin residue Cys-239 by T138067, an antitumor agent with in vivo efficacy against multidrug-resistant tumors. Proc Natl Acad Sci U S A 96:5686-5691.

Sitzmann JV, Abrams R, 1993: Improved survival for hepatocellular cancer with combination surgery and multimodality treatment. Ann Surg 217:149-154.

Soderdahl G, et al, 2003: Liver transplantation followed by adjuvant nonmyeloablative hemopoietic stem cell transplantation for advanced primary liver cancer in humans. Transplantation 75:1061-1066.

Soini Y, et al, 1996: Expression of P-glycoprotein in hepatocellular carcinoma: a potential marker of prognosis. J Clin Pathol 49:470-473.

Solt DB, et al, 1977: Rapid emergence of carcinogen-induced hyperplastic lesions in a new model for the sequential analysis of liver carcinogenesis. Am J Pathol 88:595-618.

Stuart K, et al, 1996: 5-Fluorouracil and alpha-interferon in hepatocellular carcinoma. Am J Clin Oncol 19:136-139.

Stuart K, et al, 1999: A Phase II trial of nolatrexed dihydrochloride in patients with advanced hepatocellular carcinoma. Cancer 86:410-414.

Tada M, et al, 1990: Analysis of ras gene mutations in human hepatic malignant tumors by polymerase chain reaction and direct sequencing. Cancer Res 50:1121-1124.

Takayama T, et al, 2000: Adoptive immunotherapy to lower postsurgical recurrence rates of hepatocellular carcinoma: a randomised trial. Lancet 356:802-807.

Tang ZY, et al, 1995: Cytoreduction and sequential resection for surgically verified unresectable hepatocellular carcinoma: evaluation with analysis of 72 patients. World J Surg 19:784-789.

Taylor JS, et al, 1999: MR imaging of tumor microcirculation: promise for the new millennium. J Magn Reson Imaging 10:903-907.

Vogel CL, et al, 1977: A phase II study of adriamycin (NSC 123127) in patients with hepatocellular carcinoma from Zambia and the United States. Cancer 39:1923-1929.

Webber SE, et al, 1993: Design of thymidylate synthase inhibitors using protein crystal structures: the synthesis and biological evaluation of a novel class of 5-substituted quinazolinones. J Med Chem 36:733-746.

Weihrauch M, et al, 2001: High prevalence of K-ras-2 mutations in hepatocellular carcinomas in workers exposed to vinyl chloride. Int Arch Occup Environ Health 74:405-410.

Wilhelm SM, et al, 2004: BAY 43-9006 exhibits broad spectrum oral antitumor activity and targets the RAF/MEK/ERK pathway and receptor tyrosine kinases involved in tumor progression and angiogenesis. Cancer Res 64:7099-7109.

Williams R, Melia WM, 1980: Liver tumours and their management. Clin Radiol 31:1-11.

Wu CC, et al, 1995: Preoperative transcatheter arterial chemoembolization for resectable large hepatocellular carcinoma: a reappraisal. Br J Surg 82:122-126.

Yamamoto M, et al, 1996: Adjuvant oral chemotherapy to prevent recurrence after curative resection for hepatocellular carcinoma. Br J Surg 83:336-340.

Yamasaki S, et al, 1996: A prospective randomized trial of the preventive effect of pre-operative transcatheter arterial embolization against recurrence of hepatocellular carcinoma. Jpn J Cancer Res 87:206-211.

Yeo W, et al, 2004: A phase III study of doxorubicin (A) versus cisplatin (P)/interferonα-2b (I)/doxorubicin (A)/fluorouracil (F) combination chemotherapy (PIAF) for inoperable hepatocellular carcinoma (HCC). 2004 ASCO Annual Meeting Proceedings (Post-Meeting Edition). J Clin Oncol 22:4026.

Yuh WT, 1999: An exciting and challenging role for the advanced contrast MR imaging. J Magn Reson Imaging 10:221-222.

Ziparo V, et al, 2002: Indications and results of resection for hepatocellular carcinoma. Eur J Surg Oncol 28:723-728.

77b SYSTEMIC THERAPY FOR METASTATIC COLORECTAL CANCER

G. K. ABOU-ALFA AND L. B. SALTZ

SYSTEMIC THERAPY BACKGROUND

This subchapter discusses modern approaches to systemic therapy in the management of metastatic colorectal cancer (see Ch. 73). For a discussion of adjuvant and neoadjuvant therapy, see Ch. 73a. For a discussion of intra-arterial chemotherapy, see Ch. 79. The past decade has been marked by significant changes in the options available to patients with colorectal cancer. At the beginning of 1996, one drug, 5-fluorouracil (5-FU), was approved for the treatment of this disease. In 2006, there are five new drugs on the market for the management of colorectal cancer: irinotecan, oxaliplatin, capecitabine, bevacizumab, and cetuximab. Several other potentially active agents are in the late phases of clinical development. With the availability of a broader range of options, the efficacy of treatment regimens has increased substantially. The complexity of the treatment decisions the medical oncologist must make when charting a course for a patient also has increased.

CHEMOTHERAPY—THE BACKBONE OF SYSTEMIC THERAPY

5-FU and leucovorin have remained for many years the key therapeutic regimen for metastatic colorectal cancer, with an overall survival rate close to 1 year (Anonymous, 1998). More recent improvements in response rate and survival have been noted owing to several factors, including the introduction of two new cytotoxic drugs—irinotecan and oxaliplatin—and a better understanding of 5-FU delivery. A European study showed that the biweekly infusional schedule of 5-FU and leucovorin had a better response rate, time to tumor progression, and toxicity profile than bolus 5-FU, with a strong trend toward a 5-week survival advantage that just missed statistical significance (Table 77b.1)

(de Gramont et al, 1997). Irinotecan was evaluated in two key clinical trials; both trials studied this agent when added to 5-FU, but differed in the way 5-FU was delivered. A bolus approach of irinotecan, 5-FU, and leucovorin (IFL) (Saltz et al, 2000) showed a modest, but statistically significant improvement in survival by 2.2 months compared with classic bolus 5-FU and leucovorin (14.8 months versus 12.6 months; P=.04). Adding irinotecan to a continuous infusion of 5-FU given over about 2 days (known as FOLFIRI) (Douillard et al, 2000) significantly improved survival by 3.1 months compared with a continuous infusion of 5-FU (17.4 months versus 14.1 months; P=.031). At the same time, another new drug, oxaliplatin, entered the late phases of clinical development in colorectal cancer. The road to its approval in the United States was tortuous, however, because the initial data did not show a survival advantage in the first-line setting (de Gramont et al, 2000). Things changed at the completion of a national effort, intergroup trial N9741 (Goldberg et al, 2004), which showed a survival outcome of 19.5 months for oxaliplatin combined with continuous infusion of 5-FU and leucovorin (known as FOLFOX) compared with IFL, which achieved a survival of 15 months (P=.0001). Oxaliplatin was evaluated further in a second-line setting, which did not address survival outcomes (Rothenberg et al, 2003). Two trials compared first-line oxaliplatin with first-line irinotecan in a setting of identical infusional 5-FU schedules and with the same access to active second-line agents (Table 77b.2) (Colucci et al, 2005; Tournigand et al, 2004). In these trials, the first-line efficacy of oxaliplatin versus irinotecan, in terms of response rate, progression-free survival, and overall survival, were essentially identical. It is reasonable practice to use either oxaliplatin or irinotecan in conjunction with infusional 5-FU/leucovorin as first-line therapy.

Things became a bit harder to interpret at this point, as a popular perception developed among oncologists in the United States that oxaliplatin is a superior first-line drug to irinotecan. Although this perception is not well supported by data, several reasons seems to have led to its development. First, oxaliplatin was unavailable for many years in the United States, long after

Table 77b.1 Biweekly Infusional Versus Bolus Fluorouracil/Leucovorin in Metastatic Colorectal Cancer

	Bolus 5-FU/ Leucovorin (n = 216)	Biweekly Infusional 5-FU/Leucovorin (n = 217)	P Value
Response rate	14%	33%	.0004
Progression-free survival	22 wk	28 wk	.0012
Overall survival	57 wk	62 wk	.067
Grade 3-4 toxicity	24%	11%	.0004

From de Gramont A, et al, 1997: Randomized trial comparing monthly low-dose leucovorin and fluorouracil bolus with bimonthly high-dose leucovorin and fluorouracil bolus plus continuous infusion for advanced colorectal cancer: a French intergroup study. J Clin Oncol 15:808-815.

Table 77b.2 First-line FOLFIRI Versus FOLFOX in Metastatic Colorectal Cancer

	FOLFIRI (n = 109)	FOLFOX-6 (n = 111)	P Value
Response rate	56%	54%	.68
Time to tumor progression	8.5 mo	8.1 mo	.26
Overall survival	21.5 mo	20.6 mo	.99

From Tournigand C, et al, 2004: FOLFIRI followed by FOLFOX6 or the reverse sequence in advanced colorectal cancer: a randomized GERCOR study. J Clin Oncol 22:229-237.

its efficacy had been convincingly shown in the literature. Many patients who had the means were traveling to Europe or Central America to obtain the drug. This situation created an image of oxaliplatin as the hard-to-find active drug and contributed to an aura of its being a superior agent. Second, the results of the intergroup trial N9741, in which IFL was compared directly with FOLFOX-4, have been largely misunderstood to be an indication that oxaliplatin is a superior drug to irinotecan in first-line therapy. Evidently, this is an incorrect interpretation of that trial, that 5-FU was delivered in two different ways in the trial—as a proven more active continuous infusion part of the superior FOLFOX arm versus the less active bolus form as part of the IFL comparator arm. Also, the survival data from the study have been widely misunderstood. The group that received first-line FOLFOX achieved an impressive 4.7-month median survival advantage over the group that received IFL. In addition to the potential for infusional 5-FU to account for some of that advantage, however, the availability of second-line therapy was markedly imbalanced between the arms, with all patients in the FOLFOX arm having full access to irinotecan for second-line treatment, whereas the patients in the IFL arm had limited access to oxaliplatin because it was not commercially available in the United States during the time of the study.

The major differing aspect is the very different side effect profiles, with greater gastrointestinal toxicity and alopecia with irinotecan and greater peripheral neuropathy with oxaliplatin. The neuropathy may help favor use of FOLFIRI as first-line therapy in patients for whom the neuropathy of oxaliplatin would be a potential problem. Neuropathy is not just a problem for musicians, surgeons, or calligraphers, but also for anyone who uses a computer keyboard to a large degree; individuals for whom cold sensitivity would be a major problem, such as construction workers or other manual laborers who work outside in cold climates; and diabetics who present with already established neuropathy secondary to their diabetes. Cumulative use of oxaliplatin or irinotecan also has been shown to increase the risk for chemotherapy-associated steatohepatitis (Fong & Bentrem, 2006). This potential side effect is crucial to discuss among hepatobiliary surgeons and medical oncologists, in the case of an anticipated surgical resection for liver-only metastatic disease, which may require initial chemotherapy for better control and improved surgical margins.

TARGETED THERAPEUTICS IN FIRST-LINE THERAPY

Bevacizumab is a humanized monoclonal antibody that targets a key growth factor known as vascular endothelial growth factor (VEGF) (Ferrara et al, 2004). How bevacizumab actually works in metastatic colorectal cancer is the subject of some debate. That it works is a clearly established clinical fact. Bevacizumab binds to and effectively neutralizes circulating VEGF; this may have several important actions that influence tumor growth and survival. VEGF is a centrally important component of the proangiogenic pathway. New blood vessel formation necessary to support tumor progression is potentially inhibited by the decrease or absence of circulating VEGF levels. VEGF also exerts other actions, however, which may be even more crucial to its therapeutic efficacy. In contrast to mature, long-established vasculature, the newly formed blood vessels that support a growing tumor have relatively thin walls and depend on continued growth factors, including VEGF, for support and maintenance of integrity.

Table 77b.3 Results of Pivotal Phase III Trial of Bevacizumab plus IFL Versus IFL Alone in Metastatic Colorectal Cancer

	IFL + Bevacizumab (n = 403)	IFL + Placebo (n = 412)	P Value
Overall survival	20.3 mo	15.6 mo	<.0001
Progression-free survival	10.6 mo	6.2 mo	<.0001
Response rate	45%	35%	<.001

From Hurwitz H, et al, 2004: Bevacizumab plus irinotecan, fluorouracil, and leucovorin for metastatic colorectal cancer. N Engl J Med 350:2335-2342.

In the absence of sufficient VEGF levels, these immature vessels become fragile and leaky and ultimately are degraded, leading to normalization of tumor vasculature (Jain, 2001). These changes would be anticipated to deliver other, concurrently administered, chemotherapy more effectively to the tumor tissue. Additionally, bevacizumab has been shown to lower intratumoral interstitial pressure, further facilitating transfer of other anticancer agents from the bloodstream to the tumor tissue (Willett et al, 2004). To what degree each of these mechanisms is contributing to the antitumor activity of bevacizumab is unknown at this time.

The pivotal trial that showed the utility of bevacizumab in colorectal cancer was reported by Hurwitz and colleagues (2004) (Table 77b.3). In a randomized, double-blind, placebo-controlled trial of approximately 800 patients, half received IFL, which was the standard care in the United States at that time, plus a placebo, and half received the same chemotherapy plus bevacizumab at a dose of 5 mg/kg every other week. Patients receiving bevacizumab had a median survival that was almost 5 months longer than the patients who did not receive it (20.3 months versus 15.6 months; P=.00003). Other supportive end points, such as response rate and progression-free survival, were increased as well. The subjective toxicity (i.e., toxicity the patient was overtly aware of) was essentially nil, such that a placebo control was realistically possible. That is not to say that side effects were not encountered. There was a roughly 10% increased risk of serious hypertension (that responded to oral medication), a 1.5% risk of gastrointestinal perforation, and a 2.5% increased risk of arterial thrombotic events. These represent major and potentially lethal complications. In addition, there is the critical need for dialogue between surgeons and medical oncologists with regard to the timing of potential surgery for a patient receiving bevacizumab. In general, a 4- to 6-week wait after discontinuing bevacuzimab has been recommended, although there are no clear data to support this recommendation.

Other data have corroborated the efficacy of bevacizumab in metastatic colorectal cancer. The ECOG 3200 study (Reddy, 2005) randomized 829 bevacizumab-naive patients whose cancer had failed previous chemotherapy with 5-FU and irinotecan (together or individually) to receive single-agent bevacizumab, FOLFOX, or bevacizumab plus FOLFOX. The bevacizumab-alone arm was closed early because of concerns of inferior efficacy. The final data for this arm have not been reported at the time of this writing. The overall survival benefit for the bevacizumab plus FOLFOX arm over FOLFOX alone was reported (12.5 months versus 10.7 months; P<.002) (Giantonio et al, 2005). The incidence of grade 3 neurotoxicity was increased in the bevacizumab plus FOLFOX group compared with the group receiving FOLFOX alone (14.9% versus 8.4%). Although this increase simply may be a result of the greater time on therapy leading to increased oxaliplatin exposure, the possibility of bevacizumab facilitating platinum entry into neurons and so exacerbating oxaliplatin neurotoxicity cannot be excluded at this time. It would be instructive, when data are available, to see if the neuropathy incidence over time is similar between the two arms, or if the neurotoxicity occurs earlier in the bevacizumab-containing arm. This study supports the use of bevacizumab with FOLFOX as first-line therapy, and bevacizumab has become an established component of the current first-line therapies of colorectal cancer. This study stresses again the need for careful surgical planning with the increased and common use of this antiangiogenic agent.

LESS TOXIC FIRST-LINE THERAPY

The need for an effective but less toxic regimen is an important one from the surgical standpoint because it helps keep viable surgical options available for the patient. The answer to this question has been thrown into some doubt. Although most evidence would indicate that combination chemotherapy with either FOLFIRI or FOLFOX, with concurrent bevacizumab, is the most appropriate initial therapy for most medically fit, good performance status patients, more recently two observations have offered some evidence to challenge how universally applicable this assumption might be. The first is the observation that 5-FU/leucovorin plus bevacizumab had superior activity to 5-FU/leucovorin alone (Kabbinavar et al, 2003, 2004) and seemed to have similar activity to 5-FU plus irinotecan as in IFL, suggesting that the more tolerable bevacizumab might be used with 5-FU first, possibly instead of irinotecan, allowing irinotecan and oxaliplatin to remain in reserve for second-line and salvage therapies. The FOCUS trial, so far available only in preliminary abstract form, also challenges the assumption that combination cytotoxic therapy is superior to sequential therapy for all patients (Maughan et al, 2005). In this trial, 2135 patients were randomized to one of three arms: biweekly infusional 5-FU/leucovorin followed at time of progression by irinotecan alone, biweekly infusional 5-FU/leucovorin followed at progression by continuation of 5-FU/leucovorin and addition of either irinotecan or oxaliplatin (i.e., change to FOLFIRI or FOLFOX), or initial treatment with either FOLFIRI or FOLFOX. The trial showed no benefit in terms of survival for combination therapy initially versus use of first-line 5-FU/leucovorin followed by FOLFOX or FOLFIRI as second-line therapy. This is one trial, and the results are not completely consistent with some earlier evidence. It does not settle the question definitively, but it raises the possibility of incorporating sequential strategies into standard treatment paradigms for some patients. Patients with bulky symptomatic disease or patients being treated with a goal toward subsequent curative resection most likely would not be good candidates for consideration of sequential therapy.

SECOND-LINE CHEMOTHEARPY

The optimal second-line therapy is a complicated question that depends to some degree on what chemotherapy is used in first-line therapy. Based on the data presented in the first-line therapy discussion, if FOLFOX/bevacizumab was used as initial therapy, an irinotecan-based regimen should be used subsequently. Data from the United Kingdom Medical Research Council FOCUS trial addressed the issue of continuation of second-line 5-FU after failure of first-line 5-FU (i.e., using FOLFIRI as second-line therapy instead of single-agent irinotecan) and have not shown a statistically significant benefit for second-line FOLFIRI over irinotecan alone ($P=.116$) (Maughan et al, 2005). This study may make the argument for using FOLFOX as first-line therapy, to allow for the simple and less toxic use of single-agent irinotecan as second-line therapy. Alternatively, if FOLFIRI was used first, and because oxaliplatin has been shown to be ineffective as a single agent, the cumbersome use of FOLFOX cannot be avoided in the second-line setting.

At this time, there are no data to support continuing to use bevacizumab in this second-line setting after progression with a first-line bevacizumab-containing regimen. Generally, we require evidence that an intervention is useful before it is adopted as a standard practice. Some clinicians have mistakenly interpreted the recently reported ECOG 3200 study as support for continuation of bevacizumab in second-line treatment. This study, as discussed earlier (Giantonio et al, 2005), shows a modest, but statistically significant survival advantage of patients who failed irinotecan and 5-FU who received FOLFOX plus bevacizumab versus patients who received FOLFOX alone. All of the patients who entered this trial were bevacizumab-naive when they started second-line therapy. These data say nothing about the usefulness of second-line bevacizumab in patients who already have received bevacizumab as first-line therapy.

Because virtually no data on the mechanisms of bevacizumab resistance exist, we can hardly invoke a mechanistic rationale for continuation. Bevacizumab carries with it a risk of serious and even potentially fatal toxicities in the form of gastrointestinal perforation, heart attacks, and strokes. A cautious approach against being seduced by the mild subjective toxicities of bevacizumab is recommended; just because the drug does not make patients feel unwell does not mean there is not a potentially serious down side to its continuation.

THIRD-LINE THERAPY AND BEYOND

A valuable second-line systemic therapy for metastatic colorectal cancer with a survival advantage was virtually inexistent a decade ago, and, if anything, patients used to be recommended hospice care. Now we have proof for a second-line approach, and beyond. When second-line irinotecan-based chemotherapy (or FOLFOX) has failed, medical oncolgists can start tapping into cetuximab, another novel agent licensed for colorectal cancer. Cetuximab is a chimeric immunoglobulin G1 monoclonal antibody that targets the extracellular domain of the epidermal growth factor receptor (EGFR), competitively inhibiting ligand binding and EGFR activation (Thomas & Grandis, 2004). The EGFR as a transmembrane glycoprotein binds specific ligands such as epidermal growth factor to its external domain; this leads to the dimerization of the receptor with another EGFR (homodimerization) or another member of the EGFR family (heterodimerization). This dimerization stimulates phosphorylation of the intracellular tyrosine kinases of the receptor, initiating a cascade of intracellular signaling, which ultimately regulates cell proliferation, migration, adhesion, differentiation, and survival (Carpenter & Cohen, 1990; Ciardiello & Tortora, 2001; Real et al, 1986). Cetuximab, as an inhibitor of EGFR, has shown efficacy in the refractory setting as a single agent (9%) (Saltz et al, 2004) or combined with irinotecan (20.5%) (Table 77b.4) (Cunningham et al, 2004;

Table 77b.4 Response Rate to Cetuximab plus Irinotecan in Irinotecan-Refractory Colorectal Cancer

Reference	No. Patients	EGFR Status by Immunohistochemistry	Response Rate (%)
Saltz et al, 2001	120	EGFR (+)	23
Cunningham et al, 2004	218	EGFR (+)	23
Chung et al, 2005	16*	EGFR (−)	25

*Includes 2 patients treated with cetuximab alone (no concurrent irinotecan).

Saltz et al, 2001). This is in addition to a longer time to tumor progression for the combination. No survival benefit has been unequivocally shown with cetuximab, however. As a single agent or in combination with irinotecan, the most common side effect noted secondary to the use of cetuximab has been a notorious variation in degree among patients' rash, which is attributed to the abundance of epidermal growth factors (EGFR) on the skin.

At present, there are no data regarding the use of cetuximab in non–irinotecan-refractory colorectal cancer. Some authors have made the assumption that there would be benefit to adding cetuximab with initial irinotecan. A major potential concern is, however, that irinotecan is one active regimen, and irinotecan/cetuximab is another active regimen. By adding cetuximab to the initial dose of irinotecan, one may be excluding an active regimen (single-agent irinotecan) and limiting long-term treatment options.

Second-line and third-line choice may be interchangeable. Some oncologists may favor using FOLFIRI/bevacizumab first, irinotecan/cetuximab second, and FOLFOX as a third-line regimen. Although the comparison is a nonrandomized, cross study one, the response rate of FOLFOX after irinotecan and 5-FU was 10%, whereas the response rate of irnotecan/cetuximab after failure of 5-FU, irinotecan, and oxaliplatin was 23%, suggesting that cetuximab may offer greater activity in the salvage setting than oxaliplatin. This approach permits the delay of neurotoxicity until late in the patient's treatment course, although it introduces the rash of cetuximab earlier.

A controversial and practical aspect of using cetuximab is the now-discredited need for "determining" the EGFR status of a tumor. There is no prospective clinical evidence that supports the use of this testing. In the original report of cetuximab plus irinotecan (Saltz et al, 2001), the response rates, as determined by an independent response assessment committee, for 1+, 2+, and 3+ positive patients were virtually identical. The same was found to be true in a larger confirmatory trial (Cunningham et al, 2004). In all of these studies, patients thought to be "negative" for the EGFR were excluded from treatment.

Only two reports so far specifically have explored the use of cetuximab-based therapy in EGFR-negative patients. In a small series of nine EGFR-negative patients treated with single-agent cetuximab (Lenz et al, 2004), two of the nine patients were reported by the investigators to have responded. In a larger set of patients, Chung and associates (2005) reviewed the experience with cetuximab at Memorial Sloan-Kettering Cancer Center for patients who initiated treatment with cetuximab during the first 3 months of its commercial availability. Sixteen EGFR-negative patients were identified. Fourteen had received cetuximab plus irinotecan, and two had received single-agent cetuximab alone. A review of scans by a reference radiologist identified four confirmed partial responses to cetuximab-based therapy, all of which were durable at a 6-week follow-up scan. All four responders and two additional minor responders had received cetuximab plus irinotecan (see Table 77b.4).

The idea that patients who lack immunohistochemical expression of EGFR are incapable of responding to cetuximab has been convincingly disproved. This does not mean that EGFR is not the target for cetuximab. Rather, it means that the currently available immunohistochemical techniques are seriously flawed and are essentially useless from a clinical perspective. It has been shown that immunohistochemical expression of EGFR can vary over storage time and can be influenced by the type of fixative used (Atkins et al, 2004) and vary from primary tumor to metastasis. No patient who is believed to be otherwise appropriate for cetuximab-based therapy should be excluded from such therapy solely on the basis of a negative EGFR immunohistochemical stain. A high degree of EGFR expression is likewise meaningless in terms of predicting for activity of cetuximab, in colorectal cancer or otherwise, and this should not be used as justification for cetuximab use.

For now, cetuximab is indicated only in the irinotecan-refractory setting, where definitive data for cetuximab are available. We have no randomized data to support the addition of cetuximab to first-line therapy of colorectal cancer at this time. In the refractory setting, when there are no available active agents, activity from a nonrandomized phase II trial is meaningful. In the first-line setting, when given in conjunction with active chemotherapy regimens, there is little that can be determined other than the feasibility, or lack thereof, of the combination. A promising degree of activity in a small phase II trial does not establish that a combination is appropriate for routine use, and a less than outstanding response rate in a small phase II trial does not mean that a combination is without substantial merit. In the first-line setting, only a randomized trial can establish the relative safety and efficacy of the new combination.

Several small phase II pilot trials have explored the feasibility of combining cetuximab with first-line regimens (Rosenberg et al, 2002; Rougier et al, 2004; Tabernero et al, 2004). This idea became especially intriguing with the publication of the preliminary results of a small randomized phase II trial adding bevacizumab to cetuximab and to cetuximab plus irinotecan in bevacizumab-naive patients, which suggested a strong improvement in response rate and time-to-tumor progression compared with historical controls (Saltz et al, 2005). The preliminary data for cetuximab-based first-line combinations show some encouraging response rates, especially with oxaliplatin-based combinations. These small phase II trials in well-selected patients are not a reason, however, to adopt first-line cetuximab as a part of routine practice. Rather, these studies support the conduct of randomized studies of these regimens to evaluate critically the appropriateness of incorporation of cetuximab into first-line regimens. Until the results of these studies are known, the benefits and risks of cetuximab in first-line therapy are unknown in terms of relative safety and efficacy, and routine use of these combinations in first-line therapy cannot be recommended.

SURGICAL IMPLICATIONS

The improvement from 1 year to close to 2 years in median survival with the advent of newer chemotherapeutic agents and novel therapeutics has been the catalyst for the need for more discussions between oncologic surgeons and medical oncologists. This is especially true for hepatobiliary surgeons, who know that the efficacy of a therapeutic regimen may ensure the return of the patient to the surgical table for a potentially curative resection. With the added drugs and added side effects, surgeons need to know about any toxicity that may hinder further surgical options and engage with the medical oncologist at an early point in a plan of care so that the medical oncologist can help decide which therapy may suit best in a specific scenario. It also is important for the hepatobiliary surgeon to know about previously given agents and how they may affect any planned hepatic resections.

SUMMARY

Metastatic colorectal cancer to the liver is a significant component of the practice of any hepatobiliary surgeon. Systemic therapy for colorectal cancer has improved markedly in the last 10 years with a doubling in survival for first-line therapy. Newer agents continue to be developed. There is no one standard of care for metastatic colorectal cancer today. Some practices are solidly supported by consistent data, and others are based more on reasonable extrapolations than on direct evidence. No one therapeutic approach has shown outstanding superiority over all others, especially when looked at from different perspectives, such as outcome, toxicity, and other plans of care. For this reason, a disease management team approach that involves the hepatobiliary surgeon and medical oncologist is crucial in deciding among the various therapeutic options that are now available. It is imperative that the projected plan of care, its risks, and its benefits be openly and clearly discussed with patients. The patient should be an active participant in the decision-making process when it comes to the selection of therapy.

REFERENCES

Anonymous, 1998: Efficacy of intravenous continuous infusion of fluorouracil compared with bolus administration in advanced colorectal cancer. Meta-analysis Group In Cancer. J Clin Oncol 16:301-308.

Atkins D, et al, 2004: Immunohistochemical detection of EGFR in paraffin-embedded tumor tissues: variation in staining intensity due to choice of fixative and storage time of tissue sections. J Histochem Cytochem 52: 893-901.

Carpenter G, Cohen S, 1990: Epidermal growth factor. J Biol Chem 265: 7709-7712.

Chung KY, et al, 2005: Cetuximab shows activity in colorectal cancer patients with tumors that do not express the epidermal growth factor receptor by immunohistochemistry. J Clin Oncol 23:1803-1810.

Ciardiello F, Tortora G, 2001: A novel approach in the treatment of cancer: targeting the epidermal growth factor receptor. Clin Cancer Res 7: 2958-2970.

Colucci G, et al, 2005: Phase III randomized trial of FOLFIRI versus FOLFOX4 in the treatment of advanced colorectal cancer: a multicenter study of the Gruppo Oncologico Dell'Italia Meridionale. J Clin Oncol 23:4866-4875.

Cunningham D, et al, 2004: Cetuximab monotherapy and cetuximab plus irinotecan in irinotecan-refractory metastatic colorectal cancer. N Engl J Med 351:337-345.

de Gramont A, et al, 1997: Randomized trial comparing monthly low-dose leucovorin and fluorouracil bolus with bimonthly high-dose leucovorin and fluorouracil bolus plus continuous infusion for advanced colorectal cancer: a French intergroup study. J Clin Oncol 15:808-815.

de Gramont A, et al, 2000: Leucovorin and fluorouracil with or without oxaliplatin as first-line treatment in advanced colorectal cancer. J Clin Oncol 18:2938-2947.

Douillard JY, et al, 2000: Irinotecan combined with fluorouracil compared with fluorouracil alone as first-line treatment for metastatic colorectal cancer: a multicentre randomised trial. Lancet 355:1041-1047 [erratum in Lancet 2000 Apr 15;355(9212):1372].

Ferrara N, et al, 2004: Discovery and development of bevacizumab, an anti-VEGF antibody for treating cancer. Nat Rev Drug Discov 3:391-400.

Fong Y, Bentrem DJ, 2006: CASH (Chemotherapy-Associated Steatohepatitis) costs. Ann Surg 243:8-9.

Giantonio BJ, et al, 2005: High-dose bevacizumab in combination with FOLFOX4 improves survival in pateints with previously treated advanced colorectal cancer: results from the Eastern Cooperative Oncology Group (ECOG) study 3200. Proc ASCO Gastrointestinal Cancers Symposium, p 168 (abstract 169a).

Goldberg RM, et al, 2004: A randomized controlled trial of fluorouracil plus leucovorin, irinotecan, and oxaliplatin combinations in patients with previously untreated metastatic colorectal cancer. J Clin Oncol 22:23-30.

Hurwitz H, et al, 2004: Bevacizumab plus irinotecan, fluorouracil, and leucovorin for metastatic colorectal cancer. N Engl J Med 350:2335-2342.

Jain RK, 2001: Normalizing tumor vasculature with anti-angiogenic therapy: a new paradigm for combination therapy. Nat Med 7:987-989.

Kabbinavar F, et al, 2003: Phase II, randomized trial comparing bevacizumab plus fluorouracil (FU)/leucovorin (LV) with FU/LV alone in patients with metastatic colorectal cancer. J Clin Oncol 21:60-65.

Kabbinavar FF, et al, 2004: Bevacizumab (a monoclonal antibody to vascular endothelial growth factor) to prolong progression-free survival in first-line colorectal cancer (CRC) in subjects who are not suitable candidates for first-line CPT-11. Proc ASCO 22(suppl):3516.

Lenz HJ, et al, 2004: Activity of cetuximab in patients with colorectal cancer refractory to both irinotecan and oxaliplatin. American Society of Clinical Oncology, New Orleans, June 5-8.

Maughan T, et al, 2005: Fluorouracil, oxaliplatin, CPT-11 use and sequencing in advanced colorectal cancer. The UK MRC FOCUS (CR08) trial. Proc ASCO Gastrointestinal Symposium, p 166 (abstract 165).

Real FX, et al, 1986: Expression of epidermal growth factor receptor in human cultured cells and tissues: relationship to cell lineage and stage of differentiation. Cancer Res 46:4726-4731.

Reddy GK, 2005: The addition of bevacizumab to FOLFOX4 prolongs survival in relapsed colorectal cancer: interim data from the ECOG 3200 trial. Clin Colorectal Cancer 4:300-301.

Rosenberg AH, et al, 2002: Erbitux (IMC-C225) plus weekly irinotecan (CPT-11), fluorouracil (5FU) and leucovorin (LV) in colorectal cancer (CRC) that expresses the epidermal growth factor receptor (EGFr). American Society of Clinical Oncology, Orlando, Florida.

Rothenberg ML, et al, 2003: Superiority of oxaliplatin and fluorouracil-leucovorin compared with either therapy alone in patients with progressive colorectal cancer after irinotecan and fluorouracil-leucovorin: interim results of a phase III trial. J Clin Oncol 21:2059-2069.

Rougier P, et al, 2004: Cetuximab+FOLFIRI as first-line treatment for metastatic colorectal CA. Proc Am Soc Clin Oncol 22(suppl):3513.

Saltz LB, et al, 2000: Irinotecan plus fluorouracil and leucovorin for metastatic colorectal cancer. Irinotecan Study Group. N Engl J Med 343:905-914.

Saltz LB, et al, 2001: Cetuximab (IMC-C225) plus irinotecan(CPT-11) is active in CPT-11-refractory colorectal cancer (CRC) that express epidermal growth factor receptor (EGFR). Proc Am Soc Clin Oncol (abstract 7).

Saltz LB, et al, 2004: Phase II trial of cetuximab in patients with refractory colorectal cancer that expresses the epidermal growth factor receptor. J Clin Oncol 22:1201-1208.

Saltz LB, et al, 2005: Interim report of randomized phase II trial of cetuximab/bevacizumab/irinotecan (CBI) versus cetuximab/bevacizumab (CB) in irinotecan-refractory colorectal cancer. Proc ASCO Gastrointestinal Cancers Symposium, p 169 (abstract 169b).

Tabernero JM, et al, 2004: An international phase II study of cetuximab in combination with oxaliplatin/5-fluorouracil (5-FU)/folinic acid (FA) (FOLFOX-4) in the first-line treatment of patients with metastatic colorectal cancer (CRC) expressing epidermal growth factor receptor (EGFR): preliminary results. Proc Am Soc Clin Oncol 22 (abstract 3512).

Thomas SM, Grandis JR, 2004: Pharmacokinetic and pharmacodynamic properties of EGFR inhibitors under clinical investigation. Cancer Treat Rev 30:255-268.

Tournigand C, et al, 2004: FOLFIRI followed by FOLFOX6 or the reverse sequence in advanced colorectal cancer: a randomized GERCOR study. J Clin Oncol 22:229-237.

Willett CG, et al, 2004: Direct evidence that the VEGF-specific antibody bevacizumab has antivascular effects in human rectal cancer. Nat Med 10:145-147 [erratum in Nat Med 2004 Jun;10(6):649].

78

Isolated Hepatic Perfusion for Extensive Liver Cancers

Y. KU

The rationale for regional chemotherapy is to intensify dose delivery of cytotoxic chemotherapeutic agents with a steep dose-response curve at a cancer-bearing organ, while minimizing systemic exposure to these agents. Isolated hepatic perfusion (IHP) is one modality to achieve high local chemotherapeutic concentrations in the liver for patients with unresectable liver cancers. IHP is based on several pharmacokinetic and toxicologic advantages over simple hepatic arterial infusion (HAI). First, IHP can produce tumor tissue concentrations of chemotherapeutic agents several times higher than by HAI. Second, in contrast to HAI, agents with a low hepatic extraction rate on the first pass can be used with little systemic exposure and toxicity. Third, IHP can deliver hyperthermic or hypoxic conditions selectively to the liver, which may exert synergistic effects on the tumor tissue (Miller et al, 1994).

The technique of IHP by using an oxygenated recirculating circuit was first developed in the late 1950s (Creech et al, 1958) and was first performed in humans by Ausman (1961), who treated five patients with nitrogen mustard under normothermic conditions. Interest in IHP soon waned, however, because in early clinical trials it was associated with significant morbidity and mortality, and its efficacy was not shown convincingly. Over the next 3 decades, attempts were made at a few institutions to standardize the technique of IHP and to test various chemotherapeutic agents in animal models and in patients. The lack of clearly documented efficacy of this technically demanding procedure prevented its wide acceptance in clinical use, however.

In the early 1990s (Lienard et al, 1992), strikingly high response rates of isolated limb perfusion with melphalan and tumor necrosis factor (TNF) for melanomas and soft tissue sarcomas evoked a renewed interest in IHP and led several investigators to make further technical modifications in the original procedure. These modifications include (1) the use of an external venovenous bypass circuit with a centrifugal pump instead of a passive internal shunt to allow better venous return to the heart from the portal vein and the inferior vena cava (IVC) and (2) the use of a continuous intraoperative leak monitoring system that enables perfusate leakage control during procedures. The most important refinement in the technique of IHP is a thorough vascular isolation of the liver, as performed in orthotopic liver transplantation. With such complete vascular isolation of the liver and a sensitive method to detect any perfusate leak during IHP, a low leakage rate of less than 4% is accomplished, and highly toxic bioactive agents, such as TNF, can be administered safely (Alexander et al, 1998). Under these circumstances, the major limitation of IHP is that, by virtue of its aggressive nature, it cannot be performed more than once in an individual patient. A chemotherapeutic regimen used for IHP must confer sufficient efficacy to warrant such an unrepeatable approach.

Percutaneous isolated hepatic perfusion (PIHP) was developed in the 1990s as a variation of IHP (Beheshti et al, 1992; Ku et al, 1997), in which chemotherapeutic agents are administered via a percutaneously placed HAI catheter. During drug perfusion, isolated hepatic venous hemofiltration is accomplished by using a dual-balloon catheter positioned in the retrohepatic IVC to isolate and shunt hepatic venous effluent through charcoal filters. Experimental and clinical studies by several groups have shown reproducibly that various cytotoxic chemotherapeutic agents can be eliminated effectively by the system when administered via the hepatic artery (Curley et al, 1993; Ku et al, 1990). Although PIHP does not guarantee low leakage rates, it is simple, minimally invasive, and repeatable in the same patient. Its efficacy shown in phase I and II trials treating patients with extensive liver tumors warrants further evaluation.

TECHNIQUES

Isolated Hepatic Perfusion by Surgical Isolation of the Liver

By laparotomy, the diaphragmatic attachments of the liver are divided, and the retrohepatic IVC is fully dissected from all nonhepatic venous tributaries, including the right adrenal vein and several lumbar or phrenic veins. All fibroconnective tissues at the porta hepatis are divided, and surrounding lymphatic tissue is removed to avoid possible perfusate leakage. A prophylactic cholecystectomy is performed to prevent treatment-related complications. The liver could be perfused in three ways: the hepatic artery, the portal vein, or both. In most more recent trials, the hepatic artery was used as the only site for drug perfusion. In this setting, the gastroduodenal artery is skeletonized to introduce an inflow arterial cannula at the confluence of the common hepatic artery. An outflow cannula is introduced into the retrohepatic IVC via a femoral vein or by a caval incision. These cannulae are connected with the extracorporeal perfusion circuit consisting of a membrane oxygenator and a pump/heater system. The perfusion circuit is preloaded with a mixture of packed red blood cells and a crystalloid. The venovenous bypass with a centrifugal pump connecting the portal and femoral veins with the axillary vein is established to allow decompression of the portal vein and the IVC during treatment. Temperature monitoring probes are placed in the liver. Vascular clamps are placed sequentially on the common hepatic artery and the IVC above and below the hepatic veins to accomplish a complete hepatic vascular isolation. Fig. 78.1 shows the setup of an IHP system used by investigators at the National Cancer Institute (NCI) in the United States. In most reports, perfusion time is limited to 60 minutes followed by rinsing with a crystalloid and a colloid solution through the hepatic artery and portal vein. The median operative time is 4.5 to 8.5 hours, and the median blood loss is 2.2 to 5 L.

Several different chemotherapeutic regimens have been used in IHP, often as part of a single study. In more recent IHP trials (Table 78.1), the agent most frequently used is 60 to 160 mg/body of melphalan. In addition, recombinant human TNF is administered into the perfusate at a dose of 0.2 mg/body, 0.3 mg/body, 1 mg/body, or 1.5 mg/body as a biologic agent. A phase I dose-escalating study conducted by the NCI group determined the maximum tolerated dose of TNF to be 1.5 mg. As an adjunct to chemotherapy, hyperthermia is used, with the hepatic tissue temperature maintained in the range of 39°C to 41°C.

Leakage control is a crucial issue in IHP, especially when bioactive agents such as TNF are combined with chemotherapeutic agents. The simplest quantitative method is to measure the systemic concentrations of the perfused drugs. This method does not provide a real-time measurement of the leak, however. The best online leak monitoring system uses an iodine 131–labeled human serum albumin. This method has been shown to be accurate, sensitive, and capable of identifying perfusate leaks of 1% or less (Barker et al, 1995).

Percutaneous Isolated Hepatic Perfusion by Dual-Balloon Catheter Isolation of the Liver

The venous drainage of the liver is isolated to a short segment of the IVC; this allows a minimally invasive percutaneous technique of PIHP (Fig. 78.2), which circumvents an extensive mobilization and dissection of the liver and of the IVC. The HAI catheter is placed angiographically by the Seldinger technique. A specially designed dual-balloon catheter (Fig. 78.3) is introduced into the IVC through a femoral vein cutdown above the saphenofemoral junction. The catheter has two occlusion balloons and two blood circulating lumina. The cephalad balloon is inflated above the hepatic veins, and the caudad balloon is inflated 5 cm below them, just above the renal veins. The fenestrated interballoon segment of one major lumen of the catheter collects the hepatic effluent. The isolated hepatic effluent is directed to the extracorporeal pump-filter circuit and sent back to the right atrium through the other major lumen with an opening at the distal tip of the catheter. Another PIHP technique has been described by different groups (Beheshti et al, 1992; Curley et al, 1994) who use a similar but distinct dual-balloon catheter (Bodden-Glickman catheter; Delcath Systems,

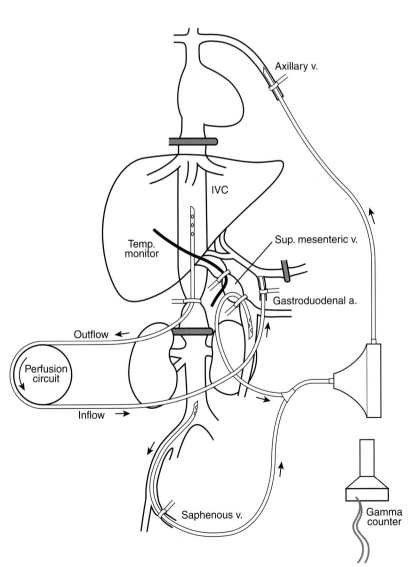

Fig. 78.1. Diagram of IHP established by investigators at the NCI. The whole procedure is performed under laparotomy. *Arrows* indicate direction of blood flow.

Axillary v.

IVC

Temp. monitor

Sup. mesenteric v.

Gastroduodenal a.

Outflow

Perfusion circuit

Inflow

Saphenous v.

Gamma counter

Table 78.1   Summary of Isolated Hepatic Perfusion Trials Since 1995

Reference	N	Etiology	Agent and Dose	Temperature (°C)	Mortality (%)	Response (%)	Median Survival (mo)
Marinelli et al, 1996	9	CLM	Mitomycin C 30 mg/m²	37	0	CR 11 PR 11	17
de Vries et al, 1998	9	CLM	Melphalan 1 mg/kg TNF 0.4-0.8 mg	≥41	33	PR 83	10
Oldhafer et al, 1998	12	6 CLM 6 others	Melphalan 60-140 mg TNF 0.2-0.3 mg	40-41	0 (2 VOD [17])	CR 8 PR 33	9
Hafström & Naredi, 1998	11	5 CLM 6 others	Melphalan 0.5 mg/kg TNF 0.03-0.2 mg	39	18	PR 27	—
Vahrmeijer et al, 2000	24	CLM	Melphalan 0.5-4 mg/kg	37	12.5	CR 6 PR 11	19
Alexander et al, 2000	22	Melanoma	Melphalan 1.5-2.5 mg/kg ± TNF 1 mg	39-40	4	≥PR 64	11
Bartlett et al, 2001	32	CLM	Melphalan 1.5 mg/kg TNF 1.0 mg	39-40	3	PR 77	16
	19	CLM	Melphalan 1.5 mg/kg	39-40	0	PR 74	27

CLM, colorectal liver metastasis; CR, complete response; PR, partial response; VOD, veno-occlusive disease.

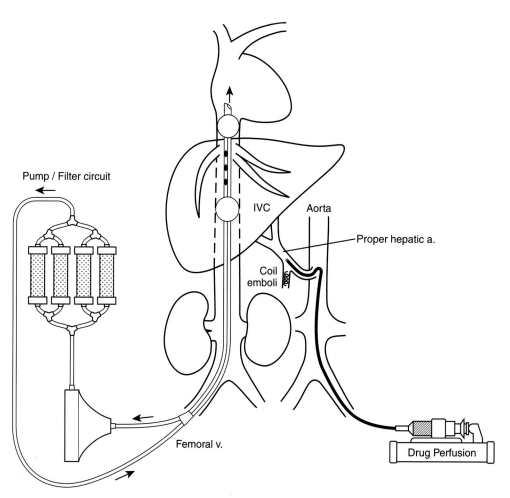

Fig. 78.2. Diagram of single catheter technique of PIHP established by Kobe group. *Arrows* indicate direction of blood flow.

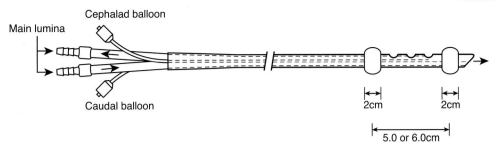

Fig. 78.3. A specially designed four-lumen/two-balloon catheter for PIHP. The catheter has two occlusion balloons and two blood circulating lumina.

New York, NY). Regardless of the design of a dual-balloon catheter, PIHP is a simple procedure and requires approximately 2 to 3 hours to complete. The liver is not completely isolated, however, from the systemic circulation by the technique; the filtered hepatic effluent returned to the systemic circulation still contains a potentially toxic drug concentration, and the portal vein and all fibroconnective tissues at the porta hepatis along with small tributaries of the hepatic segment of the IVC are unable to control. During hemofiltration of the isolated hepatic effluent, the patient receives a dose-intensified HAI of cytotoxic agents diluted in a volume of 200 to 250 mL over 15 to 40 minutes. In most reports, doxorubicin is used as a first-line chemotherapeutic agent at a dose level of 60 to120 mg/m^2.

RESULTS OF ISOLATED HEPATIC PERFUSION

Although several groups have reported their clinical results with IHP over the past 45 years, the role of IHP in the treatment of unresectable primary or metastatic liver cancers is unclear. To date, there have been no randomized studies comparing IHP with more traditional therapies. In addition, it is difficult to compare the results of one series with those of others, each of which differs in technique, chemotherapeutic regimens, and etiologic factors. Most of the IHP trials consist of small numbers of patients and lack appropriate controls. Despite these limitations, selected data of IHP for extensive liver tumors are summarized in Table 78.1 according to disease etiology.

In most IHP trials, most patients had metastatic liver cancers of mainly colorectal origin. Schwemmle and colleagues (1987) reported results of 50 patients with metastatic liver cancers, of which 45 had colorectal cancer. There were four deaths (8%). In 41 assessable colorectal cancer patients treated primarily with 5-fluorouracil alone or 5-fluorouracil and mitomycin C, the investigators observed a 22% complete response and a 68% partial response with a median survival of 14 months. Responses were determined by nonstandard criteria, however, including decreases in the serum carcinoembryonic antigen concentrations. Aigner and coworkers (1988) published their experience with IHP under hyperthermic conditions in 46 colorectal cancer patients using 5-fluorouracil as a main agent. There were three deaths (6%). Interpretation of these data is difficult because nonstandard response criteria were used, and the overall survival was not presented. Using standard response criteria, Hafström and associates (1994) reported results of IHP with melphalan and cisplatin in 29 patients. The response rate was reported to be 20% with an operative mortality rate of 14%. Taken together, response and survival data after IHP in early series failed to show a convincing improvement compared with HAI therapy.

Rekindled by spectacular results of isolated limb perfusion using melphalan and TNF, several centers in Europe and one in the United States initiated clinical IHP trials combining TNF with melphalan for treatment of metastatic liver cancers. It has been shown that TNF damages tumor-associated vascular endothelial cells, resulting in increased vascular permeability and chemotherapeutic agent concentrations in the tumors (Ruegg et al, 1998). de Vries and associates (1995) from the Netherlands reported nine patients treated with 1 mg/kg of melphalan and either 0.4 mg or 0.8 mg of TNF with inflows through the hepatic artery and portal vein. Despite a high operative mortality rate (33%), these investigators observed significant tumor responses in five of six assessable patients. The median survival time was 10 months (range 6-26 months).

Using a similar two-route inflow perfusion, a Swedish group (Hafström & Naredi, 1998) reported results in 11 patients treated with 0.5 mg/kg of melphalan and 0.03 to 0.2 mg of TNF. The treatment-related mortality rate was 18%. Except for five nonresponding colorectal cancer patients, six patients with ocular melanoma or leiomyosarcoma had a significant anti-tumor response. Oldhafer and coworkers (1998) from Hannover, Germany, reported 12 metastatic liver cancer patients treated with either 20 to 50 mg of mitomycin C alone or a combination of TNF and 60 to 140 mg of melphalan via the hepatic artery. Although no immediate postoperative deaths occurred, there were two treatment-related deaths at 2 and 4 months after IHP. In four of six assessable patients with colorectal liver cancer, two (50%) had a partial response.

The series reported by Bartlett and colleagues (2001) at the NCI represents the largest single institutional experience of IHP for the treatment of colorectal liver cancers. Among 51 patients with a 60-minute IHP with 1.5 mg/kg of melphalan and hyperthermia, 32 concomitantly received 1 mg of TNF, and 19 had melphalan alone followed by monthly HAI with 0.2 mg/kg of floxuridine and 15 mg/m^2 of leucovorin for 14 days. There was one death (2%). The partial response rate was 77% in 31 assessable patients who had TNF and melphalan, with a median survival of 16 months. For the 19 patients who underwent IHP with melphalan alone and subsequently HAI maintenance therapy, the response rate was greater than 70% and remained high. This group had a longer duration of response with a median survival of 27 months. These data suggest that adjuvant HAI seems to prolong tumor response and survival after IHP. Conversely, the same data imply that a single treatment of IHP with currently available regimens has a limited efficacy in achieving definitive local control of metastatic liver cancers. Another argument is whether TNF contributes to augmentation of the antitumor effects of melphalan seen with IHP. These issues remain to be determined by well-designed control studies.

Malignant melanoma metastatic to the liver has been the second treatment target of IHP. Investigators at the NCI (Alexander et al, 2000) reported a single institutional experience with IHP using either melphalan alone or melphalan plus TNF for ocular melanoma patients. In 22 patients, the overall response rate was 62% with 2 complete responses and 11 partial responses. The median survival was 11 months. In the subsequent series with 29 patients, IHP with melphalan alone produced a comparable response rate of 62%, but the median survival was only 1 year (Feldman et al, 2004a). These results suggest a need for new IHP regimens to improve the outlook for patients with melanoma metastatic to the liver.

IHP also seems to be attractive for the treatment of primary liver cancers. Because hepatocellular carcinoma (HCC) remains within the liver for a significant period, local control of the disease most likely affects the overall survival. HCC frequently accompanies hepatitis-associated cirrhosis, however, which precludes extensive surgical intervention such as IHP. To date, there are few IHP trials, all of which consist of only a few HCC patients. Feldman and colleagues (2004b) at the NCI reported results of hyperthermic IHP in nine patients with advanced primary liver cancer. Five patients had HCC, and four had cholangiocarcinoma. Most patients had highly advanced disease, as characterized by the averaged tumor nodules of 13, the mean percent hepatic replacement of 41%, and the mean tumor diameter of 10 cm. The overall response rate was 67% as determined by serial post-treatment magnetic resonance imaging. Although the overall median survival was limited to 13 months, the achievement of substantial tumor responses in patients with advanced tumor burden is notable and warrants further evaluation of IHP in a large cohort of patients with primary liver cancers.

RESULTS OF PERCUTANEOUS ISOLATED HEPATIC PERFUSION

Several groups have reported results of phase I and II trials of PIHP using different dual-balloon catheters for the treatment of metastatic or primary liver cancers. The data mainly come from one center in Japan, Kobe University, and two centers in the United States, Yale University and University of Texas M.D. Anderson Cancer Center (Table 78.2). Eligibility criteria were similar among these centers, including performance status of 1 or less, serum bilirubin concentration of 2 mg/dL or less, platelet count greater than 50,000/mL, and normal coagulation profile.

Beheshti and coworkers (1992) at Yale University reported a phase I dose-escalation study with the use of Bodden-Glickman catheters in eight patients with metastatic liver cancers. One patient could not tolerate balloon occlusion of the IVC; seven patients successfully underwent a total of 14 treatments using 1000 to 2000 mg/m^2 of 5-fluorouracil. Subsequently, Ravikumar and associates (1994) reported results of a phase I toxicity estimation study with either 5-fluorouracil or doxorubicin. Twenty-one patients were treated with 58 procedures. Dose-limiting toxicity was observed with 5-fluorouracil at a dose of 5000 mg/m^2 and doxorubicin at a dose of 120 mg/m^2. In a more recent trial of PIHP by the same group (Hwu et al, 1999), 18 patients with unresectable primary or metastaic liver tumors underwent a total of 57 procedures with doxorubicin. No tumor response was seen in patients treated at 50 or 75 mg/m^2 dose level of doxorubicin. In 12 patients who underwent repetitive treatments with 90 or 120 mg/m^2 of doxorubicin, the overall response rate was 58%. Curley and associates (1994) from Texas reported results of PIHP using the same dual-balloon catheter. Ten of 11 enrolled patients with unresectable HCC underwent a total of 17 treatments with 60 to 120 mg/m^2 of doxorubicin. In this phase I trial, 7 of 10 assessable patients had a partial response, and 2 of these 7 patients had a marked tumor volume reduction, which allowed a sequential hepatectomy for the remaining tumors. The investigators recommended PIHP to be used in the neoadjuvant or adjuvant setting in selected patients with HCC.

Ku and colleagues (1998) from Kobe reported long-term results of PIHP in 28 consecutive patients with multiple advanced HCC. In this group of stage IV patients, the main tumor diameter averaged 7.4 cm, and 17 of 28 patients had macroscopic vascular invasion to the portal vein. All patients successfully underwent PIHP as a total of 39 procedures with 60 to 150 mg/m^2 of doxorubicin. The overall response rate was 63% with 5 complete remissions and 12 partial responses. The overall survival rate was 67% at 1 year and 39% at 5 years. A similar tumor response rate

Table 78.2 Summary of Percutaneous Isolated Hepatic Perfusion Trials Since 1994

Reference	N	Etiology	Agent and Dose	No. of PIHP/Patient (total)	Mortality (%)	Response (%)	Survival (mo)
Curley et al, 1994	11	HCC	Doxorubicin C 60-120 mg/m^2	1-3 (17)	10	PR 70	—
Ravikumar et al, 1994	21	8 CLM 5 HCC 8 others	Doxorubicin 50-120 mg/m^2 or 5-FU 100-150 mg/m^2	2-4 (58)	0	PR 22	—
Ku et al, 1995	12	HCC	Doxorubicin 100-150 mg/m^2	1-2 (18)	13	CR 7 PR 57	—
Ku et al, 1998	15	HCC	Doxorubicin 100-150 mg/m^2	1-4 (39)	7	CR 18 PR 44	Median 16
Hwu et al, 1999	18	7 HCC 11 others	Doxorubicin 90-120 mg/m^2	1-10 (57)	0	≥ MR 66	Median; responder 23, nonresponder 8
Ku et al, 2004	25	HCC	Doxorubicin 60-120 mg/m^2 in combination with reductive hepatectomy	1-3 (39)	0	CR 45 PR 41	5-yr survival 42%

CLM, colorectal liver metastasis; CR, complete response; HCC, hepatocellular carcinoma; MR, minor response; PR, partial response.

of 64% has been reproduced by the current updating series with 79 patients (Fig. 78.4) (Ku et al, 2003), which represents the largest single institution experience with PIHP. In this expanded series, there were three deaths with a mortality rate of 4%. The 1-year and 5-year survival rates of stage IV-A patients were 81% and 20%. Because other studies did not provide the survival data, comparison among studies is difficult. Tumor response data were almost comparable among studies in three different groups.

The Kobe group (Ku et al, 2004) also reported results of repetitive PIHP combined with reductive hepatectomy for 25 patients with multiple advanced HCC previously deemed to be unresectable. This novel dual treatment strategy of surgical resection plus PIHP is based on several oncologic advantages. First, a large HCC frequently accompanies feeding arteries from adjacent organs, such as the diaphragm and the major and minor omentum. These collateral arteries, which otherwise affect drug delivery to the tumors during PIHP, could be eliminated at the time of surgical resection. Second, reductive hepatectomy results in a decreased vascular bed of the liver, which is theoretically beneficial to PIHP because the relative dose rate to the residual tumors is increased. Third, in HCC patients with tumor thrombi in the portal trunk, a life-threatening sequence of events, such as massive ascites, variceal hemorrhage, and eventually hepatic failure,

frequently occurs. Such an urgent situation could be prevented by the first stage of surgery. These hypotheses are supported by impressively increased overall response rates of 86% with several long-term survivors after the treatment (Fig. 78.5). In the updating series in 35 patients (Tominaga et al, 2004) with multiple advanced HCC, the complete response rate was 46% with a partial response rate of 36%. In patients with the disease confined to the liver, the 5-year survival rate reached 51%. These data are encouraging and warrant further evaluation in an appropriately selected group of patients with technically resectable main tumors and preserved liver function adequate for planned hepatectomy.

COMPLICATIONS AND TOXICITIES

The IHP-related mortality was significant in early series, ranging from 6% to 33%. In recent years, after improving the techniques of liver isolation and leakage control, IHP has been performed more safely with a mortality rate of less than 2% (Alexander et al, 1998; Bartlett et al, 2001). The extensive surgical insult to the liver and the use of concentrated chemotherapeutic agents with or without TNF cause significant elevations of the liver enzymes in almost all patients. These enzyme elevations are usually transient

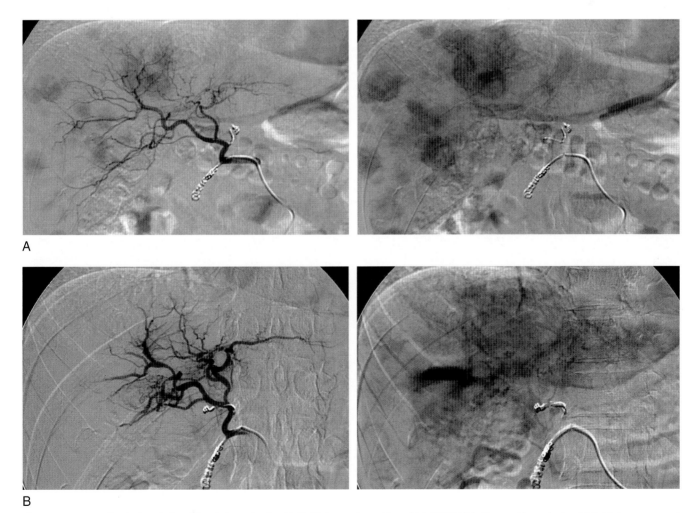

A

B

Fig. 78.4. Angiographic findings before (**A**) and 6 months after PIHP (**B**) in a patient with multiple HCC. This 52-year-old man had multiple bilobar tumors and underwent two treatments, each with 100 mg/m² of doxorubicin. He is at present disease-free 3 years after treatment. *Left side* of each panel represents early arterial phase, and *right side* of each panel represents late venous phase.

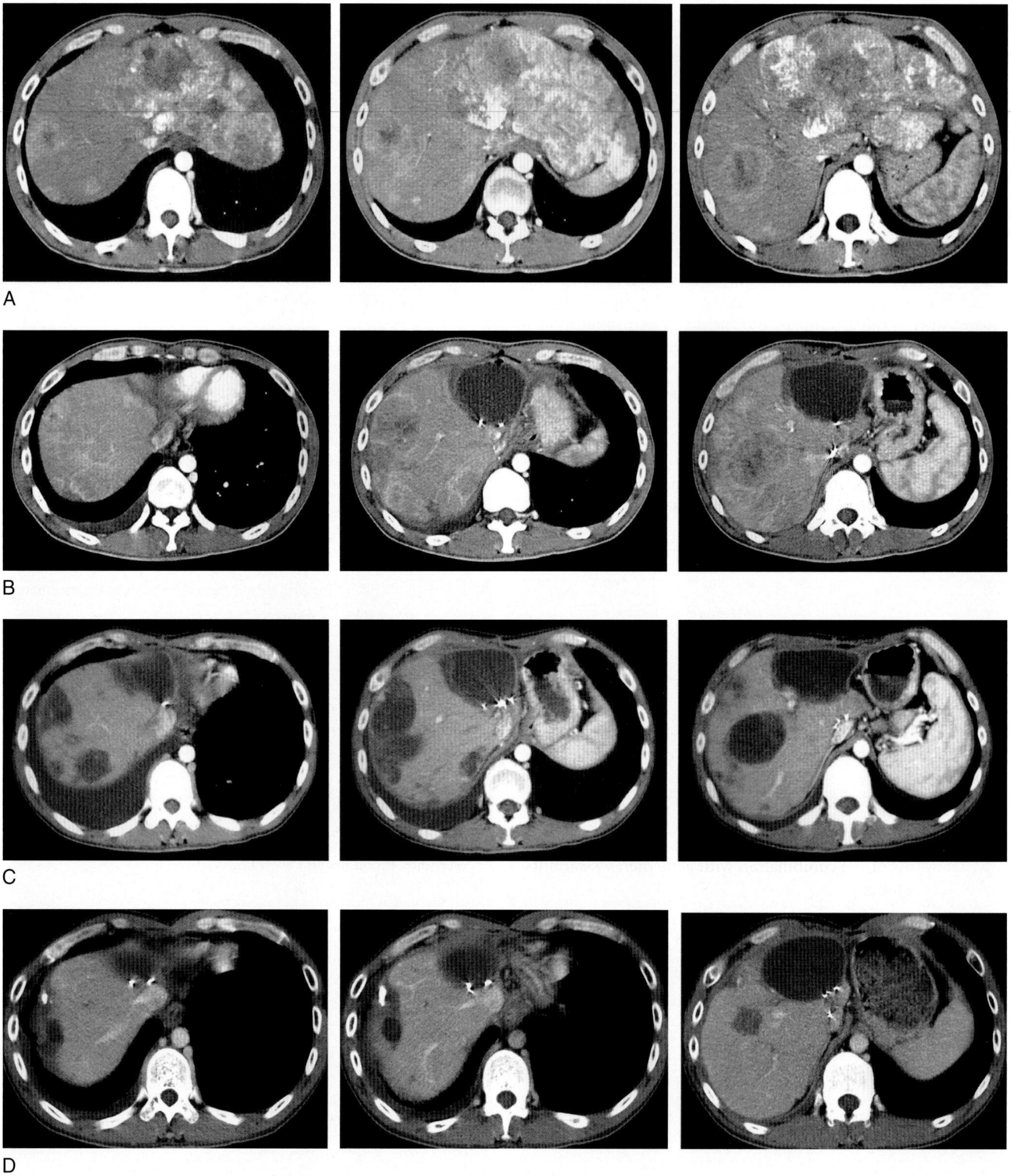

Fig. 78.5. Sequential computed tomography (CT) findings before and after dual treatment with hepatectomy plus PIHP in a patient with HCC. This 31-year-old man presented with multiple bulky tumors in the entire liver **(A)**. The patient underwent extended left lobectomy as a first-stage reductive treatment. Although residual tumors in the remnant liver enlarged in size 1 month after reductive hepatectomy **(B)**, repetitive PIHP, each time with 100 mg/m^2 of doxorubicin and 30 mg/m^2 of mitomycin C, produced significant tumor responses, as shown by CT scans 2 months **(C)** and 1 year **(D)** after reductive hepatectomy. The patient eventually died of recurrent disease with bleeding esophageal varices 28 months after the start of dual treatment.

and subside within 1 week. Hepatic toxicity is no doubt a major dose-limiting factor of chemotherapeutic agents in IHP, however. Bartlett and coworkers (2001) reported one patient with progressive hepatic veno-occlusive disease, in whom 2 mg/kg of melphalan was administered. In this regard, mitomycin C has been reported as a high-risk causative agent of veno-occlusive disease (Marinelli et al, 1996; Oldhafer et al, 1998). Other complications include bleeding, coagulopathy, pulmonary edema, and hypotension.

PIHP has lower mortality and morbidity rates compared with IHP. Hepatic toxicity as determined by serum liver enzyme and bilirubin concentrations is usually lower than the toxicity seen after IHP. PIHP has the potential risk of HAI catheter–related complications, however. Ku and colleagues (1998) reported one patient with necrotizing pancreatitis and duodenal perforation caused by drug malperfusion through the gastroduodenal artery. In addition, two patients with repetitive treatments developed progressive liver failure as a result of hepatic artery occlusion. Preventive measures to such arterial damage caused by multiple HAI of high-dose chemotherapeutic agents need to be explored. Other investigators (Curley et al, 1994) reported a death secondary to acute cardiac failure, presumably as a result of catecholamine depletion during hemofiltration. Excluding these, PIHP can be performed safely in most patients. Because of higher drug leakage rates, systemic toxicity, as represented by leukopenia or hair loss, occurs more frequently after PIHP compared with IHP.

FUTURE DIRECTIONS

Owing to recent technical refinements, IHP has become a safe procedure with acceptable treatment-related mortality in specialized centers. The development of less invasive techniques is the crucial element in allowing IHP to be a more commonly considered option for patients with extensive liver cancers. Although the use of TNF during IHP has proved to be safe, its antitumor efficacy also remains to be determined. Considering unique pharmacokinetic benefits of IHP, the use of new chemotherapeutic or bioactive agents or the combination with gene therapy warrants further investigation.

The results of several phase I and II trials are in accordance that IHP can produce significant tumor regression in patients with advanced tumor burden and in patients with refractory tumors after prior treatments. The tumor response rates are high (>70% in the large series). Although the impact on overall survival is unclear, it is reasonable to consider IHP an emerging option for the treatment of extensive primary or secondary liver cancers in currently hopeless situations. The issue of identifying patients likely to benefit from IHP is an important open question.

PIHP is a promising variation of IHP by which a dose intensified regional chemotherapy can be delivered repeatedly in an individual patient. Several investigators report high rates of tumor regression in unresectable primary and metastatic liver cancers, which are almost comparable to the rates obtained by surgical isolation and perfusion of the liver. Large series show that repetitive PIHP treatments yield long-term survival in a subset of patients with otherwise intractable HCC. Based on these encouraging data, PIHP is currently combined with reductive hepatectomy in patients with previously unresectable HCC. This dual treatment results in impressively increased response and survival rates. These results justify randomized and nonrandomized trials with PIHP in a large cohort of patients with advanced HCC.

As a future direction, IHP followed by repetitive PIHP treatments may be an interesting combination to achieve definitive local control of extensive liver cancers.

REFERENCES

Aigner KR, et al, 1988: Isolated liver perfusion with MMC/5-FU: surgical technique, pharmacokinetics, clinical results. Contrib Oncol 29:229-246.

Alexander HR Jr, et al, 1998: Isolated hepatic perfusion with tumor necrosis factor and melphalan for unresectable cancers confined to the liver. J Clin Oncol 16:1479-1489.

Alexander HR Jr, et al, 2000: A phase I-II study of isolated hepatic perfusion using melphalan with or without tumor necrosis factor for patients with ocular melanoma metastatic to liver. Clin Cancer Res 6:3062-3070.

Ausman RK, 1961: The development of a technique for isolated perfusion of the liver. New York State J Med 61:3393-3397.

Barker WC, et al, 1995: Continuous intraoperative external monitoring of perfusate leak using I-131 human serum albumin during isolated perfusion of the liver and limbs. Eur J Nucl Med 22:1242-1248.

Bartlett DL, et al, 2001: Isolated hepatic perfusion for unresectable hepatic metastases from colorectal cancer. Surgery 129:176-187.

Beheshti MV, et al, 1992: Percutaneous isolated liver perfusion for treament of hepatic malignancy: preliminary report. J Vasc Interv Radiol 3:1461-1572.

Creech O Jr, et al, 1958: Chemotherapy of cancer: regional perfusion utilizing an extracorporeal circuit. Ann Surg 148:616-632.

Curley SA, et al, 1993: Reduction of systemic drug exposure following hepatic arterial infusion of doxorubicin with complete hepatic venous isolation and extracorporeal chemofiltration. Surgery 114:579-585.

Curley SA, et al, 1994: Complete hepatic venous isolation and extracorporeal chemofiltration as treatment for human hepatocellular carcinoma: a phase I study. Ann Surg Oncol 1:389-399.

de Vries MR, et al, 1995: Soluble TNF-alpha receptor induction by isolated hepatic perfusion with TNF-alpha and melphalan. Eur Surg Res 27:108A.

de Vries MR, et al, 1998: Isolated hepatic perfusion with tumor necrosis factor alpha and melphalan: experimental studies in pigs and phase Is data from humans. Recent Results Cancer Res 147:107-119.

Feldman ED, et al, 2004a: Regional treatment options for patients with ocular melanoma metastatic to the liver. Ann Surg Oncol 11:290-297.

Feldman ED, et al, 2004b: Treatment of patients with unresectable primary hepatic malignancies using hyperthermic isolated hepatic perfusion. J Gastrointest Surg 8:200-207.

Hafström LR, Naredi PLJ, 1998: Isolated hepatic perfusion with extracorporeal oxygenation using hyperthermia TNF-alpha and melphalan: Swedish experience. Recent Results Cancer Res 147:120-126.

Hafström LR, et al, 1994: Isolated hyperthermic liver perfusion with chemotherapy for liver malignancy. Surg Oncol 3:103-108.

Hwu WJ, et al, 1999: A clinical-pharmacological evaluation of percutaneous isolated hepatic infusion of doxorubicin in patients with unresectable liver tumors. Oncol Res 11:529-537.

Ku Y, et al, 1990: Extracorporeal removal of anticancer drugs in hepatic arterial infusion: the effect of direct hemoperfusion combined with veno-venous bypass. Surgery 107:273-281.

Ku Y, et al, 1995: Clinical pilot study on high-dose intraarterial chemotherapy with direct hemoperfusion under hepatic venous isolation in patients with advanced hepatocellular carcinoma. Surgery 117:510-519.

Ku Y, et al, 1997: Single catheter technique of hepatic venous isolation and extracorporeal charcoal hemoperfusion for malignant liver tumors. Am J Surg 173:103-109.

Ku Y, et al, 1998: Induction of long-term remission in advanced hepatocellular carcinoma with percutaneous isolated liver chemoperfusion. Ann Surg 227:519-526.

Ku Y, et al, 2003: Percutaneous isolated hepatic perfusion for advanced hepatocellular carcinoma established with the aid of interventional radiology technique. Geka 65:1158-1167.

Ku Y, et al, 2004: Reductive surgery plus percutaneous isolated hepatic perfusion for multiple advanced hepatocellular carcinoma. Ann Surg 239:53-60.

Lienard D, et al, 1992: High-dose recombinant tumor necrosis factor alpha in combination with interferon gamma and melphalan in isolation perfusion of the limbs for melanoma and sarcoma. J Clin Oncol 10:52-60.

Marinelli A, et al, 1996: Phase I/II studies of isolated hepatic perfusion with mitomycin C or melphalan in patients with colorectal hepatic metastases. Jpn J Clin Oncol 26:341-350.

Miller RC, et al, 1994: Interaction of hyperthermia and chemotherapy agents: cell lethality and oncogenic potential. Int J Hyperthermia 10:89-99.

Oldhafer KJ, et al, 1998: First experience and technical aspects of isolated liver perfusion for extensive liver metastasis. Surgery 123:622-631.

Ravikumar TS, et al, 1994: Percutaneous hepatic vein isolation and high-dose hepatic arterial infusion chemotherapy for unresectable liver tumors. J Clin Oncol 12:2723-2736.

Ruegg C, et al, 1998: Evidence for the involvement of endothelial cell integrin alphaVbeta 3 in the disruption of the tumor vasculature induced by TNF and IFN-gamma. Nat Med 4:408-414.

Schwemmle K, et al, 1987: Rationale and indications for perfusion in liver tumors: current data. World J Surg 11:534-540.

Tominaga M, et al, 2004: Kobe strategy with reductive hepatectomy plus percutaneous isolated hepatic perfusion for multiple advanced hepatocellular carcinoma. Syoukakika 39:229-235.

Vahrmeijer AL, et al, 2000: Increased local cytostatic drug exposure by isolated hepatic perfusion: a phase I clinical and pharmacologic evaluation of treatment with high dose melphalan in patients with colorectal cancer confined to the liver. Br J Cancer 82:1539-1546.

79

Intra-arterial Chemotherapy for Liver Tumors

N. E. KEMENY, M. D'ANGELICA, AND P. F. SALDINGER

The liver is an organ with a rich blood supply and the destination of metastases for many tumors. The portal vein drains the entire gastrointestinal tract, and gastrointestinal malignancies frequently produce liver metastases. Because of the dual blood supply and the large blood flow to a receptive environment in the liver, extra-abdominal tumors, such as bronchogenic carcinoma, breast cancer, and malignant melanoma, which spread hematogenously, also metastasize to the liver.

This chapter discusses the use of intra-arterial chemotherapy for the treatment of liver metastases. Because colorectal cancer is one of the most common diseases to have isolated liver metastases, most major studies address liver metastases from colorectal cancer. The use of systemic therapy is not discussed in detail, but a short paragraph is provided to define the response rate and survival so that the work with intrahepatic therapy can be put in perspective.

SYSTEMIC CHEMOTHERAPY

Responses to systemic chemotherapy (SYS) vary with the type of tumor (see Chs. 73a and 77). Patients with breast metastases can have high response rates with SYS (Harris et al, 1997). Only more recently, patients with metastatic colon carcinoma have had response rates greater than 30%. With the development of new drugs, such as irinotecan and oxaliplatin, response rates have increased to 35% to 40% with median survivals of 15 to 19 months (Goldberg et al, 2002; Saltz et al, 2000). The use of antibodies against molecular targets—such as an antibody against vascular endothelial growth factor, bevacizumab—has increased survival to 20 months (Hurwitz et al, 2004). Many chemotherapy trials do not separate out patients with liver-only metastases to show how these patients respond to chemotherapy. In tumors with high response rates, such as breast carcinoma, there is a reasonable response to SYS even in patients with liver metastases, although the response is lower with liver metastases than with soft tissue metastases (George & Hoogstraten, 1978). In patients with colorectal cancer, the liver is the most common site of dissemination, with 60% (Daly & Kemeny, 1986) of patients developing liver metastases during the course of their disease.

RATIONALE FOR HEPATIC ARTERIAL CHEMOTHERAPY

The rationale for hepatic arterial chemotherapy has an anatomic and pharmacologic basis.

1. Liver metastases are perfused almost exclusively by the hepatic artery, whereas normal hepatocytes derive their blood supply from the portal vein and the hepatic artery (Breedis & Young, 1954). After the injection of floxuridine (FUDR) into either the hepatic artery or the portal vein of patients, mean liver concentrations of the drug do not differ depending on the route of injection; however, mean tumor FUDR levels are significantly increased (15-fold) when the drug is injected via the hepatic artery (Sigurdson et al, 1987).

2. The use of drugs that are largely extracted by the liver during the first pass results in high local concentrations of drug with minimal systemic toxicity. Ensminger and colleagues (1978) showed that 94% to 99% of FUDR is extracted by the liver during the first pass compared with 19% to 55% of 5-fluorouracil (5-FU). FUDR is an ideal drug for hepatic arterial chemotherapy. The pharmacologic advantage of various chemotherapeutic agents for hepatic arterial infusion (HAI) is summarized in Table 79.1 (Ensminger & Gyves, 1983).

3. Drugs with a steep dose-response curve are more useful when given by the intrahepatic route because small increases in the concentration of drug that can be given result in a large improvement in response.

4. Drugs with a high total body clearance are more useful for hepatic infusion. The area under the concentration versus time curve is a function not only of drug clearance, but also of hepatic arterial flow. Because hepatic arterial blood flow has a high regional exchange rate (100-1500 mL/min), drugs with a high clearance rate are needed (Collins, 1984). If a drug is not cleared rapidly, recirculation through the systemic circulation mitigates the advantage of intra-arterial therapy over systemic therapy (Collins, 1986).

5. Another rationale for hepatic arterial chemotherapy, especially for patients with metastatic colorectal cancer, is the concept of a stepwise pattern of metastatic progression (Weiss, 1989; Weiss et al, 1986). This theory states that hematogenous spread occurs first via the portal vein to the liver, then from the liver to the lungs, and then to other organs. Aggressive treatment of metastases confined to the liver (i.e., either resection or hepatic infusion) yields prolonged survival for some patients.

The development of a totally implantable infusion pump allowed for the safe administration of hepatic arterial chemotherapy in the outpatient setting (Blackshear et al, 1972). Early trials using an implantable pump and continuous FUDR therapy produced a median response rate of 45% and a median survival of 17 months. To show further that HAI had a therapeutic benefit, randomized studies were conducted.

One of the first randomized trials was conducted at Memorial Sloan-Kettering Cancer Center (MSKCC) (Kemeny N et al, 1987). Before randomization, patients were stratified for extent of liver involvement by tumor and baseline lactate dehydrogenase level, two factors that have been shown to be important prognostic indicators of survival (Table 79.2) (Kemeny N & Braun, 1983;

Table 79.1 Estimated Increase in Hepatic Exposure for Drugs Given by Hepatic Arterial Infusion

Drug	Half-Life (min)	Estimated Increase by Hepatic Arterial Exposure
Fluorouracil	10	5-10 fold
Floxuridine	<10	100-400 fold
Bis-chloroethyl-nitrosourea	<5	6-7 fold
Mitomycin C	<10	6-8 fold
Cisplatin	20-30	4-7 fold
Doxorubicin	60	2-fold
Dichloromethotrexate	—	6-8 fold

Kemeny N et al, 1989). This prospective randomized trial compared HAI with SYS using the same chemotherapeutic agent (FUDR), same drug schedule (a 14-day continuous infusion), and same method of administration (internal pump) in both groups.

Of the 99 evaluable patients, there were 2 complete responses and 23 partial responses (53%) in the group receiving HAI and 10 partial responses (21%) in the SYS group (P=.001). Of the patients randomized to SYS, 31 (60%) crossed over to HAI after tumor progression. Twenty-five percent of these patients went on to a partial response after the crossover, and 60% had a decrease in carcinoembryonic antigen levels.

Toxicity differed between the two groups. An increase in hepatic enzymes and serum bilirubin levels occurred in the HAI group. In the SYS group, diarrhea occurred in 70% of patients, with 9% requiring admission for intravenous hydration. Mucositis occurred in 10% of patients receiving SYS.

The median survival for the HAI and SYS groups was 17 and 12 months (P=.424). The interpretation of survival is difficult in this study because 60% of the patients in the systemic group crossed over. The patients who did not cross over usually had clots of the hepatic arterial system and had a median survival of only 8 months compared with 18 months for the patients who crossed over to hepatic infusion (P=.04). An analysis of baseline

characteristics in the crossover and noncrossover groups revealed no significant differences. Two new European randomized trials using HAI therapy have been published. The first was conducted by the Medical Research Council (MRC) and European Organization for the Research and Treatment of Cancer (EORTC) groups, which compared HAI 5-FU/leucovorin with intravenous 5-FU/leucovorin (Kerr et al, 2003). Crossover from the intravenous to the HAI arm was not allowed. Of 290 patients randomized, only 66% on the HAI arms received treatment. Response rates were 22% for HAI and 19% for intravenous 5-FU/leucovorin. This trial used subcutaneous ports rather than implantable pumps and had significant catheter-related problems (36% of HAI patients) (Kerr et al, 2003). The median survival was 14.7 months and 14.8 months in the HAI and SYS groups (P=.79).

The second trial was by a German Cooperative Group, which randomized 168 patients with unresectable liver metastases from colorectal cancer to HAI of FUDR, HAI of 5-FU/leucovorin, or intravenous 5-FU/leucovorin (Lorenz & Muller, 2000). Response rates were higher in the two HAI arms, with no significant differences in time to progression (the primary end point) or overall survival between the arms. Only 70% of patients on the HAI arms actually received assigned treatment. The study also used ports instead of pumps.

The Cancer and Leukemia Group B (CALGB) (Kemeny N et al, 2005c) completed trial 9481, which compared systemic 5-FU/leucovorin via the Mayo regimen (considered standard of care at the time of trial design) with HAI of FUDR, leucovorin, and dexamethasone, a regimen that had produced high response rates (78%) and lower toxicity (3% biliary sclerosis) in a phase II study (Kemeny N et al, 1994). No crossover was permitted. A total of 134 patients were randomized. Most patients (70%) had greater than 30% liver involvement, had synchronous metastases (78%), and were chemotherapy-naive (97%). Response rates were higher in the HAI group (48% versus 25%; P=.012), although time to progression was not significantly different (5.3 months versus 6.8 months; P=.8), with time to hepatic progression better in the HAI arm (9.8 months versus 7.3 months; P=.017) and time to extrahepatic progression better in the systemic arm (7.7 months versus 14.8 months; P=.029). Median overall survival

Table 79.2 Randomized Studies of Hepatic Arterial Infusion Versus Systemic Chemotherapy for Unresectable Hepatic Metastases

Group (Reference)	No. Patients	HAI Drug	HAI Response (%)	SYSTEMIC Drug	SYSTEMIC Response (%)	P
MSKCC (Kemeny N et al, 1987)	162	FUDR	50	FUDR	20	.001
NCOG (Chang et al, 1987)	143	FUDR	42	FUDR	10	.0001
NCI (Hohn et al, 1989)	64	FUDR	62	FUDR	17	.003
Consortium (Niederhuber, 1987)	43	FUDR	58	FU	38	—
City of Hope (Wagman et al, 1990)	41	FUDR	55	FU	20	—
Mayo Clinic (Martin et al, 1990)	69	FUDR	48	FU	12	.02
French (Rougier et al, 1992)	163	FUDR	44	FU*	—	—
German (Lorenz & Muller, 2000)	168	FUDR	43	FU + leucovorin	22	.009
EORTC (Kerr et al, 2003)	290	FU/leucovorin	22	FU + leucovorin	19	—
CALGB (Kemeny N et al, 2005c)	135	FUDR + dexamethasone + leucovorin	48	FU + leucovorin	26	.012

*Patients treated only when they became symptomatic.

was significantly better in the HAI arm (24.4 months versus 20 months; P=.0013) (Kemeny N et al, 2005b). Resource use, quality of life, and molecular markers of prognosis, such as thymidylate synthase and $p21$ gene expression, were examined prospectively in this study, and final analysis of these factors is presented.

SUMMARY OF RANDOMIZED STUDIES

There are now 11 randomized trials, with 10 showing a significantly higher response rate with HAI versus SYS in patients with hepatic metastases from colorectal carcinoma (see Table 79.2). Whether this increase in response rate translates into increased survival is controversial. Several factors complicate this issue. First, most of the trials contain relatively few patients, and the power to observe differences in survival rates is low. Second, because of early successes with intrahepatic infusion, some of these studies allowed patients in the systemic arm to cross over to intrahepatic therapy after tumor progression on systemic therapy. This crossover may have negated any difference in survival between the two groups. The studies show a survival advantage for the groups that received subsequent HAI, with a mean 1-year survival of 69% for the patients who had crossed over from SYS to HAI versus 35% for the patients who did not cross over (Table 79.3). The European studies are difficult to interpret because in the first two studies the SYS group received SYS only when they became symptomatic. The two new European studies used ports and not pumps, which allows for more technical complications. Two meta-analyses of the original seven trials were conducted, with more than 600 patients included. The Meta-Analysis Group in Cancer (1996) confirmed the increased response rates seen with HAI (41% versus 14%; P=.0009). A second meta-analysis found a 12.5% 1-year (P=.002) and 7.5% 2-year (P=.026) absolute survival difference in favor of HAI versus SYS. A new study from CALGB with pumps and no crossover showed a survival advantage (Kemeny N et al, 2005c).

TOXICITY OF INTRAHEPATIC THERAPY

Table 79.4 summarizes the gastrointestinal toxicities noted by investigators using the implantable pump. The side effects of SYS are almost never observed with HAI. Myelosuppression does not occur with intrahepatic FUDR (Kemeny N et al, 1984).

Although intrahepatic mitomycin C or bis-chloroethyl-nitrosourea may depress platelet counts, the absolute depression and frequency of depression are less than with systemic administration. Nausea, vomiting, and diarrhea do not occur with HAI of FUDR. If diarrhea does occur, shunting of the chemotherapeutic agent to the bowel should be suspected (Gluck et al, 1985). The most common problems with HAI are ulcer disease and hepatic toxicity (Hohn et al, 1985; Kemeny N et al, 1984). Severe ulcer disease results from inadvertent perfusion of the stomach and duodenum with drug via small unligated branches from the hepatic artery and can be prevented by meticulous dissection at the time of pump placement (Hohn et al, 1985). Even without radiologically visible perfusion of the stomach or duodenum, however, mild gastritis and duodenitis can occur. This toxicity can be reduced by careful dose reductions when any gastrointestinal symptoms occur. Hepatobiliary toxicity is the most problematic toxicity seen with HAI. Although there is some evidence of hepatocellular necrosis and cholestasis on liver biopsy specimens (Doria et al, 1986), most studies point to a combined ischemic and inflammatory effect on the bile ducts as the most important cause of this toxicity. The bile ducts are particularly sensitive to HAI because, similar to hepatic tumors, the bile ducts derive their blood supply almost exclusively from the hepatic artery (Northover & Terblanche, 1979).

In patients with severe toxicity, endoscopic retrograde cholangiopancreatography shows lesions resembling primary sclerosing cholangitis (Kemeny MM et al, 1985). Because the ducts are sclerotic and nondilated, ultrasound usually is not helpful. In some patients, the strictures are more focal, usually worse at the bifurcation, and drainage procedures by endoscopic or by percutaneous transhepatic intubation may be helpful. Duct obstruction from metastases should be excluded first by computed tomography (CT) of the liver.

Close monitoring of liver function tests is necessary to avoid biliary sclerosis. If the serum bilirubin becomes elevated, no further treatment should be given until the bilirubin returns to normal and then only with a small test dose (0.05 mg/kg/day). In patients who cannot tolerate even a low dose for 2 weeks, it may be possible to continue treatment by giving the FUDR infusion for 1 week, rather than the usual 2 weeks. At MSKCC, we modify treatment as outlined in Table 79.5.

In older trials, cholecystitis occurred in 33% of patients receiving HAI (Kemeny MM et al, 1986a). In more recent series, the gallbladder was removed at the time of catheter placement to prevent this complication and to avoid the confusion of these symptoms with other hepatic side effects of chemotherapy.

Table 79.3 Summary of Survival in Randomized Trials Comparing Hepatic Arterial Infusion Versus Systemic Chemotherapy

| Group (Reference) | SURVIVAL (% ALIVE) | | | | SURVIVAL (% ALIVE) | | | |
| | 1 YEAR | | 2 YEAR | | 1 YEAR | | 2 YEAR | |
	HAI	Systemic	HAI	Systemic	Crossover	No Crossover	Crossover	No Crossover
MSKCC (Kemeny N et al, 1987)	60	50	25	20	60	28	25	14
NCOG (Hohn et al, 1989)	60	42	30	20	78	42	40	17
NCI* (Chang et al, 1987)	85	60	44	13	—	—	—	—
France (Rougier et al, 1992)	61	44	22	10	—	—	—	—
Mean	66	49	30	18	69	35	37	15

*Excluding patients with metastasis to hepatic lymph nodes.

Table 79.4 Hepatic Arterial Floxuridine Infusion with Internal Pump: Toxicity

Reference	No. Patients	Gastritis (%)	Ulcer (%)	AST (%)	Bilirubin (%)	Diarrhea (%)	Biliary Sclerosis (%)
Niederhuber et al, 1984	70	56	8	32	24	—	—
Balch & Urist, 1986	50	—	6	23	23	0	—
Kemeny N et al, 1984	41	29	29	71	22	0	5
Shepard et al, 1985	53	—	20	49	24	—	—
Cohen et al, 1983	50	—	40	10	25	—	—
Weiss et al, 1983	17	50	11	80	23	23	—
Schwartz et al, 1985	23	53	—	77	20	10	—
Johnson et al, 1983	40	—	8	50	13	0	5
Kemeny MM et al, 1985	31	17	6	47	—	8	19
Hohn et al, 1989	61	35	2	0	78	11	29

AST, aspartate aminotransferase.

SURGICAL TECHNIQUE FOR HEPATIC ARTERY PUMP PLACEMENT

The arterial anatomy of the liver varies (Table 79.6) with normal anatomy present in only about two thirds of patients (Allen et al, 2002). Before consideration of pump placement, it is imperative to carry out a careful review of the arteriogram with the radiologist and formulate a plan for the management of aberrant anatomy. In the past, invasive arteriograms were required, but excellent definition now can be ascertained from CT angiography. In most cases, a pump with a single catheter is adequate to provide access to the entire hepatic arterial inflow. It is preferable not to place the catheter directly into the hepatic artery (which risks thrombosis of the vessel), but instead into an accessible side branch. The gastroduodenal artery is the preferable conduit for the catheter and provides the most reliable method of catheter implantation (Allen et al, 2002). A cholecystectomy should be performed to prevent chemotherapy-induced cholecystitis. Numerous incisions have been employed for this operation with success, including an upper midline incision, right subcostal incision, or limited right subcostal hockey-stick incision. Preoperative intravenous antibiotics at the time of incision are imperative.

For patients with unresectable disease, a staging laparoscopy is advisable to rule out occult extrahepatic disease. In our experience, approximately one third of patients are found to have occult extraheptic metastases precluding the use of a pump (Grobmyer et al, 2004). A thorough examination of the abdomen is performed at laparoscopy and at laparotomy to look for extrahepatic disease. The most common sites of extrahepatic metastases are the peritoneum and portal lymph nodes; a biopsy should be done if the lymph nodes are suspicious because their involvement generally would preclude the use of the pump. The extent of liver involvement should be assessed and documented. Any radiographically occult hepatic tumors should be documented, and the potential for future resection should be addressed specifically in the operative note.

SURGICAL TECHNIQUE FOR STANDARD HEPATIC ARTERIAL ANATOMY

A standard cholecystectomy is performed. The hepatic artery and its branches are circumferentially dissected. The common hepatic artery and the gastroduodenal artery are palpable superior to the body of the pancreas and the first portion of the duodenum. The gastroduodenal artery runs parallel to and lies immediately to the left of the common bile duct. It is advisable to start by dissecting the common hepatic artery to minimize the risk of injuring the bile duct. The right gastric artery is ligated and divided. The distal common hepatic artery, the entire gastroduodenal artery, and the proximal proper hepatic artery are dissected away from their attachments. It is important to mobilize the full length of the extrapancreatic gastroduodenal artery to facilitate insertion of the catheter. Suprapyloric side branches of the gastroduodenal artery are often encountered and must be ligated. Frequently, branches to the pancreas and duodenum arise from any of these dissected vessels, and it is essential to identify and ligate these branches to avoid perfusion of the pancreas, stomach, or duodenum. The common hepatic artery is mobilized 1 cm proximally, and the proper hepatic artery is mobilized about 2 cm distally from the origin of the gastroduodenal artery. Branches to the retroperitoneum from the right or left hepatic artery are common and should be ligated. Review of preoperative angiography to look specifically for these branches is important because they are often found in retrospect. At this point, a complete circumferential dissection of the common hepatic artery, gastroduodenal artery, and proper hepatic artery should be ensured such that no vessels to the pancreas, stomach, or duodenum are present (Fig. 79.1). The gastroduodenal artery should be temporarily occluded with palpation of the proper hepatic artery to rule out retrograde flow to the liver through the gastroduodenal artery secondary to celiac stenosis. No attempt at dissection of the common bile duct is necessary because this risks devascularization and possibly ischemic stricturing.

The pump pocket should be created in the lower abdomen so that the pump lies below the waist and avoids contact with the

Table 79.5 Dose Modification for Hepatic Toxicity

AST	Bilirubin	Alkaline Phosphatase	FUDR Dose (%)
2× baseline	—	—	80
3× baseline	or 1.5×	or 1.5×	50
>3× baseline	or 2×	or 2×	Hold

AST, aspartate aminotransferase.

Table 79.6 Summary of Reported Prevalence of Hepatic Arterial Anatomic Variants

Anatomy	Daly et al, 1984 (*n* = 200)	Michels, 1966 (*n* = 200)	Kemeny MM et al, 1986b (*n* = 100)	Curley et al, 1993 (*n* = 180)	Allen et al, 2002 (*n* = 265)
Normal	70%	55%	50%	63%	63%
Variant GDA	6%	—	9%	9%	11%
Acc RHA	4%	7%	4%	1%	1%
Rep RHA	6%	12%	16%	12%	6%
Acc LHA	3.5%	8%	1%	2%	10%
Rep LHA	4%	10%	16%	11%	4%
Other	5%	2.5%	1%	2%	5%

Acc, accessory; GDA, gastroduodenal artery; LHA, left hepatic artery; Rep, replaced; RHA, right hepatic artery.
From Allen PJ, et al, 2002: The management of variant arterial anatomy during hepatic arterial infusion pump placement. Ann Surg Oncol 9:875-880.

iliac spine and the edge of the ribs. In obese patients, placing the pump over the ribs should be considered because this may help in locating and accessing the pump. The pump and catheter should be handled carefully, avoiding contact with the patient's skin. The catheter is trimmed at a bevel just beyond the last tying ring and is tunneled into the abdominal cavity. The pump is secured to the abdominal fascia with nonabsorbable sutures. The catheter should be positioned behind the pump to prevent injury by a needle. The gastroduodenal artery is ligated with a nonabsorbable tie at its most distal point, and vascular control of the common and proper hepatic arteries is achieved with vascular clamps or vessel loops. Isolated vascular control of the gastroduodenal artery at its orifice also can be used to avoid occlusion of the hepatic artery.

An arteriotomy is made in the distal gastroduodenal artery, and the catheter is inserted up to, but not beyond, the junction with the hepatic artery (Fig. 79.2). If the catheter protrudes into the common hepatic artery, turbulence of blood flow can lead to thrombosis of the vessel. Failure to pass the catheter to the junction leaves a short segment of the gastroduodenal artery exposed to full concentrations of FUDR without the diluting effect of blood flow, potentially resulting in sclerosis, thrombosis, or

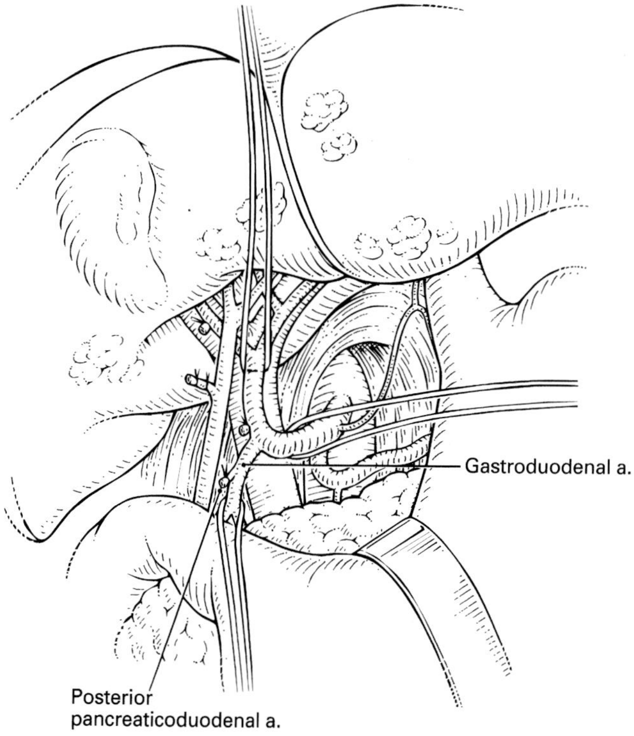

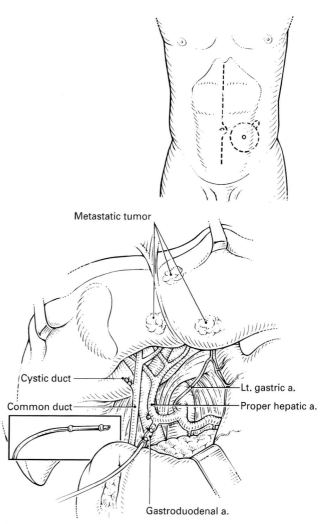

Fig. 79.1. The common hepatic, proper hepatic, and gastroduodenal arteries are completely mobilized. All branches to the stomach, duodenum, or pancreas are identified and ligated.

Fig. 79.2. The infusion pump ideally is placed in the left lower quadrant, away from the liver to avoid artifacts on subsequent CT scans. With normal anatomy, the catheter is placed in the gastroduodenal artery and secured with nonabsorbable ties. The right gastric artery is ligated. The gallbladder is removed.

late dislodgment. When positioned, the catheter should be secured two or three times with nonabsorbable ties proximal to the tying rings on the catheter. Perfusion of both lobes of the liver and lack of extrahepatic perfusion is confirmed by infusing 2 to 3 mL of half-strength fluorescein through the pump and visualization with a Wood's lamp. Half-strength methylene blue injection is an alternative method of ensuring proper perfusion. After the perfusion test, the catheter is flushed with heparinized saline, and the wounds are closed. Antibiotic coverage should be continued for 2 to 3 days postoperatively because the consequence of a pump infection is so serious. Any sign of erythema indicating a wound infection postoperatively should be treated immediately and aggressively.

SURGICAL TECHNIQUE FOR ABERRANT HEPATIC ARTERIAL ANATOMY

As discussed earlier, aberrant hepatic arterial anatomy is common, and numerous variations occur. Each anatomic situation is specifically addressed here, but first general principles in managing variant anatomy are discussed. In analyses of our extensive experience with this operation, the most consistent factor associated with catheter-related complications and decreased durability of the catheter is cannulation of a vessel other than the gastroduodenal artery. The overall preferred technique is placement of the catheter in the gastroduodenal artery with ligation of the isolated variant vessel. This method relies on intrahepatic collateral development and cross-perfusion to the liver fed by the ligated vessel. Although there have been concerns over incomplete hepatic perfusion with this technique, it is rare. In our published experience with this operation for variant anatomy, incomplete hepatic perfusion occurred once in 52 cases. This cross-perfusion sometimes can take 4 weeks to occur, and early perfusion scans may be initially abnormal and should be rechecked in a few weeks to assess for the cross-perfusion because most normalize (Allen et al, 2002; Curley et al, 1993). The only exception to this rule may be in patients with large central tumors that can act to impede cross-collateralization. Lastly, although cross-perfusion after ligation of aberrant vessels is highly reliable, it has not been proved that equal blood flow for chemotherapy delivery develops.

Aberrant Origin of the Gastroduodenal Artery

The gastroduodenal artery can arise from the right or left hepatic artery, or there can be a trifurcation in which the gastroduodenal artery, right hepatic artery, and left hepatic artery all arise simultaneously from the common hepatic artery. This anomaly occurs 6% to 11% of the time (Allen et al, 2002). In general, it is always preferable to place the catheter into the gastroduodenal artery and ligate vessels that are not receiving catheter-directed flow because this is the technique associated with the lowest rate of cather-related complications (Allen et al, 2002, 2005). In the case of a trifurcation, the catheter should be placed in the gastroduodenal artery, and perfusion should be tested with fluoroscein or methylene blue. If there is good bilobar perfusion, ligation of vessels is unnecessary. If at testing there is no perfusion of one lobe of the liver, the hepatic artery to that lobe should be ligated (most commonly the left hepatic artery) relying on cross-perfusion. The hepatic arterial tree also may be accessed through the splenic artery just to the left of the celiac axis. The catheter is placed in the splenic artery and floated across the celiac axis to lie freely in the hepatic artery, ending proximal to the bifurcation. The gastroduodenal artery and the right gastric artery are ligated, and the catheter is secured doubly in the splenic artery. This technique is technically difficult, requiring extensive dissection of the celiac axis and floating a catheter across the celiac branching. This technique also is associated with more complications, including thrombosis and extrahepatic perfusion, and is rarely used. Another option is retrograde cannulation of the common hepatic artery through the gastroduodenal artery into the common hepatic artery with an attached short, stiff, small-gauge catheter. The technique also is associated with a higher rate of complications, including arterial dissection and thrombosis, and is rarely, if ever, used.

Accessory Left Hepatic Artery

An accessory left hepatic artery arises from the left gastric artery, crosses the gastrohepatic ligament, enters the liver at the base of the umbilical fissure, and typically supplies segments II and III. The native left hepatic artery, which arises from the proper hepatic artery, also supplies the left liver (typically segment IV in this situation). This abnormality is present in 2% to 10% of cases. The simplest, safest, and most reliable option is to ligate the accessory left hepatic artery and place the pump catheter in the gastroduodenal artery because cross-perfusion is highly reliable. Another possibility is the use of two catheters (or pumps), one in the gastroduodenal artery and one in the accessory left hepatic artery. This is a cumbersome technique, however, and generally not used.

Accessory Right Hepatic Artery

Accessory right hepatic arteries arise from the superior mesenteric artery and run in the portacaval space to supply a portion of the right lobe of the liver. This abnormality is present 1% to 7% of the time. Accessory and replaced right hepatic arteries rarely have side branches adequate for cannulation. The preferred technique in this situation is placement of the catheter in the gastroduodenal artery and ligating the accessory vessel because cross-perfusion is reliable. Placing a second catheter directly in the accessory vessel is another option, but generally unnecessary and inadvisable.

Replaced Left Hepatic Artery

A replaced left hepatic artery arises from the left gastric artery and supplies the left liver. There is no native left hepatic artery. This abnormality is present 4% to 16% of the time. The preferred technique is to place the catheter in the gastroduodenal artery and ligate the replaced left hepatic artery. Initial reports on this specific situation suggested rates of incomplete cross-perfusion of 40% (Cohen et al, 1987). More recent reports, including our experience, show that incomplete cross-perfusion is uncommon in this situation and occurred in only 1 of 10 of our patients at last analysis (Allen et al, 2002; Curley et al, 1993). Other techniques, such as placing catheters in the gastroduodenal artery and in a branch of the replaced left hepatic artery, can be considered in patients with bulky disease in the left liver or with a large central tumor that may impede cross-perfusion.

Replaced Right Hepatic Artery

A replaced right hepatic artery originates from the superior mesenteric artery, runs in the portacaval space, and supplies the whole right liver. No branches to the right liver originate from the proper hepatic artery. This anatomic situation occurs 6% to 16% of the time. If the surgeon ligates the replaced right hepatic artery, cross-perfusion from the left hepatic artery occurs almost uniformly (Allen et al, 2002; Cohen et al, 1987; Curley et al, 1993). The catheter should be placed in the gastroduodenal artery, and the replaced right hepatic artery should be ligated. Other techniques, such as placing a second catheter in the replaced right hepatic artery directly through a small arteriotomy (there are no significant side branches from this vessel), have been described, but are rarely, if ever, indicated. This technique requires that the catheter be trimmed flush just beyond the tying ring, and the catheter be placed such that the ring lies just inside the vessel and the arteriotomy is closed over the ring.

PUMP PLACEMENT AFTER MAJOR HEPATECTOMY

In the event that a pump is being placed after a hepatectomy for adjuvant therapy, the anatomy to the remnant liver must be specifically considered. In general, the best results are obtained if the catheter is placed in the gastroduodenal artery. When there are replaced or accessory vessels to the remnant liver, the surgeon must consider the condition of that remnant (i.e., steatosis, congestion) and the potential risk of ligating arterial supply or risking thrombosis by directly cannulating the vessel to the remnant. One option that is often available after a hemihepatectomy is to use the stump of the artery to the removed liver as a conduit for the catheter if the anatomy allows this. If the arterial anatomy is normal, or there is a trifurcation at the gastroduodenal artery, there is generally no issue, and the catheter is placed routinely in the gastroduodenal artery. If there is a variation of the origin of the gastroduodenal artery (i.e., off of the right or left hepatic artery), care must be taken to preserve the origin such that the catheter can be placed. For a remnant right lobe, an accessory right artery generally can be ligated, unless there are major concerns about the condition of the remnant. In the case of a remnant right lobe and a replaced right hepatic artery, it is generally not recommended to place a pump because it would require direct cannulation of that artery risking thrombosis, injury, and in general a higher rate of catheter-related complications. For a remnant left lobe, an accessory left artery generally can be ligated. If the remnant left lobe is fed solely by a replaced left hepatic artery, a pump can be placed, but this requires dissection of the left gastric artery and a suitable side branch for the catheter. Special care must be taken to ensure that all branches to the stomach have been properly ligated to prevent extrahepatic perfusion.

POSTOPERATIVE ASSESSMENT

After surgery and before administering chemotherapy, the distribution of arterial perfusion is assessed by a radionuclide pump flow study. A baseline technetium 99m (^{99m}Tc) sulfur-colloid scan is obtained to identify the liver outline. Pump perfusion is assessed by infusing 3 to 5 mCi of ^{99m}Tc-labeled macroaggregated albumin (MAA) through the bolus port of the pump and into the hepatic artery. When the MAA scan produces an image that matches the sulfur-colloid liver scan, the pump is perfusing the entire liver as intended. Perfusion of extrahepatic tissues produces ^{99m}Tc signals outside of the liver image (Fig. 79.3). Incomplete perfusion of the liver produces an incomplete image of the liver on MAA scan. Misperfusion is discovered in 5% to 7% of cases and often can be corrected by surgical or angiographic intervention to occlude additional hepatic vessels missed at operation (Campbell et al, 1993). If there are no additional vessels on angiography for embolization, it is worth repeating the scan in a few weeks to allow sufficient time for intrahepatic collaterals and cross-perfusion to develop (Allen et al, 2002).

TECHNICAL COMPLICATIONS OF HEPATIC ARTERY INFUSION PUMP PLACEMENT

Surgical and technical complications of pump placement occur, and the spectrum and frequency of these complications need to be understood by the surgeon, the medical oncologist, and the patient before initiating treatment. To assess the risks of insertion and the use of an implantable pump for hepatic artery chemotherapy, we reviewed the charts of all patients who underwent pump insertion for unresectable metastases over a 15-year period (1986-2001) at MSKCC (Allen et al, 2005). During this period, 544 infusion pumps were inserted by several different surgeons for HAI of FUDR alone or in combination with other drugs for patients with isolated unresectable colorectal hepatic metastases. Variant arterial anatomy was present in 205 patients (38%), most of which (82%) involved a single vessel. A colectomy was performed in addition to the pump placement in 136 patients (25%).

Operative mortality is generally low. In our series, five patients died within 30 days of the operation (0.9% mortality rate). Early in our series, two deaths were from hepatic failure secondary to extensive metastatic disease within the liver. We now exclude patients with extensive (>70%) liver replacement from pump placement because of this risk. Generalized operative morbidity unrelated to the pump itself occurred in approximately 25% of patients in our series. The most common complications were prolonged ileus, wound complications, atelectasis, and abscesses.

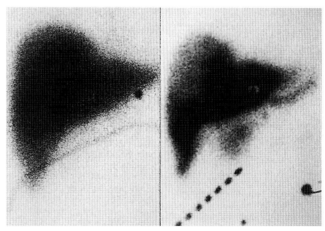

Fig. 79.3. The liver-spleen technetium sulfur-colloid scan on the left shows the normal liver. The MAA scan on the right shows extrahepatic perfusion to the duodenum and head of the pancreas.

Table 79.7 Postoperative Pump-Related Complications and Salvage Rates in 544 Hepatic Artery Infusion Pump Placements

Type of Complication	Total (N)	EARLY (<30 DAYS)		LATE (>30 DAYS)	
		n	% Salvaged	n	% Salvaged
Pump malfunction	6	6	100	—	—
Pocket					
Infection	14	4	50	10	40
Hematoma	1	1	100	—	—
Pump migration	4	1	100	3	33
Catheter					
Occlusion	11	—	—	11	36
Dislodgment	18	—	—	18	11
Erosion	4	—	—	4	0
Arterial					
Hemorrhage	1	1	100	—	—
Thrombosis	33	13	31	20	30
Extrahepatic perfusion	16	9	100	7	57
Incomplete perfusion	12	9	78	3	67
Overall	*120*	*44*	*70*	*76*	*30*

From Allen PJ, et al, 2005: Technical complications and durability of hepatic artery infusion pumps for unresectable colorectal liver metastases: an institutional experience of 544 consecutive cases. J Am Coll Surg 201:57-65.

In our series, pump-related morbidity occurred in 120 patients (22%) and is summarized in Table 79.7. Most of these complications (63%) occurred later than 30 days after pump placement. The most common complications (51%) were related to the hepatic arterial system and included thrombosis, hemorrhage, or perfusion abnormalities. Early (<30 days) pump-related morbidity occurred in only 8% of cases. All of the catheter-related complications occurred after 30 days. Overall, the pumps were salvaged from these complications 45% of the time. Salvage was much more common with early complications (70% if <30 days) than with late complications (30% if after 30 days). In a multivariate analysis, surgeon experience and the use of any vessel other than the gastroduodenal artery were independently associated with pump-related morbidity and pump survival. Pump failure was generally low and was 5% at 6 months, 9% at 1 year, 16% at 2 years, and 26% at 3 years. HAI was discontinued for pump-related complications in 9% of cases. The performance of a concomitant colorectal resection was not associated with a higher rate of complications.

Extrahepatic Perfusion

Small branches of the hepatic artery to the stomach, duodenum, and pancreas can be missed on preoperative angiography. If small vessels are not divided and ligated, perfusion of the bowel with FUDR produces severe pain, gastrointestinal ulceration, and, if the pancreas is perfused, severe pancreatitis. These complications are potentially lethal, and extrahepatic perfusion should be identified and corrected before onset of chemotherapy whenever possible.

If extrahepatic perfusion is seen on the ^{99m}Tc MAA scan, the next step is to perform an angiogram by bolus injection through the pump. The angiogram usually shows the unligated vessel that is the cause of extrahepatic perfusion. This is occasionally unsuccessful, and a transfemoral celiac or superior mesenteric artery study is needed to identify the problem (Fig. 79.4). We have used initial transfemoral angiograms for assessment of cases in which the perfusion scan shows obvious extrahepatic perfusion. This approach simplifies the process in that one procedure is

done to diagnose the problem definitively and potentially to treat it. In our review of 544 cases, 9 patients (2%) were found to have extrahepatic perfusion on the postoperative scan. The cause was identified arteriographically and in seven cases was corrected with transarterial embolization or surgical ligation. These seven patients went on to receive HAI without complication (Allen et al, 2005).

Incomplete Perfusion

In nine cases (2%), the postoperative ^{99m}Tc MAA scan showed incomplete perfusion of the liver. The causes included failure to ligate a replaced or accessory hepatic artery and failure to achieve cross-perfusion after ligation of an accessory artery (in one case).

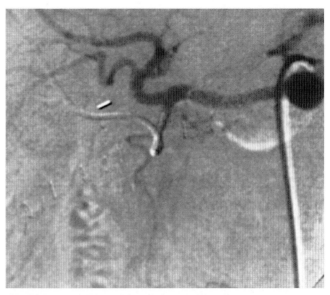

Fig. 79.4. A transfemoral celiac angiogram shows a vessel arising from the gastroduodenal artery, which had not been ligated. At operation, this vessel was found to be arising from the posterior aspect of the gastroduodenal artery.

In every case, the anatomic problem was identified by a side port or transfemoral angiogram. Overall, seven of the nine cases were corrected with embolization or surgical ligation of the accessory vessel, and chemotherapy was administered without a problem. In the instance of incomplete crossover perfusion, collateral flow developed over time to the remaining liver. A repeat MAA scan in 4 weeks confirmed the development of collateral blood flow.

Gastroduodenal Ulcers

In rare instances, the ^{99m}Tc MAA scan fails to identify subtle extrahepatic perfusion. The most frequent anomaly is a small branch to the lesser curve of the stomach. Early in our experience, we treated three patients who were clinically shown to have extrahepatic perfusion that was not apparent on ^{99m}Tc MAA scan, even in retrospect. The patients developed severe epigastric pain during the first course of chemotherapy. Endoscopy showed large ulcers in the stomach or duodenum. These patients do not respond to standard ulcer medication because the cause of their ulcer is not acid secretion, but loss of the gastroduodenal mucosa in the area perfused with FUDR. The diagnosis is confirmed by angiography, and treatment requires angiography or laparotomy

for identification and ligation of the vessel. When the ulcer has healed, chemotherapy can be given safely. If a patient develops unexplained epigastric pain during infusional chemotherapy, the pump should be emptied immediately and refilled with heparinized saline until the cause of the pain can be elucidated.

Arterial or Catheter Thrombosis

Complete dissection and thrombosis of the hepatic artery intraoperatively has been described during pump insertion, but this condition is rare. In our series, 13 cases (2%) of acute postoperative arterial thrombosis were noted. The technical problem leading to thrombosis was uncertain in most of these cases. Of these 13 cases of early thrombosis, 31% were salvaged with anticoagulation or lytic therapy. We also observed that delayed thrombosis of the hepatic artery (20 cases) was more common than acute thrombosis (13 cases). The vasculitis caused by infusional chemotherapy is thought to contribute to late arterial thrombosis. Often, arterial thrombosis manifests as extrahepatic perfusion on ^{99m}Tc MAA scan (Fig. 79.5). Catheter thrombosis was seen only as a late complication. Catheter thrombosis occurred in 11 cases (2%) and was more likely to be related to technical errors, such as not

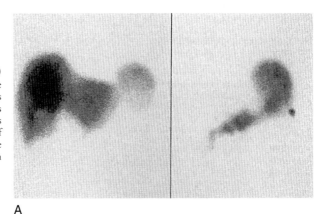

Fig. 79.5. A, When hepatic artery thrombosis occurs, the MAA scan *(right)* shows an absence of perfusion of the liver, together with perfusion of the spleen, stomach, and pancreas. **B,** Arteriogram before operation shows normal patent vessels *(left)*, but postoperative arteriography *(right)* confirms that the artery is thrombosed. The first sign of hepatic artery thrombosis may be abdominal pain occurring with chemotherapy owing to perfusion of the stomach and pancreas. If severe pain occurs during chemotherapy, the first step should be to empty the pump and replace the chemotherapy with heparinized saline.

A

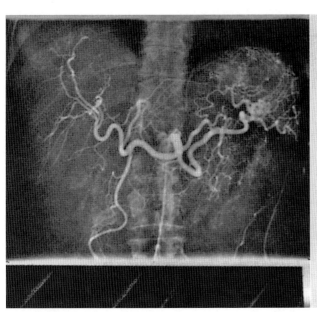

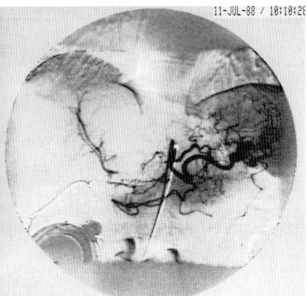

B

filling the pump frequently or allowing back-bleeding into the catheter during side port manipulation.

Infectious Complications

Infectious complications associated with any major operation may occur after laparotomy and pump placement, including pneumonia, urinary tract infections, and wound infections. Because a foreign body is inserted during this operation, particular care must be directed against wound or pump pocket infections. Technical precautions need to be taken in the operating room to limit bacterial contamination of the pump. Postoperatively, any sign of pump pocket redness should be treated early and aggressively with parenteral antibiotics.

We have not seen an increased incidence of complications in patients undergoing pump insertion during a colectomy. It is preferable to place the pump first, close the pump pocket, exclude the catheter from the rest of the procedure, and then proceed with the colectomy. In this way, the instruments and the wound have not been contaminated by the open bowel. Because this approach violates the principle of treating the primary problem first, the surgeon may choose to mobilize the bowel initially. In this manner, the colectomy can be performed rapidly and safely should the patient have difficulty on the operating table.

Hemorrhagic Complications

Two patients developed bleeding complications postoperatively. In one case, the patient developed severe abdominal pain when the pump was injected for the initial ^{99m}Tc MAA scan. On the flow scan, extrahepatic extravasation of ^{99m}Tc was seen. At laparotomy, bleeding from a suprapyloric branch that had been inadequately clipped during the operation was observed. A second patient developed bleeding into the pump pocket resulting in a hematoma. Both complications were salvaged, and the pumps were used successfully.

LAPAROSCOPIC PLACEMENT OF HEPATIC ARTERIAL INFUSION PUMPS

The necessity of a laparotomy to place HAI pumps has been and remains a hurdle for this therapy. Because a major operation is mandated as part of the therapy, many oncologists and patients have been deterred, and minimally invasive methods of pump implantation are attractive. HAI pump placement requires substantial skill, sophisticated knowledge of upper gastrointestinal anatomy, and experience, making this operation technically challenging and difficult to perform laparoscopically.

The technique of laparoscopic HAI pump placement should mimic the open operation. Review of the preoperative angiogram is crucial, and management of aberrant anatomy must be planned for in advance. A right subcostal port is placed for retraction of the liver, and a three-port working triangle is created in the left upper quadrant aiming at the porta hepatis. The dissection and isolation of the vessels is exactly the same as the open operation. Ultrasonic dissectors are helpful to divide the often dense lymphatics and keeps bleeding to a minimum. Branches to the stomach, duodenum, or pancreas can be clipped or divided with the ultrasonic dissector; patience is crucial because controlling torn branches

can be difficult. When the anatomy is dissected, the pump pocket is made in the right abdominal wall, and the catheter is placed into the peritoneal cavity under laparoscopic visualization. The distal gastroduodenal artery is ligated, and ties are left long for countertraction. Laparoscopic bulldogs are used for vascular isolation; two can be placed on the common hepatic artery and proper hepatic artery each, or a single clamp can be placed just at the orifice of the gastroduodenal artery. A tie is left around the gastroduodenal artery in anticipation of tying the catheter in, and a laparoscopic No. 11 blade is used to create an arteriotomy. Using countertraction on the gastroduodenal artery, the catheter is placed into the gastroduodenal artery up to the orifice and tied into place. The clamps are carefully removed, and hemostasis is ensured. We test perfusion with half-strength methylene blue through the pump and confirm bilobar hepatic perfusion and lack of extrahepatic perfusion.

Published experience with laparoscopic placement of HAI pumps is largely limited to small cases series (Cheng et al, 2003, 2004; Feliciotti et al, 1996; Urbach & Hansen, 2000; Urbach et al, 2001). The largest series to date was published by Cheng and coworkers and describes their experience in 38 patients (Cheng et al, 2004). Of 38 patients, 24 had additional radiofrequency ablation, and 2 had a laparosopic partial hepatectomy. There was one conversion to laparotomy, and the median time in the operating room was 5.5 hours. Overall, their results were excellent; there was one postoperative cardiac-related mortality, but no pump-related morbidity, and the median hospital stay was 3 days. Over a 2-year period at MSKCC, we have attempted laparoscopic pump placement in 13 cases. Five cases were converted for minor bleeding, severe chronic cholecystitis, bowel injury, dense adhesions, and a small gastroduodenal artery that could not be cannulated at open operation. Eight cases were completed laparoscopically with no significant moribidy, no pump-related complications, and a median hospital stay of 3.5 days (unpublished data). With limited experience, it seems that laparoscopic HAI pump placement is feasible and safe. It is crucial, however, that these cases are attempted by surgeons experienced in laparoscopic surgery and open pump placement.

NONOPERATIVE PLACEMENT OF HEPATIC ARTERIAL INFUSION PUMPS

HAI pump placement can be done safely by laparotomy with an acceptable morbidity (see earlier). Poor overall prognosis and the requirement for a laparotomy has deterred many surgeons and oncologists from using this modality, however. Several groups have worked on alternate placement methods to eliminate the laparotomy "hurdle."

Percutaneous techniques to catheterize the hepatic artery for delivery of intrahepatic chemotherapy have been developed using a variety of peripheral arteries for access (Table 79.8). Most of these techniques have been abandoned or are used only by a few specialized groups for the following reasons:

1. The insertion is technically difficult and sometimes cumbersome. The technique described by Arai and coworkers (Arai, 1988; Arai et al, 1997; Inaba et al, 1998) requires embolization of the gastroduodenal artery to anchor the catheter. The tip of the catheter remains anchored in the gastroduodenal artery, while perfusion is done through a side hole in the catheter.

Table 79.8 Peripheral Arteries Used for Catheter Placement in the Hepatic Artery

Artery	Reference
Femoral artery	Matsumada et al, 1997
Brachial artery	Cohen et al, 1980
Axillary artery	Arai, 1988; Cohen et al, 1983
Subclavian artery	Arai, 1988; Arai et al, 1997, 1998; Inaba et al, 1998
Hypogastric artery	Arai et al, 1997, 1988; Inaba et al, 1998
Intercostal artery	Castaing et al, 1998; Saldinger & Sandhu, 2004

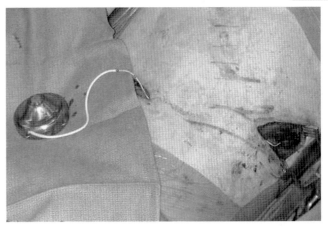

Fig. 79.6. The indwelling arterial catheter is tunneled from the insertion site at the 11th rib to the left upper quadrant, where it is connected to the catheter of the infusion pump via a connector. The pump is placed into a pocket in the subcutaneous tissue.

2. The insertion site is in a mobile part of the body, such as the arm or the leg, resulting in catheter dislocation or migration (Oberfield et al, 1979).
3. The artery used for access is "essential" to a limb, and any thrombotic complication could result in a loss of limb (see Table 79.8).

Castaing and coworkers (1998) tried to address these shortfalls by using an intercostal artery as conduit. A cutdown is performed over the 10th left rib. The intercostal artery is catheterized, and the catheter is advanced, under fluoroscopic control, across the aorta into the ostium of the celiac axis and ultimately into the proper hepatic artery just beyond the takeoff of the gastroduodenal artery. The catheter is connected to an implantable port located in the left upper quadrant. The study included 35 patients with metastatic lesions to the liver, mainly from colorectal cancer. Thirty patients (86%) underwent a successful placement. Placement was not feasible in five patients because of an unsuitable artery. There was no procedure-associated mortality. There were no thrombotic complications in either the aorta or the hepatic artery. There also was no dislocation or migration of the catheter. Follow-up was brief because most of these patients died from their disease. All of the patients had failed previous standard treatments and had advanced disease at the time of catheter placement.

This method has clear advantages because of its simplicity and the fact that the catheter is attached to an immobile part of the body excluding catheter motion. Catheter patency was less than 50% at 4 months likely as a result of a lack of continuous flow. Also, the catheter used in Castaing's study is not Food and Drug Administration approved for prolonged indwelling use, and the method is not applicable in the United States.

Our group modified Castaing's method to address these points (Saldinger & Sandhu, 2004). A 3-Fr peripherally inserted central catheter was chosen as the indwelling arterial catheter (Arrow International, Reading, PA). We used a 15-mL Codman 3000 constant flow implantable pump for access and drug delivery (Codman, Raynham, MA). The pump catheter and arterial catheter were connected via a special connector (Arrow International, Walpole, MA) (Fig. 79.6). Our method uses largely the same techniques as described by Castaing, but for a few differences.

1. A preoperative angiogram is obtained for mapping of the hepatic vessels (Fig. 79.7). The angiogram is saved and used during the procedure as a guide. Accessory hepatic arteries are embolized to optimize pump perfusion, and the gastroduodenal artery is embolized if the distance between the gastroduodenal artery and the hepatic bifurcation is deemed too short posing a risk for nondelivery of the target drug.

2. The intercostal artery is accessed by micropuncture followed by introduction of a sheath. This sheath allows repeated introduction of wires should the situation require it. A guidewire is introduced and placed into the hepatic artery (Fig. 79. 8). The 3-Fr catheter is advanced into the hepatic artery, the wire is withdrawn, and the catheter is secured (Fig. 79.9). An on-table angiogram is obtained through the catheter to confirm proper placement. We confirm catheter placement and exclude extrahepatic perfusion the next day with a perfusion scan. The pump is filled the same day with chemotherapy.

This procedure has been performed successfully in four patients with metastatic colon cancer to the liver as part of a feasibility study. All patients had failed at least two chemotherapeutic regimens and were unresectable. There were no perioperative deaths or complications. The catheters remained patent until the patient's

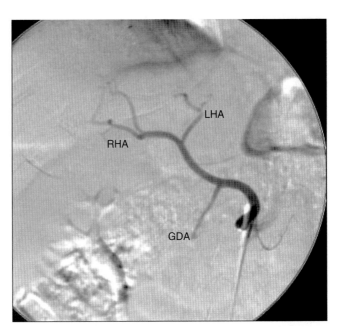

Fig. 79.7. Transfemoral celiac arteriogram mapping the hepatic arterial anatomy. GDA, gastroduodenal artery; LHA, left hepatic artery; RHA, right hepatic artery.

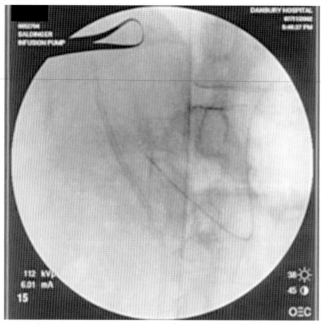

Fig. 79.8. Fluoroscopic control of guidewire placement. Note the course of the wire outlining its entrance into the aorta and exit into the celiac axis and finally hepatic artery.

death, from progression of disease, at 1, 3, 6, and 7 months. The nonoperative placement of HAI pumps is a safe method and has all the advantages of minimally invasive procedures. Its role in the armamentarium of therapies to treat metastatic colorectal cancer to the liver depends largely on the role of intra-arterial chemotherapy for liver tumors.

APPROACHES TO DECREASE HEPATIC TOXICITY

New approaches to decrease the hepatic toxicity induced by HAI FUDR are being studied. Because portal triad inflammation may lead to ischemia and stricturing of the bile ducts, the hepatic arterial administration of dexamethasone may decrease

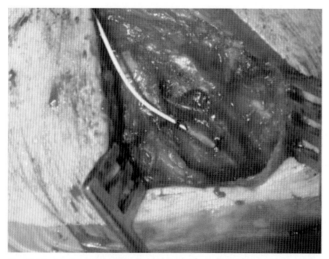

Fig. 79.9. A 3-Fr catheter secured to the intercostal artery. The inferior border of the 11th rib has been exposed allowing exposure of the intercostal artery and vein.

biliary toxicity. A prospective double-blind randomized study of intrahepatic FUDR with dexamethasone versus FUDR alone was conducted at MSKCC. The response rate in 49 evaluable patients was 71% for the FUDR plus dexamethasone group versus 40% for FUDR alone (P=.03). Survival also favored the FUDR plus dexamethasone group: 23 months versus 15 months for FUDR alone. In addition, there was a trend toward decreased bilirubin elevation in patients receiving FUDR plus dexamethasone compared with the group receiving FUDR alone (9% versus 30%; P=.07).

A second method to decrease hepatic toxicity is the use of circadian modification of hepatic intra-arterial FUDR infusion. In a retrospective, nonrandomized study (Hrushesky et al, 1990), a comparison of constant (flat) infusion versus circadian modified HAI FUDR was conducted in 50 patients. Over nine courses of treatment, the patients with circadian-modified infusion tolerated almost twice the daily dose of FUDR. Circadian-modified infusion resulted in 46% of patients having no hepatic toxicity versus 16% of patients after flat FUDR infusion. The authors did not present information on response rates achieved in both groups.

Another approach to decrease toxicity from HAI is to alternate intra-arterial FUDR with intra-arterial FU. Weekly intra-arterial bolus of FU has similar activity to intra-arterial FUDR and does not cause hepatobiliary toxicity; however, it frequently produces treatment-limiting systemic toxicity or arteritis. Stagg and colleagues (1991) used an alternating HAI FUDR and HAI FU regimen, with a response rate of 51% and median survival of 22.4 months. In contrast to the experience with single-agent HAI FUDR, no patient had treatment terminated because of drug toxicity.

METHODS TO INCREASE RESPONSE RATE

Based on the fact that systemic combination chemotherapy regimens are more effective than single agents, the potential benefit of multidrug HAI is being evaluated. In an early study using mitomycin C, bis-chloroethyl-nitrosourea, and FUDR, Cohen and associates (1985) produced a 69% partial response rate. In a randomized trial at MSKCC comparing this three-drug regimen with FUDR alone (Kemeny N et al, 1993), the response rates were 45% for the three-drug regimen and 32% for FUDR alone in the 67 patients who entered this trial. The median survivals from the initiation of HAI were 18.9 months and 14.9 months. Other trials using FUDR and leucovorin produced a 62% response rate.

METHODS TO TREAT EXTRAHEPATIC DISEASE

Extrahepatic disease develops in 40% to 70% of patients undergoing HAI. Such metastases can occur even when the patient is still responding in the liver. In many patients, extrahepatic disease is the cause of death. Safi and coworkers (1989) studied the ability of concomitant SYS to reduce the development of extrahepatic metastases in patients receiving HAI. Ninety-five patients were randomized to intra-arterial FUDR (0.2 mg/kg/day for 14 of 28 days) or a combination of intra-arterial FUDR (0.21 mg/kg/day) and intravenous FUDR (0.09 mg/kg/day) given concurrently for 14 of 28 days (intra-arterial/intravenous). The response rates were 60% for both arms of the study. The incidence of extrahepatic disease was significantly less, however, in patients receiving the intra-arterial/intravenous treatment (56%) compared with intra-arterial treatment (79%; *P*<.01). No significant difference in survival was found between the two groups (*P*=.08). The results of this trial warrant further study of combined systemic/intra-arterial regimens.

COMBINED HEPATIC ARTERIAL INFUSION AND SYSTEMIC CHEMOTHERAPY

Irinotecan is a topoisomerase I inhibitor with proven efficacy in first-line and second-line treatment of metastatic colorectal carcinoma. The activity of irinotecan is not inhibited by high thymidylate synthase activity (Saltz et al, 1998); combining systemic irinotecan with HAI therapy may result in improved control of extrahepatic disease. In a phase I study at MSKCC, 38 patients with unresectable liver metastases received HAI of FUDR/dexamethasone and systemic irinotecan in escalating doses. All patients were previously treated, and 16 had prior therapy with irinotecan. The regimen was well tolerated, with dose-limiting toxicities of diarrhea and myelosuppression. The response rate was 74%, median time to progression was 8.1 months, and median survival presently is 20 months. Thirteen of 16 patients who had previously received irinotecan had partial responses (Kemeny N et al, 2001).

Another nonrandomized study used HAI of FUDR with systemic irinotecan as adjuvant therapy after cytoreduction of unresectable hepatic colorectal carcinoma metastases. The cytoreduction was defined as using cryosurgery, radiofrequency ablation, partial resection, or some combination to treat all identifiable sites of disease. Seventy-one patients received adjuvant therapy and were compared with a historical control group receiving cytoreduction alone. Time to progression was 19 months versus 10 months and median survival was 30.6 months versus 20 months for HAI versus control groups (Bilchik et al, 2000).

Oxaliplatin is a new cytotoxic agent with a mechanism of action similar to that of other platinum derivatives, but with a different spectrum of activity and toxicity. When combined with 5-FU/leucovorin, clinical response rates have been greater than 50%, with median survival of 16.2 months in untreated patients with metastatic colorectal carcinoma (de Gramont et al, 2000; Tournigand et al, 2004). Preliminary studies using systemic oxaliplatin-based regimens combined with HAI of FUDR have shown the feasibility and safety of this approach and reveal promising early results (Pancera et al, 2002). In the MSKCC phase I study, 21 previously treated patients (74% prior irinotecan) with unresectable hepatic metastases received HAI of FUDR/dexamethasone plus systemic oxaliplatin with either 5-FU/leucovorin

or irinotecan. Both regimens have been well tolerated, and response rates are 90% and 88% (Table 79.9) (Kemeny N et al, 2005c). The high response rate and survival for second-line therapy with HAI plus SYS has not been reproduced by these new drugs alone.

ADJUVANT TREATMENT AFTER LIVER RESECTION OF COLORECTAL METASTASES

The rationale for the use of adjuvant chemotherapy after resection of liver metastases from colorectal cancer is based on this fact: Although some patients are cured, after resection many patients experience recurrence in the liver alone, some experience recurrence with extrahepatic and intrahepatic disease, and some experience recurrence with extrahepatic disease alone. An effective adjuvant treatment may have a substantial impact on recurrence and survival. The use of SYS has been formally tested in this setting only to a very limited extent with one randomized study (Portier et al, 2002), which failed to show a survival benefit with a 5-FU–based regimen. A current EORTC study is randomizing patients to preoperative and postoperative chemotherapy with 5-FU/leucovorin compared with resection alone.

Because HAI and SYS may be useful in decreasing recurrence, four reasonably large randomized trials have been conducted in this group of patients (Table 79.10). In the MSKCC study (Kemeny N et al, 1999), 156 patients with resected hepatic metastases were randomized to 6 months of systemic 5-FU/leucovorin or systemic 5-FU/leucovorin plus HAI with FUDR. Primary end points were 2-year overall and progression-free survival. Forty percent of patients received prior adjuvant chemotherapy after resection of their primary colorectal carcinoma, and 15% had received prior chemotherapy as treatment for metastatic disease. Randomization was performed intraoperatively after complete resection of metastases, and patients were stratified based on number of metastases and prior treatment history. Of patients, 92% received treatment as assigned. Two-year survival was 86% in the combined therapy group versus 72% for systemic therapy alone (*P*=.03), with median survivals of 72.2 months and 59.3 months. In an updated analysis, 10-year survival is 41% in the HAI plus SYS group, with 27% in the systemic alone group still alive (Fig. 79.10) (Kemeny & Gonen, 2005). Two-year hepatic progression-free survival was 90% for the combined group and 60% for the monotherapy group (*P*<.001). Updated hepatic progression free-survival at 10 years is 70% and 40% (*P*=.0001) (Fig. 79.11), and overall progression free-survival is 40% and 20% (*P*=.001) at 10 years. If patients with poor clinical risk scores (Fong et al, 1999) are considered, their survival is still improved when they received the HAI compared with SYS alone (Fig. 79.12).

Table 79.9 Results of Hepatic Arterial Infusion Combined with Systemic Chemotherapy in the Second-Line Setting

Drug	No. Patients	Response (%)	Median Survival from Pump Placement (mo)
FUDR + dexamethasone + sideport mitomycin C	37	70	20
FUDR + dexamethasone + SYS CPT-11	56	74	20
FUDR + dexamethasone + SYS oxaliplatin + CPT-11	21	90	28
FUDR + dexamethasone + SYS oxaliplatin + FU/leucovorin	15	88	22

CPT-11, irinotecan.
Data from Kemeny N, et al 2001, 2005a, 2005b.

Table 79.10 Randomized Trials of Adjuvant Hepatic Arterial Infusion After Resection of Liver Metastases*

	MSKCC, 1999		Intergroup, 2002		German, 1998*	
Arms	HAI + SYS	SYS	HAI + SYS	Control	HAI (port)	Control
n	74	82	53	56	113	113
Median time to progression (mo)	37.4[†]	17.2	37[‡]	18[‡]	20*	12.6*
Median time to hepatic progression (mo)	Not reached[†]	42.7	Not reached	20.2	44.8*	23.3*
Median overall survival (mo)	72.2	59.3	63.7	49.7	44.8	39.7
2-Year overall survival	86%[†]	72%	62%	53%	62%[‡]	65%[‡]
5-Year overall survival	57%[§]	48%[§]	55%[§]	37.5%[§]	—	—

*Results of treated patients are reported here.
[†]Statistically significant difference (*P*<.05) compared with control group.
[‡]Not reported, but calculated based on Kaplan-Meier curves published in original citations.
[§]Updated results.
Modified from Cohen AD, Kemeny NE, 2003: An update on hepatic arterial infusional chemotherapy for colorectal cancer. Oncologist 8:553-566.

Toxicity was increased in the combined group, with 39% of patients in the combined therapy group requiring hospitalization for diarrhea, neutropenia, mucositis, or small bowel obstruction compared with 22% in the monotherapy group (*P*=.02). Elevated bilirubin was seen in 18% of patients in the combined group. In most patients, the bilirubin returned to normal, but 6% of patients required biliary stents. In the control group, 2% had an elevation in bilirubin, and 2% required biliary stents. There was no significant difference between the groups in therapy-related deaths (one combined, two monotherapy).

The Intergroup study (Kemeny MM et al, 1999) randomized 109 patients to resection alone or resection followed by four cycles of HAI with FUDR and infusional systemic 5-FU, followed by eight more cycles of systemic 5-FU. Patients with more than three liver metastases or extrahepatic disease at laparotomy were taken off study; only 80 of 109 patients were actually included in the study. The study was designed to answer the question: Is there an increase in disease-free survival in patients receiving adjuvant therapy? When patients were analyzed as treated (*n* = 75), the

4-year disease-free survival (46% versus 25%; *P*=.04) and 4-year hepatic disease-free survival (67% versus 43%; *P*=.03) favored the HAI over the control groups. Based on an intention-to-treat analysis, there was no difference in median or 4-year overall survival between the groups. Currently, the 5-year survival is 55% versus 37.5% favoring adjuvant therapy (Kemeny M, 2005). This study was not designed to look at overall survival, however.

In the German Cooperative multicenter study (Lorenz et al, 1998), 226 patients were randomized to resection alone or resection plus 6 months of HAI with 5-FU/leucovorin (given as a 5-day continuous infusion every 28 days). The study was terminated early because an interim analysis suggested a very low chance of showing a survival benefit with adjuvant therapy. The impact of HAI in this study is difficult to assess because only 74% of patients assigned to HAI received this treatment, and only 30% completed it. No difference in time to progression, time to hepatic progression, and median overall survival was noted in an intention-to-treat analysis. When patients were analyzed "as treated," time to hepatic progression (45 months versus 23 months) and

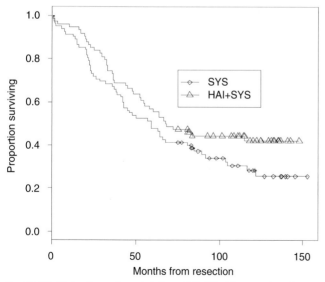

Fig. 79.10. Updated overall survival from MSKCC trial comparing adjuvant SYS with HAI plus SYS.

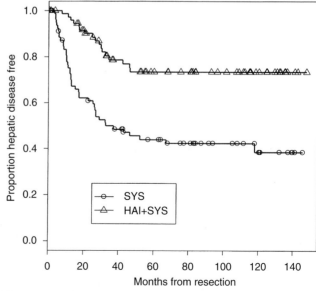

Fig. 79.11. Updated hepatic disease-free survival from MSKCC trial comparing adjuvant SYS with HAI plus SYS.

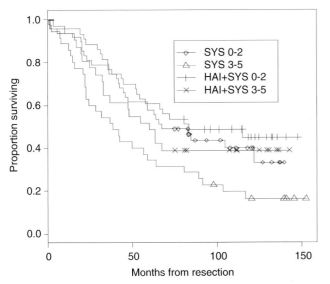

Fig. 79.12. Survival stratified by clinical risk score. A clinical risk score ranging from 0 to 5 was calculated by summing 1 point for the following clinical characteristics: tumor size >5 cm, tumor number >1, serum carcinoembryonic antigen >200 ng/mL, node positive primary tumor and disease-free interval <12 months (Fong et al, 1999).

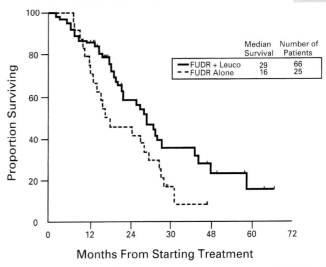

Fig. 79.13. MSKCC trial. Survival curves of patients treated with HAI of FUDR and leucovorin compared retrospectively with patients treated with HAI of FUDR alone (from the randomized study of HAI of FUDR and dexamethasone [Decadron] versus FUDR alone.) All patients had nonresectable disease.

time to progression or death (20 months versus 12.6 months) were improved in the HAI arm. Grade 3/4 toxicity, including stomatitis and nausea and vomiting, was noted in 63% of patients receiving adjuvant therapy. These findings reflected significant systemic absorption of 5-FU when given via HAI.

A study conducted in Greece on 122 patients used mitomycin C, 5-FU, and interleukin-2 by HAI and intravenous route versus intravenous route alone. The 2-year survival was 92% versus 75%, and 5-year survival was 73% versus 60% for the HAI plus SYS group versus SYS alone group. Disease-free survival was significantly longer for the HAI plus SYS group, 60% at 5 years versus 20% for the intravenous group ($P=.0012$). Hepatic disease-free survival was 85% versus 50% ($P=.0001$) (Lygidakis et al, 2001).

The two American studies showed a reduction in hepatic and extrahepatic recurrence for combined HAI plus systemic therapy after surgical resection. Of the two European studies, one showed a significant increase in survival and disease-free survival, whereas the other did not. In the MSKCC study, 2-year survival after liver resection was significantly improved with combined therapy, 86% compared with 72% with systemic therapy alone. Historical 2-year survivals (Chang et al, 1987; Fegiz et al, 1991; Jamison et al, 1997; Scheele et al, 1990) for patients treated with resection alone range from 55% to 70% (Fig. 79.13).

CONCLUSION

There are several advantages to HAI. From a pharmacologic standpoint, HAI is more effective than SYS because higher drug levels are achieved at the sites of metastatic disease. Using agents with high hepatic extraction virtually eliminates the systemic toxicity observed with "standard" therapy (intravenous 5-FU or 5-FU and leucovorin).

The 50% to 70% response rate obtained in trials of intrahepatic FUDR therapy has not been matched by any systemic therapy to date. The addition of leucovorin or dexamethasone to FUDR

has increased response rate and survival. Most randomized HAI studies do not clearly evaluate the issue of survival, mainly because a crossover was allowed in some, whereas patients with positive portal nodes were included in the HAI treated groups in other studies. Severe toxicity may occur with HAI or SYS. Although HAI therapy may produce gastrointestinal or hepatic toxicity, this toxicity may be minimized with better surgical technique, close monitoring of liver function tests, and HAI dexamethasone.

Because the liver is often the initial site of metastatic disease in patients with colorectal carcinoma, early intensive therapy with surgical resection or HAI or both at a time when the tumor burden is small may prevent the progression of metastases to other sites. Although HAI therapy is applicable only to a few patients with metastatic colorectal carcinoma (patients with only hepatic metastases), it may be the best available therapy for these patients—especially in patients who progress on first-line therapy.

REFERENCES

Allen PJ, et al, 2002: The management of variant arterial anatomy during hepatic arterial infusion pump placement. Ann Surg Oncol 9: 875-880.

Allen PJ, et al, 2005: Technical complications and durability of hepatic artery infusion pumps for unresectable colorectal liver metastases: an institutional experience of 544 consecutive cases. J Am Coll Surg 201:57-65.

Arai Y, 1988: The study of catheter placement into the hepatic artery via the left subclavian artery for hepatic infusion therapy. J Nagoya City Univ Med Assoc 39:453-464.

Arai Y, et al, 1997: Interventional techniques for hepatic arterial infusion chemotherapy. In Castaneda-Zuniga WR (ed): Interventional Radiology, vol 1. Philadelphia, Williams & Wilkins, pp 192-205.

Balch CM, Urist MM, 1986: Intraarterial chemotherapy for colorectal liver metastases and hepatomas using a totally implantable drug infusion pump. Recent Results Cancer Res 100:123-147.

Bilchik AJ, et al, 2000: Cryosurgery ablation and radiofrequency ablation for unresectable hepatic malignant neoplasms: a proposed algorithm. Arch Surg 135:657-662.

Blackshear PJ, et al, 1972: The design and initial testing of an implantable infusion pump. Surg Gynecol Obstet 134:51-56.

Breedis C, Young C, 1954: The blood supply of neoplasms in the liver. Am J Pathol 30:969.

Campbell KA, et al, 1993: Regional chemotherapy devices: effect of experience and anatomy on complications. J Clin Oncol 11:822-826.

Castaing D, et al, 1998: Implantable hepatic arterial infusion device: placement without laparotomy via an intercostal artery. J Am Coll Surg 187:565-568.

Chang AE, et al, 1987: A prospective randomized trial of regional versus systemic continuous 5-fluorodeoxyuridine chemotherapy in the treatment of colorectal liver metastases. Ann Surg 206:685-693.

Cheng J, et al, 2003: Laparoscopic radiofrequency ablation and hepatic artery infusion pump placement in the evolving treatment of colorectal hepatic metastasis. Surg Endosc 17:61-67.

Cheng J, et al, 2004: Laparoscopic placement of hepatic artery infusion pumps: technical considerations and early results. Ann Surg Oncol 11:558-559.

Cohen AD, Kemeny NE, 2003: An update on hepatic arterial infusional chemotherapy for colorectal cancer. Oncologist 8:553-566.

Cohen AM, et al, 1980: Transbrachial hepatic arterial chemotherapy using an implanted infusion pump. Dis Colon Rectum 23:223-227.

Cohen AM, et al, 1983: Regional hepatic chemotherapy using an implantable drug infusion pump. Am J Surg 145:529-533.

Cohen AM, et al, 1985: Treatment of colorectal cancer hepatic metastases by hepatic artery chemotherapy. Dis Colon Rectum 28:389-393.

Cohen AM, et al, 1987: Effect of ligation of variant hepatic arterial structures on the completeness of regional chemotherapy infusion. Am J Surg 153:378-380.

Collins JM, 1984: Pharmacologic rationale for regional drug delivery. J Clin Oncol 2:498-504.

Collins JM, 1986: Pharmacologic rationale for hepatic arterial therapy. Recent Results Cancer Res 100:140-148.

Curley SA, et al, 1993: Technical considerations and complications associated with the placement of 180 implantable hepatic arterial infusion devices. Surgery 114:928-935.

Daly J, Kemeny N, 1986: The therapy of colorectal hepatic metastases. In DeVita VT, et al (eds): Important Advances in Oncology. Philadelphia, Lippincott, pp 251-268.

Daly J, et al, 1984: Long-term hepatic arterial infusion chemotherapy. Arch Surg 119:936-941.

de Gramont A, et al, 2000: Leucovorin and fluorouracil with or without oxaliplatin as first-line treatment in advanced colorectal cancer. J Clin Oncol 18:2938-2947.

Doria MI Jr, et al, 1986: Liver pathology following hepatic arterial infusion chemotherapy: hepatic toxicity with FUDR. Cancer 58:855-861.

Ensminger WD, Gyves JW, 1983: Clinical pharmacology of hepatic arterial chemotherapy. Semin Oncol 10:176-182.

Ensminger WD, et al, 1978: A clinical pharmacological evaluation of hepatic arterial infusions of 5-fluoro-2-deoxyuridine and 5-fluorouracil. Cancer Res 38:3784-3792.

Fegiz G, et al, 1991: Hepatic resections for colorectal metatases: the Italian multicenter experience. J Surg Oncol Suppl 2:1441-1454.

Feliciotti F, et al, 1996: Laparoscoic intraarterial catheter implantation for regional chemotherapy of liver metastasis. Surg Endosc 10:449-453.

Fong Y, et al, 1999: Clinical score for predicting recurrence after hepatic resection for metastatic colorectal cancer: analysis of 1001 consecutive cases. Ann Surg 230:309-318.

George SL, Hoogstraten B, 1978: Prognostic factors in the initial response to therapy by patients with advanced breast cancer. J Natl Cancer Inst 60:731-736.

Gluck WL, et al, 1985: A reversible enteropathy complicating continuous hepatic artery infusion chemotherapy with 5-fluoro 2-deoxyuridine. Cancer 56:2424-2427.

Goldberg R, et al, 2002: Oxaliplatin (Oxal) or CPT-11 + 5-fluorouracil (5FU)/leucovorin (LV) or oxal + CPT-11 in advanced colorectal cancer (CRC). Proc Am Soc Clin Oncol 21:511.

Grobmyer SR, et al, 2004: Diagnostic laparoscopy prior to planned hepatic resection for colorectal metastases. Arch Surg 139:1326-1330.

Harris J, et al, 1997: Malignant tumors of the breast. In DeVita VT, et al (eds): Cancer: Principles and Practice of Oncology. Philadelphia, Lippincott Williams & Wilkins, pp 1557-1616.

Hohn DC, et al, 1985: Avoidance of gastroduodenal toxicity in patients receiving hepatic arterial 5-fluoro-2'-deoxyuridine. J Clin Oncol 3:1257-1260.

Hohn DC, et al, 1989: A randomized trial of continuous intravenous versus hepatic intraarterial floxuridine in patients with colorectal cancer metastatic to the liver: the Northern California Oncology Group trial. J Clin Oncol 7:1646-1654.

Hrushesky W, et al, 1990: Circadian-shaped infusions of floxuridine for progressive metastatic renal cell carcinoma. J Clin Oncol 8:1504-1513.

Hurwitz H, et al, 2004: Bevacizumab plus irinotecan, fluorouracil, and leucovorin for metastatic colorectal cancer. N Engl J Med 350:2335-2342.

Inaba Y, et al, 1998: Unnecessity of surgical approach for hepatic arterial catheter placement—minimally invasive procedures using angiographic techniques. Presented at the ASCO annual meeting, Los Angeles, Calif., 1998 (abstract 1125).

Jamison RL, et al, 1997: Hepatic resection for metastatic colorectal cancer results in cure for some patients. Arch Surg 132:505-511.

Johnson LP, et al, 1983: FUDR hepatic arterial infusion via an implantable pump for treatment of hepatic tumors. Proc Am Soc Clin Oncol 2:119.

Kemeny M: Personal communication, 2005.

Kemeny MM, et al, 1985: Sclerosing cholangitis after continuous hepatic artery infusion of FUDR. Ann Surg 202:176-181.

Kemeny MM, et al, 1986a: Results of a prospective randomized trial of continuous regional chemotherapy and hepatic resection as treatment of hepatic metastases from colorectal primaries. Cancer 57:492-498.

Kemeny MM, et al 1986b: Continuous hepatic artery infusion with an implantable pump: problems with hepatic artery anomalies. Surgery 99:501-504.

Kemeny MM, et al, 1999: Results of the Intergroup [Eastern Cooperative Oncology Group (ECOG) and Southwest Oncology Group (SWOG)] prospective randomized study of surgery alone versus continuous hepatic artery infusion of FUDR and continuous systemic infusion of 5FU after hepatic resection for colorectal liver metastases. Proc Am Soc Clin Oncol (abstract 1012).

Kemeny N, Braun DW, 1983: Prognostic factors in advanced colorectal carcinoma: the importance of lactic dehydrogenase, performance status, and white blood cell count. Am J Med 74:786-794.

Kemeny NE, Gonen M, 2005: Hepatic arterial infusion after liver resection. N Engl J Med 352:734-735.

Kemeny N, et al, 1984: Hepatic artery pump infusion toxicity and results in patients with metastatic colorectal carcinoma. J Clin Oncol 2:595-600.

Kemeny N, et al, 1987: Intrahepatic or systemic infusion of fluorodeoxyuridine in patients with liver metastases from colorectal carcinoma. Ann Intern Med 107:459-465.

Kemeny N, et al, 1989: Prognostic variables in patients with hepatic metastases from colorectal cancer: importance of medical assessment of liver involvement. Cancer 63:742-747.

Kemeny N, et al, 1993: Randomized trial of hepatic arterial floxuridine, mitomycin and carmustine versus floxuridine alone in previously treated patients with liver metastases from colorectal cancer. J Clin Oncol 11:330-335.

Kemeny N, et al, 1994: Phase II study of heptic arterial floxuridine, leucovorin, and dexamethasone for unresectable liver metastases from colorectal carcinoma. J Clin Oncol 12:2288-2295.

Kemeny N, et al, 1999: Hepatic arterial infusion of chemotherapy after resection of hepatic metastases from colorectal cancer. N Engl J Med 341:2039-2048.

Kemeny N, et al, 2001: Phase I study of hepatic arterial infusion of floxuridine and dexamethasone with systemic irinotecan for unresectable hepatic metastases from colorectal cancer. J Clin Oncol 19:2687-2695.

Kemeny N, et al, 2005a: A Phase I trial of systemic oxaliplatin combination chemotherapy with hepatic arterial infusion in patients with unresectable liver metastases from colorectal cancer. J Clin Oncol 23:4888-4896.

Kemeny N, et al, 2005b: Hepatic arterial infusion of floxuridine and dexamethasone plus high-dose Mitomycin C for patients with unresectable hepatic metastases from colorectal carcinoma. J Surg Oncol 91:97-101.

Kemeny N, et al, 2005c: Hepatic arterial infusion (HAI) versus systemic therapy for hepatic metastases from colorectal cancer: a randomized trial of efficacy, quality of life (QOL), cost effectiveness, and molecular markers. N Engl J Med 352:734-735.

Kerr DJ, et al, 2003: Intrahepatic arterial versus intravenous fluorouracil and folinic acid for colorectal cancer liver metastases: a multicentre randomized trial. Lancet 361:368-373.

Lorenz M, Muller H, 2000: Randomized, multicenter trial of fluorouracil plus leucovorin administered either via hepatic arterial or intravenous infusion versus fluorodeoxyuridine administered via hepatic arterial infusion in patients with nonresectable liver metastases from colorectal carcinoma. J Clin Oncol 18:243-254.

Lorenz M, et al, 1998: Randomized trial of surgery versus surgery followed by adjuvant hepatic arterial infusion with 5-fluorouracil and folinic acid for liver metastases of colorectal cancer. German Cooperative on Liver Metastases. Ann Surg 228:756-762.

Lygidakis NJ, et al, 2001: Metastatic liver disease of colorectal origin: the value of locoregional immunochemotherapy combined with systemic chemotherapy following liver resection: results of a prospective randomized study. Hepatogastroenterology 48:1685-1691.

Martin JK Jr, et al, 1990: Intra-arterial floxuridine vs systemic fluorouracil for hepatic metastases from colorectal cancer: a randomized trial. Arch Surg 125:1022-1027.

Matsumada T, et al, 1997: Laparotomy versus interventional radiological procedures for implantation of arterial infusion devices. Surg Today 27:398-402.

Meta-Analysis Group in Cancer, 1996: Reappraisal of hepatic arterial infusion in the treatment of nonresectable liver metastases from colorectal cancer. J Natl Cancer Inst 88:252-258.

Michels NA, 1966: Newer anatomy of the liver and its variant blood supply and collateral circulation. Am J Surg 112:337-347.

Niederhuber JE, 1987: Hepatic artery chemotherapy for colorectal cancer metastatic to the liver. Surg Annu 19:263-277.

Niederhuber JE, et al, 1984: Regional chemotherapy of colorectal cancer metastatic to the liver. Cancer 53:1336.

Northover JM, Terblanche J, 1979: A new look at the arterial supply of the bile duct in man and its surgical implications. Br J Surg 66:379-384.

Oberfield RA, et al, 1979: Prolonged and continuous percutaneous intra-arterial hepatic infusion chemotherapy in advanced metastatic liver adenocarcinoma from colorectal primary cancer. Cancer 44:414-423.

Pancera G, et al, 2002: A feasibility study of combined hepatic arterial infusion (HAI) with FUDR and systemic chemotherapy (SYS) with FOLFOX-4 in advanced colorectal cancer (CRC). Proc Am Soc Clin Oncol 21:105b (abstract 2233).

Portier G, et al, 2002: Adjuvant systemic chemotherapy (CT) using 5-fluorouracil (FU) and folinic acid (FA) after resection of liver metastases (LM) from colorectal (CRC) origin: results of an intergroup phase III study (trial FFCD-ACHBTH-AURC 9002). Proc Am Soc Clin Oncol 21:133 (abstract 528).

Rougier P, et al, 1992: Hepatic arterial infusion of floxuridine in patients with liver metastases from colorectal carcinoma: long-term results of a prospective randomized trial. J Clin Oncol 10:1112-1118.

Safi F, et al, 1989: Regional chemotherapy for hepatic metastases of colorectal carcinoma (continuous intra-arterial versus continuous intra-arterial/intravenous therapy). Cancer 64:379-387.

Saldinger PF, Sandhu F, 2004: Minimally invasive/transintercostal placement of hepatic arterial infusion pump. J Gastrointest Surg 8:167A.

Saltz L, et al, 1998: High thymidylate synthase (TS) expression does not preclude activity of CPT-11 in colorectal cancer (CRC). Proc Am Soc Clin Oncol 17:281a (abstract 1080).

Saltz LB, et al, 2000: Irinotecan plus fluorouracil and leucovorin for metastatic colorectal cancer. Irinotecan Study Group. N Engl J Med 343:905-914.

Scheele J, et al, 1990: Hepatic metastases from colorectal carcinoma: impact of surgical resection on the natural history. Br J Surg 77:1241-1246.

Schwartz SI, et al, 1985: Assessment of treatment of intrahepatic malignancies using chemotherapy via an implantable pump. Ann Surg 201:560-567.

Shepard KV, et al, 1985: Therapy for metastatic colorectal cancer with hepatic artery infusion chemotherapy using a subcutaneous implanted pump. J Clin Oncol 3:161-169.

Sigurdson ER, et al, 1987: Tumor and liver drug uptake following hepatic artery and portal vein infusion. J Clin Oncol 5:1936-1940.

Stagg RJ, et al, 1991: Alternating hepatic intra-arterial floxuridine and fluorouracil: a less toxic regimen for treatment of liver metastases from colorectal cancer. J Natl Cancer Inst 83:423-428.

Tournigand C, et al, 2004: FOLFIRI followed by FOLFOX6 versus FOLFOX or the reverse sequence in advanced colorectal cancer: a randomized GERCOR study. J Clin Oncol 22:229-237.

Urbach DR, Hansen PD, 2000: Laparoscopic placement of a continuous hepatic artery infusion pump. Semin Laparosc Surg 7:140-147.

Urbach DR, et al, 2001: Laparoscopic hepatic artery infusion pump placement. Arch Surg 136:700-704.

Wagman LD, et al, 1990: A prospective, randomized evaluation of the treatment of colorectal cancer metastatic to the liver. J Clin Oncol 8:1885-1893.

Weiss GR, et al, 1983: Long-term hepatic arterial infusion of 5-fluorodeoxyuridine for liver metastases using an implantable infusion pump. J Clin Oncol 1:337-344.

Weiss L, 1989: Metastatic inefficiency and regional therapy for liver metastases from colorectal carcinoma. Reg Cancer Treat 2:77-81.

Weiss L, et al, 1986: Haematogenous metastatic patterns in colonic carcinoma: an analysis of 1541 necropsies. J Pathol 150:195-203.

Hepatic Resection

Liver Resection for Benign Disease and for Liver and Biliary Tumors

L. H. BLUMGART AND J. BELGHITI

Addendum: Laparoscopic Techniques

M. D'ANGELICA

EXTENDED RESECTION FOR BILIARY TUMORS—AN ALTERNATIVE APPROACH

Y. NIMURA AND T. SANO

LIVER RESECTION IN LIVING RELATED DONORS

J. BELGHITI

COMPUTER-ASSISTED OPERATION PLANNING AND VIRTUAL LIVER RESECTION

H. LANG, H.-O. PEITGEN, AND C. E. BROELSCH

Hepatic resection for removal of lesions of the liver may be necessary for a wide variety of conditions (Table 80.1). Partial hepatectomy for the treatment of primary benign or malignant growths of the liver or biliary tract or secondary neoplasms is the most common indication. Hepatic resection also may be necessary in the management of complex cystic disease (see Chs. 64 and 65) involving the liver and to allow access for repair in some benign biliary strictures (see Ch. 43). Liver resection is necessary in the management of some liver injuries (see Ch. 66). More recently, liver resection in living donors has been employed in liver transplantation (see further on and Ch. 109).

The principles of segmental and subsegmental resection have been beautifully developed (Nagasue et al, 1985), more recently using ultrasound techniques (Bismuth & Castaing, 1984; Castaing et al, 1985; Scheele, 1989) to identify intrahepatic structures (see Ch. 86). This chapter discusses the major procedures of right and left hepatectomy, extended left hepatectomy, and right lobectomy (right hepatectomy extended to segment IV). More commonly used segmental resections are briefly described. A more detailed description of segment-oriented resection of the liver is provided in Ch. 83.

Hepatic resection in the cirrhotic liver is compromised by the concomitant deficit in functional hepatic reserve and the associated portal hypertension. Liver resection for the removal of gallbladder carcinoma and cholangiocarcinoma at the confluence of the bile ducts is a special subject because in this instance, resection is frequently necessary in the presence of biliary obstruction and infection. Particular difficulties arise as a result of involvement of hilar blood vessels and the caudate lobe by tumor.

GENERAL PRINCIPLES

Benign Disease

Partial hepatectomy for the removal of benign tumors or cysts of the liver generally should be performed only for symptomatic patients, in the presence of doubt as to the diagnosis, or for tumors with known malignant potential (see Ch. 70). Removal of liver tissue should be kept to a minimum, and the employment of techniques for enucleation of such tumors is often appropriate. Such enucleative methods are employed in the management of hemangioma, but sometimes may be appropriate for excision of adenoma or fibronodular hyperplasia. Enucleation also may be appropriate for tumor debulking of metastatic neuroendocrine tumors. The principles of enucleation are applied in the operation of pericystectomy for the removal of hydatid cysts of the liver (see Ch. 61).

Liver resection may be necessary in the management of some complex benign biliary strictures, especially when associated with unilateral liver atrophy (see Ch. 43), and a variety of other benign biliary conditions, including hepatic resection for the removal of intrahepatic stones sometimes in association with recurrent pyogenic cholangitis (see Ch. 62) and in congenital disease of the liver, such as Caroli's disease (see Chs. 64 and 65). In this situation, removal of liver tissue should be kept to the minimum compatible with effective operation. The place of liver resection in hydatid disease is discussed in Ch. 61. Liver resection for injury is discussed in Ch. 66.

Malignant Disease

Partial hepatectomy as treatment for malignant tumors of the liver must be guided by the principle of complete tumor removal with a margin of parenchymal transection clear of the tumor. This margin ideally should be no less than 1 cm, but frequently practical considerations, particularly in the removal of large tumors, dictate that the clearance is less than this. Because long-term survival has been recorded even with close margins, inability to obtain wide clearance should not restrain the surgeon. Despite the need to resect with clear margins, every effort should be made to minimize removal of normal liver tissue.

The main problems in achieving adequate clearance margins in wedge resections for tumors apparently situated peripherally

Table 80.1 Most Common Conditions for Which Liver Resection May Be Used for Therapy

Benign liver tumors

Hemangioma
Adenoma
Focal nodular hyperplasia
Cystadenoma

Malignant liver tumors

Primary

Hepatocellular carcinoma
Cholangiocarcinoma

Metastatic arising from

Colorectal cancer
Noncolorectal cancers and neuroendocrine tumors
Tumors directly invading the liver
    Adrenal tumors
    Renal carcinoma
    Gastric cancer
    Colonic cancer
    Retroperitoneal and IVC sarcoma

Gallbladder cancer

Hilar cholangiocarcinoma

Benign conditions

Intrahepatic biliary strictures/fistulae
Intrahepatic biliary stones
Recurrent pyogenic cholangitis
Caroli's disease
Liver cysts/polycystic liver disease
Parasitic cysts

Liver trauma

Liver resection in liver donors for transplantation

in the liver should not be underestimated. In this situation, adequate clearance often is compromised in the depth of the wedge. It has been shown that wedge resections carry an unacceptable local recurrence rate (DeMatteo et al, 2000; Gall & Scheele, 1986). Another factor that may compromise wedge resection is the presence of a very hard tumor residing in a soft and easily fractured liver; this is often the case with metastatic colorectal carcinoma. Extreme care should be taken so that at the point of closest parenchymal transection, the liver does not tear open and split along the tumor-liver interface at the time of transection. The principle of achieving clearance is best met by performing resection along anatomic lines.

Patients with metastatic neuroendocrine tumors undergoing palliative resections often have tumors that are amenable to enucleation using techniques similar to those employed for other benign lesions. Gallbladder carcinoma and cholangiocarcinoma at the confluence of the hepatic bile ducts frequently occlude biliary flow, and resection may be compromised not only by the adverse pathophysiology of obstructive jaundice, but also by infection that may have been introduced before operation as a result of interventional radiologic or endoscopic procedures. In addition, hepatic resection must be accompanied by resection of the extrahepatic biliary apparatus and by subsequent biliary reconstruction (see Chs. 51 and 52).

Liver resection is much more challenging in cirrhotic patients for several reasons. Intraoperatively, there are technical difficulties in mobilizing the liver and transecting the liver parenchyma, and there may be increased blood loss associated with portal hypertension. Postoperatively, hepatic failure and increased

susceptibility to infection are major concerns. In the cirrhotic liver, resection should be restricted to patients with good liver function; mobilization should be limited; and removal of liver tissue should allow tumor clearance, but preserve maximal residual liver (see later; see also Ch. 82).

Principal Hazards

The main hazards of hepatic resection are biliary leakage and bleeding. Biliary leakage is a particular problem with patients in whom biliary reconstruction is necessary, as, for example, in the removal of cholangiocarcinoma at the confluence of the hepatic ducts. Bleeding from the hepatic veins and the inferior vena cava (IVC) during parenchymal transection is a major concern. Bleeding is especially likely to occur during major resection for high and posteriorly placed tumors, where there is little clearance between the tumor margin and the passage of the hepatic veins into the vena cava, or when tumors are closely adherent or adjacent to the IVC (Fig. 80.1).

Postoperative Functional Hepatic Reserve

A noncirrhotic healthy liver may tolerate a resection of 80% of its volume. The enormous regenerative capacity enables functional compensation within a few weeks (see Ch. 5) (Blumgart et al, 1971). Such a favorable outcome cannot be taken for granted, however, in extended hepatic resections. Only if reduction of the functional liver parenchyma is less than 50% can the risk of clinically significant liver insufficiency be virtually disregarded. Postoperative hepatic reserve is of particular importance after extended left hepatectomy and when all of the liver to the right of the falciform ligament is removed (right lobectomy) (see later).

There is virtually no risk if most of the specimen volume has been replaced by an extensive tumor mass. In such patients, compensatory hypertrophy of the unaffected residual liver already has occurred, and the loss of functional parenchyma is limited. A comparable resection performed for multiple or unfavorably located smaller lesions carries a much greater risk, however, of postoperative liver failure. Small tumors located adjacent to the inflow or outflow vessels of multiple segments may mandate removal of large amounts of functioning parenchyma. More recent approaches have advocated the use of portal vein embolization in this situation (see Ch. 84) (Makuuchi et al, 1990). There is little evidence, however, that portal vein embolization is associated with improved postoperative results in patients with normal parenchyma (Farges et al, 2003). In a series of 1800 liver resections, we reported significant liver dysfunction with death in only 6 patients (Jarnagin et al, 2002). In this series, we did not use the indocyanine green retention test (see Ch. 2) or other test of liver function.

In patients with a *steatotic liver*, which is more common in obese patients, diabetic patients, and patients receiving chemotherapy, there is an increased risk (Behrns et al, 1998; Kooby et al, 2003). Portal vein embolization may prove to be justified in this group of patients. *Biliary obstruction with jaundice* is common in patients with hilar cholangiocarcinoma, who also are at increased risk (see later). Portal vein embolization also may be justified in some such cases (see Ch. 84) (Seyama et al, 2003).

In the cirrhotic liver, there is much less effective liver regeneration, and impairment of liver function is greater, may last longer, and may result in terminal liver failure. Liver failure is the most common cause of postoperative death after liver resection in cirrhotic patients. Postoperative liver failure and postoperative

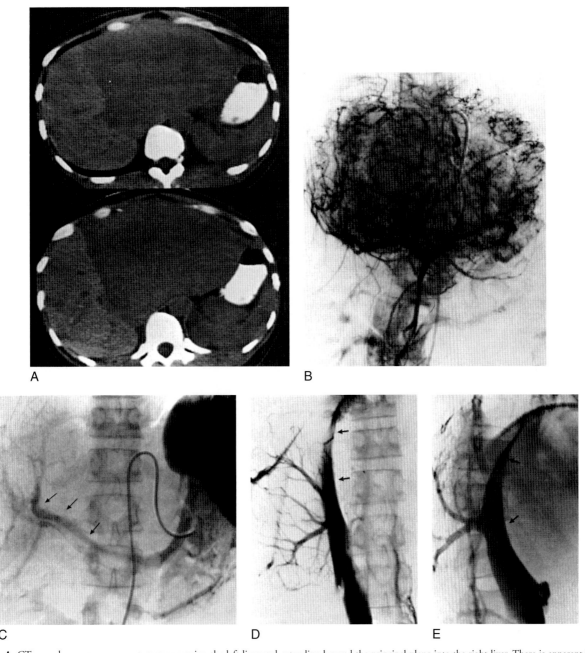

Fig. 80.1. A, CT scan shows an enormous tumor occupying the left liver and extending beyond the principal plane into the right liver. There is apparent involvement of the vena cava and of the hilar structures. **B,** Selective hepatic artery angiogram reveals the gross size of the tumor within the left liver. **C,** Late phase portogram shows gross displacement of the main trunk of the portal vein and its right branch *(arrows)*. There is no filling of the left branch of the portal vein. **D** and **E,** Anteroposterior **(D)** and lateral **(E)** views of the IVC reveal severe compression, but no tumor invasion. A collateral circulation has developed. The tumor proved to be a fibrolamellar hepatocellular carcinoma and was treated by extended left hepatectomy. *Note: Direct angiographic techniques have been supplanted by dynamic CT and MRI. The authors only rarely perform angiographic procedures (see text).*

mortality are related to the degree of preoperative liver decompensation and to the extent of nontumorous liver parenchyma removed. Liver failure may be precipitated by intraoperative bleeding, and there is a significant relationship between intraoperative blood loss, the postoperative increase in serum bilirubin, and postoperative mortality. The onset of nonspecific postoperative surgical complications, such as abdominal infection, also may trigger postoperative liver failure. Cirrhosis also predisposes to multiorgan failure after hepatectomy. Although there is evidence that major hepatic resection can be performed safely in cirrhotics with Child's A liver function (Fong et al,

1999a; Franco et al, 1990), there is some suggestion, but as yet no proof, that portal vein embolization may improve hepatic functional reserve in the remnant of the liver.

Portal Hypertension and Ascites

Liver resection leads to only a small increase in portal pressure in patients with a normal liver, but in cirrhotics, there is a further augmentation of portal hypertension related to the amount of parenchyma removed and to an incapacity of the remaining liver to drain the splanchnic bed. The increase in portal hypertension also may be related to the increased risk of variceal bleeding after liver resection in patients with cirrhosis.

Ascites is one of the most frequent complications after liver resection in cirrhotic patients, occurring in 80% of patients. Ascites is favored by the increase in portal hypertension and the severance of lymph vessels in the hepatic pedicle and liver ligaments. Postoperative ascites is a serious complication. Gross abdominal distention interferes with ventilatory function and may result in leakage and disruption of the abdominal incisions. Leakage of ascites may lead to major fluid, protein, and electrolyte loss. In addition, ascites may be infected, and this may be irreversible. Ascites also complicates liver resection and fenestration in polycystic liver disease (see Ch. 65).

Infection

Despite the frequent occurrence of fluid collections after major liver resection in noncirrhotic patients, infection is relatively infrequent. There is a serious risk of infection after liver resection in patients with biliary obstruction, especially in the presence of previous radiologic or endoscopic intubation and in cirrhotic patients. Alterations of humoral and cellular immunity and decrease of nonimmune acute responses to infection together with bacterial translocation are associated with the infective risks after abdominal surgery in cirrhotic patients. This risk is particularly high in patients with ascites or jaundice or both (Rimola et al, 1986).

Selection of Patients for Liver Resection

Careful selection, taking into account the general condition of the patient and, in particular, the liver functional status and the adaptation of the volume of resection to the size of the tumor, is important (see earlier). *Noncirrhotic* patients in whom a clearance of tumor or removal of benign lesions can be obtained without compromising hepatic arterial and portal venous inflow or biliary drainage are suitable for hepatic resection, but special care must be taken in the performance of major resections necessary for the removal of multiple or centrally situated small lesions in patients in whom compensatory hypertrophy of the residual liver has not occurred. Selection of patients with benign biliary stricture requiring hepatic resection is described in Ch. 43. Details regarding the place of liver resection in specific situations (e.g., in hilar cholangiocarcinoma and hemangioma) are detailed subsequently.

Cirrhotic patients with one or two tumors should be considered for partial resection. Resection is contraindicated in patients with multiple nodules. Besides the general condition of the patient and the extension of the cancer, *liver function is the main prognostic factor.* The Child (Child & Turcotte, 1964) and Pugh (Pugh et al, 1973) classifications are simple means of assessing liver function preoperatively. Although more sophisticated tests can be used (see Ch. 2), we find the Child classification sufficient for routine purposes. Operative mortality is much higher in patients with Child B or C than patients with grade A liver function. Liver resection is particularly hazardous in a patient with a Pugh score greater than 8. Serum bilirubin concentration may be the most important prognostic factor; *liver resection should not be carried out in patients with a serum bilirubin greater than 2 mg/mL or in the presence of clinically detectable ascites.* The extent of hepatectomy is based on tumor size, and in general one should remove as little parenchyma as possible (see later). Small nodules of tumor located deep in the bulk of the right liver are the most

challenging, and it is preferable to avoid performing a right hepatectomy in such cases. In this situation, preoperative portal vein embolization of the affected lobe may allow hypertrophy of the contralateral side (see earlier; see also Ch. 84). The advent of alternative methods for tumor control in a cirrhotic patient should be considered. Alcohol injection, transarterial chemoembolization, cryoablation, radiofrequency ablation, and liver transplantation for managing tumors of the liver are discussed in detail in Chs. 74, 76, 103, and 106.

ANATOMY AND CLASSIFICATION

Precise knowledge of the surgical anatomy of the liver, blood vessels, and biliary channels is essential for the performance of partial hepatectomy and is described in detail in Ch. 1. The liver is divided into sectors that are formed from liver segments supplied by branches of the portal triads and drained by hepatic veins. Partial hepatectomy involves removal of one or more segments by isolation of the relevant portal pedicle, severance of the relevant hepatic veins, and removal of the associated liver tissue.

The anatomic division between the right and left liver is not at the falciform ligament, but follows a line projected through a plane (the principal plane or Cantlie's line) running from the medial margin of the gallbladder bed to the left of the IVC posteriorly (Fig. 80.2) (Couinaud, 1954, 1957; Goldsmith & Woodburne, 1957; Healey & Schroy, 1953; McIndoe & Counseller, 1927). Each of these major right and left portions of the liver is divided into sectors and segments. The left liver is demarcated along the line of insertion of the ligamentum teres and the falciform ligament. The portion of the liver to the left of the ligamentum teres forms the left lobe, and the portion to the right of the ligamentum teres forms the right lobe. The portal venous and hepatic arterial branches conform to the segmental organization and run within the segments. Between the sectors, the draining hepatic veins converge posteriorly toward the vena cava and mark the main scissurae of the liver (see Fig. 80.2) within which they run (Couinaud, 1954, 1957).

Essentially and for practical purposes, there are five types of major resection (Fig. 80.3; see Fig. 80.2). The nomenclature of these operations is based on the anatomic descriptions of Couinaud (1954, 1957) and of Bismuth (1982) (Table 80.2). This classification emphasizes the importance of the scissurae of the liver and the umbilical fissure. The alternative, more commonly used terminology of Goldsmith and Woodburne (1957) also is listed in Table 80.2. A newer terminology proposed by the International Hepato-Pancreatico-Biliary Association (Strasberg et al, 2000) is referred to in Ch. 1, but is not used in this text.

The portal vein and hepatic artery divide into major right and left branches outside the liver substance below the hilus (see Fig. 80.2A). Here, when the overlying peritoneum is incised, it is possible to dissect each major branch beyond its bifurcation. The confluence of the right and left hepatic ducts also occurs outside the liver. At the delta of the portal vein, the right branch is short, and its first branch often arises posteroinferiorly close to the bifurcation, where it is easily damaged during dissection. By contrast, the left branch of the portal vein and the left hepatic duct pursue a longer, more horizontal extrahepatic course beneath the quadrate lobe and are more easily dissected.

The ligamentum teres runs sharply into the umbilical fissure of the liver, at the base of which the main vascular and biliary channels branch to the segments of the left liver. After

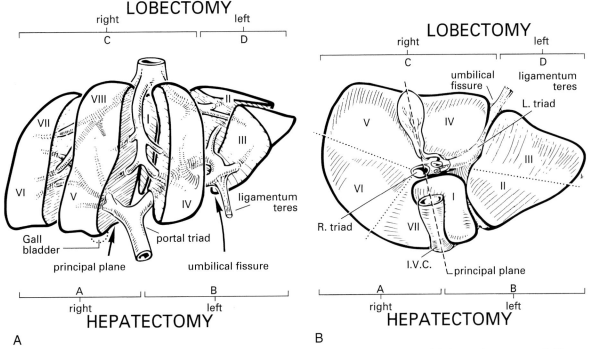

Fig. 80.2. A, Exploded view to show the sectors (separated by the major hepatic veins) and the segmental structure of the liver, each segment supplied by a portal triad. The left portal pedicle traverses beneath segment IV to the umbilical fissure, the umbilical portion of the pedicle curving ventrally and caudally in the umbilical fissure. The blood supply to segment IV is recurrent as feedback vessels. **B,** Inferior surface of the liver. Segment VIII is not seen because it lies superiorly. The anatomic division into right and left lobes by the umbilical fissure and into a right and left liver in the principal plane (along the principal scissura) is evident (see Ch. 1).

entering the umbilical fissure, the left branch of the portal vein curves caudally and gives branches not only to the left lobe (segments II and III), but also, together with branches of the left hepatic artery, gives rise to "feedback vessels" to the medial segment (segment IV; quadrate lobe) of the left liver (see Fig. 80.2A) (Goldsmith & Woodburne, 1957; Starzl et al, 1975).

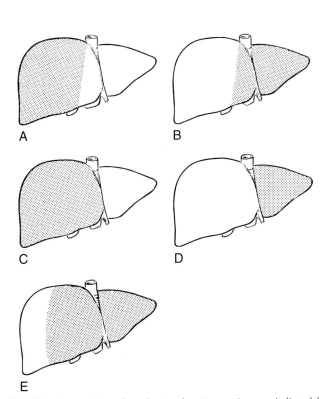

Fig. 80.3. Commonly performed major hepatic resections are indicated by *shaded areas.* **A,** Right hepatectomy. **B,** Left hepatectomy. **C,** Right lobectomy. **D,** Left lobectomy. **E,** Extended left hepatectomy. For the nomenclature of Goldsmith and Woodburne (1957), see text and Table 80.2.

Table 80.2   Nomenclature of Hepatic Resection

Couinaud (1957)	Goldsmith & Woodburne (1957)
Right hepatectomy (segments V, VI, VII, VIII)	Right hepatic lobectomy
(see Fig. 80.3A)	
Left hepatectomy (segments II, III, IV)	Left hepatic lobectomy
(see Fig. 80.3B)	
Right lobectomy (segments IV, V, VI, VII, VIII; sometimes include segment I)*	Extended right hepatic lobectomy*
(see Fig. 80.3C)	
Left lobectomy (segments II and III)	Left lateral segmentectomy
(see Fig. 80.3D)	
Extended left hepatectomy (segments II, III, IV, V, VIII; sometimes also segment I)†	Extended left lobectomy†
(see Fig. 80.3E)	

*Right lobectomy (extended right hepatic lobectomy) represents right hepatectomy extended to segment IV and has been referred to by Starzl et al (1975, 1980) as right trisegmentectomy, and this term is commonly found in the literature.
†Also referred to as left trisegmentectomy (Starzl et al, 1982).

Outside of the liver substance, there is no characterized sheath around the portal triad structures, and they must be dissected independently. The structures of the portal triad (portal vein, hepatic artery, and bile duct) take Glisson's capsule with them, however, so that within the liver they are contained in well-formed branching fibrous sheaths (pedicles). Dissection outside of the liver substance mandates individual isolation of the portal triad structures, where there are considerable variations in anatomy. Intrahepatic dissection of the pedicles, which are strong structures containing the constituents of the portal triad, allows isolation of the pedicles, however, without the need to dissect the constituents of the triad (see later) (Launois & Jamieson, 1992b).

The liver lies astride the IVC, immediately below the diaphragm, and the hepatic veins run a short course outside the liver to empty into the vena cava (see Fig. 80.2). This portion of the vena cava and the draining hepatic veins is masked behind a fold of peritoneum extending from the upper falciform ligament to the right and left triangular ligaments. The right hepatic vein emerges from the right scissura and usually enters the vena cava separately. By contrast, the left hepatic vein, which runs in the left scissura between segments II and III, frequently is joined by the middle hepatic vein, which occupies the principal scissura, before entering the vena cava separately. Several smaller veins drain from the posterior surface of the liver into the IVC, and veins from the caudate lobe, which is closely applied to the left of the vena cava, also drain directly into the cava.

An additional but important hepatic vein, the umbilical vein, runs beneath the falciform ligament and empties into the left hepatic vein. This vein is important in resections that remove segment IVa because it provides drainage of segment IVb in the presence of ligation of the middle hepatic vein (see Ch. 83).

PREOPERATIVE CONSIDERATIONS

Preoperative Investigations

Preoperative investigations should seek to determine the nature of the lesion and give an index of resectability and surgical approach.

Preoperative transcutaneous needle biopsy of liver tumor masses is not always advisable (see Ch. 22). In the presence of a strong presumptive diagnosis of a potentially resectable liver tumor, we prefer to avoid the possibility of tumor dissemination, rupture, or hemorrhage, which may occur using percutaneous methods, and to obtain a biopsy specimen at open laparotomy or at preliminary laparoscopy (Thompson et al, 1985). Laparoscopic techniques, particularly when used in combination with laparoscopic ultrasound, may give valuable information, particularly regarding the presence of lesions additional to those shown on imaging studies and the presence or absence of extrahepatic disease. This approach, by minimizing unnecessary laparotomy, has been shown to increase the resectability rate of patients submitted to laparotomy (Jarnagin et al, 2000; John et al, 1994).

The extent of tumor involvement of the liver, blood vessels, and bile ducts is important because this may influence the decision to operate and the operative approach. The major risks of hepatic resection are as follows:

1. Hemorrhage, which may arise at the porta hepatis from branches of the hepatic artery or portal vein or posteriorly from hepatic venous radicles or the IVC
2. Biliary fistula or stricture as a result of damage to the biliary apparatus

Operative complications are most likely to occur with tumors or other lesions that are large and encroach on the IVC, especially close to the junction of the major hepatic veins with the IVC (Hawkins et al, 2005) or with tumors near the hilus, at which the confluence of the hepatic ducts occurs and where the major vessels are in close proximity as they enter the liver substance. Because there are numerous anatomic variations in the vascular and biliary anatomy at the hilus of the liver, information should be obtained before elective operation in such cases.

Computed tomography (CT) gives valuable information (see Ch. 18). Peripherally placed lesions never involve the hilar structures or vena cava. CT, by showing such lesions, indicates freedom from vascular involvement and may obviate the need for further studies. More centrally situated lesions may involve major vessels close to the hilus, and appropriate CT scanning (see Ch. 18) can

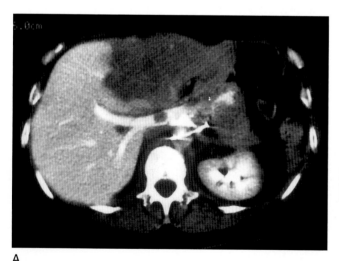
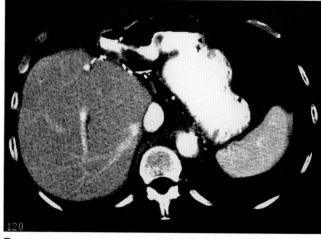

A   B

Fig. 80.4. CT portography illustrates metastatic melanoma to the liver. **A,** A large metastatic deposit of melanoma occupies segments II, III, and IV and extends into segments V and VIII. The left portal vein contains an extension of tumor that protrudes into the main portal venous trunk. **B,** Extended left hepatectomy was performed together with resection of the affected portion of the portal vein and subsequent portal vein reconstruction. Recurrent tumor in the right buttock was excised 1 year after hepatectomy. The patient was alive and well without evidence of further recurrence in the liver 10 years postoperatively.

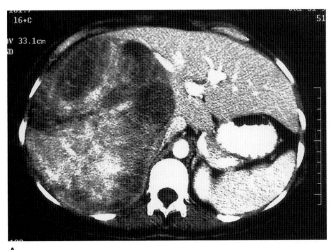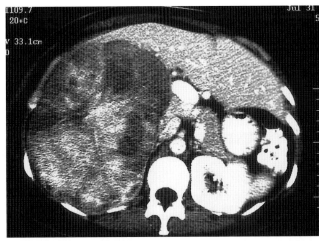

A   B

Fig. 80.5. A large well-circumscribed tumor in the right liver has expanded and is adjacent to the IVC. **A,** It has pushed the middle hepatic vein medially. **B,** The tumor protrudes by pressure effect into segment IV. Final histology revealed that this lesion was a benign fibrous tumor of the liver. Extended right hepatic lobectomy (right lobectomy) was performed without incident.

be most helpful in creating an image of the extent of disease and of vascular compromise by the tumor (Fig. 80.4). Liver tumors tend to respect intersegmental planes and to push structures away rather than to invade them directly, and such displacement not only can be shown on CT scan (Figs. 80.5 and 80.6), but also can be confirmed by angiographic methods (see Fig. 80.1) or by duplex ultrasound. Other tumors may hang from the liver in a pedunculated fashion (Baer et al, 1989) and even when very large may be attached to the liver by a relatively small base. Such "hanging" tumors may be readily shown on CT scan (Fig. 80.7). Involvement of the diaphragm also may be suggested by CT, but likewise should not deter the surgeon because such apparent diaphragmatic involvement in secondary tumors is frequently the result of adhesion at the site of previous necrosis of a tumor and not of direct invasion (Weinbren & Blumgart, 1986). Primary tumors, even if involving the diaphragm, still may be approached for resection (Foster & Berman, 1977).

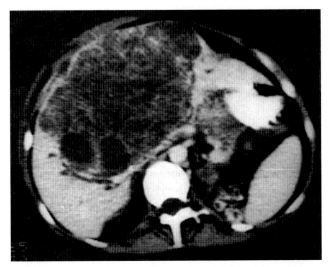

Fig. 80.6. CT scan shows a large metastatic deposit from a hypernephroma occupying segments II, III, IV, V, and VIII of the liver. The tumor is pushing the posterior sectoral triad posteriorly. A thin rim of liver tissue separates the tumor from the vessels. In this instance, the plane of transection is dictated by the tumor. Hepatic resection by extended left hepatectomy was successfully carried out. The patient was alive and well for more than 7 years.

Magnetic resonance imaging (MRI) (see Ch. 19) has become increasingly valuable in the imaging of the liver before resection. Masses are well shown, as are the presence of additional lesions sometimes not shown on CT. MRI can show major blood vessels accurately. MRI angiographic images are particularly valuable in the demonstration of the major hepatic veins and vena cava and their relationship to tumor masses (Fig. 80.8). MRI also may give an indication of the pathologic nature of the lesion.

Ultrasonography (see Ch. 15) gives information regarding the size of the tumor and extent of liver involvement and is of special value in the preoperative assessment of multiple tumors. Ultrasound also may help distinguish cysts from solid tumors. Duplex ultrasound by showing vascular structures, including the hepatic veins and vena cava, may obviate the need for other imaging techniques (Gibson et al, 1986) and is a valuable technique to define further the blood vessels after initial CT scanning (Fig. 80.9) (Hann et al, 1998). Ultrasound is of particular importance in the preoperative evaluation of hilar cholangiocarcinoma (Fig. 80.10) (Hann et al, 1997).

Hepatic angiography and *inferior venacavography* (see Ch. 21) usually are unnecessary and should not be used except in the instance of large hemangiomata in which precise information as to the arterial supply of the lesion may assist at surgery. Modern advances in duplex ultrasound and MRI have all but rendered these studies obsolete. In the event that adequate ultrasound or MRI is unavailable, there remains a place for angiography (Blumgart, 1982; Voyles et al, 1983). We have provided some figures of these angiographic techniques for illustrative purposes (Fig. 80.11; see Figs. 80.1 and 80.7), but emphasize that they are unnecessary in most patients. In our practice, the indication for hepatic angiography is usually the preoperative demonstration of *extrahepatic arterial anatomy* in patients in whom the insertion of a hepatic arterial infusion pump for postoperative adjunctive chemotherapy (see Ch. 79) is contemplated.

Other Investigations

Extrahepatic metastases should be sought by means of chest radiography or chest CT before major resection is undertaken. Positron emission tomography is being actively investigated, and initial results suggest that it is an important approach to evaluation

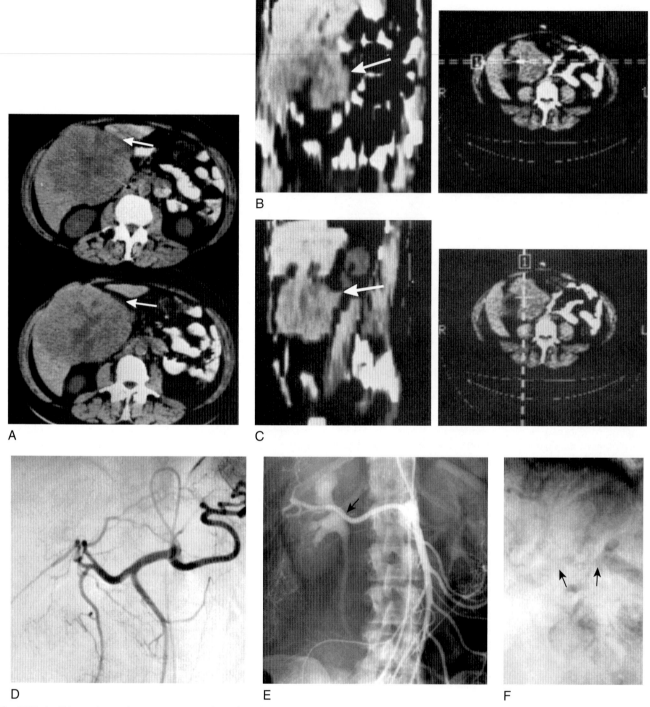

Fig. 80.7. A, CT scan shows a large tumor apparently in the right liver and extending well into the left *(top arrow)*. On the lower cut, there is a gap between the tumor and segments II and III *(bottom arrow)*. **B,** Coronal reconstruction shows that the tumor *(arrow)* is pedunculated. **C,** Sagittal reconstruction shows the pedunculated (hanging) nature of the tumor *(arrow)*, which originates from segments IV and V. **D,** Celiac axis angiogram shows the arterial supply to the tumor arising from the left hepatic artery. **E,** An accessory right hepatic artery is revealed to arise from the superior mesenteric trunk *(arrow)*. **F,** Late phase portogram obtained from selective splenic artery catheterization shows tumor involvement of the right branch of the portal vein extending to the portal venous bifurcation *(arrows)*. The tumor proved to be a primary hepatocellular carcinoma. Treatment was by right lobectomy (extended right hepatectomy). *Note:* Angiographic techniques are now rarely employed in diagnosis, but the images are retained for illustrative purposes (see text).

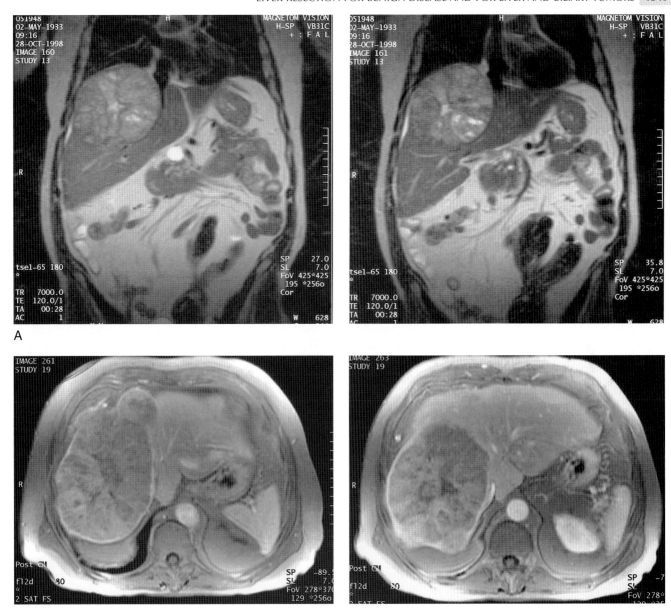

Fig. 80.8. MRI shows an extremely large, but well-demarcated hepatocellular carcinoma occupying the right liver and extending into segment IV. **A,** Coronal views show that the tumor is seriously compromising and compressing the IVC and extends upward and involves the right hepatic vein at its point of junction with the vena cava. The tumor is distorting and compressing the suprahepatic IVC and was found at operation to be causing a pressure effect without direct invasion of the diaphragm and to lie just adjacent to the IVC–right atrial junction. **B,** Transverse scans illustrate the extent of the tumor and the severe compression of the IVC. Extended right hepatic lobectomy (right lobectomy) was done. Tumor clearance was obtained. Hepatic vascular isolation was not employed. The patient was alive and well 9 months after operation.

of the extent of spread of malignant disease (see Chs. 17 and 73) (Beets et al, 1994; Fong et al, 1999a; Lai DTM et al, 1996; Schüssler-Fiorenza et al, 2004).

If jaundice is present, direct cholangiography may be carried out by endoscopic retrograde cholangiography or percutaneous transhepatic cholangiography (see Ch. 20). Hilar involvement of the bile ducts may have occurred, and there may be tumor seeding into the bile duct, or the tumor may be so widespread as to indicate irresectability. *Ultrasound and MRI cholangiography are noninvasive studies that are in many ways superior to direct cholangiography and have all but replaced endoscopic retrograde cholangiography and percutaneous transhepatic cholangiography*

for assessing hilar cholangiocarcinoma (see Fig. 80.10; see also Ch. 52).

Staging Laparoscopy

Laparoscopy and laparoscopic ultrasound are widely used now to prevent unnecessary laparotomy in patients with hepatobiliary malignancy. Staging laparoscopy significantly improves resectability. The yield is greater for detection of peritoneal metastases than for identifying additional hepatic tumors, and it often fails in identification of lymph node metastases (Jarnagin et al, 2000; John et al, 1994; Lo et al, 1998). In one study at Memorial Sloan-Kettering Cancer Center (MSKCC) (Jarnagin et al, 2000), 83% of

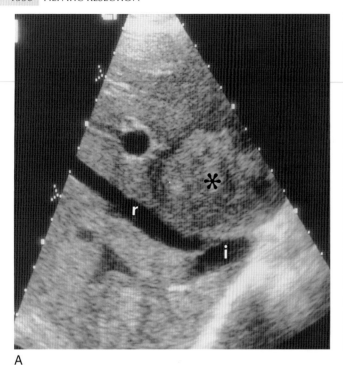
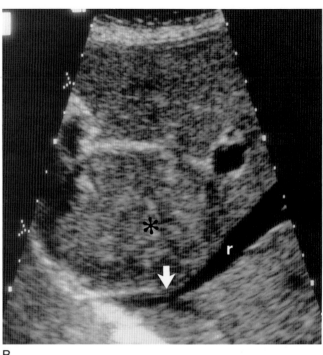

A   B

Fig. 80.9. Ultrasound defines the relationship between a colorectal metastasis and the veins at the hepatic vein confluence. **A,** Transverse ultrasound shows the metastasis *(asterisk)* contacting the IVC (i) and right hepatic vein (r). **B,** Oblique intercostal projection confirms that the right hepatic vein is compressed *(arrow)*, but not invaded by tumor *(asterisk)*.

patients subjected to laparotomy after laparoscopy underwent potentially curative resection compared with 66% of patients not staged laparoscopically (see Ch. 23).

Assessment of Resectability

An attempt should be made to assess resectability *before* operation in each case. In many instances, there are no difficulties.

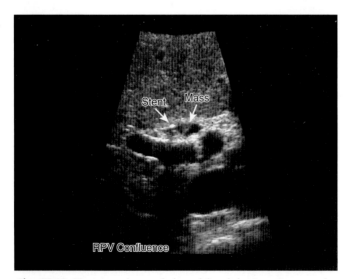

Fig. 80.10. Transverse ultrasound shows hilar cholangiocarcinoma at the confluence of the hepatic ducts. An endoscopically introduced stent is visible. The portal vein confluence immediately below the tumor is unaffected, and the portal vein is free. The tumor extended into the right hepatic duct, and an extended right hepatic lobectomy was necessary because of the tumor extent. The patient was alive, well, and tumor-free 8 months after operation.

Lesions shown on detailed preoperative investigation to be situated in the liver parenchyma at some distance from the major vascular structures and with no radiologic evidence of additional tumors come to operation defined as resectable, although a proportion may be found to have lymph node involvement or additional liver lesions at laparoscopy or open exploration. Other cases, in which there is clear evidence of multiple bilateral deposits, are nonresectable.

Major problems arise in two situations. First, tumors closely applied to the major hilar structures (see Fig. 80.7) or markedly compressing (see Fig. 80.11) or involving the vena cava can be difficult to assess preoperatively. Involvement of major structures, such as invasion of bile ducts or portal venous branches or apparent involvement of the IVC, does not preclude resection (see Fig. 80.1) (Soreide et al, 1985). Second, very large tumors, which push structures aside and have been slowly growing over a long time, are difficult to define precisely because pressure changes may mimic invasion on radiography, and considerable caution must be exercised before declaring such cases nonresectable. In patients with tumors of this nature, it is often difficult at initial exploration to be certain of resectability, and considerable dissection and mobilization is necessary before a clear-cut decision can be made. The morphologic configuration of tumors as defined on imaging studies has been shown to have a clear relationship to subsequent resectability. Tumors that expand and compress surrounding tissues ("pushing" tumors) and tumors that are pedunculated and attached to the liver by a base of variable width (hanging tumors) are nearly always resectable and can be distinguished from tumors that are irregular at the margins and clearly invasive (Baer et al, 1989).

The senior author (L.H.B.) adopted a deliberate policy of full investigation and laparotomy with a view to full exploration and possible resection in all patients with solitary large liver tumors, provided that there is no positive evidence of extrahepatic

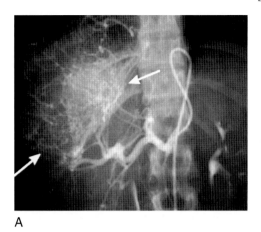 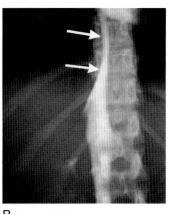 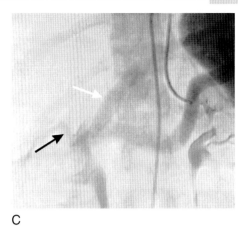

A   B   C

Fig. 80.11. A, Selective hepatic arteriogram shows a large primary hepatocellular carcinoma *(arrows).* **B,** Inferior venacavogram shows severe compression of the IVC *(arrows).* Such severe compromise of the IVC demands vena caval control and precise dissection of the right hepatic vein (see text). **C,** Selective splenic artery catheterization and late phase splenoportogram show severe compromise of the right branch of the portal vein *(black arrow).* The left branch of the portal vein is intact *(white arrow).* Treatment was by right hepatic lobectomy. Angiographic techniques are now rarely performed.

spread, patients are otherwise fit for major resective surgery, and the residual liver is noncirrhotic. Of 22 patients with primary liver cancer evaluated in an early study at the Hepatobiliary Unit, Hammersmith Hospital, London, in May 1979–December 1984, 13 patients were approached, and resection was carried out in all. Only 3 of the 13 (23%) had a classically described formal hepatic resection, the rest being submitted to extensive resections crossing the principal scissura (Cantlie's line) and necessitating extended resection (see Fig. 80.11). Two of these patients had tumor embolization before surgery to reduce vascularity and tumor size. Eight of these tumors were found to involve the right and left liver on CT scan; there was involvement by tumor extension into the main portal vein in two patients, and one patient had involvement of the right branch of the portal vein. Six patients had severe compression or involvement of the IVC (see Fig. 80.11). Extrahepatic involvement was suspected in three patients. The resections carried out were potentially curative in 12 of the 13 patients with macroscopic clearance of all tumor, but in 1 patient with fibrolamellar hepatocellular carcinoma, a deliberate extended resection was performed despite regional lymph node metastases. There were no intraoperative or in-hospital (30-day) deaths (Soreide et al, 1985). This early experience has been confirmed in our subsequent studies (Vauthey et al, 1993) and in studies by many other investigators.

The resectability rate within a specialized unit does not indicate the overall resectability rate for any particular tumor because the patient population is highly selected. It does seem, however, that an aggressive surgical policy, especially in patients with large solitary tumors, is justified. *In particular, the size of the tumor alone is not a contraindication to resection.* Other authors agree with this view (Adson & Weiland, 1981; Balasegaram & Joishy, 1981; Okamoto et al, 1984; Starzl et al, 1982; Steele et al, 1984). As pointed out earlier, radiologic demonstration of apparent involvement of major inflow and outflow vessels does not constitute an absolute contraindication to exploration for resection. Techniques are now available to deal with portal vein and IVC involvement (see later). These points are particularly applicable in the *fibrolamellar variety of hepatocellular cancer* (Berman et al, 1980; Craig et al, 1980; Hemming et al, 1997; Nagorney

et al, 1985; Soreide et al, 1986). This tumor is more easily resected and may have a more favorable prognosis. Its presence should be suspected in patients with large liver tumors with a normal α-fetoprotein and with noncirrhotic livers who may have increased neurotensin plasma levels (Collier et al, 1984) or increased vitamin B_{12}–binding capacity (Paradinas et al, 1982) or both.

Some patients with primary hepatocellular carcinoma present with *biliary tract obstruction* secondary to tumor emboli within the bile ducts. These emboli may be shown by direct cholangiography, MRI cholangiography, or ultrasound. This presentation does not preclude resection (Blumgart, 1978, 1980).

It is often stated that young patients with large nonresectable hepatocellular cancers are suitable candidates for transplantation, and many physicians and surgeons see liver transplantation as the only therapeutic alternative in such cases. This view seemed to be supported by the National Institutes of Health Consensus Development Conference Statement on Liver Transplantation (National Institutes of Health, 1983). More recent experience does not support this broad approach, however, and controversy exists regarding the place of liver transplantation for the management of liver tumors. This issue is discussed in detail in Chs. 71, 72, 82, 103, 106, and 109.

Finally, portal venous involvement in cholangiocarcinoma affecting the confluence of the bile ducts does not preclude resection (Blumgart et al, 1984; Burke et al, 1998). This topic is fully discussed subsequently and in Ch. 52.

Preoperative Preparation

Preoperative preparation involves the correction of anemia and of coagulopathy and appropriate single-dose antibiotic prophylaxis. All patients with a history of cardiorespiratory disease and all patients older than age 65 years undergo a full cardiorespiratory investigation. All patients with cirrhosis are assessed carefully as to the possibility of present or past infection with hepatitis B or C, for the presence of alcoholic cirrhosis, and for liver function according to the Child-Pugh criteria.

ANESTHETIC CONSIDERATIONS

Anesthetic techniques should take into account the possibility of major intraoperative hemorrhage. Suitable monitoring and facilities for rapid transfusion should be set up, and the possibility of a thoracoabdominal incision should be allowed. Hemorrhage during hepatic resection usually arises from the major hepatic veins or vena cava, and we have pursued a policy of deliberate retrohepatic dissection of the minor and major hepatic veins before beginning parenchymal transection. This procedure is done under anesthesia with a controlled central venous pressure that is not allowed to increase to greater than 5 mm Hg. To obviate air embolism, the dissection is done with the patient in a 15-degree Trendelenburg position. Control of the central venous pressure is maintained at the desired level using a combination of anesthetic techniques and intraoperative fluid restriction. A minimum accepted intraoperative urine output is regarded as 25 mL/hr (see Ch. 25) (Cunningham et al, 1994; Melendez et al, 1998).

We now limit intraoperative blood transfusion, the indications being a decrease in the hematocrit 24% in patients without antecedent cardiac disease or decrease to 29% in patients with cardiac disease. Other indications include a total volume blood loss estimated at 20% or more and hemodynamic instability.

Should vascular isolation of the liver be necessary, the anesthetic requirements are different and require the maintenance of cardiac output during cross-clamping of the vena cava. We rarely employ vascular isolation of the liver even during the removal of very large tumors close to or involving the hepatic veins or the IVC or both. Even tumors directly involving the vena cava may be removed without vascular isolation. Nevertheless, some authors (Bismuth et al, 1989; Huguet & Gavelli, 1994; Huguet et al, 1978, 1992a, 1992b) have advocated vascular isolation techniques during hepatic resection, especially of large tumors. Other authors employ the method for even limited resections (Kelly et al, 1996), but this seems unnecessary. Vascular isolation is discussed fully in Ch. 81.

Prolonged operation with wide abdominal exposure may result in hypothermia. The body temperature should be carefully monitored and maintained. Blood and other infusion fluids should be warmed.

OPERATIVE PROCEDURES

Position of the Patient

The patient should be positioned supine with the right arm extended at right angles to the body. It is unnecessary to place the patient in a lateral position. Tilting the operating table allows adequate exposure during operation. Electrocardiogram leads should be kept clear of the right chest wall and the presternal area. Draping should expose the lower chest and the entire upper abdomen to below the umbilicus (Fig. 80.12). This exposure is adequate for most hepatic resections. If preliminary laparoscopy is to be performed, it is done at this stage.

For large posteriorly lying tumors, a thoracoabdominal incision or median sternotomy may be necessary, and in this instance draping should expose the right chest, extending on the left to the midclavicular line and vertically from the suprasternal notch to the subumbilical area. The abdomen should be widely exposed from midaxillary line to midaxillary line to allow adequate space for a transverse incision. A cross bar or similar device should be

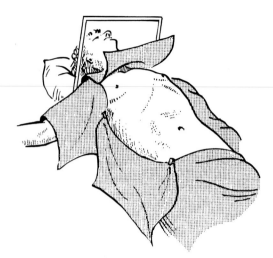

Fig. 80.12. Position of the patient on the operating table. Note the wide exposure of the abdomen and chest. The cross bar later holds a large retractor used to elevate the costal margin (see Fig. 80.14).

fitted to the table, which later holds a self-retaining retractor to elevate the costal margin (see Fig. 80.12). In patients in whom extracorporeal venovenous bypass is to be performed in conjunction with complete vascular isolation of the liver or in patients in whom resection is to be done in association with autotransplantation or in the hypothermic perfused liver (see Ch. 85), the right or left groin should be prepared to allow access to the appropriate femoral vein, and the left axilla or the left neck should be exposed to allow venous access.

Incisions

The incision depends on circumstances (Fig. 80.13). There should never be any hesitation to extend or enlarge the wound to gain adequate access. For most hepatic resections, the initial incision should be an extended right subcostal incision (*ABD* in Fig. 80.13) or a bilateral subcostal incision with a vertical extension. A limited

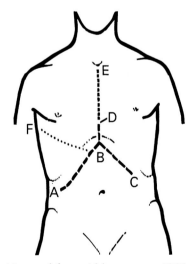

Fig. 80.13. Incisions used for partial hepatectomy. *ABCD*, rooftop incision with vertical extension; *F*, right thoracic extension; *DE*, median sternotomy. Most often an extended right subcostal incision (*ABD*) is adequate.

right-sided incision may be made first to allow preliminary exploration to exclude obviously nonresectable disease or the presence of extrahepatic disease. Assessment at this time may dictate whether it is necessary to extend the incision. Large tumors of the right side of the liver, especially lying posteriorly and possibly involving the IVC, may require extension as a right thoracoabdominal approach, but this is rarely necessary. Our experience in more than 2000 cases of liver resection dictated a thoracoabdominal incision in only 3% of cases. A median sternotomy gives good access, is rapid, and spares disruption of either pleural cavity, but it is seldom required. If median sternotomy is employed, the diaphragm may be split through the central tendon giving excellent exposure of the suprahepatic IVC and the major hepatic veins, and the open pericardium can be used to allow direct access to the intrapericardial IVC.

Exposure, Mobilization, and Assessment

When the abdomen is opened, the entire peritoneal cavity should be explored. In particular, the structures occupying the free edge of the lesser omentum and lymph nodes related to the hepatic artery and the celiac axis and the supraduodenal nodes should be assessed. There may be difficulty exploring the lower abdomen through an upper abdominal incision in patients with previous pelvic surgery (e.g., sigmoid colectomy for primary colorectal cancer). In cases in which access is limited, palpation in conjunction with previous CT and positron emission tomography scans is sufficient. As a preliminary to exploration of the liver, the ligamentum teres is divided, and the falciform ligament is incised and separated from the anterior abdominal wall (Fig. 80.14A). The falciform ligament is divided as far back as

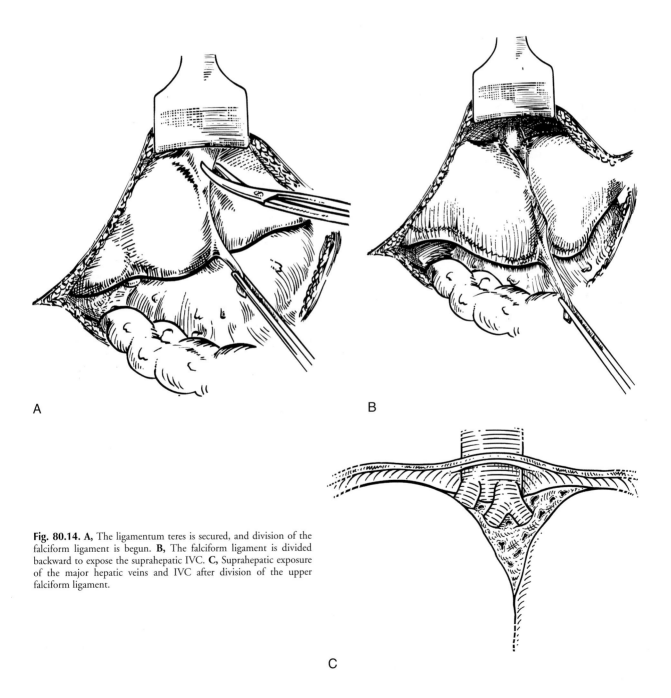

A

B

C

Fig. 80.14. A, The ligamentum teres is secured, and division of the falciform ligament is begun. **B,** The falciform ligament is divided backward to expose the suprahepatic IVC. **C,** Suprahepatic exposure of the major hepatic veins and IVC after division of the upper falciform ligament.

the subdiaphragmatic IVC (see Fig. 80.14B and C). Vessels running within the falciform ligament require careful diathermy control. A stout ligature should be left on the ligamentum teres, which acts as a useful retractor during subsequent exploration and dissection.

Exploration of the abdomen for masses in the liver should follow division of the ligamentum teres and falciform ligament. Elevation of the ligamentum teres helps expose the undersurface of the liver and the area of the hilus and umbilical fissure. Both hands should be inserted into the abdomen to allow bimanual palpation. Unless bimanual palpation is carried out, quite large lesions may be missed or underestimated. The lesser omentum should be incised, and a finger should be introduced into the lesser sac to allow adequate palpation of the caudate lobe (segment I). Complete palpation of the right lobe and particularly assessment of the right side of the vena cava require mobilization of the right liver from the diaphragm, but this may be delayed until ultrasound

examination of the liver in conjunction with initial palpation indicates that the lesions are potentially resectable, and that operation should proceed.

To mobilize the right lobe, the peritoneal reflection at the edge of the right triangular ligament is incised, and the incision is developed medially between the diaphragm and the liver until the entire bare area of the liver on the right is exposed (Fig. 80.15); this allows the liver to be turned to the left. During this dissection, the table is rotated a little to the left, and it is helpful for the surgeon to be seated on the patient's right. Complete exposure of the IVC and of the right hepatic vein requires division of the fibrous tissue (vena caval ligament), which usually obscures the right side or the upper part of the retrohepatic vena cava (see Fig. 80.15A). This division can be done with scissors (see Fig. 80.15A), or the endoscopic gastrointestinal anastomosis vascular stapler (Endo-GIA; United States Surgical Corporation, Norwalk, CT) can be used

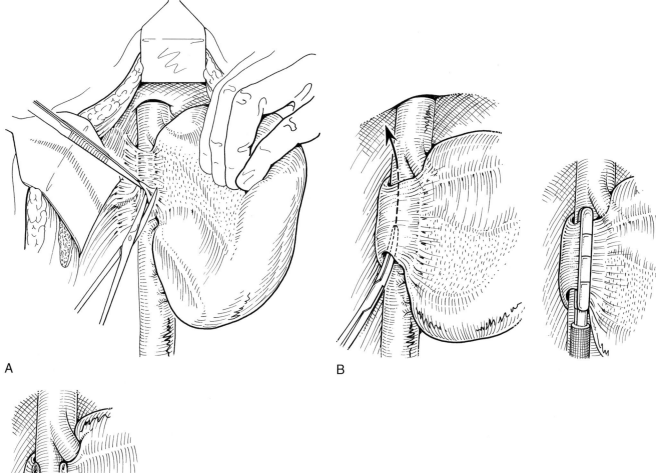

A

B

C

Fig. 80.15. A, Incision of the peritoneal reflection of the right triangular ligament allows mobilization of the right liver. The exposure is deepened to display the right lateral margin of the IVC. *Note:* If the right hepatic vein is to be exposed, the IVC ligament must be divided with scissors as illustrated. **B,** The ligament also may be mobilized, and a clamp is passed beneath it *(left)*. It is divided with the Endo-GIA vascular stapler *(right)*. **C,** The retrohepatic IVC is fully exposed.

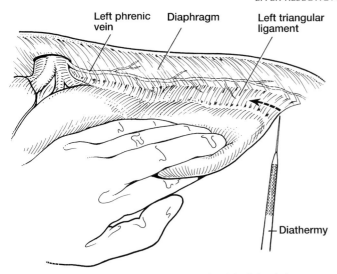

Left phrenic vein   Diaphragm   Left triangular ligament

Diathermy

Fig. 80.16. The left triangular ligament is exposed and divided with the cautery. Care should be taken not to injure the left phrenic vein.

(see Fig. 80.15B) to expose the vena cava completely (see Fig. 80.15C). The vena caval ligament also extends behind the vena cava posteriorly, embracing it and joining a similar fibrous extension from the caudate lobe on the left (see Ch. 1). Rarely, this posterior part of the ligament is replaced by a thin rim of liver tissue so that at this point the vena cava runs through a tunnel of liver parenchyma. This can be a source of difficulty, but this thin plate of liver tissue can similarly be divided to expose the IVC completely. If during mobilization of the right liver the tumor is found attached to the diaphragm, this is usually only over a limited distance, and the affected area of diaphragm is separated, or a segment of the diaphragm is excised and subsequently repaired. An anterior approach with initial transection of the parenchyma without preliminary mobilization of the right liver is valuable in many cases (see later) (Lai EC et al, 1996).

On the left side, the liver is mobilized by division of the apex of the left triangular ligament. The table is rotated a little toward the right to allow good visualization. Care must be taken not to damage the spleen at the far left of the triangular ligament. The ligament is opened, and between its anterior and posterior leaves, the upper part of the IVC and the left hepatic vein become visible (Fig. 80.16).

Intraoperative Ultrasound

We use intraoperative ultrasound to define the number and location and anatomic relationships of lesions within the liver and for the performance of guided needle biopsy of small, deeply placed lesions. Transhepatic cannulation of biliary or vascular elements for the performance of contrast studies (Hasegawa et al, 1991b) or ultrasound to guide planes of parenchymal dissection is rarely employed. A detailed description of the use of intraoperative ultrasound in liver resection is provided in Chs. 23 and 86. Essentially, examination is carried out with a B-mode real-time system. The probes for intraoperative use are waterproof and sterilizable. A T-shaped probe is used and is enclosed in a latex sheath within which a layer of contact jelly eliminates air bubbles and allows application of the probe to the liver surface. The moisture of the liver allows good contact. Regulation of the

pulse processing system is performed by the circulating nurse under the direction of the surgeon, and the images are displayed on a television monitor.

Examination should be carried out in a systematic fashion. We start with examination of the umbilical fissure, progressing to examination of the hilar structures. We follow this with a careful examination of the hepatic veins and finally of the hepatic parenchyma. In cases of doubt, further examination may be done after mobilization of the right or left liver, or the probe may be used from the inferior surface of the liver.

The information obtained at intraoperative ultrasound is frequently valuable in assessing the liver and in planning resection. We have found, however, that with modern high-quality preoperative imaging studies, intraoperative ultrasound, more frequently than not, plays a confirmatory role in diagnosis, rather than revealing features not suspected before laparotomy (Jarnagin et al, 2001b). This is particularly true in the noncirrhotic liver. High-quality laparoscopy and *laparoscopic ultrasound* are now available (see earlier), and studies at MSKCC show that the findings at intraoperative ultrasound changed the operative plan in only a few patients (see Ch. 23).

MAJOR ANATOMIC HEPATIC RESECTIONS

All major hepatic resections mandate control of the inflow vasculature to the portion of liver to be resected with maintenance of good hepatic arterial and portal venous blood supply to the remnant. This may be done by dissection of the relevant portal pedicle at the hilus and outside the liver substance (Blumgart, 1982). Alternatively, the major branches may be secured within the liver by division of the liver tissue by finger fracture (Foster & Berman, 1977; Ton That Tung & Quang, 1963), as described subsequently, or by crushing the liver substance with clamps as described by Ton That Tung (1979). More recently, Launois and Jamieson (1992a, 1992b) have advocated control of the intrahepatic pedicles, and this is detailed in this chapter. In practice, most surgeons employ a combination of techniques in hepatic resection (Fig. 80.17). Biliary drainage from the remnant must be preserved without biliary leakage and without damage to the biliary tract. The hepatic venous outflow must be controlled subsequently, and the liver parenchyma must be transected to provide tumor clearance in cases of malignancy.

Inflow Control and Preservation of the Integrity of the Biliary Tree

Control of the hepatic arterial and portal venous blood supply to the portion of liver to be removed can be obtained by extrahepatic dissection or alternatively by transecting the relevant pedicles within the liver substance. Extrahepatic vascular dissection may be accompanied by extrahepatic dissection and control of the relevant biliary radicles, but this is associated with the risk of biliary injury, especially in dissection on the right side, where anatomic variations of the major right sectoral ducts at their junction with the main biliary channel are frequent (see Ch. 1). For this reason, we reserve extrahepatic biliary dissection for patients whose tumors are close to the hilar structures and where an intrahepatic approach to the portal pedicles would be impossible without compromising tumor clearance. Extrahepatic dissection also is mandatory in dissection for hilar cholangiocarcinoma

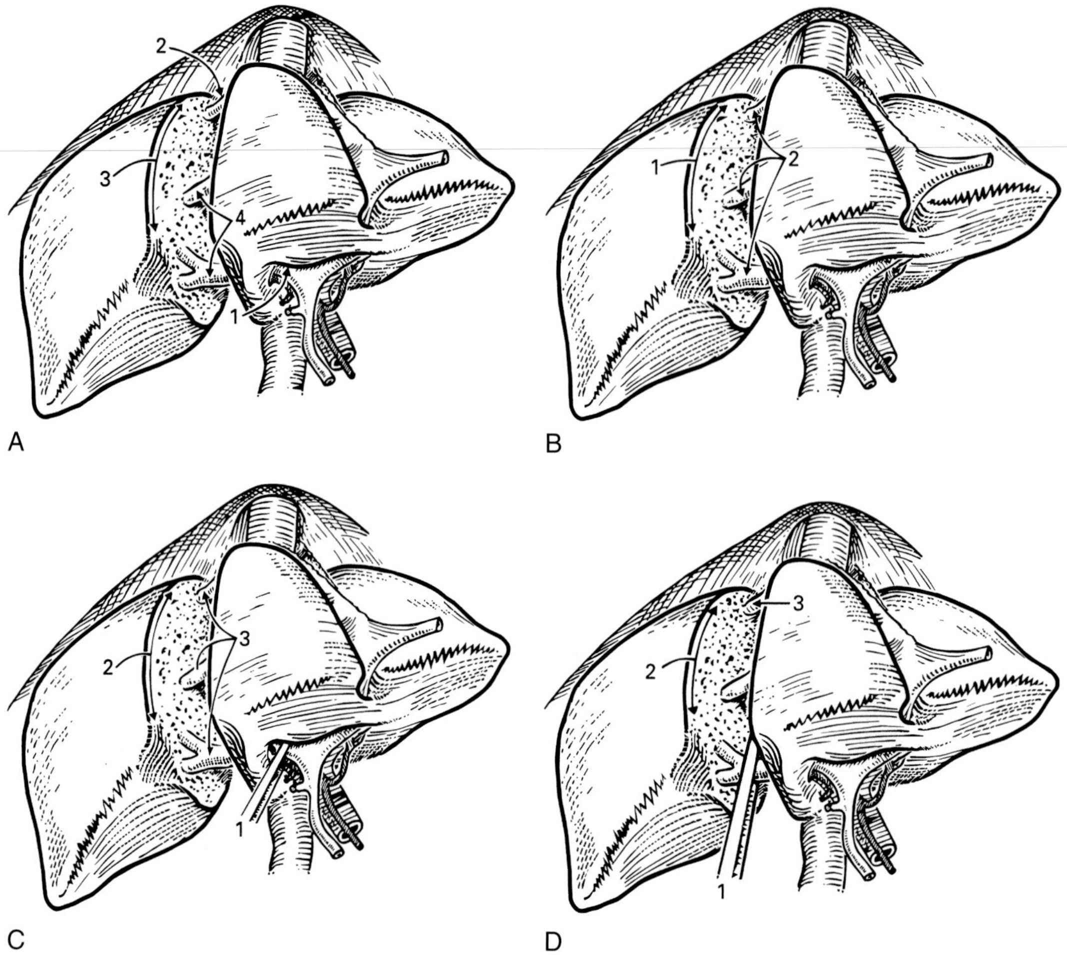

Fig. 80.17. Alternative steps in the performance of right hepatectomy. **A,** Initial division of the right portal triad *(1)* and of the right hepatic vein *(2)* and subsequent transection of the liver substance *(3)* with intrahepatic isolation of vessels *(4)*. **B,** Initial parenchymal dissection *(1)* with intrahepatic control of the vessels *(2)*. **C,** Initial dissection of the portal triad and clamp *(1)* followed by parenchymal transection *(2)* with intrahepatic control of the vessels *(3)*. **D,** Intrahepatic control of the portal pedicles *(1)* followed by parenchymal transection *(2)* with subsequent intrahepatic control of the hepatic veins *(3)*.

(see later). *Even when performing extrahepatic dissection for solid tumors, we divide the right hepatic artery and the right portal vein; however, we usually do not attempt detailed extrahepatic dissection of the biliary structures, but divide them laterally within the pedicles at the time of parenchymal transection.* For left-sided resections, although a pedicle approach is possible, we usually pursue dissection within or at the base of the umbilical fissure and well to the left of the hilar bifurcation (see later). Since the work of Launois and Jamieson (1992b, 1993), we have used pedicular control when possible and have performed more than 400 liver resections without extrahepatic dissection of the hilar structures (see later).

Outflow Control

The major danger in controlling hepatic venous outflow is the risk of hemorrhage. Some authors prefer total vascular isolation techniques to overcome this problem, especially for large tumors abutting or involving the vena cava or major hepatic venous structures (Delva et al, 1989; Emond et al, 1995; Emre et al, 1993; Hannoun et al, 1993). At MSKCC, total vascular isolation was not used in more than 1800 consecutive liver resections (Jarnagin et al, 2002).

Intrahepatic control of the hepatic veins carried out during parenchymal transection can be practiced for tumors that allow clearance superiorly with adequate tumor margins and with safe access to these vessels. *Extrahepatic dissection and control of the major hepatic veins is possible in nearly all cases, however, and for the difficult tumor lying high and posteriorly, it allows good clearance together with reliable control of hemorrhage during right or left hepatectomy.* This approach has two essential requisites:

1. Good anesthetic control of central venous pressure, which is not allowed to increase to greater than 5 mm Hg (see earlier and Ch. 25)
2. Precise extrahepatic dissection of the major hepatic veins

The dissection is done with the patient in a 15-degree Trendelenburg position to minimize the risk of air embolism. No case of clinically significant air embolism has been encountered in 496 resected cases (Melendez et al, 1998). These techniques are accompanied by an acceptable blood loss and blood transfusion rate and are simpler yet comparable to any series reported using total vascular isolation (Table 80.3) (Cunningham et al, 1994; Jones et al, 1998; Melendez et al, 1998). The method avoids the need for fluid loading and the use of pressor agents during periods of vascular isolation and the adverse biochemical

Table 80.3 Comparison of Operative Indices Between Hepatic Vascular Isolation and Low Central Venous Pressure–Aided Hepatectomy

Reference	Technique	Total Patients	Major Resections*	Mean Blood Loss (mL)[†]	Median Blood Loss (mL)	Transfusion (U or mL)[†]
Delva et al, 1989	HVI	35	35	—	—	8 ± 8.3
Emre et al, 1993	HVI	16	13	1866 ± 1683	1325	—
Hannoun et al, 1993	HVI	15	15	—	—	5.8 ± 4.7
Habib et al, 1994	HVI	56	33	1651 ± 1748	1200	930 ± 750
Cunningham et al, 1994	LCVP	100	69	1021 ± 964	1000	1.4 ± 2.1
Emond et al, 1995	HVI	48	44	1255 ± 1291	—	1.9 ± 2.6
Belghiti et al, 1996	HVI	24	24	1195 ± 1105	—	2.5 ± 3.4
Melendez et al, 1998[‡]	LCVP	496	357	849 ± 972	618	0.9 ± 1.8
Jarnagin et al, 2002	LCVP	1803	1027	—	600	4 ± 0.3[§]

*Major resections include all lobectomies and extended lobectomies.
[†]Values are reported as mean ± SD.
[‡]Series included cirrhotic patients.
[§]Total transfusion of all blood products during hospital stay.
HVI, hepatic vascular isolation; LCVP, low central venous pressure.

and hemodynamic effects that ensue when the clamps maintaining the vascular isolation are released.

In a study of 1803 patients undergoing hepatic resection at MSKCC, we showed that our approach yields an acceptable blood loss (600 mL median). Transfusion of any blood product was necessary in only 49% of patients at any time during hospital admission. Mortality was 4% in the first 5 years of the study, but decreased to 1.3% in the last 2 years, there being no deaths in the last 84 consecutive cases (Jarnagin et al, 2002).

Parenchymal Transection

The liver parenchyma may be transected using a simple crushing technique, and this is our preference. Glisson's capsule is scored with the diathermy along the line of proposed transection, and a Kelly clamp is used to crush the liver tissue and expose vessels for clipping or suture ligation. The technique is rapid and efficient, and during this phase of the operation we apply intermittent inflow occlusion (Pringle, 1908) to control blood flow to the remnant, usually maintaining inflow occlusion for periods of 5 minutes interspersed by 1-minute periods of relief to allow perfusion of the remnant and decompression of the bowel. We never employ long periods of inflow occlusion despite the fact that this has been shown to be safe (Berney et al, 1998; Hannoun et al, 1993; Huguet et al, 1978, 1992a, 1992b), and we especially avoid prolonged occlusion during hepatic resection in patients with jaundice or cirrhosis. *There is no need for prolonged portal inflow occlusion, and usually for major hepatic resections, we complete parenchymal transection in 20 minutes with three or four periods of occlusion.* During the 1-minute breaks, we use the Argon Beam Coagulator (Valley Lab Inc, Boulder, CO) to control small vessel oozing on the side of the remnant. Avitene, Surgicel, or fibrin sealants also may be applied to the cut surface of the liver to achieve final hemostasis.

The parenchyma also may be transected using an ultrasonic dissector (Hodgson & DelGuercio, 1984) or a water-jet dissector (Baer et al, 1992b). The ultrasonic dissector (Hanna et al, 1996) has become popular and has some advantages in displaying vessels, particularly in the performance of segmental and subsegmental

resections and especially in the cirrhotic liver, but it is tedious and has no apparent advantage in the performance of major resections. There are no published data to indicate that the technique is associated with improved control of blood loss. The ultrasonic machine is expensive, and reliance on its use leaves the operator insecure during periods of instrumental breakdown. The new version of the water-jet dissector (Helix Hydro-Jet ERBE; USA Inc., Marietta, GA) is much more efficient than the original version, and one of us (L.H.B.) has found it of considerable value, particularly in the exposure of major pedicles.

Several alternative techniques have been developed. Two devices, a computer-controlled bipolar cautery marketed as LigaSure (Valley Lab Inc, Boulder, CO) and a saline-linked radiofrequency ablation device called TissueLink (TissueLink Medical Inc, Dover, NH), have been used with success by some authors (Clavien et al, 2004; Sakamoto et al, 2004; Strasberg et al, 2002). The harmonic scalpel (SonoSurg; Olympus Key Med, Ltd, New York, NY) also has been used successfully, particularly in the performance of laparoscopic partial hepatectomy (see later). *We prefer to use simple crushing techniques* and to teach these approaches to our residents and fellows because they form an ideal basis from which to develop skills using alternative technical devices. More recently, we have employed stapling techniques to divide major vessels and pedicles within the liver substance and for parenchymal transection (Fong & Blumgart, 1997).

Drainage of the Abdominal Cavity

Franco and colleagues (1989) suggested that hepatic resection should be performed without drainage. After performing a controlled clinical trial (Fong et al, 1996), we no longer use drainage routinely after major hepatic resection. The institution of drainage is associated with a prolonged hospital stay, an increased possibility of infection, and in our experience no decrease in the need for postoperative interventional radiology–directed drainage. In particular, we do not drain the abdomen after resection in patients with a cirrhotic liver. When instituted, such drainage may have to be prolonged because the drain often delivers copious quantities of ascitic fluid. Drainage also is accompanied by

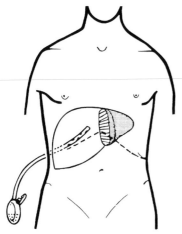

Fig. 80.18. Drainage of the right subdiaphragmatic space with simple large-bore drains connected to a closed system or to a suction apparatus. Our practice now is abdominal closure without routine drainage (see text).

an increased risk of infected ascites. The policy of avoiding drainage has been vindicated in a further study at MSKCC of more than 1000 patients.

We routinely drain the liver bed in all patients undergoing resection that is accompanied by biliary reconstruction. In such instances, we employ a single sealed suction drain, which is converted to a dependent drain within 24 hours (Fig. 80.18). The drain is removed usually within 48 to 72 hours, when drainage is reduced to less than 50 mL, and provided that there is no biliary leakage.

Right Hepatectomy

Inflow and Biliary Control

The liver is elevated to display its inferior surface and the portal structures. *We always lower the hilar plate to expose the left hepatic duct and the confluence of the bile ducts* (see Ch. 30). Division of the peritoneal reflection along the free edge of the lesser omentum exposes the lateral side of the portal vein and the common bile duct. The peritoneum overlying the common bile duct on the free edge of the lesser omentum and extending up into Calot's triangle is incised. The cystic duct and the cystic artery are exposed, ligated, and divided (Fig. 80.19). The cystic duct is transfixed before being ligated, and a tie is left on the cystic duct for later retraction.

Some surgeons now proceed to extrahepatic dissection of the right hepatic duct. We no longer advocate this approach. We proceed to dissection of the right hepatic artery and portal vein and usually leave management of the right hepatic duct until later in the operation (see later).

The right hepatic artery is dissected, ligated, and divided (Fig. 80.20). The right hepatic artery originates from the main hepatic arterial trunk and usually passes posterior to the common bile duct (see Ch. 1). It may be ligated to the right or medial to the common hepatic duct. It is important to be certain by palpation at the umbilical fissure that there is no compromise to the blood supply passing to the left lobe of the liver, and this may be done after temporary occlusion of the right hepatic artery and before ligation. We prefer to ligate the artery to the right of the common hepatic duct, and *we deliberately double-suture ligate the*

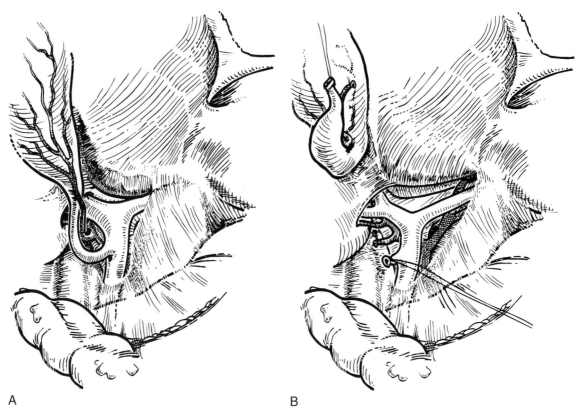

A   B

Fig. 80.19. A, The peritoneum overlying the common bile duct on the free edge of the lesser omentum and extending up into Calot's triangle is incised, and the common bile duct, common hepatic duct, and Calot's triangle are exposed. **B,** The cystic duct and cystic artery are secured. A tie is left on the cystic duct for later retraction (see text and Fig. 80.20). The hilar plate is lowered to expose the left hepatic duct and the confluence of the bile ducts, and dissection of the right hepatic duct is begun.

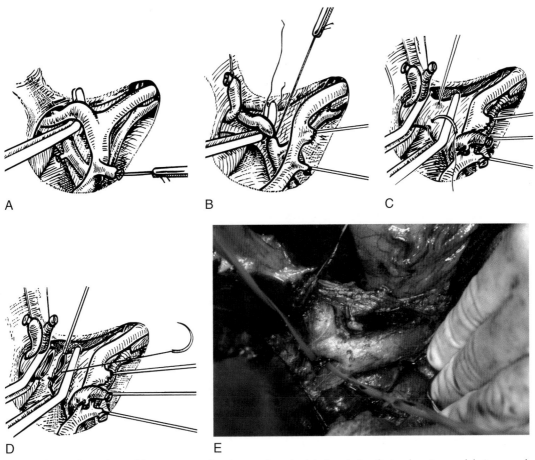

Fig. 80.20. A, The right hepatic duct is dissected (we now, more often than not, leave the right hepatic duct for intrahepatic control during parenchymal transection; see text). The confluence of the hepatic ducts and the origin of the left hepatic duct are shown. **B,** The right hepatic duct has been transfixed with absorbable suture material, divided, and ligated or oversewn. Alternatively, it simply may be divided under direct vision and then oversewn. In any event, the suture is held and retracted toward the left. Traction on the sutures attached to the cystic duct and the right hepatic duct stump allows retraction of the common hepatic duct and common bile duct to the left and assists display of the vessels beneath. The right hepatic artery is dissected, ligated, and divided usually to the right (as shown), but sometimes to the left, of the common hepatic duct. **C,** The right portal vein is dissected, and forceps are gently passed beneath it. Special care is taken not to damage the first branch of the right portal vein, which comes off early and posteroinferiorly. This branch is sought initially and ligated and divided or avoided (see text). Straight-bladed vascular clamps are applied to the right portal vein. Note retaining sutures to secure the vein before division. **D,** The vein is divided, and its proximal stump is oversewn using a vascular suture. The distal stump is transfixed with 3-0 polyglactin 910 (Vicryl) suture and ligated. Light traction on the cystic duct, right hepatic duct stump, and right hepatic artery assists display. **E,** Intraoperative photograph illustrates dissection of the portal vein and its branches seen from the patient's right. The main portal vein gives rise to the anterior and posterior sectoral branches independently. Both of these are surrounded by blue vessel loops. The left portal vein and the anterior right sectoral vein arise at the same point. It is important to recognize this variant anatomy and to identify all branches during dissection.

proximal end and hold this after division for light traction to the left, which together with traction on the cystic duct stump (see earlier) *is of considerable assistance in exposing the portal vein.*

The portal vein is exposed. The vein is approached laterally and posteriorly. The surgeon may be seated on the right and the table rotated to the left. The main portal trunk is exposed, and the left branch is revealed and preserved. Sometimes, the right anterior and posterior sectoral branches of the portal vein arise individually, and these origins may be separated by 2 cm (see Fig. 80.20E). It is important not to misidentify these branches during dissection. The right branch of the portal vein may be delivered from the hilus, and a good length usually is obtained. Curved forceps are passed gently around the right portal vein under direct vision. Special care should be taken not to damage the first posterior branch of the right portal vein, which comes off early and posteroinferiorly to supply the right portion of the caudate lobe. This branch should be deliberately sought, and the forceps, which are passed behind the right branch of the portal vein, should be introduced to avoid this vulnerable area. *If any difficulty*

is encountered, this branch should be individually ligated and divided before any instrument is passed beneath the right portal trunk.

Application of a straight-bladed vascular clamp is a safe method of transecting the right portal vein (see Fig. 80.20). It is good practice to pass two retaining sutures to secure the vein before dividing it. These sutures, if left with the needle in place, can be developed to oversew the stump when the vein has been divided (see Fig. 80.20). If the vein is short, it is inadvisable to attempt simply to ligate the right portal vein and transect it because the ligatures have a tendency to slip unless transfixed. If the vein is ligated, it should be transfixed and double ligated. We have divided the right branch of the portal vein using the Endo-GIA vascular stapler (Fong & Blumgart, 1997). Should it be found that the right anterior and posterior sectoral branches arise independently (see Fig. 80.20E), they require individual control.

If it is decided to control the right hepatic duct, this is now dissected. The confluence of the bile ducts and the origin of the infrahepatic course of the left hepatic duct should be seen clearly after lowering of the hilar plate (see Fig. 80.19B). Occasionally, and particularly if segment IV is large, it may help to divide the liver tissue that occupies the lower limits of the umbilical fissure and bridges the gap between the quadrate lobe (segment IV) and segment III of the left liver. This maneuver opens the umbilical fissure and allows better exposure of the subhepatic and the hilar area.

When the right hepatic duct is dissected, it should be transfixed, ligated, and divided (see Fig. 80.20). Absorbable suture material and not silk should be employed because silk might find its way into the biliary tree postoperatively. It may be that difficulty is encountered in passing a ligature about the right hepatic duct, in which case it may be divided under direct vision and subsequently oversewn with a 4-0 polyglactin 910 suture (Vicryl; Ethicon, Edinburgh, UK) on an atraumatic needle. In many instances, the ducts draining the anterior and posterior right sectors are found entering the confluence separately, or the posterior sectoral duct may join the left hepatic duct (see Ch. 1). In such cases, both of these major sectoral ducts should be individually identified and secured. It may be difficult to obtain a clear view of the right hepatic duct for dissection and ligation, in which case these structures are best left intact. *The duct or its major sectoral tributaries may be secured in the pedicles further laterally at the time of parenchymal dissection. We usually use this approach because it is safe and obviates precise dissection of the ducts extrahepatically.* Deliberate dissection of the hepatic duct must be carried out for tumors that approach the hilus of the liver and engulf the pedicles down to the point of entry of the portal triads into the liver substances.

Pedicle Ligation

An important alternative to extrahepatic dissection of the hilar structures is the pedicle ligation technique using the intrahepatic approach first described in Japan by Takasaki and colleagues (1986a, 1986b) and then in the West by Launois (1994) and Lanois and Jamieson (1992b, 1993). This approach is most useful for right-sided tumors located away from the hilus, which allows its use without compromising tumor clearance. *This technique allows the surgeon to dissect and clamp the required sheaths early in the operation and define the segment or segments to be removed.*

Essentially, the method relies on intrahepatic definition and control of the portal triads to the segments to be removed. The structures of the portal triad carry Glisson's capsules with them as they penetrate the liver and are contained in a well-formed sheath within the parenchyma (Fig. 80.21). The pedicular sheaths can

be exposed after appropriate hepatotomies (Fig. 80.22) and are tough enough to be dissected (Fig. 80.23), encircled, and clamped. Pedicle ligation, by eliminating the hilar dissection, saves time and obviates potential injury to the contralateral vessels and bile ducts.

We have found it important first to ligate the lowermost retrohepatic veins draining from the caudate process and lower part of the liver to the vena cava (see Fig. 80.22A). Failure to do this has resulted in hemorrhage during passage of a finger or dissector (see Figs. 80.23 and 80.24) about the right portal pedicle, and we regard this preliminary move as essential before using the right pedicle approach. Other than this cautionary note, the technique we employ is almost identical to that described by Launois (see later). Care must be taken to respect the anatomy of the pedicles, in particular the pedicle to the right posterior sector (Fig. 80.24; see Fig. 80.23). When the right pedicle has been exposed (see Fig. 80.22B and E), and trial clamping reveals the demarcation line along the Glissonian plane, we divide the pedicle. We usually use a vascular stapling device (see Fig. 80.22D and F) (Fong & Blumgart, 1997). This method also can be used to control the left sheath, but we prefer to dissect the structures within the umbilical fissure (see later).

Exposure and Control of the Right Hepatic Vein

The right hepatic vein may be controlled from within the liver during hepatic parenchymal transection or alternatively may be isolated extrahepatically before proceeding with division of the liver tissue. *Extrahepatic control of the right hepatic vein is important for large tumors lying posteriorly in segments VII and VIII adjacent to the vena cava because it is difficult to obtain tumor clearance during transparenchymal dissection in such instances and still avoid major hemorrhage arising from accidental laceration to the vein.*

To control the right hepatic vein, the liver is turned to the left, and the retrohepatic veins are ligated. Some authors pass tapes around the vena cava above and below the liver, but we usually omit this step. Tapes can be passed easily between the inferior surface of the liver and the right renal vein below and after subdiaphragmatic dissection of the IVC, above the liver. If difficulty is encountered in gaining control of the IVC below the diaphragm, and this is sometimes the case with large tumors, the surgeon should not hesitate to extend the incision to the right chest or vertically as a sternotomy. This possibility usually would have been considered on the basis of preoperative investigations. It is dangerous to persist through an abdominal incision in an attempt to mobilize a rigid right lobe of the liver containing a large tumor because the right hepatic vein may tear posteriorly. When the chest is open, the vena cava may be approached more easily. Through a median sternotomy, the pericardium can be opened and control gained after dissection of the IVC within the pericardial sac. This incision is usually unnecessary, however, and in most cases the IVC and the right hepatic vein can be dissected through an abdominal incision alone.

It is important to dissect the hepatic veins with the central venous pressure controlled at no greater than 5 mm Hg. To obviate air embolism, the patient is placed in a 15-degree Trendelenburg position (Cunningham et al, 1994). Complete posterolateral exposure of the right hepatic vein requires division of a tongue of fibrous tissue (the IVC ligament), which obscures to a variable extent the right side of the upper part of the retrohepatic vena cava. This dissection may have been done at an earlier stage in the operation, but if not it should be completed at this stage by the techniques described previously (see Fig. 80.15). The right hepatic vein is approached starting from below and working

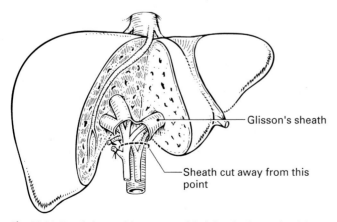

Fig. 80.21. Detailed view of the anatomy of the left and right portal pedicles at the hilus.

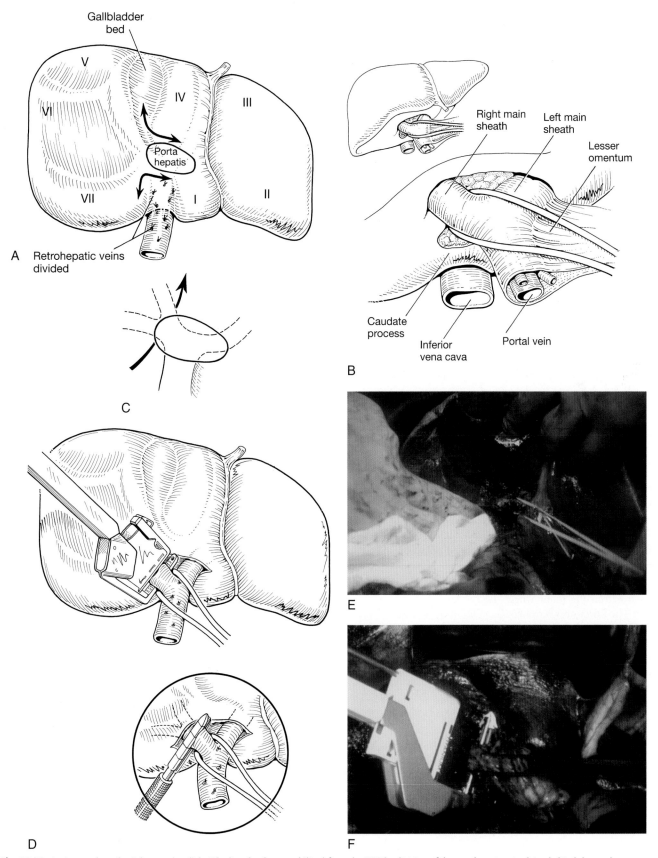

Fig. 80.22. A, Approach to the right portal pedicle. The liver has been mobilized from the IVC by division of the retrohepatic veins lying behind the caudate process. Hepatotomies have been made in the region of the gallbladder fossa and the caudate process. The *curved double-headed arrows* indicate the sites of the hepatotomies above and below the porta hepatis. The approach in the caudate process is essentially a posterior approach. **B,** A vessel loop is drawn about the right pedicle and pulled to the left to protect the left pedicular structures during control and transection of the right main sheath. **C,** The *curved arrow* indicates the path of the finger (see Fig. 80.23) or instrument during dissection of the right pedicle allowing its isolation. **D,** The right portal pedicle is controlled and subsequently divided with a vascular stapler or with the Endo-GIA vascular stapler *(inset)*. **E,** Intraoperative photograph shows the right portal pedicle exposed by finger dissection and surrounded by a yellow vessel loop, which is drawn to the patient's left (see also **B** above). The vessel loop is drawn firmly to the left, and the pedicle is divided using the stapler as shown in **D. F,** Operative photograph shows division of the right portal vein pedicle, which is encircled by a red vessel loop pulled to the left. The vascular stapler is being used to divide the pedicle as illustrated in **D.**

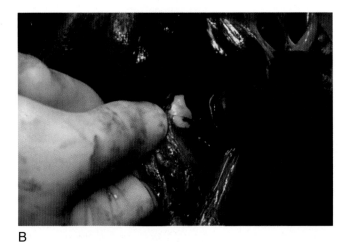

A

B

Fig. 80.23. A, Illustration shows digital isolation of the right pedicle. **B,** Operative photograph illustrates insertion of the index finger through a hepatotomy in the caudate lobe where it merges with the base of the gallbladder fossa to isolate the right portal pedicle. A vessel loop is drawn about the pedicle as shown in Fig. 80.22F.

upward from the point where the caudate process crosses the IVC. The lowermost retrohepatic veins are approached first and may be controlled by fine ligatures passed around the vessels with an aneurysm needle (Fig. 80.25). This can be tedious, and for the smaller vessels we apply two clips on the vena caval side and one on the liver side of each vessel. Larger veins and especially an inferior right hepatic vein can be controlled by formal

division between clamps or by the use of the Endo-GIA vascular stapler. It is important in approaching the right hepatic vein to perform an *extensive retrohepatic dissection and to secure all the short hepatic veins draining from the posterior aspect of the liver.* This dissection should be carried well over to the left of the IVC. Only in this way is sufficient access obtained to visualize and dissect the main right hepatic vein safely.

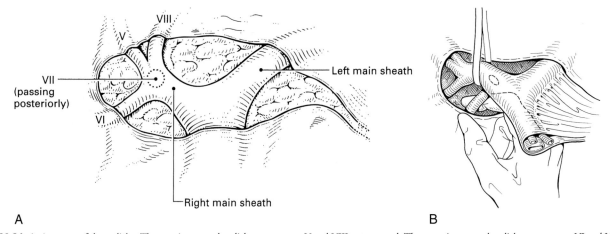

A

B

Fig. 80.24. A, Anatomy of the pedicles. The anterior sectoral pedicles to segments V and VIII pass upward. The posterior sectoral pedicles to segments VI and VII run posterolaterally (see text). **B,** This illustration shows the approach to the right posterior pedicle (right lateral pedicle).

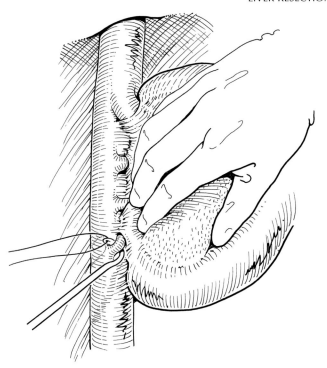

Fig. 80.25. Short hepatic veins issuing from the caudate lobe and the right liver are secured individually using aneurysm needles to pass fine sutures about the vessels, which are tied and cut. Alternatively, these vessels are clipped and divided. This procedure is carried upward beneath the liver until the right lobe is mobilized, and the vena cava is displayed up to the right hepatic vein. This is necessary for subsequent safe dissection of the right hepatic vein.

Before any attempt is made to pass an instrument about the right hepatic vein, there should be full exposure of the vein superiorly. This exposure is achieved by dissecting the filamentous fibrous tissue above the liver and anterior to the suprahepatic IVC. This dissection too may have been done as a preliminary procedure during exposure of the liver at an early stage (see Fig. 80.14). This dissection must be performed right against the exposed liver substance. It is ineffective and dangerous to wander away from the liver surface.

When the right hepatic vein is exposed, a vascular clamp is applied on the caval side. There is usually space for the application of a second clamp on the caval side and a third on the hepatic side, although this may not be always possible (Fig. 80.26A). If it is not possible to place a clamp on the hepatic side, division of the vessel does not result in great hemorrhage, provided that inflow control has been obtained previously. In any event, the vessel is now divided with a scalpel (see Fig. 80.26B). One clamp is removed, and the exposed stump is closed with an over-and-over 3-0 polypropylene vascular suture (see Fig. 80.26C). The proximal (hepatic) side of the right hepatic vein is now closed with a 3-0 polypropylene suture.

Alternatively, in more than 800 cases, we have employed the Endo-GIA (TA30) vascular stapler to divide the right hepatic vein, and in no instance has this been a problem (Fig. 80.27). The stapled approach is quick, effective, and safe (Fong & Blumgart, 1997), and we now use it routinely except for large tumors almost at the exit of the right hepatic vein into the IVC, which, by their size and rigidity, limit the entry of the stapler into the tunnel to the left of the right hepatic vein and anterior to the IVC. Extrahepatic control of the middle hepatic vein is unnecessary during right hepatectomy.

An important new approach to the right hepatic vein involves exposure by preliminary transection of the parenchyma down to

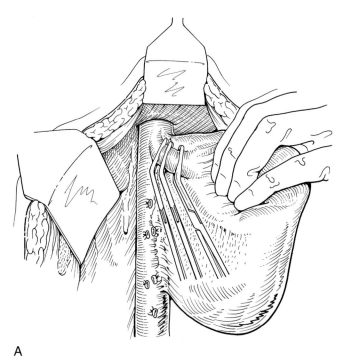

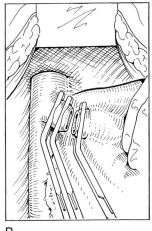

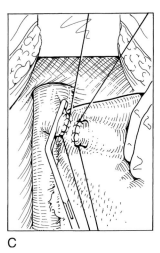

A   B   C

Fig. 80.26. A, Approach to the right hepatic vein. The right liver has been extensively mobilized and the IVC exposed up to the right hepatic vein. The right hepatic vein is dissected (see text), and a vascular clamp is applied on the caval side. A further clamp is placed on the hepatic side, although this is not essential because if the vein is divided after the portal triad at the hilus, bleeding from the exposed venous orifice can be readily controlled with a suture after division of the vein. A second clamp should be applied on the caval side before division of the vein, but if there is not a space for this, a second clamp is applied immediately after the vein is divided. **B,** The right hepatic vein has been divided. **C,** The stump is closed with an over-and-over 3-0 vascular suture.

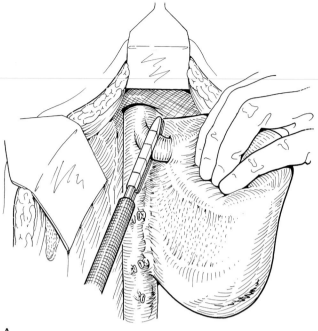

A

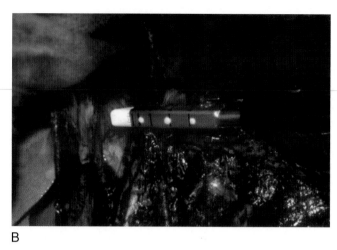

B

Fig. 80.27. A, The right hepatic vein also can be divided using the Endo-GIA vascular stapler. This method is rapid and safe. **B,** Intraoperative photograph shows division of the right hepatic vein with the Endo-GIA vascular stapler.

the anterior surface of the IVC (Lai EC et al, 1996). This so-called *anterior approach* is described later.

Parenchymal Transection

Liver tissue is divided by a tissue fracture technique as described earlier. Pringle's maneuver is performed, and the liver tissue is crushed in the line of transection using a Kelly clamp or similar instrument (Fig. 80.28), leaving the vessels intact. During this process, inflow occlusion is provided by encircling and compressing the hilar structures in a vessel loop. It may be helpful for the first assistant to compress the left liver with the hand and to pull it downward gently. Suction is applied at the blunt end of the sucker, which is used to tease the tissues away from the vessels (see Fig. 80.28).

Large vessels may be isolated easily by crushing the tissue between finger and thumb. When located, smaller vessels and

bile ducts are ligated or occluded with metal clips and divided. Large vessels may be underrun or ligated or controlled with the Endo-GIA stapler. In recent years, we have combined the crushing technique with parenchymal division using the Endo-GIA or similar stapler, which crushes tissue and staples vessels simultaneously.

As the tissue is divided, the fissure that is developed in the liver is opened; this is done by the operator, whose left hand holds the right liver. With fingers located posteriorly in the region of the vena cava, the hand elevates the right lobe opening the wound in the liver to expose its depth. As dissection proceeds, *the middle hepatic vein is displaced to the left*, the dissection proceeding along its right margin. The branches from segments V and VIII are controlled. If the right sectoral bile ducts have not previously been divided extrahepatically, they are now controlled during division of the portal triads. The right portal triad is encountered and divided close to the hilus. If the right hepatic vein has not

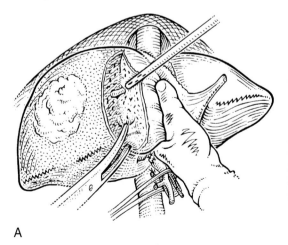

A

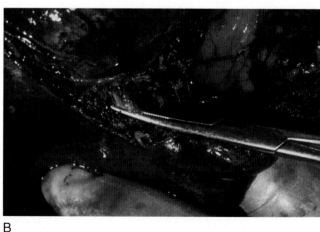

B

Fig. 80.28. A, Parenchymatous transection of the liver tissue by a fracture or crushing technique using a clamp. The portal triad to the right liver has been divided, and a line of demarcation has developed. The liver tissue is opened in this line. The assistant's left hand compresses the left liver close to the transection line. The operator opens the liver tissue, and a combination of crushing the liver between clamps, finger fracture and strong suction exposes the vessels for ligation. The parenchymal transection is done with a vessel loop occluding the hilar vessels (Pringle's maneuver). **B,** Intraoperative photograph shows the crushing of the parenchyma with exposure of vessels using a Kelly clamp.

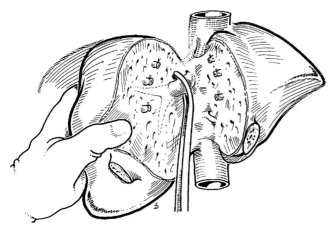

Fig. 80.29. Division of the liver tissue has progressed. The fingers of the operator's left hand are located posteriorly elevating the right lobe and opening the wound in the liver. At this stage, major hepatic veins are identified and secured within the liver substance. This is an alternative to extrahepatic isolation of the right hepatic vein.

been secured behind the liver, it is now isolated and ligated or divided with the stapler within the liver (Fig. 80.29). Alternative methods of parenchymal transection were described earlier.

Hemostasis finally is secured using the Argon Beam Coagulator and by the application of sutures to any obviously hemorrhaging small vessels. Alternatively, a fibrinogen sealant (Guthy, 1986; Scheele, 1989) may be used, but one of us (L.H.B.) prefers the Argon Beam Coagulator, which is effective and is associated with very little tissue necrosis (Postema et al, 1993). In a few cases, if oozing should continue, and particularly if it seems to be coming from divided veins, the passage of large sutures (chromic catgut) anteroposteriorly in a mattress fashion secures hemostasis. These sutures should not be so tight or so numerous as to cause tissue ischemia (Fig. 80.30). Any bleeding from the exposed undersurface of the diaphragm needs to be carefully controlled; in this respect, the Argon Beam Coagulator can be of great value.

Wound Closure and Drainage

If there has been a diaphragmatic incision, this is closed, and if any defects have been created in the diaphragm, these are similarly sutured. There is no need to attempt to close the exposed raw area of the liver with peritoneal flaps because these may cause compression of liver tissue and distortion of hilar vessels. The ligamentum teres should not be used for this purpose, and similarly, omental grafts are usually unnecessary, although any convenient omentum may be laid against the raw surface. *We do not drain the subdiaphragmatic space after liver resection except in the instance of patients in whom there has been biliary obstruction or damage to the biliary tree or biliary reconstruction necessary during the operation* (see earlier). In this instance, drainage of the subdiaphragmatic space is carried out with one or two suction drains connected to a closed system (see Fig. 80.18). The wound is closed in a single layer of looped PDS with clips to the skin. If necessary, a chest drain is placed and connected to an underwater sealed drainage system.

Anterior Approach to Right Hepatectomy

Hanging Maneuver

In right hepatectomy, complete mobilization of the liver before parenchymal transection is considered as a basic maneuver for a safe procedure (see earlier). When a huge tumor invades the

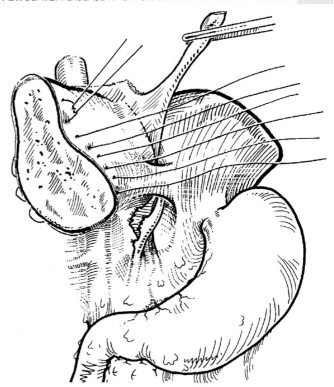

Fig. 80.30. Method of suture of the cut surface of the liver to achieve hemostasis. This technique is seldom necessary.

diaphragm or is attached to the lateral side of the vena cava at a higher level, mobilization may be difficult. In such cases, E.C. Lai and colleagues (1996) reported an anterior approach with initial parenchymal transection from the anterior surface down to the IVC (see later). Because it may be difficult to control bleeding in the deeper parenchymal plane, Belghiti and colleagues (2001) described a new technique of hanging the liver after lifting it with a tape passed between the anterior surface of the IVC and the liver parenchyma.

The most important steps in this maneuver are the definition of the anterior plane of the IVC. Initially, intraoperative ultrasound is performed to confirm the absence of tumor in contact with the anterior surface of the IVC. The upper surface of the liver is exposed up to the anterior surface of the suprahepatic IVC (see Fig. 80.14). The space between the right and the middle hepatic veins is dissected approximately 2 cm downward; we find it convenient to do this using a right angle or a renal pedicle clamp. The anterior surface of the infrahepatic IVC is exposed. The lowermost veins draining between the caudate process and the vena cava are ligated and divided. The most important step is the dissection of the plane anterior to the vena cava. A long Kelly clamp is passed gently upward posterior to the caudate lobe. If a right inferior hepatic vein is present, it is dissected, but not ligated, and the clamp is passed to its right side. With great care, the clamp is worked along the middle plane of the IVC toward the space between the right and middle hepatic veins previously dissected. The tunnel beneath the liver measures about 4 to 6 cm of blind dissection, and the clamp appears between the right and middle hepatic veins. A tape is seized in the clamp and pulled down behind the liver parenchyma. The tape then can be used to elevate the liver away from the anterior surface of the IVC.

Before parenchymal transection, the right pedicle is divided, devascularizing the right liver. The parenchymal transection is conducted from the anterior surface down to the posterior plane in front of the IVC. During the parenchymal transection, upward traction of the tape helps define the plane of transection and facilitates exposure of the deeper parenchymal plane in front of the IVC. After completing the exposure of the anterior surface of the IVC, the right side of the IVC is dissected with division and ligation of the inferior hepatic veins and IVC ligaments. Finally, the trunk of the right hepatic vein is stapled with a vascular stapler or divided between clamps and oversewn. The coronary and right triangular ligaments are transected, and the specimen is removed. The steps in the hanging maneuver are illustrated in the description of liver resection for living liver donation (see Figs. 80.85-80.103).

Anterior Approach

In some patients with very large right-sided hepatic tumors, an anterior approach, which involves initial parenchymal transection before the right hepatic lobe is mobilized, is an alternative. If this approach is adopted, the hilar inflow vessels are first controlled as described earlier. The liver parenchyma is transected from the anterior surface of the liver working posteriorly. This parenchymal transection is pursued until the anterior surface of the right hepatic vein and IVC is encountered. The hanging maneuver described earlier can offer useful definition in this approach. Venous tributaries, including the right hepatic vein, are controlled from the front (Lai EC et al, 1996). The senior author (L.H.B.) has used this approach in selected patients and has found it possible even in the presence of diaphragmatic invasion. As described later, right hepatectomy for living related donor transplantation is carried out essentially using this approach.

Right Hepatic Lobectomy

Right hepatic lobectomy involves removal of segments IV, V, VI, VII, and VIII. It is in effect a right hepatectomy extended to segment IV. In the nomenclature of Goldsmith and Woodburne (1957), it is referred to as *extended right hepatic lobectomy*. Starzl and coworkers (1975, 1980) referred to the procedure as *right trisegmentectomy*, and this term is in common use in the United States.

The initial steps in the procedure are as for right hepatectomy as described earlier, but the operation involves further dissection and mobilization before parenchymal transection. First, the quadrate lobe (segment IV of the liver) is devascularized, and second, the middle hepatic vein must be divided. Occasionally, the caudate lobe (segment I) is removed together with segments IV through VIII as part of the procedure.

After inflow control to segments V, VI, VII, and VIII by extrahepatic dissection or pedicle control as described for right hepatectomy, the next and essential step is *to display precisely the umbilical fissure* of the liver (Starzl et al, 1975). A strong ligature tied to the ligamentum teres is elevated. In many cases, the lower part of the umbilical fissure is concealed by a bridge of tissue fusing segment III of the left liver to the quadrate lobe (segment IV) (see Ch. 1). This tissue is divided easily by passing a curved director beneath it, the tissue then being divided with diathermy (Fig. 80.31). No large vessels traverse here, and hemostasis is readily secured by diathermy or the Argon Beam Coagulator.

After opening of the umbilical fissure, the ligamentum teres can be visualized running down to join the termination of the left portal vein within the umbilical fissure (see Fig. 80.31B). The triad of the left portal vein, left hepatic artery, and left hepatic duct enters at the base of the umbilical fissure. Their anatomy with the branching of the pedicles to supply segments II, III, and IV is shown in Fig. 80.32.

It is important for the safe performance of right hepatic lobectomy to be certain that the hilar plate has been lowered (Fig. 80.33) (see Ch. 30), separating the main left hepatic duct from the undersurface of segment IV. The left hepatic artery, whether arising from the common hepatic artery or from the left gastric artery, always enters the base of the umbilical fissure and is not endangered during this operation. The middle hepatic artery supplying segment IV is sometimes identifiable separately

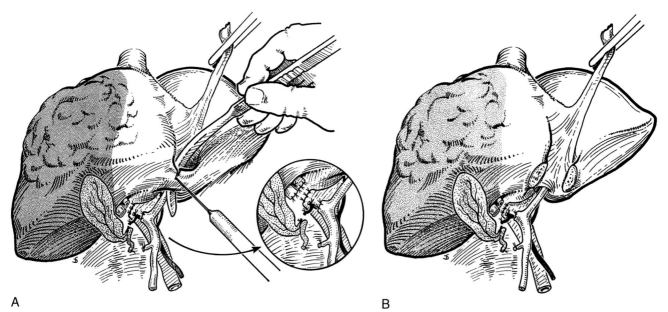

A   B

Fig. 80.31. A, Exposure of the umbilical fissure and division of the bridge of liver tissue at the base of the fissure. A director usually can be passed beneath the liver tissue, which is divided using diathermy. Note the vessels to the right liver already have been divided *(inset).* **B,** The bridge of liver tissue has been divided.

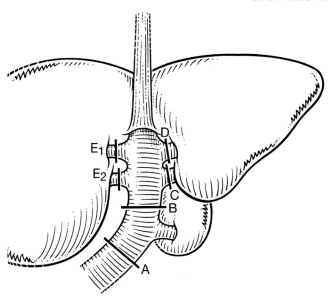

Fig. 80.32. Distribution and points of division of pedicles at the base of the left liver. A, Pedicle to left liver including segment I. B, Pedicle to left liver sparing segment I. C, Pedicle to segment II. D, Pedicle to segment III. E1, Pedicle to segment IVb. E2, Pedicle to segment IVa.

running to the right of the left hepatic artery and entering the umbilical fissure at its base and on its right (see Ch. 1).

Close to the base of the umbilical fissure, a major branch (often two branches) of the left portal triad passes posterolaterally to the caudate lobe (see Fig. 80.32). Division of these branches interrupts the portal flow to the caudate lobe, but this needs to be carried out only if the caudate lobe is to be removed together with the rest of the specimen (see later). *The vital step in the performance of right lobectomy is the division of veins and arteries that originate in the umbilical fissure of the liver from the left portal triads and "feed back" from the main left trunk to segment IVa and*

IVb (the medial segment of the left liver) (see Fig. 80.32). It is not important to attempt to divide these structures within the umbilical fissure if there is no tumor immediately adjacent to the fissure. It is easier to secure them within the liver substance just to the right of the umbilical fissure during parenchymal dissection, and it is safer to do so because there is no chance of damage to the blood supply to or biliary drainage from the left lobe. *If there is a tumor close to the umbilical fissure, however, it is necessary to control the "feedback" vessels within the right margin of the umbilical fissure.* This control can be obtained by passing a suture about these vessels and ligating them in continuity (Fig. 80.34). Alternatively, the vessels are dissected and individually ligated and divided.

The parenchymal dissection is begun anteriorly and proceeds down to the base of the umbilical fissure (Fig. 80.35A). When the feedback vessels are divided, segment IV is devascularized. Division of the liver substance is developed backward toward the vena cava just to the right of the falciform ligament (see Fig. 80.35B). *The middle hepatic vein is encountered as the dissection is deepened. When it is identified, it is easily controlled by ligation or division with the Endo-GIA vascular stapler.* If it is necessary to pursue the middle hepatic vein intrahepatically toward the vena cava to obtain tumor clearance, the index finger of the left hand can be slid gently along the upper surface of the vein (Fig. 80.36). Any minor branches, which are divided during this maneuver, are controlled by finger pressure, and the vein is ligated distal to the finger (see Fig. 80.36B). If the right hepatic vein has not previously been secured extrahepatically, it is now approached from within the liver substance, as described earlier, and appropriately controlled.

One particular difficulty may arise in the instance of a large tumor occupying segment IV and displacing the left hepatic duct

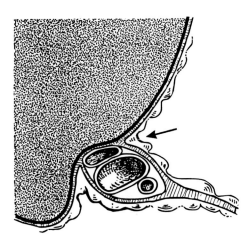

Fig. 80.33. Lowering of the hilar plate. Glisson's capsule is incised at the base of the quadrate lobe (segment IV), and the structures of the left portal triad are lowered from beneath the overhanging quadrate, exposing the left hepatic duct. This step may be carried out before opening of the umbilical fissure.

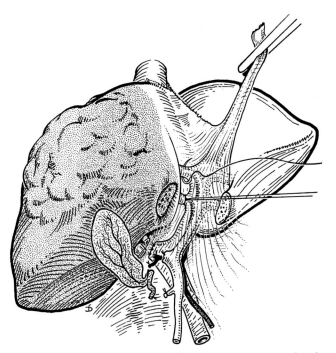

Fig. 80.34. Feedback vessels from the left portal triad may be secured in the parenchyma just a little to the right of the falciform ligament (see Fig. 80.35). This dissection must be within the umbilical fissure in the event of adjacent tumor in segment IV, but is carried out more safely within the liver tissue just to the right of the falciform ligament (see Fig. 80.32). Preliminary suture ligation within the umbilical fissure may be performed as illustrated. This procedure deprives segment IV of its blood supply.

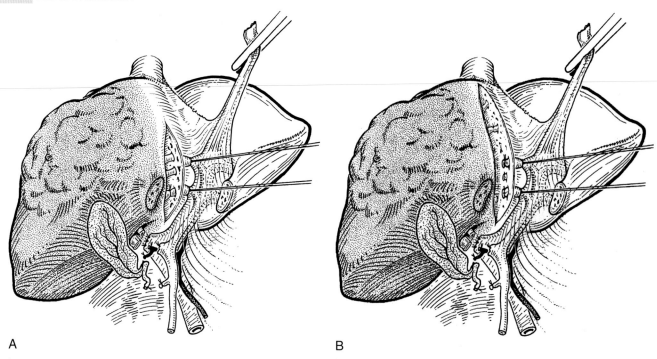

Fig. 80.35. A, Feedback vessels are secured within the parenchyma. **B,** Division of the liver substance is developed backward toward the vena cava just to the right of the falciform ligament.

at the base of segment IV and as it traverses into the umbilical fissure (Fig. 80.37). In such cases, freeing of the left hepatic duct in the hilar area and at the base of the umbilical fissure is difficult and may be impossible without deliberate excision of a portion of the left hepatic duct. In such cases, there should be no hesitation in sacrificing any necessary length of the left hepatic duct. After removal of the specimen, repair may be carried out by anastomosing the stump of the left hepatic duct to the upper end of the common hepatic duct. Alternatively, biliary-enteric

continuity may be restored by hepaticojejunostomy Roux-en-Y to the left hepatic duct (Fig. 80.38).

Left Hepatectomy

Left hepatectomy can be a difficult procedure, particularly in the presence of a large, posteriorly situated tumor close to the junction of the middle and left hepatic veins with the vena cava.

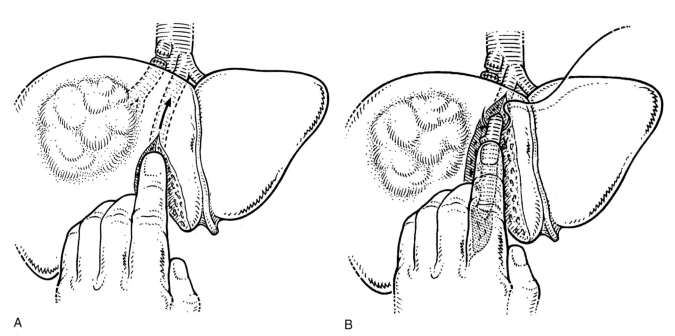

Fig. 80.36. A, The middle hepatic vein is exposed, and the index finger slides up its anterior surface to show its length. **B,** The middle hepatic vein is suture ligated.

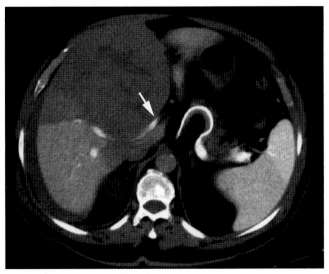 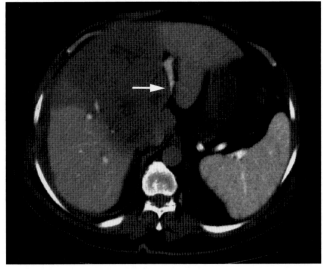

Fig. 80.37. Large metastatic carcinoma within segment IV threatens the integrity of the left hepatic duct *(arrows)*. At operation, right lobectomy was performed, and a length of the left hepatic duct was excised and repaired as illustrated in Fig. 80.38.

Inflow Control

Inflow control to the left liver is obtained by dissection at the base of the umbilical fissure. The ligamentum teres is elevated. The hilar plate is lowered as described earlier (see Fig. 80.33). The left hepatic artery is easily identified by opening the peritoneum covering the left portion of the immediate subhilar area at the base of the umbilical fissure. It is double ligated and divided. The gastrohepatic ligament is inspected, and any accessory or replaced hepatic artery arising from the left gastric artery is similarly ligated.

Dissection at the base of the umbilical fissure exposes the left portal vein as it traverses into the umbilical fissure, and *it should be controlled at this point and not at its origin from the main portal venous trunk*. This dissection allows identification of the branches to the caudate lobe, which arise just before the left portal vein enters the umbilical fissure. If the caudate lobe is to be removed together with the left lobe, the vein is secured below the takeoff of the caudate branches (see Fig. 80.32A). If the caudate lobe is to be preserved (and this is usually the case), the vein is divided distal to the takeoff of the caudate branch (see Fig. 80.32B). The left hepatic duct usually is easily identified just above and behind the left portal vein and can be encircled with a suture and divided as it curves into the umbilical fissure. These steps are illustrated in Fig. 80.39. A line of demarcation in the Glissonian plane extending from the gallbladder fossa to the left of the vena cava now is clearly visible on the liver surface (Fig. 80.40) and is marked with a diathermy. It is usually (but not always) necessary to remove the gallbladder.

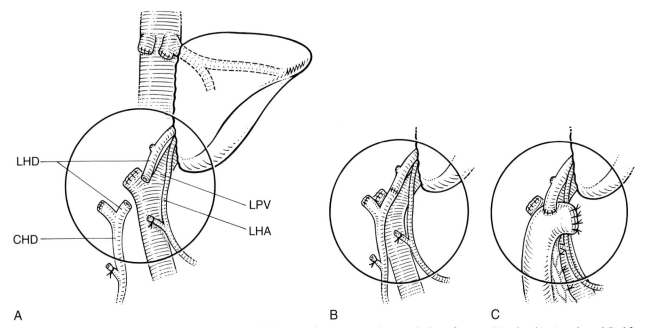

A   B   C

Fig. 80.38. The left hepatic duct may be compromised during right lobectomy for tumor extending into the base of segment IV and pushing into the umbilical fissure (see Fig. 80.37). **A,** After resection with excision of a portion of the left hepatic duct (LHD). **B,** Repair of the duct by direct end-to-end anastomosis. **C,** Repair by hepaticojejunostomy Roux-en-Y. CHD, common hepatic duct; LHA, left hepatic artery; LPV, left portal vein.

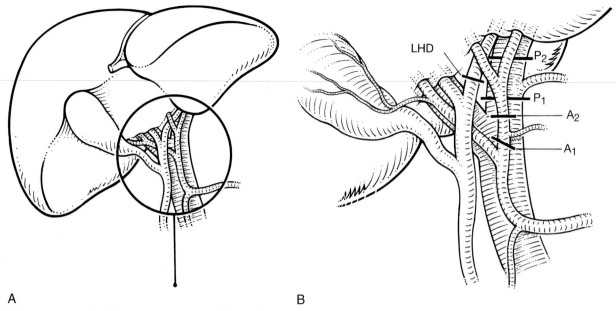

A   B

Fig. 80.39. A, Dissection for left hepatectomy at the base of the umbilical fissure. **B,** Left hepatic duct (LHD) is divided at the base of the umbilical fissure. A1, point of division of LHA for concomitant removal of caudate lobe; A2, point of division of LHA for left hepatectomy; LHA, left hepatic artery; P1, point of division of LPV for left hepatectomy and caudate lobectomy; P2, point of division of LPV for left hepatectomy alone.

Outflow Control

The left lobe of the liver (segments II and III) is now mobilized from the diaphragm by division of the left triangular ligament from its tip up to the lateral margin of the suprahepatic IVC. The upper surfaces of the left and middle hepatic veins and of the suprahepatic IVC are displayed (Fig. 80.41) (Czerniak et al, 1993). The main trunk of the middle hepatic vein usually joins the left hepatic vein, but may enter the vena cava separately. In essence, the veins are cleared below the diaphragm, and their junction with the vena cava is displayed. The left lobe of the liver (segments II and III) is turned to the right (see Fig. 80.41). The gastrohepatic ligament is fully divided, and the ligamentum venosum is identified. We divide the ligamentum venosum close to its entry into the left hepatic vein. This division opens up a triangular tunnel, the sides of which are the left hepatic vein anteriorly, the anterior surface of the vena cava posteriorly, and the upper surface of segment II inferiorly. This tunnel is developed

carefully, and an instrument is passed beneath the left and middle hepatic veins to emerge anterior to the vena cava between the middle hepatic vein and the right hepatic vein (see Fig. 80.41B).

The common trunk of the left and middle hepatic veins or each vein individually is now secured in vascular clamps, divided, and oversewn with a 3-0 polyproprylene suture. Alternatively, the Endo-GIA vascular stapler may be used to divide the veins (Fig. 80.42). *Controlling the major draining hepatic veins to the left liver is crucial in controlling hemorrhage during the removal of large left-sided tumors.*

Parenchymal Transection

A vessel loop is now passed about the hilar structures. These structures are intermittently occluded during parenchymal transection, which is carried out in the principal plane. It is important that transection is carried out so that the parenchyma is divided posteriorly just anterior to the ligamentum venosum, separating the left liver from the anterior surface of the caudate lobe.

Extended Left Hepatectomy

In some instances, a large tumor occupying the left half of the liver encroaches across the principal scissura (Cantlie's line) into segments V and VIII (the anterior sector of the right liver) (see Figs. 80.1 and 80.4). In other cases, multiple tumors occupy portions of the left liver and of segments V and VIII. In such cases, left hepatectomy can be performed with extension of the procedure to remove segments V and VIII.

The procedure is extensive, and although Couinaud (1957) described the anatomic basis for extension of a left hepatectomy to include removal of the anterior sector of the right liver, there were few reported series of successful operations. Joishy and Balasegaram (1980) referred to extended left hepatectomy done in eight patients. The nature of these operations is described as indicating a line of transection to the right of the principal

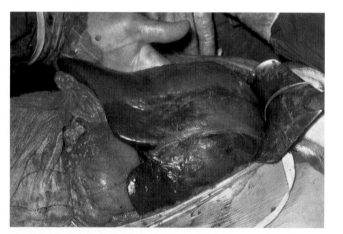

Fig. 80.40. The left liver has been devascularized before parenchymal transection for left hepatectomy.

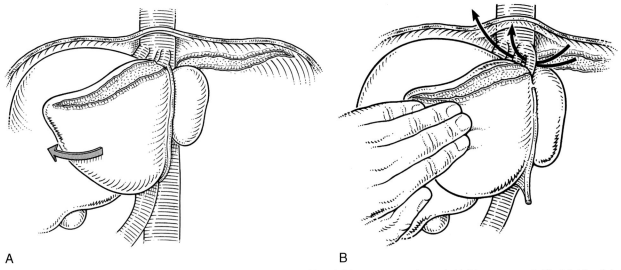

A

B

Fig. 80.41. Approach and dissection of the left and middle hepatic veins applicable to left hepatectomy and extended left hepatectomy. **A,** The left lobe of the liver (segments II and III) is completely mobilized from the diaphragm and turned to the right. The gastrohepatic ligament is divided, and the line of the ligamentum venosum is exposed. **B,** The ligamentum venosum is divided. This maneuver allows the exposure of the window between the vena cava and the left hepatic vein. By dissection in this space, it is possible to dissect free the left and middle hepatic veins separately or together *(black curved arrows)*. The left and middle hepatic veins are clamped, divided, and oversewn or divided with the Endo-GIA vascular stapler.

plane, but almost certainly not extending to the right scissura. The senior author (Blumgart, 1978) described a case of extended left hepatectomy, but it was not until Starzl and coworkers (1982) reported four cases, which they referred to as having been treated by left hepatic trisegmentectomy, that the necessary hilar dissection was described accurately. The difficulty in defining the plane of parenchymal transection on the right and of controlling hemorrhage and biliary complications was recognized. Subsequently, reports of small numbers of patients continued to appear, but perioperative problems and, in particular, biliary complications were frequent (Al-Hadeedi et al, 1990; Hasegawa et al, 1989).

Preoperative Evaluation

Anatomic assessment is paramount, and radiologic imaging should not exclude patients from operation based on the size of the tumor alone. Even patients with very large tumors that expand and compress the surrounding tissue, displacing blood vessels and bile ducts ("pushing" tumors), may be selected for laparotomy (Baer et al, 1989). CT is important in suggesting the expansile pushing form of tumor (see Fig. 80.6). Ultrasound, including Doppler imaging of the portal and hepatic vessels, is most valuable in this regard, as is MRI. These studies also show impingement of large

tumors on the vena cava. Arteriography and inferior venacavography are rarely necessary.

Operative Technique

The operation involves removal of segments II, III, IV, V, and VIII (Blumgart et al, 1993). Segment I can be included in the resection (Fig. 80.43; see Fig. 80.32). An important aspect of the operative technique is the early full mobilization of the liver not only by division of the left triangular ligament from its apex to the left of the IVC, but also by complete division and mobilization of the ligament on the right. This mobilization not only allows palpation of segment VII for the presence of unsuspected additional tumor, but also assists later in the identification of the correct plane of parenchymal dissection. Intraoperative ultrasound is performed to confirm the previously defined anatomic configuration of the tumor and of the major hepatic veins. In particular, an attempt is made to identify the presence of a large inferior right hepatic vein. Its presence augments drainage of segment VII and may allow the right main hepatic vein to be sacrificed during operation (Baer et al, 1991).

Initial dissection is identical to that for left hepatectomy. The suprahepatic bare area of the liver is fully exposed to display

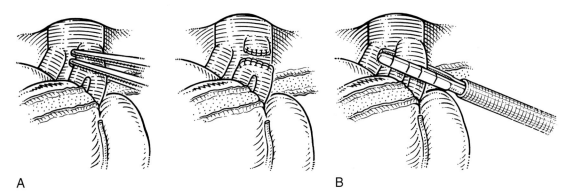

A

B

Fig. 80.42. A, The left and middle hepatic veins are clamped, divided, and oversewn. **B,** Alternatively, the veins may be divided with the Endo-GIA stapler.

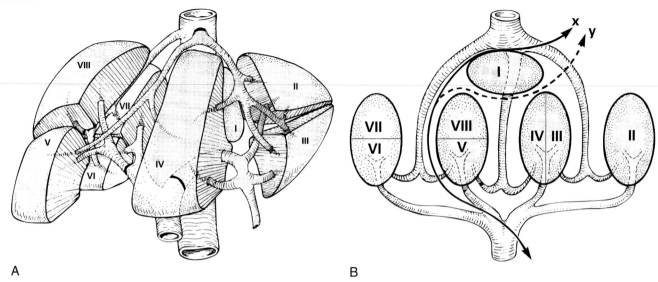

A

B

Fig. 80.43. A, Exploded view to show the sectors and segments of the liver. Extended left hepatectomy involves removal of segments II, III, IV, V, and VIII and sometimes of segment I. The segments to be removed are illustrated by *dark shading*. The *solid lines* on the right anterior sectoral pedicle and the left portal triad illustrate the devascularization necessary. The *solid line* on the middle and left hepatic veins illustrates the point of hepatic venous transection. The right posterior sectoral triad supplying segments VI and VII is preserved, as is the right hepatic vein. **B,** Schematic representation of extended left hepatectomy. Note preservation of the posterior sectoral triad supplying segments VI and VII and of the right hepatic vein. The *solid line x* illustrates the line of transection for removal of the caudate lobe, and the *dotted line y* illustrates the line of transection if the caudate lobe is to be preserved.

the suprahepatic IVC and the hepatic veins. The left liver is now turned to the right side, and the portal triad is approached from the left (Fig. 80.44). The point of ligation of the portal vessels to the left liver is dictated by the involvement of the caudate lobe (segment I) by tumor. If segment I requires resection, the left hepatic artery, bile ducts, and portal vein must be ligated close to the hilus to interrupt the blood supply to segment I and to the left liver (see Figs. 80.32 and 80.44). As described by Starzl and coworkers (1982) and Blumgart and colleagues (1993), however, when segment I is to be preserved, the structures of the left portal triad are secured in the base of the umbilical fissure to leave intact the blood supply to segment I (see Fig. 80.44).

After obtaining vascular control at the hilus, the middle and left hepatic veins and the left of the subdiaphragmatic IVC are dissected as described earlier for left hepatectomy (Czerniak et al, 1993). If the caudate lobe (segment I) is to be removed in continuity, it is mobilized from the left side and upper surface of the IVC as described for resection of the caudate lobe (see later).

The difficult aspect of the operation is the definition of the line of transection of the parenchyma, which lies well to the right of the principal scissura. The plane is horizontal, lateral to the gallbladder fossa, and parallel to and just anterior to the right scissura. In an attempt to define this plane, Starzl and coworkers (1982) described finger dissection beginning from above and anterior to the main right hepatic venous entry into the vena cava. We have avoided this approach, which may be associated with considerable hemorrhage. It is important to define the plane of parenchymal dissection, however, which passes anterior to the right hepatic venous trunk and allows division of the anterior sectoral branch of the right portal triad, while preserving and avoiding damage to the posterior sectoral triad (Fig. 80.45). Although there are no reliable surface markings, a plane passing from the anterior border of the right hepatic vein above and extending horizontally to emerge well to the right of the gallbladder fossa designates the approximate correct position within the parenchyma. *This line can be accurately defined when it is possible to clamp the anterior*

sectoral pedicle to the right liver, and this is often possible using the pedicular Glissonian approach. This approach should be possible in all cases in which the tumor does not extend so close to the right main pedicle as to make access impossible without compromising tumor clearance. The right anterior sectoral pedicle is isolated and clamped. The right posterior pedicle is left intact. A line of demarcation extending along the right scissura develops rapidly (Fig. 80.46).

The parenchymal phase is now carried out, opening the liver tissue from below upward and medially and keeping the plane of parenchymal dissection horizontal. If significant bleeding occurs, it arises from branches of the right hepatic vein. Dissection carried out under low central venous pressure (see Ch. 25) allows bleeding from the transected branches of the right vein to be visualized and controlled. Dissection proceeds, and when the right anterior sectoral pedicle has been identified, dissection is kept anterior to the right posterior pedicular structures. These structures are dense and white as opposed to the hepatic veins and are readily appreciated.

Many large expansile tumors ("pushing" tumor) produce a narrow zone of compressed atrophic liver tissue just anterior to the posterior pedicular triad. In such instances, although tumor clearance is small, it can be achieved by peeling the tumor away from the residual parenchyma in this atrophic plane. *With large tumors, the plane of dissection is dictated by the tumor* (see Fig. 80.6). *For smaller tumors, the plane of dissection can be anatomically defined.*

If the middle and left hepatic veins have not been secured previously, they are controlled when encountered within the line of transection, and the parenchymal division is completed. *It cannot be emphasized strongly enough, however, that prior control of these veins is associated with prevention of venous bleeding.*

After removal of the resected specimen, the remnant (segments VI and VII) presents an en face raw surface area (Fig. 80.47). Intermittent use of Pringle's maneuver allows identification and control of bleeding from small branches of the

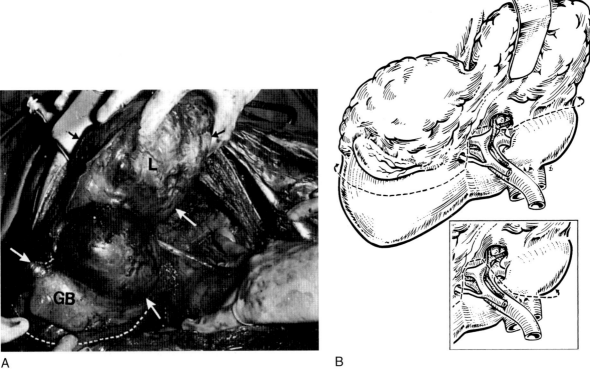

A   B

Fig. 80.44. A, Operative photograph of a large left-sided primary hepatocellular carcinoma occupying the left lobe of the liver (segments II, III, and IV) and extending into segments V and VIII beneath the gallbladder (GB). The left lobe (L) has been mobilized and turned toward the right. The extent of the tumor is indicated by the *arrows*. The line of parenchymal incision in the right liver is indicated by the *dotted line*. **B,** The situation is as depicted here. Initial approach during extended left hepatectomy allows dissection of the portal triad structures from the left posterolateral aspect. The line of future transection is indicated. If the caudate lobe is to be preserved, the left portal vein is ligated beyond its caudate branch, but if the caudate is to be removed as well, the portal vein can be ligated more proximally *(inset)*. The line of transection runs along the obliterated ligamentum venosum, then across the base of the quadrate lobe and hilus, and curves to the right extending into the right scissura lateral to the gallbladder fossa. The dissection as illustrated in the *main diagram* would preserve the caudate lobe, but in the *inset*, the caudate lobe also is removed (see also Fig. 80.43).

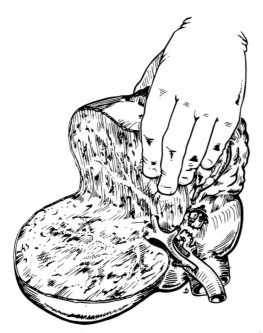

Fig. 80.45. Extended left hepatic lobectomy. The liver tissue is entered for the parenchymatous transection just anterior to the estimated lower limit of the right scissura. This plane of dissection is followed, the operator working toward the base of the gallbladder fossa and the point of entry of the right hepatic duct into the liver substance. The anterior sectoral vessel of supply and the bile ducts are identified in the liver substance *(arrow)* and can be ligated.

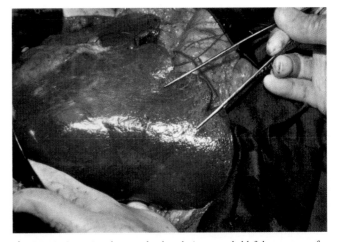

Fig. 80.46. Operative photograph taken during extended left hepatectomy for a large tumor occupying the left liver. The left liver already has been devascularized, and the anterior sector (segments V and VIII) is seen devascularized and demarcated from the posterior sector (segments VI and VII), which remains vascularized.

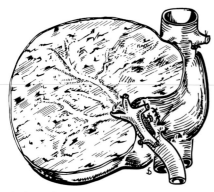

Fig. 80.47. The liver substance is removed anterior to the posterior sectoral ducts and vessels, and the upper part of this parenchymal dissection runs just anterior to the right hepatic vein and involves control of the middle and left hepatic vein. After resection, the right posterior sectoral portal triad can be seen branching on the surface of exposed liver tissue.

hepatic artery or portal vein, and any visible open bile ducts are closed with fine resorbable (Vicryl 4-0) sutures. Final hemostasis is achieved as described earlier. The omentum may be laid over the divided surface. There is a tendency for biliary fistulization after this operation. Three of the four patients initially reported by Starzl and coworkers (1982) had biliary complications (two fistulae and one bile duct stricture).

Experience: Extended Left Hepatectomy

Extended left hepatectomy has been described in some detail because large tumors arising from the left liver and extending to the right, and previously considered unresectable, can be removed successfully with complete tumor clearance and a chance of cure (Blumgart et al, 1993; Soreide et al, 1985). As stated earlier, prediction of possible resectability is difficult, but in large tumors with a clear-cut margin on CT and evidence of displacement rather than invasion of right-sided intrahepatic structures (see Fig. 80.6), exploration for excision is worthwhile (Soreide et al, 1985). Although this operation has been reported as being associated with high perioperative morbidity and mortality and poor outcome (Hasegawa et al, 1989), several small series have given support to its utility (Al-Hadeedi et al, 1990; Bismuth et al, 1989, 1992; Blumgart et al, 1993; Elias et al, 1992; Houssin et al, 1993; Huguet et al, 1994; Iwatsuki & Starzl, 1988; Starzl et al, 1982; Tsuzuki et al, 1990).

One of us (L.H.B.) reported a series of 51 patients who underwent extended left hepatectomy at MSKCC during 1992-1998 (Povoski et al, 1999). There were no intraoperative deaths. Postoperative morbidity was 53%, with biliary leak and abdominal abscess being the most commonly encountered postoperative complication. Postoperative mortality was 8%. Compared with historical controls for hepatic resection at MSKCC from 1985-1994 (Fong et al, 1995), in which overall postoperative morbidity was 40% and postoperative mortality was 4%, morbidity and mortality were greater for extended left hepatectomy, although postoperative hospital stay was identical. This operation is one of the most difficult procedures in hepatic resectional surgery.

Factors influencing resectability and oncologic efficacy, especially with regard to extensive anatomic dissections, have long been debated. In the series of patients referred to previously, the finding of positive microscopic margins or of tumor within one high-power field was associated with the largest hepatic lesions (Povoski et al, 1999).

Left Lobectomy (Left Lateral Segmentectomy)

The left lobe of the liver, which comprises segments II and III, is resected by approaching the portal triads to segments II and III in the umbilical fissure. If present, the bridge of tissue between segments IV and III is divided as described previously. The left lobe is mobilized. Dissection is carried out within the umbilical fissure to the left of the main triad. The pedicles to segments II and III usually can be dissected and controlled individually (see Fig. 80.32). This approach is important in allowing tumor clearance for lesions close to the umbilical fissure. Alternatively, the liver may be split anteroposteriorly just to the left of the ligamentum teres and the falciform ligament, and as this is done, the vessels are encountered and divided serially. The latter approach is suitable only for more peripherally placed tumors.

As the liver tissue is opened, the left hepatic vein is encountered posteriorly and can be controlled within the liver substance, and the left lobe is removed. In patients in whom there is a posteriorly situated tumor close to the junction of the left hepatic vein and the middle hepatic vein, it is best to approach the left hepatic vein extrahepatically as described previously for left hepatectomy (see Figs. 80.41 and 80.42).

HEPATIC SEGMENTECTOMY

A detailed understanding of intrahepatic anatomy and advances in imaging technology have facilitated an approach to hepatic resection based on the removal of individual hepatic segments (Billingsley et al, 1998; DeMatteo et al, 2000; Franco et al, 1988; Gazelle & Haaga, 1992; Hemming et al, 1997; Takayama & Makuuchi, 1996). Hepatic segmentectomy is discussed in detail in Ch. 83, but is briefly described here. Resection of segment I (caudate lobectomy) is discussed in detail, however, because resection of the caudate lobe is often done in combination with a major hepatectomy. The number of hepatic segments resected has been shown to be a predictor of perioperative morbidity and mortality (Jarnagin et al, 2002).

Segmental resections offer a variety of advantages over classic major resections and nonanatomic wedge resections. Segmental resections conserve functional liver parenchyma and minimize the physiologic impact of liver resection. This is of particular benefit in a cirrhotic patient with impaired hepatocellular function. Nonanatomic wedge resection has been advocated as an alternative approach for parenchymal conservation (Brown et al, 1988). Wedge resection is hampered, however, by intraoperative hemorrhage and unacceptable rates of margin positivity of 35% (Scheele et al, 1991, 1995). Segmentectomy may be regarded as a unisegmentectomy when one segment is removed or as a plurisegmentectomy when two or more segments are excised (Castaing et al, 1985; Nagasue et al, 1985). More commonly performed segmental resections include resection of segment I; resection of segment IV; and segmentectomy to remove segments IV, V, and VI (Figs. 80.48 and 80.49). Central hepatic resection comprising resection of segments IV, V, and VIII is being increasingly performed, and this may be combined with resection of segment I, the latter operation being particularly indicated in some patients with hilar cholangiocarcinoma (Ogura et al, 1998). Resection of segments VI and VII is, in effect, a posterior right sectorectomy, and resection of segments V and VIII is an anterior right sectorectomy.

Although indicated for removal of some benign liver tumors and for biliary exposure in some cases of benign biliary stricture,

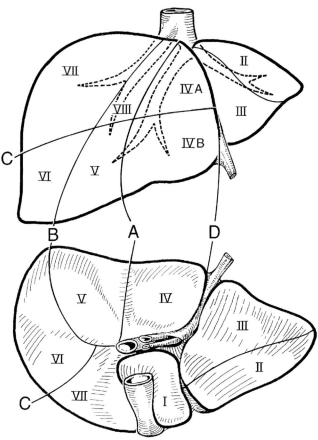

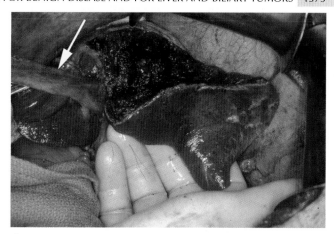

Fig. 80.50. Photograph illustrates resection of segment III. Segment II is turned forward by the operator's hand. The ligamentum teres is illustrated *(arrow)*.

Fig. 80.48. Lines of resection for excision of various segments. Resection of segments VI and VII, right posterior sectorectomy. Resection of segments V and VIII, right anterior sectorectomy. Resection of segments IV, V, and VIII, central hepatectomy. Resection of segment IV follows *A-D*.

resection of segment IV is of some value in the management of malignant lesions occupying only the quadrate lobe. Carcinoma of the gallbladder is a special case because the organ lies between segments IV and V of the liver. Resection for gallbladder cancer should involve as a minimum removal of segments IVb and V (see later). Resections of segments II and III (Fig. 80.50) are less frequently performed. Segment I may be removed on its own or

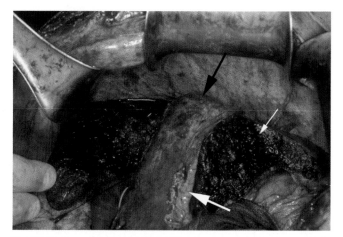

Fig. 80.49. Intraoperative photograph illustrates resection of segments III, V, and VIII. Segments II *(small white arrow)* and IV *(black arrow)* remain intact. Falciform ligament is evident *(large white arrow)*.

in continuity with right or left hepatectomy, right lobectomy, central hepatectomy, or extended left hepatectomy.

Segmentectomy I (Caudate Resection)

The caudate lobe of the liver is a frequent site of involvement in primary and secondary liver tumors. In addition, cholangiocarcinoma at the confluence of hepatic ducts frequently involves caudate bile ducts and may extend to the caudate lobe (see later). Resection of the caudate lobe of the liver is often necessary for complete tumor clearance. The procedure may be required as an isolated caudate lobe resection or as caudate resection combined with major hepatectomy. The anatomy of the caudate lobe and its close proximity to major vascular structures make resection difficult.

Anatomy

The caudate lobe (segment I) is the dorsal portion of the liver posteriorly and embraces the retrohepatic IVC. The lobe lies between major vascular structures: the IVC posteriorly and the portal triad inferiorly and the IVC and the middle and left hepatic veins superiorly (Figs. 80.51 and 80.52) (see Ch. 1). The main bulk of the lobe lies to the left of the vena cava, the left and inferior margins being free in the lesser omental bursa. The gastrohepatic omentum separates the left portion of the caudate lobe from segments II and III of the left liver as it passes between them to be attached to the ligamentum venosum. The left portion of the caudate lobe inferiorly traverses to the right between the portal vein and IVC as the caudate process where it fuses with the right lobe of the liver. Superiorly, the left portion of the caudate lobe is linked to the posterior margin of the hilum by a deep anterior portion, which passes embedded in the parenchyma immediately under the middle hepatic vein and fuses on the right side to segment VII anterolateral to the IVC. The portion of the caudate lobe on the right varies, but is usually quite small (it is often referred to by some as segment IX). The anterior surface within the parenchyma is covered by the posterior surface of segment IV, the limit being an oblique plane slanting from the left portal vein to the left hepatic vein. There is a caudate lobe (segment I) with a constantly present left portion and a right portion of variable size (see Ch. 1).

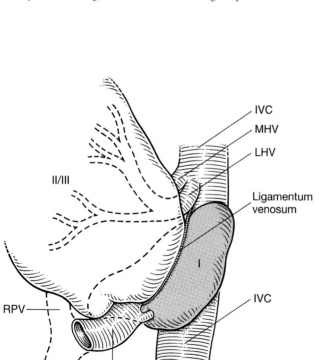

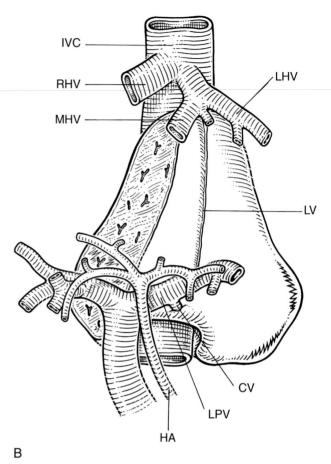

Fig. 80.51. A, Cross-sectional sketch shows caudate lobe anatomy at the level of the porta hepatis. Note principal caudate branch of left portal vein (LPV). Note (1) position of lesser omentum and ligamentum venosum; (2) middle hepatic vein (MHV), which separates segments IV and V and is close to right portion of caudate lobe; and (3) posterior ligamentous band joining segments I and VII. **B,** The relationships of the caudate lobe are illustrated. The caudate lies anterior to the IVC, but posterior to the portal venous structures. There is a right portion of the caudate lobe. Blood supply to the caudate lobe is mainly from the caudate branch (CV) of the LPV. This branch may arise from the main trunk of the portal vein in some cases. HA, hepatic artery; LHV, left hepatic vein; LV, ligamentum venosum; RHV, right hepatic vein.

Fig. 80.52. Sketch shows the position of the caudate lobe relative to surrounding structures and particularly the vena cava. Segments II and III have been rotated to the right to expose the caudate lobe. The position of the ligamentum venosum is indicated. Note the extension of the caudate lobe between the vena cava and the portal vein (PV) anteriorly and between the vena cava and the middle and left hepatic veins superiorly. Caudate portal blood supply is via a branch of the left portal vein (LPV). LHV, left hepatic vein; MHV, middle hepatic vein; RPV, right portal vein (see also Fig. 80.51).

The caudate lobe is supplied by blood vessels and drained by biliary tributaries of the right and left portal vein and the left hepatic artery close to the base of the umbilical fissure of the liver. The right portion of the caudate lobe, including the caudate process, receives predominantly portal venous blood from the right portal vein (or the bifurcation of the main portal trunk), whereas on the left side the major portal supply arises almost exclusively from the left branch of the portal vein. Similarly, the arterial supply and biliary drainage of the right portion is most commonly associated with the right posterior sectoral vessels or pedicle, and that of the left segment is associated with the left main vessels (Mizumoto & Suzuki, 1988).

The hepatic venous drainage of the caudate lobe is unique in that it is the only hepatic segment that drains directly into the IVC. The number of hepatic veins varies (one to nine; mean four) (Heloury et al, 1988). In general, the veins are short and drain from the caudate lobe directly into the anterior and left aspect of the vena cava (see Fig. 80.51A) (see Ch. 1). They can drain into the posterior aspect of the vena cava if there is a significant retrocaval caudate component.

The posterior edge of the caudate lobe on the left usually has a fibrous component, which fans out to attach to the crus of the diaphragm and extends posteriorly behind the vena cava to link with a similar component of fibrous tissue protruding from the posterior surface of segment VII and embracing the vena cava (see Fig. 80.51A). In 50% of patients, this ligament is replaced, in whole or in part, by hepatic tissue, and the caudate may completely encircle the IVC and contact segment VII on the right side. A significant retrocaval component may compromise a left-sided approach to the caudate vein.

Resection

The major problems in caudate lobe resection are dissection and control of the retrohepatic caudate veins and, in the presence of a substantial tumor, controlling bleeding from the posterior surface of the middle hepatic vein. Resection of the caudate lobe involves three major steps: (1) control of the inflow blood supply from the left portal vein and left hepatic artery at the base of the umbilical fissure and of other inflow by lowering of the hilar plate and dividing any vessels encountered; (2) dissection of the retrohepatic veins; and (3) in isolated caudate resection, dividing the liver parenchyma between the right portion of the caudate and the base of segment IV and the left side of segment VII to allow removal of the lobe.

Dissection at the base of the umbilical fissure allows identification of the caudate vessels issuing from the left side of the portal vein and the left hepatic artery before these vascular structures enter the umbilical fissure (Figs. 80.53 and 80.54). The left lobe of the liver is mobilized and turned to the right. The left lateral margin of the caudate is freed by division of the fibrous extension of the tissue as it courses posteriorly to the IVC. This division allows access to the caudate veins (see Figs. 80.51 and 80.54). During this dissection, it becomes evident whether the caudate lobe is embracing the vena cava posteriorly, in which case no further attempt is made to free the lobe on the left side, but an approach should be made from the right (see Fig. 80.54) (Hasegawa et al, 1991a; Lerut et al, 1990).

After freeing of the ligamentous attachments on the left side, the caudate can be elevated easily. Such hepatic veins as are evident may be encircled and suture-ligated or controlled with clips; working from the left side of the vena cava toward the right side, extensive and sometimes complete mobilization can be performed (see Figs. 80.51, 80.53, and 80.54). This technique is most applicable when the caudate lobe is not involved by a bulky tumor

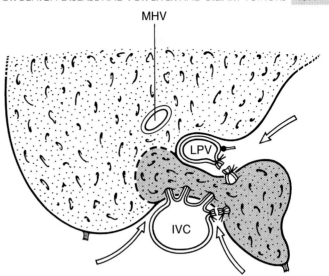

Fig. 80.54. Lines of approach *(arrows)* to free the caudate lobe. Compare with Fig. 80.51. The lesser omentum has been opened. The caudate branch of the left portal vein has been tied. The ligamentous attachments of the caudate lobe posteriorly have been opened, and dissection of the retrohepatic caudate veins can be approached from the right or left side (see text). MHV, middle hepatic vein; PV, portal vein.

(e.g., in removal of the lobe in continuity to allow clearance in left hepatectomy for hilar cholangiocarcinoma). This approach also is valuable in extended left hepatic lobectomy, during which it is our practice to attempt to use it as a routine because it allows less disturbance of the retrohepatic blood flow from the right liver.

A bulky tumor within the caudate lobe is often rigid, and upward mobilization of the caudate is difficult and hazardous. In this case, the retrohepatic veins are best approached from the right side (see Fig. 80.54) (Lerut et al, 1990). Should right hepatic resection or extended right hepatic resection be contemplated in continuity with the caudate lobe, an approach from the right is easier and is a simple extension of the retrohepatic dissection. The right lobe is turned toward the left, and the retrohepatic veins are dissected serially, beginning from below behind the caudate process and extending upward with division of all veins until the major hepatic trunks are reached (Miyagawa et al, 1992). As this dissection is carried out, it is easy to extend it over the anterior surface of the IVC to the left side until the caudate lobe is completely mobilized and freed from the vena cava (see Fig. 80.54) (Lerut et al, 1990).

For right or left hepatic resection involving division of the middle hepatic vein, the caudate lobe is easily removed without danger of tearing the middle hepatic vein because this may be controlled extrahepatically for left-sided resections or intrahepatically for right-sided resections. *In resection of the caudate lobe as an isolated procedure, and particularly should there be a bulky tumor within the caudate, it is important to recognize the danger that may arise from hemorrhage from the middle hepatic vein should this be torn posteriorly* (Colonna et al, 1993). In this instance, we have found it valuable to isolate the left and middle hepatic veins by opening up the tunnel between the left hepatic vein and the IVC at the upper end of the caudate lobe (see Figs. 80.41 and 80.53) and to pass a clamp across the left and middle hepatic veins. This practice provides temporary control during the parenchymal phase of dissection of the portion of the caudate lobe that lies anterior to the IVC and allows safe resection of large tumors (Figs. 80.55 and 80.56). Some authors have split the liver anteriorly

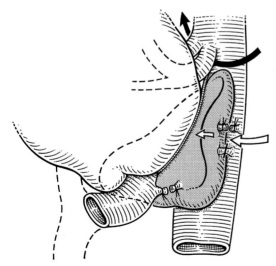

Fig. 80.53. Start of mobilization of the caudate lobe from left. The caudate branch of the portal vein has been tied. The caudate lobe has been freed from the left side of the IVC and turned medially *(small white arrow)*. Dissection is proceeding between the vena cava and the caudate lobe *(large white arrow)*. The retrocaudate hepatic veins are being tied. The *black arrow* indicates the tunnel between the middle and left hepatic veins and the IVC. Dissection of this tunnel allows placement of a clamp across the left and middle hepatic veins (see text).

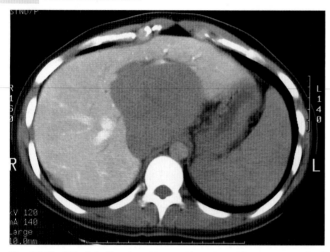

Fig. 80.55. CT of the liver in a 25-year-old woman with symptomatic focal nodular hyperplasia in the caudate lobe compressing the IVC and portal vein without invasion. Freeing of this tumor necessitated an approach to the retrohepatic veins from the right and left sides.

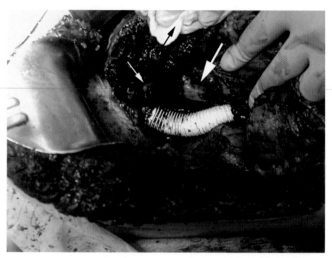

Fig. 80.57. Intraoperative photograph from the patient's right. Right lobectomy has been carried out together with excision of the caudate lobe and portion of the IVC. Segments II and III are drawn upward and to the left by the operator's hand *(black arrow)*. The middle hepatic vein coursing to join the upper IVC is seen *(large white arrow)*. The IVC has been replaced by a Dacron graft. The main trunk of the portal vein and its left branch are illustrated *(small white arrow)*. Tumor had occupied the dangerous portion of the caudate lobe lying between the right branch of the portal vein, the middle hepatic vein, and the IVC (see text).

in the Glissonian plane, separating the right and left liver and dividing the liver along the right margin of segment IV to approach the caudate lobe transhepatically (Yamamoto et al, 1992). A combination of these techniques allows preservation of middle hepatic venous flow and good control of bleeding. Approaches to caudate lobectomy depend largely on the size and location of the lesion, the type of associated resection, and the presence of scarring from previous resection. In practice, the liver frequently is rotated from side to side during the resection.

Preoperative imaging cannot differentiate accurately tumor invasion from compression of the IVC and of the portal vein, and most caudate lobe masses warrant operative exploration to

determine resectability. Many tumors thought to invade the vena cava can be dissected free of the cava in a tumor-free plane. In selected cases, the IVC can be resected in part or en bloc with the caudate lobe (Gardner et al, 1992; Takayama et al, 1991), but this is usually unnecessary. Short segments of the IVC can be repaired or reconstructed with autogenous grafts, whereas longer segments may require a prosthetic graft (Fig. 80.57). A chronically occluded IVC can be resected without reconstruction because abundant collateral vessels usually have developed (Takayama et al, 1991). Although techniques involving complete vascular isolation can be used for caudate lobe resection, one of the authors (L.H.B.) has not had recourse to use this.

Numerous series and case reports of caudate lobe resection are summarized in Table 80.4. Nimura and associates (1990b) reported a large series of caudate resections for hilar cholangiocarcinoma. They described 45 complete caudate lobe resections for microscopic involvement of caudate bile ducts, including 3 isolated caudate lobectomies. The operative mortality rate was 7%. Elias and coworkers (1992) reported 20 resections involving the caudate lobe, only 7 of which were complete caudate lobectomies. There were no operative deaths. Bartlett and colleagues (1996) reported a retrospective review of 21 consecutive complete caudate lobe resections over a 30-month period. Four of the 21 patients underwent complete isolated caudate lobectomy. The most common diagnosis was metastatic colorectal cancer in nine patients, and the most common procedure was an extended left hepatic lobectomy with en bloc caudate lobectomy. The median operative time was 5 hours. The median blood loss was 1160 mL. The major complication rate was 38% with 9.5% mortality (Bartlett et al, 1996). In a review reported from MSKCC (Hawkins et al, 2005), 150 patients underwent caudate lobectomy for cancer, including 21 isolated caudate resections (see Table 80.4). The most common indications were for metastatic colon cancer and hilar cholangiocarcinoma. Thirty patients required resection or reconstruction of the portal vein or vena cava (see Fig. 80.57). Nine patients (6%) died, and the death rate was significantly higher in patients who underwent major vascular reconstruction.

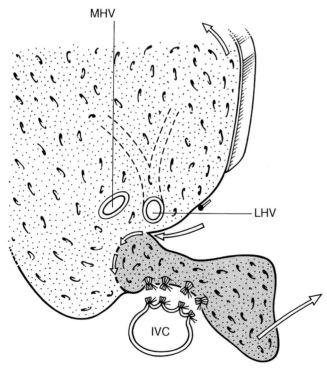

Fig. 80.56. Parenchymal phase of dissection *(arrows)*. Note proximity of the left hepatic vein (LHV) and middle hepatic vein (MHV). The right portion of the caudate lobe lies just to the left of the MHV.

Table 80.4 Literature Review of Caudate Lobe Resections Reported 1990–1996* and 2004

Reference	*n*	Diagnosis	Procedure	Comments
Takayama et al, 1990	1	Hepatoblastoma	Left hepatectomy with complete lobectomy	Neoadjuvant therapy
Lerut et al, 1990	1	Benign adenoma	Isolated caudate lobectomy	Technique: right-sided retrohepatic approach to caudate veins
Moriura et al, 1990	3	Varied	Combined IVC resection	Technique: IVC reconstruction
Nimura et al, 1990b	45	Cholangiocarcinoma	Complete en bloc caudate lobectomy and IVC resection	Advocate routine complete caudate resection for cholangiocarcinoma
Takayama et al, 1991	1	Hepatoblastoma	Extended left hepatectomy with caudate lobectomy and IVC resection	No IVC reconstruction necessary after resection for chronic occlusion
Gardner et al, 1992	1	Metastatic colonic cancer	Caudate lobectomy with IVC resection	Technique: use of Gott shunt during IVC resection
Yamamoto et al, 1992	1	Hepatoma	Isolated caudate lobectomy	Technique: transhepatic approach
Elias et al, 1992	20	Varied	7 complete, 13 partial, 1 isolated caudate lobectomy	Emphasize varied approach to caudate; no deaths
Miyagawa et al, 1992	1	Benign adenoma	Isolated caudate lobectomy	Technique: vascular occlusion with temporary caval occlusion
Iyomasa et al, 1992	1	Cholangiocarcinoma	Isolated caudate lobectomy	Technique: isolated caudate lobectomy
Colonna et al, 1993	3	FNH, metastatic colonic cancer	3 isolated caudate lobectomies	Technique: left approach to caudate veins
Shimada et al, 1994	9	Hepatocellular carcinoma	2 complete caudate lobectomies; 7 partial caudate lobectomies	High morbidity rate; high rate of early recurrence for hepatocellular carcinoma
Kosuge et al, 1994	1	Hepatoma	Isolated caudate lobectomy	Technique: counterstaining
Yanaga et al, 1994	2	Hepatoma	Isolated caudate lobectomy	Technique: vascular isolation by occlusion of hepatic veins
Bartlett et al, 1996	21	Varied	21 complete caudate lobectomies; 4 isolated caudate lobectomies	Technique: no vascular isolation (see text)
Hawkins et al, 2005	150	Varied (all malignant)	21 isolated caudate lobectomies	Technique: no vascular isolation (see text)

*Reported in Bartlett et al, 1996.
FNH, focal nodular hyperplasia.
Modified from Bartlett D, et al, 1996: Complete resection of the caudate lobe of the liver: technique and results. Br J Surg 83:1076-1081.

Resection of Segments II, III, IV, V, VI, VII and VIII

Resection of segments of the liver as monosegmentectomies or as combined resections of two or more segments depends on control of the relevant pedicles (Fig. 80.58). These resections are mentioned briefly here, but the technical details and results are fully described in Ch. 83.

Resection of Segment IV

Segment IV may be resected in its entirety (quadrate lobe resection), or a subsegmental resection of segment IVb can be done alone or in combination with an extended right hepatic resection. The procedure involves lowering of the hilar plate, exposure and control of vessels within the umbilical fissure, and parenchymal dissection to the right of the falciform ligament and along the principal scissura. Posteriorly, parenchymal transection separates segment IV from the upper surface of the right side of segment I.

Segmentectomy with Removal of Segments IV and V

The initial steps in segmentectomy with removal of segments IV and V are the same as for segment IV resection. The liver parenchyma is split to the right of the falciform ligament. After this, the liver tissue is transected in an oblique line parallel to the right scissura. This transection is carried medially toward the right portal pedicle. As this parenchymatous transection proceeds, the portal pedicle of segment V is located, secured, and divided. The parenchymatous incision is continued medially to join with the incision to the right of the falciform ligament (see Figs. 80.48 and 80.50).

Resection of Segments V and VIII

The primary indications for an isolated resection of segment VIII include small, solitary metastases and focal hepatocellular cancer in cirrhotic patients. For resection of segments V and VIII (right anterior sector), the left plane of dissection is within the principal

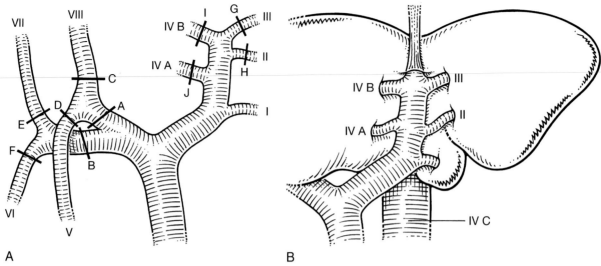

Fig. 80.58. A, Distribution of pedicles and points of control *(A-J)* for segmental resections. Note that control of the anterior *(A)* or posterior *(B)* sectoral pedicles allows anterior or posterior right sectorectomy. Control of pedicles at points *A, I,* and *J* allows central hepatectomy. **B,** Detailed diagram of the umbilical fissure of the liver (see also Fig. 80.32). After the umbilical fissure is entirely exposed, the relevant portal triads to segments II, III, and IV are exposed. If the entire segment is to be removed, all portal pedicle branches from the umbilical portion to the right are divided. If segment IVb is to be resected only, its pedicle is divided. For left lobectomy, pedicles to both segments II and III are divided. For isolated segments II and III resection only, the relevant pedicle is controlled. (See also Ch. 83 and Figs. 80.49 and 80.50.)

plane (Cantlie's line). The lateral dissection is performed within the right portal scissura. The planes of parenchymal section are as described by Makuuchi and colleagues (1993a). Inflow control is obtained by dividing the right anterior sectoral pedicle, and during parenchymal transection the right hepatic vein must be preserved to its junction with the vena cava.

Central Hepatic Resection

Central hepatic resection is a major procedure that involves en bloc resection of segments IV, V, and VIII. This procedure involves the resection of liver parenchyma that is supplied by the right and left portal pedicles. The procedure is useful in preserving normal liver parenchyma for patients with central liver tumor and may include resection of segment I, particularly in selected patients with hilar cholangiocarcinoma (Ogura et al, 1998).

The technical approach involves a combination of the techniques described for resection of segment IV and resection of the right anterior sector. During the parenchymal phase, it is necessary to ligate the middle hepatic vein because this dissection nears the vena cava. Caution must be exercised to preserve the left hepatic vein. The right hepatic vein must be carefully identified and preserved (Kanematsu et al, 1984). For large centrally placed tumors that impinge on the area of the umbilical fissure, care must be taken not to damage the left hepatic duct or the base of the liver within the hilar plate or within the umbilical fissure. This problem is illustrated in Fig. 80.38.

Resections of Segments VI and VII

For monosegmental resection of segment VI or VII, the major plane of dissection is just posterior to the right portal scissura. Inflow control is obtained by securing the segmental branches to segment VI or VII (right posterior sectoral branches) from the right posterior pedicle or by isolation of the entire right posterior pedicle (Reynaud et al, 1991). Resection of segments VI and VII together (posterior sectoral resection) also can be done with sacrifice of the right hepatic vein because venous drainage from segments V and VIII is carried by the middle hepatic vein.

Segmental Resections of the Left Lobe

Isolated resection of segment II or III (see Fig. 80.50) may be performed when it is necessary to preserve as much of the left liver as possible. This is frequently the case when patients have undergone a prior liver resection or have cirrhosis. When isolated segmental resections in this area are performed, inflow control is achieved by isolation of the pedicles to segment II or III within the umbilical fissure (Fig. 80.59; see Fig. 80.58). Ligation of the relevant pedicle provides demarcation of the parenchyma, which guides resection. In these resections, the left hepatic vein must be identified and preserved to provide venous drainage for the retained segment.

HEPATIC RESECTION FOR HILAR CHOLANGIOCARCINOMA

In the case of tumors close to the hilus of the liver or the confluence of the hepatic ducts, removal of which often requires hepatic resection, surgical approaches differ. Although the techniques described here are sometimes applicable for hepatocellular carcinoma involving hilar structures, the situation occurs more frequently when hilar cholangiocarcinoma extends into the adjacent liver or involves major vascular structures (Fig. 80.60) (see Ch. 52). In this circumstance, the added complication of biliary tract obstruction is almost always present.

Some authors, in particular Japanese surgeons, use preoperative biliary drainage and portal venous embolization extensively for hilar cholangiocarcinoma (see subsequent description by Nimura and Sano). We employ these techniques with reserve and have seldom performed preliminary drainage except in deeply jaundiced patients and have not used preoperative portal vein embolization (see Ch. 52). In a series of 226 patients submitted to extended hepatic resection at MSKCC, the important preoperative variables associated with death were the presence of cholangitis, a creatinine value greater than 1.3 mg/dL, and a total bilirubin greater than 6 mg/dL. Five of 14 patients who died had biliary reconstruction

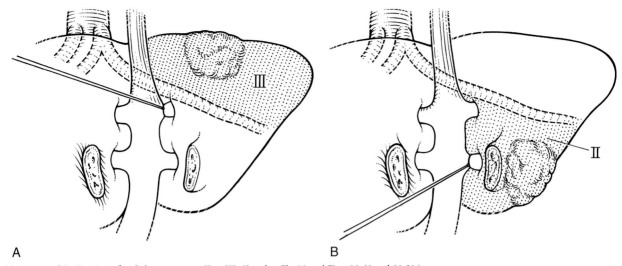

Fig. 80.59. A and **B,** Ligation of pedicles to segment II or III. (See also Ch. 83 and Figs. 80.48 and 80.50.)

(Melendez et al, 2001). Most patients referred to the Hepatobiliary Surgical Services at MSKCC had been submitted to sometimes inappropriate percutaneous or endoscopic intubation before referral. Many patients are infected, and mortality is strongly related to this infection. Similarly, in a study of 1803 consecutive liver resections done during December 1991–September 2001 at MSKCC, it was shown that patients with biliary malignancy had the highest morbidity and mortality of any patient group (Jarnagin et al, 2002). The advisability of preoperative biliary drainage requires further study, in particular, to define the criteria indicating the need for such preoperative preparations.

The major limiting factor for resection of hilar cholangiocarcinoma is related to involvement or compression of adjacent vessels and, in particular, one or other branch of the main trunk of the portal vein (Beazley et al, 1984; Blumgart et al, 1984;

Voyles et al, 1983). The pattern of vascular involvement taken in conjunction with ductal extension of tumor shown at cholangiography (see Ch. 52) gives valuable preoperative information to the surgeon deciding on resection, with regard to the extent of operation and operative strategy (Burke et al, 1998; Jarnagin et al, 2002).

Local resection for small tumors not extending into the intrahepatic bile ducts or involving major vessels may be possible, but for more advanced lesions liver resection is necessary to effect tumor clearance. Liver resection is mandatory when the lesion extends unilaterally into the right or left liver, but leaves the contralateral half of the liver free of tumor and capable of retention as a liver remnant with an intact biliary drainage and blood supply. *More recent reports suggest that hepatic resection should be used in virtually all cases because tumor clearance and*

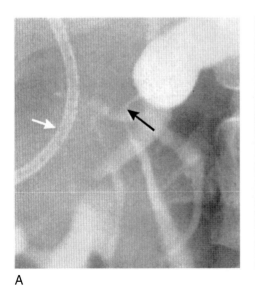

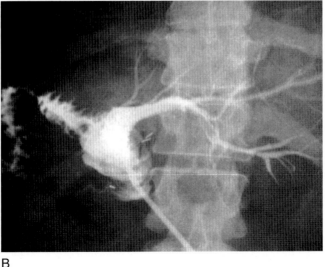

Fig. 80.60. A, Percutaneous transhepatic cholangiogram shows cholangiocarcinoma at the confluence of the bile ducts *(black arrow)*. The left hepatic duct is involved only at its origin, but distally is grossly dilated. A tube *(white arrow)* has been passed into the right hepatic ductal system using a percutaneous technique. There was involvement of the right branch of the portal vein by tumor, and the right hepatic artery was encased. Right hepatic lobectomy with tumor clearance was obtained. **B,** Tubogram in the postoperative period shows hepaticojejunostomy to the left hepatic duct at the level of the umbilical fissure. The patient was alive, well, and free of recurrence 3 years after operation.

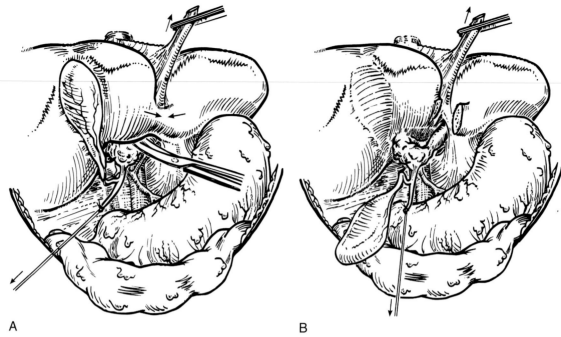

A   B

Fig. 80.61. A, Dissection to expose structures at the hilus of the liver. The ligamentum teres is strongly elevated, and the liver is turned upward. Dissection at the base of the quadrate lobe (scissors) lowers the hilar plate. The bridge of liver tissue *(arrow)* at the base of the umbilical fissure is still intact. The common bile duct is divided immediately above the duodenum, and its lower part has been separated together with the associated connective tissue and lymph nodes. **B,** The biliary confluence has been delivered by lowering of the hilar plate. The bridge of tissue at the base of the umbilical fissure has been divided.

long-term survival have been linked directly to hepatic resection (see Ch. 52) (Jarnagin et al, 2001a).

Hepatic resection in some instances may be limited to removal of the quadrate lobe (segment IV) or may include removal of segment I (caudate lobe). The procedures described subsequently relate to the more extensive resection of right or left hepatectomy or right lobectomy, however, usually necessary in these circumstances. The variation in techniques compared with the techniques described earlier relate to the dissection of the tumor at the hilus of the liver.

Preliminary laparoscopy before open exploration of the abdomen saves a proportion of patients with liver metastases or peritoneal seeding from unnecessary laparotomy (Jarnagin et al, 2000). Also of importance is the examination of the liver for extension of the tumor and biopsy of any suspicious areas (Blumgart et al, 1984). Excision biopsy with frozen section of apparently involved nodes should be performed. Evident multicentricity within the liver or spread to a distant site or lymph node involvement precludes resection, and the patient should be submitted to appropriate biliary-enteric decompression (see Ch. 30).

To be able to reach the confluence of the bile ducts and explore the related vessels, the operator must explore the area beneath the quadrate lobe. If there is no tumor invasion at this point, the hilar plate is lowered according to the technique of Hepp and Couinaud (1957) (Fig. 80.61) (see Ch. 30). If the left hepatic duct can be so lowered, the tumor is usually extending into the right hepatic duct, and right lobectomy or right hepatectomy is required. It is usually clear at this stage that sufficient left duct can be maintained beyond the line of resection to allow tumor clearance. In some cases, if the base of the quadrate lobe is involved over a limited area, the left duct may be identified further laterally. Further exploration of the hilus can be effected by splitting the liver in the Glissonian plane down to the hilus

(Fig. 80.62) (Blumgart, 1980; Goff et al, 1967; Templeton & Dodd, 1963).

Before any form of resection is undertaken, involvement of the caudate lobe must be assessed. The caudate lobe is explored by exposing the IVC below the liver. The lowermost hepatic veins are divided between ligatures to allow palpation of the caudate lobe from behind. Removal of the caudate lobe as an integral part of the operation frequently is necessary and is recommended as a routine by some authors (Mizumoto et al, 1986; Nimura et al, 1990b). Central hepatic resection involving segments IV, V, and VIII together with the caudate may be possible (Ogura et al, 1998).

The *common bile duct is transected* above the duodenum (Figs. 80.63 and 80.64) and turned upward. The curve of the duodenum is mobilized by the maneuver of Kocher, and the bile duct is transected and ligated immediately above the duodenum. The duct is turned upward and forward, clearing the vessels of fascia and lymph nodes. As dissection proceeds, *the gallbladder also is mobilized* so that the entire extrahepatic biliary apparatus is turned forward and upward (Fig. 80.65). This allows a safe approach to the retroductal structures lying at the confluence behind the tumor. The situation now encountered would be one of three.

First, in patients in whom there is no tumor involvement of the portal vein, the lesion can be freed and turned forward. If the caudate lobe is involved, it should be mobilized as described earlier and freed for removal as an integral part of the resection. The left hepatic duct, having been previously mobilized, is now located, dissected, and secured with stay sutures. It is transected, the cut duct being turned upward and to the right clear of the portal structures and allowing access for further dissection (Fig. 80.66). If the tumor extends into the left hepatic duct, it becomes necessary to transect the right duct initially and turn it

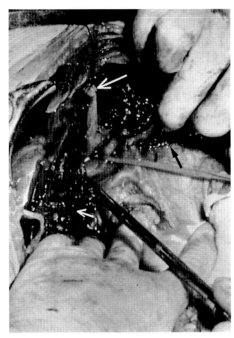

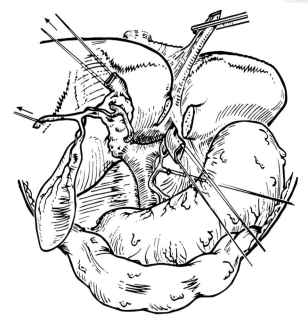

Fig. 80.62. Hepatotomy in the Glissonian plane. The left liver *(black arrow)* is separated from the right liver *(small white arrow)*. The common bile duct has been transected and is elevated on a tie *(large white arrow)*. A sling is passed about the left branch of the portal vein, which just beyond this point is involved by a cholangiocarcinoma at the confluence of the bile ducts and extending into the left hepatic duct. The hepatic artery is dissected and shown to be free of tumor involvement.

Fig. 80.64. The left hepatic duct has been divided, and the bifurcation of the portal vein has been cleared. The tumor is still attached to the right portal vein, however, and extends into the right liver. An alternative method would leave the transection division of the bile duct until a later stage during parenchymal transection.

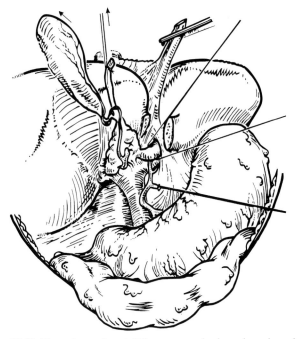

Fig. 80.63. The entire extrahepatic biliary apparatus has been elevated together with the associated connective tissue and nodes to allow dissection anterior to the bifurcation of the portal vein and elevation of the tumor, which is completely mobilized; the right hepatic artery has been tied and divided, and the portal vein has been skeletonized. The tumor is seen to extend into the right liver; stay sutures are placed in the left hepatic duct.

to the left. It is also possible, and often practiced, to dissect the duct and delay transection of the ducts until the time of parenchymal transection. In any event, when the ductal structures and the tumor are elevated, the relevant hepatic artery can be ligated, and the branch of the portal vein supplying the portion of the liver to be removed can be dealt with by clamping and oversewing in a standard fashion (see Fig. 80.65A). Hepatic resection proceeds as described previously, the liver tissue being divided from before backward with control of the hepatic veins extrahepatically or within the liver substance (see Fig. 80.65B).

Second, the tumor may involve the right or left branch of the portal vein (the area of bifurcation of the portal vein being entirely free). In this circumstance, the procedure is similar to that described earlier with the exception of the fact that transection of the affected portal branch may be difficult because of the proximity of the lesion. The caudate lobe may have to be mobilized to effect its removal at a later stage.

Third, the tumor may encroach on the portal vein bifurcation or involve the bifurcation directly. If this situation is encountered, a more extensive procedure is required. If the portal vein bifurcation is involved, and the tumor extends to involve the right ductal system, right lobectomy proceeds as follows. The common bile duct and gallbladder are mobilized and turned upward as described previously. Lowering of the hilar plate (see earlier) is done if possible, and the left hepatic duct and the left portal vein are dissected. The right hepatic artery is ligated, but the left hepatic artery is preserved. Stay sutures are placed, and the left hepatic duct is transected. The left branch of the portal vein and its main trunk are cross-clamped (see Fig. 80.66), and the affected segment of portal vein at the bifurcation is freed and turned together with the medial part of the left hepatic duct to the right (Fig. 80.67). A direct anastomosis is performed between the main trunk of the portal vein and its own left branch (Fig. 80.68). This anastomosis allows maintenance of an intact vascular supply to the left lobe.

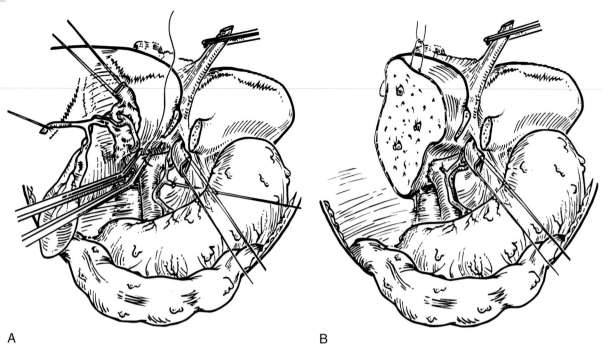

A   B

Fig. 80.65. A, Clamps are applied to the right branch of the portal vein, and a suture is passed through the vein between the clamps before the division of the vein and its subsequent suture. **B,** The right branch of the portal vein has been divided and oversewn using a 3-0 vascular suture. The right liver has been removed together with the attached biliary structures containing the tumor. The left hepatic duct is held on stay sutures ready for subsequent anastomosis.

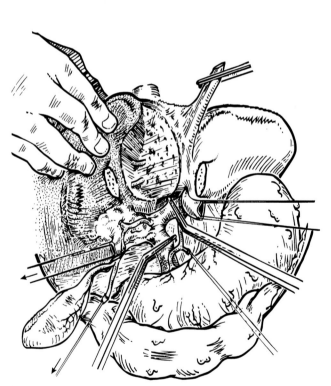

Fig. 80.66. Excision of hilar cholangiocarcinoma involving the bifurcation of the portal vein. The tumor is firmly attached to the portal vein. The initial steps are as described previously in Figs. 80.61, 80.63, and 80.64. The left hepatic duct has been identified and transected. The right hepatic artery has been divided. The main trunk of the portal vein and its left branch have been dissected and are held in clamps. The tumor is seen to be firmly attached in the region of the bifurcation of the portal vein. Resection sometimes is facilitated by starting a split of the liver substance immediately to the right of the falciform ligament dividing the feedback vessels that course to supply the quadrate lobe (segment IV).

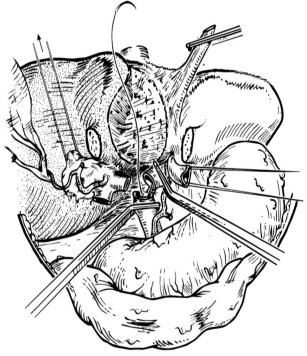

Fig. 80.67. The main trunk of the portal vein is divided, as is its left branch. The extrahepatic biliary apparatus, the confluence of the bile ducts, the tumor, and the bifurcation of the portal vein have been separated and are left attached to the right liver. The exposed ends of the main trunk of the portal vein and its left branch are approximated. End-to-end anastomosis is carried out using an over-and-over 4-0 vascular suture. When this anastomosis has been completed, the initial right hepatic lobectomy is completed, leaving a remnant of the liver comprising segments II and III and segment I (the caudate lobe) supplied by the left hepatic artery and the left branch of the portal vein and draining through the left hepatic duct. Individual caudate ducts exposed during the resection must be oversewn carefully or individually anastomosed. Alternatively, the caudate lobe may be removed (see text).

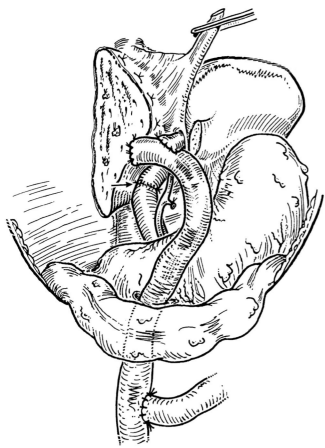

Fig. 80.68. The operation of right hepatic lobectomy has been completed, the line of resection running just to the right of the falciform ligament. The portal vein anastomosis is shown *(arrow)*. A Roux-en-Y loop of jejunum has been brought up in a retrocolic fashion and anastomosed to the exposed left hepatic duct (see also Fig. 80.60B).

Right hepatic lobectomy proceeds along standard lines as described previously. The caudate lobe is removed en bloc with the tumor and the right lobe. Biliary-enteric continuity is reconstructed by hepaticojejunostomy to a Roux-en-Y loop of jejunum (see Fig. 80.68).

If access or application of clamps is difficult, the liver may be initially split to the right of the falciform ligament, securing feedback vessels as for the initial stages of right hepatic lobectomy. Clamps are applied, the portal bifurcation is freed, and portal vein reconstruction is performed before transection of the remaining liver tissue backward to the vena cava.

Alternative methods for reconstruction of the portal vein using the splenic vein have been proposed (Longmire et al, 1973). An interposition of an autogenous venous graft may be necessary. If left hepatectomy is necessary, the principles of the procedure are as described earlier, but portal vein reconstruction is more difficult.

Resectional methods with reconstruction of the portal vein and hepatic artery are discussed subsequently by Nimura and Sano. In some cases, the division of the intrahepatic right or left hepatic ducts may be delayed until the final phase of parenchymal transection, and many surgeons prefer this approach. The selection of patients with hilar cholangio-carcinoma for liver resection and the results are discussed further in Ch. 52.

CRYOABLATION-ASSISTED HEPATIC RESECTION

Cryoablation, or the destruction of tissues by the freeze and thaw process, is a recognized approach to the treatment of malignant tumors (see Ch. 76). The destruction of hepatic tumors using cryoablation is well recorded. Most studies (Atkinson et al, 1992; Charnley et al, 1989, 1991; Horton et al, 1991; Onik et al, 1991, 1993; Ravikumar & Steele, 1989; Ravikumar et al, 1987, 1991) report in situ freezing of hepatic tumors, and this is described in detail in Ch. 76. The use of the cryoprobe as a device to assist during resection also has been suggested (Welling & Lamping, 1990) and developed (Polk et al, 1995).

Cryosurgery is used to assist resection in three particular situations. (1) Wedge resections, especially for lesions situated on the dome of the liver, are fraught with difficulty not only regarding control of hemorrhage within the depths of the wedge, but also in obtaining tumor-free margins. Wedge resections of the liver have been shown to be associated with an extremely high local recurrence rate. A major reason for the positive margin associated with wedge resections is the likelihood of fracturing the specimen along the interface of the hard tumor and soft liver. Freezing a rim of normal hepatic tissue around the tumor prevents fracture along this tumor-liver interface. (2) In many patients, major hepatic resection is required for removal of unilateral lesions, but there are accompanying minor lesions in the contralateral lobe that could be resected if only a small amount of functional hepatic tissue were removed. (3) Although cryosurgery has been used in the management of hepatocellular carcinoma (Zhou, 1992a, 1992b), it has been used in a cryoablative manner. The use of cryoablation-assisted resection in cases of hepatocellular carcinoma in the cirrhotic liver allows removal of tumors with adequate margins of clearance and maximum preservation of functional parenchymal tissue.

Technique

The liver is examined by bimanual palpation and intraoperative ultrasound using a 7.5-mHz transducer. Lesions suitable for cryoablation-assisted resection are identified. Glisson's capsule is scored with a diathermy at the point of insertion of the selected cryoprobe (Fig. 80.69), which is gently inserted using direct vision and guided by ultrasound to the center of the lesion to be resected. Laparotomy pads are placed to protect adjacent structures. We occlude vascular inflow (Pringle's maneuver) before start of the freeze cycle. The freeze cycle is initiated, and ultrasound is used to monitor freezing. The freeze margin is easily seen as a hyperechoic rim with posterior acoustic shadowing slowly developing from the center of the lesion. The freeze margin is allowed to reach a distance of approximately 1 cm outside the periphery of the tumor (see Fig. 80.69). At this point, hepatic vascular inflow occlusion is temporarily released. Two minutes are allowed for reperfusion of the liver after initial freezing, then the Pringle maneuver is reinstituted during resection of the parenchyma. To maintain the ice ball at a constant size during resection, we allow freeze and thaw cycles of 1 minute each during the resection procedures. This cycling is successful in preventing extension of the ice ball or inadvertent removal of the probe, which can be used as a "handle" to manipulate the lesion during resection. Dissection is performed directly on the ice ball or at a slight distance from it (see Fig. 80.69C). Traction on the cryoprobe and ice ball complex provides useful exposure to the line of parenchymal transection.

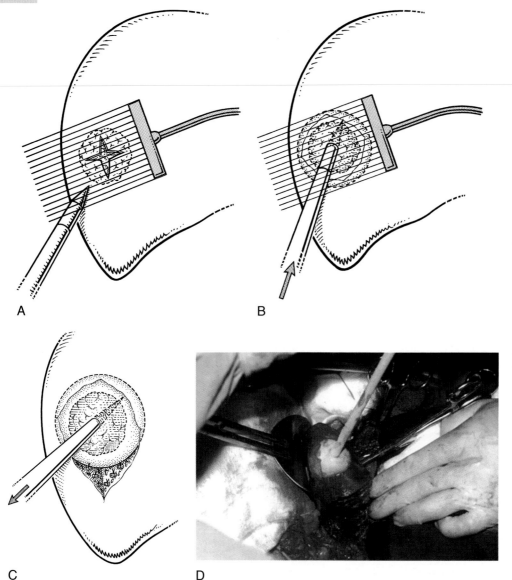

Fig. 80.69. A, Tumor is located using intraoperative ultrasound. Glisson's capsule is scored in cruciate fashion with the diathermy. **B,** The cryoprobe is introduced. The position of the cryoprobe is controlled using ultrasound guidance, and the tumor is frozen to approximately 1 cm of clearance. **C,** The cryoprobe is used as a handle to manipulate the tumor, which is excised at the ice ball edge (see text). **D,** Intraoperative photograph shows a cryoprobe inserted into a tumor in segment VI. The tumor is being removed by the cryoassisted technique (see text).

Blood vessels are easily visualized, and they are individually controlled as they are encountered. In patients in whom the tumor is shown on ultrasound to approximate a major venous structure (e.g., the right hepatic vein), preliminary mobilization of the liver from the underlying vena cava and isolation of the right hepatic vein and temporary clamping of the vein during the procedure has allowed safe resection.

The specimen is left attached to the cryoprobe (see Fig. 80.69D) and is allowed to thaw, at which time it is removed and sectioned to ensure adequate resection margins. If there is doubt as to the adequacy of the margins, a flat cryoprobe may be inserted into the cavity, and further freezing of the relevant margin can be done.

ENUCLEATION OF GIANT HEMANGIOMATA AND OTHER BENIGN LIVER TUMORS

The surgical management of giant hemangioma was described in 1942 by Schumaker, and following the advent of noninvasive imaging techniques, there has been renewed interest in the subject (Baer et al, 1987, 1992a; Iwatsuki & Starzl, 1988; Schwartz & Husser, 1987). Selective arteriography often gives additional information by showing the characteristic patchy pooling of contrast material and by defining the intrahepatic and extrahepatic vascular anatomy.

A technique of enucleation (Alper et al, 1988; Baer et al, 1987, 1992a) that can be applied to the elective management of a giant cavernous hemangioma (Fig. 80.70), ensuring minimal blood loss and the preservation of virtually all normal hepatic parenchyma, is described. We also have used this technique to enucleate adenoma, fibronodular hyperplasia, and metastatic neuroendocrine tumors. Others (Lerner et al, 2004) have confirmed that this approach offers preservation of normal parenchyma and fewer complications than hepatic lobectomy.

Technique

Depending on the site and the arterial supply of the tumor identified before operation, the right or left hepatic artery is identified

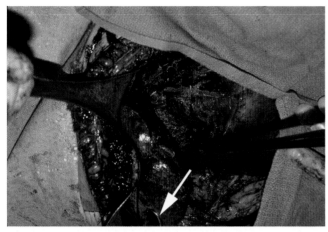

Fig. 80.70. Intraoperative photograph shows enucleation of a large hemangioma of the right lobe of the liver. The hemangioma has been compressed and can be manipulated with forceps *(arrow)*. The hemangioma is enucleated from the liver substance. A major branch of the middle hepatic vein is seen exposed in the depths of the wound. There is no sacrifice of normal liver tissue (see Fig. 80.71).

and traced back to the common hepatic artery. Bleeding from the enucleation site is controlled by prior complete extrahepatic vascular control. Ligation of the right or left hepatic artery for a major lesion of the right or left liver is usually adequate. For lesions involving segment IV, however, a more selective dissection controlling the relevant vessels within the umbilical fissure may be necessary. The lesion can be compressed and as tension

is relieved can be clamped for traction as dissection proceeds (see later). Division of only a few millimeters of liver tissue at the periphery of the hemangioma is usually all the parenchymal dissection required. At this point, a sheath of compressed liver tissue is encountered that defines the border between the cavernous tissue and the normal liver parenchyma. Dissection is now possible by gliding the surgeon's finger along this plane, following the margin of the lesion and avoiding entry into the liver parenchyma or into the tumor itself. As blood vessels or bile ducts are encountered, they are controlled by suture ligature and divided. Proceeding in this way, it is possible to shell out the hemangioma from the parenchyma without damage to major vessels or bile ducts (see Fig. 80.70). The resulting hepatic defect after enucleation can be treated in a variety of ways. Generally, the bleeding from the bed of the hemangioma is minimal and can be controlled by compression and the use of the Argon Beam Coagulator. The omentum may be mobilized and placed over the raw surface as an omentoplasty.

The technique described allows large hemangiomata to be resected with a limited disruption of the surrounding liver tissue (Fig. 80.71). The reason this is possible is shown by the histology (Baer et al, 1992a). The enucleation occurs along a relatively avascular capsular plane. The few blood vessels that do transverse the capsule are encountered, and the amount of normal functioning parenchyma removed is minimal. Even when the size of the tumor means that most of the right or left liver has been removed, the disturbance of liver function is insignificant. A similar approach to that of enucleation of benign tumors is applied to pericystectomy in the operative management of echinococcal cysts (see Ch. 61).

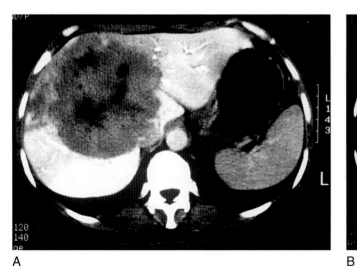
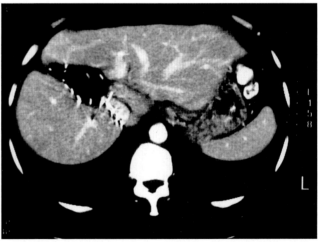

A   B

Fig. 80.71. A, CT scan shows a large symptomatic hemangioma within segments IV, V, VI, and VIII of the right liver. This hemangioma was enucleated without loss of any functional liver tissue. The large cavity was filled with an omentoplasty. **B,** CT scan after operation shows there has been no loss of parenchyma.

ADDENDUM: LAPAROSCOPIC TECHNIQUES

M. D'ANGELICA

The use of laparoscopic surgery has emerged as a viable and sometimes routine option for many general surgical operations. These include, among others, cholecystectomy, adrenalectomy, splenectomy, colectomy, Nissen fundoplication, and gastric bypass for morbid obesity. Liver resection has been a notable exception to the explosion of minimally invasive abdominal surgery. This is likely the result of numerous issues. Open hepatic surgery has become a safe proposition only since the 1980s, and rapid adoption of minimally invasive techniques was inappropriate. Fear of major hemorrhage and air embolism through open hepatic veins with a lack of good laparoscopic instrumentation for partial hepatectomy was a major concern. Lastly, many surgeons who specialize in hepatic surgery are not experts in laparoscopic surgery, and many surgeons who specialize in laparoscopic surgery are not experts in hepatic surgery. The performance of laparoscopic liver resections requires expertise in two technically challenging areas of surgery, and only more recently have a few centers developed these combined skills.

The benefits of minimally invasive surgery have been well documented since the late 1980s, when the first laparoscopic cholecystectomy was performed. From many studies, it has been shown that smaller incisions result in less pain, less postoperative ileus, shorter hospital stays, and an overall shortened recovery time. Additional theoretical benefits are decreased immunosuppression and shorter time to initiation of adjuvant medical therapies, which are particularly relevant to cancer patients (Soper et al, 1994).

Laparoscopy has a well-defined role in the staging and diagnosis of hepatobiliary malignancy and is used routinely in appropriate situations (D'Angelica et al, 2003). Laparoscopic procedures also have been used widely for the fenestration of simple hepatic cysts (Paterson-Brown & Garden, 1991) and have been described for the treatment of hydatid cysts (Fiamingo et al, 2003; Gigot et al, 2001; Khoury et al, 2000; Manterola et al, 2002). Thermoablative procedures for liver tumors also can be performed now with laparoscopic ultrasound guidance and with probes adopted for laparoscopic application (Berber, et al, 2004; Iannitti et al, 1998; Ido et al, 1997; Lezoche et al, 1998). These hepatic operations are technically simpler than hepatic resection, rendering them more amenable to laparoscopic techniques, and they have been adopted more readily. Other chapters in this book focusing on cystic diseases of the liver and ablation address the role of laparoscopic surgery for these diseases. Following is a review of the available literature and our experience with laparoscopic partial hepatectomy.

Many legitimate concerns exist regarding the performance of laparoscopic liver resections. Because these operations are performed under carbon dioxide pneumoperitoneum at an abdominal pressure of 12 to 15 mm Hg, gas embolism into the venous system is one such concern. Inability to control bleeding from the cut liver surface expeditiously is an additional concern. Lastly, and perhaps most important, is the adequacy of an oncologic operation in cases of hepatic malignancy (the most common indication for liver resection). Although there were initial concerns of wound implantation of malignancy during laparoscopic surgery, this has largely been disproved (Shoup et al, 2002). More recently,

randomized prospective trials have addressed the role of laparoscopic surgery for cancer, and two trials have shown laparoscopic and open colectomy to be equivalent in the treatment of colon cancer (Clinical Outcomes of Surgical Therapy Study Group, 2004; Lacy et al, 2002).

To date, most laparoscopic liver resections have been segmental or wedge resections of relatively peripheral tumors located in the more accessible portions of the liver (segments II, III, IVb, V, and VI). Laparoscopic major hepatectomy has been performed in limited numbers and is not widely used because of safety concerns and the significant technical challenge. The technique of laparoscopic partial hepatectomy should employ the same general principles that apply to standard open surgery. Because no palpation of the liver is possible, hepatic ultrasound is crucial to stage the patient properly, define vascular anatomy, and plan a proper anatomic operation with adequate margins. Most authors use four or five ports with a variety of port placement schemes. In general, the ports have to be placed appropriately for visualization of the area to be resected and for the angles necessary to divide the parenchyma or ligaments. Port placement varies significantly from case to case depending on the location of the tumor. Adequate retraction remains a major problem, but numerous atraumatic fan retractors are available for use.

We and others have used a hand-assisted technique (Fong et al, 1999a) in which an operator's hand can be placed through a 6- to 7-cm incision. The hand generally is used for retraction and for assistance in the case of hemorrhage. Portal clamping (Pringle's maneuver) can be employed laparoscopically with a sling or with a bulldog clamp. Liver segments can be mobilized by incising appropriate ligaments, or conversely the ligaments can be left intact and used for countertraction during the parenchymal transection. Numerous instruments have been developed that can perform parenchymal transection with minimal blood loss when the hepatic capsule has been scored with cautery. Ultrasonic dissecting shears, the LigaSure device, and the TissueLink device can divide parenchyma containing small to medium size vessels with effective coagulation. These instruments can disperse significant amounts of thermal energy and should be used with caution around major bile ducts because they can injure these structures easily. Parenchyma also can be divided with a clamp crushing technique or with a laparoscope-adapted Cavitron ultrasonic surgical aspirator (CUSA; Valleylab, Boulder, CO) exposing veins and pedicles, which can be divided with clips. Endovascular staplers are useful for well-dissected pedicles and major veins and hemostatically divide these structures. Additionally, thin pieces of parenchyma can be divided with multiple fires of an endovascular stapler with excellent hemostasis. Final hemostasis at the cut edge of the liver can be achieved with all of the above-mentioned techniques, but can be supplemented with a laparoscopic Argon Beam Coagulator.

Published experience with laparoscopic liver resection is limited. The cumulative data to date document feasibility and some basic assessments of adequacy of oncologic outcome, such as margin status. No long-term follow-up exists, and no randomized trials have been performed comparing open with laparoscopic liver resection. Additionally, as stated earlier, laparoscopic liver resection has largely been applied to small, peripheral tumors in the more accessible portions of the liver. Early reports involved resections of one or two segments located in the left lateral segment (Samama et al, 1998) and in segments IVb, V, and VI (Antonetti et al, 2002; Cherqui et al, 2000; Descottes et al,

Table 80.5   Summary of Case Control Studies Comparing Laparoscopic with Open Partial Hepatectomy

Reference	n	Disease	Operative Time (min)	Blood loss (mL)	Length of Stay (days)	Morbidity (%)	Margin <1 cm (%)
Mala et al, 2002	15 versus 14	Colorectal metastases	187 versus 185	600 versus 500	4 versus 8.5*	13 versus 29	29 versus 37
Lesurtel et al, 2003	18 versus 20	Mixed	202 versus 145	236 versus 429*	8 versus 10	11 versus 15	6 versus 0
Morino et al, 2003	30 versus 30	Mixed	150 versus 140	320 versus 479	6 versus 8*	7 versus 7	43 versus 40
Farges et al, 2002	21 versus 21	Benign	177 versus 156	218 versus 285	5 vs 6.5*,†	10 versus 10	—
Shimada et al, 2001	17 versus 28	HCC	325 versus 280	400 versus 800	12 versus 25*,†	6 versus 11	41 versus 50‡
Laurent et al, 2003	13 versus 14	HCC	267 versus 182*	620 versus 720	8 versus 12.5	No difference§	15 versus 15‡

*P<.05.
†Mean.
‡<5 mm.
§No significant difference among the specific complications analyzed.
HCC, hepatocellular carcinoma.

2000; Huscher et al, 1998; Ker et al, 2000; Rau et al, 1998; Shimada et al, 2001). A European multicenter trial has documented outcomes in 124 cases, 37 of which were for malignancy. There were no perioperative deaths, and the morbidity rate was 10% (Descottes et al, 2003; Gigot et al, 2002). In general, conversion rates to laparotomy have been 10% to 20%, and specific concerns such as wound implantation of tumor and air embolism have not been found to be a problem.

Major liver resections, such as right hemihepatectomy, have been performed, but in limited numbers. In the largest series of laparoscopic major hepatectomies to date, O'Rourke and Fielding (2004) reported on 12 laparoscopic right hepatectomies. Two cases were converted to an open procedure, five were laparoscopic-assisted procedures, and five were completed laparoscopically. There were two significant postoperative morbidities: one bile leak and one wound dehiscence (O'Rourke & Fielding, 2004).

In the European multicenter trial, five major hepatectomies were performed; there was a major left bile duct injury during a laparoscopic right hepatectomy that required formal open repair. One group also specifically described seven cases of a hand-assisted approach to tumors in the posterior sector of the right liver (Huang et al, 2003).

No prospective comparisons between open and laparoscopic hepatectomy have been performed, but numerous retrospective case-control comparisons have been published (Farges et al, 2002; Laurent et al, 2003; Lesurtel et al, 2003; Mala et al, 2002; Morino et al, 2003; Shimada et al, 2001). These studies show that laparoscopic liver resection is associated with a slightly longer operative time, less blood loss, less narcotic usage, and shorter hospital stays. Morbidity has been minimal and similar to open cases. In all series, the incidence of close margins has been similar to open cases (Table 80.5). In the study by Farges and colleagues (2002),

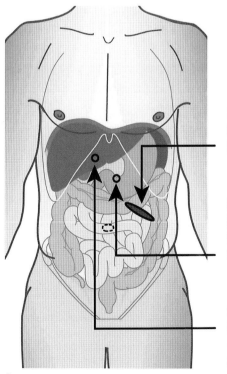

Port site No.1
Size: 10/11mm
Pneumo Sleeve

Port site No.2
Size: 10/12mm
Laparoscope
Harmonic Scalpel
Stapler

Port site No.3
Size: 10/12mm
Laparoscope
Harmonic Scalpel
Stapler

A

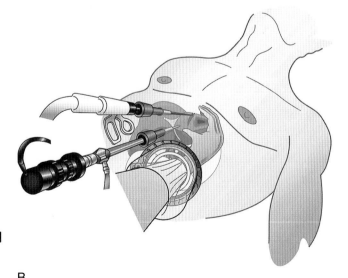

B

Fig. 80.72. **A**, Port placement for laparoscopic left lateral segmentectomy. These are the main ports necessary. Additional ports are placed as necessary. **B**, Laparoscopic left lateral segmentectomy. After complete mobilization of the left lateral segment by dividing the left triangular ligament, the liver parenchymal transection is performed using the harmonic scalpel and the vascular endoscopic stapler. The hand is used for retraction and to assess for tumor clearance. A bulldog clamp can be placed across the porta hepatis to provide for Pringle's maneuver.

patients undergoing laparoscopic hepatectomy were monitored with a Swan-Ganz catheter for hemodynamic changes. Compared with patients being treated with an open resection, there was no difference in mean arterial pressure, cardiac index, pulmonary artery pressure, or pulmonary artery wedge pressure during hepatic pedicle clamping. Additionally, there was no significant difference in end-tidal carbon dioxide or oxygen saturation throughout the cases, dispelling the fear of carbon dioxide embolism. In four patients, an intraoperative transesophageal echocardiogram also was performed, and no significant passage of gas bubbles could be detected going through the heart (Farges et al, 2002).

At MSKCC, we perform laparoscopic hepatic resections with hand assistance except for the most peripheral lesions (Fig. 80.72) (Fong et al, 2000). This approach provides numerous advantages, while maintaining a minimally invasive approach. The liver is a difficult organ to retract, and no laparoscopic instrument is perfectly suitable. The hand provides the perfect retracting instrument and provides a rapid and effective way to tamponade bleeding should this occur. At our last analysis, we had attempted a laparoscopic hepatic resection in 45 patients. No major hepatic

resections were performed laparoscopically, and these cases were confined mostly to tumors in the left lateral segment and in more accessible portions of segments IVb, V, and VI. Twelve cases were converted to laparotomy, and of the laparoscopic cases, two thirds were performed with hand assistance. The two most common diagnoses were metastatic colorectal cancer and hepatocellular carcinoma. The mean operative time was 195 ± 12 minutes, and the median estimated blood loss was 100 mL (range 5-500 mL). There were no postoperative mortalities, and postoperative morbidity was minimal. Despite a mean tumor size of 4.3 cm, there was only one positive margin in a patient with an adenoma (unpublished data).

Laparoscopic liver resection is a feasible procedure for peripheral and smaller tumors. With proper surgical judgment, this procedure can be performed safely and with sound oncologic principles. Performance of laparoscopic liver resections requires expertise, however, in open liver resection and in advanced laparoscopic techniques. With improvements in instrumentation and technique, laparoscopic surgery will undoubtedly play a larger role in the performance of liver resection in the future.

Extended Resection for Biliary Tumors—an Alternative Approach

Y. NIMURA AND T. SANO

The approach to hilar cholangiocarcinoma described here differs from that described earlier in this chapter particularly in respect to the detailed preoperative percutaneous transhepatic biliary drainage (PTBD), cholangioscopy, and vascular imaging practiced by the authors. Such approaches are favored in Japan, but rarely pursued by Western surgeons (see earlier).

PREOPERATIVE DIAGNOSIS AND MANAGEMENT OF HILAR CHOLANGIOCARCINOMA

Accurate preoperative staging using extensive investigation is indispensable before radical surgery for hilar cholangiocarcinoma (Nagino et al, 1998; Nimura, 1994, 1997; Nimura et al, 1990a, 1995b, 2000). Most cases of hilar cholangiocarcinoma are associated with obstructive jaundice as a result of obstruction of the intrahepatic bile ducts. Obstruction usually involves multiple ducts as a result of proximal spread of carcinoma along the intrahepatic segmental bile ducts. We believe multiple PTBD (Nagino et al, 1992; Nimura et al, 1995a; Takada et al, 1976), which relieves the cholestasis and restores the functional reserve of the future remnant liver, is essential before radical operation involving extensive hepatic resection. We described in the previous edition that the first step in the preoperative management was PTBD, but more recently multidetector-row CT is the first examination. Multidetector-row CT allows a rough definition as to which side of the liver should be resected. PTBD is applied by the direct anterior approach under fluoroscopic guidance (Takada et al, 1976) to relieve cholestasis of the future remnant liver. This procedure has diagnostic and therapeutic advantages (Nagino et al, 1995a).

Usually, it is not possible to define accurately the cancer extent and to determine the possibility of curative resection

using conventional percutaneous transhepatic cholangiography or endoscopic retrograde cholangiography. High-quality cholangiograms through the PTBD catheters in various positions— supine, right and left anterior oblique, right and left lateral, and cephalad-anterior–oblique (Kamiya et al, 1994)—show the tumor location clearly and provide the most reliable information of the proximal extension of hilar cholangiocarcinoma along the intrahepatic segmental bile ducts (Fig. 80.73) (Ebata et al, 2002;

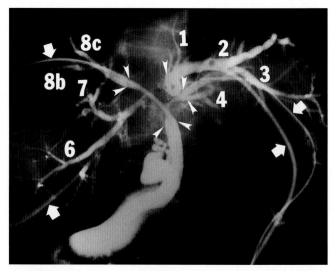

Fig. 80.73. Cholangiogram through four percutaneous transhepatic biliary drainage cathethers *(arrows)* shows the stricture at the hepatic hilum and suggests cancer extension along the intrahepatic segmental bile ducts *(arrowheads)*. Numerals refer to the Couinaud's segments of the liver. *8b* is a lateral branch of the right anterior superior segmental bile duct; *8c* is a dorsal branch of the right anterior superior segmental bile duct.

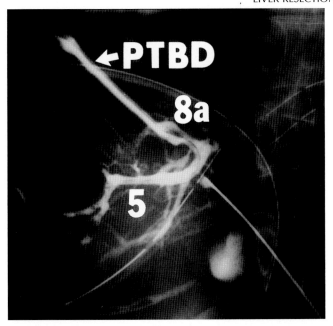

Fig. 80.74. Urgent additional PTBD to the anterior sectoral ducts was performed for intrahepatic segmental cholangitis. *5* is a branch of the right anterior inferior segmental bile duct; *8a* is a ventral branch of the right anterior superior segmental bile duct.

Sakamoto et al, 1998). When cholangiography provides insufficient information as to tumor extent, additional PTBD is performed to the remaining bile ducts. Percutaneous transhepatic cholangioscopy, after dilating the sinus tract of PTBD, also can provide reliable information of anatomic variations of the biliary tree and mucosal extension of the cancer (Kamiya et al, 1994; Nimura, 1993; Nimura et al, 1989). Superficial mucosal extension of the carcinoma often is associated with polypoid or nodular tumors of macroscopic type or both. Percutaneous transhepatic cholangioscopy with biopsy may be valuable in diagnosis of the extent of cancer (Nimura et al, 1988; Sakamoto et al, 1997). Biliary tract infection results in deterioration of the functional reserve of the liver, however. When intrahepatic segmental cholangitis develops in patients with PTBD catheters during the preoperative period, urgent additional selective PTBD to the affected segmental duct should be performed (Fig. 80.74) (Kanai et al, 1996).

Concomitant vascular resection and reconstruction is often indicated in advanced cases of hilar cholangiocarcinoma (Nimura et al, 1991). We used to perform visceral angiography, percutaneous transhepatic portography, and selective retrograde hepatic venography to assess the vascular invasion of the tumor (Nishio et al, 1999, 2003). More recently, three-dimensional multidetector-row CT using techniques of volume rendering, multiplanar reformation, and maximum intensity projection has allowed high-quality images with less invasive imaging (Fig. 80.75). We usually estimate

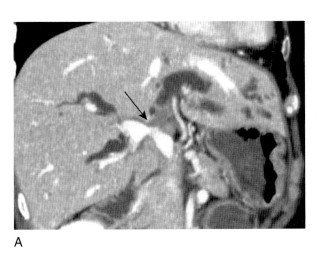

A

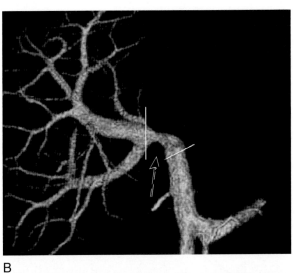

B

Fig. 80.75. Three-dimensional reconstructed images of multidetector-row CT. **A,** Coronal view multiplanar reformation image shows left hepatic duct tumor invading the portal bifurcation *(arrow).* **B,** Anteroposterior view of volume rendering image shows obstruction of the left portal vein and narrowing of the contralateral side of the portal bifurcation *(arrow).* Portal vein resection was planned at lines. **C,** Craniocaudal view of maximum intensity projection image reveals narrowing of the portal bifurcation *(arrow).* This view can be obtained by neither conventional arterial portography nor percutaneous transhepatic portography.

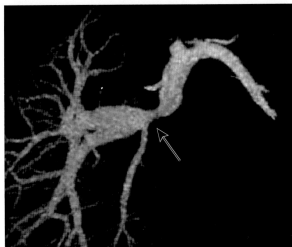

C

the relationship between one tumor and the vascular system in the hepatoduodenal ligament and diagnose the vascular involvement of the tumor on the multiplanar reformation images and plan the reconstruction method (e.g., wedge or segmental resection, direct end-to-end anastomosis, or segmental autogenous vein grafting) by volume rendering and maximum intensity projection images.

Postoperative morbidity and mortality remain considerable, particularly if extensive resection is necessary (Nagino et al, 2001). Postoperative liver failure sometimes occurs and results in death. For this reason, liver resection usually is scheduled only after the serum total bilirubin concentration decreases to less than 2 mg/dL. In addition, since 1989, we have routinely performed percutaneous transhepatic portal vein embolization (see Ch. 84) (Nagino et al, 1993, 1996, 2000) as preoperative preparation for extensive liver resection. This procedure is done to minimize the incidence of postoperative liver failure. After estimation of the resultant compensatory hypertrophy by volumetric study of a CT scan (Nagino et al, 1995b, 1995c) and of the functional reserve of the liver as assessed by the indocyanine green disappearance rate (Uesaka et al, 1996), hepatectomy is performed, usually 2 to 3 weeks after percutaneous transhepatic portal vein embolization.

RIGHT HEPATIC RESECTION WITH TOTAL CAUDATE LOBECTOMY, EXTRAHEPATIC BILE DUCT RESECTION, AND PORTAL VEIN RESECTION AND RECONSTRUCTION

Right hepatectomy with total caudate lobectomy is carried out for tumors involving the right anterior and posterior sectoral bile ducts with sparing of the left medial segmental bile duct to

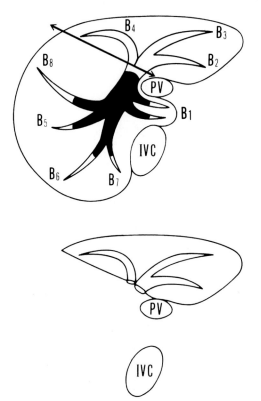

Fig. 80.76. Schematic representation of the tumor extent (*blackened area*) and the resection for right hepatectomy with total caudate lobectomy. Numerals (B1-B8) refer to Couinaud's segments of the liver. PV, portal vein.

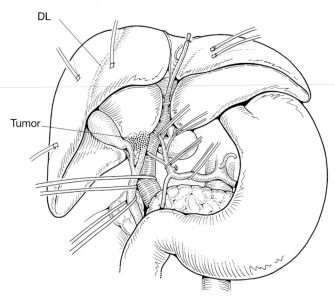

Fig. 80.77. Right hepatic resection. After laparotomy, all PTBD catheters are fixed at the liver surface for intraoperative biliary drainage. A faint demarcation line (DL) along the main portal fissure is observed owing to preoperative portal vein embolization. After retropancreatic lymph node dissection, the distal bile duct is divided in the pancreas with a histologic free margin, then skeletonization resection of the hepatoduodenal ligament is advanced up to the hepatic hilus.

segment IV (or when the right hepatic artery is also involved) (Fig. 80.76). If the cancer involves the right hepatic duct and the left medial segmental duct, right hepatic trisegmentectomy with caudate lobectomy is indicated.

At operation and after exploration of the peritoneal cavity, PTBD catheters are fixed at the liver surface to maintain intraoperative biliary drainage. The right lobe is usually atrophic to some extent, and a faint demarcation between the right and left lobe is observed as a result of the preoperative percutaneous transhepatic portal vein embolization. After retropancreatic lymph node dissection, the distal bile duct is divided in the pancreas with a histologic free margin, and the hepatoduodenal ligament is dissected, the vessels being skeletonized and removed (Bhuiya et al, 1992). The middle hepatic artery usually runs ventral to the left portal vein and enters the liver below the left medial segment branch of the portal vein. This artery is carefully preserved. The left hepatic artery enters the liver to the left of the umbilical portion of the portal vein (Fig. 80.77).

After skeletonization of the hepatoduodenal ligament, the caudate lobe is prepared by isolation, ligation, and division of the arterial branches and portal branches. The details of the technique were described previously (see Figs. 80.52-80.54 and 80.77). Although the arterial branches directly arise from the left and right hepatic arteries, they cannot be identified accurately in some cases. Two to six branches of the portal vein arise from the left portal vein, two to three branches form the right portal vein, and one to two branches arise from the main trunk or the bifurcation of the portal vein. The significance of total caudate lobectomy in cases of hilar cholangiocarcinoma is not resection of the parenchyma of the caudate lobe, but clearance of the connective tissue of the hilar plate around the caudate bile duct branches, which are often involved by cancer (Nimura et al, 1992). After complete division of the caudate arteries and portal vein branches, the right hepatic lobe is mobilized, and short retrohepatic veins are ligated and divided. The caudate lobe is completely detached from the IVC (see earlier; see Fig. 80.54). The confluence of the

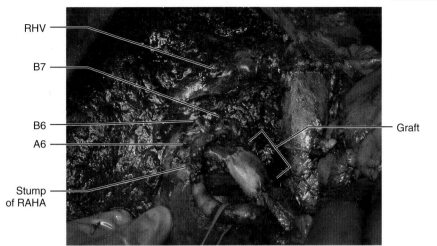

Fig. 80.78. Intraoperative photograph after the extended left hepatic resection (left trisegmentectomy) with total caudate lobectomy, extrahepatic bile duct resection, and portal vein resection and reconstruction. The vessel loop is around the right posterior sectoral artery. An autogenous graft using the right external iliac vein is shown. The right posterior superior (*B7*) and the right posterior inferior (*B6*) segmental bile ducts are divided separately above the reconstructed portal vein. *A6* is the right posterior inferior segmental hepatic artery. RHV, right hepatic vein.

right hepatic vein with the IVC is carefully encircled, clamped, divided, and closed with a running suture (see Fig. 80.26) or a vascular stapler.

In case of direct cancer invasion of the portal bifurcation, portal vein resection and reconstruction is performed before liver resection (see Fig. 80.66). Direct end-to-end anastomosis of the main trunk of the portal vein and the left branch is performed (Ebata et al, 2003; Nimura et al, 1991). Portal vein resection and reconstruction is carried out during the hilar dissection before hepatic parenchymal transection because the portal flow to the future remnant liver is easily impeded owing to kinking during operative manipulations. Direct end-to-end anastomosis between the main portal trunk and the left portal vein is usually possible during right-sided resections. Interposition of an autogenous vein graft is often required during portal vein reconstruction between the right portal vein and the main trunk during left-sided resections (Fig. 80.78) (see later). We usually harvest an external iliac vein for an autogenous vein graft by an extraperitoneal approach. The key to portal vein resection and reconstruction during right-sided hepatectomies is the feasibility of cross-clamping the root of the umbilical portion of the left portal vein. In the case of left-sided hepatectomies, isolation and clamping of the right posterior sectoral or the right anterior sectoral portal vein is the key maneuver.

After confirmation of the course of the middle hepatic vein using intraoperative ultrasound, liver transection is performed along the demarcation line that appears after ligation of the right hepatic artery. On the caudal aspect of segment IV, the liver transection line is horizontally advanced approximately 1 cm ventral to the hilar plate to achieve a free surgical margin. When the middle hepatic vein is exposed, liver transection is reduced toward the left laterally to the distal portion of the ligamentum venosum. When the caudodorsal aspect of the middle hepatic vein is completely exposed, the confluence of middle hepatic vein and IVC is seen. At this point, the caudate lobe can be turned and pulled ventrally from behind the left lateral segment. Finally, the bile duct is transected after placing a stay suture, and the right hepatic lobe is resected en bloc with the entire caudate lobe, portal bifurcation, and extrahepatic bile duct. The transected bile duct stumps—left medial segmental branch (segment IV), left lateral anterior segmental branch (segment III), and left lateral posterior segmental branch (segment II)—are noted just to the right of the umbilical portion of the left portal vein (Figs. 80.79 and 80.80).

Biliary-enteric continuity is re-established using a Roux-en-Y jejunal loop. The jejunal limb is brought to the transected hepatic ducts via the retrocolic-antegastric or the retrocolic-retrogastric route (Nagino et al, 2002). We perform hepaticojejunostomy in one layer using a 5-0 absorbable monofilament suture; a biliary drainage tube is placed across all anastomoses through the jejunal loop or transhepatically.

EXTENDED LEFT HEPATIC RESECTION WITH LEFT TRISEGMENTECTOMY, CAUDATE LOBECTOMY, EXTRAHEPATIC BILE DUCT RESECTION, AND PORTAL VEIN RESECTION AND RECONSTRUCTION

Extended left hepatic resection with caudate lobectomy is used for hilar cholangiocarcinoma that predominantly involves the left intrahepatic bile ducts in continuity with the duct to the right anterior sector (Fig. 80.81). During the subhepatic dissection of the hepatoduodenal ligament, the left hepatic artery and middle hepatic artery are ligated and divided at their origins, and the right hepatic artery is carefully isolated up to its bifurcation

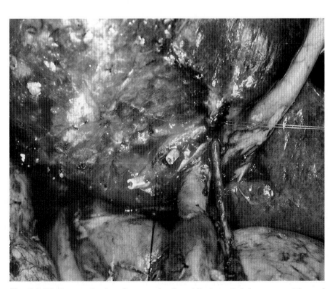

Fig. 80.79. Intraoperative photograph after right hepatic lobectomy with total caudate lobectomy, extrahepatic bile duct resection, and portal vein resection and reconstruction. Note tubes in the transected bile ducts.

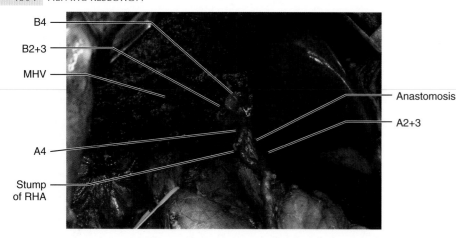

B4
B2+3
MHV

Anastomosis

A2+3

A4

Stump
of RHA

Fig. 80.80. Intraoperative photograph after right hepatic lobectomy with total caudate lobectomy, extrahepatic bile duct resection, and portal vein resection and reconstruction. Portal vein reconstruction is done by end-to-end anastomosis. The left medial hepatic artery *(A4)* originates from the right hepatic artery, which has been divided. *B2+3* is the transected left lateral segmental bile duct, *B4* is the transected left medial segmental bile duct, and *A2+3* is the left lateral segmental hepatic artery. MHV, middle hepatic vein.

into the anterior and posterior sectoral branches. Then the anterior sectoral branch and caudate lobe branches of the right hepatic artery are ligated and divided. Mobilization of the gallbladder provides a good operative view of the right posterior pedicle. The left portal vein is ligated and divided, followed by division of the right anterior branch of the right portal vein and caudate lobe branches arising from the main portal trunk and right portal vein. If cancer invasion of the portal bifurcation or the right portal vein is observed, combined portal vein resection and reconstruction is usually performed *after liver transection in the case of left-sided hepatectomies.* It can be done before liver transection in some cases, however. The caudate lobe and segments II and III are mobilized to the right, and the short retrohepatic caudate veins are ligated

and divided beginning on the left caudally and progressing cranially. When the confluence of the ligamentum venosum and the left hepatic vein or IVC is displayed, the ligament is ligated and divided. The left hepatic vein and middle hepatic vein are divided and closed with a running suture or a vascular stapler. The caudate lobe and the left lobe are completely detached from the IVC.

Subsequently, the liver is transected along a demarcation line in the right portal scissura between the right anterior and right posterior sectors. The course of the right hepatic vein is confirmed by ultrasound. After parenchymal transection, the right hepatic vein should be exposed on the raw surface of the liver. The plane of the liver transection courses between the right posterior superior segment (segment VII) and the right portion of caudate lobe and begins from the sulcus on the right side of the caudate process and advances cranially along the right margin of the IVC. Finally, the right wall of the IVC is clearly exposed (Fig. 80.82).

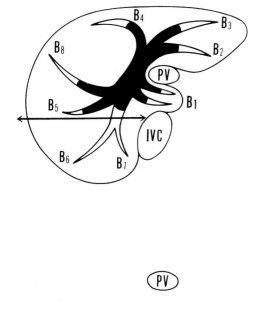

Fig. 80.81. Schematic representation of the tumor extent *(blackened space)* and resection carried out for extended left hepatectomy (left hepatic trisegmentectomy) with total caudate lobectomy. Numerals refer to the Couinaud's segments of the liver. PV, portal vein.

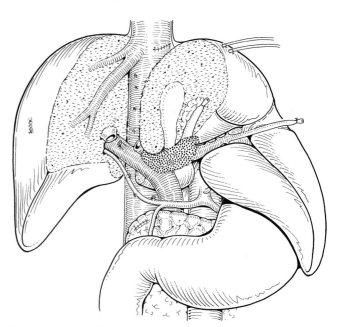

Fig. 80.82. Extended left hepatic resection, caudate lobectomy, and portal vein resection. The liver transection is between the plane of the right posterior superior segment and the right part of the caudate lobe and begins from the sulcus on the right side of the caudate process and advances cranially along the right margin of the IVC. Finally, the posterior segmental bile duct is divided, and the right wall of the IVC is clearly exposed.

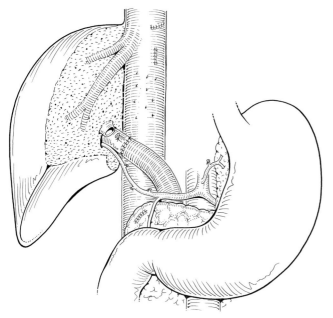

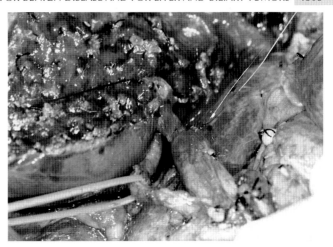

Fig. 80.84. Intraoperative photograph after the extended left hepatic resection (left trisegmentectomy) with total caudate lobectomy, extrahepatic bile duct resection, and portal vein resection and reconstruction. The vessel loop is around the right posterior sectoral artery. The transected bile duct is above the reconstructed portal vein.

Fig. 80.83. The extended left hepatic resection en bloc with entire caudate lobe, involved segment of the portal vein, and extrahepatic bile duct is complete. Portal vein reconstruction is possible without an interposition of an autogenous vein graft on rare occasions.

The right posterior sectoral bile duct is exposed cranially to the right portal vein and divided to obtain histologic free margins. Finally, vascular clamps are placed distally and proximally to the involved portal bifurcation. The distal clamp is placed obliquely to adjust the caliber of the distal portal vein to the transversely transected main portal trunk, and the specimen is resected en bloc, including the entire caudate lobe, the involved segment of the portal vein, and the extrahepatic bile duct (Figs. 80.83 and 80.84). The portal vein reconstruction between the main portal trunk and the right posterior sectoral portal branch is performed. An interposition graft of autogenous vein is often necessary (see Fig. 80.78).

Liver Resection in Living Related Donors

J. BELGHITI

The primary aim in performing living donor liver transplantation (LDLT) is to harvest a sufficient graft volume with complete inflow and outflow of blood and with minimal risk for the donor. Contrary to hepatic resectional techniques, liver bipartition in LDLT is distinguished by the fact that the remaining liver in the donor and the graft represent totally functional units in terms of inflow (portal and arterial blood supply), outflow (venous drainage), and bile duct arborization. The type of graft is selected with respect to two factors. First, graft volume is important in order to obtain 30% to 40% of the calculated standard liver volume of the recipient. Second, it is essential to obtain an autonomous graft with potential for provision of complete arterial, portal, and hepatic venous flow and with complete biliary drainage. LDLT was started in children at the end of 1980 and was rapidly accepted because the use of a left graft, which usually has single inflow and outflow vessels, can be performed with low donor risk. Adult LDLT was an important development at the beginning of the 21st century, but remains challenging, combining several volumetric and anatomic difficulties.

DONOR EVALUATION

After examination by physicians and interview by a clinical psychologist, the donor should have normal hematologic, biologic, and virology tests and the absence of an inherited procoagulation disorder (see Ch. 109). Morphologic assessment includes CT with vascular reconstruction, estimate of the volume of the liver segments, and display of the vascular anatomy. The graft choice is based on volumetric and vascular anatomy of the liver segments with an emphasis on the importance of the hepatic venous outflow. Biliary tree anatomy is preoperatively estimated by MRI cholangiography. Although anatomic abnormalities are often present, all are surmountable if the surgeon is fully cognizant of intrahepatic and extrahepatic anatomy and its variations. LDLT should be performed by well-trained liver surgeons who are accustomed to the use of intraoperative ultrasound. Contraindications for living donation are not clearly established, but donor safety leads many centers to eliminate donors with the characteristics listed in Table 80.6.

Table 80.6   Contraindications to Living Donation

Association of hepatic arterial, portal venous, and biliary abnormalities
Steatosis >20%
Donor remnant liver volume <30% of the whole liver volume
Body mass index >30
Donor age >60 yr

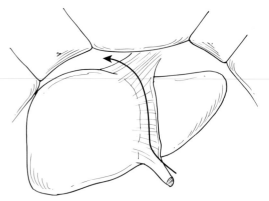

Fig. 80.85. Transection line of the falciform ligament. The falciform ligament is cut close to the diaphragm to allow fixation in the recipient.

CHOICE OF GRAFT

The graft volume obtained from healthy donors without steatosis should be more than 30% to 40% of the standard liver volume of the recipient (or >0.8% of the recipient's body weight) (Kiuchi et al, 1999). The left lateral graft (segments II and III) is sufficient for a pediatric recipient weighing 30 kg. Children weighing more than 30 kg and small adults weighing 50 kg can be transplanted with a left liver graft (segments I-IV) (Broelsch et al, 1991; Makuuchi et al, 1993b). In most cases, adults require a right graft (segments V-VIII) (Lo et al, 1997). Occasionally, posterior sectoral grafts (segments VI and VII) (Sugawara et al, 2002) or two left hemiliver grafts (including left lobectomy—segments II and III—or left hepatectomy—segments II-IV) (Lee et al, 2001) are used in adult LDLT. An increased graft volume (>1% of the recipient's body weight) is necessary, however, in the following situations:

1. The recipient is in poor general condition
2. There is severe liver failure
3. The graft has an incomplete venous outflow
4. A combination of these factors

Similarly, a reduced graft volume can be accepted (<0.8% of the body weight) if the recipient is in good general condition without liver insufficiency and the graft has complete and adequate venous drainage.

SURGICAL TECHNIQUE FOR LEFT LIVER HARVESTING: LEFT LOBECTOMY (SEGMENTS II AND III) AND LEFT HEPATECTOMY (SEGMENTS II, III, AND IV)

A similar initial procedure is used for left lobe harvesting (segments II and III), which is the most frequent graft used in pediatric transplantation, and left hepatectomy harvesting (segments II-IV) (Broelsch et al, 1991; Kawasaki et al, 1998; Makuuchi et al, 1993b; Tanaka & Inomata, 1997; Tanaka et al, 2003). Although the graft volume is small with good access to its pedicles, we nevertheless advocate a large incision for two reasons. First, in case of sudden bleeding, a good exposure allows rapid control of inflow and outflow vessels. Second, the manipulation of the graft should be minimized, avoiding parenchymal compression. Except in some donors with a narrow costal margin in whom a long epigastric midline incision is performed, a bilateral subcostal incision is usually used. After ligation and division of the round ligament, the falciform ligament is cut close to the diaphragm to allow sufficient tissue for subsequent fixation in the recipient (Fig. 80.85).

After examination and palpation of the liver, intraoperative ultrasound is performed with particular attention to the configuration of the junction of the middle hepatic vein and the left hepatic vein. After detaching the left triangular ligament, requiring in some cases ligation of the left phrenic vein, the anterior surface of the left hepatic vein and middle hepatic vein are dissected. After verifying the absence of an accessory or replaced left hepatic artery, the lesser omentum is incised close to the liver. When a single left artery originating from the left gastric artery is present, this artery is dissected sometimes up to the celiac trunk (Fig. 80.86). When an accessory left hepatic artery is present, this is usually clamped and ligated after checking by intraoperative Doppler ultrasound the presence of left arterial flow (Tanaka & Inomata, 1997).

The venous outflow can be easily controlled extraparenchymally. After rotation of the left lateral liver to the right, the Arantius ligament (ligamentum venosum) is encircled, ligated, and divided near the IVC to expose the left side of the IVC and the posterior surface of the common trunk of middle hepatic vein and left hepatic vein (Fig. 80.87). The common trunk of these two veins can be encircled by passing a clamp through the space between the right hepatic vein and the common trunk toward the left and in front of the IVC (Figs. 80.86 and 80.87).

In both harvesting procedures (left lobectomy and left hepatectomy), the dissection of the hepatic pedicle starts with the dissection of the cystic duct. Cholecystectomy with intraoperative cholangiography is systematically performed. After encircling the pedicle with a tape, the trunk of the hepatic artery is dissected from the lower part of the pedicle up to the bifurcation of the right hepatic artery.

Left Lobectomy

After the bifurcation of the hepatic artery, the left branch divides into middle hepatic artery and left hepatic artery. This left branch passes along the left side of the hepatoduodenal ligament. The middle hepatic artery is often a small branch to segment IV and usually is sacrificed to harvest a long hepatic artery with the graft. The left branch of the hepatic artery is encircled with a vessel loop. Then the portal vein can be displayed. The left portal vein is easily controlled and encircled just beyond the bifurcation of the portal vein (Fig. 80.88). The hilar plate containing the left main bile duct is exposed.

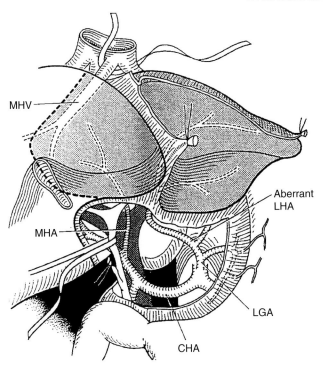

Fig. 80.86. The lesser omentum is incised close to the liver. The presence of a single left artery originating from the left gastric artery is illustrated (see text). CHA, common hepatic artery; LGA, left gastric artery; LHA, left hepatic artery; MHA, middle hepatic artery; MHV, middle hepatic vein.

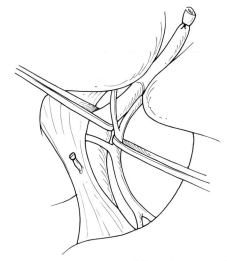

Fig. 80.88. The left hepatic artery and the left portal vein are encircled.

The identification of the left hepatic duct in the hilar plate may be difficult. It should be isolated and transected during dissection of the parenchyma after location of the resection line and with reference to cholangiography.

The parenchymal transection starts 1 cm to the right side of the falciform ligament (Fig. 80.89). The harvesting of this slice of segment IV is aimed at preserving the umbilical fissure vein (also called the scissural vein), which can drain a part of segment III. Although the parenchymal dissection generally is performed without vascular inflow control, there is no deleterious effect of

two or three 15-minute periods of intermittent clamping (Imamura et al, 2002). The liver is incised with a cautery knife, and the parenchyma is dissected with an ultrasonic dissector, whereas small vessels on the cut surface are coagulated on both sides with a bipolar cautery; larger vessels are clipped or sutured. During the parenchymal transection, all vessels of segment IV are ligated, including the biliary duct of this segment. The sacrifice of segment IV pedicle results in partial postoperative ischemia with a high level of transaminase and atrophy of segment IV. Although patients can experience some "unexplained" postoperative fever during the first 3 postoperative days, this procedure had no deleterious outcome for the donor. When the parenchymal transection reaches the hepatic hilar plate, the anterior surface of left hilar plate is encountered and dissected (Fig. 80.90). The left hepatic duct is cut, and the stump of the main duct is closed with 5-0 PDS suture, while the left hepatic duct is left open. Should the orifice of the hepatic duct arising from segment I or IV appear on the transection line, it is simply closed by suture.

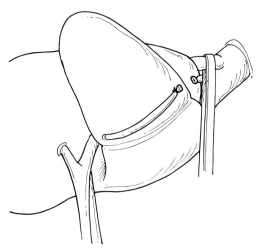

Fig. 80.87. The common trunk of the middle hepatic vein (MHV) and left hepatic vein (LHV) can be encircled by passing a clamp in the space between the right hepatic vein and the trunk of the MHV and the LHV toward the left and in front of the IVC (see also Fig. 80.41).

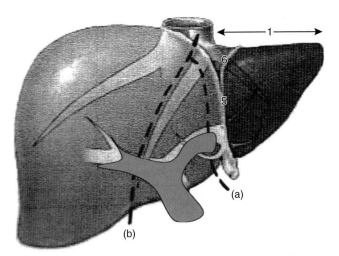

Fig. 80.89. The parenchymal transection lines for left liver harvest vary from 1 cm on the right side of the falciform ligament *(a)* to the right side of the middle hepatic vein *(b)*. *a*, transection line for harvesting of segments II and III; *b*, transection line for harvesting of segments II, III, and IV. 1 indicates the left lateral segment (segments II and III) and 5 and 6 indicate the falciform ligament.

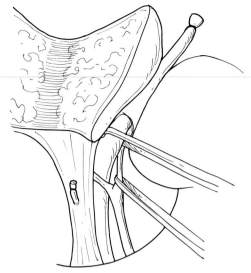

Fig. 80.90. When the parenchymal transection meets the hepatic hilar plate, the anterior surface of the left hilar plate is encountered and exposed.

The posterior part of the parenchymal dissection can be facilitated by a hanging maneuver (see earlier) using a large clamp inserted behind the left pedicle in front of the caudate lobe toward the common trunk of the left hepatic vein and middle hepatic vein (Fig. 80.91) (Belghiti et al, 2001). When the parenchymal dissection reaches the tissue around the hepatic veins, the level of transection should be examined carefully with respect to the venous anatomy. Although the left hepatic vein is usually the only vessel of the left lateral segment, some variations should be taken into account. These variations, which are easily identified preoperatively on CT scan, require intraoperative assessment with intraoperative ultrasound. Such variations include drainage of the umbilical vein into the left hepatic vein and the presence of an independent drainage vein from segment III into the middle hepatic vein.

The graft removal starts with the clamping and division of the left hepatic artery and left branch of the portal vein. Another clamp is placed on the left hepatic vein. After transection of the left hepatic vein, the graft is placed immediately on the back table. After removing the graft, the surgeon responsible for the harvesting should concentrate on the donor operation without thinking further about the graft. The stump of the hepatic vein is closed with a running 4-0 polypropylene suture, and the portal stump is closed with a running 5-0 suture. The hepatic artery stump is ligated. After confirming the absence of biliary leak with blue dye injection through the cystic duct drain, this drain is removed, and the cystic duct is closed with a 4-0 PDS suture. The abdomen can be closed without drain.

Left Hepatectomy

The left liver (segments II-IV) is a functional liver unit with one portal vein, usually one main artery, and an autonomous venous drainage ensured by left hepatic vein and middle hepatic vein through their common trunk. The pedicular dissection is performed similarly to left lobectomy. After identification of the bifurcation between the right hepatic artery and left hepatic artery, the trunk of the left hepatic artery should be encircled with the middle hepatic artery, which vascularizes segment IV. The left portal vein is encircled just beyond the bifurcation of the portal vein.

The section line of the parenchymal transection is identified by the discoloration of the left liver after a temporary and short clamping of left arterial and portal vessels. The parenchymal transection starts in the middle of the gallbladder bed following Cantlie's line on the right side of the middle hepatic vein. During the parenchymal transection, all veins from segments V and VIII are ligated. When the parenchymal transection reaches the hepatic hilar plate, the anterior surface of the left hilar plate is encountered and dissected. The hilar plate containing the left main bile duct is exposed. To preserve the posterior right biliary duct, the transection of the left bile duct should not be performed

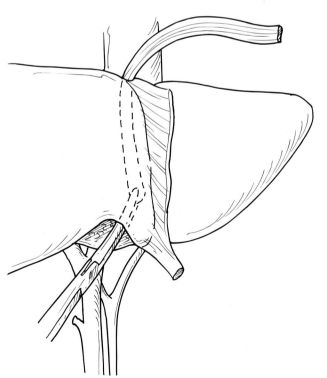

Fig. 80.91. The posterior part of the parenchymal transection can be facilitated by a hanging maneuver. A large clamp is inserted in front of the caudate lobe toward the common trunk of the left hepatic vein and middle hepatic vein.

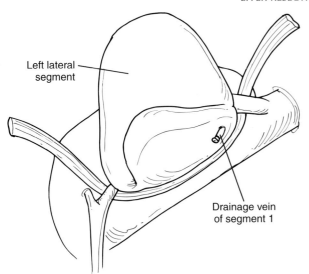

Fig. 80.92. After detaching the left side of the caudate lobe from the IVC, the posterior parenchymal transection is facilitated by a hanging maneuver using a tape in front of the IVC.

without reference to the operative cholangiography. The left hepatic duct is cut, and the stump of the main duct is closed. Similarly, the posterior part of the parenchymal dissection can be facilitated by a hanging maneuver using a tape inserted behind the common trunk of the left hepatic vein and middle hepatic vein in front of the caudate lobe. When the parenchymal dissection reaches the right side of the common trunk of the left hepatic vein and middle hepatic vein, this trunk should be exposed and dissected up to the vena cava.

Because the left liver is not usually large enough to avoid small-for-size syndrome in the recipients, Miyagawa and colleagues (1998) reported the safe use of the left liver including segment I when the liver volume represented more than one third of the standard volume of the recipient's liver. The technique consists of a left hemihepatectomy including the middle hepatic vein and the caudate lobe. After detaching the caudate lobe from the IVC, the posterior parenchymal transection is facilitated by a hanging maneuver using a tape in front of the IVC (Fig. 80.92). Among all veins from the caudate lobe, the largest one should be preserved. The technique of graft removal is similar to left lobectomy.

TECHNIQUE FOR RIGHT LOBE GRAFTS

The donor procedure consists of a right hepatectomy (segments V-VIII) (Lo et al, 1997; Tanaka et al, 2003). Right hepatectomy should provide a graft not only with adequate portal and arterial inflow, but also with complete hepatic venous outflow. In more than two thirds of cases, the anterior sector of the right liver (segments V and VIII) is drained mainly through the middle hepatic vein. To avoid venous congestion, which impairs early graft function, several reports have proposed that there should be venous reconstruction to segments V and VIII veins using jump grafts or harvesting of the middle hepatic vein in the donor. The harvesting of the middle hepatic vein is considered technically demanding, and it could have some detrimental effect on the venous drainage of segment IV in donor. We describe in this chapter a right hepatectomy without and with middle hepatic vein harvesting.

A bilateral subcostal incision is usually used. After ligation and dissection of the round ligament, the falciform ligament is cut close to the diaphragm to facilitate fixation of the left remnant liver in its anatomic position after right hepatectomy (see Fig. 80.84). Intraoperative ultrasound examination identifies major vascular structures, especially the right and middle hepatic veins, and all major portal branches.

After opening the anterior leaf of the coronary ligament and the anterior part of the right triangular ligament, the suprahepatic IVC is exposed. The space located between the right hepatic vein and middle hepatic vein is dissected. Then the right liver is retracted toward the left to mobilize the right liver to expose the right side of the IVC (see Figs. 80.14 and 80.15). The dissection of the hepatic veins requires full exposure of the IVC. Dissection of the IVC starts from the caudate process passing upward toward the right hepatic vein. The inferior right hepatic vein, which is frequently present, can be ligated if its diameter is less than 5 mm. Otherwise, it should be encircled and preserved. Before reaching the right hepatic vein level, the IVC ligament is transected from caudal to cranial as described previously for right hepatectomy (see Fig. 80.15). After insertion of a clamp between the ligament and the IVC, this ligament is clamped and transected. This ligament, which contains small veins, should be closed with a running suture. It also may be divided using a stapling device (see Fig. 80.15). The right hepatic vein is easily encircled by a clamp passing on the anterior surface of the IVC toward the space between right hepatic vein and middle hepatic vein as described for right hepatectomy (see earlier). To facilitate the subsequent parenchymal dissection, a tape is inserted behind the right hepatic vein and passed along the anterior surface of the IVC (Fig. 80.93). Then the right liver is released to lie in its anatomic position. The hanging maneuver allows easy mobilization of the right liver and minimizes the parenchymal injury induced by the compression of left and right livers. Using this maneuver, the dissection of the right hepatic vein is performed later via an anterior approach

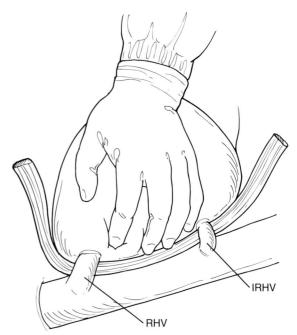

Fig. 80.93. After mobilization of the right liver, a tape is passed on the anterior surface of the IVC, as described in the text. This tape passes behind the right hepatic vein (RHV) and the inferior right hepatic vein (IRHV).

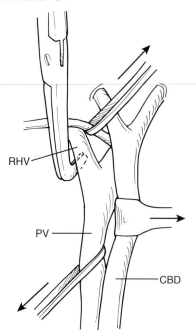

Fig. 80.94. After exposing and encircling the portal trunk, the dissection of the anterior surface of the portal bifurcation is facilitated by pulling down the portal loop as indicated by the *arrow*. The other *arrows* indicate the direction of traction to expose the portal bifurcation. CBD, common bile duct; PV, portal vein; RHA, right hepatic artery.

and after the anterior part of the IVC is completely exposed by the parenchymal transection.

The hilar dissection starts with a cholecystectomy and the cannulation of the cystic duct. Biliary tree opacification by intraoperative cholangiography can be performed at this stage to check the "real" anatomy, to evaluate the length of the right bile duct, and to localize the future transection plane with the placement of a clip or a small clamp on the right bile duct. The bile duct is

not dissected to avoid biliary injury and devascularization. The right hepatic artery is identified behind the common bile duct and dissected toward the bifurcation of the anterior and posterior sectoral branches. The arterial bifurcation is dissected to the right of the bile duct and identified to allow harvest of the maximal length of right hepatic artery. A vessel loop is passed about the right hepatic artery. Although the right portal vein is easily identified after preparation of the right hepatic artery, its complete dissection may be difficult when this artery is preserved. After exposing and encircling the portal trunk, the anterior surface of the portal bifurcation is dissected while the assistant pulls down the portal loop on the main trunk. This maneuver facilitates the exposure of the portal bifurcation (Fig. 80.94).

Care must be taken concerning a small portal vein branch to the right side of the caudate lobe, which should be ligated and transected. If the anterior and the posterior sectoral branches of the right portal vein arise independently, they should be encircled separately. The presence of an intact contralateral arterial and portal flow is checked using Doppler control during temporary occlusion of right hilar vessels. The proximal area of the right bile duct is not dissected at this step. The advantages of the hanging maneuver in the harvesting procedure include a facilitation of the transection plane following the proper plane along the right or the left side of the middle hepatic vein (depending on whether or not the middle hepatic vein is harvested).

After opening the anterior leaf of the coronary ligament and the anterior part of the right triangular ligament, the suprahepatic IVC is exposed. The space between the right and the middle hepatic vein is dissected 3 cm in the caudal direction using a vascular clamp (Fig. 80.95). This blind dissection of the anterior part of the suprahepatic IVC prepares the upper part of the hanging maneuver. The lower part of this maneuver includes a dissection of the IVC above the origin of the right renal vein. After elevating the caudal edge of the caudate lobe, one or two short caudate vessels are ligated (Fig. 80.96A). The middle plane of the IVC is dissected toward the space between the right hepatic vein and the middle hepatic vein using scissors for 4 or 5 cm and then

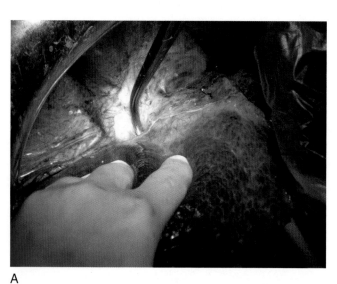

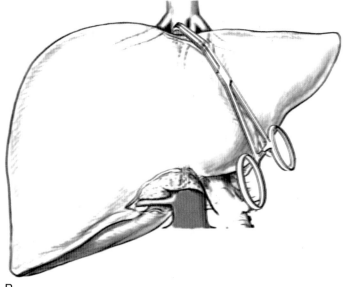

A   B

Fig. 80.95. A and **B,** The space located between the right and middle hepatic vein trunk is dissected 3 cm in a caudal direction using a vascular clamp. This prepares the upper part of the hanging maneuver (see text).

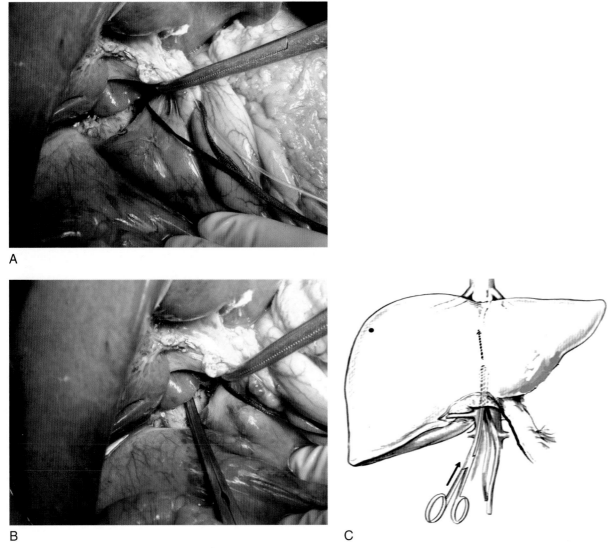

A

B   C

Fig. 80.96. A, After elevating the edge of the caudate process, one or two short caudate veins are ligated. **B** and **C,** The retrohepatic space along the middle plane of the IVC is dissected aiming toward the space between the right and the middle hepatic veins using scissors for 4 or 5 cm and then pursuing the dissection with a long, curved aortic clamp.

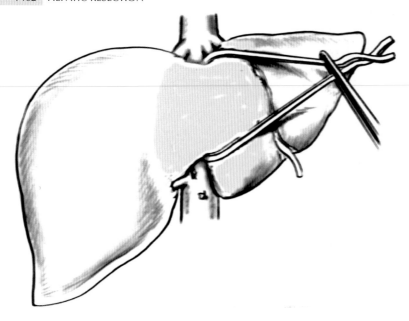

Fig. 80.97. A tape is seized with the protruding clamp and drawn down between the anterior surface of the IVC and the posterior surface of the liver parenchyma.

a long curved aortic clamp. This clamp is passed through the "avascular plane" located just along the anterior surface of the IVC (Fig. 80.96B). When the clamp is passed in the space previously dissected between right hepatic vein and middle hepatic vein (Fig. 80.97), a tape is seized with the clamp and passed between the anterior surface of the IVC and the posterior surface of the liver parenchyma. Using a slight traction on the lower part of the tape, the thin hepatic parenchyma on the lower edge of the caudate lobe is exposed and divided toward the posterior surface of the hilar plate (Fig. 80.98).

The section line of the parenchymal transection is identified by the discoloration of the right liver after a temporary and short clamping of both the right arterial and portal vessels. The proper plane of transection is facilitated by pulling the upper part of the tape from the right side of the middle hepatic vein from the top

of the dome of the liver toward the gallbladder bed. The resection line on the inferior surface of the liver is marked by connecting the lower end of the anterior surface line to the level of the right bile duct. Parenchymal transection, which can be performed with or without intermittent pedicle clamping, starts at the lower part of the liver in the gallbladder bed progressing toward the right pedicle. The ultrasonic dissector allows precise dissection. Vessels smaller than 3 mm diameter are coagulated using irrigated bipolar forceps. Vessels larger than 3 mm are ligated on both sides using sutures or clips.

After ligation of some veins in the gallbladder bed, the first important vessel encountered is the drainage vein of segment V, which should be isolated and clamped on the graft side if the diameter is greater than 5 mm. The stump of this vein on the left side is ligated. Division of the parenchyma at this level allows the

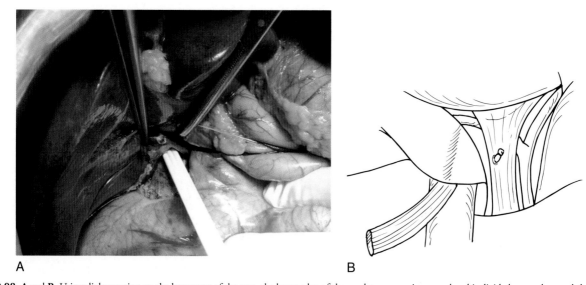

A   B

Fig. 80.98. A and **B,** Using slight traction on the lower part of the tape, the lower edge of the caudate process is exposed and is divided upward toward the posterior surface of the hilar plate.

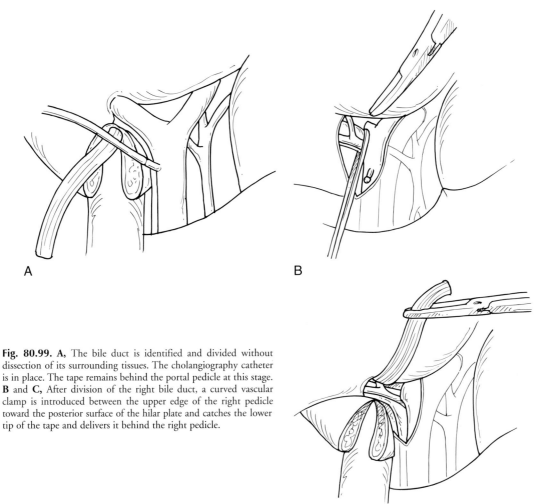

Fig. 80.99. A, The bile duct is identified and divided without dissection of its surrounding tissues. The cholangiography catheter is in place. The tape remains behind the portal pedicle at this stage. **B** and **C,** After division of the right bile duct, a curved vascular clamp is introduced between the upper edge of the right pedicle toward the posterior surface of the hilar plate and catches the lower tip of the tape and delivers it behind the right pedicle.

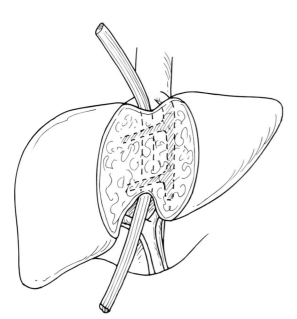

Fig. 80.100. Right graft harvest without the middle hepatic vein. The drainage veins of segments V and VIII are isolated, clamped, and preserved on the graft side if the diameter is greater than 5 mm.

exposure of the anterior plane of the right bile duct. The bile duct is divided, without full dissection of its surrounding tissue and only after checking the cholangiogram (Fig. 80.99A and B). After division of the right bile duct, a curved vascular clamp is introduced between the upper edge of the right pedicle and passed toward the posterior surface of the hilar plate and catching the lower tip of the tape, which is then pulled behind the pedicle (see Fig. 80.99C). The liver parenchymal transection on the right side of the middle hepatic vein is facilitated by the traction on the tape, which preserves the trunk of the middle hepatic vein. The tape elevates the liver and provides excellent exposure of the remaining parenchyma.

When two thirds of the parenchymal dissection has been conducted, the vein of segment VIII is isolated and clamped on the graft side if the diameter is greater than 5 mm. Alternatively, the tape can be passed behind the vein of segment VIII after division of the cranial part of the caudate lobe (Fig. 80.100). The anterior part of the IVC is completely exposed, and the graft is almost completely separated leaving the right lobe attached by the right hepatic artery, the right portal vein, and the right hepatic vein and the inferior hepatic veins in some cases. After dissection of the right part of the IVC, preserving an inferior right hepatic vein if the diameter is greater than 5 mm, the right hepatic vein is encircled and taped (Fig. 80.101).

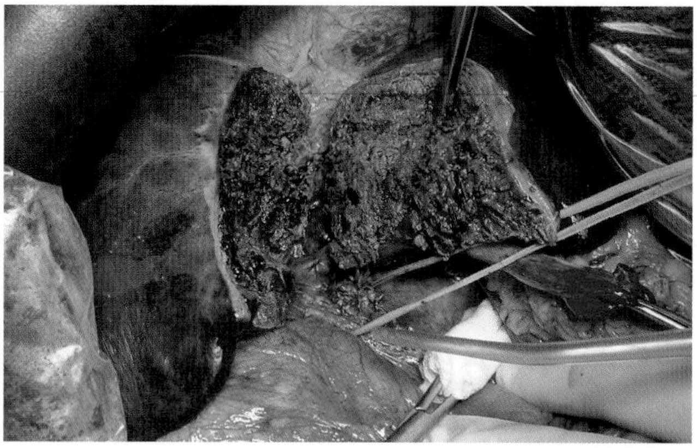

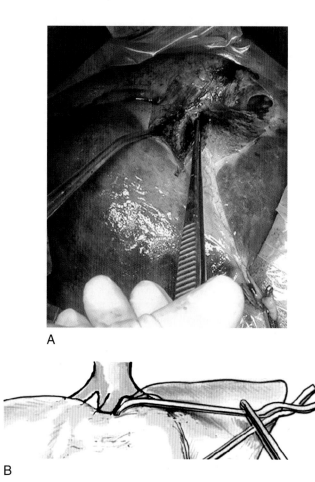

Fig. 80.101. A and **B,** The anterior part of the IVC is completely exposed, and the graft is completely separated leaving the right lobe attached by the right hepatic artery, the right portal vein, the right hepatic vein, and the anterior right hepatic vein.

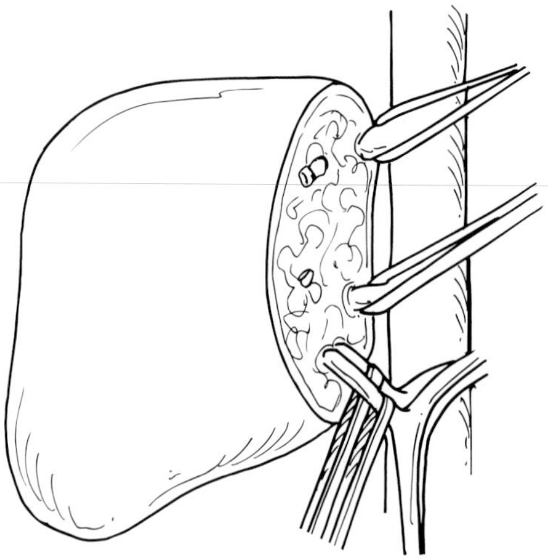

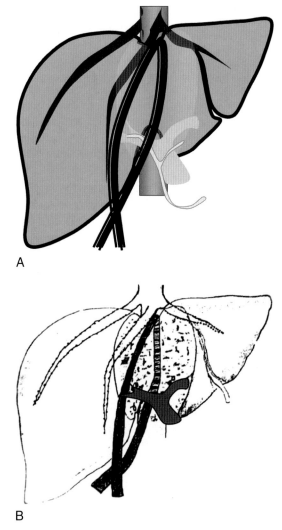

Fig. 80.102. A and **B,** In cases in which it is decided to harvest the middle hepatic vein (MHV), the parenchyma is dissected for 2 cm downward exposing the left hepatic vein (LHV) and the MHV junction. The space between these two veins is dissected and opened, and a clamp is passed behind the MHV. The tape is drawn between the MHV and the LHV.

Fig. 80.103. A and **B,** Right vein graft with harvesting of the middle hepatic vein (MHV). The deeper plane of the parenchymal dissection is determined by the tape pulled from its upper part on the left side of the MHV toward the gallbladder bed.

Graft removal starts with the clamping and division of the right hepatic artery. The right branch of the portal vein is clamped with a vascular clamp placed a few millimeters distal to the bifurcation so as not to compromise the left portal flow. Another portal clamp is placed on the graft side. If there is a significant inferior right hepatic vein, it too is clamped, the clamp being placed on the IVC to allow a cuff for subsequent suture in the recipient. The right hepatic vein is clamped with a large vascular clamp, and the vein is transected. The graft is placed immediately on the back table. After removing the graft, the surgeon responsible for the harvesting should concentrate on the donor operation without thinking further about the graft. The stump of the hepatic vein is closed with a running 4-0 polypropylene suture, and the portal stump is closed vertically with a running 5-0 suture to prevent an angulation of the left portal vein. The hepatic artery stump is ligated, and the biliary stump is closed using a continuous 6-0 PDS suture. After confirming the absence of biliary leak with blue dye injected through the cystic duct drain, this drain is removed, and the cystic duct is closed with a 4-0 PDS suture. The remnant liver is fixed in its anatomic position to ensure an efficient outflow (Ogata et al, 2005). The abdomen is closed after placing a drain in the right subphrenic space.

It may be necessary to harvest the middle hepatic vein. The aim of harvesting the right liver with the middle hepatic vein is not to increase the volume of the graft, but to prevent the congestion of the anterior sector of the transplantation. The hanging maneuver is adapted to define the transection plane along the left side of the middle hepatic vein (Belghiti et al, 2001; Kokudo et al, 2003). After passing the tape on the right side of the middle hepatic vein, parenchymal transection is carried out from the upper part of the liver in front of the median hepatic venous trunk. The parenchyma is dissected for 2 cm toward the left hepatic vein and middle hepatic vein junction. The space between these two veins is dissected, and the clamp is passed behind the middle hepatic vein (Fig. 80.102). The tape is seized and switched from the right to the left side of the middle hepatic vein. The surface plane of transection also is determined by the discoloration line after a transitory clamping of the inflow pedicle as described earlier. The deeper plane is determined by the tape pulled from its upper part on the left side of the middle hepatic vein toward the gallbladder bed (Fig. 80.103). The parenchymal transection procedure is similar to that described earlier, but follows the left side of the middle hepatic vein. Some veins of segment IV are encountered, and they are ligated on both sides.

Computer-Assisted Operation Planning and Virtual Liver Resection

H. LANG, H.-O. PEITGEN, AND C. E. BROELSCH

Computer-aided diagnosis and intervention planning is one of the most exciting and promising developments in surgery, but it has yet to gain widespread use in liver surgery (Marescaux et al, 1998; Rau et al, 2000; Wigmore et al, 2001). Currently, patient selection and preoperative planning for liver resection are based mainly on the knowledge of a schematic model of the vascular anatomy of the liver, as first described by Couinaud in 1954, and on two-dimensional imaging by CT (see Ch. 18) and, to a lesser extent, MRI (see Ch. 19) (Bismuth, 1982; Blumgart & Hann, 2000; Couinaud, 1957; Strasberg et al, 2000). Data provided by these imaging modalities allow the identification of the number, the extent, and the localization of intrahepatic tumors and a calculation of liver volume. In most circumstances, this information is sufficient for operative planning purposes.

In recent years, the use of more specialized image processing techniques has played a greater role, in particular, in extended liver resections in which a small liver remnant may be insufficient for postoperative liver function and recovery. Because the reasons for liver failure after hepatic resection are multifactorial and may vary from case to case, the minimum amount of remaining liver tissue to preserve liver function is hard to predict (Melendez et al, 2001; Povoski et al, 1999; Yigitler et al, 2003). Studies have shown that in noncirrhotic livers, postoperative morbidity correlates well with the number of segments resected (Jarnagin et al, 2002), and a functional liver volume of only 20% to 25% of total liver volume is assumed to be the critical size of the remnant (Vauthey et al, 2000). Extended liver resection

may be challenging because of the complex anatomic hepatic structure with three different vascular systems and one excretory ductal system supplying or draining the liver: the portal vein, hepatic artery, hepatic veins, and biliary ducts. A successful operation requires enough remaining liver tissue supplied or drained by all three vascular trees and by an unimpaired excretory system (Abdalla et al, 2004; Blumgart et al, 2000).

Although current imaging modalities and basic image processing techniques provide excellent visualization of the intrahepatic structures, the extent and exact localization of their dependent vascular or biliary territories cannot be determined definitely by use of these techniques (Fasel et al, 1998). More importantly, the widespread application of Couinaud's model is questionable because the postulated segmentation is based on a regular portal venous and hepatic venous distribution that (as shown in a variety of anatomic studies) does not exist uniformly, but includes several variations (Fischer et al, 2002; Lamadé et al, 2000; Platzer & Maurer, 1966; Soyer et al, 1995). The number and size of independent portal segments and hepatic venous territories and their distribution on the liver surface show great variation. This variation makes intraoperative identification of hepatic segmentation almost impossible because there are few markings on the liver surface. Based only on the information given by two-dimensional slices of CT or MRI, it is difficult for the surgeon to reconstruct mentally the three-dimensional vascular anatomy of the liver and to estimate which part of the liver would be devascularized during surgery. This is particularly true in tumor resections, in which complete tumor removal together with an adequate safety margin may require the dissection of major intrahepatic vascular or biliary structures. Although the volume of the future liver remnant can be determined by current imaging techniques, operative planning may be imprecise with regard to the calculation of the remaining vascularized liver parenchyma. The use of pedicular control during operation does allow better definition of portal territories, however.

More recent developments in image-based computer assistance allow improved visualization of the distribution of the intrahepatic vascular branches and a better prediction of their dependent parenchymal territories. A reliable preoperative assessment of the number and individual extent of portal venous territories and their relation to hepatic veins is now possible (Van Ooijen et al, 2003; Zahlten et al, 1995). In addition, the results of vascular analysis and liver segmentation can be combined to calculate the individual volume of any vascular system and of any parenchymal territory (Fig. 80-104) (Schenk et al, 2000; Selle et al, 2002). Using the three-dimensional model, it is possible to perform virtual liver resections under realistic anatomic conditions and to

take into account the individual vascular and segmental structure of the liver and the localization and extent of the tumors. The software tools (MeVis LiverAnalyzer and MeVis LiverExplorer) are able to provide fully automatic resection models with different safety margins and the option to define virtual resection manually (Figs. 80-105 and 80-106) (Bourquain et al, 2002; Preim et al, 2002). The influence of various resection planes on blood supply and hepatic venous drainage within the remaining liver parenchyma can be calculated by computer-assisted risk analysis (Fig. 80-107). Because these techniques are based on standard two-dimensional CT scans, they cannot provide any additional information with regard to the number and the size of detected liver lesions.

Initial reports evaluating the influence of an individual three-dimensional hepatic model and further use of computer assistance on operative planning of liver resections compared with standard imaging techniques, such as two-dimensional CT, show promising results (Lang et al, 2005a). The most important finding of this investigation was that, in many partial hepatectomies, operative planning based on two-dimensional CT resulted in an amount of potentially devascularized liver tissue of 20% to 40% of the future liver remnant; this is mainly due to venous congestion, rather than to impaired portal venous perfusion. Based on these volumetric results, intrahepatic venous reconstructions were performed to avoid large areas of liver tissue without venous drainage (Fig. 80-108). These data are interesting because, so far, the decision for reconstruction of hepatic veins in partial hepatectomy was based mainly on two-dimensional imaging and on the knowledge of the typical distribution pattern of hepatic veins, but without a precise visualization and volumetric calculation (Hemming et al, 2002; Kaneoka et al, 2000; Ozeki et al, 1995; Yamamoto et al, 2001). Now, with progress in computer assistance, it is possible to consider the need for intrahepatic vascular reconstruction depending on the results of a reliable preoperative calculation of the volume of venously congested or potentially devascularized liver tissue for each dissected vessel (Lang et al, 2004). This is clinically relevant, especially because ischemic areas may not always be identified intraoperatively. Signs of compromised venous drainage or impaired blood supply sometimes develop over time and need not be present during operation.

As is the case with most developments, computer-assisted risk analysis introduces new questions. To date, there is no conclusive evidence that reconstruction of hepatic veins to avoid partial congestion is mandatory for hepatic functional recovery. The need for a sufficient portal venous blood supply or hepatic venous drainage to the entire remnant liver is self-evident, but it is unknown if impairment of either one of these vascular systems has an impact on the hepatic function of the involved area. The development of collateral flow and the capacity of the liver to compensate for impaired portal venous flow by the hepatic artery (or vice versa) play important roles and must be taken into account. Currently, there is little precise knowledge of these pathways. The importance of an optimal hepatic venous outflow for sufficient postoperative hepatic function may be anticipated best by the experience with segmental liver transplantation, in particular with LDLT of the right lobe (Lo et al, 2003; Malagó et al, 2005). Although hepatic circulation after segmental liver transplantation and partial hepatectomy is difficult to compare (because of different pathophysiologic pathways, such as cold or warm ischemic time, hemodynamic changes in the splanchnic system in patients with liver cirrhosis, or total denervation of transplants), it is likely that, after liver resection, impairment of

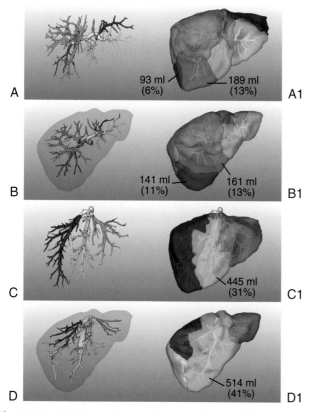

Fig. 80.104. Calculation of individual vascular liver territories based on preoperative CT data. **A/A1** and **B/B1,** Analysis of two different portal venous systems (**A** and **B**) and visualization of the corresponding vascular territories (**A1** and **B1**). The extent of the different segments on the liver surface varies considerably between the two visualized livers. Main branches of supply are classified according to Couinaud: P I, P II, P III, P IVa, P IVb, P V, P VI, P VII, and P VIII. **C/C1** and **D/D1,** Analysis of two hepatic venous systems (**C** and **D**) and visualization of the corresponding venous territories (**C1** and **D1**). **D/D1** shows a liver with a small right hepatic vein *(red)*, a large inferior right hepatic vein *(yellow)*, and a dominant middle hepatic vein *(light blue)*. The latter two are draining large parts of the inferior right lobe. Also shown are left hepatic vein *(light brown)*, segment I veins *(magenta)*, and a small additional inferior right vein *(green)*. The corresponding volumes of the vascular territories are calculated. The absolute volumes and the relative volumes for the two portal venous territories (P V and P VI) and for the middle hepatic venous territories are shown.

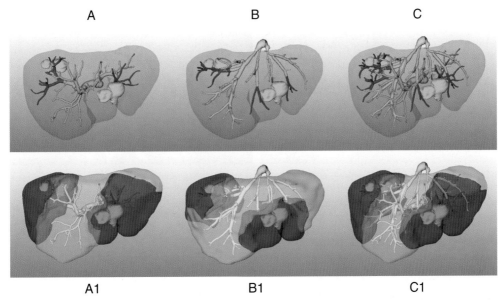

Fig. 80.105. Vascular risk analyses for four tumors in the right and left liver lobes, calculated for a safety margin of 1 cm. **A-C,** The risk analysis for the portal venous system (**A**), for the hepatic venous system (**B**), and combined for both vascular systems (**C**). The branches affected by a resection with a 1-cm safety margin are labeled *red*. Colorization indicates the branches of the corresponding vessel that would be separated from the main vascular system. **A1-C1,** The vascular territories at risk, supplied or drained by the labeled vessels above, for the portal venous system (**A1**), hepatic venous system (**B1**), and both systems combined (**C1**).

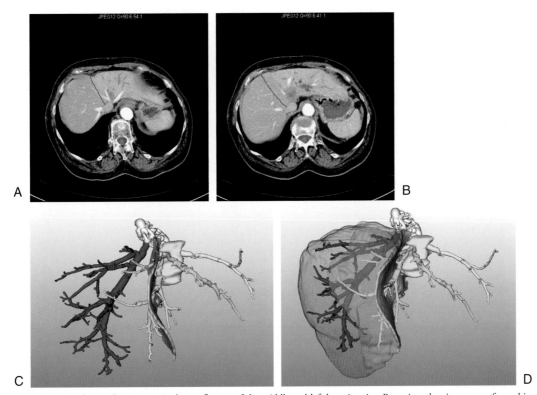

Fig. 80.106. A and **B,** CT scan shows a liver tumor in the confluence of the middle and left hepatic veins. Resection planning was performed in two-dimensional CT by drawing lines of dissection manually within several axial CT slices. The operation planned is a left hepatectomy including caudate lobectomy (segments I-IV). **C,** Transfer of the resection plane as defined in two-dimensional CT into the three-dimensional reconstructed hepatic venous system showing that large sub-branches of the middle hepatic vein running out of the right lobe would be dissected.

Continued

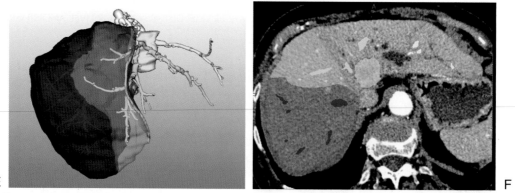

Fig. 80.106, cont'd. **D** and **E,** Visualization of the volume at risk for impaired hepatic venous outflow *(blue)*. This territory accounts for 23% of the entire remaining tissue. The territory of the remnant having a preserved venous drainage via the right hepatic vein is colored *red*. **F,** Two-dimensional CT shows the area at risk for impaired venous outflow *(blue)*, as identified in computer-assisted risk analysis.

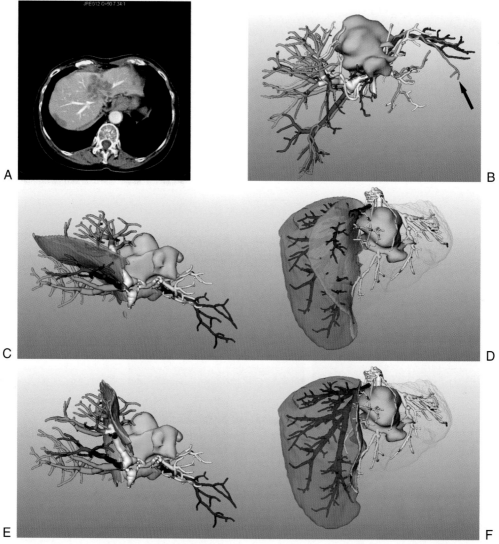

Fig. 80.107. **A,** CT scan with a liver tumor infiltrating all three major hepatic veins. Resection of the tumor has to include the dissection and reconstruction of the right hepatic vein. **B,** Three-dimensional reconstruction of hepatic artery and portal vein shows that the tumor involves segment VIII *(brown)*, but does not infiltrate the main anterolateral pedicle of the portal vein. There is an accessory left hepatic artery *(pink)*. In the right liver lobe, the hepatic artery parallels the portal vein, indicating that both structures may be considered together when planning the operation. **C** and **D,** Virtual left trisectionectomy. The resection plane is between the anterolateral and the posterolateral portal venous territories, preserving only segments VI *(blue)* and VII *(green)*. Transfer of the resection plane into the venous system **(D)** shows that the entire remnant *(red)* is drained via the right hepatic vein. The calculated volume is 403 mL. **E** and **F,** Virtual left hepatectomy (segments I-IV) plus partial resection of segments V and VIII. The resection plane runs through segments V and VIII, but does not impair the main anterolateral pedicle of the portal vein. Transfer of the resection plane into the venous system **(F)**. The volume of the remnant is 680 mL. With the exception of a very small territory (see tiny *blue* branch of the middle hepatic vein), the entire remnant is drained via the right hepatic vein *(red)*. The reconstruction clearly shows that the right hepatic vein has to be dissected at the junction of the two main branches shortly before reaching the IVC. *Comment:* The tumor was resected according to the proposed transsegmental approach (see Fig. 80-108), achieving tumor-free margins. The right hepatic vein was dissected and reconstructed.

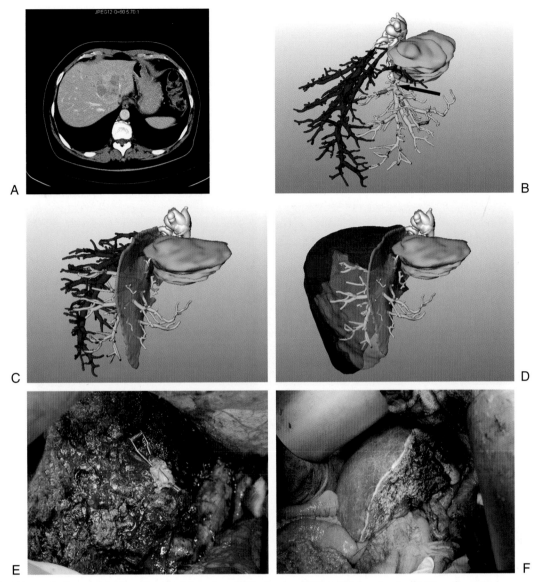

Fig. 80.108. A, CT scan of a liver tumor with a diameter of about 8 cm infiltrating the middle and left hepatic veins. **B,** Three-dimensional reconstruction of hepatic veins shows that the middle hepatic vein *(arrow)* is draining large parts of the right liver lobe. **C** and **D,** Virtual resection in the three-dimensional reconstructed hepatic venous system **(C)** includes the dissection of the middle hepatic vein at the position marked with an *arrow* in **B. D** shows the remnant liver with the territory at risk *(blue)* for impaired venous outflow. The total volume of the remnant is 890 mL. The amount of remaining tissue with impaired venous drainage is 368 mL, accounting for 41% of the entire remnant. **E,** Operative situs after left hepatectomy and resection of the superior part of the middle hepatic vein. The trunk of the dissected vein is temporarily clamped. **F,** Situs after reconstruction of the middle hepatic vein to the IVC by interpositioning of a venous allograft. The remaining liver tissue, in particular the inferior part, is homogeneous without signs of venous congestion.

liver function also could be caused by an insufficient hepatic venous outflow. Besides functional considerations, areas with venous congestion or compromised vascular blood supply are at risk for necrosis and are a potential source for infectious complications. Regardless of the fact that there is always a certain amount of necrosis at the cut surface, large ischemic areas of parenchyma should be avoided by resection of these areas or by reconstruction of the corresponding vessels. As already stated, intraoperative identification of potentially devascularized tissue may be difficult because decolorization may not develop immediately. The preoperative knowledge of potentially affected areas may be of particular help for operative planning (Lang et al, 2004).

The resections most likely to be at risk for large amounts of devascularized tissue are extended left hepatectomies, central hepatectomies, or left hepatectomies combined with additional partial resection of the right lobe (Lang et al, 2005a), clinical circumstances in which operative results always have been associated with the highest complication rate (Nishio et al, 2005; Povoski et al, 1999). This is not a surprising finding, mainly because of the difficulty in visualizing segmental boundaries owing to the absence of liver surface markers and the often unpredictable intrahepatic vascular structure of the right lobe. In particular, the distribution of the right and middle hepatic veins shows a great variability and often differs significantly from the regular hepatic venous anatomy as postulated by Couinaud

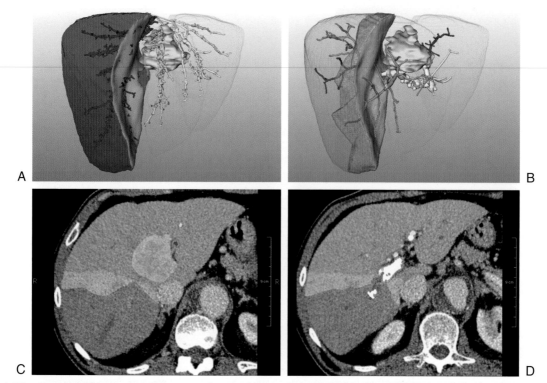

Fig. 80.109. A, Virtual extended left hepatectomy for resection of a tumor located in the confluence of the left and middle hepatic veins. The resection line is guided along the right hepatic vein. The remnant *(red)* has a volume of 702 mL, accounting for 38% of the total liver volume. **B,** Vascular risk analysis of the remnant with respect to the portal vein. The territory colored *brown* has been supplied by the dissected segment V *(light red)* and segment VIII branches *(brown)* and is exposed to devascularization after resection. This territory has a volume of 141 mL, equal to 20% of the remaining tissue. The remaining volume without vascular impairment is 561 mL, accounting for 30% of total liver volume only. **C** and **D,** A transfer of the resection line as defined in **A,** showing the posterior venous sector in two-dimensional CT. The area colored *dark red* belongs to the portal venous segments VI and VII; the *brown* area is the tissue at risk for devascularization as it is supplied by the portal venous branches of segments V and VIII.

(Radtke et al, 2005). These variations can be visualized and quantitatively calculated by computer-assisted planning. This technique seems to be useful for the preoperative assessment of postresectional functional reserve in extended hepatectomies that are at risk for the development of large ischemic areas. This assumption is endorsed from clinical experience after extended left hepatectomy. Despite a sufficiently large remnant (posterior venous sector) usually being present, these resections are associated with a distinctly higher complication rate than extended right resections in which the liver remnant (segments II and III) is often considerably smaller (Fig. 80-109) (Abdalla et al, 2004). This higher complication rate suggests that the truly functional parenchymal mass, rather than the volume of the remaining tissue, is one of the key factors for postoperative functional recovery.

Computer assistance provides little additional information in planning for extended right hepatectomy (Lang et al, 2005a), in contrast to extended left hepatectomy, because of the more predictable left portal venous inflow and hepatic venous outflow related to the anatomic landmark of the falciform ligament. This statement is confirmed by the experience with segmental liver transplantation of the left lateral lobe, which is a well-defined anatomic unit with independent vascular supply and complete venous and biliary drainage (see Ch. 107) (Broering et al, 2004; Goss et al, 1998).

Most of the clinical experience with computer-assisted operative planning refers to first liver resections and focuses on analysis of the portal venous and hepatic venous systems (Fuchs et al, 2005; Lang et al, 2005a). Nevertheless, the hepatic artery and the biliary tree have to be taken into consideration. The amount of liver tissue with impaired vascularization or drainage is likely to be larger when taking these structures into account. More recent advances have shown that it is possible not only to visualize all four hepatic nonparenchymal structural systems simultaneously, but also to compute their hepatic territories. With ongoing progress, operative planning will continue to improve by taking into account the entire Glisson triads and the hepatic venous system.

Similarly, it is likely that the potential use of three-dimensional reconstruction and computer-assisted resection planning will be valuable in repeat hepatectomy. In such cases, there may be a distorted vascular system as a result of previous vascular dissection and liver regeneration. This seems to be particularly true in operative planning after previous left or right hepatectomy, when there is often only one draining hepatic vein for the entire remnant. Compensatory hypertrophy of the remaining liver also may lead to a sometimes unpredictable anatomic organization of the vascular tree. In these situations, preoperative three-dimensional reconstruction and computer-assisted operative planning is able to give much more detailed information of the

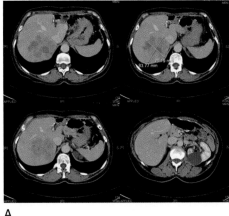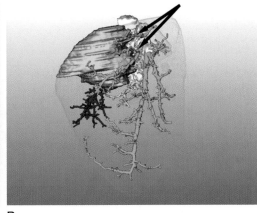

A   B

Fig. 80.110. A, Two-dimensional CT scans of recurrent colorectal metastases in the right liver lobe with obstruction of the right hepatic vein after prior left lateral resection. The inferior parts of the liver are tumor-free. The middle hepatic vein is patent and runs out of the inferior and lateral portions of the right lobe. **B,** Three-dimensional reconstruction of hepatic venous anatomy shows that the inferior part of the right liver lobe is almost completely drained via the middle hepatic vein *(blue)*. The right hepatic vein *(red)* is small and contributes to the drainage of the superior portion of the right lobe only. An inferior right hepatic vein is colored *yellow.* According to virtual resection including computer-assisted risk analysis (figure not shown), the resection of the tumor with a safety margin of 1 cm is possible, requiring the dissection of the right hepatic vein and of some smaller tributaries to the middle hepatic vein *(arrows)*. The middle hepatic vein and the inferior right hepatic vein can be preserved. The calculated volume of the remaining liver tissue with unimpaired venous outflow is 768 mL. *Comment:* The metastases could be resected completely with tumor-free margins. Postoperatively, there was no evidence for liver failure at any time.

individual anatomy than is possible by conventional imaging techniques (Lang et al, 2005b). In such circumstances, the knowledge of the distribution pattern of the remaining vascular branches may contribute considerably to preoperative assessment of postresectional functional reserve and to the safety of the operation (Fig. 80-110).

Although operative planning is improved by the use of three-dimensional reconstruction and further computer assistance in marginal cases with small liver remnants, the preoperatively collected additional information is still difficult to apply during operation. This difficulty is at least partially due to the absence of reliable markers on the liver surface representing the intrahepatic vascular territories. Currently, intraoperative realization of the results of computer-assisted planning is based on the visualization of hepatic vascular anatomy by intraoperative ultrasound and on the surgeon's ability to transfer the preoperative figures into the operative situs; this is even more difficult in the mobilized and exposed liver because there is frequently tremendous alteration of liver shape. In these situations, the surgeon sometimes has to rely mainly on tactile orientation when handling the liver together with the tumor. Navigation systems or techniques that ensure the preoperative planned resection line is applied accurately in the liver are under intense investigation but are not available as yet.

Developments in image-based computer assistance provide improved visualization of the intrahepatic vascular branching system in a virtual three-dimensional model of the liver, allowing a quantitative assessment of any vascular territory. Because these imaging techniques are based on standard two-dimensional CT scans, they do not provide additional information with regard to the number and the size of detected liver lesions. To date, the advantages of computer-assisted resection planning refer to a better preoperative assessment of functional resectability in areas at risk for devascularization or impaired drainage. In selected

cases, this information may have considerable influence on operative planning, especially with regard to the extent of resection or the need for vascular reconstruction; this is important in case of a marginal liver remnant or in repeat hepatectomy when intrahepatic vascular anatomy may be distorted.

As with most developments, computer-assisted operative planning gives rise to new questions. Although the importance of a sufficient blood supply or hepatic venous drainage to the entire remnant liver is self-evident, it is not yet known if impairment of either one of these vascular systems has a major impact on hepatic function of the involved area. In addition, intraoperative application of the preoperative findings of computer-assisted risk analysis is still difficult because of the absence of reliable liver surface markers corresponding with hepatic segmentation. Navigation techniques to ensure the accurate application of the preoperative planned resection line are under investigation, but not available yet.

REFERENCES

Abdalla EK, et al, 2004: Total and segmental liver volume variations: implications for liver surgery. Surgery 135:404-410.

Adson MA, Weiland LH, 1981: Resection of primary solid hepatic tumours. Am J Surg 141:8.

Al-Hadeedi S, et al, 1990: Extended left hepatectomy for hepatocellular carcinoma. Br J Surg 77:1247-1250.

Alper A, et al, 1988: Treatment of liver hemangiomas by enucleation. Arch Surg 123:600-661.

Antonetti MC, et al, 2002: Hand-assisted laparoscopic liver surgery. Arch Surg 137:407-412.

Atkinson D, et al, 1992: Hepatic cryosurgery for metastatic carcinoma. Proc Am Soc Clin Oncol 11:A473.

Baer HU, et al, 1987: Klinik, diagnostik and therapie von, "grossen" leberhamangiomen. Helv Chir Acta 54:387-389.

Baer HU, et al, 1989: Resectability of large focal liver lesions. Br J Surg 76: 1042-1044.

Baer HU, et al, 1991: Subtotal hepatectomy: a new procedure based on the inferior right hepatic vein. Br J Surg 78:1221-1222.

Baer HU, et al, 1992a: Enucleation of giant hemangiomas of the liver: technical and pathologic aspects of a neglected procedure. Ann Surg 216:673-676.

Baer HU, et al, 1992b: Water-jet dissection in hepatic surgery. Minim Invasive Ther 1:169-172.

Balasegaram M, Joishy SK, 1981: Hepatic resection: pillars of success built on a foundation of 15 years of experience. Am J Surg 141:360-365.

Bartlett D, et al, 1996: Complete resection of the caudate lobe of the liver: technique and results. Br J Surg 83:1076-1081.

Beazley RM, et al, 1984: Clinicopathological aspects of high bile duct cancer: experience with resection and bypass surgical treatment. Ann Surg 199:1-14.

Beets G, et al, 1994: Clinical value of whole-body positron emission tomography with [18F]fluorodeoxyglucose in recurrent colorectal cancer. Br J Surg 81: 1666-1670.

Behrns KE, et al, 1998: Hepatic steatosis as a potential risk factor for major hepatic resection. J Gastrointest Surg 2:292-298.

Belghiti J, et al, 1996: Portal triad clamping of hepatic vascular exclusion for major liver resection—a controlled study. Ann Surg 224:155-161.

Belghiti J, et al, 2001: Liver hanging maneuver: a safe approach to right hepatectomy without liver mobilization. J Am Coll Surg 193:109-111.

Berber E, et al, 2004: Laparoscopic radiofrequency ablation of hepatic tumors: prospective clinical evaluation of ablation size comparing two treatment algorithms. Surg Endosc 18:390-396.

Berman MM, et al, 1980: Hepatocellular carcinoma: polygonal cell type with fibrous stroma—an atypical variant with a favourable prognosis. Cancer 46:1448.

Berney T, et al, 1998: Total vascular exclusion of the liver for the resection of lesions in contact with the vena cava or the hepatic veins. Br J Surg 85: 485-488.

Bhuiya M, et al, 1992: Clinicopathological studies on perineural invasion of bile duct carcinoma. Ann Surg 215:344-349.

Billingsley KG, et al, 1998: Segment-oriented hepatic resection in the management of malignant neoplasms of the liver. J Am Coll Surg 187:471-481.

Bismuth H, 1982: Surgical anatomy and anatomic surgery of the liver. World J Surg 6:3-9.

Bismuth H, Castaing D, 1984: L'Echographe per-operatoire dans le chirurgie hepato-biliaire. Bull Acad Natl Med 168:98-103.

Bismuth H, et al, 1989: Major hepatic resection under total vascular exclusion. Ann Surg 210:13-19.

Bismuth H, et al, 1992: Management strategies in resection for hilar cholangiocarcinoma. Ann Surg 215:31-38.

Blumgart LH, 1978: Biliary tract obstruction—new approaches to old problems. Am J Surg 135:19-31

Blumgart LH, 1980: Hepatic resection. In Taylor S (ed): Recent Advances in Surgery. Edinburgh, Churchill Livingstone, pp 1-26.

Blumgart LH, 1982: Hepatic resection. In Dudley HA, Pories WJ (eds): Operative Surgery, 4th ed. Kent, UK, Butterworth, pp 477-499.

Blumgart LH, Hann LE, 2000: Surgical and radiological anatomy of the liver and biliary tract. In Blumgart LH, Fong Y (eds): Surgery of the Liver and Biliary Tract, 3rd ed. Philadelphia, Saunders, pp 3-34.

Blumgart LH, et al, 1971: Observations on liver regeneration after right hepatic lobectomy. Gut 12:922-1028.

Blumgart LH, et al, 1984: Surgical approaches to cholangiocarcinoma at confluence of hepatic ducts. Lancet 1:66-70.

Blumgart LH, et al, 1993: Extended left hepatectomy: technical aspects of an evolving procedure. Br J Surg 80:903-906.

Blumgart LH, et al, 2000: Liver resection for benign disease and for liver and biliary tumors. In Blumgart LH, Fong Y (eds): Surgery of the Liver and Biliary Tract, 3rd ed. Philadelphia, Saunders, pp 1639-1714.

Bourquain H, et al, 2002: HepaVision 2: A Software Assistant for Preoperative Planning in Living-Related Liver Transplantation and Oncologic Liver Surgery. Springer, Proc CARS, pp 341-346.

Broelsch CE, et al, 1991: Liver transplantation in children from living related donors: surgical techniques and results. Ann Surg 214:428-439.

Broering DC, et al, 2004: One hundred thirty-two consecutive pediatric liver transplants without hospital mortality: lessons learned and outlook for the future. Ann Surg 240:1002-1012.

Brown DA, et al, 1988: Nonanatomic hepatic resection for secondary hepatic tumors with special reference to hemostatic technique. Arch Surg 123: 1063-1066.

Burke EC, et al, 1998: Hilar cholangiocarcinoma: patterns of spread, the importance of hepatic resection for curative operation, and a presurgical clinical staging system. Ann Surg 228:385-394.

Castaing D, et al, 1985: Intraoperative ultrasound study of the liver: methodology and anatomical results. Am J Surg 149:676-682.

Charnley RM, et al, 1989: Cryotherapy for liver metastases: a new approach. Br J Surg 76:1040-1041.

Charnley RM, et al, 1991: Effect of hepatic cryotherapy on serum CEA concentration in patients with multiple inoperable hepatic metastases from colorectal cancer. Aust N Z J Surg 61:55-58.

Cherqui D, et al, 2000: Laparoscopic liver resections: a feasibility study in 30 patients. Ann Surg 232:753-762.

Child CG, Turcotte JG, 1964: Surgery and portal hypertension. In Dunphy JE (ed): The Liver and Portal Hypertension. Philadelphia, Saunders, pp 50-52.

Clavien P-A, et al, 2004: Protection of the liver during hepatic surgery. J Gastrointest Surg 8:313-327.

Clinical Outcomes of Surgical Therapy Study Group, 2004: A comparison of laparoscopically assisted and open colectomy for colon cancer. N Engl J Med 350:2050-2059.

Collier NA, et al, 1984: Neurotensin secretion by fibrolamellar carcinoma of the liver. Lancet 1:538-540.

Colonna JO, et al, 1993: Resection of the caudate lobe through 'bloody gultch.' Surg Gynecol Obstet 176:401-402.

Couinaud CL, 1954: Bases anatomiques des hepatectomies gauche et droite reglees. J Chir 70:933-966.

Couinaud CL, 1957: Etudes Anatomiques et Chirurgicales. Mason, Paris.

Craig JR, et al, 1980: Fibrolamellar carcinoma of the liver: a tumour of adolescents and young adults with distinctive clinico-pathologic features. Cancer 46:372.

Cunningham JD, et al, 1994: One hundred consecutive hepatic resections: blood loss, transfusion and operative technique. Arch Surg 129:1050-1056.

Czerniak A, et al, 1993: A direct approach to the left and middle hepatic veins during left-sided hepatectomy. Surg Gynecol Obstet 177:303-306.

D'Angelica M, et al, 2003: The role of staging laparoscopy in hepatobiliary malignancy: prospective analysis of 401 cases. Ann Surg Oncol 10:183-189.

Delva E, et al, 1989: Vascular occlusions for liver resections: operative management and tolerance to hepatic ischemia: 142 cases. Ann Surg 209:211-218.

DeMatteo RP, et al, 2000: Anatomic segmental hepatic resection. J Gastrointest Surg 4:178-184.

Descottes B, et al, 2000: Early experience with laparoscopic approach for solid liver tumors: initial 16 cases. Ann Surg 232:641-645.

Descottes B, et al, 2003: Laparoscopic liver resection of benign liver tumors. Surg Endosc 17:23-30.

Ebata T, et al, 2002: Pathological appraisal of lines of resection for bile duct carcinoma. Br J Surg 89:1260-1267.

Ebata T, et al, 2003: Hepatectomy with portal vein resection for hilar cholangiocarcinoma: audit of 52 consecutive cases. Ann Surg 238:720-727.

Elias D, et al, 1992: Surgical approach to segment I for malignant tumors of the liver. Surg Gynecol Obstet 175:17-24.

Emond J, et al, 1995: Total vascular exclusion for major hepatectomy in patients with abnormal liver parenchyma. Arch Surg 130:824-831.

Emre S, et al, 1993: Liver resection under total vascular isolation—variations on a theme. Ann Surg 217:15-19.

Farges O, et al, 2002: Prospective assessment of the safety and benefit of laparoscopic liver resections. J Hepatobiliary Pancreat Surg 9:242-248.

Farges O, et al, 2003: Portal vein embolization before right hepatectomy—prospective clinical trial. Ann Surg 237:208-217.

Fasel JHD, et al, 1998: Segmental anatomy of the liver: poor correlation with CT. Radiology 206:151-156.

Fiamingo P, et al, 2003: Laparoscopic treatment of simple hepatic cysts and polycystic liver disease. Surg Endosc 17:623-626.

Fischer L, et al, 2002: Limits of Couinaud's liver segment classification: a quantitative computer-based three-dimensional analysis. J Comp Assist Tomogr 26:962-967.

Fong Y, Blumgart LH, 1997: Useful stapling techniques in liver surgery. J Am Coll Surg 185:100.

Fong Y, et al, 1995: Pancreatic or liver resection for malignancy is safe and effective for the elderly. Ann Surg 222:426-437.

Fong Y, et al, 1996: Drainage is unnecessary after elective liver resection. Am J Surg 171:158-162.

Fong Y, et al, 1999a: Utility of 18F-FDG positron emission tomography scanning on selection of patients for resection of hepatic colorectal metastases. Am J Surg 178:282-287.

Fong Y, et al, 1999b: An analysis of 412 cases of hepatocellular carcinoma at a Western center. Ann Surg 229:790-799.

Fong Y, et al, 2000: Hand-assisted laparoscopic liver resection: lessons from an initial experience. Arch Surg 135:854-859.

Foster J, Berman M, 1977: Solid liver tumors. In Ebert P (ed): Major Problems in Clinical Surgery. Philadelphia, Saunders, pp 209-234.

Franco D, et al, 1988: Segmentectomies in the management of liver tumors. Arch Surg 123:519-522.

Franco D, et al, 1989: Hepatectomy without abdominal drainage. Ann Surg 210:748-750.

Franco D, et al, 1990: Resection of hepatocellular carcinomas: results in 72 European patients with cirrhosis. Gastroenterology 98:733-738.

Fuchs J, et al, 2005: Three-dimensional visualization and virtual simulation of resection in pediatric solid tumors. J Pediatr Surg 40:364-370.

Gall FP, Scheele J, 1986: Die operative Therapie von Lebermetastasen. In Schildberg FW (ed): Chirurgische Behandlung von Tumormetastasen. Federal Republic of Germany, Bibliomed, Melsungen, pp 223-240.

Gardner B, et al, 1992: En bloc caudate lobe and partial vena cava resection using a Gott shunt for retrohepatic caval bypass. J Surg Oncol 109: 208-213.

Gazelle GS, Haaga JR, 1992: Hepatic neoplasms: surgically relevant segmental anatomy and imaging techniques. AJR Am J Roentgenol 158:1015-1018.

Gibson RN, et al, 1986: Bile duct obstruction: radiologic evaluation of level, cause and tumor resectability. Radiology 160:43-47.

Gigot JF, et al, 2001: The surgical management of congenital liver cysts. Surg Endosc 15:357-363.

Gigot JF, et al, 2002: Laparoscopic liver resection for malignant liver tumors: preliminary results of a multicenter European study. Ann Surg 236:90-97.

Goff RD, et al, 1967: Interlobar intrahepatic approach to biliary tract reconstruction. Ann Surg 165:624-627.

Goldsmith NA, Woodburne RT, 1957: The surgical anatomy pertaining to liver resection. Surg Gynecol Obstet 105:310-318.

Goss JA, et al, 1998: Long-term results of pediatric liver transplantation: an analysis of 569 transplants. Ann Surg 228:411-420.

Guthy E, 1986: Die infrarotkontaktkoagulation. In Reifferscheid M (ed): Neue Techniken der Operativen Medizin. Berlin, Springer-Verlag.

Habib N, et al, 1994: Liver resection with total vascular occlusion for malignant tumors. Br J Surg 81:1181-1184.

Hann LE, et al, 1997: Cholangiocarcinoma at the hepatic hilus: sonographic findings. AJR Am J Roentgenol 168:985-989.

Hann LE, et al, 1998: Tumor involvement in hepatic veins: comparison of MR imaging and US for preoperative assessment. Radiology 206: 651-656.

Hanna SS, et al, 1996: Liver resection by ultrasonic dissection and intraoperative ultrasonography. HPB Surg 9:121-128.

Hannoun L, et al, 1993: Liver resection with normothermic ischaemia exceeding 1 h. Br J Surg 80:1161-1165.

Hasegawa H, et al, 1989: Poor prognoses following left hepatic trisegmentectomies for cancer. Jpn J Clin Oncol 19:271-275.

Hasegawa H, et al, 1991a: Surgical strategy for hepatocellular carcinoma of the caudate lobe. J Chir 128:533-540.

Hasegawa H, et al, 1991b: Segmentectomy under echographic control on cirrhotic liver. J Chir 128:343-350.

Hawkins W, et al, 2005: Caudate hepatectomy for cancer: a single institution experience with 150 patients. J Am Coll Surg 200:345-352.

Healey JE, Schroy PC, 1953: Anatomy of the biliary ducts within the human liver. Arch Surg 66:599-616.

Heloury Y, et al, 1988: The caudate lobe of the liver. Surg Radiol 10:83-91.

Hemming AW, et al, 1997: Aggressive surgical management of fibrolamellar hepatocellular carcinoma. J Gastrointest Surg 1:342-346.

Hemming AW, et al, 2002: Hepatic vein reconstruction for resection of hepatic tumors. Ann Surg 235:850-858.

Hepp J, Couinaud C, 1957: L'abord et l'utilisation du canal hepatique gauche dans le separation de la voie biliare principale. Presse Med 64:947-948.

Hodgson WJ, DelGuercio LR, 1984: Preliminary experience in liver surgery using the ultrasonic scalpel. Surgery 95:230-234.

Horton MD, et al, 1991: Hepatic artery cytotoxic perfusion therapy after cryotherapy: a single patient control trial? Med J Aust 155:849 (letter).

Houssin D, et al, 1993: Resection d'au moins six segments anatomiques en un temps pour tumeur du foie. Gastroenterol Clin Biol 17:750.

Huang M, et al, 2003: Hand-assisted laparoscopic hepatectomy for solitary tumor in the posterior portion of the right lobe: initial experience. Ann Surg 238:674-679.

Huguet C, Gavelli A, 1994: Experience with total vascular isolation of the liver. Semin Liver Dis 14:115-119.

Huguet C, et al, 1978: Normothermic hepatic vascular occlusion for extensive hepatectomy. Surg Gynecol Obstet 147:689-693.

Huguet C, et al, 1992a: Technique of hepatic vascular exclusion for extensive liver resection. Am J Surg 163:602-605.

Huguet C, et al, 1992b: Liver ischemia for hepatic resection: where is the limit? Surgery 111:251-259.

Huguet C, et al, 1994: Extended left hepatectomy with vascular exclusion. J Am Coll Surg 178:288.

Huscher CG, et al, 1998: Laparoscopic liver resections. Semin Laparosc Surg 5:204-210.

Iannitti DA, et al, 1998: Laparoscopic cryoablation of hepatic metastases. Arch Surg 133:1011-1015.

Ido K, et al, 1997: Laparoscopic microwave coagulation therapy for solitary hepatocellular carcinoma performed under laparocopic ultrasonography. Gastrointest Endosc 45:415-420.

Imamura H, et al, 2002: Pringle's manoeuvre in living donors. Lancet 360: 2049-2050.

Iwatsuki S, Starzl TE, 1988: Personal experience with 411 hepatic resections. Ann Surg 208:421-434.

Iyomasa S, et al, 1992: Cholangiocellular carcinoma in the caudate lobe with intraluminal growth in the extrahepatic bile duct. Hepatogastroenterology 39:570-573.

Jarnagin WR, et al, 2000: A prospective analysis of staging laparoscopy in patients with hepatobiliary primary and secondary malignancies. J Gastrointest Surg 4:34-43.

Jarnagin W, et al, 2001a: Staging, resectability, and outcome in 225 patients with hilar cholangiocarcinoma. Ann Surg 234:507-517.

Jarnagin W, et al, 2001b: What is the yield of intraoperative ultrasonography during partial hepatectomy for malignant disease? J Am Coll Surg 192: 577-583.

Jarnagin W, et al, 2002: Improvement in perioperative outcome after hepatic resection: analysis of 1,803 consecutive cases over the past decade. Ann Surg 236:397-407.

John T, et al, 1994: Superior staging of liver tumors with laparoscopy and laparoscopic ultrasound. Ann Surg 220:711-719.

Joishy SK, Balasegaram M, 1980: Hepatic resection for malignant tumors of the liver: essentials for a unified surgical approach. Am J Surg 139:360-369.

Jones RM, et al, 1998: Central venous pressure and its effect on blood loss during liver resection. Br J Surg 85:1058-1060.

Kamiya J, et al, 1994: Preoperative cholangiography of the caudate lobe: surgical anatomy and staging for biliary carcinoma. J Hepatobiliary Pancreat Surg 4:385-389.

Kanai M, et al, 1996: Preoperative intrahepatic segmental cholangitis in patients with advanced carcinoma involving the hepatic hilus. Surgery 119:498-504.

Kanematsu T, et al, 1984: Limited hepatic resection effective for selected cirrhotic patients with primary liver cancer. Ann Surg 199:51-56.

Kaneoka Y, et al, 2000: Hepatic vein reconstruction by external iliac vein grafting using vascular clips. World J Surg 24:377-382.

Kawasaki S, et al, 1998: Living related liver transplantation in adults. Ann Surg 227:269-274.

Kelly D, et al, 1996: Resection of benign hepatic lesions with selective use of total vascular isolation. J Am Coll Surg 183:113-116.

Ker CG, et al, 2000: Laparoscopic subsegmentectomy for hepatocellular carcinoma with cirrhosis. Hepatogastroenterology 47:1260-1263.

Khoury G, et al, 2000: Laparoscopic treatment of hydatid cysts of the liver and spleen. Surg Endosc 14:243-245.

Kiuchi T, et al, 1999: Impact of graft size mismatching on graft prognosis in liver transplantation from living donors. Transplantation 67:321-327.

Kokudo N, et al, 2003: Sling suspension of the liver in donor operation: a gradual tape-repositioning technique. Transplantation 76:803-807.

Kooby D, et al, 2003: Hepatic steatosis is associated with increased complications following major liver resection for cancer but does not impact survival. Gastroenterology 124:A794.

Kosuge T, et al, 1994: An isolated, complete resection of the caudate lobe, including the paracaval portion, for hepatocellular carcinoma. Arch Surg 129:280-284.

Lacy AM, et al, 2002: Laparoscopy-assisted colectomy versus open colectomy for treatment of non metastatic colon cancer: a randomized trial. Lancet 359:2224-2229.

Lai DTM, et al, 1996: The role of whole body positron emission tomography with [18F] fluorodeoxyglucose in identifying operable colorectal cancer metastases. Arch Surg 131:703-707.

Lai EC, et al, 1996: Anterior approach for difficult major right hepatectomy. World J Surg 20:314-318.

Lamadé W, et al, 2000: The impact of 3-dimensional reconstruction on operation planning in liver surgery. Arch Surg 135:1256-1261.

Lang H, et al, 2004: Extended left hepatectomy—modified operation planning based on three-dimensional visualization of liver anatomy. Langenbecks Arch Surg 389:306-310.

Lang H, et al, 2005a: Impact of virtual tumor resection and computer-assisted risk analysis on operation planning and intraoperative strategy in major hepatic resection. Arch Surg 140:629-638.

Lang H, et al, 2005b: Improved assessment of functional resectability in repeated hepatectomy by computer-assisted risk analysis operation planning. Hepatogastroenterology 52:1645-1648.

Launois B, 1994: Comment to liver resection—liver and biliary tumors. In Blumgart LH (ed): Surgery of the Liver and Biliary Tract, 2nd en. Edinburgh, Churchill Livingstone, pp 1495-1537.

Launois B, Jamieson GG, 1992a: The importance of Glisson's capsule and its sheath in the intrahepatic approach to resection of the liver. Surg Gynecol Obstet 174:7-10.

Launois B, Jamieson GG, 1992b: The posterior intrahepatic approach for hepatectomy or removal of segments of the liver. Surg Gynecol Obstet 174:155-158.

Launois B, Jamieson GG, 1993: Modern Operative Techniques in Liver Surgery. Edinburgh, Churchill Livingstone.

Laurent A, et al, 2003: Laparoscopic liver resection for subcapsular hepatocellular carcinoma complicating chronic liver disease. Arch Surg 138:763-769.

Lee S, et al, 2001: An adult-to-adult living donor liver transplant using dual left lobe grafts. Surgery 129:647-650.

Lerner S, et al, 2004: Giant cavernous liver hemangiomas. Arch Surg 139:818-823.

Lerut J, et al, 1990: Resection of the caudate lobe of the liver. Surg Gynecol Obstet 171:160-162.

Lesurtel M, et al, 2003: Laparoscopic versus open left lateral hepatic lobectomy: a case-control study. J Am Coll Surg 196:236-242.

Lezoche E, et al, 1998: Ultrasound-guided laparoscopic cryoablation of hepatic tumors: preliminary report. World J Surg 22:829-835.

Lo CM, et al, 1997: Adult-to-adult living donor liver transplantation using extended right lobe grafts. Ann Surg 226:261-270.

Lo CM, et al, 1998: Laparoscopy and laparoscopic ultrasonography avoid exploratory laparotomy in patients with hepatocellular carcinoma. Ann Surg 227:527-532.

Lo CM, et al, 2003: Hepatic venoplasty in living-donor liver transplantation using right lobe graft with middle hepatic vein. Transplantation 75:358-360.

Longmire WP Jr, et al, 1973: Carcinoma of the extrahepatic biliary tract. Ann Surg 178:333-345.

Makuuchi M, et al, 1990: Preoperative portal embolization to increase safety of major hepatectomy for hilar bile-duct carcinoma—a preliminary report. Surgery 107:521.

Makuuchi M, et al, 1993a: Personal experience of right anterior segmentectomy (segments V and VIII) for hepatic malignancies. Surgery 114:52-58.

Makuuchi M, et al, 1993b: Donor hepatectomy for living related partial liver transplantation. Surgery 113:395-402.

Mala T, et al, 2002: A comparative study of the short-term outcome following open and laparoscopic liver resection of colorectal metastases. Surg Endosc 16:1059-1063.

Malagó M, et al, 2005: Hepatic venous outflow reconstruction in the right live donor liver transplantation. Transplantation 11:364-365.

Manterola C, et al, 2002: Laparoscopic pericystectomy for liver hydatid cysts. Surg Endosc 16:521-524.

Marescaux J, et al, 1998: Virtual reality applied to hepatic surgery simulation: the next revolution. Ann Surg 228:627-634.

McIndoe AH, Counseller VS, 1927: The bilaterality of the liver. Arch Surg 15:589-594.

Melendez JA, et al, 1998: Perioperative outcomes of major hepatic resections under low central venous pressure anesthesia: blood loss, blood transfusion, and the risk of postoperative renal dysfunction. J Am Coll Surg 187:620-625.

Melendez J, et al, 2001: Extended hepatic resection: a 6-year retrospective study of risk factors for perioperative mortality. J Am Coll Surg 192:47-53.

Miyagawa S, et al, 1992: Resection of a large liver cell adenoma originating in the caudate lobe. Hepatogastroenterology 39:173-176.

Miyagawa S, et al, 1998: Concomitant caudate lobe resection as an option for donor hepatectomy in adult living related liver transplantation. Transplantation 66:661-663.

Mizumoto R, Suzuki H, 1988: Surgical anatomy of the hepatic hilum with special reference to the caudate lobe. World J Surg 12:2-10.

Mizumoto R, et al, 1986: Surgical treatment of hilar cholangiocarcinoma of the bile duct. Surg Gynecol Obstet 162:153-158.

Morino M, et al, 2003: Laparoscopic vs open hepatic resection. Surg Endosc 17:1914-1918.

Moriura S, et al, 1990: Combined resection of the superior vena cava for hepatobiliary and pancreatic malignancies. Hepatogastroenterology 37:253-255.

Nagasue N, et al, 1985: Segmental and subsegmental resections of the cirrhotic liver under hepatic inflow and outflow occlusion. Br J Surg 72:565-568.

Nagino M, et al, 1992: Percutaneous transhepatic biliary drainage in patients with malignant biliary obstruction of the hepatic confluence. Hepatogastroenterology 39:297-300.

Nagino M, et al, 1993: Percutaneous transhepatic portal embolization using newly devised catheters: preliminary report. World J Surg 17:520-524.

Nagino M, et al, 1995a: Preoperative management of hilar cholangiocarcinoma. J Hepatobiliary Pancreat Surg 2:215-223.

Nagino M, et al, 1995b: Changes in hepatic lobe volume in biliary tract cancer patients after right portal vein embolization. Hepatology 21:434-439.

Nagino M, et al, 1995c: Right or left trisegment portal vein embolization before hepatic trisegmentectomy for hilar bile duct carcinoma. Surgery 117:677-681.

Nagino M, et al, 1996: Selective percutaneous transhepatic embolization of the portal vein in preparation for extensive liver resection: the ipsilateral approach. Radiology 200:559-563.

Nagino M, et al, 1998: Segmental liver resections for hilar cholangiocarcinoma. Hepatogastroenterology 45:7-13.

Nagino M, et al, 2000: Right trisegment portal vein embolization for biliary tract carcinoma: technique and clinical utility. Surgery 127:155-160.

Nagino M, et al, 2001: Complications of hepatectomy for hilar cholangiocarcinoma. World J Surg 25:1277-1283.

Nagino M, et al, 2002: Hepaticojejunostomy using Roux-en-Y jejunal limb via retrocolic-retrogastric route. Langenbecks Arch Surg 387:188-189.

Nagorney DM, et al, 1985: Fibrolamellar hepatoma. Am J Surg 149:113.

National Institutes of Health, 1983: Liver transplantation. NIH Consensus Statement 4:1-15.

Nimura Y, 1993: Staging of biliary carcinoma: cholangiography and cholangioscopy. Endoscopy 25:76-80.

Nimura Y, 1994: Hepatectomy for proximal bile duct cancer. In Braasch JW, Tompkins RG (eds): Surgical Disease of the Biliary Tract and Pancreas. St Louis, Mosby–Year Book, pp 251-261.

Nimura Y, 1997: Surgical anatomy of the biliary ducts. In Rossi P, Bezzi M (eds): Medical Radiology: Biliary Tract Radiology. Berlin, Springer-Verlag, pp 21-30.

Nimura Y, et al, 1988: Value of percutaneous transhepatic cholangioscopy (PTCS). Surg Endosc 2:213-219.

Nimura Y, et al, 1989: Cholangioscopic differentiation of biliary stricture and polyps. Endoscopy 21:351-356.

Nimura Y, et al, 1990a: Cholangioscopic differentiation of biliary stricture and polyps. World J Surg 14:533-544.

Nimura Y, et al, 1990b: Hepatic segmentectomy with caudate lobe resection for bile duct carcinoma of the hepatic hilus. World J Surg 14:533-544.

Nimura Y, et al, 1991: Combined portal vein and liver resection for carcinoma of the biliary tract. Br J Surg 78:727-731.

Nimura Y, et al, 1992: Hepatic segmentectomy with caudate lobe resection for bile duct carcinoma of the hepatic hilus. World J Surg 14:535-543.

Nimura Y, et al, 1995a: Technique of inserting multiple biliary drains and management. Hepatogastoenterology 42:323-331.

Nimura Y, et al, 1995b: Hilar cholangiocarcinoma—surgical anatomy and curative resection. J Hepatobiliary Pancreat Surg 2:239-248.

Nimura Y, et al, 2000: Aggressive preoperative management and extended surgery for hilar cholangiocarcinoma: Nagoya experience. J Hepatobiliary Pancreat Surg 7:155-162.

Nishio H, et al, 1999: Value of percutaneous transhepatic portography before hepatectomy for hilar cholangiocarcinoma. Br J Surg 86:1415-1421.

Nishio H, et al, 2003: Most informative projection for portography: quantitative analysis of 47 percutaneous transhepatic portograms. World J Surg 27:433-436.

Nishio H, et al, 2005: Left hepatic trisectionectomy for hepatobiliary malignancy—results and an appraisal of its current role. Ann Surg 242:267-275.

Ogata S, et al, 2005: Doppler assessment after right hepatectomy confirms the necessity to fix the left remnant liver in the anatomical position. Br J Surg 92:592-595.

Ogura Y, et al, 1998: Central bisegmentectomy of liver plus caudate lobectomy for carcinoma of the gallbladder. Dig Surg 15:218-223.

Okamoto E, et al, 1984: Results of surgical treatments of primary hepatocellular carcinoma: some aspects to improve long-term survival. World J Surg 8:360-366.

Onik G, et al, 1991: Ultrasound-guided hepatic cryosurgery in the treatment of metastatic colon carcinoma: preliminary results. Cancer 67:901-907.

Onik GM, et al, 1993: Hepatic cryosurgery with and without the Bair Hugger. J Surg Oncol 52:185-187.

O'Rourke N, Fielding G, 2004: Laparoscopic right hepatectomy: surgical technique. J Gastrointest Surg 8:213-216.

Ozeki Y, et al, 1995: Extended left hepatic trisegmentectomy with resection of main right hepatic vein and preservation of middle and inferior hepatic veins. Surgery 117:715-717.

Paradinas FJ, et al, 1982: High serum vitamin B12 binding capacity as a marker of the fibrolamellar variant of hepatocellular carcinoma. BMJ 285:840-842.

Paterson-Brown S, Garden OJ, 1991: Laser-assisted laparoscopic excision of liver cysts. Br J Surg 78:1047.

Platzer W, Maurer H, 1966: Zur Segmenteinteilung der Leber. Acta Anat 63: 8-31.

Polk W, et al, 1995: A technique for the use of cryosurgery to assist hepatectomy. J Am Coll Surg 180:171-176.

Postema RR, et al, 1993: Less hepatic tissue necrosis after argon beam coagulator than after conventional electrocoagulation. Surg Gynecol Obstet 176: 177-180.

Povoski SP, et al, 1999: Extended left hepatectomy. World J Surg 23:1289-1293.

Preim B, et al, 2002: Resection Proposals for Oncologic Liver Surgery Based on Vascular Territories. Springer, Proc CARS, pp 353-358.

Pringle JH, 1908: Notes on the arrest of hepatic hemorrhage due to trauma. Ann Surg 48:514-519.

Pugh RNH, et al, 1973: Transection of the oesophagus for bleeding oesophageal varices. Br J Surg 60:646-649.

Radtke A, et al, 2005: Anatomical and physiological comparison of liver volumes among three frequent types of parenchymal transection in live donor transplantation. Hepatogastroenterology 52:333-338.

Rau HC, et al, 1998: Laparoscopic liver resection compared with conventional partial hepatectomy—a prospective analysis. Hepatogastroenterology 45: 2333-2338.

Rau HG, et al, 2000: Impact of virtual reality imaging on hepatic liver tumor resection: calculation of risk. Langenbecks Arch Surg 385:162-170.

Ravikumar TS, Steele GD Jr, 1989: Hepatic cryosurgery. Surg Clin North Am 69:433-440.

Ravikumar TS, et al, 1987: Hepatic cryosurgery with intraoperative ultrasound monitoring for patients with metastatic colon carcinoma. Arch Surg 122:403-409.

Ravikumar TS, et al, 1991: A 5-year study of cryosurgery in the treatment of liver tumors. Arch Surg 126:1520-1524.

Reynaud BH, et al, 1991: Basis to improve several hepatectomy techniques involving the surgical anatomy of incisura dextra of Gans. Surg Gynecol Obstet 172:490-492.

Rimola A, et al, 1986: Infective complications in acute and chronic liver failure: basis and control. In Williams R (ed): Liver Failure: Clinics in Critical Care Medicine. Edinburgh, Churchill Livingstone, pp 93-111.

Sakamoto E, et al, 1997: Clinicopathological studies of mucin-producing cholangiocarcinoma. J Hepatobiliary Pancreat Surg 4:157-162.

Sakamoto E, et al, 1998: The pattern of infiltration at the proximal border of hilar bile duct carcinoma. Ann Surg 227:405-411.

Sakamoto Y, et al, 2004: Bloodless liver resection using the monopolar floating ball plus ligature diathermy: preliminary results of 16 liver resections. World J Surg 28:166-172.

Samama G, et al, 1998: Laparoscopic anatomical hepatic resection: report of four left lobectomies for solid tumors. Surg Endosc 12:76-78.

Scheele J, 1989: Segment oriented resection of the liver: rationale and technique in hepato-biliary and pancreatic malignancies. In Lygidakis NJ, Tytgat GNJ (eds): Hepatobiliary and Pancreatic Malignancies: Diagnosis, Medical and Surgical Therapy. Stuttgart, Thieme, pp 219-246.

Scheele J, et al, 1991: Indicators of prognosis after hepatic resection for colorectal secondaries. Surgery 110:13-19.

Scheele J, et al, 1995: Resection of colorectal liver metastases. World J Surg 19:59-71.

Schenk A, et al, 2000: Efficient semiautomatic segmentation of 3D objects in medical images. In Scott L, et al (eds): Medical Image Computing and Computer-Assisted Intervention. Berlin, Springer, pp 186-195.

Schumaker HB Jr, 1942: Hemangioma of the liver. Surgery 11:209-222.

Schüssler-Fiorenza C, et al, 2004: Clinical risk score correlates with yield of PET scan in patients with colorectal hepatic metastases. J Gastrointest Surg 8: 150-158.

Schwartz SI, Husser WC, 1987: Cavernous hemangioma of the liver: a single institution report of 16 resections. Ann Surg 205:456.

Selle D, et al, 2002: Analysis of vasculature for liver surgery planning. IEEE Trans Med Imaging 21:1344-1357.

Seyama Y, et al, 2003: Long-term outcome of extended hemihepatectomy for hilar bile duct cancer with no mortality and high survival rate. Ann Surg 238:73-83.

Shimada M, et al, 1994: Characteristics of hepatocellular carcinoma originating in the caudate lobe. Hepatology 19:911-915.

Shimada M, et al, 2001: Laparoscopic hepatectomy for hepatocellular carcinoma. Surg Endosc 14:541-544.

Shoup M, et al, 2002: Port site metastasis after diagnostic laparoscopy for upper gastrointestinal tract malignancies: an uncommon entity. Ann Surg Oncol 9:632-636.

Soper NJ, et al, 1994: Laparoscopic general surgery. N Engl J Med 330: 409-419.

Soreide O, et al, 1985: Larger hepatocellular cancers: resection or liver transplant—which treatment when. BMJ 291:853-857.

Soreide O, et al, 1986: Characteristics of fibrolamellar hepatocellular carcinoma: an experience of 9 cases and a review of the literature. Am J Surg 151: 518-523.

Soyer P, et al, 1995: Variations in the intrahepatic portions of the hepatic and portal veins: findings on helical scans during arterial portography. AJR Am J Roentgenol 164:103-108.

Starzl TE, et al, 1975: Hepatic trisegmentectomy and other liver resections. Surg Gynecol Obstet 141:429-438.

Starzl TE, et al, 1980: Right trisegmentectomy for hepatic neoplasms. Surg Gynecol Obstet 150:208-214.

Starzl TE, et al, 1982: Left hepatic trisegmentectomy. Surg Gynecol Obstet 155:21-27.

Steele G, et al, 1984: Patterns of failure after surgical cure of large liver tumors. Am J Surg 147:554-559.

Strasberg SM, et al, 2000: The Brisbane 2000 terminology of liver anatomy and resections. HPB Surg 2:333-339.

Strasberg S, et al, 2002: Use of a bipolar vessel-sealing device for parenchymal transection during liver surgery. J Gastrointest Surg 6:569-574.

Sugawara Y, et al, 2002: Right lateral sector graft in adult living-related liver transplantation. Transplantation 73:111-114.

Takada T, et al, 1976: Percutaneous transhepatic cholanigal drainage: direct approach under fluoroscopic control. J Surg Oncol 8:83-97.

Takasaki K, et al, 1986a: New developed systematized hepatectomy by Glissonean pedicle transection method. Kyujutu (Operation) 40:7-14.

Takasaki K, et al, 1986b: Highly selected hepatic resection by Glissonean sheath binding method. Dig Surg 3:121.

Takayama T, Makuuchi M, 1996: Intraoperative ultrasonography and other techniques for segmental resections. Surg Oncol Clin North Am 5:261-269.

Takayama T, et al, 1990: Resection after intra-arterial chemotherapy of a hepatoblastoma originating in the caudate lobe. Surgery 107:231-235.

Takayama T, et al, 1991: A hepatoblastoma originating in the caudate lobe radically resected with the inferior vena cava. Surgery 109:208-213.

Tanaka K, Inomata Y, 1997: Present status and prospects of living-related liver transplantation. J Hepatobiliary Pancreat Surg 4:51-70.

Tanaka K, et al, 2003: Living-donor liver transplantation: surgical techniques and innovations. Barcelona, Spain, Prous Science.

Templeton JY, Dodd GD, 1963: Anatomical separation of the right and left lobes of the liver for intrahepatic anastomosis of the biliary ducts. Ann Surg 157:287-291.

Thompson JN, et al, 1985: Focal liver lesion: a plan for management. BMJ 290:1643-1644.

Ton That Tung, 1979: Les Resections Majeures et Mineures du Foie. Paris, Masson.

Ton That Tung, Quang ND, 1963: A new technique for operation on the liver. Lancet 1:192-193.

Tsuzuki T, et al, 1990: Hepatic resection for hepatocellular carcinoma. Surgery 107:511-520.

Uesaka K, et al, 1996: Changes in hepatic lobar function after right portal vein embolization. Ann Surg 223:77-83.

Van Ooijen PMA, et al, 2003: Recent developments in organ-selective reconstruction and analysis of multiphase liver CT. Imaging Decisions 7:37-43.

Vauthey JN, et al, 1993: Comparison of outcome between extended and nonextended liver resections for neoplasms. Surgery 114:968-975.

Vauthey JN, et al, 2000: Standardized measurement of the future liver remnant prior to extended liver resection: methodology and clinical associations. Surgery 127:512-519.

Voyles CR, et al, 1983: Carcinoma of the proximal extrahepatic biliary tree radiologic assessment and therapeutic alternatives. Ann Surg 197:188-194.

Weinbren HK, Blumgart LH, 1986: Pathological changes in the liver and computed tomography. Recent Results Cancer Res 100:58-67.

Welling RE, Lamping K, 1990: Cryoprobe as a 'handle' for resection of metastatic liver tumors. J Surg Oncol 45:227-228.

Wigmore SJ, et al, 2001: Virtual hepatic resection using three-dimensional reconstruction of helical computed tomography angio-portograms. Ann Surg 233:221-226.

Yamamoto J, et al, 1992: An isolated caudate lobectomy by the transhepatic approach for hepatocellular cancer. Surgery 111:699-702.

Yamamoto Y, et al, 2001: In situ pedicle resection in left trisegmentectomy of the liver combined with reconstruction of the right hepatic vein to an inferior vena caval segment transpositioned from the infrahepatic portion. J Am Coll Surg 92:137-141.

Yanaga K, et al, 1994: Isolated hepatic caudate lobectomy. Surgery 115: 757-761.

Yigitler C, et al, 2003: The small remnant liver after major liver resection: how common and how relevant? Liver Transplant 9:18-25.

Zahlten C, et al, 1995: Portal vein reconstruction based on topology. Eur J Radiol 19:96-100.

Zhou XD, 1992a: Cryosurgery for primary hepatic cancer of 87 patients (Chinese). Chung-Hua Wai Ko Tsa Chih 30:334-336.

Zhou XD, 1992b: Improved cryosurgery for primary liver cancer (Chinese). Chung-Hua Chung Liu Tsa Chih 14:61-63.

Vascular Isolation Techniques in Liver Resection

J. BELGHITI, O. SCATTON, AND D. VARMA

Bleeding and subsequent blood transfusions are the main causes of mortality and morbidity of hepatectomies. In addition, there is evidence that blood transfusion may be associated with an increased risk of recurrence of malignancy, through impairment of the patient's immune response (Asahara et al, 1999; Blumberg et al, 1986; Tung-Ping Poon et al, 2000). Vascular clamping, regardless of its modality, minimizes the risk of bleeding during liver resection. Liver cell injury induced by ischemia and reperfusion is the major drawback of clamping. Long duration of clamping carries a risk of postoperative liver failure, especially in patients with abnormal liver parenchyma (Huguet et al, 1992a).

With technical improvements in liver surgery, increasing numbers of patients with various underlying liver conditions (fibrosis, steatosis, or chemotherapy-induced injury) are undergoing complex and extensive liver resections (Belghiti et al, 2000; Poon et al, 2002). In this regard, pedicular intermittent clamping, which alternates short periods of clamping with intervals of restoration of blood flow, has shown to be the best-tolerated clamping modality, especially in patients with diseased liver parenchyma (Belghiti et al, 1999; Man et al, 1997). Similarly, ischemic preconditioning, which initiates a short period of clamping and restoration of blood flow followed by continuous clamping, seems to be an attractive concept (Clavien et al, 2000). Better understanding of vascular anatomy (particularly venous tributaries), better anesthesiologic management with perioperative low venous pressure, and the development of modern tools of transection coagulation (ultrasonic dissector and bipolar coagulation) have made possible major liver resection without vascular clamping. Vascular clamping needs to be applied balancing its efficacy to control bleeding with the risk of liver injury. This chapter describes techniques, benefits, drawbacks, and hemodynamic monitoring of vascular control so that the clinician uses the most appropriate technique to each patient's requirements.

ANATOMIC BASIS FOR VASCULAR CONTROL
(see Ch. 1)

The liver receives a dual vascular inflow providing approximately one quarter of the total cardiac output, or a blood flow of 1500 mL/min. The portal vein provides 75% of the total hepatic blood flow, and the hepatic artery provides the remaining 25%. The portal vein originates behind the neck of the pancreas as the confluence of the superior mesenteric and splenic veins and courses posterior to the bile duct and hepatic artery in the free edge of the lesser omentum. At the hilum of the liver, the vein divides into a shorter, more vertically oriented right branch and longer, horizontally oriented left branch. The right portal branch may be absent when the right anterior and posterior sectoral veins originate directly from the trunk of the portal vein. The right portal branch can be more difficult to dissect and control than the left portal branch.

Although highly variable, the hepatic artery arises most commonly as a branch of the celiac axis and enters the hepatoduodenal ligament after providing the right gastric and gastroduodenal arteries. The right and left branches usually lie on a plane posterior to the bile ducts at the hilum of the liver. This classic branching pattern is found in only 50% of patients. The accessory or replaced arteries pertinent to vascular clamping include a left artery, which can arise from the left gastric artery (25-30%), and a right artery, which can arise from the superior mesenteric artery (17-20%).

The three large hepatic veins that lie posterosuperior to the liver just below the diaphragm form the major drainage of the liver (Fig. 81.1). The right hepatic vein is formed as a short wide trunk by the convergence of an anterior trunk situated in the right portal fissure, which drains mainly segments V and VI, and a posterior trunk, which drains mainly segment VII. The right hepatic vein also drains part of segment VIII. The middle hepatic vein is situated in the plane of the principal portal fissure. It drains the entire central sector. It receives the veins from segments V and VIII at its right border and the veins of segment IV at its left border. The middle hepatic vein forms the major drainage vein of segment IV and part of segments V and VIII. The left hepatic vein arises from the confluence of segment II and III veins. It often receives drainage from the posterior part of segment IV, and it terminates as a short common trunk with the middle hepatic vein in most individuals. In 10% to 20% of cases, a significant right inferior hepatic vein may be found (>5 mm diameter), which mainly drains segment VI. In addition to these, there are two groups of accessory hepatic veins, the right and the left. The right accessory veins drain the posterior part of the dorsal sector. On the left, they are formed by the veins of the caudate lobe. In half of individuals, a large solitary vein terminates in the inferior vena cava (IVC), and in the other half, two or three veins are present, and they end in a staged fashion at the left border of the IVC. These anatomic variations are important in the context of vascular clamping because the presence of large drainage veins can result in inability to achieve complete vascular control during the clamping procedure.

HEMODYNAMIC RESPONSE TO DIFFERENT TYPES OF CLAMPING

The hemodynamic changes are proportional to the type and extent of vascular interruption. Hemodynamic changes also depend on several other factors, including the level of anesthesia, quantity and rapidity of bleeding, vascular filling, and spontaneous adaptation

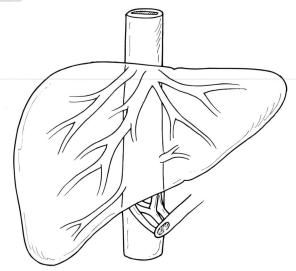

Fig. 81.1. Venous drainage of the liver depicting the major hepatic veins and their tributaries.

of the circulatory system to the reduction of venous return. Pedicle clamping is nearly always well tolerated, whereas the addition of caval clamping is followed by major hemodynamic consequences.

Hemodynamic Response to Pedicle Clamping

Pedicle clamping, which leads to a moderate decrease in cardiac preload with a 5% decrease in pulmonary artery pressure and a 10% decrease in cardiac index, is paradoxically associated with a 10% increase in mean arterial pressure (Belghiti et al, 1996; Delva et al, 1987). This phenomenon is the result of a sympathetic reflex inducing a significant increase in systemic vascular resistance (Belghiti et al, 1996; Delva et al, 1984). These hemodynamic changes are depicted in Table 81.1. Isolated pedicle clamping usually is well tolerated and does not require specific anesthetic management. The blood pressure is restored to normal or shows an increase from the baseline during the period of declamping. It is a frequently observed phenomenon, however, that as the cycle of clamping and declamping progresses, declamping causes more significant hypotension. This phenomenon, which can be observed when the cumulative period of clamping exceeds 1 hour, could be attributed to the reperfusion syndrome, owing to the long-term ischemia of liver

parenchyma and splanchnic release of toxic vasodilators. It is recommended to increase the duration of declamping during each cycle if the cumulative duration is prolonged more than 1 hour, especially in patients with diseased liver (Imamura et al, 2003).

Hemodynamic Consequences and Limitations of Hepatic Vascular Exclusion

The hemodynamic consequences of the addition of total caval clamping to pedicle clamping are more profound (see Table 81.1). Hepatic vascular exclusion (HVE), which leads to severe decrease in cardiac preload with 25% decrease in pulmonary artery pressure and 40% to 50% decrease in cardiac index, is associated with a 10% decrease in mean arterial blood pressure despite a 50% increase of heart rate and a significant increase in systemic vascular resistance. Reduced venous return produces a marked reduction in left ventricular and diastolic volume that can be monitored precisely by transesophageal echocardiography (Eyraud et al, 2002). The sequence of HVE includes initial inflow occlusion followed by infrahepatic caval clamping and suprahepatic caval clamping. The compensatory cardiac response to maintain the blood pressure requires approximately 5 minutes to occur and is facilitated by "preloading" the patient with intravenous fluids. A decrease in mean arterial pressure to less than 80 mm Hg, suggesting intolerance to HVE, should lead to consideration of caval declamping. Causes of this hemodynamic intolerance to HVE include (1) inadequate fluid loading, (2) hepatic congestion as a result of persistent inflow (see later), and (3) inadequate cardiovascular response. Insufficient fluid loading is likely to occur in the case of fluid restriction and unexpected need for caval occlusion without adequate preparation of the patient. The 10% of patients who are unable to increase their cardiac output are difficult to identify preoperatively.

ANESTHETIC CONSIDERATIONS

Historically, liver resections were associated with significant hemorrhage. Anesthesiologists tend to overload patients with intravenous fluids to minimize the hemodynamic consequences of blood loss. This approach paradoxically has aggravated operative blood loss even during pedicle clamping. This occurs as a consequence of backflow bleeding from the hepatic veins and is increased by elevated central venous pressure (CVP). A major advance in the 1990s was the ability of anesthesiologists to maintain a low CVP during hepatectomy (see Chs. 25 and 80).

Table 81.1   Hemodynamic Changes Observed during Various Methods of Clamping

Clamping Procedure	Portal Pressure	Caval Pressure	Pulmonary Artery Pressure	Cardiac Index	Vascular Resistance	Arterial Pressure
Pedicle clamping	↑↑↑	—	↓	↓	↑↑	↑
HVE	↑↑↑	↑↑	↓↓	↓↓	↑↑↑	↓
HVE with preservation of caval flow	↑↑↑	—	↓↓	↓	↑↑	—

HVE, hepatic vascular exclusion.
↑↑↑, severe increase; ↑↑, moderate increase; ↑, slight increase; ↓↓, moderate decrease; ↓, slight decrease; —, no change.

Low Central Venous Pressure Anesthesia (see Ch. 25)

Maintaining a low CVP during hepatic transection reduces the distention of hepatic veins and significantly decreases bleeding (Jones et al, 1998). It also avoids vena caval distention and facilitates safe dissection of retrohepatic vena cava and major hepatic veins. Because the blood loss resulting from a vascular injury is proportional to the pressure gradient across the vessel wall and the fourth power of the radius of the injury, lowering the CVP to one fifth decreases the blood loss by a factor greater than 5 (Melendez et al, 1998). Lowering the CVP lessens the pressure component and the radius component (owing to decrease in distention of the vein). Use of low CVP anesthesia during hepatic surgery has been shown to reduce intraoperative blood loss and the postoperative morbidity related to blood transfusion (Chen et al, 2000; Cunningham et al, 1994; Jones et al, 1998; Melendez et al, 1998).

The two drawbacks of low CVP anesthesia are the possibilities of postoperative renal failure and air embolism. The risk of renal failure occurs only when there is an unexpected hemorrhage in a patient who could not be brought back rapidly to euvolemia (Redai et al, 2004). Postoperative renal failure has never been significant, however, in clinical studies of liver resections, including major resections, under low CVP anesthesia (Melendez et al, 1998). Although the actual risk has not been quantified, there are clinical reports of air embolism. This risk can be reduced by (1) operating on the patient in 15 degrees head low position and (2) using an ideal anesthetic gas mixture (isoflurane delivered in oxygen) (Melendez et al, 1998; Redai et al, 2004).

How to Maintain Low Central Venous Pressure

The anesthesiologist can maintain a low CVP by several methods. Most frequently, low CVP is maintained by intentional underhydration of the patient by restricting intravenous fluids before, during, and after induction. Intravenous fluids are given at a rate of 0.5 to 1 mL/kg/hr until the hepatic resection is completed. The patient is brought back to euvolemia at the end of surgery, and hemostasis is ensured. Although low tidal volume ventilation was considered to reduce backflow bleeding, there is no evidence that this maneuver reduces the quantity of blood loss during hepatic transection phase (Hasegawa et al, 2002). Other methods commonly employed are the use of anesthetic gases, such as isoflurane, which has vasodilatory properties with minimal cardiac depression, and the use of certain drugs with vasodilatory effects. The surgeon can decrease the CVP by clamping the infrahepatic IVC, which leads to decreased venous return and has been shown to have no deleterious effect on renal function, even with a clamping time of 1 hour (Otsubo et al, 2004).

Special Considerations During Hepatic Vascular Exclusion

Application of vascular isolation techniques mandates a high level of anesthetic expertise. Intraoperative management of patients undergoing vascular exclusion should include the use of pulmonary artery catheterization and occasionally transesophageal echocardiography. When a major hepatectomy using HVE is planned, anesthetic management is adjusted to anticipate

the reduction in venous return, sudden decrease in cardiac output, and increase in afterload. Volume expansion usually is required for patients undergoing HVE. Volume expansion is achieved by rapid infusion of 500 mL of colloids before cross-clamping of the vena cava. In patients who do not tolerate caval cross-clamping, even after volume expansion, vasopressor agents, such as dopamine or norephinephrine, are added (Redai et al, 2004). Persistent hypotension or low cardiac index, which can occur in 10% to 20% of patients, should be considered as intolerance to HVE and is an indication for caval declamping or consideration of the use of venovenous bypass (Redai et al, 2004).

SURGICAL ASPECTS OF VASCULAR CLAMPING

The easiest procedure to reduce bleeding during liver resection is inflow control. Pedicle clamping, which controls the inflow, has few hemodynamic consequences and has the greatest efficiency in association with a low CVP. Continuous clamping, which increases ischemic injury of the liver parenchyma, also induces splanchnic congestion. Intermittent clamping has supplanted the use of selective pedicle clamping to overcome these two drawbacks. Patients with large tumors involving caval-hepatic confluence may require additional outflow vascular control.

Inflow Vascular Clamping

Hepatic pedicle clamping (Pringle's maneuver), which interrupts the arterial and portal venous inflow to the liver, is a standard in hepatic surgery.

Total Inflow Control

Inflow control implies encirclement of the hepatic pedicle (Fig. 81.2). Adhesions to the gallbladder are freed, and the lesser omentum is opened at the level of the pars flaccida, taking care to avoid injury to the right gastric pedicle. A finger or a blunt dissector thereafter may be passed easily through Winslow's foramen, and the hepatoduodenal ligament is encircled with a tape.

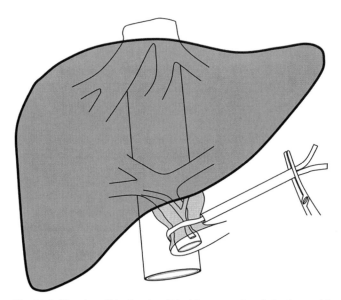

Fig. 81.2. Hepatic pedicle clamping (Pringle's maneuver) occludes the arterial and portal inflow of the liver.

Clamping is achieved easily by a vascular clamp or tourniquet, which should be closed until the pulse in the hepatic artery distal to the clamp is stopped. Excessive closure should be avoided because it otherwise may result in arterial or biliary injury. Care should be taken to avoid lymph nodes of the hepatoduodenal ligament (these may be large in cirrhotic patients or in patients with a long-standing cholestasis). A search for a left hepatic artery originating from the left gastric artery is mandatory to prevent persistent bleeding during parenchymal transection. When a left hepatic artery exists, simultaneous occlusion of this artery should be performed to complete the vascular inflow control.

In patients who have undergone previous abdominal surgery, there may be dense adhesions between the right lateral and posterior aspects of the hepatoduodenal ligament (in particular the portal vein) and the anterior surface of the IVC and segment I. Adhesions may form between the duodenum, greater omentum, and anterior aspect of the hepatoduodenal ligament. All of these adhesions should be lysed before pedicle clamping to avoid accidental injury to vena cava or the duodenum. A safe approach is to expose the IVC in its retropancreatic portion by a Kocher maneuver and to progress cranially.

Continuous Clamping. Continuous clamping implies interruption of inflow continuously during the hepatic transection phase, without intermittent release to allow reperfusion. Although conceptually efficient to control bleeding, continuous clamping is not used frequently because it is not universally effective, and it has several disadvantages (Table 81.2). The efficacy is limited by the inability of continuous clamping to control the backflow bleeding, which is increased if the CVP is high and when the patient has large hepatic tumors compressing hepatic veins associated with multiple venous collaterals.

Disadvantages of continuous clamping include splanchnic congestion and prolonged parenchymal ischemia. The splanchnic congestion and fluid sequestration in the visceral compartment cause bowel edema, which takes a long time to subside, leading to difficulties in the closure of the abdominal cavity at the end of the operation and prolonged postoperative ileus. A difficult closure of

the abdomen can lead to abdominal compartment syndrome with subsequent effects on the intra-abdominal organs (Moore et al, 2004). Development of edema is detrimental to bowel anastomoses, especially in the context of synchronous hepatic resections for colorectal malignancies (Elias et al, 1995a). Continuous clamping has been shown to induce hyperamylasemia and can lead to clinically significant pancreatitis in some patients (Miyagawa et al, 1994, 1996). Interruption of splenic venous return without arterial interruption poses a risk for spontaneous splenic rupture during prolonged continuous clamping (Emree et al, 1993).

Continuous clamping causes prolonged ischemia to the liver. Normal liver can tolerate inflow occlusion under normothermic conditions for 60 minutes (Delva et al, 1989; Huguet et al, 1992b). Diseased livers tolerate a much shorter duration of ischemia. Continuous clamping cannot be applied to diseased livers for a long time. Restoration of blood flow after prolonged clamping can cause reperfusion syndrome characterized by hemodynamic disturbances, owing to the release of toxic metabolites and vasodilators from the liver and the splanchnic bed (Kim, 2003; Kim et al, 2002). Intermittent clamping has been introduced to overcome these drawbacks of continuous clamping.

Intermittent Clamping. Intermittent inflow occlusion with intervals of reperfusion reduces the consequences of splanchnic congestion and decreases the ischemic injury to the liver parenchyma. After a short period of pedicle clamping (10-20 minutes), the inflow is restored for 5 to 10 minutes according to the duration of the transection, to the underlying liver status, and to the surgeon's preference (Imamura et al, 2003). Classically, each cycle comprises 15 minutes of clamping followed by 5 minutes of reperfusion (Belghiti et al, 1999; Hardy et al, 1995; Man et al, 1997; Takayama et al, 1998). Genuine intermittent clamping requires a true period of unclamping. "True" period of unclamping implies that the surgeon should not continue transection during the period of unclamping. This period, during which the surgeon applies gentle compression of the transected surface, can be used to re-examine the adequacy of the transection line with respect to the vascularization and the oncologic margin. The period of revascularization gives the

Table 81.2 Comparison of Relative Technical Difficulty, Control of Blood Loss, and Physiologic Tolerance for Various Clamping Techniques

Clamping Technique	Technical Difficulty	Hemodynamic Tolerance	Hepatic Tolerance	Prevention of Bleeding	Contraindications	Complications
No clamping	—	+++	+++	+	—	Bleeding requiring transfusion
Intermittent hepatic pedicle clamping	+	+++	++	++	—	—
Continuous hepatic pedicle clamping	+	+++	+	++	Diseased liver	Splanchnic congestion
Hepatic pedicle and infrahepatic IVC clamping	+	++	++*	+++	Low CVP	—
Partial pedicle clamping	++	+++	+++	+	Pedicular involvement	—
HVE (classic)	++	+	+	+++	Diseased liver; cardiac disease	Splanchnic congestion; renal dysfunction
Intermittent HVE with preservation of caval flow	+++	++	++	+++	Juxtacaval tumors	—

*If, intermittent.
+, least; ++, intermediate; +++, most.

surgeon an opportunity to visualize the healthy color of the remnant liver. Intraoperative ultrasonography can be performed to confirm the adequacy of inflow and outflow of the remnant liver and to examine the progress and direction of transection in relation to tumor margin.

Intermittent pedicle clamping, which is the most commonly used vascular clamping modality, has gained wide acceptance because it is technically simple, effective in control of hemorrhage, and well tolerated, above all, by diseased liver. Intermittent clamping in diseased liver has not been shown to cause significant deleterious effects even if the cumulative clamping time is 1 hour (Takayama et al, 1998). In a controlled study comparing continuous versus intermittent portal triad clamping, we found that although there was significantly more bleeding in the intermittent group during parenchymal transection, there was no statistical difference in the total operative blood loss. The most important result was the better tolerance of the liver to intermittent clamping (Belghiti et al, 1999). The application of intermittent clamping in normal livers has prolonged the total clamping duration (3 hours) and has enabled the surgeon to perform even complex hepatic resection with minimal blood loss (Sakamoto et al, 1999). The wide safety margin of intermittent pedicle clamping currently has promoted its safe use in donor hepatectomy in living donor liver transplantation. This clamping has neither jeopardized donor safety nor compromised graft function (Imamura et al, 2002, 2004). The use of intermittent clamping enables a bloodless resection, and it adds to donor safety, suggesting that the surgeon should not hesitate to use this during the living donor operation (Imamura et al, 2002, 2004). The better tolerance of intermittent ischemia has stimulated investigators to explore the concept of *preconditioning*.

Preconditioning. A newer perspective on inflow vascular clamping has emerged from study of the biologic response to ischemia-reperfusion (Clavien et al, 2000; Hardy et al, 1996). Realization that a period of ischemia followed by reperfusion of the liver not only protects the liver from the negative effects of a subsequent period of ischemia, but also may protect distant organs from the systemic effects of organ ischemia led to a study of this technique in humans. Clavien and coworkers (2000) revealed that an initial period of ischemia (10 minutes) followed by reperfusion (10 minutes) protects the liver against subsequent prolonged ischemia and postulated that some of the benefits of intermittent clamping may result from the impact of the first clamp-unclamp sequence as a preconditioning treatment. Preconditioning followed by continuous clamping may have the advantage of avoidance of blood loss during the unclamped period, although no major differences have been shown in terms of blood loss between the continuous versus intermittent clamping approaches.

This protective strategy against hepatic ischemia was shown to be efficient, especially in the presence of steatosis, in a prospective clinical randomized study (Clavien et al, 2003). The beneficial effect of preconditioning was shown only for 30 minutes of continuous clamping, however, and for small-volume liver resection (Clavien et al, 2003). Although the theoretical advantage of hepatoprotective effect of preconditioning is definitely attractive, in practice this procedure has not shown significant advantages over intermittent clamping. In controlled studies, the application of this principle in the setting of liver transplantation has not been shown to be beneficial compared with conventional liver harvesting methods either for deceased or for living donors (Azoulay et al, 2005; Koneru et al, 2005).

Topical Hypothermia. Because hepatic inflow occlusion carries a serious risk of ischemic injury to the remnant liver, induction of hypothermia was proposed to reduce the injury, particularly in patients with underlying liver disease (Kim et al, 1994, 2004). The adverse hemodynamic effects of systemic hypothermia led some authors to use topical cooling by placing ice packs or ice slush on the liver surface (Imakita et al, 2000; Yamanaka et al, 1998). Ischemic time could be prolonged to more than 1 hour in diseased livers, especially if hepatic core temperature decreased to less than 30°C (Kim et al, 2004).

Selective Inflow Control (see Ch. 80)

Selective inflow control selectively interrupts the arterial and portal venous inflow to the hemiliver to be resected. The advantages of this procedure include (1) clear demarcation of the limits of resection, (2) absence of ischemic injury of the remnant liver, and (3) absence of splanchnic congestion and hemodynamic disturbances. Selective inflow control was devised specifically for segmental and subsegmental resections for small hepatocellular carcinoma in diseased liver (Castaing et al, 1989; Shimamura et al, 1986). Additional clamping of the ipsilateral hepatic vein can be performed along with this procedure for better vascular control (Fig. 81.3) (Makuuchi et al, 1987). With the wider use of intermittent clamping, selective clamping techniques have not gained wide acceptance because this is more technically demanding and has no obvious beneficial effects compared with genuine intermittent clamping. In a prospective controlled study including patients who underwent minor resection, both techniques were associated with similar blood loss and postoperative complications (Figueras et al, 2005). Induction of less cytolysis was observed in the cirrhotic patients, however, who underwent selective clamping (Figueras et al, 2005).

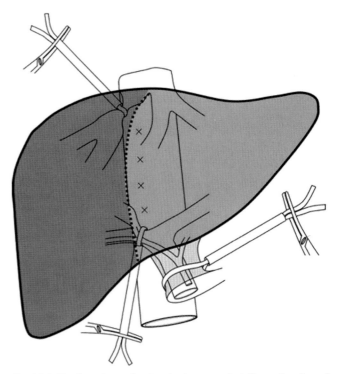

Fig. 81.3. Hemihepatic vascular clamping interrupts the inflow and outflow of the hemiliver to be resected.

After encircling the pedicle and performing cholecystectomy, the portal vein is approached posterolaterally from the right to avoid devascularization of the common bile duct. Care must be taken to avoid inadvertent injury to a right hepatic artery arising from the superior mesenteric artery. The main portal vein is dissected caudally to cranially on its anterior surface up to the bifurcation. During the dissection of its posterior surface, the consistent branch from the right posterior face of the right portal vein to the paracaval portion of the caudate lobe is ligated. After isolation and retraction of the right branch of the hepatic artery, the portal bifurcation is identified. The posterior passage of the curved dissector in the bifurcation is facilitated by a slight caudal traction of the main portal trunk. The bifurcation of the portal vein usually is accessed from the right side. When the caudate lobe is preserved, the dissection of the left branch of the portal vein should be accessed from the left side of the portal pedicle, with attention to one or two small portal branches to the left part of the caudate lobe. The right or left branch of the hepatic artery is identified and encircled. We do not advocate extrahepatic biliary dissection before parenchymal transection because of the risk for biliary injury (Launois & Jamieson, 1992a). The branches of the portal vein and hepatic artery supplying the liver that are to be resected can be cross-clamped or ligated.

The intrahepatic posterior approach described by Launois and Jamieson (1992a, 1992b) allows extra-Glissonian vascular control of the right pedicle without dissecting its structures individually. This technique includes division of the hepatic parenchyma anterior and posterior to the glissonian pedicle, and passage of a large curved clamp encircles the glissonian pedicle allowing its clamping. The caudal traction of the right pedicle facilitates the exposure of the anterior and posterior segmental branches of the right pedicle (see Ch. 80). The Launois procedure, which had a great initial success, is now usually reserved for patients who had previous hilar dissection or inflammation.

Segmental selective clamping can be useful for delineating the territory of some tumors that require difficult segmental or subsegmental resection. Sectoral territories can be delineated by extraparenchymal pedicle control of the respective sectors. Isolated control of a single segment is more difficult, requiring balloon occlusion of the portal flow. Under ultrasound guidance, the portal branch is punctured followed by introduction of a balloon catheter. Inflation of the balloon along with pedicular arterial clamping can delineate the portal territory. The injection of methylene blue into the portal catheter can allow more precise identification of the territory of interest.

Inflow and Outflow Vascular Control

Hepatic Vascular Exclusion

HVE combines total inflow and outflow vascular occlusion of the liver. Total isolation of the liver from the systemic circulation is intended during resection of large tumors adjacent to or involving the major hepatic veins or the IVC or both. This procedure also can be considered when significant backflow bleeding occurs because of persistently elevated CVP despite efficient hepatic pedicle clamping (i.e., patient with tricuspid insufficiency). This procedure, which requires prolonged continuous clamping, cannot be tolerated in patients with diseased liver and can cause significant hemodynamic disturbance in some patients (see Table 81.2). Two refinements have been proposed to overcome these drawbacks: (1) HVE with preservation of caval

flow to minimize the hemodynamic impact and (2) hypothermic perfusion to decrease parenchymal injury related to prolonged warm ischemia.

Effective HVE requires complete mobilization of the liver from its ligamentous attachments and all surrounding adhesions. The IVC is completely freed from the retroperitoneum, which requires ligation of the right adrenal vein. The IVC is mobilized above and below the liver and encircled. The hepatoduodenal ligament is encircled, as described earlier, and a careful search is made for accessory or replaced hepatic arteries (Fig. 81.4). Clamps are applied in the following order: (1) hepatoduodenal ligament, (2) infrahepatic IVC, and (3) suprahepatic IVC. When the surgeon and the anesthesiologist agree that clamping would be tolerated, clamps are reapplied for a duration of 60 minutes in patients with normal liver. After completion of the parenchymal transection and before removing the clamps, the clamp on the infrahepatic vena cava can be partially released to flush air that might have been trapped and to test for caval integrity. The clamps are removed in the reverse order in which they were placed.

Inadequate HVE technique results in the progressive congestion of the liver as a result of (1) inadequate clamping of the portal pedicle or the IVC, (2) persistent arterial inflow through an unrecognized left hepatic artery or hypervascular perihepatic adhesions, or (3) persistent entry of venous blood into the excluded retrohepatic IVC via anatomic (right adrenal vein) or pathologic (tumor adhesions) veins. Patients with huge tumors with diaphragmatic and peritoneal adhesions (who could be the best candidates for HVE) could experience hepatic congestion after suprahepatic caval clamping. This congestion, which is revealed by increase in liver size and change in color and consistency of the liver, is always associated with hemodynamic intolerance, which immediately reverses after release of the suprahepatic clamp.

Flow through retrocaval veins may fill the liver when every connection from the cava to the liver is not controlled (Huguet et al, 1992a). Supracaval declamping provides the path of least resistance for blood from the liver toward the heart, rather than backward into the surgical field. Although concomitant

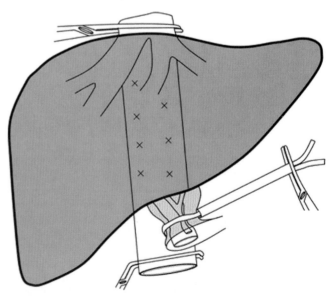

Fig. 81.4. HVE.

supraceliac aortic clamping (Stephen et al, 1996) has been proposed in this situation, the technique has not been widely adopted.

Hepatic Vascular Exclusion with Caval Flow Preservation

Historically, extraparenchymal control of the main hepatic veins was considered to be dangerous because a tear in this part of the vein would risk massive blood loss and air embolism. Better understanding of intrahepatic anatomy and advances in surgical techniques allow many liver surgeons to expose safely and control the three main hepatic veins. In the absence of tumor involvement of the hepatocaval junction, HVE with caval flow preservation can be considered. The association of inflow occlusion (hepatic pedicle clamping) and outflow occlusion by extraparenchymal clamping of the three main hepatic veins (Fig. 81.5) enables complete vascular isolation without interruption of the IVC flow (Cherqui et al, 1999; Elias et al, 1995b). The indication for this procedure is restricted, however, to patients without tumor involvement of the hepatocaval junction. In addition, the presence of large veins draining the caudate lobe may render this procedure inefficient. Caudate lobe veins that are not isolated in this technique and that can communicate intraparenchymally with other major veins cause persistent backflow bleeding. The technical sequence of HVE with preserved caval flow includes total pedicle clamping with subsequent clamping of the three major hepatic veins at their confluence with the IVC. This clamping procedure can be applied either continuously or intermittently.

Extrahepatic control of the right hepatic vein requires complete mobilization of the right liver. Division of the falciform ligament is extended cranially to the upper peritoneal folds of the right and left triangular ligaments. The gutter between the liver, the right hepatic vein, and the middle hepatic vein is dissected

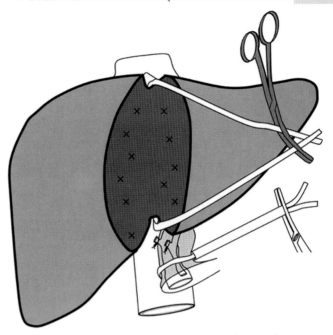

Fig. 81.6. Liver hanging maneuver facilitates to guide the direction of transection.

free to the anterior surface of the IVC. At this stage, dissection of a major hepatic vein from above is considered hazardous and should not be continued. After mobilization of the right lobe and complete exposure of the right and anterior sides of the IVC, the liver is retracted medially and upward. The right half of the IVC is dissected caudally to cranially with ligation of short and small retrohepatic veins. When a significant right inferior hepatic vein is present, it is encircled or ligated and divided according to type of resection. Before reaching the right hepatic vein level, the IVC ligament is encountered. This ligament is dissected and divided between clamps. This ligament, which contains small veins, should be closed with a running suture. Only after this closure has been completed should the right hepatic vein be encircled and taped. The right hepatic vein is encircled easily by a clamp passing on the anterior surface of the IVC toward the space between right hepatic vein and middle hepatic vein. To facilitate the subsequent parenchymal dissection, a tape is inserted behind the right hepatic vein and passed along the anterior surface of the IVC (Fig. 81.6). The right liver is released to lie in its anatomic position. This tape, which elevates the precaval space ("hanging maneuver"), facilitates subsequent division and hemostasis of the parenchyma (Belghiti et al, 2001).

The extrahepatic control of the middle and left hepatic veins requires exposure of the left border of the IVC. The left upper aspect of the IVC is exposed by division of the peritoneal reflection above the caudate lobe, and the ligamentum venosum is ligated and divided exposing the junction of the left hepatic vein and the IVC (Majno et al, 2002). When the left phrenic vein drains directly into the left hepatic vein, it is ligated and divided. A dissector is inserted from above in the previously dissected gutter between the right and middle hepatic veins and passed in close contact with the anterior surface of the IVC beneath the middle hepatic vein. The common trunk is encircled with a tape. When the confluence of the middle and left hepatic veins

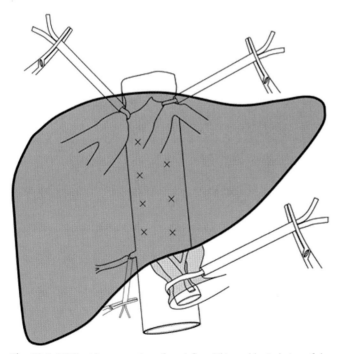

Fig. 81.5. HVE with preservation of caval flow. This enables isolation of the liver from the systemic circulation, avoiding the hemodynamic disturbances of HVE as the vena caval flow is maintained.

is extrahepatic, it is possible to encircle these two vessels separately; otherwise, the common trunk of the middle and left hepatic veins can be encircled as a unit.

Hepatic Vascular Exclusion with Refrigeration

Initially described by Fortner and coworkers (1974), the technique of HVE with refrigeration was re-evaluated by Azoulay and associates (2005), especially when HVE was longer than 60 minutes (Azoulay et al, 2005). Compared with standard HVE, these investigators showed that hypothermic perfusion of the liver was associated with better postoperative liver and renal functions and a lower morbidity, especially in patients requiring HVE for longer than 60 minutes. The technical aspect requires systemic venovenous bypass. Refrigeration is performed using 2 to 4 L of University of Wisconsin solution chilled at 4°C, perfused through the portal vein and let out through a cavotomy above the inferior caval clamp. This renewed procedure, applicable in difficult and complex liver resection in patients with diseased liver, needs to be added to the armamentarium of modern surgery.

Isolated Caval Clamping

Infrahepatic Caval Clamping

The major impact of caval pressure on blood loss during liver resection has led some surgeons to propose isolated IVC clamping to decrease the CVP (Fig. 81.7) (Abdalla et al, 2004; Otsubo et al, 2004). The technique is simple and usually hemodynamically well tolerated. The technique, which decreases the CVP by approximately 4 cm H_2O, can be used alone when liver resection is performed without pedicle clamping or along with pedicle clamping. When it is used in fluid-loaded patients, the hemodynamic consequences on arterial pressure and postoperative renal function are minimal (Otsubo et al, 2004). Surgeons should consider this method especially when the anesthesiologist cannot maintain a low CVP.

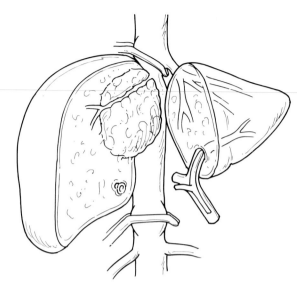

Fig. 81.8. The vena cava is isolated, while the hepatic flow is maintained through the remnant liver.

Isolated Total Caval Clamping

When a suprahepatic venous trunk is not involved by tumor that otherwise involves the vena cava, total caval clamping is feasible maintaining the hepatic flow through the remnant liver. This technique of caval clamping is indicated in patients with tumors in contact with the vena cava or near the cavohepatic junction, which necessitates en bloc resection of the IVC or cavohepatic junction. In this maneuver, the vena cava alone is clamped leaving the inflow and outflow of the remnant liver intact. This procedure requires the control of the infrahepatic vena cava and of the uninvolved venous trunk. The initial phase of the procedure consists of parenchymal transection by an anterior approach, usually under intermittent clamping, after ligation of the hepatic pedicle to the tumor-bearing hemiliver. When the parenchymal transection reaches the anterior surface of the vena cava, the tape that encircled the uninvolved venous trunk is passed behind the suprahepatic IVC. The IVC is clamped at the site of this caval tape after clamping the infrahepatic vena cava. The vena cava is isolated, while the hepatic flow is maintained through the remnant liver (Fig. 81.8). The maintenance of the flow to the suprahepatic vein through the "liver shunt" avoids splanchnic congestion, hemodynamic disturbances, and liver ischemia. The total caval clamping without liver ischemia allows comfortable caval resection and reconstruction. This procedure, which is especially indicated and efficient when there is involvement and resection of the caudate lobe, further reduces the indications for HVE to exceptional patients.

No-Clamping Technique

The ideal alternative to clamping would be to perform hepatectomy without clamping and without significant blood loss. This ideal approach is considered by many surgeons faced with major resection on underlying diseased parenchyma, living donor harvesting, and combined digestive operation to avoid splanchnic congestion on bowel anastomoses. Several conditions should be satisfied to perform a hepatectomy without clamping: (1) a low CVP; (2) completely preserved remnant liver venous drainage

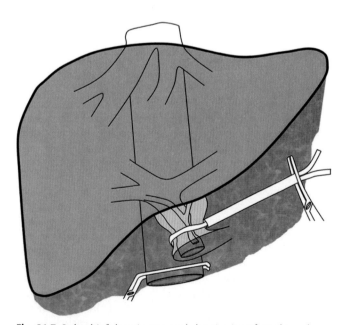

Fig. 81.7. Isolated infrahepatic vena caval clamping is performed to reduce a persistently elevated CVP.

assessed preoperatively with computed tomography scan and intraoperatively by Doppler ultrasound, and (3) possession of modern tools of parenchymal transection. Bleeding from the transection surface is minimized when the remnant liver has a patent venous drainage. Nonclamping technique should be considered essentially in major anatomic resection that preserves complete venous drainage of the remnant liver. The nonclamping technique increases liver transection time, which can be reduced by the use of several technical refinements, including ultrasonic dissector, bipolar scissors, or water-irrigated bipolar forceps. Because minimizing blood loss remains the major objective, the pedicle should be controlled and clamped if the blood loss approaches 20 mL/kg (Scatton et al, 2004).

CONCLUSION

Each vascular occlusion technique has a place in major and minor hepatic resectional surgery, based on the tumor location, presence of associated underlying liver disease, patient cardiovascular status, and experience of the operating surgeon. Understanding of the potential application of different techniques, anticipation of the expected and potential hemodynamic responses, and knowledge of the limitations of each technique are fundamental to appropriate surgical planning adapted to each patient. Experience with the various clamping methods enables an aggressive but safe approach to surgical treatment of hepatobiliary diseases, with acceptable blood loss and transfusion requirements. In all cases, surgical strategy should be defined with the anesthesiologist, particularly in regard to hemodynamic monitoring, to optimize perioperative patient management and to minimize the risk of complications, such as bleeding and air embolism.

Randomized study has shown that the added dissection, operative, and postoperative risks associated with HVE are not balanced by decreased blood loss compared with hepatic pedicle clamping except in exceptional cases when tumors involve the major hepatic veins or vena cava. In addition, dissection in preparation for clamping may be used as a safe approach technique to tumors in difficult locations, even when eventual clamping is not performed. Similarly, the liver hanging maneuver enables resection without mobilization, compression, and manipulation of large tumors.

REFERENCES

Abdalla EK, et al, 2004: Hepatic vascular occlusion: which technique? Surg Clin North Am 84:563-585.

Asahara T, et al, 1999: Perioperative blood transfusion as a prognostic indicator in patients with hepatocellular carcinoma. World J Surg 23:676-680.

Azoulay D, et al, 2005: In situ hypothermic perfusion of the liver versus standard total vascular exclusion for complex liver resection. Ann Surg 24:277-285.

Belghiti J, et al, 1996: Portal triad clamping or hepatic vascular exclusion for major liver resection: a controlled study. Ann Surg 224:155-161.

Belghiti J, et al, 1999: Continuous versus intermittent portal triad clamping for liver resection: a controlled study. Ann Surg 229:369-375.

Belghiti J, et al, 2000: Seven hundred forty-seven hepatectomies in the 1990s: an update to evaluate the actual risk of liver resection. J Am Coll Surg 191:38-46.

Belghiti J, et al, 2001: Liver hanging maneuver: a safe approach to right hepatectomy without liver mobilization. J Am Coll Surg 193:109-111.

Blumberg N, et al, 1986: Association between transfusion of whole blood and recurrence of cancer. BMJ 293:530-533.

Castaing D, et al, 1989: Segmental liver resection using ultrasound-guided selective portal venous occlusion. Ann Surg 210:20-23.

Chen H, et al, 2000: Hepatic resection using intermittent vascular inflow occlusion and low central venous pressure anesthesia improves morbidity and mortality. J Gastrointest Surg 4:162-167.

Cherqui D, et al, 1999: Hepatic vascular exclusion with preservation of the caval flow for liver resections. Ann Surg 230:24-30.

Clavien PA, et al, 2000: Protective effects of ischemic preconditioning for liver resection performed under inflow occlusion in humans. Ann Surg 232:155-162.

Clavien PA, et al, 2003: A prospective randomized study in 100 consecutive patients undergoing major liver resection with versus without ischemic preconditioning. Ann Surg 238:843-852.

Cunningham JD, et al, 1994: One hundred consecutive hepatic resections: blood loss, transfusion, and operative technique. Arch Surg 129:1050-1056.

Delva E, et al, 1984: Hemodynamic and biochemical monitoring during major liver resection with use of hepatic vascular exclusion. Surgery 95:309-318.

Delva E, et al, 1987: Hemodynamic effects of portal triad clamping in humans. Anesth Analg 66:864-868.

Delva E, et al, 1989: Vascular occlusions for liver resections: operative management and tolerance to hepatic ischemia: 142 cases. Ann Surg 209:211-218.

Elias D, et al, 1995a: Is simultaneous hepatectomy and intestinal anastomosis safe? Am J Surg 169:254-260.

Elias D, et al, 1995b: Intermittent vascular exclusion of the liver (without vena cava clamping) during major hepatectomy. Br J Surg 82:1535-1539.

Emree S, et al, 1993: Liver resection under total vascular isolation, variations on a theme. Ann Surg 217:15-19.

Eyraud D, et al, 2002: Hemodynamic and hormonal responses to the sudden interruption of caval flow: insights from a prospective study of hepatic vascular exclusion during major liver resections. Anesth Analg 95:1173-1178.

Figueras J, et al, 2005: Complete versus selective portal triad clamping for minor liver resection: a prospective randomized trial. Ann Surg 241:852-890.

Fortner JG, et al, 1974: Major hepatic resection using vascular isolation and hypothermic perfusion. Ann Surg 180:644-652.

Hardy KJ, et al, 1995: Comparison of continuous versus intermittent ischaemia-reperfusion during liver resection in an experimental model. Br J Surg 82:833-836.

Hardy KJ, et al, 1996: Ischaemic preconditioning of the liver: a preliminary study. Aust N Z J Surg 66:707-710.

Hasegawa K, et al, 2002: Effect of hypoventilation on bleeding during hepatic resection: a randomized controlled trial. Arch Surg 137:311-315.

Huguet C, et al, 1992a: Technique of hepatic vascular exclusion for extensive liver resection. Am J Surg 163:602-605.

Huguet C, et al, 1992b: Liver ischemia for hepatic resection: where is the limit? Surgery 111:251-259.

Imakita M, et al, 2000: Does topical cooling alleviate ischemia/reperfusion injury during inflow occlusion in hepatectomy? Results of an experimental and clinical study. Surg Today 30:795-804.

Imamura H, et al, 2002: Pringle's manoeuvre in living donors. Lancet 360:2049-2050.

Imamura H, et al, 2003: One thousand fifty-six hepatectomies without mortality in 8 years. Arch Surg 138:1198-1206.

Imamura H, et al, 2004: Pringle's maneuver and selective inflow occlusion in living donor liver hepatectomy. Liver Transpl 10:771-778.

Jones RM, et al, 1998: Central venous pressure and its effect on blood loss during liver resection. Br J Surg 85:1058-1060.

Kim YI, 2003: Ischemia-reperfusion injury of the human liver during hepatic resection. J Hepatobiliary Pancreat Surg 10:195-199.

Kim YI, et al, 1994: In situ and surface liver cooling with prolonged inflow occlusion during hepatectomy in patients with chronic liver disease: Arch Surg 129:620-624.

Kim YI, et al, 2002: Enhanced inflammatory cytokine production at ischemia/reperfusion in human liver resection. Hepatogastroenterology 49:1077-1082.

Kim YI, et al, 2004: 101 hepatectomies under continuous inflow occlusion following simple in-situ liver cooling in patients with chronic liver diseases. Hepatogastroenterology 51:1093-1098.

Koneru B, et al, 2005: Ischemic preconditioning in deceased donor liver transplantation: a prospective randomized clinical trial of safety and efficacy. Liver Transpl 11:196-202.

Launois B, Jamieson GG, 1992a: The importance of Glisson's capsule and its sheaths in the intrahepatic approach to resection of the liver. Surg Gynecol Obstet 174:7-10.

Launois B, Jamieson GG, 1992b: The posterior intrahepatic approach for hepatectomy or removal of segments of the liver. Surg Gynecol Obstet 174:155-158.

Majno PE, et al, 2002: Arantius' ligament approach to the left hepatic vein and to the common trunk. J Am Coll Surg 195:737-739.

Makuuchi M, et al, 1987: Safety of hemihepatic vascular occlusion during resection of the liver. Surg Gynecol Obstet 164:155-158.

Man K, et al, 1997: Prospective evaluation of Pringle maneuver in hepatectomy for liver tumors by a randomized study. Ann Surg 226:704-713.

Melendez JA, et al, 1998: Perioperative outcomes of major hepatic resections under low central venous pressure anesthesia: blood loss, blood transfusion and the risk of postoperative renal dysfunction. J Am Coll Surg 187:620-625.

Miyagawa S, et al, 1994: Changes in serum amylase level following hepatic resection in chronic liver disease. Arch Surg 129:634-638.

Miyagawa S, et al, 1996: Serum amylase elevation following hepatic resection in patients with chronic liver disease. Am J Surg 171:235-238.

Moore AF, et al, 2004: Intra-abdominal hypertension and the abdominal compartment syndrome. Br J Surg 91:1102-1110.

Otsubo T, et al, 2004: Bleeding during hepatectomy can be reduced by clamping the inferior vena cava below the liver. Surgery 135:67-73.

Poon RT, et al, 2002: Extended hepatic resection for hepatocellular carcinoma in patients with cirrhosis: is it justified? Ann Surg 236:602-611.

Redai I, et al, 2004: Anesthetic considerations during liver surgery. Surg Clin North Am 84:401-411.

Sakamoto Y, et al, 1999: Pringle's maneuver lasting 322 min. Hepatogastroenterology 46:457-458.

Scatton O, et al, 2004: Major liver resection without clamping: a prospective reappraisal in the era of modern surgical tools. J Am Coll Surg 199:702-708.

Shimamura Y, et al, 1986: Selective portal branch occlusion by balloon catheter during liver resection. Surgery 100:938-941.

Stephen MS, et al, 1996: Hepatic resection with vascular isolation and routine supraceliac aortic clamping. Am J Surg 171:351-355.

Takayama T, et al, 1998: Selective and unselective clamping in cirrhotic liver. Hepatogastroenterology 45:376-380.

Tung-Ping Poon R, et al, 2000: Risk factors, prevention, and management of postoperative recurrence after resection of hepatocellular carcinoma. Ann Surg 232:10-24.

Yamanaka N, et al, 1998: Historical evolution of hypothermic liver surgery. World J Surg 22:1104-1107.

Liver Resection in Cirrhosis of the Liver

R. T. POON AND S. T. FAN

Over the past 2 decades, partial hepatectomy has evolved from a hasty, bloody procedure with high operative mortality to a controlled and relatively bloodless operation with an acceptable mortality rate in experienced hands (see Ch. 80). Hepatectomy in the cirrhotic liver remains a difficult operation, however, with a substantial operative risk. In a study of 747 hepatectomies performed in the 1990s in a high volume center, the operative mortality among cirrhotic patients was 8.7% compared with an operative mortality of 1% in patients with normal livers (Belghiti et al, 2000).

Hepatectomy in the cirrhotic liver is performed most commonly in patients with hepatocellular carcinoma (HCC), which is one of the most common malignancies in the world. Most patients with HCC have underlying cirrhosis related to hepatitis B or C viral infection. The presence of cirrhosis not only increases the operative risk of liver resection, but also contributes to a higher risk of tumor recurrence after resection because of increased multicentric hepatocarcinogenesis in the cirrhotic liver. Nonetheless, hepatic resection remains the mainstay of potentially curative treatment for HCC. Liver transplantation offers a prospect of cure for HCC and underlying cirrhosis in a selected group of patients with early HCC (Mazzaferro et al, 1996). Its application is restricted, however, by the worldwide shortage of liver donors. Local ablative treatments, such as radiofrequency ablation (see Ch. 76c), have been used to treat small HCC (<5 cm in diameter) in the cirrhotic liver. Although ablation may be safer than hepatic resection in patients with cirrhotic livers, it is still unclear whether it could achieve long-term disease-free and overall survival results similar to those of hepatic resection. Hepatic resection should be considered the treatment of choice for patients with HCC associated with cirrhotic livers, provided that the liver function reserve is satisfactory. With appropriate attention to preoperative patient selection, operative techniques, and perioperative management, hepatectomy now can be performed in the cirrhotic liver with acceptable operative morbidity and mortality in major centers.

RISKS OF HEPATECTOMY IN THE CIRRHOTIC LIVER

Hepatectomy in cirrhotic patients is associated with increased operative risk compared with patients with a normal liver because of the increased risk of intraoperative bleeding, postoperative liver failure, ascites, and malnutrition.

Intraoperative Bleeding

The increased risk of bleeding during hepatectomy in the cirrhotic liver is related to several factors, including (1) distorted anatomy,

(2) portal hypertension, (3) difficulty in liver mobilization and transection secondary to firm liver texture, and (4) bleeding tendency. As a result of liver fibrosis and atrophy, the anatomy of cirrhotic livers is often distorted, making it difficult to identify the usual anatomic landmarks and intrahepatic vascular anatomy. The presence of large thin-walled collateral vessels in the liver ligaments and peritoneum also increases the risk of bleeding, especially when mobilization is hampered by the firm texture of the cirrhotic liver. The most difficult part of hepatic resection in the cirrhotic liver is liver transection, however. The firm liver texture hinders the exposure of the transection plane, and dissection of the fibrotic parenchyma is more challenging regardless of the techniques used. If adequate exposure cannot be achieved in the deep transection plane when performing a right or left hepatectomy, major bleeding from the middle hepatic vein branches is a frequent event. It also is more difficult to isolate such venous branches clearly in the presence of fibrotic parenchyma, making them more vulnerable during transection. In patients who have more severe cirrhosis, bleeding tendency secondary to thrombocytopenia or coagulopathy adds further challenge to the surgeon in hemostasis during liver resection.

Liver Failure

Patients with a cirrhotic liver have decreased liver function reserve and limited capacity of liver regeneration (see Ch. 80). As a result, major hepatectomy in the cirrhotic liver is associated with a significant risk of liver failure. Liver failure could occur primarily as a result of inadequate liver remnant, but more often it is precipitated by massive bleeding or septic complications. Despite improved safety of hepatectomy in recent years, postoperative liver failure still occurs in about 3% to 10% of patients after resection for HCC (Kubo et al, 2004; Osada & Saji, 2004). Liver failure is associated with a high mortality rate and is the most common cause of hospital mortality after hepatic resection in the cirrhotic liver (Belghiti et al, 2000; Wu et al, 2001). Cirrhotic patients also are prone to gradual hepatic decompensation with long-term follow-up, especially after major hepatic resection for large HCC (Huo et al, 2004).

Ascites

In the presence of significant portal hypertension, ascites is common after hepatectomy in the cirrhotic liver even when the patient does not have ascites before operation. Leakage of ascites through the wound is a common complication, which not only results in loss of electrolytes and protein, but also increases the risk of intra-abdominal infection. Gross ascites also restricts ventilation and increases the risk of pulmonary complications. Careful perioperative management is crucial in reducing the adverse impact of ascites on postoperative outcome.

Malnutrition

Cirrhosis commonly is associated with a state of protein calorie malnutrition, which may be present in 60% of cirrhotic patients and is multifactorial in etiology (Caregaro et al, 1996) (see Ch. 24). Contributing factors include reduced dietary intake, malabsorption related to small bowel dysfunction and decreased bile salts, reduced hepatic protein synthesis, and pancreatic exocrine insufficiency (Fan & Poon, 2001). Malnutrition has an important implication in cirrhotic patients undergoing hepatectomy. Patients with malnutrition are more susceptible to impaired wound healing and septic complications because of the compromise in immune function. Malnutrition may impair liver regeneration, which already is reduced in cirrhotic patients.

PREOPERATIVE ASSESSMENT AND PATIENT SELECTION

Tumor Status

The main indication for hepatectomy in the cirrhotic liver is HCC. Careful preoperative evaluation of the tumor status is essential for the selection of appropriate patients with HCC for hepatic resection. In our center, we routinely perform chest x-ray, ultrasonography, and helical contrast computed tomography (CT) for workup of patients with a potentially resectable HCC. Modern helical contrast CT provides a good assessment of the relationship of the tumor to major intrahepatic vessels; any satellite tumor nodules; and tumor invasion of the inferior vena cava (IVC), main portal vein, or intrahepatic venous branches. Magnetic resonance imaging is an alternative imaging modality for HCC used in some centers. Hepatic arteriography is performed occasionally for diagnostic purposes in patients with uncertain diagnosis of HCC on the CT scan.

The usual criteria for hepatic resection with regard to the tumor status include absence of extrahepatic metastasis and absence of tumor thrombus in the IVC or main portal vein. Although hepatic resection with removal of tumor thrombus in the IVC or main portal vein has been advocated by some authors (Konishi et al, 2001; Shirabe et al, 2001), most liver surgeons consider the presence of tumor thrombus in the IVC or main portal vein a contraindication for hepatic resection because the prognosis is usually poor even with such an aggressive approach. Hepatic resection for patients with tumor invasion of the hepatic veins or major intrahepatic branches of the portal vein is justified, however, because favorable survival results may be expected compared with nonsurgical treatment (Minigawa et al, 2001; Poon et al, 2003). Large tumor size alone should not be considered a contraindication for hepatic resection (Poon et al, 2002a; Regimbeau et al, 1999). Even in the presence of cirrhotic liver, extended hepatectomy for large HCC is justified on the condition that the liver function reserve remains satisfactory (Poon et al, 2002b).

The role of hepatic resection for bilobar HCC is more controversial. Bilobar HCC may represent advanced disease with intrahepatic metastasis from one lobe to the contralateral lobe or may represent multifocal HCC derived from multicentric hepatocarcinogenesis. Clinically, it is sometimes difficult to differentiate these two situations. Major hepatectomy in one lobe combined with wedge resection for a smaller lesion in the other lobe is possible in some cases. Alternatively, hepatic resection in one lobe can be combined with local ablation of a smaller lesion in the other lobe using ablative modalities, such as radiofrequency ablation. In a study by our group, hepatic resection for patients with bilobar HCC resulted in a better survival outcome than therapies that did not include resection (Liu et al, 2003). We recommended that hepatic resection should be considered in selected patients with bilobar HCC, especially patients with small solitary lesions in the contralateral lobe that are amenable to wedge resection or local ablative therapy.

For small HCC (≤5 cm in diameter) without macroscopic vascular invasion in a Child's A cirrhotic patient, there is controversy regarding whether hepatic resection or liver transplantation should be offered (see Chs. 71 and 103). Liver transplantation results in a better disease-free survival compared with hepatic resection, yet the overall survival results seem comparable after the two treatments (Figueras et al, 2000; Otto et al, 1998; Pichlmayr et al, 1998). In the presence of severe graft shortage, some authors, including our group, advocate hepatic resection as the first-line treatment for cirrhotic patients with small HCC and preserved liver function and reserve salvage transplantation for recurrence or deterioration of liver function after hepatic resection, which seems to be a feasible and rational strategy (Belghiti et al, 2003; Poon et al, 2002c).

Assessment of Liver Function Reserve

Careful assessment of the liver function reserve is crucial in patient selection for hepatectomy in the cirrhotic liver to avoid postoperative liver failure and mortality (see Ch. 2). Some centers rely on liver biochemistry and Child's classification alone in determining the liver function of patients. Major hepatectomy with removal of three segments or more should be performed in Child's A cirrhotic patients only, whereas minor hepatectomy of two or fewer segments may be safe in selected cases of Child's B cirrhotic patients. Child's C cirrhosis should be considered an absolute contraindication for hepatic resection.

Other centers use more sophisticated quantitative liver function tests, such as indocyanine green (ICG) clearance test (Imamura et al, 2003), galactose elimination capacity (Redaelli et al, 2002), and lidocaine test (Ravaioli et al, 2003), to predict the risk of postoperative liver failure in patients with cirrhosis. We routinely perform ICG clearance test for all patients undergoing hepatic resection for HCC. We showed in a multivariate analysis in a previous study that of many liver function tests, ICG clearance was the best test in predicting hospital mortality after major hepatectomy for HCC (Lau et al, 1997). Based on our experience of hepatectomy for HCC in the early 1990s, ICG retention at 15 minutes of less than 14% was identified as the safety limit for major hepatic resection in a study in the mid-1990s (Fan et al, 1995). With improved surgical techniques and perioperative care, however, we found that the limit could be extended. In a more recent study, the postoperative results after major hepatectomy of selected patients with ICG retention at 15 minutes higher than 14% were found to be comparable to the results of patients having ICG retention at 15 minutes less than 14% (Lam et al, 1999). Currently, we have shifted the

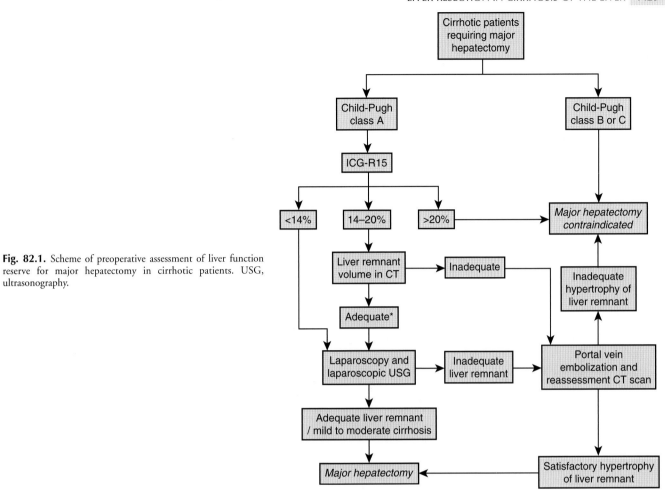

Fig. 82.1. Scheme of preoperative assessment of liver function reserve for major hepatectomy in cirrhotic patients. USG, ultrasonography.

upper limit of ICG retention at 15 minutes to 20% for major hepatectomy. For patients with borderline ICG retention at 15 minutes of 14% to 20%, attention to the size of liver remnant and severity of the cirrhosis is important to avoid postoperative liver failure.

Measurement of the volume of the remnant liver after planned resection by CT volumetry has been shown to be helpful in selecting patients for major hepatic resection. A small liver remnant volume was associated with worse postoperative liver function and a higher complication rate after extended hepatectomy (Vauthey et al, 2000). The safety limit for the remnant liver volume in patients with normal liver is controversial, however, ranging from 25% to 40% of the total nontumorous or functional liver volume as suggested by different studies (Kubota et al, 1997; Vauthey et al, 2000; Yigitler et al, 2003). The safety limit in terms of remnant liver volume in patients with cirrhosis has not been clearly documented; it would vary depending on the severity of cirrhosis. In general, a higher volume of remnant liver is required in the presence of cirrhosis, and we would not consider major hepatectomy in cirrhotic patients with a remnant liver volume less than 30% of the estimated standard liver volume. Some authors have advocated preoperative evaluation of the severity of cirrhosis by biopsy of the nontumorous liver for histologic grading of fibrosis or measurement of portal pressure, but these are not widely practiced because of the

invasiveness of these investigations (Bruix et al, 1996; Farges et al, 1999). In addition to these measures, we found the use of laparoscopy for assessment of the severity of cirrhosis and the size of the liver remnant helpful in determining the resectability of HCC in cirrhotic patients (Lo et al, 2000). Laparoscopic ultrasound can be used to evaluate any tumor nodules in the contralateral lobe of the liver or any tumor thrombus in the portal vein or the hepatic vein. Laparoscopic assessment is subjective, however, and depends on the experience of the surgeon. Fig. 82.1 summarizes the assessment of liver function reserve in cirrhotic patients planned for major hepatectomy in our center.

General Status of Patients

Attention to the general medical fitness of patients is paramount in selecting patients with HCC for hepatic resection, especially in cirrhotic patients who are at higher risk of postoperative complications. With the improved accuracy of assessment of liver function in recent years, comorbid illness has become a major factor in predicting the mortality of patients undergoing hepatectomy. In an analysis of the risk factors for postoperative mortality after extended hepatectomy for HCC in our institution, the presence of comorbid illness was one of the two independent factors predictive of perioperative mortality (Wei et al, 2003). Although the presence of severe comorbid illnesses, such as congestive heart failure and chronic renal failure, is a definite contraindication for hepatectomy for HCC, patients with less severe comorbid illnesses still may benefit from hepatic resection accompanied by meticulous perioperative care. One example is diabetes mellitus, which is a common comorbid illness in cirrhotic patients. Our previous study showed that postoperative morbidity and mortality after hepatectomy for HCC in patients with diabetes mellitus were similar to those of patients without diabetes mellitus, as long as optimal perioperative control of blood glucose level and postoperative care were provided (Poon et al, 2002d).

ROLE OF PREOPERATIVE PORTAL VEIN EMBOLIZATION

For patients who require major or extended hepatectomy, but have inadequate remnant liver volume, preoperative portal vein embolization could be used to induce hypertrophy of the remnant liver (Makuuchi et al, 1990; Vauthey et al, 2000) (see Ch. 84a). There is a general concern that preoperative portal vein embolization may be less effective in the cirrhotic liver compared with normal liver because of the impaired regenerative capacity of the cirrhotic liver as shown in an early study (Nagasue et al, 1987). A few studies have shown, however, that preoperative portal vein embolization is effective in inducing hypertrophy of remnant liver and decreasing postoperative complications in patients with cirrhotic livers undergoing hepatic resection for HCC (Azoulay et al, 2000; Farges et al, 2003). Our center also employed portal vein embolization in selected patients with cirrhosis with inadequate remnant liver volume (Fig. 82.2). There is a limitation of portal vein embolization, however, for extension of indications for hepatectomy in cirrhotic patients with HCC because the response to portal vein embolization varies according to the severity of cirrhosis (Hirohashi et al, 2004). Currently, there is no accurate predictor of the efficacy of portal vein embolization in cirrhotic patients. Some authors have suggested the use of surrogate serum markers of severity of cirrhosis, such as hyaluronic acid and procollagen

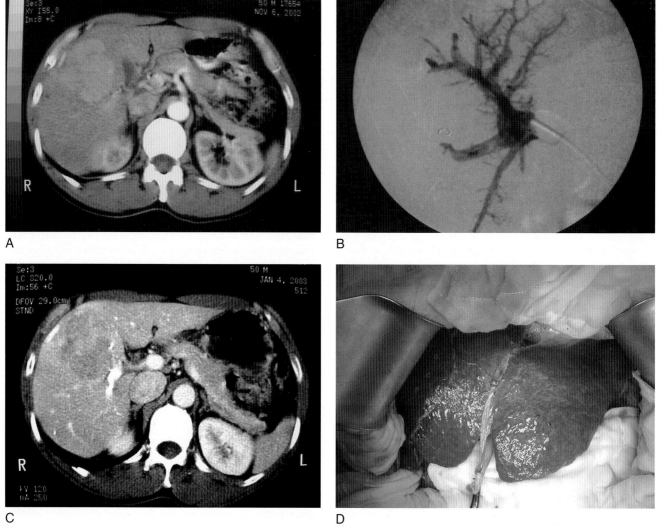

A

B

C

D

Fig. 82.2. A, Cirrhotic patient with a right lobe tumor requiring right hepatectomy, but a small left lobe (272 cm³ by CT volumetry, 24% of estimated standard liver volume). **B,** Open right portal vein embolization by a minilaparotomy via the transileocolic vein using a triple lumen balloon catheter, injecting a mixture of fibrin glue and lipiodol. **C,** Left lobe enlarged to 358 cm³ (30% of estimated standard liver volume by CT volumetry) 4 weeks after portal vein embolization. **D,** Operative photograph shows the enlarged left lobe of the liver.

type III peptide, as predictors (Hirohashi et al, 2004), but these are not widely available clinically. The possible influence of portal vein embolization on the growth of occult tumor nodules in the contralateral lobe of the liver is a theoretical concern that remains to be clarified.

OPERATIVE TECHNIQUES

The general techniques of liver resection are described in Ch. 80. This chapter focuses mainly on operative techniques specifically related to the cirrhotic liver.

Skin Incision

Bilateral subcostal incision with an upward midline extension is the standard incision for hepatic resection and is adequate for most cases of hepatectomy (Fig. 82.3A). The presence of cirrhosis frequently leads to difficulty in mobilization of a large right lobe tumor or tumors located in segment VII or VIII. In such a situation, adequate exposure can be achieved by a thoracoabdominal approach using a J-incision (see Fig. 82.3B) or a right subcostal incision with a perpendicular extension in the seventh or eighth intercostal space (see Fig. 82.3C), with the diaphragm incised. This approach also facilitates parenchymal transection by making the transection plane perpendicular to the wound. A previous study by our group showed that a thoracoabdominal approach for right-sided hepatectomy does not increase operative

morbidity compared with an abdominal approach alone and may help reduce blood loss and transfusion requirements (Xia et al, 2003). For cirrhotic patients with HCC in the superior segments of the liver located underneath the right diaphragm, an exclusive transthoracic approach has been described, but this approach allows only limited resection with a high risk of positive margin (Pocard et al, 2002). This approach was particularly advocated by Pocard and colleagues (2002) for patients with previous upper abdominal surgery or patients undergoing resection as a bridge therapy before liver transplantation.

Intraoperative Ultrasound

Intraoperative ultrasound (see Ch. 86) is an invaluable tool in hepatic resection. The proximity of the tumor to major portal or hepatic veins can be assessed, which is important in determining the extent of liver resection. Any tumor thrombus in the portal vein or hepatic vein should be noted. The use of color Doppler ultrasonography enhances the detection of tumor thrombus. Intraoperative ultrasound allows detection of additional nodules not found in the preoperative imaging studies, although sometimes it may be difficult to differentiate regenerative or dysplastic nodules from early HCC nodules by ultrasound. Intraoperative ultrasound also enables accurate marking of the transection line to ensure an adequate tumor-free margin. The use of intraoperative ultrasound helps optimize the balance between oncologic radicality and sparing of the largest amount of functioning liver parenchyma in the cirrhotic liver.

Liver Mobilization

Liver mobilization in the cirrhotic liver is technically more demanding because of the firm texture of the fibrotic liver. The collateral vessels formed secondary to portal hypertension may increase the risk of bleeding during liver mobilization. Prolonged forceful rotation of the liver increases the risk of avulsion injury to the hepatic veins and may twist the inflow and outflow vascular pedicles, resulting in ischemic damage to the remnant liver. Care should be taken to avoid prolonged rotation of the liver. Intermittent release of the liver back to the original position may help avoid ischemic damage to the liver.

In patients with a large right lobe tumor, the anterior approach (see Ch. 80) can avoid the problems of difficult mobilization of the right lobe (Liu et al, 2000). In this approach, the liver is transected from the anterior surface down to the IVC without prior mobilization of the right lobe and extrahepatic control of the right hepatic vein (Fig. 82.4). The caudate lobe, if it is to be included in the resection, is detached from the IVC. The right hepatic vein and other branches between the IVC and the liver are controlled and divided. Mobilization of the right lobe is performed by division of the triangular ligament. In the anterior approach, the liver is mobilized only after complete division of all the inflow and outflow vessels, and this has a theoretical advantage of reducing the risk of tumor cell dissemination resulting from compression of a large right lobe tumor in the conventional approach to right hepatectomy. In a retrospective analysis, we observed that patients with large right lobe HCC operated by the anterior approach were associated with a significantly better overall and disease-free survival compared with

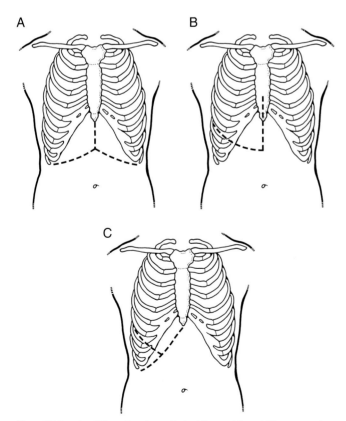

Fig. 82.3. A, Bilateral subcostal incision with midline extension. **B,** Thoracoabdominal approach by J-incision. **C,** Thoracoabdominal approach by a thoracotomy extension from the subcostal incision. An extension of the right subcostal wound to the left side may be needed in some cases.

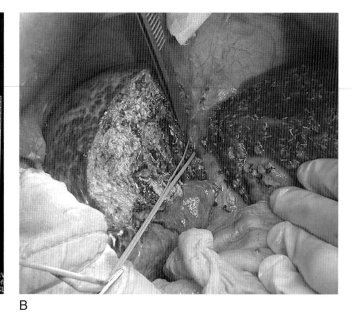

A   B

Fig. 82.4. A, Large right lobe tumor resected by right hepatectomy using the anterior approach. **B,** Transection of the liver is performed without prior mobilization of the right lobe or extrahepatic control of the right hepatic vein. Operative photograph shows completion of transection down to the IVC, with the right hepatic vein slinged.

patients operated by the conventional approach, in addition to less blood loss and lower hospital mortality (Liu et al, 2000).

Anatomic and Nonanatomic Resections

One of the major dilemmas in resection of HCC in the cirrhotic liver is the need for parenchyma preservation versus the need for adequate resection margin. Many surgeons advocate at least a 1-cm resection margin (Shi et al, 2004). There is not a strict biologic basis for choosing this cutoff value, however. In a previous study by our center, we found that a positive histologic margin, but not the width of resection margin, was a significant risk factor for an increase in the recurrence rate (Poon et al, 2000a). The need to obtain a wide margin should be balanced carefully against the need to preserve functional parenchyma in the cirrhotic liver based on individual consideration for each specific patient. Although the optimal width of resection margin is a controversial subject, most surgeons consider segmental resection superior to nonanatomic resections in oncologic clearance of HCC because of the potential intrahepatic metastasis via the segmental portal vein branch (Billingsley et al, 1998). Removal of the territory of segmental portal vein branch allows removal of potential metastatic nodules. In general, anatomic resection is preferred, but nonanatomic resections may be indicated in some patients with poor liver function reserve.

The choice of the types of anatomic resection depends on the size and location of the tumor. For large tumors in one lobe of the liver in Child's A cirrhotic patients, major hepatectomy is generally safe. The volume of nontumorous liver removed may not be substantial in the presence of a large tumor. If the remnant liver volume seems small, preoperative portal vein embolization can be used. The presence of a small HCC in the center of the right lobe or in close proximity to the right portal vein or right hepatic vein may require a right hepatectomy for complete tumor removal. This situation poses a dilemma in patients with cirrhosis because the volume of functional liver parenchyma removed is substantial. Nonetheless, in carefully

selected patients, our group has shown that major hepatectomy for small HCC is safe in patients with Child's A cirrhosis (Lang et al, 2003). For patients with more peripherally located small HCC, removal of one or two segments is the procedure of choice. Any single segment of the liver can be removed alone or in combination with adjacent segments. Central tumors located between the right and left lobes are most difficult to treat. An extended hepatectomy may sacrifice a lot of functional parenchyma. For such tumors, bisegmentectomy IV and VIII and trisegmentectomy IV, V, and VIII are safe approaches that allow preservation of functional parenchyma (Chouillard et al, 2003).

Different techniques of segmental resection exist. Intraoperative ultrasound could be used to localize vascular pedicles. Together with the help of landmarks provided by liver scissurae, the surface border of the segment could be outlined. This is a simple technique, but the exact border of the segment may not be well defined, and there is a substantial risk of bleeding in controlling the vascular pedicles deep in the transection plane. Some surgeons use ultrasound-guided injection of dye, such as methylene blue, to produce thrombosis of the portal vein, to delineate the liver territory supplied by the portal vein branch (Makuuchi et al, 1985). The success of this technique depends, however, on the expertise of the operating surgeon in interventional ultrasonography. Another approach is to control the vascular pedicles of the segment to be removed before starting liver transection, especially for right lobe tumors. This approach allows more precise delineation of the border of the segments and reduces the risk of bleeding during transection. The dissection of the vascular pedicles can be difficult in cirrhotic livers. Details of surgical techniques of different segmentectomies are described in Chs. 80 and 83.

Techniques of Liver Transection

The main difficulty of hepatic resection in the cirrhotic liver lies in the control of bleeding during transection of the liver. Hepatic transection is particularly challenging in the cirrhotic

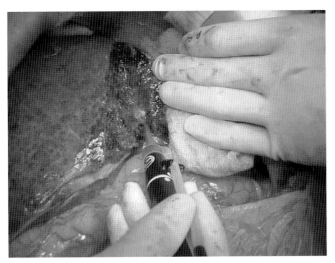

Fig. 82.5. Liver transection using an ultrasonic dissector.

liver because of the fibrotic nature of the liver tissue. Finger fracture and clamp crushing are the conventional methods of liver transection that still are used in some centers (Imamura et al, 2003; Jarnagin et al, 2002). Cavitron ultrasonic aspirator (CUSA) has become the standard technique of liver transection in many centers (Fig. 82.5). With CUSA, the liver tissue is fragmented with ultrasound and sucked off, exposing the vascular and ductal structures, which can be ligated or clipped with titanium hemoclips. A previous study from our center showed that ultrasonic dissector resulted in reduced blood loss compared with the clamp crushing technique (Fan et al, 1996). In our experience, a wider tumor-free margin could be achieved by ultrasonic dissection because of the more precise transection plane. In centers experienced in the clamp crushing technique, however, ultrasonic dissection may not offer a significant advantage in reduction of blood loss (Takayama et al, 2001).

Water jet is another technique of liver resection that works on a similar principle as CUSA in exposing the vascular and ductal structures by fragmenting softer liver tissue. This technique has not become as popular as CUSA, however. One limitation of using either CUSA or water jet in liver transection is the long transection time because of the need for ligation or clipping of individual vessels.

New technologies that allow sealing of small vessels at the same time during transection of liver parenchyma have been developed, with an aim to reduce blood loss and transection time. Such technologies may have a particular role in transection of the cirrhotic liver. One technology is Harmonic Scalpel (Ethicon Endo-Surgery, Cincinnati, OH), which employs ultrasonically activated shears to seal small vessels between the vibrating blades. The coagulation effect is caused by protein denaturation, which occurs as a result of destruction of the hydrogen bonds in proteins and generation of heat in vibrating tissue. There is some concern, however, regarding the effectiveness of sealing small intrahepatic bile ducts with this technique. A study comparing Harmonic Scalpel with the conventional clamp crushing method showed that although the Harmonic Scalpel reduced operative time, it was associated with a significantly increased rate of postoperative bile leak (Kim et al, 2003).

Weber and colleagues (2002) have described a technique of bloodless liver transection using radiofrequency thermocoagulation. In this technique, a Cool-tip radiofrequency electrode (Radionics Inc, Burlington, MA) is inserted along the transection

plane serially 1 to 2 cm apart, and radiofrequency energy is applied for 1 to 2 minutes to create overlapping cylinders of coagulated tissues, followed by transection of the coagulated liver using a simple scalpel. In the preliminary study of 15 cases of mainly segmental or wedge resection reported by Weber and colleagues (2002), the mean blood loss was only 30 ± 10 mL, and no complications, such as bile leak, were observed. Another group reported favorable results with minimal blood loss using this technique of liver resection (Stella et al, 2003). This technique has not yet been compared with CUSA or clamp crushing, but it seems to be a promising technique for wedge or segmental resection, especially in patients with cirrhosis when transection using the conventional techniques is relatively difficult. The technique is mastered easily by surgeons with the availability of the radiofrequency system. One potential disadvantage of this technique is the need to sacrifice parenchymal tissue in the liver remnant because of thermocoagulation of tissues at the transection margin, which may be a concern in cirrhotic patients requiring major liver resection. The additional 1-cm-wide tissue necrosis along the transection margin enlarges the actual resection margin, which may be an advantage in liver resection for cancers. The use of this technique in major hepatectomy is limited, however, by the possible thermal injury to the hilar structures and hepatic veins.

A new technology employing saline-linked radiofrequency energy for liver transection has become available. Compared with the technique of thermocoagulation using the Cool-tip electrode, it has a theoretical advantage in inducing a thinner zone of tissue necrosis of about 0.5 cm on each side of transection. The saline running to the tip of the electrode transmits radiofrequency energy to the liver surface and causes thermocoagulation. Our group has used a TissueLink radiofrequency dissecting sealer (TissueLink DS3.5C dissecting sealer; TissueLink Medical Inc, Dover, NH) for liver transection without the aid of any other devices, such as CUSA, in a few cases (Fig. 82.6). This device allows transection and sealing of vessels at the same time. In a preliminary experience of 10 cases, including 2 cases of right hepatectomy, the median blood loss was 100 mL (range 30-700 mL), and no postoperative bile leakage was observed. Further studies to compare this technique with CUSA or clamp crushing are needed to clarify the benefit of this new technology in liver resection. The role of this technology probably is limited to segmental or wedge excision because of the potential risk of bile duct injury when using this instrument near the liver hilum and its inability to control bleeding from large venous branches.

Use of Vascular Staplers

Staplers can be used in liver surgery for control of inflow and outflow vessels (see Ch. 80). In our center, it is now a routine practice to use an endoscopic gastrointestinal anastomosis vascular stapler to divide hepatic veins extrahepatically or during liver transection (Fig. 82.7). The use of the vascular stapler helps to reduce blood loss, especially in situations in which a big tumor in the right or left lobe hinders exposure of the right or left hepatic vein or during control of the middle hepatic vein deep in the transection plane. Exposure is particularly difficult in the presence of a cirrhotic liver. In such circumstances, there is a risk of slipping of the clamp or tearing of suture resulting in massive blood loss using the conventional technique of applying vascular clamp followed by suturing.

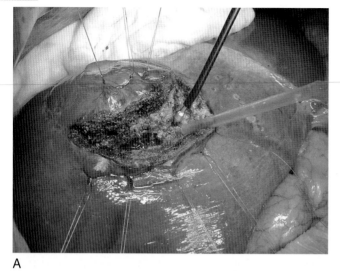

A

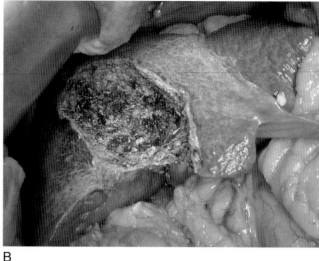

B

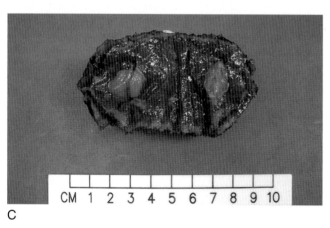

C

Fig. 82.6. A, Resection of a segment VIII tumor using a TissueLink dissecting sealer in a noncirrhotic liver. B, Transection area with secure hemostasis after a wedge excision of segment V tumor using the TissueLink dissector sealer. C, Specimen showing a 0.5-cm zone of necrosis caused by radiofrequency thermocoagulation, which theoretically may be beneficial by increasing the resection margin.

The vascular stapler also can be used to divide the hepatic duct pedicle in right or left hepatectomy. In our experience, we prefer dividing the hepatic duct pedicle during hepatic transection instead of dividing the duct extrahepatically to avoid leaving an ischemic stump of the hepatic duct, which may increase the risk of biliary fistula. The use of a vascular stapler to divide the hepatic duct saves time from suturing, but care has to be exercised not to narrow the hepatic duct confluence, especially during a right or left extended hepatectomy (Wang & Fan, 2003).

Inflow and Outflow Vascular Control

Clamping of the portal triad (Pringle's maneuver) is used frequently to reduce bleeding during hepatic transection. A previous prospective randomized trial conducted in our center showed that the use of intermittent Pringle's maneuver during liver transection was effective in reducing blood loss (Man et al, 1997). There is a limit, however, to the duration of Pringle's maneuver that can be applied. Prolonged application of Pringle's maneuver for more than 120 minutes may have a deleterious effect on liver function (Man et al, 1999).

Other authors have used total hepatic vascular exclusion instead of Pringle's maneuver to reduce blood loss in major liver resection. The relative advantage of each technique is controversial. One randomized trial showed that hepatic vascular exclusion

was associated with unpredictable hemodynamic intolerance and increased postoperative complications compared with Pringle's maneuver (Belghiti et al, 1996). Another randomized trial showed that selective hepatic vascular exclusion was well tolerated by patients and was associated with less intraoperative blood loss, better postoperative liver function, and shorter

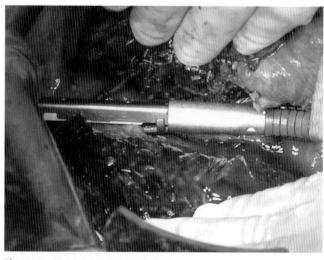

Fig. 82.7. A vascular stapler is used to divide the middle hepatic vein during liver transection in an extended right hepatectomy.

hospital stay compared with Pringle's maneuver (Smyrniotis et al, 2003).

In our experience of more than 1200 cases of hepatic resection over 14 years, total vascular exclusion has never been employed (Poon et al, 2004). Other authors also have reported that hepatic resection even for tumors close to the hepatocaval junction could be performed without total vascular exclusion (Torzilli et al, 2001). In recent years in our center, most hepatic resections were performed without Pringle's maneuver because of increased experience of the surgeons in liver resection. Despite reduced use of Pringle's maneuver, there has been a significant decrease in intraoperative blood loss in recent years, with perioperative blood transfusion rates of less than 5% (Poon et al, 2004). With the advent of new technologies of liver transection that help reduce blood loss during liver transection, it is likely that the role of Pringle's maneuver in liver resection will decline in the future.

Low Central Venous Pressure

The main source of bleeding during liver transection often comes from the hepatic venous branches, which could not be reduced even with the use of Pringle's maneuver. Such bleeding may be difficult to control with a high central venous pressure. A high central venous pressure also can lead to increased bleeding from the venous branches entering directly from the posterior aspect of the liver into the IVC during mobilization of the liver. A high central venous pressure makes repair of injury to the hepatic vein or IVC difficult.

An important advance that has contributed to reduced blood loss during liver resection in recent years is the practice of low central venous pressure anesthesia (see Ch. 80), which is achieved mainly by fluid restriction and, if necessary, morphine infusion. Isoflurane is the preferred anesthetic agent for low central venous pressure anesthesia because it produces vasodilation and only minor myocardial depression. The central venous pressure should be lowered to less than 5 mm Hg, provided that the hemodynamic status is stable. The patient is placed in 15 degrees of Trendelenburg position to counteract iatrogenic hypovolemia and to help protect the kidney. The patient should be observed carefully for the possibility of air embolism, the risk of which is increased as a result of the low filling pressure of the hepatic veins and IVC. Volume replacement can be started when hepatic transection is completed. Low central venous pressure anesthesia is well tolerated by most patients and is effective in reducing blood loss (Melendez et al, 1998) (see Ch. 25).

Role of Drainage

Ascites is common after hepatic resection in the cirrhotic liver. It is a conventional practice of many surgeons to insert an abdominal drain after hepatic resection to drain the ascitic fluid. A randomized controlled trial performed by our center showed, however, that the placement of the abdominal drain after hepatic resection in the cirrhotic liver was associated with increased wound complications, septic complications, and prolonged hospital stay (Liu et al, 2004). The drain provides a route for ascending infection and results in loss of protein and electrolytes. It is now our routine practice not to insert a drain after hepatic resection even in cirrhotic patients. Another possible function of an abdominal drain after hepatic resection is to drain bile in case of bile leakage. With the advance in the technique of liver transection, the bile leakage rate is generally low in experienced centers (Poon et al, 2004). Even if bile leakage does occur, it can be drained percutaneously under ultrasound or CT guidance.

Role of Concomitant Splenectomy

In cirrhotic patients with significant portal hypertension and hypersplenic thrombocytopenia, hepatic resection is risky. A low platelet count often is considered a contraindication for hepatic resection. Some authors advocated concomitant splenectomy in cirrhotic patients with severe hypersplenic thrombocytopenia (platelet count $<80 \times 10^9/L$) requiring hepatic resection (Oh et al, 2003; Wu et al, 2004). In one study of 41 cirrhotic patients with severe hypersplenic thrombocytopenia who underwent concomitant hepatic resection and splenectomy, there was only 1 operative mortality (2.4%), and the mortality and morbidity were not significantly different from patients who underwent hepatectomy without concomitant splenectomy in the same institution (Wu et al, 2004). The platelet count of all patients with hypersplenic thrombocytopenia returned to normal in the postoperative period after splenectomy. The long-term survival of the group with concomitant splenectomy was similar to that of patients who underwent hepatic resection without splenectomy. In that study, 40 of the 41 patients had minor hepatic resection, and the tumors in the splenectomy group were earlier tumors with smaller tumor size and less vascular invasion. Concomitant splenectomy and liver resection may be able to extend indications for hepatic resection to include patients with severe hypersplenism, but its role is confined to minor hepatic resection for small tumors. The presence of severe hypersplenic thrombocytopenia indicates severe cirrhosis, and major hepatectomy is contraindicated.

Laparoscopic Liver Resection

The application of laparoscopic surgery to liver resection (see Ch. 80) has been hindered by the limited accessibility of the liver, the difficulty in retraction of the liver, and the problem of major hemorrhage during liver transection. These problems are particularly obvious in patients with cirrhotic livers. There also is a concern of carbon dioxide embolism if a major hepatic vein is injured. In recent years, several technologic developments have made laparoscopic liver resection feasible. The development of better laparoscopic ultrasound with higher resolution and maneuverability allows accurate examination of the liver without palpation. The use of a hand port has been advocated by some groups to overcome some of the potential problems of laparoscopic liver resection (Fong et al, 2000; Huang et al, 2003). The hand port allows palpation and better retraction of the liver. More importantly, manual compression of the liver can be performed during liver transection to control hemorrhage and prevent carbon dioxide embolism in case a major intrahepatic vessel is divided. Hemorrhage during liver transection is a particularly difficult issue in laparoscopic liver resection. Not only does it risk major blood loss, but it also obscures the view for proper hemostasis. The small incision for a hand port does not diminish greatly the benefits accrued from laparoscopic surgery. The hand port site can be used to deliver a relatively large specimen intact.

CUSA dissection and water jet dissection have been employed for laparoscopic liver resection. These techniques, which are used frequently in open surgery, are not easy to apply in the laparoscopic setting, however. When CUSA is used, there is a problem of maintaining the pneumoperitoneum because of the suction. Various other laparoscopic instruments have been employed in laparoscopic liver resection, such as endostaplers, harmonic scalpel, and microwave tissue coagulator. Our group has employed the technique of radiofrequency thermocoagulation of the transection plane using the Cool-tip radiofrequency electrode, followed by transection using a simple diathermy, in laparoscopic liver resection. This is an appealing technique for minor liver resection in the laparoscopic setting. Currently, the literature contains no reports comparing the various techniques of laparoscopic liver resection. The choice of techniques is based mainly on the surgeon's personal experience and availability of instruments. Argon beam coagulator is an instrument frequently used for hemostasis in liver resection during open surgery. It also can be applied during laparoscopic liver resection. When using the argon beam coagulator in the laparoscopic setting, however, it is necessary to prevent excessive intra-abdominal pressure owing to the flow of argon gas, which may cause gas embolism when a hepatic vein is injured. To overcome the potential risk of gas embolism, some authors suggested laparoscopic liver resection using a gasless lift-up system (Itamoto et al, 2002).

To date, the use of laparoscopic liver resection generally is limited to wedge or segmental resection of lesions in the anterior and inferior segments of the liver or the left lateral segments in most centers that perform this procedure. More recently, some authors have reported successful laparoscopic resection of tumors in the right posterior segments (Huang et al, 2003). With the improvement in laparoscopic techniques of liver transection that helps to reduce the risk of major bleeding, laparoscopic liver resection is gaining popularity. Few data are available on the long-term survival outcome after laparoscopic liver resection for malignant tumors. One study showed a significantly higher 3-year survival after laparoscopic liver resection for HCC associated with chronic liver disease compared with open liver resection, whereas the tumor recurrence rates were similar between the two groups (Laurent et al, 2003). In that study, laparoscopic surgery resulted in a lower rate of decompensation of liver function after liver resection compared with the open approach. The exact mechanism was unclear, but the authors suggested that preservation of portosystemic venous collaterals in the abdominal wall and less liver trauma from manipulation of the liver could be the contributing factors. The laparoscopic approach may extend the indication of liver resection to cirrhotic patients with some evidence of liver failure that would contraindicate open surgery (Abdel-Atty et al, 1999).

POSTOPERATIVE MANAGEMENT

General Postoperative Care

Cirrhotic patients with major hepatic resection should be monitored in the intensive care unit in the immediate postoperative period. Management aims at adequate oxygenation and perfusion to ensure optimal function and regeneration of the remnant liver. With current techniques of hepatic resection, postoperative mechanical ventilation usually is not required unless there is massive intraoperative hemorrhage or significant comorbid illnesses. Adequate pain control should be provided by continuous intravenous morphine infusion if the patient requires

mechanical ventilation; otherwise, pain control should be provided by patient-controlled intravenous infusion of morphine. Adequate pain control is an important factor in reducing the incidence of pulmonary complications in our experience of hepatic resection for HCC (Poon et al, 2004).

Intravenous Fluid

Crystalloid solution (dextrose and saline) is used for maintenance of intravenous fluid. In some centers, fresh frozen plasma is used routinely for fluid replacement during and after the operation (Imamura et al, 2003). In our center, fresh frozen plasma is seldom used. Instead, we give intravenous albumin, 20 g twice daily for 3 to 5 days. Avoidance of excessive fluid is important to prevent elevation of central venous pressure, which could cause congestion of the remnant liver and impaired liver function.

Antibiotics

Prophylactic antibiotics are essential because cirrhotic patients are immunocompromised. The risk of infection is aggravated further by the prolonged operation and the high frequency of ascites. Septic complications, especially wound infection, are the most common complications after hepatectomy for HCC (Fan et al, 1999a). There is no randomized trial suggesting the optimal regimen of antibiotics. We give a broad-spectrum antibiotic on induction and for 3 days after surgery.

Nutritional Support

Because of the prevalence of malnutrition in cirrhotic patients, nutritional support is important to enhance postoperative recovery and liver regeneration. Caution should be taken to prevent central line infection when giving parenteral nutrition because sepsis is a common cause of secondary liver failure in cirrhotic patients after hepatic resection. A Broviac catheter can be inserted at the end of the operation for postoperative parenteral nutrition. A formula enriched with branched chain amino acids and medium-chain triglyceride is given for 5 to 7 days after the operation. When parenteral nutrition is given, other intravenous fluid should be withheld to avoid fluid overload and congestion of the liver. Since a randomized controlled trial published in 1994 (Fan et al, 1994) showed the benefit of parenteral nutrition in reducing postoperative morbidity, postoperative parenteral nutrition has become a routine practice in many centers for patients with cirrhosis undergoing major hepatic resection. Oral feeding is started usually on postoperative day 1 if the patient does not manifest signs of liver failure; in cirrhotic patients, an oral preparation of branched chain amino acid–enriched solution (Aminoleban EN; Otsuka Pharmaceutical Co, Ltd, Seoul, Korea) is given as a supplement to the usual diet.

PERIOPERATIVE OUTCOME

Hepatic resection for HCC in the presence of cirrhosis is a major operation associated with a significant risk of mortality. In the 1980s, the mortality rate after liver resection in cirrhotic patients was typically 15% to 30%, and liver resections in cirrhotic patients were largely restricted to segmental or subsegmental resections (Bismuth et al, 1986; Matsumata et al, 1990). Substantial improvement in the surgical techniques of hepatic resection has led to a dramatic decline in the operative mortality of hepatic resection for HCC and allowed hepatectomy in cirrhotic patients with improved outcome. We reported that even extended right or left hepatectomy could be performed in cirrhotic patients with acceptable morbidity and mortality, which were not significantly different from rates of patients with lesser resection (Poon et al, 2002a). The hospital mortality rate after hepatic resection for HCC in the cirrhotic liver reported in the recent literature ranged from 0% to 8.7% (Belghiti et al, 2000; Capussotti et al, 2004; Grazi et al, 2001; Imamura et al, 2003; Poon et al, 2004; Wu et al, 2001). The operative morbidity in these studies after hepatic resection in the cirrhotic liver remained high (30-40%), however. Further effort is required to reduce the operative morbidity.

LONG-TERM OUTCOME

In addition to reduced operative mortality, long-term survival results after resection of HCC have improved (Grazi et al, 2001; Poon et al, 2001). In a study comparing the long-term outcome of patients with hepatic resection for HCC in our institution in the years 1989-1993 and 1994-1999, we found that the overall and disease-free survival results improved significantly in the more recent period (Poon et al, 2001). In an analysis of the factors responsible for the improved outcome, we observed that a significantly reduced perioperative transfusion rate was a major contributing factor for the better long-term survival, in addition to an increased proportion of subclinical HCC detected by screening. Perioperative blood transfusion is known to induce immune suppression, which could result in an enhanced risk of tumor recurrence. The surgeon's performance in controlling bleeding and reducing blood transfusion requirement influences not only the operative mortality, but also the long-term survival (Fan et al, 1999b).

Currently, the overall 5-year survival after resection of HCC in our center is about 50% (Poon et al, 2001). Even among cirrhotic patients, the 5-year survival rate is about 45% (Poon et al, 2000b). Other centers have reported a 5-year survival rate of 32% to 49% after resection of HCC in the cirrhotic liver (Capussotti et al, 2004; Grazi et al, 2001; Yeh et al, 2002). The disease-free survival after partial hepatectomy remains unsatisfactory, however, owing to a high incidence of intrahepatic recurrence. The 5-year disease-free survival after resection of HCC in the cirrhotic liver is 22% to 28% in more recent studies (Grazi et al, 2001; Poon et al, 2001; Yeh et al, 2002). Although tumor factors, such as tumor size, presence of venous invasion, and microsatellite nodules, are important aspects determining the risk of tumor recurrence (Poon et al, 2001; Yeh et al, 2002), cirrhosis itself also is a risk factor for tumor recurrence because of the propensity of multicentric HCC development (Ko et al, 2002; Tanaka et al, 2003). Liver fibrosis or cirrhosis has a particularly prominent prognostic impact in predicting the chance of long-term survival beyond 5 years when the influence of tumor factors becomes less obvious (Bilimoria et al, 2001). Apart from the degree of fibrosis, the activity of the underlying hepatitis as reflected by preoperative serum aspartate aminotransferase also is identified as a prognostic factor for survival after resection of HCC.

In addition to the predisposing effect of cirrhosis on multicentric HCC and tumor recurrence, long-term deterioration of liver function after hepatic resection can occur, leading to complications such as variceal bleeding and spontaneous bacterial peritonitis, which have an adverse impact on prognosis (Huo et al, 2004; Poon et al, 2000b). Tumor recurrence remains the major limiting factor, however, for long-term survival among cirrhotic patients with resection of HCC because most cirrhotic patients died as a result of tumor recurrence rather than cirrhotic complications after resection of HCC (Poon et al, 2000b). Because there is no established adjuvant therapy that has been well proven to be effective in the prevention of recurrence after resection of HCC, vigilant detection and aggressive management of recurrences using various modalities, including surgical repeat resection, transarterial chemoembolization, and local ablation, is currently the most practical approach to prolong survival after resection of HCC. The improved management of intrahepatic recurrent tumors in recent years has contributed to the better survival outcome in cirrhotic patients with HCC treated by resection (Grazi et al, 2001). Nevertheless, more active research is mandatory to identify an effective neoadjuvant or adjuvant therapy, further improving the survival outcome of cirrhotic patients after hepatectomy for HCC.

REFERENCES

Abdel-Atty MY, et al, 1999: Laparoscopy extends the indications for liver resection in patients with cirrhosis. Br J Surg 86:1397-1400.

Azoulay D, et al, 2000: Percutaneous portal vein embolization increases the feasibility and safety of major liver resection for hepatocellular carcinoma in injured liver. Ann Surg 232:665-672.

Belghiti J, et al, 1996: Portal triad clamping or hepatic vascular exclusion for major liver resection: a controlled study. Ann Surg 224:155-161.

Belghiti J, et al, 2000: Seven hundred forty-seven hepatectomies in the 1990s: an update to evaluate the actual risk of liver resection. J Am Coll Surg 191:48-46.

Belghiti J, et al, 2003: Resection prior to liver transplantation for hepatocellular carcinoma. Ann Surg 238:885-893.

Bilimoria MM, et al, 2001: Underlying liver disease, not tumor factors, predicts long-term survival after resection of hepatocellular carcinoma. Arch Surg 136:528-535.

Billingsley KG, et al, 1998: Segment-oriented hepatic resection in the management of malignant neoplasms of the liver. J Am Coll Surg 187:471-481.

Bismuth H, et al, 1986: Liver resections in cirrhotic patients: a Western experience. World J Surg 10:311-317.

Bruix J, et al, 1996: Surgical resection of hepatocellular carcinoma in cirrhotic patients: prognostic value of preoperative portal pressure. Gastroenterology 111:1018-1022.

Capussotti L, et al, 2004: Major liver resections for hepatocellular carcinoma on cirrhosis: early and long-term outcomes. Liver Transpl 10(2 suppl 1): S64-S68.

Caregaro L, et al, 1996: Malnutrition in alcoholic and virus-related cirrhosis. Am J Clin Nutr 63:602-609.

Chouillard E, et al, 2003: Anatomical bi- and trisegmentectomies as alternatives to extensive liver resections. Ann Surg 238:29-34.

Fan ST, Poon RT, 2001: Liver disease and parenteral nutrition. In Rombeau JL, Rolandelli RH (eds): Clinical Nutrition: Parenteral Nutrition, 3rd ed. Philadelphia, Saunders, pp 392-406.

Fan ST, et al, 1994: Perioperative nutritional support in patients undergoing hepatectomy for hepatocellular carcinoma. N Engl J Med 331:1547-1552.

Fan ST, et al, 1995: Hospital mortality of major hepatectomy for hepatocellular carcinoma associated with cirrhosis. Arch Surg 130:198-203.

Fan ST, et al, 1996: Hepatectomy with an ultrasonic dissector for hepatocellular carcinoma. Br J Surg 83:117-120.

Fan ST, et al, 1999a: Hepatectomy for hepatocellular carcinoma: toward zero hospital deaths. Ann Surg 229:322-330.

Fan ST, et al, 1999b: Hepatectomy for hepatocellular carcinoma: the surgeon's role in long-term survival. Arch Surg 134:1124-1130.

Farges O, et al, 1999: Risk of major liver resection in patients with underlying chronic liver disease: a reappraisal. Ann Surg 229:210-215.

Farges O, et al, 2003: Portal vein embolization before right hepatectomy: prospective clinical trial. Ann Surg 237:208-217.

Figueras J, et al, 2000: Resection or transplantation for hepatocellular carcinoma in cirrhotic patients: outcomes based on indicated treatment strategy. J Am Coll Surg 190:580-587.

Fong Y, et al, 2000: Hand-assisted laparoscopic liver resection: lessons from an initial experience. Arch Surg 135:854-859.

Grazi GL, et al, 2001: Improved results of liver resection for hepatocellular carcinoma on cirrhosis give the procedure added value. Ann Surg 234:71-78.

Hirohashi K, et al, 2004: Limitation of portal vein embolization for extension of hepatectomy indication in patients with hepatocellular carcinoma. Hepatogastroenterology 51:1084-1087.

Huang MT, et al, 2003: Hand-assisted laparoscopic hepatectomy for solid tumor in the posterior portion of the right lobe: initial experience. Ann Surg 238:674-679.

Huo TI, et al, 2004: Deterioration of hepatic functional reserve in patients with hepatocellular carcinoma after resection: incidence, risk factors, and association with intrahepatic tumor recurrence. World J Surg 28:258-262.

Imamura H, et al, 2003: One thousand fifty-six hepatectomies without mortality in 8 years. Arch Surg 138:1198-1206.

Itamoto T, et al, 2002: Gasless laparoscopic hepatic resection for cirrhotic patients with solid liver tumors. Surg Laparosc Endosc Percutan Tech 12:325-330.

Jarnagin WR, et al, 2002: Improvement in perioperative outcome after hepatic resection: analysis of 1,803 consecutive cases over the past decade. Ann Surg 236:397-406.

Kim J, et al, 2003: Increased biliary fistulas after liver resection with the harmonic scalpel. Am Surg 69:815-819.

Ko S, et al, 2002: Liver fibrosis increases the risk of intrahepatic recurrence after hepatectomy for hepatocellular carcinoma. Br J Surg 89:57-62.

Konishi M, et al, 2001: Surgical treatment of hepatocellular carcinoma with direct removal of the tumor thrombus in the main portal vein. Hepatogastroenterology 48:1421-1424.

Kubo S, et al, 2004: Correlation between preoperative serum concentration of type IV collagen 7s domain and hepatic failure following resection of hepatocellular carcinoma. Ann Surg 239:186-193.

Kubota K, et al, 1997: Measurement of liver volume and hepatic functional reserve as a guide to decision-making in resectional surgery for hepatic tumors. Hepatology 26:1176-1181.

Lam CM, et al, 1999: Major hepatectomy for hepatocellular carcinoma in patients with an unsatisfactory indocyanine green clearance test. Br J Surg 86:1012-1017.

Lang BH, et al, 2003: Perioperative and long-term outcome of major hepatic resection for small solitary hepatocellular carcinoma in patients with cirrhosis. Arch Surg 138:1207-1213.

Lau H, et al, 1997: Evaluation of preoperative hepatic function in patients with hepatocellular carcinoma undergoing hepatectomy. Br J Surg 84:1255-1259.

Laurent A, et al, 2003: Laparoscopic liver resection for subcapsular hepatocellular carcinoma complicating chronic liver disease. Arch Surg 138:763-769.

Liu CL, et al, 2000: Anterior approach for major right hepatic resection for large hepatocellular carcinoma. Ann Surg 232:25-31.

Liu CL, et al, 2003: Hepatic resection for bilobar hepatocellular carcinoma: is it justified? Arch Surg 138:100-104.

Liu CL, et al, 2004: Abdominal drainage after hepatic resection is contraindicated in patients with chronic liver diseases. Ann Surg 239:194-201.

Lo CM, et al, 2000: Determining resectability for hepatocellular carcinoma: the role of laparoscopy and laparoscopic ultrasonography. J Hepatobiliary Pancreat Surg 7:260-264.

Makuuchi M, et al, 1985: Ultrasonically guided subsegmentectomy. Surg Gynecol Obstet 161:346-350.

Makuuchi M, et al, 1990: Preoperative portal embolization to increase safety of major hepatectomy for hilar bile duct carcinoma: a preliminary report. Surgery 107:521-527.

Man K, et al, 1997: Prospective evaluation of Pringle maneuver in hepatectomy for liver tumors by a randomized study. Ann Surg 226:704-713.

Man K, et al, 1999: Tolerance of the liver to intermittent Pringle maneuver in hepatectomy for liver tumors. Arch Surg 134:533-539.

Matsumata T, et al, 1990: Decreased morbidity and mortality rates in surgical patients with hepatocellular carcinoma. Br J Surg 77:677-680.

Mazzaferro V, et al, 1996: Liver transplantation for the treatment of small hepatocellular carcinoma in patients with cirrhosis. N Engl J Med 334:693-699.

Melendez JA, et al, 1998: Perioperative outcomes of major hepatic resections under low central venous pressure anesthesia: blood loss, blood transfusion, and the risk of postoperative renal dysfunction. J Am Coll Surg 187:620-625.

Minagawa M, et al, 2001: Selection criteria for hepatectomy in patients with hepatocellular carcinoma and portal vein tumor thrombus. Ann Surg 233:379-384.

Nagasue N, et al, 1987: Human liver regeneration after major hepatic resection: a study of normal liver and livers with chronic hepatitis and cirrhosis. Ann Surg 206:30-36.

Oh JW, et al, 2003: The role of splenectomy in patients with hepatocellular carcinoma and secondary hypersplenism. Yonsei Med J 44:1053-1058.

Osada S, Saji S, 2004: The clinical significance of monitoring alkaline phosphatase level to estimate postoperative liver failure after hepatectomy. Hepatogastroenterology 51:1434-1438.

Otto G, et al, 1998: Survival and recurrence after liver transplantation versus liver resection for hepatocellular carcinoma: a retrospective analysis. Ann Surg 227:424-432.

Pichlmayr R, et al, 1998: Appraisal of transplantation for malignant tumours of the liver with special reference to early stage hepatocellular carcinoma. Eur J Surg Oncol 24:60-67.

Pocard M, et al, 2002: Limits and benefits of exclusive transthoracic hepatectomy approach for patients with hepatocellular carcinoma. Hepatogastroenterology 49:32-35.

Poon RT, et al, 2000a: Significance of resection margin in hepatectomy for hepatocellular carcinoma: a critical reappraisal. Ann Surg 231:544-551.

Poon RT, et al, 2000b: Long-term prognosis after resection of hepatocellular carcinoma complicating hepatitis B–related cirrhosis. J Clin Oncol 18:1094-1101.

Poon RT, et al, 2001: Improving survival results after resection of hepatocellular carcinoma: a prospective study of 377 patients. Ann Surg 234:63-70.

Poon RT, et al, 2002a: Selection criteria for hepatic resection in patients with large hepatocellular carcinoma larger than 10 cm in diameter. J Am Coll Surg 194:592-602.

Poon RT, et al, 2002b: Extended hepatic resection for hepatocellular carcinoma in patients with cirrhosis: is it justified? Ann Surg 236:602-611.

Poon RT, et al, 2002c: Long-term survival and pattern of recurrence after resection of small hepatocellular carcinoma in patients with preserved liver function: implications for a strategy of salvage transplantation. Ann Surg 235:373-382.

Poon RT, et al, 2002d: Does diabetes mellitus influence the perioperative outcome or long-term prognosis after resection of hepatocellular carcinoma? Am J Gastroenterol 97:1480-1488.

Poon RT, et al, 2003: Prognosis after hepatic resection for stage IVA hepatocellular carcinoma: a need for reclassification. Ann Surg 237:376-383.

Poon RT, et al, 2004: Improving perioperative outcome expands the role of hepatectomy in management of benign and malignant hepatobiliary diseases: analysis of 1222 consecutive patients from a prospective database. Ann Surg 240:698-708.

Ravaioli M, et al, 2003: Operative risk by the lidocaine test (MEGX) in resected patients for HCC on cirrhosis. Hepatogastroenterology 50:1552-1555.

Redaelli CA, et al, 2002: Preoperative galactose elimination capacity predicts complications and survival after hepatic resection. Ann Surg 235:77-85.

Regimbeau JM, et al, 1999: Is surgery for large hepatocellular carcinoma justified? J Hepatol 31:1062-1068.

Shi M, et al, 2004: Micrometastases of solitary hepatocellular carcinoma and appropriate resection margin. World J Surg 28:376-381.

Shirabe K, et al, 2001: Thrombectomy before hepatic resection for hepatocellular carcinoma with a tumor thrombus extending to the inferior vena cava. Int Surg 86:141-143.

Smyrniotis VE, et al, 2003: Selective hepatic vascular exclusion versus Pringle maneuver in major liver resections: prospective study. World J Surg 27:765-769.

Stella M, et al, 2003: Radiofrequency-assisted liver resection. J Gastrointest Surg 7:797-801.

Takayama T, et al, 2001: Randomized comparison of ultrasonic vs clamp transection of the liver. Arch Surg 136:922-928.

Tanaka Y, et al, 2003: Accompanying liver cirrhosis as a risk factor for recurrence after resection of solitary hepatocellular carcinoma. Hepatogastroenterology 50:1991-1995.

Torzilli G, et al, 2001: Liver resection without total vascular exclusion: hazardous or beneficial? An analysis of our experience. Ann Surg 233: 167-175.

Vauthey JN, et al, 2000: Standardized measurement of the future liver remnant prior to extended liver resection: methodology and clinical associations. Surgery 127:512-519.

Wang WX, Fan ST, 2003: Use of the Endo-GIA vascular stapler for hepatic resection. Asian J Surg 26:193-196.

Weber JC, et al, 2002: New technique for liver resection using heat coagulative necrosis. Ann Surg 236:560-563.

Wei AC, et al, 2003: Risk factors for perioperative morbidity and mortality after extended hepatectomy for hepatocellular carcinoma. Br J Surg 90:33-41.

Wu CC, et al, 2001: Improving operative safety for cirrhotic liver resection. Br J Surg 88:210-215.

Wu CC, et al, 2004: Appraisal of concomitant splenectomy in liver resection for hepatocellular carcinoma in cirrhotic patients with hypersplenic thrombocytopenia. Surgery 136:660-668.

Xia F, et al, 2003: Thoracoabdominal approach for right-sided hepatic resection for hepatocellular carcinoma. J Am Coll Surg 196:418-427.

Yeh CN, et al, 2002: Prognostic factors of hepatic resection for hepatocellular carcinoma with cirrhosis: univariate and multivariate analysis. J Surg Oncol 81:195-202.

Yigitler C, et al, 2003: The small remnant liver after major liver resection: how common and how relevant? Liver Transpl 9:S18-S25.

83

Segment-Oriented Anatomic Liver Resections

K. H. LIAU AND R. P. DEMATTEO

Segment-oriented hepatectomy is defined as the removal of one or more of the eight anatomic segments of the liver. The techniques of segment-oriented anatomic liver resection are based on the pioneering work of Couinaud (1957), who identified intrahepatic anatomy by creating vascular and biliary casts of the liver. Couinaud (1957) established that the liver is subdivided into eight autonomous segments, each having its own biliary drainage and vascular inflow and outflow. Anatomic resection originally was described by Lortat-Jacob and Robert in 1952 and subsequently by Pack and Miller (1961) and McBride and Wallace (1972). Because each liver segment has an individual function, each segment can be removed without affecting the others (Bismuth et al, 1982). Segment-oriented liver resection is now refined and allows the surgeon to resect the liver in a variety of ways to remove pathology and preserve normal liver parenchyma (see Ch. 80).

INDICATIONS

Segment-oriented hepatectomy can be performed for benign liver processes, malignant primary liver tumors, malignant gallbladder and biliary tumors, and secondary liver neoplasms. Other indications include donor hepatectomy in living related liver transplantation and liver trauma. Patient selection for segment-oriented liver resection is based on physiologic and oncologic considerations. The main physiologic indication is to spare normal parenchyma, especially when there is a need to remove bilateral or noncontiguous segments, or when the patient has liver cirrhosis (Maddern et al, 1995). Isolated segmentectomy may be used for a small tumor in segment VII or VIII when the liver is cirrhotic and it is necessary to conserve parenchyma to minimize the risk of postoperative liver failure (Lui et al, 1995). There are also oncologic reasons to perform a segment-oriented liver resection. In primary liver tumors, initial vascular inflow control reduces the dissemination of malignant cells (Takayama & Makuuchi, 1996). In secondary liver tumors, following anatomic boundaries is more likely to achieve tumor clearance, as opposed to wedge excision, which risks fracture of the plane between the tumor and normal liver (Polk et al, 1995). Segment-oriented liver resection also offers better operative visibility because it minimizes the chance of major hemorrhage and increases the likelihood of attaining a negative microscopic margin.

TERMINOLOGY

The terminology used in this chapter follows the nomenclature based on the anatomic descriptions of Couinaud (1954, 1957) and of Bismuth (1982). Right anterior sectorectomy includes segments V and VIII, and right posterior sectorectomy includes segments VI and VII (see Ch. 1).

GENERAL OPERATIVE PRINCIPLES

Anesthesia

Liver resections generally are best performed under low central venous pressure general anesthesia (see Ch. 25). Maintaining the central venous pressure at less than 5 mm Hg during liver mobilization and parenchymal transection minimizes intraoperative blood loss (Jones et al, 1998; Melendez et al, 1998). Low central venous pressure is established by positioning the patient in Trendelenburg position at 15 degrees below horizontal, minimizing fluid infusion, and restricting intraoperative blood transfusion unless more than 25% of the blood volume is lost (Melendez et al, 1998). Systolic blood pressure is maintained at greater than 90 mm Hg, and intraoperative urine output is maintained at about 25 mL/hr. Occasionally, nitroglycerin is required when the aforementioned measures prove ineffective (Rees et al, 1996). Although low central venous pressure might expose patients to the potential risk of inadequate organ perfusion intraoperatively, the incidence of perioperative renal failure was not higher compared with historical data (Melendez et al, 1998).

Exposure

A variety of incisions can be used in liver surgery (Fig. 83.1) (see Ch. 80). Generally, a hockey stick–shaped incision or J-incision affords wide exposure for most segment-oriented liver resections. Left-sided resections can be performed through a midline incision. A right thoracic extension is rarely required, unless there is axial rotation of the liver because of liver atrophy and hypertrophy. A bilateral subcostal incision with an upward midline extension (Mercedes incision) or alone (Gable or Chevron incision) may be useful in bilateral segment-oriented liver resection, caudate resection for large tumors, and resection in large patients. Mechanical retractors, such as the Omni-tract (Omni Tract Surgical, Minneapolis, MN), Bookwalter (Codman, MA), or Ulmer retractor (Ulrich, Ulm, Germany) are generally preferred.

Adequate mobilization of the liver is mandatory for proper intraoperative assessment and subsequent performance of safe liver resection. The round ligament is divided, and the falciform ligament is taken down to its posterior limit, just anterior to the inferior vena cava (IVC). The superior ligamentous attachments are divided on the side of the segmental resection. For left-sided resections, the gastrohepatic and left triangular ligaments are divided. The gastrohepatic ligament should be inspected for a replaced left hepatic artery, which occurs in 15% to 20% of patients. For right-sided resections, the right triangular ligament should be divided. The right adrenal gland should be separated from the inferior surface of the liver after dividing the peritoneal reflection with electrocautery or a pair of dissection scissors.

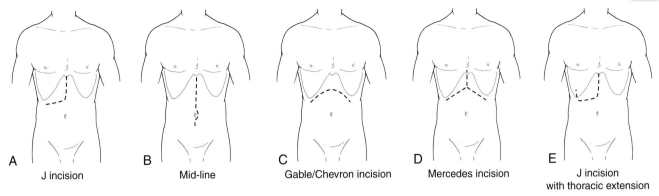

Fig. 83.1. Incisions used in partial hepatectomy. **A,** We prefer a hockey stick–shaped incision for most hepatic resections. **B,** A midline incision is adequate for thin patients or left-sided resections. **C** and **D,** Gable/Chevron (**C**) and Mercedes (**D**) incisions are needed occasionally in larger patients. **E,** A hockey stick–shaped incision with lateral thoracic extension affords generous access. It is particularly valuable when there is portal axis rotation secondary to atrophy and hypertrophy of the liver or for large tumors near the hepatic vein confluence.

Extra care must be taken during the adrenal gland dissection because the tiny adrenal veins are vulnerable to avulsion. The assistant surgeon has the important task of maintaining adequate retraction of the right liver by gradually rotating it to the left as its attachments are divided. Dissection continues until the IVC is exposed. To free the liver from the IVC, the retrohepatic venules are divided, and the dorsal ligament is transected with a pair of scissors or a vascular stapler.

Intraoperative Assessment

After the liver has been satisfactorily mobilized, it should be inspected and palpated with both hands. Next, ultrasonography should be performed to localize the lesion precisely and exclude other intrahepatic pathology (Makuuchi et al, 1987, 1991). This is a standard practice, and it may alter the planned operation in 50% of patients (Hanna et al, 1996; Kane et al, 1994; Ravikumar, 1996), although we have found that it usually does not alter the procedure when adequate preoperative radiologic assessment has been performed (Jarnagin et al, 2001). Intraoperative ultrasound may reveal the presence of tumor thrombus, tumor vascular invasion, and intrahepatic vessel patency of the portal veins and hepatic veins (Patel & Roh, 2004). In addition, intraoperative ultrasound mapping may be used in a few cases, in which early inflow control proves hazardous, to estimate the segmental boundary for parenchymal transection. Based on preoperative imaging and intraoperative findings, it is important to establish the spatial orientation of the pathology in relation to the intrahepatic vasculature and resection margin before deciding on the type of liver resection (Castaing et al, 1989; Takayama & Makuuchi, 1996).

INFLOW CONTROL

Concepts

There are three stages of performing a segment-oriented liver resection—inflow control, outflow control, and parenchymal transection. Each stage is considered in detail. Hepatic inflow derives from the hepatic artery and portal vein. Early inflow control has four primary advantages. First, as alluded to earlier, the chance of intrahepatic tumor dissemination through the

portal vein during tumor manipulation is minimized (Matsumata et al, 1989; Yamanaka et al, 1992). The second advantage is that intraoperative blood loss is minimized; this facilitates parenchymal transection and improves perioperative outcome and long-term survival (Fan et al, 1999; Jamieson et al, 1992). The other important components of minimizing intraoperative blood loss, in addition to the Trendelenburg position and low central venous pressure anesthesia, are intermittent Pringle's portal occlusion in 10- to 20-minute intervals and the use of hemostatic adjuncts, such as 3% hydrogen peroxide, the argon beam coagulator, and vascular staplers. The third benefit to inflow control is that the anatomic segmental boundaries are demarcated by the differential color change between the perfused and ischemic liver. Fourth, extrahepatic vascular and biliary variations often can be avoided by dividing the intrahepatic pedicles.

Technique

There are two primary techniques to achieve inflow control. Sectoral branches can be ligated individually outside of the liver, but it is considerably easier to divide them en masse within the glissonian sheath. In the original approach used by Lortat-Jacob and Robert (1952), the anterior peritoneum of the hepatoduodenal ligament is incised, and the common bile duct is identified before the arterial and portal confluences are exposed and their bifurcations are isolated. The alternative technique was popularized by Launois and Jamieson (1992a) and is known as the *Glissonian approach*. The Glissonian approach can be performed via a posterior intrahepatic approach or via an anterior intrahepatic approach (Launois, 1997; Launois & Jamieson, 1992b, 1992c, 1993a, 1993b). We usually prefer to achieve inflow control with the Glissonian approach using small hepatotomies or in combination with splitting the liver in the midline.

Another method of inflow control relies on the injection of methylene blue dye into a segmental or portal pedicle under intraoperative ultrasound guidance. The resultant dye staining of the segment demarcates the boundary for resection (Makuuchi et al, 1985). A last option is to use a balloon catheter to occlude the segmental portal pedicle to outline its borders (Bismuth & Dennison, 1993).

The Glissonian sheaths are divided en masse by either suture ligation or stapling. The use of endoscopic gastrointestinal anastomosis (endo-GIA [US Surgical, Norwalk, CT]) vascular staplers allows expedient and precise transection of the inflow pedicle (DeMatteo et al, 2000a; Fong & Blumgart, 1997) (see Ch. 80). Generally, the intrahepatic approach is safer in situations in which it is hazardous to control the inflow outside the liver, such as with portal hypertension where there are collateral vessels, or dense adhesions around the hepatoduodenal ligament from previous upper abdominal surgery or biliary stenting (Blumgart, 2000). The right and left hepatic pedicles usually can be isolated and divided en masse after detaching and lowering the hilar plate (Hepp & Couinaud, 1956). Isolation of the sectoral pedicles en masse may be challenging, however, unless the pedicles take off early from the main hepatic pedicle. In situations in which selective dissection of the inflow portal pedicles is difficult, one can create two small linear or cruciate hepatotomies on each side of the pedicle on the inferior surface of the liver to enable the pedicle to be encircled with a finger or a clamp (Galperin & Karagiulian, 1991). Sometimes it may be helpful to localize the pedicle with ultrasound and make a minor dissection of the parenchyma along the Glissonian sheath with an ultrasound dissector or a hydrojet device (Matsumata et al, 1992). The forceps delivers a nylon tape to encircle the Glissonian pedicle for traction to facilitate subsequent inflow control using either a vascular stapler or suture ligation. For safe and successful extrahepatic inflow control, factors for consideration include classic vascular anatomy, ability to lower the hilar plate adequately, tumor location being away from the proximal inflow pedicle or the hilum, and the absence of tumor thrombus. The various techniques to control the right or left pedicle are discussed in Ch. 80.

OUTFLOW CONTROL

Technique

Hepatic outflow consists primarily of the right, middle, and left hepatic veins. Additional venous outflow is provided by the short retrohepatic veins, umbilical fissure vein, and, in some patients, an inferior or accessory hepatic vein. The three major hepatic veins each have an extrahepatic length of 0.5 to 1.5 cm (Skandalakis et al, 2004). Almost invariably, the right hepatic vein drains independently into the IVC, whereas in about 60% of individuals, the middle and left hepatic veins unite to form a common trunk (Healey & Schwartz, 1964). In the remaining individuals, the middle and the left hepatic veins enter directly into the IVC without a common trunk. The roots of the right hepatic vein and the common trunk can be approached extrahepatically and stapled with an endo-GIA vascular stapler (Ramacciato et al, 1996; Voyles & Vogel, 1989). If the confluence of the middle hepatic vein, left hepatic vein, and umbilical fissure vein is deep in the parenchyma, an intrahepatic approach is necessary for selective conservation of the outflow.

Short Retrohepatic Veins

Dividing the retrohepatic veins is necessary to mobilize the right hemiliver completely. This step allows the liver to be separated from the anterior wall of the IVC. To avoid inadvertent avulsion of these fragile veins, the assistant surgeon gently retracts the right hemiliver to the left, while the retrohepatic veins are clipped or ligated and divided systematically in a caudad-to-cephalad

direction until the right hepatic vein is reached. In the vicinity of the right hepatic vein, clips should be avoided if an endo-GIA vascular stapler is to be employed (Fong & Blumgart, 1997). Visualization can be improved by rotating the operating table to the left with the operating surgeon sitting down so that the operative field is at eye level. An additional light source to enhance the operation field illumination may be helpful.

Right Hepatic Vein

Exposure of the right hepatic vein at the junction of IVC requires complete division of the dorsal retrocaval ligament that bridges the caudate and segment VII. A vascular stapler may be used to divide the ligament. Subsequently, a tunnel between the right hepatic vein and the posterior surface of the liver is created. A notch on the superior border of the liver marks the right hepatic vein anteriorly. A vascular clamp or vessel loop is used to encircle it for temporary occlusion during liver transection. This maneuver minimizes backflow bleeding during transection. When the vein has to be sacrificed, it can be divided with a vascular stapler or suture ligation. It is usually necessary to preserve the right hepatic vein during right anterior sectorectomy, whereas preservation is optional in right posterior sectorectomy or resection of segment VII. Whether the right hepatic vein is to be preserved or sacrificed, it is often advisable to gain vascular control of the right hepatic vein whenever difficult resections of segment VII or VIII or a right posterior sectorectomy is planned.

Left Hepatic Vein

The left hepatic vein is preserved in isolated resection of segment II or III, and extrahepatic control of the vein is usually unnecessary if the central venous pressure is low. In left lateral segmentectomy, the left hepatic vein can be approached and stapled within the liver. If the tumor is situated near the proximal left hepatic vein, extrahepatic control of the vein before parenchymal transection is advocated as a safety measure. To show the main trunk of the left hepatic vein, the liver is first rotated to the right after full mobilization of the left hemiliver. The crucial step here is to identify the tunnel that exists behind the left hepatic vein and in front of the IVC. This angle is best exposed by dividing the cephalad portion of the ligamentum venosum and dropping the top of the caudate off of the IVC (see Ch. 80). When the middle and left hepatic veins join within the liver parenchyma, it is easier to gain control of both veins en masse.

Middle Hepatic Vein

The middle hepatic vein is ligated and divided during a central liver resection. Here, the middle hepatic vein is stapled at the completion of the parenchymal transection. At this stage, the danger exists of tearing the thin-walled middle hepatic vein when handling the mobile central liver. In monosegmentectomy, the middle hepatic vein is rarely sacrificed, unless it is necessary for oncologic clearance in resection of segment IV. The decision to preserve or sacrifice the middle hepatic vein in right anterior sectorectomy depends on the proximity of tumor to the vein. Sacrificing the middle hepatic vein seldom affects segment IV because of the collateral drainage provided by the umbilical fissure vein. Extrahepatic control of the middle hepatic vein may not be necessary, unless the tumor is near its trunk. In that case, it may be safer to encircle the middle hepatic vein together with the left hepatic vein en masse as previously described.

Inferior or Accessory Hepatic Vein

About 25% of patients have an accessory right hepatic vein (also known as an inferior right hepatic vein) that drains directly into the IVC (Baer et al, 1991a; Makuuchi et al, 1985). This vein is identified and divided during a right posterior sectorectomy. In resection of segment VII, the right hepatic vein may be sacrificed without the fear of postoperative congestion of segment VI if collateral venous drainage of segment VI through a right accessory vein or variant segment VI drainage from the middle hepatic vein is present (Makuuchi et al, 1983, 2002). In isolated caudate resection, the right accessory hepatic vein is ligated and divided to free the caudate from the IVC.

PARENCHYMAL TRANSECTION

Techniques (see Ch. 80)

The liver parenchyma can be divided by a variety of methods, including finger fracture (Lin et al, 1958); crushing with a clamp (Lin, 1973), such as a Storm-Longmire clamp (Storm & Longmire, 1971) or nowadays a Kelly clamp; Cavitron ultrasonic aspirator (Fasulo et al, 1992; Storck et al, 1991); hydrojet (Baer et al, 1991b; Rau et al, 1995a, 1995b); or thermal disruption, such as electrocautery or the harmonic scalpel (Hodgson & DelGuercio, 1984; Kokudo et al, 2000). First, electrocautery is used to score the liver capsule along the line of demarcation outlined by clamping or ligation of the vascular inflow. Stay sutures are placed at the liver edges to provide traction and exposure during parenchymal transection. Transection begins from the free edge of the liver, where it is relatively thin. For liver parenchymal division, we prefer the stapler-assisted parenchymal transection technique (Fong & Blumgart, 1997). First, repeated steps of parenchyma crushing are carried out using a pair of Kelly forceps (Lin, 1974); next, any small intervening vessels are clipped and divided. Larger vessels are stapled with an endo-GIA vascular stapler. Intermittent Pringle's portal occlusion of 10- to 20-minute intervals with 5 minutes of restored flow is used (Cunningham et al, 1994; Man et al, 1997). Even in the noncirrhotic liver, which can tolerate warm ischemia for 60 minutes, intermittent Pringle's portal occlusion still is preferred because it allows decompression of the mesenteric veins during the parenchymal transection phase and minimizes bowel congestion and postoperative ileus.

Hemostasis and Biliary Control

Intraoperative hemorrhage usually should be dealt with immediately because deferring hemostasis may result in excessive and unnecessary blood loss. A variety of techniques are available. Bleeding from small, transverse branches can be controlled with clips or electrocautery. Bleeding from a large or main hepatic vein often requires a stitch or use of a vascular stapler. Suturing the liver substance in a blind fashion is often ineffective, unless

part of a nearby portal structure or the liver capsule can be included. Oozing from the raw liver surface is controlled with microfibrillar collagen hemostat (Avitene Hemostat) and the argon-beam coagulator, which produces a surface coagulum to plug the vessels (Postema et al, 1993).

Control of bile duct leakage also must be achieved at the conclusion of a segment-oriented hepatectomy. Overall, bile leak from the cut end of the liver, in the absence of a biliary reconstruction, develops infrequently. An onlay omental flap can be used to reduce biliary leakage. If a bile leak is suspected to come from a main bile duct, it must be sought and repaired. When the source of a bile leak cannot be identified by inspection, intraoperative cholangiogram or infusion of water or dye into the cystic duct may be helpful. Placing a piece of white gauze over the raw liver surface is an alternative method to uncover a minor bile leak, which may be localized through bile staining on the gauze. Some authors advocate fibrin glue to seal the liver surface (Kohno et al, 1992). Drains are unnecessary for routine segment-oriented liver resection, unless concomitant biliary resection and reconstruction have been performed (Fong et al, 1996; Liu et al, 2004).

SPECIAL CONSIDERATIONS

Anatomic Variability

Variability in the hepatic vasculature and ductal anatomy is common (see Ch. 1). Liver surgeons must be vigilant in looking for anatomic variants. Preoperative imaging using computed tomography (CT) and CT angiography may identify nonstandard anatomy. In 30% of patients, the right posterior sectoral duct or the right anterior sectoral duct drains directly into the main left hepatic duct (Healey & Schroy, 1953). Injury to aberrant bile ducts may cause major morbidity. Whenever there is uncertainty regarding hepatic pedicle anatomy, it may be better to avoid early ligation of major structures. Hepatic and sectoral pedicles always can be identified after parenchymal transection, when the major ducts at the level of the hilar plate are defined. Other vascular and anatomic variations that influence the planning of segment-oriented liver resection include outflow of segment VI draining mainly into the middle hepatic vein and the right posterior sectoral pedicle supplying only segment VI.

Coexisting Pathology

Segment-oriented liver resection is generally safe except in the presence of portal hypertension with associated collaterals, previous right upper abdominal surgery accompanied by dense adhesions, rich neovascularization around an exophytic tumor, or polycystic liver. Dissection at the hilum may prove hazardous in these situations. In addition, liver cirrhosis and preoperative portal vein embolization may distort liver anatomy. Anatomic distortion secondary to hypertrophy and atrophy of the liver may present special challenges in inflow and outflow control. The structures in the porta hepatis often are rotated in a hypertrophied or atrophied liver. These factors generally can be anticipated based on cross-sectional imaging and should be taken into account during preoperative planning. A right thoracoabdominal incision may be necessary to access the hilum when the liver has rotated markedly because of right hemiliver atrophy.

Location of Pathology

As mentioned earlier, the location of a lesion dictates the surgical approach. If a tumor is located near the proximal inflow pedicles, the pedicle ligation approach is contraindicated. Likewise, when a tumor is located near the trunks of the hepatic veins, segmental resection may not allow tumor clearance, and a more extensive liver resection may be necessary.

Tumor Thrombus

Tumor thrombus sometimes is encountered with malignant tumors, such as hepatocellular carcinoma. If tumor resection with portal vein thrombectomy is planned, an extrahepatic dissection of the portal structures is performed, and the portal vein is opened to remove the thrombus.

SPECIFIC SEGMENTAL PROCEDURES

Monosegmentectomy

Segment I (see Ch. 80)

The caudate receives blood from the left and right hepatic arteries and portal veins. Care should be exercised in dividing the short branches from the posterior aspects of the right and left main lobar vessels. The inflow from the left portal vein and

left hepatic artery is accessible at the base of the umbilical fissure when approached from the left side of the liver. To ensure adequate exposure, it is necessary to divide the gastrohepatic ligament and transect the ligamentum venosum at the root of the hepatic vein, which is facilitated by lifting the left lateral segment anteriorly. A constant venule arises from the lateral portion of the right portal vein and enters segment VI.

Numerous, small, retrohepatic veins constitute the outflow of the caudate. To gain access to these veins from the left side (Fig. 83.2), the gastrohepatic ligament and the fibrous retrocaval ligament between the caudate and the left side of the IVC have to be divided (Takayama & Makuuchi, 1996). For a small tumor in the caudate, these veins can be exposed from the left side without having to mobilize completely the right hemiliver. Access from the left side is often limited with a large and bulky tumor located in the caudate, however, and it is generally safer to mobilize the right liver and approach the outflow from the right side (Fig. 83.3) (Lerut et al, 1990).

When the caudate is fully mobilized and devitalized, the parenchymal bridge joining the caudate to segments VI and VII is clearly displayed. To deliver the caudate specimen, it is necessary to transect this tissue (Bartlett et al, 1996; Lerut et al, 1990). This maneuver is particularly challenging if the caudate tumor is large because there is limited space in which to work. Approaching the caudate from both sides often is required. When transecting the anterior boundary of the caudate lobe, great care must be taken to avoid injuring the middle and left hepatic veins. With a large tumor, it may be prudent to control the left

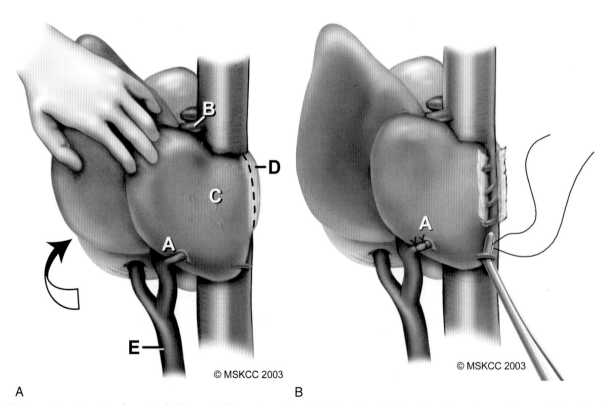

A   B

Fig. 83.2. Approach to the caudate from the left. The portal inflow to the caudate *(A)*, left hepatic vein *(B)*, caudate *(C)*, caudate-caval ligament *(D)*, and main portal vein *(E)* is shown. **A,** The left liver is mobilized by dividing the gastrohepatic and left triangular ligaments. The caudate and caudate-caval ligament are exposed by rotating the left lateral segment to the right side. The caudate-caval ligament is divided. **B,** The portal inflow is divided. Multiple venules are ligated and divided from below upward to detach the caudate from the IVC.
(From Liau KH, et al, 2004: Segment-oriented approach to liver resection. Surg Clin North Am 84:543-561.)

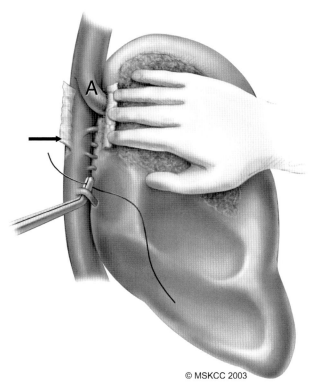

Fig. 83.3. Approach to the caudate from the right. The right liver is mobilized by dividing the right triangular ligament and the inferior peritoneal attachments. The liver is rotated to the left to expose the dorsal ligament *(arrow)*, which is divided to expose the right hepatic vein *(A)*. The short draining veins of the caudate are clipped or tied and divided.
(From Liau KH, et al, 2004: Segment-oriented approach to liver resection. Surg Clin North Am 84:543-561.)

and middle hepatic veins outside the liver and occasionally the suprahepatic IVC as well. The split liver technique, described by Yamamoto and colleagues (1992, 1999), is sometimes useful because it provides direct visualization of the middle hepatic vein, reducing the chance of injury to it (Fig. 83.4) (Liau et al, 2004).

Segments II and III (see also "Left Lateral Segmentectomy")

The segment II and III inflow pedicles arise directly from the umbilical portion of the left main portal vein in the umbilical fissure (Fig. 83.5). To isolate these pedicles, it is necessary to lift the left hemiliver with traction on the divided falciform ligament. The parenchymal bridge (if present) between segments III and IV and anterior to the umbilical fissure is divided with an endo-GIA stapler or electrocautery. Dissection to the left of the umbilical fissure allows for isolation of the segment II and III pedicles. When a tumor is distant from the umbilical fissure, these pedicles can be accessed and ligated via minor hepatotomies; otherwise, the main left portal pedicle must be dissected.

The transection plane between segments II and III is oriented in an oblique anterocranial plane. During transection along this plane, the left hepatic vein is encountered and should be preserved. The medial extent of a segment III resection lies just to the left of the umbilical fissure.

Segment IV

Segment IV is supplied by various pedicles arising from the left main portal pedicle with the liver. The segment IV pedicles can be approached directly just to the right of the umbilical fissure. If a tumor is not located near the umbilical fissure, the transection plane can be slightly more to the right, to avoid inadvertent injury to the left pedicle (Fig. 83.6). The right extent of a segment IV resection corresponds to the line of Cantlie. Transection can occur on the medial or lateral side of the middle hepatic vein. Overall, the sequence of parenchymal transection begins on the left side, then the right side, and finally a transverse resection of the superior boundary is used to detach segment IV from the caudate posteriorly.

Segments V and VI

The inflow to segment V arises as a branch from the anterior sectoral pedicle. The direction of the glissonian sheath is often anteroposterior and straight. To gain control and ligate the segment V pedicle early, the right anterior sectoral pedicle is dissected at the hilum (Fig. 83.7). This dissection may prove technically difficult, however, if the right anterior and posterior

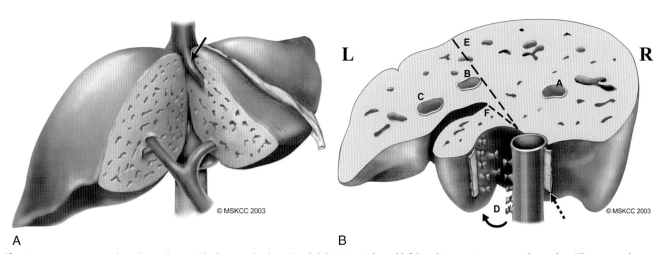

A   B

Fig. 83.4. Anterior approach to the caudate. **A,** The liver is split along Cantlie's line into right and left hemilivers to gain access to the caudate. The correct plane can be approximated by the line connecting the gallbladder fossa to the left border of the IVC cephalad. This approach allows direct visualization of the middle hepatic vein *(arrow)*, minimizing the risk of iatrogenic vascular injury. **B,** Posterior view of the liver in cross-section shows that the caudate is separated from the IVC after ligation and division of the caudate veins *(D)*. The caudate-caval ligament has been divided *(broken arrow)*. The line of transection of the caudate *(broken line at F)* and Cantlie's line *(broken line at E)* are shown. The right *(A)*, middle *(B)*, and left *(C)* hepatic veins also are shown.
(From Liau KH, et al, 2004: Segment-oriented approach to liver resection. Surg Clin North Am 84:543-561.)

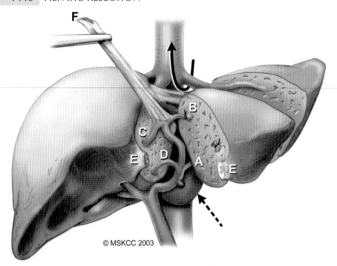

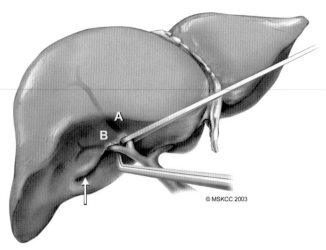

Fig. 83.5. Resection of segment III. The bridge of liver tissue *(E)* concealing the base of the umbilical fissure is divided with cautery. The falciform ligament *(F)* is retracted upward to display the umbilical fissure. The caudate lobe *(broken arrow)* and the pedicles to segment II *(A)*, segment III *(B)*, and segment IV *(C and D)* are shown. The segment III inflow pedicle is ligated at the umbilical fissure where it branches directly from the umbilical portion of the left main portal pedicle, which should be carefully preserved. The left hepatic vein may be isolated by tunneling behind it as shown by a *curved solid arrow.* In most patients, the left hepatic vein and middle hepatic vein join within the liver, so selective isolation of the left hepatic vein outside the liver may be impossible. The plane of transection is just to the left of the umbilical fissure and in an oblique anterocranial plane adjacent to segment II. Care should be taken to preserve the inflow and outflow of segment II.
(From Liau KH, et al, 2004: Segment-oriented approach to liver resection. Surg Clin North Am 84:543-561.)

Fig. 83.7. Isolation of the right anterior and posterior sectoral pedicles. The right anterior *(A)* and right posterior *(B)* sectoral pedicles can be traced from the porta hepatis, or if the tumor is at a distance from their origin, the sectoral pedicles can be isolated through the use of hepatotomies. The fissure of Ganz *(arrow)* marks the location of the right posterior sectoral pedicle in about 70% of patients.
(From Liau KH, et al, 2004: Segment-oriented approach to liver resection. Surg Clin North Am 84:543-561.)

sectoral pedicles branch distally within the liver parenchyma. In this situation, minor hepatotomies to approach the right anterior sectoral pedicle or the intrahepatic approach to gain access to the segment V pedicle is necessary.

The segment VI inflow pedicle is identified by first isolating the right posterior sectoral pedicle at the hilum. The pedicle is

sought during parenchymal transection through the plane of segment VI. Alternatively, if hilar dissection is hazardous, ultrasound can be used to guide the transection plane and ligate the pedicle within the liver.

The right sagittal transection plane of segment V corresponds to the left transection plane of segment VI. The left plane of segment V is along Cantlie's line. These resection planes can be precisely demarcated by selectively clamping the right anterior sectoral pedicle. Cholecystectomy is performed to facilitate transection of this plane. The superior extent of resection is a transverse plane that crosses the hepatic hilum.

Segment VII
The deep inflow pedicles and the anatomic location of segment VII high up beneath the diaphragm make it technically difficult to approach. This pedicle is best approached intrahepatically after fully mobilizing the right hemiliver. The liver is transected along the transverse plane through the hilum. The segment VII inflow pedicle, a branch from the right posterior sectoral pedicle, is identified by its upward course and secured within the parenchyma. The final step is to transect the medial boundary in the plane just lateral to the right hepatic vein. This plane also may be outlined early in the operation by selectively clamping the right posterior sectoral pedicle located in the fissure of Ganz, also known as the *recessus dextra of Ganz*.

Segment VIII
Similar to the segment VII vascular pedicle, the segment VIII vascular pedicle is best approached within the liver. To isolate this pedicle, the liver is first split in the principal plane through Cantlie's line, leaving the middle hepatic vein on the left hemiliver. Cantlie's line can be estimated by connecting a line through the gallbladder fossa and the left border of the IVC. A more precise delineation is made by clamping the right sectoral pedicle or the right main portal pedicle. In resection of segment VIII, it is technically more advantageous to clamp the right anterior sectoral pedicle because it demarcates the right and left resection boundaries of segment VIII.

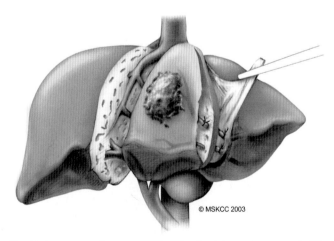

Fig. 83.6. Resection of segment IV. The hilar plate is lowered to protect the bile duct confluence. The left boundary of the parenchymal transection is just a few millimeters to the right of the umbilical fissure. The right parenchymal transection boundary is along Cantlie's line. The segment IV inflow pedicles are ligated at the umbilical fissure as they emerge from the umbilical portion of the left hepatic pedicle.
(From Liau KH, et al, 2004: Segment-oriented approach to liver resection. Surg Clin North Am 84:543-561.)

Segment VIII resection has four resection planes—right, left, inferior, and posterior. The left parenchymal transection plane is accomplished when the liver is split along Cantlie's line, which minimizes the risk of damaging vascular structures (Mazziotti et al, 2000). As the incision deepens toward the IVC, a large transversely running tributary, the vein of segment VIII, is ligated. The second step involves parenchymal transection of the inferior boundary of segment VIII, which corresponds to the transverse plane through the liver hilum. During transection of this plane, the segment VIII vascular pedicle is sought (Fig. 83.8). Care should be taken to preserve the right anterior and posterior sectoral pedicles and the segment VII vascular pedicle. After control of the inflow, the right boundary, which is in the plane just to the left of the right hepatic vein, is dissected. The parenchymal transection is completed by detaching the posterior boundary from the anterior surface of the IVC, between the main trunks of the middle and right hepatic veins.

In segment VIII resection, the limited operative space between the right and middle hepatic veins makes it difficult for the surgeon to control a major hemorrhage. It is imperative to pay careful attention to preserving the right and middle hepatic veins during parenchymal dissection at the posterior boundary. If the tumor is situated at the crotch of these hepatic veins, a more extensive resection should be considered because there is a tendency not to go deep enough into the liver, and an oncologic resection may not be achieved.

Bisegmentectomy

Right Anterior Sectorectomy
After cholecystectomy, the right main portal pedicle can be isolated by first lowering the hilar plate and then dissecting proximally until it bifurcates into the right anterior and right posterior sectoral pedicles. The right anterior sectoral pedicle can be encircled with a nylon tape, if its origin is not too distal. In that case, minor hepatotomies to allow access to the origin of the sectoral pedicle may be helpful. Caution should be taken to avoid injuring the right posterior sectoral pedicle.

The right posterior biliary duct hooks around the right posterior sectoral portal vein, in an area known as *Hjortsjo's crook* (Hjortsjo, 1951). To avoid compromising the duct, the right anterior sectoral pedicle must be divided as far distally as possible. It should be a routine practice to check the vascularity of segments VI and VII at the end of right anterior sectorectomy because segment VI sometimes drains mainly via the middle hepatic vein.

Liver transection begins along the sagittal plane through Cantlie's line, then follows the plane through the right hepatic vein. These two planes meet anterior to the IVC (Fig. 83.9). It is wise to stay a few millimeters away from the right and middle hepatic veins if they are to be conserved.

Right Posterior Sectorectomy
The left transection plane is demarcated by clamping the right posterior sectoral pedicle. The fissure of Ganz (recessus dextra of Ganz) is a helpful surface landmark in locating the right posterior sectoral pedicle and is present in 70% of patients. The pedicle may be visualized and controlled at the base of the fissure of Ganz. Otherwise, it can be isolated by minor hepatotomies (Raynaud et al, 1991) or by lowering the hilar plate and pedicle dissection. After isolating the pedicle, a nylon tape is placed around it for countertraction during application of the stapler for division. Demarcation of the liver surface is outlined with cautery. Dissection should be on either side of the right hepatic vein depending on whether it is to be sacrificed. Complete right hemiliver mobilization is crucial for these maneuvers.

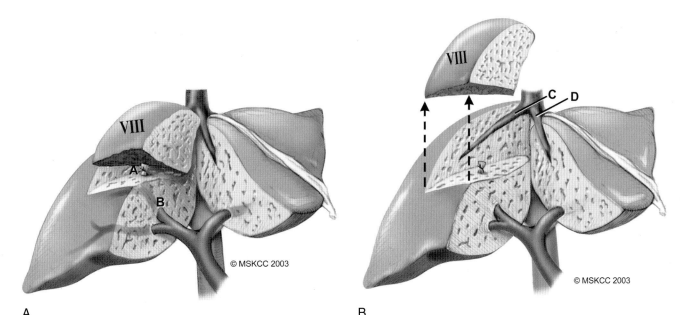

A   **B**

Fig. 83.8. Resection of segment VIII. **A,** Segment VIII resection begins with splitting the liver through the line of Cantlie. Next, parenchymal transection is performed in the horizontal plane that passes through the hilum to expose the segment VIII pedicle (A). Care should be taken to preserve the right anterior (B) and right posterior sectoral pedicles. **B,** The resection is completed by dividing the liver just to the left of the right hepatic vein (C). The middle hepatic vein (D) is resected if necessary, depending on the location of the tumor.
(From Liau KH, et al, 2004: Segment-oriented approach to liver resection. Surg Clin North Am 84:543-561.)

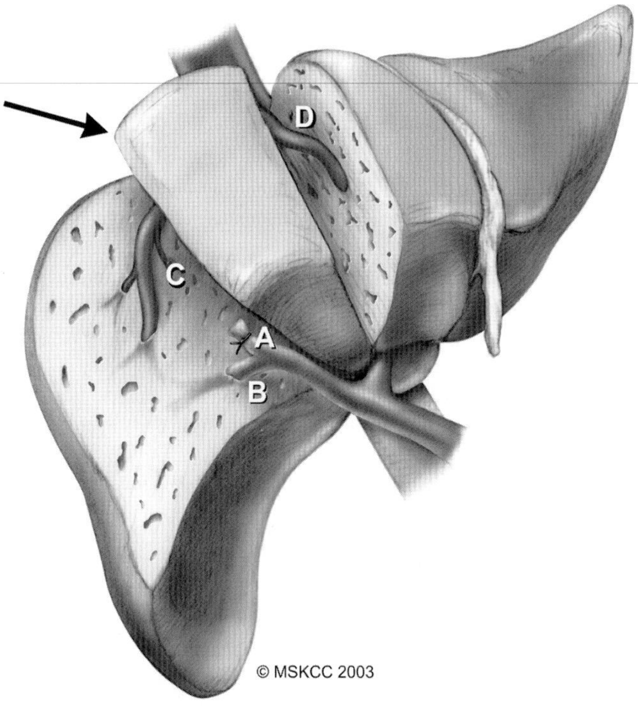

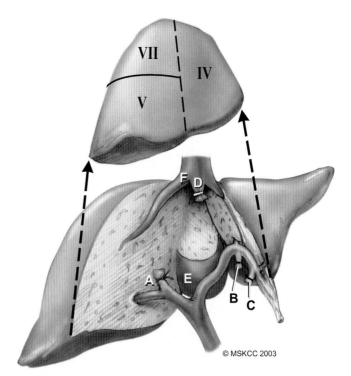

Fig. 83.9. Right anterior sectorectomy. After the hilar plate is lowered, the right anterior sectoral pedicle *(A)* is isolated by following the extrahepatic main right portal pedicle or by using hepatotomies. The pedicle is clamped to demarcate the anterior sector *(arrow)*. The right posterior sectoral pedicle *(B)* is identified and preserved. The planes of transection are just to the left of the right hepatic vein *(C)* and through the line of Cantlie. The middle hepatic vein *(D)* may be sacrificed if the tumor lies near it.
(From Liau KH, et al, 2004: Segment-oriented approach to liver resection. Surg Clin North Am 84:543-561.)

Left Lateral Segmentectomy (see also "Segments I and II")

Inflow to the left lateral segment consists of the segment II and III vascular pedicles. The location of the tumor in relation to its proximity to the umbilical fissure influences the choice of the approach to inflow control. When the tumor is located peripherally, the inflow pedicles can be taken within the liver at some distance from their origin. Otherwise, dissection of the umbilical fissure is required. Parenchymal division is performed in the sagittal plane to the left of the umbilical fissure. Demarcation is unnecessary because the umbilical fissure is a reliable landmark. The liver usually can be divided directly under inflow control using Pringle's maneuver. If the umbilical fissure vein is to be preserved, the transection plane is placed 5 to 10 mm away to the left of the umbilical fissure. In the intrahepatic approach to inflow and outflow control, the first major pedicle encountered is the segment III inflow pedicle, and the segment II inflow pedicle is about 1 inch deeper. The left hepatic vein lies cephalad and is superficial to the liver capsule.

Multisegmentectomy

Central Liver Resection (Mesohepatectomy)

The inflow of the central liver derives from the right and left main hepatic pedicles. After cholecystectomy, the hilum and umbilical fissure are dissected. Segment IV vascular pedicles are divided first (Fig. 83.10). Parenchymal division continues cephalad to the

main trunk of the middle hepatic vein. The right anterior sectoral pedicle is isolated. Next, liver transection proceeds in the plane of the right hepatic vein up to the top. The central liver is now freely attached to the middle hepatic vein. If the middle hepatic vein has not been controlled extrahepatically, it should be taken carefully within the liver. While stapling the middle hepatic vein, excessive traction on the vein should be avoided to prevent avulsion injury. On stapling the middle hepatic vein, the specimen is removed.

RESULTS

Mortality and Morbidity

When we reviewed 79 patients treated with segment-oriented resection for metastatic neoplasms or hepatocellular carcinoma, the overall rate of postoperative morbidity was 26% (Billingsley et al, 1998). Pulmonary complications, including atelectasis, pneumonia, and pulmonary failure, were the most common. The overall mortality rate was 2.5%, and mortality occurred only in patients with hepatocellular carcinoma and cirrhosis. The median hospital stay was 8 days. Our results are consistent with the results of others (Redaelli et al, 2002). In caudate resection, one (5%) bile leak and no perioperative deaths were reported in a series of 19 patients in one study (Sarmiento et al, 2002). In another series of 21 patients who had an isolated caudate

Fig. 83.10. Central liver resection. In central liver resection, first the inflow pedicles to segment IV *(B and C)* are ligated and divided along the umbilical fissure, then the right anterior sectoral pedicle *(A)* is divided. The parenchymal transection proceeds from the left side and then the right side until these two planes unite just anterior to the IVC. The right hepatic vein *(F)* is preserved. The middle hepatic vein *(D)* is stapled with an endo-GIA stapler. Segments IV, V, and VIII are removed en masse.
(From Liau KH, et al, 2004: Segment-oriented approach to liver resection. Surg Clin North Am 84:543-561.)

resection during 1992-2004, there was no operative mortality, and the median hospital stay was 7 days (Hawkins et al, 2005).

Intraoperative Blood Loss

Segment-oriented liver resection minimizes intraoperative blood loss by using low central venous pressure anesthesia and early devascularization techniques. The median estimated blood loss for isolated caudate resection was 600 mL in a cohort of 21 patients (Hawkins et al, 2005). In another study of 19 patients with caudate resection, the mean estimated blood loss was 760 ± 150 mL (Sarmiento et al, 2002). In our center, the mean transfusion requirement was 1 ± 0.3 U of packed red blood cells (Billingsley et al, 1998). Patients with hepatocellular carcinoma required more transfusions (2.7 ± 1.3 U versus 0.6 ± 0.2 U). Median blood loss for colorectal metastases in a group of 148 patients undergoing segment-oriented liver resection was 530 ± 60 mL (DeMatteo et al, 2000b). In a European study of 90 patients with liver malignancy treated over a 7-year period, the median blood loss was 965 mL (Redaelli et al, 2002). Segment-oriented liver resection can be performed with less than 1 L of blood loss.

Oncologic Efficacy

Resection Margin and Recurrence

Anatomic segment-oriented hepatectomy has been shown to be a superior oncologic operation that has a survival advantage over simple wedge resection. In 267 patients with solitary colorectal liver metastases who were treated with wedge resection or segment-oriented liver resection, wedge resection resulted in a positive margin rate of 16% (DeMatteo et al, 2000b), and it has been reported to be 30% (Scheele et al, 1995). In contrast, only 2% of the segment-oriented liver resections were associated with a positive margin. Billingsley and coworkers (1998) reported an overall positive margin rate of 8% (6 of 79), and half of these patients underwent repeat liver resection for their recurrence. We had a positive microscopic margin in 3 (14%) of 21 patients with a median tumor size of 2.7 cm in their caudate (Hawkins et al, 2005). In hepatocellular carcinoma, local recurrence was observed more frequently after nonanatomic resection than after segment-oriented resections (50% versus 10%) (Regimbeau et al, 2002). Hepatocellular carcinoma has the proclivity to invade the portal veins and disseminate along its intrasegmental branches (Makuuchi et al, 2002; Scheele & Stangl, 2000).

Long-Term Survival

In caudate resection for colorectal hepatic metastases, the overall median survival was 64 months, and 5-year survival was 50% in a group of 12 patients (Sarmiento et al, 2002). In a larger series of 150 patients, the median overall survivals for patients with colorectal hepatic metastasis, cholangiocarcinoma, and hepatocellular carcinoma were 37 months, 28 months, and 32 months. The cohort comprised patients with caudate alone resection and caudate plus other segments resection. The median overall survival for all patients with malignancy was 34 months with a 5-year actuarial survival rate of 28% (Hawkins et al, 2005).

In hepatocellular carcinoma, the 5-year overall survival rate after nonanatomic resection was 35% versus 54% for segment-oriented resection (Regimbeau et al, 2002). Patients undergoing segment-oriented resection also had a superior 5-year disease-free

survival rate—45% versus 26% for patients with nonanatomic liver resection. Surgery for colorectal hepatic metastasis showed a similar trend. Segment-oriented hepatectomy resulted in longer survival with a median of 53 months versus 38 months for wedge hepatectomy in a study of 148 and 119 patients (DeMatteo et al, 2000b). The median survival after segment-oriented liver resection for 29 patients with hepatocellular carcinoma and 25 patients with colorectal hepatic metastases was 42 months and 40 months with 3-year actuarial survival of 62% for both (Redaelli et al, 2002). Although to date there are no randomized prospective data to support the superiority of segmental resection over the other procedures, patients who had oncologic segment-oriented liver resection have a reasonably good long-term survival.

RECENT ADVANCES

With the advent of laparoscopic surgery and innovations in laparoscopic instrumentation, it is now possible to perform laparoscopic and hand-assisted laparoscopic segment-oriented liver resection, particularly for the peripheral liver segments (Fong et al, 2000; Hashizume et al, 2000; Huscher et al, 1997) (see Ch. 80). In a series of 17 cases of laparoscopic hepatectomy, ranging from single segment to right hepatectomy, the mean blood loss was 288 mL, median length of stay was 3 days, and mean operative time was 2.8 hours (Buell et al, 2004). There was one death from hepatic failure. Complications included two cases of postoperative hemorrhage requiring reoperation and one bile leak. Although laparoscopic resection is feasible, careful patient selection is paramount. There are issues relating to compliance to the tenets of oncologic surgery. Also, improvement is needed in the techniques for laparoscopic control of bleeding and bile leak before laparoscopic segmental resection can be widely accepted. With the advent of nanotechnology and telesurgery, the future is likely to include progress in minimal access and robotic liver surgery in segment-oriented liver resection (Satava, 1999).

REFERENCES

Baer HU, et al, 1991a: Subtotal hepatectomy: a new procedure based on the inferior right hepatic vein. Br J Surg 78:1221-1222.

Baer HU, et al, 1991b: New water-jet dissector: initial experience in hepatic surgery. Br J Surg 78:502-503.

Bartlett D, et al, 1996: Complete resection of the caudate lobe of the liver: technique and results. Br J Surg 83:1076-1081.

Billingsley KG, et al, 1998: Segment-oriented hepatic resection in the management of malignant neoplasms of the liver. J Am Coll Surg 187:471-481.

Bismuth H, 1982: Surgical anatomy and anatomic surgery of the liver. World J Surg 6:3-9.

Bismuth H, Dennison AR, 1993: Segmental liver resection. Adv Surg 26:189-208.

Bismuth H, et al, 1982: Major and minor segmentectomies "reglees" in liver surgery. World J Surg 6:10.

Blumgart LH, 2000: Liver resection for benign disease and for liver and biliary tumors. In Blumgart LH, Fong Y (eds): Surgery of the Liver and Biliary Tract, 3rd ed. London, Saunders, pp 1639-1713.

Buell JF, et al, 2004: An initial experience and evolution of laparoscopic hepatic resectional surgery. Surgery 136:804-811.

Castaing D, et al, 1989: Segmental liver resection using ultrasound-guided selective portal venous occlusion. Ann Surg 210:20-23.

Couinaud CL, 1954: Bases anatomiques des hépatectomies gauche et droite réglées. J Chir 70:933-966.

Couinaud CL, 1957: Le Foie: Etude Anatomique et Chirurgicales. Paris, Masson.

Cunningham JD, et al, 1994: One hundred consecutive hepatic resections: blood loss, transfusion and operative technique. Arch Surg 129:1050-1056.

DeMatteo RP, et al, 2000a: Recent advances in hepatic resection. Semin Surg Oncol 19:200-207.

DeMatteo RP, et al, 2000b: Anatomic segmental hepatic resection is superior to wedge resection as an oncologic operation for colorectal liver metastases. J Gastrointest Surg 4:178-184.

Fan ST, et al, 1999: Hepatectomy for hepatocellular carcinoma: toward zero hospital deaths. Ann Surg 229:322-330.

Fasulo F, et al, 1992: Cavitron ultrasonic surgical aspirator (CUSA) in liver resection. Int Surg 77:64-66.

Fong Y, Blumgart LH, 1997: Useful stapling techniques in liver surgery. J Am Coll Surg 185:93-100.

Fong Y, et al, 1996: Drainage is unnecessary after elective liver resection. Am J Surg 171:158-162.

Fong Y, et al, 2000: Hand-assisted laparoscopic liver resection: lessons from an initial experience. Arch Surg 135:854-859.

Galperin EI, Karagiulian SR, 1991: A new simplified method of selective exposure of hepatic pedicles for controlled hepatectomies. HPB Surg 1:119-130.

Hanna SS, et al, 1996: Liver resection by ultrasonic dissection and intraoperative ultrasonography. HPB Surg 9:121-128.

Hashizume M, et al, 2000: Laparoscopic hepatectomy: new approach for hepatocellular carcinoma. J Hepatobiliary Pancreat Surg 7:270-275.

Hawkins WG, et al, 2005: Caudate hepatectomy for cancer: a single institution experience with 150 patients. J Am Coll Surg 200:345-352.

Healey JE Jr, Schroy PC, 1953: Anatomy of the biliary ducts within the human liver: analysis of the prevailing pattern of branchings and the major variations of the biliary ducts. Arch Surg 66:599.

Healey JE Jr, Schwartz SI, 1964: Surgical anatomy. In Schwartz SI (ed): Diseases of the Liver. New York, McGraw-Hill.

Hepp J, Couinaud C, 1956: L'abord et l'utilisation du canal hépatique gauche dans les réparations de la voie biliaire principale. Presse Med 64:947-948.

Hjortsjo CH, 1951: The topography of the intrahepatic duct system. Acta Anat 11:599-615.

Hodgson W, DelGuercio L, 1984: Preliminary experience in liver resection using the ultrasonic scalpel. Surgery 95:230-234.

Huscher CG, et al, 1997: Current position of advanced laparoscopic surgery of the liver. J R Coll Surg Edinb 42:219-225.

Jamieson GG, et al, 1992: Major liver resection without a blood transfusion—is it a realistic objective. Surgery 112:32-36.

Jarnagin WR, et al, 2001: What is the yield of intraoperative ultrasonography during partial hepatectomy for malignant disease? J Am Coll Surg 192:577-583.

Jones RM, et al, 1998: Central venous pressure and its effects on blood loss during liver resection. Br J Surg 85:1058-1060.

Kane R, et al, 1994: The impact of intraoperative ultrasonography on surgery for liver neoplasms. J Ultrasound Med 13:1.

Kohno H, et al, 1992: Comparison of topical hemostatic agents in elective hepatic resection: a clinical prospective randomized trial. World J Surg 16:966-970.

Kokudo N, et al, 2000: Hepatic parenchymal transection using ultrasonic coagulating shears: a preliminary report. J Hepatobiliary Pancreat Surg 7:295-298.

Launois B, 1997: Hepatectomy: the posterior intrahepatic approach. Br J Surg 84:291-292.

Launois B, Jamieson GG, 1992a: The intrahepatic Glissonian approach to resection of the liver. Surg Gynecol Obstet 174:7-10.

Launois B, Jamieson GG, 1992b: The posterior intrahepatic approach for hepatectomy or removal of segments of liver. Surg Gynecol Obstet 174:155-158.

Launois B, Jamieson GG, 1992c: The importance of Glisson's capsule and its sheaths in the intrahepatic approach to resection of the liver. Surg Gynecol 174:7-10.

Launois B, Jamieson GG, 1993a: General principles of liver surgery. In Modern Operative Techniques in Liver Surgery (Clinical Surgery International), Vol 18. New York, Churchill Livingstone, pp 23-26.

Launois B, Jamieson GG, 1993b: Segmentectomy procedures: the left liver. In Modern Operative Techniques in Liver Surgery (Clinical Surgery International), Vol 18. New York, Churchill Livingstone, pp 51-65.

Lerut J, et al, 1990: Resection of the caudate lobe of the liver. Surg Gynecol Obstet 171:160-162.

Liau KH, et al, 2004: Segment-oriented approach to liver resection. Surg Clin North Am 84:543-561.

Lin TY, 1973: Results in 107 hepatic lobectomies with a preliminary report on the use of a clamp to reduce blood loss. Ann Surg 177:413-421.

Lin TY, 1974: A simplified technique for hepatic resection: the crush method. Ann Surg 180:285-290.

Lin TY, et al, 1958: Study of a lobectomy of liver. J Formos Med Assoc 57:742-759.

Liu CL, et al, 2004: Abdominal drainage after hepatic resection is contraindicated in patients with chronic liver diseases. Ann Surg 239:194-201.

Lortat-Jacob JL, Robert HG, 1952: Hépatectomie droite réglée. Presse Med 60:549-551.

Lui WY, et al, 1995: Hepatic segmentectomy for curative resection of primary hepatocellular carcinoma. Arch Surg 130:1090-1097.

Maddern GJ, et al, 1995: Clinical experience with the intrahepatic posterior approach of the portal triad for right hepatectomy and right segmental resection. World J Surg 19:764-767.

Makuuchi M, et al, 1983: The inferior right hepatic vein: ultrasonic demonstration. Radiology 148:213-217.

Makuuchi M, et al, 1985: Ultrasonically guided subsegmentectomy. Surg Gynecol Obstet 161:346-350.

Makuuchi M, et al, 1987: The use of operative ultrasound as an aid to liver resection in patients with hepatocellular carcinoma. World J Surg 11:615-621.

Makuuchi M, et al, 1991: The value of ultrasonography for hepatic surgery. Hepatogastroenterology 38:64-70.

Makuuchi M, et al, 2002: Progress in surgical treatment of hepatocellular carcinoma. Oncology 62(suppl 1):74-81.

Man K, et al, 1997: Prospective evaluation of Pringle maneuver in hepatectomy for liver tumors by a randomized study. Ann Surg 226:704-711.

Matsumata T, et al, 1989: Lack of intrahepatic recurrence of hepatocellular carcinoma by temporary portal venous embolization with starch microspheres. Surgery 105:188-191.

Matsumata T, et al, 1992: Simplified hilar division in controlled right hepatectomy. Am J Surg 163:339.

Mazziotti A, et al, 2000: Isolated resection of segment 8 for liver tumor: a new approach for anatomical segmentectomy. Arch Surg 135:1224-1229.

McBride CM, Wallace S, 1972: Cancer of the right lobe of the liver: a variety of operative procedures. Arch Surg 105:289-296.

Melendez JA, et al, 1998: Perioperative outcomes of major hepatic resections under low central venous pressure anesthesia: blood loss, blood transfusion, and the risk of postoperative renal dysfunction. J Am Coll Surg 187:620-625.

Pack GT, Miller TR, 1961: Middle hepatic lobectomy for cancer. Cancer 14:1295-1300.

Patel NA, Roh MS, 2004: Utility of intraoperative liver ultrasound. Surg Clin North Am 84:513-524.

Polk W, et al, 1995: A technique for the use of cryosurgery to assist hepatic resection. J Am Coll Surg 180:171-176.

Postema RR, et al, 1993: Haemostasis after partial hepatectomy using argon beam coagulation. Br J Surg 80:1563-1565.

Ramacciato G, et al, 1996: Vascular endostapler as aid to hepatic vein control during hepatic resections. Am J Surg 172:358-362.

Rau HG, et al, 1995a: Laparoscopic liver resection with the water-jet dissector. Surg Endosc 9:1009-1012.

Rau HG, et al, 1995b: A comparison of different techniques for liver resection: blunt dissection, ultrasonic aspirator and jet-cutter. Eur J Surg Oncol 21:183-187.

Ravikumar T, 1996: Laparoscopic staging and intraoperative ultrasonography for liver tumor management. Surg Oncol Clin North Am 5:271.

Raynaud BH, et al, 1991: Basis to improve several hepatectomy techniques involving the surgical anatomy of insura dextra of Gans. Surg Gynecol Obstet 172:490-492.

Redaelli CA, et al, 2002: Liver surgery in the era of tissue-preserving resections: early and late outcome in patients with primary and secondary hepatic tumors. World J Surg 26:1126-1132.

Rees M, et al, 1996: One hundred and fifty hepatic resections: evolution of technique towards bloodless surgery. Br J Surg 83:1562-1569.

Regimbeau JM, et al, 2002: Extent of liver resection influences the outcome in patients with cirrhosis and small hepatocellular carcinoma. Surgery 131:311-317.

Sarmiento JM, et al, 2002: Surgical outcomes of isolated caudate lobe resection: a single series of 19 patients. Surgery 132:697-709.

Satava RM, 1999: Emerging technologies for surgery in the 21st century. Arch Surg 134:1197-1202.

Scheele J, Stangl R, 2000: Segment-oriented anatomical liver resections. In Blumgart LH, Fong Y (eds): Surgery of the Liver and Biliary Tract, 3rd ed. London, Saunders, pp 1743-1764.

Scheele J, et al, 1995: Resection of colorectal liver metastases. World J Surg 19:59-71.

Skandalakis JE, et al, 2004: Hepatic surgical anatomy. Surg Clin North Am 84:413-435.

Storck BH, et al, 1991: The impact of CUSA ultrasonic dissection device on major liver resection. Neth J Surg 43:99-101.

Storm FK, Longmire WP Jr, 1971: A simplified clamp for hepatic resection. Surg Gynecol Obstet 133:103-104.

Takayama T, Makuuchi M, 1996: Intraoperative ultrasonography and other techniques for segmental resections. Surg Oncol Clin North Am 5:261-269.

Voyles CR, Vogel SB, 1989: Hepatic resection using stapling devices to control the hepatic veins. Am J Surg 158:459-460.

Yamamoto J, et al, 1992: An isolated caudate lobectomy by the transhepatic approach for hepatocellular carcinoma in cirrhotic liver. Surgery 111:699-702.

Yamamoto J, et al, 1999: Anterior transhepatic approach for isolated resection of the caudate lobe of the liver. World J Surg 23:97-101.

Yamanaka N, et al, 1992: Do the tumor cells of hepatocellular carcinomas dislodge into the portal venous stream during hepatic resection? Cancer 70:2263-2267.

Portal Vein Embolization

84a PLACE OF PORTAL VEIN EMBOLIZATION

H. IMAMURA, T. TAKAYAMA, AND M. MAKUUCHI

Extensive liver resection often results in more than 70% of the functioning liver parenchyma being lost, along with an abrupt increase in portal venous pressure. Both changes may contribute to an increased rate of postoperative morbidity associated with cholestasis, ascites, and impaired synthetic function. These conditions all may lead to a prolonged recovery time and hospitalization and eventually can culminate in, albeit rarely, fatal liver failure. These concerns are particularly serious in patients with obstructive jaundice or underlying liver disease.

In 1982, we first carried out preoperative portal vein embolization (PVE) in a patient with hilar bile duct carcinoma with the intention of increasing the operative safety under these circumstances (Makuuchi et al, 1984, 1990). This approach is based on the concept of the *hepatic atrophy-hypertrophy complex* (see Ch. 5). We attempted to induce atrophy in the embolized part of the liver to be resected, with compensatory hypertrophy of the nonembolized future liver remnant (FLR) after hepatectomy. Satisfactory initial outcomes led us to extend the indications for PVE to patients with metastatic liver tumors of colorectal origin (Kawasaki et al, 1994a) and patients undergoing hepatopancreaticoduodenectomy (Kawasaki et al, 1994b). Because of its technical simplicity and the consistent attainment of liver hypertrophy after the procedure, PVE has become a standard preoperative intervention worldwide, and its indications have been expanded to patients with hepatocellular carcinoma (HCC) (Aoki et al, 2004; Azoulay et al, 2000a; Lee et al, 1993; Tanaka et al, 2000; Yamakado et al, 1997).

HISTORICAL BACKGROUND

The hepatic atrophy-hypertrophy complex concept dates back to 1920, when Rous and Larimore (1920) showed ligation of a major branch of the rabbit portal vein to result in atrophy of the ipsilateral hepatic lobe and hypertrophy of the contralateral lobe. The same phenomenon was observed in experiments involving long-term bile duct obstruction (McMaster & Rous, 1921). In contrast to the predictable response to portal venous occlusion, however, the magnitude of the response to bile duct obstruction differs substantially among species (cat, rat, rabbit, and human) (Braasch et al, 1972; Schalm et al, 1956; Steiner & Martinez Batiz, 1962; Stewart et al, 1937).

In 1975, Honjo and colleagues ligated the ipsilateral portal venous branch in patients with HCC in an effort to suppress tumor growth. Although this approach did not succeed in preventing tumor growth, it did produce marked atrophy of the occluded hemiliver. Likewise, our patients experienced an uneventful postoperative clinical course after extensive hepatectomy for hilar bile duct carcinoma involving a branch of the portal vein, causing hemiliver atrophy and corresponding hypertrophy of the contralateral hemiliver (Takayasu et al, 1986). These clinical observations led one of us (M.M.) to attempt PVE application as an adjunct to major hepatectomy.

TECHNIQUE

PVE can be performed by direct catheterization of the ileocolic vein at laparotomy or via percutaneous transhepatic approach under ultrasound guidance. The ileocolic approach allows evaluation of the extent of the tumor at the time of PVE, including peritoneal dissemination and hilar lymph node metastases (Imamura et al, 1999a). Catheterization of all portal tributaries is simple even in cases with anatomic variations and can be applied when the transhepatic approach is difficult because of the location of the hepatic tumor. Open laparotomy under general anesthesia is required, however, and this technique is not recommended in patients with a history of prior lower abdominal surgery. Intestinal ileus has been reported to occur (Imamura et al, 1999a).

The transhepatic procedure can be performed under local anesthesia with or without intravenous sedatives. The contralateral approach is technically easier than the ipsilateral approach, especially in the presence of anatomic variations (De Baere et al, 1996). The shortcoming of this method is that the portal vein in the FLR is punctured. We experienced bleeding from the portal venous wall at the puncture site during hilar dissection in a case of hilar bile duct carcinoma. Iatrogenic lesions of the FLR lobe, including hematoma, portal vein wall dissection, and portal vein thrombosis, were described in a multicenter review (Di Stefano et al, 2005). The ipsilateral approach was proposed as a means of possibly avoiding FLR injury (Nagino et al, 1996). Embolization materials can be placed along the puncture line at completion of the procedure to prevent post-PVE hemorrhage. This approach is theoretically superior to the contralateral procedure in terms of safety, but is technically demanding, particularly when there is severe angulation between portal branches to right paramedian (segments V/VIII) and lateral (segments VI/VII) sectors. The rate of recanalization is higher than with the contralateral approach, and an appropriate puncture line sometimes cannot be secured because of the location of the liver tumor. Post-PVE portography or portal pressure measurement to confirm the efficacy of embolization cannot be performed with this procedure.

Fig. 84a.1 shows computed tomography (CT) before and 2 weeks after right liver PVE. Fig. 84a.2 shows each step of right

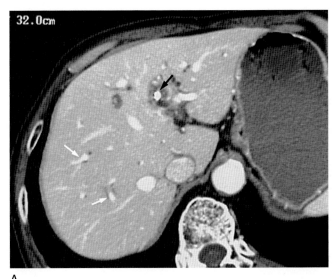 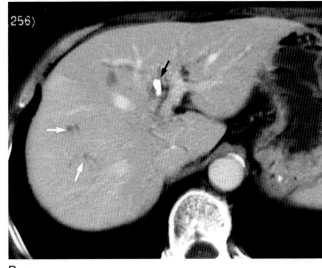

A B

Fig. 84a.1. CT of a 70-year-old woman with hilar bile duct carcinoma before (**A**) and 2 weeks after (**B**) PVE to right liver with Gelfoam particles and thrombin. Coil was not used in this patient. *Black arrows* indicate percutaneous transhepatic biliary drainage catheter. *White arrows* indicate portal tributaries to segment VIII. Note the cessation of portal flow and attenuation difference by hepatic arterial buffer response in the right liver after PVE.

liver PVE by the ipsilateral approach. For every procedure, portal vein anomalies should be investigated by CT before PVE and by direct portography at the start of embolization, paying particular attention to whether or not second-order branches originate close to, or independently of, the main portal trunk. Right anterolateral fluoroscopy is recommended during embolization of branches to the right lateral sector (segments VI/VII). The success of this technique is nearly 100%. Rare technical failures usually are associated with catheterization difficulty because of severe angulations between portal branches and migration of embolization materials to the FLR. The use of a balloon-tipped catheter is advocated to avoid the latter complication.

EMBOLIZATION MATERIALS

There is no general consensus regarding the ideal embolization material to be used for PVE (Table 84a.1). Biomaterials including absorbable gelatin sponge (Gelfoam) particles with thrombin (Imamura et al, 1999a; Makuuchi et al, 1984, 1990) and fibrin glue (combination of fibrinogen and thrombin) (Nagino et al, 1995, 1996), synthetic glue (*N*-butyl-2-cyanoacrylate) (De Baere et al, 1996), synthetic embolization particles (polyvinyl alcohol) (Abdalla et al, 2002; Madoff et al, 2003), coils, iodized oil, and absolute ethanol (Shimamura et al, 1997) are used. Biomaterials are absorbable and allow recanalization, a theoretical drawback associated with these substances. Conversely, unwanted outcomes induced by migration of embolization materials into portal branches of the FLR are minimal or absent (Imamura et al, 1999a). *N*-butyl-2-cyanoacrylate has a permanent embolizing effect and has been used for obliteration of the gastric coronary vein and esophageal varices. Because it immediately polymerizes on contact with blood, this agent cannot be used for the ipsilateral transhepatic procedure. Despite a long-lasting embolization effect, accompanying massive fibrosis of the perivascular connective tissue and portal vein casting (De Baere et al, 1996) may lead to difficulty with hilar dissection or discrimination of tumor invasion (Elias et al, 2002). Polyvinyl alcohol particles are

used for uterine artery embolization for symptomatic uterine fibrosis. The particles have a smaller diameter (150-100 μm) than the Gelfoam (500-1000 μm). This material is selected because of its safety, minimal periportal reaction, and enduring embolization effect when used in combination with coils (Madoff et al, 2003). Coils and iodized oil usually are used in combination with these materials. In particular, iodized oil produces a long-lasting "portal cast," which can be viewed on follow-up CT scans.

All of these agents reportedly yield a similar extent of hypertrophy in the FLR, 2 to 4 weeks after PVE (see Table 84a.1). PVE with absolute ethanol has been proposed because of its strong coagulation effect (Shimamura et al, 1997). The hypertrophy seemed to be more significant than with other materials (see Table 84a.1), but PVE with absolute ethanol was associated with marked increases in serum aspartate transaminase (AST) and alanine transaminase (ALT) levels, secondary to liver necrosis (Shimamura et al, 1997).

HEMODYNAMIC CONSEQUENCES

Total portal venous flow (mL/min) is thought to be unchanged after PVE because the liver does not have an intrinsic ability to modulate portal flow, which is a function of extrahepatic (i.e., splanchnic and systemic) factors (see Ch. 3). This principle was confirmed in a study using a rat model of hemihepatic portal vein ligation and radioactive microsphere technique (Rocheleau et al, 1999) and in a human PVE study using Doppler ultrasound (Denys et al, 2000). The same volume of portal flow as before PVE is assumed to enter exclusively the nonembolized hemiliver after PVE. Portal pressure in the nonembolized hemiliver is elevated immediately after PVE by 4.9 ± 2.7 cm H_2O (Takayama et al, 1997). Despite the higher baseline portal pressure, a similar increment was observed in patients with cirrhosis (Aoki et al, 2004). Information on chronologic alterations in portal pressure after PVE is unavailable, but the elevation is thought to be transient, with pressure gradually returning to the baseline value in 2 to 3 weeks, as indicated by the portal flow

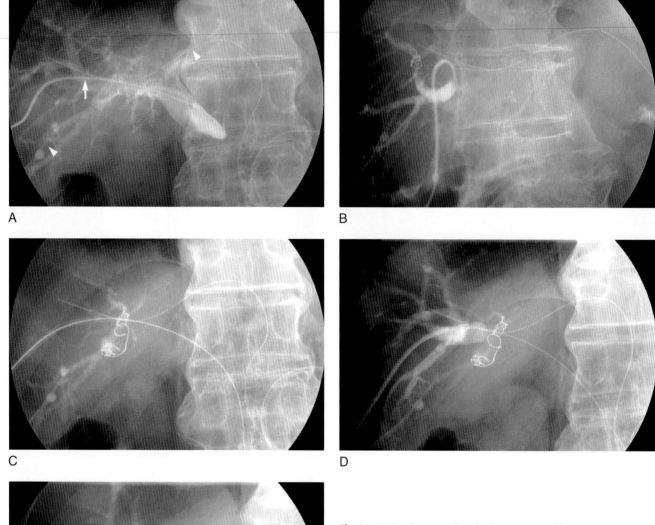

Fig. 84a.2. Transhepatic ipsilateral right PVE with Gelfoam particles, thrombin, and coils in a 72-year-old man with hilar bile duct carcinoma. **A,** Anteroposterior flush portogram obtained before right PVE with use of a 6-Fr vascular sheath in segment V portal branch and a 5-Fr flush catheter in the main portal vein *(arrow)*. *Arrowheads* indicate percutaneous transhepatic biliary drainage catheters. **B,** Embolization was begun from portal branch to segment VII with a reverse-curve catheter with distal end hole under right anterolateral fluoroscopy. **C,** Completion of embolization to portal branches to segments VI and VII. The tip of the catheter was placed in the main portal vein. Anteroposterior fluoroscopy view. **D,** Embolization of portal branches to segments V and VIII with proximal side hole–type catheter. **E,** Completion of PVE. Coils were placed at the root of portal branches to segments V, VI, VII, and VIII.

velocity (cm/sec) changes measured by Doppler ultrasound (Goto et al, 1998).

Our concern that an abrupt increase in portal venous pressure after major hepatectomy may result in liver damage is one of two reasons we attempted PVE. This concern seems to have been given less attention than the concern that an excessively small liver may not meet the metabolic demand after resection. More recent studies on living donor liver transplantation have focused on portal pressure and the small-for-size syndrome. Attempts were made to attenuate this problem by splenic arterial ligation or portacaval shunt (Boillot et al, 2002; Man et al, 2003; Troisi et al, 2003, 2005).

In contrast to portal flow, the liver is known to have an intrinsic regulatory mechanism to compensate for, albeit partially, the alteration in portal flow, which is referred to as the *hepatic arterial buffer response* (Lautt, 1985). In the case of PVE with hemihepatic portal vein occlusion, hepatic arterial buffer response is thought to operate still in the nonembolized liver based on studies using dynamic CT (see Fig. 84a.1) (Nagino et al, 1998; Wakabayashi et al, 2001) or Doppler ultrasound (Denys et al, 2000; Kito et al, 2001), and these findings are in line with the findings of a study using a rat model (Rocheleau et al, 1999). Controversy exists, however, regarding the maintenance of hepatic arterial buffer

Table 84a.1 Hypertrophy of Left Liver After Right Liver Portal Vein Embolization

Reference	Underlying Liver	Embolizing Material	Interval (wk)	Volume Increase (%)*
Nagino et al, 1995	Normal	Fibrinogen + thrombin + iodized oil	2	11
Shimamura et al, 1997	Fibrosis F1-F4	Absolute alcohol	4	27
Imamura et al, 1999a	Normal	Gelatin sponge + thrombin + iodized oil	2	10
Azoulay et al, 2000a[†]	Fibrosis F1-F4	N-butyl-2-cyanoacrylate + iodized oil	4	16
Azoulay et al, 2000b	Normal	N-butyl-2-cyanoacrylate + iodized oil	4	11
Wakabayashi et al, 2002	Normal Fibrosis F1-F4	Gelatin sponge	3	11 9
Elias et al, 2002	Normal	N-butyl-2-cyanoacrylate + iodized oil	4	13
Abdalla et al, 2002	Normal	Polyvinyl alcohol + coils	4-6	8
Farges et al, 2003	Normal Fibrosis F3-F4	N-butyl-2-cyanoacrylate + iodized oil	3-7	16 9

*Increase in the FLRV/TLV ratio.
[†]Combined with TAE.
Fibrosis is graduated from F1 (nonextensive portal fibrosis) to F4 (cirrhosis).

response in the nonembolized hemiliver (Denys et al, 2000; Kito et al, 2001; Rocheleau et al, 1999; Wakabayashi et al, 2001). Total liver blood flow, as estimated by a pharmacologic method, remained unchanged throughout the post-PVE period in our previous study (Shimada et al, 2002). In summary, arterial flow in the embolized hemiliver is increased after PVE, in part to compensate for the cessation of portal flow; it is unclear whether arterial flow in the nonembolized hemiliver remains stable or decreases in response to the increment in portal flow. These factors may be a major concern when considering tumor growth in these hemilivers after PVE.

Because hepatic arterial buffer response is a partial compensation, hyperperfusion in the nonembolized hemiliver, in contrast to hypoperfusion in the embolized hemiliver, as expressed per gram of liver tissue, occurs after PVE. Rocheleau and colleagues (1999) reported, in a rat model of hemihepatic portal vein ligation, the hepatic atrophy-hypertrophy complex process (i.e., liver weight changes in the ligated and the nonligated lobes) continues until total lobar flow per gram of liver tissue is restored. Uesaka and coworkers (1996) observed in a human PVE study that patients with obstructive jaundice showed biliary indocyanine green (ICG) excretion from the nonembolized lobe to be increased from the baseline value 10 to 16 days after PVE, and that this increment was more significant than the volume increase. Taking into account that the ICG extraction ratio in the noncirrhotic liver is 0.7 to 0.8, ICG transport from hepatocyte to bile canaliculi is extremely fast, and, accordingly, its biliary excretion is highly flow dependent, this human result is thought to be equivalent to that of the rat study reported by Rocheleau and colleagues (1999) and suggests that the hepatic atrophy-hypertrophy complex process is still under way 2 weeks after PVE. Although this study is often considered to suggest the gain in function to be faster than that in volume after PVE, the results appropriately should be interpreted relating to hemodynamic changes after PVE considering the pharmacokinetic properties of ICG.

CLINICAL COURSE AFTER PORTAL VEIN EMBOLIZATION

In contrast to transcatheter arterial embolization (TAE), signs and symptoms of postembolization syndrome, such as pain,

nausea, and vomiting, are minimal. Most patients experience a mild fever after PVE, which subsides within 2 to 3 days. Changes in liver function, as reflected by an increased total bilirubin value and prolonged prothrombin time, are mild and transient, returning to their baseline values 2 to 3 days after PVE. Serum AST and ALT values are stable in half of patients and are mildly elevated (1.5 to 3 times the pre-PVE values) on day 1, returning to baseline values in 4 to 7 days after PVE, in the remaining patients regardless of the embolization materials used (Fig. 84a.3). These findings suggest that inflammatory and necrotic reactions after PVE are minimal, if present (Imamura et al, 1999a). The exceptions are when absolute ethanol is used (Shimamura et al, 1997) for embolization and when PVE is carried out after TAE (Aoki et al, 2004). In both situations, PVE is followed by marked AST and ALT elevations, although both have returned to baseline values by the time of the scheduled hepatectomy (see Fig. 84a.3).

VOLUMETRIC CONSEQUENCES OF PORTAL VEIN EMBOLIZATION

CT scan with contrast enhancement is the most commonly used method of calculating total liver volume (TLV) and FLR volume

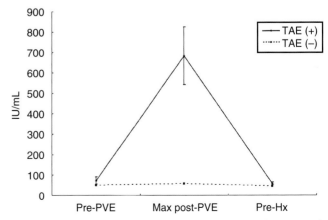

Fig. 84a.3. Chronologic alterations in serum AST values after PVE with (TAE [+]) and without (TAE [−]) prior TAE. Means ± SEM.

(FLRV) (see Fig. 84a.1). The nontumorous FLRV/(TLV − tumor volume) (FLRV/TLV) ratio is a widely used parameter to determine whether PVE is necessary before hepatic resection and to assess the degree of FLR hypertrophy. Vauthey and associates (2002) proposed the use of standard liver volume (SLV), a concept first applied to the clinical situation by us in 1995 (Urata et al, 1995). SLV is an alternative method of estimating the TLV from a linear regression formula correlating body surface area or body weight and TLV in healthy subjects (Urata et al, 1995; Vauthey et al, 2002). This formula is based on the concept that the optimal liver-to-body mass ratio in healthy subjects is constant. We first referred to this optimal liver volume as SLV and have proposed the application of SLV to recipients of living donor liver transplantation and patients with end-stage liver disease, whose actual liver volumes are extremely large or small in terms of the ideal liver volume to be grafted, such as in cases of primary biliary cirrhosis or fulminant hepatic failure (Urata et al, 1995).

Vauthey and associates (2002) (see later) emphasized the importance of SLV in determining the indications for PVE because it can be applied to patients with pathologic liver or obstructive jaundice with dilated bile ducts and can be calculated even in patients with multiple liver metastases (see Ch. 84b). Nevertheless, we adhere to the use of actual TLV based on several considerations. First, SLV is a virtual volume estimated employing a formula and varies among investigators using different formulas; r^2 in the equation of Vauthey and associates (2002) is 0.49, indicating that their formula explains only half of interindividual variations in TLV even in healthy subjects. Second, patients with extremely large or small livers in terms of SLV, secondary to underlying liver diseases, cannot be candidates for liver resection even after PVE. Finally, in the present era, multislice helical CT with contrast administration allows accurate volumetric measurement by subtracting small tumor volumes and vasculobiliary structures, even to Couinaud's segment level.

PVE leads to an increased segmental volume in the nonembolized hemiliver and a decrease in segmental volume of the embolized hemiliver, homogeneously maintaining a constant TLV. In the case of right hemiliver PVE, the regeneration rate in the noncirrhotic liver was 12 cm²/day 2 weeks after PVE (Lee et al, 1993; Nagino et al, 1995), then decreased to 11 cm²/day at 4 weeks (Nagino et al, 1995) and 6 cm²/day at 32 days (De Baere et al, 1996). In cirrhotic patients, the regeneration rate is reportedly slower, 9 cm²/day at 2 weeks (De Baere et al, 1996; Lee et al, 1993). In noncirrhotic and cirrhotic livers, regeneration processes are thought to be blunted by approximately 50% compared with after hepatectomy (Yamanaka et al, 1993).

Various factors have been reported to affect the regeneration rate after PVE. The regeneration rate depends on the embolized hemiliver volume (Imamura et al, 1999a; Yamakado et al, 1997); in other words, the greater the FLRV before PVE, the smaller the volume increase after PVE. Various materials used for embolization resulted in the different magnitudes of hypertrophy (see Table 84a.1). Hypertrophy seemed to be modest when biologic materials, such as Gelfoam and fibrin glue, were used, most probably as a result of the progressive recanalization that occurred. Absolute alcohol was reported to achieve the highest degree of regeneration, but at the expense of marked increases in AST and ALT levels, secondary to liver necrosis. Among disorders related to background patient characteristics, diabetes, obstructive jaundice, active hepatitis, and cirrhosis (see earlier) have been reported to hamper the regeneration process (Imamura et al, 1999a; Nagino et al, 1995; Tanaka et al, 2000). In general, a 30% increase in

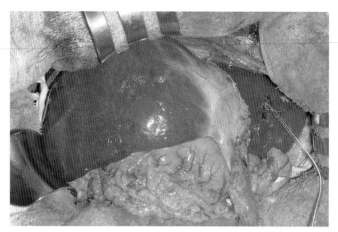

Fig. 84a.4. Gross appearance of the liver of a 67-year-old man with hilar bile duct carcinoma after right PVE. Left liver was hypertrophied; right liver was atrophied with darkened color and wrinkled surface.

nonembolized hemiliver volume, as an absolute value, and a 10% increase, as expressed by the FLRV/TLV ratio, are seen 2 weeks after right hemiliver PVE (Fig. 84a.4).

HISTOLOGIC CONSEQUENCES OF PORTAL VEIN EMBOLIZATION

Human liver tissue obtained 3 weeks after PVE showed almost normal microscopic structures in the embolized and the nonembolized lobes. In the embolized lobe, dilation of sinusoids with decreased hepatocyte density and hepatocyte apoptosis, especially in the pericentral area, were observed (Harada et al, 1997). Nevertheless, there were no signs of necrosis or inflammation except when embolizing material was absolute ethanol, with tissue showing clear evidence of necrosis (Shimamura et al, 1997), or cyanoacrylate, which produces peribiliary fibrosis (De Baere et al, 1996). In contrast, microscopic findings in the nonembolized hemiliver showed hepatocyte replication as evidenced by the increased mitotic figures and other parameters of cell proliferation, such as proliferative cell nuclear antigen and Ki-67 (Harada et al, 1997; Kusaka et al, 2006). Hepatocytes in this hemiliver were histologically characterized by basophilic cytoplasm and abundant binuclear cells, and they were small. These observations provide indirect evidence of hepatocyte proliferation (Harada et al, 1997).

Taking the above-described laboratory and volumetric data together, the embolized hemiliver seems to atrophy (see Fig. 84a.4) through apoptosis and subsequent cell deletion, as already suggested by Kerr and associates (1972), who coined the term *shrinkage necrosis*. In contrast, the volume increase in the nonembolized hemiliver is explained by hyperplasia (i.e., a net increase in cell number, rather than cellular hypertrophy), such as in the case of *foie gras de canard*.

FUNCTIONAL CONSEQUENCES OF PORTAL VEIN EMBOLIZATION

Cellular hyperplasia and the resulting hemiliver hypertrophy do not signify functional gain in the corresponding hemiliver, considering that proliferating isolated hepatocytes lose their differentiated hepatocyte-specific functions. Most former reports investigating liver function after PVE assessed whole liver function, including the embolized and the nonembolized lobe. Overall, functional hepatocyte number, as estimated by the clearance of antipyrine, a prototype of low-extractable drugs, showed similar values before and 2 weeks after PVE (Shimada et al, 2002). The adenosine triphosphate concentrations and hepatic energy reserves per gram of liver tissue, assessed in the nonembolized lobe 3 weeks after PVE, were similar to those of control tissue (Chijiiwa et al, 2000). Likewise, the nonembolized lobe uptake of technetium 99m–galactosyl human serum albumin (^{99m}Tc-GSA), a ligand bound to asialoglycoprotein receptors on the hepatocyte cell membrane, showed a rapid increase 1 to 2 weeks after PVE (Hirai et al, 2003; Nishiguchi et al, 2000). These findings showed the volume increase in the nonembolized lobe to be accompanied by a parallel increment in liver function in the corresponding lobe.

INDICATIONS

Cholangiocarcinoma

PVE is indicated most frequently for cholangiocarcinoma because extended right hepatectomy together with caudate lobe resection is often necessary for curative resection (Kawasaki et al, 2003; Makuuchi et al, 1984, 1990; Nagino et al, 2001; Seyama et al, 2003). Most patients have obstructive jaundice and cholestasis-induced impairment of liver function. Associated pancreaticoduodenectomy is necessary in cases of widespread bile duct carcinoma of the main bile duct, as a scheduled procedure or as a result of intraoperative frozen section pathology to obtain a negative surgical margin. These factors favor the application of PVE to achieve safe hepatic resection. Unilateral biliary decompression of the FLR lobe is recommended before PVE to improve function in the portion of the liver that will remain after hepatectomy. We favor a unilateral approach even when the communication between the right and left bile ducts is interrupted by tumor progression, in view of the enhanced atrophy-hypertrophy process and the volume gain in the FLR lobe (Braasch et al, 1972; Kawasaki et al, 2003; Kyokane et al, 2003; Seyama et al, 2003). Also, the rate of catheter-related infection reportedly increases with the number of stents (Neuhaus et al, 1999). It is important not to carry out an unnecessary cholangiography after biliary drainage until hepatectomy. When PVE by the transhepatic contralateral approach is scheduled, biliary decompression before PVE decreases the risk of portobiliary fistula. Not all authors agree with this approach (see Ch. 52).

Liver Metastases

Liver resection offers the only chance for cure with possible long-term survival for patients with liver metastases of colorectal origin, including bilateral metastases (see Ch. 73a) (Weber et al, 2000). In patients with massive liver tumors occupying the right liver, extended right hepatectomy does not result in a marked decrease in normally functioning hepatic mass. When similar extensive surgical procedures are indicated for small multiple metastases in the right hemiliver, with a solitary tumor located adjacent to the hilum of the liver, or with bilateral tumors, a large amount of functional hepatic mass must be removed.

PVE may be done under these circumstances to expand the operative indications to patients whose tumor otherwise would be unresectable owing to a small FLRV, or to increase operative safety (Azoulay et al, 2000b; Elias et al, 2002; Kawasaki et al, 1994a). PVE also is recommended when major hepatectomy is planned with a simultaneous major gastrointestinal procedure (e.g., when hepatic metastases are removed synchronously with the primary colorectal lesion) and when liver injury is suspected because of preceding systemic or locoregional chemotherapy (Farges et al, 2003). One major concern is whether PVE enhances tumor growth, especially in the nonembolized lobe (Elias et al, 1999, Kokudo et al, 2001). This concern is based on the observation of three to five patients who had tumors in the nonembolized lobe, however, and long-term results have been reported to be similar regardless of whether or not PVE was conducted (Azoulay et al, 2000b; Elias et al, 2002). No definitive conclusion can be drawn at present. With this possible shortcoming in mind, several authors have proposed two-stage procedures to avoid possible tumor growth in the nonembolized FLR lobe in patients with bilobar metastases. As a first step, resection of the primary tumor, if necessary, left liver limited metastasectomies, and right portal vein ligation or PVE are carried out. After an interval of several weeks, (extended) right hepatectomy is performed (Jaeck et al, 2004; Kianmanesh et al, 2003a).

Hepatocellular Carcinoma

Hepatectomy remains the sole treatment for large HCC, and major hepatic resection is often required for curative resection. Likewise, segment-oriented anatomic resection is recommended even for small HCC to prevent postoperative recurrence (Hasegawa et al, 2005; Imamura et al, 1999b; Makuuchi et al, 1985; Regimbeau et al, 2002). Ninety percent of HCC patients have impaired hepatic functional reserve, however, because of hepatitis B virus–associated or hepatitis C virus–associated liver fibrosis/cirrhosis, which is the main obstacle to performing hepatic resection (see Ch. 82). Shirabe and coworkers (1999) reported an increased rate of postoperative liver failure with a smaller FLRV in HCC patients. PVE triggered liver regeneration in 80% to 90% of HCC patients with chronic liver disease, but the process was hampered compared with that in patients with normal livers (Aoki et al, 2004; Azoulay et al, 2000a; Farges et al, 2003; Wakabayashi et al, 2002).

We combine selective TAE with PVE before performing major hepatic resection in HCC patients (Aoki et al, 2004; Kubota et al, 1997). This double preparation aims at (1) using TAE to prevent tumor progression during the period between PVE and the planned hepatectomy, in view of the fact that most HCCs are hypervascular tumors fed exclusively by arterial blood flow, and (2) enhancing the effect of PVE by first embolizing the possible arterioportal shunt, which is frequently found in cirrhotic livers and HCC tumors, using TAE. Others also advocate this double preparation (Azoulay et al, 2000a; Ogata et al, 2005; Wakabayashi et al, 2002; Yamakado et al, 1997). We perform PVE when liver function test results stabilize, usually 7 to 10 days after the TAE procedure in most cases. In contrast to cases with PVE alone, PVE performed after TAE resulted in marked elevations of AST and ALT values reflecting necrotic and inflammatory reactions after embolization (see Fig. 84a.3). These values had returned to baseline by the time of the planned hepatectomy. The bilirubin level remained essentially stable after PVE (Aoki et al, 2004).

Ogata and colleagues (2005) reported that, compared with PVE alone, the combination with TAE resulted in superior FLR hypertrophy and better long-term survival. Ten percent to 20% of patients failed to show FLR hypertrophy after PVE (see earlier), and hepatectomy was abandoned. The lack of hypertrophy, despite a technically successful PVE, most probably is explained by failure to increase portal flow to the FLR because of the presence or development of collateral vessels to the systemic circulation.

Our group and others have reported similar phenomena after embolization in patients with portal hypertension (Hasegawa et al, 2004; Nagino et al, 2002). Based on these observations, Kianmanesh and associates (2003b) proposed that in Child-Turcotte-Pugh A patients, PVE preoperatively tests the capacity of the injured liver to regenerate, and that the absence of hypertrophy after PVE is a contraindication for major hepatic resection in these patients. Wakabayashi and colleagues (2002) also recognized a close relationship between the success or failure of hypertrophy and short-term outcome. Based on their results, Farges and coworkers (2003) asserted that, contrary to the views of Azoulay and colleagues (2000a), in most patients showing adequate hypertrophy, the actual period between PVE and resection can be less than 4 weeks. Our opinion is in line with Farges and coworkers (2003) because one of the aims of conducting PVE is to avoid the sudden increase of portal venous pressure after major hepatectomy, and portal pressure, although elevated immediately after PVE, is supposed to decrease gradually in 1 to 2 weeks.

General Indications

Under what circumstances does PVE become necessary? General indications for PVE are based on the size of the FLR, underlying liver disease, and the extent or complexity of the procedure. Intuitively, patients with liver pathology (e.g., fibrosis or cirrhosis, cholestasis, steatosis, and prior chemotherapy) require a larger FLRV than patients with a normal liver. The same holds true for patients requiring a synchronous additional surgery, such as pancreaticoduodenectomy or low anterior resection for rectal carcinoma. Few data exist, however, regarding the hepatic volume to support life and prevent complications. In living donor liver transplantation, the lower limit of residual liver volume/TLV allowing a patient to be a donor candidate is thought to be 30% (Fan et al, 2000; Kokudo et al, 2005). The FLRV/TLV ratio indicated for PVE is determined arbitrarily in various institutions and ranges from 25% to 40% (Azoulay et al, 2000a, 2000b; Elias et al, 2002; Hemming et al, 2003; Imamura et al, 1999a).

We advocate PVE for (1) patients with a normal liver (i.e., ICG retention rate at 15 minutes [ICG R15] ≤ 10%) if FLRV/TLV is less than 40% and (2) patients with an injured liver (i.e., 10% ICG R15 ≤ 20%) if FLRV/TLV is less than 50%. If ICG R15 exceeds 20%, major hepatectomy is contraindicated even after PVE (Kubota et al, 1997). Farges and coworkers (2003) reported that the induction of PVE resulted in an increase in the FLRV/TLV ratio from 31% to 47% in patients with normal liver parenchyma ($n = 13$), but these patients showed postoperative courses similar to those of patients undergoing hepatectomy without PVE ($n = 14$; FLRV/TLV = 30%) in terms of total bilirubin, prothrombin time, and hospital stay. In contrast, these investigators obtained improvements in these parameters by conducting PVE in patients with chronic liver disease ($n = 14$ each; FLRV/TLV ratio increased by 9% in PVE group) (Farges et al, 2003).

Based on these findings, they recommended routine application of PVE in patients with diseased livers, but considered this procedure to be unnecessary in patients with a normal liver except in patients undergoing extensive resection, a major synchronous surgical procedure, or minor hepatectomies involving the FLR lobe (Belghiti, 2003; Farges et al, 2003).

Indications for PVE should be discussed with special emphasis on the medical cost and complications associated with this procedure. The complication rate particularly depends on technical expertise. Assuming these factors to be negligible, we favor our criteria (see earlier). Although fatal complications, such as liver insufficiency, are rare, hepatic dysfunction as assessed by prothrombin time prolongation and bilirubin elevation, the overall complication rate, and mean hospital stay were correlated closely with the FLRV/TLV ratio (Abdalla et al, 2002; Belghiti, 2004; Shoup et al, 2003). In parallel, in living donor liver transplantation, although the clinically significant complication rate did not differ among various types of grafts, the residual liver volume fraction showed a close correlation with peak prothrombin international normalized ratio and total bilirubin levels (Kokudo et al, 2005; Salamé et al, 2002). These figures strongly suggest that Heinrich's theory (Heinrich et al, 1982), first proposed in 1941, can be applied to the indication criteria for PVE. That is, for one fatal or serious accident (i.e., mortality or liver failure), there were 29 accidents (i.e., minor complication or long hospital stay) and 300 potential incidents involving a high probability of causing injuries (i.e., clinically insignificant prothrombin time prolongation and bilirubin elevation). This issue is anticipated to be a matter of future debate.

CONCLUSION

PVE induces the atrophy of the embolized hemiliver to be resected, with compensatory hypertrophy of the hemiliver to be preserved, with TLV being constant in 2 to 4 weeks. By decreasing the risk of liver failure, complication rate, and hospital stay, PVE is thought to increase the safety of resection and to expand the indication for liver resection for patients who otherwise are poor candidates for hepatectomy owing to inadequate estimated liver size and function after hepatectomy. It is particularly of value in patients with chronic liver disease, including obstructive jaundice and steatosis; with concomitant resection of major organs; or with bilateral liver tumors. The cutoff residual liver volume indicated for PVE ranges from 25% to 40% according to published reports. Because a randomized trial to verify the patients with the lowest residual liver volume who can be candidates for liver resection without PVE would be unethical, continued prospective examination of PVE with defined end points, such as postoperative liver function, operative complications, and length of hospital stay, should clarify the benefits obtained by PVE.

REFERENCES

Abdalla EK, et al, 2002: Extended hepatectomy in patients with hepatobiliary malignancies with and without preoperative portal vein embolization. Arch Surg 137:675-681.

Aoki T, et al, 2004: Sequential preoperative arterial and portal venous embolizations in patients with hepatocellular carcinoma. Arch Surg 139:766-774.

Azoulay D, et al, 2000a: Percutaneous portal vein embolization increases the feasibility and safety of major liver resection for hepatocellular carcinoma in injured liver. Ann Surg 232:665-672.

Azoulay D, et al, 2000b: Resection of nonresectable liver metastases from colorectal cancer after percutaneous portal vein embolization. Ann Surg 231:480-486.

Belghiti J, 2004: Arguments for a selective approach of preoperative portal vein embolization before major hepatic resection. J Hepatobiliary Pancreat Surg 11:21-24.

Boillot O, et al, 2002: Small-for-size partial liver graft in an adult recipient: a new transplant technique. Lancet 359:406-407.

Braasch JW, et al, 1972: Segmental obstruction of the bile duct. Surg Gynecol Obstet 134:915-920.

Chijiiwa K, et al, 2000: Effect of preoperative portal vein embolization on liver volume and hepatic energy status of the nonembolized liver lobe in humans. Eur Surg Res 32:94-99.

De Baere T, et al, 1996: Preoperative portal vein embolization for extension of hepatectomy indications. Hepatology 24:1386-1391.

Denys AL, et al, 2000: Intrahepatic hemodynamic changes following portal vein embolization: a prospective Doppler study. Eur Radiol 10:1703-1707.

Di Stefano DR, et al, 2005: Preoperative percutaneous portal vein embolization: evaluation of adverse events in 188 patients. Radiology 234:625-630.

Elias D, et al, 1999: During liver regeneration following right portal embolization the growth rate of liver metastases is more rapid than that of the liver parenchyma. Br J Surg 86:784-788.

Elias D, et al, 2002: Preoperative selective portal vein embolization before hepatectomy for liver metastases: long-term results and impact on survival. Surgery 131:294-299.

Fan ST, et al, 2000: Safety of donors in live donor liver transplantation using right lobe grafts. Arch Surg 135:336-340.

Farges O, et al, 2003: Portal vein embolization before right hepatectomy: prospective clinical trial. Ann Surg 237:208-217.

Goto Y, et al, 1998: Doppler estimation of portal blood flow after percutaneous transhepatic portal vein embolization. Ann Surg 228:209-213.

Harada H, et al, 1997: Fate of the human liver after hemihepatic portal vein embolization: cell kinetic and morphometric study. Hepatology 26:1162-1170.

Hasegawa K, et al, 2004: Administration of iodized oil resulted in impaired liver function due to enhanced portosystemic shunting. Cardiovasc Interv Radiol 27:282-284.

Hasegawa K, et al, 2005: Prognostic impact of anatomic resection for hepatocellular carcinoma. Ann Surg 242:252-259.

Heinrich HW, et al, 1982: Industrial Accident Prevention, 5th ed. New York, McGraw-Hill.

Hemming AW, et al, 2003: Preoperative portal vein embolization for extended hepatectomy. Ann Surg 237:686-691.

Hirai I, et al, 2003: Evaluation of preoperative portal vein embolization for safe hepatectomy, with special reference to assessment of nonembolized lobe function with 99mTc-GSA SPECT scintigraphy. Surgery 133:495-506.

Honjo I, et al, 1975: Ligation of a branch of the portal vein for carcinoma of the liver. Am J Surg 130:296-302.

Imamura H, et al, 1999a: Preoperative portal vein embolization: an audit of 84 patients. Hepatology 29:1099-1105.

Imamura H, et al, 1999b: Prognostic significance of anatomical resection and des-γ-carboxy prothrombin in patients with hepatocellular carcinoma. Br J Surg 86:1032-1038.

Jaeck D, et al, 2004: A two-stage hepatectomy procedure combined with portal vein embolization to achieve curative resection for initially unresectable multiple and bilobar colorectal liver metastases. Ann Surg 240:1037-1051.

Kawasaki S, et al, 1994a: Resection for multiple metastatic liver tumors after portal embolization. Surgery 115:674-677.

Kawasaki S, et al, 1994b: Radical operation after portal embolization for tumor of hilar bile duct. J Am Coll Surg 178:480-486.

Kawasaki S, et al, 2003: Results of surgical resection for patients with hilar bile duct cancer: application of extended hepatectomy after biliary drainage and hemihepatic portal vein embolization. Ann Surg 238:84-92.

Kerr JF, et al, 1972: Apoptosis: a basic biological phenomenon with wide-ranging implications in tissue kinetics. Br J Cancer 26:239-257.

Kianmanesh R, et al, 2003a: Right portal vein ligation: a new planned two-step all-surgical approach for complete resection of primary gastrointestinal tumors with multiple bilateral liver metastases. J Am Coll Surg 197:164-170.

Kianmanesh R, et al, 2003b: Selective approach to major hepatic resection for hepatocellular carcinoma in chronic liver disease Surg Oncol Clin N Am 12:51-63.

Kito Y, et al, 2001: Doppler sonography of hepatic arterial blood flow velocity after percutaneous transhepatic portal vein embolization. AJR Am J Roentgenol 176:909-912.

Kokudo N, et al, 2001: Proliferative activity of intrahepatic colorectal metastases after preoperative hemihepatic portal vein embolization. Hepatology 34:267-272.

Kokudo N, et al, 2005: Tailoring the type of donor hepatectomy for adult living donor liver transplantation. Am J Transplant 5:1694-1703.

Kubota K, et al, 1997: Measurement of liver volume and hepatic functional reserve as a guide to decision-making in resectional surgery for hepatic tumors. Hepatology 26:1176-1181.

Kusaka K, et al, 2006: Expression of transforming growth factor α and β in hepatic lobes after hemihepatic portal vein embolization. Dig Dis Sci., in press.

Kyokane T, et al, 2003: Simultaneous segmental obstruction of bile duct and portal vein markedly changes a population of biliary and hepatic cells in human liver. Langenbeck Arch Surg 388:270-275.

Lautt WW, 1985: Mechanism and role of intrinsic regulation of hepatic arterial blood flow: hepatic arterial buffer response. Am J Physiol 249: G549-G556.

Lee KC, et al, 1993: Extension of surgical indications for hepatocellular carcinoma by portal vein embolization. World J Surg 17:109-115.

Madoff DC, et al, 2003: Portal vein embolization with polyvinyl alcohol particles and coils in preparation for major liver resection for hepatobiliary malignancy: safety and effectiveness—study in 26 patients. Radiology 227:251-260.

Makuuchi M, et al, 1984: Preoperative transcatheter embolization of the portal venous branch for patients receiving extended lobectomy due to the bile duct carcinoma. J Jpn Surg Assoc 45:1558-1564.

Makuuchi M, et al, 1985: Ultrasonically guided subsegmentectomy. Surg Gynecol Obstet 161:346-350.

Makuuchi M, et al, 1990: Preoperative portal embolization to increase safety of major hepatectomy for hilar bile duct carcinoma: a preliminary report. Surgery 107:521-527.

Man K, et al, 2003: Graft injury in relation to graft size in right lobe live donor liver transplantation. Ann Surg 237:256-264.

McMaster PD, Rous P, 1921: The biliary obstruction required to produce jaundice. J Exp Med 33:731-750.

Nagino M, et al, 1995: Changes in hepatic lobe volume in biliary tract cancer patients after right portal vein embolizaiton. Hepatology 21:434-439.

Nagino M, et al, 1996: Selective percutaneous transhepatic embolization of the portal vein in preparation for extensive liver resection: the ipsilateral approach. Radiology 200:559-563.

Nagino M, et al, 1998: Immediate increase in arterial blood flow in embolized hepatic segments after portal vein embolization: CT demonstration. AJR Am J Roentgenol 171:1037-1039.

Nagino M, et al, 2001: Liver regeneration after major hepatectomy for biliary cancer. Br J Surg 88:1084-1091.

Nagino M, et al, 2002: Acute hypersplenism with splenomegaly after portal vein embolization. Surgery 131:695.

Neuhaus P, et al, 1999: Extended resection for hilar cholangiocarcinoma. Ann Surg 230:808-819.

Nishiguchi S, et al, 2000: Course before and after percutaneous transhepatic portal vein embolization of a patient with cholangiocarcinoma monitored by scintigraphy with Tc-99m galactosyl human serum albumin. Ann Nucl Med 14:231-234.

Ogata S, et al, 2005: Preoperative arterial chemoembolization combined with portal vein embolization improves long-term survival in cirrhotic patients with HCC. Hepatology 42(suppl 1):296A.

Regimbeau JM, et al, 2002: Extent of liver resection influences the outcome in patients with cirrhosis and small hepatocellular carcinoma. Surgery 131:311-317.

Rocheleau B, et al, 1999: Hepatic artery buffer response following left portal vein ligation: its role in liver tissue homeostasis. Am J Physiol 277: G1000-1007.

Rous P, Larimore LD, 1920: Relation of the portal blood to liver maintenance: a demonstration of liver atrophy conditional on compensation. J Exp Med 31:609-632.

Salamé E, et al, 2002: Analysis of donor risk in living-donor hepatectomy: the impact of resection type on clinical outcome. Am J Transplant 2:780-788.

Schalm L, et al, 1956: Atrophy of the liver after occlusion of the bile ducts or portal vein compensatory hypertrophy of the unoccluded portion and its clinical importance. Gastroenterology 31:131-155.

Seyama Y, et al, 2003: Long-term outcome of extended hemihepatectomy for bile duct cancer with no mortality and high survival rate. Ann Surg 238:73-83.

Shimada R, et al, 2002: Changes in blood flow and function of the liver after right portal vein embolization. Arch Surg 137:1384-1388.

Shimamura T, et al, 1997: Efficacy and safety of preoperative percutaneous transhepatic portal embolization with absolute ethanol: a clinical study. Surgery 121:135-141.

Shirabe K, et al, 1999: Postoperative liver failure after major hepatic resection for hepatocellular carcinoma in the modern era with special reference to remnant liver volume. J Am Coll Surg 188:304-309.

Shoup M, et al, 2003: Volumetric analysis predicts hepatic dysfunction in patients undergoing major liver resection. J Gastrointest Surg 7:325-330.

Steiner PE, Martinez Batiz J, 1962: Effects on the rat liver of bile duct, portal vein and hepatic artery ligations. Am J Pathol 39:257-289.

Stewart HL, et al, 1937: Changes in the liver of the cat following ligation of simple hepatic ducts. Arch Pathol 23:641-652.

Takayama T, et al, 1997: Preoperative portal vein embolization. Ann Ital Chir 68:745-750.

Takayasu K, et al, 1986: Hepatic lobar atrophy following obstruction of the ipsilateral portal vein from cholangiocarcinoma. Radiology 160:389-393.

Tanaka H, et al, 2000: Preoperative portal vein embolization improves prognosis after right hepatectomy for hepatocellular carcinoma in patients with impaired hepatic function. Br J Surg 87:879-882.

Troisi R, et al, 2003: Modulation of portal graft inflow: a necessity in adult living-donor liver transplantation? Ann Surg 237:429-436.

Troisi R, et al, 2005: Effects of hemi-portocaval shunts for inflow modulation on the outcome of small-for-size grafts in living donor liver transplantation. Am J Transplant 5:1397-1404.

Uesaka K, et al, 1996: Changes in hepatic lobar function after right portal vein embolization: an appraisal by biliary indocyanine green excretion. Ann Surg 223:77-83.

Urata K, et al, 1995: Calculation of child and adult standard liver volume for liver transplantation. Hepatology 21:1317-1321.

Vauthey JN, et al, 2002: Body surface area and body weight predict total liver volume in Western adults. Liver Transpl 8:233-240.

Wakabayashi H, et al, 2001: Changes in arterial and portal perfusion in embolized and nonembolized hepatic lobes after portal vein embolization evaluated by helical computed tomography. Surg Today 31:991-995.

Wakabayashi H, et al, 2002: Application of preoperative portal vein embolization before major hepatic resection in patients with normal or abnormal liver parenchyma. Surgery 131:26-33.

Weber SM, et al, 2000: Survival after resection of multiple hepatic colorectal metastases. Ann Surg Oncol 7:643-650.

Yamakado K, et al, 1997: Regeneration of the un-embolized liver parenchyma following portal vein embolization. J Hepatol 27:871-880.

Yamanaka N, et al, 1993: Dynamics of normal and injured human liver regeneration after hepatectomy as assessed on the basis of computed tomography and liver function. Hepatology 18:79-85.

84b PREOPERATIVE PORTAL VEIN EMBOLIZATION—A WESTERN PERSPECTIVE

J.-N. VAUTHEY, D. C. MADOFF, AND E. K. ABDALLA

With improvements in perioperative care, major liver resections are increasingly performed for primary or metastatic liver cancer. Major technical complications and fatal liver failure after hepatic resection are rare. Complications associated with cholestasis, fluid retention, and impaired synthetic function contribute to extended hospital stay and protracted recovery after major resection, however (Belghiti et al, 2000; Jarnagin et al, 2002; Vauthey et al, 1993). To overcome these nontechnical factors, portal vein embolization (PVE) was proposed to initiate hypertrophy of the future liver remnant before resection. This concept emerged on recognition that portal invasion by tumor leads to ipsilateral hepatic lobar atrophy and contralateral lobar hypertrophy (see Ch. 5).

Experience has provided insight into the role of PVE, but the technique and embolic substances, the method of measurement of the future liver remnant (FLR) and its function, and the specific indications for PVE remain controversial (Madoff et al, 2005a, 2005b). There is no consensus as to the extent of liver that can be resected safely, with resection ranging from 60% to 90% (Kubota et al, 1997; Soyer et al, 1992) and 80% to 90% (Nagasue et al, 1987). This disagreement regarding the extent of resection results from variability in the size and quality of the FLR and from a lack of standardization in the volumetric assessment of the liver before resection (Abdalla et al, 2004a; Vauthey et al, 2000).

In this chapter, we advocate a standardized, translatable approach to patient selection for PVE based on careful assessment of the FLR using a technique that integrates variations in liver size and patient size. The specific indications for PVE depend on the presence or absence and the degree of underlying liver disease and the planned operation. This approach includes embolization of the entire tumor-bearing liver to maximize hypertrophy and to minimize the risk for tumor progression during the FLR growth period. Analysis of existing data, including data validating this approach, are presented.

LIVER HYPERTROPHY

Hepatocyte regeneration (see Ch. 4) occurs early after partial hepatectomy, PVE, or liver injury. Resection of more than 10% of the liver volume results in proliferation of cells throughout the entire remaining liver (Bucher & Swaffield, 1964). When more than 50% of the liver is resected, a second peak in hepatocyte replication occurs within 2 to 7 days and slows by day 12 (Duncan et al, 1999). The overall hepatocyte proliferative response is proportional to the magnitude of the stimulus.

The mechanisms underlying the atrophy-hypertrophy complex are poorly understood. Components essential for hypertrophy include signals to initiate, sustain, and arrest regeneration. The most important and powerful known stimulus for regeneration is hepatocyte growth factor, which has a mitogenic effect on hepatocytes (see Ch. 4) (Michalopoulos & DeFrances, 1997; Michalopoulos & Zarnegav, 1992). Hepatocyte growth factor is released from hepatocytes in response to priming factors (probably proteases) after hepatocellular injury. In concert with primary mitogenic factors (hepatocyte growth factor, epidermal growth factor, and transforming growth factor-α) (Michalopoulos & DeFrances, 1997), essential cytokine comitogenic signals and transcription factors (Rudnick, 2005) lead to gene induction within 30 minutes of a stimulus, such as partial hepatectomy (Taub, 1996). DNA synthesis begins within 24 hours of the hypertrophy stimulus and peaks 24 to 96 hours later (Fabrikant, 1968; Francavilla et al, 1978). Hepatocytes clonally expand, leading to increase in cell number, not just cell mass. The mitotic index, DNA synthesis, and the number and function of mitochondria increase (Ozawa et al, 1974). With regard to mitochondrial function, compensatory hypertrophy is analogous whether PVE or hepatic resection is the stimulus (Katoh et al, 1991; Nagino et al, 1989; Ozawa et al, 1971). Insulin (Starzl et al, 1978), norepinepherine (Cruise et al, 1985), and specifically portal (not arterial) hormones are comitogenic with hepatocyte growth factor (Michalopoulos & DeFrances, 1997). Slower hypertrophy in diabetics compared with nondiabetics shows the clinical significance of insulin in this process (Nagino et al, 1995a). The presumed "stop" signals are even less well understood. Transforming growth factor-β is one of several candidates for signals that lead to the arrest of cellular expansion when appropriate liver mass for a patient or animal is regained (Carr et al, 1986).

Although severely damaged livers may not have the capacity to regenerate, some cirrhotic livers do regenerate. Cirrhosis often is diagnosed or suggested based on radiologic findings of *hypertrophy* of the left and caudate liver (Vitellas et al, 2001). The magnitude and rate of the regenerative response to resection (or embolization) in diseased livers are less than in normal livers. Normal livers regenerate the fastest, whereas patients with diabetes or cirrhosis have been found to have slower rates of regeneration (Nagino et al, 1995a; Shimamura et al, 1997; Yamanaka et al, 1993). In cirrhosis, this slower regeneration may be the result of the diminished capacity of hepatocytes to respond to hepatotropic factors or the result of parenchymal damage, such as fibrosis, which leads to slower portal blood flow rates (Goto et al, 1998).

Steatosis experimentally seems to impair liver regeneration, but regeneration still may be possible after PVE (Anderson et al, 2004). At this time, the severity of steatosis that is clinically significant is unknown. In laboratory animals, a high-fat diet was shown to impair liver regeneration after partial hepatectomy and to be associated with increased expression of the inhibitor of nuclear factor κB and decreased activation of nuclear factor κB. Exposure to a high-fat diet was associated with increased hepatocellular apoptosis. A high-fat diet not only may impair liver regeneration, but also may increase the risk for hepatic injury (steatohepatitis) (DeAngelis et al, 2005).

PATHOPHYSIOLOGY OF PORTAL VEIN EMBOLIZATION

Major hepatic resection results in removal of functional hepatic parenchyma, physical manipulation of the liver remnant, and an abrupt increase in portal pressure, which together contribute to hepatocellular injury and possibly hepatic congestion postresection (see Ch. 84a) (Makuuchi et al, 1990). Preoperative PVE permits adaptation of the remnant liver to the changed portal pressure and flow and dissociates this event from the mechanical hepatocellular injury incurred at the time of actual resection (Makuuchi et al, 1991). Immediately after embolization, portal blood flow to the unembolized liver measured by transcutaneous Doppler ultrasound increases significantly, then decreases to approach the baseline value after 11 days (see Ch. 3) (Goto et al, 1998). The resulting hypertrophy rate correlates with flow rate measurements. In addition, functional hepatic mass is increased before resection, providing a larger buffer of safety to reduce the risk of postresection metabolic changes and liver dysfunction.

Alterations in liver function tests are minor and transient after PVE in patients with normal values before embolization. If transaminases or prothrombin time rise, they typically peak at a level less than three times baseline 1 to 3 days after embolization and return to baseline by 7 to 10 days after embolization (Abdalla et al, 2001, Madoff, 2001, Vauthey et al, 2000). Minimal changes in total bilirubin and white blood cell count are seen.

PVE is not associated with the postembolization syndrome seen after arterial embolization; nausea and vomiting are rare, and fever and pain are minimal. Few side effects occur after PVE because there is no distortion of anatomy, minimal inflammation except immediately around the embolized vein, and minimal, if any, parenchymal or tumor necrosis (Vauthey et al, 2000). Animal studies indicate that hepatocytes undergo apoptosis, rather than necrosis, after portal occlusion (Duncan et al, 1999; Nagino et al, 2000).

LIVER VOLUME DETERMINATION

The rationale for PVE is based on existing data indicating that an increase in FLRV is associated with an improvement in its function as shown by an increase in biliary excretion (Ijichi et al, 2001; Uesaka et al, 1996), an increase in technetium-99m-galactosyl human serum albumin (^{99m}Tc-GSA) uptake (Hirai et al, 2003), and a significant improvement in postoperative liver function tests after PVE compared with no PVE (Vauthey et al, 2000). The aim of "measurement" of the liver volume is not simply to assess the actual volume of the FLR, but rather to provide a tool to predict FLR function after removal of the tumor-bearing liver. Several methods for liver volume determination have been proposed. Most use CT, which is essential for planning hepatic resection (Denys et al, 2002; Vauthey et al, 2000). Three-dimensional CT volumetric measurements are acquired by outlining the hepatic segmental contours and calculating volumes from each of the slice areas. CT must be performed with intravenous contrast agent administration in several phases to demarcate the vascular landmarks of the hepatic segments. Using this technique, a

highly accurate and reproducible FLRV can be calculated within minutes of scanning with error less than ±5% (Heymsfield et al, 1979; Soyer et al, 1992). FLR can be standardized to total liver volume (TLV) to determine the %TLV that will remain after hepatic resection.

Measurement of the TLV is possible with CT; however, direct measurement of the TLV may not be relevant to surgical planning for several reasons. First, in patients with large tumors, the total volume of the liver is altered, and attempts to subtract tumor volume from TLV require additional time to calculate and lead to additive mathematical errors in volume calculation (TLV − tumor volume) (Abdalla et al, 2001). These errors are greater in patients with multiple tumors or biliary dilation in the liver to be resected. Cirrhotic patients often have enlarged livers or shrunken livers, and the measured TLV may not be useful as an index to which FLRV is standardized.

A simpler, more accurate, and more reproducible method uses the estimated TLV, calculated from a formula that relates TLV to body weight or body surface area (Vauthey et al, 2000). It has long been known that liver size and patient size are related in a relatively linear fashion (Urata et al, 1995; Vauthey et al, 2000, 2002), and this association has been the cornerstone of determination of the appropriate graft size for recipients of partial liver grafts from living donors (Kawasaki et al, 1998; Kiuchi et al, 1999; Nishizaki et al, 2001). Using data from major centers in Europe and the United States, we have established a formula that correlates body surface area and TLV (Vauthey et al, 2002). This formula was evaluated in a meta-analysis comparing 12 different formulas and was recommended as one of the least biased and most precise for estimation of the TLV (Johnson et al, 2005). Using this approach, the FLRV is measured by three-dimensional CT, and the estimated TLV is calculated from the formula: estimated TLV = −794.41 + 1267.28 × body surface area (Fig. 84b.1) (Vauthey et al, 2002). The resulting FLR/estimated TLV ratio is calculated to provide a volumetric *estimate* of function of the FLR. Similar methods of measurements based on body surface area are used for the administration of chemotherapy agents and in pharmacokinetic models of hepatic drug clearance (Johnson et al, 2005). At our institution, CT scans are performed immediately before PVE and approximately 3 to 4 weeks after PVE to assess the degree of FLR

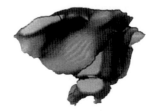

Segments I+II+III = 266 cm^3
BSA = 1.8 m^2

$$\frac{\text{Measured FLR volume}}{\text{Calculated TLV*}} = \frac{266}{1686} = 16 \text{ \% of TLV}$$

*Total Liver Volume based on Body Surface Area (BSA):
TLV = -794 + 1267 x BSA

Fig. 84b.1. Standardized FLR defined as the ratio of the CT three-dimensional measured FLR/calculated TLV. Formula for calculating TLV is based on body surface area.
(Modified from Vauthey JN, et al, 2002: Body surface area and body weight predict total liver volume in Western adults. Liver Transpl 8:233-240.)

Pre-PVE

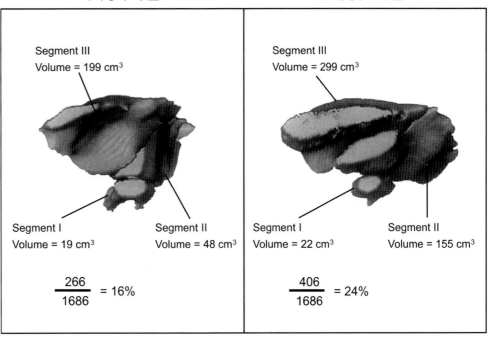

Fig. 84b.2. Hypertrophy of the FLR after PVE determined by three-dimensional reconstruction of CT images. Before embolization, the volume of segments I, II, and III is 266 cm³, or 16% of the TLV (1686 cm³). After embolization, the volume of segments I, II, and III is 406 cm³, or 24% of the TLV (increase of 8%).
(Modified from Vauthey JN, et al, 2000: Standardized measurement of the future liver remnant prior to extended liver resection: methodology and clinical associations. Surgery 127:512-519.)

Segment III
Volume = 199 cm³

Segment I
Volume = 19 cm³

Segment II
Volume = 48 cm³

$$\frac{266}{1686} = 16\%$$

Post-PVE

Segment III
Volume = 299 cm³

Segment I
Volume = 22 cm³

Segment II
Volume = 155 cm³

$$\frac{406}{1686} = 24\%$$

hypertrophy (Fig. 84b.2). From this method of calculation, called *standardized FLR measurement*, a correlation between the anticipated liver remnant and postoperative outcome has been established (Abdalla et al, 2002; Vauthey et al, 2000, 2004).

INDICATIONS FOR PORTAL VEIN EMBOLIZATION

Indications for PVE depend on several key factors. First, the presence or absence of underlying liver disease has a major impact on the volume of liver remnant needed for adequate function. Second, patient size must be considered—large patients require larger liver remnants; small patients, smaller liver remnants. Third, the extent and complexity of the planned resection and the probability that simultaneous nonhepatic surgery will be performed at the time of liver resection (e.g., hepatectomy plus pancreaticoduodenectomy) must be considered. These three major factors must be considered in the setting of the patient's age and comorbidities that may have an impact on regeneration, such as diabetes. When the procedure type and extent of resection necessary to treat the patient have been determined, appropriate liver volumetry can be performed. The volumetry technique detailed earlier integrates assessment of the actual FLRV with patient size so that the standardized FLRV expressed as a percentage of the estimated TLV (see section on liver volume determination and Figs. 84b.1 and 84b.2) can be used to determine the need for PVE based on resection extent planned and, importantly, the degree of underlying liver disease.

The true volume limit may never be known exactly, but likely varies from patient to patient. Guidelines have evolved, however, from recognition of the importance of the presence or absence of liver disease and proper attention to liver volume and patient size (Fig. 84b.3). In patients with an otherwise normal liver, PVE is indicated when the standardized FLRV is 20% or less.

This cutoff was determined by analysis of complications in 42 patients, all of whom had normal underlying liver and underwent extended right hepatectomy (resection of Couinaud segments IV-VIII) (Abdalla et al, 2002). The complication rate was prolonged in patients with FLRV 20% or less compared with patients with FLRV greater than 20% (Fig. 84b.4). The 20% cutoff FLRV provides a margin of safety or a buffer volume, as no patient died in the 20% or less group, including a patient with an 11% FLRV, although the 20% cutoff point determined which patients were at risk for a complicated postoperative course. This approach was validated in a subsequent study in which standardized FLRV was calculated, and PVE was used based on these criteria. Among 127 consecutive patients who underwent extended hepatectomy, hepatic complications occurred in 19% (including perihepatic collection or abscess, bile leak, or hepatic insufficiency) with an overall complication rate of 31%, all of which resolved. Only 1 perioperative death (0.8%) occurred in the entire series.

It is important to recognize and individualize the indication for PVE by using a standardized volume cutoff because of the normal variations in segmental liver volume. Liver volume analysis has revealed that the lateral left liver (segments II and III) contributes 20% or less of the TLV in more than 75% of patients in the absence of compensatory hypertrophy (Fig. 84b.5). The left liver (segments II, III, and IV) contributes 20% or less

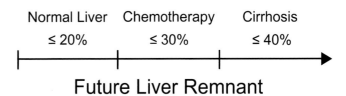

Normal Liver	Chemotherapy	Cirrhosis
≤ 20%	≤ 30%	≤ 40%

Future Liver Remnant

Fig. 84b.3. Proposed indications for PVE according to the extent of underlying liver disease.

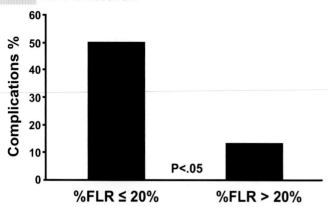

Fig. 84b.4. Complication rate stratified by standardized FLRV. Patients with an FLR of 20% or less had significantly more complications than patients with an FLR greater than 20%.
(Adapted from Abdalla EK, et al, 2004: Total and segmental liver volume variations: implications for liver surgery. Surgery 135:404-410.)

Liver injury can occur among patients who receive extensive chemotherapy before hepatic resection (Vauthey et al, 2006). The clinical significance of chemotherapy-related liver injury is not well defined, although hepatic steatosis (Behrns et al, 1998; Kooby et al, 2003) is known to increase the risk of postoperative complications (but not death) after hepatectomy, and chemotherapy-associated steatohepatitis may increase the 90-day mortality after liver surgery (Vauthey et al, 2006). The physiologic basis for this problem is likely related to the increased risk for hepatic injury described in preclinical models (see Ch. 4) (DeAngelis et al, 2005). A continuum of hepatic injuries, including steatohepatitis and sinusoidal dilation, seems to be related to oxaliplatin-based and irinotecan-based fluoropyrimidine chemotherapy (Fernandez et al, 2005; Rubbia-Brandt et al, 2004; Vauthey et al, 2006). Some authors have recommended the use of a larger buffer of safety when performing extended resection in selected patients who have received preoperative systemic chemotherapy. In this group, although less well studied than patients with normal liver, PVE may be indicated when the FLR is 30% or less of the TLV (Adam et al, 2004; Azoulay et al, 2000a).

of the TLV in more than 10% of patients (Abdalla et al, 2004a). FLR/TLV ratio less than 20% can be expected in most patients who do not develop compensatory hypertrophy from tumor growth and require an extended right hepatectomy. Left PVE is rarely necessary, however; Nagino and colleagues (1995b) showed that a left trisegmentectomy with caudate lobectomy results in resection of only 67% of the liver, leaving FLR of 33%—the same residual volume after right hepatectomy in a normal liver. Volumetric analysis of normal livers also confirms the consistently large volume of the posterior right liver (segments VI and VII) (Abdalla et al, 2004a; Leelaudomlipi et al, 2002).

Major resection can be performed safely in some cirrhotic patients (see Ch. 82), although extended hepatectomy is rarely an option. In contrast to patients with normal liver, patients with marginal liver remnants and cirrhosis are not only at risk for complications, but also are at significantly increased risk for death from liver failure (Shirabe et al, 1999). In carefully selected patients with preserved liver function (Child classification A) and normal ICG retention at 15 minutes (ICG R15 <10%), major resection can be performed safely. In this subgroup with chronic liver disease, PVE is indicated when the FLRV is less than 40% of the TLV (Kubota et al, 1997). This guideline is supported

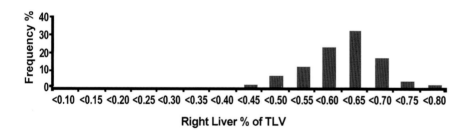

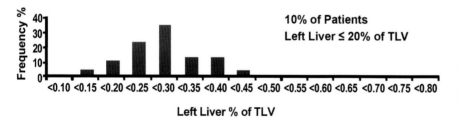

Fig. 84b.5. Variability in volume contributions of the right liver, left liver, and segments II and III (left lateral section) based on CT volumetry in 102 patients. (Adapted from Abdalla EK, et al, 2004: Total and segmental liver volume variations: implications for liver surgery. Surgery 135:404-410.)

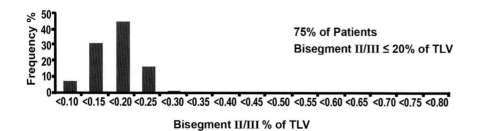

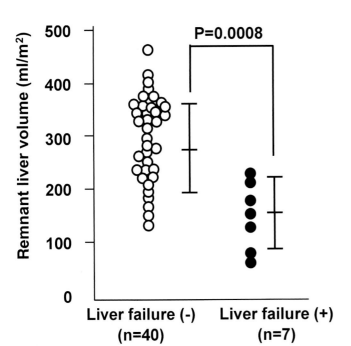

P=0.0008

Fig. 84b.6. Small liver volume standardized using body surface area correlates with poor outcome in patients with chronic liver disease. In this study, although an overlap in remnant liver volumes is noted between patients who died and patients who did not die from liver failure after surgery, all deaths occurred in patients with future liver remnants less than 300 mL/m².
(From Shirabe K, et al, 1999: Postoperative liver failure after major hepatic resection for hepatocellular carcinoma in the modern era with special reference to remnant liver volume. J Am Coll Surg 188:304-309.)

by the finding that when liver volume is standardized to body surface area, standardized FLRV predicts death from liver failure after hepatectomy in chronic liver disease (Fig. 84b.6) (Shirabe et al, 1999).

A randomized study also indicated that patients with chronic liver disease who underwent right hepatectomy after PVE had fewer complications and shorter intensive care unit stays than patients with chronic liver disease who underwent right hepatectomy without PVE (Farges et al, 2003). This guideline has been expanded to include patients in whom the liver is compromised by biliary obstruction who require extended hepatectomy (Abdalla et al, 2001; Makuuchi et al, 1990; Nagino et al, 1995a; Vauthey et al, 2000), but is not recommended by all (see Ch. 80). Highly selected patients with advanced liver disease also might undergo safe resection. Specifically, in cirrhotic patients with a moderately abnormal ICG retention (10-20%), but with preserved liver function, a sequence of transarterial chemoembolization followed by PVE has been proposed to maximize the atrophy/hypertrophy complex (Aoki et al, 2004). Because of the continuum of liver disease, the specific indications for PVE in patients with chronic liver disease remain to be defined precisely and require an individualized approach (see Fig. 84b.3). It is anticipated that refined criteria will be developed with the accrual of more experience with the standardized measurement of FLR.

CONTRAINDICATIONS TO PORTAL VEIN EMBOLIZATION

Contraindications to PVE include adequate liver volume based on the aforementioned criteria and tumor invasion of the portal vein to be resected because portal flow is already diverted. Relative contraindications to PVE include tumor extension to the FLR, uncorrectable coagulopathy, biliary dilation in the FLR (if the biliary tree is obstructed, drainage is recommended), portal hypertension, and renal failure. The presence of an ipsilateral tumor may preclude safe ipsilateral transhepatic access if the tumor burden is great. If access to an adequate portal vein branch for PVE is impossible, the contralateral approach can be considered.

TECHNICAL CONSIDERATIONS

See also Ch. 84a for discussion of technical considerations for PVE.

Approaches

PVE is performed to redirect portal blood flow toward the hepatic segments that will remain after surgery (i.e., FLR). To ensure adequate hypertrophy, embolization of portal branches must be as complete as possible so that recanalization of the occluded portal system is minimized. The entire portal tree to be resected must be occluded to avoid the development of intrahepatic portoportal collaterals that may limit regeneration (Denys et al, 1999; Madoff et al, 2003). The magnitude of regeneration is proportional to the magnitude of the hypertrophy stimulus.

PVE can be performed by any of three standard approaches: transhepatic contralateral (i.e., portal access via the FLR), transhepatic ipsilateral (i.e., portal access via the liver to be resected), and intraoperative transileocolic venous approaches. These approaches are chosen on the basis of operator preference, type of hepatic resection planned, extent of embolization (e.g., right PVE with or without extension to segment IV), and type of embolic agent used.

The transhepatic ipsilateral approach, first described by Nagino and colleagues (1996) in the mid-1990s, is currently being advocated by additional investigators, including those in our group (Madoff et al, 2003, 2005a). For this approach, a peripheral portal vein branch in the liver *to be resected* is accessed, through which liquid embolic material is injected. Because Nagino's ipsilateral approach requires the use of specialized balloon catheters unavailable outside of Japan, modifications of the ipsilateral technique have been developed. At M.D. Anderson Cancer Center, we modified Nagino's technique to use standard angiographic catheters for combined particulate and coil embolization (Fig. 84b.7) (Madoff et al, 2002, 2003, 2005a). When right hepatectomy is planned, right PVE (RPVE) is performed in the interventional radiology suite. RPVE is performed via access to a distal right portal vein branch.

When extended right hepatectomy is planned, RPVE is extended to segment IV (RPVE + IV). After right portal vein puncture, the segment IV embolization is performed first so as not to manipulate catheters through previously embolized segments. A microcatheter is advanced coaxially through an angled catheter into the portal vein branches supplying segment IV so that small particles and then coils can be delivered. When segment IV embolization is completed, a reverse-curved catheter is used for RPVE. After complete occlusion of the right portal vein (with or without segment IV), embolization of the access tract is performed with coils to reduce the risk of perihepatic hemorrhage at

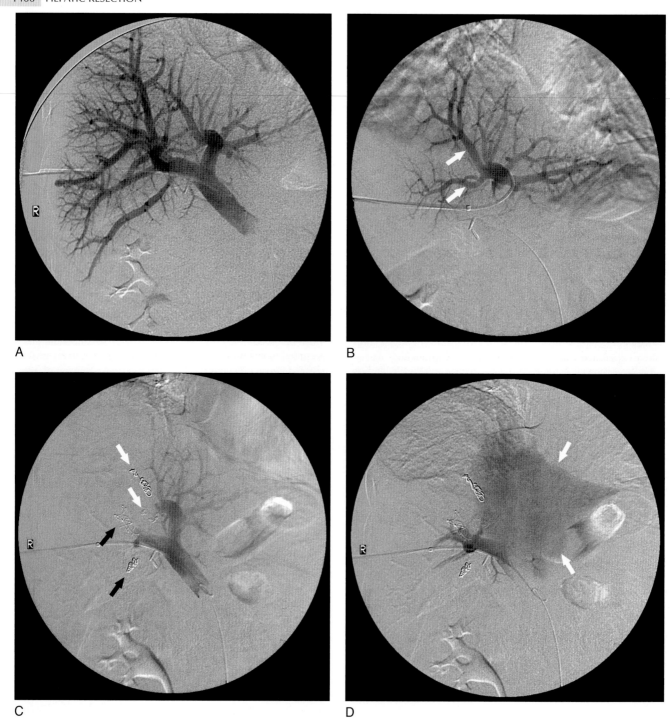

Fig. 84b.7. Transhepatic ipsilateral right PVE + IV with tris-acryl particles and coils performed in a 73-year-old woman with carcinoid disease metastatic to the liver. **A,** Anteroposterior flush portogram obtained before right PVE + IV with use of a 6-Fr vascular sheath in a right portal vein branch and a 5-Fr flush catheter in the main portal vein. **B,** Selective left portogram shows the veins that supply segment IV *(arrows)*. **C,** Postprocedural portogram shows occlusion of segments IV through VIII portal veins *(white arrows* show coils within segment IV portal veins, and *black arrows* show coils within proximal anterior and posterior sector right portal veins) with continued patency of the veins supplying the left lateral bisegment II/III. **D,** Later phase of postprocedural portogram shows normal parenchymal flow to left lateral bisegment II/III *(white arrows)* with complete absence of flow to segments IV through VIII.
(From Madoff DC, et al, 2005: Transhepatic ipsilateral right portal vein embolization extended to segment IV: improving hypertrophy and resection outcomes with spherical particles and coils. J Vasc Interv Radiol 16:215-225.)

the puncture site. This modified approach respects the FLR (avoiding puncture) and uses standard angiographic catheters and readily available embolic agents (Madoff et al, 2005a). In our experience with 101 consecutive PVEs, the ipsilateral approach was used in all patients but one. This includes 99 RPVEs, of which 79 were extended to segment IV.

The transhepatic contralateral approach, developed by Kinoshita and associates (1986), is the most commonly used technique worldwide. The FLR is punctured directly, which provides straight access to the right portal branches, making the procedure technically straightforward (De Baere et al, 1996). The disadvantage of this technique is the risk of injury to the FLR parenchyma and the left portal vein. A multicenter European study of 188 patients who underwent contralateral PVE (Di Stefano et al, 2004) reported 24 adverse events (12.8%), including migration of embolic material to the FLR in 10 patients (5.3%), occlusion of a major portal branch requiring intervention in 3 patients (1.6%), bleeding in 5 patients (2.7%) (hemobilia, $n = 1$; hemoperitoneum, $n = 1$; rupture of gallbladder metastasis, $n = 1$; subcapsular hematoma, $n = 2$), and transient liver failure in 6 patients (3.2%). These adverse events associated with the migration of embolic material and use of the contralateral approach may compromise the integrity of the FLR and may make the planned resection more difficult or impossible.

The transileocolic venous approach is performed during laparotomy by direct cannulation of the ileocolic vein and advancement of a balloon catheter into the portal vein for subsequent embolization (Makuuchi et al, 1990). This approach is preferred by some groups and often is performed when an interventional radiology suite is unavailable, when a percutaneous approach is not feasible, or when additional treatment is needed during the same surgical exploration. Disadvantages of this method are the need for general anesthesia and laparotomy, with their inherent risks, and the inferior imaging equipment often available in an operating room setting compared with the state-of-the-art imaging equipment available in most interventional radiology suites.

Some centers have recommended intraoperative portal vein ligation during the first step of two-stage planned hepatectomy (see Ch. 80) in lieu of PVE (Kianmanesh et al, 2003). We generally do not recommend this approach because regeneration is not optimized without segment IV occlusion (Nagino et al, 2000), and tumor growth in segment IV may be accelerated (Elias et al, 1999b; Kokudo et al, 2001). Portal vein ligation results in inferior rates of hypertrophy of the FLR compared with PVE (Broering et al, 2002), and recanalization through portoportal collaterals has been reported (Denys et al, 1999).

Extent of Portal Vein Embolization

The optimal extent of PVE is debated. Left embolization is rarely necessary because of the consistently large volume of the right posterior sector (Abdalla et al, 2004a; Leelaudomlipi et al, 2002; Nagino et al, 1995b). Currently, several investigators who use PVE to prepare for extended right hepatectomy embolize only the branches of the right portal vein and leave the portal veins supplying segment IV patent despite the need to resect segment IV (Capussotti et al, 2005; De Baere et al, 1993; Farges et al, 2003). Although hypertrophy of the FLR does occur, full diversion of portal flow to segments II and III with or without segment I ensures the maximal stimulus for hypertrophy of the true FLR (Nagino et al, 1995b, 2000). In addition, incomplete

embolization of the liver to be resected (i.e., RPVE only) leads to hypertrophy of segment IV and the true FLR.

Segment IV hypertrophy is not desired for extended right hepatectomy because of the larger area of intraoperative parenchymal transection across this hypertrophic segment. Nagino and colleagues (2000), using liquid embolics, first showed that greater left lateral bisegment hypertrophy occurs after RPVE + IV (50% increase in FLRV) than after RPVE only (31% increase; $P<.0005$). We reported similar results for RPVE + IV with polyvinyl alcohol particles and coils. We found the absolute FLR increased 45.5% and the FLR/TLV increased 6.9%, and the subsequent resection rate was 57%. The development of small spherical particulate embolics led us to refine our technique for RPVE + IV further by using a stepwise infusion of small (100-300 μm) tris-acryl microspheres followed by larger spheres (700 μm) and coils to ensure complete outflow and inflow occlusion. This approach led to an absolute increase in FLR of 69%, FLR/TLV increase of 9.7%, and subsequent resection rate of 86% (Madoff et al, 2005a). Extension of embolization to segment IV prior to extended right hepatectomy with this refined technique led not only to improved hypertrophy but increased resection rates after PVE.

From an oncologic standpoint, a potential benefit of RPVE + IV is that the entire tumor-bearing liver is systematically embolized, including segment IV, to minimize the risk of tumor growth that may result from increased portal blood flow and hepatotropic factors. Tumor growth in the nonembolized liver has been discussed on analysis of a limited number of patients with primary and secondary liver tumors after RPVE alone (although no comparison to pre-PVE tumor growth rate was made, so the true impact of PVE on tumor growth could not be proved) (Elias et al, 1999b; Kokudo et al, 2001). In contrast, we have analyzed reasons for failure to resect after PVE and found that change in tumor size after complete embolization of the entire tumor-bearing liver does not affect subsequent resectability (Abdalla et al, 2004b). Liver hypertrophy occurs quickly in patients with normal liver (patients with severely diseased livers rarely undergo extended hepatectomy, so embolization of the right portal branches plus segment IV does not apply to that group); resection can be undertaken in patients with multiple colorectal metastases within 3 to 4 weeks of PVE in most cases. We occasionally have administered chemotherapy in the interim between PVE and resection, and this combined approach does not seem to affect hypertrophy or outcome (unpublished data).

Complications

As with all percutaneous transhepatic procedures, technical complications can occur from PVE and include subcapsular hematoma, hemobilia, pseudoaneurysm, arteriovenous fistula, arterioportal shunts, portal vein thrombosis, pneumothorax, and sepsis. In 2002, Kodama and coworkers reported on a series in which 7 (15%) of 47 patients had complications: 2 pneumothoraces, 2 subcapsular hematomas, 1 arterial puncture, 1 pseudoaneurysm (in a patient who also had a subcapsular hematoma), 1 hemobilia, and 1 portal vein thrombosis. Because most technical complications occurred in the punctured lobe, Kodama and coworkers (2002) recommended that the transhepatic ipsilateral approach be tried first. In our series of 101 consecutive PVEs, 13 (13%) complications occurred, but only 1 (1%) precluded subsequent resection. Using embolization of the entire tumor-bearing liver, misplaced coils in the FLR

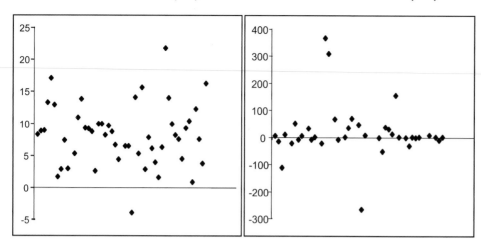

FLR volume (%)   **Tumor volume (cc)**

Fig. 84b.8. Changes in FLR *(left panel)* and tumor volume *(right panel)* after PVE. The FLR increased by a median of 8.7%, whereas the tumor volume did not significantly change (median 0 mL).
(From Abdalla EK, et al, 2004: Portal vein embolization of the entire tumor-bearing liver prior to major hepatectomy is not associated with significant tumor growth. HPB Surg 6:6 [abstract 18].)

occurred in only 3 patients (2.9%), and we found no significant tumor growth despite a consistent increase in FLRV (Fig. 84b.8).

The close interaction between surgeons and radiologists in our institution has allowed us to develop this approach to protect the liver remnant from injury. Similar to Kodama and coworkers (2002), we strongly advocate the ipsilateral approach to PVE to maximize the probability of optimal FLR hypertrophy and operative outcome.

OUTCOMES AFTER PORTAL VEIN EMBOLIZATION AND HEPATECTOMY

Chronic Liver Disease

In patients with chronic liver disease (chronic hepatitis, fibrosis, or cirrhosis), the magnitude and rate of volume increase after PVE are less than in patients with normal underlying liver.

As with other procedures in patients with cirrhosis, the complication rates after PVE are higher in patients with chronic liver disease than in patients with an otherwise normal liver because of the increased risk of secondary portal vein thrombosis, presumably from slow flow in the portal vein trunk after PVE (Azoulay et al, 2000a). The combination of transarterial chemoembolization (TACE) of the tumor followed by PVE within 2 weeks may optimize outcome for some patients who have HCC in the presence of chronic liver disease and require major resection (Fig. 84b.9) (Aoki et al, 2004). At M.D. Anderson Cancer Center, portal pressures are measured routinely during pre-embolization portography, and if pressures are frankly elevated, PVE is not performed. Mild elevation of portal pressure has not led us to abandon PVE as an option. We do not consider patients with overt portal hypertension (splenomegaly, low platelets, imaging evidence of varices) for PVE or surgery, however.

The appropriate use of PVE significantly decreases the number and severity of complications and the incidence of postoperative

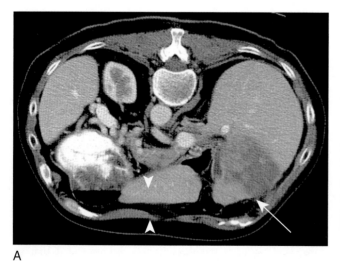

A

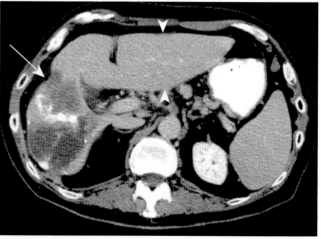

B

Fig. 84b.9. A 74-year-old man with HCC. **A,** A large HCC (12.5 cm) arising in a background of hepatitis C and chronic liver disease with involvement of segments V through VIII of the liver. **B,** After sequential TACE and right PVE, left liver volume increased from 27% to 47% of the total estimated liver volume with a decrease in size of the tumor mass. Complete necrosis with no viable tumor was found at pathologic examination after right hepatectomy. *(Arrows* indicate tumor before and after embolizations; *arrowheads* show left liver before and after embolizations.)

liver failure and death after major hepatic resection in patients with chronic liver disease (De Baere et al, 1996; Imamura et al, 1999; Nagino et al, 1995b). A prospective study corroborated this significant benefit of PVE in patients with chronic liver disease before right hepatectomy (Farges et al, 2003).

Oncologic outcome after resection in cirrhosis post-PVE is similar to outcome after resection without PVE. Azoulay and associates (2000b) found that major resection for HCC after PVE (performed when FLR was predicted to be ≤40%) could be performed without death or liver failure in any of 10 embolized patients, whereas 3 of 19 patients resected without PVE had liver failure, and one patient died postoperatively. Disease-free and overall survivals were similar in the PVE and no-PVE groups (Azoulay et al, 2000b).

In a larger study, Tanaka and colleagues (2000) found similar disease-free survival after resection with PVE as after resection without PVE. The overall survival was longer in the PVE group, however. A larger proportion of patients with recurrence in the PVE group were candidates for a second potentially curative treatment, an additional potential benefit of PVE in the long term.

No Chronic Liver Disease

Optimal preparation of the FLR for extended resection requires complete diversion of portal flow to the intended liver remnant, segments II and III (see Fig. 84b.7). Technical aspects of PVE (Madoff, 2001; Madoff et al, 2003, 2005b) are important to maximize the hypertrophy stimulus and minimize the risk for tumor growth after PVE before resection (Madoff et al, 2005a, 2005b).

We reported our experience with 127 consecutive extended hepatectomies using standardized liver volume calculations to select patients for PVE (Vauthey et al, 2004). In this series, 31 (24.4%) patients underwent PVE before extended hepatectomy. Of 127 patients, only 6 (5%) experienced significant postoperative liver insufficiency (total bilirubin level >10 mg/dL or international normalized ratio >2). The postoperative complication rate was 30.9% (39 of 127), and only 1 patient (0.8%) died after extended hepatectomy. The median survival was 41.9 months, and the overall 5-year survival rate was 26% for the entire group. The low mortality rate of extended hepatectomy reflects many factors, among which were the systematic attention to FLR and the use of PVE based on the aforementioned indications.

Several other studies have validated residual volume as the key to prediction of postoperative liver function and posthepatectomy course. Shoup and colleagues (2003), in a retrospective analysis of outcome after resection of colorectal cancer liver metastases, found that FLRV of 25% or less was an independent predictor of postoperative complications and increased length of hospital stay and recommended FLR assessment before consideration of PVE. Elias and associates (1999a) showed that patients considered to have unresectable tumors owing to inadequate liver volume at presentation could undergo complete resection after treatment with PVE, with an associated 5-year overall survival rate of 29%. Azoulay and colleagues (2000a) showed that the 5-year overall survival rate after resection in patients with colorectal liver metastases who required PVE was similar to that in patients who did not have PVE (40% versus 38%).

PVE has an important role in the preoperative preparation of patients with normal underlying liver and an inadequate liver remnant before extended hepatectomy. Proper patient selection (FLR <20% of the TLV) and technical aspects of the performance of PVE can affect the degree and rate of hypertrophy of the liver remnant. Although changes in tumor size related to PVE seem not to have clinical significance, increases in tumor size can be avoided, and FLR hypertrophy can be maximized if the entire tumor-bearing liver is systematically embolized, including the right liver and segment IV, before extended right hepatectomy.

CONCLUSION

PVE increases the safety of resection in appropriately selected patients and expands the indications for liver resection. Using a standardized method of measurement, we have shown that the FLR correlates with postoperative hepatic function and outcome. Complete embolization of the tumor-bearing liver maximizes FLR growth and minimizes tumor growth. The combination of microspheres and coils seems to improve hepatic regeneration and resectability after PVE. A period of 3 to 4 weeks is sufficient to enable adequate hypertrophy in patients with normal livers, minimizing the delay to resection. Longer periods (6-8 weeks) may be necessary to permit adequate hypertrophy in patients with cirrhosis and diabetes.

A randomized trial cannot be recommended to test the efficacy of PVE, for it would be unethical to deny the benefit of the technique and safer resection to patients who are otherwise poor candidates for resection based on inadequate liver size or function. Continued prospective examination of PVE and liver volumetric measurement, with defined end points such as liver function, operative complications, and length of stay, should clarify the additional benefits provided by preoperative embolization.

REFERENCES

Abdalla EK, et al, 2001: Portal vein embolization: rationale, technique and future prospects. Br J Surg 88:165-175.

Abdalla EK, et al, 2002: Extended hepatectomy in patients with hepatobiliary malignancies with and without preoperative portal vein embolization. Arch Surg 137:675-680.

Abdalla EK, et al, 2004a: Total and segmental liver volume variations: implications for liver surgery. Surgery 135:404-410.

Abdalla EK, et al, 2004b: Portal vein embolization of the entire tumor-bearing liver prior to major hepatectomy is not associated with significant tumor growth. HPB Surg 6:6 (abstract 18).

Adam R, et al, 2004: Rescue surgery for unresectable colorectal liver metastases downstaged by chemotherapy: a model to predict long-term survival. Ann Surg 240:644-657.

Anderson CD, et al, 2004: Contralateral portal vein embolization for hepatectomy in the setting of hepatic steatosis. Am Surg 70:609-612.

Aoki T, et al, 2004: Sequential preoperative arterial and portal venous embolizations in patients with hepatocellular carcinoma. Arch Surg 139:766-774.

Azoulay D, et al, 2000a: Percutaneous portal vein embolization increases the feasibility and safety of major liver resection for hepatocellular carcinoma in injured liver. Ann Surg 232:665-672.

Azoulay D, et al, 2000b: Resection of nonresectable liver metastases from colorectal cancer after percutaneous portal vein embolization. Ann Surg 231:480-486.

Behrns KE, et al, 1998: Hepatic steatosis as a potential risk factor for major hepatic resection. J Gastrointest Surg 2:292-298.

Belghiti J, et al, 2000: Seven hundred forty-seven hepatectomies in the 1990s: an update to evaluate the actual risk of liver resection. J Am Coll Surg 191:38-46.

Broering DC, et al, 2002: Portal vein embolization vs. portal vein ligation for induction of hypertrophy of the future liver remnant. J Gastrointest Surg 6:905-913.

Bucher NL, Swaffield MN, 1964: The rate of incorporation of labeled thymidine into the deoxyribonucleic acid of regenerating rat liver in relation to the amount of liver excised. Cancer Res 24:1611-1625.

Capussotti L, et al, 2005: Extension of right portal vein embolization to segment IV portal branches. Arch Surg 140:1100-1103.

Carr BI, et al, 1986: Inhibition of DNA synthesis in rat hepatocytes by platelet-derived type beta transforming growth factor. Cancer Res 46:2330-2334.

Cruise JL, et al, 1985: Induction of DNA synthesis in cultured rat hepatocytes through stimulation of alpha 1 adrenoreceptor by norepinephrine. Science 227:749-751.

DeAngelis RA, et al, 2005: A high-fat diet impairs liver regeneration in C57BL/6 mice through overexpression of the NF-kappaB inhibitor, IkappaBalpha. Hepatology 42:1148-1157.

De Baere T, et al, 1993: Portal vein embolization: utility for inducing left hepatic lobe hypertrophy before surgery. Radiology 188:73-77.

De Baere T, et al, 1996: Preoperative portal vein embolization for extension of hepatectomy indications. Hepatology 24:1386-1391.

Denys AL, et al, 1999: Failure of right portal vein ligation to induce left lobe hypertrophy due to intrahepatic portoportal collaterals: successful treatment with portal vein embolization. AJR Am J Roentgenol 173:633-635.

Denys A, et al, 2002: Indications for and limitations of portal vein embolization before major hepatic resection for hepatobiliary malignancy. Surg Oncol Clin N Am 11:955-968.

Di Stefano DR, et al, 2004: Preoperative percutaneous portal vein embolization: evaluation of adverse events in 188 patients. Radiology 234:625-630.

Duncan JR, et al, 1999: Embolization of portal vein branches induces hepatocyte replication in swine: a potential step in hepatic gene therapy. Radiology 210:467-477.

Elias D, et al, 1999a: [Long-term oncological results of hepatectomy performed after selective portal embolization]. Ann Chir 53:559-564.

Elias D, et al, 1999b: During liver regeneration following right portal embolization the growth rate of liver metastases is more rapid than that of the liver parenchyma. Br J Surg 86:784-788.

Fabrikant JI, 1968: The kinetics of cellular proliferation in regenerating liver. J Cell Biol 36:551-565.

Farges O, et al, 2003: Portal vein embolization before right hepatectomy: prospective clinical trial. Ann Surg 237:208-217.

Fernandez FG, et al, 2005: Effect of steatohepatitis associated with irinotecan or oxaliplatin pretreatment on resectability of hepatic colorectal metastases. J Am Coll Surg 200:845-853.

Francavilla A, et al, 1978: Liver regeneration in dogs: morphologic and chemical changes. J Surg Res 25:409-419.

Goto Y, et al, 1998: Doppler estimation of portal blood flow after percutaneous transhepatic portal vein embolization. Ann Surg 228:209-213.

Heymsfield SB, et al, 1979: Accurate measurement of liver, kidney, and spleen volume and mass by computerized axial tomography. Ann Intern Med 90:185-187.

Hirai I, et al, 2003: Evaluation of preoperative portal embolization for safe hepatectomy, with special reference to assessment of nonembolized lobe function with 99mTc-GSA SPECT scintigraphy. Surgery 133:495-506.

Ijichi M, et al, 2001: Portal embolization relieves persistent jaundice after complete biliary drainage. Surgery 130:116-118.

Imamura H, et al, 1999: Preoperative portal vein embolization: an audit of 84 patients. Hepatology 29:1099-1105.

Jarnagin WR, et al, 2002: Improvement in perioperative outcome after hepatic resection: analysis of 1,803 consecutive cases over the past decade. Ann Surg 236:397-406.

Johnson TN, et al, 2005: Changes in liver volume from birth to adulthood: a meta-analysis. Liver Transpl 11:1481-1493.

Katoh T, et al, 1991: Enhancement of rat liver mitochondrial function by portal branch ligation secures subsequent extended hepatectomy. Biochem Int 24:107-116.

Kawasaki S, et al, 1998: Living related liver transplantation in adults. Ann Surg 227:269-274.

Kianmanesh R, et al, 2003: Right portal vein ligation: a new planned two-step all-surgical approach for complete resection of primary gastrointestinal tumors with multiple bilateral liver metastases. J Am Coll Surg 197:164-170.

Kinoshita H, et al, 1986: Preoperative portal vein embolization for hepatocellular carcinoma. World J Surg 10:803-808.

Kiuchi T, et al, 1999: Impact of graft size mismatching on graft prognosis in liver transplantation from living donors. Transplantation 67:321-327.

Kodama Y, et al, 2002: Complications of percutaneous transhepatic portal vein embolization. J Vasc Interv Radiol 13:1233-1237.

Kokudo N, et al, 2001: Proliferative activity of intrahepatic colorectal metastases after preoperative hemihepatic portal vein embolization. Hepatology 34:267-272.

Kooby DA, et al, 2003: Impact of steatosis on perioperative outcome following hepatic resection. J Gastrointest Surg 7:1034-1044.

Kubota K, et al, 1997: Measurement of liver volume and hepatic functional reserve as a guide to decision-making in resectional surgery for hepatic tumors. Hepatology 26:1176-1181.

Leelaudomlipi S, et al, 2002: Volumetric analysis of liver segments in 155 living donors. Liver Transpl 8:612-614.

Madoff DC, 2001: Portal vein embolization using polyvinyl alcohol and coils in preparation for major liver resection in patients with advanced hepatobiliary malignancy. J Vasc Interv Radiol 12: S39.

Madoff DC, et al, 2002: Transhepatic portal vein embolization: anatomy, indications, and technical considerations. Radiographics 22:1063-1076.

Madoff DC, et al, 2003: Portal vein embolization with polyvinyl alcohol particles and coils in preparation for major liver resection for hepatobiliary malignancy: safety and effectiveness—study in 26 patients. Radiology 227:251-260.

Madoff DC, et al, 2005a: Transhepatic ipsilateral right portal vein embolization extended to segment IV: improving hypertrophy and resection outcomes with spherical particles and coils. J Vasc Interv Radiol 16:215-225.

Madoff DC, et al, 2005b: Portal vein embolization in preparation for major hepatic resection: evolution of a new standard of care. J Vasc Interv Radiol 16:779-790.

Makuuchi M, et al, 1990: Preoperative portal embolization to increase safety of major hepatectomy for hilar bile duct carcinoma: a preliminary report. Surgery 107:521-527.

Makuuchi M, et al, 1991: New possibilities for major liver surgery in patients with Klatskin tumors or primary hepatocellular carcinoma—an old problem revisited. Hepatogastroenterology 38:329-336.

Michalopoulos GK, DeFrances MC, 1997: Liver regeneration. Science 276:60-66.

Michalopoulos GK, Zarnegav R, 1992: Hepatocyte growth factor. Hepatology 15:149-155.

Nagasue N, et al, 1987: Human liver regeneration after major hepatic resection. A study of normal liver and livers with chronic hepatitis and cirrhosis. Ann Surg 206:30-39.

Nagino M, et al, 1989: Stimulated rat liver mitochondrial biogenesis after partial hepatectomy. Cancer Res 49:4913-4918.

Nagino M, et al, 1995a: Changes in hepatic lobe volume in biliary tract cancer patients after right portal vein embolization. Hepatology 21:434-439.

Nagino M, et al, 1995b: Right or left trisegment portal vein embolization before hepatic trisegmentectomy for hilar bile duct carcinoma. Surgery 117:677-681.

Nagino M, et al, 1996: Selective percutaneous transhepatic embolization of the portal vein in preparation for extensive liver resection: the ipsilateral approach. Radiology 200:559-563.

Nagino M, et al, 2000: Right trisegment portal vein embolization for biliary tract carcinoma: technique and clinical utility. Surgery 127:155-160.

Nishizaki T, et al, 2001: Small graft for living donor liver transplantation. Ann Surg 233:575-580.

Ozawa K, et al, 1971: Effect of ligation of portal vein on liver mitochondrial metabolism. J Biochem 70:755-764.

Ozawa K, et al, 1974: Clinical application of cytochrome a (plus a3) assay of mitochondria from liver specimens: an aid in determining metabolic tolerance of liver remnant for hepatic resection. Ann Surg 180:868-876.

Rubbia-Brandt L, et al, 2004: Severe hepatic sinusoidal obstruction associated with oxaliplatin-based chemotherapy in patients with metastatic colorectal cancer. Ann Oncol 15:460-466.

Rudnick DA, 2005: Trimming the fat from liver regeneration. Hepatology 42:1001-1003.

Shimamura T, et al, 1997: Efficacy and safety of preoperative percutaneous transhepatic portal embolization with absolute ethanol: a clinical study. Surgery 121:135-141.

Shirabe K, et al, 1999: Postoperative liver failure after major hepatic resection for hepatocellular carcinoma in the modern era with special reference to remnant liver volume. J Am Coll Surg 188:304-309.

Shoup M, et al, 2003: Volumetric analysis predicts hepatic dysfunction in patients undergoing major liver resection. J Gastrointest Surg 7:325-330.

Soyer P, et al, 1992: Hepatic metastases from colorectal cancer: influence of hepatic volumetric analysis on surgical decision making. Radiology 184:695-697.

Starzl TE, et al, 1978: The effect of splanchnic viscera removal upon canine liver regeneration. Surg Gynecol Obstet 147:193-207.

Tanaka H, et al, 2000: Preoperative portal vein embolization improves prognosis after right hepatectomy for hepatocellular carcinoma in patients with impaired hepatic function. Br J Surg 87:879-882.

Taub R, 1996: Liver regeneration in health and disease. Clin Lab Med 16:341-360.

Uesaka K, et al, 1996: Changes in hepatic lobar function after right portal vein embolization: an appraisal by biliary indocyanine green excretion. Ann Surg 223:77-83.

Urata K, et al, 1995: Calculation of child and adult standard liver volume for liver transplantation. Hepatology 21:1317-1321.

Vauthey JN, et al, 1993: Comparison of outcome between extended and nonextended liver resections for neoplasms. Surgery 114:968-975.

Vauthey JN, et al, 2000: Standardized measurement of the future liver remnant prior to extended liver resection: methodology and clinical associations. Surgery 127:512-519.

Vauthey JN, et al, 2002: Body surface area and body weight predict total liver volume in Western adults. Liver Transpl 8:233-240.

Vauthey JN, et al, 2004: Is extended hepatectomy for hepatobiliary malignancy justified? Ann Surg 239:722-732.

Vauthey JN, et al, 2006: Chemotherapy regimen predicts steatohepatitis and an increase in ninety-day mortality after surgery for hepatic colorectal metastases. J Clin Oncol 24:2065-2072.

Vitellas KM, et al, 2001: Cirrhosis: spectrum of findings on unenhanced and dynamic gadolinium-enhanced MR imaging. Abdom Imaging 26:601-615.

Yamanaka N, et al, 1993: Dynamics of normal and injured human liver regeneration after hepatectomy as assessed on the basis of computed tomography and liver function. Hepatology 18:79-85.

Ex Vivo and In Situ Hypothermic Hepatic Resection

A. W. HEMMING

Liver surgery has progressed to become a distinct area of specialization. Extended right and left hepatectomies, previously considered to be pushing the boundaries of resection, have become relatively standard procedures for experienced liver surgeons. The use of strategies such as preoperative portal vein embolization (see Ch. 84) to allow growth of the planned liver remnant allows even more aggressive resections to be performed with morbidity similar to less extensive resections. Advances in surgical technique have been paralleled by advances in hepatic imaging, giving the liver surgeon greater ability to assess tumor position in relation to the intrahepatic vascular and biliary structures. Over the same period, liver transplantation has thrived and proliferated. The success of liver transplantation led to an increasing shortage of cadaveric donor organs for patients who might benefit from transplantation. The development of living donor liver transplantation in response to this organ shortage has led to a variety of techniques that also can be applied in nontransplant liver surgery. Resection and reconstruction of portal venous, hepatic arterial, biliary, and hepatic venous structures, all standard components of living donor liver transplant surgery, now are considered more commonly for resection of hepatic tumors by surgeons experienced with liver resection and transplantation techniques.

Vascular reconstruction during hepatic resection leads to varying degrees and duration of hepatic ischemia. During standard liver resections, the use of hepatic inflow occlusion is often used during the parenchymal transection to control excessive blood loss. The use of a combination of inflow occlusion with maintenance of low central venous pressure allows relatively bloodless transection of the liver. The normal liver can tolerate 60 minutes of continuous inflow occlusion and warm ischemia (Huguet et al, 1994). Patients with cirrhosis or altered liver function from biliary obstruction or prolonged chemotherapy may tolerate significantly less ischemic insult before sustaining irreversible injury (Hannoun et al, 1996). Intermittent hepatic inflow occlusion for 15 minutes with 5 minutes of reperfusion at the end of each 15-minute interval has been suggested to reduce the degree of liver injury (Man et al, 1997) and may be particularly useful in more complex resections, in which the parenchymal transection may be prolonged or which may require hepatic venous reconstruction at the completion of the liver transection. The use of ischemic preconditioning seems to protect the liver from subsequent ischemic injury (Clavien et al, 2003). Ischemic preconditioning is performed by applying Pringle's maneuver for 10 minutes, then reperfusing the liver for at least 10 minutes before reapplying inflow occlusion. The mechanisms by which ischemic preconditioning protects the liver from subsequent ischemia has not been fully elucidated.

Tumors that involve the retrohepatic inferior vena cava (IVC) or that involve the hepatic veins at their junction with the vena cava may require total vascular isolation (see Ch. 81). There is some evidence that hepatic venous blood backdiffusion into the liver plays a role in minimizing ischemic injury, and that total vascular isolation increases the degree of ischemic liver injury (Smyrniotis et al, 2003). In most cases, however, the procedure can be planned such that most of the hepatic parenchymal division is performed without total vascular exclusion, and cava clamping is reserved for the relatively short time that is required to deal with the IVC or hepatic veins. Tumors that involve hilar vessels usually can be dealt with by temporary occlusion of the hepatic artery or portal vein with relatively short ischemic times. Blood flow to the liver is maintained by the artery if the portal vein is reconstructed or the portal vein if the artery is reconstructed. In the rare case that the hepatic artery and the portal vein require reconstruction, the reconstructions can be performed sequentially, maintaining flow through one vessel or the other.

Based on the previous information, it seems that standard liver resection techniques could be applied to almost every liver resection, without the need to consider the use of techniques that require hypothermic perfusion. Occasionally, however, patients have lesions that seem truly unresectable by any conventional technique. Lesions that are centrally placed and involve all three main hepatic veins, with or without involvement of the retrohepatic IVC, are essentially unresectable using standard liver resection techniques. The few patients who require complex reconstruction of hepatic venous outflow may benefit from ex vivo or in situ hypothermic perfusion of the liver with subsequent hepatic resection and vascular reconstruction.

Fortner and colleagues (1974) first described the use of hypothermic perfusion during liver resection to protect the liver from ischemic injury in a series of 29 patients. Technical improvements in liver surgery over the next 2 decades along with the growing understanding of the liver's ability to tolerate normothermic ischemia made the use of hypothermic perfusion unnecessary in most cases. During the same period, liver transplantation had been applied to technically unresectable primary and secondary liver malignancy with dismal results. Although the procedure was technically feasible, transplantation for large unresectable primary liver tumors and especially metastatic lesions resulted in the recurrence of malignancy, either in the new liver or elsewhere, shortly after transplantation.

In response to these patients with tumors that were assessed to be unresectable and yet who were considered inappropriate for liver transplantation, Pichlmayr and associates (1988) developed hypothermic perfusion with ex vivo liver resection. During ex vivo liver resection, the liver is removed completely from the body and perfused with cold preservation solution on the back table. The liver resection is performed on the back table through a completely bloodless field, allowing reconstruction of hepatic venous outflow to be performed under ideal conditions. The development of in situ hypothermic perfusion techniques, including the so-called in situ and ante situm procedures, followed. In situ hypothermic perfusion is performed using standard liver resection mobilization techniques; however, the liver is cold perfused via the portal vein. In the ante situm procedure, the liver is cold perfused via the portal vein, and the hilar structures are left otherwise intact. The suprahepatic IVC is divided, and the liver is rotated forward, allowing improved access to the area of the liver and IVC centered around the hepatic vein confluence. The procedure and role for each technique are described subsequently.

IN SITU HYPOTHERMIC PERFUSION

In situ hypothermic perfusion is technically the least demanding of hypothermic perfusion techniques. In situ perfusion has been recommended (Hannoun et al, 1996) for liver resections that require total vascular isolation for periods exceeding 1 hour. The need for total vascular isolation infers that patients have tumors in close proximity to or involving the hepatic veins or retrohepatic IVC or both. In initial descriptions, the entire hepatic parenchymal transection was performed after cold perfusion of the liver, allowing precise dissection of the hepatic veins and IVC to occur under bloodless conditions. If cava or hepatic vein resection was required during resection of the tumor, hepatic hypothermia safely allowed the additional ischemic time to perform reconstruction of the vascular structures.

To perform in situ cold perfusion, the liver is mobilized as for total vascular isolation (see Ch. 81) with control of suprahepatic and infrahepatic IVC and the portal structures. The main portal vein is dissected out for insertion of a perfusion catheter. Although the portal vein can be dissected from the right of the bile duct, for in situ perfusion, it is usually easier to dissect it from the left of the bile duct after dissecting out the hepatic artery. The hepatic artery eventually requires control in any event. A sufficient length of portal vein (3-4 cm) is exposed to place a perfusion catheter and place the portal venous cannula of venovenous bypass if used. Most patients tolerate total vascular isolation without venovenous bypass; however, the standard use of bypass reduces the time pressure that is involved in these cases and reduces the gut edema associated with prolonged portal clamping. The infrahepatic cava is clamped, and the patient is placed on the cava portion of venovenous bypass.

It is generally advisable, although not absolutely necessary, to ligate and divide the right adrenal vein before clamping the infrahepatic IVC because it otherwise has a tendency to become avulsed during some particularly inconvenient portion of the procedure. A portal clamp is placed relatively superiorly on the portal vein with bypass instituted below. The portal cannula can be inserted down toward the superior mesenteric vein after complete division of the portal vein or by dividing just the anterior wall of the portal vein and sliding the cannula down the back wall. Full venovenous bypass is started. The liver side of the portal vein is cannulated with the perfusion solution tubing, and the hepatic artery is clamped. The suprahepatic cava is clamped, and a transverse venotomy is created in the infrahepatic IVC just above the clamp. Cold perfusion of the liver is begun with preservation solution, and the effluent is suctioned from the venotomy in the infrahepatic cava (Fig. 85.1).

Preservation solution is either histidine-tryptophan-ketoglutarate (Gubernatis et al, 1990) or University of Wisconsin solution (Kalayoglu et al, 1988). The liver resection proceeds

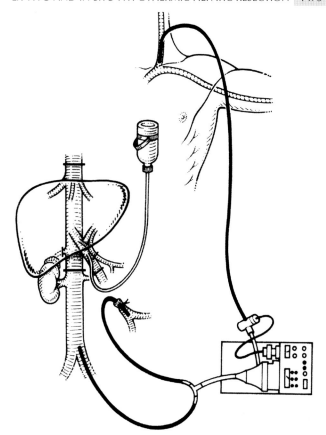

Fig. 85.1. In situ cold perfusion. The patient is placed on venovenous bypass. Cold perfusion solution is infused through the portal vein and vented through a venotomy in the infrahepatic IVC.

in a bloodless field with excellent visualization of intrahepatic structures. The liver can be cooled continuously throughout the parenchymal transection by slow infusion of cooling solution or can be cooled intermittently every 30 minutes by bolus infusion. At completion of the liver resection, the liver should be flushed of cold preservation solution. This can be done by flushing the portal vein with cold 5% albumin before restoring flow to the liver or by allowing the initial 300 to 500 mL of venous effluent from the reperfused liver to be vented out the infrahepatic cava venotomy after reperfusion, but before removing the suprahepatic cava clamp.

The portal bypass cannula is removed, and the portal vein is repaired or reanastomosed if divided. If the liver has been flushed with 5% albumin, the infrahepatic venotomy is closed, and the suprahepatic cava clamp is removed to assess hepatic venous bleeding, which is controlled if present. Portal and hepatic arterial inflow is re-established. If the liver is warm flushed with the initial blood flow through the liver, the sequence is altered slightly to prevent flushing of cold, high potassium solution into the cardiac return. If a warm flush technique is employed, the portal vein is repaired, and the infrahepatic venotomy is closed with a running suture left loose and untied. Portal flow is established with the suprahepatic cava clamp in place. The initial 300 to 500 mL of blood is suctioned from the infrahepatic cava venotomy, and the suture is secured. The suprahepatic cava clamp is removed. We cold flush the liver with 5% albumin because it can be done in unhurried fashion and allows sequential removal of clamps with separate assessment of hepatic venous and portal bleeding on reperfusion. The patient is decannulated from cava bypass.

We rarely use in situ perfusion as just described. The advent of living donor liver transplantation (see Chs. 80 and 109) and the more frequent use of the anterior approach (Liu et al, 2000) to liver resection have improved the ability to divide the liver parenchyma and dissect along the hepatic veins without the need for extensive periods of inflow occlusion. In cases in which a single hepatic vein, or perhaps the vena cava, requires reconstruction, most of the parenchymal transection can be performed without inflow occlusion under low central venous pressure conditions. As the parenchymal transection is near completion, total vascular isolation is applied to divide and reconstruct the vascular structures only. This practice results in substantially shorter periods of hepatic ischemia and allows a different method of applying in situ cold perfusion that is simpler and generally does not require bypass.

In this technique, the liver is mobilized as for total vascular isolation. The portal vein is dissected to the right and left branches, and perfusion tubing is placed into the portal vein branch on the side of the liver to be removed (Fig. 85.2). The branch is divided, maintaining portal flow to the side of the liver to be left in, while allowing access for cold perfusion. As much of the hepatic parenchyma as possible is divided under low central venous pressure conditions, while maintaining hepatic perfusion until it becomes necessary to divide the hepatic veins or IVC that requires reconstruction. At this point, the patient is volume loaded, and clamps are placed sequentially on the infrahepatic cava, the portal vein, hepatic artery, and the suprahepatic IVC. If only the hepatic vein requires reconstruction, cava flow can be maintained by controlling the offending hepatic vein by placing a clamp tangentially down onto the IVC, across the hepatic vein orifice, but only partially occluding the IVC (Fig. 85.3). The anterior wall of the IVC or hepatic vein is incised, and cold perfusion of the liver is instituted through the portal cannula. Only the side of

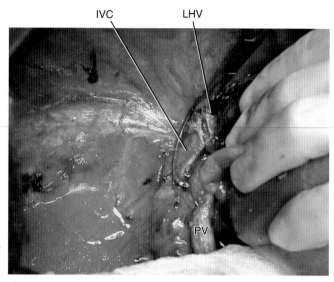

Fig. 85.3. A vascular clamp can be placed tangentially on the IVC, occluding the implantation site of the hepatic vein, but allowing maintenance of cava flow. This maneuver may allow in situ perfusion to be performed without the need for venovenous bypass. LHV, left hepatic vein.

the liver remaining in place is perfused. The vessels are transected, and the specimen is removed. The vessels, the hepatic veins or IVC, can be reconstructed in a bloodless field, without time pressure. Before completing the anastomoses, the liver is flushed with cold 5% albumin. At completion of the vascular anastomoses, portal and hepatic arterial flow is re-established. With the shorter ischemic periods involved, we have not had to use venovenous bypass with this technique (Hemming et al, 2002, 2004).

ANTE SITUM PROCEDURE

The ante situm technique of liver resection can be used in cases in which resection of the IVC and hepatic veins is expected to be difficult, and in which improved access to the hepatic veins and IVC is required. We have used this technique when combined cava and hepatic vein reconstruction is required. The ante situm technique employs the same technique as in situ cold perfusion with several caveats. The suprahepatic IVC requires more extensive dissection to achieve enough length to place a clamp on, divide, and subsequently reanastomose. Greater exposure of the suprahepatic cava can be obtained by dividing the phrenic veins and gently dissecting the IVC away from the diaphragm (Fig. 85.4). We frequently also open the pericardium directly anterior to the IVC and loop the intrapericardial vena cava.

Control of the intrapericardial cava allows placement of the clamp on the vena cava within the pericardium as a primary option or as a secondary option in case technical difficulties arise with placement of the original suprahepatic cava clamp. We perform as much of the liver transection as possible without inflow occlusion before cold perfusing the liver. Venovenous bypass is recommended for this procedure; however, many patients tolerate cava clamping without difficulty. Institution of cold perfusion is as originally described for in situ perfusion; however, the venotomy to vent the perfusate is in the suprahepatic IVC because the suprahepatic cava is divided at completion of perfusion. Dividing the suprahepatic IVC allows the liver to be rotated forward and upward toward the abdominal wall, enabling greater access to the area

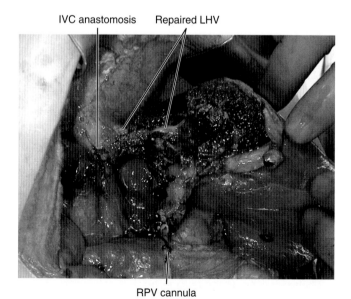

Fig. 85.2. A portal cannula is inserted in the right portal vein (RPV) branch allowing in situ perfusion of the remaining segments II and III in an infant undergoing resection for hepatoblastoma. Cold perfusion allows resection of the IVC and resection and repair of the medial aspect of the left hepatic vein (LHV) to be done in a controlled fashion.

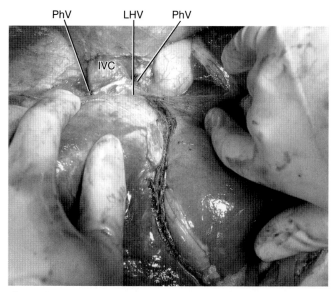

Fig. 85.4. The phrenic veins (PhV) are divided, and the suprahepatic IVC is dissected away from the diaphragm to allow adequate length for placement of a suprahepatic cava clamp. This allows division of the suprahepatic vena cava with enough length to allow reanastomosis. LHV, left hepatic vein.

immediately around the IVC–hepatic vein junction (Figs. 85.5 and 85.6).

If further access is required, the infrahepatic vena cava can be divided, allowing the liver to be rotated completely up onto the abdominal wall. With this technique, we have found that continuous slow cold perfusion is required after the initial flush to prevent excessive warming of the liver. The liver transection is completed,

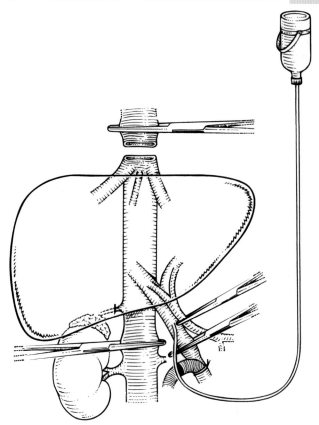

Fig. 85.6. Venovenous bypass can be used during ante situm perfusion. If more exposure is required to the retrohepatic IVC than is provided by dividing the suprahepatic IVC alone, the infrahepatic IVC also can be divided, allowing the liver to be rotated completely up onto the abdominal wall.

dividing the hepatic vein within the liver and resecting the origin of the junction of the IVC and hepatic vein en bloc with the tumor. If extension grafts are required, vascular reconstruction can be performed, with the hepatic vein anastomoses (which are the most tenuous) performed while the liver is rotated onto the abdominal wall. The liver is replaced, and the cava anastomosis is performed. The liver is flushed with 5% albumin before reperfusion.

The ante situm approach gives better access to the cava–hepatic vein junction than does simple in situ cold perfusion. It does not give as good exposure, however, as a complete ex vivo approach. The advantage to the ante situm approach is that biliary and hepatic arterial anastomoses are not required, reducing the ischemic time to the liver and reducing the potential for complications resulting from these additional anastomoses. Currently, we use the ante situm approach when a combination of cava resection and hepatic vein reconstruction is required, and we expect only a single hepatic vein orifice would require reimplantation into the cava (Figs. 85.7-85.9). If the reconstruction is expected to be more complex, we use a complete ex vivo approach.

EX VIVO LIVER RESECTION

Patients who have tumors that involve the IVC and hepatic veins that require complex venous repair or patients with combined hepatic vein and hilar involvement may be candidates for ex vivo resection. During ex vivo resection, the liver is removed completely

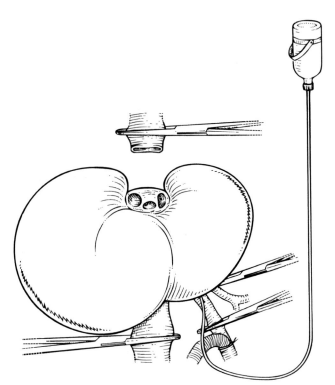

Fig. 85.5. Ante situm cold perfusion. The suprahepatic IVC is divided allowing the liver to be rotated forward. The region of the hepatic vein–IVC confluence can be visualized better.

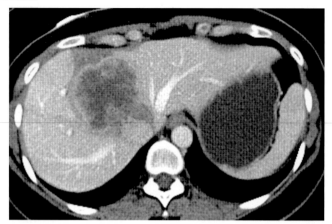

Fig. 85.7. CT scan showing a cholangiocarcinoma that is centered on all three hepatic veins at the junction of the IVC. Right portal structures also were involved. A right trisegmentectomy with reconstruction of the left hepatic vein was planned.

from the patient and perfused with cold preservation solution on the back table. The hepatic resection is performed in a bloodless field, and vascular reconstructions are performed before reimplanting the remnant liver into the patient.

Patient Selection and Preoperative Workup

In principle, any patient with liver malignancy that is unresectable by other means can be assessed for ex vivo liver surgery. In practice, almost all liver resections can be performed without the need for an ex vivo approach. Patients with tumors that involve the junction of the IVC and hepatic veins, such that complex, prolonged vascular reconstruction is required, or patients with combined vascular involvement of the hepatic veins and hilar structures

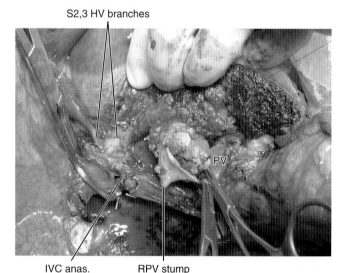

Fig. 85.8. Parenchymal division along a right trisegmentectomy plane was performed crossing into segments II and III superiorly. A cannula was placed in the stump of the right portal vein (RPV) for cold perfusion with University of Wisconsin solution. A short segment of the IVC at the level of the hepatic veins and the first 3 cm of the left hepatic vein origin were resected, and the liver was rotated anteriorly. The IVC was reconstructed end to end with the left hepatic vein reimplanted above the cava anastomosis. IVC anas, IVC anastomosis; S2, S3 HV, segments II and III hepatic vein branches.

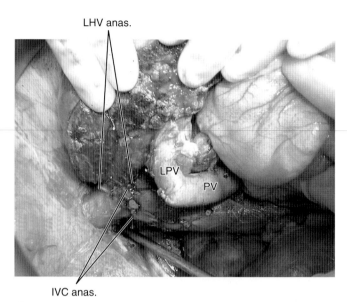

Fig. 85.9. Reimplanted segments II and III from Fig. 85.8. The left hepatic duct was reconstructed later using a Roux-en-Y limb. IVC anas, IVC anastomosis; LHV, left hepatic vein; LPV, left portal vein; PV, portal vein.

may benefit, however, from a planned ex vivo approach. One of the benefits of planning the ex vivo approach is that frequently at operation what initially was thought to be unresectable by any method short of complete removal of the liver is found to be resectable with a less complex procedure. General assessment of the patient is similar to that for liver transplantation, with particular assessment of cardiac risk factors. In patients older than 50 years of age or with any cardiac abnormalities, a functional stress test, such as dobutamine stress echocardiogram, is performed. Any significant cardiac abnormalities would be a contraindication. Even mild renal dysfunction has been shown to increase the risk of standard extended hepatectomy (Melendez et al, 2001), and a creatinine level greater than 1.3 mg/dL would be a contraindication. Ex vivo liver resection should be attempted only in otherwise healthy, well-selected patients.

Preoperative imaging is crucial to stage the tumor and to assess its position in relation to hepatic vascular anatomy. Our current standard is triphasic spiral computed tomography (CT) with three-dimensional reconstructions to assess the liver anatomy and tumor position and CT of the chest and pelvis. In some instances, magnetic resonance imaging (MRI) (including MRI angiography and MRI venography) is required, particularly when all three hepatic veins are involved, and there is some degree of hepatic venous obstruction that prevents adequate flow of contrast material into the hepatic veins during CT. With the combination of CT and MRI and the present availability of three-dimensional reconstruction, invasive angiography usually is unnecessary. Remnant liver volume assessment can be performed as for extended hepatectomy. Usually 25% of total liver volume after resection would be considered adequate for resection without the need for preoperative portal vein embolization (see Ch. 84). With cold preservation and reperfusion, an additional ischemic injury occurs over and above what happens during standard liver resection. We arbitrarily have chosen a projected liver remnant of 40% of total liver volume as a cutoff for consideration for preoperative portal vein embolization in patients requiring extended hepatectomy who may need complex vascular reconstruction and cold perfusion techniques (Hemming et al, 2003). Positron emission tomography also is performed on all patients to assess for the possibility of otherwise undetected extrahepatic disease.

Accurate imaging of the intrahepatic architecture is paramount to assess the possibilities for reconstruction. Three-dimensional imaging techniques occasionally may discover unusual anatomy that makes vascular reconstruction unnecessary, such as the presence of a large inferior hepatic vein that makes reconstruction of the main right hepatic vein unnecessary. Alternatively, anatomy may be discovered that requires additional reconstruction, such as a large segment VI vein that drains into the middle hepatic vein (Lang et al, 2004).

Anesthesia

Anesthetic management for ex vivo liver resections is similar as for liver transplantation. Maintaining patient temperature is a key component of anesthesia management and includes the use of forced air warming blankets and warming of all fluids. In addition to standard monitoring for liver resection, a Swan-Ganz catheter is inserted for hemodynamic monitoring and assessment of blood temperature in the pulmonary artery. Access for venovenous bypass, which originally was achieved by cutdowns, has been simplified by percutaneous insertion techniques. Most cases begin with maintenance of low central venous pressure as would be standard for most liver resections because most cases do not proceed to ex vivo techniques. Percutaneous catheters are placed in the internal jugular vein or subclavian vein and the femoral vein for the cava portion of the bypass circuit when an ex vivo procedure is decided on. At that time, the patient subsequently can be volume loaded. The portal limb of the circuit is placed directly into the portal vein by the surgeon.

The anhepatic phase lasts 2 to 4 hours, and attention must be paid to coagulation during this period. We give fresh frozen plasma to meet volume requirements during this time and to attempt to minimize any crystalloid that is given. Glucose levels are monitored with constant glucose infusion required.

On reperfusion of the cold autograft, the temperature of the blood in the pulmonary artery can drop precipitously. For liver transplantation and ex vivo liver resection, we manually compress the portal inflow temporarily when pulmonary artery blood temperature decreases to less than 34.5°C. Portal occlusion for 10 seconds allows the pulmonary artery blood temperature to increase to 36°C, after which portal compression is released. Pulmonary artery blood temperature commonly decreases to 32°C to 33°C without portal compression on reperfusion. In our experience, avoiding this precipitous drop in pulmonary artery blood temperature seems to reduce the cardiac dysfunction that occurs on reperfusion of the liver.

Surgical Procedure

Pichlmayr and Hauss (1994) described the procedure of ex vivo liver resection in the second edition of this textbook; they appropriately described the procedure in terms similar to liver transplantation. The following description of technique is taken largely from Pichylmayr's original description in this textbook with some minor modifications by this author. There are three phases to the procedure: (1) assessment of resectability and removal of

the liver, (2) liver resection and vascular reconstruction on the back table, and (3) reimplantation of the liver autograft.

Assessment of Resectability and Removal of the Liver

An initial assessment of resectability is undertaken via laparoscopy or a limited abdominal incision. Laparoscopy assesses the presence of peritoneal disease that would preclude proceeding with resection. Even after a negative laparoscopy, we perform a limited abdominal incision and assess the abdominal cavity. It is common to have a negative laparoscopy only to find additional small lesions in the liver or elsewhere that would be a contraindication. The incision is lengthened to some variation of a bilateral subcostal incision, with or without a midline extension.

The liver is assessed for resectability. Because the indication for ex vivo resection is involvement of the hepatic veins with or without cava involvement, the liver may be venous congested, and care must be taken not to injure the liver during mobilization because any small breach of the liver capsule becomes an outflow route for the obstructed venous flow, and bleeding can be torrential. Venous congestion of the liver is not a contraindication to resection because the planned resection should relieve the venous outflow obstruction. Large tumors may restrict the ability to rotate the liver without undue tension, and in these cases it is prudent to make an early decision regarding ex vivo resection before attempting elevation of the liver off of the IVC. Intraoperative ultrasound is used to assess the level of vascular involvement and to confirm vascular anatomy originally identified on preoperative imaging. If a decision is made to proceed with an ex vivo approach, the following steps are performed.

1. The hilar structures are prepared. The arterial anatomy is dissected out, and an appropriate site is chosen for planned division. This usually is at the level of the common hepatic artery–gastroduodenal artery junction. If there is aberrant arterial anatomy, an alternative site may be required depending on the particular anatomy and portion of the liver that remains after the resection. The artery is not dissected high into the hilum in most cases to preserve small arterial communications to the biliary tree. If the tumor involves the hilar structures, the artery must be dissected far enough to determine that there is a usable, tumor-free portion of the respective hepatic artery branch to reconstruct. The portal vein is identified, and the common bile duct is encircled without skeletonization. A cholecystectomy is performed. The bile duct is reflected off the portal vein taking care to preserve the blood supply, and the neural and lymphatic tissue around the portal vein is cleared.

2. The infrahepatic IVC is dissected out down to the level of the renal veins and encircled. Planned vascular clamp placement is immediately above the renal veins, although division of the vena cava may be substantially more cephalad. The right adrenal vein should be ligated and divided. Small caudate veins should be divided if accessible. The large size of the tumor may make access to the caudate veins difficult, in which case they can be dealt with on the back table.

3. The liver is freed from surrounding attachments. If the tumor is infiltrating the diaphragm, the portion of the diaphragm involved is resected en bloc with the tumor.

4. The suprahepatic IVC is prepared. The phrenic veins are divided, allowing the diaphragm to be dissected away from the IVC and providing an increased length of intra-abdominal IVC to be available for subsequent clamping and reconstruction. We currently also open the pericardium directly anterior to

the IVC and loop the intrapericardial IVC. Control of the intrapericardial IVC allows placement of the clamp on the vena cava within the pericardium as a primary option for tumors that are very large or as a secondary option in case technical difficulties arise with placement of the original suprahepatic cava clamp.

5. Clamp placement and subsequent transection lines are assessed. The need for vascular conduits for reconstruction is assessed, and alternatives for reconstruction are contemplated before removing the liver. Hepatic venous branches may be reconstructed using hepatic vein or portal vein segments from the side of the liver resected or from autologous vein grafts, such as superficial femoral vein, proximal left renal vein, gonadal vein, or saphenous vein panel grafts. Cryopreserved femoral vein grafts can be used for reconstruction of long segments of hepatic veins or IVC; however, the issue of long-term patency is currently unclear. The IVC alternatively can be replaced with 20-mm ringed polytetrafluoroethylene (Gore-Tex) tube graft. Planning for these eventualities should occur before placement of clamps and removal of the liver.

6. Percutaneous access of the internal jugular vein and femoral vein is achieved, the IVC is clamped, and the cava portion of bypass is started. The portal vein is clamped just below the bifurcation, and the portal cannula is inserted down toward the superior mesenteric vein and secured. The portal vein is completely transected approximately 1.5 to 2 cm below the bifurcation, and the portal flow is added to the bypass circuit. The liver continues to be perfused by arterial blood at this time.

7. The liver is removed. The bile duct is transected sharply approximately 1 to 1.5 cm below the bifurcation. We do not ligate either end because we may elect to perform a duct-to-duct anastomosis on reimplantation. The gastroduodenal artery is ligated and divided. The common hepatic artery is clamped, and the hepatic artery is transected at the takeoff of the gastroduodenal artery, such that a branch patch is formed on either side of the arterial transection if possible. The suprahepatic IVC is clamped either below the diaphragm or within the pericardium, and the suprahepatic vena cava is transected far enough away from tumor to provide an adequate oncologic margin, but leaving enough room to perform the suprahepatic cava anastomosis at the time of reimplantation. If the vena cava has been freed of its posterior attachments before clamp placement, the infrahepatic IVC is divided as cephalad as possible, and the liver is removed and placed in an ice bath. Cold perfusion through the portal vein and hepatic artery is initiated on the back bench. Cold perfusion can be with either histidine-tryptophan-ketoglutarate solution or University of Wisconsin solution. If the retrohepatic IVC has not been freed up previously because of the large tumor size and difficulty with access, the liver can be cold perfused via the portal vein after the suprahepatic IVC is divided. The liver is rotated forward as in the ante situm approach, and the retrohepatic IVC is freed of attachments. The infrahepatic IVC is divided, and the liver is removed and placed in the ice bath.

8. Bleeding is controlled, and the bypass circuit is assessed. Flows of 3 to 6 L/min would be expected on total bypass (see Fig. 85.1). The abdomen is loosely packed and covered, and attention is turned to the back table.

An alternative method can be performed in cases that have complex hepatic vein involvement without IVC involvement with tumor. If access allows, the liver can be mobilized completely off

of the retrohepatic IVC until suspended only by the hepatic veins. The hilar structures are divided as for standard ex vivo resection, but the patient is not placed on bypass. A vascular clamp is placed partially across the IVC, occluding the hepatic vein orifices, but allowing cava flow to remain uninterrupted. The hepatic veins are transected, and the liver is removed and cold flushed on the back table. A temporary portacava shunt (Fig. 85.10) is constructed decompressing the enteric circulation. This option avoids bypass, but can be used only when there is no IVC involvement and when the IVC can be preserved in situ. It is worth assessing whether the tumor can be dissected away from the IVC in most patients because preoperative imaging can be inaccurate in determining true IVC involvement (Okada et al, 2003).

Ex Situ Liver Resection

After it is removed from the patient, the liver is placed immediately in an ice bath and perfused with preservation solution through the portal vein. We use University of Wisconsin solution because it is also the preservation solution we use for cadaveric and living donor liver transplantation; histidine-tryptophan-ketoglutarate solution also is a reasonable choice. After the initial 500 to 1000 mL of solution has been flushed through the liver, the effluent from the IVC should be clear. The hepatic artery and biliary tree also are flushed with another 200 to 300 mL of preservation solution. The liver is immersed in cold University of Wisconsin solution, and the resection is performed.

Hilar structures are dissected out and divided. Great care must be taken not to divide segmental arteries to portions of the liver that are to remain because their caliber is too small to reconstruct with confidence. Main segmental divisions of the portal vein usually can be repaired and reconstructed. Parenchymal transection can be performed using a variety of techniques, including ultrasonic dissection and water jet, or the parenchyma can be divided sharply with a knife. Small bile ducts and vessels are ligated or oversewn. Large hepatic veins are cut sharply and later

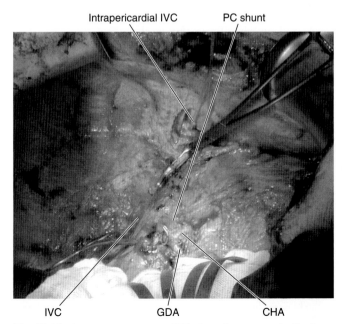

Fig. 85.10. A temporary portacava (PC) shunt is constructed, allowing a prolonged anhepatic phase without the need for venovenous bypass. The intrapericardial IVC has been encircled. CHA, common hepatic artery; GDA, gastroduodenal artery.

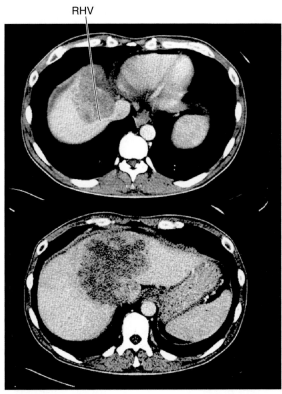

Fig. 85.11. A single colorectal metastasis involving all three hepatic veins. RHV, right hepatic vein.

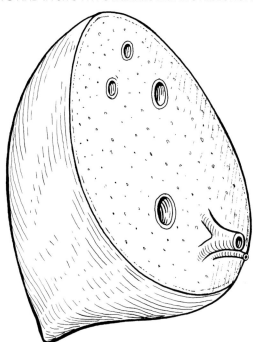

Fig. 85.13. Back table transection of the liver results in multiple branches of the right hepatic vein requiring reconstruction. A large segment VI branch that enters the middle hepatic vein also requires reimplantation.

assessed for reconstruction (Figs. 85.11-85.14). The surgical tumor margin should not be compromised to minimize the subsequent complexity of vascular reconstruction. A key advantage to the ex vivo approach is the ability to extend the resection to obtain negative margins, while providing the necessary time and exposure for complex reconstructions. At completion of the resection, it is helpful to flush the portal vein, hepatic artery, and bile duct with University of Wisconsin solution to identify leaks from the cut surface of the liver, which can be repaired before reimplantation. Fibrin glue may be sprayed on the cut surface of the liver to minimize bleeding.

Hepatic Vein and Inferior Vena Cava Reconstruction

Hepatic vein reconstruction, with or without IVC reconstruction, is the *raison d'être* for ex vivo liver resection. The hepatic veins

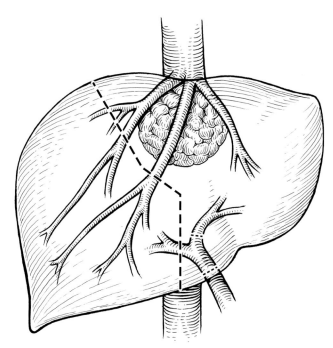

Fig. 85.12. The planned hepatic transection line for the tumor shown in Fig. 85.11. Multiple hepatic vein branches require reconstruction.

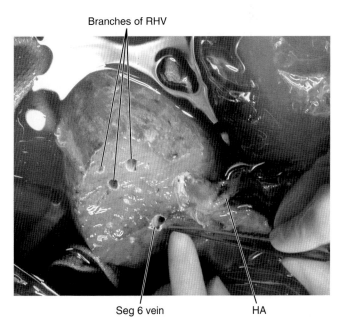

Fig. 85.14. Completed transection on the back table. HA, hepatic artery; RHV, right hepatic vein; Seg 6, segment VI.

are relatively thick walled and straightforward to reconstruct within 2 to 3 cm of their merging with the IVC. For reconstructions of hepatic veins transected relatively close to the IVC, the liver parenchyma can be trimmed back such that direct reimplantation of the hepatic vein into the IVC or the IVC replacement can be performed. Multiple orifices of hepatic veins can be "plastied" together or implanted into venous conduits (Figs. 85.15-85.17). The farther away from the IVC that the hepatic vein is transected, the thinner the wall of the hepatic vein, and the more difficult it is to reimplant the vein directly into the IVC. We have harvested the portal vein bifurcation, reversed it, and used it to reconstruct multiple hepatic vein branches into a single outflow vessel on several occasions (Figs. 85.18-85.20) (Hemming & Cattral, 1999). Saphenous vein, superficial femoral vein, internal jugular vein, and cryopreserved vein grafts all have been used to reconstruct hepatic veins (Dong et al, 2004; Kaneoka et al, 2000; Kishi et al, 2004; Kubota et al, 1997, 1998). Segments of uninvolved hepatic vein from the side of the liver resected can be salvaged and used for grafts, or patches. Venous grafts should be kept as short as possible, and great care must be taken to place the grafts such that they do not kink. For extension grafts, the hepatic vein–to-graft anastomosis is performed first with subsequent reimplantation of the graft into the IVC.

If possible, it is preferential to reimplant the hepatic veins into native vena cava. Frequently, a large portion of the vena cava that was removed initially with the liver can be salvaged and moved superiorly with the hepatic veins reimplanted into this newly situated portion of IVC. Ringed 20-mm Gore-Tex tube graft can be used to make a composite cava graft with the Gore-Tex graft placed inferiorly. Alternatively, a section of the IVC remaining in the patient immediately above the renal veins can be harvested and used as the segment of IVC into which the hepatic veins are reimplanted. Ringed 20-mm Gore-Tex tube

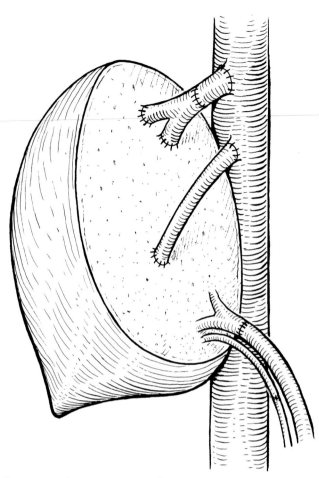

Fig. 85.16. The prepared autograft is reimplanted into the patient as diagrammed. Reimplantation is done in similar fashion as for living donor right lobe transplantation.

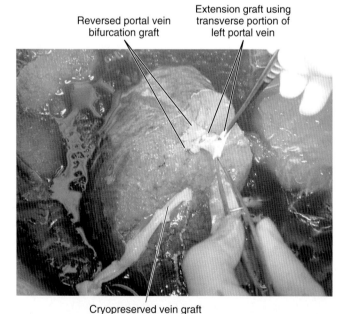

Fig. 85.15. Joining two of the three right hepatic vein branches together and implanting the resulting two orifices into the reversed portal vein bifurcation taken from the patient's hilum allows reconstruction of the right hepatic vein branches. The transverse portion of the left portal vein is added to allow the graft to reach the IVC without tension. A cryopreserved femoral vein graft is used to extend the segment VI vein to the IVC.

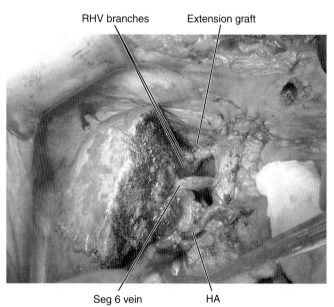

Fig. 85.17. The reimplanted liver as in Fig. 85.16. HA, hepatic artery; RHV, right hepatic vein; Seg 6, segment VI vein.

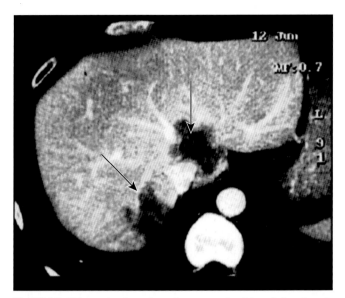

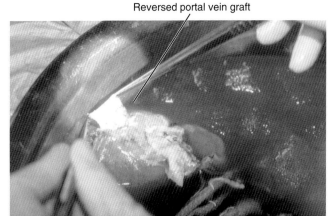

Reversed portal vein graft

Fig. 85.20. A reversed portal vein bifurcation graft taken from the patient's hilum is used to reconstruct the left hepatic vein outflow.

Fig. 85.18. CT scan showing colorectal metastases involving all three hepatic veins. *Arrows* indicate tumor.

graft is used to replace the segment of IVC immediately above the renal veins. In some circumstances, it is necessary to reimplant the hepatic veins directly into a relatively stiff Gore-Tex graft that is replacing the IVC (Figs. 85.21 and 85.22). In this situation, it is important to make a larger opening in the Gore-Tex than one might expect and to triangulate the anastomosis to prevent anastomotic stricturing (Lodge et al, 2000).

At completion of the back bench reconstruction, one has an autograft that is similar to that of a reduced size or split liver allograft. Total cold ischemic time is 2 to 6 hours. This time is well within acceptable limits when comparing cold ischemic times for split liver or reduced size liver transplantation.

Reimplantation

Reimplantation is similar as for reduced size liver transplantation. The suprahepatic IVC anastomosis is performed first. If a Gore-Tex graft has been used to reconstruct the IVC, it is shortened

such that it does not kink on implantation. When the back wall of the infrahepatic vena cava anastomosis has been completed, the portal vein is flushed with 500 mL of cold 5% albumin, which is vented through the infrahepatic cava anastomosis. The infrahepatic vena cava anastomosis is then completed. The cold rinse washes the University of Wisconsin solution out of the liver before reperfusion. University of Wisconsin solution contains high levels of potassium and adenosine, which can cause dramatic cardiac dysfunction or arrest if allowed into the circulation on reperfusion. An alternative to cold flushing the liver before reperfusion is to leave the lower cava anastomosis open until after portal reperfusion, venting the initial 300 mL of blood before removing the suprahepatic cava clamp. There is little solid evidence to support one technique over the other. We prefer the cold flush technique only because it reduces the number of possible bleeding sites at the time of reperfusion. After the infrahepatic cava anastomosis is performed, the portal limb of the bypass circuit is clamped and removed from the portal vein. The portal venous anastomosis is performed.

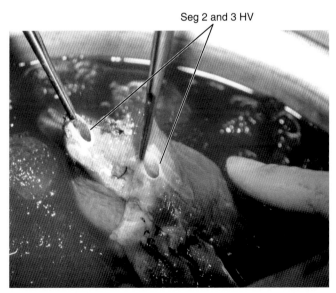

Seg 2 and 3 HV

Fig. 85.19. Remnant liver after ex vivo resection of tumor seen in Fig. 85.18. Seg 2 and 3 HV, segments II and III hepatic vein branches.

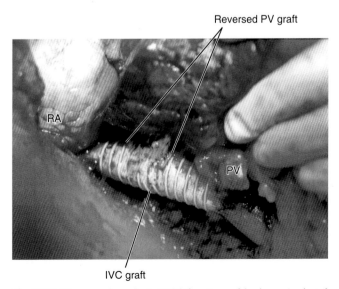

Reversed PV graft

RA

PV

IVC graft

Fig. 85.21. The reversed portal vein (PV) bifurcation graft has been reimplanted directly into a segment of ringed 20-mm polytetrafluoroethylene (Gore-Tex) that replaces the IVC. RA, right atrium.

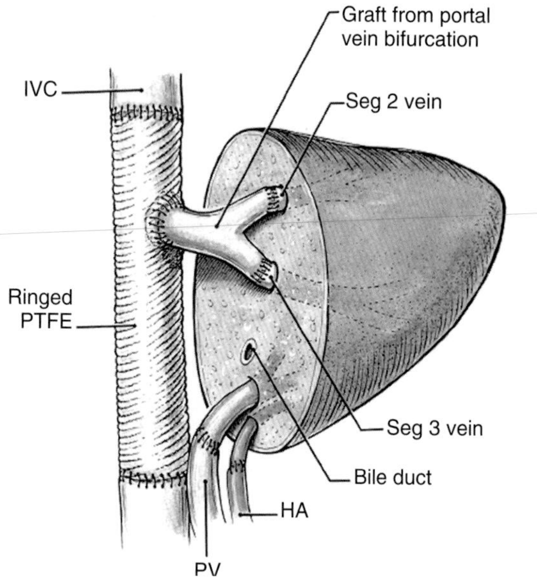

Fig. 85.22. Diagrammatic representation of Fig. 85.21. HA, hepatic artery; PTFE, polytetrafluoroethylene (Gore-Tex); PV, portal vein; Seg, segment.

The suprahepatic cava clamp is removed, and the liver is allowed to back perfuse through the hepatic veins. Any major bleeding is controlled before re-establishing the portal flow. The portal venous clamp is removed, and the liver is reperfused. Any bleeding from the cut surface of the liver is controlled. The patient is then taken off cava bypass.

The arterial anastomosis is performed, and the liver is reperfused with arterial blood. Total warm ischemic time is 20 to 40 minutes. After hemostasis has been achieved, the biliary anastomosis is performed. In the first few ex vivo liver resections that we performed, our preference was to perform a Roux-en-Y choledochojejunostomy. Our more recent cases have been duct-to-duct anastomoses over an internal stent. This experience mirrors our larger experience with living donor right lobe transplantation.

Postoperative Course

Postoperative care is similar to any major liver resection or liver transplantation. Ultrasound with Doppler assessment is performed on postoperative day 1 to assess liver blood flow. Transaminases in the 200 to 1000 IU/L range are standard, but return to near normal by 1 week. Hyperbilirubinemia is common and, as one might expect, seems to be worse the smaller the size of the liver remnant. Hyperbilirubinemia by itself is not concerning if other markers of liver function are improving. An early sign that the autograft is functioning is the return of lactate levels to baseline in the first 12 to 24 hours after surgery. Maintenance of coagulation parameters, in particular prothrombin time or international normalized ratio, suggests recovery of liver function. It is frequently necessary, however, to give fresh frozen plasma for the first few days to maintain an international normalized ratio target less than 2 (Martin et al, 2003). Hypophosphatemia can occur between postoperative days 1 and 3 as the liver regenerates. This occurrence is actually encouraging, but the hypophosphatemia may be profound and require constant intravenous replacement. Without much evidence as to its effectiveness, we have used low-dose intravenous heparin (500 U/hr) perioperatively and attempt to maintain the hematocrit between 30% and 35%. Patients who

have Gore-Tex grafts placed are started on low-dose aspirin before discharge, and this is maintained for life.

Current Role of Ex Vivo Liver Resection

The role of such an extensive procedure in advanced malignancies is open for discussion. Although almost 2 decades have passed since Pichlmayr and colleagues (1988) described the first ex vivo liver resection, relatively few surgeons have attempted the procedure. The largest reported series from Pichlmayr's own group consists of only 22 patients (Oldhafer et al, 2000). There may be several reasons behind the lack of adoption of this technique.

The technique requires a surgeon who is familiar with advanced techniques in liver resection and liver transplantation, which restricts the procedure to relatively few individuals. Many patients who may be candidates for ex vivo resection are called "unresectable" by competent hepatic surgeons and not referred on. Perhaps the most compelling reason for the lack of adoption of this technique is the relatively high risk-to-benefit ratio that the procedure offers. Most of the literature on ex vivo liver resections has been case reports that describe aspects of technique, and long-term follow-up is not available. Perioperative mortality even in well-selected patients is between 10% and 30%. At best, the 5-year survival for ex vivo resections performed for malignancy is 15% to 30%. In Oldhafer's series (2000), the six patients who underwent ex vivo resection for colorectal metastases had a median survival of 21 months.

Although it may seem that there is limited benefit to performing ex vivo liver resection, there is no doubt that the occasional patient is cured by this aggressive procedure One patient with resection for cholangiocarcinoma in Oldhafer's series was alive and disease-free at 3.5 years after resection, whereas one of our own patients undergoing ex vivo resection for hepatocellular carcinoma is alive and disease-free at 5 years (Hemming et al, 2000). Other patients may benefit by being considered for ex vivo liver resection simply because a surgeon prepared to perform ex vivo resection realizes that the resection can be performed using a less aggressive technique, such as in situ cold perfusion or standard vascular reconstruction. Standard liver resection for malignancy was considered questionable several decades ago. Improvements in surgical technique and perioperative care transformed liver resection for malignancy from a technique that many thought bordered on lunacy into an accepted therapy. Further advances in surgical technique along with advances in adjuvant oncologic therapies may do the same for ex vivo liver resection. Currently, it seems reasonable to consider highly selected patients for ex vivo liver resection on a case-by-case basis.

REFERENCES

Clavien PA, et al, 2003: A prospective randomized study in 100 consecutive patients undergoing major liver resection with versus without ischemic preconditioning. Ann Surg 238:843-852.

Dong G, et al, 2004: Cadaver iliac vein outflow reconstruction in living donor right lobe liver transplantation. J Am Coll Surg 199:504-507.

Fortner JG, et al, 1974: Major hepatic resection using vascular isolation and hypothermic perfusion. Ann Surg 180:644-652.

Gubernatis G, et al, 1990: HTK-solution (Bretschneider) for human liver transplantation: first clinical experiences. Langenbecks Arch Chir 375:66-70.

Hannoun L, et al, 1996: Major extended hepatic resections in diseased livers using hypothermic protection: preliminary results from the first 12 patients treated with this new technique. J Am Coll Surg 183:597-605.

Hemming AW, Cattral MS, 1999: Ex vivo liver resection with replacement of the inferior vena cava and hepatic vein replacement by transposition of the portal vein. J Am Coll Surg 189:523-526.

Hemming AW, et al, 2000: Ex vivo liver resection. Can J Surg 43:222-224.

Hemming AW, et al, 2002: Hepatic vein reconstruction for resection of hepatic tumors. Ann Surg 235:850-858.

Hemming AW, et al, 2003: Preoperative portal vein embolization for extended hepatectomy. Ann Surg 237:686-693.

Hemming AW, et al, 2004: Combined resection of the liver and inferior vena cava for hepatic malignancy. Ann Surg 239:712-721.

Huguet C, et al, 1994: Hepatic resection with ischemia of the liver exceeding one hour. J Am Coll Surg 178:454-458.

Kalayoglu M, et al, 1988: Extended preservation of the liver for clinical transplantation. Lancet 1:617-619.

Kaneoka Y, et al, 2000: Hepatic vein reconstruction by external iliac vein graft using vascular clips. World J Surg 24:377-382.

Kishi Y, et al, 2004: Sharing the middle hepatic vein between donor and recipient: left liver graft procurement preserving a large segment VIII branch in donor. Liver Transpl 10:1208-1212.

Kubota K, et al, 1997: Reconstruction of the inferior vena cava using a hepatic venous patch obtained from resected liver. Hepatogastroenterology 44: 378-379.

Kubota K, et al, 1998: Reconstruction of the hepatic and portal veins using a patch graft from the right ovarian vein. Am J Surg 176:295-297.

Lang H, et al, 2004: Extended left hepatectomy—modified operation planning based on three-dimensional visualization of liver anatomy. Langenbecks Arch Surg 389:306-310.

Liu CL, et al, 2000: Anterior approach for major right hepatic resection for large hepatocellular carcinoma. Ann Surg 232:25-31.

Lodge JP, et al, 2000: Ex vivo and in situ resection of inferior vena cava with hepatectomy for colorectal metastases. Ann Surg 231:471-479.

Man K, et al, 1997: Prospective evaluation of Pringle maneuver in hepatectomy for liver tumors by a randomized study. Ann Surg 226:704-713.

Martin RC 2nd, et al, 2003: The use of fresh frozen plasma after major hepatic resection for colorectal metastasis: is there a standard for transfusion? J Am Coll Surg 196:402-409.

Melendez J, et al, 2001: Extended hepatic resection: a 6-year retrospective study of risk factors for perioperative mortality. J Am Coll Surg 192:47-53.

Okada Y, et al, 2003: Diagnosis and treatment of inferior vena cava invasion by hepatic cancer. World J Surg 27:689-694.

Oldhafer KJ, et al, 2000: Long-term experience after ex situ liver surgery. Surgery 127:520-527.

Pichlmayr R, Hauss J, 1994: Autotransplantation of the liver and resection in the hypothermic perfused liver. In Blumgart LH (ed): Surgery of the Liver and Biliary Tract, 2nd ed. New York, Churchill Livingstone, pp 1857-1862.

Pichlmayr R, et al, 1988: [Ex situ operation on the liver: a new possibility in liver surgery]. Langenbecks Arch Chir 373:122-126.

Smyrniotis V, et al, 2003: Effects of hepatovenous back flow on ischemic-reperfusion injuries in liver resections with the Pringle maneuver. J Am Coll Surg 197:949-954.

86

Intraoperative Ultrasound of the Liver: Techniques for Liver Resection and Transplantation

R. B. ADAMS

Intraoperative ultrasound (see Ch. 23) has become a firmly established and essential tool for hepatic surgery. It is a crucial modality for the evaluation and management of liver diseases amenable to surgical therapy. Intraoperative ultrasound has the advantage of being the only real-time, intraoperative technique for hepatic imaging available in the operating room. To make full use of intraoperative ultrasound, the surgeon must understand basic and advanced ultrasound principles and have a fundamental knowledge of three-dimensional hepatic anatomy. Together, these offer greater flexibility in managing hepatic neoplasms and other liver diseases and allow the surgeon to perform diagnostic and therapeutic procedures intraoperatively.

Before the introduction of intraoperative ultrasound in the late 1970s by Makuuchi (Makuuchi et al, 1977, 1981a), the location of nonpalpable liver lesions and intrahepatic anatomic relationships were inferred by preoperative imaging studies and surface landmarks on the liver. With growing experience and widespread use, the applications for intraoperative ultrasound in hepatic surgery have expanded dramatically (Table 86.1). Intraoperative ultrasound provides detailed information regarding lesions diagnosed by preoperative imaging. Occult lesions missed preoperatively or during intraoperative inspection and palpation can be detected. Intrahepatic anatomy can be mapped clearly, and the relationship of hepatic tumors to intrahepatic structures can be defined precisely. The ultrasound features of hepatic lesions can aid in the differential diagnosis of these tumors, and intraoperative ultrasound allows targeted biopsy of lesions when necessary. Intraoperative ultrasound facilitates intraoperative decision making and has enabled the development of numerous novel hepatectomy techniques. Nonresectional treatments for tumors, such as cryotherapy and radiofrequency thermal ablation, have become feasible with intraoperative ultrasound guidance.

This chapter describes the general uses of intraoperative ultrasound during hepatic surgery. Specific scanning techniques for examining the liver during resection and transplantation are reviewed in detail in this chapter. Normal hepatic anatomy as viewed during intraoperative ultrasound and the intraoperative ultrasound features of hepatic pathology are discussed and illustrated here. The use of intraoperative ultrasound to guide interventions during liver surgery is detailed. Intraoperative ultrasound of the liver during open surgery (laparotomy) is described. The use of ultrasound during laparoscopy (laparoscopic ultrasound) for liver diseases is discussed in Chs. 15 and 23. Transabdominal ultrasound is reviewed in Ch. 15. A detailed understanding of normal hepatic anatomy as described in Ch. 1

is essential to interpreting these intraoperative ultrasound images.

INDICATIONS

The main indications for intraoperative ultrasound of the liver are screening for known and occult metastatic lesions; evaluating hepatic neoplasms for resectability; planning of the appropriate intervention based on the position of the mass relative to the intrahepatic anatomy; and providing image guidance for interventions such as needle biopsy, ablation, or resection. Detection of metastatic lesions is important, despite improvements in preoperative imaging. Although the detection limits for computed tomography, magnetic resonance imaging, and positron emission tomography have continued to improve, and these modalities can detect lesions between 5 and 10 mm, intraoperative ultrasound is the most sensitive screening method for metastases (Bloed et al, 2000; Boldrini et al, 1987; Clarke et al, 1989; Gunven et al, 1985; Machi et al, 1987; Olsen, 1990; Zacherl et al, 2002). Intraoperative ultrasound detects lesions 3 to 5 mm (Clouse, 1989). When combined with inspection and palpation, intraoperative ultrasound detects metastases with greater than 90% sensitivity (Knol et al, 1993; Parker et al, 1989; Soyer et al, 1992). Intraoperative ultrasound is excellent at detecting occult metastases (Bloed et al, 2000; Clarke et al, 1989; Machi et al, 1987, 1991; Ravikumar et al, 1994; Stone et al, 1994) and additional tumors in patients with known metastatic disease (Bloed et al, 2000; Jarnagin et al, 2001; Kane et al, 1994; Machi et al, 1987; Staren et al, 1997). When planning therapy, intraoperative ultrasound can aid in determining the optimal approach for treatment and frequently changes the initial plan that was developed based on preoperative imaging (Boutkan et al, 1992; Brower et al, 1989; Carter et al, 1996; Castaing et al, 1986;

Table 86.1   Intraoperative Liver Ultrasound

Allows real-time hepatic imaging

Highly sensitive and accurate
  Detects small lesions, 3-5 mm (e.g., occult lesions)

Acquires new information and confirms known data
  Defines intrahepatic anatomy and relationship to lesions

Rapid and repetitive use during procedures

Guides performance of intraoperative procedures

Jarnagin et al, 2001; Kane et al, 1994; Parker et al, 1989; Rifkin et al, 1987; Salminen et al, 1990; Solomon et al, 1994; Zacherl et al, 2002). Intraoperative ultrasound continues to be important in the diagnosis and treatment of metastatic lesions.

Intraoperative ultrasound plays a principal role in managing primary hepatic malignancies, particularly hepatocellular carcinoma (see Ch. 71). Liver fibrosis and cirrhosis result in a stiff liver, and palpation of hepatic masses in this situation is difficult; only 50% to 67% of tumors less than 5 cm can be identified intraoperatively by inspection and palpation alone (Makuuchi et al, 1991; Nagasue et al, 1984; Sheu et al, 1985b). Intraoperative ultrasound is crucial for the identification and localization of these lesions (Gozzetti et al, 1988; Kokudo et al, 1996; Nagasue et al, 1989; Salminen et al, 1990). Detail not clearly evident by preoperative imaging also is attained by intraoperative ultrasound providing a more accurate assessment of tumor extent, intrahepatic metastases (satellite or daughter nodules), and vascular involvement or tumor thrombus (Gozzetti et al, 1986, 1988; Hayashi et al, 1987; Makuuchi et al, 1983b, 1983c, 1991). Finally, data confirm improved survival at centers that routinely use intraoperative ultrasound in this setting compared with centers that do not (Gozzetti et al, 1992).

Many intraoperative hepatic procedures depend on intraoperative ultrasound for their conduct. Accurate needle placement for biopsy is guided by intraoperative ultrasound for tumors that are not palpable or are deep within the parenchyma (Castaing et al, 1986). Likewise, intraoperative ultrasound is essential for accurate targeting and successful ablation of tumors by ethanol injection, cryotherapy, or radiofrequency thermal ablation (Machi, 1999; Machi et al, 1990; Montorsi et al, 2002; Rozycki, 1998; Wong et al, 2001) (see Ch. 76). Hepatic resections can be guided by intraoperative ultrasound, ensuring adequate margins, while minimizing resection of normal parenchyma (Lau et al, 1993). Finally, numerous novel hepatic resection techniques have been developed that depend on intraoperative ultrasound (Fan &

Chang, 2002; Makuuchi et al, 1983a, 1985, 1987a, 1987b, 1993; Montorsi et al, 2002; Torzilli & Makuuchi, 2001; Torzilli et al, 1999, 2002).

INSTRUMENTATION AND SCANNING TECHNIQUES

A flat, side-viewing, linear array probe facilitates liver scanning. This probe gives a rectangular image of the underlying structures, and its long footprint results in efficient scanning of the whole organ (Fig. 86.1). Its low profile allows access in the limited space between the anterior abdominal wall or diaphragm and the liver. A 7.5-MHz probe has the widest application for liver scanning, giving superb detail of intrahepatic structures, while allowing adequate sound penetration to permit viewing of the entire liver. When a fatty liver, cirrhosis, or a large organ is encountered, a 5-MHz probe with its deeper sound penetration may be necessary to scan the depths of the parenchyma (Fig. 86.2).

An overriding concept for intraoperative ultrasound of the liver is for the surgeon to develop a systematic scanning approach that addresses the issues outlined in this section. To ensure an adequate and thorough examination, this system should be followed fastidiously every time intraoperative ultrasound of the liver is performed. This approach initially identifies the segmental anatomy of the liver. When this anatomy is understood, the next step is to evaluate known lesions and their location and relationship to the segmental anatomy. The final step is to survey the remaining liver for occult lesions.

Contact scanning, in which the probe is placed directly on the liver surface, is the most common initial approach for hepatic imaging (Fig. 86.3). This approach is excellent for all parts of the liver except masses or structures within 5 to 10 mm of the liver surface at the site of scanning (Fig. 86.4). These superficial areas directly under the probe represent a "blind spot" during contact scanning. In addition, contact scanning is difficult on

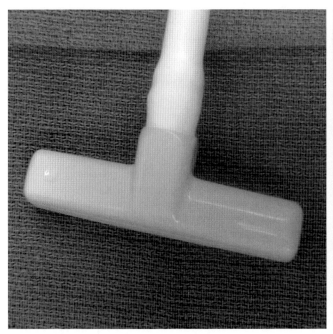

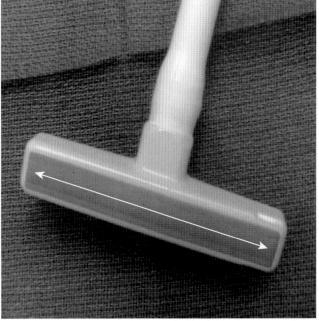

A   B

Fig. 86.1. Intraoperative ultrasound T-probe (Aloka, Tokyo, Japan). **A,** Top view. **B,** Transducer (7.5 MHz linear) view. *Line with arrowheads* marks the crystal array.

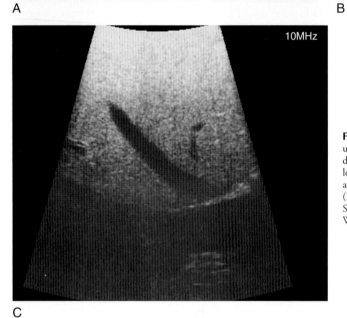

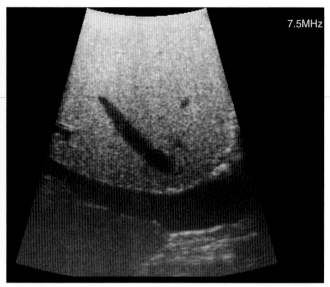

Fig. 86.2. Diffuse fatty infiltration scanned by intraoperative ultrasound using 5-MHz (**A**), 7.5-MHz (**B**), and 10-MHz (**C**) frequencies. To delineate deep areas of the liver in patients with steatosis, cirrhosis, or a large organ, a lower frequency is required. The steatotic liver has increased echogenicity with a fine granular pattern as shown here. RHV, right hepatic vein; VC, vena cava. (From Adams RB, 2005: Intraoperative ultrasound of the liver. In Machi J, Staren ED [eds]: Ultrasound for Surgeons. Philadelphia, Lippincott Williams & Wilkins, pp 315-359.)

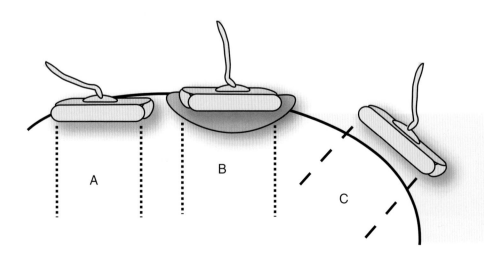

Fig. 86.3. Probe placement for liver scanning. **A,** For contact scanning, probe is placed directly on the liver surface. **B,** Probe standoff scanning using a saline-filled bag or glove as an acoustic interface. This holds the probe away from the liver surface to allow adequate viewing of superficial structures or lesions. **C,** Probe standoff scanning using the saline immersion technique. The organ is immersed in saline *(gray area)*, and the probe is held away from the surface of the organ while immersed within the saline bath. (Original art by RB Adams.)

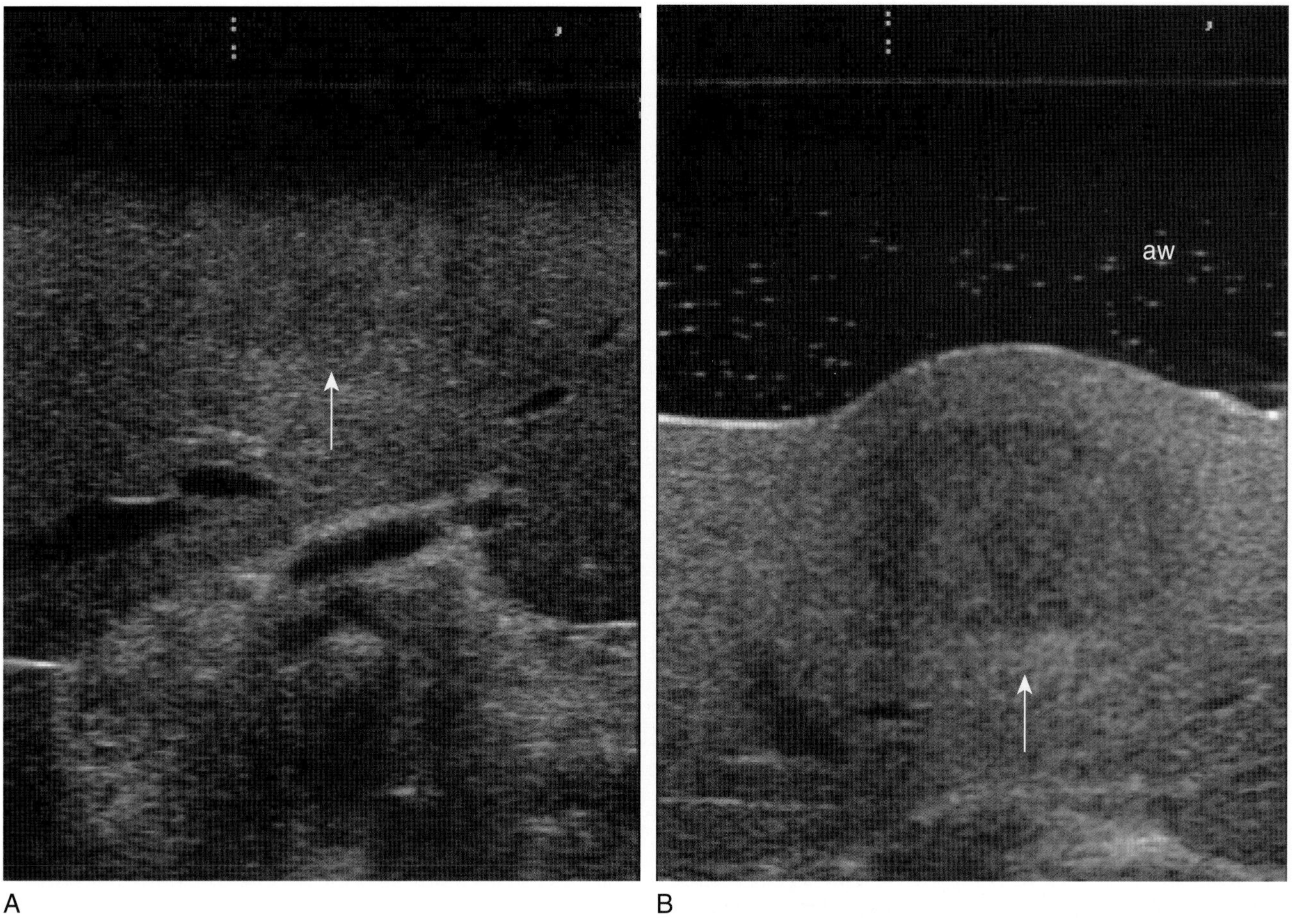

Fig. 86.4. Examination of a mass *(arrows)* adjacent to the liver surface is facilitated by the probe standoff technique. **A,** Direct probe contact on the liver surface. **B,** Probe standoff technique using saline immersion showing improved imaging of this superficial lesion. Acoustic window (aw) using saline.

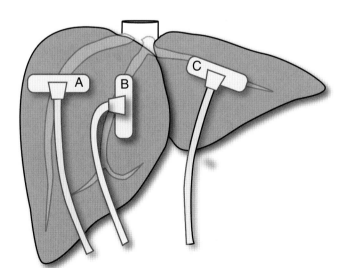

Fig. 86.5. Basic probe positions for contact scanning of the liver. **A,** Transverse. **B,** Longitudinal. **C,** Oblique.
(Original art by RB Adams. From Adams RB, 2005: Intraoperative ultrasound of the liver. In Machi J, Staren ED [eds]: Ultrasound for Surgeons. Philadelphia, Lippincott Williams & Wilkins, pp 315-359.)

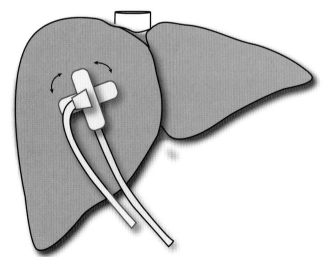

Fig. 86.6. Rotating maneuver for liver scanning. Rotation of the probe on a fixed point allows examination of a structure in two planes.
(Original art by RB Adams. From Adams RB, 2005: Intraoperative ultrasound of the liver. In Machi J, Staren ED [eds]: Ultrasound for Surgeons. Philadelphia, Lippincott Williams & Wilkins, pp 315-359.)

irregular surfaces, such as the cirrhotic liver. These limitations are overcome by using a *probe standoff* scanning technique (see Figs. 86.3 and 86.4). Using saline as an interface (acoustic window) between the probe and the liver surface, scanning is done with the probe held away from the liver; this allows better delineation of superficial structures or scanning of an irregular surface. The probe standoff technique can be done by filling the abdomen with saline so that the liver is submerged or by using a saline-filled glove or bag interposed between the probe and the liver surface. Difficulty imaging superficial or surface lesions with intraoperative ultrasound reinforces the important role of intraoperative inspection and palpation because these techniques are complementary to intraoperative ultrasound. All of these procedures must be done to ensure complete evaluation of the liver.

Transverse scanning is the basic technique for intraoperative ultrasound of the liver and is used in conjunction with longitudinal and oblique scanning to define intrahepatic structures and to verify lesions by showing their presence in two or more planes (Fig. 86.5). Probe rotation over a fixed point allows the area of interest to be examined in several planes, an important technique to ensure that a structure is not an imaging artifact (Fig. 86.6). Rocking or tilting the probe at a fixed point increases the field of view and allows the relationship of structures in close proximity to one another to be delineated (Fig. 86.7). When combined with saline immersion, rocking or tilting provides an excellent view of the superior segments of the liver at the dome and diaphragm (Fig. 86.8).

A systematic approach to liver scanning can be broken down into several steps (Table 86.2). For a screening examination, the liver can be examined fully without mobilization. When resection or another intervention is planned, it is useful to scan the liver before mobilization. This practice minimizes artifacts such as air, which can result from the mobilization and may obscure the field of vision. Scanning is repeated after complete liver mobilization. The two major goals of liver scanning are (1) evaluation of the hepatic vasculature and definition of the segmental anatomy and

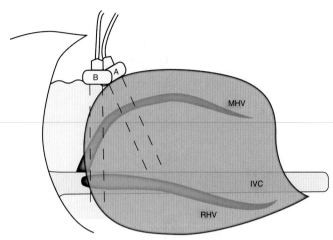

Fig. 86.8. Rocking or tilting maneuver and saline immersion combined to allow examination of the superior portion of the liver. **A,** Direct probe contact allows examination of the central liver and the middle hepatic vein (MHV), but examination of the confluence of the hepatic veins with the inferior vena cava (IVC) using this method is sometimes difficult. **B,** Combining saline immersion with probe rocking or tilting at the same position allows excellent imaging of the confluence of the hepatic veins with the vena cava. The same maneuver is valuable for scanning the dome of the liver or the superior portion of segment VII. RHV, right hepatic vein.
(Original art by RB Adams. From Adams RB, 2005: Intraoperative ultrasound of the liver. In Machi J, Staren ED [eds]: Ultrasound for Surgeons. Philadelphia, Lippincott Williams & Wilkins, pp 315-359.)

(2) systematic scanning of the hepatic parenchyma. The initial scan should focus on the following:

1. Delineate the intrahepatic vascular anatomy. The segmental anatomy of the liver is defined by the hepatic veins and portal pedicles and should be mapped first. This defines the surgical anatomy of the liver (see Ch. 1).
   a. Define the confluence of the major hepatic veins into the vena cava at the superior border of the liver. Follow these veins out to their terminal branches in both lobes. The hepatic veins lie between segments of the liver. Identify any anomalous hepatic veins, which are quite common. Identify vascular involvement by tumors.
   b. Define the portal vein branches from the transverse portion of the portal vein to its terminal branches. Identify vascular or biliary tract involvement by tumors.

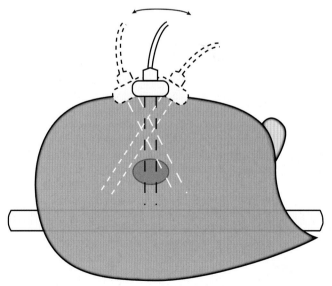

Fig. 86.7. Rocking or tilting maneuver for liver scanning. Rocking or tilting the probe at a fixed point on the liver surface, while maintaining contact, allows examination of a wide area of liver around a point of interest.
(Original art by RB Adams. From Adams RB, 2005: Intraoperative ultrasound of the liver. In Machi J, Staren ED [eds]: Ultrasound for Surgeons. Philadelphia, Lippincott Williams & Wilkins, pp 315-359.)

Table 86.2 Stepwise Approach to Liver Scanning

Scan liver
Before mobilization
Repeat scanning after liver mobilization
Identify hepatic veins
Find junction with vena cava
Follow to terminal branches
Identify anomalous branches
Identify portal branches
Find main, right, and left portal veins
Follow each into its segmental branches
Systematic liver scan
Develop standard scanning routine
View all of the parenchyma
Note tumor location, size, and features
Note vasculobiliary involvement or thrombosis

2. Systematically scan the entire liver parenchyma noting the primary or preoperatively known tumors and any other occult tumors or lesions. The liver should be scanned from various directions, including from the inferior surface, as necessary to delineate fully any masses.
3. Establish the relationship between the portal and hepatic veins and all the tumors noted on the systematic parenchymal scan, with particular attention to understanding their exact segmental locations.

After liver mobilization for resection or other purposes, intraoperative ultrasound is repeated to assess the following points:

1. Systematically scan the parenchyma with particular focus on segment VII (posterior-superior segment) and deeper portions of the liver that might not have been seen adequately on the initial survey.
2. Confirm the spatial relationship of the anatomic segments and the tumors. Re-evaluate the tumor's relationship to, or involvement with, the local hepatic vasculature. Understand these anatomic relationships as the liver is manipulated into position in preparation for resection because the ultrasound features will be altered as the position of the liver changes.

Examination of the intrahepatic vasculature begins with contact scanning on the anterior surface of the liver. The three major hepatic veins are identified at the superior-most portion (diaphragmatic surface) of the liver over the area of the falciform ligament. At this point, their entry into the vena cava can be evaluated (Fig. 86.9), and each hepatic vein can be followed

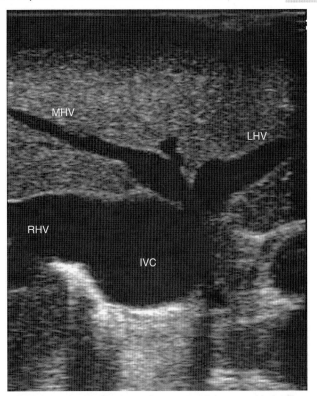

Fig. 86.9. Hepatic vein confluence with the inferior vena cava (IVC). Junction of the right hepatic vein (RHV) with the IVC. The middle hepatic vein (MHV) and left hepatic vein (LHV) are seen just as they form a common trunk. This common trunk joins the IVC.

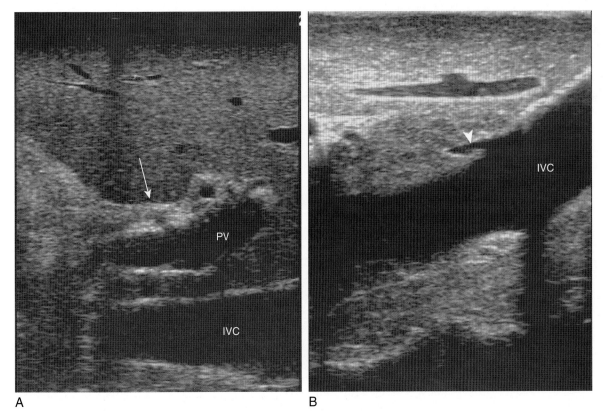

A B

Fig. 86.10. Longitudinal view of the inferior vena cava (IVC). **A,** View through inferior edge of the liver. *Arrow* shows the posterior-inferior aspect of segment IVb as it sits on the anterior surface of the hepatoduodenal ligament. **B,** Longitudinal view of IVC with small branch *(arrowhead)* draining directly into it. A branch of the middle hepatic vein can be seen anterior to the IVC. The superior border of the hepatic hilum can be seen at the left edge of the photograph. PV, portal vein at the hepatic hilum, longitudinal view.

peripherally to its terminal branches. Gentle probe placement allows these veins to be seen; they easily disappear with too much probe pressure. Next, a longitudinal (sagittal) scan is done, and the vascular structures are re-evaluated and confirmed. The retrohepatic vena cava can be evaluated along its full length in this fashion (Fig. 86.10).

Contact scanning at the inferior aspect of the liver allows evaluation of the hepatic hilum. Initial scanning is done transversely (Fig. 86.11) to identify the transverse portion of the portal vein. From this point, the main right branch can be followed to its division into the anterior (segments V and VIII) and posterior (segments VI and VII) sectoral branches (Fig. 86.12). Each sectoral branch is followed to its superior or inferior segmental branch (Fig. 86.13). This allows mapping of the entire inflow to the right lobe. Next, the transverse portion of the left portal vein is traced to the base of the umbilical fissure. Here it ascends anteriorly and inferiorly within the umbilical fissure. At this point, the ascending portion has the appearance of a tree trunk with branches coming off of the main trunk to its left and right. The branches followed to the right of the falciform ligament supply the medial segment of the left lobe (segment IV). Vessels traveling to the left of the falciform ligament go to the lateral portion of the anterior (or inferior) segment of the left lobe (segment III) and the posterior (or superior) segment of the left lobe (segment II), which is posterior-superior to the left hepatic vein (Fig. 86.14).

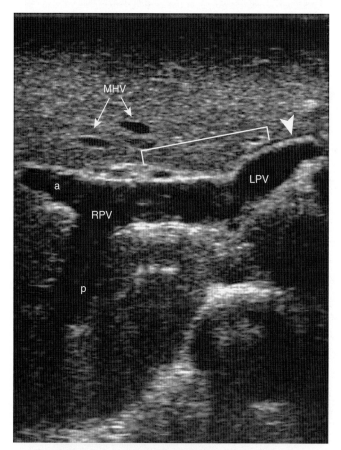

Fig. 86.11. Transverse view of the hepatic hilum illustrating the main portal vein as it branches into the right portal vein (RPV) and the left portal vein (LPV). The relationship of the terminal branches of the middle hepatic vein (MHV) to the hepatic hilum is shown. The *bracketed line* illustrates the transverse portion of the LPV. The base of the umbilical fissure where the LPV ascends anteriorly is noted *(arrowhead)*. Sectoral branches of the RPV are shown. a, anterior sectoral branch; p, posterior sectoral branch.

At this point, the intrahepatic vasculature and segmental anatomy has been defined, and a systematic survey of the parenchyma is begun. This part of the examination seeks to evaluate the parenchyma for diffuse and focal abnormalities, such as hepatic masses. Lesions known from the preoperative studies are identified and evaluated. Simultaneously, the presence of occult lesions is sought. Systematic scanning is performed by contact scanning on the anterior or diaphragmatic liver surfaces. Regardless of where one begins, the same approach should be used in every case to ensure that all segments of the liver are scanned. Scanning should be completed in the transverse and longitudinal planes. Adequate examination of segment VII may require alternate scanning methods, such as rocking or tilting the probe or a probe standoff technique. Evaluation of the deepest portions of segments VI and VII may require scanning from the inferior or right lateral liver surfaces. Similarly, segment I may require scanning from the inferior or posterior surfaces.

Careful and routine use of this systematic approach to liver scanning allows the outlined goals for liver scanning to be accomplished. These techniques, coupled with an understanding of intrahepatic anatomy, allow the surgeon to localize accurately any structure or mass within the liver. This localization facilitates intraoperative diagnosis of hepatic pathology and decision making regarding the appropriate therapeutic approach.

ULTRASOUND ANATOMY OF THE NORMAL LIVER

A principal advantage of intraoperative ultrasound is the ability to combine the visual surface anatomy of the liver with the intrahepatic structures seen by ultrasound to define hepatic segmental anatomy precisely. This section reviews normal ultrasound anatomy of the liver to facilitate recognition of the structures crucial for defining segmental anatomy. The hepatic parenchyma normally has a uniform and homogeneous echo appearance by intraoperative ultrasound. Compared with the adjacent right renal cortex, the liver is more echogenic (brighter) by intraoperative ultrasound (Fig. 86.15). Less commonly, one can observe similar echogenicity between the liver and renal cortex. Changes in liver echogenicity can occur with steatosis, fibrosis, and cirrhosis.

Hepatic veins and portal triads are distinguishable from each other by their ultrasound appearance. As portal triads enter the liver, they are surrounded by Glisson's capsule; this results in an echogenic (bright white) border on intraoperative ultrasound that appears to encircle the portal triads. In contrast, hepatic veins are thin walled because they lack this investing tissue. Hepatic veins are much less echogenic and appear to be black holes within the liver parenchyma (Fig. 86.16). Occasionally, larger hepatic veins can show some echogenicity, particularly when the ultrasound beam is directed perpendicular to the hepatic vein wall. If the nature of the structure is in question, it can be followed to the main portal vein or the vena cava depending on the type of structure it represents.

As noted in Ch. 1, hepatic anatomy is described as sections (sectors) and segments, defined by the intrahepatic vascular anatomy (Anonymous, 2000). In general, the portal vein branches are within the various segments (intrasegmental), whereas the hepatic veins are between segments (intersegmental). Initially, the vascular anatomy is defined by identifying the three major hepatic veins—the right, middle, and left—as they drain into the vena cava. Typically, the right hepatic vein joins the vena cava

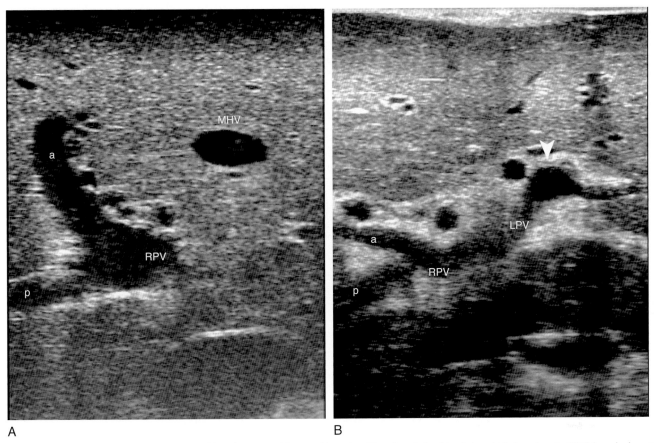

Fig. 86.12. A, Right portal vein (RPV). Anterior (a) and posterior (p) sectoral branches. Note the relationship of the middle hepatic vein (MHV) to the hepatic hilum. RPV anterior and posterior sectoral branches as seen in a transverse view of the hepatic hilum. **B,** Left portal vein (LPV). *Arrowhead* denotes base of umbilical fissure where the LPV ascends anteriorly.

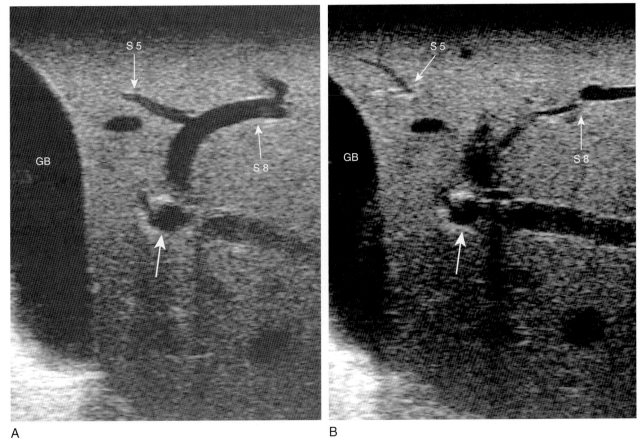

Fig. 86.13. A and **B,** Right anterior sectoral portal vein branch *(arrow)*. This gives rise to the anterior inferior segmental branches (segment V [S 5]) and the anterior superior segmental branches (segment VIII [S 8]). GB, gallbladder.

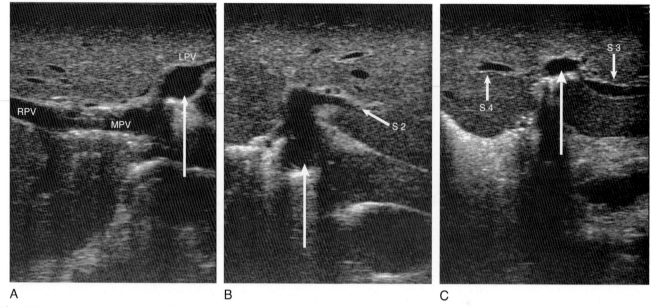

A   B   C

Fig. 86.14. Ascending portion *(arrows)* of the left portal vein (LPV). **A,** *Arrow* points to the base of the umbilical fissure, noting the origin of the ascending portion of the LPV off the relatively short transverse portion of the LPV. **B,** Origin of ascending portion of the LPV at the base of the umbilical fissure *(arrow)* with a branch going to segment II (S 2), to the left of the umbilical fissure. **C,** Terminal portion of ascending LPV *(arrow)* giving rise to branches to segments III (S 3) and IV (S 4). MPV, main portal vein.

separately and to the right lateral side, whereas the middle and left veins join each other just before their entry into the vena cava, where they enter as a common orifice (>50% of the population) (Fig. 86.17; see also Fig. 86.9). Anterior to the hepatic hilum, branches draining segments IVb and V join to form the initial part of the middle hepatic vein.

Variations in hepatic venous anatomy are common, and one of the primary advantages of intraoperative ultrasound is identifying these before intervention. All three major hepatic veins can enter the vena cava separately. More than three major hepatic veins can be present. Recognized variants include large right or left marginal veins that drain into one of the main hepatic veins. The anterior sector (segments V and VIII) can be drained by a large branch entering directly into the middle hepatic vein (Fig. 86.18). A large draining branch from segment IV can drain into the left hepatic vein or alternately into the middle hepatic vein. Less commonly, this segment IV branch can drain directly into the vena cava (called the *umbilical vein*). The inferior right hepatic vein, a large accessory right hepatic vein, can drain segment VI directly into the vena cava in 20% of the population (Makuuchi et al, 1983c; Nakamura & Tsuzuki, 1981). It can be seen by intraoperative ultrasound almost directly posterior to the main right portal vein as it enters the right anterolateral portion of the retrohepatic vena cava (Fig. 86.19). Intraoperative ultrasound can readily identify these hepatic vein abnormalities.

Moving the probe caudally along the liver allows the hepatic veins to be followed into the liver parenchyma. In this fashion, the hepatic and portal veins can be captured together on the same image (Fig. 86.20). Demonstration of this relationship facilitates identification of the hepatic segments and aids planning for hepatic resection.

After defining the hepatic venous anatomy, the main portal vein is identified at the base of segment IV. At this point, its division into the main right and left portal veins can be found (Fig. 86.21). With the probe in the transverse position at the

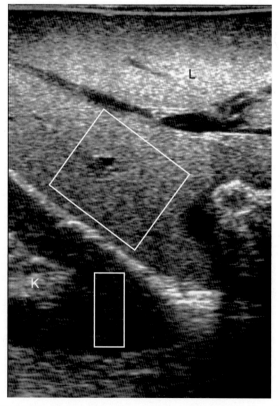

Fig. 86.15. Normal liver echogenicity. The liver (L) parenchyma *(large box)* is typically more echogenic than the renal (K) cortex *(small box)*.

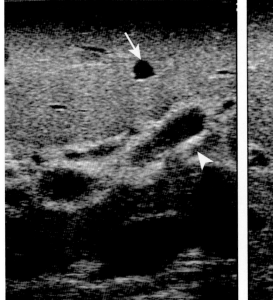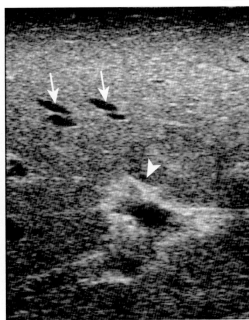

Fig. 86.16. Echogenicity of portal veins and hepatic veins. Portal veins *(arrowheads)* have a thicker, more echogenic appearance compared with the thinner walled hepatic veins *(arrows)*, which have little echogenicity around their circumference.

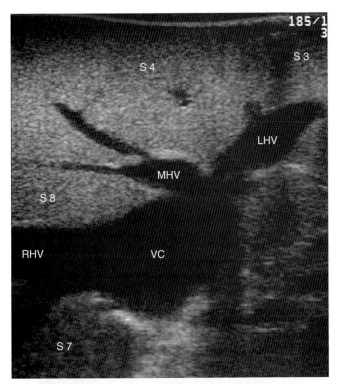

Fig. 86.17. Vascular anatomy defined by the hepatic veins. The right hepatic vein (RHV) drains separately into the vena cava (VC). Posterior to the RHV lies segment VII (S 7). The middle hepatic vein (MHV) and left hepatic vein (LHV) most commonly join to form a common trunk, as shown here, before draining into the VC. Segment VIII (S 8) lies between the RHV and the MHV. Segment IV (S 4) lies to the left of the MHV and the right of the falciform ligament. Segment III (S 3) lies to the left of the falciform ligament and anterior inferior to the LHV.

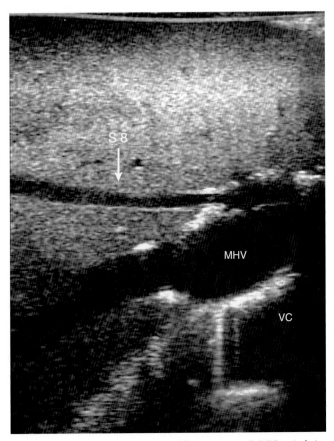

Fig. 86.18. Longitudinal view of the middle hepatic vein (MHV) as it drains into the vena cava (VC). A large draining branch of segment VIII (S 8) is shown joining the MHV.

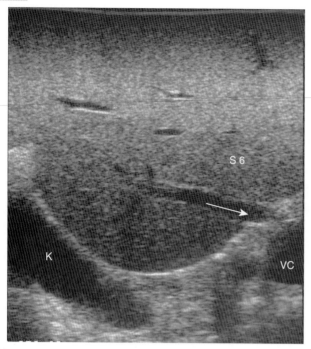

Fig. 86.19. Inferior right hepatic vein (*arrow* within the vein) draining into the vena cava (VC). This accessory vein drains segment VI (S 6), typically joining the VC in the right anterolateral position at a level directly posterior to the hepatic hilum. K, right kidney.

inferior edge of segment IV, the portal vein, hepatic artery, and bile duct can be seen together in cross-section. The portal vein is the largest circular structure of the three, and the most posterior. The bile duct and hepatic artery lie anterior to the portal vein in this position (Fig. 86.22). At the inferior-most part of the hepatoduodenal ligament, the proper hepatic artery lies anterior and to the patient's left of the portal vein. Similarly, the bile duct is anterior to the portal vein. This is the third circular structure in the ligament, lying to the right of the proper hepatic artery and the patient's portal vein (Fig. 86.23). This ultrasound image is in a configuration that has been referred to as the Mickey Mouse view. Because hepatic arterial anatomy is frequently aberrant, color Doppler imaging can be used to distinguish the hepatic artery quickly from the bile duct in the hepatoduodenal ligament or the liver.

Scanning toward the right liver, the main right portal triad divides into the anterior (segments V and VIII) and posterior sectoral branches (segments VI and VII) (Fig. 86.24). The anterior sectoral branch supplies superior branches to segment VIII (Fig. 86.25; see also Fig. 86.13) and inferior branches to segment V (see Figs. 86.13 and 86.25). Segment VIII typically receives two branches, a ventral and dorsal, with the ventral branch frequently coming from the segment V pedicle. Segment V can consist of three to five branches arising from the anterior sectoral pedicle. The posterior sectoral pedicle supplies segment

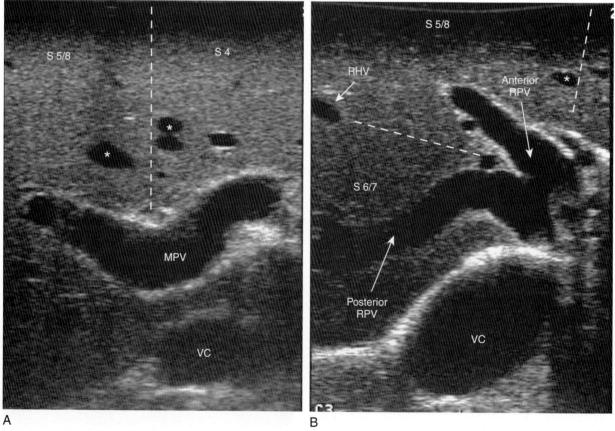

Fig. 86.20. Intrahepatic relationships of hepatic and portal veins define segmental anatomy. **A,** The middle hepatic vein (*asterisks* denote terminal branches of middle vein) lies directly anterior to the transverse portion of the main portal vein (MPV) at the hepatic hilum. To the left of the middle hepatic vein is segment IV (S 4); to its right are segments V and VIII (S 5/8). The *dotted line* shows the division along the middle hepatic vein (Cantlie's line) that separates the right and left hemiliver. **B,** The right hepatic vein (RHV) lies between the anterior and posterior sectoral branches of the right portal vein (RPV). Anterior to the RHV and to the right of the middle hepatic vein (*asterisk*) are segments V and VIII (S 5/8). Posterior to the RHV are segments VI and VII (S 6/7). VC, vena cava.

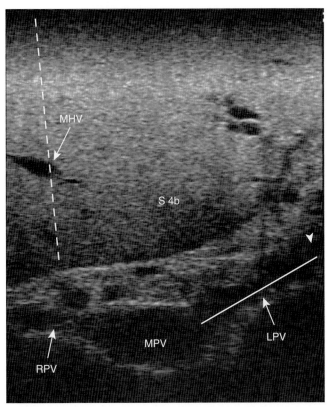

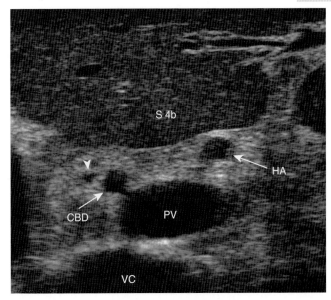

Fig. 86.21. Transverse segment of the left portal vein (hypoechoic tubular structure shown by the *line*) as it runs along the base of segment IVb (S 4b). The extrahepatic portion of the left portal vein is typically longer than the right portal vein (RPV) as illustrated here. The *arrowhead* indicates the transverse segment of the left portal vein at the point where it turns anteriorly to become the ascending portion of the left portal vein. *Dotted line* denotes the division between the right and left hemiliver. MHV, middle hepatic vein; MPV, main portal vein.

Fig. 86.23. Relationships in the inferior hepatoduodenal ligament. Segment IVb (S 4b) lies over the anterior hepatoduodenal ligament and functions as an acoustic window to the structures in the ligament. The vena cava (VC) is the posterior-most hypoechoic structure in this typical view. The structures in the hepatoduodenal ligament are shown in their most typical configuration, the so-called Mickey Mouse view. *Arrowhead* denotes the cystic duct. CBD, common bile duct; HA, proper hepatic artery; PV, main portal vein.

VII, which usually consists of a single (superior) branch to segment VII (see Fig. 86.25). Segment VI is supplied by one or two inferior branches off the posterior sectoral branch (see Fig. 86.25).

Scanning toward the left liver, the main left portal can be seen as it branches off the main portal vein. From the bifurcation to the base of the umbilical fissure, the left portal vein travels a much longer transverse (parallel to the ultrasound probe) and extrahepatic course than the right portal vein (Fig. 86.26). At the base of the umbilical fissure, the transverse portion of the left vein turns abruptly anteriorly (toward the probe) as it ascends into the umbilical fissure. This branch of the portal vein is unique because it is intersegmental (running between

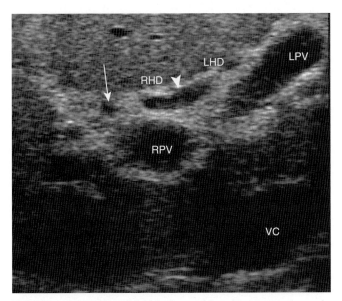

Fig. 86.22. Relationship of the bile duct and hepatic artery anterior to the portal vein at the level of the hepatic hilum. *Arrow* denotes right hepatic artery. *Arrowhead* shows the septum at the junction of the right and left hepatic ducts. The junction of these ducts typically sits just cranial to the division of the portal vein into the right and left branches. LHD, left hepatic duct; LPV, left portal vein; RHD, right hepatic duct; RPV, right portal vein; VC, vena cava.

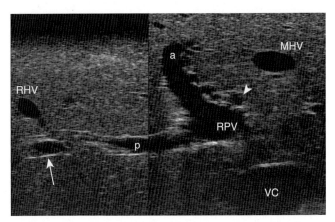

Fig. 86.24. The right portal vein (RPV) divides into an anterior (a) and posterior (p) sectoral branch, which can be shown as the probe is moved from the transverse view of the hepatic hilum to the right liver. *Arrowhead* shows right hepatic duct. *Arrow* denotes segment VI pedicle. MHV, middle hepatic vein; RHV, right hepatic vein; VC, vena cava.

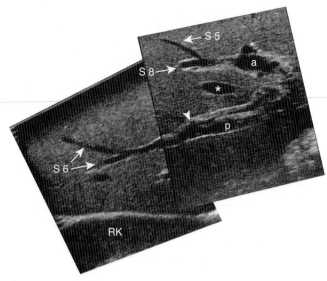

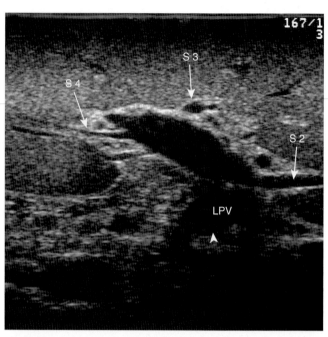

Fig. 86.25. Right portal branches. The anterior (a) sectoral branch of the right portal vein lies anterior to the right hepatic vein *(asterisk)* and supplies segment V (S 5) inferiorly and segment VIII (S 8) superiorly. The posterior (p) sectoral branch lies posterior to the right hepatic vein and supplies segment VI (S 6) inferiorly and segment VII superiorly. The *arrowhead* marks the takeoff of the segment VII branch. RK, right kidney.

Fig. 86.27. Left portal vein (LPV) in the umbilical fissure. *Arrowhead* marks the base of the umbilical fissure. The LPV ascends in the umbilical fissure with the initial branch traveling to the left into segment II (S 2). More anteriorly, it branches to the left again, to segment III (S 3), and to the right, supplying segment IV (S 4).

segments IV and II/III), in contrast to the other portal branches. As the portal triad ascends into the umbilical fissure, it has the appearance of a tree trunk with branches extending to the right and left (Fig. 86.27; see also Fig. 86.14). At the base of the umbilical fissure (off the bottom of the tree trunk), intraoperative ultrasound frequently shows a branch passing posteriorly to supply the left portion of segment I (caudate) (Fig. 86.28). Just after the

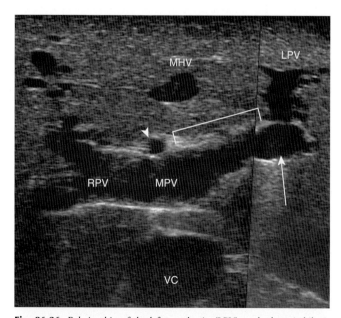

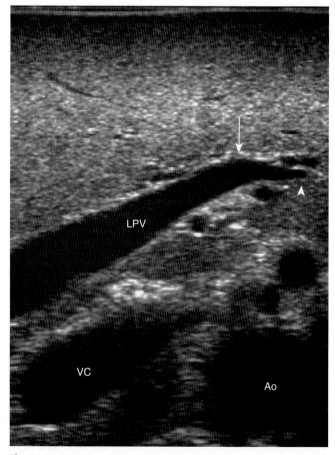

Fig. 86.26. Relationship of the left portal vein (LPV) to the hepatic hilum. Scanning toward the left liver, the main LPV branches off the main portal vein (MPV). The long transverse, extrahepatic portion of the LPV is shown by the *bracketed line*. This runs to the base of the umbilical fissure *(arrow)*, then turns abruptly anteriorly (toward the probe) as it ascends into the umbilical fissure. In this view, it has the appearance of a tree trunk with multiple side branches to the left and right. *Arrowhead* illustrates the common hepatic duct. MHV, middle hepatic vein; MPV, main portal vein; RPV, right portal vein; VC, vena cava.

Fig. 86.28. Portal branch to segment I *(arrowhead)*. As the transverse portion of the left portal vein (LPV) transitions into the ascending portion *(arrow)*, a posterior branch can be identified coming off at this site and supplying segment I. Ao, aorta; VC, vena cava.

branch to segment I, a branch arises off the base of the portal triad (base of the tree trunk) and passes to the patient's left supplying segment II (lateral-superior branch) (see Fig. 86.27). At the top of the tree (close to the probe), a branch or branches extend to the right to supply segment IV, and one branch to the left supplies segment III (lateral-inferior) (Fig. 86.29).

Portal venous anatomy, in contrast to the hepatic vein, rarely deviates from its usual configuration. Occasionally, portal vein anomalies are seen, such as a portal vein trifurcation. In this case, separate right anterior and posterior sectoral branches come off the main portal vein. A main right portal vein is lacking in these patients. An analogous situation may occur on the left. In this case, the transverse portion of the left portal vein is absent, and the ascending portion of this vein arises almost directly off the main portal vein bifurcation. Finally, one of the right sectoral pedicles can arise from the left portal pedicle, rather than from its standard position on the right (Fig. 86.30).

Many ligaments associated with the liver can be detected by intraoperative ultrasound. The ligamentum teres lies along the posterior edge of the inferior portion of the falciform ligament. Followed superiorly, the ligamentum teres enters the umbilical fissure. Within the ligamentum teres is the round ligament, the remnant of the obliterated umbilical vein. The round ligament passes into the umbilical fissure, where it joins the terminus of the left portal vein. The round ligament can be recognized as a thickened, hyperechoic band that appears to abut or join the terminal part of the left portal vein as it ascends into the umbilical fissure (Fig. 86.31). This structure lies between and separates segment IV from segment II/III. The ligamentum venosum, the obliterated ductus venosus remnant, is a thin, linear, hyperechoic band that runs almost parallel to the transducer. It appears to emanate from the left side of the left portal vein as it transitions from the transverse portion of the left portal vein to the ascending portion (Fig. 86.32). A thin echogenic band, parallel to the transducer, is seen to the left of the ligamentum venosum. This is the gastrohepatic ligament.

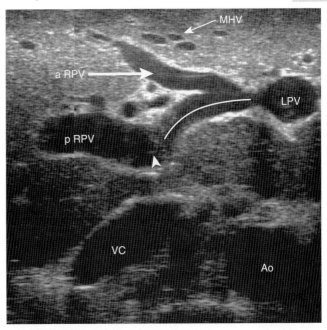

Fig. 86.30. Aberrant portal vein anatomy. The anterior sectoral branch of the right portal vein (a RPV) arises from the transverse portion (denoted by *curved white line*) of the left portal vein (LPV). The posterior sectoral branch of the right portal vein (p RPV) arises from the main portal vein *(arrowhead)*. Ao, aorta; MHV, middle hepatic vein; VC, vena cava.

The surrounding vascular structures and the ligamentum venosum identify the boundaries of segment I (caudate lobe) (Fig. 86.33). The transverse portion of the left portal vein denotes the anterior limit of segment I. Further to the left of the portal vein is the thin hyperechoic ligamentum venosum and gastrohepatic omentum, which separates segment I from segment II/III. Anterior to the ligamentum venosum are segments II and III; posterior to it is segment I. Longitudinal scanning over this area also shows these relationships (Fig. 86.34). Posterior to segment I is the vena cava, which defines the posterior aspect of segment I. Occasionally, segment I or a fibrous band can extend posterior to the vena cava and encircle it (Fig. 86.35). Toward the right hemiliver, the caudate fuses with the right lobe of the liver. More superiorly in the liver, the caudate lobe is limited anteriorly by the middle vein. Segment I can be defined by these anatomic structures readily identified and mapped by intraoperative ultrasound.

ULTRASOUND CHARACTERISTICS OF HEPATIC PATHOLOGY AND FINDINGS THAT MODIFY THE OPERATIVE STRATEGY

The most common use of intraoperative ultrasound in hepatic surgery is to identify and characterize mass lesions in the liver and to define their relationship to intrahepatic structures. Numerous mass lesions may be identified within the liver (Table 86.3). Intraoperative ultrasound can distinguish easily among many of these lesions, particularly lesions that are cystic and solid. A detailed review of the ultrasound characteristics of hepatic lesions is available elsewhere (Adams, 2005). This section reviews some highlights of these features and findings that might affect the planned surgical strategy.

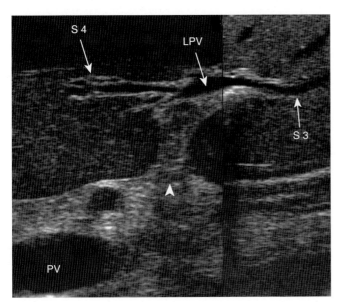

Fig. 86.29. Left portal vein (LPV) terminal branches. As the LPV passes anteriorly in the umbilical fissure *(arrowhead)*, it supplies segment III (S 3) to the left and segment IV (S 4) to the right. PV, main portal vein.

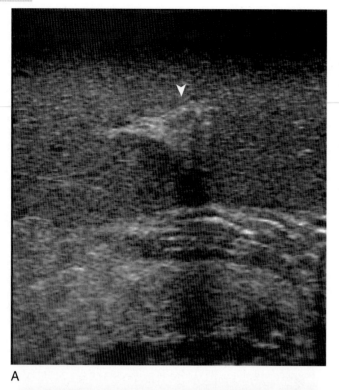

A

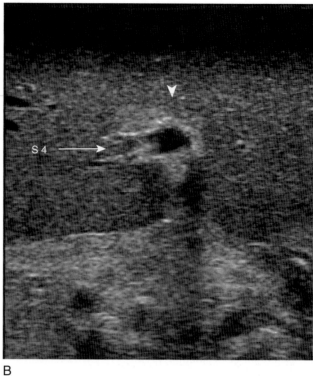

B

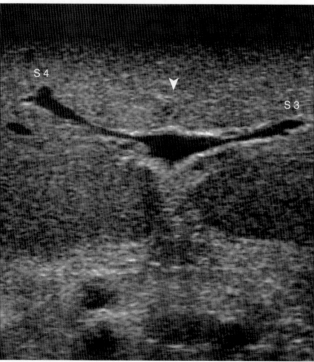

C

Fig. 86.31. Ligamentum teres and its relationship to the left portal vein. **A,** Scanning from the inferior edge of the liver to more superiorly over the umbilical fissure, the round ligament *(arrowhead)* can be seen entering the hepatic parenchyma. **B,** As the probe is moved superiorly, the junction of the round ligament with the inferior-most portion of the left portal vein can be identified *(arrowhead)*. Branches supplying segment IV (S 4) can be identified at this point. **C,** As the probe is moved further superiorly, the ascending portion of the left portal vein *(arrowhead)* becomes more prominent and gives off branches supplying segment III (S 3) and segment IV (S 4).

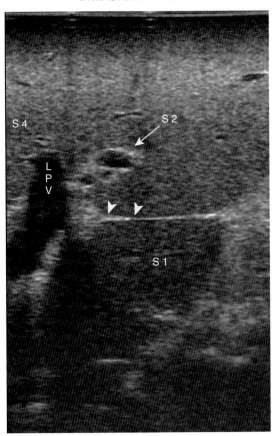

Fig. 86.32. Ligamentum venosum and surrounding structures. The ligamentum venosum lies at the junction of the transition between the transverse and ascending portions of the left portal vein (LPV) and the gastrohepatic ligament *(arrowheads)*. The ligamentum venosum and gastrohepatic ligament separate segment I (S 1) from segment II/III (S 2). Segment IV (S 4) lies to the right of the umbilical fissure/falciform ligament.

The ultrasound features of hepatic lesions contribute to their characterization by taking advantage of the echogenicity and echo patterns typical of specific lesions (Choji et al, 1988; Hung et al, 2001; Mirk et al, 1982; Shamsi et al, 1993; Vilgrain et al, 2000). The echogenicity of a lesion is described relative to the surrounding hepatic parenchyma. Lesions can be hyperechoic (brighter, whiter), isoechoic (similar gray scale appearance), or hypoechoic (darker, blacker) compared with the surrounding liver tissue (Fig. 86.36). Masses may appear heterogeneous, having a mixture of echo characteristics within them (Fig. 86.37). The shape of the lesion and the nature of its borders can help characterize the cause of the mass. Shadowing deep to the lateral edges of the mass (lateral or edge shadowing) or directly behind (deep to) the lesion (posterior shadowing) is present in many lesions (Fig. 86.38). Conversely, enhancement (brighter echoes) posterior to the mass (posterior enhancement) may be seen (Fig. 86.39). A hypoechoic ring (halo, bull's eye, or target pattern) surrounding a solid mass is a typical feature of malignant liver tumors (Fig. 86.40). Displacement of surrounding vasculature or other structures is consistent with a mass effect from a liver lesion (Fig. 86.41). Vascular invasion occurs with some tumors (Fig. 86.42), or they may be associated with tumor thrombus within the vascular or biliary lumen (Figs. 86.43 and 86.44). Some lesions, such as focal fatty changes, appear to be masses, but cause no mass effect as the vessels can be seen passing through them unaltered (Fig. 86.45) (Aubin et al, 1995; Caturelli et al, 1992; Dietrich et al, 1997). All of these characteristics can vary with the size of the mass. The smaller (<2 cm) or larger (>10 cm) the lesion, the more difficult the diagnosis based on ultrasound features alone.

Features characteristic of hepatic cystic lesions (see Chs. 64 and 65) are shown in Table 86.4. Although most cystic lesions in the liver are simple hepatic cysts, the differential diagnosis can

Fig. 86.33. Segment I (caudate lobe). Intraoperative ultrasound identifies the structures delineating the boundaries of the caudate lobe. **A,** Segment I (S 1) is surrounded by the *solid line.* Anteriorly, its boundary is the right and left portal veins (RPV and LPV) at the hepatic hilum. Posteriorly, its boundary is the vena cava (VC). Adjacent structures are the aorta (Ao), segment II/III (S 2/3), and segment IV (S 4). **B,** The left side of segment I (S 1) is delineated anteriorly by the ligamentum venosum *(arrows),* which separates segment I from segment II/III. Toward the right, the anterior border is the LPV and the hepatic hilum. *Arrowheads* outline segment I. Adjacent structures include the ascending portion of the LPV, the VC, Ao, and segment III (S 3) and IV (S 4).

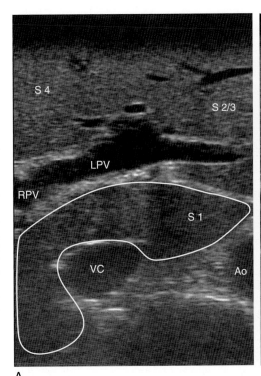

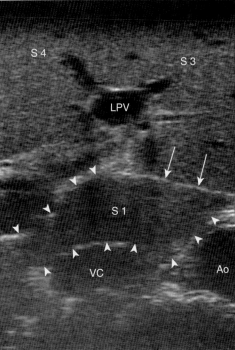

A

B

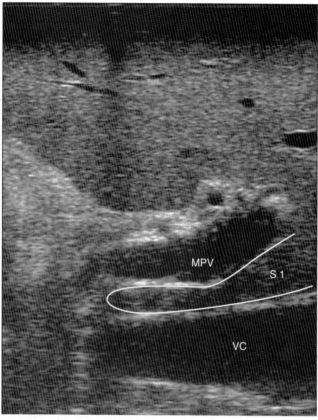

Fig. 86.34. Segment I (S 1), longitudinal view. The main portal vein (MPV), the hepatic hilum, and the ligamentum venosum (not shown in this view) lie anterior to segment I. The vena cava (VC) lies posterior to segment I.

be complex (Table 86.5). The intraoperative ultrasound findings must be placed in the appropriate clinical context to narrow the differential diagnosis. One of the major advantages of intraoperative ultrasound is the ability to characterize a lesion clearly as cystic, rather than solid, when preoperative imaging fails to distinguish the two (Fig. 86.46).

Although intraoperative ultrasound is excellent at distinguishing cystic from solid masses in the liver, determining whether a solid mass is benign or malignant is more difficult. The clinical context is important for narrowing the diagnostic possibilities. Although characteristic ultrasound features of specific mass lesions have been described in an effort to identify them, biopsy generally is required for definitive diagnosis.

The ability to detect a solid mass in the liver by intraoperative ultrasound depends on differences in contrast between the mass and the surrounding liver parenchyma. Hypoechoic and hyperechoic masses are readily seen, whereas isoechoic masses, particularly small ones, may be difficult to discern from the surrounding liver (Fig. 86.47; see also Figs. 86.36B and E and 86.40). Clues to the presence of isoechoic masses include the existence of a hypoechoic rim and secondary signs, such as distortion of surrounding structures (Fig. 86.48). Another clue is the presence of vascular invasion or thrombosis, which raises the suspicion of a mass lesion (see Figs. 86.42 to 86.44 and 86.48B). Difficulty characterizing lesions occurs with conditions such as hepatic steatosis that alter the echogenicity (increased or brighter) of the liver parenchyma. Consequently, detection of hypoechoic mass lesions may be easier, whereas detection of hyperechoic lesions can be more difficult.

Benign hepatic tumors (see Ch. 70) are relatively uncommon except for hemangioma, the most frequent benign liver tumor. Less frequent benign liver masses include focal nodular hyperplasia, hepatic adenoma, regenerative nodules, and focal fatty changes. In Western countries, metastatic disease (see Ch. 73) is the most common solid liver mass. In the United States, metastatic tumors are 10 to 20 times more common than primary liver cancers. In other parts of the world, hepatocellular carcinoma is the most frequent solid hepatic tumor. The likely cause of a solid

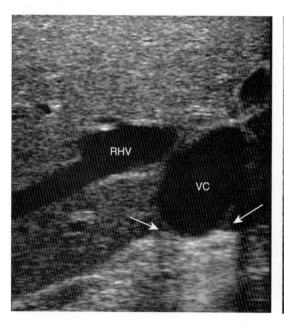

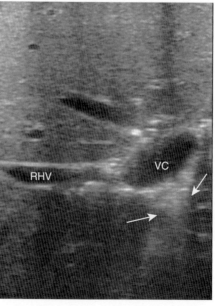

Fig. 86.35. Segment I and the posterior right hepatic lobe often are fused posterior to the vena cava (VC) by a bridge of hepatic parenchyma or a fibrous band of tissue *(arrows)*. RHV, right hepatic vein.

Table 86.3   Common Mass Lesions in the Liver

Cystic

Simple, multiple, or complex cysts
Infectious cysts
Cystic tumors

Solid

Benign tumors
Malignant tumors
Regenerative nodules
Fatty infiltration

liver mass depends on the clinical scenario. Other solid malignancies in the liver, such as intrahepatic cholangiocarcinoma, are less frequent. All of these diagnoses must be considered in the differential diagnosis (Table 86.6) because the intraoperative ultrasound features of benign and malignant lesions frequently overlap. Table 86.7 summarizes the ultrasound features of liver tumors. Characteristic features that suggest malignant liver tumors are listed in Table 86.8.

Liver metastasis can have a range of appearances by intraoperative ultrasound (Marchal et al, 1985a). The echogenicity and echo pattern typically vary with the size of metastatic tumors. Metastases larger than 1 to 2 cm from gastrointestinal primary tumors are frequently isoechoic to hyperechoic and surrounded by

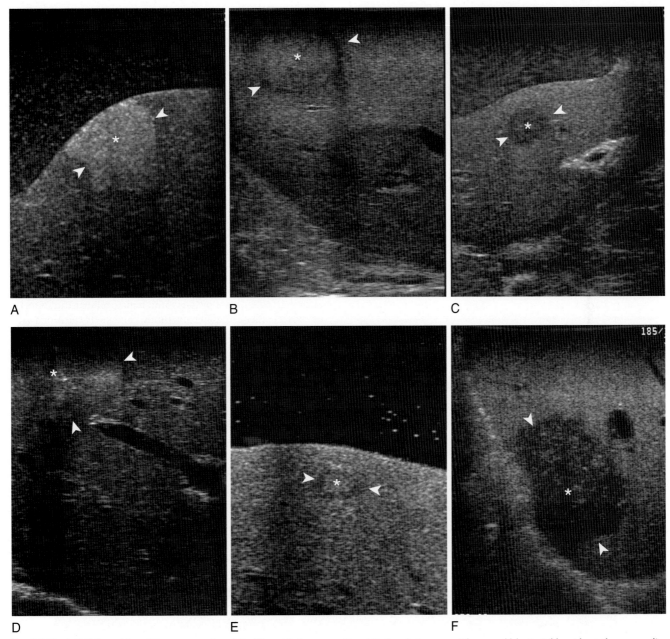

Fig. 86.36. A-F, Echogenicity of liver masses. **A** and **D,** Hyperechoic masses. **B** and **E,** Isoechoic masses. These would be invisible without the surrounding hypoechoic ring around the masses. **C** and **F,** Hypoechoic masses. *Asterisk* marks the central portion of the mass, and *arrowheads* indicate the periphery.

Text continued on p. 1507

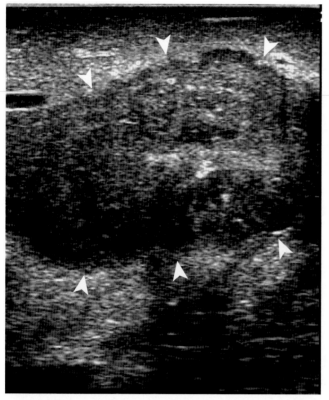

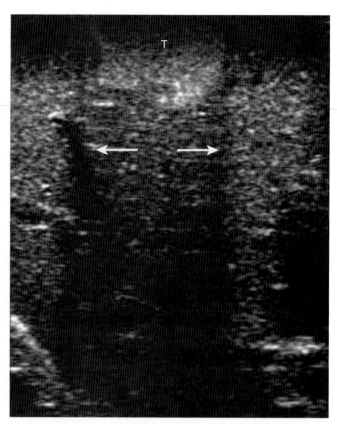

Fig. 86.37. Heterogeneous liver mass. This mostly hypoechoic mass has hyper-echoic and isoechoic regions mixed within its interior. *Arrowheads* mark the tumor's margins.

Fig. 86.38. Tumor (T) is associated with lateral shadowing *(arrows)*.

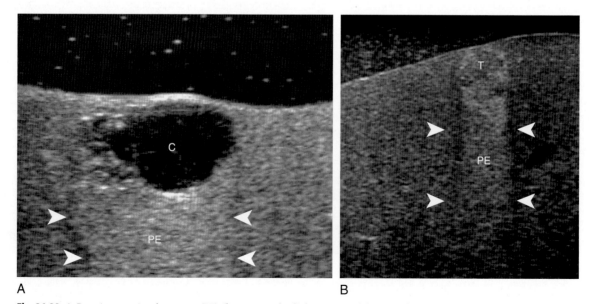

A   B

Fig. 86.39. A, Posterior acoustic enhancement (PE) *(between arrowheads)* deep to a cyst (C). **B,** PE *(between arrowheads)* deep to a solid mass (T).

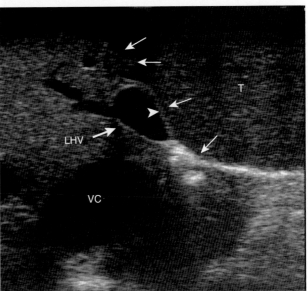

Fig. 86.40. Tumor halo. A hypoechoic ring *(arrowheads)* frequently surrounds malignant liver masses (T). Both masses are isoechoic and would be nearly invisible without the tumor halo.

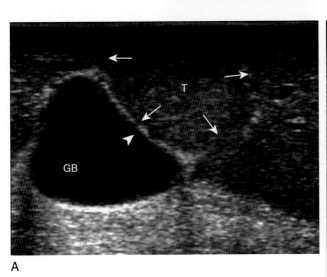

A

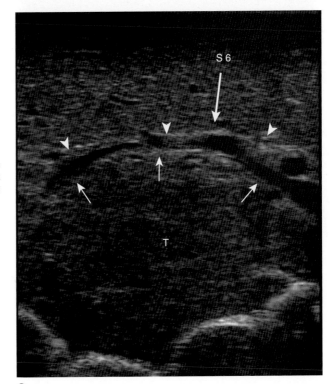

B

C

Fig. 86.41. Tumor mass effect. Tumor (T) impinging *(arrowheads)* on the gallbladder (GB) **(A),** left hepatic vein (LHV) just before it joins the vena cava (VC) **(B),** and segment VI (S 6) pedicle **(C).** *Arrows* mark the margins of the tumor.

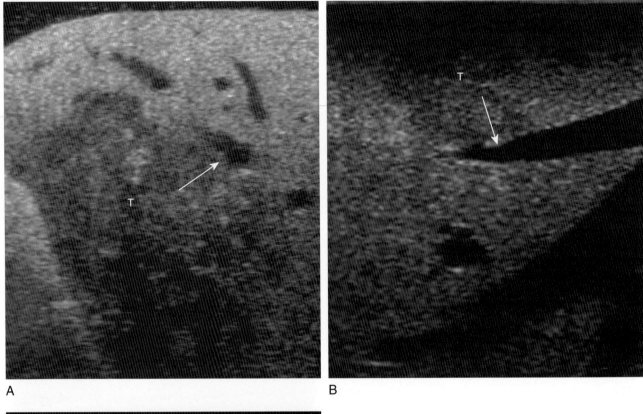

A

B

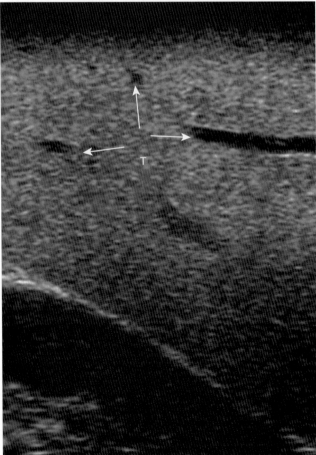

C

Fig. 86.42. Vascular invasion by malignant tumor. Tumor (T) invading peripheral veins **(A)**, a major branch of the right hepatic vein **(B)**, and the terminal branches of the segment VI pedicle **(C)**. *Arrows* show sites of invasion.

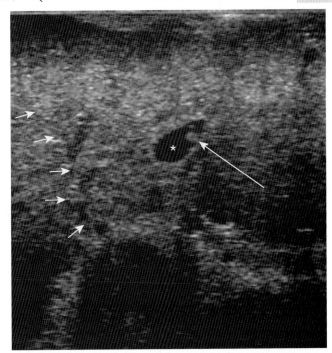

Fig. 86.43. Tumor thrombus *(long arrow)* within the left hepatic vein *(asterisk)*. A subtle, diffuse, poorly seen hepatocellular carcinoma is invading the liver (leading edge of tumor noted by *arrows*) resulting in the tumor thrombus.

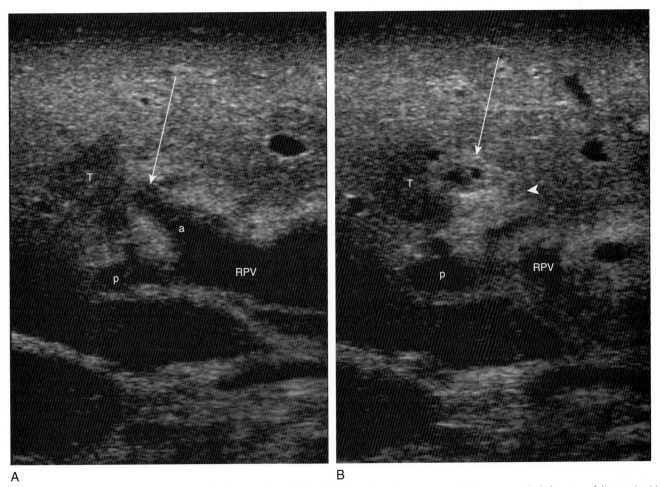

A   B

Fig. 86.44. Tumor thrombus within the anterior (a) right portal vein (RPV). **A,** An invasive gallbladder tumor (T) is present at the bifurcation of the anterior (a) and posterior (p) branches of the RPV. *Arrow* denotes tumor invasion of the anterior branch. **B,** This image is immediately to the right of the one in **A** and shows tumor (T) thrombus within the anterior RPV *(arrow)*. *Arrowhead* illustrates the echogenic investing fascia around the portal pedicle.

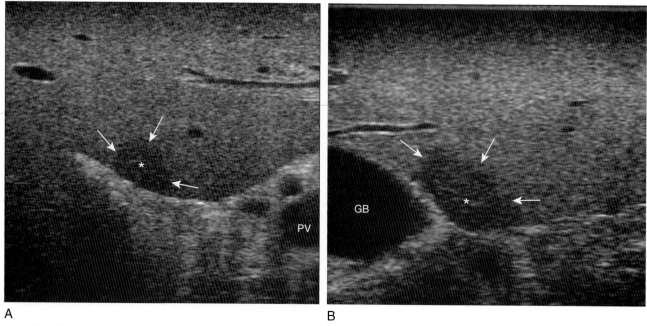

A

B

Fig. 86.45. Diffuse fatty liver parenchyma with a focal area of sparing. Areas of sparing *(asterisk)* can appear as masses within the liver and commonly occur adjacent to the hepatic hilum (portal plate) **(A)** and the gallbladder (GB) fossa **(B).** Another common site is along the ligamentum teres. *Arrows* note the margins of the spared areas. PV, portal vein.

Table 86.4   Typical Characteristics of Cystic Liver Lesions

Anechoic (black within lesion)

Sharp well-circumscribed borders

Lateral shadowing

Posterior enhancement (brighter deep to lesion)

Fine, delicate internal septa in some

Table 86.5   Etiology of Cystic Liver Lesions

Simple cyst

Polycystic liver disease

Pyogenic abscess

Amebic abscess

Echinococcal disease

Resolving hematoma

Cystic adenoma

Cystic adenocarcinoma

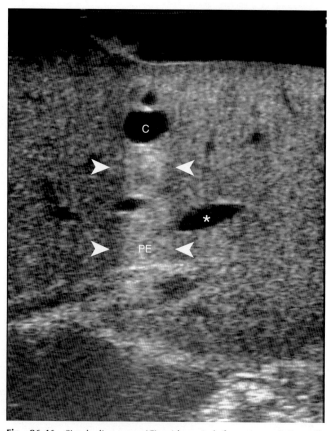

Fig. 86.46. Simple liver cyst (C) with typical features: anechoic, well-circumscribed borders, posterior enhancement (PE), and lateral shadowing *(arrowheads)*. *Asterisk* denotes hepatic vein. The hepatic vein, although anechoic, does not have the other features of the cyst.

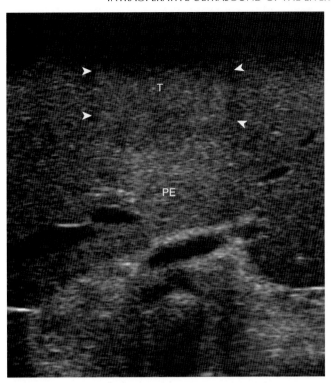

Fig. 86.47. Isoechoic liver tumor (T). This tumor is identifiable owing to the surrounding hypoechoic ring *(arrowheads)* and posterior enhancement (PE).

a hypoechoic ring or halo (target or bull's eye lesion) (Fig. 86.49; see also Figs. 86.36, 86.40, 86.47, and 86.48) (Marchal et al, 1985b). Distortion of surrounding structures is seen frequently as a result of the mass effect of the tumor. Although vascular or biliary invasion occurs occasionally, these lesions tend to push structures aside, resulting in displacement, rather than invasion, of intrahepatic vessels (Fig. 86.50). Mapping of metastatic lesions and identification of vascular or biliary involvement are ways in which intraoperative ultrasound findings may alter the operative plan. If any uncertainty persists regarding the nature of the lesion, a core needle biopsy should be done.

Occult metastases often are detected by intraoperative ultrasound. Because preoperative imaging is excellent, most of these occult lesions are smaller than 1 cm in size. These small lesions identified by intraoperative ultrasound pose a difficult diagnostic problem. When less than 1 to 2 cm in diameter, lesions tend to be hypoechoic and lack the features characteristic of metastatic lesions (Fig. 86.51) (Itai et al, 1987). They may retain the hypoechoic halo, however, a feature highly suggestive of malignancy (Fig. 86.52; see also Fig. 86.36E). Identification of occult malignant lesions outside the planned resection area affect the planned operative approach. When it would alter the surgical approach, biopsy of these small lesions is generally necessary for definitive diagnosis.

The most common primary malignancy of the liver is hepatocellular carcinoma (see Ch. 71). Intraoperative ultrasound has become essential for the intraoperative treatment of hepatocellular carcinoma. It is important for detecting occult hepatocellular

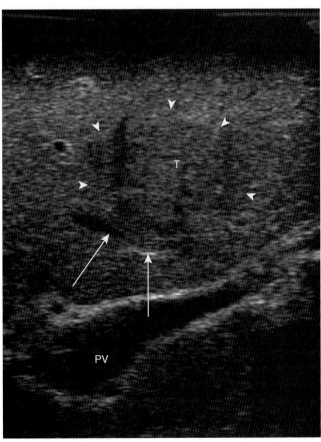

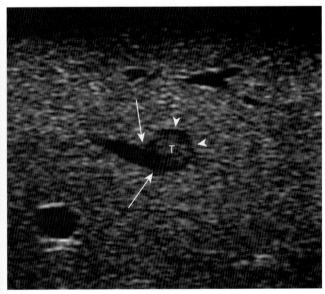

Fig. 86.48. Isoechoic tumor (T). **A,** Tumor is distinguishable from the surrounding liver parenchyma by the subtle hypoechoic ring *(arrowheads)* and nearly complete compression of the adjacent middle hepatic vein *(arrows)*. PV, portal vein. **B,** Tumor is distinguishable by the hypoechoic halo *(arrowheads)* and invasion of the adjacent hepatic vein *(arrows)*.

A

Table 86.6 Etiology of Common Solid Liver Lesions

Benign

Hemangioma
Focal nodular hyperplasia
Hepatic adenoma
Regenerative nodule
Focal fatty changes

Malignant

Metastatic disease
Hepatocellular carcinoma
Intrahepatic cholangiocarcinoma

Table 86.8 Ultrasound Features of Malignant Liver Tumors

Hypoechoic halo (dark ring)
  Target or bull's eye pattern

Displacement of intrahepatic structures (mass effect)

Local invasion—vascular or biliary structures
  Tumor thrombus

Loss of vascular flow (Doppler or color signal)

Biliary dilation

carcinomas and associated daughter nodules and for planning operative therapy, particularly in the cirrhotic patient. Small lesions within the cirrhotic liver missed by preoperative studies can be detected by intraoperative ultrasound (Gozzetti et al, 1988; Nagasue et al, 1984; Sheu et al, 1985b).

Characteristic traits of hepatocellular carcinoma, such as vascular invasion, are detectable by intraoperative ultrasound better than with preoperative studies (Makuuchi et al, 1991). Hepatocellular carcinomas have widely variable ultrasound characteristics. Two primary forms of hepatocellular carcinoma are recognized, nodular and diffuse. Each form has differing qualities on intraoperative ultrasound. Nodular tumors are more common and appear as single or multiple discrete masses. Diffuse tumors can be difficult to see because they have infiltrative, indistinct borders that tend to blend in with the surrounding heterogeneous cirrhotic parenchyma. Hints to the presence of a diffuse tumor are secondary signs, such as vascular displacement or invasion (Fig. 86.53). Nodular tumors are reported to have echo characteristics suggestive of a diagnosis of hepatocellular carcinoma. In addition, several studies have examined the differing ultrasound characteristics of these tumors and correlated them with the pathologic findings. Hepatocellular carcinomas less than 2 cm in diameter typically are uniformly hypoechoic (Fig. 86.54) (Itai et al, 1987; Sheu et al, 1984). As the size of the tumor increases, the echogenicity changes (Sheu et al, 1985a). Larger lesions are more echogenic, having a hypoechoic halo (Fig. 86.55). Often, a variegated or mosaic pattern is seen within tumors ranging in size from 2.1 to 5 cm. A thin hypoechoic halo, posterior enhancement, and lateral shadowing also can be present (Fig. 86.56). Larger tumors have these qualities more frequently than tumors smaller than 2 cm (Makuuchi et al, 1981b). Finally, as hepatocellular carcinomas enlarge to more than 5 cm, they develop into hyperechoic lesions often with heterogeneous features (Fig. 86.57) (Cottone et al, 1983; Ebara et al, 1986). The most likely explanation for the increased echogenicity and heterogeneity in these larger tumors seems to be tumor hemorrhage or necrosis, based on pathologic studies.

Other mass lesions occur in cirrhotic patients and should be considered in the differential diagnosis. Regenerative nodules are seen as discrete nodules by intraoperative ultrasound. Often small and hypoechoic, they can be mistaken for hepatocellular carcinomas (Fig. 86.58). Distinguishing regenerative nodules from hepatocellular carcinoma based on intraoperative ultrasound characteristics alone is difficult (Kanematsu et al, 1999). Likewise, hemangiomata (see Ch. 70) can be mistaken for hepatocellular carcinoma (Caturelli et al, 2001). The most reliable findings that suggest hepatocellular carcinoma are signs of a mass effect with effacement or invasion of surrounding intrahepatic structures and a thin hypoechoic halo surrounding the lesion. These findings are often absent, making a definitive diagnosis difficult. In these situations, core needle biopsy is necessary to establish the diagnosis.

Cystic and solid liver masses can have varying and overlapping appearances when viewed by intraoperative ultrasound. A broad differential diagnosis for a discovered lesion must be kept in mind. When the discovered lesion is placed into the current clinical context for the particular patient, the differential diagnosis can be narrowed considerably. Using intraoperative ultrasound to define these lesions provides an excellent depiction of the liver mass. Clues to help differentiate a malignant tumor from a benign one include the following:

1. The presence of effacement or invasion of intrahepatic structures. This finding is highly suggestive of a malignant lesion.

Table 86.7 Characteristic Ultrasound Features of Liver Tumors

Tumor Type	Shape	Boundary	Internal Echoes	Marginal Hypoechoic Zone	Posterior Echoes	Lateral Shadow
Metastatic carcinoma or cholangiocarcinoma	Cauliflower-like	Coarsely irregular	Vary	Present; thick	Attenuated or even	Absent
Metastatic sarcoma or carcinoid	Round	Sharp and smooth	Vary	Absent	Even or enhanced	Absent
Hepatocellular carcinoma	Round	Sharp and smooth	Vary; mosaic pattern	Present; thin	Enhanced	Occasionally present
Hemangioma	Round	Finely irregular	Echogenic or mixed	Absent	Even or enhanced	Absent

From Adams RB, 2005: Intraoperative ultrasound of the liver. In Machi J, Staren ED (eds): Ultrasound for Surgeons. Philadelphia, Lippincott Williams & Wilkins, pp 315-359.

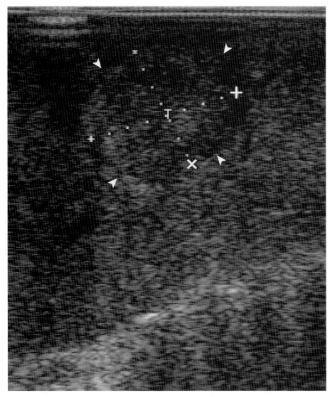

Fig. 86.49. Hypoechoic halo *(arrowheads)* around tumors (T) is characteristic of malignant lesions. These also are called bull's eye or target lesions.

If present, this finding is important in determining resectability of a tumor and selecting the type of resection necessary (Figs. 86.59 and 86.60).

2. The presence of a hypoechoic ring (target or bull's eye lesion) around the mass. This finding is highly correlated with malignancy, particularly if the patient has a primary extrahepatic malignancy or in the presence of cirrhosis. Although this finding is commonly described in the literature as being correlated with malignancy, its sensitivity and specificity are not well studied (Marchal et al, 1985b; Wernecke et al, 1992).

3. The presence of multiple tumors in the setting of a known extrahepatic malignancy. This finding suggests metastatic disease.

4. The presence of a well-circumscribed, hyperechoic lesion less than 2 to 3 cm in diameter. This lesion suggests a hemangioma (Fig. 86.61).

Finally, when the imaging characteristics are such that the diagnosis of a hepatic mass lesion is uncertain, fine-needle or core needle biopsy is necessary. Intraoperative ultrasound can precisely guide the biopsy procedure.

Because intraoperative ultrasound is the most sensitive method to detect and characterize hepatic lesions, it can uncover numerous findings not evident from preoperative imaging, potentially altering the surgical approach. In patients with primary extrahepatic malignancies, the discovery of occult metastases may modify the surgical approach or preclude it altogether. If an occult lesion appears different from the known metastasis, its diagnosis should be confirmed by biopsy if the lesion will be left in the liver remnant after resection. As previously noted, in patients with cirrhosis, intraoperative ultrasound is crucial in examining the liver for occult lesions because only 50% of lesions less than 5 cm can be identified by palpation. Liver biopsy is essential for determining whether occult lesions in the cirrhotic liver are malignant. Intraoperative ultrasound–guided biopsy can be done safely, precisely, and with a high degree of accuracy (Kokudo et al, 1996). Similarly, intraoperative ultrasound is more sensitive in detecting satellite nodules associated with hepatocellular carcinoma and any associated vascular invasion or thrombosis (Makuuchi et al, 1991).

The planned surgical approach to a lesion may be altered after mapping in relationship to surrounding intrahepatic structures. Intraoperative ultrasound allows superb detail and spatial mapping compared with other imaging techniques. Demonstration of an adequate dissection plane between a portal

Fig. 86.50. Vessel displacement *(arrows)* by metastatic tumor (T). Vessel is denoted by *asterisk*. *Arrowheads* indicate tumor boundaries.

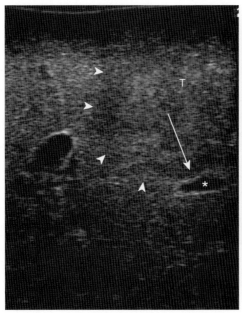
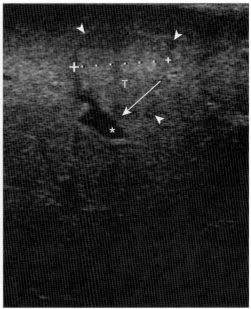

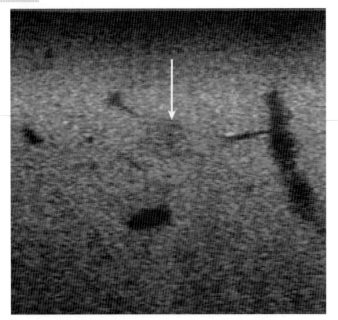

Fig. 86.51. Small occult colon metastasis *(arrow)* measuring 9 mm. Small lesions often are hypoechoic and lack the surrounding tumor halo.

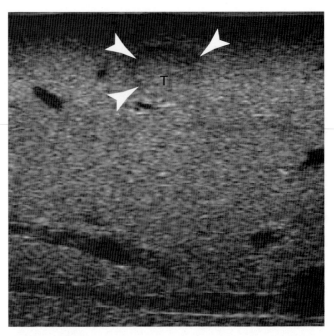

Fig. 86.52. Small occult carcinoid metastatic tumor (T) measuring 11 mm with a hypoechoic tumor halo *(arrowheads)*.

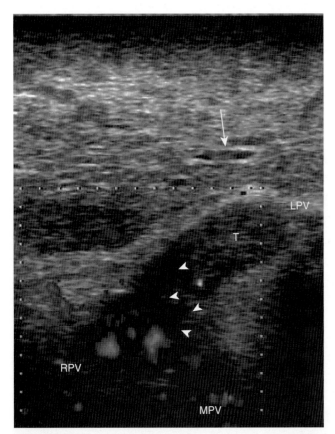

Fig. 86.53. Tumor invasion with thrombosis of the main left portal vein. *Arrowheads* denote the edge of the tumor thrombus (T) in the left portal vein. *Arrow* indicates a small vein with echogenic tumor thrombus within it. The main portal vein (MPV) and right portal vein (RPV) have flow by color Doppler imaging.

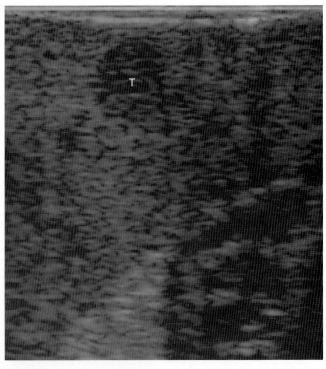

Fig. 86.54. Small hepatocellular carcinoma (T) exhibiting hypoechoic features.

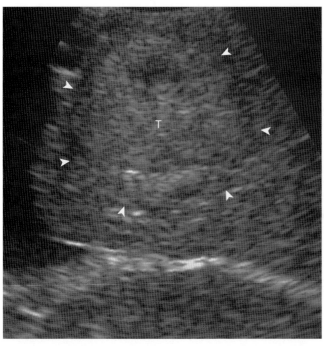

Fig. 86.55. Hepatocellular carcinoma (T) with increased echogenic features, including a variegated or mosaic pattern with a hypoechoic halo *(arrowheads)*.

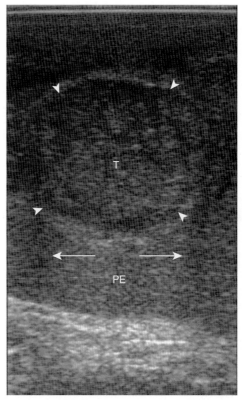

Fig. 86.56. Large hepatocellular carcinoma (T) with specific features, including hypoechoic halo *(arrowheads)*, posterior enhancement (PE), and lateral shadowing *(arrows)*.

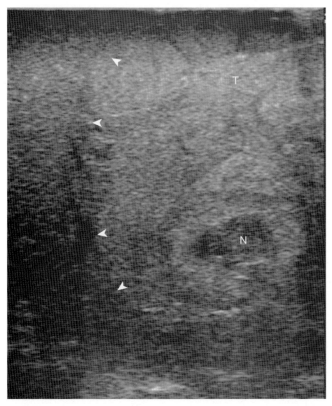

Fig. 86.57. Large hepatocellular carcinoma (T) with hyperechoic, heterogeneous features, including an area of tumor necrosis (N). *Arrowheads* note tumor edges.

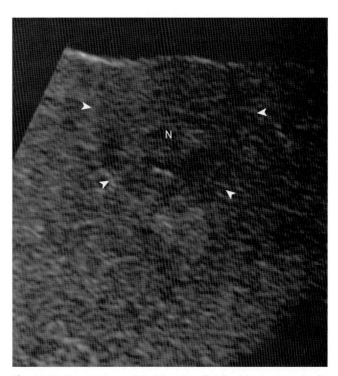

Fig. 86.58. Regenerative nodule (N) with well-defined border *(arrowheads)*. These nodules often appear as a small hypoechoic mass and can mimic small hepatocellular carcinomas. Intraoperative biopsy is required to make a diagnosis.

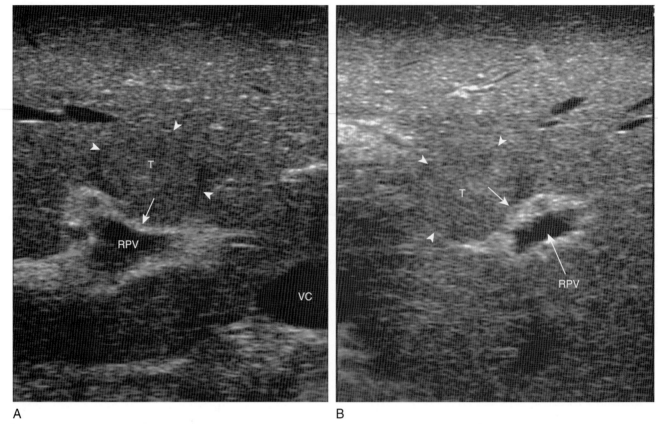

A   B

Fig. 86.59. Colon metastasis (T) abutting the right portal pedicle (RPV). Transverse **(A)** and longitudinal **(B)** views of the tumor (*arrowheads* define tumor border). Intraoperative ultrasound is the optimal imaging modality to define this relationship. VC, vena cava.

pedicle or hepatic vein and the lesion may allow a parenchymal sparing resection. Conversely, if no clear margin is present, if satellite lesions are evident in the portal segment, or if vascular invasion is present, an alternative approach, such as a segmental or lobar resection, can be planned. Intraoperative ultrasound has utility in planning and altering the surgical strategy based on findings evident only on this type of examination. Although difficult to define, reports suggest that 30% of planned procedures are altered by intraoperative ultrasound findings (Carter et al, 1996; Castaing et al, 1986; Gozzetti et al, 1986; Luck & Maddern, 1999; Machi & Sigel, 1996; Machi et al, 1993; Parker et al, 1989; Salminen et al, 1990; Staren et al, 1997).

ULTRASOUND GUIDANCE FOR HEPATIC INTERVENTIONS

Intraoperative ultrasound has become indispensable for image-guided procedures during hepatic surgery. Detection of small or deep lesions is facilitated by intraoperative ultrasound, whether the liver is normal or cirrhotic. Additionally, intraoperative ultrasound improves the accuracy of needle placement for biopsy or treatment, probe positioning for ablation therapies, and image guidance for tissue dissection and hepatectomies (Table 86.9). Its use to determine the transection plane during hepatectomy results in greater negative resection margins compared with procedures not using intraoperative ultrasound (Lau et al, 1993).

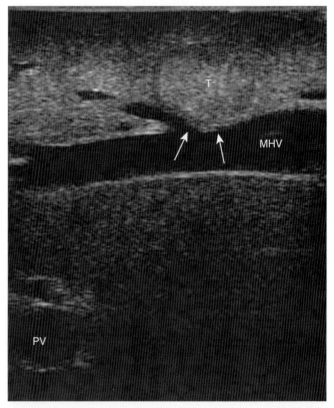

Fig. 86.60. Colon metastatic tumor (T) impinging (*arrows*) on the middle hepatic vein (MHV). Intraoperative ultrasound shows this relationship and confirms the necessity of resection including this portion of the MHV. PV, portal vein.

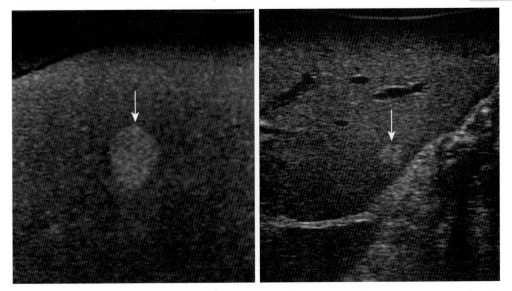

Fig. 86.61. Hemangiomata *(arrows).* Typical appearance by intraoperative ultrasound includes a well-circumscribed, round lesion that is hyperechoic and less than 2 to 3 cm in diameter.

Needle Guidance and Probe Placement Using Intraoperative Ultrasound

Precise guidance of a needle or probe into a liver lesion or a vessel is best accomplished by intraoperative ultrasound. Although a needle guidance system that attaches to the ultrasound probe (Fig. 86.62) can be used, the freehand technique is more versatile. The guidance system is easier to learn and use because it fixes the needle into a position that keeps it in the scanning plane, allowing precise guidance of the needle into the target. The guidance system is bulky, however, limiting its utility in tight working spaces or in situations in which the needle needs to be placed remotely. The alternative is the freehand technique (Fig. 86.63). The freehand technique, although more difficult to master, is ultimately more versatile than the guidance system. A key to becoming skilled at the freehand technique is identifying and maintaining the needle in the scanning plane; this is best done by placing the needle into the tissue directly beneath and parallel to the long axis of the transducer (Fig. 86.64). As the needle advances under the transducer, it appears as a fine hyperechoic line, typically with posterior shadowing or reverberation artifacts (Figs. 86.65 and 86.66). Visibility of the needle can be increased by scratching it with a knife blade or twisting it within the lightly closed jaws of a needle holder. The roughened surface of the needle is more echogenic and more easily seen. While the operator initially is learning biopsy techniques, the needle guidance system is helpful. When the operator is experienced, the freehand technique can be used in all situations.

Needle guidance to diagnose hepatic lesions discovered at the time of surgery is an important use of intraoperative ultrasound. Fluid sampling or therapeutic drainage of cystic lesions or abscesses is readily accomplished under ultrasound guidance. Needle biopsy, either fine-needle aspiration or core biopsy, is the most common use of intraoperative ultrasound, particularly for newly discovered lesions that are not palpable. A core biopsy is appropriate for most solid lesions because histology is typically necessary to distinguish between the many potential hepatic lesions. If the issue is simply the presence of malignant cells (e.g., is it a metastatic lesion?), however, fine-needle aspiration is sufficient. An important distinction when doing a core biopsy

compared with fine-needle aspiration is needle excursion. During fine-needle aspiration, there is no needle excursion; the tip of the needle seen under intraoperative ultrasound is the site of the biopsy. This is not the case during core needle biopsy. The final biopsy site is approximately 1.5 to 2.5 cm distal to the initial location of the core needle tip. Needle excursion must be taken into account during core needle biopsy; ultrasound guidance ensures the needle is positioned the appropriate distance away from the lesion before biopsy (see Fig. 86.65A), and that the needle is within the lesion after needle excursion (see Fig. 86.65B). After biopsy, intraoperative ultrasound can show a hyperechoic needle tract. If this is within the lesion, it confirms accurate targeting of the lesion (see Fig. 86.65C). Finally, intraoperative ultrasound facilitates needle cannulation of intrahepatic or extrahepatic bile ducts for intraoperative cholangiography. Similarly, intraoperative ultrasound guidance allows placement of transhepatic catheters into the intrahepatic biliary system for biliary drainage.

Numerous treatments for hepatic malignancies not involving resection require accurate needle or probe placement. Intraoperative ultrasound guidance is ideal for all of these modalities.

Table 86.9 Utility of Intraoperative Ultrasound for Hepatic Procedures

Needle guidance and placement
   Mass or liver biopsy
   Cyst or cavity aspiration
   Ethanol injection for tumor ablation
   Biliary cannulation (cholangiography or drainage)

Ablation probe placement
   Cryoablation or thermal ablation

Resection guidance
   Margin measurement and marking
   Maintain margin during liver transection

Techniques for segmental resections
   Defining segmental anatomy
   Marking segmental inflow
   Systematic subsegmentectomy

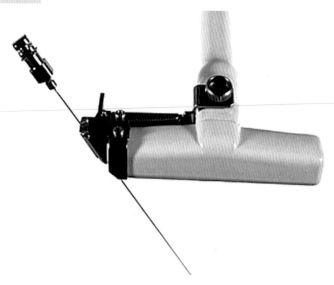

Fig. 86.62. Needle guidance system for intraoperative ultrasound probe. (From Adams RB, 2005: Intraoperative ultrasound of the liver. In Machi J, Staren ED [eds]: Ultrasound for Surgeons. Philadelphia, Lippincott Williams & Wilkins, pp 315-359.)

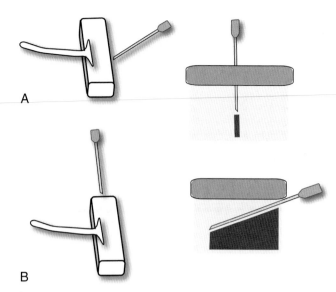

Fig. 86.64. Needle placement under intraoperative ultrasound guidance. Top view on the *left*, and view beneath the probe on the *right*. **A,** Needle placement perpendicular to the crystal array results in a small needle profile seen in the scanning plane. It is difficult to see the needle in this position. **B,** Proper needle placement is parallel to the crystal array, giving a long and easily seen needle image beneath the ultrasound probe.
(Original art by RB Adams)

A common and simple therapy is ethanol ablation of hepatocellular carcinomas (see Ch. 76a) (Huang et al, 2004; Livraghi, 1992; Mazzanti et al, 2004). Although most ethanol ablation is done percutaneously, newly discovered lesions at the time of laparoscopy or laparotomy that are not amenable to resection are candidates for intraoperative ultrasound–guided ethanol ablation. In addition to accurate needle placement, intraoperative ultrasound allows real-time monitoring to ensure complete ethanol dispersion throughout the lesion. This monitoring facilitates decision making when determining the necessity of additional treatments.

Cryoablation relies on accurate probe placement for satisfactory tumor ablation and to monitor its completeness (see Ch. 76b) (Onik et al, 1991). Single or multiple probes can be introduced precisely into the lesion by intraoperative ultrasound (Gaitini et al, 2001). As tissue freezing begins, an ablation zone develops. This zone is apparent as a hyperechoic leading edge, which is monitored in real time by intraoperative ultrasound as it advances into the normal liver parenchyma. The area within the "ice ball" is hypoechoic or anechoic. It is accompanied by posterior shadowing, preventing structures within the ablation zone from being seen. The sharp transition zone seen on intraoperative

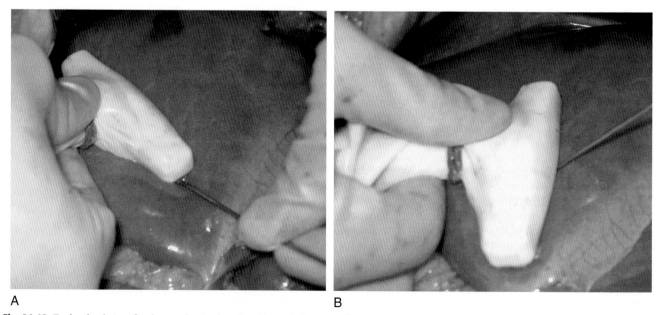

Fig. 86.63. Freehand technique for ultrasound-assisted needle guidance. **A,** Proper needle orientation, parallel to the transducer crystal. **B,** Improper needle orientation, perpendicular to the transducer crystal. This orientation makes it difficult to locate the needle by ultrasound.

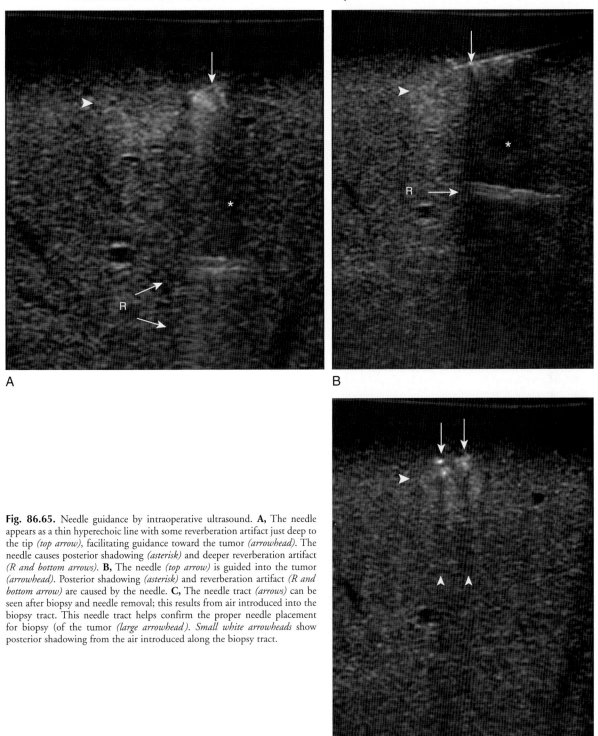

A

B

C

Fig. 86.65. Needle guidance by intraoperative ultrasound. **A,** The needle appears as a thin hyperechoic line with some reverberation artifact just deep to the tip *(top arrow),* facilitating guidance toward the tumor *(arrowhead).* The needle causes posterior shadowing *(asterisk)* and deeper reverberation artifact *(R and bottom arrows).* **B,** The needle *(top arrow)* is guided into the tumor *(arrowhead).* Posterior shadowing *(asterisk)* and reverberation artifact *(R and bottom arrow)* are caused by the needle. **C,** The needle tract *(arrows)* can be seen after biopsy and needle removal; this results from air introduced into the biopsy tract. This needle tract helps confirm the proper needle placement for biopsy (of the tumor *(large arrowhead). Small white arrowheads* show posterior shadowing from the air introduced along the biopsy tract.

ultrasound between the ice ball and normal liver allows precise delineation of the ablation zone. Observation under intraoperative ultrasound of the lesion as it disappears into the ablation zone ensures that the zone adequately covers the target.

Thermal ablation is the most recently developed technique for treating unresectable liver tumors (see Ch. 76c). Intraoperative ultrasound is essential for its successful use, including probe placement and ablation monitoring (Machi et al, 2001, 2002).

Similar to the cryotherapy probe, the thermal probe is guided into the lesion using intraoperative ultrasound. With real-time intraoperative ultrasound, the multiple retractable tines of the probe are deployed to ensure accurate placement within the lesion (Fig. 86.67). Accurate probe placement before the beginning of ablation is crucial. After ablation begins, the field of vision is obscured, and the lesion no longer remains visible (Fig. 86.68). This difficulty arises during ablation because the treatment site

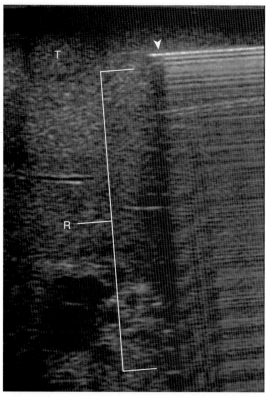

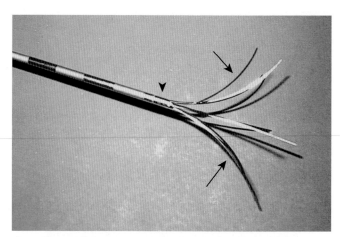

Fig. 86.67. Radiofrequency ablation probe *(arrowhead)* with retractable tines deployed *(arrows)*.

Fig. 86.66. Reverberation artifact. Needle *(arrowhead)* placement into a tumor (T) often is accompanied by reverberation artifact (R). This artifact facilitates needle identification for image-guided needle placement.

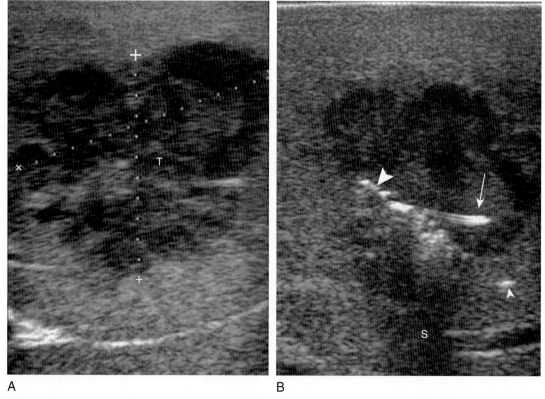

A   B

Fig. 86.68. Radiofrequency probe placement by intraoperative ultrasound guidance. **A,** Hypoechoic hepatocellular carcinoma (T). Tumor margins noted by caliper marks. **B,** Intraoperative ultrasound was used to guide the radiofrequency probe *(large arrowhead)* into the tumor. The tines *(arrow)* were deployed under ultrasound guidance to ensure the entire tumor was encompassed by the ablation zone. *Large arrowhead* and *arrow* correspond to those in Figure 86.67. Accurate initial probe placement is crucial because the tumor becomes obscured by the needle and subsequent ablation. During and after ablation, posterior shadowing (S) and tissue gas *(small arrowhead)* formation mask the tumor and tissue deep to the ablation site.

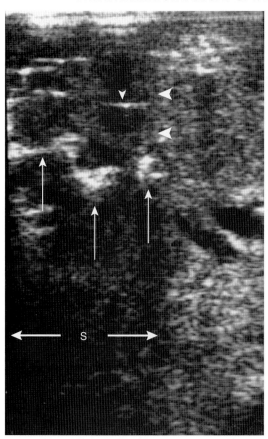

is obliterated by diffuse, irregular, hyperechoic changes resulting from tissue gas formation. The acoustic interface between the gas and tissue causes hyperreflective changes that obscure the lesion (Fig. 86.69). Because these tissue changes are diffuse, the ablation zone is not sharply demarcated similar to that seen during cryotherapy. The precise ablation margins are difficult to discern. After completion of ablation, the zone remains hyperechoic with posterior shadowing for 10 to 20 minutes, with slow resolution after that period, obscuring tissue deep to the ablation zone for a prolonged period. These technical challenges are the reason that accurate probe placement is imperative before the initiation of the ablation (Leyendecker et al, 2002). Monitoring during ablation may be improved by the use of contrast-enhanced ultrasound techniques (Solbiati et al, 2004).

Resection Techniques Using Intraoperative Ultrasound

Intraoperative ultrasound is an indispensable aid during hepatic resection (see Chs. 80, 82, and 83). It is used to identify deep lesions and plan the appropriate resection. A combination of intraoperative ultrasound and palpation allows lesion identification and resection planning (Fig. 86.70). Another simple use is to identify and mark a resection margin around the lesion of interest. The margin distance from the lesion can be measured precisely by intraoperative ultrasound and marked on the liver surface with electrocautery. The scored capsule appears as a hypoechoic linear shadow perpendicular to the ultrasound probe when viewed by intraoperative ultrasound, allowing verification of the surgical margin's position and width from the lesion before parenchymal transection (Fig. 86.71). Similarly, the hepatic veins and portal triads can be identified by intraoperative ultrasound and marked on the liver surface to guide the dissection (Fig. 86.72). As the hepatic parenchyma is divided,

Fig. 86.69. Tissue changes after radiofrequency ablation. The edge of the ablation zone can be seen laterally *(large black arrowheads)*. The probe tine is seen within the ablation zone *(small white arrowhead)*. Tissue within and posterior to the ablation zone is obscured by the hyperreflective changes *(arrows)* and posterior shadowing (S) resulting from the ablation. In contrast to cryoablation, the thermal ablation margins are not well defined.

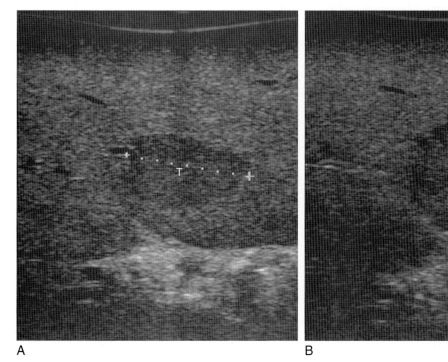

A   B

Fig. 86.70. Intraoperative ultrasound and palpation are complementary techniques. **A,** A 26-mm tumor (T) is identified by intraoperative ultrasound. **B,** Palpation under intraoperative ultrasound guidance facilitates tumor identification and treatment planning. F, surgeon's finger.

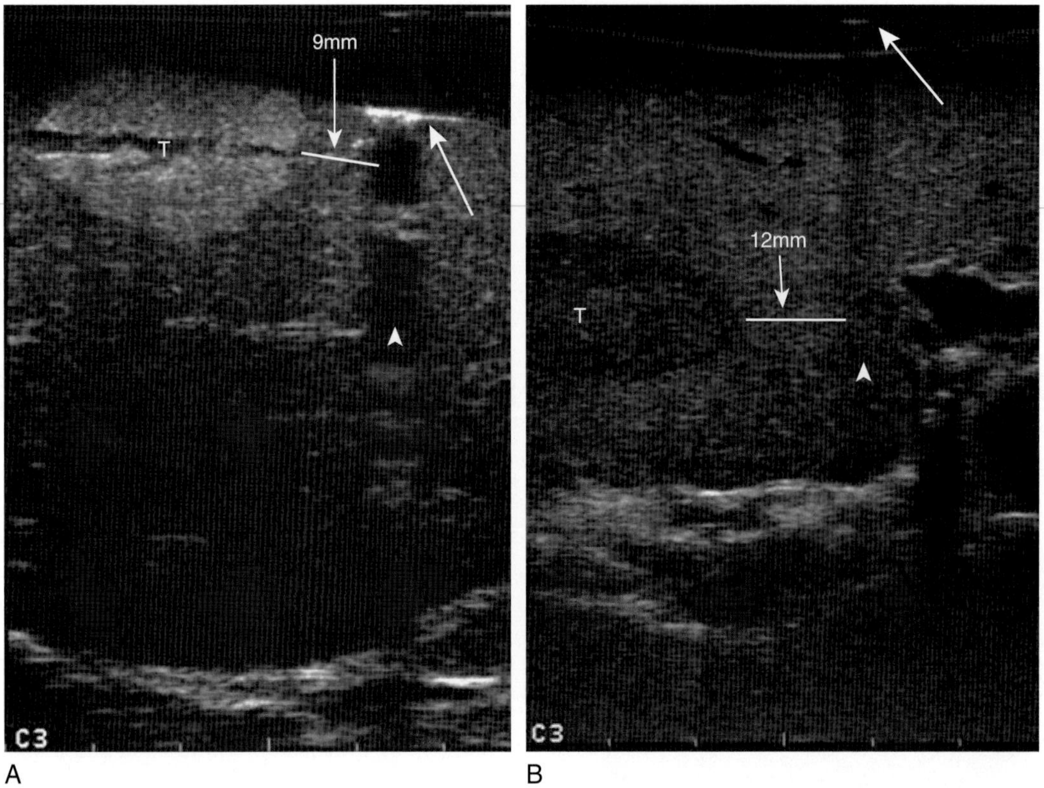

Fig. 86.71. Intraoperative ultrasound–guided liver resection. **A** and **B,** The liver capsule is scored *(arrow)* with electrocautery while using ultrasound guidance to determine accurately the resection margin from the tumor (T). The scored capsule appears as a hypoechoic linear shadow beneath the scored site *(arrowhead).*

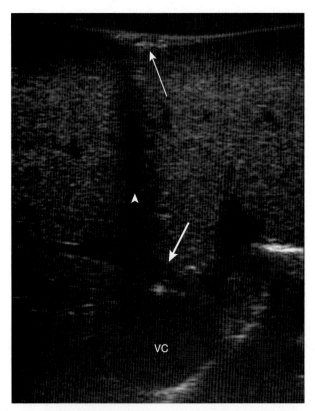

Fig. 86.72. Intraoperative ultrasound–guided identification and marking of intrahepatic structures. The position of the middle hepatic vein *(thick arrow)* is identified as it joins the vena cava (VC). The liver capsule is scored *(thin arrow)* over this site, resulting in a hypoechoic linear shadow *(arrowhead).* In this fashion, intraoperative ultrasound can be used to guide the resection plane.

the resection margin can be monitored during the dissection by repeated scans with intraoperative ultrasound. The dissection plane is visualized as a hyperechoic line, which results from the air introduced into the dissection plane. Echogenic material, such as a sponge or instrument, can be placed in the resection plane to accentuate the transection margin and confirm the relationship to the tumor. Used in this fashion, intraoperative ultrasound guides the direction of the incision and verifies its position in relationship to the lesion and the surrounding intrahepatic structures (Fig. 86.73). Using intraoperative ultrasound to monitor the transection plane intermittently allows corrections in the direction or depth of the incision if needed.

The development of liver resection based on its segmental anatomy became a reality with the availability of intraoperative ultrasound. Many elegant hepatic resection techniques were developed taking advantage of this technology. These surgical approaches were driven by the desire to spare hepatic parenchyma, particularly in patients with limited hepatic reserve. In addition, precise pedicle identification allowed control of the segmental blood supply, diminishing blood loss during resection. Finally, intraoperative ultrasound allowed identification and resection of the portal territory of hepatocellular carcinoma, allowing complete resection of local portal metastases. Most of these techniques originally were applicable for patients with hepatocellular carcinoma and concomitant fibrosis or cirrhosis. More recently, these techniques have gained acceptance in a variety of situations that do not involve cirrhosis or hepatocellular carcinoma (Torzilli & Makuuchi, 2003). Two primary techniques have been developed, each with the similar end result of identifying a specific anatomic distribution within the liver. One technique, called *systematic subsegmentectomy,* employs intraoperative

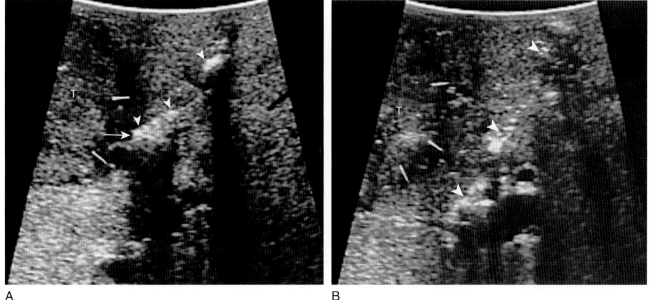

Fig. 86.73. Correction of dissection direction by intraoperative ultrasound guidance. **A,** During resection of a tumor (T), intraoperative ultrasound was used repeatedly to guide the transection plane *(thick arrowheads)*. This image shows the plane *(arrow)* heading toward the tumor *(thin white lines)*. **B,** The direction of dissection was changed and rechecked by intraoperative ultrasound. This image shows the new dissection plane *(thick arrowheads)* heading away from the tumor margin *(thin arrowheads)*.
(From Adams RB, 2005: Intraoperative ultrasound of the liver. In Machi J, Staren ED [eds]: Ultrasound for Surgeons. Philadelphia, Lippincott Williams & Wilkins, pp 315-359.)

ultrasound to guide a staining or tattooing technique to mark the segmental anatomy (Fig. 86.74) (Makuuchi et al, 1985, 1991). The second technique uses balloon catheter occlusion of the segmental portal vein to identify the segment for resection (Fig. 86.75) (Castaing et al, 1989; Igawa et al, 1985; Shimamura et al, 1986).

In systematic subsegmentectomy, intraoperative ultrasound is used to guide a needle into the portal vein supplying the area of the tumor (Makuuchi et al, 1985, 1991). Several milliliters

(typically 5 mL is sufficient to stain a segment) of dye (methylene blue or indigo carmine) are injected (Fig. 86.76). Portal vein cannulation is done just distal to the origin of the segmental portal vein of interest, to avoid reflux of dye into adjacent segmental branches. The hepatic parenchyma supplied by this portal pedicle is stained by the dye, and the surface of the liver is marked, defining the area for resection. Electrocautery is used to score the interface of the stained liver and its junction with the unstained liver. Electrocautery must be done fairly quickly

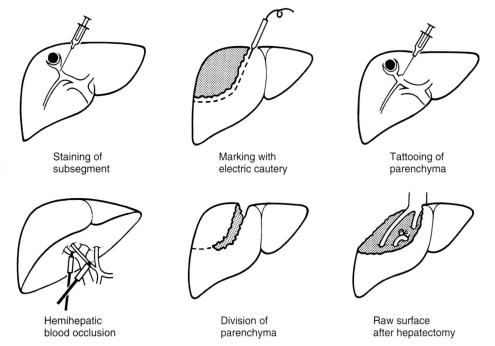

Fig. 86.74. Systematic subsegmentectomy. Operative steps for completion of subsegmentectomy.
(Courtesy of Dr. Masatoshi Makuuchi.)

Staining of subsegment

Marking with electric cautery

Tattooing of parenchyma

Hemihepatic blood occlusion

Division of parenchyma

Raw surface after hepatectomy

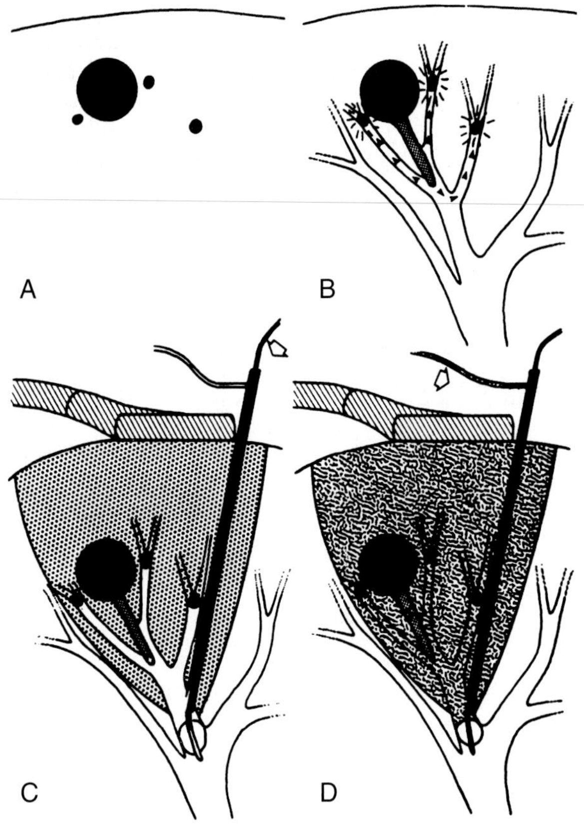

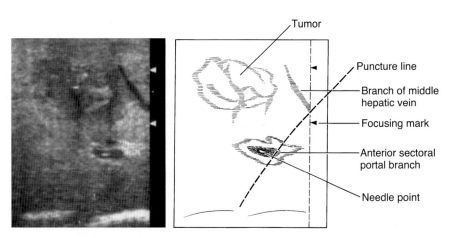

Fig. 86.75. Rationale for segmental resection in hepatocellular carcinoma and technique of balloon occlusion of a portal vein branch. **A,** Classic appearance of a primary liver cancer surrounded by satellite nodules. **B,** Pathogenesis of satellite nodules and mode of spread of the primary tumor. Intrahepatic dissemination occurs by invasion of the tributary portal branches and tumor emboli seeding into neighboring branches in the same segment. **C,** With ultrasound guidance, the portal branch proximal to the tumor is entered retrogradely and occluded with a balloon catheter. Alternatively, a portal branch in a neighboring segment can be entered and the catheter threaded antegradely into the portal branch to be resected (e.g., segment V for a tumor in segment VIII). **D,** The territory at risk for intrahepatic metastasis can be marked with dye to mark the planned resection. Keeping the balloon inflated (i.e., with a tie on the piston of the Fogarty syringe) and occluding the corresponding branch of the hepatic artery considerably decreases bleeding during the resection. The remaining segments are perfused by the portal vein on the ipsilateral side and by the portal vein and the hepatic artery on the contralateral side.
(Courtesy of Dr. Henri Bismuth.)

because staining can fade after injection. In patients with cirrhosis, slower portal flow may result in less effective staining. Staining may be improved by clamping the portal pedicle followed by injection of the segmental portal vein. Alternatively, a similar technique has been developed that counterstains the parenchyma around the segment of interest to define the resection margins (Takayama et al, 1991). Likewise, intraoperative ultrasound can be used to identify and mark the portal triad, within the hepatic parenchyma, to identify its site of ligation at the time of tissue dissection. The ligation site is tattooed by injecting blue dye into the liver parenchyma just anterior to the vessels, guiding needle placement to the tattoo site by intraoperative ultrasound (Makuuchi et al, 1981a). As the parenchymal dissection proceeds, this ligation site can be identified by the blue staining. Intraparenchymal tattooing also can be used to mark a hepatic vein to be preserved along the resection margin (Takayama et al, 1994). If portal vein embolization of the area of interest has been done preoperatively, direct staining of this portal distribution is not feasible. In these cases, the counterstaining method can be used (Takayama et al, 1991). Through a combination of staining techniques, segmental and subsegmental anatomy can be defined to allow precise resections.

The balloon occlusion technique is similar to staining, allowing identification of the area supplied by a specific portal pedicle (see Fig. 86.75). This technique relies on ischemic changes on the liver surface to demarcate the segmental area of interest. As originally described and used by others, a balloon catheter is used to occlude the portal vein to the area of interest (Castaing et al, 1989; Igawa et al, 1985; Shimamura et al, 1986). This catheter is coupled with occlusion of the hepatic artery supplying the ipsilateral hemiliver. The resulting ischemic demarcation on the liver surface can be marked with electrocautery. This zone of demarcation defines the resection margin. An advantage of this technique is the presumed decreased blood loss because of ischemia in the resection area. Proper placement of the occlusion balloon is important to allow pedicle ligation distal to the occlusion site, avoiding the balloon catheter. Similar to staining, segmental ischemic changes can be used to define the resection margins for segmental or subsegmental hepatic resections.

Other techniques have been described that use intraoperative ultrasound to assist in defining resection margins. Needles or small plastic cannulae can be inserted along the border of the resection margins under intraoperative ultrasound guidance (Izumi et al, 1993). The authors reported that a clear resection margin

Fig. 86.76. Puncture of portal vein branch to the anterior sector in a patient with hepatocellular carcinoma in segment V. The *white spot* in the lumen of the vessel is the tip of a standard lumbar puncture needle. The echogenicity of the needle tip is increased by scratching it within the bites of a needle holder by a gentle twisting movement. The superficial setting of the focusing (*triangular arrows*) allows one to follow the needle tip from its entry in the liver, and the deviation from the puncture marks (*small white dots*) sometimes is experienced when puncturing the hard cirrhotic liver.
(Courtesy of Dr. Henri Bismuth.)

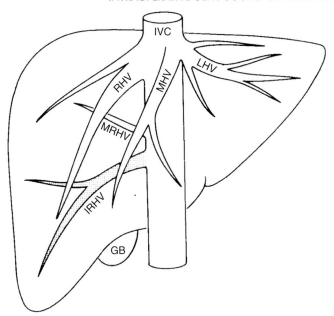

Fig. 86.77. Inferior right hepatic vein (IRHV) in relationship to the inferior vena cava (IVC), right hepatic vein (RHV), marginal right hepatic vein (MRHV), and middle hepatic vein (MHV). GB, gallbladder; LHV, left hepatic vein.
(From Makuuchi M, et al, 1983c: The inferior right hepatic vein: ultrasonic demonstration. Radiology 148:213-217.)

can be defined in this manner, eliminating repeated ultrasound imaging during the dissection and saving time. Another more recent technique involves a "hooking" method using intraoperative ultrasound to define the intrahepatic structures of interest (Torzilli et al, 1999). In this manner, precise intrahepatic ligation sites can be identified for individual portal pedicles. Finally, intraoperative ultrasound–guided finger compression has been described to assist segmental anatomy delineation (Torzilli & Makuuchi, 2004).

An inferior right hepatic vein (draining vein of segment VI) is a common variant of hepatic vein anatomy. It is reportedly present in approximately 20% of patients (Figs. 86.77 and 86.78)

(Nakamura & Tsuzuki, 1981). Identification and mapping of this structure by intraoperative ultrasound allow the successful performance of many specific hepatectomies that rely on this structure for venous drainage. Four procedures have been described that allow resection of the right hepatic vein and preservation of the inferior right hepatic vein (e.g., segment VII/VIII resection while preserving segment VI in situ) (Fig. 86.79) (Baer et al, 1991; Makuuchi et al, 1987a).

Intraoperative Ultrasound Use in Systematic Subsegmentectomy

Using intraoperative ultrasound–guided techniques, each Couinaud's segment, or a portion thereof, can be anatomically resected. Several examples outlining the technique for segmental resection (see Chs. 80 and 83) are described here.

Segment VIII Resection

The right lobe is fully mobilized, and the right hepatic vein is exposed. Segment VIII is supplied by two main portal vein branches, dorsal and ventral, in about 90% of patients. The ventral branch typically arises from a shared pedicle with one to three branches of segment V in approximately 60% of patients. Initially, the dorsal branch is cannulated with intraoperative ultrasound guidance and injected with several milliliters of indigo carmine. The area stained by this dorsal injection is marked on the liver capsule with electrocautery. Next, the ventral branch is cannulated and treated in a similar manner. The margins of segment VIII can be identified using this intraoperative ultrasound–guided approach. If a single portal pedicle supplies all of segment VIII, it is cannulated, and the margins are marked with electrocautery. The dissection begins by hemihepatic occlusion of the left hepatic artery and portal vein. This occlusion demarcates the liver parenchyma of the left margin of the resection, between segments IV and VIII, allowing parenchymal division at this site. This dissection exposes the distal two thirds of the middle hepatic vein. When defined, the left vessels are unclamped. Next, the right hepatic artery and

Fig. 86.78. Inferior right hepatic vein (IRHV). The IRHV *(thin white arrow)* typically enters the vena cava (VC) in an anterolateral position. **A,** The IRHV typically can be identified entering the VC at a level posterior to the right portal vein triad (RPV). **B,** Tumor *(arrowheads)* invading the liver parenchyma and an IRHV *(thin white arrow)*. *Thick black arrows* show branches of the middle hepatic vein.

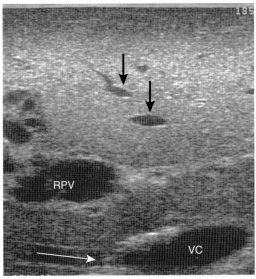

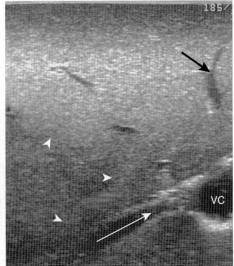

A

B

portal vein are occluded, and the parenchyma along the inferior (caudal) border of segment VIII (between segments V and VIII) is divided down to the investing connective tissue of the anterior surface of the portal pedicle. Intraoperative ultrasound–guided tattooing of this area can be used as needed. With exposure of the portal pedicle, the ventral and dorsal branches are identified and ligated; this occludes the inflow to segment VIII. Along the right resection margin, the right hepatic vein is exposed from caudal to cranial, up to its confluence with the inferior vena cava. The remaining posterior parenchyma is divided completing the segmental resection. During the parenchymal dissection, the middle and right hepatic veins and the anterior portal vein branches are located using intraoperative ultrasound to guide the direction of the dissection.

Segment V Resection

Because segment V frequently has three to five portal vein branches, it is difficult to puncture all of these. The "counterstaining" technique can be employed for the resection of this segment. Staining of the segment VIII ventral branch and the segment VI branch defines the cranial and right borders of segment V.

The left margin is identified by the ischemic changes seen with the hemihepatic occlusion technique of the left lobe vasculature. Resection is begun along the left border ischemic zone, exposing the right branch of the middle hepatic vein. This branch is divided, and the left vessels are unclamped. Dissection along the superior (cranial) border is done along the line defined by staining segment VIII. Dissection along this plane exposes the portal pedicle branches of segment V. Working ventrally to dorsally, these are divided until the primary anterior pedicle of the right lobe is identified. These branches are individually ligated, occluding the inflow to segment V. Division of the right lateral margin completes the resection of segment V.

Other Resections

Similar techniques allow anatomic resections of segments VI or VII to be accomplished. The left medial segment (segment IV) and the left lateral inferior and superior areas (segments II and III) can be resected by conventional hepatectomy procedures. Intraoperative ultrasound–guided systematic subsegmentectomy is possible, however, when the superior or inferior part of segments IV, II, or III or another smaller area requires resection.

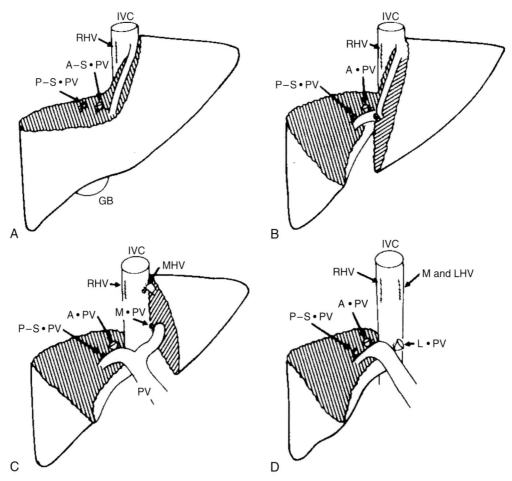

Fig. 86.79. Four types of hepatectomies based on preservation of the inferior right hepatic vein. **A,** Resection of the right anterosuperior (A-S • PV; segment VIII) and posterior-superior (P-S • PV; segment VII) segments. **B,** Resection of the right anterior sector (A • PV; segments V and VIII) and the right posterior-superior segment (P-S • PV; segment VII). **C,** Resection of the left medial (M • PV; segment IV) and right anterior sector (A • PV; segments V and VIII) and the right posterior-superior segment (P-S • PV; segment VII), an extended central bisegmentectomy. **D,** Resection of the left lobe (L • PV; segments I-IV), right anterior section (A • PV; segments V and VIII), and right posterior-superior segment (P-S • PV, segment VII), an extended left trisegmentectomy. GB, gallbladder; IVC, inferior vena cava; LHV, left hepatic vein; MHV, middle hepatic vein; RHV, right hepatic vein.
(From Makuuchi M, et al, 1987a: Four new hepatectomy procedures for resection of the right hepatic vein and preservation of the inferior right hepatic vein. Surg Gynecol Obstet 164:68-72.)

By combining these staining techniques, multisegmental resections can be achieved in a similar fashion to that described for single segments (e.g., segment V plus segment VI, segment V plus segment IVb). Although prospective studies of segmental resections compared with standard resections have not been done, many studies suggest this approach is reasonable, safe, and effective (Billingsley et al, 1998; Takayama & Makuuchi, 1996).

Intraoperative Ultrasound Use in Liver Transplantation

Intraoperative ultrasound has become crucial for the conduct of hepatectomies for living donor liver transplantation (see Ch. 109). Intraoperative ultrasound defines the intrahepatic vasculature of the segments for transplant, defines the direction of the resection plane, and guides the parenchymal transection throughout the procedure (Kasai et al, 1992). Aberrant hepatic venous and portal pedicle anatomy can be identified by intraoperative ultrasound and may alter the resection approach. In right liver donors, accessory right hepatic veins may be present, requiring separate anastomosis to prevent outflow obstruction and graft congestion (Gondolesi et al, 2002; Huang et al, 2001; Lo et al, 1997). For left liver donors with resection of segment IV, the left medial vein can be defined as it inserts into the left hepatic vein (common), the middle hepatic vein, or directly into the inferior vena cava. Intraoperative ultrasound allows its course to be mapped for inclusion in the donor resection (Kawasaki et al, 1996). Bile duct patency and the segmental course of the ducts have been mapped by intraoperative ultrasound (Harihara et al, 1997). Finally, spectral analysis of the Doppler waveform has been used after implantation of the donor liver to screen for and identify potential vascular problems, including inflow and outflow, which might impair graft function (Cheng et al, 1998; Fujimoto et al, 1997; Someda et al, 1995). As a result of its utility in predicting graft dysfunction, many institutions now use intraoperative ultrasound and Doppler studies to evaluate graft performance at the end of the recipient procedure.

REFERENCES

Adams RB, 2005: Intraoperative ultrasound of the liver. In Machi J, Staren ED (eds): Ultrasound for Surgeons. Philadelphia, Lippincott Williams & Wilkins, pp 315-359.

Anonymous, 2000: The Brisbane 2000 terminology of hepatic anatomy and resections. HPB Surg 2:333-339.

Aubin B, et al, 1995: Focal sparing of liver parenchyma in steatosis: role of the gallbladder and its vessels. J Ultrasound Med 14:77-80.

Baer HU, et al, 1991: Subtotal hepatectomy: a new procedure based on the inferior right hepatic vein. Br J Surg 78:1221-1222.

Billingsley KG, et al, 1998: Segment-oriented hepatic resection in the management of malignant neoplasms of the liver. J Am Coll Surg 187:471-481.

Bloed W, et al, 2000: Role of intraoperative ultrasound of the liver with improved preoperative hepatic imaging. Eur J Surg 166:691-695.

Boldrini G, et al, 1987: The systematic use of operative ultrasound for detection of liver metastases during colorectal surgery. World J Surg 11:622-627.

Boutkan H, et al, 1992: The impact of intraoperative ultrasonography of the liver on the surgical strategy of patients with gastrointestinal malignancies and hepatic metastases. Eur J Surg Oncol 18:342-346.

Brower ST, et al, 1989: Operative ultrasound establishes resectability of metastases by major hepatic resection. World J Surg 13:649-657.

Carter R, et al, 1996: A prospective study of six methods for detection of hepatic colorectal metastases. Ann R Coll Surg Engl 78:27-30.

Castaing D, et al, 1986: Utility of operative ultrasound in the surgical management of liver tumors. Ann Surg 204:600-605.

Castaing D, et al, 1989: Segmental liver resection using ultrasound-guided selective portal venous occlusion. Ann Surg 210:20-23.

Caturelli E, et al, 1992: Hypoechoic lesions in the "bright liver": a reliable indicator of fatty change: a prospective study. J Gastroenterol Hepatol 7:469-472.

Caturelli E, et al, 2001: Hemangioma-like lesions in chronic liver disease: diagnostic evaluation in patients. Radiology 220:337-342.

Cheng YF, et al, 1998: Intraoperative Doppler ultrasound in liver transplantation. Clin Transplant 12:292-299.

Choji K, et al, 1988: Significant reduction of the echogenicity of the compressed cavernous hemangioma. Acta Radiol 29:317-320.

Clarke MP, et al, 1989: Prospective comparison of preoperative imaging and intraoperative ultrasonography in the detection of liver tumors. Surgery 106:849-855.

Clouse ME, 1989: Current diagnostic imaging modalities of the liver. Surg Clin North Am 69:193-234.

Cottone M, et al, 1983: Ultrasound in the diagnosis of hepatocellular carcinoma associated with cirrhosis. Radiology 147:517-519.

Dietrich CF, et al, 1997: Sonographic detection of focal changes in the liver hilus in patients receiving corticosteroid therapy. Z Gastroenterol 35:1051-1057.

Ebara M, et al, 1986: Natural history of minute hepatocellular carcinoma smaller than three centimeters complicating cirrhosis: a study in 22 patients. Gastroenterology 90:289-298.

Fan MH, Chang AE, 2002: Resection of liver tumors: technical aspects. Surg Oncol 10:139-152.

Fujimoto M, et al, 1997: Hepatic arterial complications in pediatric segmental liver transplantations from living donors: assessment with color Doppler ultrasonography. Clin Transplant 11(5 pt 1):380-386.

Gaitini D, et al, 2001: Impact of intraoperative sonography on resection and cryoablation of liver tumors. J Clin Ultrasound 29:265-272.

Gondolesi GE, et al, 2002: Venous hemodynamics in living donor right lobe liver transplantation. Liver Transpl 8:809-813.

Gozzetti G, et al, 1986: Intraoperative ultrasonography in surgery for liver tumors. Surgery 99:523-530.

Gozzetti G, et al, 1988: Clinical experience with hepatic resections for hepatocellular carcinoma in patients with cirrhosis. Surg Gynecol Obstet 166:503-510.

Gozzetti G, et al, 1992: Liver resection for hepatocellular carcinoma in cirrhotic patients. Ital J Gastroenterol 24:105-110.

Gunven P, et al, 1985: Preoperative imaging of liver metastases: comparison of angiography, CT scan, and ultrasonography. Ann Surg 202:573-579.

Harihara Y, et al, 1997: A simple method to confirm patency of the graft bile duct during living-related partial liver transplantation. Transplantation 64:535-537.

Hayashi N, et al, 1987: Metastatic nodules of hepatocellular carcinoma: detection with angiography, CT, and US. Radiology 165:61-63.

Huang GT, et al, 2004: Current role of local ablative treatments for hepatocellular carcinoma. J Formos Med Assoc 103:403-410.

Huang TL, et al, 2001: Hepatic outflow insults in living-related liver transplantation: by Doppler sonography. Transplant Proc 33:3464-3465.

Hung CH, et al, 2001: Sonographic features of hepatic adenomas with pathologic correlation. Abdom Imaging 26:500-506.

Igawa S, et al, 1985: Intraoperative sonography: clinical usefulness in liver surgery. Radiology 156:473-478.

Itai Y, et al, 1987: Ultrasonography of small hepatic tumors. Radiat Med 5:14-19.

Izumi R, et al, 1993: Hepatic resection guided by needles inserted under ultrasonographic guidance. Surgery 114:497-501.

Jarnagin WR, et al, 2001: What is the yield of intraoperative ultrasonography during partial hepatectomy for malignant disease? J Am Coll Surg 192:577-583.

Kane RA, et al, 1994: The impact of intraoperative ultrasonography on surgery for liver neoplasms. J Ultrasound Med 13:1-6.

Kanematsu M, et al, 1999: Small hepatic nodules in cirrhosis: ultrasonographic, CT, and MR imaging findings. Abdom Imaging 24:47-55.

Kasai H, et al, 1992: Intraoperative color Doppler ultrasonography for partial-liver transplantation from the living donor in pediatric patients. Transplantation 54:173-175.

Kawasaki S, et al, 1996: Extended lateral segmentectomy using intraoperative ultrasound to obtain a partial liver graft. Am J Surg 171:286-288.

Knol JA, et al, 1993: Comparisons of dynamic infusion and delayed computed tomography, intraoperative ultrasound, and palpation in the diagnosis of liver metastases. Am J Surg 165:81-87.

Kokudo N, et al, 1996: Management of new hepatic nodules detected by intraoperative ultrasonography during hepatic resection for hepatocellular carcinoma. Surgery 119:634-640.

Lau WY, et al, 1993: Ultrasonography during liver resection for hepatocellular carcinoma. Br J Surg 80:493-494.

Leyendecker JR, et al, 2002: Sonographically observed echogenic response during intraoperative radiofrequency ablation of cirrhotic livers: pathologic correlation. AJR Am J Roentgenol 178:1147-1151.

Livraghi T, 1992: Percutaneous ethanol injection of hepatocellular carcinoma. Ital J Gastroenterol 24:72-74.

Lo CM, et al, 1997: Adult-to-adult living donor liver transplantation using extended right lobe grafts. Ann Surg 226:261-270.

Luck AJ, Maddern GJ, 1999: Intraoperative abdominal ultrasonography. Br J Surg 86:5-16.

Machi J, 1999: Intraoperative and laparoscopic ultrasound. Surg Oncol Clin N Am 8:205-226.

Machi J, Sigel B, 1996: Operative ultrasound in general surgery. Am J Surg 172:15-20.

Machi J, et al, 1987: Intraoperative ultrasonography in screening for liver metastases from colorectal cancer: comparative accuracy with traditional procedures. Surgery 101:678-684.

Machi J, et al, 1990: Operative ultrasound guidance for various surgical procedures. Ultrasound Med Biol 16:37-42.

Machi J, et al, 1991: Accuracy of intraoperative ultrasonography in diagnosing liver metastasis from colorectal cancer: evaluation with postoperative follow-up results. World J Surg 15:551-557.

Machi J, et al, 1993: Operative ultrasonography during hepatobiliary and pancreatic surgery. World J Surg 17:640-646.

Machi J, et al, 2001: Ultrasound-guided radiofrequency thermal ablation of liver tumors: percutaneous, laparoscopic, and open surgical approaches. J Gastrointest Surg 5:477-489.

Machi J, et al, 2002: Hand-assisted laparoscopic ultrasound-guided radiofrequency thermal ablation of liver tumors: a technical report. Surg Laparosc Endosc Percutan Techniques 12:160-164.

Makuuchi M, et al, 1977: Ultrasonic examination by electronic scanning during operation. Proceedings of the 32nd Meeting of the Japan Society of Ultrasonics in Medicine, pp 129-130.

Makuuchi M, et al, 1981a: Intraoperative ultrasonic examination for hepatectomy. Jpn J Clin Oncol 11:367-390.

Makuuchi M, et al, 1981b: Ultrasonic characteristics of the small hepatocellular carcinoma less than five centimeters in diameter, mosaic pattern of internal echoes and posterior echo enhancement. Acta Hepatol Jpn 22:1740.

Makuuchi M, et al, 1983a: [Development in segmentectomy and subsegmentectomy of the liver due to introduction of ultrasonography]. Nippon Geka Gakkai Zasshi 84:913-917.

Makuuchi M, et al, 1983b: Intraoperative ultrasonic examination for hepatectomy. Ultrasound Med Biol 2(suppl):493-497.

Makuuchi M, et al, 1983c: The inferior right hepatic vein: ultrasonic demonstration. Radiology 148:213-217.

Makuuchi M, et al, 1985: Ultrasonically guided subsegmentectomy. Surg Gynecol Obstet 161:346-350.

Makuuchi M, et al, 1987a: Four new hepatectomy procedures for resection of the right hepatic vein and preservation of the inferior right hepatic vein. Surg Gynecol Obstet 164:68-72.

Makuuchi M, et al, 1987b: The use of operative ultrasound as an aid to liver resection in patients with hepatocellular carcinoma. World J Surg 11:615-621.

Makuuchi M, et al, 1991: The value of ultrasonography for hepatic surgery. Hepatogastroenterology 38:64-70.

Makuuchi M, et al, 1993: Surgery for small liver cancers. Semin Surg Oncol 9:298-304.

Marchal GJ, et al, 1985a: Correlation of sonographic patterns in liver metastases with histology and microangiography. Invest Radiol 20:79-84.

Marchal GJ, et al, 1985b: Anechoic halo in solid liver tumors: sonographic, microangiographic, and histologic correlation. Radiology 156:479-483.

Mazzanti R, et al, 2004: Survival and prognostic factors in patients with hepatocellular carcinoma treated by percutaneous ethanol injection: a 10-year experience. Can J Gastroenterol 18:611-618.

Mirk P, et al, 1982: Ultrasonographic patterns in hepatic hemangiomas. J Clin Ultrasound 10:373-378.

Montorsi M, et al, 2002: Perspectives and drawbacks of minimally invasive surgery for hepatocellular carcinoma. Hepatogastroenterology 49:56-61.

Nagasue N, et al, 1984: Intraoperative ultrasonography in the surgical treatment of hepatic tumors. Acta Chir Scand 150:311-316.

Nagasue N, et al, 1989: Intraoperative ultrasonography in resection of small hepatocellular carcinoma associated with cirrhosis. Am J Surg 158:40-42.

Nakamura S, Tsuzuki T, 1981: Surgical anatomy of the hepatic veins and the inferior vena cava. Surg Gynecol Obstet 152:43-50.

Olsen AK, 1990: Intraoperative ultrasonography and the detection of liver metastases in patients with colorectal cancer. Br J Surg 77:998-999.

Onik G, et al, 1991: Ultrasound-guided hepatic cryosurgery in the treatment of metastatic colon carcinoma: preliminary results. Cancer 67:901-907.

Parker GA, et al, 1989: Intraoperative ultrasound of the liver affects operative decision making. Ann Surg 209:569-577.

Ravikumar TS, et al, 1994: Intraoperative ultrasonography of liver: detection of occult liver tumors and treatment by cryosurgery. Cancer Detect Prev 18:131-138.

Rifkin MD, et al, 1987: Intraoperative ultrasound of the liver: an important adjunctive tool for decision making in the operating room. Ann Surg 205:466-472.

Rozycki GS, 1998: Surgeon-performed ultrasound: its use in clinical practice. Ann Surg 228:16-28.

Salminen PM, 1990: Intraoperative ultrasound as an aid to surgical strategy in liver tumor. Acta Chir Scand 156:329-332.

Shamsi K, et al, 1993: Focal nodular hyperplasia of the liver: radiologic findings. Abdom Imaging 18:32-38.

Sheu JC, et al, 1984: Ultrasonography of small hepatic tumors using high-resolution linear-array real-time instruments. Radiology 150:797-802.

Sheu JC, et al, 1985a: Hepatocellular carcinoma: US evolution in the early stage. Radiology 155:463-467.

Sheu JC, et al, 1985b: Intraoperative hepatic ultrasonography—an indispensable procedure in resection of small hepatocellular carcinomas. Surgery 97:97-103.

Shimamura Y, et al, 1986: Selective portal branch occlusion by balloon catheter during liver resection. Surgery 100:938-941.

Solbiati L, et al, 2004: Guidance and monitoring of radiofrequency liver tumor ablation with contrast-enhanced ultrasound. Eur J Radiol 51(suppl):S19-S23.

Solomon MJ, et al, 1994: Does intraoperative hepatic ultrasonography change surgical decision making during liver resection? Am J Surg 168:307-310.

Someda H, et al, 1995: Vascular complications in living related liver transplantation detected with intraoperative and postoperative Doppler US. J Hepatol 22:623-632.

Soyer P, et al, 1992: Detection of liver metastases from colorectal cancer: comparison of intraoperative US and CT during arterial portography. Radiology 183:541-544.

Staren ED, et al, 1997: Intraoperative ultrasound in the management of liver neoplasms. Am Surg 63:591-597.

Stone MD, et al, 1994: Intraoperative ultrasound imaging of the liver at the time of colorectal cancer resection. Arch Surg 129:431-436.

Takayama T, Makuuchi M, 1996: Intraoperative ultrasonography and other techniques for segmental resections. Surg Oncol Clin N Am 5:261-269.

Takayama T, et al, 1991: A new method for mapping hepatic subsegment: counterstaining identification technique. Surgery 109:226-229.

Takayama T, et al, 1994: High dorsal resection of the liver. J Am Coll Surg 179:72-75.

Torzilli G, Makuuchi M, 2001: Ultrasound-guided liver subsegmentectomy: the peculiarity of segment 4. J Am Coll Surg 193:706-708.

Torzilli G, Makuuchi M, 2003: Tricks for ultrasound-guided resection of colorectal liver metastases. Hepatogastroenterology 50:1-3.

Torzilli G, Makuuchi M, 2004: Ultrasound-guided finger compression in liver subsegmentectomy for hepatocellular carcinoma. Surg Endosc 18:136-139.

Torzilli G, et al, 1999: A new technical aspect of ultrasound-guided liver surgery. Am J Surg 178:341-343.

Torzilli G, et al, 2002: Ultrasound-guided liver resections for hepatocellular carcinoma. Hepatogastroenterology 49:21-27.

Vilgrain V, et al, 2000: Imaging of atypical hemangiomas of the liver with pathologic correlation. Radiographics 20:379-397.

Wernecke K, et al, 1992: Pathologic explanation for hypoechoic halo seen on sonograms of malignant liver tumors: an in vitro correlative study. AJR Am J Roentgenol 159:1011-1016.

Wong SL, et al, 2001: Radiofrequency ablation for unresectable hepatic tumors. Am J Surg 182:552-557.

Zacherl J, et al, 2002: Current value of intraoperative sonography during surgery for hepatic neoplasms. World J Surg 26:550-554.

Cirrhosis and Portal Hypertension

87

Cirrhosis and Portal Hypertension: Pathologic Aspects

H. L. WANG AND E. M. BRUNT

Cirrhosis is the end stage of a variety of chronic diseases involving the liver. It is characterized by diffusely nodular replacement and remodeling of the normal hepatic architecture as a result of septum formation separating nodules of regenerative hepatocytes. Biochemically, the cirrhotic liver functions less efficiently than the normal liver. Decompensated cirrhosis manifests as portal hypertension and liver failure, both of which are associated with numerous clinically important complications (see Chs. 88 and 90). In addition, cirrhosis is a major predisposing condition to the development of hepatocellular carcinoma (Suriawinata & Xu, 2004). Portal hypertension secondary to cirrhosis develops as a result of alterations of the hepatic microcirculatory system. Infrequently, portal hypertension occurs in the absence of cirrhosis (noncirrhotic portal hypertension); this condition may be idiopathic or associated with a variety of prehepatic, intrahepatic, or posthepatic conditions. This chapter focuses on pathology of cirrhosis and noncirrhotic portal hypertension and many of the conditions that result in portal hypertension.

CIRRHOSIS

The true prevalence of cirrhosis in the United States is unknown because many patients with compensated cirrhosis do not exhibit symptoms or signs of liver failure, but cirrhosis is among the top 10 causes of death in the Western world. In autopsy series, cirrhosis is documented in 5% to 10% of cases, but autopsy subjects may not be representative of the general population (Karsan et al, 2004). Currently, the only available and definitive treatment for established cirrhosis is liver transplantation.

Pathogenesis and Reversibility

The transformation from normal hepatic architecture to cirrhosis ultimately is due to progressive deposition of fibrous tissue and vascular remodeling, regardless of different underlying etiologies. Fibrogenesis is a dynamic and complex process triggered by liver injury and mediated by complex interplay of cellular necrosis, inflammation, apoptosis, and various cytokines. Transforming growth factor-β seems to be a major fibrogenic mediator that activates perisinusoidal hepatic stellate cells (Ito cells) and portal fibroblasts (myofibroblasts) to produce collagens and other types of extracellular matrix and degradatory products (Canbay et al, 2004; Friedman, 2000; Pinzani & Marra, 2001; Ramadori & Saile, 2004). Recent work has shown the fibrogenic nature of leptin, the anorectic hormone produced

in adipose tissue (LeClercq et al, 2002). During pathologic fibrogenesis, prevention of matrix degradation by metalloproteinases is orchestrated by the release of potent tissue metalloproteinase inhibitors; apoptosis of fibrogenic hepatic stellate cells also is inhibited. Scar formation ultimately is the consequence of imbalanced collagen synthesis, deposition, and degradation.

Established cirrhosis traditionally is considered irreversible. Accumulating clinical and experimental evidence suggests, however, that reversal or regression of liver fibrosis and cirrhosis may be possible (Fallowfield & Iredale, 2004). A study by Poynard and coworkers (2002) analyzed 3010 patients with chronic hepatitis C virus (HCV) included in four major clinical trials to receive randomized treatment regimens with interferon or pegylated interferon, with or without additional ribavirin. Reversal of cirrhosis was reported in 75 (49%) of 153 patients with baseline cirrhosis. More recently, Pol and associates (2004) examined 64 immunocompetent patients with HCV-related cirrhosis and found that cirrhosis disappeared in 5 patients (7.8%) on followup biopsies with a mean interval of 4.6 years. In addition, three of four patients on dialysis showed reversal of cirrhosis secondary to HCV infection. Resolution of cirrhosis was shown in two cases by examining the whole liver explants at the time of transplantation.

Regression of cirrhosis has been reported in patients with diverse chronic liver diseases, such as hepatitis B virus (HBV), alcoholism, hemochromatosis, autoimmune hepatitis, and primary biliary cirrhosis (Arthur, 2002; Fallowfield & Iredale, 2004; Wanless et al, 2000). Spontaneous resolution of fibrosis also has been described in rats treated with carbon tetrachloride (Iredale et al, 1998; Issa et al, 2004). The proposed mechanisms for breakdown and remodeling of liver fibrosis include loss of activated stellate cells via apoptosis, decreased expression of metalloproteinase inhibitors, and increased production and activity of metalloproteinases or collagenases (Arthur, 2002; Benyon & Arthur, 2001; Fallowfield & Iredale, 2004). It is unclear, however, how these molecular and cellular events are initiated and regulated.

Currently, whether cirrhosis is truly reversible is the subject of debate (Arthur, 2002; Chedid, 2000; Desmet & Roskams, 2003; Geller, 2000; Ray, 2000). Many important questions remain to be answered. Even if scar tissue is resorbed, can normal hepatic architecture be completely restored? Were there sampling differences or interpretation errors on biopsies in the studies showing reversibility? Was there a possibility that some of the reversed cases might have undergone a conversion of micronodular to macronodular cirrhosis as shown in animal models (Issa et al, 2004), a condition that made the diagnosis of cirrhosis more difficult on a needle core biopsy sample (Desmet & Roskams, 2003)? Nevertheless, this discussion may have important clinical implications. Many liver diseases progress insidiously, and patients may seek medical attention only at the advanced stage when treatment choice is limited. If cirrhosis is truly reversible, many patients with advanced liver disease still may benefit from medical treatment for specific etiologies, particularly with the discovery of new drug therapies.

Role of Liver Biopsy

In modern medicine, investigation of patients with chronic liver disease and cirrhosis involves multiple disciplines, including radiology, chemistry, biochemistry, virology, serology, and molecular biology. Liver biopsy evaluation remains the primary diagnostic tool despite the drawback of invasiveness. For cirrhotic patients, liver biopsy can serve several important roles, such as establishing or confirming the diagnosis; assessing the possible cause; analyzing the grade of ongoing necroinflammatory activity; detecting dysplastic lesions or hepatocellular carcinoma; and providing tissue for chemical, biochemical, molecular, or ultrastructural studies (Brunt, 2000a).

There are two types of biopsy to sample liver tissue: needle biopsy and wedge biopsy. Needle biopsy has proved to be the most useful technique to obtain representative liver tissue for analysis. This procedure can be done percutaneously, transjugularly, or during open surgery or laparoscopy, using a cutting needle or the Menghini aspiration needle, although the former usually generates a better biopsy specimen than the latter. The size of the needle biopsy specimen is important in avoiding sampling error. Traditionally, it has been recommended that an adequate biopsy specimen should be no smaller than 20-gauge and at least 1.5 cm in length or should contain at least five portal tracts (Afdhal & Nunes, 2004). It has been suggested more recently, however, that for accurate and reliable grading and staging of chronic viral hepatitis, a biopsy specimen of 2 cm in length or longer containing at least 11 complete portal tracts is needed (Guido & Rugge, 2004).

Wedge biopsy, usually performed during open surgery or laparoscopy, is discouraged for evaluation of diffuse parenchymal liver diseases because this technique primarily samples the subcapsular liver parenchyma, which may contain misleading fibrous septa extended from the capsule, mimicking cirrhosis or bridging fibrosis. In addition, nonspecific necroinflammatory change can occur quickly in the subcapsular region during surgical procedures, which may confuse the histology further. A wedge biopsy is more suitable for focal lesions present on or immediately below the capsule. Even during open surgery, a needle biopsy to sample deep liver parenchyma is preferred (Guido & Rugge, 2004).

Prompt fixation of the liver biopsy specimen in buffered formalin is vital to high-quality histology. Many special stains and analyses, such as iron or copper quantitation, can be performed on formalin-fixed tissue nowadays. If a metabolic disorder is suspected, and electron microscopic examination is expected, additional tissue should be fixed in glutaraldehyde. If fresh tissue is submitted for molecular analyses, it should never be dry or be immersed in saline. The appropriate method is to place the tissue on a piece of saline-moistened gauze in a container. Consultation with a pathologist before the biopsy procedure is encouraged to help avoid inappropriate tissue handling.

Histopathologic interpretation of liver biopsy specimens can be challenging. The importance of communication among surgeons, hepatologists, and pathologists cannot be overemphasized. Clinicians should provide sufficient clinical information when submitting a liver biopsy specimen for pathologists to analyze histologic findings in the appropriate clinical setting.

Morphology

Grossly, established cirrhosis exhibits a nodular appearance and involves the entire liver (Fig. 87.1). Microscopically, the liver parenchyma is divided by variable-sized fibrovascular septa into rounded nodules that typically no longer retain a terminal hepatic venule or portal tracts. The normal portal-to-central relationship is completely effaced. The hepatocytes within the nodules may appear morphologically normal or show evidence of regeneration. The latter may be characterized by thickened cell plates with two to three cell layers, anisonucleosis, large cell change, or small, crowded cells. The reticulin stain is useful to show cord thickening. In the fibrovascular septa, there are usually a variable number of increased ductular profiles (ductular proliferation), referred to as "ductular reaction" (Roskams et al, 2004). This ductular reaction is accompanied by a variable degree of inflammatory cell infiltration, the nature and amount of which may indicate an ongoing necroinflammatory process; some cases may show interface hepatitis.

According to the size of the nodules, cirrhosis has been classified as micronodular if nearly all the nodules are less than 0.3 cm in diameter and macronodular if greater than 0.3 cm. Mixed micronodular and macronodular cirrhosis is defined by the presence of relatively equal numbers of small and large nodules. Although this morphologic classification may provide clues to the underlying etiology in some cases, it is not recommended for clinical practice because micronodular cirrhosis may progress to a macronodular pattern over time. Mixed micronodular and macronodular cirrhosis is common in end-stage liver disease regardless of the underlying etiology.

Biliary cirrhosis is caused by many disorders, such as primary biliary cirrhosis, primary or secondary sclerosing cholangitis, and biliary atresia. This type of cirrhosis exhibits unique morphologic features characterized by a highly irregular, "jigsaw puzzle" or "geographic" nodular pattern (Fig. 87.2) (see Ch. 43). Loss or effacement of native bile ducts by lymphoid aggregates or scar

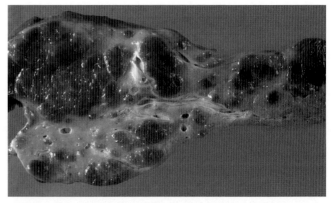

Fig. 87.1. Gross appearance of cirrhosis showing diffuse involvement of the entire liver by regenerative nodules and broad fibrous bands.

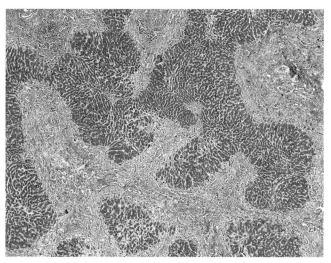

Fig. 87.2. Biliary cirrhosis exhibiting a "jigsaw puzzle" pattern. (Masson trichrome stain.)

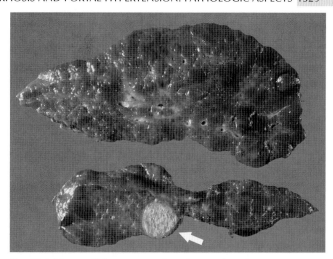

Fig. 87.4. Hepatocellular carcinoma *(arrow)* in a cirrhotic liver.

tissue may be evident. Ductular reaction (proliferation) may be more pronounced than that seen in other types of cirrhosis. A characteristic clue to biliary cirrhosis is the constellation of findings in periseptal hepatocytes referred to as cholate stasis. These findings include periseptal hepatocyte ballooning, Mallory hyalin, and copper deposition. In addition, foam cell aggregates may be seen in the nodules. Some authors have attributed large cell change to chronic cholestasis. Another subtle histologic clue to biliary cirrhosis is the presence of nodular regenerative hyperplasia in the regenerative nodules.

Recognition of cirrhosis is usually straightforward even on hematoxylin and eosin–stained sections when an explant or an adequate biopsy specimen is examined. It may be helpful to use Masson trichrome stain to highlight the fibrous septa in difficult cases, particularly for needle biopsy specimens (Fig. 87.3). Fragmentation of the specimen noted at the time of biopsy should raise the suspicion of cirrhosis. On histologic sections, a thin layer of collagen, better appreciated on trichrome and reticulin stains, tends to adhere to the surface of detached nodules. Cirrhosis also may be difficult to diagnose on needle biopsy

specimens when a macronodule is sampled, or when cirrhosis is incomplete (incomplete septal cirrhosis). In the latter case, the morphologic features of cirrhosis are not exhibited, but vascular relationships are markedly altered, and ectatic portal veins may be noted. Additional stains considered "routine" by liver pathologists include the iron stain and periodic acid–Schiff stain after diastase digestion (PAS-d). The former is useful in detecting small amounts of hepatocellular or reticuloendothelial iron and highlighting intracanalicular bile plugs, and the latter is useful in detecting PAS-d "globules" characteristic of α_1-antitrypsin deficiency. PAS-d also is quite helpful in noting bile duct basement membranes, perisinusoidal basement membranes, and the PAS-d–laden Kupffer cells and septal macrophages that are characteristic of recent necroinflammatory activity.

Cancer Risk

The most common cancer that arises in cirrhotic livers is hepatocellular carcinoma (Fig. 87.4) (see Ch. 71). Although this cancer may occur in cirrhosis of any etiology, it is a particular risk in cirrhosis attributed to HBV and HCV infection and alcoholic liver disease. Grossly, hepatocellular carcinoma may be multifocal or grow as a well-circumscribed mass. It may show evidence of necrosis or possess different color and texture from background cirrhotic nodules. It also may bulge from the cut surface on sectioning. Most cases of hepatocellular carcinoma arising in cirrhotic livers are found in nodules larger than 1 cm (Bruix et al, 2001). Studies have shown, however, that nodules smaller than 1 cm can be malignant in the setting of cirrhosis (Caturelli et al, 2004). Premalignant lesions, or dysplastic nodules, may be indistinguishable from hepatocellular carcinoma by gross examination.

Cholangiocarcinoma in cirrhosis usually develops in the setting of primary sclerosing cholangitis and is seen more commonly in noncirrhotic livers (see Ch. 42). The tumor may infiltrate the liver diffusely or present as a mass lesion that can be intrahepatic or extrahepatic. Rarely, cholangiocarcinoma is detected in cirrhosis and attributed to a nonbiliary cause, such as viral hepatitis, and may be confused with benign florid bile ductular proliferation commonly seen in cirrhotic livers. The cirrhotic liver is extremely resistant to metastatic tumors.

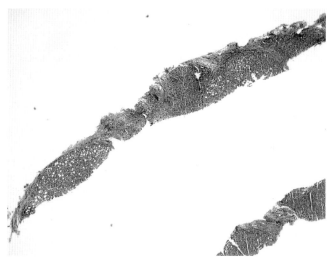

Fig. 87.3. Cirrhosis visible on a needle biopsy specimen. (Masson trichrome stain.)

Not all large nodules detected in cirrhotic livers are hepatocellular carcinoma. A macroregenerative nodule or large regenerative nodule usually measures 0.5 to 1.5 cm (rarely ≥5 cm) in diameter (International Working Party, 1995). It is seen more commonly in macronodular cirrhosis and may be distinct from surrounding cirrhotic nodules on gross examination. Histologically, a macroregenerative nodule may contain portal structures or fibrovascular septa. The hepatocytes within the nodule are similar to the hepatocytes in smaller cirrhotic nodules, but almost always exhibit hyperplastic change evidenced by plates of two to three cells thick. The clonal nature of the macroregenerative nodule has been shown in studies; its malignant potential is an area of ongoing discussion (Bailey & Brunt, 2002).

A dysplastic nodule is a premalignant lesion usually measuring greater than 0.5 cm (International Working Party, 1995). Evolution to hepatocellular carcinoma within months or a few years has been well documented (Hytiroglou, 2004). Morphologic separation of a low-grade dysplastic nodule from a macroregenerative nodule is challenging, if possible. A high-grade dysplastic nodule exhibits more clear-cut architectural or cytologic atypia, such as bulging or maplike clonal growth; pseudoglandular formation; unpaired arteries; and small cell change characterized by increased cell density, high nuclear-to-cytoplasmic ratio, and nuclear hyperchromasia. These morphologic changes are insufficient, however, for the diagnosis of hepatocellular carcinoma because a dysplastic nodule does not invade the stroma or blood vessels and maintains cell plates no more than three cells wide (Roncalli, 2004). Distinguishing a high-grade dysplastic nodule from well-differentiated hepatocellular carcinoma can be extremely difficult or impossible on a needle biopsy specimen, although it may be less ambiguous when an explant is examined (Kojiro, 2004). Clinical management of patients with cirrhosis and dysplasia in biopsy specimens is challenging.

Assessment of Underlying Etiology

Cirrhosis is best classified by its underlying etiology (Table 87.1), which can be determined by clinical history and laboratory investigation in many, but not all, cases. Morphologic examination may help establish the diagnosis or guide the clinical investigation. In the following discussion, the morphologic features characteristic of many chronic liver diseases commonly causing cirrhosis are illustrated. At the end stage of liver disease, however, the histopathologic findings may be nonspecific and indiscriminate even to experienced hepatopathologists. Many cases of "cryptogenic" cirrhosis represent "burned-out" processes for which no identifying clinical or morphologic features remain.

Alcoholic Liver Disease

Excessive alcohol consumption is the leading cause of liver disease in the Western world, which encompasses a clinicopathologic spectrum that includes fatty liver, alcoholic hepatitis, and alcoholic cirrhosis (Haber et al, 2003; Menon et al, 2001; O'Connor & Schottenfeld, 1998; Tome & Lucey, 2004). Alcoholic cirrhosis (Laënnec's cirrhosis) is classically micronodular and may retain some of the features of alcoholic hepatitis at the initial stage. The liver may appear pale or yellow, enlarged, and greasy on gross examination. Histologically, the lesions predominate in the perivenular region (zone 3) of the acinus and

Table 87.1   Causes of Cirrhosis

Drugs and toxins
  Alcohol
  Methotrexate
  Isoniazid
  Methyldopa
  Amiodarone

Infections
  HBV
  HCV
  Hepatitis D
  Schistosomiasis

Autoimmune disorders
  Autoimmune hepatitis
  Primary biliary cirrhosis
  Primary sclerosing cholangitis

Inherited metabolic defects
  Hemochromatosis
  Wilson's disease
  α_1-Antitrypsin deficiency
  Galactosemia
  Tyrosinemia
  Glycogen storage disease
  Hereditary fructose intolerance
  Urea cycle disorders
  Abetalipoproteinemia
  Progressive familial intrahepatic cholestasis
  Cystic fibrosis

Acquired bile duct diseases
  Biliary atresia
  Gallstone obstruction
  Common bile duct stricture

Vascular disorders
  Budd-Chiari syndrome
  Veno-occlusive disease
  Congestive heart failure
  Hereditary hemorrhagic telangiectasia

Miscellaneous
  Nonalcoholic steatohepatitis
  Total parenteral nutrition
  Indian childhood cirrhosis
  Intestinal bypass surgery
  Hypervitaminosis A
  Sarcoidosis

Cryptogenic

Modified from MaeSween RNM, et al, 2002: Pathology of the Liver, 4th ed. London, Churchill Livingstone.

include various combinations of steatosis (fatty change), ballooning, Mallory hyalin (or body), and satellitosis. Steatosis may be predominantly macrovesicular, defined by the presence of large fat droplets in the cytoplasm of hepatocytes displacing the nuclei. Microvesicular steatosis, characterized by fine fat droplets surrounding the central nuclei, also can be seen. Inflammatory infiltrate in alcoholic hepatitis is typically rich in neutrophils, most frequently distributed in the lobules adjacent to Mallory hyalin–containing hepatocytes (Fig. 87.5). Lymphocytes and histiocytes also may be present, sometimes in the form of lipogranulomas. Megamitochondria also may be evident. In the portal and periportal regions, ductular reaction with numerous neutrophils may occur. Cholangiolitis and canalicular bile plugs are worrisome lesions for pancreatitis.

The patterns of fibrosis in alcoholic hepatitis are characteristic. Fibrosis usually involves the terminal hepatic venules, leading to the thickening of the wall; luminal occlusion may be seen with

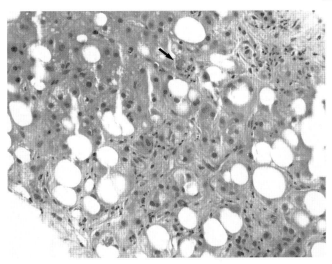

Fig. 87.5. Alcoholic hepatitis characterized by macrovesicular steatosis, hepatocyte ballooning, lobular neutrophilic infiltration, and presence of Mallory bodies. One of the hepatocytes containing a Mallory body is surrounded partially by neutrophils *(arrow).*

necrosis of adjacent hepatocytes and Mallory hyalin in a lesion referred to as *central hyaline necrosis.* Subendothelial fibrosis is a veno-occlusive lesion of alcoholism that may be noted even in end-stage cirrhotic livers. Fibrosis may extend into the lobules in perisinusoidal spaces as delicate or dense strands, giving rise to a distinctive "chicken wire" pericellular (perisinusoidal) distribution (Brunt, 2002). Trichrome stain is particularly useful in recognizing this unique form of fibrosis. With time, the liver may be replaced by micronodular cirrhosis; often, the septa of alcoholic liver disease are quite broad as manifestations of the microvascular obliteration.

As alcoholic cirrhosis progresses, the aforementioned morphologic features may become less obvious. The liver may shrink, and the cirrhosis may evolve into a macronodular or mixed nodular architecture. Steatosis, ballooning, and Mallory hyalin may not be discernible, especially in patients who have remained abstinent for several months.

Nonalcoholic Fatty Liver Disease

Nonalcoholic fatty liver disease is increasingly recognized as a significant form of potentially progressive liver disease. Prevalence studies estimate that approximately 20% to 25% of the U.S. population is affected by fatty liver; of these individuals, a small percentage is at risk for progression to cirrhosis (Angulo, 2002). The lesions noted in liver tissue may resemble many of the features of alcohol-induced liver damage in individuals who are not heavy drinkers (Brunt, 2004; Salt, 2004; te Sligte et al, 2004; Zafrani, 2004). The disease is etiologically attributed primarily to insulin resistance and is considered the hepatic manifestation of the metabolic syndrome, a constellation of obesity, hypertension, diabetes, and hyperlipidemia (Marchesini et al, 2001). Studies have correlated the lesions of nonalcoholic steatohepatitis (NASH) with features of metabolic syndrome.

Most, but not all, of the histopathologic features described for alcoholic hepatitis can be found in NASH. These mainly include steatosis, which is predominantly macrovesicular and commonly of zone 3 (centrilobular) distribution; hepatocyte

ballooning; lobular inflammation, which is usually mild and includes neutrophils; small lipogranulomas; and patchy perisinusoidal fibrosis (Fig. 87.6). Hepatocytes also may exhibit prominent glycogenated nuclei in NASH, particularly when associated with diabetes. Portal inflammation may be present in some cases, but is usually mild and less intense than lobular inflammation. The presence of heavy portal inflammation, particularly when accompanied by lymphoid aggregates or abundant plasma cells, should raise the suspicion of overlapping disease, such as chronic viral hepatitis or autoimmune hepatitis (Brunt et al, 2003). In addition, Mallory hyalin may or may not be seen in NASH and may be poorly formed if present. In contrast to alcoholic liver disease, in which Mallory hyalin may be present in apoptotic hepatocytes, in NASH, Mallory hyalin is restricted to ballooned hepatocytes. Immunohistochemical stains are available for confirmation of Mallory hyalin, if that is required. If numerous Mallory bodies are present in the background of steatohepatitis, an alcoholic origin is more likely (Brunt, 2002, 2004).

Fibrosis in NASH begins in the pericentral perisinusoidal spaces and eventually may extend to involve the portal tracts, leading to bridging fibrosis and cirrhosis, but typically does not obliterate the terminal hepatic venules, a feature dissimilar to alcoholic hepatitis. A grading and staging system has been proposed for NASH primarily based on the extent and severity of the constellation of steatosis, ballooning change, lobular and portal inflammation (grade), and fibrosis and remodeling (stage) (Brunt, 2004; Brunt et al, 1999). Similar to the widespread use of grading and staging in other forms of chronic liver disease, this proposal was made in recognition of the unique features of steatohepatitis to facilitate further reproducible evaluation for clinical and laboratory investigation.

Chronic Hepatitis C

A high proportion of patients infected with HCV develop cirrhosis (Poynard et al, 2003), particularly patients with a long duration of infection, concurrent alcohol consumption, coinfection with HBV or human immunodeficiency virus, nonresponse

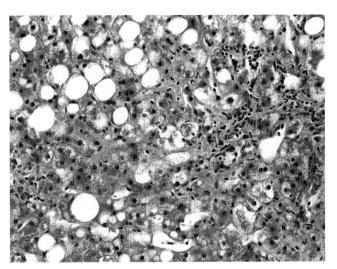

Fig. 87.6. Zone 3 chicken wire perisinusoidal fibrosis; this feature can be seen in nonalcoholic and alcoholic steatohepatitis. (Masson trichrome stain.)

to antiviral therapy, and male gender (de Torres & Poynard, 2003; McCaughan & George, 2004). HCV-related cirrhosis is virtually always macronodular or mixed macronodular and micronodular. The fibrovascular septa vary in width and usually are infiltrated by mononuclear cells, predominantly lymphocytes, but also including plasma cells and eosinophils. Lymphoid aggregates, often with well-formed germinal centers, are characteristic, although not pathognomonic (Fig. 87.7). A mild degree of bile duct damage (the Poulsen lesion) also may be seen in some cases. Interface hepatitis may be present. The lobular inflammation is typically spotty and mild, with or without acidophilic bodies. Subendothelial inflammation in portal veins, identical to endotheliitis, also may occur in HCV infection. There has been no reliable antibody for immunohistochemical detection of HCV proteins.

Steatosis is a common histologic finding in chronic HCV and may be a manifestation of host phenotype (increased body weight, presence of the metabolic syndrome) or viral cytopathic effect, as in genotype 3. Although a small subset of the patients concurrently may have steatohepatitis of either nonalcoholic or alcoholic origin (Brunt et al, 2003; Ramalho, 2003), viral proteins have been shown to promote fat accumulation in hepatocytes directly (Lai, 2002; Lonardo et al, 2004; Ramalho, 2003). Accumulating evidence indicates that steatosis contributes to fibrosis progression, particularly in patients infected with genotype 3 HCV (Brunt & Tiniakos, 2002; Ramalho, 2003; Rubbia-Brandt et al, 2004).

Liver biopsy has a central role in assessing the grade of necroinflammation and the portal-based progression of fibrosis and evaluating the effect of antiviral therapy. Numerous grading and staging systems for chronic hepatitis have been developed; these systems share the assessment of portal and lobular inflammation and necrosis for grade and portal-based fibrosis for stage (Brunt, 2000b).

Chronic Hepatitis B

Chronic hepatitis secondary to HBV infection is another common cause of cirrhosis (Fattovich, 2003; Ganem & Prince, 2004; Lai et al, 2003). Compared with HCV, HBV hepatitis may exhibit more severe portal and lobular necroinflammation, particularly

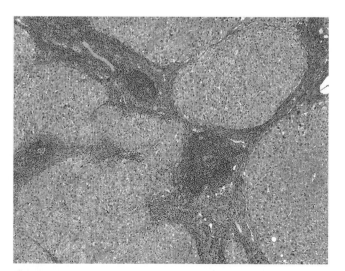

Fig. 87.7. HCV cirrhosis with septal lymphoid aggregates that are characteristic of HCV.

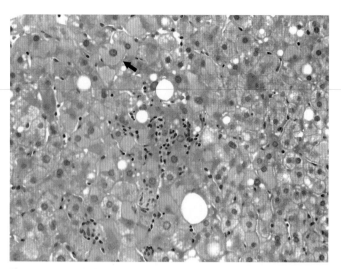

Fig. 87.8. Ground-glass hepatocytes in chronic HBV hepatitis, one of which is highlighted by an *arrow*.

when there is an acute exacerbation. Confluent or multiacinar bridging necrosis with collapse of the lobular framework may be seen. A relatively specific finding in chronic HBV hepatitis is the presence of "ground-glass" inclusions within hepatocytes, which are uniform, pale or eosinophilic cytoplasmic alterations resulting from enriched smooth endoplasmic reticulum filled with hepatitis B surface antigen (Fig. 87.8). A definitive diagnosis can be established by histochemical stains (orcein, Victoria blue) or immunohistochemical detection of hepatitis B surface antigen in the cytoplasm and hepatitis B core antigen in the nucleus.

Coinfection or superinfection with hepatitis D virus in HBV patients usually causes more severe liver damage and accelerates the development of cirrhosis (Farci, 2003). Immunohistochemical detection of hepatitis D virus intranuclear antigen is helpful in establishing the diagnosis.

Autoimmune Hepatitis

The diagnosis of autoimmune hepatitis relies on a constellation of clinical, laboratory, and histopathologic findings, none of which alone is considered specific (Alvarez et al, 1999; McFarlane, 2002a; 2002b; Vergani & Mieli-Vergani, 2003). Histopathologic examination of liver tissue serves important roles in confirming the clinical concern and excluding diseases secondary to other etiologies (Carpenter & Czaja, 2002). Classic autoimmune hepatitis exhibits a dense portal, septal, and lobular mononuclear cell infiltrate, with marked periportal or periseptal interface hepatitis enriched in plasma cells. The presence of numerous plasma cells in portal inflammation and within lobular foci of necrosis and the formation of "hepatitic rosettes" are characteristic (Fig. 87.9). In severe cases, confluent or bridging necrosis may be seen, sometimes accompanied by pseudoacinar formation. Predominantly centrilobular necrosis with relatively mild portal inflammation also has been described in autoimmune hepatitis (Misdraji et al, 2004). Fibrosis usually develops rapidly in untreated patients. At the cirrhotic stage, the liver parenchyma is divided by broad fibrous bands into variable-sized nodules, similar to that caused by alcoholic or chronic viral hepatitis. Plasma cells and rosettes may become less prominent. Burned-out autoimmune hepatitis may be a cause of "cryptogenic" cirrhosis.

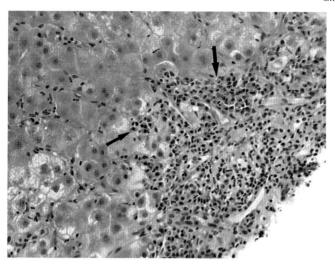

Fig. 87.9. Autoimmune hepatitis may be characterized by hepatitic rosettes and numerous plasma cells *(arrows)* in the portal tracts and lobules.

Morphologic features do not separate different types of autoimmune hepatitis classified by either autoantibody profiles or immunogenetic markers (McFarlane, 2002a).

Primary Biliary Cirrhosis

Primary biliary cirrhosis is an autoimmune disorder that leads to progressive destruction of intrahepatic bile ducts (Leuschner, 2003; Selmi et al, 2004). In the early stage, the disease is characterized by mixed portal chronic inflammation with lymphocytes, plasma cells, and eosinophils and the pathognomonic lesion, the florid duct lesion. The florid duct lesion is characterized by lymphocytic or granulomatous bile duct infiltration (Fig. 87.10). Ductular reaction and interface hepatitis may be seen in more advanced cases. In the setting of positive serum antimitochondrial antibody (AMA), the florid duct lesion is essentially diagnostic. The affected duct may rupture, or the duct epithelium may exhibit degenerative change. It is recommended that even in the setting of AMA, epithelioid granulomas be

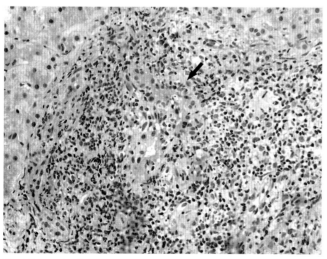

Fig. 87.10. Florid duct lesion with granulomatous portal inflammation and damaged bile duct *(arrow)* in early stage primary biliary cirrhosis.

evaluated with routine stains for fungal and acid-fast organisms. With disease progression, ductopenia becomes evident. The native ducts may be absent or obscured by lymphoid aggregates or collections of foamy macrophages. Cholate stasis, as described previously, may be an initial clue to the diagnosis. Features of autoimmune hepatitis also may occur in AMA-positive primary biliary cirrhosis, referred to as "overlap syndrome" (Dienes et al, 2002; Durazzo et al, 2003).

Cirrhosis is seen only at the late stage of primary biliary cirrhosis, is commonly inhomogeneously distributed, and may be micronodular. Florid duct lesion and granulomas may continue to exist in regions where native bile ducts have not been completely destroyed. Canalicular cholestasis with bile plugs may be seen in the late stage and is regarded as a sign of poor prognosis.

The term *autoimmune cholangiopathy* (also *antinuclear antibody–positive, AMA-negative primary biliary cirrhosis*) has been used to describe a small subset of patients who present with typical clinical and histopathologic findings of primary biliary cirrhosis, but are seronegative for AMA. These patients may have other autoantibodies, such as antinuclear antibody and anti–smooth muscle antibody, as seen in autoimmune hepatitis. Accumulating evidence suggests that autoimmune cholangiopathy and primary biliary cirrhosis are likely to be a single disease with variations in the type and concentration of autoantibodies (Vierling, 2004).

Primary Sclerosing Cholangitis

Primary sclerosing cholangitis is also an autoimmune inflammatory and fibrosing process that segmentally affects the extrahepatic and intrahepatic biliary tree, leading to biliary strictures and cirrhosis (Cullen & Chapman, 2003; Mendes & Lindor, 2004; Rodriguez & Bass, 2003). It is strongly associated with inflammatory bowel disease, particularly ulcerative colitis, and with the development of cholangiocarcinoma. The definitive diagnosis of primary sclerosing cholangitis rests on characteristic cholangiographic findings. Histopathologic examination of a liver biopsy specimen may or may not reveal diagnostic features because of the patchy nature of the disease. Mild portal lymphocytic infiltration and mild bile ductular reaction may be the only observations. The relatively specific finding of concentric periductal fibrosis with an "onionskin" appearance indicates chronic biliary obstruction and is not pathognomonic of primary sclerosing cholangitis. The duct epithelium usually exhibits atrophic and degenerative changes, and a characteristic fibro-obliterative scar eventually replaces the bile duct (Fig. 87.11). As in other forms of biliary cirrhosis, inhomogeneity of cirrhosis and histologic evidence of cholate stasis are recognized features in primary sclerosing cholangitis. Careful evaluation of explant livers for occult cholangiocarcinoma is recommended.

Hereditary Hemochromatosis

Hereditary hemochromatosis is an autosomal recessive iron overload disorder, primarily associated with mutation of the *HFE* gene (Limdi & Crampton, 2004; Pietrangelo, 2004). Iron deposition initially occurs in zone 1 (periportal) hepatocytes with a decreasing gradient toward the centrilobular area; the iron granules are concentrated along the border of the canaliculi; this is best shown by Perls' Prussian blue stain (Fig. 87.12).

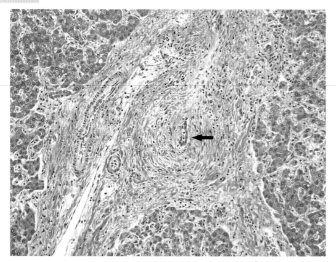

Fig. 87.11. Characteristic concentric onionskin periductal fibrosis in primary sclerosing cholangitis. The residual duct epithelial cells show atrophic and degenerative changes *(arrow)*. (Masson trichrome stain.)

With progression, untreated hereditary hemochromatosis results in iron deposition throughout the entire lobule, and iron granules are seen not only in hepatocytes, but also in Kupffer cells, biliary epithelial cells, and portal macrophages. Kupffer cell clusters, siderotic nodules, are common. There is usually little to no significant inflammation. This pattern of iron deposition is not restricted to hereditary hemochromatosis, so the diagnosis rests with genetic testing.

Fibrosis in hereditary hemochromatosis is portal based. When cirrhosis develops, it is typically micronodular, with retention of the terminal hepatic venules. Hepatocytes in cirrhotic nodules also are loaded with iron, which may exhibit a periseptal distribution pattern. Occurrence of iron-free nodules or foci is of concern for dysplasia or hepatocellular carcinoma.

Secondary iron overload in the liver is a common finding in a variety of conditions, including cirrhosis (Limdi & Crampton, 2004). Iron deposition secondary to transfusion can be heavy, but initially principally involves Kupffer cells in the sinusoids.

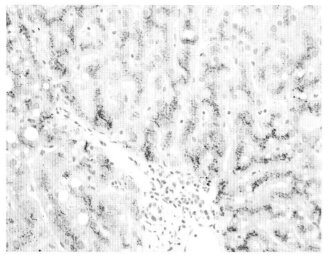

Fig. 87.12. Hepatocellular iron deposition in pericanalicular location in periportal (zone 1) hepatocytes in hereditary hemochromatosis. (Perls' Prussian blue stain.)

Significant amounts of stainable iron may be detected in chronic HCV and HBV hepatitis, alcoholic steatohepatitis and NASH, and cirrhosis unrelated to hereditary hemochromatosis or the above-mentioned chronic liver diseases. Iron deposition in these conditions is usually mild and rarely exceeds 2+ when a 1-4 scale semiquantitative histologic score is used. Iron granules may be found in hepatocytes, Kupffer cells and endothelial cells. If a higher score is appreciated in hepatocytes (e.g., 3+ or 4+, which is more commonly associated with hereditary hemochromatosis), age-adjusted chemical quantitation of iron concentration in dry hepatic tissue, the hepatic iron index, or genetic testing for *HFE* mutations should be performed. A hepatic iron index greater than 2 was developed to distinguish hereditary hemochromatosis from iron overload secondary to alcoholic siderosis, but this is not considered a diagnostic test for hereditary hemochromatosis (Bacon, 2001). Patients with chronic viral hepatitis or steatohepatitis who also have an increased liver iron content have a higher chance to harbor *HFE* mutations. It has been suggested that these patients are less likely to respond to therapy and more prone to develop fibrosis and cirrhosis (Bonkovsky et al, 2003). Other genetic markers have been developed to correlate with non-*HFE* iron overload (Pietrangelo, 2004).

Wilson's Disease

Wilson's disease is an autosomal recessive inherited metabolic disorder of copper metabolism. Any young patient with unexplained chronic or fulminant liver disease should be investigated for Wilson's disease (Ferenci, 2004; Gitlin, 2003). Morphologic features in the liver vary widely at different stages of the disease and lack specificity. At the precirrhotic stage, there may be lymphocytic portal inflammation with interface hepatitis, mimicking chronic viral hepatitis or autoimmune hepatitis. Hepatocytes may show variable degrees of steatosis, necrosis, anisocytosis, and anisonucleosis. In later stages, atypical lipofuscin, canalicular cholestasis, and Kupffer cell iron accumulation may be noted. Periportal hepatocytes may contain glycogenated nuclei and Mallory hyalin. Cirrhosis is usually micronodular.

Copper and copper binding protein accumulation may be shown on tissue sections by histochemical techniques, such as rhodanine, rubeanic acid, orcein, or Victoria blue stains (Fig. 87.13). Copper deposition also may be seen in other chronic cholestatic liver diseases, such as primary biliary cirrhosis or primary sclerosing cholangitis, usually in zone 1 or periseptal hepatocytes; alternatively, the absence of stainable copper does not exclude the diagnosis of Wilson's disease. Copper quantitation in hepatic tissue is the diagnostic test and can be performed reliably on formalin-fixed, paraffin-embedded tissue. A value of greater than 250 µg/g dry hepatic tissue has been used as a cutoff. Currently, genetic testing has not yet become practical for clinical diagnosis.

α₁-Antitrypsin Deficiency

Liver injury in α_1-antitrypsin deficiency, an autosomal recessive inherited metabolic disorder, results from retention of mutant α_1-antitrypsin molecules in hepatocytes (Carrell & Lomas, 2002; Perlmutter, 2000). The histopathologic hallmark of the disease is the presence of eosinophilic globules of varying sizes in zone 1 hepatocytes in subjects older than infants. These globules are

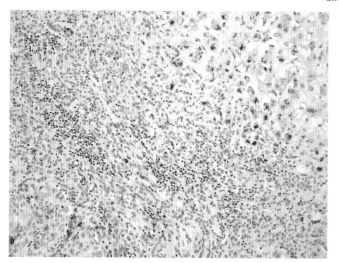

Fig. 87.13. Abundant copper deposition in a case of Wilson's disease. (Rhodanine stain.)

best shown by PAS-d stain (Fig. 87.14). Immunohistochemical stain may confirm the diagnosis. The globules can be seen in homozygous (PiZZ) and heterozygous (PiMZ) phenotypes, which may be determined by serum protein electrophoresis, but homozygous patients seem to be more likely to develop liver disease and cirrhosis. Other morphologic findings in the liver are relatively nonspecific, which may or may not include hepatitic inflammatory infiltration. When chronic hepatitis is seen in α_1-antitrypsin deficiency, other causes, such as HCV or alcohol, should be excluded (Ishak, 2002). Cirrhosis developing from α_1-antitrypsin deficiency can be micronodular, macronodular, biliary, or mixed in pattern.

Cryptogenic Cirrhosis

Cryptogenic cirrhosis refers to cases with no clinically or pathologically identifiable cause and is a diagnosis of exclusion. There is accumulating evidence, however, to suggest that a large

proportion of cryptogenic cirrhosis may represent burned-out nonalcoholic fatty liver disease. This suggestion is based on reported biopsy series of diagnosed NASH followed by subsequent cryptogenic cirrhosis with complete loss of the features of active steatohepatitis. In addition, several authors have shown that many of these patients have type 2 diabetes or obesity or both compared with patients with cirrhosis of other etiologies (Ayata et al, 2002; Caldwell et al, 1999; Ong et al, 2001; Poonawala et al, 2000; Sakugawa et al, 2003; Sanjeevi et al, 2003). Development of post-transplant nonalcoholic fatty liver disease also is frequent in this group of patients (Ong et al, 2001; Sanjeevi et al, 2003), but whether this represents actual recurrence of NASH or de novo NASH is an area of discussion (Czaja, 1997).

An autoimmune etiology also has been proposed based on clinical and histopathologic findings (Ayata et al, 2002; Kaymakoglu et al, 1998), but autoantibodies no longer may be detectable in these cases (Carpenter & Czaja, 2002). Primary sclerosing cholangitis and alcoholic cirrhosis may present as cryptogenic cirrhosis, and a case report documented prior biopsy-proven Budd-Chiari syndrome presenting as cryptogenic cirrhosis 34 years later (Havlioglu et al, 2003). Finally, the possibility of an as yet unknown viral infection or metabolic condition cannot be excluded in cryptogenic cirrhosis. Evaluation of patients with unexplained cirrhosis should include careful review of all prior liver biopsy specimens, especially those from several years prior.

NONCIRRHOTIC PORTAL HYPERTENSION

An increase in the pressure of the portal venous system can be seen in a heterogeneous group of prehepatic, intrahepatic, and posthepatic conditions in the absence of cirrhosis (Table 87.2). The etiopathogenetic mechanisms leading to portal hypertension in these conditions, the clinical presentation, and the prognosis vary widely (Molina and Reddy, 2001; Okuda, 2002). Portal hypertension in Budd-Chiari syndrome (see Ch. 100) is secondary to posthepatic vein obstruction and may have an acute or subacute clinical course with liver failure. Portal hypertension

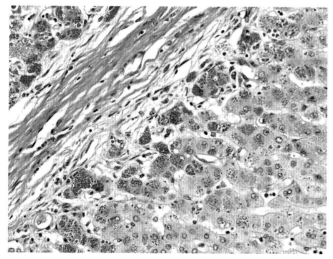

Fig. 87.14. Varying sized and shaped diastase-resistant hyaline globules in periseptal hepatocytes in α_1-antitrypsin deficiency. (PAS-d.)

Table 87.2 Causes of Noncirrhotic Portal Hypertension

Prehepatic
    Portal or splenic vein thrombosis
    Arterioportal shunt
    Tropical splenomegaly

Intrahepatic
    Nodular regenerative hyperplasia
    Partial nodular transformation
    Alcoholic hepatitis
    Drugs and toxins
    Sarcoidosis
    Schistosomiasis
    Veno-occlusive disease
    Hematologic disorders
    Congenital hepatic fibrosis
    Hereditary hemorrhagic telangiectasia
    Idiopathic portal hypertension

Posthepatic
    Budd-Chiari syndrome
    Congestive heart failure

Modified from Geller SA, Petrovic LM, 2004: Biopsy Interpretation of the Liver. Philadelphia, Lippincott Williams & Wilkins.

associated with infiltrative hematologic disorders, such as leukemia, mastocytosis, and Gaucher's disease, is believed to occur primarily at the intrahepatic sinusoidal level. Precirrhotic alcoholic hepatitis also may cause portal hypertension because of hepatocyte swelling, sinusoidal fibrosis, and central sclerosis, which may be more insidious clinically. Liver biopsy not only functions to confirm the absence of cirrhosis, but also helps to establish or suggest the diagnosis (Roskams et al, 2003). The histopathologic features of several selected entities associated with noncirrhotic portal hypertension are discussed briefly.

Nodular Regenerative Hyperplasia

Portal hypertension has been reported in about half of patients with nodular regenerative hyperplasia (Al-Mukhaizeem et al, 2004). It is associated with a wide range of conditions, mainly including hematologic disorders, connective tissue diseases, and medications. The pathogenesis is unclear, but may involve portal venous thrombosis leading to microcirculatory disturbance in the liver, which causes localized nonlethal ischemia and compensatory hyperplasia. The liver may be normal in size or enlarged when associated with a hematologic disease. On cut surface, the liver is diffusely nodular in appearance, with nodules ranging from 0.1 to 1 cm in diameter. Microscopically, the nodular appearance is best appreciated with reticulin stain (Fig. 87.15), which highlights regenerative hepatocytes within the nodules and atrophic hepatocytes at the edges of the nodules. Nodular regenerative hyperplasia differs from cirrhosis in that there is no or only minimal fibrosis, and the portal tract architecture is usually unaltered. These characteristic features may be shown more easily on a wedge biopsy specimen and may be difficult to appreciate on a needle biopsy specimen.

Partial nodular transformation is a rare condition with underlying pathogenesis similar to that proposed for nodular regenerative hyperplasia. Partial nodular transformation is a localized lesion almost always seen in the perihilar region. The hyperplastic hepatocyte nodules are larger than those of nodular regenerative hyperplasia, often well defined and surrounded by fibrous tissue.

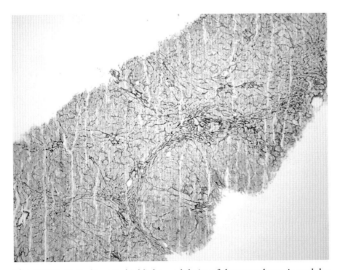

Fig. 87.15. Reticulin stain highlights nodularity of the parenchyma in nodular regenerative hyperplasia; no scar tissue (fibrous septum) is present (Sweet's reticulin.)

Venous Outflow Obstruction

Obstruction of hepatic venous outflow increases sinusoidal pressure and results in subsequent portal hypertension. Etiologically, it ranges from congestive heart failure, narrowing or occlusion of large hepatic veins (Budd-Chiari syndrome), to obliteration of the terminal or sublobular hepatic veins. Liver injury caused by congestive heart failure is characterized by zone 3 sinusoidal dilation and congestion and, when severe or acute, extravasation of red blood cells under the space of Disse into the hepatic cords. Hepatocellular necrosis is usually uncommon, but may become evident if accompanied by systemic hypotension and hypoperfusion. The portal tracts are typically unremarkable and devoid of significant inflammatory cell infiltration. In long-standing cases, zone 3 hepatocytes exhibit atrophic change with markedly attenuated cell plates. Lipofuscin pigment and sinusoidal lining cell iron may accrue. Perivenular fibrosis and bridging fibrosis also may develop and rarely may eventuate in septa formation, reverse lobulation, and cardiac cirrhosis.

Budd-Chiari syndrome results from obstruction at any level of the hepatic venous system between the liver and the inferior vena cava or the right atrium. It involves a variety of thrombotic and nonthrombotic causes, among which hypercoagulable states secondary to myeloproliferative disorders are the most common (Menon et al, 2004). The histopathologic features of Budd-Chiari syndrome are similar to those of congestive heart failure, but acute onset also may give rise to a hemorrhagic appearance at zone 3, with extravasation of red blood cells under the space of Disse to replace hepatocytes within the cords and more significant hepatocyte necrosis. If unrelieved, Budd-Chiari syndrome results in substantial fibrosis with eventual cirrhosis.

In contrast to Budd-Chiari syndrome, veno-occlusive disease rarely results in cirrhosis and has variable clinical manifestations ranging from elevation of liver function tests to life-threatening ascites and liver failure. This process affects the intrahepatic portion of the hepatic venous system and the terminal hepatic and sublobular veins. It has been stressed that the injury in this process is to the sinusoids and surrounding hepatocytes. DeLeve and colleagues (2002) recommended nomenclature change to *sinusoidal obstruction syndrome*. It is common after bone marrow or hematopoietic stem cell transplantation, is more likely to occur in HCV-infected subjects, and is associated with chemotherapeutic agents and hepatic radiation (Coppell et al, 2003; Kumar et al, 2003; Wadleigh et al, 2003). The lesion initially manifests subendothelial edema, zone 3 sinusoidal dilation, congestion, hemorrhage, and perivenular hepatocyte necrosis, followed by collagen deposition in the subendothelial space and sinusoids. As a result, the terminal hepatic veins become thickened, narrowed, and eventually obliterated by fibrosis (Fig. 87.16). Bridging fibrosis, cirrhosis, or nodular regenerative hyperplasia may ensue in more advanced cases.

Sarcoidosis

The histopathologic hallmark of hepatic sarcoidosis is the presence of multiple granulomas, composed of well-defined, rounded collections of epithelioid histiocytes rimmed by variable amounts of lymphocytes, multinucleated giant cells, plasma cells, and eosinophils (Ishak, 1998). The giant cells sometimes contain Schaumann and asteroid bodies. Small areas of central fibrinoid necrosis may be noted, but caseating necrosis as seen

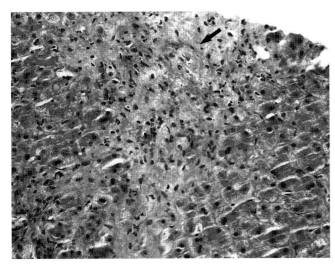

Fig. 87.16. This connective tissue stain highlights the lesions of veno-occlusive disease (sinusoidal obstruction syndrome). The remnants of the wall of the terminal hepatic venule are seen *(arrow)*; necrosis and dropout of the perivenular, zone 3 hepatocytes is appreciated. (Masson trichrome stain.)

able to differentiate them (Gaya et al, 2003; Valla & Benhamou, 2000). Common examples include primary biliary cirrhosis, HCV hepatitis, autoimmune hepatitis, mycobacterial or fungal infection, schistosomiasis, drug reaction, Hodgkin's lymphoma, and idiopathic granulomatous hepatitis. A diagnosis of hepatic sarcoidosis requires correlation with clinical, radiologic, and laboratory findings and cannot be rendered solely based on histopathologic examination.

Schistosomiasis

In endemic areas, infestation by *Schistosoma japonicum* or *Schistosoma mansoni* is a frequent cause of portal hypertension (Bica et al, 2000; Okuda, 2002). The mechanism involves ova deposition in the portal venules, which incites granulomatous inflammatory response and extensive, so-called clay pipestem fibrosis, leading to hemodynamic disturbance. Definitive diagnosis can be made by showing the presence of schistosomal ova.

Congenital Hepatic Fibrosis

Congenital hepatic fibrosis is a developmental disorder of the ductal plate predominantly seen in children and only rarely in adults. It is inherited in an autosomal recessive or, less commonly, autosomal dominant fashion and may be part of the spectrum of polycystic kidney disease (Kamath & Piccoli, 2003). The affected patient may present with portal hypertension. The liver is usually enlarged and of firm consistency. Microscopically, the portal tracts are expanded by fibrous tissue and may show portal-to-portal bridging fibrosis. An increased number of aberrant duct profiles is distributed at the periphery of the portal tracts, which are believed to represent remnants of incompletely remodeled ductal plates (Fig. 87.18). Inspissated bile may be noted in the lumina. The portal vein branches may be hypoplastic or decreased in number, but the branches of hepatic artery may be hypertrophic and abnormally numerous (Desmet, 1992), suggesting arteriovenous anastomosis.

in tuberculosis is never present. The granulomas typically are traversed by reticulin fibers and surrounded in a concentric fashion by collagen. They are noted scattered throughout the liver, but tend to be more frequent in the portal and periportal regions (Fig. 87.17). They may coalesce to become confluent masslike lesions. Portal hypertension may develop in some patients as a result of extensive fibrosis or cirrhosis, which may or may not be related directly to fibrous conversion and hyalinization of the granulomas. Portal hypertension also occurs in the absence of marked fibrosis, possibly as a result of compression of portal vein branches and sinusoids by granulomatous inflammation (Blich & Edoute, 2004; Valla & Benhamou, 2000). Nodular regenerative hyperplasia and Budd-Chiari syndrome also have been proposed as potential mechanisms.

Noncaseating granulomas can be identified in the liver in a wide variety of disorders, and the pathologist may not always be

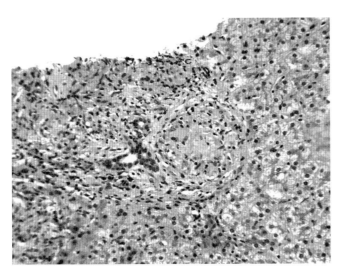

Fig. 87.17. Noncaseating, non-necrotizing epithelioid granulomas in a case of hepatic sarcoidosis.

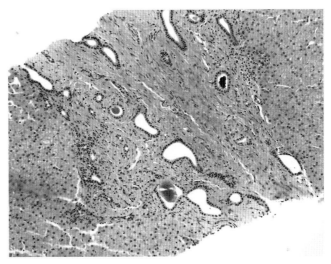

Fig. 87.18. Congenital hepatic fibrosis. The duct plate abnormality is manifested by remnant ductal profiles along the limiting plate; some of the duct structures contain inspissated bile.

Drugs and Toxins

Chronic liver injury by drugs and toxins may cause extensive fibrosis and cirrhosis, leading to portal hypertension. Examples include methotrexate toxicity, long-term exposure to arsenic or vinyl chloride, and chronic hypervitaminosis A. Drugs and toxins also induce noncirrhotic portal hypertension via different mechanisms, such as veno-occlusive disease, Budd-Chiari syndrome, and nodular regenerative hyperplasia. Herbal medicines have been increasingly recognized as hepatotoxic agents in recent years (Stedman, 2002). A classic example is pyrrolizidine alkaloids found in a variety of herbal medicines causing veno-occlusive disease and portal hypertension.

Idiopathic Portal Hypertension

As the name implies, idiopathic portal hypertension is a disorder of unknown etiology, characterized by splenomegaly, anemia, and long-standing portal hypertension in the absence of cirrhosis (Nakanuma et al, 2001; Okudaira et al, 2002). It is primarily a disorder of middle-aged adults and generally has a better prognosis than cirrhotic portal hypertension because the liver function is usually preserved. It is also called hepatoportal sclerosis and noncirrhotic portal fibrosis in the literature (Dhiman et al, 2002). Subtle differences may exist among these terms, however, which may reflect different underlying etiologies (Sarin & Kapoor, 2002).

Although the etiology is obscure, idiopathic portal hypertension frequently is associated with autoimmune disorders. Immunologic disturbance is thought to be involved in pathogenesis. Bacterial infection leading to repeated stimulation also has been proposed as a candidate mechanism, but remains speculative. In addition, some authors (Hillaire et al, 2002; Nakanuma et al, 2001; Sarin & Kapoor, 2002) suggest that prothrombotic disorders and thromboembolism play a role in etiopathogenesis, but this hypothesis has not been accepted by others (Okudaira et al, 2002).

Because idiopathic portal hypertension is essentially a diagnosis of exclusion, morphologic examination of liver tissue is imperative to rule out the presence of cirrhosis or other known etiology. The pathologic changes in idiopathic portal hypertension are believed to represent the effects of long-standing portal venous insufficiency, which may or may not be related to the initiating factors (Nakanuma et al, 2001). They are subtle, heterogeneous, and nonpathognomonic and may be missed on a needle biopsy specimen. Macroscopically, the liver may have a reduced weight, and the surface may be irregularly undulant or finely wrinkled, owing to subcapsular parenchymal atrophy. The cut surface may show portal and perivascular fibrosis, dilation and wall thickening of the veins, and unusual distribution and approximation of the portal and vascular structures. Microscopically, the normal relationship between the portal and central areas is distorted. The portal tracts are either abnormally approximated to each other or widely separated. The terminal hepatic vein may be eccentrically located in the lobule adjacent to a portal tract, and sometimes multiple ectatic tributaries are seen in a single lobule. Conspicuous fibrosis usually is present in the portal tracts, which may extend into the periportal areas and the lobules in a pericellular fashion. The portal veins may show loss of the normal muscle coat or marked wall thickening, and luminal narrowing or obliteration (Fig. 87.19).

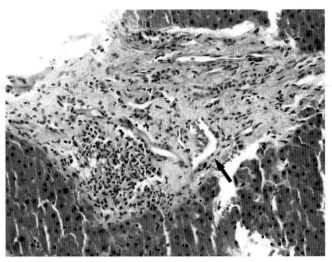

Fig. 87.19. Portal fibrosis in hepatoportal sclerosis (idiopathic portal hypertension). The portal vein *(arrow)* is small and has a narrowed lumen. (Masson trichrome stain.)

CONCLUSION

Long-standing portal hypertension causes serious extrahepatic complications. Common presentations include esophageal varices with variceal bleeding, portal hypertensive gastropathy, congestive splenomegaly with hypersplenism, and ascites with spontaneous bacterial peritonitis. Portal hypertension also contributes to the development of hepatic encephalopathy and hepatorenal syndrome. In general, portal hypertension secondary to a noncirrhotic etiology has a better prognosis than portal hypertension caused by liver cirrhosis because of maintained synthetic function. The characteristic morphologic features of many commonly encountered disorders underlying cirrhosis and noncirrhotic portal hypertension have been discussed in this chapter. Pathologic recognition of these entities would help in clinical management of patients with cirrhosis and portal hypertension.

REFERENCES

Afdhal NH, Nunes D, 2004: Evaluation of liver fibrosis: a concise review. Am J Gastroenterol 99:1160-1174.

Al-Mukhaizeem KA, et al, 2004: Nodular regenerative hyperplasia of the liver: an under-recognized cause of portal hypertension in hematological disorders. Am J Hematol 75:225-230.

Alvarez F, et al, 1999: International Autoimmune Hepatitis Group Report: review of criteria for diagnosis of autoimmune hepatitis. J Hepatol 31:929-938.

Angulo P, 2002: Nonalcoholic fatty liver disease. N Engl J Med 346:1221-1231.

Arthur MJ, 2002: Reversibility of liver fibrosis and cirrhosis following treatment for hepatitis C. Gastroenterology 122:1525-1528.

Ayata G, et al, 2002: Cryptogenic cirrhosis: clinicopathologic findings at and after liver transplantation. Hum Pathol 33:1098-1104.

Bacon BR, 2001: Hemochromatosis: diagnosis and management. Gastroenterology 120:718-725.

Bailey MA, Brunt EM, 2002: Hepatocellular carcinoma: predisposing conditions and precursor lesions. Gastroenterol Clin North Am 31:641-662.

Benyon RC, Arthur MJ, 2001: Extracellular matrix degradation and the role of hepatic stellate cells. Semin Liver Dis 21:373-384.

Bica I, et al, 2000: Hepatic schistosomiasis. Infect Dis Clin North Am 14:583-604.

Blich M, Edoute Y, 2004: Clinical manifestations of sarcoid liver disease. J Gastroenterol Hepatol 19:732-737.

Bonkovsky HL, et al, 2003: Iron as a co-morbid factor in nonhemochromatotic liver disease. Alcohol 30:137-144.

Bruix J, et al, 2001: Clinical management of hepatocellular carcinoma: conclusions of the Barcelona-2000 EASL conference. J Hepatol 35:421-430.

Brunt EM, 2000a: Liver biopsy interpretation for the gastroenterologist. Curr Gastroenterol Rep 2:27-32.

Brunt EM, 2000b: Grading and staging the histopathological lesions of chronic hepatitis: the Knodell histology activity index and beyond. Hepatology 31:241-246.

Brunt EM, 2002: Alcoholic and nonalcoholic steatohepatitis. Clin Liver Dis 6:399-420.

Brunt EM, 2004: Nonalcoholic steatohepatitis. Semin Liver Dis 24:3-20.

Brunt EM, Tiniakos DG, 2002: Steatosis, steatohepatitis: review of effects on chronic hepatitis C. Curr Hepatitis Rep 1:38-44.

Brunt EM, et al, 1999: Nonalcoholic steatohepatitis: a proposal for grading and staging the histological lesions. Am J Gastroenterol 94:2467-2474.

Brunt EM, et al, 2003: Concurrence of histologic features of steatohepatitis with other forms of chronic liver disease. Mod Pathol 16:49-56.

Caldwell SH, 1999: Cryptogenic cirrhosis: clinical characterization and risk factors for underlying disease. Hepatology 29:664-669.

Canbay A, et al, 2004: Apoptosis: the nexus of liver injury and fibrosis. Hepatology 39:273-278.

Carpenter HA, Czaja AJ, 2002: The role of histologic evaluation in the diagnosis and management of autoimmune hepatitis and its variants. Clin Liver Dis 6:397-417.

Carrell RW, Lomas DA, 2002: Alpha₁-antitrypsin deficiency: a model for conformational diseases. N Engl J Med 346:45-53.

Caturelli E, et al, 2004: Ultrasound-guided fine needle biopsy of early hepatocellular carcinoma complicating liver cirrhosis: a multicentre study. Gut 53:1356-1362.

Chedid A, 2000: Regression of human cirrhosis. Arch Pathol Lab Med 124:1591.

Coppell JA, et al, 2003: Veno-occlusive disease: cytokines, genetics, and haemostasis. Blood Rev 17:63-70.

Cullen S, Chapman R, 2003: Primary sclerosing cholangitis. Autoimmun Rev 2:305-312.

Czaja AJ, 1997: Recurrence of nonalcoholic steatohepatitis after liver transplantation. Liver Transpl Surg 3:185-186.

DeLeve LD, et al, 2002: Toxic injury to hepatic sinusoids: sinusoidal obstruction syndrome (veno-occlusive disease). Semin Liver Dis 22:27-42.

Desmet VJ, 1992: What is congenital hepatic fibrosis? Histopathology 20:465-477.

Desmet VJ, Roskams T, 2003: Reversal of cirrhosis: evidence-based medicine? Gastroenterology 125:629-630.

de Torres M, Poynard T, 2003: Risk factors for liver fibrosis progression in patients with chronic hepatitis C. Ann Hepatol 2:5-11.

Dhiman RK, et al, 2002: Non-cirrhotic portal fibrosis (idiopathic portal hypertension): experience with 151 patients and a review of the literature. J Gastroenterol Hepatol 17:6-16.

Dienes HP, et al, 2002: Autoimmune hepatitis and overlap syndromes. Clin Liver Dis 6:349-362.

Durazzo M, et al, 2003: Overlap syndromes of autoimmune hepatitis: what is known so far. Dig Dis Sci 48:423-430.

Fallowfield JA, Iredale JP, 2004: Reversal of liver fibrosis and cirrhosis—an emerging reality. Scott Med J 49:3-6.

Farci P, 2003: Delta hepatitis: an update. J Hepatol 39:S212-S219.

Fattovich G, 2003: Natural history and prognosis of hepatitis B. Semin Liver Dis 23:47-58.

Ferenci P, 2004: Diagnosis and current therapy of Wilson's disease. Aliment Pharmacol Ther 19:157-165.

Friedman SL, 2000: Molecular regulation of hepatic fibrosis, an integrated cellular response to tissue injury. J Biol Chem 275:2247-2250.

Ganem D, Prince AM, 2004: Hepatitis B virus infection: natural history and clinical consequences. N Engl J Med 350:1118-1129.

Gaya DR, et al, 2003: Hepatic granulomas: a 10 year single centre experience. J Clin Pathol 56:850-853.

Geller SA, 2000: Coming or going? What is cirrhosis? Arch Pathol Lab Med 124:1587-1588.

Gitlin JD, 2003: Wilson disease. Gastroenterology 125:1868-1877.

Guido M, Rugge M, 2004: Liver biopsy sampling in chronic viral hepatitis. Semin Liver Dis 24:89-97.

Haber PS, et al, 2003: Pathogenesis and management of alcoholic hepatitis. J Gastroenterol Hepatol 18:1332-1344.

Havlioglu N, et al, 2003: Budd-Chiari syndrome and hepatocellular carcinoma: a case report and review of the literature. Am J Gastroenterol 98:201-204.

Hillaire S, et al, 2002: Idiopathic non-cirrhotic intrahepatic portal hypertension in the West: a re-evaluation in 28 patients. Gut 51:275-280.

Hytiroglou P, 2004: Morphological changes of early human hepatocarcinogenesis. Semin Liver Dis 24:65-75.

International Working Party, 1995: Terminology of nodular hepatocellular lesions. Hepatology 22:983-993.

Iredale JP, et al, 1998: Mechanisms of spontaneous resolution of rat liver fibrosis: hepatic stellate cell apoptosis and reduced hepatic expression of metalloproteinase inhibitors. J Clin Invest 102:538-549.

Ishak KG, 1998: Sarcoidosis of the liver and bile ducts. Mayo Clin Proc 73:467-472.

Ishak KG, 2002: Inherited metabolic diseases of the liver. Clin Liver Dis 6:455-479.

Issa R, et al, 2004: Spontaneous recovery from micronodular cirrhosis: evidence for incomplete resolution associated with matrix cross-linking. Gastroenterology 126:1795-1808.

Kamath BM, Piccoli DA, 2003: Heritable disorders of the bile ducts. Gastroenterol Clin North Am 32:857-875.

Karsan HA, et al, 2004: Primary prevention of cirrhosis: public health strategies that can make a difference. Postgrad Med 115:25-30.

Kaymakoglu S, et al, 1998: Is severe cryptogenic chronic hepatitis similar to autoimmune hepatitis? J Hepatol 28:78-83.

Kojiro M, 2004: Focus on dysplastic nodules and early hepatocellular carcinoma: an Eastern point of view. Liver Transpl 10:S3-S8.

Kumar S, et al, 2003: Hepatic veno-occlusive disease (sinusoidal obstruction syndrome) after hematopoietic stem cell transplantation. Mayo Clin Proc 78:589-598.

Lai CL, et al, 2003: Viral hepatitis B. Lancet 362:2089-2094.

Lai MM, 2002: Hepatitis C virus proteins: direct link to hepatic oxidative stress, steatosis, carcinogenesis and more. Gastroenterology 122:568-571.

LeClercq IA, et al, 2002: Leptin is essential for the hepatic fibrogenic response to chronic liver injury. J Hepatol 37:206-213.

Leuschner U, 2003: Primary biliary cirrhosis: presentation and diagnosis. Clin Liver Dis 7:741-758.

Limdi JK, Crampton JR, 2004: Hereditary haemochromatosis. QJM 97:315-324.

Lonardo A, et al, 2004: Steatosis and hepatitis C virus: mechanisms and significance for hepatic and extrahepatic disease. Gastroenterology 126:586-597.

Marchesini G, et al, 2001: Nonalcoholic fatty liver disease: a feature of the metabolic syndrome. Diabetes 50:1844-1850.

McCaughan GW, George J, 2004: Fibrosis progression in chronic hepatitis C virus infection. Gut 53:318-321.

McFarlane IG, 2002a: Autoimmune hepatitis: diagnostic criteria, subclassifications, and clinical features. Clin Liver Dis 6:317-333.

McFarlane IG, 2002b: Definition and classification of autoimmune hepatitis. Semin Liver Dis 22:317-324.

Mendes FD, Lindor KD, 2004: Primary sclerosing cholangitis. Clin Liver Dis 8:195-211.

Menon KV, et al, 2001: Pathogenesis, diagnosis, and treatment of alcoholic liver disease. Mayo Clin Proc 76:1021-1029.

Menon KV, et al, 2004: The Budd-Chiari syndrome. N Engl J Med 350:578-585.

Misdraji J, et al, 2004: Autoimmune hepatitis with centrilobular necrosis. Am J Surg Pathol 28:471-478.

Molina E, Reddy KR, 2001: Noncirrhotic portal hypertension. Clin Liver Dis 5:769-787.

Nakanuma Y, et al, 2001: Pathology and pathogenesis of idiopathic portal hypertension with an emphasis on the liver. Pathol Res Pract 197:65-76.

O'Connor PG, Schottenfeld RS, 1998: Patients with alcohol problems. N Engl J Med 338:592-602.

Okuda K, 2002: Non-cirrhotic portal hypertension versus idiopathic portal hypertension. J Gastroenterol Hepatol 17:S204-S213.

Okudaira M, et al, 2002: Idiopathic portal hypertension and its pathology. Semin Liver Dis 22:59-72.

Ong J, et al, 2001: Cryptogenic cirrhosis and posttransplantation nonalcoholic fatty liver disease. Liver Transpl 7:797-801.

Perlmutter DH, 2000: Liver injury in alpha 1-antitrypsin deficiency. Clin Liver Dis 4:387-408.

Pietrangelo A, 2004: Hereditary hemochromatosis: a new look at an old disease. N Engl J Med 350:2383-2397.

Pinzani M, Marra F, 2001: Cytokine receptors and signaling in hepatic stellate cells. Semin Liver Dis 21:397-416.

Pol S, et al, 2004: Reversibility of hepatitis C virus-related cirrhosis. Hum Pathol 35:107-112.

Poonawala A, et al, 2000: Prevalence of obesity and diabetes in patients with cryptogenic cirrhosis: a case-control study. Hepatology 32:689-692.

Poynard T, et al, 2002: Impact of pegylated interferon alfa-2b and ribavirin on liver fibrosis in patients with chronic hepatitis C. Gastroenterology 122:1303-1313.

Poynard T, et al, 2003: Viral hepatitis C. Lancet 362:2095-2100.

Ramadori G, Saile B, 2004: Portal tract fibrogenesis in the liver. Lab Invest 84:153-159.

Ramalho F, 2003: Hepatitis C virus infection and liver steatosis. Antiviral Res 60:125-127.

Ray MB, 2000: Regression of cirrhosis: a timely topic. Arch Pathol Lab Med 124:1589-1590.

Rodriguez HJ, Bass NM, 2003: Primary sclerosing cholangitis. Semin Gastrointest Dis 14:189-198.

Roncalli M, 2004: Hepatocellular nodules in cirrhosis: focus on diagnostic criteria on liver biopsy: a Western experience. Liver Transpl 10:S9-S15.

Roskams TA, et al, 2003: Histopathology of portal hypertension: a practical guideline. Histopathology 42:2-13.

Roskams TA, et al, 2004: Nomenclature of the finer branches of the biliary tree: canals, ductules, and ductular reactions in human livers. Hepatology 39:1739-1745.

Rubbia-Brandt L, et al, 2004: Steatosis affects chronic hepatitis C progression in a genotype specific way. Gut 53:406-412.

Sakugawa H, et al, 2003: Clinical characteristics of patients with cryptogenic liver cirrhosis in Okinawa, Japan. Hepatogastroenterology 50:2005-2008.

Salt WB II, 2004: Nonalcoholic fatty liver disease (NAFLD): a comprehensive review. J Insur Med 36:27-41.

Sanjeevi A, et al, 2003: Outcomes of liver transplantation for cryptogenic cirrhosis: a single-center study of 71 patients. Transplant Proc 35:2977-2980.

Sarin SK, Kapoor D, 2002: Non-cirrhotic portal fibrosis: current concepts and management. J Gastroenterol Hepatol 17:526-534.

Selmi C, et al, 2004: Epidemiology and pathogenesis of primary biliary cirrhosis. J Clin Gastroenterol 38:264-271.

Stedman C, 2002: Herbal hepatotoxicity. Semin Liver Dis 22:195-206.

Suriawinata A, Xu R, 2004: An update on the molecular genetics of hepatocellular carcinoma. Semin Liver Dis 24:77-88.

te Sligte K, et al, 2004: Nonalcoholic steatohepatitis: review of a growing medical problem. Eur J Intern Med 15:10-21.

Tome S, Lucey MR, 2004: Current management of alcoholic liver disease. Aliment Pharmacol Ther 19:707-714.

Valla DC, Benhamou JP, 2000: Hepatic granulomas and hepatic sarcoidosis. Clin Liver Dis 4:269-285.

Vergani D, Mieli-Vergani G, 2003: Autoimmune hepatitis. Autoimmun Rev 2:241-247.

Vierling JM, 2004: Primary biliary cirrhosis and autoimmune cholangiopathy. Clin Liver Dis 8:177-194.

Wadleigh M, et al, 2003: Hepatic veno-occlusive disease: pathogenesis, diagnosis and treatment. Curr Opin Hematol 10:451-462.

Wanless IR, et al, 2000: Regression of human cirrhosis: morphologic features and the genesis of incomplete septal cirrhosis. Arch Pathol Lab Med 124:1599-1607.

Zafrani ES, 2004: Nonalcoholic fatty liver disease: an emerging pathological spectrum. Virchows Arch 444:3-12.

Management of Liver Failure

88

J. G. O'GRADY

Liver failure presents as one of two distinct clinical problems—the specific entity of *acute liver failure* (a term that is used interchangeably with *fulminant hepatic failure*) and the more frequently encountered scenario of an episode of acute decompensation of established chronic liver disease, called *acute-on-chronic liver failure*. Acute liver failure evolves after a catastrophic insult to the liver and results in the development of encephalopathy within days or weeks of the liver injury. Acute-on-chronic liver failure usually occurs in patients with cirrhosis and often is precipitated by infection or gastrointestinal hemorrhage. The principles of management are similar in some respects (e.g., encephalopathy, coagulopathy), but very different in others (e.g., cerebral edema is observed almost exclusively in acute liver failure). This chapter focuses mainly on acute liver failure unless otherwise specified.

Acute liver failure is a heterogeneous condition that incorporates a range of clinical syndromes. The dominant factors that give rise to this heterogeneity are the underlying etiology (which varies significantly from country to country [Table 88.1]), the age of the patient, and the duration of time over which the disease evolves. Natural history studies indicate that survival rates without liver transplantation range from 10% to 90%, with the best outcomes seen in patients with pregnancy-related syndromes, acetaminophen overdose, and hepatitis A. Survival rates are poor in older patients and possibly in very young children. The rate of progression of the disease is used to subclassify patients into groups with differing clinical problems and outcomes. There is a lack of universal agreement on terminology, but the terms *hyperacute liver failure* (encephalopathy within 7 days of the onset of jaundice), *acute liver failure* (encephalopathy within 8-28 days of the onset of jaundice), and *subacute liver failure* (encephalopathy >28 days of the onset of jaundice) are used in this chapter.

ETIOLOGY OF ACUTE LIVER FAILURE

Viruses and drugs account for most cases of acute liver failure, although many patients have no definable cause. The latter condition is referred to as *seronegative hepatitis* in this chapter, but is also known as *non-A–E hepatitis* and *acute liver failure of indeterminate etiology*. The overall incidence of acute liver failure complicating acute hepatitis in the United States is 0.9%, and this equates to about 2000 deaths annually. Most drug-induced cases are rare idiosyncratic reactions, but some, such as acetaminophen, are at least in part dose-related toxic events.

Viral

Acute liver failure is a rare complication of hepatitis A infection, occurring in 0.14% to 0.35% of hospitalized cases and in 0.4% of all cases seen in the United States. The incidence of acute liver failure after hepatitis B is 1% to 4% of hospitalized patients.

In early studies, hepatitis D coinfection or superinfection was thought to increase the risk because it was found in 34% to 43% of patients with acute liver failure secondary to hepatitis B compared with 4% to 19% of less severe cases. The prevalence of hepatitis D seems to have decreased dramatically in recent years, however. Vaccination and antiviral therapy with drugs such as lamivudine and adefovir should alter the observed pattern of hepatitis B–related acute liver failure (Sjogren, 2003). The risk of developing acute liver failure after exposure to hepatitis C seems to be very low. Hepatitis E is common in parts of Asia and Africa, and the risk of developing acute liver failure ranges from 0.6% to 2.8% to greater than 20% in pregnant women, being particularly high during the third trimester. Hepatitis E also is encountered in Europe and the United States and may account for 8% of cases that previously would have been described as seronegative hepatitis.

Seronegative hepatitis is a common cause of acute liver failure in some parts of the Western world. It is doubtful this is a viral infection because most cases are sporadic; unidentified toxins or autoimmune processes may be the true underlying mechanisms. Middle-aged women are affected most frequently, and the risk of developing acute liver failure has been calculated at 2.3% to 4.7% of hospitalized cases.

Drugs

Acetaminophen (paracetamol) overdose is the most common cause of acute liver failure in the United Kingdom and the United States (Bernal, 2003; Lee, 2003). The drug usually is taken with suicidal or parasuicidal intent, but 8% to 30% of cases of acute liver failure follow the therapeutic use of acetaminophen. This is because of unintentional overdosing or accelerated metabolism in individuals with liver enzyme induction as a consequence of antiepileptic therapy or regular alcohol usage.

Estimates of the risk of developing acute liver failure as a result of an idiosyncratic reaction range from 0.001% for nonsteroidal

Table 88.1 Geographic Variation in the Etiology of Acute Liver Failure*

	U.K.	U.S.	France	India
Acetaminophen (paracetamol)	54	40	2	—
Drug reactions	7	12	15	5
Seronegative hepatitis	17	17	18	24
Hepatitis A or B	14	12	49	33
Hepatitis E	—	—	—	38
Other causes	8	19	16	—

*All values in table are percentages.

anti-inflammatory drugs to 1% for the isoniazid/rifampicin combination. The diagnosis is made on the basis of a temporal relationship between exposure to the drug and the development of acute liver failure; common offending drugs are listed in Table 88.2. Most cases develop during the first exposure to the drug, but some, such as with halothane, occur in sensitized individuals on the second or subsequent exposure. Nontherapeutic drugs also cause acute liver failure (e.g., Ecstasy [3,4-methylene-dioxymethamphetamine], which has been associated with numerous clinical syndromes ranging from rapidly progressive acute liver failure associated with malignant hyperpyrexia to subacute liver failure.

Other Etiologies

Acute liver failure associated with pregnancy tends to occur during the third trimester. Three discrete entities have been described, although considerable overlap is frequently observed. Acute fatty liver of pregnancy usually occurs in primagravid women carrying a male fetus and is characterized by severe microvesicular steatosis. The *HELLP* syndrome is defined as the combination of *h*emolysis, *e*levated *l*iver enzymes and *l*ow *p*latelets. Acute liver failure complicating preeclampsia or eclampsia typically exhibits high serum transaminase levels and abnormal tissue perfusion patterns on computed tomography that reflect the microvascular infarction characteristic of this condition.

Wilson's disease may present as acute liver failure, usually during the teens. It is characterized clinically by a Coombs' negative hemolytic anemia and demonstrable Kayser-Fleischer rings in most cases. The serum ceruloplasmin levels are usually, but not invariably, low, and the serum and urinary copper levels are increased. Poisoning with *Amanita phalloides* (mushrooms) is seen most commonly in central Europe, South Africa, and the West coast of the United States. Severe diarrhea, often with vomiting, is a typical feature and starts 5 or more hours after ingestion of the mushrooms; liver failure develops 4 to 5 days later. Autoimmune chronic hepatitis may present as acute liver failure, but by then it is usually beyond treatment with corticosteroid or other immunosuppressive therapy. Budd-Chiari syndrome may present with acute liver failure; the diagnosis is suggested by hepatomegaly and confirmed by the demonstration of hepatic vein thrombosis. Malignancy infiltration, especially with lymphoma, is another rare cause of acute liver failure that typically is associated with hepatomegaly. Ischemic hepatitis is increasingly recognized as a cause of acute liver failure, especially in older patients. Other unusual causes of acute liver failure include heatstroke and sepsis.

Pediatric Causes

Children are at risk of developing most of the causes of acute liver failure already discussed, but also have some unique underlying causes, especially in the category of metabolic disease. Neonatal hemochromatosis presents within the first few weeks of life and has been treated by liver transplantation at 5 days of age (Rodrigues et al, 2005). Acute liver failure secondary to mitochondrial disorders may be triggered by bacterial infections and is characterized by high lactate levels in blood. Other metabolic causes include tyrosinemia, galactosemia, and fructose intolerance. Young infants can develop acute liver failure with viral infections, such as adenovirus, coxsackievirus, and cytomegalovirus.

DIAGNOSIS

The diagnosis of acute liver failure is a clinical one based on the detection of evidence of encephalopathy in patients with acute liver disease. The diagnosis of encephalopathy is made on overt clinical criteria, but psychometric testing may be useful in patients with subacute liver failure to detect subtle changes to mental state. Commonly, hypoglycemia and, unusually, uremia may mimic hepatic encephalopathy in patients with acute liver failure, and these need to be excluded before the diagnosis is confirmed.

The cause of acute liver failure must be identified accurately. Tables 88.3 and 88.4 outline the key essential investigations and the investigations that are relevant in certain circumstances. Imaging of the liver assesses the size and shape of the liver and screens for portal hypertension. The detection of portal hypertension does not always indicate chronic liver disease because

Table 88.2 Drugs That Cause Acute Liver Failure

Category 1—Common Causes

Acetaminophen (paracetamol)
Halothane
Isoniazid/rifampicin
Nonsteroidal anti-inflammatory drugs
Sulfonamides
Flutamide
Sodium valproate
Carbamazepine
Ecstasy (3,4-methylenedioxymethamphetamine)

Category 2—Rare Causes

Benoxaprofen
Phenytoin
Isoflurane
Enflurane
Tetracycline
Allopurinol
Ketoconazole
Monoamine oxidase inhibitors
Disulfiram
Methyldopa
Amiodarone
Tricyclic antidepressants
Propylthiouracil
Gold
Dideoxyinosine

Table 88.3 Core Investigation of Cause of Acute Liver Failure

Cause	Investigation
Hepatitis A virus	IgM anti–hepatitis A virus
Hepatitis B virus and hepatitis D virus	IgM anti-core, hepatitis B virus DNA*
Hepatitis E virus	Anti–hepatitis E virus
Paracetamol	Drug levels in blood

*Hepatitis B surface antigen may be negative.

Table 88.4   Extended Investigation of the Cause of Acute Liver Failure

Cause	Investigation
Idiosyncratic drug reactions	Eosinophil count, histology
Autoimmune	Autoantibodies, immunoglobulins
Pregnancy-related syndromes	
Fatty liver	Ultrasound, uric acid, histology
HELLP syndrome	Platelet count
Toxemia	Serum transaminases
Wilson's disease	Urinary copper, ceruloplasmin, slit lamp examination
Budd-Chiari syndrome	Ultrasound or venography
Malignancy	Imaging, histology
Ischemic hepatitis	Transaminases

Table 88.5   Findings That Suggest Acute Alcoholic Hepatitis

Hepatomegaly
Marked elevation of gamma-glutamyltransferase
Elevated white blood cell count not responding to antibiotics
Elevated IgA level
Appearance of fatty infiltration on ultrasound

ascites or splenomegaly or both may be seen in subacute liver failure and acute Wilson's disease.

Histologic assessment of liver tissue may aid in the diagnosis of the cause of acute liver failure. Confluent necrosis is the most common histologic finding, and this may be zonal or involve all of the parenchyma. Necrosis that is zonal within the acinus and coagulative or eosinophilic is more likely to be secondary to a toxic insult or ischemia. The features of necrosis and parenchymal collapse may be interspersed with evidence of regeneration, occurring in a diffuse pattern of small areas throughout the liver or in random larger nodules that give the "maplike pattern" that has been described in this condition. The latter pattern is seen most commonly in patients with subacute liver failure.

Histologic features may suggest specific diagnoses, including sodium valproate toxicity, malignant infiltration, Wilson's disease, pregnancy-related syndromes, and Budd-Chiari syndrome. Sodium valproate toxicity is characterized by microvesicular steatosis. Screening for malignant infiltration as the cause of acute liver failure is a strong indication for performing a liver biopsy in this condition. Patients with Wilson's disease who present with acute liver failure usually have established cirrhosis, commonly associated with interface hepatitis resembling autoimmune disease, hepatocyte ballooning, and steatosis. Liver histology may be useful in making a precise diagnosis within the spectrum of pregnancy-related liver diseases. The histologic features of Budd-Chiari syndrome are extreme sinusoidal dilation, congestion, and coagulative necrosis.

Liver biopsy also may assist differentiating acute liver failure from established cirrhosis and from acute alcoholic hepatitis, whether or not it is associated with cirrhosis. The former scenario usually can be distinguished on clinical grounds, but acute alcoholic hepatitis can present with clinical features similar to subacute liver failure. A history of high alcohol consumption may not be available, but the diagnosis of acute alcoholic hepatitis is suggested by the investigational findings outlined in Table 88.5.

PROGNOSIS

In acute liver failure, the grade of encephalopathy correlates strongly with outcome, and this is true for the grade of encephalopathy at the time of presentation to a specialist unit and the maximum grade attained. The prognosis deteriorates further when grade 4 encephalopathy is complicated by cerebral edema and further still when the latter coexists with renal failure. Other patients with acute liver failure have a very poor prognosis, however, despite the absence of cerebral edema and renal failure. This is especially true of patients with subacute liver failure, who, in addition, often do not manifest severely abnormal coagulation parameters.

The use of transplantation intensified the need for early indicators of prognosis so that patients in need of this intervention could be identified as quickly as possible. The King's College criteria, with some modifications, still are widely used to identify patients most in need of liver transplantation (Tables 88.6 and 88.7). The acetaminophen criteria have been found to be specific, but lack adequate sensitivity. Serum lactate levels (levels >3.5 mg/dL before resuscitation and >3 mg/dL after resuscitation) have been suggested as an alternative or supplementary assessment of prognosis in these patients (Bernal et al, 2002). Another problem with these criteria is the difficulty applying the coagulation parameters outside the United Kingdom. The scale on which prothrombin times are reported in the United States is dramatically shorter than in the United Kingdom reflecting differences in technique and the reagents used, and the implementation of the international normalized ratio has not resolved this problem entirely because of loss of accuracy at higher readings. In France, factor V levels are used in preference to prothrombin time or international normalized ratio. Factor V levels less than 20% in patients younger than 30 years and less than 30% in older patients indicate a poor prognosis when encephalopathy develops.

Assessment of the volume of viable hepatocytes by histologic examination is considered by some investigators to be of prognostic value, but the potential for sampling error is considerable. The critical mass that suggests a good prognosis has been calculated at between 25% and 40%. A small liver on clinical or radiologic assessment or more particularly a liver that is found to be shrinking rapidly is another poor prognostic indicator that is especially useful in subacute liver failure.

Table 88.6   Indicators of a Poor Prognosis in Acetaminophen-Induced Acute Liver Failure

Arterial pH <7.25 >24 hr after drug ingestion and after adequate fluid resuscitation
Serum lactate >3.5 mg/dL or >3 mg/dL after adequate fluid resuscitation

All of the following concomitantly:
  Prothrombin time >100 sec or international normalized ratio >6.5
  Creatinine >3.5 mg/dL or anuria
  Grade 3-4 encephalopathy

Table 88.7 Indicators of Poor Prognosis in Nonacetaminophen Causes of Acute Liver Failure

Prothrombin time >100 sec or international normalized ratio >6.7
Any 3 of the following:
Unfavorable etiology (seronegative hepatitis or drug reaction)
Age <10 or >40 yr
Acute or subacute categories (i.e., jaundiced >7 days)
Serum bilirubin >17 mg/dL
Prothrombin time >50 sec or international normalized ratio >3.5
Acute presentation of Wilson's disease

MANAGEMENT

Overall Strategy

In acute liver failure, the overall strategy is a combination of intensive medical care, liver transplantation in selected patients (see Ch. 105), and, to some degree, the use of a liver support device (see Ch. 89). Management starts with identification of etiology and an initial assessment of prognosis, which is progressively updated. Appropriate patients should be referred to specialist centers where monitoring is instituted and a decision on the need for immediate liver transplantation is made. Patients are monitored for the complications that may develop, and these are treated as they emerge to the point of recovery, death, or transplantation.

Patients with acute-on-chronic liver failure often require, and benefit from, intensive monitoring. This monitoring is especially appropriate when the deterioration has been triggered by a specific reversible complication. It also is appropriate in patients who are active candidates for liver transplantation. Liver support systems (particularly molecular absorbent recirculation system) are being increasingly used in this situation. Ascites and bleeding varices are frequently important components of the clinical problem; the management of these is discussed in Chs. 90-92.

General Measures in Liver Failure

Many drugs have well-defined roles in specific etiologies of acute liver failure. N-acetyl cysteine is established as an antedote to acetaminophen hepatotoxicity when given within 16 to 24 hours of the overdose, but it also has been shown to be beneficial in reducing mortality and cerebral edema when started up to 36 hours after the overdose. Even later, N-acetyl cysteine may improve tissue oxygen delivery and consumption. A trial of N-acetyl cysteine in other etiologies of acute liver failure is in progress in the United States. Penicillin, and possibly silymarin, should be added at the earliest opportunity to the standard supportive measures in patients with A. phalloides (mushroom) toxicity. Patients with Wilson's disease or autoimmune hepatitis presenting with acute liver failure rarely respond to penicillamine or immunosuppressive therapy, respectively. Patients with severe acute alcoholic hepatitis may benefit from corticosteroid therapy or treatment with pentoxifylline. Neither corticosteroids nor pentoxifylline is indicated in acute-on-chronic episodes of alcoholic cirrhosis in the absence of the component of alcoholic hepatitis.

MANAGEMENT OF SPECIFIC COMPLICATIONS

Neurologic Complications

Encephalopathy is invariably present in acute liver failure and often present in acute-on-chronic liver failure. Patients with grades 1 and 2 encephalopathy exhibit degrees of drowsiness or disorientation, but they can be roused, and they respond appropriately to verbal stimuli. Patients with chronic liver disease usually have a hepatic flap and fetor hepaticus, but these classic features of encephalopathy are usually absent in patients with acute liver failure and an equivalent degree of encephalopathy. In acute liver failure, progression to grade 3 encephalopathy often is heralded by a short period of extreme agitation before the patient becomes confused and at best obeys simple commands. Grade 4 encephalopathy signifies deep coma with the patient being responsive at best to painful stimuli. Most patients in this situation require intubation and supported ventilation.

Cerebral edema is common in acute liver failure, especially hyperacute and subacute liver failure, but has been described in only a few patients with cirrhosis. There is some evidence that the incidence of cerebral edema is decreasing with modern management protocols, but the precise reason for this change has not been specified. Nevertheless, it remains a major cause of death and frequently disqualifies patients from transplantation. The clinical features of cerebral edema include systemic hypertension, decerebrate posturing, hyperventilation, abnormal pupillary reflexes, and ultimately impairment of brainstem reflexes and functions. Papilledema is rarely seen, however. Cerebral edema can be life-threatening by means of classic brainstem herniation or hypoxic brain damage.

Encephalopathy with acute-on-chronic liver failure is managed with dietary protein restriction, lactulose, and phosphate enemas, usually with good effect. Treatment of triggering events also is important (Table 88.8). In contrast, specific management options for encephalopathy are limited in acute liver failure. Patients with subacute liver failure may benefit from the measures used in chronic liver disease. These approaches are ineffective, however, in the treatment of the more rapidly progressive encephalopathy characteristic of the hyperacute and acute syndromes. No convincing data have emerged to support the use of branched chain amino acids or flumazenil.

Mannitol is the mainstay of treatment of surges in intracranial pressure that may compromise brainstem function. A rapid bolus of 0.3 to 1 g/kg is recommended to achieve the maximal diuretic effect, and in anuric patients diuresis is simulated by ultrafiltrating 3× the administered volume over the subsequent 30 minutes. This process is repeated as determined by the pattern

Table 88.8 Common Precipitants of Acute-on-Chronic Hepatic Encephalopathy

Infection
Constipation
Gastrointestinal bleed
Large dietary protein intake
Narcotic drugs
Benzodiazepines

of clinical relapses until the serum osmolarity exceeds 320 mOsm. More recent studies showed that the administration of mannitol was followed by an increase in cerebral blood flow associated with an increase in cerebral metabolic rate for oxygen and reduced brain lactate formation. Sodium thiopentone (phenobarbitone) was shown to control cerebral edema that had become unresponsive to mannitol in an uncontrolled study, but has not been subjected to a controlled trial and has not been shown to improve the survival rate. Acute, but not chronic, hyperventilation was reported to be beneficial in reducing critical surges in intracranial hypertension. Nevertheless, hyperventilation to Pco_2 levels less than 25 mm Hg is routinely incorporated as a first-line treatment in the United States. Hypothermia and hypertonic saline infusions also have been shown in small studies to be useful adjuncts in the management of intracranial hypertension (Murphy et al, 2004).

In the later stages of neurologic complications, the emphasis of management changes to the preservation of cerebral perfusion pressure, increased oxygen delivery to the brain, and manipulation of the neuronal microcirculation to promote cerebral oxygen extraction. The patient should be nursed with the trunk at a 0 to 10 degrees to the horizontal. The options for increasing the mean arterial pressure and consequently improving cerebral perfusion pressure are outlined in the section dealing with hemodynamics. These adjustments are made to maintain a cerebral perfusion pressure greater than 50 mm Hg when possible. At this stage of the complication, spontaneous recovery is unlikely without liver transplantation, and hepatectomy is useful to secure transient improvement. Occult seizure activity may contribute to neurologic instability in patients with grade 4 encephalopathy. Phenytoin and diazepam are effective therapies, despite the theoretical consideration that the latter may aggravate the underlying encephalopathy.

The use of intracranial pressure monitoring is controversial and has not been subjected to clinical trials. Early detection of cerebral edema and the facility to monitor this complication constantly help to optimize therapeutic interventions. Intracranial pressure monitoring allows earlier and more accurate detection of pressure changes, especially in a ventilated patient in whom most of the clinical signs are masked, and it facilitates careful monitoring of the intracranial pressure during high-risk therapeutic interventions, such as hemodialysis and tracheal suctioning. It also is considered valuable during orthotopic liver transplantation because increases in intracranial pressure often occur during the dissection and reperfusion phases of the transplant operation. The most commonly used system places transducers on or through a small nick in the dura. The risk of intracranial hemorrhage is a deterrent, although the studies that systematically addressed safety favored the use of intracranial pressure monitoring, especially using fiberoptic extradural or subdural devices. Proponents argue that it has been shown to be effective and relatively safe, despite the attendant coagulopathy. Epidural transducers were associated with a low complication rate at 3.8%, but subdural and parenchymal devices had higher complication rates at 20% and 22%.

Infection

Infection is a prominent complication in all varieties of liver failure. In acute liver failure, it is one of the most common causes of death and has an integral role in the evolving cycle of hemodynamic instability and multisystem failure (Rolando et al, 2000). It also frequently disqualifies potential candidates from emergency liver transplantation. Infection may be difficult to detect with confidence because there is a poor correlation between the presence of infection and body temperature or white blood cell counts. Bacterial infection occurs in 80% of cases, whereas fungal infection occurs in 30%. Systemic fungal infection is notoriously difficult to diagnose in the setting of acute liver failure, and a high index of suspicion is required, especially in high-risk patients and in cases in which there is a very high white blood cell count or an arrest in the normalization of the parameters of coagulation activity. Risk factors for bacterial and fungal sepsis include coexisting renal failure, cholestasis, treatment with thiopentone, and liver transplantation. Surveillance cultures are required on a regular basis.

Clinical trials of prophylactic antibiotics showed that systemic antibiotics reduced the incidence of culture-positive bacterial infection by half, but this strategy was associated with the emergence of highly resistant organisms in 10% of cases. This reduction in infection rates was not accompanied by a significant impact on major clinical outcomes (mortality, progression to transplantation) or economic considerations (duration of intensive care unit and hospital stay, overall cost of antimicrobials). Small bowel decontamination was not effective in altering the pattern of infection. Systemic antibiotics are recommended when infection is suspected, and the precise regimens used are determined by local antibiotic policy.

In chronic liver disease, infection of an apparent trivial nature can be the trigger for an episode of acute-on-chronic liver failure, and as a result antibiotic therapy is a standard component of the management of this condition. Spontaneous bacterial peritonitis is a particularly important infection to consider in this setting, and the diagnosis can be excluded with confidence only if the white blood cell count in ascites is less than 250/mm³. Patients with a history of spontaneous bacterial peritonitis should be maintained on low-dose antibiotic prophylaxis (e.g., with norfloxacin 400 mg daily).

Hemodynamic Instability and Oxygen Debt

The hemodynamic changes in liver failure are similar to the changes observed in the systemic inflammatory response syndrome. The early hemodynamic profile reflects a hyperdynamic circulation with increased cardiac output and reduced systemic peripheral vascular resistance. Profound vasodilation may cause relative hypovolemia, and invasive monitoring is used to determine appropriate fluid regimens and adequate intravascular volumes. Progressive disease leads to circulatory failure as a result of a falling cardiac output or an inability to maintain an adequate mean arterial pressure. This is a common mode of death in liver failure.

Circulatory failure is managed initially with appropriate combinations of colloid, crystalline fluids, and blood products. Hypotension occurring despite adequate intravascular volumes is treated with vasopressor agents, using norepinephrine if the cardiac index exceeds 4.5 L/min/m² or epinephrine if the cardiac output needs to be boosted above this threshold. The initial stabilizing dose to achieve a mean arterial pressure greater than 60 mm Hg is 0.2 to 1.8 mg/kg/min of epinephrine and 0.2 to 2 mg/kg/min of norepinephrine. Vasopressor agents may cause or aggravate an oxygen debt, and prostacyclin and N-acetyl cysteine have been shown to improve these parameters in patients receiving vasopressors. Some patients with acute liver failure who develop resistance to inotropes may have a hypoadrenal profile that responds to hydrocortisone (Harry et al, 2002).

Renal Failure

Renal failure occurs in 75% of patients developing grade 4 encephalopathy after an acetaminophen overdose and 30% of patients with other etiologies of acute liver failure. Renal failure after an acetaminophen overdose is a consequence of direct renal toxicity and develops early in the course of the illness. Early renal dysfunction also is seen in Wilson's disease and pregnancy-related syndromes. In the other etiologies, renal impairment develops relatively late and progresses from a stage of functional or prerenal failure (urinary sodium <10 mmol/L, urine-to-plasma osmolarity ratio >1.1) to acute tubular necrosis. Urea synthesis is impaired in acute liver failure, and serum creatinine levels are preferred for the purposes of monitoring renal function.

Hepatorenal failure is a serious complication of acute-on-chronic liver failure. Two types are recognized: Type 1 hepatorenal syndrome is characterized by a rapidly progressive decline in renal function leading to a doubling of the initial serum creatinine to greater than 2.5 mg/dL or a 50% reduction of creatinine clearance to less than 20 mL/min over a period of no longer than 2 weeks. Type 2 hepatorenal syndrome is characterized by renal failure not fulfilling the above-mentioned parameters. Hepatorenal syndrome can improve dramatically after liver transplantation reflecting the role of vasospasm in the pathogenesis of the condition. True hepatorenal syndrome can progress imperceptibly to acute tubular injury, however, which does not resolve as quickly.

Optimization of intravascular filling is essential in patients with deteriorating renal function. The prophylactic use of dopamine has been common practice, but its benefits have been challenged, especially in the setting of profound vasodilation that is typical of acute liver failure. The metabolic complexity of combined liver and renal failure suggests that early intervention with hemodialysis, preempting standard indications, is prudent in the setting of acute liver failure. Continuous filtration systems are associated with less hemodynamic instability and run a lower risk of aggravating latent or established cerebral edema than intermittent hemodialysis. The role for renal support therapy is less well defined in acute-on-chronic liver failure. Molecular absorbent recirculation system therapy may be especially useful in deeply jaundiced patients with renal dysfunction.

Metabolic Abnormalities

Hypoglycemia is common in acute liver failure and can induce reversible impairment of consciousness before the onset of classic encephalopathy. The signs and symptoms of hypoglycemia are often masked, and regular blood glucose monitoring is required. Metabolic acidosis is present in 30% of patients developing acute liver failure after an acetaminophen overdose and is associated with a particularly high mortality—greater than 90% if the pH of arterial blood is less than 7.30 on the second or subsequent days after the overdose. This acidosis precedes the onset of encephalopathy and is independent of renal function. In contrast, a metabolic acidosis is found in 5% of patients with other etiologies of acute liver failure, occurring later in the disease

process and associated with a poor outcome. Increased serum lactate levels have been documented in patients with a metabolic acidosis, and these correlate inversely with mean arterial pressure, systemic vascular resistance, and oxygen extraction ratios. The hyperlactatemia possibly reflects tissue hypoxia resulting from impaired oxygen extraction as a result of microvascular shunting of blood away from actively respiring tissues. In most etiologies of acute liver failure, alkalosis is the dominant acid-base abnormality, and it may be associated with hypokalemia. Hyponatremia may reflect sodium depletion in patients with vomiting, or it may be dilutional owing to excessive antidiuretic hormone secretion or intracellular sodium shifts. Hypophosphatemia is encountered most frequently in acetaminophen-induced acute liver failure when renal function is preserved.

Hyponatremia is the dominant abnormality seen in acute-on-chronic liver failure. Hyponatremia does not reflect sodium depletion because total body sodium levels are almost always above normal in these patients. The hyponatremia may be diuretic induced in patients with ascites, and withdrawal of diuretic therapy is advised if the serum sodium is less than 130 mEq/L. Refractory hyponatremia is managed by fluid restriction of 800 to 1500 mL/day depending on severity. Hemofiltration may be used to correct hyponatremia in severe cases or when the serum sodium is less than 120 mEq/L immediately before liver transplantation (to reduce the risk of central pontine myelinolysis associated with the rapid increase in serum sodium levels that inevitably occurs).

Coagulopathy

The liver is responsible for the synthesis of most of the coagulation factors (except factor VIII, which is produced by endothelial cells) and some of the inhibitors of coagulation and fibrinolysis. In acute liver failure, circulating levels of fibrinogen; prothrombin; and factors V, VII, IX, and X are reduced, and the prothrombin time is widely used as an indicator of the severity of liver damage. In addition to decreased synthesis of coagulation factors by the liver, there is evidence of increased peripheral consumption. Overt disseminated intravascular coagulation is observed occasionally, especially in pregnancy-related syndromes, but sensitive investigative techniques point to the presence of a low-grade process in most patients. Quantitative and qualitative defects in platelet function are well described in acute liver failure, and platelet counts of less than 100×10^9/L are seen in 70% of patients. Platelet aggregation is impaired, but there is an increase in platelet adhesiveness, a pattern that may be due to increased levels of circulating von Willebrand factor. There is a fairly poor correlation between the laboratory and clinical manifestations of the coagulopathy, and the highest risk of bleeding is seen in patients with an associated thrombocytopenia or a frank disseminated intravascular coagulation syndrome, rather than in patients with isolated severe prolongations of prothrombin time. Management of the coagulopathy is repletion of the appropriate combination of clotting factors and platelets. The practice of prophylactic repletion of clotting factors is controversial because it may interfere with assessment of prognosis, especially in patients being considered for liver transplantation. Limited data are available on the utility of recombinant activated factor VII in this setting (Caldwell et al, 2004).

The abnormality of coagulation is usually less severe in acute-on-chronic liver failure, and thrombocytopenia in this setting is usually due to hypersplenism. Patients with protracted cholestasis may have a component to the coagulopathy that responds to parenteral vitamin K. The management of the coagulopathy follows the same principles as in acute liver failure.

NUTRITION

Although patients with acute liver failure usually are well nourished at the onset of the illness, it is important to institute nutritional support as soon as possible. The catabolic rate increases in patients with acute liver failure, and this is most apparent in patients with complicating sepsis and patients undergoing liver transplantation. The theoretical problems that limit nutritional options include gastrointestinal ileus, desire to minimize gastrointestinal protein, difficulty maintaining isoglycemia, fluid restriction secondary to renal failure, theoretical role of amino acid ratios in mediating encephalopathy, difficulty handling lipids, and aggravation of sepsis by intravenous feeding. Despite all of these considerations, adequate nutritional support can be obtained in most patients. An element of enteral nutrition is desirable to help maintain the integrity of the small intestine mucosa, and this is titrated against the volume of gastric aspirate and the development of diarrhea.

Nutritional support in acute-on-chronic liver failure is equally as important, but subject to more constraints. In contrast to patients with acute liver failure, these patients frequently are undernourished before the onset of the episode of acute-on-chronic liver failure. Protein intake should not exceed 60 g/day in patients with encephalopathy. There also may be restrictions on fluid volume and the sodium content of feeds. A substantial proportion of patients have some degree of insulin resistance that may lead to hyperglycemia with high carbohydrate intake. Finally, patients with problematic varices may not tolerate the presence of nasogastric tubes.

REFERENCES

Bernal B, 2003: Changing patterns of causation and the use of transplantation in the United Kingdom. Semin Liver Dis 23:227-237.

Bernal W, et al, 2002: Blood lactate as an early indicator of outcome in paracetamol-induced acute liver failure. Lancet 359:558-563.

Caldwell SH, et al, 2004: Recombinant activated factor VII (rFVII) as a hemostatic agent in liver disease: a break from convention in need of controlled trials. Hepatology 39:592-598.

Harry R, et al, 2002: The clinical importance of adrenal insufficiency in acute hepatic dysfunction. Hepatology 36:395-402.

Lee WM, 2003: Acute liver failure in the United States. Semin Liver Dis 23:217-226.

Murphy N, et al, 2004: The effect of hypertonic sodium chloride on intracranial pressure in patients with acute liver failure. Hepatology 39:464-470.

Rodrigues F, et al, 2005: Neonatal hemochromatosis—medical management vs. transplantation: the King's experience. Liver Transpl 11:1417-1424.

Rolando N, et al, 2000: The systemic inflammatory response syndrome in acute liver failure. Hepatology 32:734-739.

Sjogren M, 2003: Immunization and the decline of viral hepatitis as a cause of acute liver failure. Hepatology 38:554-556.

Support of the Failing Liver

89

A. A. DEMETRIOU

Acute hepatic failure is associated with high morbidity and mortality (Lee, 1993). The complexity of the liver is so great, and the number of physiologic, biochemical, and metabolic functions it performs so large, that to date no realistic alternative to liver transplantation for permanent liver replacement has been developed (see Ch. 103). Liver transplantation as a treatment for acute hepatic failure is restricted primarily by limited organ availability. In recent years, indications for liver transplantation have expanded, patients with small hepatocellular carcinomas are undergoing transplantation, the age range for recipients has been extended at both ends of the age spectrum, and patients with more than one failing organ are being offered multiorgan transplants. Organ availability for transplantation has not kept pace with increased demand.

There is a need for temporary liver support in acute hepatic failure to support patients with borderline functional mass until their livers recover or until a donor liver becomes available for transplantation. The major limitation to the provision of effective liver support is lack of a clear understanding of the pathophysiology of acute hepatic failure and the mechanism of development of cerebral edema, the major cause of death in these patients. Various toxic factors have been implicated, and this has led to development of therapies designed to remove a broad range of toxins (Arnaout & Demetriou, 2000). In acute hepatic failure, the primary goal of plasma detoxification is to remove toxins responsible for the development of cerebral edema. It is unknown, however, whether toxins are the cause of the syndrome. It is difficult to predict whether removal of a specific factor would have a positive or negative effect. A specific cytokine may have toxic effects on hepatocytes in vitro and in vivo; however, it also may be a potent stimulus of liver regeneration. The picture becomes even more complex when one realizes that some of the potentially relevant compounds have inhibitory or stimulatory effects depending on their plasma and tissue levels.

Some investigators argue that the major therapeutic goal in acute hepatic failure simply should be to provide additional liver mass. Liver transplantation, which involves replacing the diseased liver with a healthy one, is effective. Auxiliary liver transplantation, which provides a substantial increase in liver mass, has not emerged as a successful therapy in acute hepatic failure, however. Similarly, in experimental animals with acute liver failure, treatment with a small number of cells in a liver support system can result in profound changes in the regenerative response pattern of the native liver and reduction in serum levels of a liver regeneration inhibitor (Suh et al, 1999). The relevant findings from the research and clinical literature are confusing and often conflicting. Against this background, investigators are attempting to design rational liver support systems using biologic and nonbiologic components.

MEDICAL THERAPY

Medical management of acute hepatic failure has to be multidisciplinary because of the complexity of the underlying disease and its progression to multiple organ failure (see Ch. 88). Hemodynamic and respiratory support and prevention and treatment of cerebral edema are the major goals of therapy in these severely ill patients. Patients with acute hepatic failure are managed in an intensive care unit. General measures are instituted with invasive monitoring, including placement of a pulmonary artery catheter for cardiovascular pressure and mixed oxygen measurements, arterial line, continuous pulse oximetry, urinary catheter, and nasogastric tube. Patients in stage III/IV encephalopathy (Trey & Davidson, 1970) with brainstem dysfunction are placed on ventilatory support and may have an intracranial pressure monitor installed at the bedside for intracranial pressure and cerebral perfusion pressure monitoring. The head of the bed is elevated, noise in the room is kept to a minimum, and lighting is sparingly used to avoid agitating the patient. Vital signs, neurologic assessment, intravenous input, and body fluid output are recorded hourly. In patients with neurologic dysfunction, a head computed tomography scan is obtained whenever possible. Liver function tests, coagulation tests, complete blood cell count, serum electrolytes, ammonia, lactate, blood urea nitrogen, and creatinine levels are determined at regular time intervals. Arterial gases are determined serially.

Standard medical therapy includes hyperventilation and administration of mannitol and lactulose. Supportive measures are initiated to correct electrolyte (e.g., hypocalcemia, hypophosphatemia, hypokalemia) and acid-base (e.g., lactic acidemia) imbalances; hypoglycemia; and respiratory, coagulation, and hemodynamic abnormalities. Renal dialysis and filtration are used, as needed (Watanabe & Rosenthal, 1996). Infection poses a serious threat to acute hepatic failure patients by placing them at risk for sepsis and by being a contraindication to liver transplantation. Although prophylactic antibiotic administration is not advocated without suspicion of active infection, the threshold for starting antibiotics should be low because the usual clinical presentation with fever and leukocytosis may be absent in 30% of fulminant hepatic failure patients (Rolando et al, 1990).

NONBIOLOGIC SYSTEMS

Plasma Exchange

Plasma exchange was a natural outgrowth of the less effective and more risky blood exchange transfusion technique. The goals of this therapy in acute hepatic failure are to reduce the level of circulating toxins and to replace deficient essential factors (e.g., clotting factors) manufactured by the liver. Plasma exchange is achieved by plasmapheresis, removal of the patient's plasma, and replacement with normal plasma. The results of early clinical trials were discouraging. Therapeutic gains (e.g., reduction in serum bilirubin, partial recovery from coma) were short-lived and were seen predominantly in patients with drug-induced liver failure (Freeman & Matthewsson, 1986; Lepore et al, 1972; Sabin & Merritt, 1968). In acute hepatic failure, the overall survival rate remained less than 50% (Takahashi et al, 1991). In addition, there was a significant complication rate, including reports of chemical toxicity, viral infections, and deaths from lung and brain complications (Brunner & Losgen, 1987). The effect of repeated, high-volume plasma exchange in patients with acute hepatic failure was studied; there were some beneficial effects that need to be confirmed in a prospective trial (Kondrup et al, 1992). More recently, Clemmesen and coworkers (1999) investigated the effect of repeated, high-volume (15% of the body weight) plasma exchange in 23 patients (14 with acute hepatic failure and 9 with acute-on-chronic liver disease). In the acute hepatic failure group, only one patient of eight who developed acute hepatic failure after paracetamol overdose died. Only four of these patients fulfilled the King's College criteria of fulminant hepatic failure (predicted mortality of 90% without a transplant), however. In the acute-on-chronic liver disease group, only two of five survivors required transplantation. Despite its limitations and unproven efficacy, plasma exchange continues to be the most frequently used method of liver support in patients with acute hepatic failure. It is used primarily for the correction of coagulopathy.

Blood Purification

Throughout the 1960s and 1970s, it was believed that toxins that cause coma in hepatic failure are small (<5 KD) dialyzable molecules (Kiley et al, 1956; Opolon, 1979). As a result, numerous attempts were made to treat acute hepatic failure patients using hemodialysis (Kiley et al, 1958; Merrill et al, 1950). At the same time, electrolytes, nutrients, drugs, and other substances were delivered concurrently to patients. Subsequently, recognition of the role of so-called middle molecules (<15 KD; e.g., bilirubin, bile acids, barbiturates) and protein-bound neurotoxins in the pathogenesis of acute hepatic failure led to the development of hemofiltration and hemadsorption techniques using hollow-fiber membranes and various specific and nonspecific adsorption columns (Denis et al, 1979; Gimson et al, 1982; Schechter et al, 1958; Yatzidis & Oreopoulos, 1976). A major disadvantage of the latter approach was that direct contact between blood and sorbents resulted in loss of platelets, leukocytes, clotting factors, humoral mediators, and other important plasma components. Coating of the sorbent particles with a semipermeable membrane (e.g., cellulose nitrate, cellulose acetate, esters of methacrylic acid, albumin) has decreased or even eliminated some of these losses, but at the cost of lower efficacy.

No blood purification measures, including the most widely used hemoperfusion through charcoal (Gimson et al, 1982; O'Grady et al, 1988), have been shown to reverse hepatic encephalopathy and improve survival in acute hepatic failure patients. Results of removal of middle molecules and protein-bound compounds using "less tight" dialysis membranes (Silk et al, 1977), postdilution

hemofiltration (Rakela et al, 1988), and a combination of hemofiltration and plasma exchange (Matsubara et al, 1990; Yoshiba et al, 1993) have been equally disappointing. In a prospective study by Matsubara and colleagues (1990), hemofiltration using a high-performance membrane was performed in 16 patients with acute liver failure. Of these patients, 10 were in grade 3 or 4 coma, and 8 had acute hepatic failure. The procedure was conducted between plasma exchanges for more than 20 hours. The replacement fluid used contained electrolytes, lactate, bicarbonates, and glucose. The total fluid volume filtered was 10 to 15 L per session. Half of the patients experienced improvement in level of consciousness and were weaned successfully from therapy. Although there were only 3 long-term survivors (1 with acute hepatic failure), 13 patients lived an average of 15 days. It is difficult to interpret these findings because of inability to determine the relative contribution of the two components of this therapy (hemofiltration and plasma exchange). Similar reservations apply to a study by Yoshiba and associates (1996), who reported a 55% survival rate in 67 acute hepatic failure patients with viral hepatitis treated with a combination of plasma exchange and hemodiafiltration. In this series, patients with acute hepatic failure secondary to acute hepatitis A or B infection responded to treatment better than hepatitis B carriers and individuals with non-A, non-B fulminant hepatitis.

A dual approach (i.e., a combination of hemofiltration and plasma exchange) may have a potential use as a bridge to transplantation in patients with acute hepatic failure. Equally appealing is the idea of using plasma ultrafiltration selectively to remove neurotoxins, endotoxin, and cytokines from the ultrafiltrate (Cohen et al, 1987; Nagaki et al, 1992).

Ash and colleagues (1993) developed a system using a parallel plate cellulose membrane dialyzer (BioLogic DT HemoCleanse, Inc., Lafayette, IN), in which blood is circulated against a proprietary mixture of finely powdered sorbents. Preliminary clinical studies indicated that the system had significant capacity to remove drugs and small molecular weight toxins. In a prospective, controlled study, 37 patients with acute or acute-on-chronic liver failure were randomized to receive three to five daily hemodiabsorption treatments or standard of care. Significant improvement was observed in neurologic status regardless of the cause of hepatic failure. Outcome, which was defined as survival to discharge, survival to liver transplantation, or survival for 5 days, was improved in patients with acute exacerbation of chronic liver disease, but not in acute hepatic failure patients.

Stange and associates (1993) developed a dialysis system called molecular absorbents recirculation system (MARS, Gambro, Rostock, Germany), which reportedly facilitates rapid and efficient transport of albumin-bound substances, such as bilirubin. The MARS device uses a highly permeable membrane impregnated with albumin, which also is added to the dialysate solution and is "regenerated" during continuous recirculation in a closed loop system through adsorbents (charcoal, resin). The MARS system has been studied in a series of limited uncontrolled clinical trials in Europe and the United States with promising results (Schmidt et al, 2001; Steiner & Mitzner, 2002). One prospective, randomized and controlled trial showed significant improvement in survival in patients with hepatorenal syndrome (Mitzner et al, 2000). In acute hepatic failure, the MARS system has not been shown to have clinically significant effects.

BIOLOGIC LIVER SUPPORT SYSTEMS

In acute hepatic failure, an effective liver support system should enhance or replace all essential functions of the liver (i.e., detoxification, biotransformation, and synthesis). Such a system would result in correction of coagulopathy and other metabolic and physiologic derangements and a decrease in the operative and perioperative risks associated with extended hepatectomy and liver transplantation. Because the leading cause of death in acute hepatic failure is brainstem compression caused by tonsillar or uncal herniation, an effective therapy should either arrest or reverse cerebral edema and development of intracranial hypertension. It has been hypothesized that these therapeutic goals could be achieved only by employing biologically active liver tissue preparations. The approaches tried to date clinically, and which have showed the greatest promise, include ex vivo liver perfusion and use of extracorporeal devices loaded with isolated hepatocytes arranged in a monolayer or three-dimensional aggregates.

Ex Vivo Liver Perfusion

Multiple attempts have been made to support acute hepatic failure patients using whole blood perfusion through baboon, porcine, dog, bovine, and calf livers (Abouna et al, 1970; Chari et al, 1994; Eiseman et al, 1965; Parbhoo et al, 1971). In most instances, only transient improvement in encephalopathy and blood chemistry was noted. Additionally, hyperacute rejection of the xenogeneic organ resulted in cessation of function, bleeding into the perfused liver, hemolysis, and thrombocytopenia (Chari et al, 1994). Although use of livers from transgenic pigs with reduced immunogenicity may solve the problem of early loss of function, the procedure itself remains cumbersome and costly. Human livers unsuitable for transplantation have been used for ex vivo perfusion (Fox et al, 1993). This strategy seems impractical, however, because of inability to obtain the organ on short notice. One also could question whether a liver capable of providing metabolic support ex vivo should not be transplanted. Cadaveric human livers have been used for extracorporeal blood perfusion, but no acute hepatic failure patients survived longer than 48 hours (Sen et al, 1966).

Hepatocyte Transplantation

Studies in experimental models of hepatic failure and genetic defects of liver metabolism indicate that transplanted hepatocytes can assume the full range of functions of intact whole livers (Arkadopoulos et al, 1998; Demetriou et al, 1986; Rozga et al, 1994b). For a hepatocyte transplantation method to be useful, the technique must be simple, result in early engraftment, and allow transplantation of an adequate number of hepatocytes, and transplanted hepatocytes should maintain differentiated functions for a prolonged period (Moscioni et al, 1996). In searching for optimal transplantation techniques, hepatocytes have been introduced virtually into every body site, including the liver, spleen, thymus, testes, lungs, kidneys, peritoneal cavity, subcutaneous tissues, fat pads, dorsal fascia, and other locations (Demetriou et al, 1986; Groth et al, 1977; Matas et al, 1976; Mito et al, 1978; Selden et al, 1984; Vroemen et al, 1988). Currently, two techniques that have gained general acceptance

are intrasplenic and intraportal injection of isolated hepatocytes. The spleen, because its outflow tract, joins the portal vein, and the patient's own liver could help excrete bile produced by intrasplenically transplanted cells. Additionally, the spleen parenchyma is rich in cytokines, including growth stimulatory factors; this may help explain why at other ectopic locations transplanted hepatocytes undergo atrophy, whereas in the spleen they may increase in number (Mito et al, 1978). The intraportal route seems to be better because transplanted cells integrate with hepatic cell plates (Moscioni et al, 1996; Rozga et al, 1994b). This allows interaction with other hepatocytes and nonparenchymal liver cells and secretion of bile into the biliary tree. In addition, this technique allows injection of cells into selective liver lobes, allowing portal decompression, repeated injections using an indwelling catheter, and expansion of the transplanted cell population under a liver regeneration response (Moscioni et al, 1996).

Clinical experience with hepatocyte transplantation is limited (Bilir et al, 1996; Fox et al, 1998; Grossman et al, 1994; Habibullah et al, 1994; Mito & Kusano 1993; Muraca et al, 2002). Additionally, convincing evidence of transplanted cell function is lacking because the number of the transplanted cells was small (Bilir et al, 1996; Grossman et al, 1994; Mito et al, 1993). Allogeneic hepatocyte transplantation is hampered by lack of donor organs because harvested normal livers are being used for whole organ transplantation. Techniques need to be developed for isolation of cells suitable for transplantation from cadaveric livers and livers rejected for whole organ transplantation. Another option would be to transplant liver stem cells. In that case, however, we would need to learn how to expand them in culture and convert them into differentiated mature hepatocytes.

Extracorporeal Hepatocyte Systems

The concept of *artificial liver* was introduced by Sorrentino (1956), who showed that fresh liver tissue homogenates could metabolize ketone bodies, barbiturate, salicylic acid, and ammonia. Pioneering work was carried out in Japan, where in 1959 Kimoto performed short-term (55 minutes) cross-hemodialysis between a comatose patient and a dog. The treatment lowered blood ammonia levels, and the patient rapidly regained consciousness. A few years later, using a similar approach, Nose and colleagues (1963) found that hemodialysis against various canine liver tissue preparations (homogenate, fresh liver slices, and freeze-dried granules of liver tissue) had beneficial effects on glucose homeostasis, hyperlactemia, and hyperammonemia. Four patients were treated with extracorporeal perfusion of freeze-dried granulated canine liver. Two patients with moderate liver dysfunction improved remarkably. Two patients who had severe acute hepatic failure showed only temporary improvement and died shortly after treatment. No additional studies followed these preliminary clinical reports.

The next steps were taken by Wolf and Munkelt (1975) and by Hager and colleagues (1978, 1983), who placed Reuber hepatoma cells (Wolf & Munkelt, 1975) and adult and fetal human hepatocytes (Hager et al, 1978, 1983) on the outer surface of synthetic capillaries. Eiseman and coworkers (1976) and Olumide and associates (1977) tested hepatocyte function in several devices, including a centrifuge, a dialyzer, and a perfusion chamber. Other investigators tried to employ isolated liver enzymes (Brunner et al, 1979), cellular components (Denti & Luboz, 1974), and liver slices (Kimura et al, 1980) to develop a variety of liver support systems. In 1988, Uchino and coworkers described a device in which 80 g of liver cells was cultured on 200 collagen-coated borosilicated glass plates. Altogether, during the past 30 years, multiple hepatocyte-based artificial livers were developed and tested (Kamohara et al, 1998). Among these designs, the most interesting are those developed by Nyberg and colleagues (1993), Gerlach and colleagues (1994), Miyoshi and associates (1994), Bader and coworkers (1995), and Flendrig and associates (1997).

In general, it has been shown that protein synthesis, gluconeogenesis, ureagenesis, cytochrome P-450 activity, and conjugation can be carried out in vitro by hepatocyte-based systems. This work is encouraging, especially if one considers that cells are cut off from most regulatory mechanisms that control hepatocyte function in vivo. Additionally, most investigators have provided evidence that hepatocytes remain functional and viable in their systems for relatively long periods, and that their "biolivers" are able to provide metabolic and physiologic support in animals with experimentally induced acute liver failure. Problems facing further development in the field include difficulty to scale-up systems previously tested in small animals and difficulty in overcoming financial, organizational, and regulatory (quality control) problems associated with implementation and execution of prospective, controlled clinical trials.

Patient data on the use of hepatocyte-based liver support systems are limited. In 1987, Matsumura and coworkers added a cryopreserved rabbit liver cell suspension to a dialysis chamber. A patient in hepatic failure secondary to an inoperable cholangiocarcinoma underwent two cycles of hemodialysis, and on each occasion, serum bilirubin levels decreased. Margulis and associates (1989) treated 59 patients with liver failure with daily 6-hour hemoperfusions through a 20-mL capsule in which activated charcoal was mixed with 0.5 g of porcine hepatocytes. A control group of 67 patients underwent standard medical therapy. Survival in the treated group was improved, but no evidence was provided to substantiate the conclusion that the bioartificial liver was functional.

Sussman and colleagues (1992) developed an extracorporeal liver assist device that used cells from a clonally derived human hepatoma cell line. Cells were grown in hollow-fiber cartridges and reportedly retained normal hepatocyte differentiated function, while maintaining a short population doubling time and showing contact inhibition. In the initial group of 10 treated patients, no significant effect on disease outcome was noted with only one survivor (Sussman & Kelly, 1993). The system was tested further at King's College Hospital in London in two groups of patients with acetaminophen-induced acute hepatic failure: patients who had a potential for recovery and patients listed for emergent liver transplantation. The results of this trial were negative (Ellis et al, 1996). Although the concept of growing hepatocytes in a hollow-fiber cartridge is valid, the use of hepatoma-derived cells raises safety issues. Nyberg and coworkers (1994) noted extracapillary passage of HepG2 cells through a hollow-fiber wall even though there was no physical damage to the bioreactor. Establishment of a transformed cell line using media conditioned by HepG2 cells also has been reported (Roberts et al, 1994). The consequences of both events may be serious in an acute hepatic failure patient undergoing liver transplantation and maintained on lifelong immunosuppression.

Porcine hepatocytes show remarkable morphologic and functional homology with human hepatocytes and outperform all current liver cell lines as the source of biotransformation functions (Nyberg et al, 1994).

van de Kerkhove and colleagues (2004) summarized the status of the liver support device field in a comprehensive review. Only bioartificial liver devices used in clinical trials were included. Eleven systems were used clinically in acute hepatic failure. The systems generally were shown to be safe. The authors concluded that the results of the studies were promising and recommended that the devices could be improved further by using human hepatocytes. Large-scale availability of fully functional human hepatocytes or clinical use at this time remains elusive, however.

To date, there has only been one large, multicenter, international, prospective, randomized clinical trial of a bioartificial liver (HepatAssist; Circe Biomedical, Inc, Lexington, MA) in acute hepatic failure (Demetriou et al, 2004). Early versions of this bioartificial liver system initially were tested in clinical trials involving 51 patients (Watanabe et al, 1997). The design of the bioartificial liver system used in the current multicenter clinical trial has evolved from a series of in vitro and in vivo experimental animal and pilot clinical studies carried out over several years (Fig. 89.1). Blood is removed from a patient through a double lumen catheter placed in the superficial femoral vein and

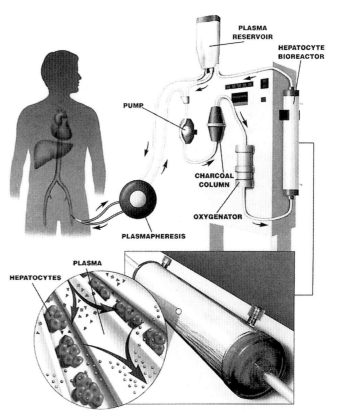

Fig. 89.1. Schematic representation of a bioartificial liver (HepatAssist 2000; Circe Biomedical, Lexington, MA). A transmission reservoir allows high recirculation flow through the circuit. An oxygenator and a heater are placed in the bioartificial liver circuit to supply hepatocytes with 30% oxygen/5% carbon dioxide and to maintain them at 37°C.
(From Kamohara Y, et al, 1998: Artificial liver: review and Cedars-Sinai experience. J Hepatobiliary Pancreat Surg 5:273-285.)

separated into blood cells and plasma by the apheresis unit. The plasma is delivered at 50 mL/min to the bioartificial liver recirculation loop consisting of a reservoir, a column loaded with activated cellulose-coated charcoal, an oxygenator, a heater, and a hollow-fiber module containing approximately 7 billion viable microcarrier (dextran)-attached porcine hepatocytes. Plasma circulates through the fibers at 400 mL/min, and after return from the bioartificial liver, it is reconstituted with blood cells and delivered to the patient. Sodium citrate is used as an anticoagulant to prevent thrombosis within the circuit. Plasma ionized calcium levels are measured hourly during bioartificial liver treatment, and calcium chloride infusion is administered to prevent ionized hypocalcemia secondary to the calcium-chelating effect of citrate.

In the trial of the HepatAssist system (Demetriou et al, 2004), 171 patients (86 control and 85 bioartificial liver) were enrolled. Patients with fulminant/subfulminant hepatic failure ($n = 147$) and primary nonfunction after transplantation ($n = 24$) were included. Data were analyzed with and without accounting for the following confounding factors: liver transplantation, time to transplantation, disease etiology, disease severity, and treatment site. For the entire patient population, survival at 30 days was 71% for bioartificial liver versus 62% for control ($P = .26$). After exclusion of the primary nonfunction patients, survival was 73% for bioartificial liver versus 59% for control ($P = .12$). When survival was analyzed taking into account the aforementioned confounding factors, in the entire patient population there was no significant difference between the two groups (risk ratio 0.67; $P = .13$). Survival in fulminant/subfulminant hepatic failure patients was significantly higher, however, in the bioartificial liver group compared with the control group (risk ratio 0.56; $P = .048$). This trial showed safety and improved survival in patients with fulminant/subfulminant hepatic failure. This is the first time that a biologic-type liver support system has been shown to have a significant beneficial effect on survival in a major group of acute hepatic failure patients. It provides "proof of concept" that hepatocyte-based liver support therapy can improve survival in these patients. With further refinements, this and other such systems should become part of the therapeutic armamentarium for acute hepatic failure. For now, the main therapeutic objective for severely ill acute hepatic failure patients is liver transplantation. This study confirmed that the most important predictor of survival in acute hepatic failure patients is liver transplantation.

SUMMARY

The ability to support the acutely failing liver has been enhanced through improvements in critical care and liver transplantation. Significant progress has been achieved in the area of liver support system development. The ultimate goal of a liver support system is to treat patients early and repeatedly to allow their livers to recover normal function without need for transplantation. Major technical challenges remain, but with advances in hepatocyte isolation and cryopreservation, the promise of stem cell research, improved hepatocyte scale-up methods, and application of creative engineering approaches, effective and widely used liver support therapy may become a reality in the near future.

REFERENCES

Abouna GM, et al, 1970: Long-term hepatic support by intermittent multi species liver perfusion. Lancet 2:391-396.

Arkadopoulos N, et al, 1998: Intrasplenic transplantation of allogeneic hepatocytes prolongs survival in anhepatic rats. Hepatology 28:1365-1370.

Arnaout WS, Demetriou AA, 2000: Liver: hepatic support and the bioartificial liver. In Baue AE, et al (eds): Multiple Organ Failure. New York, Springer-Verlag, pp 462-473.

Ash SR, et al, 1993: Effect of sorbent-based dialytic therapy with Biologic-DT on an experimental model of hepatic failure. ASAIO J 39:M675-M680.

Bader A, et al, 1995: A novel bioreactor design for in vitro reconstruction of in vivo liver characteristics. Artif Organs 19:368-374.

Bilir B, et al, 1996: Transjugular intra-portal transplantation of cryopreserved human hepatocytes in a patient with acute liver failure. Hepatology 24:308A.

Brunner G, Losgen H, 1987: Benefits and dangers of plasma exchange in patients with fulminant hepatic failure. In Oda T, Shiokawa Y, Inoue N (eds): Therapeutic Plasmapheresis. Cleveland, ISAO Press, pp 187-191.

Brunner G, et al, 1979: The application of immobilized enzymes in an artificial liver support system. Artif Organs 3:27-30.

Chari RS, et al, 1994: Brief report: treatment of hepatic failure with ex vivo pig-liver perfusion followed by liver transplantation. N Engl J Med 331:234-237.

Clemmesen JO, et al, 1999: Hepatic blood flow and splanchnic oxygen consumption in patients with liver failure: effect of high-volume plasmapheresis. Hepatology 29:347-355.

Cohen J, et al, 1987: Protection from endotoxemia: a rat model of plasmapheresis and specific adsorption with polymyxin B. J Infect Dis 155:690-695.

Demetriou AA, et al, 1986: Replacement of liver function by transplantation of microcarrier-attached hepatocytes. Science 233:1190-1192.

Demetriou AA, et al, 2004: Prospective, randomized, multicenter, controlled trial of a Bioartificial Liver in treating acute liver failure. Ann Surg 239:660-670.

Denis J, et al, 1979: Long-term extra-corporeal assistance by continuous haemofiltration during fulminant hepatic failure. Gastroenterol Clin Biol 3:337-348.

Denti E, Luboz MP, 1974: Preparation and properties of gel entrapped liver cell microsomes. In Williams R, Murray-Lyon IM (eds): Artificial Liver Support. Kent, UK, Pitman Medical, pp 148-152.

Eiseman B, et al, 1965: Heterologous liver perfusion in treatment of hepatic failure. Ann Surg 162:329-345.

Eiseman B, et al, 1976: Hepatocyte perfusion within a centrifuge. Surg Gynecol Obstet 142:21-28.

Ellis AJ, et al, 1996: Pilot-controlled trial of the extracorporeal liver assist device in acute liver failure. Hepatology 24:1446-1451.

Flendrig LM, et al, 1997: In vivo investigation of a novel bioartificial liver based on porcine hepatocytes. Hepatology 26:168A.

Fox IJ, et al, 1993: Successful application of extracorporeal liver perfusion for the treatment of fulminant hepatic failure: a technology whose time has come. Am J Gastroenterol 88:1876-1881.

Fox IJ, et al, 1998: Treatment of the Crigler-Najjar syndrome type I with hepatocyte transplantation. N Engl J Med 338:1422-1426.

Freeman JG, Matthewsson K, 1986: Plasmapheresis in acute liver failure. Int J Artif Organs 9:433-438.

Gerlach J, et al, 1994: Hybrid liver support system in a short term application on hepatectomized pig. Int J Artif Organs 17:549-553.

Gimson AES, et al, 1982: Earlier charcoal haemoperfusion in fulminant hepatic failure. Lancet 2:681-683.

Grossman M, et al, 1994: Successful ex vivo gene therapy directed to liver in a patient with familial hypercholesterolemia. Nat Genet 6:335-341.

Groth CG, et al, 1977: Correction of hyperbilirubinemia in the glucuronyltransferase deficient rat by intraportal transplantation. Transplant Proc 9:313-316.

Habibullah CM, et al, 1994: Human fetal hepatocyte transplantation in patients with fulminant hepatic failure. Transplantation 58:951-977.

Hager JC, et al, 1978: A prototype for a hybrid artificial liver. ASAIO Trans 24:250-253.

Hager JC, et al, 1983: Neonatal hepatocyte culture on artificial capillaries: a model for drug metabolism and artificial liver. ASAIO J 6:26-35.

Kamohara Y, et al, 1998: Artificial liver: review and Cedars-Sinai experience. J Hepatobiliary Pancreat Surg 5:273-285.

Kiley JE, et al, 1956: Removal of blood ammonia by hemodialysis. Proc Soc Exp Biol Med 91:489-490.

Kiley JE, et al, 1958: Ammonia intoxication treated by hemodialysis. N Engl J Med 259:1156-1161.

Kimoto S, 1959: The artificial liver experiments and clinical application. ASAIO Trans 5:102-110.

Kimura K, et al, 1980: Hemoperfusion over small liver pieces for liver support. Artif Organs 4:297-301.

Kondrup J, et al, 1992: High volume plasma exchange in fulminant hepatic failure. Int J Artif Organs 15:669-676.

Lee WM, 1993: Acute liver failure. N Engl J Med 329:1862-1868.

Lepore MJ, et al, 1972: Plasmapheresis with plasma exchange in hepatic coma. Arch Intern Med 129:900-907.

Margulis MS, et al, 1989: Temporary organ substitution by hemoperfusion through suspension of active donor hepatocytes in a total complex of intensive therapy in patients with acute hepatic insufficiency. Resuscitation 18:85-94.

Matas A, et al, 1976: Hepatocellular transplantation for metabolic deficiencies: decrease of plasma bilirubin in Gunn rats. Science 192:892-894.

Matsubara S, et al, 1990: Continuous removal of middle molecules by hemofiltration in patient with acute liver failure. Crit Care Med 18:1331-1338.

Matsumura KN, et al, 1987: Hybrid bioartificial liver in hepatic failure: preliminary clinical report. Surgery 101:99-103.

Merrill JP, et al, 1950: The use of an artificial kidney: II. clinical experience. J Clin Invest 29:452-458.

Mito M, Kusano M, 1993: Hepatocyte transplantation in man. Cell Transplant 2:65-74.

Mito M, et al, 1978: Hepatocellular transplantation. Gastroenterol Jpn 13:480-485.

Mito M, et al, 1993: Hepatocyte transplantation for hepatic failure. Transpl Rev 7:35-43.

Mitzner SR, et al, 2000: Improvement of hepatorenal syndrome with extracorporeal albumin dialysis MARS: results of a prospective, randomized, controlled clinical trial. Liver Transpl 6:277-286.

Miyoshi H, et al, 1994: Long-term continuous culture of hepatocytes in a packed-bed reactor utilizing porous resin. Biotechnol Bioeng 43:635-644.

Moscioni AD, et al, 1996: Long-term correction of albumin levels in the Nagase analbuminemic rat: repopulation of the liver by transplanted normal hepatocytes under a regeneration response. Cell Transplant 5:499-503.

Muraca M, et al, 2002: Hepatocyte transplantation as a treatment for glycogen storage disease type 1a. Lancet 359:317-318.

Nagaki M, et al, 1992: In vitro plasma perfusion through adsorbents and plasma ultrafiltration to remove endotoxin and cytokines. Circ Shock 38:182-188.

Nose Y, et al, 1963: An experimental artificial liver utilizing extracorporeal metabolism with sliced or granulated canine liver. ASAIO Trans 9:358-362.

Nyberg SL, et al, 1993: Evaluation of a hepatocyte entrapment hollow fiber bioreactor, a potential use bioartificial liver. Biotechnol Bioeng 41:194-203.

Nyberg SL, et al, 1994: Primary hepatocytes outperform HepG2 cells as the source of biotransformation functions in bioartificial liver. Ann Surg 220:59-67.

O'Grady JG, et al, 1988: Controlled trials of charcoal hemoperfusion and prognostic factors in fulminant hepatic failure. Gastroenterology 94:1186-1192.

Olumide F, et al, 1977: Hepatic support with hepatocyte suspension in a permeable membrane dialyzer. Surgery 82:599-606.

Opolon P, 1979: High permeability membrane hemodialysis and hemofiltration in acute hepatic coma: experimental and clinical results. Artif Organs 3:354-360.

Parbhoo SP, et al, 1971: Extracorporeal pig-liver perfusion in treatment of hepatic coma due to fulminant hepatitis. Lancet 2:659-665.

Rakela J, et al, 1988: Postdilution hemofiltration in the management of acute hepatic failure: a pilot study. Mayo Clin Proc 63:113-118.

Roberts EA, et al, 1994: Characterization of human hepatocyte lines derived from normal liver tissue. Hepatology 19:1390-1399.

Rolando N, et al, 1990: Prospective study of bacterial infections in acute liver failure: an analysis of fifty patients. Hepatology 11:49-53.

Rozga J, et al, 1993a: Development of bioartificial liver: properties and function of a hollow-fiber module inoculated with liver cells. Hepatology 17:258-265.

Rozga J, et al, 1993b: Control of cerebral oedema by total hepatectomy and extracorporeal liver support in fulminant hepatic failure. Lancet 342:898-899.

Rozga J, et al, 1994a: Clinical use of a bioartificial liver to treat fulminant hepatic failure. Ann Surg 219:538-546.

Rozga J, et al, 1994b: Repeated intraportal hepatocyte transplantation in rats. Cell Transplant 4:237-243.

Sabin S, Merritt JA, 1968: Treatment of hepatic coma in cirrhosis by plasmapheresis and plasma infusion (plasma exchange). Ann Intern Med 68:1-7.

Schechter DC, et al, 1958: A simple extracorporeal device for reducing elevated blood ammonia levels. Surgery 44:892-897.

Schmidt LE, et al, 2001: Hemodynamic changes during a single treatment with the MARS in patients with acute-on-chronic liver failure. Liver Transpl 7:1034-1039.

Selden AC, et al, 1984: The pulmonary vascular bed as a site for implantation of isolated liver cells in inbred rats. Transplantation 38:81-83.

Sen PK, et al, 1966: Use of isolated perfused cadaveric liver in the management of hepatic failure. Surgery 59:774-781.

Silk DBA, et al, 1977: Treatment of fulminant hepatic failure by polyacrylo-nitrile membrane hemodialysis. Lancet 1:1-3.

Sorrentino F, 1956: Prime ricerche per la realizzazione di un fegato artificiale. Chir Patol Speriment 4:1401-1414.

Stange J, et al, 1993: A new procedure for the removal of protein bound drugs and toxins. ASAIO J 39:M621-625.

Steiner C, Mitzner S, 2002: Experiences with MARS liver support therapy in liver failure: analysis of 176 patients of the International MARS Registry. Liver 22(suppl 2):20-25.

Suh KS, et al, 1999: Bioartificial liver treatment in rats with fulminant hepatic failure: effect on DNA-binding activity of liver-enriched and growth-associated transcription factors. J Surg Res 85:243-250.

Sussman NL, Kelly JH, 1993: Improved liver function following treatment with an extracorporeal liver assist device. ASAIO Trans 17:27-30.

Sussman NL, et al, 1992: Reversal of fulminant hepatic failure using an extracorporeal liver assist device. Hepatology 16:60-65.

Takahashi T, et al, 1991: Artificial liver: state of the art. Dig Dis Sci 36:1327-1340.

Trey C, Davidson C, 1970: The management of fulminant hepatic failure. In Popper H, Schaffner F (eds): Progress in Liver Disease. New York, Grune & Stratton, pp 282-298.

Uchino J, et al, 1988: A hybrid bioartificial composed of multiplated hepatocyte monolayers. ASAIO Trans 34:972-977.

van de Kekhove MP, et al, 2004: Clinical application of Bioartificial Liver support systems. Ann Surg 240:216-228.

Vroemen JPMA, et al, 1988: Transplantation of isolated hepatocytes into the pancreas. Eur Surg Res 20:1-11.

Watanabe FD, Rosenthal P, 1996: Medical therapy. In Demetriou AA (ed): Support of the Acutely Failing Liver. Austin, TX, RG Landes Co, pp 22-32.

Watanabe FD, et al, 1997: Clinical experience with a bioartificial liver in the treatment of severe liver failure. Ann Surg 225:484-494.

Wolf CFW, Munkelt BE, 1975: Bilirubin conjugation by an artificial liver composed of cultured cells and synthetic capillaries. ASAIO Trans 21:16-26.

Yatzidis H, Oreopoulos D, 1976: Early clinical trials with sorbents. Kidney Int 7:S215-S217.

Yoshiba M, et al, 1993: Development of reliable artificial liver support (ALS) plasma exchange in combination with hemodiafiltration using high-performance membrane. Dig Dis Sci 38:469-476.

Yoshiba M, et al, 1996: Favorable effect of new artificial liver support on survival of patients with fulminant hepatic failure. Artif Organs 20:1169-1172.

Management of Ascites in Cirrhosis and Portal Hypertension

J. P. AHLUWALIA AND D. R. LABRECQUE

Ascites is one of three serious complications secondary to portal hypertension in patients with cirrhosis of the liver. Along with variceal hemorrhage and hepatic encephalopathy, ascites is a harbinger of a poor outcome in patients with cirrhosis. Among patients with cirrhosis, 40% develop ascites within 10 years (Gines et al, 1987b). Thirty percent to 50% die within 1 year of ascites onset, and 60% to 80% die within 5 years (D'Amico et al, 1986; Gines et al, 1987b; Powell & Klatskin, 1968; Saunders et al, 1981). If the ascites is refractory to treatment, less than 50% of patients survive 1 year (Salerno et al, 1993). Intractable ascites is a common indication for liver transplantation, although it is not accounted for in the current Model for End-stage Liver Disease classification of patients awaiting liver transplant.

The association of ascites and liver disease was recognized in the Indian Ayurveda 5000 years ago, is depicted in Mayan figures, and was well described by Hippocrates and Galen in 300 to 400 B.C. Paracentesis was the preferred form of therapy then and remained so into the middle of the 20th century (Runyon, 1997). The crucial role of sodium in maintaining plasma volume and the role of the sodium concentration in the passive determination of water movement were defined in the 1930s (Darrow & Yannet, 1935; Hastings & Eichelberger, 1937). These seminal findings led to the use of sodium restriction and the development of ever more powerful diuretics for the medical treatment of ascites and the gradual demise of the "paracentesis clinic" (Brater, 1998; Eisenmenger et al, 1948, 1950; Faloon et al, 1948; Layne & Schemm, 1947; Morrison, 1997).

Attempts to eliminate minor amounts of ascites, detectable only by ultrasound or computed tomography, may produce more complications from the treatment than benefits, and the ascites may be better left alone after its cause has been elucidated. Large amounts of tense ascites often produce serious consequences, however, including spontaneous bacterial peritonitis (SBP); development of hernias with incarceration or rupture; and impairment of food intake, respiratory function, and physical activity. Major complications (e.g., variceal bleeding, hepatic encephalopathy, and hepatorenal syndrome) are much more common in patients with severe ascites. Although not a direct consequence of the ascites, the refractoriness of ascites to medical therapy is an indication of the seriousness of the underlying disease. Conversely, overaggressive treatment of ascites also can lead to complications, including hyponatremia, hypovolemia, and hepatic encephalopathy. In the surgical patient, the presence of ascites presents special problems, first, as an indication of severely compromised hepatic function with its attendant increased risks for general anesthesia and surgery in general,

and second, because of the fluid and electrolyte management problems it poses.

In approaching a patient with ascites, it is crucial to remember that the mere presence of ascites does not equate to liver cirrhosis. In the United States, 20% of cases are due to another cause, including cardiac, renal, pancreatic, infectious, and malignant causes (Reynolds, 2000; Runyon et al, 1992). The percentage of cases secondary to noncirrhotic causes may be even higher in less developed parts of the world. Determining the cause of the ascites is the first step in managing a patient with ascites (Garcia-Tsao, 2001; Runyon, 2004; Runyon et al, 1992). This chapter focuses on the stepwise approach to managing cirrhotic ascites, based on an understanding of the pathophysiologic basis of cirrhotic ascites (Table 90.1).

NONPHARMACOLOGIC THERAPY

Sodium Restriction

In cirrhosis, the kidney avidly retains sodium. If dietary intake of sodium exceeds urinary and insensible losses of sodium, excess fluid is retained with the development of ascites or peripheral edema or both. The simple concept, *water follows sodium,* is the cornerstone of successful treatment of ascites. *Weight loss occurs because of sodium restriction, not fluid restriction.* The goal is to make sodium output exceed sodium input. This produces contraction of extracellular fluid volume with loss of peripheral edema and ascites. Insensible losses of sodium, primarily from the skin and gut, are usually less than 10 mmol/day (Eisenmenger et al, 1948, 1950). All other sodium must be cleared through the kidneys. Even in the complete absence of renal sodium clearance, dietary restriction of sodium to less than 10 mmol/day controls ascites (Eisenmenger et al, 1948, 1950). Such a diet is neither palatable nor practical.

A reasonable restriction is 87 mmol/day (2 g sodium). This requires that patients avoid most commercially prepared foods, canned soups and vegetables, and fast food restaurants and read all labels conscientiously. The patient and the individual who prepares the patient's food should meet with a dietitian to give a complete diet history and to receive detailed instructions on the new diet. Avoidance of salt substitutes, especially "white" ones (containing potassium with or without sodium salts), is essential. Spices without salt (herbal or "colored" substitutes) should be encouraged. Diligence also is necessary to avoid inadvertent use of "healthy" high salt foods (e.g., tomato and V8 juices [800-1000 mg sodium per 8 oz/240 mL]), other high-salt substances

Table 90.1 Stepwise Approach to the Treatment of Ascites in Cirrhotic Patients

Treatment	Success Rate
Sodium restriction	10-20%
Sodium restriction plus spironolactone	>50%
Sodium restriction plus spironolactone plus loop diuretic	90%

Table 90.2 Nonpharmacologic Cornerstones of Therapy for Cirrhotic Ascites

First treat the underlying disease		
Modality	Prescription	Comments
Sodium restriction	87 mmol (2 g)/day	Cornerstone of therapy. Follow compliance with daily weights and spot urine Na:K ratio (should be >1)
Fluid restriction	1200-1500 mL/day	Only if serum sodium is <125-130 mmol/L
Patience is the key to successful therapy		

(e.g., chewing tobacco [900-1200 mg per plug]), and medical therapies (e.g., Shohl's solution [1 mmol/mL] or sodium bicarbonate [11.8 mmol/g]). Shohl's solution and sodium bicarbonate may be prescribed for the mild acidosis frequently seen in these patients.

Compliance is crucial, and documentation of actual urinary sodium excretion and daily body weight is the most useful way to ascertain compliance. Although the most accurate measure of sodium output is a 24-hour urine sodium, properly confirmed as a complete collection by an appropriate 24-hour clearance of creatinine, this is not practical, especially on an outpatient basis. In contrast, a spot urinary sodium-to-potassium ratio (Na:K) is easy to obtain in the office or clinic. A low urinary Na:K ratio correlates with high mineralocorticoid activity (Alexander et al, 1977), and a random urinary Na:K ratio of greater than 1 is associated with a 24-hour urinary sodium excretion of greater than 78 mmol/day in 95% of samples (Runyon & Heck, 1996). Eggert (1970) found that patients with a Na:K ratio greater than 1 usually diuresed well with spironolactone. We have observed that patients who convert their urinary Na:K ratios from less than 1 to greater than 1 diurese successfully, whereas patients who do not convert their urinary Na:K ratios fail to diurese. This simple test is invaluable when initiating therapy and in following patients in clinic.

If a patient fails to diurese, or ascites fluid increases, despite a 2 g/day (87 mmol/day) sodium diet and a urinary sodium excretion of greater than 78 mmol/day (plus 10 mmol/day insensible losses), and has a urine Na:K of greater than 1, the patient is noncompliant with the diet. *Patients should not be labeled as having intractable ascites if they are merely noncompliant.* Such patients may require at least brief hospitalization to document that diuresis is possible on a controlled dietary (with or without diuretic) regimen and to allow for intensive dietary education.

Fluid Restriction

Although most patients are placed routinely on a 1 to 1.5 L/day fluid restriction, this is usually not necessary because free water excretion only follows sodium excretion. Fluid restriction should not be considered unless the serum sodium is less than 130 mmol/L. Some experts do not restrict fluids until the serum sodium is less than 125 mmol/L or 120 mmol/L (Caldwell, 1999; Runyon, 1998).

Bed Rest

Diuresis is enhanced by bed rest, which may explain the better response of patients initiated on ascites therapy while hospitalized. The stricter control of diet while hospitalized is probably also a factor. Pressor systems are triggered on standing, however, which worsen renal function and the response to diuretics (Bernardi et al, 1985; Palmer, 1999; Ring-Larsen et al, 1986; Salo et al, 1997). *Adherence to a sodium-restricted diet alone produces diuresis and ascites resolution in 20% of patients* (Table 90.2) (Gregory et al, 1977).

DIURETIC THERAPY

Most patients require the addition of one or more diuretics to achieve an adequate natriuresis. The key diuretic to long-term management is spironolactone (Table 90.3).

Spironolactone

Aldosterone produces avid reabsorption of sodium in exchange for potassium in the collecting duct of the nephron, the final arbiter of urine composition (Palmer, 1999). Hyperaldosteronism is common in cirrhotics owing to reduced metabolism of aldosterone by the liver. This condition produces fluid retention and the severe, total body potassium deficit commonly seen in cirrhotics with ascites. Spironolactone reverses this abnormality by competing directly with aldosterone for the mineralocorticoid-sensitive receptor (Brater, 1998; Morrison, 1997; Palmer, 1999).

Table 90.3 Diuretic Use in Cirrhotic Ascites*

Drug	Daily Dose (mg)	Comments
Primary		
Spironolactone	100-400	Can use as monotherapy; hyperkalemia, gynecomastia can be a problem
Amiloride	10-40	Can substitute for spironolactone if gynecomastia troublesome
Adjunct		
Loop diuretic (furosemide)	40-160	Not primary or monotherapy; use only with spironolactone. Do not use intravenously
Thiazide diuretics (hydrochlorothiazide, metolazone)	Hydrochlorothiazide: 25-100 Metolazone: 10-100	Use with furosemide for synergistic effect

*Patients must be on 87 mmol (2 g)/day sodium restriction.

In contrast to loop and thiazide diuretics, which require secretion into the proximal tubule lumen from which they travel down the nephron to their respective sites of action, spironolactone requires no tubular secretion, but is delivered directly to the collecting duct cells by the bloodstream. Efficacy is not impaired in cirrhosis, which may produce reduced renal blood flow with resultant decreased tubular secretion of other diuretics (Palmer, 1999).

As a result of a very long half-life, it takes 3 to 4 days to achieve steady-state drug levels of spironolactone, so the onset of action is slow, and the dose should not be adjusted more frequently than every 3 to 4 days to observe the effects of the drug at steady state (Brater, 1998; Gregory et al, 1977; Ochs et al, 1978; Sungaila et al, 1992). The starting dose is usually 50 to 100 mg, increasing to a maximum of 400 mg/day. Hyperkalemia may become a problem in patients on monotherapy, especially greater than 200 mg/day. Some patients, particularly men, may not tolerate spironolactone, most often because of the development of tender and disfiguring gynecomastia caused by this C-17 substituted steroid compound (Rose et al, 1977). Amiloride is an acceptable substitute (10 mg amiloride is approximately equal to 100 mg spironolactone). *Spironolactone monotherapy, combined with sodium restriction, produces a satisfactory diuresis in more than 50% of patients with ascites secondary to cirrhosis* (Gregory et al, 1977; Palmer, 1999; Stanley et al, 1989).

Loop and Thiazide Diuretics

Loop and thiazide diuretics are the mainstays in the management of fluid retention secondary to cardiac and renal diseases. They are much less effective than spironolactone as monotherapies for cirrhotic ascites, however. Spironolactone produced a diuresis in 18 of 19 cirrhotic patients in one study compared with only 11 of 21 patients in response to furosemide monotherapy. Nine of 10 patients who did not respond to furosemide subsequently diuresed on spironolactone therapy (Perez-Ayuso et al, 1983).

Cirrhotic patients show a reduced responsiveness to maximally effective doses of furosemide (25-30 mmol sodium excreted per day versus 200-250 mmol/day in normals), and increased doses are no more effective (Brater, 1998). A more avid, rebound sodium retention may occur because of the short half-life of furosemide, so more frequent dosing may prove to be effective (Brater, 1998; Ellison, 1991). In addition, hypertrophy of distal tubule nephron segments may lead to increased distal reabsorption of sodium, negating the proximal blockade produced by the furosemide. Thiazide diuretics can be used to block this distal reabsorption, providing a significant synergistic benefit when used in conjunction with furosemide (Brater, 1998; Ellison, 1991; Sica & Gehr, 1996). In contrast to spironolactone, both classes of drug promote heavy potassium loss with its attendant potential effects of increased renal ammonia synthesis, increased intestinal absorption of ammonia owing to decreased intestinal motility and increased ammonia trapping owing to decreased intracellular pH because of K^+/H^+ exchange, all leading to hepatic encephalopathy. A decrease in plasma sodium and plasma volume also may occur (Brater, 1998; Morrison, 1997).

In contrast to the success of continuous intravenous infusions of furosemide in renal and cardiac failure patients, intravenous furosemide produced acute reductions in glomerular filtration rates owing to vasoconstriction in more than 50% of patients studied (Daskalopoulos et al, 1987). Oral bioavailability is excellent in cirrhotics, and intravenous use is to be discouraged (Sawhney et al, 1981). Standard initial dosing would be 40 mg of furosemide and 100 mg of spironolactone, escalating to a maximum of 160 mg and 400 mg, respectively, before adding a thiazide. *Using this stepwise approach of sodium restriction plus titrated doses of spironolactone and furosemide, 90% of cirrhotic ascites patients can be diuresed successfully* (Stanley et al, 1989).

ALBUMIN

Hypoalbuminemia is frequently a problem in postoperative patients as a result of protein removal during frequent paracenteses, surgical and wound losses, inadequate preoperative and postoperative nutrition, and a hypercatabolic state. Plasma albumin makes crucial contributions to the oncotic pressure, which retains fluids intravascularly. In hospitalized patients whose ascites was relatively resistant to sodium restriction plus combination diuretic therapy, the addition of daily infusions of 12.5 g of albumin was shown to be beneficial and cost-effective. A combination of daily albumin, octreotide, and the α-adrenergic agent midodrine may help to reverse renal failure in some patients with hepatorenal syndrome (Angeli et al, 1999).

TREATMENT FOR REFRACTORY ASCITES

Ascites that is unresponsive to dietary sodium restriction (2 g/day) and high-dose diuretics (furosemide, 160 mg, and spironolactone, 400 mg/day), or ascites that recurs rapidly after a large therapeutic paracentesis despite the aforementioned measures, is referred to as *refractory ascites* (Arroyo et al, 1996). Refractory ascites occurs in less than 10% of cirrhotic patients being treated for ascites with standard medical therapy (Arroyo et al, 1996; Salerno et al, 1993). Patients developing hepatic encephalopathy, hyponatremia, hyperkalemia, or azotemia on lower doses of diuretics also are considered to have refractory ascites.

It is important to avoid nonsteroidal anti-inflammatory drugs in patients with cirrhotic ascites because these drugs have the potential of converting diuretic-responsive ascites to refractory ascites as a result of a reduction of urinary sodium excretion secondary to a block in compensatory prostaglandin synthesis (Boyer et al, 1979). Use of nonsteroidal anti-inflammatory drugs in cirrhotic patients with ascites carries the risk of inducing azotemia. Treatment options for refractory ascites include repeated large-volume paracentesis (LVP), a transjugular intrahepatic portosystemic stent (TIPS), peritoneovenous shunt (PVS), and liver transplantation. The first three treatment options are discussed in detail.

Therapeutic Paracentesis

Therapeutic paracentesis or LVP was reintroduced in 1987 when Gines and colleagues (1987a) reported a comparison of paracentesis with diuretics in a randomized study. LVP involves serial peritoneal taps with removal of 4 to 6 L of ascitic fluid at a time every 2 to 4 weeks until the patient is dry. This procedure can be performed in the outpatient setting. LVP does not affect the underlying mechanisms responsible for production of ascites.

Recurrence of ascites is inevitable and requires repeat paracenteses with the interval determined by the rapidity of reaccumulation of tense ascites.

Removal of 5 L of ascites without any colloid infusion has been shown to be safe in patients with diuretic-resistant tense ascites (Peltekian et al, 1997). Comparison of five 1-L paracenteses repeated daily versus a single total 5-L paracentesis has shown that total paracentesis is as effective and safe as repeated partial paracenteses (Tito et al, 1990). LVP or total paracentesis shortens the length of hospitalization and allows for outpatient intervention in treating refractory ascites (Gines et al, 1987a).

A randomized trial compared LVP involving removal of 4 to 6 L of ascitic fluid daily along with intravenous albumin infusion (40 g per paracentesis) with standard diuretic therapy comprising furosemide and spironolactone in cirrhotic patients with tense ascites admitted to the hospital (Gines et al, 1987a). This study, along with other randomized controlled trials published thereafter (Salerno et al, 1987; Sola et al, 1994; Tito et al, 1990), concluded that LVP is more effective than diuretics in eliminating ascites and shortening hospital stay without inducing any significant hepatic or renal dysfunction, serum electrolyte abnormalities, activation of endogenous neurohumoral systems, hyponatremia, or hepatic encephalopathy. LVP did not affect mortality rate, however, which remained at 50% at 2 years (Gines et al, 1987a). *The success of LVP requires sodium restriction and administration of diuretics to prevent reaccumulation of ascitic fluid* (Gines et al, 1987a). Continuation of diuretic use in patients subjected to LVP decreases the recurrence of ascites from 93% to 18% (Fernandez-Esparrach et al, 1997).

Although LVP with plasma volume expansion is considered to be a first-line treatment of tense ascites for patients with cirrhosis, paracentesis without volume expansion results in multiple complications, including renal function impairment, rapid recurrence of ascites, shorter time to first readmission, and shorter survival (Gines et al, 1996). Because any LVP can result in hypovolemia hours or days after the procedure, volume expansion with colloids is recommended after completion of paracentesis (Panos et al, 1990).

Several randomized studies have been conducted to determine the best and most economical agent for plasma volume expansion after LVP. One study compared dextran 70 with albumin given at a rate of 6 g/L of ascitic fluid removed in 20 and 21 patients after daily paracentesis of 5 L until patients were dry (Fassio et al, 1992). No significant differences were noted in liver or kidney function or the probability of survival and readmission to the hospital between the two groups (Fassio et al, 1992). Another randomized trial compared therapeutic paracentesis with or without intravenous albumin in patients with cirrhotic ascites using the same protocol of daily paracentesis and albumin infusion (Gines et al, 1988). Although paracentesis was effective, as expected, in eliminating ascites equally well in both groups, paracentesis without albumin infusion resulted in a significant renal impairment, increased plasma renin activity and plasma aldosterone concentration, and hyponatremia, but no change in the probability of survival in the two groups after entry into the study (Gines et al, 1988).

A larger study from Spain assessed the efficacy of albumin, dextran 70, and polygeline as volume expanders after LVP in 289 cirrhotic patients with ascites (Gines et al, 1996). All agents were given at a rate of 8 g/L of ascitic fluid removed with 50% of the dose given within the first 2 hours and 50% given within 6 to 8 hours after paracentesis (Gines et al, 1996). Marked

activation of the renin-angiotensin-aldosterone system, also known as paracentesis-induced circulatory dysfunction, occurred more frequently in patients treated with dextran 70 (34.4%) or polygeline (37.8%) compared with patients who received albumin (18.5%) (Gines et al, 1996). Because paracentesis-induced circulatory dysfunction is associated with shorter survival, albumin now is thought to be the plasma expander of choice. Albumin also has been shown to improve the response of cirrhotic patients with ascites to diuretics, with respect to rate of response and prevention of recurrence of ascites (Gentilini et al, 1999). LVP involving removal of more than 5 L of ascitic fluid is a safe and effective treatment of ascites in patients with cirrhosis when combined with albumin infusion at a rate of 6 to 8 g/L of ascitic fluid removed. LVP is recommended in patients with refractory ascites and for temporary relief in patients with ascites sensitive to diuretics while awaiting their effects.

The main complications of LVP include subcutaneous or intraperitoneal hemorrhage and paracentesis-induced circulatory dysfunction (Arnold et al, 1997; Gines et al, 1996; Sola-Vera et al, 2003), although the incidence of paracentesis-induced circulatory dysfunction can be minimized with albumin infusion whenever more than 5 to 6 L of ascitic fluid is removed (Sola-Vera et al, 2003). Use of LVP as a therapeutic modality does not obviate the need for concomitant salt restriction and diuretic therapy to minimize recurrence of ascites.

Peritoneovenous Surgical Shunts

PVSs became available for treatment of refractory ascites with the introduction of the LeVeen shunt, which permitted one-way passage of ascitic fluid into the systemic circulation, and were popularized in the 1970s (LeVeen et al, 1974). A variety of PVSs have been described. The LeVeen, Denver, and Minnesota shunts all work by draining the ascitic fluid directly into the central venous system. The LeVeen shunt has been used more commonly in patients with refractory ascites and hepatic hydrothorax.

Initially, PVSs were shown to be superior to medical management in removing tense ascites more rapidly, decreasing the length of hospitalization (Bories et al, 1986; Stanley et al, 1989). One of the largest studies evaluating the use of PVS, the Veterans Administration Cooperative Study on Patients with Alcoholic Cirrhosis with Ascites, compared intensive medical therapy with peritoneovenous shunting using a LeVeen shunt and reported the median time to the resolution of ascites to be 5.4 weeks versus 3 weeks for patients treated medically or with a LeVeen shunt (Stanley et al, 1989). The median time to the recurrence of ascites also was significantly longer and median hospitalization shorter in patients undergoing surgical shunting versus intensive medical therapy (Stanley et al, 1989). Median survival time was similar, however, for medical and surgical patients in all risk groups divided according to the severity of underlying liver disease, and the length of survival was determined by the severity of illness at the time of randomization (Stanley et al, 1989). At least three other prospective randomized trials have assessed outcome in patients with cirrhotic ascites using conventional therapy with medications or surgical portovenous shunting (Bories et al, 1986; Ring-Larsen et al, 1989; Wapnick et al, 1979). Although one study suggested an improvement in survival and shorter hospitalization in the surgical group that received LeVeen shunts compared with the medical group (Wapnick et al, 1979), the other studies concluded that PVS did not influence survival in patients with cirrhosis and ascites deemed refractory to diuretic therapy.

PVSs are associated with multiple complications and significant postoperative overall mortality (Foley et al, 1984; Moskovitz, 1990). Early complications include pulmonary edema and increased risk of variceal bleeding owing to rapid plasma volume expansion (Samanta & Leevy, 1989; Stanley et al, 1989; Vons et al, 1991). Technical problems related to shunt placement can account for failure in 40% of patients within the first year owing to shunt thrombosis, kinking, and clogging of the valve (Arroyo et al, 1992). Postshunt coagulopathy, including disseminated intravascular coagulation, has been reported in 10% to 60% of patients, and late peritonitis, likely related to transient bacteremia, can be seen in 10% of the patients with surgical shunts. Hepatic encephalopathy also occurs in about 15% of these patients (Gines et al, 1991). One of the most serious complications involves thrombosis of the superior vena cava, which can be seen in 23% of cases with 8% developing pulmonary emboli (Foley et al, 1984). Cardiac tamponade also has been reported to occur with placement of PVS (Dulai et al, 1998).

PVSs do not offer any long-term survival benefits (Bories et al, 1986; Gines et al, 1991; Stanley et al, 1989). Thirty-day and 1-year survivals were lower in the surgical group versus the medical group (Bories et al, 1986). PVS should not be considered in several groups of patients, including patients with hepatorenal syndrome and severely decompensated cirrhosis, because of increased morbidity and mortality (Moskovitz, 1990; Scholz et al, 1989).

With the advent of TIPS, peritoneovenous shunting currently is considered to play little role in the treatment of refractory ascites. The use of these shunts has been abandoned because of a significant rate of complications (Gines et al, 1991). These shunts may play a useful role, however, in patients with mild to moderate, but not severe, liver dysfunction who are not candidates for orthotopic liver transplantation.

Transjugular Intrahepatic Portosystemic Shunts (TIPS)

TIPS (see Ch. 96) creates a communication between the central hepatic vein and an intrahepatic branch of the portal vein, decompressing the portal system. TIPS achieves portal decompression without the usual surgical risks. It is a nonsurgical side-to-side portocaval shunt with a procedure-related complication rate of less than 10% (Rossle et al, 1994). It was performed initially in the late 1980s in a cirrhotic patient with continued variceal bleeding despite numerous therapies (Rossle et al, 1989).

Insertion of a TIPS shunt results in a marked increase in cardiac output with a resultant decrease in systemic vascular resistance and an increase in effective arterial blood volume (Huonker et al, 1999). TIPS placement has been shown to improve sodium secretion and renal function after 4 weeks (Wong et al, 1997). One study by Rossle's group reported an improvement in serum creatinine from 1.5 mg/dL to 0.9 mg/dL in patients with refractory ascites after shunt placement (Ochs et al, 1995).

Five prospective randomized clinical trials have compared TIPS with LVP (Gines et al, 2002; Lebrec et al, 1996; Rossle et al, 2000; Salerno et al, 2004; Sanyal et al, 2003). All of these studies indicated that TIPS is more effective in controlling ascites than LVP at 3 months and at 12 months of follow-up. No significant improvement in survival or improvement in

quality of life was noted, however, in patients treated with TIPS versus LVP. In the latest North American multicenter randomized controlled trial involving a total of 109 patients, TIPS was much more effective in controlling ascites at 1-year follow-up (30 of 52 versus 9 of 57) (Sanyal et al, 2003). Control of ascites was defined as recurrence of tense ascites requiring therapeutic paracentesis in either group. LVP was performed in both groups whenever tense ascites developed with albumin infused at a rate of 6 to 8 g/L of ascites removed at the time of LVP. Although the median transplant-free survival time was longer in patients receiving TIPS (19.6 months versus 12.4 months), this was not significant ($P = .77$ by log-rank test) (Sanyal et al, 2003). A more recent European multicenter randomized controlled trial comparing TIPS with LVP showed an increased probability of survival without transplantation ($P = .021$) in the TIPS group at 1 year (77% versus 52%) and at 2 years (59% versus 29%) after randomization into the study (Salerno et al, 2004). The improved survival in this patient population may be partially due to the exclusion of patients with Child-Pugh score greater than 11 (Salerno et al, 2004).

TIPS-related complications include immediate complications associated with the procedure and late complications related to the shunt. Immediate complications include capsule puncture and intra-abdominal bleeding (Rossle & Grandt, 2004). Rare complications resulting in death include cardiac perforations and caval and portal lacerations (Rossle & Grandt, 2004). Hemobilia, resulting from an arterial-biliary fistula manifesting as right upper quadrant colicky pain, jaundice, and elevated liver enzymes with a cholestatic pattern, also is reported as a complication of the procedure (Rossle & Grandt, 2004). Late complications include shunt stenosis secondary to intimal proliferation. This is a major shunt-related complication that occurs in approximately 50% of patients after 6 to 12 months (Boyer, 2003). A sudden worsening of refractory ascites, or an improvement in hepatic encephalopathy without any interval change in medical regimen or salt restriction, suggests the possibility of shunt stenosis. This situation requires evaluation of the shunt with duplex Doppler studies and shunt revision if it is stenosed. Shunt stenosis may be minimized by the use of polytetrafluoroethylene-coated stents; two randomized studies reported significantly superior shunt patency in polytetrafluoroethylene-coated stents than uncoated stents (Bureau et al, 2004; Hernandez-Guerra et al, 2004). Other complications involve displacement of the shunt with protrusion into the portal or caval veins or into the right atrium or pulmonary artery or migration through a wall (Rossle & Grandt, 2004).

The most important clinical complications related to the shunt are deterioration in liver function and worsening of hepatic encephalopathy. The latter seems to be related to shunt size and the degree of reduction in the portal pressure gradient (Casado et al, 1998). Individual reduction in portal gradient pressure by about 40% to 50% compared with the baseline has been recommended (Rossle et al, 2001). As expected, the incidence of post-TIPS hepatic encephalopathy also depends on the Child-Pugh score and the presence of encephalopathy before shunt placement (Nolte et al, 1998).

TIPS is contraindicated in patients with advanced liver failure, especially in the presence of renal failure. Malinchoc and Kamath and colleagues (Kamath et al, 2001; Malinchoc et al, 2000) reported a median survival of 3 months or less after elective TIPS placement for prevention of variceal bleeding or for treatment of refractory ascites in patients with Model for End-stage Liver Disease score greater than 18 (R score >1.8). TIPS is best in patients with severe refractory ascites and relatively preserved liver function. It is a procedure that serves as a bridge to liver transplantation, the ultimate treatment for refractory ascites.

TREATMENT FOR HEPATIC HYDROTHORAX

The presence of a large pleural effusion in a patient with cirrhosis and portal hypertension in the absence of coexistent cardiopulmonary disease is referred to as hepatic hydrothorax. Hepatic hydrothorax occurs in 9% of cirrhotic patients with ascites, and it is often massive. It is right-sided in about 85% of cases, but can be left-sided or bilateral (Cardenas et al, 2004). As expected, isolated observation of hepatic hydrothorax usually accompanies biochemical and other evidence of chronic liver disease. Numerous different pathophysiologic mechanisms have been proposed to explain the development of hepatic hydrothorax, including hypoalbuminemia with a decreased colloid osmotic pressure, leakage of plasma from hypertensive azygos veins that serve as collaterals between the portal and the azygos venous system, lymphatic leakage from the thoracic duct, transfer of ascitic fluid from the peritoneal cavity to the pleural space via diaphragmatic lymphatic channels, and direct passage of ascites into the pleural space via diaphragmatic defects (Strauss & Boyer, 1997).

Clinical manifestations of hepatic hydrothorax are varied, with many patients reporting no pulmonary symptoms. Hepatic hydrothorax should be suspected in cirrhotic patients presenting with unilateral pleural effusions. Biochemical abnormalities and signs and symptoms of cirrhosis and ascites are common findings. As a result of negative intrathoracic pressure favoring unidirectional transfer of fluid across the diaphragmatic defect, hepatic hydrothorax can be present without ascites, confusing the clinician and leading to an extensive diagnostic evaluation for causes of pleural effusion (Cardenas et al, 2004; Rubinstein et al, 1985; Strauss & Boyer, 1997). Depending on the size of the hydrothorax, shortness of breath, cough, and hypoxemia may be the pulmonary symptoms encountered in these patients. Chest discomfort also may be present. Other physical and radiographic findings in hepatic hydrothorax are identical to the findings commonly seen in other patients presenting with pleural effusions. Rarely, patients present with acute tension hydrothorax resulting in dyspnea and hypotension (Castellote et al, 2002).

Diagnosis of hepatic hydrothorax largely is based on clinical presentation. A thoracentesis is not always necessary to establish the diagnosis in asymptomatic cirrhotic patients with ascites presenting with pleural effusion. Thoracentesis should be performed in patients presenting with left-sided hydrothorax, fever, pleuritic chest pain, shortness of breath, or lack of ascites to exclude other diagnoses, including spontaneous bacterial empyema, which carries a poor prognosis (Xiol et al, 1996). Biochemical analysis of pleural fluid in hepatic hydrothorax reveals the fluid to be transudative with serum-to-ascites protein ratio less than 0.5, serum-to-ascites lactic dehydrogenase ratio less than 0.6, and total protein concentration usually less than or equal to 2.5 g/dL. Definitive diagnosis of hepatic hydrothorax involves the demonstration of a communication between the peritoneal cavity and pleural space. This usually is accomplished by instillation of technetium 99m-labeled sulfur colloid into the peritoneal cavity following which movement of the radiotracer to the pleural space is detected by scintigraphy (Bhattacharya et al, 2001). In the absence of ascites, 500 mL of saline can be injected into the peritoneal space under ultrasound or computed tomography guidance followed by radiolabeled colloid injection (Strauss & Boyer, 1997). A thoracentesis should be performed immediately before injecting radiolabeled colloid into the peritoneal cavity to increase the rate of movement of the radiotracer into the pleural space.

Medical management of hepatic hydrothorax is aimed at the origin of the fluid (i.e., ascites resulting from complications of cirrhosis). The mainstay of treatment involves a combination of sodium-restricted diet and diuretics to attain a negative sodium balance. Accumulation of large-volume hepatic hydrothorax resulting in shortness of breath requires additional therapies. Shortness of breath at rest warrants a large volume thoracentesis, but placement of a chest tube is relatively contraindicated because of the risk of life-threatening fluid depletion (Runyon et al, 1986). TIPS to lower the pressure in the portal circulation has been shown to be an effective way to control refractory ascites (Ochs et al, 1995), and it is recommended in patients with hepatic hydrothorax requiring repeated thoracenteses for symptom control (Boyer, 2003). In a landmark study describing the outcome of 24 patients with refractory ascites treated with TIPS insertion, relief or improvement was noted in 79% of the cases (Gordon et al, 1997).

The encouraging results are counterbalanced by the development of TIPS-related complications, including hepatic encephalopathy and sudden worsening of liver function leading to death in 20% of the patients (Gordon et al, 1997). In another more recent study involving 40 patients with hepatic hydrothorax refractory to diuretic therapy, pleurocentesis or pleurodesis reportedly improved hydrothorax in 82% of patients with resolution in 71% of the patients (Siegerstetter et al, 2001). TIPS may be a good option for patients with refractory hepatic hydrothorax who do not have critically deteriorated liver function. Pleurodesis often fails because of a rapid passage of ascites from the peritoneal cavity to the pleural space (Ikard & Sawyers, 1980). Video-assisted thoracoscopy to repair diaphragmatic defects combined with pleurodesis has been reported to be a successful treatment modality (Ferrante et al, 2002; Milanez et al, 2000; Mouroux et al, 1996). The newest technique involves thoracoscopic pleurodesis using argon plasma coagulation, fibrin glue, and minocycline. This procedure was shown to be effective in nine patients with only two recurrences in 4 months of follow-up (Takayama et al, 2004). These procedures generally are associated with high morbidity and mortality.

LIVER TRANSPLANTATION

None of the aforementioned therapies for refractory ascites has been shown to prolong life expectancy. At best, they should be viewed as temporizing measures while awaiting liver transplantation in patients who qualify for a transplant. Survival in patients with refractory ascites, as already noted, is poor, with 1-year survival of 64% and relapse-free 1-year survival of only 35% in one series (Siegerstetter et al, 2001). Liver transplantation is the only option for curative treatment of refractory ascites with an expectation of prolonging of life (see Ch. 103).

TREATMENT FOR SPONTANEOUS BACTERIAL PERITONITIS

SBP is a potentially life-threatening complication in patients with cirrhosis. It is characterized by spontaneous infection of ascitic fluid in the absence of any overt intra-abdominal source of infection. Prevalence of SBP in patients with ascites ranges from 10% to 30% (Rimola et al, 2000) with an annual risk of 10% (Garcia-Tsao, 2001). Despite antibiotic therapy, in-hospital mortality related to SBP is still high at greater than 20% (Garcia-Tsao, 2001).

In most studies assessing bacterial infections in cirrhosis performed in the 1980s, the most common infections were urinary tract infection, pneumonia, and SBP. Most of these infections were community acquired with 70% to 80% of the isolated organisms being gram-negative bacilli. Depressed immunity with defective leukocyte chemotaxis, hypocomplementemia, and impaired reticuloendothelial activity in conjunction with decreased clearance of bacteria owing to the presence of shunting from portosystemic collaterals are some of the proposed mechanisms for the development of SBP in patients with cirrhosis (Rimola et al, 2000). SBP is thought to be caused by bacterial translocation across the intestinal wall to the mesenteric lymph nodes (Llovet et al, 1998). Bacteria are thought to translocate from these lymph nodes to the bloodstream and to the ascitic fluid (Llovet et al, 1998). SBP develops in patients with low protein concentration ascitic fluid, secondary to decreased opsonic activity (Runyon, 1986).

Signs and symptoms of SBP include abdominal pain, fever, and impairment of liver function, such as unexplained hepatic encephalopathy. Renal failure and alteration in gastrointestinal motility also have been described. SBP frequently is associated with only minor symptoms, however, or may be completely asymptomatic. A high index of suspicion needs to be exercised in patients with cirrhosis and ascites, especially patients admitted to the hospital. SBP also is more common in patients presenting with gastrointestinal hemorrhage (Rimola et al, 2000).

Diagnostic evaluation starts with a paracentesis and sending the fluid for cell count with white blood cell differential. Ascitic fluid culture yield is improved by inoculating aerobic and anaerobic culture bottles at the bedside with a minimum of 10 mL of ascites inoculated in each bottle. The presence of greater than 250 polymorphonuclear cells (PMN)/mm^3 of ascitic fluid is consistent with SBP, even before culture results are available, and needs to be treated accordingly (Runyon, 2004). Typically, ascitic fluid cultures grow single organisms. Very high ascitic fluid white blood cell count, ascitic fluid culture growing multiple organisms, or growth of anaerobic organisms in ascitic fluid culture should raise suspicion of perforated bowel, intra-abdominal abscess, or a surgical source of infection. Culture-negative neutrocytic ascites is diagnosed when an ascitic fluid PMN count of greater than 250/mm^3 is unaccompanied by a positive ascitic fluid culture. Culture-negative neutrocytic ascites carries a similar prognosis to SBP and is managed similarly (Garcia-Tsao, 2001).

Ascites also should be sent for cytology and for acid-fast bacillus smear and culture in cases in which malignancy or intraperitoneal tuberculosis is suspected. Triglyceride analysis of chylous-appearing ascitic fluid can help confirm the diagnosis of chylous ascites. Determination of total protein in ascitic fluid is helpful on the initial diagnostic paracentesis to help establish the underlying etiology. Ascites with high total protein (>2.5 mg/dL) suggests ascites related to cardiac disease, Budd-Chiari syndrome,

veno-occlusive disease, and myxedema, among other possibilities. Gram stain of ascitic fluid usually is not helpful. Rapid and automated cell count testing is being investigated currently to expedite the detection of SBP. These tests include use of reagent strip testing for leukocyte esterase similar to that used for urinalysis (Castellote et al, 2003) and automated blood cell counter for determination of PMN count (Angeloni et al, 2003).

SBP can be treated with cefotaxime, 2 g intravenously every 8 hours for 5 days (Garcia-Tsao, 2001; Rimola et al, 2000). Cefotaxime, a third-generation cephalosporin, covers 95% of flora seen in SBP, including *Escherichia coli, Klebsiella pneumonia,* and pneumococcus (Felisart et al, 1985). Cefotaxime treatment for 5 days has been shown to be as effective as 10 days of therapy in a randomized controlled trial of 100 patients (Runyon et al, 1991). In patients allergic to penicillin or cephalosporins, aztreonam and vancomycin can be used as guided by the ascitic fluid cultures. Repeat diagnostic paracentesis is indicated after 48 hours of appropriate antibiotic therapy only if there is a lack of clinical improvement or in cases of secondary bacterial peritonitis (Rimola et al, 2000). An increase in PMN count on repeat paracentesis 48 hours after antibiotic treatment suggests (1) SBP resistant to currently used antibiotic regimen; (2) noninfectious cause of neutrocytic ascites, including pancreatic ascites; or (3) secondary bacterial peritonitis.

One controlled randomized trial assessed use of albumin infusion in addition to cefotaxime for treatment of hospitalized patients with SBP (Sort et al, 1999). Patients were randomized to receive cefotaxime alone or cefotaxime plus albumin, 1.5 g/kg body weight within 6 hours of enrollment into the study and 1 g/kg body weight on day 3. This study showed a reduction in in-hospital mortality from 29% to 10% (Sort et al, 1999). Based on this study, use of albumin with this dosing regimen is now recommended by the American Association for the Study of Liver Diseases Practice Guidelines (Runyon, 2004).

Prevention of SBP is indicated in patients with risk factors for development of SBP, including patients with low ascitic fluid total protein concentration less than 1 g/dL, gastrointestinal hemorrhage, or a prior history of SBP, especially during a hospitalization. Randomized controlled trials have shown that norfloxacin, 400 mg twice daily for 7 days, decreases the incidence of SBP in patients with variceal bleeding (Soriano et al, 1992) and in patients with low-protein ascites (Soriano et al, 1991). Selective intestinal decontamination with norfloxacin, 400 mg twice daily, has been shown to reduce the recurrence of SBP in patients with a prior history of SBP (Gines et al, 1990). Trimethoprim/sulfamethoxazole, one double strength tablet daily 5 times/week, is reported to be effective in preventing SBP in cirrhotic patients with ascites (Singh et al, 1995). Ciprofloxacin, 750 mg dosed once per week, also has been shown in a prospective controlled trial to prevent SBP (Rolachon et al, 1995). A meta-analysis showed that norfloxacin prophylaxis for SBP improved survival (Bernard et al, 1998). Continued use of prophylactic antibiotics is recommended in patients with a history of SBP after discharge from the hospital because of poor survival in these patients (Jepsen et al, 2003).

Prevalence of SBP in a population of 427 cirrhotic outpatients was reported to be 3.5% (Evans et al, 2003). Patients not receiving antibiotics for neutrocytic ascites (≥250 PMN/mm^3) did as well as patients who received antibiotics. In addition, organisms cultured from ascitic fluid in these cirrhotic outpatients were predominantly gram-positive, similar to a previous report from Spain (Fernandez et al, 2002). In the latter study, there was a significantly higher percentage of patients with SBP owing to quinolone-resistant, gram-negative bacillus in the group receiving long-term norfloxacin versus patients who were not receiving norfloxacin, raising a concern for the development of quinolone resistance as an emergent problem in patients on long-term norfloxacin prophylaxis (Fernandez et al, 2002). Of patients with quinolone-resistant, gram-negative bacillus SBP, 68% also were resistant to trimethoprim-sulfamethoxazole (Fernandez et al, 2002), indicating a need for new prophylactic treatment options in SBP in the future.

REFERENCES

Alexander WD, et al, 1977: The urinary sodium:potassium ratio and response to diuretics in resistant oedema. Postgrad Med J 53:117-121.

Angeli P, et al, 1999: Reversal of type 1 hepatorenal syndrome with the administration of midodrine and octreotide. Hepatology 29:1690-1697.

Angeloni S, et al, 2003: Validation of automated blood cell counter for the determination of polymorphonuclear cell count in the ascitic fluid of cirrhotic patients with or without spontaneous bacterial peritonitis. Am J Gastroenterol 98:1844-1848.

Arnold C, et al, 1997: Acute hemoperitoneum after large-volume paracentesis. Gastroenterology 113:978-982.

Arroyo V, et al, 1992: Treatment of ascites in cirrhosis: diuretics, peritoneovenous shunt, and large-volume paracentesis. Gastroenterol Clin North Am 21:237-256.

Arroyo V, et al, 1996: Definition and diagnostic criteria of refractory ascites and hepatorenal syndrome in cirrhosis. International Ascites Club. Hepatology 23:164-176.

Bernard B, et al, 1998: Antibiotic prophylaxis for the prevention of bacterial infections in cirrhotic patients with ascites: a meta-analysis. Digestion 59(suppl 2):54-57.

Bernardi M, et al, 1985: Renal function impairment induced by change in posture in patients with cirrhosis and ascites. Gut 26:629-635.

Bhattacharya A, et al, 2001: Radioisotope scintigraphy in the diagnosis of hepatic hydrothorax. J Gastroenterol Hepatol 16:317-321.

Bories P, et al, 1986: The treatment of refractory ascites by the LeVeen shunt: a multi-centre controlled trial (57 patients). J Hepatol 3:212-218.

Boyer TD, 2003: Transjugular intrahepatic portosystemic shunt: current status. Gastroenterology 124:1700-1710.

Boyer TD, et al, 1979: Effect of indomethacin and prostaglandin A1 on renal function and plasma renin activity in alcoholic liver disease. Gastroenterology 77:215-222.

Brater DC, 1998: Diuretic therapy. N Engl J Med 339:387-395.

Bureau C, et al, 2004: Improved clinical outcome using polytetrafluoroethylene-coated stents for TIPS: results of a randomized study. Gastroenterology 126:469-475.

Caldwell SH, 1999: Ascites and spontaneous bacterial peritonitis. In Schiff ER, et al (eds): Schiff's Diseases of the Liver. Philadelphia, Lippincott-Raven, pp 503-544.

Cardenas A, et al, 2004: Review article: hepatic hydrothorax. Aliment Pharmacol Ther 20:271-279.

Casado M, et al, 1998: Clinical events after transjugular intrahepatic portosystemic shunt: correlation with hemodynamic findings. Gastroenterology 114:1296-1303.

Castellote J, et al, 2002: Acute tension hydrothorax: a life-threatening complication of cirrhosis. J Clin Gastroenterol 34:588-589.

Castellote J, et al, 2003: Rapid diagnosis of spontaneous bacterial peritonitis by use of reagent strips. Hepatology 37:893-896.

D'Amico G, et al, 1986: Survival and prognostic indicators in compensated and decompensated cirrhosis. Dig Dis Sci 31:468-475.

Darrow DC, Yannet H, 1935: The changes in the distribution of body water accompanying increase and decrease in extracellular electrolyte. J Clin Invest 14:266-275.

Daskalopoulos G, et al, 1987: Immediate effects of furosemide on renal hemodynamics in chronic liver disease with ascites. Gastroenterology 92:1859-1863.

Dulai G, et al, 1998: A novel complication of peritoneovenous shunt: cardiac tamponade. Am J Gastroenterol 93:1379-1380.

Eggert RC, 1970: Spironolactone diuresis in patients with cirrhosis and ascites. BMJ 4:401-403.

Eisenmenger WJ, et al, 1948: The effect of rigid sodium restriction in patients with cirrhosis of the liver and ascites. J Lab Clin Med 34:1029-1038.

Eisenmenger WJ, et al, 1950: Electrolyte studies on patients with cirrhosis of the liver. J Clin Invest 29:1491-1499.

Ellison DH, 1991: The physiologic basis of diuretic synergism: its role in treating diuretic resistance. Ann Intern Med 114:886-894.

Evans LT, et al, 2003: Spontaneous bacterial peritonitis in asymptomatic outpatients with cirrhotic ascites. Hepatology 37:897-901.

Faloon WW, et al, 1948: The effect of human serum albumin, mercurial diuretics, and a low sodium diet on sodium excretion in patients with cirrhosis of the liver. J Clin Invest 28:595-602.

Fassio E, et al, 1992: Paracentesis with dextran-70 vs paracentesis with albumin in cirrhosis with tense ascites—results of a randomized study. J Hepatol 14:310-316.

Felisart J, et al, 1985: Cefotaxime is more effective than is ampicillin-tobramycin in cirrhotics with severe infections. Hepatology 5:457-462.

Fernandez J, et al, 2002: Bacterial infections in cirrhosis: epidemiological changes with invasive procedures and norfloxacin prophylaxis. Hepatology 35:140-148.

Fernandez-Esparrach G, et al, 1997: Diuretic requirements after therapeutic paracentesis in non-azotemic patients with cirrhosis: a randomized double-blind trial of spironolactone versus placebo. J Hepatol 26:614-620.

Ferrante D, et al, 2002: Video-assisted thoracoscopic surgery with talc pleurodesis in the management of symptomatic hepatic hydrothorax. Am J Gastroenterol 97:3172-3175.

Foley WJ, et al, 1984: Central venous thrombosis and embolism associated with peritoneovenous shunts. Arch Surg 119:713-720.

Garcia-Tsao G, 2001: Current management of the complications of cirrhosis and portal hypertension: variceal hemorrhage, ascites, and spontaneous bacterial peritonitis. Gastroenterology 120:726-748.

Gentilini P, et al, 1999: Albumin improves the response to diuretics in patients with cirrhosis and ascites: results of a randomized, controlled trial. J Hepatol 30:639-645.

Gines A, et al, 1996: Randomized trial comparing albumin, dextran 70, and polygeline in cirrhotic patients with ascites treated by paracentesis. Gastroenterology 111:1002-1010.

Gines P, et al, 1987a: Comparison of paracentesis and diuretics in the treatment of cirrhotics with tense ascites—results of a randomized study. Gastroenterology 93:234-241.

Gines P, et al, 1987b: Compensated cirrhosis: natural history and prognostic factors. Hepatology 7:122-128.

Gines P, et al, 1988: Randomized comparative-study of therapeutic paracentesis with and without intravenous albumin in cirrhosis. Gastroenterology 94:1493-1502.

Gines P, et al, 1990: Norfloxacin prevents spontaneous bacterial peritonitis recurrence in cirrhosis—results of a double-blind, placebo-controlled trial. Hepatology 12:716-724.

Gines P, et al, 1991: Paracentesis with intravenous-infusion of albumin as compared with peritoneovenous shunting in cirrhosis with refractory ascites. N Engl J Med 325:829-835.

Gines P, et al, 2002: Transjugular intrahepatic portosystemic shunting versus paracentesis plus albumin for refractory ascites in cirrhosis. Gastroenterology 123:1839-1847.

Gordon FD, et al, 1997: The successful treatment of symptomatic, refractory hepatic hydrothorax with transjugular intrahepatic portosystemic shunt. Hepatology 25:1366-1369.

Gregory PB, et al, 1977: Complications of diuresis in the alcoholic patient with ascites: a controlled trial. Gastroenterology 73:534-538.

Hastings AB, Eichelberger L, 1937: The exchange of salt and water between muscle and blood. J Biol Chem 117:73-93.

Hernandez-Guerra M, et al, 2004: PTFE-covered stents improve TIPS patency in Budd-Chiari syndrome. Hepatology 40:1197-1202.

Huonker M, et al, 1999: Cardiac function and haemodynamics in alcoholic cirrhosis and effects of the transjugular intrahepatic portosystemic stent shunt. Gut 44:743-748.

Ikard RW, Sawyers JL, 1980: Persistent hepatic hydrothorax after peritoneojugular shunt. Arch Surg 115:1125-1127.

Jepsen P, et al, 2003: Prognosis of patients with liver cirrhosis and spontaneous bacterial peritonitis. Hepatogastroenterology 50:2133-2136.

Kamath PS, et al, 2001: A model to predict survival in patients with end-stage liver disease. Hepatology 33:464-470.

Layne JA, Schemm ER, 1947: The use of a high fluid intake and a low sodium acid-ash diet in the management of portal cirrhosis with ascites. Gastroenterology 9:705-717.

Lebrec D, et al, 1996: Transjugular intrahepatic portosystemic shunts: comparison with paracentesis in patients with cirrhosis and refractory ascites: a randomized trial. French Group of Clinicians and a Group of Biologists. J Hepatol 25:135-144.

LeVeen HH, et al, 1974: Peritoneo-venous shunting for ascites. Ann Surg 180:580-591.

Llovet JM, et al, 1998: Translocated intestinal bacteria cause spontaneous bacterial peritonitis in cirrhotic rats: molecular epidemiologic evidence. J Hepatol 28:307-313.

Malinchoc M, et al, 2000: A model to predict poor survival in patients undergoing transjugular intrahepatic portosystemic shunts. Hepatology 31:864-871.

Milanez DC Jr, et al, 2000: Thoracoscopy and talc poudrage in the management of hepatic hydrothorax. Chest 118:13-17.

Morrison RT, 1997: Edema and principles of diuretic use. Med Clin North Am 81:689-704.

Moskovitz M, 1990: The peritoneovenous shunt: expectations and reality. Am J Gastroenterol 85:917-929.

Mouroux J, et al, 1996: Management of pleural effusion of cirrhotic origin. Chest 109:1093-1096.

Nolte W, et al, 1998: Portosystemic hepatic encephalopathy after transjugular intrahepatic portosystemic shunt in patients with cirrhosis: clinical, laboratory, psychometric, and electroencephalographic investigations. Hepatology 28:1215-1225.

Ochs A, et al, 1995: The transjugular intrahepatic portosystemic stent-shunt procedure for refractory ascites. N Engl J Med 332:1192-1197.

Ochs HR, et al, 1978: Spironolactone. Am Heart J 96:389-400.

Palmer BF, 1999: Pathogenesis of ascites and renal salt retention in cirrhosis. J Invest Med 47:183-202.

Panos MZ, et al, 1990: Single, total paracentesis for tense ascites: sequential hemodynamic changes and right atrial size. Hepatology 11:662-667.

Peltekian KM, et al, 1997: Cardiovascular, renal, and neurohumoral responses to single large-volume paracentesis in patients with cirrhosis and diuretic-resistant ascites. Am J Gastroenterol 92:394-399.

Perez-Ayuso RM, et al, 1983: Randomized comparative study of efficacy of furosemide versus spironolactone in nonazotemic cirrhosis with ascites: relationship between the diuretic response and the activity of the renin-aldosterone system. Gastroenterology 84:961-968.

Powell WJ Jr, Klatskin G, 1968: Duration of survival in patients with Laennec's cirrhosis: influence of alcohol withdrawal, and possible effects of recent changes in general management of the disease. Am J Med 44:406-420.

Reynolds TB, 2000: Ascites. Clin Liver Dis 4:151-168.

Rimola A, et al, 2000: Diagnosis, treatment and prophylaxis of spontaneous bacterial peritonitis: a consensus document. International Ascites Club. J Hepatol 32:142-153.

Ring-Larsen H, et al, 1986: Diuretic treatment in decompensated cirrhosis and congestive heart failure: effect of posture. BMJ (Clin Res Educ) 292:1351-1353.

Ring-Larsen H, et al, 1989: Denver shunt in the treatment of refractory ascites in cirrhosis: a randomized control trial. Gastroenterology 96:A649.

Rolachon A, et al, 1995: Ciprofloxacin and long-term prevention of spontaneous bacterial peritonitis: results of a prospective controlled trial. Hepatology 22:1171-1174.

Rose LI, et al, 1977: Pathophysiology of spironolactone-induced gynecomastia. Ann Intern Med 87:398-403.

Rossle M, Grandt D, 2004: TIPS: an update. Best Pract Res Clin Gastroenterol 18:99-123.

Rossle M, et al, 1989: New non-operative treatment for variceal haemorrhage. Lancet 2:153.

Rossle M, et al, 1994: The transjugular intrahepatic portosystemic stent-shunt procedure for variceal bleeding. N Engl J Med 330:165-171.

Rossle M, et al, 2000: A comparison of paracentesis and transjugular intrahepatic portosystemic shunting in patients with ascites. N Engl J Med 342:1701-1707.

Rossle M, et al, 2001: How much reduction in portal pressure is necessary to prevent variceal rebleeding? A longitudinal study in 225 patients with transjugular intrahepatic portosystemic shunts. Am J Gastroenterol 96:3379-3383.

Rubinstein D, et al, 1985: Hepatic hydrothorax in the absence of clinical ascites: diagnosis and management. Gastroenterology 88:188-191.

Runyon BA, 1986: Low-protein-concentration ascitic fluid is predisposed to spontaneous bacterial peritonitis. Gastroenterology 91:1343-1346.

Runyon BA, 1997: Historical aspects of treatment of patients with cirrhosis and ascites. Semin Liver Dis 17:163-173.

Runyon BA, 1998: Management of adult patients with ascites caused by cirrhosis. Hepatology 27:264-272.

Runyon BA, 2004: Management of adult patients with ascites due to cirrhosis. Hepatology 39:841-856.

Runyon BA, Heck M, 1996: Utility of 24 hour urine sodium collections and urine Na/K ratios in the management of patients with cirrhosis and ascites. Hepatology 24:571A.

Runyon BA, et al, 1986: Hepatic hydrothorax is a relative contraindication to chest tube insertion. Am J Gastroenterol 81:566-567.

Runyon BA, et al, 1991: Short-course versus long-course antibiotic treatment of spontaneous bacterial peritonitis: a randomized controlled study of 100 patients. Gastroenterology 100:1737-1742.

Runyon BA, et al, 1992: The serum-ascites albumin gradient is superior to the exudate-transudate concept in the differential-diagnosis of ascites. Ann Intern Med 117:215-220.

Salerno F, et al, 1987: Repeated paracentesis and i.v. albumin infusion to treat 'tense' ascites in cirrhotic patients: a safe alternative therapy. J Hepatol 5:102-108.

Salerno F, et al, 1993: Survival and prognostic factors of cirrhotic patients with ascites: a study of 134 outpatients. Am J Gastroenterol 88:514-519.

Salerno F, et al, 2004: Randomized controlled study of TIPS versus paracentesis plus albumin in cirrhosis with severe ascites. Hepatology 40:629-635.

Salo J, et al, 1997: Impairment of renal function during moderate physical exercise in cirrhotic patients with ascites: relationship with the activity of neurohormonal systems. Hepatology 25:1338-1342.

Samanta AK, Leevy CM, 1989: Effect of peritoneo-venous shunt on portal pressure. Gut 30:86-89.

Sanyal AJ, et al, 2003: The North American study for the treatment of refractory ascites. Gastroenterology 124:634-641.

Saunders JB, et al, 1981: A 20-year prospective study of cirrhosis. BMJ (Clin Res Educ) 282:263-266.

Sawhney VK, et al, 1981: Furosemide disposition in cirrhotic patients. Gastroenterology 81:1012-1016.

Scholz DG, et al, 1989: Poor outcome from peritoneovenous shunts for refractory ascites. Am J Gastroenterol 84:540-543.

Sica DA, Gehr TW, 1996: Diuretic combinations in refractory oedema states: pharmacokinetic-pharmacodynamic relationships. Clin Pharmacokinet 30:229-249.

Siegerstetter V, et al, 2001: Treatment of refractory hepatic hydrothorax with transjugular intrahepatic portosystemic shunt: long-term results in 40 patients. Eur J Gastroenterol Hepatol 13:529-534.

Singh N, et al, 1995: Trimethoprim-sulfamethoxazole for the prevention of spontaneous bacterial peritonitis in cirrhosis: a randomized trial. Ann Intern Med 122:595-598.

Sola R, et al, 1994: Total paracentesis with dextran 40 vs diuretics in the treatment of ascites in cirrhosis: a randomized controlled study. J Hepatol 20:282-288.

Sola-Vera J, et al, 2003: Randomized trial comparing albumin and saline in the prevention of paracentesis-induced circulatory dysfunction in cirrhotic patients with ascites. Hepatology 37:1147-1153.

Soriano G, et al, 1991: Selective intestinal decontamination prevents spontaneous bacterial peritonitis. Gastroenterology 100:477-481.

Soriano G, et al, 1992: Norfloxacin prevents bacterial infection in cirrhotics with gastrointestinal hemorrhage. Gastroenterology 103:1267-1272.

Sort P, et al, 1999: Effect of intravenous albumin on renal impairment and mortality in patients with cirrhosis and spontaneous bacterial peritonitis. N Engl J Med 341:403-409.

Stanley MM, et al, 1989: Peritoneovenous shunting as compared with medical treatment in patients with alcoholic cirrhosis and massive ascites. Veterans Administration Cooperative Study on Treatment of Alcoholic Cirrhosis with Ascites. N Engl J Med 321:1632-1638.

Strauss RM, Boyer TD, 1997: Hepatic hydrothorax. Semin Liver Dis 17:227-232.

Sungaila I, et al, 1992: Spironolactone pharmacokinetics and pharmacodynamics in patients with cirrhotic ascites. Gastroenterology 102:1680-1685.

Takayama T, et al, 2004: A new technique of thoracoscopic pleurodesis for refractory hepatic hydrothorax. Surg Endosc 18:140-143.

Tito L, et al, 1990: Total paracentesis associated with intravenous albumin management of patients with cirrhosis and ascites. Gastroenterology 98:146-151.

Vons C, et al, 1991: Splanchnic and systemic hemodynamics in cirrhotic patients with refractory ascites: effect of peritoneovenous shunting. HPB Surg 3:259-267.

Wapnick S, et al, 1979: Randomized prospective matched pair study comparing peritoneovenous shunt and conventional therapy in massive ascites. Br J Surg 66:667-670.

Wong F, et al, 1997: The mechanism of the initial natriuresis after transjugular intrahepatic portosystemic shunt. Gastroenterology 112:899-907.

Xiol X, et al, 1996: Spontaneous bacterial empyema in cirrhotic patients: a prospective study. Hepatology 23:719-723.

Medical Management of Bleeding Varices

D. N. SAMONAKIS, C. K. TRIANTOS, J. GOULIS, AND A. K. BURROUGHS

Variceal bleeding is the most serious complication in patients with cirrhosis and portal hypertension. Mortality rates have declined in recent years (D'Amico et al, 2003; McCormick & O'Keefe, 2001), which is also reported in individual centers, to around 20% (Carbonell et al, 2004), but variceal bleeding continues to be a leading cause of death in these patients. The optimal management of bleeding esophagogastric varices and bleeding from portal hypertensive gastropathy depends first on general measures related to the cirrhosis per se and second on specific measures to treat the bleeding. The reduction in hospital mortality of patients with cirrhosis and variceal bleeding has occurred with the use of early and combined pharmacologic and endoscopic therapies and short-term antibiotic prophylaxis. Knowledge of how to deal with this life-threatening emergency is important for general surgeons and physicians. Close liaison between hepatologists, endoscopists, radiologists, and surgeons is essential. Patients are best managed by a team approach in specialized intensive care units.

DIAGNOSIS

Variceal bleeding may vary from a single life-threatening hematemesis with cardiovascular collapse to asymptomatic anemia. The reported frequency of variceal bleeding differs according to the population studied. In the United States, 11% of patients undergoing routine endoscopy for upper gastrointestinal bleeding were thought to have bled from esophageal varices (Silverstein et al, 1981), whereas in the United Kingdom, 2% to 5% are diagnosed at endoscopy as bleeding from varices (Atkinson, 1981; Dronfield et al, 1982). In cirrhotics, ruptured esophageal varices cause 60% to 70% of all upper gastrointestinal bleeding episodes (D'Amico et al, 2003).

Certain clinical features should lead to a suspicion of bleeding from varices. In the history, the following should be elicited: a history of chronic liver disease or portal hypertension, jaundice, excessive alcohol consumption, recent ingestion of nonsteroidal anti-inflammatory drugs or aspirin, previous episodes of variceal hemorrhage, past abdominal sepsis or surgery, umbilical vein sepsis or catheterization (for portal vein thrombosis), or a family history of liver disease. The pattern of bleeding is more frequently a presentation with hematemesis and less often that of coffee-ground vomiting or only melena. There are no specific features of the hemorrhage, however, that clearly indicate that varices have been the source.

All patients with upper gastrointestinal bleeding should be examined for cutaneous signs of chronic liver disease, hepatosplenomegaly, hepatic bruits, ascites, hepatic encephalopathy, and distended periumbilical veins because these signs suggest the possibility of bleeding varices (see Ch. 14). Bleeding resulting from portal hypertension may occur in the absence of these clinical findings, however, more frequently with extrahepatic splanchnic vein thrombosis than with chronic liver disease. Upper gastrointestinal endoscopy is essential to establish an accurate diagnosis of bleeding from varices. If necessary, endoscopy is performed under general anesthesia and in some rare cases just before emergency laparotomy when this is being performed for exsanguinating hemorrhage; potentially inappropriate surgery is avoided because balloon tamponade can be used to arrest the bleeding.

In patients with chronic liver disease and portal hypertension in whom varices have been shown by endoscopy, bleeding may occur from nonvariceal sites—26% to 56% of cases in one series (Mitchell et al, 1982) and 30% to 40% in another (D'Amico et al, 2003). Bleeding from portal hypertensive gastropathy and peptic ulcers is common. Definitive endoscopic diagnosis during or shortly after upper gastrointestinal bleeding is difficult and subjective, even in the hands of the most experienced endoscopist. When the view is restricted by hemorrhage, a bleeding point cannot always be identified, and the usual finding is of bright red blood around the gastroesophageal junction and in the gastric fundus in the presence of esophageal varices. A diagnosis of bleeding varices is accepted when a venous spurt (nonpulsatile) is seen, or fresh bleeding from the gastroesophageal junction is identified in the presence of varices. In the absence of active bleeding (approximately 50-70% of cases), the presence of varices in the absence of other lesions or a "white nipple sign"—a platelet plug on the surface of a varix—is acceptable evidence (Siringo et al, 1991). Endoscopy should be performed as soon as resuscitation is adequate, preferably within 6 hours of admission. Mitchell and colleagues (1982) showed that when a repeat endoscopy is performed during rebleeding, active bleeding from varices is seen in greater than 75% of patients in whom the initial endoscopy failed to show a precise source of hemorrhage. Repeat endoscopy in patients with portal hypertension often diagnoses the source of hemorrhage. If rebleeding occurs in the absence of an initial diagnosis, repeat endoscopy is mandatory. Bleeding from gastric varices, particularly from fundal varices, may be difficult to diagnose because of pooling of blood in the fundus. Performing endoscopy with the patient on the right side with the head up may help. If the diagnosis still is not made, splanchnic angiography can establish the presence of varices and may display the bleeding site if the patient is actively bleeding.

RESUSCITATION

Many patients with bleeding varices are severely hypovolemic when first seen and require emergency resuscitative measures. In addition, problems related to compromised hepatic function require urgent attention. The following scheme can be used as a clinical guideline for the resuscitation of such patients.

1. Perform a rapid clinical assessment of the degree of hypovolemia by noting the patient's appearance, pulse rate, blood pressure, and peripheral perfusion. If blood pressure is well maintained in the supine position, the appearance of tachycardia and a decrease in diastolic blood pressure in the sitting or erect position confirm hypovolemia. Cirrhotic patients, particularly when decompensated, may have a reduced peripheral vasoconstrictor response because of the established peripheral arterial vasodilatory state of cirrhosis and portal hypertension (Schrier et al, 1988), a disturbed baroreceptor reflex with an attenuated response to adrenaline (Moreau et al, 1989), and the presence of an autonomic neuropathy, particularly in alcoholics.

2. Ensure protection of the airway during general resuscitation. Lung aspiration of gastric contents and blood is a particular danger, especially in encephalopathic patients, who may have depressed pharyngeal reflexes. This risk is exacerbated further by endoscopic procedures, for which some sedation still may be required. Endotracheal intubation is mandatory if there is any concern about the safety of the airway.

3. Ensure adequate intravenous access, and assess cardiovascular status. Access to the circulation should be peripheral and central. Insert one or more intravenous lines, preferably with a large-gauge cannula. A central venous line is usually necessary to gauge fluid replacement, but this should be inserted by an experienced operator and preferably under ultrasound guidance. In this case, an internal jugular line is safer than a subclavian approach because the carotid artery can be compressed in the case of accidental puncture, whereas the subclavian cannot. The presence of coagulopathy and thrombocytopenia is not a contraindication to central venous access. In the presence of ascites, higher readings are seen owing to compression of the right atrium (Panos et al, 1990). In patients with cardiac disease, pulmonary wedge pressure may need to be monitored.

4. Take blood for laboratory analysis for a complete blood count, urea, electrolytes, creatinine, liver function tests, prothrombin time, blood glucose, blood cultures, blood gases, hepatitis B surface antigen and anti–hepatitis C virus, and crossmatching for 6 U of blood. Order a diagnostic ascitic tap, blood cultures, a chest x-ray, and an electrocardiogram. Start infusion of plasma or a colloidal preparation (human albumin fraction or gelatin-based colloid is recommended) according to the degree of hypovolemia. Use universal donor blood if necessary (group O, rhesus negative).

5. Initiate blood transfusion to achieve a hematocrit of 30% or a hemoglobin of 10 g/dL. Overtransfusion should be avoided because it may exacerbate increases in portal and variceal pressure (Zimmon & Kessler, 1974), although the effect of transfusion on portal pressure in humans is controversial (Vlavianos et al, 1999). Clotting deficiencies may be ameliorated with fresh frozen plasma; the administration of 2 U of fresh frozen plasma for every 4 U of blood and when the prothrombin time is greater than 20 seconds is recommended. Cryoprecipitate is indicated when the fibrinogen level is less than 0.2 g/L and has the advantage of not containing fibrinolytic factors. Platelet transfusions may be necessary to prevent a dilutional decrease during massive transfusion and improve primary hemostasis and should be used if the baseline count is $50 \times 10^9/L$ or less. It also is routine to give intravenous vitamin K to cirrhotic patients with variceal bleeding, but no more than three doses of 10 mg is required, and it is likely to have little benefit except in biliary-type cirrhosis.

6. Correct abnormalities of blood glucose and electrolytes, particularly hypoglycemia and hypokalemia, which may precipitate encephalopathy. Avoid infusion of sodium-containing electrolyte and antibiotic solutions.

7. When volume depletion is corrected, arrange urgent diagnostic endoscopy. Pulse oximetry and oxygen are essential during endoscopy. Staff must be adequate to provide optimal suction and to ensure airway protection.

8. Ensure that medical, radiologic, and surgical teams are involved or that the gastrointestinal bleeding team is informed. Referring centers should refer patients early, particularly if local expertise is not available.

9. If life-threatening hemorrhage continues in the absence of a definite diagnosis, but bleeding from varices is strongly suspected, insert a modified four lumen Sengstaken-Blakemore tube (SBT) preferably with the airway protected by an endotracheal tube under a short general anesthetic because the risk of aspiration is very high, particularly in unskilled hands (Vlanianos et al, 1989) (see later). If blood is still coming up the gastric aspiration lumen, varices are less likely to be the cause of blood loss, although gastric fundal varices are not always controlled by tamponade. Whenever this situation occurs, and the position of the SBT has been checked and adequate traction applied, the diagnosis of variceal bleeding should be questioned, and emergency angiography should be performed.

Other Early Measures

The presence of infection always should be sought. Apart from blood and urine cultures, a chest x-ray and an ascitic tap for white blood cell count and ascitic fluid culture in blood culture bottles should be obtained routinely. Meta-analysis of studies using prophylactic antibiotics has shown that bacterial infections are significantly reduced and mortality is reduced regardless of underlying risk factors (Soares-Weiser et al, 2003). Prophylactic antibiotic therapy (usually with a quinolone) is recommended immediately after patient admission for variceal bleeding. Our group has shown that bacterial infection, diagnosed on admission, is an independent prognostic factor of failure to control bleeding or early rebleeding (Goulis et al, 1998). These data may support a role of bacterial infection in the initiation of variceal bleeding (Goulis et al, 1999). This theory is confirmed by the results of a randomized trial in which antibiotic prophylaxis prevented not only infection, but also early rebleeding and reduced the amount of blood transfusion requirement in cirrhotics with variceal bleeding after endoscopic treatment (Hou et al, 2004).

Hepatic encephalopathy frequently complicates upper gastrointestinal bleeding in patients with chronic liver disease. Hypokalemia, hypomagnesemia, and hypoglycemia may precipitate encephalopathy and should be aggressively corrected. As soon as the patient tolerates oral fluid, lactulose, 5 to 10 mL four times daily, can be started. Antibiotics, including non-absorbable antibiotics, are at least as effective as lactulose (Als-Nielsen et al, 2004). Phosphate enemas also are useful. Management of hepatic encephalopathy has been dealt with in detail elsewhere. In patients with alcoholic liver disease, acute withdrawal of alcohol may precipitate delirium tremens. Chlormethiazole (Heminevrin) via infusion or administered orally and chlorodiazepoxide can be titrated easily to treat or prevent delirium tremens. Vitamin deficiencies also are common, and intravenous thiamine and folic acid should be given.

Treatment for ascites and fluid retention follows standard protocols (Moore et al, 2003). Paracentesis may be needed to treat tense ascites; this lowers portal pressure (Luca et al, 1993). Salt intake should be restricted. Daily weighing, when possible, and urinary sodium excretion are the best indicators for managing fluid retention in cirrhotics.

Careful attention is required to ensure optimal renal function because bleeding may be the initial step in the development of hepatorenal failure. The intravascular volume should be maintained with the administration of human albumin solution or blood initially. Dextrose solution is used for maintenance fluid avoiding overload. Nephrotoxic drugs, especially aminoglycosides and nonsteroidal drugs, should be avoided. Oliguria needs to be intensively managed; if hypovolemia has been corrected, the differential diagnosis is usually acute tubular necrosis or the initial stage of hepatorenal syndrome; in this clinical setting, it is difficult to separate them. Hepatorenal syndrome is treated with terlipressin, 1 to 2 mg every 4 to 6 hours; coadministration with albumin improves the therapeutic response (Gines et al, 2004). Terlipressin with albumin also may benefit renal failure in cirrhosis, independently of whether or not hepatorenal syndrome criteria are fulfilled (Triantos et al, 2004).

Feeding with a low-sodium diet should be restarted as soon as possible, usually after no more than 24 hours of stable vital signs. Enteral feeding may be useful in the presence of severe encephalopathy and makes fluid management easier. Parenteral feeding is necessary only if enteral absorption is impaired.

An ultrasound scan (see Ch. 15) of the liver and portal vein should be performed soon after admission to establish if there is a hepatocellular carcinoma or portal vein thrombosis or both, which may alter the overall management of the patient. If available, obtain a Doppler ultrasound scan of the portal vein to show patency, particularly if a transjugular intrahepatic portosystemic stent (TIPS) (see Ch. 96) is being considered.

PROGNOSIS OF ACUTE VARICEAL HEMORRHAGE

Acute variceal bleeding is characterized by a high mortality and a high rate of early rebleeding, which is a distinct characteristic of variceal bleeding (Burroughs et al, 1989). Mortality secondary to variceal bleeding is related to the degree of hepatic decompensation (Burroughs et al, 1989; Graham & Smith, 1981). The average mortality of the first hemorrhage is reduced to 20% in most studies (D'Amico et al, 2003), but in grade C patients mortality still can be 50%. Renal dysfunction has been reported to be independently predictive of survival using serum creatinine (Christensen et al, 1989; Garden et al, 1985). The criteria used in the Child-Pugh classification (i.e., serum bilirubin, albumin, prothrombin time, ascites, and hepatic encephalopathy) in a linear-regression model have been found to be superior to other published scoring systems in predicting 30-day or 6-week mortality (Ohmann et al, 1990). Other prognostic factors for survival include a portohepatic gradient measured 2 weeks after hemorrhage (it is unclear if this is independently predictive of the degree of liver cell dysfunction) (Vinel et al, 1986); measurement of hepatic venous pressure gradient (HVPG) within 48 hours, when 20 mm Hg or greater also correlates with early mortality (Moitinho et al, 1999; Monescillo et al, 2004); early rebleeding or continued bleeding within 5 days (Cardin et al, 1990); and active bleeding in most studies (oozing or spurting from the ruptured varix) at endoscopy (Ben-Ari et al, 1999; Cardin et al, 1990).

Severity of liver disease and active bleeding at endoscopy have been found to be risk factors for early rebleeding (≤5 days) (Cardin et al, 1990; Goulis et al, 1998). Bacterial infection diagnosed on admission or shortly after admission is an independent predictive factor of early rebleeding (Goulis et al, 1998; Hou et al, 2004). Ready and coworkers (1991a, 1991b) found in an elegant study that a higher HVPG was associated with continued bleeding or early rebleeding when measured on day 1 or 2 after admission for bleeding in 21 alcoholic cirrhotics. Patients whose HVPG was 16 mm Hg or greater on day 1 had more than a 50% chance of continued bleeding or rebleeding. By convention, the definition of failure to control bleeding is divided into time frames (De Franchis, 2004a): (1) within 6 hours, any of the following factors: need to transfuse 4 U or more of blood, inability to increase systolic pressure by 20 mm Hg or to 70 mm Hg, or failure to reduce pulse to 100 beats/min or less or by 20 beats/min from baseline; (2) any of the following: occurrence of hematemesis, systolic blood pressure reduction greater than 20 mm Hg from 6-hour point or increase of pulse rate of greater than 20 beats/min from 6-hour point or both on two consecutive readings 1 hour apart, or transfusion of 2 U or more of blood (over and above the previous transfusions) required to increase the hematocrit to greater than 27% or hemoglobin to greater than 9 g/dL.

The risk of very early rebleeding and the risk of death decrease rapidly after admission (Burroughs et al, 1989; Thomsen et al, 1994). When expressed as a hazard function, it can be seen that the risk of death becomes virtually constant about 6 weeks after bleeding (Burroughs et al, 1989; Graham & Smith, 1981); this occurs earlier for patients with well-compensated cirrhosis (Burroughs et al, 1989). This risk has implications for the potential therapeutic impact of techniques to prevent early rebleeding. Unless such measures are used and are efficacious within this high-risk interval, they are unlikely to affect survival with respect to bleeding, given that all therapeutic measures except liver transplantation have no beneficial effect on liver function itself. This issue was addressed in a randomized study in which emergency TIPS within 24 hours of admission was used in patients with a baseline HVPG 20 mm Hg or greater and in whom (compared with patients randomized to no TIPS) rebleeding and mortality were significantly reduced (Monescillo et al, 2004). HVPG 20 mm Hg or greater was associated with Child C cirrhosis and active bleeding on endoscopy, both of which were independent predictors of mortality.

DRUGS FOR ACUTE VARICEAL BLEEDING

Vasopressin with or without Nitrovasodilators

Vasopressin has been used widely for more than 30 years in the management of acute variceal bleeding. It has been compared with nonactive treatment or placebo, however, in only four randomized controlled trials (Conn et al, 1975; Fogel et al, 1982; Mallory et al, 1980; Merigan et al, 1962), including 157 patients. Using meta-analysis, there was a significant heterogeneity in the evaluation of failure to control bleeding between these studies. There was a clear trend in favor of vasopressin, but the result was not statistically significant by the Der Simonian and Laird method (odds ratio [OR] 0.23; 95% confidence interval [CI] 0.05-1.02). There was no difference in mortality (OR 0.98; 95% CI 0.47-2.1). Vasopressin was compared with somatostatin in a randomized trial in which no difference in efficacy was shown, but complications were significantly less in the somatostatin group (Lee et al, 2003).

Vasopressin administration is associated with serious side effects in about 25% of patients, some of which are fatal, such as myocardial infarction, gut ischemia, and local gangrene. To minimize the systemic side effects of vasopressin, nitroglycerin has been added to the regimen. Three randomized controlled trials compared vasopressin alone with vasopressin plus nitroglycerin transdermally (Bosch et al, 1989), sublingually (Tsai et al, 1986), and intravenously (Gimson et al, 1986), including 176 patients. Failure to control bleeding was significantly less

common with vasopressin plus nitroglycerin (OR 0.39; 95% CI 0.21-0.72), but there was no difference in mortality (OR 0.94; 95% CI 0.49-1.79). In two of the trials (Gimson et al, 1986; Tsai et al, 1986), side effects were significantly reduced with the combination treatment. Vasopressin (0.4 U/min for 24-48 hours) should always be used with nitroglycerin (4-hourly sublingual), keeping the systolic pressure greater than 100 mm Hg. Nitroglycerin, because of portocollateral shunting, bypasses the liver, however, and can cause significant systemic effects. This combination therapy must be monitored closely and is less applicable as an immediate therapy.

Terlipressin

Terlipressin is a synthetic analogue of vasopressin (triglycyl lysine vasopressin) with a prolonged biologic half-life so that a continuous intravenous infusion is unnecessary. The standard dose is 2 mg every 4 hours for the initial 24 hours and 1 mg every 4 hours for the next 24 hours. Terlipressin was statistically significantly more effective than placebo in the prevention of failure to control bleeding in the meta-analysis of six randomized controlled studies (Freeman et al, 1989; Levacher et al, 1995; Patch et al, 1999; Pauwels et al, 1994; Soderlund et al, 1990; Walker et al, 1986) including 388 patients (OR 0.49; 95% CI 0.33-0.75) (Table 91.1). In one of these studies, the drug was given before arriving at the hospital (Levacher et al, 1995). Terlipressin is the only vasoconstrictor that significantly reduces mortality (OR 0.51; 95% CI 0.33-0.79). There is some

Table 91.1 Randomized Controlled Trials of Terlipressin, Somatostatin, and Octreotide Compared with Placebo for Treatment of an Acute Bleeding Episode

Study/Reference	No. Patients (C/T)	Child C (%)	Failure to Control Bleeding (n; C/T)	Death (n; C/T)
Terlipressin versus Placebo				
Walker et al, 1986	25/25*	50	12/5	8/3
Freeman et al, 1989	16/15	29	10/6	4/3
Soderlund et al, 1990	29/31	33	13/5	11/3
Pauwels et al, 1994	14/17	NR	6/7	5/6
Levacher et al, 1995	43/41	81	23/12	20/12
Patch et al, 1999	66/66	62	40/37	28/22
POR (95% CI)			*0.49 (0.33-0.75)*	*0.51 (0.33-0.79)*
Somatostatin versus Placebo or Inactive Treatment				
Flati et al, 1986	16/19	40	9/2	7/4
Testoni et al, 1986	14/15	17	1/1	0/1
Loperfido et al, 1987	25/22	19	21/17	7/6
Valenzuela et al, 1989	36/48	32	9/21	10/15
Burroughs et al, 1990	59/61	41	35/22	7/9
Gotzsche et al, 1995	44/42	NR	NR	16/16
POR (95% CI)			*0.6 (0.21-1.65)†*	*1.2 (0.6-1.6)*
Octreotide versus Placebo				
Burroughs et al, 1996	139/123	40	85/71	37/35
Variceal bleeding only	109/88	40	75/56	32/24
Octreotide versus Placebo for Early Rebleeding				
Primignani et al, 1995	32/26	46	10/9‡	7/5‡
D'Amico et al, 1998	131/131	31	37/31§	20/26

*Bleeding episodes in a total 34 patients.
†Der Simonian and Laird method.
‡Evaluation at 30 days.
§Evaluation at 15 days.
C/T, control versus treatment; NR, not reported; POR, pooled odds ratio.

criticism of these studies, however. The sample sizes were not large enough, and in the study in which terlipressin or placebo was administered before arriving at the hospital (Levacher et al, 1995), the drug was given only as three doses up to 8 hours, with no difference in transfusion requirements at 12 hours and no hemodynamic improvement. The causal link between early administration of terlipressin and reduction in mortality must be reproduced in further studies.

Terlipressin was as effective as vasopressin in five unblinded studies (Chiu et al, 1990; D'Amico et al, 1994; Desaint et al, 1987; Freeman et al, 1982; Lee et al, 1988). In two of these studies, vasopressin was combined with nitroglycerin (D'Amico et al, 1994; Lee et al, 1988) for failure to control bleeding (OR 0.64; 95% CI 0.36-1.14) and mortality (OR 1.48; 95% CI 0.85-2.57) (Table 91.2). The complication rate was significantly lower with terlipressin even when vasopressin was combined with nitroglycerin.

The comparison of terlipressin with balloon tamponade in three randomized controlled trials showed no statistically significant difference in any outcome examined. Comparison with somatostatin in another three randomized controlled trials failed to show any difference between the two drugs (Ioannou et al, 2003a).

Meta-analysis of three randomized controlled trials comparing terlipressin with octreotide found no statistically significant difference in mortality, rebleeding, or procedures required for uncontrolled bleeding or rebleeding (Ioannou et al, 2003b).

Terlipressin administered for 5 to 7 days was as effective as sclerotherapy in arresting acute variceal bleeding and preventing early rebleeding in a single, large, multicenter randomized clinical trial involving 219 patients (Escorsell et al, 2000). There was no significant difference in 6-week mortality and incidence of complications between the two treatment groups, although terlipressin was better tolerated. Finally, the combination of terlipressin with sclerotherapy has been reported to be more effective than sclerotherapy alone for the prevention of failure to control bleeding in an unblinded, small study, published in abstract form (Brunati et al, 1996). There was no difference in mortality between the two groups.

Currently, terlipressin is one of the agents of first choice for the treatment of acute variceal bleeding. The most robust evidence for therapeutic benefit is for terlipressin, including survival benefit versus nonvasoactive therapy. Its benefit in hepatorenal syndrome suggests that it may have some renal protective effects, which may make it the drug of choice in variceal bleeding

Table 91.2 Randomized Controlled Trials of Comparisons Between Drugs for Treatment of an Acute Bleeding Episode

Study/Reference	No. Patients (C/T)	Child C (%)	Failure to Control Bleeding (n; C/T)	Death (n; C/T)	Complications (n; C/T)
Vasopressin versus Vasopressin plus Nitroglycerin					
Tsai et al 1986	20/19	34	11/15	11/11	—
Gimson et al 1986	38/34	61	12/19	9/9	—
Bosch et al 1989	30/35	51	8/16	9/10	—
POR (95% CI)			*0.39 (0.21-0.72)*	*0.94 (0.49-1.8)*	—
Terlipressin versus Vasopressin					
Freeman et al, 1982	11/10	15	10/3	3/2	—
Desaint et al, 1987	6/10	43	1/2	2/3	—
Lee et al, 1988	24/21	27	16/17	8/10	—
Chiu et al, 1990	28/26	60	13/13	10/12	—
D'Amico et al, 1994	55/56	9	13/5	9/14	—
POR (95% CI)			*0.64 (0.36-1.14)*	*1.48 (0.85-2.6)*	—
Somatostatin versus Vasopressin*					
Kravetz et al, 1984	31/30	41	13/14	17/16	22/3
Jenkins et al, 1985	12/10	54	8/3	4/2	2/0
Bagarani et al, 1987	25/24	69	17/8	10/6	3/1
Cardona et al, 1989	18/20	26	8/12	3/6	15/6
Hsia et al, 1990	24/22	65	15/10	15/14	11/4
Saari et al, 1990	22/32	46	10/11	15/22	11/1
Rodriguez-Moreno et al, 1991	16/15	30	6/9	3/3	11/0
POR (95% CI)			*0.74 (0.47-1.16)*	*0.9 (0.6-1.5)*	*0.1 (0.07-0.2)*
Somatostatin versus Terlipressin					
Feu et al, 1996	80/81	29	16/13	13/13	31/19
Walker et al, 1996[†]	53/53	12	5/10	11/11	0/3
Pauwels et al, 1994	18/17	NR	4/7	7/6	—
Octreotide versus Vasopressin*					
Hwang et al, 1992	24/24	44	13/9	12/11	11/3
Huang et al, 1992	20/21	—	8/14	5/9	—
Octreotide versus Terlipressin*					
Silvain et al, 1993	41/46	47	17/10	11/10	31/19
Pedretti et al, 1994	30/30	—	7/14	3/4	—

*References in De Franchis, 2004b.
†Bleeding episodes.
C/T, control versus treatment; NR, not reported; POR, pooled odds ratio.

if nonhypovolemic oliguria develops (Gines et al, 2003). The drug cannot be given in every patient, however, because it is contraindicated in patients with ischemic heart disease, cerebrovascular accidents, or peripheral vascular disease (Nevens, 2004).

Somatostatin

Somatostatin has been used in the pharmacologic treatment of variceal bleeding because of its reported ability to reduce splanchnic blood flow (Sonnenburg et al, 1981), portal pressure, and azygos blood flow (Bosch et al, 1981) in cirrhotic patients, although only the findings regarding the reduction in azygos flow are consistent. Bolus injections of somatostatin seem to have greater hemodynamic effects compared with continuous infusion. The standard dose for a bolus injection is 250 µg; 250 to 500 µg/hr is given as a continuous infusion. Higher doses of somatostatin (500 µg/hr) increased the success rate in controlling bleeding, particularly in patients with active bleeding at endoscopy, and improved survival (Moitinho et al, 2001).

Three placebo-controlled studies of somatostatin exhibit divergent results (see Table 91.1) (Burroughs et al, 1990; Gotzsche et al, 1995; Valenzuela et al, 1989). The trials by Valenzuela and associates (1989) and Gotzsche and colleagues (1995) suggested that somatostatin was no more effective than placebo. Both studies had a long recruitment period, suggesting marked patient selection. Gotzsche and colleagues (1995) did not evaluate the end point of failure to control bleeding, whereas Valenzuela and associates (1989) reported an extremely high response rate (83%) in the placebo group (the highest ever reported). In contrast, the study by Burroughs and coworkers (1990) reported a statistically significant benefit for somatostatin in controlling variceal bleeding over 5 days using time to failure as an end point.

Most randomized clinical trials evaluating somatostatin show that it has an efficacy of about 65%, and that it is equivalent to vasopressin, vasopressin combined with nitroglycerin, terlipressin, or balloon tamponade in the prevention of failure to control bleeding and short-term mortality (see Table 91.2) (De Franchis, 2004b). The addition of isosorbide mononitrate did not improve therapeutic efficacy, inducing more side effects (Junquera et al, 2000). Side effects were significantly less frequent with somatostatin in most of these trials.

Five trials (Chen et al, 2004; DiFebo et al, 1990; Planas et al, 1992; Ramires et al, 2000; Shields et al, 1992) including 345 patients compared somatostatin with endotherapy in the control of variceal hemorrhage. Meta-analysis showed that somatostatin was less efficacious than endotherapy (relative risk −12%; 95% CI −4% to −20%; $P<.003$) with regard to control of bleeding, with no difference in mortality (CI +6% to −9%; $P=.7$). Somatostatin in combination with sclerotherapy was more effective than sclerotherapy alone for control of bleeding in two randomized studies (Avgerinos et al, 1997; Signorelli et al, 1996) with 215 patients. There was no difference, however, in short-term mortality or in the incidence of complications. The results show that somatostatin can be used safely as adjuvant therapy to sclerotherapy during the crucial 5-day period after variceal bleeding. After the initial control of acute variceal bleeding, a randomized trial (Escorsell et al, 1998) of somatostatin versus sclerotherapy showed that continuous somatostatin infusion was as effective as sclerotherapy in preventing subsequent early

variceal rebleeding, with similar mortality but a lower complication rate.

Octreotide

Octreotide is a synthetic octapeptide analogue of somatostatin that has a longer biologic half-life (1-2 hours). Octreotide has been reported to cause a reduction in portal pressure (Jenkins et al, 1988) and a transient decrease in azygos blood flow (McCormick et al, 1992), but some studies did not confirm these data, using similar or even greater doses of the drug (Escorcell et al, 1996). The recommended dose is as a continuous infusion of 25 to 50 µg/hr, but this is not well established. In some trials, a bolus of 50 to 100 µg is used followed by an infusion.

The efficacy of octreotide treatment for acute variceal bleeding has not been evaluated adequately. There is only one double-blind trial of octreotide versus placebo, currently available only in abstract form (Burroughs et al, 1996), the largest ever carried out to evaluate the efficacy of a vasoactive drug ($n = 262$ patients) in the management of acute variceal bleeding. In this study, a continuous 5-day infusion of 50 µg/hr of octreotide, starting as soon as possible after admission, did not differ in efficacy from placebo, whether or not injection sclerotherapy was needed for active bleeding or drug failure. Two other studies (D'Amico et al, 1998; Primignani et al, 1995) using octreotide (100 µg 8-hourly subcutaneously) or placebo after the control of the initial bleeding episode failed to show any difference in early rebleeding or mortality between the two treatment groups.

In contrast, octreotide was found to be comparable to balloon tamponade in one study ($n = 40$ patients) (McKee 1990), to vasopressin in two small studies (in total 87 patients) (Huang et al, 1992; Hwang et al, 1992), to terlipressin plus nitroglycerin in another study ($n = 48$ patients) (Silvain et al, 1993), and to terlipressin alone in a final study (Pedretti et al, 1994), but the sample sizes were small and the end points not clear, indicating that these results should be interpreted with caution. Nine clinical trials (Bildozola et al, 2000; El-Jackie et al, 1998; Freitas et al, 2000; Jenkins et al, 1997; Lopez et al, 1999; Poo et al, 1996; Sivri et al, 2000; Sung et al, 1993; Yousuf et al, 2000) including 804 patients compared the efficacy of octreotide continuous infusion with sclerotherapy. Sclerotherapy was superior to octreotide for control of bleeding (relative risk 5.6%; 95% CI 0.1-11%; $P=.04$), but with no difference in mortality.

Several clinical trials have used octreotide in combination with endoscopic therapy—sclerotherapy in five trials (Besson et al, 1995; Brunati et al, 1996; Freitas et al, 2000; Signorelli et al, 1997; Zuberi & Baloch, 2000), variceal ligation in one trial (Sung et al, 1995), and vapreotide in one trial (Cales et al, 2001) versus sclerotherapy or band ligation or, in cases of gastric varices, glue with or without ligation—and compared this treatment with endoscopic therapy alone. The meta-analysis of these studies including 786 patients showed that combined therapy was superior to endotherapy alone with regard to the control of bleeding (pooled odds ratio [POR] 0.135; 95% CI 0.08-0.19), although there was heterogeneity (one study showed sclerotherapy to be better compared with six studies that showed combination to be better). The comparison for mortality showed no significant difference.

Antibiotics

Bacterial infections, regardless of the etiology, have been recognized as a severe complication of decompensated cirrhosis and, although frequently asymptomatic, account for longer hospital stays and increased mortality (Borzio et al, 2001). The incidence of bacterial infections in patients with acute variceal bleeding is well documented, with rates of 35% to 66% within 14 days (Ferguson et al, 2003). Two meta-analyses (Bernard et al, 1999; Soares-Weiser et al, 2003) documented that antibiotic prophylaxis in cirrhotic patients with gastrointestinal bleeding reduces the incidence of bacterial infections and increases short-term survival. A prospective study in more than 200 cirrhotics showed that bacterial infections significantly increase the risk for early rebleeding and 6-week mortality (Vlachogiannakos et al, 2004). A randomized trial (Hou et al, 2004) of antibiotic prophylaxis versus on-demand antibiotics showed that prophylaxis was more effective in preventing infection and rebleeding and decreasing transfusion requirements. A causative link between infection-related events (endotoxin-related increased intrahepatic vascular resistance and inhibition of platelet aggregation resulting in further deterioration of primary hemostasis) and initiation of acute variceal bleeding has been postulated (Goulis et al, 1999). The understanding of the consequences of bacterial infections and bacterial products on the portal and systemic hemodynamics in cirrhosis and the extensive amount of clinical data on infection gathered from retrospective and prospective studies in variceal bleeding have been followed by clinical evidence of the efficacy of antibiotic treatment in reversing systemic vasodilation and the prevention of early variceal rebleeding (Thalheimer et al, 2005). Antibiotics and terlipressin are the only drugs proved to improve survival in acute variceal bleeding.

BALLOON TAMPONADE

The SBT (Sengstaken & Blakemore, 1950) is the most frequently used tube for tamponade of bleeding varices. In addition to two lumina for inflation and deflation of the balloons, this tube has a central lumen for gastric aspiration and is referred to as the three lumen SBT. Addition of a simple nasogastric tube to aspirate hypopharyngeal secretions was described by Boyce (1962), and this is the four lumen SBT. This fourth lumen has now been incorporated into the design of the tube (Minnesota tube) (Fig. 91.1) (see Ch. 97). Linton (1966) described an alternative tube design. This tube has a single large-volume gastric balloon (600 mL compared with 150-200 mL for the SBT). There is no esophageal balloon, lumina are provided for aspiration of the stomach and the lower esophagus, and the tube is more effective for gastric varices (Teres et al, 1978).

Tamponade is an effective means of arresting active bleeding in 90% or more of patients (Panes et al, 1988). Tamponade should be used only for exsanguinating hemorrhage or when endoscopic treatment is unavailable or for transport of the patient when medical care for bleeding might be suboptimal or unavailable. Infrequent use of tamponade leads to a high rate of complications because of inexperience. The most frequent complication is aspiration pneumonia (Vlanianos et al, 1989). Protection of the airway, if necessary with an endotracheal tube, is paramount, particularly in patients with encephalopathy.

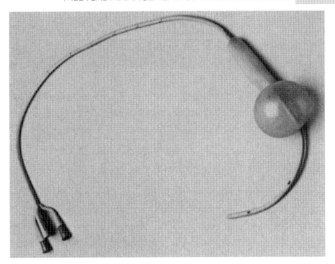

Fig. 91.1. The Minnesota tube.

Definitive therapy must follow removal of the tube. The few randomized comparisons with vasoactive therapy that have been made are difficult to interpret because of the different indications for these two treatments. Balloon tamponade is effective only as a temporary measure, however, because of the high frequency of rebleeding in the 24 hours after removal (Conn, 1971).

Technique for Passage of a Sengstaken-Blakemore Tube

1. When possible, empty the stomach before passage of the tube (e.g., suction of gastric contents at endoscopy). The patient should be kept head down. It is easier to introduce the tube with the patient lying on his or her side, with an endoscopy mouth guard and nasal oxygen prongs.
2. Use a new tube for each patient. We prefer the four lumen (Minnesota) tube (see Fig. 91.1). Easy passage is facilitated if the tube is used immediately after removal from a refrigerator. The cold stiffens the tube and prevents coiling in the pharynx or esophagus.
3. Pass the tube orally with suction applied to the esophageal aspiration lumen into the stomach. An assistant should be ready with a second suction catheter to aspirate blood from the mouth and pharynx.
4. Inflate the gastric balloon with 300 mL of air. If inflation is difficult, or the patient is in pain, deflate immediately, and check that the tube is in the stomach. Withdraw the tube until resistance is met as the gastric balloon impinges on the fundus of the stomach. This is usually at 35 to 40 cm from the mouth. Tape the tube in position to the side of the mouth, with no additional traction.
5. Inflate the esophageal balloon with air to a pressure of 30 to 40 mm Hg.
6. Double clamp the gastric and esophageal balloons.
7. Maintain the gastric aspiration lumen on free drainage and the esophageal aspiration lumen on constant low pressure suction (5-10 mm Hg).
8. Check the position of the tube by radiography.

Management of a Sengstaken-Blakemore Tube

1. Check the pressure in the esophageal balloon hourly.
2. Give nothing by mouth when the tube is in position.
3. Ensure the patient is attended constantly by experienced nursing staff.
4. If bleeding is controlled, deflate the esophageal balloon after 12 hours, and observe. In the event of further bleeding, reinflate the esophageal balloon. If no further bleeding occurs, remove the tube after no more than 24 hours. Always fully deflate both balloons before removal of the tube.
5. If bleeding is not controlled, check the position of the balloon by radiography. It is imperative that the gastric balloon is positioned in the fundus of the stomach. If the tube is in the correct position, and hemorrhage continues, apply 300-g traction to the proximal end of the tube. Always be prepared to consider an alternative diagnosis in these circumstances.
6. If the tube is in situ for prolonged periods, check its position by radiography daily. Never leave the esophageal balloon inflated for longer than is necessary.
7. In the event of sudden respiratory distress related to proximal displacement of the tube, deflate both balloons as rapidly as possible, and remove the tube. Use scissors to cut across the tube if deflation cannot be achieved by suction.

LONG-TERM DRUG THERAPY

Among various treatments for portal hypertension for primary or secondary prevention of variceal bleeding, medical treatment is, by nature, simpler and cheaper to administer than long-term sclerotherapy or variceal ligation, surgery, or TIPS. Lebrec and colleagues (1980) first described long-term medical treatment in a seminal article. The aim of long-term medical treatment of portal hypertension is to reduce portal pressure and prevent bleeding. Portal pressure can be reduced in three ways: (1) by diminishing the portal inflow using vasoconstrictors, (2) by reducing the intrahepatic vascular resistance, or (3) by reducing the resistance in the collateral circulation using vasodilators. Theoretically, the development of portal hypertension and varices might be prevented in this way; this has been shown with β-blockers in various animal models of portal hypertension. Many drugs have been evaluated in cirrhotics with portal hypertension (Lebrec, 1998), but patients with noncirrhotic portal hypertension have seldom been studied.

β-Blockers

Numerous clinical investigations and experimental studies have shown that β-blockers significantly reduce portal pressure by decreasing splanchnic inflow. It has been shown that propranolol reduces intravariceal pressure compared with placebo (Feu et al, 1991). Pressure at the site of rupture can be reduced. These reductions are due to a decreased cardiac output and extracardiac factors, such as the unopposed splanchnic vasoconstriction. There is no relationship between the effect of propranolol and the height of portal pressure, severity of liver disease, or presence of ascites and variceal size (Poynard et al, 1991). There are nonresponders to β-blockers, however, in terms of portal pressure reduction. Bendtsen and coworkers (1991) defined nonresponders as patients exhibiting less than 10% reduction

in portal pressure after an oral dose of 80 mg of propranolol. They compared the hemodynamic indices of responders and nonresponders. All patients had evidence of adequate β blockade with plasma propranolol levels greater than 50 ng/mL and a decrease in cardiac output. The nonresponders had a lower baseline cardiac index and a higher systemic vascular resistance (i.e., the circulation was less hyperdynamic).

Studies have been done to evaluate factors associated with a marked reduction in portal pressure and HVPG or with a target threshold portal pressure below which the risk of bleeding or rebleeding is substantially reduced. From the analysis of the Barcelona-Boston-New Haven Primary Prophylaxis trial (Groszmann et al, 1990), it was concluded that variceal bleeding did not occur with HVPG less than 12 mm Hg, in patients with predominantly sinusoidal portal hypertension. An additional hemodynamic index has been proposed by Feu and colleagues (1995). Patients who had a percentage reduction of HVPG of 20% or more from baseline or an absolute reduction 12 mm Hg or more in HVPG had a rebleeding rate of 15% compared with 50% in patients who did not achieve this hemodynamic target. Although other studies with one exception (McCormick et al, 1998) seem to confirm these findings, there is a debate as to its clinical applicabiltiy (Thalheimer et al, 2004a); in particular, no prospective study has evaluated early remeasurement at 2 weeks from the bleeding episode and assessed if the pressure was high and whether a change in therapy from β-blockers to banding ligation results in less rebleeding (Thalheimer et al, 2004b).

Combination of β-Blockers with Other Drugs

Drugs reported to reduce portal pressure through different mechanisms have been combined in an attempt to provoke additive portal hypotensive effects in responders or to induce a portal hypotensive effect in nonresponders. It has been shown that oral isosorbide mononitrate when added to β-blockers induces a greater decrease in portal pressure than β-blockers alone (Garcia Pagan et al, 1991). Isosorbide mononitrate was especially effective for patients who did not respond to propranolol. Other drugs that may work in combination with β-blockers include molsidomine (a nitric oxide donor) (Vinel et al, 1990) and serotonin antagonists (Vorobioff et al, 1989), but as yet these drugs have not been evaluated in randomized clinical trials to establish if there is any effect in the reduction of rebleeding.

RISK OF FIRST BLEEDING

The incidence of variceal bleeding is approximately 4% per year in nonselected patients who have never bled at the time of diagnosis. The risk is about 2% in patients without varices at diagnosis and increases to about 5% per year in patients with small varices and 15% in patients with medium to large varices (D'Amico & Luca, 1997). At the time of diagnosis of cirrhosis, varices are present in about 60% of decompensated and 30% of compensated patients (D'Amico et al, 1995). Mortality of the first bleeding episode continues to be higher, however, than for subsequent bleeding episodes (Graham & Smith, 1981). The identification of patients with varices who will bleed before they do so is important to offer effective prophylactic therapy to patients who need it and avoid it in patients who do not, particularly if the therapy is invasive or costly.

The risk factors for the first episode of variceal bleeding in cirrhotic patients are the severity of liver dysfunction, large size of varices, and presence of endoscopic red color signs. The combination of these three factors is the basis of the North Italian Endoscopic Club (NIEC) index for the prediction of the first variceal bleeding (NIEC, 1988). Only a third of patients who present with variceal hemorrhage have the aforementioned risk factors, however (Grace et al, 1998). There is a need to define new predictive factors that could be combined in the NIEC index to improve its validity. The main interest has been in the identification of hemodynamic factors that could reflect more readily the pathophysiologic changes that lead to variceal bleeding. It is now well accepted that no bleeding occurs if HVPG decreases to less than 12 mm Hg (Armonis et al, 1997); in addition, the height of HVPG has been shown to be an independent risk factor of bleeding (Merkel & Gatta, 1991). The tension on the variceal wall, which is related to the radius of the varix, and the intravariceal pressure are believed to be crucial in the pathogenesis of variceal rupture (Polio & Groszmann, 1986). Variceal pressure has been shown, in a prospective study, to be an independent predictive factor for the first variceal bleeding, and its addition to NIEC index could result in a significant gain in prognostic accuracy (Nevens et al, 1998).

RISK OF REBLEEDING

Patients surviving the first episode of variceal bleeding are at very high risk of recurrent bleeding ($\geq$70%) and death (30-50%), with the highest risk period occurring within 6 weeks of the index bleed (D'Amico et al, 2003). There is a general consensus that all patients who previously have bled from varices should have secondary therapy to prevent further variceal bleeding (Grace et al, 1998). Severity of liver disease (Pagliaro et al, 1994), continued alcohol abuse (Vorobioff et al, 1996), and variceal size have been associated with variceal rebleeding. In addition, the inability to achieve the proposed hemodynamic targets of an absolute reduction of HVPG to 12 mm Hg or less or a reduction of 20% or greater from baseline, significantly increases the risk of rebleeding. Nevertheless, the absolute reduction of HVPG to 12 mm Hg or less is rare even in the studies, whereas for the reduction of 20% or greater from baseline, there are several difficulties in interpreting its clinical validity from the published studies (Thalheimer et al, 2004b). This, together with the increased cost of target HVPG monitoring, suggests that there is need for solid evidence for better therapeutic efficacy and clinical applicability of this approach.

RANDOMIZED TRIALS OF PRIMARY PROPHYLAXIS

β-Blockers and Isosorbide Mononitrate

Primary prophylaxis is prevention of the first portal hypertensive bleeding episode in cirrhotics, whether from varices or portal hypertensive gastropathy. The ideal regimen, considering patients are asymptomatic relative to their portal hypertension, should be effective and have minimal side effects. Nonselective β-adrenergic blockers meet these criteria better than endoscopic techniques. The benefit is proved only for cirrhotics with moderate or large varices, regardless of the severity of liver dysfunction (Poynard et al, 1991). Prevention of progression of small varices

to large ones with reduction of bleeding and mortality has been shown in a placebo-controlled trial of nadolol (Merkel et al, 2004). Regression of varices also was shown, but this occurred only in alcoholic cirrhotics who abstained. Further studies are awaited to confirm these results. β-Blockers should be continued for life because their withdrawal returns the risk for bleeding to that of the untreated population (Abraczinskas et al, 2001).

Nine primary prophylaxis trials have been performed, including 996 patients. Seven trials were carried out with propranolol and two with nadolol, which showed that the incidence of first bleeding is reduced significantly by *β-blockers compared with no treatment*. There was no statistical heterogeneity (i.e., the variation in treatment effect is consistent with "normal" biologic variability). The pooled OR of bleeding with β-blockers is almost half that of placebo: 0.54 (95% CI 0.39-0.74; *P*<.001), with only one Australian trial showing an increased risk of bleeding with propranolol. The number of patients who need to be treated to prevent one adverse bleeding event is 10 (95% CI 8-18). The mortality rate also is reduced, but not significantly so: 0.75 (95% CI 0.57-1.06) (D'Amico et al, 1999). The same conclusion was reached by using individual patient data, rather than trial group outcomes, in a meta-analysis of four of the trials comprising 589 patients (Poynard et al, 1991). Prevention of fatal bleeding by β-blockers was highly significant (*P*<.004)— 8 lives were saved among 100 patients followed for 2 years. Finally, propranolol has been shown to prevent acute and chronic bleeding from portal hypertensive gastropathy in a single blind randomized study (Perez-Ayuso et al, 1991). Side effects of β-blockers usually are reversible after discontinuation of the drug, and no fatal complications have been reported. Because of relative or absolute contraindications, *15% to 20% of cirrhotics cannot tolerate β-blockers* (Garcia Pagan et al, 2001). Alternative approaches have been sought, particularly with isosorbide mononitrate (Garcia Pagan et al, 1990).

Merkel and colleagues (2000) evaluated the combination of isosorbide mononitrate and nadolol and found the combination to be more effective in reducing bleeding, with only a small increase in side effects. A double-blind, placebo-controlled trial by Garcia Pagan and coworkers (2003) comprising 349 patients found no difference in 2-year actuarial probability of variceal bleeding or survival, with adverse effects being more frequent in the combination group. Preliminary results of another trial (Pietrosi et al, 1999) report less bleeding with a similar survival in the combination group, but higher side effects.

A study assessing nitrates used alone was associated with a higher long-term mortality compared with propranolol (Angelico et al, 1997). Currently, there is scanty clinical evidence to support the use of combination therapy. The combination of spironolactone (which decreases portal pressure by reducing increased plasma volume in cirrhosis) and nadolol versus nadolol alone in cirrhotics without ascites (Abecasis et al, 2003) resulted in no significant difference in variceal bleeding, development of ascites, or survival.

β-Blockers Alone or Combined with Endoscopic Therapy versus Endoscopic Therapy

More recent trials have compared *endoscopic therapy with β-blockers alone or in combination with endoscopic treatment*. Endoscopic sclerotherapy (see Ch. 92) has been used in combination with propranolol versus propranolol alone (Avgerinos et al, 2000), in which no significant differences in bleeding and mortality were found, but there was a significantly increased complication rate in the combination group. Nine randomized trials, involving 645 patients, compared *endoscopic band ligation of high-risk esophageal varices with propranolol* (Chen et al, 1998; De et al, 1999; De la Mora et al, 2000; Jutabha et al, 2001; Lui et al, 2002; Psilopoulos et al, 2002; Sarin et al, 1999; Schepke et al, 2004) or nadolol (Lo et al, 2004) (Table 91.3). Meta-analysis showed that variceal ligation significantly reduced the risk of first bleeding compared with propranolol (POR 0.56; 95% CI 0.36-0.86), but there was no difference in terms of mortality (POR 1.03; 95% CI, 0.68-1.55). The absence of any effect on mortality, owing to the risk of fatal bleeding induced by banding (Schepke et al, 2004), still justifies using nonselective β-blockers as the treatment of first choice and reserving banding if there is a contraindication or intolerance to β-blockers.

Screening for moderate and large varices in cirrhotics should become part of routine clinical practice (Cales et al, 1990), and if these are found, β-blockers should be given to reduce the incidence of bleeding and death from variceal bleeding and bleeding from portal hypertensive gastropathy. Propranolol, which is very inexpensive, also should be used in cirrhotics with small varices, particularly patients with progressive liver disease, because the risk of first bleeding is still relatively high (NIEC, 1988; Samonakis et al, 2004).

Prevention of Bleeding from Portal Hypertensive Gastropathy

The natural history of portal hypertensive gastropathy is that it worsens with increasing severity of liver disease and of portal hypertension; acute bleeding is infrequent, but may be severe and is associated in almost all cases with the severe form (petechiae in the mucosa). Chronic anemia is more common with mild portal hypertensive gastropathy (Merli et al, 2004; Primignani et al, 2000). Propranolol has been shown to prevent acute and chronic bleeding in a single blind randomized study (Perez-Ayuso et al, 1991). The actuarial percentages of patients free of rebleeding from portal hypertensive gastropathy at 12 months were 65% versus 38% (*P*<.05) and at 30 months were 52% versus 7% (*P*<.05). There also were fewer episodes of acute rebleeding (mean episodes per patient/month = 0.01 versus 0.12).

Pre–Primary Prophylaxis

Pre–primary prophylaxis refers to the prevention of varices. Two randomized studies, one of propranolol in the prevention of development of large varices in cirrhotics with no or small varices (Cales et al, 1999) and the second of timolol in prevention of development of varices or variceal hemorrhage in cirrhotics without varices (Groszmann et al, 2003), failed to show benefit with nonselective β-blockers in these populations. The discouraging results mean that pharmacologic prevention of varices is not possible at present.

PREVENTION OF REBLEEDING FROM VARICES

Patients surviving the first episode of variceal bleeding are at very high risk of recurrent bleeding (>70% at 1 year, the highest risk period being within 6 weeks of the index bleed) and death (30-50%) (Grace et al, 1998). Treatment to prevent recurrent hemorrhage is considered mandatory and should be initiated as soon as the patient is stable.

There are 12 trials of *β-blockers compared with placebo or no treatment* comprising 769 patients. A comprehensive meta-analysis of these trials (Bernard et al, 1997a) showed a significant heterogeneity in the evaluation of rebleeding (*P*<.01), but only in the magnitude and not direction of treatment effect. Treatment with β-blockers has decreased significantly the risk of rebleeding (Der Simonian and Laird method: POR 21%; 95% CI 10-32%). The number of patients needed to treat to prevent one rebleeding episode is five. Survival also was improved significantly in patients treated with β-blockers to prevent rebleeding (Der Simonian and Laird method: POR 5.4%; 95% CI 0-11%), although there was significant heterogeneity in this analysis (*P*<.01). Fourteen patients would need to be treated to prevent one death.

Studies of *β-blockers plus isosorbide mononitrate versus β-blockers* had their impetus from an article showing that about one third of hemodynamic nonresponders to β-blockers become responders after addition of isosorbide mononitrate (Garcia Pagan et al, 1991), such that more reduced their portal pressure by greater than 10% from baseline. There are two trials; one showed reduced rates of bleeding (Gournay et al, 2000), and one (published in abstract form) did not show reduced bleeding (Pasta et al, 2001). The limited data do not support the use of the combination therapy. It is believed that patients who respond to β-blockers hemodynamically on their own do not benefit from the addition of isosorbide mononitrate (Bosch & Garcia Pagan, 2003).

β-Blockers have been compared with sclerotherapy in 11 trials comprising 971 patients—propranolol in 10 and nadolol plus isosorbide mononitrate in 1 (Table 91.4). Meta-analysis showed

Table 91.3 Randomized Controlled Trials of β-Blockers Compared with Variceal Band Ligation for Prevention of First Bleeding Episode

Reference	No. Patients (D/L)	Child C (%)	Rebleeding (*n*; D/L)	Death (*n*; D/L)
Chen et al, 1998	28/26	NR	2/1	3/3
Sarin et al, 1999	44/45	31.5	12/4	5/5
De et al, 1999	15/15	13	1/2	NR
De la Mora et al, 2000	12/12	NR	2/1	1/0
Jutabha et al, 2001	25/26	NR	5/1	NR
Psilopoulos et al, 2002	14/21	20	1/1	0/1
Lui et al, 2002	66/44	34	9/3	18/11
Lo et al, 2004	50/50	16	13/8	11/12
Schepke et al, 2004	75/77	9.5	22/19	33/34
POR (95% CI)			0.56 (0.36-0.86)*	1.03 (0.68-1.55)

*Der Simonian and Laird method.
D/L, drugs cirrsus ligaton; NR, not reported; POR, pooled odds ratio.

Table 91.4 Randomized Controlled Trials of Sclerotherapy Compared with β-Blockers for Prevention of Rebleeding

Reference*	No. Patients (D/S)	Child C (%)	Rebleeding (n; D/S)	Death (n; D/S)	Adverse Events (n; D/S)
Alexandrino et al, 1988[†]	34/31	—	25/17	11/9	24/28
Dollet et al, 1988[†]	27/28	27	11/18	12/15	0/10
Fleig et al, 1988[†]	57/58	NR	26/26	16/20	NR
Westaby et al, 1990[†]	52/56	—	29/28	22/21	4/0
Liu et al, 1990[†]	58/60	NR	33/20	27/17	NR
Martin et al, 1991[†]	34/42	24	18/23	8/13	0/19
Rossi et al, 1991[†]	27/26	38	13/13	7/6	3/8
Andreani et al, 1990[†]	35/40	35	12/17	9/17	NR
Dasarathy et al, 1992[†]	53/51	34	31/19	19/10	5/9
Teres et al, 1993[†]	58/58	14	37/26	23/21	10/23
Villanueva et al, 1996[‡]	43/43		11/23	4/9	
POR (95% CI)			0.88 (0.58-1.32)	0.95 (0.72-1.25)	

*References in Bernard et al, 1997b.
[†]Propranolol.
[‡]Nadolol plus isosorbide mononitrate.
D/S, drug versus sclerotherapy; NR, not reported; POR, pooled odds ratio.

that the two therapies are equivalent, with a POR of 0.95 (95% CI 0.58-1.32) for mortality and 0.88 (95% CI 0.58-1.32) for rebleeding, although there was significant heterogeneity in the latter analysis ($P=.004$). The number of patients free of adverse events was significantly higher in the drug group compared with the sclerotherapy group. There have been no reports of fatal complications of β-blockers in cirrhotic patients. Withdrawal because of the expected side effects (e.g., heart failure or asthma) is infrequent. Occasionally, hepatic encephalopathy may be precipitated by propranolol, but the effect is reversible. Only one randomized trial compared histocryl obliteration with propranolol in 41 patients; there was no difference in rebleeding or survival, but there were more complications with injection of glue (Evrard et al, 2003).

There are 12 trials of *sclerotherapy combined with drugs* (propranolol in 8, nadolol in 3, and isosorbide mononitrate in 1) *versus sclerotherapy alone,* comprising 853 patients (Table 91.5). Theoretically, the drug might prevent rebleeding before variceal obliteration, and the β-blockers have been given short-term only. Only one group showed rebleeding to be significantly decreased before and after eradication (Jensen & Krarup, 1989). POR showed that there was statistically significantly less rebleeding in the combined treatment arm (Der Simonian and Laird method: POR 0.54; 95% CI 0.34-0.86), although there was statistically significant heterogeneity caused by differences between studies in the direction and the size of the effect of treatment. There was no statistically significant heterogeneity in the evaluation of survival. There were fewer statistically significant deaths in the combined treatment arm (POR 0.65; 95% CI 0.43-0.97).

In the study of *drugs versus banding,* a meta-analysis of six trials with 761 patients (Agrawall et al, 2002; Lo et al, 2002; Patch et al, 2002; Romero et al, 2004; Shiha et al, 2005; Villanueva et al, 2001) comparing drugs (propranolol, propranolol plus isosorbide, nadolol plus isosorbide) with elective long-term ligation showed no significant difference for rebleeding (POR 0.78; 95% CI 0.46-1.33; $P=.06$) or for mortality (POR 1.14; 95% CI 0.82-1.6) (Table 91.6). There was heterogeneity in the degree of rebleeding, however, in these studies.

Regarding *variceal ligation plus β-blockers versus variceal ligation,* a randomized trial (Lo et al, 2000) compared esophageal variceal ligation with sucralfate and nadolol with variceal ligation alone. The combination was more effective than ligation alone in terms of preventing variceal recurrence, upper gastrointestinal bleeding, and variceal rebleeding. Mortality was 16.7% for patients receiving combination therapy compared with 32.3% for patients treated with ligation ($P=.08$). It is likely that sucralfate may be unnecessary, but this study indicates that combination

Table 91.5 Randomized Controlled Trials of Sclerotherapy plus Drugs Compared with Sclerotherapy Alone for Prevention of Rebleeding

Reference*	No. Patients (S/S+D)	Child C (%)	Bleeding (n; S/S+D)	Death (n; S/S+D)
Westaby et al, 1986	27/26	41	8/7	7/9
Jensen & Krarup, 1989	26/25	29	12/3	1/1
Lundell et al, 1990	22/19	51	11/12	NR
Bertoni et al, 1990	14/14	36	4/1	3/1
Gerunda et al, 1990	30/30	NR	7/6	3/1
Vinel, 1992	35/39	NR	14/7	5/5
Avgerinos et al, 1993	40/45	7	21/14	9/8
Villanueva et al, 1993	18/22	NR	7/12	0/2
Acharya et al, 1993	56/58	NR	12/10	7/5
Vickers et al, 1994	34/39	34	14/17	9/9
Bertoni, 1994	37/39	—	15/4	9/2
El-Sayed, 1996	87/91	—	34/13	10/11
POR (95% CI)			0.54 (0.34-0.86)[†]	0.65 (0.43-0.97)

*References in D'Amico et al, 1995.
[†]Der Simonian and Laird method.
S/S+D, sclerotherapy versus sclerotherapy plus drugs; NR, not reported; POR, pooled odds ratio.

Table 91.6   Randomized Controlled Trials of Drugs Compared with Variceal Band Ligation for Prevention of Rebleeding

Reference	No. Patients (D/L)	Child C (%)	Rebleeding (n; D/L)	Death (n; D/L)
Villaneuva et al, 2001*	72/72	22	24/35	23/30
Agrawall et al, 2002[†]	51/53	NR	13/10	7/7
Lo et al, 2002*	61/60	21	26/12	8/15
Patch et al, 2002[‡]	51/51	51	19/27	17/17
Romero et al, 2004*	57/52	NR	47/46§	11/10
Shiha et al, 2005[‡]	60/61	NR	31/17	11/8
Shiha et al, 2005[†]	60/61	NR	25/17	9/8
POR (95% CI)			0.77 (0.45-1.33)¶	1.14 (0.819-1.599)

*Nadolol + isosorbide mononitrate.
[†]Propranolol + isosorbide mononitrate.
[‡]Propranolol.
§Ligation plus low volume sclerotherapy.
¶Der Simonian and Laird method.
D/L, drugs versus ligation; NR, not reported; POR, pooled odds ratio.

of ligation and nonselective β-blockers may be the best strategy for prevention of rebleeding.

A trial by Escorsell and colleagues (2002) *comparing TIPS with drug therapy* found that the 2-year rebleeding rate was significantly lower in the TIPS group. Patients in the drug group experienced less encephalopathy and more frequent improvement in the Child-Pugh score, however, with lower associated costs.

On this basis, β-blockers would be the treatment of first choice for the prevention of rebleeding, barring contraindications. β-Blockers are less expensive and less invasive, and they do not increase endoscopy workload. At present, variceal ligation should be used for patients with intolerance or noncompliance to drugs.

HEMODYNAMIC MONITORING

Pharmacologic therapy of portal hypertension using nonselective β-blockers is effective in reducing bleeding rates in primary and secondary prophylaxis and is at least equivalent to banding for the secondary prevention of variceal bleeding. Some centers have advocated monitoring of HVPG (HVPG= wedge hepatic venous pressure − free hepatic venous pressure) to assess target reductions of portal pressure. HVPG measurement is the most reproducible and reliable method of assessing the portal pressure in cirrhosis (Groszmann & Wongcharatrawee, 2004). Wedge hepatic venous pressure is equivalent to portal venous pressure in cirrhosis where the major site of resistance is sinusoidal or presinusoidal (alcoholic and viral [hepatitis B, C]) or both. A decrease in HVPG 20% or greater from baseline or to 12 mm Hg or less has been shown to correlate with a significant reduction in bleeding. The issue is the applicability of routinely measuring HVPG, however, because many patients rebled early (Thalheimer et al, 2004a), and studies supporting measurement had a second measurement on average between 1 and 3 months. Remeasurement probably needs to be done at 2 weeks. Undoubtedly a valuable tool, the applicability of HVPG needs further prospective evaluation in future studies.

FUTURE DRUG THERAPY FOR MANAGEMENT OF PORTAL HYPERTENSION

In acute variceal bleeding, drug therapy is the only treatment that is immediately available and is not dependent on skilled staff—in contrast to endoscopic therapies. Its future role will be in combination with the latter, to prevent the early rebleeding that is frequently seen in such patients. To date, the drugs of choice are terlipressin and somatostatin. Another potential approach is hemostatic therapy. Recombinant activated factor VII was shown to normalize prothrombin time in cirrhotics with variceal bleeding (Ejlersen et al, 2001) and to achieve hemostasis in bleeding esophageal varices unresponsive to standard treatment (Romero-Castro et al, 2004). A randomized study was performed in 245 cirrhotics with upper gastrointestinal bleeding: variceal (66%), nonvariceal (29%), and unknown source (5%) (eight doses of recombinant activated factor VII, 100 μg/kg, or placebo) in addition to combined endoscopic and pharmacologic therapy. There were no significant differences in control of bleeding, blood transfusion requirements, or mortality. In Child-Pugh B/C patients with variceal bleeding, however, recombinant activated factor VII significantly reduced a combined end point for control of bleeding (Bosch et al, 2004). Further studies are in progress.

Carvedilol is a vasodilating nonselective β-blocker with weak intrinsic anti–α-adrenergic activity. Carvedilol administration causes significant reductions in HVPG after single or multiple doses, equal or enhanced efficacy compared with propranolol; nevertheless, it was reported to be associated with substantial symptomatic hypotension in patients with decompensated cirrhosis (Hemstreet, 2004). A randomized hemodynamic study compared oral administration of carvedilol with the combination of propranolol and isosorbide mononitrate and HVPG at baseline and 90 minutes after administration. Carvedilol proved more effective in reduction of HVPG, increasing hepatic blood flow; the decrease in mean arterial pressure did not differ between the two groups (Lin et al, 2004). Further studies are needed.

Activation of the renin-angiotensin-aldosterone system is a frequent finding in cirrhotics. Angiotensin II has been shown to induce contraction of activated human hepatic stellate cells and to be mitogenic acting through an angiotensin II type 1 receptor subtype (Battaler et al, 2000). The use of angiotensin-converting enzyme inhibitors and angiotensin II antagonists in cirrhosis is hampered, however, by the deleterious effects on renal hemodynamics (Vlachogiannakos et al, 2001). Angiotensin II inhibitors could be useful drugs for patients with chronic hepatitis without significant portal hypertension, to postpone the development of portal hypertension because they might have an antifibrotic effect. This needs to be established.

The future long-term management of portal hypertension will increasingly be based on drug therapy. Drug combinations will be used as in systemic hypertension. At present, it is impossible to prevent the development of varices. Further studies need to be performed to prevent the growth of small varices. Antifibrotic drugs may achieve the same result. The current problem is the lack of a simple "splanchnic sphygmomanometer," however, which could be used to monitor therapy precisely. Measurement of hepatic venous pressure is invasive and not routinely available. More work needs to be done to establish a baseline clinical or hemodynamic index that can be measured before therapy, and that would reliably predict the therapeutic efficacy. Gradient changes in hepatic venous pressure after drug administration may predict the therapeutic response, but repeat measurements need to be done at 2 weeks from bleeding to capture most patients still at risk. Variceal pressure measurements (Gertsch, 1994; Nevens et al, 1996) may prove valuable in the future. Future studies will be directed at simple ways of establishing individual patient response to portal hypotensive agents in relation to the targeted reduction of pressure.

Preclinical data suggest that selectively delivering therapeutic quantities of nitric oxide to the liver microcirculation without significant effects on systemic and splanchnic circulation, such as using NCX-1000 (a stable compound obtained by adding a nitric oxide–releasing moiety to ursodeoxycholic acid) may provide a novel therapy for the treatment of patients with portal hypertension (Fiorucci et al, 2003). Hepatic gene transfer of the endothelial and neuronal isoforms of nitric oxide synthase (endothelial nitric oxide synthase) in two different animal models of portal hypertension enhanced nitric oxide synthase expression and nitric oxide synthesis and reduced portal pressure (Albillos, 2004). Simvastatin was found to increase hepatosplenic output of nitric oxide products and decrease hepatic resistance in cirrhotics (Zafra et al, 2004). In an animal model, inhibition of portosystemic collateral vessel formation was shown by blocking of vascular endothelial growth factor signaling pathway (with anti–vascular endothelial growth factor receptor-2 monoclonal antibody) (Fernandez et al, 2004).

REFERENCES

Abecasis R, et al, 2003: Nadolol plus spironolactone in the prophylaxis of first variceal bleed in non ascitic cirrhotic patients: a preliminary study. Hepatology 37:359-365.

Abraczinskas DR, et al, 2001: Propranolol for the prevention of first esophageal variceal hemorrhage: a lifetime commitment? Hepatology 34:1096-1102.

Agrawall SR, et al, 2002: Comparable efficacy of propranolol plus isosorbide mononitrate and endoscopic variceal ligation in the prevention of variceal rebleed. J Hepatol 36:631A.

Albillos A, 2004: Therapeutic tools in portal hypertension: drugs. In Groszmann RJ, Bosch J (eds): Portal Hypertension in the 21st Century. Dordrecht, Kluwer, pp 175-184.

Als-Nielsen B, et al, 2004: Non-absorbable disaccharides for hepatic encephalopathy: systematic review of randomised trials. BMJ 328:1046.

Angelico M, et al, 1997: Effects of isosorbide-5-mononitrate compared with propranolol on first bleeding and long-term survival in cirrhosis. Gastroenterology 113:1632-1639.

Armonis A, et al, 1997: Hepatic venous pressure measurement: an old test as new prognostic marker in cirrhosis? Hepatology 25:245-248.

Atkinson M, 1981: Bleeding from the esophagus. In Dykes P, Keighley M (eds): Gastrointestinal Hemorrhage. Bristol, England, J Wright, p 29.

Avgerinos A, et al, 1993: Propranolol in the prevention of recurrent upper gastrointestinal bleeding in patients with cirrhosis undergoing endoscopic sclerotherapy—a randomized controlled trial. J Hepatol 19:301-311.

Avgerinos A, et al, 1997: Early administration of somatostatin and efficacy of sclerotherapy in acute esophageal variceal bleeds: the European Acute Bleeding Esophageal Variceal Episodes (ABOVE) randomised trial. The ABOVE Study Group. Lancet 350:1495-1499.

Avgerinos A, et al, 2000: Endoscopic sclerotherapy plus propranolol versus propranolol alone in the primary prevention of bleeding in high risk cirrhotic patients with esophageal varices: a prospective multicenter randomized trial. Gastrointest Endosc 51:652-658.

Battaler R, et al, 2000: Angiotensin II induces contraction and proliferation of human hepatic stellate cells. Gastroenterology 118:1149-1156.

Ben-Ari Z, et al, 1999: A predictive model for failure to control bleeding during acute variceal haemorrhage. J Hepatol 31:443-450.

Bendtsen F, et al, 1991: Propranolol and haemodynamic response in cirrhosis. J Hepatol 13:144-148.

Bernard B, et al, 1997a: Beta-adrenergic antagonists in the prevention of gastrointestinal rebleeding in patients with cirrhosis: a meta-analysis. Hepatology 25:63-70.

Bernard B, et al, 1997b: Propranolol and sclerotherapy in the prevention of gastrointestinal rebleeding in patients with cirrhosis: a meta-analysis. J Hepatol 26:312-314.

Bernard B, et al, 1999: Antibiotic prophylaxis for the prevention of bacterial infections in cirrhotic patients with gastrointestinal bleeding: a meta-analysis. Hepatology 29:1655-1661.

Besson I, et al, 1995: Sclerotherapy with or without octreotide for acute variceal bleeding. N Engl J Med 333:555-560.

Bildozola M, et al, 2000: Efficacy of octreotide and sclerotherapy in the treatment of acute variceal bleeding in cirrhotic patients: a prospective, multicentric and randomized clinical trial. Scand J Gastroenterol 35:419-425.

Borzio M, et al, 2001: Bacterial infection in patients with advanced cirrhosis: a multicentre prospective study. Dig Liver Dis 33:41-48.

Bosch J, Garcia-Pagan JC, 2003: Prevention of variceal rebleeding. Lancet 361:952-954.

Bosch J, et al, 1981: Effects of somatostatin on hepatic and systemic haemodynamics in patients with cirrhosis of the liver: comparison with vasopressin. Gastroenterology 80:518-525.

Bosch J, et al, 1989: Association of transdermal nitroglycerin to vasopressin infusion in the treatment of variceal hemorrhage: a placebo-controlled clinical trial. Hepatology 10:962-968.

Bosch J, et al, 2004: Recombinant factor VIIIa for upper gastrointestinal bleeding in patients with cirrhosis: a randomized double-blind trial. Gastroenterology 127:1123-1130.

Boyce HW Jr, 1962: Modification of the Sengstaken-Blakemore balloon tube. N Engl J Med 267:195-196.

Brunati S, et al, 1996: Sclerotherapy alone vs sclerotherapy plus terlipressin vs sclerotherapy plus octreotide in the treatment of acute variceal hemorrhage. Hepatology 24:207A (abstract).

Burroughs AK, et al, 1989: Cirrhotics with variceal hemorrhage: the importance of the time interval between admission and the start of the analysis for survival and rebleeding rates. Hepatology 9:801-807.

Burroughs AK, et al, 1990: Randomised double-blind placebo controlled trial of somatostatin for variceal bleeding: emergency control and prevention of early variceal rebleeding. Gastroenterology 99:1388-1395.

Burroughs AK, et al, 1996: Double blind RCT of 5 day octreotide versus placebo, associated with sclerotherapy for trial failures. International Octreotide Varices Study Group. Hepatology 24:352A (abstract).

Cales P, et al, 1990: Incidence of large esophageal varices in patients with cirrhosis: application to prophylaxis of first bleeding. Gut 31:1298-1302.

Cales P, et al, 1999: Lack of effect of propranolol in the prevention of large oesophageal varices in patients with cirrhosis: a randomized French-Speaking Club for the Study of Portal Hypertension. Eur J Gastroenterol Hepatol 11:741-745.

Cales P, et al, 2001: Early administration of vapreotide for variceal bleeding in patients with cirrhosis. French Club for the Study of Portal Hypertension. N Engl J Med 344:23-28.

Carbonell N, et al, 2004: Improved survival after variceal bleeding in patients with cirrhosis over the past two decades. Hepatology 40:652-659.

Cardin F, et al, 1990: A predictive model for very early rebleeding from varices. Gut 31:A1204 (abstract).

Chen CY, et al, 1998: Prophylactic endoscopic variceal ligation (EVL) with multiple band ligator for esophageal varices. Gastroenterology 114:A1224.

Chen WC, et al, 2004: Emergency endoscopic variceal ligation versus somatostatin for acute esophageal variceal bleeding. Hepatology 40:626A (abstract).

Chiu WK, et al, 1990: A controlled study of glypressin versus vasopressin in the control of bleeding from esophageal varices. J Gastroenterol Hepatol 5:549-553.

Christensen E, et al, 1989: Prognosis after the first episode of gastrointestinal bleeding or coma in cirrhosis. Scand J Gastroenterol 24:999-1006.

Conn HO, 1971: Sengstaken-Blakemore tube revisited. Gastroenterology 61:398-400.

Conn HO, et al, 1975: Intraarterial vasopressin in the treatment of upper gastrointestinal hemorrhage: a prospective, controlled clinical trial. Gastroenterology 68:211-221.

D'Amico G, Luca A, 1997: Natural history: clinical-haemodynamic correlations: prediction of the risk of bleeding. Baillieres Clin Gastroenterol 11:243-256.

D'Amico G, et al, 1994: Terlipressin or vasopressin plus transdermal nitroglycerin in a treatment strategy for digestive bleeding in cirrhosis: a randomized clinical trial. J Hepatol 20:206-212.

D'Amico G, et al, 1995: The treatment of portal hypertension: a meta-analytic review. Hepatology 22:332-354.

D'Amico G, et al, 1998: Octreotide compared with placebo in a treatment strategy for early rebleeding in cirrhosis: a double blind, randomized pragmatic trial. Hepatology 28:1206-1214.

D'Amico G, et al, 1999: Pharmacological treatment of portal hypertension: an evidence-based approach. Semin Liver Dis 19:475-505.

D'Amico G, et al, 2003: Upper digestive bleeding in cirrhosis: post-therapeutic outcome and prognostic indicators. Cooperative Study Group. Hepatology 38:599-612.

De BK, et al, 1999: Endoscopic variceal ligation for the primary prophylaxis of oesophageal variceal bleed: preliminary report of a randomized controlled trial. J Gastroenterol Hepatol 14:220-224.

De Franchis R, 2004a: Review article: definition and diagnosis in portal hypertension—continued problems with the Baveno consensus? Aliment Pharmacol Therap 3(suppl):2-6.

De Franchis R, 2004b: Somatostatin, somatostatin analogues and other vasoactive drugs in the treatment of bleeding oesophageal varices. Dig Liver Dis 36(suppl 1):S93-S100.

De la Mora J, et al, 2000: Ligation vs propranolol for primary prophylaxis of variceal bleeding using a multiple band ligator and objective measurements of treatment adequacy: preliminary results. Gastroenterology 118:6512.

Desaint B, et al, 1987: A randomized trial of triglycyl-lysine vasopressin versus lysine vasopressin in active cirrhotic variceal hemorrhage. In Lebrec D, Blei AT (eds): Vasopressin analogs and portal hypertension. Paris, John Libbey Eurotext, pp 155-157.

DiFebo G, et al, 1990: Somatostatin and urgent sclerotherapy in active esophageal variceal bleeding. Gastroenterology 98:A583 (abstract).

Dronfield MW, et al, 1982: Outcome of endoscopy and barium radiography for acute upper gastrointestinal bleeding: controlled trial in 1037 patients. BMJ 284:545-548.

Ejlersen E, et al, 2001: Recombinant activated factor VII (rFVIIa) acutely normalizes prothrombin time in patients with cirrhosis during bleeding from oesophageal varices. Scand J Gastroenterol 36:1081-1085.

El-Jackie A, et al, 1998: Octreotide vs. sclerotherapy in the control of acute variceal bleeding in schistosomal portal hypertension: a randomized trial. Hepatology 28:533A (abstract).

Escorsell A, et al, 1996: Desensitation to the effects of intravenous octreotide in cirrhotic patients with portal hypertension. Hepatology 24:322.

Escorsell A, et al, 1998: Randomized controlled trial of sclerotherapy versus somatostatin infusion in the prevention of early rebleeding following acute variceal hemorrhage in patients with cirrhosis. Variceal Bleeding Study Group. J Hepatol 29:779-788.

Escorsell A, et al, 2000: Multicenter randomized controlled trial of terlipressin versus sclerotherapy in the treatment of acute variceal bleeding: the TEST study. Hepatology 32:471-476.

Escorsell A, et al, 2002: TIPS versus drug therapy in preventing variceal rebleeding in advanced cirrhosis: a randomized controlled trial. Hepatology 35:385-392.

Evrard S, et al, 2003: Endoscopic histoacryl obliteration vs. propranolol in the prevention of esophagogastric variceal rebleeding: a randomized trial. Endoscopy 35:729-735.

Ferguson JW, et al, 2003: Review article: the management of acute variceal bleeding. Aliment Pharmacol Therap 18:253-262.

Fernandez M, et al, 2004: Anti-VEGF receptor-2 monoclonal antibody prevents portal systemic collateral vessel formation in portal hypertensive mice. Gastroenterology 126:886-894.

Feu F, et al, 1991: Double-blind investigation of the effects of propranolol and placebo on the pressure of esophageal varices in patients with portal hypertension. Hepatology 13:917-922.

Feu F, et al, 1995: Relation between portal pressure response to pharmacotherapy and risk of recurrent variceal hemorrhage in patients with cirrhosis. Lancet 346:1056-1059.

Feu F, et al, 1996: Double-blind randomized controlled trial comparing terlipressin and somatostatin for acute variceal hemorrhage. Gastroenterology 111:1291-1299.

Fiorrucci S, et al, 2003: NCX-100, a nitric oxide–releasing derivative of ursodeoxycholic acid, ameliorates portal hypertension and lowers norepinephrine-induced intrahepatic resistance in the isolated and perfused rat liver. J Hepatol 39:932-939.

Flati G, et al, 1986: [Somatostatin: massive upper digestive hemorrhage in portal hypertension: results of a controlled study] [Spanish]. Rev Esp Enferm Dig 70:411-414.

Fogel MR, et al, 1982: Continuous intravenous vasopressin in active upper gastrointestinal bleeding. Ann Intern Med 96:565-569.

Freeman JG, et al, 1982: Controlled trial of terlipressin (glypressin) versus vasopressin in the early treatment of esophageal varices. Lancet 2:66-68.

Freeman JG, et al, 1989: Placebo controlled trial of terlipressin (glypressin) in the management of acute variceal bleeding. J Clin Gastroenterol 11:58-60.

Freitas DS, et al, 2000: Octreotide in acute bleeding esophageal varices: a prospective randomized study. Hepatogastroenterology 47:1310-1314.

Garcia-Pagan JC, et al, 1990: Long-term haemodynamic effects of isosorbide 5 mononitrate in patients with cirrhosis and portal hypertension. J Hepatol 11:189-195.

Garcia-Pagan JC, et al, 1991: Propranolol compared with propranolol plus isosorbide 5 mononitrate for portal hypertension in cirrhosis: a randomized controlled study. Ann Intern Med 114:869-873.

Garcia-Pagan JC, et al, 2001: Isosorbide mononitrate in the prevention of first variceal bleeding in patients who cannot receive beta-blockers. Gastroenterology 121:908-914.

Garcia-Pagan JC, et al, 2003: Propranolol plus placebo versus propranolol plus isosorbide mononitrate in the prevention of a first variceal bleed: a double-blind RCT. Hepatology 37:1260-1266.

Garden OJ, et al, 1985: Prediction of outcome following acute variceal hemorrhage. Br J Surg 72:91-95.

Gertsch PH, 1994: Measurement of variceal pressure. In Blumgart LH (ed): Surgery of the Liver and Biliary Tract, 2nd ed. Edinburgh, Churchill Livingstone, pp 1613-1618.

Gimson AES, et al, 1986: A randomized trial of vasopressin and vasopressin plus nitroglycerin in the control of acute variceal hemorrhage. Hepatology 6:410-413.

Gines P, et al, 2003: Hepatorenal syndrome. Lancet 362:1819-1827.

Gines P, et al, 2004: Review article: pharmacological treatment of hepatorenal syndrome. Aliment Pharmacol Therap 3(suppl):57-62.

Gotzsche PC, et al, 1995: Somatostatin v placebo in bleeding esophageal-varices—randomised trial and meta-analysis. BMJ 310:1495-1498.

Goulis J, et al, 1998: Bacterial infection is independently associated with failure to control bleeding in cirrhotic patients with gastrointestinal hemorrhage. Hepatology 27:1207-1212.

Goulis J, et al, 1999: The role of bacterial infection in the pathogenesis of variceal bleeding. Lancet 353:139-142.

Gournay J, et al, 2000: Isosorbide mononitrate and propranolol compared with propranolol alone for the prevention of variceal rebleeding. Hepatology 31:1239-1245.

Grace ND, et al, 1998: Portal hypertension and variceal bleeding: an AASLD single topic symposium. Hepatology 28:868-880.

Graham DY, Smith JL, 1981: The course of patients after variceal hemorrhage. Gastroenterology 80:800-809.

Groszmann RJ, Wongcharatrawee S, 2004: The hepatic venous pressure gradient: anything worth doing should be done right. Hepatology 39:280-282.

Groszmann RJ, et al, 1990: Hemodynamic events in a prospective randomized trial of propranolol versus placebo in the prevention of a first variceal hemorrhage. Gastroenterology 99:1401-1407.

Groszmann RJ, et al, 2003: Multicenter randomized placebo controlled trial of non-selective beta-blockers in the prevention of the complications of portal hypertension: final results and identification of a predictive factor. Hepatology 38(suppl 1):206A.

Hemstreet BA, 2004: Evaluation of carvedilol for the treatment of portal hypertension. Pharmacotherapy 24:94-104.

Hou MC, et al, 2004: Antibiotic prophylaxis after endoscopic therapy prevents rebleeding in acute variceal hemorrhage: a randomized trial. Hepatology 39:746-753.

Huang CC, et al, 1992: A prospective randomized controlled trial of somato-statin and vasopressin in the management of acute bleeding esophageal varices. Changgeng Yi Xue Za Zhi 15:78-83.

Hwang SJ, et al, 1992: A randomized controlled trial comparing octreotide and vasopressin in the control of acute esophageal variceal bleeding. J Hepatol 16:320-325.

Ioannou GN, et al, 2003a: Systematic review: terlipressin in acute oesophageal variceal hemorrhage. Aliment Pharmacol Therap 17:53-64.

Ioannou GN, et al, 2003b: Terlipressin for acute esophageal variceal hemorrhage. Cochrane Database Systematic Reviews 1:CD002147.

Jenkins SA, et al, 1988: The effects of somatostatin and SMS 201-995 on hepatic haemodynamics in patients with cirrhosis and portal hypertension. Fibrinolysis 2:48-50.

Jenkins SA, et al, 1997: A multicentre randomised trial comparing octreotide and injection sclerotherapy in the management and outcome of acute variceal hemorrhage. Gut 41:526-533.

Jensen LS, Krarup N, 1989: Propranolol in prevention of rebleeding from oesophageal varices during the course of endoscopic sclerotherapy. Scand J Gastroenterol 24:339-345.

Junquera F, et al, 2000: Somatostatin plus isosorbide 5-mononitrate versus somatostatin in the control of acute gastro-oesophageal variceal bleeding: a double blind, randomised, placebo controlled trial. Gut 46:127-132.

Jutabha R, et al, 2001: A randomized, prospective study of prophylactic rubber band ligation compared to propranolol for the prevention of first variceal hemorrhage in cirrhotics with large esophageal varices. Gastrointest Endosc 53:568.

Lebrec D, 1998: Pharmacological treatment of portal hypertension: present and future. J Hepatol 28:896-907.

Lebrec D, 1980: Propranolol—a medical treatment for portal hypertension. Lancet 2:180-182.

Lee FY, et al, 1988: A randomised controlled study of triglycyl-vasopressin and vasopressin plus nitroglycerin in the control of acute esophageal variceal hemorrhage. Chin J Gastroenterol 5:131-138.

Lee HY, et al, 2003: A prospective randomized controlled clinical trial comparing effects of somatostatin and vasopressin for control of acute variceal bleeding in the patients with liver cirrhosis. Korean J Intern Med 18:161-166.

Levacher S, et al, 1995: Early administration of terlipressin plus glyceryl trinitrate to control active upper gastrointestinal bleeding in cirrhotic patients. Lancet 346:865-868.

Lin HC, et al, 2004: Acute administration of carvedilol is more effective than propranolol plus isosorbide-5-mononitrate in the reduction of portal pressure in patients with viral cirrhosis. Am J Gastroenterol 99:1953-1958.

Linton RR, 1966: The treatment of esophageal varices. Surg Clin North Am 46:485-498.

Lo GH, et al, 2000: Endoscopic variceal ligation plus nadolol and sucralfate compared with ligation alone for the prevention of variceal rebleeding: a prospective randomized trial. Hepatology 32:461-465.

Lo GH, et al, 2002: Banding ligation versus nadolol and isosorbide monitrate for the prevention of esophageal variceal rebleeding. Gastroenterology 123:728-734.

Lo GH, et al, 2004: Endoscopic ligation vs. nadolol in the prevention of first variceal bleeding in patients with cirrhosis. Gastrointest Endosc 59:333-338.

Loperfido S, et al, 1987: Somatostatin in the treatment of bleeding oesophagogastric varices: controlled clinical trial in comparison with ranitidine [Italian]. Rec Progress Med 78:82-86.

Lopez F, et al, 1999: Octreotide vs sclerotherapy in the treatment of acute variceal bleeding. Hepatology 30:574A (abstract).

Luca A, et al, 1993: Hemodynamic effects of acute changes in intra-abdominal pressure in patients with cirrhosis. Gastroenterology 104:222-227.

Lui HF, et al, 2002: Primary prophylaxis of variceal hemorrhage: a randomized controlled trial comparing band ligation, propranolol and isosorbide mononitrate. Gastroenterology 123:735-744.

Mallory A, et al, 1980: Selective intra-arterial vasopressin infusion for upper gastrointestinal tract hemorrhage: a controlled trial. Arch Surg 115:30-32.

McCormick PA, O'Keefe C, 2001: Improving prognosis following a first variceal haemorrhage over four decades. Gut 49:682-685.

McCormick PA, et al, 1992: Octreotide inhibits the meal-induced increases in portal venous pressure in cirrhotic patients with portal hypertension: a double-blind placebo-controlled study. Hepatology 16:1180-1186.

McCormick PA, et al, 1998: Clinical vs haemodynamic response to drugs in portal hypertension. J Hepatol 28:1015-1019.

McKee R, 1990: A study of octreotide in esophageal varices. Digestion 45(suppl 1):60-65.

Merigan TC, et al, 1962: Effect of intravenously administered posterior pituitary extract on hemorrhage from bleeding esophageal varices: a controlled evaluation. N Engl J Med 266:134-135.

Merkel C, Gatta A, 1991: Can we predict the 1st variceal bleeding in the individual patient with cirrhosis and esophageal varices. J Hepatol 13:378.

Merkel C, et al, 2000: Long-term results of a clinical trial of nadolol with or without isosorbide mononitrate for primary prophylaxis of variceal bleeding in cirrhosis. Hepatology 31:324-329.

Merkel C, et al, 2004: A placebo-controlled clinical trial of nadolol in the prophylaxis of growth of small esophageal varices in cirrhosis. Gastroenterology 127:476-484.

Merli M, et al, 2004: The natural history of portal hypertensive gastropathy in patients with liver cirrhosis and mild hypertensive gastropathy. Am J Gastroenterol 99:1959-1965.

Mitchell K, et al, 1982: Endoscopy in patients with portal hypertension and upper gastrointestinal bleeding. In Westaby D, et al (eds): Variceal Bleeding. London, Pitman, pp 62-67.

Moitinho E, et al, 1999: Prognostic value of early measurements of portal pressure in acute variceal bleeding. Gastroenterology 117:626-631.

Moitinho E, et al, 2001: Multicenter randomized controlled trial comparing different schedules of somatostatin in the treatment of acute variceal bleeding. J Hepatol 35:712-718.

Monescillo A, et al, 2004: Influence of portal hypertension and its early decompression by TIPS placement on the outcome of variceal bleeding. Hepatology 40:793-801.

Moore KP, et al, 2003: The management of ascites in cirrhosis: report on the consensus conference on the International Ascites Club. Hepatology 38:258-266.

Moreau R, et al, 1989: Low dose of nitroglycerin failed to improve splanchnic hemodynamics in patients with cirrhosis: evidence for an impaired cardiopulmonary baroreflex function. Hepatology 10:93-97.

Nevens F, 2004: Review article: a critical comparison of drug therapies in currently used therapeutic strategies for variceal haemorrhage. Aliment Pharmacol Therap 3(suppl):18-22.

Nevens F, et al, 1996: The effect of long-term treatment with spironolactone on variceal pressure in patients with portal hypertension without ascites. Hepatology 23:1047-1052.

Nevens F, et al, 1998: Variceal pressure is a factor predicting the risk of a first variceal bleeding: a prospective cohort study in cirrhotic patients. Hepatology 27:15-19.

North Italian Endoscopic Club (NIEC) for the Study and Treatment of Esophageal Varices, 1988: Prediction of the first variceal hemorrhage in patients with cirrhosis of the liver and esophageal varices: a prospective study. N Engl J Med 319:983-989.

Ohmann C, et al, 1990: Prognostic scores in esophageal or gastric variceal bleeding. Scand J Gastroenterol 25:501-512.

Pagliaro L, et al, 1994: Portal hypertension in cirrhosis: natural history. In Bosch J, Groszmann R (eds): Portal Hypertension: Pathophysiology and Treatment. Cambridge, MA, Blackwell Scientific, pp 72-92.

Panes J, et al, 1988: Efficacy of balloon tamponade in treatment of bleeding gastric and esophageal varices: results in 151 episodes. Dig Dis Sci 33:454-459.

Panos M, et al, 1990: Sequential haemodynamic changes during single total paracentesis and right atrial size in patients with tense ascites. Hepatology 11:662-667.

Pasta L, et al, 2001: Isosorbide mononitrate with nadolol compared to nadolol alone for the prevention of recurrent bleeding in cirrhosis: a double blind placebo controlled randomized trial. Gastroenterology 120:A375 (abstract).

Patch D, et al, 1999: Randomized double blind controlled trial of 5 day terlipressin vs placebo in acute variceal hemorrhage. J Hepatol 30:55 (abstract).

Patch D, et al, 2002: A randomized, controlled trial of medical therapy versus endoscopic ligation for the prevention of variceal rebleeding in patients with cirrhosis. Gastroenterology 123:1013-1019.

Pauwels A, et al, 1994: Terlipressin and somatostatin in the treatment of hemorrhages from rupture of esophageal varices. Gastroenterol Clin Biol 18:388-389 (letter).

Pedretti G, et al, 1994: Octreotide versus terlipressin in acute variceal hemorrhage in liver cirrhosis. Emergency control and prevention of early rebleeding. Clin Invest 72:653-659.

Perez-Ayuso R, et al, 1991: Propranolol in prevention of recurrent bleeding from severe portal hypertensive gastropathy in cirrhosis. Lancet 337:1431-1434.

Pietrosi G, et al, 1999: Isosorbide mononitrate with nadolol compared to nadolol alone for prevention of first bleeding in cirrhosis, a double blind placebo-controlled randomised trial. J Hepatol 30(suppl 1):66A.

Planas R, et al, 1992: A prospective randomised trial comparing somatostatin and sclerotherapy in the treatment of acute variceal bleeding. Gastroenterology 102:A869 (abstract).

Polio J, Groszmann RJ, 1986: Haemodynamic factors involved in the development and rupture of esophageal varices: a pathophysiological approach to treatment. Semin Liver Dis 6:318-328.

Poo JL, et al, 1996: Octreotide versus emergency sclerotherapy in acute variceal hemorrhage in liver cirrhosis. Gastroenterology 110:1297A (abstract).

Poynard T, et al, 1991: Beta-adrenergic antagonist drugs in the prevention of gastro-intestinal bleeding in patients with cirrhosis and esophageal varices. N Engl J Med 324:1532-1538.

Primignani M, et al, 1995: Sclerotherapy plus octreotide versus sclerotherapy alone in the prevention of early rebleeding from esophageal-varices—a randomized, double-blind, placebo-controlled, multicenter trial. Hepatology 21:1322-1327.

Primignani M, et al, 2000: Natural history of portal hypertensive gastropathy in patients with liver cirrhosis. The New Italian Endoscopic Club for the study and treatment of esophageal varices (NIEC). Gastroenterology 119:181-187.

Psilopoulos D, et al, 2002: A randomized trial comparing endoscopic variceal ligation (EVL) with propranolol for primary prevention of variceal bleeding (preliminary report). Gastrointest Endosc 55:T1897.

Ramires RP, et al, 2000: [Sclerotherapy versus somatostatin in the treatment of upper digestive hemorrhage caused by rupture of eosophageal varices]. Arq Gastroenterol 37:148-154.

Ready JB, et al, 1991a: Effects of vasopressin on portal pressure during hemorrhage from esophageal varices. Gastroenterology 100:1411-1416.

Ready JB, et al, 1991b: Assessment of risk of bleeding from esophageal varices by continuous monitoring of portal pressure. Gastroenterology 100:1403-1410.

Romero G, et al, 2004: Nadolol plus isosorbide mononitrate compared to banding plus low volume sclerotherapy for prevention of variceal rebleeding in patients with cirrhosis. Hepatology 40:204A (abstract).

Romero-Castro R, et al, 2004: Recombinant-activated factor VII as hemostatic therapy in eight cases of severe hemorrhage from esophageal varices. Clin Gastroenterol Hepatol 2:78-84.

Samonakis DN, et al, 2004: Management of portal hypertension. Postgrad Med J 80:634-641.

Sarin SK, et al, 1999: Comparison of endoscopic ligation and propranolol for the primary prevention of variceal bleeding. N Engl J Med 340:988-993.

Schepke M, et al, 2004: Ligation versus propranolol for the primary prophylaxis of variceal bleeding in cirrhosis. Hepatology 40:65-72.

Schrier RW, et al, 1988: Peripheral arterial vasodilation hypothesis: a proposal for the initiation of renal sodium and water retention in cirrhosis. Hepatology 8:1151-1157.

Sengstaken RW, Blakemore AH, 1950: Balloon tamponade for the control of hemorrhage from oesophageal varices. Ann Surg 131:781-789.

Shields R, et al, 1992: A prospective randomised controlled trial comparing the efficacy of somatostatin with injection sclerotherapy in the control of bleeding oesophageal varices. J Hepatol 16:128-137.

Shiha G, et al, 2006: Endoscopic ligation compared with propranolol and combined isosorbide mononitrates (ISMN) and propranolol to prevent recurrent variceal bleeding: a prospective randomized trial. Gut, in press.

Signorelli S, et al, 1996: Sclerotherapy with or without somatostatin or octreotide in the treatment of acute variceal haemorrhage: our experience. Gastroenterology 110:1326A (abstract).

Signorelli S, et al, 1997: Esophageal varices bleeding: comparison between treatment with sclerotherapy alone vs sclerotherapy plus octreotide. Hepatology 26:137A (abstract).

Silvain C, et al, 1993: Terlipressin plus transdermal nitroglycerin vs. octreotide in the control of acute bleeding from esophageal varices: a multicenter randomized trial. Hepatology 18:61-65.

Silverstein F, et al, 1981: The national ASGE survey on upper gastrointestinal bleeding. Parts 1-3. Gastrointest Endosc 27:73-102.

Siringo S, et al, 1991: Prognostic significance of the white nipple sign in variceal bleeding. Gastrointest Endosc 37:5-55.

Sivri B, et al, 2000: A prospective randomized trial from Turkey comparing octreotide versus injection sclerotherapy in acute variceal bleeding. Hepatogastroenterology 47:168-173.

Soares-Weiser K, et al, 2003: Antibiotic prophylaxis of bacterial infections in cirrhotic inpatients: a meta-analysis of randomized controlled trials. Scand J Gastroenterol 38:193-200.

Soderlund C, et al, 1990: Terlipressin (triglycyl-lysine vasopressin) controls acute bleeding oesophageal varices: a double blind randomised placebo controlled trial. Scand J Gastroenterol 25:622-630.

Sonnenburg GE, et al, 1981: Effect of somatostatin on splanchnic haemodynamics. Gastroenterology 80:5226-5232.

Sung JJ, et al, 1993: Octreotide infusion or emergency sclerotherapy for variceal haemorrhage. Lancet 324:637-641.

Sung JJY, et al, 1995: Prospective randomized study of effect of octreotide on rebleeding from oesophageal varices after endoscopic ligation. Lancet 346:1666-1669.

Teres J, et al, 1978: Esophageal tamponade for bleeding varices: controlled trial between the Sengstaken-Blakemore tube and the Linton-Nachlas tube. Gastroenterology 75:566-569.

Testoni PA, et al, 1986: Comparison of somatostatin and cimetidine in the treatment of acute esophageal variceal bleeding. Curr Theor Res 39:759-766.

Thalheimer U, et al, 2004a: Monitoring target reduction in hepatic venous pressure gradient during pharmacological therapy of portal hypertension: a close look at the evidence. Gut 53:143-148.

Thalheimer U, et al, 2004b: Targeting portal pressure measurements: a critical reappraisal. Hepatology 39:286-290.

Thalheimer U, et al, 2005: Infection, coagulation and variceal bleeding in cirrhosis: a review. Gut 54:556-563.

Thomsen BL, et al, 1994: Optimized analysis of recurrent bleeding and death in patients with cirrhosis and esophageal varices. Copenhagen Esophageal Varices Sclerotherapy Project. J Hepatol 21:367-375.

Triantos CK, et al, 2004: Terlipressin for renal failure in cirrhosis: a single centre review. Hepatology 40:646A (abstract).

Tsai Y-T, et al, 1986: Controlled trial of vasopressin plus nitroglycerin versus vasopressin alone in the treatment of bleeding esophageal varices. Hepatology 6:406-409.

Valenzuela JE, et al, 1989: A multicentre, randomized double-blind trial of somatostatin in the management of acute hemorrhage from esophageal varices. Hepatology 10:958-961.

Villanueva C, et al, 2001: Endoscopic ligation compared with combined treatment with nadolol and isosorbide monitrate to prevent recurrent variceal bleeding. N Engl J Med 345:647-655.

Vinel JP, et al, 1986: Assessment of short-term prognosis after variceal bleeding in patients with alcoholic cirrhosis by early measurement of portohepatic gradient. Hepatology 6:116-117.

Vinel JP, et al, 1990: Hemodynamic evaluation of molsidomine—a vasodilator with antianginal properties in patients with alcoholic cirrhosis. Hepatology 11:239-242.

Vlachogiannakos J, et al, 2001: Angiotensin enzyme inhibitors and angiotensin II antagonists as therapy in chronic liver disease. Gut 49:303-308.

Vlachogiannakos J, et al, 2004: Increased mortality and early rebleeding in the presence of bacterial infection in cirrhotic patients with upper gastrointestinal bleeding: a prospective single center study. Hepatology 40:628A (abstract).

Vlanianos P, et al, 1989: Balloon tamponade in variceal bleeding: use and misuse. BMJ 298:1158-1159.

Vlavianos P, et al, 1999: Splanchnic and systemic haemodynamic response to volume changes in patients with cirrhosis and portal hypertension. Clin Sci (Lond) 96:475-481.

Vorobioff J, et al, 1989: Long-term hemodynamic effects of ketanserin, a 5-hydroxytryptamine blocker, in portal hypertensive patients. Hepatology 9:88-91.

Vorobioff J, et al, 1996: Prognostic value of hepatic venous pressure gradient measurements in alcoholic cirrhosis: a 10-year prospective study. Gastroenterology 111:701-709.

Walker S, et al, 1986: Terlipressin in bleeding esophageal varices: a placebo-controlled, double-blind study. Hepatology 6:112-115.

Walker S, et al, 1992: Terlipressin vs somatostatin in bleeding esophageal varices: a controlled double-blind study. Hepatology 15:1023-1030.

Walker S, et al, 1996: Terlipresin (glypressin) versus somatostatin in the treatment of bleeding eosophageal varices—final report of a placebo-controlled, double-blind study. Z Gastroenterol 16:320-325.

Yousuf MH, et al, 2000: Initial management of acute variceal haemorrhage: comparison of octreotide and sclerotherapy. J Coll Physicians Surg Pakistan 10:95-97.

Zafra C, et al, 2004: Simvastatin enhances hepatic nitric oxide production and decreases the hepatic vascular tone in patients with cirrhosis. Gastroenterology 126:749-755.

Zimmon DS, Kessler RE, 1974: The portal pressure–blood volume relationship in cirrhosis. Gut 15:99-101.

Zuberi BF, Baloch Q, 2000: Comparison of endoscopic variceal sclerotherapy alone and in combination with octreotide in controlling acute variceal hemorrhage and early rebleeding in patients with low risk cirrhosis. Am J Gastroenterol 95:768-771.

Endoscopic Therapy in the Management of Esophageal Varices: Injection Sclerotherapy and Variceal Ligation

J. E. J. KRIGE AND P. C. BORNMAN

Variceal bleeding is the most serious life-threatening complication of portal hypertension and accounts for half of all deaths in patients with advanced liver disease and portal hypertension. Survival after variceal bleeding depends largely on the cause of portal hypertension, the presence and severity of underlying liver disease, and hepatic functional reserve. Patients with noncirrhotic portal hypertension (see Ch. 87) and normal hepatic function tolerate hemorrhage better than patients with decompensated cirrhosis, who have a high mortality rate. The risk of death is greatest during the first few days after onset of variceal hemorrhage. In addition, the probability of variceal rebleeding is greater than 70%. Most patients who have recurrent hemorrhage rebleed within 6 weeks of the initial episode, and the risk of recurrence gradually decreases thereafter (Bornman et al, 1994).

The quality and efficacy of emergency medical treatment in the management of esophageal variceal hemorrhage are crucial because the initial bleeding episode has a mortality rate of 30% to 50%, depending on the degree of liver decompensation, and requires an intensive multidisciplinary approach. The treatment of variceal hemorrhage is evolving rapidly. No single modality is applicable to all patients, and knowledge of the alternatives allows a well-informed clinician to choose the appropriate therapy. The key to effective management of acute and recurrent variceal bleeding is to choose the right treatment for the right patient at the right time. A careful and coordinated team approach is essential. Each of the available therapies may be required at different stages and for different patients. The management of acute, persistent variceal bleeding is best accomplished by a skilled, knowledgeable, and well-equipped unit that can offer the whole spectrum of treatment methods. The use of new treatment modalities, including endoscopic therapy, vasoactive drugs, and antibiotic prophylaxis, has resulted in a threefold decrease in hospital mortality of patients with variceal bleeding since the 1980s (Carbonell et al, 2004). In this chapter, the role of endoscopic therapy in the management of acute variceal bleeding and the prevention of subsequent rebleeding is discussed, and endoscopic therapy is compared with other currently available alternative therapies. The technical details of balloon tube insertion, endoscopic injection sclerotherapy (EIS), and endoscopic variceal ligation (EVL) are presented in detail.

MANAGEMENT OF ACUTE VARICEAL BLEEDING

The possibility of variceal bleeding should be considered in all patients with known risk factors for chronic liver disease or clinical evidence of portal hypertension. In Western countries, variceal bleeding accounts for approximately 7% of gastrointestinal bleeding episodes, although this varies (11% in the United States, 5% in the United Kingdom) according to the prevalence of alcohol-related liver disease.

Modern management for controlling acute variceal bleeding requires the availability of a variety of therapeutic options, which may be used sequentially or can be combined in the individual patient (Table 92.1). Several important considerations influence the choice of therapy and prognosis in individual patients, including the natural history of the disease causing portal hypertension, location of the bleeding varices, residual

Table 92.1 Management of Acute Variceal Bleeding

Pharmacologic agents
  Somatostatin
  Terlipressin
  Octreotide
  Vasopressin

Endoscopic therapy
  Band ligation
  Injection sclerotherapy
    Sclerosants
    Cyanoacrylate ("superglue")
    Thrombin

Balloon tamponade

TIPS

Surgery
  Shunt procedure
  Esophageal transection

hepatic function, presence of associated systemic disease, continuing drug or alcohol abuse, patency of major splanchnic veins, and response to each specific treatment.

PRIMARY MANAGEMENT OF BLEEDING VARICES

General Strategy

All patients with suspected acute variceal bleeding require hospitalization. The immediate aims of emergency medical treatment involve hemodynamic stabilization, blood volume replacement, control of bleeding, support of vital organ function, and prevention of complications resulting from hypovolemic shock and impending liver failure (see Ch. 91). Patients should be nursed in an intensive care unit (ICU), and standard resuscitation for major hemorrhage should be instituted. Although variceal bleeding stops spontaneously in 60% of patients, it is impossible to predict continued bleeding. Patients should be transferred

to a center with appropriate facilities and expertise as soon as they have been adequately resuscitated and are stable. A suggested management algorithm is shown in Fig. 92.1.

Initial Measures

Many patients with acute variceal hemorrhage have liver decompensation with encephalopathy, ascites, coagulopathy, bacteremia, and malnutrition. The aim of treatment is to resuscitate the patient effectively and to control the bleeding as quickly and reliably as possible using methods with the fewest possible side effects. The extent and urgency of initial therapy depends on the severity of bleeding. Stable patients with intermittent bleeding are candidates for endoscopic therapy, whereas exsanguinating bleeding may require balloon tamponade to control bleeding before endoscopy is performed.

Maintenance of a secure airway and prompt resuscitation with restoration of circulating blood volume are vital and

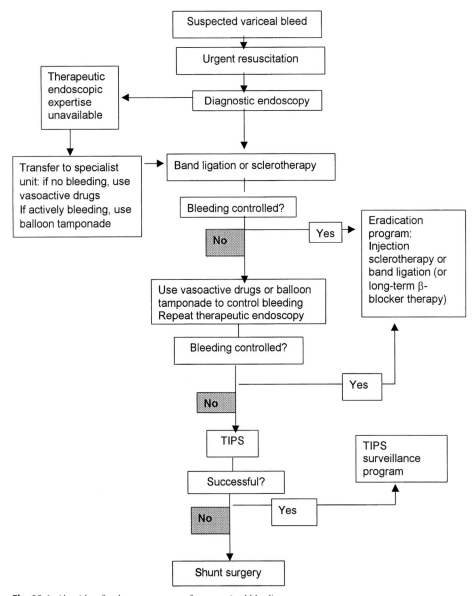

Fig. 92.1. Algorithm for the management of acute variceal bleeding.

precede any diagnostic studies. Intravenous access is obtained via a central venous cannula. While blood is being crossmatched, crystalloid solution is infused rapidly until blood pressure is restored and urine output is adequate. Saline infusions may aggravate ascites and must be avoided. Overzealous expansion of circulating volume may precipitate further bleeding (Stanley & Hayes, 1997). Central venous pressure should be maintained at 2 to 5 cm H_2O measured from the sternal angle. Patients who are hemodynamically unstable, are elderly, or have concomitant cardiac or pulmonary disease should be monitored using a pulmonary artery catheter because injudicious administration of crystalloids, combined with vasoactive drugs, may lead to the rapid onset of edema, ascites, and hyponatremia. Clotting factors are often deficient, and fresh blood, fresh frozen plasma, and vitamin K_1 should be given. Platelet transfusions may be necessary. Sedatives should be avoided.

Pharmacologic therapy should be started when a diagnosis of variceal bleeding is suspected and before performing emergency endoscopy (see Ch. 91). This policy has the theoretical advantage of controlling bleeding before the initial endoscopy, which should make diagnosis and immediate endoscopic therapy easier.

Emergency Endoscopy and Immediate Endoscopic Therapy

Emergency diagnostic endoscopy is mandatory to confirm that a patient is bleeding from esophageal varices. Patients shown to have varices on endoscopy fall into one of three groups, although the differentiation may be difficult during active bleeding: (1) patients with actively bleeding varices; (2) patients whose varices have stopped bleeding; and (3) patients who have varices, but are bleeding from another lesion. At endoscopy, varices are presumed to be the source of bleeding if adherent blood clots are noted on a varix or when varices are present in a patient with upper gastrointestinal bleeding in whom panendoscopy shows no other cause of bleeding.

Emergency endoscopy should be performed in the endoscopy unit where all the necessary equipment is available. Many units have a fully equipped emergency endoscopy trolley, and if necessary this can be taken into the operating room or the ICU. It is imperative that full resuscitative facilities are available together with skilled staff experienced in dealing with emergencies. Two endoscopy assistants should be present throughout. Adequate monitoring is necessary during the procedure. Emergency endoscopy should not begin until satisfactory venous access and central venous pressure measurement are established, and volume replacement and resuscitation procedures with blood transfusions are initiated to correct hypovolemia. If bleeding is profuse, endotracheal intubation is essential before endoscopy to protect the airway and avoid aspiration. Patients in shock and uncooperative patients are best treated in the operating room with full anesthetic support.

Patients who have endoscopically proven active variceal bleeding or in whom variceal bleeding has stopped should have immediate sclerotherapy or variceal ligation (see Fig. 92.1). If sclerotherapy or variceal ligation is deferred in patients who have stopped bleeding, there is a distinct danger of further major bleeding during the interval period. If acute or recurrent major variceal bleeding continues despite endoscopic and pharmacologic therapy, mechanical control by balloon tamponade is used.

The efficacy of emergency sclerotherapy in controlling acute variceal bleeding has been compared with pharmacologic treatment in 15 randomized controlled trials. A cumulative meta-analysis of these trials shows the superiority of sclerotherapy for control of acute variceal bleeding (Triantos et al, 2004).

After control of the index variceal bleed, all patients are considered for subsequent definitive management. Definitive management usually comprises repeat variceal ligation or sclerotherapy. The justification is the high recurrent bleeding rate in the early postprocedure period. Although the risk lessens with time, each individual bleed is associated with significant morbidity and mortality.

Balloon Tube Control

A correctly placed balloon tube (Fig. 92.2) can control acute variceal bleeding temporarily. The balloon tube is inserted when massive variceal bleeding obscures visibility during emergency endoscopic therapy, or when patients have continued active bleeding despite attempted control by emergency endoscopic sclerotherapy or band ligation. In our experience, these circumstances are uncommon. Balloon tube tamponade also has proved to be lifesaving during the transfer of patients from smaller peripheral hospitals to a major center. Balloon tube tamponade also is used to control a subsequent major bleed while awaiting emergency endoscopy or to stop variceal bleeding while preparing for alternative therapy when endoscopic therapy fails (i.e., a further major acute variceal bleed after two emergency endoscopic treatments during a single hospital admission).

The balloon tube always should be inserted by an experienced staff member familiar with the technique. The technical details are presented later. The tube should be left in place for as short a time as possible, while the patient is being resuscitated and preparations are made for endoscopic treatment. If bleeding

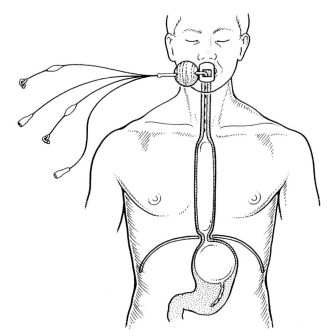

Fig. 92.2. Four lumen balloon tube. The gastric balloon, which is filled with air, is held firmly against the esophagogastric junction by fixing a split tennis ball to the tube at the patient's mouth.

continues after a balloon tube has been inserted, an experienced staff member should assess whether the tube has been inserted and secured correctly or whether to repeat the emergency endoscopy. Endoscopy usually reveals a bleeding lesion below the balloon in the distal stomach or duodenum that was missed at the first diagnostic endoscopy (Terblanche & Krige, 1994).

ALTERNATIVE EMERGENCY MANAGEMENT OPTIONS

The main alternatives to pharmacologic and endoscopic therapy for acute variceal bleeding are transjugular intrahepatic portosystemic shunt (TIPS) (see Ch. 96), surgical portosystemic shunts (see Ch. 95), and esophageal transection operations (see Ch. 94). In patients with recurrent bleeding, it is crucial to identify the cause and site of bleeding because the management of injection-induced esophageal ulceration, recurrent variceal bleeding, gastric varices, and portal hypertensive gastropathy differs.

TIPS is now the emergency procedure of choice for patients with failed endoscopic therapy. More recent data confirm the utility and efficacy of TIPS as a salvage procedure for refractory variceal bleeding unresponsive to endoscopic and pharmacologic treatment (Rosado & Kamath, 2003). Immediate control of variceal bleeding was achieved in greater than 90% of patients in a review of 15 publications (Vangeli et al, 2002). TIPS in uncontrolled variceal bleeding still has a high mortality, however. Prognosis is poor if patients have developed sepsis, have required inotropic support and ventilation (often owing to aspiration), and have deteriorating liver and renal function. Established renal failure in a decompensated cirrhotic patient with uncontrolled bleeding is a contraindication to TIPS placement in most units (Samonakis et al, 2004).

The use of emergency major surgical procedures to control acute variceal bleeding has diminished dramatically. The role of emergency surgical shunting procedures is now reserved for failures of TIPS. A successful emergency shunt effectively stops acute variceal bleeding and prevents recurrent bleeds.

Various devascularization and transection operations have been devised that disconnect the high-pressure portal system from the esophageal varices. As a basic principle, the simplest procedure should be used. Simple esophageal transection using a staple gun is the preferred procedure for patients in whom endoscopic therapy has failed and TIPS or an operative shunt is not feasible. Previous sclerotherapy may increase the difficulties and risk of performing the operation because of sclerosant-induced ulceration and periesophageal fibrosis. Esophageal transection combined with an extensive esophageal and gastric devascularization procedure is not justified in the emergency setting. Four trials have compared sclerotherapy with esophageal transection, and one compared sclerotherapy with portacaval shunt after failure of medical treatment (D'Amico et al, 1995). Failure to control bleeding was higher with sclerotherapy, significantly in one. Rebleeding, assessed in three trials, was significantly higher with injection sclerotherapy. No significant differences in mortality were found (D'Amico et al, 1995).

Emergency liver transplantation has been advocated. In our view, however, liver transplantation is best performed in a stable patient after initial control of bleeding, preferably using an endoscopic technique because this would interfere least with a subsequent transplant. For failures of endoscopic therapy in potential transplant recipients, we advocate an urgent TIPS procedure. The cost of treating patients with end-stage alcoholic liver disease and refractory bleeding is substantial. Unless patients are potential liver transplant candidates, the decision whether to proceed with expensive and often fruitless salvage procedures becomes a difficult ethical and moral dilemma.

FAILURE OF EMERGENCY ENDOSCOPIC THERAPY

Endoscopic sclerotherapy is successful in controlling acute variceal bleeding in 90% to 95% of patients after one or two injection treatments. Current evidence suggests that variceal ligation is as effective with a similar success rate after one or two treatment sessions (Tait et al, 1999). A recurrent acute variceal bleed is defined as an acute episode of variceal bleeding that occurs within hours or days after emergency sclerotherapy or emergency variceal ligation and that requires blood transfusion and subsequent emergency management.

Any patient who rebleeds after two successive emergency sclerotherapy treatments during a single hospital admission has a prohibitively high mortality if sclerotherapy treatment is pursued. This situation is defined as sclerotherapy failure, and these patients should have the bleeding controlled by balloon tube tamponade, be resuscitated, and be treated by an alternative technique. A similar definition is used for failure of variceal ligation.

The management of patients with complex or recurrent variceal bleeding who have failed endoscopic therapy has been simplified by the radiologic placement of emergency salvage or rescue TIPS. An emergency H-graft portosystemic surgical shunt (see Ch. 95), in preference to an end-to-side or side-to-side portacaval shunt, is reserved for the unusual situation where TIPS fails. If for any reason, an operative shunt is not possible, a staple-gun esophageal transection is used to control bleeding.

LONG-TERM MANAGEMENT OF PATIENTS AFTER A VARICEAL BLEED

When the acute bleeding episode has been controlled, and the patient is stabilized, a detailed evaluation is undertaken to identify the cause of the portal hypertension, the severity of any underlying liver disease, and the likely natural history and location and extent of the varices. Only then can accurate and informed decisions be made about the available treatment choices (Henderson et al, 1998). The assessment and comparison of various forms of therapy in patients with portal hypertension are complicated, however, by numerous problems, including a geographic variation in the incidence of the underlying pathology and the varied prognosis depending on the etiology. A comparison of treatments by controlled trials from different institutions is difficult. In addition, an important factor, often overlooked, is that although most surgical treatments of portal hypertension have become standardized, endoscopic therapy, especially injection sclerotherapy, varies widely in technique and application.

Although the chances of a recurrent variceal bleed diminish with time, 70% of patients have a further variceal bleed during their lifetime. For this reason, we recommend that all patients who have had a variceal bleed be considered for long-term

Table 92.2 Long-Term Management to Prevent Variceal Rebleeding

Endoscopic therapy
    Variceal band ligation
    Injection sclerotherapy
Pharmacotherapy
    β-Blockers
Surgery
    Shunt
        DSRS
        Portacaval
    Nonshunt
        Esophageal transection and gastric devascularization
        Splenectomy for gastric varices secondary to splenic vein thrombosis
TIPS
Liver transplantation

DSRS, distal splenorenal shunt.

management aimed at preventing further bleeding (Table 92.2). The options are detailed subsequently.

ENDOSCOPIC THERAPY

The most widely used endoscopic management for patients who have esophageal varices that have bled is repeat variceal ligation. Some endoscopists prefer injection sclerotherapy for actively bleeding varices because the injection can be performed immediately without first removing the endoscope to attach the ligation device. In addition, the endoscopic view is reduced, and blood clot in the ligating chamber interferes with visibility and the accurate deployment of the variceal bands. Injection sclerotherapy also is technically easier to perform than ligation when varices are small and difficult to suck into the ligation chamber.

Injection Sclerotherapy

Three different endoscopic techniques are used for injection sclerotherapy. Bleeding from esophageal varices may be controlled by injecting the sclerosant directly into the venous channel (i.e., intravariceal method), beside the channel (i.e., paravariceal method), or a combination of both. Most endoscopists in the United States favor intravariceal injection. Usually, 1 to 5 mL of sclerosant, depending on the size of the varix, is injected directly into the variceal lumen just above the gastroesophageal junction, with an additional injection into the same variceal column more proximally, if the varix is large. The goal of this technique is thrombosis of the varix and eventual obliteration of all channels in the distal 5 cm of the esophagus. The paravariceal technique, widely used in Europe, is performed by placing multiple injections using 0.5 to 1.5 mL of 0.5% or 1% polidocanol at each site beside the varices, starting at the esophagogastric junction and proceeding upward in a helical fashion, raising a wheal at each injection site. The theory is that paravariceal injection produces edema to stop acute variceal bleeding and to provoke fibrogenesis, which subsequently causes thickening of the submucosa with a protective fibrous cover to sheathe the varices and prevent them from rupturing, while preserving them as collateral channels. Both techniques seem satisfactory for treatment of

variceal hemorrhage. Many groups use a combination of these two techniques. Injections should be avoided in the mid or proximal esophagus, however, because sclerosant may escape rapidly from a large varix into the azygos system and into the pulmonary circulation.

Most endoscopists perform sclerotherapy as described previously using no special equipment other than the endoscope and injector needle (*freehand technique*). Various ancillary devices, including flexible endoscopic overtubes and balloons, have been used in the past to improve visibility and accuracy of sclerosant injection. In general, such devices have not been associated with results superior to freehand injection for control of acute bleeding, and the routine use of postsclerotherapy balloon tamponade has not been shown to improve outcome for treatment of active bleeding. With few exceptions, sclerotherapy is performed using the fiberoptic endoscope and a freehand technique without an oversheath.

A wide variety of sclerosant agents are available with different mechanisms of action and varying complication rates. Sodium tetradecyl (1-3% solution), sodium morrhuate (5% solution), and ethanolamine oleate (5% solution) are the most commonly used sclerosing agents in the United States. Outside North America, ethanolamine oleate (5% solution) and polidocanol (1% solution) are used; polidocanol is usually employed for paravariceal injections. The best sclerosant and the best route of administration have yet to be defined, although the few controlled trials available tend to favor ethanolamine oleate for intravariceal or combined therapy.

Sclerotherapy is performed with different levels of skill and in protocols using various frequencies of injections and endoscopic review. Several technical variables may affect the outcome of any individual sclerotherapy session or clinical trial. These variables include the nature and concentration of the sclerosing agent, injection site, injection volume, type of injector, frequency of injections, and the use of variceal compression. Despite the widespread popularity of the procedure for control of acute variceal bleeding, sclerotherapy technique remains, to a great extent, empiric and individualized. Several basic issues of methodology remain largely unanswered. It is not surprising that controlled trials comparing sclerotherapy with other specific therapies, including variceal ligation, have yielded conflicting results (Krige et al, 2000).

We prefer a combined paravariceal and intravariceal technique for the management of acute variceal bleeding and use a predominantly intravariceal technique for long-term management. Our sclerosant of choice is 5% ethanolamine oleate. Injection treatments are continued at weekly intervals until the varices have been eradicated. Thereafter, the patient is assessed with surveillance endoscopy at 3 months and subsequently at 6-month intervals. Whenever recurrent varices are found, a repeat course of weekly sclerotherapy is undertaken until repeat eradication is achieved (Terblanche & Krige, 1997).

Serial EIS has been compared with medical management for long-term treatment of variceal hemorrhage in eight trials (D'Amico et al, 1995). The incidence of recurrent bleeding was less in patients treated with sclerotherapy in four of the eight trials. Long-term survival in the sclerotherapy patients was significantly better than in the patients receiving conventional treatment in five of the studies. Meta-analysis of seven of the long-term studies showed a significant 25% overall reduction in mortality in patients receiving endoscopic sclerotherapy compared with medical management. Cumulative significant nonbleeding complications associated with sclerotherapy in these trials totaled 23% per patient. Failure of long-term treatment is defined as repeated life-threatening bleeds during the course of sclerotherapy or varices that are difficult to eradicate. Repeat endoscopic therapy using either variceal banding or sclerotherapy is the preferred first-line therapy, with long-term pharmacologic therapy with propranolol the major alternative option.

Tissue Adhesives

Two types of tissue adhesives, Histoacryl and bucrylate, have been used to treat variceal bleeding. These "superglues" have proved effective in the control of bleeding with 90% success rates. The adhesives harden within 20 seconds when activated by water and more rapidly on contact with blood. Adhesives potentially offer immediate control of bleeding. Their injection, via an endoscope, uses a similar technique to traditional sclerosants, but with slight modifications. There are risks of equipment damage by tissue adhesives in inexperienced hands. Care must be taken to ensure that the adhesive does not come into contact with the endoscope and block the channels of the instrument. This problem can be minimized by the application of silicone oil to the tip of the instrument and by mixing the adhesive with Lipiodol to delay premature hardening. A further precaution is to ensure that the endoscope needle is placed correctly within the varix before injection. When the needle is in position, the tissue adhesive is injected in 0.5- to 1-mL aliquots; if the adhesive leaks, the endoscope should be withdrawn and cleaned before the polymer can set (de Franchis et al, 1998). The use of tissue adhesives is reserved for gastric varices or complex recurrent bleeding from esophageal varices.

Thrombin

In initial experimental studies, control of variceal bleeding also has been achieved using either human or bovine thrombin, as components of a thrombogenic mixture, to thrombose the bleeding varices. Thrombin injection is technically easy to perform, using the same freehand injection technique as sclerotherapy, without the technical difficulties associated with the use of tissue adhesives. Uncontrolled trials have shown that thrombin is equally effective in controlling bleeding from either esophageal or gastric varices (de Franchis et al, 1998).

ESOPHAGEAL VARICEAL LIGATION

The use of endoscopic band ligation represents an important development in endoscopic treatment of varices. The concept of EVL is similar in principle to the technique used for treating hemorrhoids. Hemostasis is achieved by physical constriction of the varix by the rubber band. Ischemic necrosis of the strangulated mucosa and submucosa trapped within the band develops, followed by sloughing of the bands. The resulting shallow mucosal ulcer completely re-epithelializes over the next 14 to 21 days, with replacement of the varix by maturing scar tissue (Stiegmann, 1996). Two different types of ligating devices are used. The original Stiegmann apparatus allows the placement of one band at a time and requires the use of an overtube to allow multiple withdrawals and reinsertions of the endoscope. The newer multibanding apparatus allows the placement of eight bands during a single insertion of the endoscope, obviating the need for an overtube. The band ligation procedure is repeated at 7- to 14-day intervals until the varices are obliterated.

Analysis of data from prospective randomized studies indicates that EVL is as effective as EIS in the early management of bleeding esophageal varices (Tait et al, 1999). Variceal eradication with EVL requires fewer endoscopic treatment sessions and causes substantially fewer local complications in the lower esophagus. There are clear advantages for using EVL in preference to EIS, and EVL should be considered the endoscopic treatment of choice for variceal hemorrhage (Krige & Bornman, 2000).

Esophageal Variceal Ligation Compared with Endoscopic Injection Sclerotherapy

Ten prospective randomized studies have compared the efficacy of EVL and EIS. The key results of these 10 trials are summarized in Table 92.3, and significant differences between the treatment groups are indicated. Stiegmann and colleagues (1992) found no difference in the rates of early variceal rebleeding or treatment-induced bleeding. Eradication rates were similar, and a similar number of treatment sessions were required to achieve eradication. The number of treatment-related complications was significantly less with EVL.

Laine and coworkers (1993) reported similar rebleeding rates and variceal eradication rates for EIS and EVL. Variceal eradication was achieved in fewer sessions with EVL, however, and was associated with fewer complications overall. In a British study, rebleeding was significantly less in the banding group (Gimson et al, 1993). Eradication was achieved significantly more rapidly with banding and in fewer endoscopic sessions.

A significant reduction in rebleeding rates after variceal band ligation was found by Lo and associates (1995), with a significant improvement in overall survival in patients treated by EVL. The study by Hou and colleagues (1995) reported similar eradication rates, although fewer endoscopic sessions were required to achieve eradication with banding, and rebleeding rates were significantly greater in patients treated by EIS.

An increase in variceal recurrence rates after EVL was reported in two prospective randomized studies. Sarin and colleagues (1997) reported similar eradication rates in fewer sessions with EVL and a reduced risk of rebleeding after ligation, although this did not influence patient survival. Significantly more variceal recurrences occurred after EVL, however. The Italian study achieved similar eradication rates, with fewer endoscopic sessions required with EVL (Baroncini et al, 1997). Eradication took longer with EVL, and variceal recurrences were significantly greater in patients treated by band ligation.

Avgerinos and associates (1997) reported a complication rate of 60% in the sclerotherapy group compared with 35% in the ligation group. Sarin and colleagues (1997) showed a faster eradiction rate requiring fewer sessions with ligation compared with the sclerotherapy group (4.1 ± 1.2 versus 5.2 ± 1.8). Although recurrence of varices was higher after EVL (28.7% versus 7.5%), fewer patients rebled (3 versus 10) than with EIS. Masci and coworkers (1999) achieved similar eradication rates with EVL and EIS (88% versus 82%), but ligation required fewer sessions (3.4 versus 5.3), and the complication rate was lower (18% versus 38%). Rebleeding before variceal eradication

Table 92.3 Randomized Trials Comparing Endoscopic Sclerotherapy with Band Ligation

Study	N	Arm	Sessions	Rebleed (%)	Variceal Bleeding (%)	Complications (%)	Recurrence (%)	Eradication (%)	Survival (%)
Stiegmann et al, 1992 (n = 129)	65	EIS	5 ± 2	48	52	**22**	50	56	55
	64	EVL	4 ± 2	36	48	**2**	33	55	72
Laine et al, 1993 (n = 77)	39	EIS	**6.2 ± 0.4**	44	31	**56**	NA	69	85
	38	EVL	**4.1 ± 0.3**	26	24	**24**	NA	59	89
Gimson et al, 1993 (n = 103)	49	EIS	**4.9**	53	51	57	NA	71	37
	54	EVL	**3.4**	30	24	67	NA	82	52
Lo et al, 1995 (n = 120)	59	EIS	**6.5 ± 1.2**	51	36	**19**	NA	63	**68**
	61	EVL	**3.8 ± 0.4**	33	13	**3**	NA	74	**84**
Hou et al, 1995 (n = 134)	67	EIS	**4.6 ± 1.6**	33	43	**22**	**30**	79	84
	67	EVL	**3.5 ± 1.6**	18	38	**5**	**48**	87	79
Sarin et al, 1997 (n = 95)	48	EIS	**4.5 ± 1.8**	21	NA	**50**	**8**	92	94
	47	EVL	**4.1 ± 1.2**	6	NA	**45**	**29**	96	94
Baroncini et al, 1997 (n = 111)	54	EIS	**4 ± 0.1**	19	30	**31**	**13**	93	78
	57	EVL	**3.5 ± 0.1**	16	22	**11**	**30**	93	79
Avgerinos et al, 1997 (n = 77)	40	EIS	**5.8 ± 2.7**	47	25	**60**	44	97	80
	37	EVL	**3.7 ± 1.9**	27	14	**35**	31	93	78
Sarin et al, 1997 (n = 95)	48	EIS	5.2 ± 1.8	21	NA	**10**	8	92	NA
	47	EVL	4.1 ± 1.2	6	NA	**0**	29	96	NA
Hou et al, 1999 (n = 168)	84	EIS	5.1 ± 2.2	38	32	NA	NA	86	NA
	84	EVL	3.7 ± 1.7	24	43	NA	NA	88	NA
Masci et al, 1999 (n = 100)	50	EIS	**5.3**	**42**	10	38	27	82	NA
	50	EVL	**3.4**	**12**	14	18	32	88	NA

Significant differences between EVL and EIS highlighted in **bold type**.
NA, not available.

was significantly more frequent in the EIS group; there was, however, no difference after eradication. There were significantly more major complications of chronic esophageal ulcers and strictures with sclerotherapy (36% versus 10%).

Esophageal Variceal Ligation for Control of Active Bleeding

Band deployment during variceal ligation can be difficult in patients with active bleeding because the outer banding cylinder decreases the field of view, and blood and clot may fill the cylinder, further obscuring the endoscopist's view. Stiegmann and coworkers (1992) achieved control of acute bleeding in 12 of 14 patients (86%) with EVL compared with 10 of 13 patients (77%) with EIS. Gimson and coworkers (1993) reported control of acute bleeding in 19 of 21 patients (91%) with EVL and 21 of 23 patients (92%) with EIS. Laine and colleagues (1993), Lo and associates (1995), Hou and colleagues (1995), and Sarin and colleagues (1997) reported similar results with control of acute bleeding in 80% to 100% of patients with EVL and 77% to 86% in patients with EIS.

A prospective study designed specifically to evaluate the efficacy of EVL in acute bleeding was reported by Lo and associates (1997). Cessation of bleeding was defined as no further bleeding within 72 hours and was achieved in 97% with EVL and 76% with EIS. At 1-month follow-up, rebleeding occurred in 17% with EVL and 33% with EIS. Morbidity was significantly lower with EVL (5% versus 29%).

Combination Endoscopic Therapy After Variceal Bleeding

Injection sclerotherapy of large varices may present technical difficulties. Large varices generally require greater sclerosant volumes, more commonly have needle puncture bleeding, require more endoscopy sessions, and have increased risks of serious complications. Banding is ideally suited to large varices. Small varices are easily injected, but are often unsuitable for banding because less tissue is available to trap in the O-rings. The concept of combining banding with sclerotherapy when varices are large and converting to injection sclerotherapy when smaller is appealing. EVL combined with low-dose injection sclerotherapy might achieve more rapid variceal eradication and reduce the likelihood of rebleeding.

Seven randomized controlled trials compared the effects of synchronous combined endoscopic ligation and sclerotherapy with endoscopic ligation alone in terms of prevention of variceal rebleeding, long-term survival, and complications related to the procedure. A meta-analysis of these seven studies showed no significant difference in cessation of actively bleeding varices (odds ratio 1.01; 95% confidence interval 0.43-2.36), variceal rebleeding (odds ratio 1.12; 95% confidence interval 0.69-1.81), and mortality (odds ratio 1.1; 95% confidence interval 0.70-1.74) in patients with variceal ligation versus patients receiving the combination treatment of ligation and sclerotherapy (Singh et al, 2002). Treatment sessions required to achieve complete variceal eradication were similar in the two treatment arms. A significantly higher incidence of esophageal stricture was seen in combination therapy (*P*<.001). The authors concluded that the combination of ligation and sclerotherapy offers no advantages over ligation alone in preventing rebleeding and in reducing mortality.

Three randomized controlled studies compared sclerotherapy with ligation combined with metachronous sclerotherapy performed later when varices were reduced in size. Bhargava and Pokharna (1997) reported higher eradication (87% versus 24%) and lower rebleeding (19% versus 22%) with combination therapy, although the number of sessions required (5.9 ± 2.3 versus 4.3 ± 1.8) and the overall complication rate (44% versus 31%) were higher. Lo and coworkers (1995) reported a similar eradication rate and number of sessions needed in both groups. The mortality (2.7% versus 8.6%), rebleeding (8% versus 31%), and variceal recurrence (14% versus 43%) rates were lower, however, with combination therapy than with ligation alone. Garg and associates (1999) found similar variceal eradication rates and number of endoscopic sessions required in both groups. They noticed more complications (20% versus 3%) and rebleeding (16% versus 3%) with sclerotherapy, whereas the variceal recurrence and the cumulative probability of survival did not differ.

Failures of Variceal Ligation

Failure of variceal ligation is defined as a further bleeding episode after two ligation sessions during a single admission for acute variceal bleeding. Such patients should have a balloon tube inserted and should undergo an alternative procedure, usually a TIPS. Failure of long-term management with variceal ligation is similarly defined as for long-term sclerotherapy failure. Patients who have repeated major variceal bleeds during the course of banding before eradication or patients in whom varices are difficult to eradicate should have an alternative procedure.

ALTERNATIVE LONG-TERM MANAGEMENT OPTIONS

Although variceal ligation and sclerotherapy are the most widely used endoscopic options in most patients, pharmacologic therapy, with propranolol alone or propranolol in combination with other drugs, is an acceptable alternative in long-term management to prevent recurrent bleeding (see Ch. 91). Alternative long-term management options available if rebleeding continues despite endoscopic and pharmacologic therapy are TIPS, surgical shunt, liver transplantation, and nonshunt operations.

Transjugular Intrahepatic Portosystemic Shunt

In the past, major surgery was the only method of achieving a portosystemic shunt. TIPS is a nonoperative interventional radiologic procedure that creates an intrahepatic portosystemic shunt by placing a stent connecting the hepatic and portal veins through the liver. Ch. 96 provides a detailed analysis of TIPS. TIPS remains a short-term solution for failure of endoscopic hemostasis or the prevention of recurrent hemorrhage in patients with end-stage liver disease who are unsuitable for an operative shunt and are candidates for liver transplantation. The great advantage of TIPS is that it can be performed nonoperatively

with low morbidity by an expert radiologist, even in poor-risk patients.

Liver Transplantation

The role of liver transplantation (see Ch. 103) in the management of portal hypertension has altered dramatically the outcome for patients with advanced liver disease. Liver transplantation is the only treatment that cures the underlying liver disease and eradicates the portal hypertension. Liver transplantation is indicated for end-stage liver disease and always should be considered in patients with advanced cirrhosis who have bled. The indication for liver transplantation remains end-stage liver disease, however, rather than portal hypertension. The limitation in donor liver supply, the high cost of the procedure, and the risks of immunosuppression must be considered. Liver transplantation prevents recurrent variceal bleeding and, if successful, restores hepatocellular function to normal. In potential transplant candidates with acute variceal bleeding, emergency endoscopic therapy is considered the treatment of choice. If endoscopic therapy fails to control active variceal bleeding, and if a donor liver is not immediately available, an emergency TIPS should be performed. When the patient has recovered from the acute variceal bleed, early transplantation should be performed in patients whose liver function and general condition merit a liver transplant. Patients with good liver function should be considered for a distal splenorenal shunt, rather than a transplant. Liver transplantation has now eclipsed the use of operative shunts as the most common surgical procedure performed for the complications of portal hypertension.

Surgical Shunts

Surgical shunts (see Ch. 95) can be constructed as total, partial, or selective shunts. All surgical shunts have a greater than 90% effectiveness in controlling bleeding. The difference between the types of surgical shunt is the degree of diversion of portal flow. Total diversion of portal flow increases the risk of encephalopathy to approximately 30% to 50% and accelerates liver failure. Partial shunts (8 mm diameter) maintain some prograde portal flow to the liver, and the encephalopathy rate decreases to 10% to 15%. Selective shunting with a distal splenorenal shunt decompresses the stomach, spleen, and gastroesophageal junction, whereas portal hypertension is maintained in the splanchnic bed and liver theoretically to maintain portal flow to the cirrhotic liver. Selective and interposition portacaval or mesocaval surgical shunts provide durable portal decompression and control of bleeding and are considered in patients who are good risk Child A or B and have failed endoscopic therapy or do not have access to a readily available tertiary care facility to deal with recurrent variceal bleeding.

Devascularization and Transection Operations

To be effective in long-term management, an extensive gastric and lower esophageal devascularization together with transection of the lower esophagus is required (see Ch. 94). It is insufficient to perform simple staple-gun esophageal transection, which is frequently advocated and successful in acute bleed management. We use transabdominal extensive upper gastric devascularization without splenectomy combined with lower third esophageal devascularization and a staple-gun lower esophageal transection, with the anastomosis being protected with a "floppy" Nissen fundoplication in good risk patients who have failed endoscopic therapy and are not candidates for TIPS or a surgical shunt. The extensive abdominothoracic Sugiura operation, popular in Japan, has been replaced by a transabdominal procedure in most institutions.

No Therapy: Observation Only

Patients with end-stage liver disease who present with major esophageal variceal bleeding complicated by multiorgan failure should not be subjected to major emergency procedures. Withholding treatment in these circumstances is a difficult clinical and ethical decision, but one that must be considered and accepted, if necessary, in today's cost-conscious medical environment.

TECHNIQUE OF BALLOON TUBE INSERTION

Acute esophageal variceal bleeding can be temporarily controlled in most patients by balloon tube tamponade with a correctly placed balloon (see Fig. 92.2). The four lumen Minnesota tube is used in our institution. Its use allows time for resuscitation and management planning. Although the initial bleeding episode is effectively controlled, if no additional measures are used, 60% of patients have a further variceal bleed after removal of the tube, with a high associated mortality rate. Either injection sclerotherapy or variceal ligation should be performed when removing the tube.

Before the balloon tube is inserted in an agitated or encephalopathic patient, the airway should be protected by placing an endotracheal tube to prevent aspiration. A new tube should always be used, and the balloons should be tested by inflating them under water to confirm a complete air seal. The deflated lubricated tube is passed via the mouth through a biteguard, placed between the teeth, after adequate topical pharyngeal anesthesia. Awake patients are instructed to swallow while the tube is being passed. In a stuporous patient, the index finger placed in the mouth helps to guide the tip of the tube over the posterior tongue and through the cricopharyngeus and prevents the tube coiling in the pharynx. It may be difficult to negotiate the tube through the cricopharyngeus, particularly in patients with an endotracheal tube in place. Under these circumstances, a McGill forceps and laryngoscope are used, and the tube is passed under direct vision. The tube is inserted as far as possible. The epigastrium is auscultated, while instilling air via the aspirating lumen of the gastric tube using a 50-mL syringe, to confirm its position in the stomach. If there is doubt or uncertainty whether the gastric balloon is in the stomach, the patient should be x-rayed to confirm that the tube, which is radiopaque, is in the stomach, or an endoscope can be used to visualize the gastric balloon in the stomach. Thereafter, the gastric balloon is cautiously inflated via its lumen with 50-mL increments of air until a total of 250 mL has been inserted. Air should be easy to insert; if the tube is curled in the esophagus, resistance is felt, and the inflation must be stopped immediately, or the esophagus may be damaged. The use of water or oily contrast media to inflate the balloon is contraindicated because they are difficult to inject via the narrow lumen of the tube and are difficult to retrieve before the tube is removed.

The tube is pulled up until the inflated gastric balloon is seated firmly against the esophagogastric junction. The tension in the tube is maintained by a split tennis ball strapped to the tube at the mouthguard (see Fig. 92.2). Adequate tension on the gastric balloon can be checked regularly at the mouth. The mouthguard protects the patient's lips from the pressure of the tennis ball. Inflation of the esophageal balloon is not usually necessary because traction on the gastric balloon is generally sufficient. If esophageal balloon inflation is required, a three-way tap and a blood pressure manometer are used to inflate the esophageal balloon to 40 mm Hg before clamping the tube. This pressure needs to be checked regularly. The fourth lumen, which opens in the esophagus, is placed on constant suction, while the gastric lumen is used for suction and to administer medication, such as lactulose.

Patients with a balloon tube in place are monitored carefully in an ICU to avoid complications. The position of the gastric balloon is checked by a flat radiograph of the abdomen, which confirms the correct position of the air-filled gastric balloon in the upper stomach. When the balloon tube has been inserted and fixed, and bleeding has been arrested, resuscitation is continued, clotting defects are corrected, and the patient is made as fit as possible for the necessary subsequent management. The balloon tube should be removed after 6 to 12 hours, with a maximum time of 24 hours. We usually perform injection sclerotherapy or variceal banding at the time of removing the tube.

If bleeding persists after insertion of the tube, a senior staff member should check the tube. If the tube is found to be correctly situated, a further diagnostic endoscopy is required. A nonvariceal bleeding source, missed during initial endoscopy, usually is found.

INJECTION SCLEROTHERAPY TECHNIQUES

Trained assistants are essential, and adequate resuscitative facilities must be available. A flexible endoscope is used without general anesthesia. Standard single or twin channeled endoscopes are suitable, but the double channel endoscope is preferred. An end-viewing or side-viewing instrument can be used. The end-viewing instrument is more versatile for diagnosis and therapy, although the oblique-viewing instrument has the advantage of better visualization of the greater and lesser curves of the stomach, whereas the built-in forceps elevator helps to aim the injector, particularly for small varices during elective sclerotherapy. Several disposable sclerotherapy injectors with retractable needles within a polytetrafluoroethylene (Teflon)-coated plastic sheath are commercially available and are preferable to the flexible, reusable, metal injectors. Injectors have a 23-gauge or 25-gauge needle attached. The larger needle is preferred because this facilitates injection of the viscous sclerosant solution (Krige & Terblanche, 1994).

Stuporous or comatose patients must have the airway protected by prior endotracheal intubation. If the patient has a balloon tube in situ, the balloons should be deflated and the tube removed only when the team is ready to begin endoscopy and ligation or sclerotherapy. When the varix that was bleeding has been controlled, the remaining varices are banded or injected, and the diagnostic endoscopy is completed.

ELECTIVE SCLEROTHERAPY TECHNIQUE

Elective sclerotherapy is performed in an outpatient clinic with two assistants trained in endoscopy techniques. One assistant reassures the patient, provides suction of the patient's mouth to avoid aspiration, and ensures that the biteguard is not dislodged. The other assistant, usually a nurse, advances and retracts the injector needle and administers the sclerosant under the direction of the endoscopist.

The patient is placed in the left lateral decubitus position on the endoscopy bed with the head on a pillow and the neck slightly flexed. The pharynx and posterior tongue are anesthetized with 10% lidocaine (Xylocaine) topical spray. A small butterfly needle is inserted into a superficial hand vein for administration of sedation. We use small incremental doses of midazolam (2.5 mg). All instruments, including the endoscope, are checked before use, and commands such as "advance needle" and "retract needle" are rehearsed if an inexperienced assistant is present. Each time an injection is required, this is called for by the endoscopist and acknowledged by the assistant. The assistant is instructed to comment if resistance is encountered during injection because this may indicate that the varix is thrombosed or that the needle is not positioned correctly.

The endoscope is inserted through the mouthguard and passed through the cricopharynx into the esophagus. Small amounts of air are insufflated intermittently to maintain sufficient distention of the lumen for adequate visibility. Mucus and fluid are removed through the suction channel, and the lens is cleared with a water jet when necessary. The entire esophagus is examined, and the presence of esophageal varices is noted. The number, size, and extent of varices and the presence of endoscopic variceal stigmata (cherry red spots and red wheal marks) are documented. During elective endoscopy, the varices usually are not bleeding, and a full diagnostic panendoscopy is performed to exclude other lesions before injecting the varices. The presence and extent of gastric varices and portal hypertensive gastropathy are noted and documented.

On completion of the panendoscopy, the endoscope is withdrawn partially into the lower esophagus and positioned above the esophagogastric junction so that the varices in the lower 5 cm of the esophagus can be injected. The endoscope tip is maneuvered into position, and the target varix is identified. The endoscopist passes the injecting catheter through the biopsy channel into the field of view, and the tip of the catheter is positioned 2 cm beyond the end of the endoscope. To prevent the needle damaging the injector sheath or the endoscope channel, the injecting catheter should be passed only when the endoscope tip is in a nonflexed position. The needle should remain in the retracted position until the tip of the injecting catheter has passed through the endoscope and is visible to the endoscopist. All movements and manipulations of the injector are performed only by the endoscopist. A practice aiming pass of the catheter, with the needle retracted within the sheath before the first injection, is useful to determine the precise direction of the advancing needle in relation to the target varix.

The assistant advances the needle on instruction, and a small volume of sclerosant solution is discarded into the lumen of the esophagus to ensure that the injecting catheter is filled with sclerosant, and that residual air has been expelled. The endoscopist inserts the needle directly into the center of the most prominent part of the varix, near the esophagogastric junction, by advancing the injector a further 5 mm. When the needle has been placed

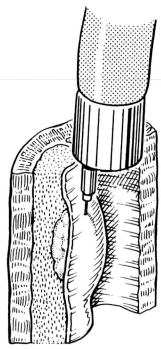

Fig. 92.3. Intravariceal injection technique. After an initial test injection of 1 mL of sclerosant, 5 mL of ethanolamine oleate is injected directly into the varix.

satisfactorily within the lumen of the varix, the assistant is instructed to inject 1 mL of sclerosant (Fig. 92.3). If this injection is achieved without resistance, further sclerosant is injected under instruction. The varix should be seen to blanch and distend above and below the injection site. A total volume of no more than 5 mL of ethanolamine oleate is usually sufficient for a large varix. Smaller varices require less sclerosant. Thereafter, any additional varices are injected at the same level. A second injection is placed 2 to 3 cm higher in large varices. Usually, only 2 to 3 mL of sclerosant is injected into the upper site (Krige & Terblanche, 1994).

Accurate positioning and placement of the needle is crucial to achieve effective and accurate delivery of sclerosant and to avoid complications that may follow incorrect injection. A flat angle for needle insertion is preferable and avoids a deep injection; a perpendicular approach may transfix the varix and penetrate the underlying esophageal wall, resulting in an intramural injection of sclerosant. In this situation, the assistant notes increased resistance to injection, and no blanching or distention of the varix occurs. The needle should be withdrawn, and a further injection performed after accurate placement of the needle. Only the needle should enter the varix. Care must be taken to ensure that neither the needle hub nor the injecting sheath is inadvertently pushed through the variceal wall because this would leave a large defect, which may give rise to troublesome bleeding. No attempt should be made to inject the varices while the patient is restless or heaving. Uncontrolled injections may result in laceration of the varix by the needle with resultant major bleeding (Krige & Terblanche, 1996).

After the procedure, the patient is observed in the outpatient endoscopy suite recovery room until fully awake and then is discharged home. It is unusual for bleeding to complicate an elective sclerotherapy session. Subsequent sclerotherapy injections are performed at weekly intervals until all the varices have been eradicated. Severe local esophageal mucosal ulceration may delay injection of a specific underlying varix, but the other variceal channels can be injected. When varices have been eradicated, a further endoscopic assessment is performed at 3 months to confirm eradication. Further evaluations are performed at 6-month intervals or annually for life. If recurrent varices are noted during surveillance endoscopy, these are injected, and repeat endoscopy and injections are performed at weekly intervals until the varices have been re-eradicated (Terblanche & Krige, 1997).

EMERGENCY SCLEROTHERAPY TECHNIQUE

The initial resuscitative measures required were presented earlier. The patient should be as stable as possible before starting sclerotherapy. The procedure usually is performed in a specially equipped endoscopy suite. If the patient is obtunded or severely encephalopathic, an endotracheal tube will have been inserted. Severely ill patients should have the injection treatment performed in the ICU. When major bleeding is present, the endoscopy is performed in the operating room, where full resuscitative facilities, appropriate monitoring, intubation equipment, and experienced anesthetic assistance are available.

The patient usually is placed in the left lateral decubitus position, as for elective sclerotherapy. If active bleeding is present and visibility is obscured, however, the table head is elevated to 30 degrees to improve visualization. The lower esophagus is flushed with saline through the irrigation channel, and residual blood and fluid are aspirated through the suction channel. Further insufflation usually provides adequate visualization to perform the first injection.

Intravariceal Injection

Active variceal bleeding is dealt with immediately by controlling the bleed with intravariceal sclerotherapy. Urgent control of bleeding with accurate placement of the needle and sclerosant injection should be performed without delay while there is adequate visibility. No attempt should be made to insert the needle into the bleeding point because this may enlarge the hole and aggravate bleeding with extravasation and loss of sclerosant. A technique similar to elective intravariceal sclerotherapy is used with needle insertion immediately proximal to the bleeding site (Fig. 92.4). A total volume of 5 mL of sclerosant is usually sufficient. Distention and blanching of the varix indicate that the needle is in the correct position, and that the appropriate volume of sclerosant has been injected. After the bleeding has been controlled, the other variceal channels are sclerosed. A second series of injections usually is performed at a higher level. Panendoscopy is undertaken on completion of sclerotherapy to exclude other lesions.

Combined Paravariceal and Intravariceal Injection Technique

We prefer combined paravariceal and intravariceal injection to control active variceal bleeding. The needle is inserted into the submucosa in a paravariceal position, and 5% ethanolamine oleate is injected proximal to the bleeding point to compress the bleeding site by raising a wheal (Fig. 92.5A and B). Sufficient sclerosant is injected to control the bleeding. If this injection does not completely control the acute bleeding, the paravariceal injection is repeated alongside the bleeding point. The procedure

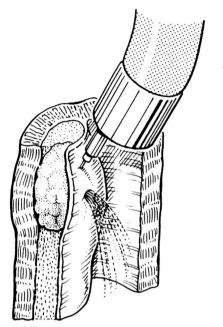

Fig. 92.4. Emergency sclerotherapy. An intravariceal injection technique is used to treat an actively bleeding varix.

is completed by injecting the varix intravariceally (see Fig. 92.5C). The volume injected paravariceally should not exceed 1 mL at each site to avoid ulceration of mucosa. The remaining variceal channels are sclerosed.

If variceal bleeding is profuse, vigorous lavage through the endoscope channel and elevation of the head of the table to 30 degrees usually improves visibility and allows identification of the bleeding site. No blind attempts at injection should be used. If immediate sclerotherapy cannot be performed because of lack of expertise or inadequate visibility, bleeding should be controlled first by balloon tube tamponade before the patient has further sclerotherapy.

Most patients (70%) respond to a single injection treatment and have no further bleeds. If bleeding does recur, intravenous somatostatin is resumed, and the patient undergoes repeat endoscopy. Further bleeding varices are treated as before. If bleeding results from an injection site esophageal ulcer, somatostatin infusion is continued, and oral sucralfate is administered. The success rate of a single injection treatment is 70%. Approximately 30% of patients have a further bleed and require an additional injection treatment. Two injection treatments usually control variceal bleeding in more than 95% of patients. Subsequently, repeat sclerotherapy sessions are undertaken at weekly intervals until all varices have been eradicated.

If further bleeding occurs after two injection treatments during a single hospital admission, this is defined as failure of emergency endoscopic therapy. The patient should have a Sengstaken or Minnesota balloon tube inserted. After resuscitation, the patient should undergo an alternative procedure, usually TIPS.

COMPLICATIONS ASSOCIATED WITH INJECTION SCLEROTHERAPY

The reported frequency of complications of sclerotherapy varies widely among trials and is related to the experience of endoscopists and the frequency and completeness of follow-up evaluation. Minor complications are regarded as technique-related

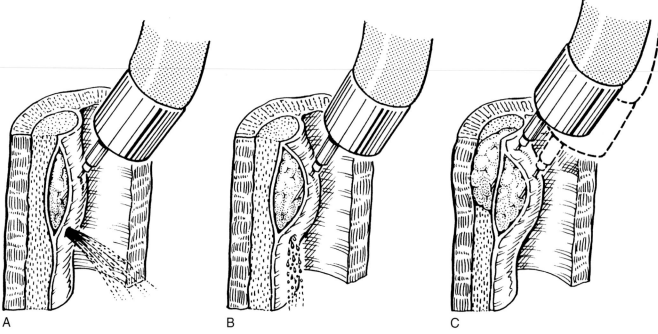

Fig. 92.5. Emergency sclerotherapy—combined paravariceal and intravariceal technique. **A,** Initial paravariceal injection immediately proximal to the bleeding point. **B,** Bleeding controlled by the paravariceal injection. **C,** An intravariceal injection completes the procedure.

side effects owing to sclerosant injection and occur in 30% to 40% of patients. Minor complications that occur within the first 24 to 48 hours of treatment include low-grade fever, retrosternal chest pain, temporary dysphagia, and asymptomatic pleural effusions, which do not generally require intervention. Esophageal complications of injection sclerotherapy are invariably a consequence of excessive sclerosant-induced submucosal or transmural necrosis (Krige et al, 1999). Mucosal ulceration is a common consequence of sclerotherapy, occurring in up to 40% of patients. The prevalence and extent of ulceration depends on the type and volume of sclerosant injected, method of injection, interval between injections, and size of varices (Krige et al, 1999). Ulcers heal rapidly in most cases and are regarded by many as a desired consequence of the healing process, rather than a complication. More significant complications occur in approximately 20% of patients after injection sclerotherapy, and the procedure-related mortality is 0% to 3%. Esophageal perforation may occur from direct iatrogenic injury or esophageal necrosis, and development of esophageal strictures is reported in 7% to 59% of patients. Dissemination of sclerosant beyond the esophagus may cause pleural effusions, pneumonia, systemic inflammatory response syndrome, and septicemia (Krige et al, 1999).

ENDOSCOPIC VARICEAL LIGATION TECHNIQUES

Single-Shot Band Application

EVL uses an ingenious device attached to the tip of a flexible endoscope to ensnare an esophageal varix with a rubber band. The endoscopic variceal banding device (C.R. Bard, Tewksberry, MA) consists of an outer housing cylinder, an inner banding cylinder, a trip wire, and a single elastic O-ring (Fig. 92.6). The outer housing cylinder attaches to the end of the endoscope by

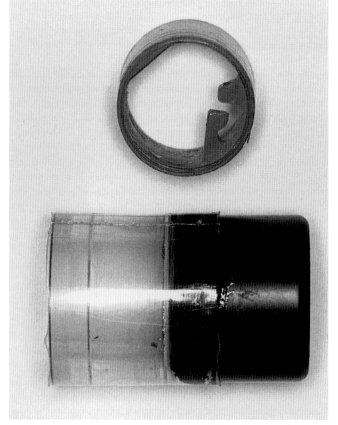

Fig. 92.6. Single-shot endoscopic banding device. Inner banding cylinder illustrated with loaded O-ring ready for application and unstretched band for comparison.

means of a Silastic friction mount. The banding cylinder is a smaller cylinder fitted with an inner clasp that allows attachment of the trip wire. The banding cylinder is constructed to fit snugly, yet slide smoothly, within the housing cylinder. The monofilament trip wire has a flange at the distal end, which attaches to the clasp inside the banding cylinder. The small elastic O-ring is stretched and mounted on the banding cylinder (see Fig. 92.6).

After completion of diagnostic panendoscopy, confirmation of bleeding varices, and the need for variceal banding, the endoscope is removed, and the banding device is attached by sliding the Silastic friction ring onto the tip of the endoscope to secure the outer housing cylinder to the tip firmly. The trip wire is passed through the vacuum lock of the biopsy channel entry port and exits through the biopsy channel opening at the tip of the scope. The trip wire is secured to the clasp in the banding cylinder, and the banding cylinder carrying a mounted O-ring is loaded into the housing cylinder. The banding cylinder is positioned so that approximately 1 mm of the cylinder protrudes beyond the O-ring, which is seated against the end of the housing cylinder.

In contrast to injection sclerotherapy, the technique of variceal ligation is standardized. To facilitate repeated esophageal intubation and passage of the gastroscope and banding device, a flexible plastic overtube is passed through the oropharynx into the upper esophagus. The overtube is backloaded onto the endoscope, and when the gastroscope has been passed into the stomach, the lubricated overtube is advanced over the scope by gentle rotation through the oropharynx into the upper esophagus to minimize trauma to the oropharynx and upper esophagus. The target varix is identified, and the banding cylinder is applied to the varix (Fig. 92.7A), which is sucked into the banding chamber (see Fig. 92.7B). When the chamber is completely filled by the varix, which is evident by a complete "red-out" and loss of endoscopic visibility, the trip wire is pulled (see Fig. 92.7C); this releases the elastic band over the entrapped varix (see Fig. 92.7D). The endoscope is removed, and the inner cylinder is reloaded with a fresh O-ring for further variceal banding.

The treatment of varices begins with ligation of the most distal variceal columns in the esophagus just above the gastroesophageal junction, starting with the bleeding varix, if present. Subsequent ligations of the remaining varices are performed at increasingly higher levels proceeding upward in a spiral fashion to avoid circumferential placement of bands at the same level. Large varices have further bands placed more proximally within the distal 10 cm of the esophagus, and all visible variceal channels are ligated at least once at each banding session. A 2-cm mucosal space between adjacent bands is necessary to avoid excessive mucosal necrosis and dysphagia. On average, a total of six to nine bands are applied at the initial session, and progressively fewer bands are required at subsequent sessions as the varices decrease in size. Repeat treatments are performed at 1- to 2-week intervals on an outpatient basis (Tait et al, 1999).

The major limitation of the original banding technique is that only a single band can be applied per firing. The gastroscope must be removed to reload a new band after each variceal ligation. Overtube insertion combined with repeated reinsertion of the endoscope can injure the esophagus and is the principal disadvantage of this technique. Several refinements in equipment have since occurred. The original opaque outer cylinder at the tip of the endoscope substantially reduced visibility and

blinded the endoscopist's view. Replacement of these by transparent outer cylinders has improved the endoscopic view and targeting of varices. Some experienced endoscopists prefer to pass the endoscope without an overtube when applying single-shot bands during elective ligation, avoiding the risks and discomfort of the overtube.

Multishot Band Application

A subsequent innovation has been the multiband ligator capable of carrying 5, 6, 8, or 10 bands (Fig. 92.8). The multishot banding device has multiple rubber bands, which are singly activated by a drawstring that passes from the ligator through the biopsy channel and is attached to a trigger unit mounted on the biopsy channel port of the endoscope, which allows repeated individual firing of the bands. The multishot system obviates the need for an overtube, but does limit access to the biopsy port of the endoscope and requires a special adaptor for irrigation if active bleeding occurs while using the multiband ligator. The multishot variceal band ligator is a significant technical advance over the single-shot device, but because the unit is disposable and cannot be reused, the current retail cost of $200 per unit may limit the universal use of the multishot banding device.

Complications with Endoscopic Variceal Ligation

The esophageal ulceration that occurs when the thrombosed varix and band slough off after endoscopic band ligation is more superficial and resolves faster than sclerotherapy-induced ulcers. Esophageal band ligation–induced bacteremia occurs less often than with sclerotherapy and is associated with fewer episodes of significant infectious sequelae, such as spontaneous bacterial peritonitis or pneumonia. Complications associated with the use of the overtube have included esophageal mucosal tears, variceal rupture with massive bleeding, and esophageal perforation. Banding also has been associated with food impaction (Tait et al, 1999).

Despite the spectrum of EVL-induced complications, the incidence is substantially less than in EIS. Stiegmann and colleagues (1992) reported a 2% complication rate with EVL and a 22% complication rate with EIS (see Table 92.4). Fewer strictures and infective complications were noted after EVL, although neither was statistically significant, and rebleeding rates were similar in the two groups. The study by Laine and coworkers (1993) did not show a reduction in rebleeding with EVL, but showed a significant reduction in stricture formation (0% versus 33%), although infective complications were similar. Two subsequent studies reported a reduction in variceal rebleeding rates after EVL, although this benefit was offset by the associated increased risk of rebleeding from ectopic varices and congestive gastropathy after EVL. The benefits reported by Lo and colleagues (1995) (3.3% versus 19%) and Baroncini and associates (1997) (11% versus 33%) were primarily a reduction in stricture formation. A significant reduction in procedure-related complications has been shown with EVL, and this alone is probably sufficient reason to recommend EVL in preference to EIS because 50% of the iatrogenic strictures induced by sclerotherapy cause significant morbidity and require repeat treatment by dilation therapy.

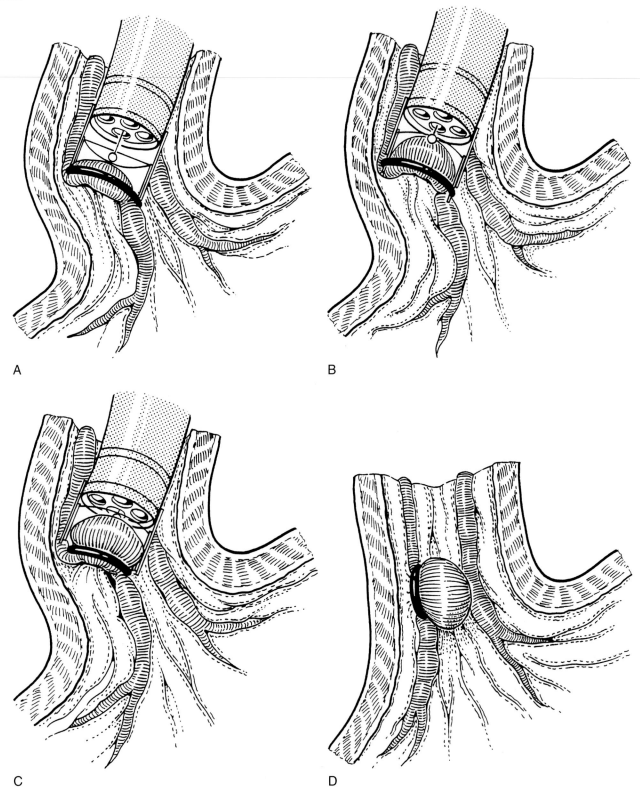

A

B

C

D

Fig. 92.7. Endoscopic ligation of esophageal varices using the flexible single-shot endoscope. **A,** Varix is approached under direct vision by the endoscopist. Full contact is made between the end of the ligating device and the tissue to be ligated. **B,** Endoscopist activates the endoscopic suction, which results in aspiration of esophageal mucosa, submucosa, and the varix into the ligating device. **C,** Trip wire (which runs through the biopsy channel of the endoscope) is pulled, which moves the inner cylinder (over which the elastic O-ring is stretched) toward the endoscope, displacing the small elastic band. **D,** Elastic band encircles the neck of the now ligated tissue, resulting in strangulation and thrombosis.

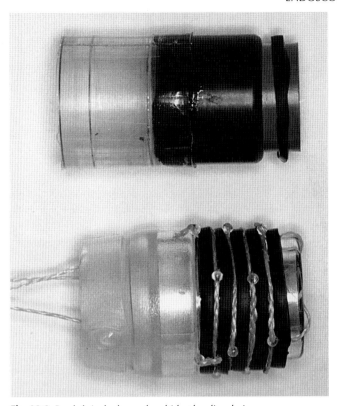

Fig. 92.8. Loaded single-shot and multishot banding devices.

ACKNOWLEDGMENTS

This study was supported by a grant from the South African Medical Research Council and the Liver Research Centre at the University of Cape Town.

REFERENCES

Avgerinos A, et al, 1997: Endoscopic sclerotherapy versus variceal ligation in the long-term management of patients with cirrhosis after variceal bleeding: a prospective randomized study. J Hepatol 26:1034-1041.

Baroncini D, et al, 1997: A prospective randomized trial of sclerotherapy versus ligation in the elective treatment of bleeding esophageal varices. Endoscopy 29:235-240.

Bhargava DK, Pokharna R, 1997: Endoscopic variceal ligation versus endoscopic variceal ligation and endoscopic sclerotherapy: a prospective randomized study. Am J Gastroenterol 92:950-953.

Bornman PC, et al, 1994: Management of esophageal varices. Lancet 343: 1079-1084.

Carbonell N, et al, 2004: Improved survival after variceal bleeding in patients with cirrhosis over the past two decades. Hepatology 40:652-659.

D'Amico G, et al, 1995: The treatment of portal hypertension: a meta-analytic review. Hepatology 22:332-354.

de Franchis R, et al, 1998: Emergency endoscopy strategies for improved outcomes. Scand J Gastroenterol Suppl 226:25-36.

Garg PK, et al, 1999: Comparison of endoscopic variceal sclerotherapy with sequential endoscopic band ligation plus low-dose sclerotherapy for secondary prophylaxis of variceal hemorrhage: a prospective randomized study. Gastrointest Endosc 50:369-373.

Gimson AES, et al, 1993: Randomised trial of variceal banding ligation versus injection sclerotherapy for bleeding esophageal varices. Lancet 342:391-394.

Henderson JM, et al, 1998: Portal hypertension. Curr Prob Surg 35:381-452.

Hou MC, et al, 1995: Comparison of endoscopic variceal injection sclerotherapy and ligation for the treatment of esophageal variceal hemorrhage: a prospective randomized trial. Hepatology 21:1517-1522.

Hou MC, et al, 1999: The rebleeding course and long-term outcome of esophageal variceal hemorrhage after ligation: comparison with sclerotherapy. Scand J Gastroenterol 34:1071-1076.

Krige JE, Bornman PC, 2000: Endoscopic treatment of oesophageal varices. S Afr J Surg 38:82-88.

Krige JEJ, Terblanche J, 1994: Injection sclerotherapy of oesophageal varices. In Jamieson GG, DeBas HT (eds): Rob and Smith's Operative Surgery: Surgery of the Upper Gastrointestinal Tract, 5th ed. London, Chapman & Hall Medical, pp 10-20.

Krige JEJ, Terblanche J, 1996: Injection sclerotherapy of oesophageal varices. In Carter D, et al (eds): Rob and Smith's Operative Surgery: Surgery of the Liver, Pancreas and Bile Ducts, 5th ed. London, Chapman & Hall Medical, pp 163-172.

Krige JEJ, et al, 1999: Complications of endoscopic variceal sclerotherapy. In Sivak MV (ed): Gastroenterologic Endoscopy, 2nd ed. Philadelphia, Saunders.

Krige JEJ, et al, 2000: Variceal rebleeding and recurrence after endoscopic injection sclerotherapy: a prospective evaluation in 204 patients. Arch Surg 135:1315-1322.

Laine L, et al, 1993: Endoscopic ligation compared with sclerotherapy for the treatment of bleeding esophageal varices. Ann Intern Med 119:1-7.

Lo G-H, et al, 1995: A prospective, randomized trial of sclerotherapy versus ligation in the management of bleeding esophageal varices. Hepatology 22: 466-471.

Lo G-H, et al, 1997: Emergency banding ligation versus sclerotherapy for the control of active bleeding from esophageal varices. Hepatology 25: 1101-1104.

Masci E, et al, 1999: Prospective multicenter randomized trial comparing banding ligation with sclerotherapy of esophageal varices. Hepatogastroenterology 46:1769-1773.

Rosado B, Kamath PS, 2003: Transjugular intrahepatic portosystemic shunts: an update. Liver Transpl 9:207-217.

Samonakis DN, et al, 2004: Management of portal hypertension. Postgrad Med J 80:634-641.

Sarin SK, et al, 1997: Prospective randomized trial of endoscopic sclerotherapy versus variceal band ligation for esophageal varices: influence on gastropathy, gastric varices and variceal recurrence. Hepatology 26:826-832.

Singh P, et al, 2002: Combined ligation and sclerotherapy versus ligation alone for secondary prophylaxis of esophageal variceal bleeding: a meta-analysis. Am J Gastroenterol 97:623-629.

Stanley AJ, Hayes PC, 1997: Portal hypertension and variceal haemorrhage. Lancet 350:1235-1239.

Stiegmann GV, 1996: Endoscopic management of esophageal varices. In Green FL, Ponsky JL (eds): Endoscopic Surgery. Philadelphia, Saunders, pp 113-124.

Stiegmann GV, et al, 1992: Endoscopic sclerotherapy as compared with endoscopic ligation for bleeding esophageal varices. N Engl J Med 326:1527-1532.

Tait IS, et al, 1999: Endoscopic band ligation of oesophageal varices. Br J Surg 86:812-817.

Terblanche J, Krige JEJ, 1994: Emergency sclerotherapy. In Bosch J, Groszman RJ (eds): Portal Hypertension: Pathophysiology and Treatment. Oxford, Blackwell Scientific Publications, pp 140-153.

Terblanche J, Krige JEJ, 1997: Endoscopic therapy in the management of esophageal varices: injection sclerotherapy and variceal ligation. In Nyhus LM, et al, (eds): Mastery of Surgery, 3rd ed. Boston, Little, Brown, pp 1329-1339.

Triantos C, et al, 2004: Sclerotherapy versus vasoactive drugs: are all meta-analyses the same? Gastroenterology 127:358-359.

Vangeli M, et al, 2002: Salvage tips for uncontrolled variceal bleeding. J Hepatol 37:703-704.

Portal Hypertension in Children

R. W. SHEPHERD

SPECIAL FEATURES OF PORTAL HYPERTENSION IN CHILDREN

As in adults, portal hypertension in children is a major cause of morbidity and mortality secondary to chronic liver disease and a range of prehepatic and posthepatic vascular conditions. The predominance of congenital etiologies and growth and developmental considerations provide different challenges, however, in understanding and management of portal hypertension in children. In general, portal hypertension is the result of a combination of increased portal blood flow and increased portal resistance and occurs when portal pressure increases to approximately greater than 10 mm Hg. Signs and symptoms are primarily the result of decompression of this elevated portal blood pressure through portosystemic collaterals, but special developmental vascular alterations may apply in children (Fig. 93.1). The major problems in children are bleeding from esophageal and other varices, ascites, and nutritional disturbances. Encephalopathy, portopulmonary hypertension, and hepatorenal syndrome, although important when they do occur, are seen less frequently in children. Splenomegaly and hypersplenism rarely require specific intervention.

CAUSES OF PORTAL HYPERTENSION IN CHILDREN

Portal hypertension may arise as a result of extrahepatic (portal vein), posthepatic (hepatic vein), or intrahepatic block, in which the block may be presinusoidal, sinusoidal, or postsinusoidal. Causes in children are shown in Table 93.1.

Extrahepatic Causes

Although possibly declining in frequency, extrahepatic portal venous obstruction, caused by a congenital thrombotic or atretic process, is an important cause of noncirrhotic portal hypertension, especially in, but not confined to, Third World countries (Sarin & Agarwal, 2002). Septic or traumatic umbilical vein injury from omphalitis or catheterization or both accounts for some cases, but most are idiopathic or perhaps a congenital malformation of the hepatic venous system. Portal vein stenosis or thrombosis also may occur in the context of portal vein anastomosis in liver transplantation in children. In the congenital form, the portal vein is transformed into a cavernoma, resulting in portal hypertension and esophagogastric varices. From a therapy standpoint, splenic vein or more extensive vein involvement causes different hemodynamics with a preponderance of gastric varices (Shah et al, 2003). In addition, an extensive collateral circulation develops, involving paracholecystic, paracholedochal, and pancreaticoduodenal veins resulting in formation of ectopic varices. Besides variceal bleeding, which is the most common presentation, some patients may have symptomatic portal biliary obstruction. Hypersplenism is common, and anemia and easy bruising from thrombocytopenia and abdominal pain may be presenting features. Growth retardation secondary to malabsorption, resulting from failure of the enteropancreatic and enterohepatic circulation, has been reported. Encephalopathy secondary to shunting seems uncommon, but subclinical signs may occur. Although the liver may seem normal, reversible decompensation may be seen after an acute variceal hemorrhage, and functional compromise may develop in the long term. The natural occurrence of shunts over time may reduce the risk of variceal bleeding, which remains the most important consequence.

Intrahepatic Causes

Portal hypertension may result from a range of presinusoidal, sinusoidal, and postsinusoidal causes of increased portal bed resistance within the liver. Presinusoidal conditions, such as *congenital hepatic fibrosis*, do not result in impaired liver function. Congenital hepatic fibrosis is a developmental disorder that belongs to the family of hepatic ductal plate malformations and is characterized histologically by a variable degree of periportal fibrosis and irregularly shaped proliferating bile ducts (Summerfield et al, 1986). In most patients, the first manifestations of the disease are signs or symptoms related to portal hypertension, especially splenomegaly and varices, often with spontaneous gastrointestinal bleeding, ranging from early childhood to sometimes adulthood. Liver biopsy is highly specific for the diagnosis.

Increased sinusoidal resistance and portal hypertension occurs almost invariably in causes of *cirrhosis in children*. In children, common causes include forms of infant cholestasis, such as biliary atresia, and a range of metabolic disorders, infections, toxins, vascular disease, and nutritional diseases. Cirrhosis is a chronic diffuse disease characterized by irreversible widespread hepatic fibrosis with regenerative nodule formation. The prominent fibrous tissue contains vascular anastomoses, which cause hemodynamic alterations and portosystemic shunting. This diffuse pathology superimposes on the primary liver disease, often obscuring the nature of the original insult. The major pathophysiologic consequences are the result of impaired hepatic function and portal hypertension. Progression to cirrhosis and its complications in pediatric liver disease is highly variable, an important consideration in management, particularly when considering surgical options that may compromise later outcomes. In some conditions, such as neonatal extrahepatic biliary atresia, the development of cirrhosis can be extraordinarily rapid, occurring by 12 to 16 weeks of age, and liver failure can develop by 24 weeks of age.

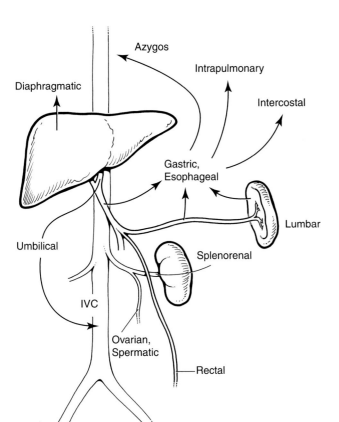

Fig. 93.1. Sites of portosystemic shunts in children with portal hypertension. IVC, inferior vena cava.

Early diagnosis and surgical treatment by portoenterostomy improve outcome, but in most cases, liver transplant is the only available treatment option. Other disorders, such as cystic fibrosis–associated focal biliary cirrhosis, can be compatible with normal liver function for many years, with patients presenting with signs of portal hypertension in the second decade of life.

Postsinusoidal intrahepatic conditions, such as *veno-occlusive disease*, are rare in children. These conditions occur in the context of chemotherapy for childhood cancers (Bouligand et al, 2003) or occasionally related to toxin ingestion (e.g., bush teas).

Table 93.1 Causes of Portal Hypertension in Children

Extrahepatic

Extrahepatic portal vein obstruction/thrombosis
   Congenital
   Acquired
     Dehydration
     Anastomotic (post–liver transplant)
Portal vein stenosis

Intrahepatic

Presinusoidal—congenital hepatic fibrosis
Sinusoidal—cirrhosis (biliary atresia, metabolic hepatopathies)
Postsinusoidal—veno-occlusive diseases

Posthepatic

Budd-Chiari syndrome (webs, thrombophilia, idiopathic)
Anastomotic (post–liver transplant)
Constrictive pericarditis
Post–Fontan procedure

Posthepatic Portal Hypertension

Posthepatic portal hypertension is an important condition in children (see Table 93.1). Obstruction to hepatic venous outflow can occur after liver transplantation (hepatic vein anastomotic stenosis), with Budd-Chiari syndrome (see Ch. 100), or secondary to cardiac lesions resulting in increased right atrial pressure or chronic systemic venous hypertension. Acute Budd-Chiari syndrome is rare in children. It may occur with some thrombophilic disorders, but is usually idiopathic and not associated with the causes seen in adults, such as myeloproliferative disorders. Of note are the effects of a *Fontan procedure*, a cavopulmonary or atriopulmonary shunt that allows lifesaving systemic-to-pulmonary blood flow for single ventricle syndromes in neonates, but results in chronic systemic venous hypertension (pressures may be >20 mm Hg) and eventually portal hypertension (Narkewicz et al, 2003).

EFFECTS OF PORTAL HYPERTENSION IN CHILDREN

An understanding of portal hypertension requires knowledge of the anatomy and physiology of the portal system in infants and children. Portal capillaries originate in the mesentery of the intestine and spleen and in the hepatic sinusoids. Capillaries of the superior mesenteric and splenic veins supply the portal vein with nutrient-rich and hormone-rich blood supply. At the hilum of the liver, the portal vein divides into two major trunks supplying the right and left lobes of the liver, and these trunks undergo a series of divisions supplying segments of the liver terminating in small branches, which pierce the limiting plate of the portal tract and enter the sinusoids through short channels. In fetal life, the ductus venosus connects the umbilical vein and the inferior vena cava, and the umbilical vein joins the left branch of the portal vein. These connections may persist or remain patent in some situations postnatally. The partly oxygenated portal venous blood supplements the oxygenated hepatic arterial blood flow to give the liver unique protection against hypoxia. Blood flow from the hepatic artery and the portal vein is well regulated allowing the liver to withstand thrombosis of either one of these major vessels.

The major pathologic effect from portal hypertension is the development of collaterals carrying blood from the portal venous system to the systemic circulation in the upper part of the stomach, the esophagus, the rectum, and the falciform ligament. These collaterals may drain into the inferior vena cava via the umbilical vein remnant or the left renal vein (see Fig. 93.1). Absence or disconnection of the inferior vena cava or interruption to the azygos system, such as occurs in some cases of biliary atresia, may cause special concern. Similarly, in extrahepatic portal venous malformations, the splenic vein can be small or thrombosed.

Only the submucosal collaterals, such as in the esophagus and stomach and rarely in some parts of the intestine, are associated with gastrointestinal bleeding. Collaterals in other parts of the intestine are more frequently likely to occur at sites of previous surgery along the gastrointestinal tract, particularly from stoma and anastomotic sites. Portal hypertensive gastropathy, which is suggested by dilated mucosal veins and capillaries and mucosal congestion in the stomach, develops particularly in patients with cavernous transformation of the portal vein and may occur after esophageal variceal obliteration.

Although changes in vascular resistance to blood flow between the splanchnic bed and the right atrium seem to be the initial events in the development of portal hypertension, many other hemodynamic changes contribute to and amplify the increased portal blood pressure. There is a hyperdynamic circulatory state with increased cardiac and decreased splanchnic arteriolar tone, both of which increase portal inflow. Changes in intravascular volume also play an important role, as do alterations in adrenergic tone in the splanchnic system. These observations have led to new experimental and clinical studies suggesting possible pharmacologic treatments for portal hypertension (Boyer, 2001). Because the major clinical effect is bleeding from esophageal varices, however, direct treatment of variceal hemorrhage or, in selected cases, shunt surgery remains the major approach except when liver decompensation coexists, when the treatment of choice is liver transplantation.

CLINICAL FEATURES

The main clinical features are splenomegaly; the occurrence of esophageal, gastric, and rectal varices; and the development of ascites (Table 93.2). In extrahepatic portal hypertension or when there is compensated liver disease, there may be no symptoms. The first indication of portal hypertension may be a gastrointestinal bleed, an incidental finding of splenomegaly alone, or anemia or thrombocytopenia secondary to hypersplenism. Commonly the liver is small and impalpable, but if there is an intrahepatic cause, in some patients it can be enlarged, hard, or nodular with a small right lobe or splenomegaly or both. Cutaneous features, such as spider angiomata, prominent periumbilical veins (caput medusae), and palmar erythema, may provide a clue to the presence of liver disease. Spider angiomata may occur in healthy children younger than age 5 years and are not pathognomonic of liver diseases in children, but the appearance of new spider angiomata or more than five or six may be indicative. Spider angiomata frequently are observed in the vascular drainage of the superior vena cava and feature a central arteriole from which radiates numerous fine vessels (2-5 mm in diameter). Other cutaneous features include easy bruising; fine telangiectasia on the face and upper back; white spots, most often on buttocks and arms, which when examined with a lens show the beginnings of spider angiomata; and clubbing of the fingers. On intranasal examination, prominent telangiectasia of Little's area is common, associated with recurrent epistaxis.

Although compensated cirrhosis in adults is mostly cryptogenic, metabolic liver diseases, such as Wilson's disease, cystic fibrosis, and α_1-antitrypsin deficiency, may manifest with compensated

Table 93.2 Clinical Features of Portal Hypertension in Children

Splenomegaly

Esophageal varices with bleeding

Portal gastropathy with bleeding

Recurrent epistaxis, easy bruising

Ascites

Malabsorption

Protein-losing enteropathy

Growth failure

Anemia, thrombocytopenia

cirrhosis in children. In Wilson's disease, specific features include hemolytic anemia; subtle signs of encephalopathy, such as personality changes, loss of memory, or school failure; and Kayser-Fleischer rings, sought by an experienced examiner using a slit lamp. Children with cholestatic liver disease have predominant signs or symptoms of persisting jaundice or pruritus. The liver is usually enlarged, and xanthelasma, malnutrition, and deficiency of fat-soluble vitamins (particularly vitamins D and K) may be prominent features.

Decompensated liver disease is characterized by clinical and laboratory findings of liver synthetic failure and the occurrence of complications. In addition to the features mentioned earlier, the major features include malnutrition, ascites, peripheral edema, coagulopathy, and gastrointestinal bleeding.

Signs of hepatic encephalopathy are subtle and uncommon in children with portal hypertension. Malnutrition with reduced lean tissue and fat stores and poor linear growth is a well-recognized and important feature secondary to malabsorption and impaired protein synthesis (Chin et al, 1992). Spontaneous bruising is caused by impaired hepatic production of clotting factors and thrombocytopenia secondary to hypersplenism and is a sign of advanced disease. Cirrhosis with decompensation also may be associated with changes in the systemic and pulmonary circulations, arteriolar vasodilation, increased blood volume, a hyperdynamic circulatory state, and cyanosis secondary to intrapulmonary shunting. Renal failure is a late but serious event.

DIAGNOSIS

Confirmation of the diagnosis of portal hypertension is based on the suggestive clinical findings discussed previously with or without signs of chronic liver disease and on four investigations: ultrasonography, endoscopy, liver biopsy, and angiography. In all forms of suspected liver disease, confirmation ultimately may rest with the interpretation of liver biopsy findings, which may confirm the presence, type, and degree of activity of cirrhosis and contribute to a diagnosis of the cause of the liver disease. A full range of laboratory and imaging investigations should be done, however, before performing a liver biopsy. These investigations may be diagnostic for the underlying cause and may allow appropriate handling of the liver biopsy specimen with respect to specific histologic and biochemical analysis, particularly for metabolic disorders.

Ultrasonography

Ultrasonography (see Ch. 15) allows visualization and measurement of the size, patency, and flow of the portal vein; determination of the occurrence of a cavernoma; and information about liver size and homogeneity. Renal cysts on ultrasound or a suggestive family history may provide a clue to the diagnosis of congenital hepatic fibrosis. Echocardiography is useful to exclude primary cardiac causes of hepatic venous outflow obstruction.

Endoscopy

Endoscopy should be performed to evaluate the size and occurrence of varices and occurrence of cherry red spots (which correlate with risk of rupture) and visualize and perhaps treat the source of bleeding varices. Other features, such as portal gastropathy and exclusion of other sources of gastrointestinal bleeding, can be visualized.

Liver Biopsy

Liver biopsy excludes liver disease, in the case of extrahepatic obstruction, or aids in the diagnosis of cirrhosis. Differentiation between cirrhosis and presinusoidal and extrahepatic causes of portal hypertension, such as congenital hepatic fibrosis and extrahepatic portal hypertension, sometimes can cause diagnostic difficulties. In both of these latter conditions, there are no signs of chronic liver disease, and transaminases and synthetic function are normal. In congenital hepatic fibrosis, the liver is enlarged and hard, and histologically hepatocytes are normal; there are prominent abnormal bile ducts in wide bands of fibrous tissue, but no nodules. In extrahepatic portal hypertension caused by portal vein malformation or obstruction, the liver is small but histologically normal. There may be mild derangement of coagulation parameters secondary to an underlying coagulation disorder (e.g., protein C or S deficiency). Obstruction to hepatic venous outflow causes centrilobular hemorrhagic necrosis, with fibrosis extending from central veins to portal tracts.

Angiography

Angiography (see Ch. 21) with direct venography or computed tomography angiography can provide important information about the site of block, the size and patency of major veins in the portal system, and relationship to the cardioesophageal or other varices. Suspected obstruction to hepatic venous outflow requires venography or cardiac catheterization or both; these are the diagnostic procedures of choice in such cases. Pressure gradient measurements may be useful across venous blocks and to determine the magnitude of the portal pressure.

MANAGEMENT

Therapy of portal hypertension is directed primarily at the major complication (i.e., the prevention or management of variceal hemorrhage) except in cases of hepatic venous outflow block, in which directly treatable causes, such as vena caval webs or constrictive pericarditis, need to be considered, and in cases of end-stage liver disease, in which liver transplantation (see Ch. 103) is the primary therapy. Encephalopathy rarely requires specific therapy. Ascites can be a major problem and often requires specific treatment. Hypersplenism, although common, rarely results in morbidity or mortality. The management of these and other complications of portal hypertension in children is primarily medical and beyond the scope of this chapter.

In most cases, direct therapy of varices is indicated before considering surgery because the various options for creation of a surgical shunt are indirect treatments for varices via reduction in portal pressure. The risk of variceal bleeding, the potential evolution of spontaneous shunts over time, the presence or absence of liver disease, and the portal vascular anatomy are the four main factors influencing any decision for the application of shunt surgery in children.

Variceal hemorrhage clinically manifests as a need for emergency therapy or as a need for prophylaxis of initial or subsequent rebleeding. Most of the data concerning the management of variceal hemorrhage have come from large controlled trials in adults. The pediatric literature is generally descriptive or anecdotal, with some exceptions.

Emergency Therapy

Bleeding esophageal varices (see Ch. 91) in children require emergency treatment (Fig. 93.2). However small the hemorrhage, admission to the nearest hospital with blood transfusion facilities is advised. As soon as the patient has blood transfusion available and a secure intravenous infusion line and is hemodynamically stable, referral to a tertiary center with experience in the management of variceal hemorrhage in children is recommended. An initial melena or sentinel bleed may precede sudden hematemesis and shock, requiring rapid blood transfusion to prevent death. Significant bleeding with hypotension impairs hepatic perfusion, often causes deterioration of liver function, and precipitates ascites and encephalopathy. Initial fluid management in the form of crystalloids followed by red blood cell transfusion is important, and any coagulopathy should be corrected with vitamin K and fresh frozen plasma. Pharmacologic therapy with a short-acting splanchnic vasoconstrictor may be useful (Boyer, 2001). Octreotide (maximum dose 1 μg/kg/hr intravenously or 2-4 μg/kg/dose subcutaneously every 8 hours for 24 hours or until the bleeding

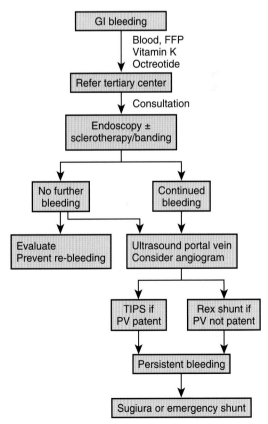

Fig. 93.2. Management of acute variceal bleeding in children. FFP, fresh frozen plasma; GI, gastrointestinal; PV, portal vein; TIPS, transjugular intrahepatic portosystemic shunt.

has ceased) is the drug of choice in this circumstance because of fewer side effects (Moitinho et al, 2001). Alternatives are vasopressin (0.3 U/kg as a bolus over 20 minutes followed by continuous infusion of the same amount on an hourly basis) or its inactive precursor terlipressin (0.01 mg/kg bolus every 4-6 hours or 0.05 mg/kg infusion over 6 hours for 24-48 hours). Common side effects include skin pallor, abdominal colic, and chest pain. Studies in adults have indicated that an adjunctive vasodilator, such as nitroglycerin in the form of a 10-mg patch, may reduce these hemodynamic complications. Nasogastric intubation is an essential part of management, allowing the documentation of ongoing bleeding and the removal of blood that might precipitate encephalopathy.

When hemodynamically stable, endoscopy is indicated. A significant percentage of patients with known varices have bleeding from sources other than varices, including duodenal/gastric ulceration. In addition, a meta-analysis of multiple controlled adult studies showed that endoscopic treatment (see Ch. 92) plus pharmacologic treatment is currently the best measure to achieve initial control of significant acute variceal bleeding (Banares et al, 2002).

Endoscopic Treatment of Acute Variceal Bleeding

Episodes of minor variceal hemorrhage may terminate spontaneously, but endoscopic treatment by sclerotherapy or band ligation is often necessary (see Ch. 92). Both techniques are well described in children (Goenka et al, 1993; Goncalves et al, 2000; Zargar et al, 2004). In adults, comparative trials of sclerotherapy and ligation indicate equal efficacy in controlling bleeding, reducing rebleeding, and ablating varices, but fewer adverse effects with banding. The two procedures can be complementary, however, and access to both procedures may be warranted. Ligation may be technically difficult in an esophagus awash with blood or for small varices, particularly in small infants, where entrapment of part of the esophageal wall with perforation or bleeding can occur. In these circumstances, sclerotherapy is more appropriate. Sclerotherapy involves injection of sclerosant (ethanolamine or tetradecyl sulfate) paravariceally or intravariceally, in volumes of 0.5 to 1 mL just above the gastroesophageal junction. Care should be taken to avoid injecting too high above the cardia because this can increase bleeding from a distal varix. This procedure is associated with bacteremia, and broad-spectrum antibiotics should be prescribed (amoxicillin, cefuroxime, and metronidazole). Complications, which should be uncommon in experienced centers, include esophageal ulceration, stricture, and pain.

Sengstaken-Blakemore Tube

For rare cases, if the aforementioned measures fail to control bleeding, temporary cessation of bleeding can be achieved employing mechanical compression of esophageal and gastric varices using a pediatric Sengstaken-Blakemore tube or a Linton tube. These devices are best inserted under anesthesia at the time of attempted sclerotherapy, but should not be used for longer than 24 or 48 hours because of the risk of ulceration, particularly in the esophagus. There is a high incidence of rebleeding when the tubes are removed.

Emergency Surgical Approaches and Emergency Portosystemic Shunts

Emergency creation of portosystemic shunts (see Ch. 95) or other surgical therapy is usually a last resort for persisting exsanguinating acute variceal hemorrhage. Patients who come to emergency shunts often have gastric variceal bleeding. Considerations in these circumstances include potential mortality and the range of techniques available, including transjugular intrahepatic portosystemic shunt (TIPS) (see Ch. 96), surgical shunts, esophageal transection, and esophagogastric devascularization with splenectomy (see Chs. 94 and 95). TIPS is an attractive approach because it does not require major surgery. TIPS has been used effectively in critically ill adults to control bleeding before liver transplantation and in some children with bleeding stomal varices (Lagier et al, 1994). The procedure seems to decrease portal pressure acutely, although 60% occlude within 3 to 12 months, so it is best viewed as a bridging procedure only. Pediatric application is limited by size constraints, but in experienced hands in selected children older than age 2 to 5 years, TIPS has application and is preferable to major shunt surgery for hepatic causes of portal hypertension.

Prophylaxis Against First Gastrointestinal Bleed

In recognized cases of portal hypertension with varices, controversy exists as to whether any therapy reduces the risk or prevents the occurrence of gastrointestinal bleeding. In all cases, it is reasonable to be prepared for the possibility by ensuring that the child's caregivers understand the importance of seeking early medical advice by going to the nearest hospital for blood crossmatching and appropriate referral to a tertiary unit. β-Blockers, such as propranolol and the more selective atenolol, reduce hepatic arterial and portal vein blood flow and have been studied with respect to reduction in portal pressures to less than 12 mm Hg, reducing the risk of an initial bleed in adults (Lebrec, 2001; Shasidhar et al, 1999). There may be a case under certain circumstances for prophylactic sclerotherapy, but the potential for bleeding of known varices that have never bled in children is conjectural. Goncalves and associates (2000) compared sclerotherapy with no treatment in a controlled clinical trial in children and found a reduced risk of bleeding, but an increase in portal gastropathy.

Prevention of Recurrent Gastrointestinal Bleeding

Intrahepatic Causes of Portal Hypertension

Direct Obliteration of Varices. When bleeding has occurred secondary to intrahepatic causes of portal vein obstruction, direct obliteration of the varices is the initial treatment of choice, although consideration of the underlying liver disease is the major determinant of long-term management. Randomized controlled trials in adults have shown a reduction in the frequency of bleeding and improved survival. Although no randomized controlled trials have been performed in children, several large studies of sclerotherapy versus banding in children with portal hypertension indicate that this procedure is safe and reduces the chance of rebleeding (Fox et al, 1995; Goenka et al, 1993; McKiernan et al, 2002; Zargar et al, 2002). Neither sclerotherapy nor banding reduces portal pressure, but they do obliterate the dangerous varices (Fig. 93.3). These procedures (described earlier) may cause some interference with the vascular hemodynamics. Hypersplenism and portal gastropathy temporarily worsen, but ultimately with time spontaneous portosystemic shunts can arise, reducing portal pressures.

Several vasoactive drugs also have been documented in multiple controlled trials in adults to reduce the risk of rebleeding by reducing portal and systemic pressures (Boyer, 2001). At present,

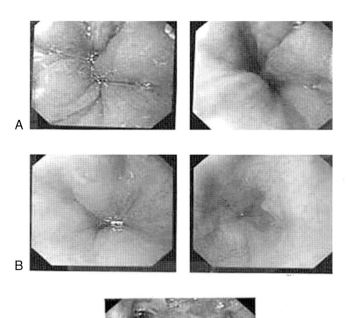

Fig. 93.3. A-C, Ablation of esophageal varices by sclerotherapy in a 6-year-old patient with portal hypertension following a Fontan procedure for congenital heart disease.

Table 93.3 Surgical Options for Portal Hypertension in Children

Devascularization
    Sugiura procedure

Nonselective shunts
    Mesocaval—"H" graft or direct
    Portacaval
    Central splenorenal
    TIPS

Selective shunts
    Distal splenorenal
    Splenoadrenal

Restorative shunt
    Rex shunt (mesenteric–left portal vein bypass)

Anatomic repair
    Hepatic or portal webs, stenosis

Orthotopic liver transplantation

a combination of a nonselective β-blocker and certain nitrates (e.g., isosorbide 5-mononitrate) is the drug regimen of choice, aiming at a 25% reduction in resting heart rate. Major adverse effects of β-blockers include reactive airway disease and heart block, in which they are contraindicated.

Surgery. When there is active liver disease, but a significant risk of mortality from bleeding, surgical management of portal hypertension is a major consideration (Table 93.3). Patients ideally should be evaluated and treated in a transplant center, where the range of surgical options can be assessed. *Surgical portosystemic shunts* may reduce the risk of gastrointestinal bleeding, but they decrease portal blood flow; decrease hepatic perfusion; and carry the risk of hepatic decompensation, hepatic encephalopathy, and precluding or enhancing difficulty with liver transplantation. Randomized controlled trials in adult patients have not shown any significant improvement in survival with portosystemic shunts in patients with intrahepatic causes of portal hypertension. If a shunt operation is contemplated in critically ill patients, the use of a *TIPS* as a bridging procedure is probably the procedure of choice. Ultimately, the surgical procedure of choice for uncontrolled portal hypertension resulting from intrahepatic disease is *liver transplantation.* In nonshunt, nontransplant candidates, a Sugiura procedure (esophageal disconnection/devascularization procedure) may be lifesaving, with the added advantage of a low risk of encephalopathy (see Ch. 94).

Special consideration should be given to shunt surgery in some cases of cystic fibrosis–associated liver disease, in which there is a slow evolution of hepatic dysfunction (Debray et al, 1999), and in congenital hepatic fibrosis, which is a presinusoidal cause of

portal hypertension not associated with the occurrence of liver synthetic dysfunction. In these cases, the choice of the type of shunt is determined by the vascular anatomy, the size of the veins, the risk of thrombosis and failure, and the risk of encephalopathy. *Selective shunts* (see Chs. 98 and 99), such as distal splenorenal or distal splenoadrenal, are preferred (Kato et al, 2000; Valayer et al, 1985); the latter often allows better size matching of the splenic and enlarged adrenal vein, avoiding renal vein clamping.

Extrahepatic Portal Venous Obstruction
Portal hypertension secondary to extrahepatic portal venous obstruction in children is associated with a better long-term prognosis and quality of life than portal hypertension associated with intrahepatic diseases, and management considerations differ. Acute variceal bleeding is usually well tolerated because of normal liver function, but recurrent variceal bleeds can be associated with significant morbidity (Zargar et al, 2004). Although long-term outcomes of individual center approaches are documented (Bambini, 2000; Orloff et al, 2002; Zargar et al, 2004), no controlled trials exist comparing long-term outcomes from the two main approaches to therapy—direct variceal ablation and shunt surgery. Some patients never bleed at all, and anecdotal and published data suggest that some patients develop spontaneous decompression of varices over time (Goenka et al, 1993; Lykavieris et al, 2000).

Direct Variceal Ablation. Endoscopic therapy has gained increasing acceptance in the treatment of bleeding esophageal varices in children with extrahepatic portal hypertension. Zargar and colleagues (2004) reported a 15-year follow-up of 69 children. Almost 90% of patients had no rebleeding after eradication, which was achieved in 90% of patients. Maksoud (1991) reported that 42 of 123 cases failed sclerotherapy and subsequently underwent shunt surgery. Stringer and Howard (1994) reported that only 4 of 36 cases required shunt surgery after variceal sclerotherapy over 8 years of follow-up. All of these studies had little or no morbidity or mortality, but several repeat sessions of sclerotherapy were necessary during follow-up for complete variceal eradication. The main reason for long-term failure was the occurrence of gastric varices, but this does not occur in all cases, and some studies suggest that the occurrence of spontaneous shunts after successful sclerotherapy negates the need for shunt surgery at all (Goenka et al, 1993).

Surgery. Surgery may be required for patients with extrahepatic portal hypertension with preserved liver function for recurrent bleeding or rarely for massive hypersplenism. Surgical options in the management of extrahepatic portal venous obstruction include *portosystemic shunts, Rex shunts, devascularization,* and *transection* (see Table 93.3). Although earlier outcomes of portosystemic shunts were disappointing, some more recent reports have shown recurrence of bleeding in 2.5% to 10%, low mortality, a continued shunt thrombosis rate of 7% to 13%, and an apparently low risk of encephalopathy (Botha et al, 2004; Kato et al, 2000; Orloff et al, 2002). *Nonselective mesocaval shunts and more selective distal splenorenal shunts* have been the procedures of choice in the past, although a *central splenorenal shunt with splenectomy* sometimes is advocated if there is massive hypersplenism and pain from splenic infarcts. These shunts may not be technically possible, however, because of thrombotic involvement of splenic or mesenteric veins, and in some cases, particularly when varices are derived from the cavernoma, certain shunts may not alter variceal pressures derived from the cardioesophageal veins.

The *Rex shunt,* usually an internal jugular vein graft mesenteric–left portal vein bypass, has the major theoretical advantages of restoring portal flow to the liver and reducing risk of encephalopathy, and it obviates technical problems associated with splenic vein thrombosis (Bambini, 2000; de Ville de Goyet et al, 1999). First introduced for portal vein thrombosis after liver transplant, this procedure may become the surgical procedure of choice for all causes of extrahepatic portal vein obstruction. Thrombosis and stenosis rates seem similar to portosystemic shunts. Patency of the left portal-to-right portal system is difficult to prove before the procedure. Of importance when performing any type of shunt surgery for extrahepatic venous obstruction, particularly when there is a cavernoma, is the use of a postprocedure portal venogram to ensure patency antegrade to the liver and consider selective division of the portal system (e.g., coronary branch) when there are residual collaterals.

SUMMARY

Therapeutic options for children with portal hypertension include a broad range of pharmacologic, endoscopic, radiologic, and surgical procedures, the last-mentioned being mainly indicated in pediatric patients with high risk for recurrent variceal bleeding. Thorough assessment of the causes, effects, and venous anatomy and consequent selective application of some or all of these options can improve quality of life, reduce the complications of portal hypertension, and decrease mortality.

Children with variceal bleeding resulting from extrahepatic portal hypertension, in whom there is preserved liver function, usually can be managed effectively and safely with initial direct variceal ablation by sclerotherapy or banding, which in many cases can alter the natural history and reduce or eliminate the risk of rebleeding. The development of portal hypertensive gastropathy or rebleeding or both after these palliative procedures can be definitively managed by shunt surgery, preferably the more physiologic Rex shunt. Children with intrahepatic portal hypertension who are transplant candidates are best palliated with endoscopic treatment or occasionally TIPS. Children who are not candidates for transplant or who have failed nonsurgical treatments can have good outcomes with selective portosystemic shunts. Well-planned definitive surgical treatments will continue to be important components in the treatment of children with portal hypertensive complications or progressive liver disease.

REFERENCES

Bambini DA, et al, 2000: Experience with the Rex shunt (mesenterico-left portal bypass) in children with extrahepatic portal hypertension. J Pediatr Surg 35:13-18.

Banares R, et al, 2002: Endoscopic treatment versus endoscopic plus pharmacologic treatment for acute variceal bleeding: a meta-analysis. Hepatology 35:609-615.

Botha JF, et al, 2004: Portosystemic shunts in children: a 15-year experience. J Am Coll Surg 199:179-185.

Bouligand J, et al, 2003: In children and adolescents, the pharmacodynamics of high-dose busulfan is dependent on the second alkylating agent used in the combined regimen (melphalan or thiotepa). Bone Marrow Transplant 32:979-986.

Boyer TD, 2001: Pharmacologic treatment of portal hypertension: past, present, and future. Hepatology 34(4 pt 1):834-839.

Chin SE, et al, 1992: The nature of malnutrition in children with end-stage liver disease awaiting orthotopic liver transplantation. Am J Clin Nutr 56:164-168.

Debray D, et al, 1999: Outcome of cystic fibrosis-associated liver cirrhosis: management of portal hypertension. J Hepatol 31:77-83.

de Ville de Goyet J, et al, 1999: Treatment of extrahepatic portal hypertension in children by mesenteric-to-left portal vein bypass: a new physiological procedure. Eur J Surg 165:777-781.

Fox VL, et al, 1995: Endoscopic ligation of esophageal varices in children. J Pediatr Gastroenterol Nutr 20:202-208.

Goenka AS, et al, 1993: Therapeutic upper gastrointestinal endoscopy in children: an audit of 443 procedures. J Gastroenterol Hepatol 8:44-57.

Goncalves ME, et al, 2000: Prophylactic sclerotherapy in children with esophageal varices: long-term results of a controlled prospective randomized trial. J Pediatr Surg 35:401-405.

Kato T, et al, 2000: Portosystemic shunting in children during the era of endoscopic therapy improved postoperative growth parameters. J Pediatr Gastroenterol Nutr 30:419-425.

Lagier E, et al, 1994: Treatment of bleeding stomal varices using transjugular intrahepatic portosystemic shunt. J Pediatr Gastroenterol Nutr 18:501-503.

Lebrec D, 2001: Drug therapy for portal hypertension. Gut 49:441-442.

Lykavieris P, et al, 2000: Risk of gastrointestinal bleeding during adolescence and early adulthood in children with portal vein obstruction. J Pediatr 136:805-808.

Maksoud JG, et al, 1991: The endoscopic and surgical management of portal hypertension in children: analysis of 123 cases. J Pediatr Surg 26:178-181.

McKiernan PJ, et al, 2002: A prospective study of endoscopic esophageal variceal ligation using a multiband ligator. J Pediatr Gastroenterol Nutr 34:207-211.

Moitinho E, et al, 2001: Multicenter randomized controlled trial comparing different schedules of somatostatin in the treatment of acute variceal bleeding. J Hepatol 35:712-718.

Narkewicz MR, et al, 2003: Hepatic dysfunction following the Fontan procedure. J Pediatr Gastroenterol Nutr 36:352-357.

Orloff MJ, et al, 2002: Bleeding esophagogastric varices from extrahepatic portal hypertension: 40 years' experience with portal-systemic shunt. J Am Coll Surg 194:717-728.

Sarin SK, Agarwal SR, 2002: Extrahepatic portal vein obstruction. Semin Liver Dis 22:43-58.

Shah SR, et al, 2003: Extensive portal and splenic vein thrombosis: differences in hemodynamics and management. Hepatogastroenterology 50:1085-1089.

Shasidhar H, et al, 1999: Propranolol in prevention of portal hypertensive hemorrhage in children: a pilot study. J Pediatr Gastroenterol Nutr 29:12-17.

Stringer MD, Howard ER, 1994: Longterm outcome after injection sclerotherapy for oesophageal varices in children with extrahepatic portal hypertension. Gut 35:257-259.

Summerfield JA, et al, 1986: Hepatobiliary fibropolycystic diseases: a clinical and histological review of 51 patients. J Hepatol 2:141-156.

Valayer J, et al, 1985: Shunt surgery for treatment of portal hypertension in children. World J Surg 9:258-268.

Zargar SA, et al, 2002: Endoscopic ligation compared with sclerotherapy for bleeding esophageal varices in children with extrahepatic portal venous obstruction. Hepatology 36:666-672.

Zargar SA, et al, 2004: Fifteen-year follow up of endoscopic injection sclerotherapy in children with extrahepatic portal venous obstruction. J Gastroenterol Hepatol 19:139-145.

Operative Devascularization and Esophageal Transection

C. SMAJDA AND A. CARLONI

Surgery to manage bleeding esophageal varices is in a sharp decline, especially surgical procedures for selective and nonselective portosystemic shunts, because of the potential risk of postoperative hepatic encephalopathy (Franco & Smadja, 1985) and because of the increased use of transjugular intrahepatic portosystemic shunt. Despite the widespread use of interventional endoscopy, however, failure of conservative therapeutic techniques in patients with bleeding varices raises the problem of the surgical prevention of recurrent variceal bleeding when liver replacement is not indicated. In such a situation, despite interest in the small diameter portacaval shunt popularized by Sarfeh and Rypins (1986) or transjugular intrahepatic portosystemic shunt, nonshunting procedures that do not carry the risk of hepatic encephalopathy are appealing. The lack of hepatic encephalopathy after nonshunting procedures is most likely linked to the long-term maintenance of splanchnic and systemic hemodynamics in patients with cirrhosis (Vons et al, 1996). For anatomic reasons, nonshunting procedures cannot be achieved by simple means. Multiple surgical procedures have been described that obliterate varices or disconnect the esophageal veins draining blood flow toward the azygos vein from the portal tributaries. Of these approaches, the procedure described by Sugiura and Futagawa (1973) and modified procedures are of particular interest.

DIRECT OPERATION ON ESOPHAGEAL VARICES

The suppression of varices has long tempted surgeons with special expertise in the field of portal hypertension. The rationale for these operations is based on anatomic features. The coronary vein and gastric veins are anastomosed with tributaries of the superior vena cava by collateral channels in the submucosa of the esophagus, between the two muscular layers, and in the periesophageal region. In portal hypertension, blood is flowing abnormally upward into these channels. At the level of the diaphragm, the narrowing of the hiatus does not allow periesophageal channels to enlarge. Most of the blood flow goes through the submucosal varices. In portal hypertension, the increased venous pressure can produce varices throughout the length of the esophagus and down into the upper stomach. It is rare for bleeding to occur, however, except in the lowest 5 cm of the esophagus, and it is believed that a difference in the venous anatomy in the distal segment of the esophagus accounts for the occurrence of bleeding at this site.

Using a computerized image analysis system to study the venous anatomy of the esophagus, Spence (1984) found an abrupt change in the venous pattern at the esophagogastric junction and again at a point about 2 to 5 cm proximally. In the lowest segment of the esophagus, the intrinsic esophageal veins lie mainly in the lamina propria, that is, between the muscularis mucosa and the basement membrane of the epithelium. In a normal patient, there is a sevenfold increase in the area occupied by veins in the lamina propria of the lowest segment of the esophagus compared with the corresponding area of the stomach; in patients with esophageal varices, a ninefold increase was noted (Spence, 1984). In addition, serial sections have shown that these large vessels in the lamina propria communicate directly with dilated intraepithelial blood channels via the epithelial papillae (Spence et al, 1983). These intraepithelial channels seen histologically represent the cherry-red spots viewed endoscopically. The deep intrinsic veins form the varices in portal hypertension (Spence & Terblanche, 1987). A technique that would produce permanent obliteration of the varices in this vulnerable segment of the esophagus would seem to be the ideal treatment of direct attack of bleeding esophageal varices.

HISTORY OF ESOPHAGEAL TRANSECTION AND DEVASCULARIZATION PROCEDURES

Crile (1950) proposed transthoracic ligation of esophageal varices, and subsequently many modifications of his technique have been devised. Walker (1964) used a vertical incision for the muscle layers of the esophagus and a transverse division of the mucosa and submucosa to reduce the risk of post-transection leakage. About the same time, Tanner (1961) proposed a subcardiac portoazygos disconnection with gastric transection. Boerema (1949) and Vosschulte (1957) introduced the simple button technique for transabdominal esophageal transection. This method was a major source of stricture formation (Johnston & Kelly 1976). Hassab (1967) found that in patients with bleeding esophageal varices secondary to schistosomiasis he could do an adequate gastroesophageal devascularization procedure via the abdomen. This technique included splenectomy, but not esophageal or gastric transection, and yet Hassab (1998) reported a remarkably low rate of rebleeding. Japanese surgeons devised an extensive transthoracic paraesophageal devascularization and esophageal transection combined with an abdominal component consisting of splenectomy, devascularization of the upper stomach, vagotomy, and pyloroplasty (Sugiura & Futagawa, 1973). In 1974, Vankemmel published the first report of the use of a circular stapling gun for esophageal transection. This technique removes approximately 1 cm of full-thickness esophageal wall, provides a safe suture line, and reduces the risk of stricture formation. Yamamoto and colleagues (1976) believed that the whole of this vulnerable segment of the esophagus should be resected, and they advocated proximal esophagogastric resection together with splenectomy. Hirashima and colleagues (1982) described a modified Walker's procedure via the abdomen in which only the mucosal layer is transected with the stapling gun, preserving the lower esophageal sphincter mechanism.

ESOPHAGEAL TRANSECTION

Operative Technique

The patient is positioned in a supine position. A 30-degree, head-up tilt improves the exposure of the operative field. A midline epigastric incision is generally used. The left lobe of the liver is retracted. In case of left lobe hypertrophy in cirrhotic patients, division of the left lobe ligaments may be useful. The operation is begun by dividing the gastrohepatic ligament in the area where it is thin and usually transparent, exposing the right crus of the esophageal hiatus. The incision is carried out superiorly over the anterior aspect of the esophagus, dividing the reflection of the parietal peritoneum at the junction between the esophagus and the diaphragm. The incision is pursued down the left side of the esophagus until the left crus of the esophageal hiatus is identified. The posterior vagal trunk is exposed. The abdominal esophagus is isolated by circumferential dissection. A tape is passed around the esophagus, excluding the posterior vagal trunk and the anterior vagal nerve when present as a nerve trunk (Fig. 94.1). In the absence of an anterior vagal trunk, its branches are sacrificed during the esophageal transection.

The sling is retracted to displace the esophagus to the left, and the fibrous tissue posterior to the esophagus is divided. The abdominal esophagus is completely freed and mobilized. During this maneuver, great care should be taken to secure hemostasis of the small peritoneal vessels and periesophageal collateral veins.

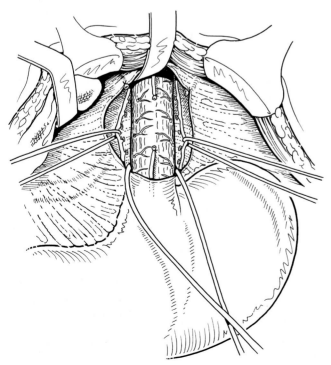

Fig. 94.1. Exposure of the abdominal esophagus. A tape has been placed around the esophagus. The vagal nerves have been retracted.

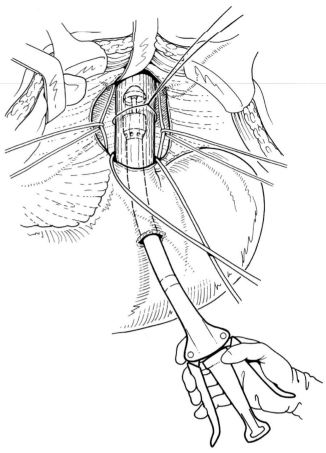

Fig. 94.2. Esophageal transection. The circular stapler has been opened, and the ligature has been tied just above the cardia.

Esophageal mobilization may be hazardous in cases of severe portal hypertension, especially in patients with portal vein thrombosis, or if there is periesophagitis as a result of previous injection sclerotherapy. A 0 monothread ligature is passed around the esophagus, taking care that vagal nerves lie outside the ligature. A small horizontal gastrotomy is made. Esophageal dilation can be performed gently using Hegar dilators. The diameter of the esophagus is measured with an obturator sizer to determine the largest size of the circular stapler to be used. The circular stapler instrument is guided into the distal esophagus. The instrument is opened over a distance of 4 to 5 cm, and the ligature is tied just above the cardia (Fig. 94.2). The head of the circular stapler is closed, and the trigger is pulled to complete the esophageal anastomosis (Fig. 94.3). The head of the circular stapler is opened, and the instrument is withdrawn. The excised tissue is examined for completeness, to confirm a satisfactory transection. A finger is introduced through the gastrotomy to check the integrity of the suture line and to direct a nasogastric tube into the stomach for postoperative drainage. The gastrotomy is sutured in one layer. The abdomen is closed without drainage.

Results

Simple transection of the esophagus using a mechanical stapler is effective for the control of variceal bleeding. In all reported cases, bleeding immediately stopped (Cello et al, 1982; Cooperman et al, 1980; Kuzmak, 1981; Wexler, 1980). Transection was proposed

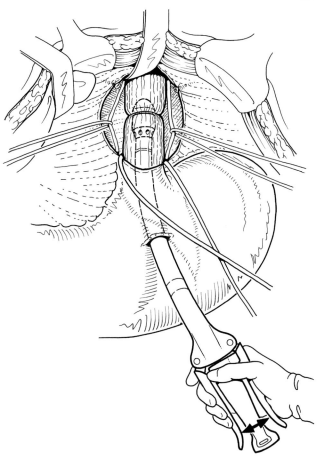

Fig. 94.3. Completion of the anastomosis. The head of the circular stapler has been closed, and the esophageal anastomosis has been completed.

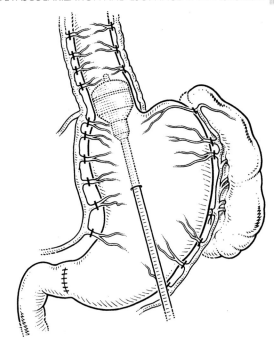

Fig. 94.4. Diagrammatic representation of the Sugiura procedure. Esophageal devascularization should include only the transverse vessels (perforating veins) connecting the adventitial veins to the submucosal veins. This makes ligation of 30 to 50 perforating veins necessary.

as an elective treatment of esophageal varices (Wexler, 1980). The rate of rebleeding was high, however—17.8% in the series of Koyama and associates (1980) and 37.7% in the series of Johnston (1994). Koyama and associates (1980) showed that to reduce the rebleeding rate significantly, esophageal transection should be combined with splenectomy and esophagogastric devascularization.

SUGIURA AND MODIFIED SUGIURA PROCEDURE

Operative Technique

The Sugiura procedure is a sophisticated nonshunting technique aimed at the eradication of esophageal varices. The operation consists of an extensive paraesophagogastric devascularization with esophageal transection and splenectomy through successive thoracic and abdominal incisions. The results obtained by Sugiura and Futagawa (1973, 1984) in Japan were impressive and led some authors to evaluate the efficacy of the operation in Western countries. In the West, the Sugiura procedure was believed to be technically complex and time-consuming and was largely ignored or abandoned. Interest was renewed when simplified procedures using an exclusive abdominal approach and stapled transection (Peracchia et al, 1980) were described. The original procedure proposed by Sugiura and Futagawa (1973) and the modified procedure described by Ginsberg and

coworkers (1982) and Umeyama and colleagues (1983), which we routinely use (Mariette et al, 1994), are described.

Sugiura Procedure

The original Sugiura procedure (Sugiura & Futagawa, 1973) is performed in two steps—a thoracic approach first, followed by an abdominal procedure 4 to 6 weeks after the initial thoracic operation. The thoracic procedure is carried out through a left lateral thoracotomy using the sixth or seventh intercostal space. The mediastinal pleura over the esophagus is opened longitudinally. The lower part of the thoracic esophagus is surrounded by dilated veins (adventitial veins), which form a plexus. These adventitial veins run parallel to the esophageal wall and communicate with the submucosal veins (variceal channels) via large perforating veins (Fig. 94.4). All of these perforating veins must be completely and systematically ligated and divided to devascularize the esophagus. Great care must be taken not to damage the adventitial veins, which represent a spontaneous portacaval shunt. Usually, there are 30 to 50 perforating veins to be ligated, over a 12- to 18-cm length of the thoracic esophagus. At the level of the hiatus, periesophageal channels are bulky, and esophageal varices predominate. Thorough devascularization of this region is paramount. It prepares the area for esophageal transection. After completion of the devascularization, esophageal transection is performed at the level of the diaphragm. The anterior muscular layer and the mucosal layer of the esophagus are completely divided, and the posterior muscular layer is left intact (Fig. 94.5A). The esophageal varices are not ligated because this often causes stenosis of the lumen. The mucosal layer of the esophagus is reconstructed by placing 70 to 90 interrupted stitches of 5-0 nonresorbable sutures (see Fig. 94.5B). During this step, esophageal varices are electively occluded with sutures. The muscular layer is reconstructed using resorbable 4-0 sutures. A nasogastric tube is left in the stomach. The thorax is closed with appropriate drainage.

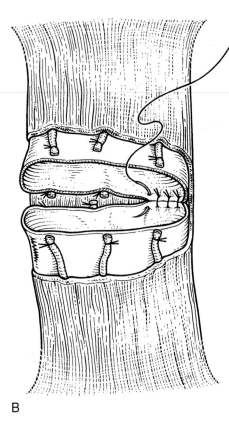

A   B

Fig. 94.5. Technique of esophageal transection according to Sugiura and Futagawa. **A,** The posterior muscular layer has been left intact. **B,** Reconstruction of the esophageal continuity requires at least 70 interrupted sutures.

The abdominal procedure subsequently is performed through an upper midline or left subcostal laparotomy. Splenectomy is performed. The abdominal esophagus and the cardia are devascularized, as are the greater curvature and the posterior aspect of the stomach. The posterior vagus nerve is divided (Sugiura & Futagawa, 1973), and devascularization of the lesser curvature of the stomach follows, as for selective vagotomy. The cardioesophageal branches of the left gastric vessels are ligated and divided. Devascularization is performed over more than 7 cm of gastric wall from the cardia (Sugiura & Futagawa, 1973), the esophagus and the cardia being completely mobilized and freed from the adjacent anatomic structures. Devascularization is facilitated by the division of the anterior vagus nerve, and because of this, pyloroplasty is performed. The abdominal incision is closed. Both steps of the procedure may be performed during the same operative session by using synchronous incisions. If such an option is elected, the abdominal procedure is carried out through a left subcostal incision.

Modified Sugiura Procedure

The whole operation is performed through a left S-shaped subcostal laparotomy extending posteriorly to the tip of the 10th rib and 4 to 8 cm across the midline. The patient is slightly rotated to the right. Strong mechanical retractors lift the costal margin cephalad, exposing the left subphrenic space.

The procedure is started by splenectomy. Removal of the spleen, which is usually enlarged, improves dramatically the exposure of the abdominal esophagus and facilitates paraesophagogastric devascularization. Gastric devascularization is begun at the greater curvature of the stomach and continues along its upper part (see Fig. 94.4). Devascularization is performed adjacent to the stomach wall. Completion of the greater curvature

devascularization at the cardia is facilitated by placing a tape around the abdominal esophagus. This maneuver is not always easy in the presence of portal hypertension, especially when extrahepatic portal venous occlusion is a feature, and is difficult in patients who have had previous sclerotherapy. The posterior aspect of the upper part of the stomach, including the esophagogastric branches of the left gastric vessels, is devascularized. Devascularization is likewise pursued along the lesser curvature. The surgical technique used is similar to that of proximal gastric vagotomy. The heel of the crow's foot of Latarjet's nerve is divided, and devascularization is carried up to the esophagus.

To improve the exposure of the esophagus, the diaphragmatic orifice of the esophagus is opened (Fig. 94.6). The pericardium is freed from the upper aspect of the diaphragm, which is divided sagittally. Esophageal devascularization is performed close to the esophageal wall by dividing only the vessels running transversely (perforating veins) and coursing to perforate the esophageal wall (see Fig. 94.6). Devascularization is pursued over a distance of 10 to 12 cm. This step of the operation is facilitated by using resorbable clips. We routinely perform bilateral truncal vagotomy. Vagal nerve division lengthens the esophagus, facilitating esophageal devascularization. In cases with previous sclerotherapy with periesophageal fibrosis, completely safe devascularization may be technically impossible, but should be done within the limits of safety to avoid damaging the esophagus. The degree of difficulty during this step of the procedure most likely is linked to the type of sclerosant used and the number of sclerotherapy sessions carried out before surgery (Alam et al, 1996; Chaudhary & Aranya, 1991).

Esophageal transection is performed using a mechanical stapler introduced via a short gastrotomy. The technique used is similar to that described earlier. In cases of previous sclerotherapy, thickness of the lower end of the esophagus and inflammatory changes

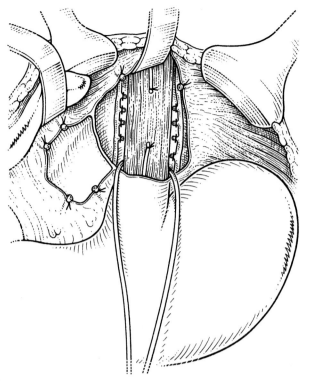

Fig. 94.6. Technique of esophageal exposure for devascularization. The diaphragm has been severed sagittally, and the pericardium has been freed from the diaphragm. A tape has been placed around the esophagus. The vagus nerves have been divided.

preclude the use of a large size stapler. In our practice, a 29-mm circular stapler is most frequently used. A smaller stapler (25 mm) is indicated in patients treated by previous sclerotherapy (Mariette et al, 1994). We routinely conclude paraesophagogastric devascularization by performing a Nissen fundoplication to prevent reflux, which might be caused by extensive dissection of the cardia. Fundoplication allows wrapping of the transection line. Pyloroplasty, which can be achieved without mucosal opening, is performed because both vagus nerves have been divided. Wedge liver biopsy is performed. A nasogastric tube is left in the antrum, and the abdominal incision is closed without drainage.

In the postoperative period, total parenteral nutrition is instituted and administered for 7 days. On postoperative day 7, the patient is administered a meglumine diatrizoate meal to check the patency of the transection line and the lack of fistulae. Endoscopic examination of the esophagus is systematically performed 3 weeks postoperatively, and dilation of any stricture is performed as required.

Results

Operative Mortality

The operative mortality of the Sugiura procedure performed electively varies from 0% to 22% (average 8%). This rate compares favorably with the operative mortality of various other abdominal operations performed in cirrhotic patients (Franzetta et al, 2003; Sirinek et al, 1987). When the operation is performed as an emergency procedure, however, the operative mortality increases dramatically to 36% (range 5-62%) (Table 94.1).

Table 94.1   Operative Mortality After the Sugiura Procedure

Reference	NO. PATIENTS			Cirrhotic Patients (%)	OPERATIVE MORTALITY (%)		
	Total	Elective	Emergency		Total	Elective	Emergency
Peracchia et al, 1980	15	—	—	100	6	—	—
Ginsberg et al, 1982	20	13	7	95	20	—	57
Sugiura & Futagawa, 1984	671*	363	105	74	5	3	13
Al-Kraida et al, 1989	50	16	34	2	10	—	—
Kitano et al, 1992	32	32	0	84	—	—	—
Orozco et al, 1992	88	88	0	69	22	22	—
Triger et al, 1992	46	46	0	86	20†	20	—
Dagenais et al, 1994	21	12	9	62	10	—	22
Mariette et al, 1994	39	39	0	79	0	—	—
Mathur et al, 1997	65	0	65	31	28	—	28
Mercado et al, 1998	83	83	0	45	4	4	—
Kapoor et al, 1999	18‡	3	15	67	16.7	—	—
Mathur et al, 1999	68	30	38	0§	4.4	3	5
Mercado et al, 1999	14	14	0	100‖	21.4	—	—
Shah et al, 1999	14‖	9	5	0	0	—	—
Selzner et al, 2001	15¶	12	3	47	6.7	—	—

*Prophylatic procedure in 203 patients; these cases were excluded for analysis of the results.
†In the first 3 postoperative months.
‡Underunning of eosophageal varices instead of esophageal transection.
§Portal vein thrombosis in 46 patients and noncirrhotic portal fibrosis in 22 patients.
‖Portal vein thrombosis in all cases.
¶Portal vein thrombosis in 8 patients.

Table 94.2 Postoperative Complications After the Sugiura Procedure

Reference	Ascites (%)	Portal Vein Thrombosis (%)	Esophageal Fistulae (%)	Esophageal Stricture (%)
Hirashima et al, 1982	—	2	—	—
Koyama et al, 1980	11	—	—	—
Peracchia et al, 1980	—	6	—	28
Ginsberg et al, 1982	—	—	—	20
Sugiura & Futagawa, 1984	—	1	6	2
Abouna et al, 1987	—	—	8	8
Barbot & Rosato, 1987	18	—	14	11
Al-Kraida et al, 1989	—	—	—	13
Ancona et al, 1989	28	4	3	23
Orozco et al, 1991	—	—	11	—
Dagenais et al, 1994	—	—	14	24
Mariette et al, 1994	18	18*	0	28
Mathur et al, 1997	—	—	—	13
Mercado et al, 1998	—	—	7	11
Shah et al, 1999	—	—	7	14
Selzner et al, 2001	3.3	—	15.7	21

*Detected by systematic ultrasound.

Morbidity

Specific complications linked to the procedure are related mainly to cirrhosis (ascites formation and portal vein thrombosis) and esophageal transection (anastomotic leak and stricture). To avoid gastric and gut disorders after vagotomy, some authors have proposed to preserve pneumogastric nerves during the devascularization stage with good results (Dong et al, 2004). Postoperative ascites has been inconstantly and variably reported. The incidence of postoperative ascites ranges from 3.3% to 28% (Table 94.2).

In our experience, 2.6% of patients required a secondary peritoneovenous shunt. The risk of portal vein thrombosis after the Sugiura procedure has been emphasized by several authors (Hirashima et al, 1982; Kahwaji et al, 1986; Peracchia et al, 1980; Sugiura & Futagawa, 1984). Portal vein thrombosis may be linked to thrombocythemia or to a decrease in portal blood flow after splenectomy (Takenaka et al, 1990). The incidence ranges from 1% to 6% (see Table 94.2). In the literature, only symptomatic cases have been recognized, and these are

Table 94.3 Rebleeding Rate, Chronic Encephalopathy, and 5-Year Survival Rate After the Sugiura Procedure

Reference	Rebleeding Rate (%)	Chronic Encephalopathy (%)	Survival Rate (%)
Kitano et al, 1992	6*	—	84[†]
Orozco et al, 1992	6	3	70
Triger et al, 1992	32	—	58
Dagenais et al, 1994	26	0	100[‡]
Mariette et al, 1994	24*	0	70*
Mathur et al, 1997	6[§]	4	—
Mercado et al, 1998	14	—	82
Kapoor et al, 1999	17	7	72[‖]
Mathur et al, 1999	5	0	88[¶]
Mercado et al, 1999	11**	33	30
Shah et al, 1999	8.7	—	100[††]
Selzner et al, 2001	7	—	93

*At 5 years.
[†]At 40 months.
[‡]In Child A patients.
[§]At 33 months.
[‖]At 30 months.
[¶]Actuarial.
**At 36 months.
[††]At 38 months.

lethal (Mariette et al, 1994). The rate of esophageal fistulae ranges from 0% to 15.7% (see Table 94.2), and mortality is 15%. To decrease the risk of fistula, Sugiura and Futagawa (1984) advocated avoidance of esophageal transection in the days immediately after endoscopic sclerotherapy. Other authors (Alam et al, 1996) reported that one or two sessions of sclerotherapy before operation do not increase intraoperative difficulty or the postoperative leak rate. Mercado and colleagues (1998) proposed a modified transection by placing a circumferential running suture without opening the mucosa. The incidence of esophageal stricture varies and ranges from 2% to 28% (see Table 94.2). As stressed by Spence and Johnston (1985), and in our experience, stricture does not seem to be related to the extent of esophagogastric devascularization or to the size of the head of the stapler used (Mariette et al, 1994). In our practice, esophageal dilation is efficient therapy. We prefer to detect stricture endoscopically 3 weeks postoperatively and to dilate the anastomosis regardless of the severity of the stricture.

Eradication of Esophageal Varices and Rebleeding

The rate of endoscopic eradication of esophageal varices 3 months after the Sugiura procedure ranges from 50% to 91% (Abouna et al, 1987; Hosking & Johnson, 1987; Koyama et al, 1980; Koyanagi et al, 1988; Mariette et al, 1994). According to Koyanagi and coworkers (1988), esophageal varices recur in about 60% of cases at 3 years, and recurrence was 63% in our series (Mariette et al, 1994). The recurrent bleeding rate has not been reported clearly in the literature (Table 94.3). In our personal experience, the cumulative 5-year rate of patients free from variceal bleeding was 76%. No author has reproduced in a large series the low rebleeding rate of 1.5% originally reported by Sugiura and Futagawa (1984).

Chronic Encephalopathy and Survival

Chronic encephalopathy is an uncommon complication of this procedure except in the experience of Mercado and colleagues (1999) (see Table 94.3). The survival rate is good after the Sugiura procedure (58-100% at 5 years) (see Table 94.3). In our series, liver failure was a minor cause of late death, which indicates that the Sugiura procedure does not alter liver function significantly in cirrhotic patients (Mariette et al, 1994). Results of a prospective controlled trial conducted by our team and comparing the Sugiura procedure with side-to-side portacaval shunt in the elective treatment of recurrent variceal bleeding showed that the Sugiura procedure was equivalent to noncalibrated portacaval shunt in the prevention of variceal bleeding in cirrhotic patients, but it significantly prolonged survival (Borgonovo et al, 1996).

DIRECT OPERATION ON FUNDAL VARICES

Fundal varices usually are treated by esophagogastric devascularization and splenectomy, when a direct approach has been selected. This approach provides satisfactory results. In the experience of Tomikawa and associates (2000), in patients with cirrhosis, no major complication occurred, and gastric varices were eradicated in all patients. The 5-year survival rate was 76%. Han and coworkers (2004) reported an original technique for fundal variceal bleeding, combining fundectomy with periesophagogastric devascularization. In essence, splenectomy is performed through a left subcostal incision, followed by a periesophageal and perigastric devascularization. In addition, the left gastric vein and

artery are ligated at their origin. According to Han and coworkers (2004), the extent of the fundal resection is determined by palpation of the fundal varices under direct vision after the opening of the gastric wall. To avoid subsequent narrowing of the distal esophagus, the proximal limit of the fundal resection should remain 1 to 2 cm from the cardia. The fundectomy incision is closed with a two-layer suture. In the hands of Han and coworkers (2004), when the procedure was performed electively, the operative mortality was 18.2% in cirrhotic patients. It was 33% in urgent cases. With a mean follow-up of 32 ± 27 months, there was no recurrent bleeding. The 5-year survival rate was 76%.

REFERENCES

Abouna GM, et al, 1987: The place of Sugiura operation for portal hypertension and bleeding esophageal varices. Surgery 110:91-98.

Alam MK, et al, 1996: Effect of previous sclerotherapy on the outcome of gastro-esophageal devascularization and esophageal transection in bleeding esophageal varices. Br J Surg 83:1702-1705.

Al-Kraida A, et al, 1989: Transabdominal gastro-esophageal devascularization and esophageal transection for bleeding esophageal varices. Br J Surg 76:943-945.

Ancona E, et al, 1989: Risultati precoci e a distanza dell'intervento di devascolirizzazione esofago gastrica con transezione esofagea usato nella cura delle varici esofagee sanguinanti. Minerva Chir 44:117-122.

Barbot DJ, Rosato EF, 1987: Experience with the esophagogastric devascularization procedure. Surgery 101:685-690.

Boerema I, 1949: Surgical therapy of bleeding varices of esophagus during hepatic cirrhosis and Banti's disease. Ned Tijdschr Geneeskd 93:4174-4182.

Borgonovo G, et al, 1996: Comparison of a modified Sugiura procedure with portal systemic shunt for prevention of recurrent variceal bleeding in cirrhosis. Surgery 119:214-221.

Cello JP, et al, 1982: Endoscopic sclerotherapy versus esophageal transection in Child's class C patients with variceal hemorrhage: comparison with results of portacaval shunt: preliminary report. Surgery 91:333-338.

Chaudhary A, Aranya RC, 1991: Devascularization following endoscopic sclerotherapy of esophageal varices: dangers and difficulties. Br J Surg 78:1249-1251.

Cooperman M, et al, 1980: EEA esophageal stapling for control of bleeding esophageal varices. Am J Surg 140:821-824.

Crile G, 1950: Transesophageal ligation of bleeding esophageal varices. Arch Surg 61:654-660.

Dagenais M, et al, 1994: Experience with radical esophagogastric devascularization procedures (Sugiura) for variceal bleeding outside Japan. World J Surg 18:222-228.

Dong YH, et al, 2004: Clinical analysis of pericardial devascularization by preserving vagus trunks in 42 patients with portal hypertension. Asian J Surg 27:108-113.

Franco D, Smadja C, 1985: Prevention of recurrent variceal bleeding: surgical procedures. Clin Gastroenterol 14:233-257.

Franzetta M, et al, 2003: Prognostic factors of cirrhotic patients in extra-hepatic surgery. Minerva Chir 58:541-544.

Ginsberg RJ, et al, 1982: A modified Sugiura procedure. Ann Thorac Surg 34:258-264.

Han HS, et al, 2004: New operative method for fundal variceal bleeding: fundectomy with periesophagogastric devascularization. World J Surg 28:406-410.

Hassab MA, 1967: Gastro-esophageal decongestion and splenectomy in the treatment of esophageal varices in bilharzial cirrhosis: further studies with a report on 355 operations. Surgery 61:169-176.

Hassab MA, 1998: Gastro-esophageal decongestion and splenectomy GEDS (Hassab), in the management of bleeding varices. Int Surg 83:38-41.

Hirashima T, et al, 1982: A new stapling technique in esophageal varices in bilharzial cirrhosis: further studies with a report on 355 operations. Surgery 61:169-176.

Hosking SW, Johnson AG, 1987: What happens to esophageal varices after transection and devascularization? Surgery 101:531-534.

Johnston GW, 1994: Operative devascularization and esophageal transection. In Blumgart LH (ed): Surgery of the Liver and Biliary Tract, 2nd ed, vol 2. New York: Churchill-Livingstone, pp 1663-1674.

Johnston GW, Kelly JM, 1976: Early experience with the Boerema button for bleeding esophageal varices. Br J Surg 63:117-121.

Kahwaji F, et al, 1986: L'intervention de Sugiura: une exclusivité japonaise? Gastroenterol Clin Biol 10:633-636.

Kapoor R, et al, 1999: Transabdominal gastroesophageal devascularization without esophageal transection for emergency treatment of variceal hemorrhage. Indian J Gastroenterol 18:149-151.

Kitano S, et al, 1992: Sclerotherapy vs. esophageal transection vs. distal splenorenal shunt for the clinical management of esophageal varices in patients with Child class A and B liver function: a prospective randomized trial. Hepatology 15:63-68.

Koyama K, et al, 1980: Results of esophageal transection for esophageal varices: experience in 100 cases. Am J Surg 139:204-209.

Koyanagi N, et al, 1988: Recurrence of varices after esophageal transection: intraoperative and postoperative assessment by endoscopy. Br J Surg 75:9-11.

Kuzmak LI, 1981: Use of EEA stapler in transection of esophagus in severe hemorrhage from esophageal varices. Am J Surg 141:387-390.

Mariette D, et al, 1994: The Sugiura procedure: a prospective experience. Surgery 115:282-289.

Mathur SK, et al, 1997: Transabdominal extensive esophagogastric devascularization with gastro-esophageal stapling in the management of acute variceal bleeding. Br J Surg 84:413-417.

Mathur SK, et al, 1999: Transabdominal extensive esophagogastric devascularization with gastroesophageal stapling for management of noncirrhotic portal hypertension: long-term results. World J Surg 23:1168-1175.

Mercado MA, et al, 1998: Comparative study of 2 variants of a modified esophageal transection in the Sugiura-Futagawa operation. Arch Surg 133:1046-1049.

Mercado MA, et al, 1999: Results of surgical treatment (modified Sugiura-Futagawa operation) of portal hypertension associated to complete splenomesoportal thrombosis and cirrhosis. HPB Surg 11:157-162.

Orozco H, et al, 1991: The Sugiura procedure for patients with hemorrhagic portal hypertension secondary to extrahepatic portal vein thrombosis. Surg Gynecol Obstet 173:45-48.

Orozco H, et al, 1992: Elective treatment of bleeding varices with the Sugiura operation over 10 years. Am J Surg 163:585-589.

Peracchia A, et al, 1980: A new technique for the treatment of esophageal bleeding in portal hypertension. Int Surg 65:401-404.

Sarfeh IJ, Rypins EB, 1986: The emergency portacaval shunt H graft in alcoholic cirrhotic patients: influence of shunt diameter on clinical outcome. Am J Surg 152:290-293.

Selzner M, et al, 2001: Current indication of a modified Sugiura procedure in the management of variceal bleeding. J Am Coll Surg 193:166-173.

Shah SR, et al, 1999: Results of a modified Sugiura's devascularization in the management of unshuntable portal hypertension. HPB Surg 11:235-239.

Sirinek KR, et al, 1987: Improving survival in patients with cirrhosis undergoing major abdominal operations. Arch Surg 122:271-273.

Spence RAJ, 1984: The venous anatomy of the lower esophagus in normal subjects and in patients with varices: an image analysis study. Br J Surg 71:739-744.

Spence RAJ, Johnston GW, 1985: Results in 100 consecutive patients with stapled esophageal transection for varices. Surg Gynecol Obstet 160:323-329.

Spence RAJ, Terblanche J, 1987: Venous anatomy of the lower esophagus: a new perspective on varices. Br J Surg 74:659-660.

Spence RAJ, et al, 1983: Oesphageal mucosal changes in patients with varices. Gut 24:1024-1029.

Sugiura M, Futagawa S, 1973: A new technique for treating esophageal varices. J Thorac Cardiovasc Surg 66:677-685.

Sugiura M, Futagawa S, 1984: Esophageal transection with para-esophagogastric devascularization (the Sugiura procedure) in the treatment of esophageal varices. World J Surg 8:673-682.

Takenaka H, et al, 1990: Hemodynamic study after devascularization procedure in patients with esophageal varices. Surgery 107:55-62.

Tanner NC, 1961: Direct operations in the treatment of complications of portal hypertension. J Int Coll Surg 36:308-314.

Tomikawa M, et al, 2000: Effectiveness of gastric devascularization and splenectomy for patients with gastric varices. J Am Coll Surg 191:498-503.

Triger DR, et al, 1992: A prospective trial of endoscopic sclerotherapy v. esophageal transection and gastric devascularisation in the long term management of bleeding esophageal varices. Gut 33:1553-1558.

Umeyama K, et al, 1983: Transabdominal esophageal transection for esophageal varices: experience in 101 patients. Br J Surg 70:419-422.

Vankemmel M, 1974: Resection-anastomose de l'esophage sus-cardial pour rupture de varices esophagiennes. Nouv Presse Med 5:1123-1124.

Vons C, et al, 1996: Long-term hemodynamic effects of portocaval shunt and Sugiura procedure in patients with cirrhosis. HPB Surg 9:209-213.

Vosschulte K, 1957: Place de la section par ligature de l'esophage dans le traitement de l'hypertension portale. Lyon Chir 53:519-525.

Walker RM, 1964: Esophageal transection for bleeding varices. Surg Gynecol Obstet 118:323-329.

Wexler MJ, 1980: Treatment of bleeding esophageal varices by transabdominal esophageal transection with the EEA stapling instrument. Surgery 88:406-416.

Yamamoto S, et al, 1976: The late results of esophagoproximal gastrectomy (TERG) with extensive devascularisation and splenectomy for bleeding esophageal varices in cirrhosis. Surgery 80:106-114.

95

The Place of Portosystemic Shunting

S. J. KNECHTLE AND L. F. RIKKERS

Esophageal varices develop in patients with portal hypertension most commonly secondary to hepatic cirrhosis. They occur most frequently in the distal esophagus, although they may be accompanied by gastric varices. Rupture of varices is associated with massive upper gastrointestinal bleeding with attendant high mortality. Therapy aimed at the prevention and treatment of bleeding varices has included pharmacologic, endoscopic, radiologic, and surgical strategies. All of these therapies have evolved technically, and increasing clinical experience has resulted in more accurate definition of the role of each treatment modality. This chapter discusses the appropriate role of surgical shunts for the management of bleeding esophageal varices. An understanding of the role of surgical therapy also requires an understanding of the context in which it is applied, however. The natural history of bleeding esophageal varices is discussed first followed by a description of the roles of alternative therapies. In current medical practice, it is most appropriate to apply surgical shunts within the context of pharmacologic (see Ch. 91) and endoscopic therapy (see Ch. 92), transjugular intrahepatic portosystemic shunts (TIPS) (see Ch. 96), and liver transplantation (see Ch. 103). Many patients are treated sequentially with more than one modality. Algorithms are presented to help establish the appropriate clinical context for surgical shunt therapy.

NATURAL HISTORY OF ESOPHAGEAL VARICES

Esophageal varices may produce massive upper gastrointestinal bleeding that is difficult to control. Not all patients with varices bleed, and not all patients with cirrhosis or portal hypertension develop esophageal varices. Clinical studies sometimes have included control groups without medical intervention, and analysis of these trials has helped define the natural history of esophageal varices. In one series, 46% of 819 subjects with biopsy or clinical evidence of cirrhosis and no history of bleeding had esophageal varices by endoscopy (PROVA Study Group, 1991). Over time, varices may appear, disappear, or change in size depending on alterations in patient physiology. A study of 84 cirrhotics without previous bleeding who were followed by serial endoscopy over 2 years showed that 31% of patients without varices progressed to large varices over 2 years, whereas in 70% of patients with small varices, the varices enlarged after 2 years (Cales et al, 1990). Dagradi (1972) studied the influence of alcohol on varices in patients with cirrhosis and found that variceal length increased in 65% of drinking cirrhotics, but decreased in 80% of abstinent cirrhotics. Baker and colleagues (1959) reported that varices regress in 25%, disappear in 32%, and progress in 21% of patients with cirrhosis and varices followed by endoscopy.

Most bleeding episodes in long-term studies occur during the first 1 to 2 years after identification of varices (Baker et al, 1959; Groszmann et al, 1990; Siringo et al, 1994; Triger et al, 1991).

Average mortality after bleeding from esophageal varices is 23% at 1 year, 34% at 2 years, and 58% at 3 years. About one third of deaths in patients with known esophageal varices are due to upper gastrointestinal bleeding. A larger proportion die as a result of liver failure. The mortality directly attributable to variceal hemorrhage is 10% to 17% for cirrhotic patients (Baker et al, 1959; Sauerbruch et al, 1988; Triger et al, 1991). In patients with varices, upper gastrointestinal bleeding is due to variceal hemorrhage in roughly two thirds of patients (Gebhard, 1998). Most patients who bleed from varices do so within 2 years of the time that varices were identified. Clinical parameters associated with increased risk of hemorrhage and mortality from esophageal varices include large varices, varices with cherry red spots (Dagradi, 1972), concurrent gastric varices (Kleber et al, 1991), Child classification, and continued alcohol use (Dagradi, 1972). Mortality correlates more closely with Child classification (Merkel et al, 1989) than with any other parameter studied.

Rebleeding and mortality markedly increase after varices bleed. Studies have reported rebleeding rates to be 30% within 6 weeks of an initial variceal hemorrhage (Graham & Smith, 1981; The Copenhagen Esophageal Varices Sclerotherapy Project, 1984) and 60% to 75% within 1 year (Baker et al, 1959; Graham & Smith, 1981). Esophageal varices are the cause of bleeding in approximately 16% of hospital admissions for upper gastrointestinal bleeding (De Franchis et al, 1991). Mortality rates from all causes within 1 year of initial hemorrhage have been estimated at 40% to 66% (Burroughs et al, 1989; Graham & Smith, 1981; Le Moine et al, 1992; The Copenhagen Esophageal Varices Sclerotherapy Project, 1984). The risk of dying increases as the interval between initial and second hemorrhage decreases (Gebhard, 1998). If patients survive for more than 12 weeks after a variceal hemorrhage, the risk of rebleeding or dying returns to that of patients who have never bled (Gebhard, 1998).

PHARMACOLOGIC MANAGEMENT OF PORTAL HYPERTENSION

Prophylaxis

β-Blocker therapy has been studied to test its efficacy in preventing primary variceal hemorrhage in patients with known varices (see Ch. 91). Nadolol (Corgard; Bristol-Myers Squibb, Princeton, NJ) is a nonselective β-blocker (blocks β_1 and β_2 receptors); patients given nadolol were compared with untreated controls. The incidence of bleeding was reduced by nadolol from 35% ± 3% to 12% ± 3%, and the incidence of fatal bleeds was reduced from 18% ± 3% to 10% ± 2%. There was no difference in overall mortality (Poynard et al, 1991). This study is used to support the use of prophylactic β blockade to prevent a first variceal hemorrhage.

Nitrates are vasodilators whose action is mediated by nitric oxide on vascular smooth muscle. Nitroglycerin decreases portal pressure in patients with cirrhosis when high doses are used (Moreau et al, 1989). In animal studies, nitroglycerin lowered portal pressure 13%, and systemic blood pressure decreased 25%. This drug lowers portal pressure less than systemic pressure. Nitrates in combination with β blockade may offer prophylaxis against an initial variceal bleed.

Randomized controlled clinical trials comparing nonselective β-blockers, propranolol or nadolol, versus no therapy in cirrhotic patients showed that drug treatment effectively reduced the risk of a first variceal hemorrhage (Poynard et al, 1991). The combination of isosorbide mononitrate and β blockade further reduces portal pressure and has been shown in three studies to reduce effectively the risk of a first variceal bleed compared with β blockade alone (Garcia-Pagan et al, 1990; Villanueva et al, 1996; Vorobioff et al, 1993). These investigations have noted, however, the difficult problem of compliance, particularly in patients with alcoholism. In addition, fatigue may be a side effect of therapy with β blockade, and, even more seriously, if patients do bleed, their ability to compensate for blood loss by tachycardia is compromised.

Acute Variceal Hemorrhage

The posterior pituitary hormone vasopressin (Pitressin; Parke-Davis, Morris Plains, NJ) causes splanchnic arteriolar vasoconstriction, reducing portal blood pressure by about 15% when given intra-arterially or intravenously (Chojkier et al, 1979; Huet et al, 1987). Intravenous use is preferred for safety and convenience. The optimal dose of the drug is 0.3 to 0.4 U/min intravenously. As a result of simultaneous vasoconstrictive effects on the cardiac, mesenteric, and cerebral circulations, the complications increase when doses of 0.5 to 0.7 U/min are administered. It is not necessary to taper the dose. The infusion can be stopped when the therapeutic end point is reached. In a controlled study comparing vasopressin with no therapy, approximately half of patients on vasopressin stopped bleeding, but this result did not differ from control subjects (Chojkier et al, 1979; Fogel et al, 1982).

Octreotide reduces bleeding (D'Amico et al, 1995) and enhances the results of sclerotherapy (Besson et al, 1995). Somatostatin and octreotide (Sandostatin; Sandoz, East Hanover, NJ) are endogenous peptides that act by reducing splanchnic, hepatic, and azygos blood flow (Bosch et al, 1981). Their principal advantage over vasopressin is that they do not cause vasoconstriction of the myocardial and cerebral circulations. Somatostatin and octreotide should be administered continuously at 250 μg/hr and increased to 500 μg/hr if bleeding continues. Preliminary studies showed that octreotide helped arrest acute variceal bleeding in six of six patients (Thulin et al, 1979; Tyden et al, 1978). Randomized controlled trials comparing somatostatin or octreotide with vasopressin versus no infusion have given equivocal results, which suggest that vasopressin and somatostatin have similar efficacy (Burroughs, 1996; Burroughs et al, 1990; Imperiale et al, 1995). Neither vasopressin nor somatostatin has been approved by the U.S. Food and Drug Administration for treatment of variceal bleeding, although both agents are commonly used for this purpose (Korula, 1998). A prospective randomized trial showed equivalence of somatostatin and sclerotherapy in the treatment of acute variceal bleeding (Planas et al, 1994).

Prevention of Rebleeding after Initial Control

Propranolol (Inderal; Wyeth-Ayerst, Philadelphia, PA) was shown by Lebrec and colleagues (1980, 1981) to reduce rebleeding significantly after acute variceal hemorrhage. This effect may be mediated by a decrease in cardiac output (β_1 blockade), increased splanchnic arteriolar resistance (β_2 blockade), and consequent decrease in portal blood flow (Lebrec et al, 1982) and collateral blood flow via the azygos venous system (Feu et al, 1993). β blockade is not widely used in the United States to prevent rebleeding after an episode of variceal hemorrhage because endoscopic sclerotherapy and ligation are preferred. β blockade after acute bleeding has not been shown to reduce mortality (Pagliaro et al, 1989). Meta-analysis comparing β blockade with endoscopic sclerotherapy showed a nonstatistically significant decrease in pooled relative risk for bleeding in the sclerotherapy group and no difference in mortality between the two groups (D'Amico et al, 1995). A randomized controlled study showed, however, that isosorbide mononitrate (80 mg/day) in combination with nadolol (80 mg/day) was more effective than sclerotherapy in reducing rebleeding (Villanueva et al, 1996). Complications were less frequent in the group treated with drugs (16% versus 37%). If this study is confirmed by other investigators, pharmacologic therapy may play a larger role in the United States in prevention of rebleeding than it currently does.

ENDOSCOPIC THERAPY OF VARICEAL HEMORRHAGE

Prophylaxis

The use of sclerotherapy prophylactically to prevent a first hemorrhage was studied in three meta-analyses (see Ch. 92) (Fardy & Laupacis, 1994; Pagliaro et al, 1989; Van Ruiswyk & Byrd, 1992). One study concluded that paravariceal injection with polidocanol decreased mortality (Fardy & Laupacis, 1994). The other two reports found that prophylactic sclerotherapy did not reduce bleeding or mortality and concluded that sclerotherapy was not indicated in this setting (D'Amico et al, 1995; Pagliaro et al, 1989; Van Ruiswyk & Byrd, 1992). The largest trial of prophylactic sclerotherapy was the Veterans Affairs (VA) cooperative trial. This trial, which included 281 patients, was prematurely closed because of excess mortality in the sclerotherapy group (The Veterans Affairs Cooperative Variceal Sclerotherapy Group, 1991). Sclerotherapy prevented variceal hemorrhage, but substituted bleeding from sclerotherapy-induced ulceration. This study effectively ended the use of prophylactic sclerotherapy in the United States.

Acute Variceal Hemorrhage

When it became apparent that emergency surgical shunts, the previously dominant therapy for variceal hemorrhage, were not improving survival, but rather substituting death from liver failure for death from bleeding, endoscopic variceal injection was evaluated as a less invasive therapy. In 1980, a prospective randomized trial in 107 patients from King's College Hospital showed control of bleeding by sclerotherapy in 57% of 51 treated patients compared with 25% of 56 patients treated medically (MacDougall et al, 1982). Two years later, a follow-up study

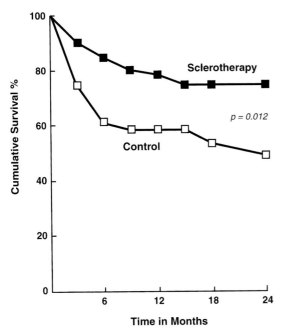

Fig. 95.1. Effect of sclerotherapy on survival in patients with cirrhosis: the King's College Hospital and Medical School Trial. Cumulative survivals in sclerotherapy patients ($n = 51$) and controls ($n = 56$) are shown. Control group patients received standard medical treatment, including blood transfusions, vasopressin, and Sengstaken-Blakemore tubes when necessary. (From MacDougall BR, et al, 1982: Increased long-term survival in variceal haemorrhage using injection sclerotherapy: results of a controlled trial. Lancet 1:124-127.)

showed improved patient survival with sclerotherapy compared with controls who received blood transfusions, vasopressin, and a Sengstaken-Blakemore tube when necessary (Fig. 95.1).

It is important when interpreting this trial and subsequent trials to understand that the King's College trial had more non-alcoholic patients than alcoholic patients (60 versus 47) and had patients with relatively mild liver failure (74 Child A and B; 33 Child C). The more patients in any study of variceal hemorrhage who are alcoholic or who have Child C liver disease, the more difficult it is to show a survival advantage of therapy. Death from bleeding in such patients tends to be replaced by death from liver failure (Block & Reichelderfer, 1998). The VA cooperative study showed no reduction of long-term survival when acute hemorrhage was treated with sclerotherapy (The Veterans Affairs Cooperative Variceal Sclerotherapy Group, 1994).

Sclerotherapy has been shown to stop acute variceal hemorrhage effectively (Gregory, 1990; Westaby et al, 1989). Meta-analysis of 20 trials of emergency sclerotherapy versus a variety of alternative therapies supported the superiority of sclerotherapy with a success rate of 71% to 100%. The complication rate was high (18%), however, with 2.7% of patients dying as a direct result of sclerotherapy (D'Amico et al, 1995).

Endoscopic variceal ligation (EVL) has been developed as an endoscopic alternative to sclerotherapy, potentially lowering the risk of ulceration and perforation of the esophagus. Seven prospective randomized controlled trials compared EVL with endoscopic sclerotherapy (Gimson et al, 1993; Hashizume et al, 1993; Hou et al, 1995; Laine et al, 1993; Lo et al, 1995, 1997; Stiegmann et al, 1992). In all studies, EVL and sclerotherapy were equally effective in controlling active bleeding. Complications were significantly lower with EVL in all studies. No esophageal strictures

were seen in patients treated with EVL compared with 5% to 33% of patients treated with sclerotherapy.

Prevention of Rebleeding

Although sclerotherapy effectively stops acute variceal bleeding, rebleeding remains a problem, and intermediate (2-5 year) survival is not improved in many trials. A confounding variable confusing interpretation of the results in many of these trials is continued alcoholism. Alcohol abstinence for 6 months, Child score, and aspartate aminotransferase level all were independent predictors of survival in the VA trial (The Veterans Affairs Cooperative Variceal Sclerotherapy Group, 1994). Meta-analyses of trials comparing sclerotherapy with pharmacologic management have shown sclerotherapy to prevent rebleeding more effectively and sometimes to improve survival (D'Amico et al, 1995; Infante-Rivard et al, 1989). When EVL was compared with sclerotherapy, rebleeding rates were significantly decreased with EVL in three studies (Gimson et al, 1993; Hou et al, 1995; Lo et al, 1995), and mortality rates were significantly lower in three studies (Hou et al, 1995; Lo et al, 1995; Stiegmann et al, 1992). EVL seems to be at least as effective as sclerotherapy in preventing rebleeding.

TRANSJUGULAR INTRAHEPATIC PORTOSYSTEMIC SHUNT

The development and clinical use of TIPS in the treatment of portal hypertension first occurred in the 1990s, and its use for the treatment of variceal hemorrhage has expanded (see Ch. 96) (LaBerge et al, 1992; McCormick et al, 1994). TIPS is used electively far more often than in the emergency setting. The broad application of TIPS is shown by the fact that over 10 years at our institution, more than 400 TIPS have been placed; during the same time period, less than 50 surgical shunts and more than 1000 liver transplants have been performed. In short, TIPS has been used extensively and has reduced the number of surgical shunts performed. Despite the effectiveness of TIPS in abruptly stopping variceal hemorrhage, overall patient mortality remains high (Smith & Graham, 1982). Death often is related to multisystem organ failure, progressive liver failure or sepsis, or disseminated intravascular coagulation, reflecting the use of TIPS in patients with end-stage disease. Complications usually are related to the underlying cirrhosis and associated comorbidities. In addition to relieving variceal hemorrhage, TIPS effectively relieves ascites in these patients (Crenshaw et al, 1996; Martin M et al, 1993) because TIPS is functionally a nonselective side-to-side portacaval shunt. In contrast to all surgical shunts, TIPS creates a shunt to the suprahepatic inferior vena cava (Fig. 95.2).

TIPS has developed as a minimally invasive procedure performed by radiologists using fluoroscopic imaging to place a noncompressible stent between the portal vein and hepatic vein. Successful TIPS lowers portal pressure, and the procedure is typically well tolerated even in very sick patients. Complications include encephalopathy secondary to portosystemic shunting, shunt stenosis and occlusion, inability to place a TIPS, and intraperitoneal bleeding if the liver capsule is punctured. Mortality at 30 days has been reported at 20%, but half of these deaths were unrelated to the procedure itself (Darcy et al, 1993). Thirty-day mortality of 67% has been reported in patients with

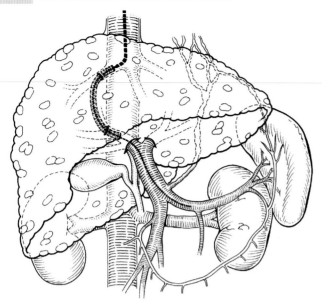

Fig. 95.2. TIPS creates an intrahepatic portosystemic shunt from the portal vein to the hepatic vein, held open by a titanium stent.

Child C cirrhosis (Martin L et al, 1993; Martin M et al, 1993). In a lower risk population of 100 patients, a 30-day mortality of 5.3% was reported (Richter et al, 1994).

Primary patency (patency without radiologic intervention to revise the TIPS) has been reported to be 46% to 85% in the first 3 to 6 months (Richter et al, 1994; Saxon et al, 1993; Sterling & Darcy, 1995) and 27% to 57% at 1 year (Haskal et al, 1994; Malisch et al, 1993; Saxon et al, 1993; Sterling & Darcy, 1995). Primary assisted patency (meaning patency after revision) has been reported at 85% (Haskal et al, 1994). La Berge and colleagues (1995) reported shunt stenosis or occlusion in 47% of 90 TIPS patients over a 2-year period. Shunt stenosis occurs in many patients because the shunt itself, which is held open by a Wallstent, is not lined by endothelium and undergoes progressive fibrosis with narrowing. Efforts are under way to develop methods of covering the lumen of the shunt with an endothelial lining. If post-TIPS ultrasound shows narrowing or thrombosis of the shunt, patency can be restored by repeat balloon dilation and stenting or by thrombectomy. Color Doppler ultrasound of TIPS is routinely performed at 1-month and at 6-month intervals postprocedure to evaluate luminal narrowing or increased flow velocity, which would suggest impending thrombosis of the TIPS. The rate of TIPS restenosis or occlusion is higher than the rate of recurrent symptoms because in some patients occlusion does not produce symptoms. Nevertheless, recurrent variceal hemorrhage occurs in about 50% of patients with TIPS stenosis or occlusion. A multicenter trial of TIPS involving 100 patients reported that 16% of patients had rebleeding by 6 months, and 5 of these were from nonvariceal sources (Coldwell et al, 1995). Similarly, La Berge and colleagues (1995) reported variceal rebleeding in 32% of 90 patients at 2 years.

Prophylaxis of Bleeding with Transjugular Intrahepatic Portosystemic Shunt

The ability of TIPS to prevent an initial variceal hemorrhage has not been studied. Patients awaiting liver transplantation who have intractable ascites are often treated with TIPS, however, as a means of bridging to liver transplantation. Although not a true study of prophylaxis, such patients seem to be at low risk of bleeding.

Acute Variceal Bleeding and Transjugular Intrahepatic Portosystemic Shunt

TIPS may be used effectively in the control of acute variceal hemorrhage when medical management or sclerotherapy or both are ineffective. Barton and coworkers (1995) found that TIPS controlled acute variceal bleeding in 91% of patients, whereas Helton and associates (1993) reported control in 17 of 23 (74%) patients. A report by Encarnacion and colleagues (1995) summarized 65 patients with acute variceal bleeding unresponsive to sclerotherapy or not treated with sclerotherapy because of recurrent massive hemorrhage. Acute bleeding stopped before the TIPS procedure in 26 patients, but not in 39 patients. Of the 65 patients, 64 had successful placement of TIPS, and all of these patients stopped bleeding within 3 days. The 30-day survival of patients who stopped bleeding before TIPS was 96%, but only 69% for patients actively bleeding at the time of TIPS. Survival also was linked to Child class with 91% 30-day survival for Child A ($n = 2$) and Child B ($n = 32$) patients, but 71% survival for Child C ($n = 31$) patients.

When used as primary therapy for acute variceal bleeding, TIPS may reduce treatment failure and mortality in high-risk patients. Monescillo and coworkers (2004) reported that in patients defined as high risk by hepatic venous pressure gradient greater than 20 mm Hg, and randomized to treatment with TIPS ($n = 26$) versus non-TIPS ($n = 26$), the non-TIPS group required more transfusions ($n = 0.002$), needed more intensive care unit care, had more treatment failures, and had poorer survival ($P < .05$). Non-TIPS patients were treated with β-blockers, variceal banding, or sclerotherapy.

Prevention of Rebleeding by Transjugular Intrahepatic Portosystemic Shunt

TIPS has been used most frequently to prevent recurrent variceal hemorrhage. The results of four large series are shown in Table 95.1 (Henderson et al, 1998). Rebleeding rates are similar in these series and are approximately 25% at 1 year. Thirty-day mortality rates were 14% to 16% except for the Rossle series (Rossle et al, 1994). Most deaths within 30 days were due to multisystem organ failure, whereas most later deaths were due to progressive liver failure. Because TIPS is a nonselective shunt, encephalopathy rates were relatively high at 25%, although in most patients, this was not debilitating.

Most episodes of rebleeding after TIPS were related to stenosis or thrombosis of the shunt. In addition, many asymptomatic patients had shunt stenosis or thrombosis detected by ultrasound. Primary patency was 40% to 67% at 1 year, which improved to 79% to 88% with revision of stenotic stents (assisted primary patency). Secondary patency, referring to patency after TIPS thrombectomy or revision, was 95% to 100% at 1 year (Coldwell et al, 1995; Fillmore et al, 1996; LaBerge et al, 1995; Rossle et al, 1994).

In a short time, TIPS has had a dramatic impact on the treatment of variceal hemorrhage. In addition to its use in preventing variceal hemorrhage, TIPS has the added benefit of often

Table 95.1 Patency of Transjugular Intrahepatic Portosystemic Shunt for Prevention of Recurrent Bleeding

Reference	Mean Follow-up Time	No. Patients (Child C)	Technical Success (%)	Procedure Deaths	Encephalopathy (%)	30-Day Mortality Rate (%)	Survival Rate (%)	Rebleed (%)	Primary Patency (%)	Assisted Primary Patency* (%)	Secondary Patency (%)†
Coldwell et al, 1995	6 mo	96 (34)	100	2	29	14	77‡	16‡	67	88	—‡
LaBerge et al, 1995	1.2 yr	94 (42)	95	0	25	16	60§ 51‖	26§ 32‖	66 42	83 79	96§ 90‖
Rossle et al, 1994	1 yr	100 (22)	93	1	25	3	85§	8‡ 18§	67	—	100§
Fillmore et al, 1996	8 mo	53 (21)	94	0	8	16	72¶	24**	40 16	— —	100‡ 95§

*Includes revised stenotic stents.
†Includes revised stenotic and thrombosed stents.
‡At 6 months.
§At 1 year.
‖At 2 years.
¶At 3 months.
**At 8 months.
From Henderson JM, et al, 1998: Portal hypertension. Curr Probl Surg 35:384-452.

improving overall liver function as measured by Child status and effectively bridging a patient to liver transplantation (Aboujoud et al, 1995; Menegaux et al, 1994; Millis et al, 1995; Odorico, 1998; Suc et al, 1995). Despite the suggestion that TIPS may reduce operative time and blood loss during liver transplantation, data are not yet available to support this contention. Nevertheless, it has been shown that the TIPS procedure effectively prevents rebleeding (D'Amico et al, 1995; Ring et al, 1992).

TIPS has been compared with endoscopic therapy for the long-term prevention of recurrent bleeding. In a meta-analysis of 11 randomized trials, fewer patients rebled after TIPS (19%) than after endoscopic therapy (47%), and encephalopathy was more common after TIPS (34%). TIPS dysfunction developed in 50% of patients overall (Papatheodoridis et al, 1999).

TIPS also has been compared with shunt surgery. The distal splenorenal shunt showed lower rates of rebleeding, encephalopathy, and shunt thrombosis than TIPS, but ascites was less common after TIPS (Khaitiyar et al, 2000). A multi-institutional, randomized trial compared TIPS with the distal splenorenal shunt in Child A and B cirrhotic patients (Henderson et al, 2004). Initial analysis of the results showed no significant differences between TIPS and the distal splenorenal shunt in variceal rebleeding, shunt occlusion, and survival. Of TIPS patients, 80% required reintervention to maintain shunt patency, however, and close surveillance was required.

TIPS also has been compared with the small-diameter interposition shunt. In this controlled trial, shunt occlusion, death from hepatic failure, and the need for liver transplantation all were significantly more common after TIPS (Rosemurgy et al, 2000). Indications for TIPS supported by current data include (1) continued variceal hemorrhage in a patient after sclerotherapy or banding, (2) prevention of rebleeding (or treatment of ascites) in a patient awaiting liver transplantation, and (3) prevention of rebleeding in a patient who is not a candidate for a surgical shunt or for liver transplantation because of expected short survival.

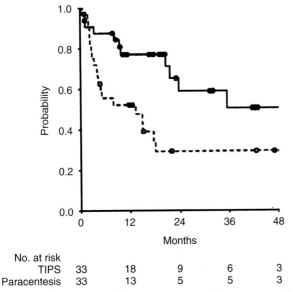

Fig. 95.3. Probability of survival without transplantation in patients assigned to TIPS treatment *(continuous line)* and patients assigned to paracentesis plus albumin *(dotted line).* The probability was superior in patients treated with TIPS (*P*=.021).
(From Salerno F, et al, 2004: Randomized controlled study of TIPS versus paracentesis plus albumin in cirrhosis with severe ascites. Hepatology 40:629-635.)

Treatment of Ascites with Transjugular Intrahepatic Portosystemic Shunt

TIPS has been used effectively to relieve ascites in patients refractory to pharmacologic therapy with diuretics. Salerno and associates (2004) reported a multicenter, randomized, controlled trial comparing TIPS (*n* = 33) with paracentesis plus albumin (*n* = 33) in patients with Child-Pugh B and C cirrhosis. Survival without liver transplantation was superior in patients treated with TIPS (*P*=.021) (Fig. 95.3). By multivariate analysis, a higher MELD (Model End-stage Liver Disease) score and paracentesis independently predicted death. Treatment failure was more common in patients treated with paracentesis, although encephalopathy occurred more commonly in patients receiving TIPS (Salerno et al, 2004).

SURGICAL SHUNTS FOR BLEEDING ESOPHAGEAL VARICES

Prophylactic Surgery

Early trials of prophylaxis for variceal bleeding compared portacaval shunts with medical therapy. Although bleeding was effectively prevented, survival was not enhanced significantly with surgery because of a marked increase in deaths secondary to accelerated hepatic failure (Grace, 1992). Because only one third of patients with varices eventually bleed, surgery cannot be justified as prophylaxis and is not recommended in this setting.

In a prospective controlled study to evaluate prophylactic surgery in 112 patients with portal hypertension and esophageal varices, Inokuchi (1984) found the bleeding rates were 19.2% in the medical group and 0% in the surgical group. There was no difference in the survival rate between the two groups at the time of 2-year follow-up. Prophylactic surgery led to a prevention of esophageal bleeding without any increase in the mortality rates. This is the only study to support a role for prophylactic surgery.

Acute Variceal Hemorrhage

At most U.S. centers, endoscopic therapy is the first option used to treat bleeding esophageal varices. An exception is the series reported by Orloff and coworkers (1994), who employed portacaval shunts as first-line therapy with excellent results. At most other centers, patients who fail sclerotherapy are referred for consideration of a TIPS or possibly a surgical shunt. Emergency surgical shunts prevent bleeding more effectively than sclerotherapy, but overall mortality is equivalent (Cello et al, 1987; D'Amico et al, 1995).

Although nonoperative therapies are useful for initial management of bleeding esophageal varices, if these measures fail to control bleeding, emergency surgery should be done promptly (Rikkers & Jin, 1994). Emergency surgical shunts normalize portal pressure immediately and effectively control variceal hemorrhage. Emergency surgery has been associated, however, with a mortality rate of 20% to 55% (Cello et al, 1987; D'Amico et al, 1995). The high risk of dying after an emergency shunt presumably is related to the frequent decompensation of liver function and associated comorbidity at the time of an acute bleed. Outcomes correlate with Child classification rather than with the type of shunt performed. Liver failure and encephalopathy often ensue and are the proximate causes of mortality associated with emergency surgery in most series.

In choosing which surgical shunt to use for emergency control of bleeding, the portacaval shunt (see Ch. 97) is an acceptable choice because it effectively decompresses the portal venous system and usually can be rapidly constructed. An end-to-side portacaval shunt is adequate, although patients with ascites should have a side-to-side portacaval shunt (see Chs. 99 and 100) to relieve their ascites as well. Orloff and coworkers' (1994) series showed the usefulness of the portacaval shunt in the emergency setting. Other functional side-to-side shunts, such as the mesocaval shunt (see Ch. 99) and proximal splenorenal shunt (see Ch. 98), also effectively decompress the portal vein and relieve esophageal variceal bleeding. In contrast to portacaval shunts, these shunts do not require dissection in the porta hepatis and do not complicate future liver transplantation. In appropriately selected patients, a distal splenorenal shunt also may be used in the emergency setting to relieve variceal hemorrhage in patients with a large patent splenic vein and absent or medically controlled ascites (Rikkers & Jin, 1995).

Prevention of Rebleeding after Initial Control

In view of the disadvantages of emergency shunts, the more attractive role of surgical shunts is in the elective setting to prevent recurrent variceal hemorrhage. Because the natural history of variceal hemorrhage places patients who have bled once at high risk for rebleeding, definitive therapy ought to be considered after control of the acute hemorrhage. In an appropriately selected patient, surgical shunts substantially reduce the risk of recurrent bleeding, maintain stable liver function, and obviate repeated endoscopic procedures. Depending on whether shunts completely divert, partially divert, or compartmentalize the portal venous circulation, they are characterized as nonselective, partial, or selective. Relative to nonselective shunts, the goal of partial and selective shunts is to preserve hepatic portal perfusion and minimize the risk of progressive liver failure and encephalopathy, while preventing variceal bleeding.

General Aspects of Nonselective Shunts

The end-to-side portacaval shunt (see Ch. 97) was the first experimental shunt performed in dogs by Eck (Konstantinov, 1997). This shunt is the prototype of the nonselective shunt and has been compared in randomized controlled trials with conventional medical management for the treatment of portal hypertension and its complications (Rikkers et al, 1992). Fig. 95.4 shows combined data of four controlled studies of the portacaval shunt comparing shunted patients with medically managed patients according to survival. No survival advantage could be shown for shunt patients, although the four studies all were biased in favor of medical management because failures of medical management were crossed over to surgical therapy. Bleeding was effectively stopped in shunt patients, whereas more than 70% of medically treated patients rebled. Encephalopathy occurred in 20% to 40% of shunted patients.

When the end-to-side portacaval shunt was compared with the side-to-side shunt in a controlled trial, no significant clinical differences were noted between these two shunts (Resnick et al, 1974). The interposition mesocaval shunt (see Ch. 99), also a nonselective

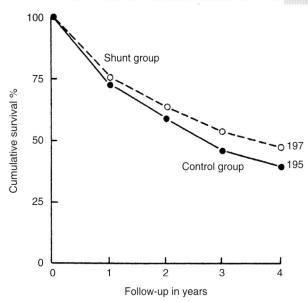

Fig. 95.4. Cumulative survival data from four controlled trials of portacaval shunt versus conventional medical management.
(Courtesy of HO Conn.)
(From Boyer TD, 1982: Portal hypertension and its complications: bleeding esophageal varices, ascites, and spontaneous bacterial peritonitis. In Zakim D, Boyer TD (eds): Hepatology: A Textbook of Liver Disease. Philadelphia, Saunders, pp 464-499.)

shunt, was studied in a randomized trial comparing it with the direct side-to-side portacaval shunt, with no clinical or hemodynamic differences shown in this study (Stipa et al, 1981). The same series documented a high graft thrombosis rate after the mesocaval shunt (Stipa et al, 1981). Nevertheless, the mesocaval shunt avoids dissection in the porta hepatis, which is an advantage for future liver transplant candidates. An additional option is a central or proximal splenorenal shunt with splenectomy. In the current era, indications for a nonselective shunt include an emergency shunt for variceal hemorrhage, an elective shunt in the presence of significant ascites, and treatment of Budd-Chiari syndrome. In some patients not suited for a selective shunt, a nonselective shunt might serve as a long-term bridge to hepatic transplantation when bleeding is not controlled endoscopically or by TIPS.

Budd-Chiari syndrome (see Ch. 100) with ascites, abdominal pain, and portal hypertension is an indication for a side-to-side portacaval shunt. A side-to-side shunt is necessary because the portal vein serves as the major efferent conduit in this syndrome. If the disease is fulminant or if cirrhosis has developed secondary to long-standing hepatic venous occlusion, liver transplantation is a preferable option. If liver transplantation is not anticipated, a side-to-side portacaval shunt may be the ideal procedure. Often the caudate lobe enlarges after occlusion of the major hepatic veins because the caudate lobe communicates directly with the vena cava and may become the major route of venous outflow from the liver. Massive hypertrophy of the caudate lobe may prevent a side-to-side portacaval shunt from being technically possible owing to caudal expansion of the caudate lobe, which is interposed between the portal vein and the inferior vena cava, preventing their side-to-side anastomosis. A mesocaval shunt may be technically more feasible in this setting. In situations in which Budd-Chiari syndrome involves occlusion of the hepatic portion of the inferior vena cava, the infrahepatic vena cava develops collaterals to the azygos venous system.

These collaterals permit the portal circulation to be decompressed into the inferior vena cava via a mesocaval shunt, and a mesoatrial shunt generally is not required in such patients. Although a mesoatrial shunt circumvents an occluded inferior vena cava, it is a long shunt with a poor patency rate and has been associated with poor outcomes. Successful management of Budd-Chiari syndrome requires accurate diagnosis and treatment of the underlying hypercoagulable state. Anticoagulation is necessary to prevent shunt thrombosis.

General Aspects of Distal Splenorenal Shunt

Warren and colleagues (1967) introduced the distal splenorenal shunt (see Ch. 98) with the goal of preserving hepatopetal blood flow in the portal vein, while decompressing esophageal varices. The distal splenic vein is anastomosed to the left renal vein, and collateral vessels, such as coronary and gastroepiploic veins connecting the superior mesenteric and gastrosplenic components of the splanchnic venous circulation, are ligated (Fig. 95.5). This procedure compartmentalizes the portal venous circulation into a high-pressure superior mesenteric venous system perfusing the liver and a decompressed gastrosplenic venous system to avoid variceal bleeding.

In patients with advanced ascites, the distal splenorenal shunt is contraindicated because lymphatics are transected during the dissection of the left renal vein, and the liver continues to have elevated sinusoidal pressures. In such patients, the distal splenorenal shunt may worsen rather than relieve ascites. Warren's claim that the operation effectively accomplishes its goal of preserving hepatic function better compared with nonselective shunts

Ligated coronary vein

Distal splenorenal shunt

Ligated inferior mesenteric vein

Ligated right gastroepiploic vein

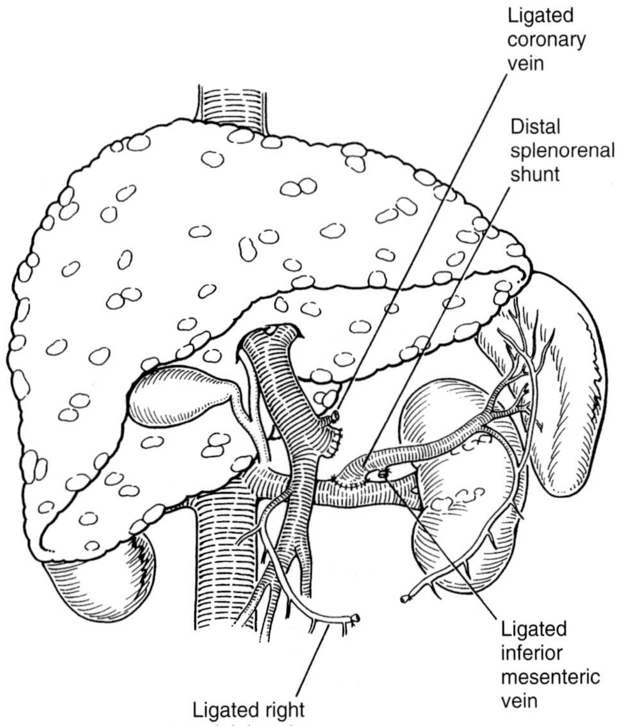

Fig. 95.5. Distal splenorenal shunt requires ligation of the coronary vein. Drainage of the splenic vein is into the left renal vein. The right gastroepiploic vein also is ligated and divided.
(From Knechtle SJ, 1998: Surgical shunts for portal hypertension. In Knechtle SJ (ed): Portal Hypertension: A Multidisciplinary Approach to Current Clinical Management. Armonk, NY, Futura, pp 175-202.)

remains controversial. Controlled trials have shown decreased postshunt portosystemic encephalopathy after the distal splenorenal shunt. Henderson and associates (1983) showed that portal flow is maintained in most patients with nonalcoholic cirrhosis and noncirrhotic portal hypertension, but that portal flow rapidly collateralizes to the shunt in patients with alcoholic cirrhosis. Failure to ligate the coronary vein results in early loss of hepatopetal portal flow. Despite surgical interruption of collaterals connecting the superior mesenteric venous system to the gastrosplenic system, collaterals gradually develop through a pancreatic network termed the *pancreatic siphon*. Surgical splenopancreatic disconnection improves selectivity of the distal splenorenal shunt, especially in alcoholic cirrhotics, but clinical benefits of this extension of the procedure have not been clearly shown.

Visceral angiography or computed tomography angiography should be done in any patient being considered for a surgical shunt, especially before a distal splenorenal shunt. A distal splenorenal shunt requires a patent splenic vein, preferably at least 7 mm in diameter. Patients who have undergone splenectomy or who have a thrombosed splenic vein are not candidates for this shunt procedure.

Controlled trials comparing the distal splenorenal with nonselective shunts have evaluated mostly alcoholic cirrhotic patients in six of the seven studies and are summarized by Jin and Rikkers (1991). None of these trials showed a survival advantage of either procedure. Four of the seven trials showed less encephalopathy after a selective shunt, whereas the other trials showed no difference in encephalopathy rates. Rebleeding rates did not differ between the two shunt groups, although one trial noted a higher rate of rebleeding after distal splenorenal shunt.

When the distal splenorenal shunt was compared with repeated endoscopic therapy, rebleeding was less frequent with selective shunts, but hepatic portal perfusion was better maintained by sclerotherapy. Encephalopathy rates were similar in both groups (Henderson et al, 1990; Rikkers et al, 1993). These two studies suggest that sclerotherapy effectively controls initial bleeding, but that patients who fail sclerotherapy should undergo surgery promptly. Another indication for surgery rather than sclerotherapy is in patients with poor access to advanced medical care. Such patients benefit from an initial selective shunt rather than long-term sclerotherapy because the latter requires multiple visits to a medical center.

Partial Shunt

The partial shunt proposed by Sarfeh and colleagues (1986) is a means of decompressing varices while preserving hepatic portal perfusion. An 8- or 10-mm polytetrafluoroethylene graft is interposed between the portal vein and inferior vena cava. A prospective randomized trial of partial (8-mm diameter) and nonselective (16-mm diameter) interposition portacaval shunts showed a lower frequency of encephalopathy after the partial shunt, but similar survival after both types of shunts (Sarfeh & Rypins, 1994).

TYPES OF SHUNTS: TECHNICAL ASPECTS

Portacaval Shunt

Nonselective portacaval shunts can be performed using a side-to-side method, an end-to-side method, or an interposition graft to create a functional side-to-side shunt (see Ch. 97).

Side-to-side shunts have the advantage of relieving ascites by reducing intrahepatic sinusoidal pressure in addition to decreasing the portal venous pressure gradient. They also are effective in decompressing varices and preventing recurrent bleeding from varices. The current recommended indication for a portacaval shunt would be a patient with significant ascites and bleeding varices unresponsive to nonsurgical treatment who would not be a future candidate for a liver transplant. Patients in whom a liver transplant eventually may be done ideally should not be treated with such a shunt, but rather a shunt in which the dissection is performed outside of the porta hepatis. Portacaval shunts involving dissection in the hilum of the liver inevitably result in postoperative scarring in the hilum and make subsequent liver transplantation more difficult with added potential morbidity and mortality. Nevertheless, liver transplantation in patients with previous portacaval shunts can be done safely. If liver transplantation is not anticipated as a future option, a portacaval shunt is technically more straightforward than a distal splenorenal shunt and is a shorter operation in an unstable, actively bleeding patient.

A side-to-side portacaval shunt (see Ch. 100) is performed through a transverse upper abdominal incision. The common bile duct is encircled and retracted to the patient's left. If a replaced right hepatic artery arises from the superior mesenteric artery, this too needs to be encircled and retracted to the left (and makes the exposure of the portal vein more difficult). The portal vein is dissected and encircled with a vessel loop. The inferior vena cava between the lower edge of the liver and the right renal vein is dissected and encircled with a vessel loop. Partially occluding vascular clamps are placed on the inferior vena cava and portal vein, and the two are approximated. A venotomy is made longitudinally in each vein approximately 2 cm in length, and stay sutures of 6-0 polypropylene are placed at the corners. These stay sutures are tied down, and the anastomosis is performed using a running technique. Vascular clamps are removed, and the wound is checked for hemostasis. The completed anastomosis is shown in Fig. 95.6.

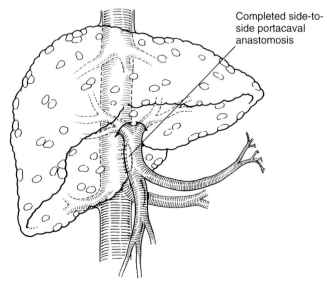

Completed side-to-side portacaval anastomosis

Fig. 95.6. The completed anastomosis normalizes portal pressures and results in hepatofugal blood flow through the shunt.
(From Knechtle SJ, 1998: Surgical shunts for portal hypertension. In Knechtle SJ (ed): Portal Hypertension: A Multidisciplinary Approach to Current Clinical Management. Armonk, NY, Futura, pp 175-202.)

Mesocaval Shunt

A mesocaval shunt may be indicated as a long-term bridge to liver transplantation or as definitive therapy in patients whose bleeding is not controlled by endoscopic methods or who have failed TIPS placement (see Ch. 99). Although a polytetrafluoroethylene or Dacron graft is commonly used as a conduit between the superior mesenteric vein and inferior vena cava, we have used an internal jugular vein autograft for this purpose. The better long-term patency rate for a vein graft favors the use of autologous vein over prosthetic material. We have had no complications from removal of one internal jugular vein and have had no shunt thromboses. Such shunts are not difficult technically and have the advantage of keeping the area of dissection away from the porta hepatis, which is an advantage if liver transplantation is a future consideration.

The mesocaval shunt is performed through a transverse upper abdominal incision. By elevating the transverse colon, the middle colic vein can be identified as it courses toward its junction with the superior mesenteric vein. The superior mesenteric vein is anterior and to the right of the superior mesenteric artery. After dividing overlying peritoneum and fat, there is generally a segment about 2 or 3 cm in length that is free of other venous tributaries. This segment of the superior mesenteric vein is dissected free and encircled. The inferior vena cava can be dissected through the right colon mesentery. It is optimal to dissect a segment of inferior vena cava that is caudal to the duodenum so that the duodenum does not interfere with shunt placement. The inferior vena cava is encircled with a vessel loop. The mesocaval shunt should take a straight path from superior mesenteric vein to vena cava, rather than coursing around the duodenum.

When using a jugular vein conduit, the left neck generally is preferred because the left jugular vein is often slightly longer than the right jugular vein (Fig. 95.7, inset). An incision similar to a carotid endarterectomy incision is made along the anterior border of the sternocleidomastoid muscle. The platysma muscle is divided, and the jugular vein is identified. Branches are doubly ligated and divided, and the jugular vein is dissected free from the clavicle to the mastoid. It is ligated with silk ties proximally and distally, and the graft segment is excised. The graft is placed in sterile saline until it is used. The neck wound is closed. The proximal end of the jugular vein graft is anastomosed end-to-side to the superior mesenteric vein using running 6-0 polypropylene (see Fig. 95.7). The distal end of the graft is anastomosed end-to-side to the inferior vena cava also using running 6-0 polypropylene. Partial occlusion clamps are placed on the superior mesenteric vein and inferior vena cava during construction of the anastomoses. After completion of the anastomoses, the clamps are removed, and shunt flow is assessed using an electromagnetic or ultrasonic flowmeter. Flow should be 1 to 2 L/min. Significantly lower flows should prompt inspection of the graft for technical problems.

Distal Splenorenal Shunt

A distal splenorenal shunt is performed through a transverse upper abdominal incision (see Ch. 98). The gastrocolic omentum is taken down such that the right gastroepiploic vein is divided, but the short gastric veins are left intact. The splenic flexure of the colon is mobilized and retracted caudally. The inferior border of the pancreas is retracted anteriorly and cranially to expose the posterior aspect of the pancreas and the splenic vein. The splenic vein is dissected free from the pancreas, and all tributaries are

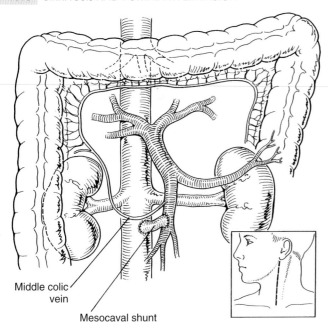

Middle colic vein

Mesocaval shunt

Fig. 95.7. The left jugular vein provides an ideal autologous endothelialized vein graft for a mesocaval shunt and is approached through the incision shown *(inset)*. The vein can be excised from the clavicle to the angle of the mandible. The proximal end of the vein should be anastomosed to the superior mesenteric vein. The completed mesocaval shunt uses an 8- to 10-cm graft to decompress the superior mesenteric vein into the vena cava.

(From Knechtle SJ, 1998: Surgical shunts for portal hypertension. In Knechtle SJ (ed): Portal Hypertension: A Multidisciplinary Approach to Current Clinical Management. Armonk, NY, Futura, pp 175-202.)

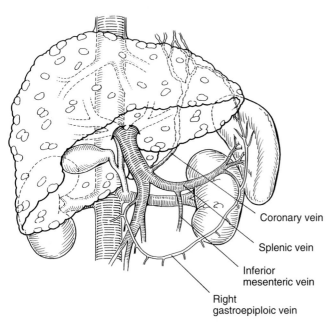

Coronary vein

Splenic vein

Inferior mesenteric vein

Right gastroepiploic vein

Fig. 95.8. The relevant anatomy exposed for a distal splenorenal shunt is shown. The short gastric veins are left intact. The coronary vein and right gastroepiploic veins are ligated.

(From Knechtle SJ, 1998: Surgical shunts for portal hypertension. In Knechtle SJ (ed): Portal Hypertension: A Multidisciplinary Approach to Current Clinical Management. Armonk, NY, Futura, pp 175-202.)

ligated and divided. The coronary vein may be one of its branches or may enter the portal vein. The splenic vein dissection is generally the most challenging aspect of the procedure and may be particularly difficult in patients with pancreatic fibrosis from chronic pancreatitis. The splenic vein is dissected medially to its confluence with the superior mesenteric vein and laterally to a point that allows the vein to be brought down to the renal vein without kinking or tension. If splenopancreatic dissection is a goal of the procedure, the dissection continues all the way to the spleen such that all pancreatic tributaries are ligated and divided (Fig. 95.8).

The left renal vein is dissected, and adjacent lymphatics are ligated to avoid the complication of chylous ascites. A vessel loop is placed around the left renal vein. An adequate length of splenic vein should be dissected such that when it is divided at the portal vein it can reach the left renal vein easily without tension. Identification and ligation of the coronary vein is an essential component of the operation. It is preferable to ligate the coronary vein at its junction with the portal vein or splenic vein. This vein also can be ligated at the superior border of the pancreas just before it extends along the lesser curvature of the stomach. It is generally large and attenuated and must be ligated if the shunt is to be selective. Blood flow through the completed shunt (see Fig. 95.5) can be measured using a flowmeter and is generally 300 to 1000 mL/min.

DEVASCULARIZATION PROCEDURES FOR BLEEDING ESOPHAGEAL VARICES

Surgical devascularization procedures were developed with the intent of disconnecting varices from the hypertensive portal venous system, decreasing the risk of variceal hemorrhage (see Ch. 94). In contrast to most shunts, these procedures avoid encephalopathy by preserving hepatic portal perfusion. The "gold standard" of devascularization procedures has become the Sugiura operation, which consists of thoracic esophageal transection and devascularization followed weeks later by laparotomy to control bleeding from esophageal varices (Sugiura & Futagawa, 1973). The Sugiura procedure differs from other devascularization procedures in that extensive esophageal and gastric devascularization is performed in a manner that preserves the venous collaterals connecting the coronary vein to the azygos system, discouraging reformation of varices. The initial report by Sugiura and Futagawa (1973) comprising 276 patients described an operative mortality rate of 4.3% and reoccurrence of varices in 2.3% after follow-up of 1 to 10 years. Actuarial survival was 83%. Survival according to Child classification was 95% for A, 87% for B, and 57% for C. Survival was better after an elective procedure than after an emergency operation.

The outstanding results achieved in the Japanese series have not been duplicated elsewhere. Many surgeons outside Japan have used modifications of the Sugiura procedure to control bleeding esophageal varices, particularly in patients with extensive mesenteric venous thrombosis or with a previous failed surgical shunt. Orozco and associates (1992) reported a 10-year experience with the elective Sugiura procedure using a one-stage transabdominal approach. Mortality correlated with Child status. The Toronto experience with the modified Sugiura procedure was reported by Dagena is in 1994 and included a 22% operative mortality rate when the procedure was used in the emergency setting. Five-year survival was 100% for Child A, 43% for Child B, and

25% for Child C patients (Dagenais et al, 1994). In a series of 32 patients undergoing transabdominal esophagogastric devascularization for variceal bleeding, 11 of the 12 patients without liver disease survived more than 10 years. The other 20 patients with cirrhosis had a 5-year survival of 51% (Jin & Rikkers, 1996). This experience suggests that esophagogastric devascularization is an effective alternative to shunt surgery, particularly in patients whose underlying condition is diffuse splanchnic venous thrombosis in the absence of liver disease. The only prospective randomized clinical trial comparing the Sugiura procedure with selective or total shunts was performed in patients with bilharzial cirrhosis and bleeding varices (da Silva et al, 1986). This trial concluded that patients treated with devascularization were more likely to survive longer without encephalopathy compared with patients treated with a shunt (da Silva et al, 1986; Raia et al, 1991).

Patients with portal venous anatomy unsuitable for surgical shunts or shunt failures who fail medical management may be considered for devascularization procedures. Patients who progress to Child C liver failure should be considered for liver transplantation. Devascularization procedures should be reserved for the rare patients with bleeding varices refractory to medical management and who also are ineligible for TIPS, a surgical shunt, or liver transplantation.

LIVER TRANSPLANTATION FOR BLEEDING ESOPHAGEAL VARICES

Definitive therapy for patients with advanced liver failure (Child B or C) is liver transplantation (see Ch. 103). Variceal hemorrhage is the most common clinical manifestation of portal hypertension prompting liver transplant evaluation. The acute management of variceal hemorrhage in liver transplant candidates begins with endoscopic diagnosis and sclerotherapy or ligation where feasible in combination with pharmacologic therapy or TIPS or both for failures of endoscopic management. In view of the strong correlation between Child classification and long-term outcome seen with virtually every form of therapy for bleeding varices, there is compelling evidence that liver transplantation should be the treatment of choice for such patients with advanced liver disease. In the current era, each of the treatments discussed so far, including surgical shunts, should be used in a complementary fashion, and many patients require sequential application of the various modalities. Naturally, liver transplantation is the ultimate solution to cirrhosis and end-stage liver failure when this is the underlying cause of portal hypertension and variceal hemorrhage.

Because of the disparity between the number of patients awaiting liver transplantation and the supply of donor livers, transplantation generally is accompanied by an unpredictable waiting period that varies depending on the supply of donor livers. Average waiting times for a liver transplant in the United States vary from 6 months to more than 2 years depending on blood type (U.S. Department of Health and Human Services, United Network for Organ Sharing, University Renal Research and Education Association, 2003). Operative morbidity and mortality associated with liver transplantation correlate with the preoperative condition of the recipient. For this reason, it is advisable to use alternative measures to arrest variceal hemorrhage and to optimize the medical condition of the patient before proceeding to liver transplantation. Liver transplant programs in the United States preclude active alcoholics from liver transplantation and require at least a 6-month period of abstinence. This therapy is

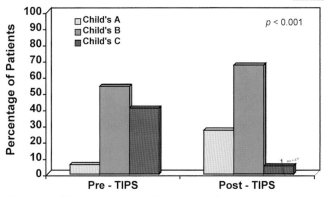

Fig. 95.9. Effect of TIPS on modified Child-Pugh score. TIPS resulted in a significant shift toward improved recipient Child-Pugh score and pretransplant status ($P<.001$).
(From Odorico JS, 1998: Impact of transjugular intrahepatic portosystemic shunt on liver transplantation. In Knechtle SJ (ed): Portal Hypertension: A Multidisciplinary Approach to Current Clinical Management. Armonk, NY, Futura, pp 253-263.)

generally unavailable to active alcoholics with variceal hemorrhage, and such patients may need to be considered for surgical shunts. Because of immediate normalization of portal pressure, liver transplantation is effective therapy for bleeding esophageal varices resulting from underlying portal hypertension (Ewaga et al, 1994).

A portacaval shunt or surgical shunt involving dissection in the porta hepatis makes a subsequent liver transplant more difficult technically. If a liver transplant is anticipated after a surgical shunt, a shunt should be performed outside of the porta hepatis whenever possible. Distal splenorenal and mesocaval shunts are preferred shunts for such patients (Knechtle et al, 1994; Shaked & Busuttil, 1991). A surgical shunt is an attractive means of controlling variceal hemorrhage in a patient who may not need a liver transplant for several years. Most patients eligible for liver transplantation with Child C cirrhosis require transplantation in the short-term and are managed more appropriately with TIPS as a bridge to liver transplantation. TIPS may improve the Child classification significantly and reduce morbidity while awaiting liver transplantation (Fig. 95.9) (Odorico, 1998).

PRESENT ROLE OF SURGICAL SHUNTS

A shunt often may serve as a long-term bridge to liver transplantation in patients who are deemed to be acceptable candidates for liver transplantation. In a report comparing liver transplantation, shunts (82% distal splenorenal shunts) in patients as future candidates for liver transplantation, and shunts in patients without the future prospect of liver transplantation, we found that the operative mortality was best in the two shunt groups (5% and 7% versus 19% in liver transplant patients). This finding was attributed to more advanced disease in the liver transplant cohort. The patients not considered for liver transplantation were excluded because of active alcoholism or advanced age. Kaplan-Meier survival analysis showed better survival in shunt patients who were transplant candidates (7 of 44 patients had progressed to liver transplantation) than either the liver transplant group or the shunt group without prospective liver transplantation during the first 5 years of follow-up, but by 10 years, there was no difference between the groups (Fig. 95.10). These results suggest

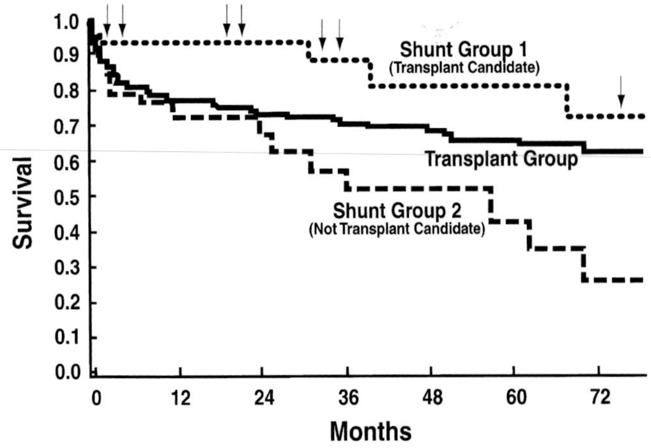

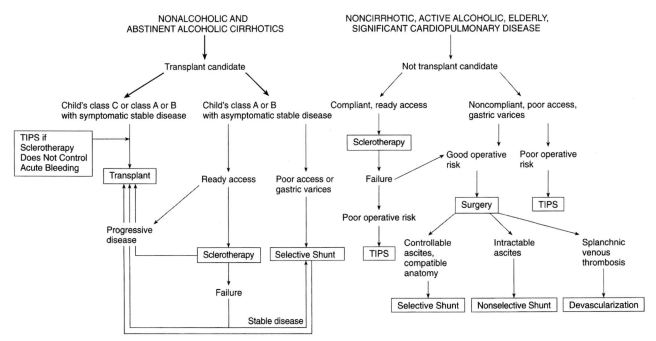

Fig. 95.10. Kaplan-Meier survival analysis of shunt group 1 *(dotted line)*, transplant group *(solid line)*, and shunt group 2 *(hyphens)*. The *arrows* on the shunt group 1 curve indicate when patients from that group underwent liver transplantation. Survival of shunt group 1 is significantly different from survival of the transplant group *(P=.003)* and shunt group 2 *(P=.018)* at 1 year (log-rank test). At 5 years, the shunt group 1 and transplant group curves are no longer different, but both are significantly different from the shunt group 2 curve *(P=.006 and P=.029).*
(From Rikkers LF, et al, 1997: Shunt surgery during the era of liver transplantation. Ann Surg 226:51-57.)

that patients with Child A or early B cirrhosis who are not actively drinking and are not too elderly or medically unfit benefit from shunt surgery most. Because it is complicated less frequently by encephalopathy and because it has an excellent long-term patency rate, distal splenorenal shunt is a good choice for such patients. If they progress to end-stage liver failure, they can be salvaged with transplantation (Rikkers et al, 1997). During the period studied, distal splenorenal shunts and nonselective shunts were more protective against rebleeding than was esophagogastric devascularization (Rikkers et al, 1997).

Consistent with the aforementioned observations, surgical shunts at the University of Wisconsin generally are reserved for patients with good hepatic reserve and variceal bleeding. Excellent results are achieved in this setting (Knechtle et al, 1999).

An algorithm summarizing current decision making in the management of variceal hemorrhage is shown in Fig. 95.11. Patients are divided into patients potentially eligible for a liver transplant versus patients who are not transplant candidates. The sequential use of various modalities is illustrated. The current use of procedures performed for variceal hemorrhage suggests that although sclerotherapy and banding continue to be used frequently, TIPS has increased dramatically in use, as has liver transplantation. Nonselective shunts are rarely used today, whereas selective shunts are performed in a highly select group of patients.

During the past 18 years, one of the authors (L.R.) has surgically treated 263 patients with portal hypertensive bleeding. During this period, liver transplantation and TIPS have evolved into effective therapies and substantially affected management of this problem and indirectly changed the risk status (Child class) of patients undergoing shunts. Analysis of this group of patients showed that, in recent years, the Child class has progressively improved, whereas the need for emergency surgery has declined. The use of nonselective shunts declined because of the development of effective alternatives, such as sclerotherapy and TIPS, and because advanced liver failure with ascites was managed by liver transplantation (sometimes preceded by TIPS). Consequently, better risk patients were selected to undergo elective shunts for treatment of variceal bleeding. The incidence of postoperative encephalopathy decreased, and long-term (10-year) survival improved, especially because shunt patients could be salvaged if they developed liver failure postoperatively (Rikkers, 1998).

Another role for portosystemic surgical shunts is in children with variceal hemorrhage after endoscopic therapy. Excellent results have been achieved in children using distal splenorenal shunts and mesocaval shunts to prevent bleeding (Botha et al, 2004).

Fig. 95.11. Algorithm for definitive therapy of variceal hemorrhage.
(From Rikkers LF, 1995: Portal hypertension. In Levine BA, et al (eds): Current Practice of Surgery, vol 3. New York, Churchill Livingstone, pp 1-22.)

SUMMARY

The clinical management of bleeding esophageal varices has changed radically over the past 20 years. Changes currently in progress include a shift away from endoscopic variceal sclerotherapy toward EVL. The excellent efficacy of EVL and its lower complication rate favor its increased use. Similarly, the minimally invasive nature of the TIPS procedure and its successful implementation by invasive radiologists have reduced further the need for surgical shunts. TIPS is being increasingly used when endoscopic intervention has failed. Liver transplantation is routinely recommended for patients with advanced liver failure. Surgical shunts are used more selectively, but with better results than in an earlier era, when they were more commonly performed. A multidisciplinary approach to evaluation and treatment of variceal hemorrhage has improved the outcomes of these patients. Selective use of each of the therapies, alone or in combination with other modalities, results in improved outcomes.

We consider the current role of surgical shunts to be (1) less frequent than in the previous era; (2) in the emergency setting when other modalities, including medical therapy, endoscopic control, or TIPS, have failed; (3) in the elective setting as a long-term bridge to liver transplantation; (4) in the elective setting as definitive therapy for patients with noncirrhotic portal hypertension or Child A cirrhosis; and (5) as treatment for Budd-Chiari syndrome. We prefer the selective distal splenorenal shunt in patients without ascites because of its lower risk of portosystemic encephalopathy and its potential for preserving portal blood flow.

REFERENCES

Abouljoud MS, et al, 1995: A comparison of treatment with transjugular intrahepatic portosystemic shunt or distal splenorenal shunt in the management of variceal bleeding prior to liver transplantation. Transplantation 59:226-229.

Baker LA, et al, 1959: The natural history of esophageal varices: a study of 115 cirrhotic patients in whom varices were diagnosed prior to bleeding. Am J Med 26:228-237.

Barton RE, et al, 1995: TIPS: short- and long-term results: a survey of 1750 patients. Semin Interv Radiol 12:364-367.

Besson I, et al, 1995: Sclerotherapy with or without octreotide for acute variceal bleeding. N Engl J Med 333:555-560.

Block KP, Reichelderfer M, 1998: Endoscopic therapy of variceal hemorrhage. In Knechtle SJ (ed): Portal Hypertension: A Multidisciplinary Approach to Current Clinical Management. Armonk, NY, Futura, pp 27-55.

Bosch J, et al, 1981: Effects of somatostatin on hepatic and systemic hemodynamics in patients with cirrhosis of the liver: comparison with vasopressin. Gastroenterology 80:518-525.

Botha JF, et al, 2004: Portosystemic shunts in children: a 15-year experience. J Am Coll Surg 199:179-185.

Boyer TD, 1982: Portal hypertension and its complications: bleeding esophageal varices, ascites, and spontaneous bacterial peritonitis. In Zakim D, Boyer TD (eds): Hepatology: A Textbook of Liver Disease. Philadelphia, Saunders, pp 464-499.

Burroughs AK, et al, 1989: Cirrhotics with variceal hemorrhage: the importance of the time interval between admission and the start of analysis for survival and rebleeding rates. Hepatology 9:801-807.

Burroughs AK, et al, 1990: Randomized, double-blind, placebo-controlled trial of emergency control and prevention of early variceal rebleeding. Gastroenterology 99:1388-1395.

Burroughs AK, 1996: Double blind RCT of 5 day octreotide versus placebo associated with sclerotherapy for trial failures. International Octreotide Varices Study Group. Hepatology 24:352A.

Cales P, et al, 1990: Incidence of large oesophageal varices in patients with cirrhosis: application to prophylaxis of first bleeding. Gut 31:1298-1302.

Cello JP, et al, 1987: Endoscopic sclerotherapy versus portacaval shunt in patients with severe cirrhosis and acute variceal hemorrhage: long-term follow-up. N Engl J Med 316:11-15.

Chojkier M, et al, 1979: A controlled comparison of continuous intraarterial and intravenous infusions of vasopressin in hemorrhage from esophageal varices. Gastroenterology 77:540-546.

Coldwell DM, et al, 1995: Multicenter investigation of the role of transjugular intrahepatic portosystemic shunt in management of portal hypertension. Radiology 196:335-340.

Crenshaw WB, et al, 1996: Severe ascites: efficacy of the transjugular intrahepatic portosystemic shunt in treatment. Radiology 200:185-192.

Dagenais M, et al, 1994: Experience with radical esophagogastric devascularization procedures (Sugiura) for variceal bleeding outside of Japan. World J Surg 18:222-228.

Dagradi AE, 1972: The natural history of esophageal varices in patients with alcoholic liver cirrhosis: an endoscopic and clinical study. Am J Gastroenterol 57:520-540.

D'Amico G, et al, 1995: The treatment of portal hypertension: a meta-analytic review. Hepatology 22:332-354.

Darcy M, et al, 1993: Efficacy and complications of transjugular intrahepatic portosystemic shunts. Radiology 189(suppl):227.

da Silva LC, et al, 1986: A randomized trial for the study of the elective surgical treatment of portal hypertension in mansonic schistosomiasis. Ann Surg 204:148-153.

De Franchis R, et al, 1991: Prophylactic sclerotherapy in high-risk cirrhotics selected by endoscopic criteria: a multicenter randomized controlled trial. Gastroenterology 101:1087-1093.

Encarnacion CE, et al, 1995: Transjugular intrahepatic portosystemic shunt placement for variceal bleeding: predictors of mortality. J Vasc Interv Radiol 6:687-694.

Ewaga H, et al, 1994: Liver transplantation for uncontrollable variceal bleeding. Am J Gastroenterol 89:1823-1826.

Fardy JM, Laupacis A, 1994: A meta-analysis of prophylactic endoscopic sclerotherapy for esophageal varices. Am J Gastroenterol 89:1938-1948.

Feu F, et al, 1993: Reduction of variceal pressure by propranolol: comparison of the effects on portal pressure and azygos blood flow in patients with cirrhosis. Hepatology 18:1082-1089.

Fillmore DJ, et al, 1996: Transjugular intrahepatic portosystemic shunt: midterm clinical and angiographic follow-up. J Vasc Interv Radiol 7:255-261.

Fogel MR, et al, 1982: Continuous intravenous vasopressin in active upper gastrointestinal bleeding: a placebo controlled trial. Ann Intern Med 96:565-569.

Garcia-Pagan JC, et al, 1990: Enhancement of portal pressure reduction by the association of isosorbide mononitrate to propranolol administration in patients with cirrhosis. Hepatology 11:230-238.

Gebhard RL, 1998: Natural history of esophageal varices. In Knechtle SJ (ed): Portal Hypertension: A Multidisciplinary Approach to Current Clinical Management. Armonk, NY, Futura, pp 1-8.

Gimson AE, et al, 1993: Randomised trial of variceal banding ligation versus injection sclerotherapy for bleeding oesophageal varices. Lancet 342:391-394.

Grace ND, 1992: Prevention of initial variceal hemorrhage. Gastroenterol Clin North Am 21:149-161.

Graham D, Smith JL, 1981: The course of patients after variceal hemorrhage. Gastroenterology 80:800-809.

Gregory PB, 1990: Sclerotherapy for actively bleeding esophageal varices in male alcoholics with cirrhosis: results of a randomized, multicenter clinical trial. VA Cooperative Variceal Sclerotherapy Group. Gastroenterology 98:A53.

Groszmann RJ, et al, 1990: Hemodynamic events in a prospective randomized trial of propranolol versus placebo in the prevention of a first variceal hemorrhage. Gastroenterology 99:1401-1407.

Hashizume M, et al, 1993: Endoscopic ligation of esophageal varices compared with injection sclerotherapy: a prospective randomized trial. Gastrointest Endosc 39:123-126.

Haskal ZJ, et al, 1994: Transjugular intrahepatic portosystemic shunt stenosis and revision: early and midterm results. AJR Am J Roentgenol 163:439-444.

Helton WS, et al, 1993: Critical appraisal of the angiographic portacaval shunt (TIPS). Am J Surg 165:566-571.

Henderson JM, et al, 1983: Hemodynamic differences between alcoholic and nonalcoholic cirrhotics following distal splenorenal shunt—effect on survival? Ann Surg 198:325-334.

Henderson JM, et al, 1990: Endoscopic variceal sclerosis compared with distal splenorenal shunt to prevent recurrent variceal bleeding in cirrhosis: a prospective, randomized trial. Ann Intern Med 112:262-269.

Henderson JM, et al, 1998: Portal hypertension. Curr Probl Surg 35:384-452.

Henderson JM, et al, 2004: DSRS or TIPS for refractory variceal bleeding: a prospective randomized controlled trial. Hepatology 40(suppl 1):725A.

Hou MC, et al, 1995: Comparison of endoscopic variceal injection sclerotherapy and ligation for the treatment of esophageal variceal hemorrhage: a prospective randomized trial. Hepatology 21:1517-1522.

Huet PM, et al, 1987: Hemodynamic effects of vasopressin in cirrhotic patients. In Lebrec D, Blei AT (eds): Vasopressin Analogues and Portal Hypertension. Paris, John Libbey Eurotext, pp 83-94.

Imperiale TF, et al, 1995: A meta-analysis of somatostatin versus vasopressin in the management of acute esophageal variceal hemorrhage. Gastroenterology 109:1289-1294.

Infante-Rivard C, et al, 1989: Role of endoscopic variceal sclerotherapy in the long-term management of variceal bleeding: a meta-analysis. Gastroenterology 96:1087-1092.

Inokuchi K, 1984: Prophylactic portal nondecompression surgery in patients with esophageal varices: an interim report. Cooperative Study of Portal Hypertension of Japan. Ann Surg 200:61-65.

Jin GL, Rikkers LF, 1991: Selective variceal decompression: current status. HPB Surg 5:1-15.

Jin G, Rikkers LF, 1996: Transabdominal esophagogastric devascularization as treatment for variceal hemorrhage. Surgery 120:641-649.

Khaitiyar JS, et al, 2000: Transjugular intrahepatic portosystemic shunt versus distal splenorenal shunt—a comparative study. Hepatogastroenterology 47:492-497.

Kleber G, et al, 1991: Prediction of variceal hemorrhage in cirrhosis: a prospective follow-up study. Gastroenterology 100:1332-1337.

Knechtle SJ, 1998: Surgical shunts for portal hypertension. In Knechtle SJ (ed): Portal Hypertension: A Multidisciplinary Approach to Current Clinical Management. Armonk, NY, Futura, pp 175-202.

Knechtle SJ, et al, 1994: Portal hypertension: surgical management in the 1990s. Surgery 116:687-695.

Knechtle SJ, et al, 1999: Surgical portosystemic shunts for treatment of portal hypertensive bleeding: outcome and effect on liver function. Surgery 126:708-711.

Korula J, 1998: Medical management of portal hypertension. In Knechtle SJ (ed) Portal Hypertension: A Multidisciplinary Approach to Current Clinical Management. Armonk, NY, Futura, pp 9-26.

Konstantinov IE, 1997: Eck-Paulov shunt: the 120th anniversary of the first vascular anastomosis. Surgery 121:640-645.

LaBerge JM, et al, 1992: Transjugular intrahepatic portosystemic shunts: preliminary results in 25 patients. J Vasc Surg 16:258-267.

LaBerge JM, et al, 1995: Two-year outcome following transjugular intrahepatic portosystemic shunt for variceal bleeding: results in 90 patients. Gastroenterology 108:1143-1151.

Laine L, et al, 1993: Endoscopic ligation compared with sclerotherapy for the treatment of bleeding esophageal varices. Ann Intern Med 119:1-7.

Lebrec D, et al, 1980: Propranolol—a medical treatment for portal hypertension? Lancet 2:180-182.

Lebrec D, et al, 1981: Propranolol for prevention of recurrent gastrointestinal bleeding in patients with cirrhosis: a controlled study. N Engl J Med 305:1371-1374.

Lebrec D, et al, 1982: The effect of propranolol on portal hypertension in patients with cirrhosis: a hemodynamic study. Hepatology 2:523-527.

Le Moine O, et al, 1992: Factors related to early mortality in cirrhotic patients bleeding from varices and treated by urgent sclerotherapy. Gut 33:1381-1385.

Lo GH, et al, 1995: A prospective, randomized trial of sclerotherapy versus ligation in the management of bleeding esophageal varices. Hepatology 22:466-471.

Lo GH, et al, 1997: Emergency banding ligation versus sclerotherapy for the control of active bleeding from esophageal varices. Hepatology 25:1101-1104.

MacDougall BR, et al, 1982: Increased long-term survival in variceal haemorrhage using injection sclerotherapy: results of a controlled trial. Lancet 1:124-127.

Malisch T, et al, 1993: Life-table analysis of middle-term patency of transjugular intrahepatic portosystemic stent. Radiology 189(suppl):227.

Martin L, et al, 1993: Is transjugular intrahepatic portosystemic shunt the treatment of choice for Class C cirrhotic patients with uncontrolled hemorrhage? Radiology 189(suppl):253.

Martin M, et al, 1993: Transjugular intrahepatic portosystemic shunt in the management of variceal bleeding: indications and clinical results. Surgery 114:719-727.

McCormick PA, et al, 1994: Emergency transjugular intrahepatic portasystemic stent shunting as salvage treatment for uncontrolled variceal bleeding. Br J Surg 81:1324-1327.

Menegaux F, et al, 1994: Comparison of transjugular and surgical portosystemic shunts on the outcome of liver transplantation. Arch Surg 129:1018-1024.

Merkel C, et al, 1989: Prognostic indicators of survival in patients with cirrhosis and esophageal varices, without previous bleeding. Am J Gastroenterol 84:717-722.

Millis M, et al, 1995: TIPS: impact on liver transplantation. Transplant Proc 27:1252-1253.

Monescillo A, et al, 2004: Influence of portal hypertension and its early decompression by TIPS placement on the outcome of variceal bleeding. Hepatology 40:793-801.

Moreau R, et al, 1989: Low dose of nitroglycerin failed to improve splanchnic hemodynamics in patients with cirrhosis: evidence for an impaired cardiopulmonary baroreflex function. Hepatology 10:93-97.

Odorico JS, 1998: Impact of transjugular intrahepatic portosystemic shunt on liver transplantation. In Knechtle SJ (ed): Portal Hypertension: A Multidisciplinary Approach to Current Clinical Management. Armonk, NY, Futura, pp 253-263.

Orloff MJ, et al, 1994: Prospective randomized trial of emergency portacaval shunt and emergency medical therapy in unselected cirrhotic patients with bleeding varices. Hepatology 20:863-872.

Orozco H, et al, 1992: Elective treatment of bleeding varices with the Sugiura operation over ten years. Am J Surg 163:585-589.

Pagliaro L, et al, 1989: Therapeutic controversies and randomized controlled trials (RCTs): prevention of bleeding and rebleeding in cirrhosis. Gastroenterol Int 2:71-84.

Papatheodoridis GV, et al, 1999: Transjugular intrahepatic portosystemic shunt compared with endoscopic treatment for prevention of variceal rebleeding: a meta-analysis. Hepatology 30:612-622.

Planas R, et al, 1994: A prospective randomized trial comparing somatostatin and sclerotherapy in the treatment of acute variceal bleeding. Hepatology 20:370-375.

Poynard T, et al, 1991: Beta-adrenergic-antagonist drugs in the prevention of gastrointestinal bleeding in patients with cirrhosis and esophageal varices: an analysis of data and prognostic factors in 589 patients from four randomized clinical trials. Franco-Italian Multicenter Study Group. N Engl J Med 324:1532-1538.

PROVA Study Group, 1991: Prophylaxis of first hemorrhage from esophageal varices by sclerotherapy, propranolol or both in cirrhotic patients: a randomized multicenter trial. Hepatology 14:1016-1024.

Raia S, et al, 1991: Portal hypertension in mansonic schistosomiasis. World J Surg 15:176-187.

Resnick RH, et al, 1974: A controlled study of the therapeutic portacaval shunt. Gastroenterology 67:843-857.

Richter G, et al, 1994: Six-year results of transjugular intrahepatic portosystemic shunt stent placement: essentials for success. Radiology 193(suppl):130.

Rikkers LF, 1995: Portal hypertension. In Levine BA, et al (eds): Current Practice of Surgery, vol 3. New York, Churchill Livingstone, pp 1-22.

Rikkers LF, 1998: The changing spectrum of treatment for variceal bleeding. Ann Surg 228:536-546.

Rikkers LF, Jin G, 1994: Surgical management of acute variceal hemorrhage. World J Surg 18:193-199.

Rikkers LF, Jin G, 1995: Emergency shunt: role in the present management of variceal bleeding. Arch Surg 130:472-477.

Rikkers LF, et al, 1992: Which portosystemic shunt is best? Gastroenterol Clin North Am 21:179-196.

Rikkers LF, et al, 1993: Shunt surgery versus endoscopic sclerotherapy for variceal hemorrhage: late results of a randomized trial. Am J Surg 165:27-33.

Rikkers LF, et al, 1997: Shunt surgery during the era of liver transplantation. Ann Surg 226:51-57.

Ring EJ, et al, 1992: Using transjugular intrahepatic portosystemic shunts to control variceal bleeding before liver transplantation. Ann Intern Med 116:304-309.

Rosemurgy AS, et al, 2000: Transjugular intrahepatic portosystemic shunt vs. small-diameter prosthetic H-graft portacaval shunt: extended follow-up of an expanded randomized prospective trial. J Gastrointest Surg 4:589-597.

Rossle M, et al, 1994: The transjugular intrahepatic portosystemic stent-shunt procedure for variceal bleeding. N Engl J Med 330:165-171.

Salerno F, et al, 2004: Randomized controlled study of TIPS versus paracentesis plus albumin in cirrhosis with severe ascites. Hepatology 40:629-635.

Sarfeh IJ, Rypins EB, 1994: Partial versus total portacaval shunt in alcoholic cirrhosis: results of a prospective, randomized clinical trial. Ann Surg 219:353-361.

Sarfeh IJ, et al, 1986: A systematic appraisal of portacaval H-graft diameters: clinical and hemodynamic perspectives. Ann Surg 204:356-363.

Sauerbruch T, et al, 1988: Prophylactic sclerotherapy before the first episode of variceal hemorrhage in patients with cirrhosis. N Engl J Med 319:8-15.

Saxon R, et al, 1993: Transjugular intrahepatic portosystemic shunt: middle-term shunt patency. Radiology 189(suppl):227.

Shaked A, Busuttil RW, 1991: Liver transplantation in patients with portal vein thrombosis and central portacaval shunts. Ann Surg 214:696-702.

Siringo S, et al, 1994: Timing of the first variceal hemorrhage in cirrhotic patients: prospective evaluation of Doppler flowmetry, endoscopy and clinical parameters. Hepatology 20:66-73.

Smith JL, Graham DY, 1982: Variceal hemorrhage: a critical evaluation of survival analysis. Gastroenterology 82:968-973.

Sterling K, Darcy M, 1995: Transjugular intrahepatic portosystemic shunts stenosis: incidence and management. AJR Am J Roentgenol 164(suppl):96A.

Stiegmann GV, et al, 1992: Endoscopic sclerotherapy as compared with endoscopic ligation for bleeding esophageal varices. N Engl J Med 326:1527-1532.

Stipa S, et al, 1981: A randomized controlled trial of mesentericocaval shunt with autologous jugular vein. Surg Gynecol Obstet 153:353-356.

Suc B, et al, 1995: Intrahepatic portocaval shunt in patients waiting for transplantation. Transplant Proc 27:1715-1716.

Sugiura M, Futagawa S, 1973: A new technique for treating esophageal varices. J Thorac Cardiovasc Surg 66:677-685.

Sugiura M, Futagawa S, 1977: Further evaluation of the Sugiura procedure in the treatment of esophageal varices. Arch Surg 112:1317-1321.

The Copenhagen Esophageal Varices Sclerotherapy Project, 1984: Sclerotherapy after first variceal hemorrhage in cirrhosis: a randomized multicenter trial. N Engl J Med 311:1594-1600.

The Veterans Affairs Cooperative Variceal Sclerotherapy Group, 1991: Prophylactic sclerotherapy for esophageal varices in men with alcoholic liver disease: a randomized, single-blind, multicenter clinical trial. N Engl J Med 324:1779-1784.

The Veterans Affairs Cooperative Variceal Sclerotherapy Group, 1994: Sclerotherapy for male alcoholic cirrhotic patients who have bled from esophageal varices: results of a randomized, multicenter clinical trial. Hepatology 20:618-625.

Thulin L, et al, 1979: Treatment of bleeding oesophageal varices with somatostatin. Acta Chir Scand 145:395-398.

Triger DR, et al, 1991: Prophylactic sclerotherapy for esophageal varices: long-term results of a single-center trial. Hepatology 13:117-123.

Tyden G, et al, 1978: Treatment of bleeding esophageal varices with somatostatin. N Engl J Med 299:1466-1467.

U.S. Department of Health and Human Services, United Network for Organ Sharing, University Renal Research and Education Association, 2003: Annual Report of the U.S. Organ Procurement and Transplantation Network and the Scientific Registry of Transplant Recipients: Transplant Data 1993-2002. U.S. Department of Health and Human Services, Health Resources and Services Administration, Office of Special Programs, Division of Transplantation, Rockville, MD; United Network for Organ Sharing, Richmond, VA; University Renal Research and Education Association, Ann Arbor, MI. Available at www.ustransplant.org.

Van Ruiswyk J, Byrd JC, 1992: Efficacy of prophylactic sclerotherapy for prevention of a first variceal hemorrhage. Gastroenterology 102:587-597.

Villanueva C, et al, 1996: Nadolol plus isosorbide mononitrate compared with sclerotherapy for the prevention of variceal bleeding. N Engl J Med 334:1624-1629.

Vorobioff J, et al, 1993: Propranolol compared with propranolol plus isosorbide dinitrate in portal-hypertensive patients: long-term hemodynamic and renal effects. Hepatology 18:477-484.

Warren WD, et al, 1967: Selective trans-splenic decompression of gastro-esophageal varices by distal splenorenal shunt. Ann Surg 166:437-455.

Westaby D, et al, 1989: Controlled clinical trial of injection sclerotherapy for active variceal bleeding. Hepatology 9:274-277.

96

The Place of Transjugular Intrahepatic Portosystemic Shunting

A. M. SMITH AND J. M. HENDERSON

TECHNIQUE OF TRANSJUGULAR INTRAHEPATIC PORTOSYSTEMIC SHUNT PLACEMENT

M. DARCY

The transjugular intrahepatic portosystemic shunt (TIPS) leads to portal decompression by creation of a low-resistance channel between a central hepatic vein and an intrahepatic branch of the portal vein. The procedure was first performed in 1988 in a patient with advanced cirrhosis who had continued variceal bleeding despite numerous sclerotherapies. The technique (described in detail later) consists of transjugular puncture of an intrahepatic branch of the portal vein, balloon dilation of the parenchymal tract between the two venous systems, and implantation of a metallic stent to improve long-term patency of the channel. The relative ease of performance and immediate lowering of the portal to hepatic vein gradient to less than 12 mm Hg in at least 90% of patients has led to the rapid acceptance of TIPS into clinical practice. In addition, TIPS placement does not alter the extra-hepatic anatomy in patients who are transplant candidates.

TIPS has been used primarily to treat the major consequences of portal hypertension: acute variceal bleeding, variceal rebleed-ing (second-line treatment), and refractory ascites. TIPS, as with most new technologies, has continued to evolve since its intro-duction (see later). The ability to place TIPS has improved, and it has become widely available as more interventional radiologists have gained experience. Procedural complications occur in less than 10%; capsular rupture is the most life-threatening complication. A vascular injury to the hepatic artery can lead to lobe infarction. Perforation of a bile duct radicle carries with it the risk of early thrombosis of the TIPS shunt. Infection ("TIPSitis") has been described and is difficult to treat. Covered stents seem to be better than uncovered stents (Bureau et al, 2004) with a lower stenosis/thrombosis rate. Successful TIPS diverts portal flow, but overall the encephalopathy associated with this has proved relatively easy to manage. This chapter discusses the evidence for the role of TIPS in variceal bleeding, ascites, and other less commonly encountered problems in which the consensus for deployment is less clear.

ACUTE VARICEAL BLEEDING

TIPS is indicated in 10% to 20% of patients for ongoing acute bleeding. Acute bleeding from ruptured esophageal varices is seen in 30% of patients with portal hypertension. The first-line treatment for acute variceal bleeding consists of octreotide or terlipressin and endoscopic variceal band ligation. Failure of this

first-line treatment may lead to the need for urgent TIPS. Failure to control an episode of acute variceal bleeding was defined by the Baveno consensus conference as the continuation of bleeding or when one clinically significant bleed occurs within 48 hours (De Franchis, 2001). A clinically significant bleed is defined by (1) decrease in hemoglobin greater than 2 g/dL, (2) greater than 2 blood units transfused per 24 hours, and (3) pulse rate greater than 100 beats/min and systolic blood pressure less than 100 mm Hg. Balloon tamponade indicates failure to stop the acute bleeding by first-line treatments, almost always controls acute bleeding, and may be used to bridge patients to TIPS. Such patients have a mortality rate of 80%, and they are poor candidates for a surgical procedure. Jalan and colleagues (1995) compared TIPS with esophageal transection in a retrospective analysis that showed TIPS was superior for stopping bleeding and reducing mortality. No randomized studies have been performed to assess the effect of TIPS on acute variceal bleeding, but many nonrandomized studies, comprising 383 patients, have been published, which showed in summary that TIPS stopped active bleeding in 90% to 100% of cases, with an early rebleeding rate of 16% to 30% and mortality rate of 16% to 55%. Most patients who underwent TIPS in these studies had Child C cirrhosis (Azoulay et al, 2001; Banares et al, 1998; McCormick et al, 1994; Patch et al, 1998).

In the acute situation, the contraindications to TIPS differ from the elective situation. Encephalopathy may be the result of acute bleeding and may not reflect poor underlying liver function and so is not a contraindication. Several groups have attempted to create selection criteria. Defined risk factors for poor outcomes were mechanical ventilation, renal failure, and sepsis. A predictive index was developed based on elevated white blood cell count, prolonged partial thromboplastin time, decreased platelet count, elevated serum creatinine, the need for ventilation, and the pres-ence of ascites. An elevated score predicts early mortality, and TIPS in the acute situation should be avoided in patients requir-ing ventilation and with evidence of sepsis and renal failure (Patch et al, 1998).

TIPS also may be effective as a rescue treatment for acute bleed-ing gastric varices, and there are anecdotal reports for its role in ectopic varices. Some reports have suggested that the efficacy of TIPS in the acute scenario may be improved with the addition of transjugular intravascular embolization of varices with coils or tissue adhesive as adjuncts to reduce variceal flow.

PREVENTION OF REBLEEDING FROM VARICES

Seventy-five percent of patients with esophagogastric varices rebled if they do not have specific therapy for the varices to reduce that risk. Standard practice for all patients who have had a variceal bleed is to undergo treatment to prevent further bleeding. First-line treatment is endoscopic band ligation or β blockade or both. With this therapy, there is still a significant rebleed rate, however, of about 18% to 20%. TIPS has been assessed for primary prevention of rebleeding compared with endoscopic therapy. In a meta-analysis of 13 randomized clinical studies comprising 948 patients (Burroughs & Vangeli, 2002), TIPS reduced rebleeding significantly better than endoscopic therapy (19% versus 47%; odds ratio [OR] 3.28; 95% confidence interval [CI] 2.3-4.7) at the cost of an increased incidence in hepatic encephalopathy—34% after TIPS compared with 19% after sclerotherapy (OR 0.48; 95% CI 0.34-0.67). There was no difference in mortality (OR 0.88; 95% CI 0.65-1.17). The results were similar comparing TIPS with endoscopic treatment with and without propranolol. Although mortality was comparable in the two treatment arms, TIPS is not regarded as a first-line treatment because the higher rate of encephalopathy after TIPS is considered to be a greater disadvantage than the higher rate of rebleeding after endoscopic treatment.

The major question regarding decompression of varices when endoscopy and β blockade (first-line treatment) fail is whether TIPS is the appropriate next step. Which patients should receive TIPS, and which patients should receive a surgical shunt? Two uncontrolled studies compared TIPS with surgical shunt in different patient populations. One group (Henderson et al, 2000) described the outcome of 149 TIPS and 62 distal splenorenal shunts (DSRS) performed in patients with refractory bleeding. Fifty percent of the TIPS patients were Child C, whereas all of the DSRS patients were Child A or B. The 30-day mortality rate was 0% for surgical shunts and 26% for TIPS; the overall survival rate was 86% (median follow-up 36 months) for surgical shunts and 53% (median follow-up 40 months) for TIPS. Surgical shunts had a rebleeding rate of 6.3%, whereas TIPS rebleeding rate was 25.5%. Encephalopathy was severe in 3.1% and mild in 17.5% of the shunt group, but was not systematically evaluated in the TIPS patients.

A second uncontrolled study (Helton et al, 2001), performed retrospectively, compared 20 elective Child A and B patients having TIPS with 20 comparable patients having a surgical shunt. The procedural (30-day) mortality in the TIPS group was 20%, and overall 50% of patients rebled, whereas in the surgical group the 30-day mortality was only 10%, and 5% rebled. Surgical shunts performed much better in all clinical end points and costs.

Two prospective randomized trials compared TIPS with surgical shunts, providing some level 1 evidence regarding the relative efficacy of both approaches. Rosemurgy and colleagues (2000) compared TIPS with small-diameter (8-mm) portocaval H-shunts. This study included "all comers" of patients who rebled through endoscopic therapy. There were 66 patients randomized to each group. Half of patients entered were Child C, and two thirds had alcoholic liver disease. Although there were no statistically significant differences in the two groups randomized, the proportion of urgent or emergent interventions was higher in the TIPS group (37%) compared with the surgical shunt group (20%), and more TIPS patients had encephalopathy (37% versus 23%) before randomization. Surgical shunt was significantly better for rebleeding (11 TIPS versus 2 H-graft; P<.01); need for transplant (5 TIPS versus 0 H-graft; P<.01); and overall failure, which was defined as inability to do the shunt, irreversible shunt occlusion, major variceal rebleed, liver transplant, or death (42 TIPS versus 23 H-graft; P<.01). Rosemurgy and colleagues (2000) concluded that 8-mm surgical H-graft was significantly superior to TIPS for refractory variceal bleeding in this population. A later follow-up of survival in this trial showed actual 5-year survivals of 41% for H-graft and 20% for TIPS with median survivals of 56 and 30 months (P=.07).

The second randomized trial compared TIPS with DSRS and has been published only in abstract form to date (Henderson et al, 2004). This study randomized 140 Child A and B patients (73 DSRS and 67 TIPS) with bleeding refractory to endoscopic and pharmacologic therapy. Patients were well matched, being stratified by Child score and disease etiology. Median follow-up was 42 months (range 0-91 months). The follow-up for patients still alive when the trial was closed was 30 months. Preliminary data analysis showed no significant difference in variceal rebleeding rates—6% for DSRS and 9% for TIPS—but a significantly higher reintervention rate for TIPS at 82% compared with 11% for DSRS (P<.001) to maintain a functional shunt and variceal decompression. Hepatic encephalopathy and mortality were not significantly different in the two groups. The authors concluded that in Child A and B patients with refractory variceal bleeding, TIPS and DSRS are equivalent choices for efficacy in controlling bleeding, but significantly more reinterventions are required for TIPS patients.

REFRACTORY ASCITES

Ascites is the most common complication of cirrhosis (see Ch. 88). It occurs with acute events, such as a variceal bleed. When ascites is refractory to medical measures, however, it is usually a sign of progressive deterioration in hepatic function and is associated with an unfavorable prognosis. Ascites is caused by the increase in transsinusoidal filtration pressure secondary to portal hypertension and a decreased oncotic pressure secondary to low albumin. Refractory ascites is defined as ascites that cannot be mobilized by dietary sodium restriction and intensive diuretic treatment. Treatment options include repeated large-volume paracentesis, peritoneovenous shunts, total portosystemic shunts, and liver transplantation. TIPS is a good treatment for some patients. It corrects sinusoidal hypertension and constitutes rational therapy for such patients. TIPS also may increase urinary sodium excretion in such patients, via mechanisms presumably related to improved hemodynamics.

Several randomized trials have evaluated TIPS compared with large-volume paracentesis in treatment of refractory ascites. The North American Study for the Treatment of Refractory Ascites (Sanyal et al, 2003) was a multicenter National Institutes of Health–funded trial completed in 2002. This study showed significantly (P<.001) better control of ascites with TIPS, but a higher rate of moderate or severe encephalopathy—12 of 57 in paracentesis versus 20 of 52 in the TIPS group (P=.058). There were no significant differences in survival, liver failure, transplant, variceal bleed, or quality of life.

A systematic review of the Cochrane database examined the literature to determine whether TIPS or paracentesis is the preferred method for the management of refractory ascites. Saab and associates (2004) evaluated the methodologic quality of the randomized clinical trials and included four trials in their analysis comprising 264 patients. The methodologic quality of the studies was moderate. There was no significant difference in the 30-day mortality (OR 1.00; 95% CI 0.10-10.06; *P*=1.0) and 24-month mortality (OR 1.17; 95% CI 0.52-2.66; *P*=.70) between TIPS and paracentesis. TIPS significantly reduced ascites reaccumulation at 3-month follow-up (OR 0.07; 95% CI 0.03-0.18; *P*<.00001) and at 12-month follow-up (OR 0.14; 95% CI 0.06-0.28; *P*<.00001). Hepatic encephalopathy occurred significantly more often in the TIPS group (OR 2.11; 95% CI 1.22-3.66; *P*=.008). Gastrointestinal bleeding, acute renal failure, septicemia/infection, and disseminated intravascular coagulation did not differ significantly between groups.

Other studies have evaluated the quality of life between TIPS and paracentesis. Using a Spitzer quality of life scale, Gulberg and colleagues (2002) showed a significant improvement in the index score for TIPS compared with paracentesis. Three other studies showed a significant improvement in the nutritional status after TIPS, which also may have an impact on quality of life.

The place for TIPS in the algorithm for the treatment of refractory ascites is uncertain. Because 20% of refractory ascites require only a single large-volume paracentesis, TIPS should not be offered as first-line management. TIPS should be considered when frequent paracenteses are required and when concurrent problems arise, such as hepatic hydrothorax.

OTHER POTENTIAL INDICATIONS FOR TRANSJUGULAR INTRAHEPATIC PORTOSYSTEMIC SHUNT

Hepatorenal Syndrome

Within 1 to 5 years after development of ascites in patients with cirrhosis, about 30% progress to hepatorenal syndrome. When this complication occurs, the life expectancy is measured in weeks to months. TIPS improves type I (progressive) and type II (steady) hepatorenal patients and may buy time for liver transplantation. Sodium excretion is increased, and renin and aldosterone concentrations are reduced after TIPS deployment. Brensing and coworkers (1997) in a small cohort of 16 hepatorenal patients showed that 2 weeks after TIPS insertion there was an approximate doubling of the creatinine clearance. There was further modest improvement over the next 8 weeks. There were three nonresponders, and all three died within 6 weeks after TIPS.

Refractory Hepatic Hydrothorax

Refractory hepatic hydrothorax is another rare complication in patients with cirrhosis in whom ascitic fluid migrates into the thoracic cavity along a pressure gradient. These patients usually have only moderate ascites, but need frequent thoracenteses to remove the pleural effusion and restore pulmonary function. Several studies on TIPS treatment of hepatic hydrothorax have been published, showing good efficacy in relieving this complication in about 70% and a 1-year survival comparable to patients with refractory ascites without hydrothorax.

Budd-Chiari Syndrome

TIPS is used increasingly in managing some patients with Budd-Chiari syndrome (Menon et al, 2004) (see Ch. 100). There are

pros and cons to using TIPS for such patients: on the pro side, TIPS offers a less invasive option than a portacaval shunt to decompress the congested liver of acute Budd-Chiari syndrome that has ongoing hepatocyte necrosis. Equally, TIPS may be a good option for patients with Budd-Chiari syndrome later in their course who have fibrosis in the liver, ascites, and portal hypertension, and it may serve as a useful bridge to transplant. On the con side, most patients with Budd-Chiari syndrome have a hypercoagulable state, so the use of TIPS, in which thrombosis and stenosis are a major issue, can be expected to lead to an increased risk of such complications. Available data seem to favor the pro rather than con side of this balance.

TIPS is an appropriate way for providing portal (and sinusoidal) decompression in Budd-Chiari syndrome patients who need this. TIPS must be accompanied by careful hematologic evaluation and management to reduce the risk of further thrombosis.

Hepatic Veno-occlusive Disease

Veno-occlusive disease of the liver is an important complication of bone marrow transplantation. The pathophysiology of this condition is related to increased sinusoidal pressure from occlusion of microscopic hepatic venules and central veins in the hepatic lobules. Insertion of TIPS has been performed in a few patients with veno-occlusive disease, and some had regression of the hepatic and renal symptoms. Patients with milder disease seem to be more likely to respond, but long-term survival seems to be uncommon. It is unclear whether these patients would have improved spontaneously. At present, the use of TIPS for veno-occlusive disease should be considered experimental.

Portal Hypertensive Gastropathy

In portal hypertension, venous and capillary ectasia is seen within the stomach, but can occur in the colon and other parts of the gastrointestinal tract. Occasionally, this disorder requires frequent transfusions with bleeding as severe as occurs with varices. Treatment options include β-blockers, shunt surgery, and TIPS. In a series of 40 patients, Kamath and colleagues (2000) showed TIPS was associated with an improvement in endoscopic findings and a decrease in transfusion requirement in 89% and 75% of patients with mild and severe portal hypertensive gastropathy. Endoscopic improvement in patients with mild gastropathy was visible within 6 weeks in most patients. The response was slower in patients with severe gastropathy. More than two thirds had endoscopic improvement by 3 months, however. TIPS is a reasonable option in patients with ongoing bleeding from portal gastropathy who do not respond to therapeutic doses of β-blockers.

CONTRAINDICATIONS TO TRANSJUGULAR INTRAHEPATIC PORTOSYSTEMIC SHUNT

Pulmonary Hypertension and Hepatopulmonary Syndrome

Cirrhosis sometimes is complicated by the development of pulmonary hypertension. The pathogenesis of this syndrome is obscure, but it seems more common with long-standing portosystemic shunting. The hepatopulmonary syndrome is a separate condition that is characterized by arteriovenous shunting within the pulmonary bed, producing a right-to-left shunt and systemic hypoxemia, usually in the absence of pulmonary hypertension.

The effect of TIPS on the pulmonary circulation is multifactorial and depends on the interaction of the changes in venous return, effective circulating volume, systemic vascular resistance, and myocardial reserve. After TIPS insertion, there is an immediate increase in venous return to the heart. Concurrently, systemic vascular resistance decreases, further worsening the hyperdynamic circulatory state. Cardiac output increases in response to these changes. When the heart's ability to handle this volume overload is exceeded, pulmonary venous pressures increase, with increasing ventilation-perfusion mismatch, hypoxia, and pulmonary vasoconstriction; pulmonary edema may ensue.

The varying effects of TIPS on patients with cirrhosis and pulmonary hypertension or hepatopulmonary syndrome are due to differences in the interactions between the aforementioned variables. TIPS should not be performed for these conditions. The outcome is unpredictable, and TIPS may be detrimental.

Prehepatic Portal Hypertension

Prehepatic portal hypertension results most commonly from portal vein thrombosis or tumors at the porta hepatis. Several anecdotal reports have documented that TIPS can be placed into a collateral vein—so-called cavernous transformation. Because TIPS placed in such collaterals may not reach the site of obstruction, however, it is unlikely to decompress the portal system and control bleeding adequately. The data do not justify placing TIPS for this indication. The exception may be a patient with an acute portal or superior mesenteric venous thrombus. TIPS provides the least invasive way to access these vessels for thrombectomy or lytic therapy or both. Increased sophistication of methods to do both of these has led to exploring this option. Data on efficacy are lacking.

Portal Hypertension Associated with Caroli's Disease and Polycystic Liver Disease

Polycystic liver disease and Caroli's disease may be complicated by portal hypertension and variceal hemorrhage. The creation of an intrahepatic tract may involve traversal of a cyst or a dilated biliary radicle; this is associated with a risk of hemorrhage or infection. TIPS is best avoided in such patients.

CONCLUSION

Since its introduction in 1988, TIPS has gone from being a novelty to being an important therapeutic modality in acute variceal bleeding refractory to endoscopic management. Its role in prevention of rebleeding is for patients who need decompression because they are refractory to first-line treatment. Data suggest bleeding control is equivalent to surgical shunt. TIPS has a role in the management of other conditions, such as refractory ascites, hepatic hydrothorax, and hepatorenal syndrome. Hepatic encephalopathy is increased after TIPS placement, but usually is controlled with medical therapy. Shunt malfunction is the main limitation of TIPS, is usually asymptomatic, and can lead to rebleeding. Recurrence of variceal bleeding in approximately 20% of patients and of ascites almost always is associated with shunt malfunction and mandates the need for intensive follow-up after TIPS placement.

Technique of Transjugular Intrahepatic Portosystemic Shunt Placement

M. DARCY

TIPS is a challenging procedure in interventional radiology. Although major complications can occur at any step of the procedure, with complete knowledge of the technique and solid understanding of imaging principles, it is possible to do TIPS with greater than 95% technical success, high clinical success (Fig. 96.1), and less than 1% direct procedural mortality.

PREPARATION FOR TRANSJUGULAR INTRAHEPATIC PORTOSYSTEMIC SHUNT

Before TIPS, careful evaluation is necessary to ensure a safe procedure. Assuming there are good indications for TIPS, contraindications must be excluded. Right heart dysfunction can be a relative contraindication because the increased venous return caused by the shunt can precipitate right heart failure. Although TIPS can be done in the presence of acute or subacute portal vein thrombosis, cavernous transformation with obliteration of the main portal vein is a relative contraindication because the chance of technical success is exceedingly low. For this reason, portal vein patency should be assessed (usually by Doppler ultrasound) before TIPS.

Severe hepatic dysfunction is another relative contraindication because shunting portal blood flow can worsen liver function. Serum bilirubin, Child-Pugh class, and several other schemes have been used to stratify patients into those who should and should not receive TIPS. The MELD (Model for End-stage Liver Disease) score has gained increased acceptance as a prognostic value. A study found good correlation between MELD and mortality (Ferral et al, 2004). The 30-day mortality was 18% for patients with a score of 18 to 25, and it increased to 43% if the MELD score was greater than 25. In cases of uncontrolled variceal hemorrhage, TIPS may be the patient's only chance for survival, however, and even with a high MELD score TIPS may be undertaken, rather than let the patient exsanguinate. It also is useful to know if the patient is a liver transplant candidate. This situation can alter the tone of the consent process if transplantation is not an available option should hepatic function deteriorate.

When the decision has been made to proceed, several steps need to be taken to optimize the patient's condition. Because puncture

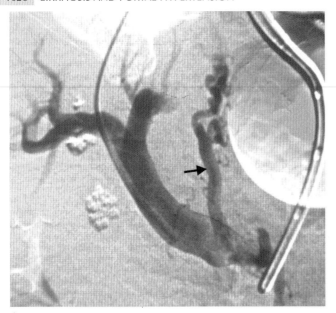

A

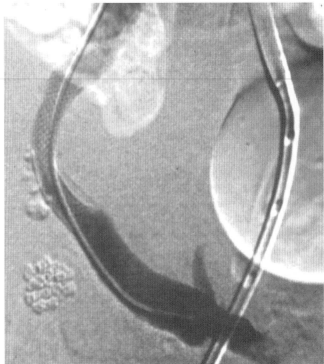

B

Fig. 96.1. A, Portal venogram (before dilating tract) in a patient with uncontrollable variceal hemorrhage shows flow up the coronary vein *(arrow)* to large varices despite the presence of a gastroesophageal tamponade balloon. **B,** Post-TIPS venogram shows good flow through the shunt and no further filling of the coronary vein or varices. The variceal hemorrhage ceased.

of the liver capsule and hemoperitoneum are potential complications, attempts should be made to correct any severe coagulopathy or thrombocytopenia. Although life-threatening hemoperitoneum is rare, it may be advisable to screen the patient's blood type for possible transfusion. The respiratory status must be assessed carefully because TIPS requires moderate to heavy sedation, and if the respiratory status is compromised, elective endotracheal intubation or general anesthesia may be warranted. Because the procedure involves passage of large stiff devices through the right atrium to the inferior vena cava (IVC), any conditions (e.g., hypokalemia) that might predispose to arrhythmias should be corrected. Prophylactic antibiotics targeting skin flora should be administered because bacteremia has been reported, and TIPS can become infected (Armstrong & MacLeod, 2003; DeSimone et al, 2000; Sanyal & Reddy, 1998). Infection is of special concern because polytetrafluoroethylene (PTFE)-covered devices are being used with increasing frequency.

INITIAL ACCESS

Initial venous access typically is through the right internal jugular vein because this is the shortest and most direct path to catheterize the hepatic veins. If the right internal jugular vein is occluded, there are two options. First, the left internal jugular vein can be used. Care must be taken, however, when passing equipment around the curved path from the left brachiocephalic vein to the hepatic veins because right atrial perforation may occur. Second, it may be possible to use a collateral vein around the right internal jugular vein or recanalize the occluded right internal jugular vein. Rarely, femoral vein access has been used as a starting point when the superior vena cava is completely occluded

(LaBerge et al, 1991). The problem with this approach is that when the portal vein has been entered, the caudal-to-cephalad trajectory makes it difficult to direct the stents down into the main portal vein, and instead they point out into the periphery.

The next step is to catheterize and evaluate the hepatic veins. The right hepatic vein is most commonly used because it is the largest hepatic vein and usually has the most favorable orientation. When the liver is shrunken and pushed cephalad, however, the angle into the right hepatic vein from the IVC becomes acute, which makes catheterization difficult. In this setting, the middle hepatic vein may be a better choice. Although it is often a smaller vein, if the access from the IVC is less acutely angled, it may present a more favorable starting point for the shunt.

Whichever vein is used, it is crucial for the clinician to identify from which vein he or she is starting. From the right hepatic vein, the needle is turned anteriorly to aim toward the right main portal trunk. If the clinician fails to realize he or she is in a middle hepatic vein, turning the needle anteriorly directs the needle away from the desired target. Although seemingly straightforward, the middle hepatic vein may be confused for the right hepatic vein on venography done only in the anteroposterior plane (Fig. 96.2). Obtaining a second view (usually right anterior oblique) helps distinguish the more posterior course of the right hepatic vein.

In Budd-Chiari syndrome, in which the hepatic veins are obliterated, there are still several options. If the hepatic vein thrombus is relatively fresh it still may be possible to advance a wire into the vein and use it as a starting point for the shunt (Fig. 96.3). When the hepatic veins are obliterated, the transhepatic puncture can be started from the stump of the hepatic veins or directly from the IVC. Punctures from the IVC should be confined to the intrahepatic segment of the IVC to limit the potential for intraperitoneal hemorrhage.

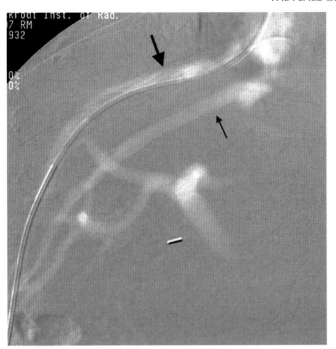

Fig. 96.2. Wedged hepatic venogram in the anteroposterior projection done to localize the portal vein. The right *(large arrow)* and middle *(small arrow)* hepatic veins have a similar course in this projection, but the middle hepatic vein drains more medially.

LOCALIZATION OF THE PORTAL VEIN

Before making the transhepatic needle passes, it is helpful to localize the portal vein because without contrast the portal vein is fluoroscopically indistinguishable from the surrounding parenchyma. The original clinical description of TIPS involved percutaneous transhepatic puncture into the portal vein and placement of a snare in the portal vein to act as a target for the needle being directed from the hepatic vein (Richter et al, 1989). The major problem with this technique is the potential for hemorrhage from the transcapsular puncture, especially because these patients often have coagulopathy. Intraperitoneal hemorrhage in this setting can be severe enough to be fatal.

More recently, various modifications have been described using smaller gauge needle systems to place small wires into the portal vein or coils adjacent to the portal vein to act as a target (Khabiri et al, 1994; Roizental et al, 1995). The smaller caliber needles have not eliminated the risk of significant intraperitoneal hemorrhage, however. Color flow ultrasound using an external probe on the anterior abdominal wall has been employed to provide noninvasive, real-time guidance to the portal vein. It can be technically challenging, however, to visualize the needle tip, and it requires coordination of two physicians. This technique is not widely used.

The noninvasive localization technique that provides the best combination of simplicity and effectiveness is wedged hepatic venography. This technique involves injecting contrast media retrograde from the hepatic vein through the sinusoids. The injection is best performed using a balloon occlusion catheter and carbon dioxide as the contrast media (Fig. 96.4). Balloon catheters decrease the risk because capsular rupture can occur with an end-hole catheter wedged very peripherally. The use of carbon dioxide improves portal opacification because it passes

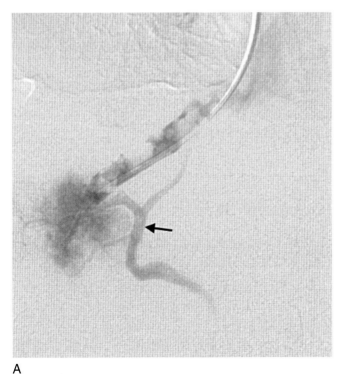

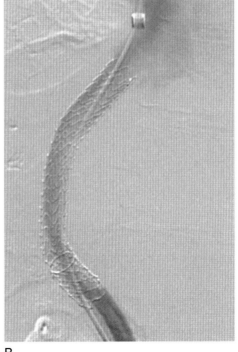

A   B

Fig. 96.3. A, Hepatic venogram in a patient with Budd-Chiari syndrome. The hepatic vein is diffusely thrombosed causing the filling defects seen in the hepatic vein. There is slight filling of a portal vein branch *(arrow).* This thrombosed vein was used as the starting point for TIPS. **B,** Portal venogram shows well-functioning TIPS despite the initial hepatic vein thrombosis.

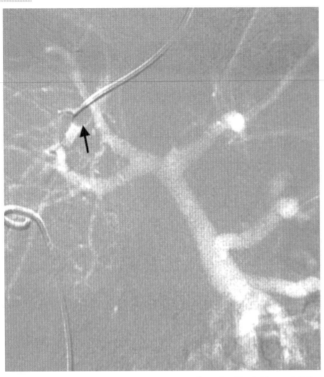

Fig. 96.4. Wedged hepatic venogram using carbon dioxide yields good delineation of the portal anatomy. The *arrow* points to the balloon occlusion catheter in the hepatic vein.

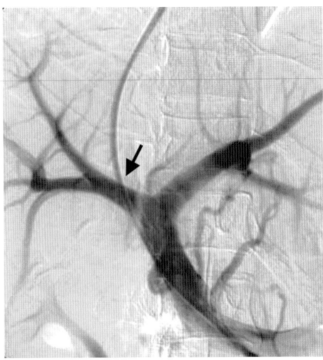

Fig. 96.5. Portal venogram at the start of TIPS shows good access *(arrow)* into the main trunk of the right portal vein. The portal vein should be intrahepatic at this point, but the tract still forms a gentle curve.

through the sinusoids better owing to its lower viscosity compared with liquid contrast agents. If done in multiple projections, carbon dioxide venography provides a good guide to the location of the portal vein. The primary disadvantage is that the carbon dioxide quickly dissipates, and wedged venography does not provide real-time guidance during needle passes.

ACCESSING THE PORTAL VEIN

The needle system is advanced into the hepatic vein, and passes are made across the hepatic parenchyma to access the portal vein. Several needle systems are available, some with larger 14-gauge needles and some with smaller 21-gauge needles. Haskal and colleagues (1995) showed that the smaller needle systems did not lead to reduced complications. The sets also have various combinations of outer catheters and sheaths. The choice of needle system is mostly a matter of physician preference.

The target is usually the main trunk of the right portal vein (Fig. 96.5). Puncturing the portal bifurcation itself increases the risk of accessing the extrahepatic portion of the portal vein. Too peripheral of a portal puncture leads to an excessively curved tract; this causes problems advancing catheters or stents, may lead to decreased efficacy of portal decompression, and may lead to lower patency. Good localization of the portal vein with carbon dioxide wedged venography helps to direct the needle passes in the right direction toward the right hepatic trunk. The clinician should limit the extent of the needle excursion to avoid capsular puncture and possible intra-abdominal hemorrhage.

After advancing the needle, it is withdrawn while aspirating or injecting contrast material. If using one of the fine needle sets, it can be difficult to aspirate blood up the long needle

catheter system. If blood is aspirated, the position of the needle tip within a portal vein needs to be confirmed with contrast injection before passing a guidewire. Blood also may be aspirated if the needle tip is in an arterial or hepatic venous branch. Alternatively, contrast material may be injected while withdrawing the needle similar to a transhepatic cholangiogram. Although it can be easier to recognize when a portal branch has been entered (compared with aspiration technique), injection of large amounts of contrast material can obscure visualization.

When the portal branch has been entered, a guidewire is passed into the portal system. A floppy wire such as a Bentson can be advantageous because this wire can be pushed until it buckles without damaging the vein; this is particularly useful if the wire first tends to go out toward the periphery. Continued pushing often buckles the wire down into the main portal trunk. A steerable hydrophilic wire, such as an angled Glidewire (Boston Scientific), can be used directing the wire in the proper direction toward the main portal vein; however, care must be taken not to pull the wire hard against the needle bevel because the outer coating of the wire may shear off. If a 21-gauge needle was used to gain portal access, a smaller 0.018-inch wire should be used. Regardless of the wire that is used, gentle probing with the wire is crucial to avoid dissection of the portal vein. Portal vein dissection can be difficult to recognize, and if the stent is deployed under the dissection flap, the shunt functions poorly.

CREATING THE TRACT

A 5-Fr catheter is advanced into the portal vein for venography and measuring pre-TIPS pressures. A portal venogram before dilating the parenchymal tract is crucial. This venogram provides confirmation that the portal vein has been accessed. If a hepatic artery puncture is not recognized by the needle contrast injection, the wire can be advanced inadvertently into a hepatic artery branch, and the course of the wire can perfectly mimic portal placement if the right hepatic artery is congenitally replaced to the superior mesenteric artery. There has been at least one case reported of dilating and stenting a tract between the hepatic artery and hepatic vein with disastrous results (Pattynama et al, 1995). This problem can be prevented by performing a portal venogram before dilating the tract.

The venogram is performed with a marking catheter to allow measurement of the length of the parenchymal tract and the distance to the hepatic vein–caval junction. Modern stent grafts used for TIPS come in different lengths. The expense of these devices makes it preferable to measure the length accurately and use only one device, rather than having to overlap multiple devices. It also is important to extend the TIPS right to the hepatic-caval junction, which requires accurate measurement, because even with bare metallic stents, patency is worse when a portion of the hepatic vein is left unstented (Clark et al, 2004). Also, almost all the stenoses that have developed after TIPS created with stent grafts have occurred in uncovered segments of the hepatic vein (Fig. 96.6) (Angeloni et al, 2004; Hausegger et al, 2004; Rossi et al, 2004). The measurement is taken from the entry point into the portal vein back to the hepatic-caval junction. If the tract is curved, an extra 1 cm is added to the measured length to compensate for the fact that the stent graft will conform more to the curves.

The parenchymal tract is dilated in preparation for stent deployment. Usually, an 8-mm standard balloon is used because larger, higher pressure balloons are difficult to advance across the periportal fibrosis into the portal vein before the tract has been dilated. Distinct waists are seen in the balloon as the portal and hepatic vein margins are dilated. Observing where these waists occur helps define the margins of the parenchymal tract. After dilatation, the access sheath is advanced into the portal vein for delivery of the stent.

STENTS AND STENT-GRAFTS

In the initial description of TIPS (Richter et al, 1989), the shunts were created with Palmaz balloon expandable stents. The Palmaz stent is rigid, however, and does not conform well to the curved tracts that often result during the puncture into the portal vein. Since then, TIPS have been created with almost every type of stent devised, but for many years the Wallstent was most commonly used. The Wallstent was easy to use, was flexible enough to work well around curves, had good radial strength, and had a Food and Drug Administration–approved indication for TIPS.

Although the Wallstent has been used with high technical and clinical success, patency has been a problem. In many series, at 1 year post-TIPS, primary patency is only 22% to 57% (Angeloni et al, 2004; ter Borg et al, 2004; Tripathi et al, 2004). About half of the stenoses occur in the hepatic vein, and half are due to intimal hyperplasia in the parenchymal segment. Many of these stenoses are asymptomatic and discovered by ultrasound screening; however, this high rate of stenosis led to the search for better devices. There is some evidence that this pseudointimal hyperplasia relates to communication with transected bile ducts (LaBerge et al, 1993), and it was logical to investigate the use of covered stents.

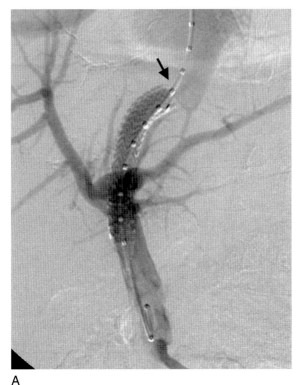

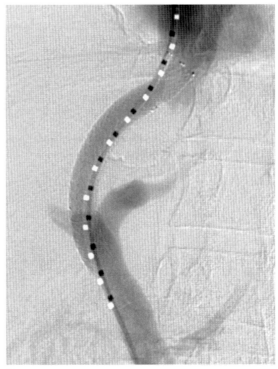

A

B

Fig. 96.6. A, Portal venogram 3 months post-TIPS shows a stenosis *(arrow)* in the short segment of hepatic vein that was not stented. The prominent opacification of the intrahepatic portal branches correlates with the elevated portal pressures caused by this stenosis. **B,** Postrevision portal venogram after extending a stent across the hepatic vein stenosis into the IVC. The decreased portal branch perfusion is angiographic evidence of improved portal decompression.

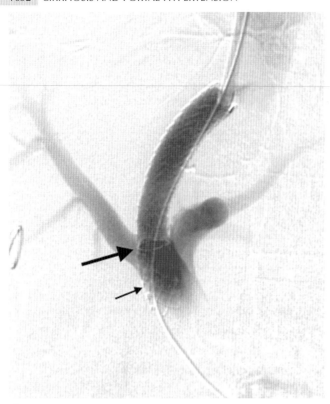

Fig. 96.7. Portal venogram in a patient with a Viatorr device in place. The radiopaque ring *(large arrow)* marks the junction between the uncovered portion of the stent *(small arrow)* that sits in the portal vein and the PTFE-covered portion in the parenchymal tract.

Several types of covered stents are commercially available, but only some are appropriate for TIPS. The polyethylene terephthalate–covered Wallgraft has been shown to be too porous, does not prevent bile leak into the shunt, and does not improve patency (Haskal et al, 2002). The Viatorr (W.L. Gore, Flagstaff, AZ) is a stent-graft specifically designed for TIPS, and it is rapidly becoming the standard device used in TIPS. This device has a 2-cm-long bare stent segment that sits in the portal vein and allows flow through the interstices to maintain portal patency (Fig. 96.7). The covered portion consists of three PTFE layers, one of which is an impermeable film to prevent bile leak into the shunt. In several series, this device has been shown to have significantly improved patency compared with uncovered stents (Angeloni et al, 2004; Hausegger et al, 2004; Otal et al, 2002; Rossi et al, 2004). Because the Viatorr comes in various lengths, its use requires accurately measuring the length of the tract from the portal vein to the hepatic vein–caval junction. The initial venograms must be done with a catheter with markers. At least one study found that the improved shunt patency of stent-grafts also translated into improved patient survival (Angermayr et al, 2003).

After inserting the chosen stent, the portal end is deployed first. With Wallstents, it is important to ensure the stents curve around toward the main portal vein so that the sharp ends do not protrude against the wall of the portal branch, a position that can lead to loss of patency and difficult future catheterizations. The stents should not extend too far into the main portal vein, however, because that may damage the portal vein and require use of an interposition graft during subsequent liver transplantation. A final venographic check right before stent deployment can be

useful to ensure proper positioning. With Viatorr devices, this is less of an issue. The device is positioned so that the junction between the bare intraportal segment and the PTFE-covered segment is situated right at the margin between the portal vein and the parenchymal tract. The uncovered intraportal segment of the Viatorr is always 2 cm long, preventing excessive extension down into the portal vein. In the past, stents were carried just high enough into the hepatic vein to prevent retraction into the tract. Because stenosis can develop in an unstented segment of the hepatic vein, it is now common practice to extend the stents or stent-graft all the way to the IVC.

After the stent has been deployed, it is usually balloon dilated to achieve the desired diameter. Although Wallstents and Viatorrs are self-expanding devices, the dense periportal fibrosis would prevent them from reaching their nominal diameter without assistance. Typically, a high-pressure balloon capable of handling 20 atm of pressure is needed to open the stent fully in the periportal region.

ASSESSING RESULTS

After creating the TIPS, venography should be repeated to ensure there is good flow through the shunt with no further filling of varices. One must be wary of artifacts. Inflow of unopacified blood from the portal branches may simulate the appearance of a stenosis at the portal end of the shunt. Forceful injection with the catheter tip pointed toward the origin of the coronary vein can simulate continued filling of the varices. If it is unclear if there is still flow into the varices, the catheter should be positioned in the splenic vein peripheral to the coronary vein so that a repeat venogram shows if the flow into the varices was spontaneous or caused by the force of injection. Confirmation of good portal decompression is obtained by measuring the portosystemic gradient, with the target being less than 12 mm Hg because this is the threshold below which varices are unlikely to bleed. If the gradient is still greater than 12 mm Hg, and no clear cause is seen by venography, careful pullback pressures can help identify if there is a focal correctable problem.

Stent morphology and position also must be assessed before ending the procedure. Any areas of residual stenosis may need to be dilated again, especially if there is a persistent high gradient. Because stenting to the IVC improves patency, identifying that the stents extend right to the hepatic vein–caval junction is important. This identification can be difficult because the high flow in the cava prevents good opacification of this junction. Injecting contrast material through the access sheath positioned at the top of the stent improves visualization of this region. If the initial stent does not extend far enough, a second stent can be placed overlapping the first one and extending more cephalad.

ANCILLARY PROCEDURES

Embolization

If the post-TIPS venogram shows persistent flow into varices, one first must look for a mechanical problem with the TIPS, such as narrowing of the stent or incomplete coverage of the parenchymal tract. Large varices may continue to have flow into them, however, even if the TIPS is wide open and the portosystemic gradient is less than 12 mm Hg. Originally, the common

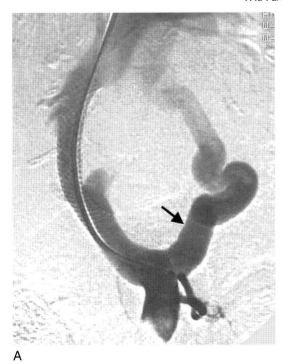
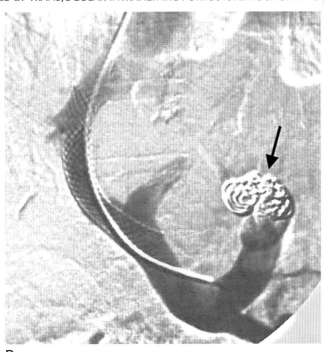

A   B

Fig. 96.8. A, Post-TIPS portal venogram shows that despite a patent TIPS, there is persistent flow to varices through the coronary vein *(arrow)*. This is due to the huge size of the coronary vein. **B,** After embolization of the coronary vein with Gianturco coils *(arrow)*, there is no further flow to the varices, and the patient had no more variceal bleeding.

opinion was that varices did not need to be embolized if the portosystemic gradient was lowered appropriately; however, bleeding from varices has been reported to occur despite a low gradient, especially when dealing with ectopic varices (Vangeli et al, 2004).

When TIPS is being performed to treat variceal hemorrhage, and the varices are still filling after creation of an adequate shunt, embolization is advisable. Embolization can be accomplished by advancing an angiographic catheter into the vessel supplying the varices and deploying Gianturco coils (Fig. 96.8). Usually the veins are large enough that a nest of different size coils is required to occlude the vein effectively. Larger coils that do not migrate down the vein are placed first to provide a framework for subsequent placement of smaller coils.

Ascites Drainage

In patients with intractable ascites, drainage of the ascites can be a useful adjunctive procedure. Draining ascites during the case is easily performed. A catheter can be inserted percutaneously at the start of the TIPS procedure; the catheter is then placed to gravity drainage. The ascites drains while the TIPS is being created. There are several benefits to doing this procedure. First, it gives the patient a head start on resolution of ascites, rather than waiting for it to resolve on its own. Second, draining the ascites makes placement of the TIPS easier by allowing the liver to relax down into a more normal position. This position makes the angle between the cava and hepatic vein less acute and easier to work through. Improved fluoroscopic visualization is another benefit because it can be difficult to obtain a good fluoroscopic image in an abdomen that is grossly distended with ascites. The ascites drainage catheter also is useful to monitor for complications

because capsular hemorrhage from needle passes causes the draining ascites to become bloody.

CONCLUSION

Basic TIPS can be a technically challenging procedure. More advanced techniques (beyond the scope of this chapter) are available to allow the experienced interventional radiologist to tackle more difficult cases, such as patients with occluded jugular access, Budd-Chiari syndrome, or portal vein thrombosis.

REFERENCES

Angeloni S, et al, 2004: Polytetrafluoroethylene-covered stent grafts for TIPS procedure: 1-year patency and clinical results. Am J Gastroenterol 99:280-285.

Angermayr B, et al, 2003: Survival in patients undergoing transjugular intrahepatic portosystemic shunt: ePTFE-covered stentgrafts versus bare stents. Hepatology 38:1043-1050.

Armstrong PK, MacLeod C, 2003: Infection of transjugular intrahepatic portosystemic shunt devices: three cases and a review of the literature. Clin Infect Dis 36:407-412.

Azoulay D, et al, 2001: Salvage transjugular intrahepatic portosystemic shunt for uncontrolled variceal bleeding in patients with decompensated cirrhosis. J Hepatol 35:658-660.

Banares R, et al, 1998: Urgent transjugular intrahepatic portosystemic shunt for control of acute variceal bleeding. Am J Gastroenterol 93:75-79.

Brensing KA, et al, 1997: Transjugular intrahepatic portosystemic stent-shunt for hepatorenal syndrome. Lancet 349:697.

Bureau C, et al, 2004: Improved clinical outcome using polytetrafluoroethylene-coated stents for TIPS: results of a randomized study. Gastroenterology 126:469-475.

Burroughs AK, Vangeli M, 2002: Transjugular intrahepatic portosystemic shunt versus endoscopic therapy: randomized trials for secondary prophylaxis of variceal bleeding: an updated meta-analysis. Scand J Gastroenterol 37: 249-252.

Clark TW, et al, 2004: The effect of initial shunt outflow position on patency of transjugular intrahepatic portosystemic shunts. J Vasc Interv Radiol 15: 147-152.

De Franchis R, 2001: What have we accomplished? In De Franchis R (ed): Portal Hypertension III. Proceedings of the Third Baveno International Consensus Workshop on Definitions, Methodology, and Therapeutic Strategies. Oxford, Blackwell, pp 1-12.

DeSimone JA, et al, 2000: Sustained bacteremia associated with transjugular intrahepatic portosystemic shunt (TIPS). Clin Infect Dis 30:384-386.

Ferral H, et al, 2004: Survival after elective transjugular intrahepatic portosystemic shunt creation: prediction with model for end-stage liver disease score. Radiology 231:231-236.

Gulberg V, et al, 2002: Improved quality of life in patients with refractory or recidivant ascites after insertion of transjugular intrahepatic portosystemic shunts. Digestion 66:127-130.

Haag K, et al, 1993: Der transjuguläre intrahepatische portosystemische Stent-Shunt (TIPS) in der Notfallbehandlung der portalen Hypertension. Intensivmedizin 30:479-483.

Haskal ZJ, et al, 1995: Transjugular intrahepatic portosystemic shunt-related arterial injuries—prospective comparison of large- and small-gauge needle systems. J Vasc Interv Radiol 6:911-915.

Haskal ZJ, et al, 2002: Recurrent TIPS thrombosis after polyethylene stent-graft use and salvage with polytetrafluoroethylene stent-grafts. J Vasc Interv Radiol 13:1255-1259.

Hausegger KA, et al, 2004: Transjugular intrahepatic portosystemic shunt creation with the Viatorr expanded polytetrafluoroethylene-covered stent-graft. J Vasc Interv Radiol 15:239-248.

Helton WS, et al, 2001: Transjugular intrahepatic portosystemic shunt vs surgical shunt in good-risk cirrhotic patients. Arch Surg 136:17-20.

Henderson JM, et al, 2000: Surgical shunts and TIPS for variceal decompression in the 1990s. Surgery 128:540-547.

Henderson JM, et al, 2004: DSRS vs. TIPS for refractory variceal bleeding: a prospective randomized controlled trial. The DIVERT study group. Hepatology 40:725A (abstract).

Jalan R, et al, 1995: A comparative study of emergency transjugular intrahepatic portosystemic stent-shunt and oesophageal transection in the management of uncontrolled variceal haemorrhage. Am J Gastroenterol 90:1932-1937.

Kamath PS, et al, 2000: Gastric mucosal responses to intrahepatic portosytemic shunting in patients with cirrhosis. Gastroenterology 118:905.

Khabiri H, et al, 1994: CT-guided localization of the portal vein before creation of a transjugular intrahepatic portosystemic shunt. AJR Am J Roentgenol 163:746-747 (letter).

LaBerge JM, et al, 1991: Percutaneous intrahepatic portosystemic shunt created via a femoral vein approach. Radiology 181:679-681.

LaBerge JM, et al, 1993: Histopathologic study of stenotic and occluded transjugular intrahepatic portosystemic shunts. J Vasc Interv Radiol 4:779-786.

McCormick PA, et al, 1994: Emergency transjugular intrahepatic portosystemic stent-shunting as salvage treatment for uncontrolled variceal bleeding. Br J Surg 81:1324-1327.

Menon KV, et al, 2004: The Budd-Chiari syndrome. N Engl J Med 350: 578-585.

Otal P, et al, 2002: Preliminary results of a new expanded-polytetrafluoroethylene-covered stent-graft for transjugular intrahepatic portosystemic shunt procedures. AJR Am J Roentgenol 178:141-147.

Patch D, et al, 1998: Factors related to early mortality after transjugular intrahepatic portosystemic shunt for failed endoscopic therapy in acute variceal bleeding. J Hepatol 28:454-460.

Pattynama PM, et al, 1995: Inadvertent arteriovenous stenting during transjugular intrahepatic portosystemic shunt procedure and the importance of hepatic artery perfusion. Cardiovasc Interv Radiol 18:192-195.

Richter GM, et al, 1989: Intrahepatic stent-assisted portosystemic shunt: new nonoperative transjugular and percutaneous method. Radiologe 29: 406-411.

Roizental M, et al, 1995: Portal vein: US-guided localization prior to transjugular intrahepatic portosystemic shunt placement. Radiology 196: 868-870.

Rosemurgy AS, et al, 2000: Transjugular intrahepatic portosystemic shunt vs. small-diameter prosthetic H-graft portacaval shunt: extended follow-up of an expanded randomized prospective trial. J Gastrointest Surg 4: 589-597.

Rossi P, et al, 2004: Polytetrafluoroethylene-covered nitinol stent-graft for transjugular intrahepatic portosystemic shunt creation: 3-year experience. Radiology 231:820-830.

Saab S, et al, 2004: TIPS versus paracentesis for cirrhotic patients with refractory ascites. Cochrane Database Syst Rev 3:CD004889.

Salerno F, et al, 2004: Randomized controlled study of TIPS versus paracentesis plus albumin in cirrhosis with severe ascites. Hepatology 40:629-635.

Sanyal AJ, Reddy KR, 1998: Vegetative infection of transjugular intrahepatic portosystemic shunts. Gastroenterology 115:110-115.

Sanyal AJ, et al, 2003: The North American Study for Treatment of Refractory Ascites. The North American Study for the Treatment of Refractory Ascites Group. Gastroenterology 124:634-641.

ter Borg PC, et al, 2004: Transjugular intrahepatic portosystemic shunts: long-term patency and clinical results in a patient cohort observed for 3-9 years. Radiology 231:537-545.

Tripathi D, et al, 2004: Ten years' follow-up of 472 patients following transjugular intrahepatic portosystemic stent-shunt insertion at a single centre. Eur J Gastroenterol Hepatol 16:9-18.

Vangeli M, et al, 2004: Bleeding ectopic varices—treatment with transjugular intrahepatic porto-systemic shunt (TIPS) and embolisation. J Hepatol 41:560-566.

97

The Technique of Portacaval Shunt*

L. H. BLUMGART

A portacaval shunt is a yardstick with which all other operations and nonoperative measures for the treatment of portal hypertension should be compared. Its primary objective is the prevention of recurrent variceal hemorrhage, and in this, it is most successful. Its disadvantage is that in about a quarter of patients, significant encephalopathy may follow the operation, spoiling an otherwise good result.

The chief indication for the operation is the elective treatment of esophageal varices, in patients who have recovered from an episode of variceal bleeding, to reduce the chances of further hemorrhage. The operation should not be performed to prevent bleeding in patients whose varices have not yet bled (prophylactic shunt). Only rarely should portacaval shunt be undertaken in an emergency, in patients whose bleeding has not responded to other measures (see Chs. 91, 92, and 95). The operation is contraindicated if hepatic function is severely impaired, as evidenced by persistent jaundice, intractable ascites, and spontaneous bouts of encephalopathy. The indications for portacaval shunt are considered further and details of the preoperative investigations and intraoperative measures are given in Ch. 95.

End-to-side and H-graft partial portacaval shunts are described. There is little evidence that the variants (e.g., side-to-side shunt) are superior, and they present technical difficulties. A side-to-side portacaval shunt has a place in the treatment of the Budd-Chiari syndrome (see Ch. 100), in which there is severe outflow block. At one time, conventional splenorenal shunt was performed as frequently as the portacaval shunt. The advantages of the proximal splenorenal shunt, which is technically more difficult to perform than portacaval shunt, are not apparent, however, and there are few surgeons who now include it in their repertoire of portosystemic shunts. The sole indication of the proximal splenorenal shunt may be in a patient whose spleen has to be removed at the same time. The main rival to portacaval shunt is distal splenorenal shunt (see Ch. 98). The techniques for side-to-side portacaval shunt and interposition mesentericocaval shunt are described in Chs. 99 and 100.

TECHNIQUE

Position on Table

Because a long, right, subcostal incision is preferred, the patient is placed on his or her back on the operating table, with the right side elevated 20 to 30 degrees to the table. The right arm is suspended, with the usual precautions, in front of the patient and the left arm, abducted to 90 degrees, is supported on an accessory table. The table is broken at the level of the costal margin. The body is placed level on the central part of the table, and the patient is in the head-down position (Fig. 97.1).

Incision

A long, right subcostal incision, two finger-breadths below the right costal margin, extending from just to the left of the midline well into the right flank, is preferred (Fig. 97.2). Other incisions have been described. The midline and right paramedian incisions do not provide good access. A right thoracoabdominal incision gives good access, but postoperative complications are common, and if ascites is present, persistent right pleural effusion can present problems after operation.

Meticulous hemostasis is important. A slight ooze from the wound edge during the operation produces a pool of blood in the depths of the wound, at the site of the vascular anastomosis.

The peritoneum should be incised carefully. Intra-abdominal adhesions, which under normal conditions could be swept aside easily with a sponge, must be carefully identified, ligated, and divided because large venous collaterals may have developed within them.

Exposure

An inexperienced surgeon can be discouraged by the sight of a large spleen, markedly diseased liver that is hard and stiff to the touch, and the many venous collaterals between the viscera and the parietal peritoneum. Great patience is required to develop the exposure. Only occasionally it becomes necessary to abandon the operation because of thick, vascular adhesions in the right upper quadrant, following a previous operation at this site. Under these circumstances, another portosystemic shunt (e.g., mesocaval shunt or distal splenorenal shunt [see Chs. 98 and 99]) should be attempted. Exposure is achieved by systematic and measured dissection. Hepatocellular carcinoma occurs in 5% to 10% of patients with long-standing cirrhosis, and this should be borne in mind, especially if preoperative axial imaging has not been performed. A catheter is inserted into the splanchnic circulation to measure portal venous pressure before and after shunting to determine the effectiveness of the shunt. A fine polyethylene catheter is inserted into a jejunal mesenteric vein that has been mobilized and held between ligatures. The tip of the catheter is advanced until it lies within a major mesenteric vein or the portal vein itself. The catheter system is filled with heparinized saline and attached to a simple central venous catheter set or,

*Adapted from Shields R, Blumgart LH, 2000: The technique of portacaval shunt. In Surgery of the Liver and Biliary Tract, 3rd ed. Philadelphia, Saunders, pp 1955-1962.

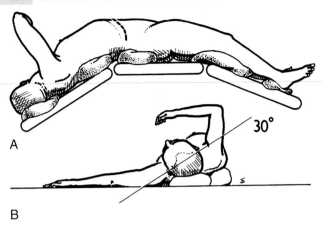

Fig. 97.1. A and **B,** Patient's position on table.

if available, a strain gauge manometer. The point of zero reference for the venous manometer is adjusted to the level of the right atrium. The mean portal pressure is recorded. Through this catheter, venous angiography can be performed, if previous studies have been unsatisfactory.

The surgeon should avoid the temptation to dissect directly into the porta hepatis. The approach should always be from the periphery, coming in from above and below, from the right and left side, establishing planes of cleavage between adjacent viscera.

The hepatic flexure of the colon is mobilized and retracted downward (Fig. 97.3). The correct plane is identified by mobilizing the lateral side of the ascending colon from below, carefully dissecting the hepatic flexure from the undersurface of the liver, gallbladder, and duodenum. If any difficulty is encountered, a second plane of cleavage can be established on the left side, along the transverse colon, detaching it from the liver and the stomach. By this combined approach, the colon can be retracted out of the operative field with a retractor placed over a swab.

The falciform ligament of the liver is divided. The liver should now be reflected cranially with a broad-blade retractor placed on its undersurface at the level of the gallbladder. A distended gallbladder should be emptied by compression. Adhesions between the gallbladder and adjacent viscera should be divided between ligatures. A plane should be established on the right side between the undersurface of the liver and the second part of the duodenum and on the left side between the undersurface of the liver and the stomach. Ultimately, the liver and the gallbladder can be reflected up from the operative field (Fig. 97.4).

The first and second parts of the duodenum lie centrally in the operative field. Many venous collaterals run to the posterior

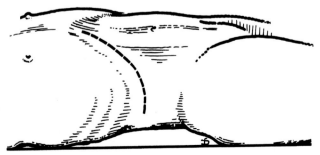

Fig. 97.2. Patient rotated 30 degrees to the left, illustrating the right subcostal incision.

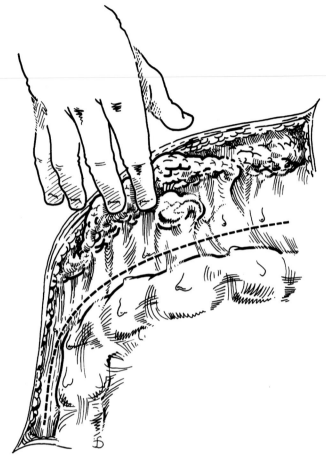

Fig. 97.3. Cirrhotic liver and gallbladder above with the colon plastered by vascular lesions to its undersurface. The *dotted line* indicates the plane of cleavage to separate the colon from the liver.

and lateral abdominal wall. To mobilize the second part of the duodenum, the posterior peritoneum on the right side of the second part of the duodenum is carefully divided. It is thicker, more vascular, and more edematous than normal, and it should be divided by a combination of cautery to smaller vessels and ligature of larger collaterals. The mobilization of the duodenum is usually easy, but should extend from the pylorus above to the first inch or so of the third part of the duodenum below so that the inferior vena cava (IVC) can be displayed in the depth of the wound.

The duodenum should be reflected to the left. The anterior and lateral surface of the IVC is exposed from the renal vessels below to the liver above (Fig. 97.5). In these patients, the peritoneum lying over the IVC is often thick. It should be lifted up between clips, incised and divided by sharp dissection. Bleeding collaterals should be cauterized again. It is crucial that the IVC is cleanly exposed in the depths of the wound: all periadventitial tissue should be removed. With end-to-side shunt, it is not necessary to mobilize the entire circumference of the IVC. It adds greatly to the complexity of the operation to do so because several small venous tributaries entering the posterior surface of the IVC have to be identified, ligated, and divided. At least two thirds of the anterior circumference of the IVC should be dissected, however (Fig. 97.6).

The free edge of the lesser omentum should be approached to mobilize the portal vein. Although it is important to know where

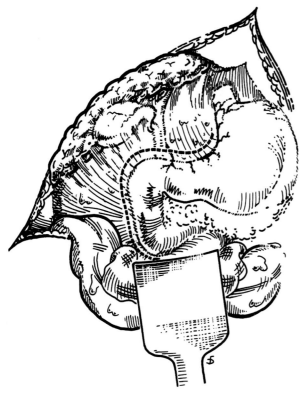

Fig. 97.4. The colon has been retracted caudally, and the illustration shows the next stage of the dissection, which is to separate the stomach and the duodenum from the undersurface of the liver.

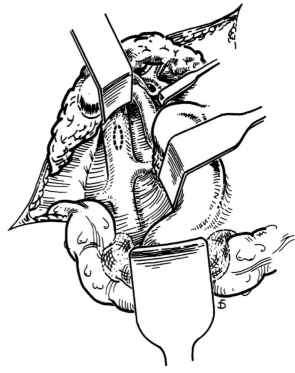

Fig. 97.6. The IVC is displayed in the depth of the wound, and a retractor is shown reflecting the mobilized free edge of the hepatic duodenal ligament to the left. This free edge of the lesser omentum contains the bile ducts (as shown); the hepatic artery and the portal vein are more deeply placed.

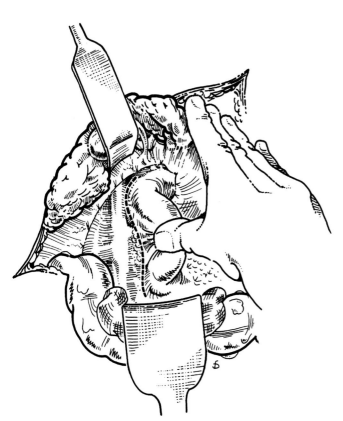

Fig. 97.5. The IVC in the depth of the wound is now displayed from the renal veins below to the undersurface of the liver above.

the common bile duct and the hepatic artery lie, the surgeon need not attempt to mobilize these separately; this would entail an unnecessarily hazardous dissection. When the positions of these two structures have been identified, the portal vein should be approached from behind in the posterolateral aspect of the free edge of the lesser omentum. The posterolateral approach is facilitated by the 20-degree to 30-degree rotation of the patient to the left. In this part of the hepatoduodenal ligament, there are few portal venous tributaries. Fatty connective tissue containing lymph nodes and lymphatics has to be divided. Some difficulty may be encountered because of the thickness of the edematous fibrofatty tissue. The portal vein may be obscured by a lymph node, which has to be dissected free. It is useful to know that, apart from the portal vein, the only other small vessels in this vicinity are those associated with the lymph node. The portal vein is recognized easily by its characteristic blue, bulging appearance. Occasionally, an accessory or replaced right hepatic artery, which has taken origin from the superior mesenteric artery, is present posterolateral to the common bile duct (see Ch. 1), and this should be preserved.

The portal vein should be mobilized throughout its entire length (see Fig. 97.6). The greater the length of portal vein exposed, the fewer problems there will be with the anastomosis. The vein should be exposed above up to its bifurcation and entry into the liver and inferiorly behind the pancreas so that its formation by the union of the superior mesenteric and the splenic veins is displayed. The vein should be freed of all periadventitial tissue.

The dissection of the medial wall of the portal vein may present some difficulty. The vein should be mobilized circumferentially at its midpoint, that is, halfway between its start and bifurcation. This process should be performed gently and slowly, until it is

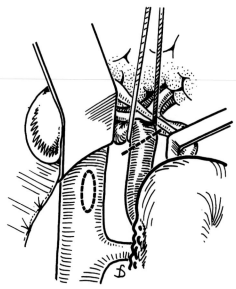

Fig. 97.7. The portal vein is displayed further. The *dotted oval* on the IVC shows the ideal position of the window.

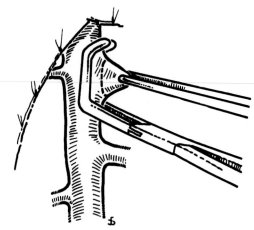

Fig. 97.8. The Satinsky clamp is placed on the anteromedial aspect of the IVC, a segment of which is drawn into the jaws of the clamp with a DeBakey dissector.

possible to slip a Lahey clamp under vision around the portal vein. Under no circumstances should the mobilization of the vein and the insertion of the clamp be performed roughly because a segment of the portal vein may be damaged, or one of the posterior or medial tributaries of the portal vein may be torn. A vessel loop is drawn around the portal vein, and the portal vein can be lifted from its bed. The entire length of the portal vein from the upper edge of the pancreas to its bifurcation is completely mobilized. At the pancreatic edge, the posterolateral tissue should be divided so as to free the portal vein completely and avoid kinking after anastomosis. Any small tributaries are identified, ligated, and divided (Fig. 97.7).

Occasionally, a prominent caudate lobe of the liver can lie between the upper portion of the portal vein and the IVC and make the approximation of the vessels difficult. Careful upward retraction is usually sufficient to allow anastomosis, however. Excision of this tissue is usually unnecessary and may be difficult, resulting in troublesome bleeding that may obscure the anastomotic site. The portal venous pressure should be measured, and the patency of the catheter should be maintained. The IVC is now prepared. An occluding Satinsky clamp is placed on the anterior medial surface of the IVC, approximately 30 degrees to the left of the midline of the cava, at a level designed to avoid any kinking, or angulation, of the portal vein. The clamp should be placed neither too high, so that the divided portal vein would be put in stretch, nor too low, at or near the renal veins, for the portal vein would be excessively angled. There is a tendency to place the clamp too far to the right on the circumference of the IVC so that the portal vein may be kinked when the anastomosis is complete.

The clamp is placed loosely in the desired position, and a segment of the IVC is drawn up with nontoothed dissectors, to provide a sufficient segment of the IVC to make a window (Fig. 97.8). The clamp is closed, and a 1.5- to 2-cm segment of the IVC is excised (Fig. 97.9). A simple incision of the IVC is insufficient. A 4-0 vascular suture is inserted in the midpoint of the right side of the window of the IVC to retract it out of the way so that the posterior layer of the anastomosis can be made easily.

A Potts clamp is placed on the portal vein as low as possible and preferably just at the junction of the superior mesenteric

vein and the splenic vein. A second clamp is placed on the portal vein close to its bifurcation (see Fig. 97.9), and the vein is divided. The portal vein stump is ligated and allowed to retract into the hilum of the liver. The portal vein is divided at an angle, to increase the caliber of the anastomosis and to prevent kinking of the vein. The lumen of the portal vein and the IVC are cleared of clots by washing with heparinized saline.

The portal vein and the IVC are approximated by stay sutures placed into the upper and lower angles of the anastomosis (Fig. 97.10). Throughout the anastomosis, 4-0 or 5-0 vascular sutures are used. An end-to-side anastomosis is performed, beginning with the posterior row and using an over suture technique.

The vein walls may be quite fragile, so the sutures should be well lubricated and eased gently through the vessel wall. Unless this is done, small holes and tears in the vessel wall may occur, which, when the anastomosis is complete and the clamps removed, bleed copiously. The posterior layer is completed (Fig. 97.11). The running suture may be anchored at this time. Alternatively, the needle may be brought out through the wall of the IVC and

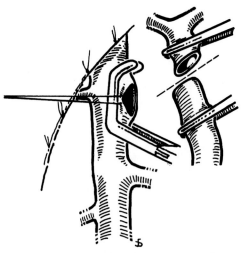

Fig. 97.9. An incision has been made in the IVC, and a small segment of vein has been excised to form a window. The portal vein has been divided obliquely between the clamps after it has been completely mobilized. The lower clamp is placed just above the junction of the splenic vein and the superior mesenteric vein, and the upper clamp is placed close to the hilum of the liver at the bifurcation of the portal vein.

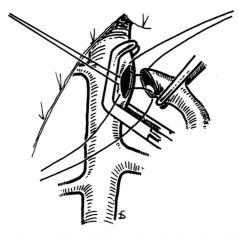

Fig. 97.10. The cut angled end of the portal vein has been brought down close to the window of the occluded segment of the IVC, and stay sutures have been applied.

the anterior layer completed by over-and-over sutures. Care should be taken to tighten the sutures gently and ease the portal vein down on to the IVC to avoid tearing. The surgeon should avoid inadvertently picking up the posterior layer while completing the anterior layer. Throughout the anastomosis, twisting, kinking, or angulation of the portal vein must be avoided to prevent occlusion of the portal vein or the anastomosis. The aim should be that, at the end of the operation, the portal vein curves gently to join the IVC.

The anterior part of the anastomosis should be inspected, if possible along with the posterior layer, particularly at the angles, to determine that there are no major tears or holes. The Satinsky clamp on the IVC is loosened temporarily. Bleeding discloses holes in the vein or gaps in the anastomosis. If the bleeding does not stop spontaneously with gentle pressure using a small gauze tamponade, these holes should be closed by well-placed interrupted

4-0 sutures. An anastomosis that is functioning effectively usually bleeds very little. The clamps can be removed, and a swab can be placed over the anastomosis for a few minutes.

The pressure within the splanchnic circulation must be measured again. The decrease in pressure should be to normal, or at least to 20% above normal; this indicates a satisfactory result. If there is no change in the portal pressure, the anastomosis in the portal vein should be inspected carefully for angulation or kinking. Under no circumstances should the operation be completed with an unchanged portal pressure. Failure to produce a significant reduction would lead to further esophageal variceal hemorrhage, early and catastrophically in the postoperative period. If the surgeon is not sure why the portal pressure has not decreased, angiography can be done by injecting contrast medium through the catheter.

There are usually two reasons for a functionally ineffective anastomosis. First, there may be angulation at the site of the anastomosis. This may be corrected by further mobilization of the portal vein, or it may be necessary to take down the anastomosis and refashion it. Another reason is kinking or angulation of the portal vein near its origin at the head of the pancreas. This kinking often can be eased by further mobilization of the portal vein, superior mesenteric vein, and splenic vein at this site (see earlier).

The surgeon can recognize an effective anastomosis quickly because there is usually little or no bleeding from it, and the oozing from adjacent venous collaterals stops immediately. A palpable thrill in the area also may indicate a satisfactory anastomosis. The completed operation is shown Fig. 97.12.

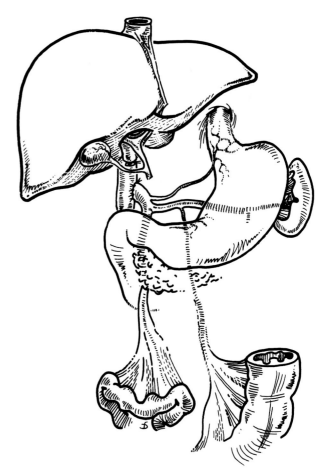

Fig. 97.12. The completed operation. Common bile duct is not illustrated.

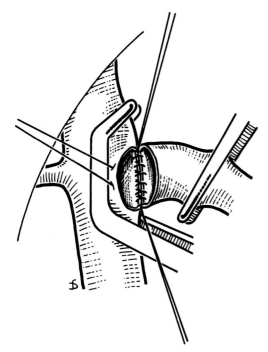

Fig. 97.11. The posterior layer of anastomosis has been completed.

Closure

Closure should be performed without drainage to avoid continuous and substantial loss of ascitic fluid. The surgeon's usual type of closure of abdominal wounds can be used. We prefer a single through-and-through one-layer closure with No. 1 unabsorbable suture with clips to the skin.

POSTOPERATIVE CARE

Patients must be observed closely after the operation, as after any major abdominal surgery. Vital functions must be monitored carefully for 1 to 2 days. Fluid intake should be given largely in the form of 10% dextrose to ensure an adequate supply of carbohydrate to the liver. Oxygen may have to be given as advised by an anesthetist.

Broad-spectrum antibiotics, which should have started preoperatively, are continued for 36 to 48 hours after the operation. The nasogastric tube can be removed on postoperative day 2 or 3, and a light diet, low in protein and sodium, is begun on postoperative day 4 or 5. Liver function should be monitored carefully, and the patient should be weighed daily to detect the onset of ascites or peripheral edema. Patients usually can be discharged on postoperative day 10 or 12.

More serious postoperative complications are observed after an emergency portacaval shunt because patients usually have been ravaged by their disease and repeated gastrointestinal hemorrhage. Great care to avoid pulmonary complications and hepatic and renal failure must be exercised. Occasionally, alcoholic patients may show delirium tremens.

Distal Splenorenal Shunt

J. M. HENDERSON

Distal splenorenal shunt (DSRS) is the prototype of selective variceal decompression that has been used since 1966. The goal of selective decompression of gastroesophageal varices is to combine the benefit of a decompressive shunt to control variceal bleeding with maintenance of portal hypertension and portal flow to the cirrhotic liver. The latter is important to help maintain liver function. Although DSRS has been most widely used, the alternative is a coronary caval shunt.

Warren and colleagues (1967) published their classic article on selective variceal decompression describing the animal work leading up to the initial clinical data on DSRS. It was the differing backgrounds of Warren and Zeppa that led to the evolution of this concept. Warren had seen the effectiveness of total portosystemic shunt in controlling variceal bleeding, but at the cost of liver failure, whereas Zeppa (1978) knew that portal perfusion and liver function were well maintained after devascularization procedures, but there was a significant risk of rebleeding. The concept of creating a low-pressure gastroesophageal and splenic decompression pathway to the left renal vein was shown to be feasible in animal studies. Concurrent with this idea, the superior mesenteric and portal venous pathway to the liver was left intact, and flow could be maintained in these animal studies. Having established this principle, the work rapidly advanced to successful outcomes in humans.

Over the next 4 decades, DSRS became a widely used technique for management of variceal bleeding. It is the most commonly used surgical shunt as shown by the current worldwide literature and is the operation of choice for decompression of varices when surgery is needed. The technique has continued to evolve. Choice of patients has improved, and the role of DSRS in the overall scheme of management of patients with variceal bleeding has been better defined. This chapter addresses these areas.

PATIENT EVALUATION

Not every patient with variceal bleeding needs or is a candidate for DSRS. It is indicated for some good risk patients with continued bleeding or persistent high-risk varices after adequate endoscopic therapy. The risk of rebleeding from varices after an initial bleed is 75%; first-line treatment to reduce this risk is with pharmacologic and endoscopic therapy. The risk of rebleeding through this first-line therapy is reduced to 25% to 30%. In addition, some good risk patients in whom varices cannot be obliterated with endoscopic therapy may be candidates for surgical decompression. The selection of patients for DSRS requires full evaluation to define the following:

1. Cause of the portal hypertension
2. Size, extent, and risk factors of the varices
3. Status of liver function/damage
4. Vascular anatomy

Most patients in the United States and Europe with variceal bleeding have cirrhosis as the underlying cause of portal hypertension. In these patients, the first question to be addressed is whether the patient now or in the future is a candidate for liver transplantation. If the patient is likely to need a transplant in the next 1 to 2 years, surgical shunt is not indicated. If the patient has good liver function and is unlikely to need a transplant in the near future, DSRS may be a good option.

Which patients are candidates for DSRS? Although surgical decompression is being used less frequently, it can provide an excellent outcome for an ideal candidate. Such patients have good liver function, have stable liver disease, and have suitable venous anatomy. The tests necessary to define such ideal candidates are endoscopy, Doppler ultrasound, clinical and laboratory assessment for liver disease, and visceral angiography for final anatomic definition.

Upper gastrointestinal endoscopy is indicated at the time of an acute variceal bleed as a diagnostic and therapeutic modality. Elective evaluation when the patient is stabilized requires repeat endoscopy to assess variceal size, red color signs, location, and extent. Larger varices with multiple risk factors, particularly when they extend into the gastric fundus, are more likely to need surgical decompression.

Liver function is assessed from clinical findings and laboratory studies. Jaundice, ascites, and encephalopathy are the three cardinal clinical signs and symptoms of advanced liver disease, and their presence indicates that patients are unlikely to be candidates for surgical decompression. Laboratory measurements of serum bilirubin, albumin, and prothrombin time prolongation are the most useful studies to assess the status of cirrhosis. Combining the clinical and laboratory parameters to calculate a Child score gives an objective assessment of risk (Table 98.1). More sophisticated testing to measure quantitative liver function has been shown to be valuable in selection of patients for DSRS (Henderson et al, 1992).

Doppler ultrasound of portal venous anatomy should be performed as part of the evaluation of patients after their initial variceal bleed. The splenic vein, superior mesenteric vein, and portal vein usually can be visualized, as can the hepatic veins for liver outflow. Early identification of thrombosis may alter the whole approach in the management of the patient. Ultrasound also should examine liver morphology, particularly for evidence of focal lesions suggesting hepatocellular carcinoma.

Arteriography is required for final definition of the veins before surgical intervention. The components of this evaluation include the following:

1. Hepatic venous pressure gradient
2. Left renal vein anatomy and drainage (this is abnormal in 20% of the population)
3. Superior mesenteric, portal, and splenic vein patency, flow direction, and venous anatomy on the venous phase of the arterial study
4. Major variceal inflow paths on the same study as in 3

Table 98.1 Child-Pugh Classification

	NO. POINTS		
	1	2	3
Bilirubin (mg/dL)	<2	2-3	>3
Albumin (g/dL)	>3.5	2.8-3.5	<2.8
Prothrombin time increase (sec prolonged)	1-3	4-6	>6
Ascites	None	Slight	Moderate
Encephalopathy	None	1-2	3-4

Grade A—5-6 points.
Grade B—7-9 points.
Grade C—10-15 points.

This combination of venous and arterial angiographic study gives information not available with ultrasound, computed tomography, or magnetic resonance imaging. Candidates for DSRS are Child A and B7 or B8 (Child-Turcotle-Pugh score 7 or 8 points) patients, usually without ascites, who are considered to have stable liver disease and are unlikely to need liver transplant in the next 5 years.

TECHNIQUE FOR DISTAL SPLENORENAL SHUNT

Perioperative and postoperative monitoring and management of a patient undergoing DSRS are crucial to a successful outcome. Monitoring requires an arterial line and a central venous catheter. In some patients, a Swan-Ganz monitoring catheter may be required. A urinary catheter should be placed. Good venous access should be obtained in case rapid transfusion is required.

Blood and blood products should be available with 4 U of packed red blood cells crossmatched. Fresh frozen plasma and platelets may be required if there is a preexisting deficit, or major intraoperative blood loss occurs. A cell saver can be used in higher risk patients and may reduce blood bank requirements.

The patient is positioned on the operating table with the left arm at the side and the left side slightly elevated. Hyperextending the operating table to open the angle between the left lower ribs and iliac crest aids in exposure and access to the tail of the pancreas. The primary operating surgeon is on the patient's right. The operation is more easily completed when the first assistant (on the left of the table) also has experience with the procedure.

The steps in DSRS are illustrated in Figs. 98.1 to 98.10. The incision is a long left subcostal incision, extended across the right rectus muscle (Fig. 98.1). The coagulating diathermy is used extensively in patients with portal hypertension to achieve hemostasis in dividing tissues. When the peritoneum is opened, ascites should be aspirated and cultured, and its total volume should be removed and measured. With complete exploration of the abdominal cavity, the liver should be inspected and a biopsy specimen obtained to document its status at the time of the procedure.

The initial steps of this procedure provide access to the vessels. The initial access is through exposure of the pancreas, which is done by opening the lesser sac (Fig. 98.2). The gastroepiploic arcade is interrupted from the pylorus to the first short gastric vessels. The lesser sac is opened further, and exposure is greatly enhanced by taking down the splenic flexure of the colon from

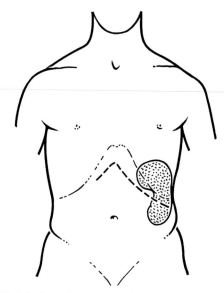

Fig. 98.1. The left subcostal incision extends across the midline and right rectus muscle.

the lower pole of the spleen. This is done most easily by initially mobilizing the left side of the splenic flexure of the colon, then identifying the plane from this site up to the lesser sac at the tail of the pancreas. The splenocolic ligament is taken down; this gives excellent exposure to the inferior margin of the pancreas from the mesenteric vessels to the splenic hilus. The pancreas should be fully mobilized along its inferior border over its entire length so that it is turned completely on its side; this is achieved with a combination of Bovie coagulation and ligature of tissues

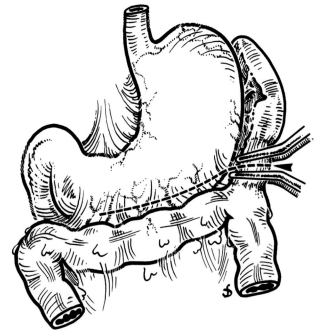

Fig. 98.2. Access to the pancreas is through the gastrocolic omentum. Dividing the splenocolic ligament improves exposure and divides collateral varices to the splenic hilus.

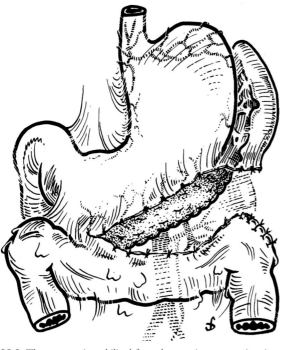

Fig. 98.3. The pancreas is mobilized from the superior mesenteric vein to the spleen by dividing the posterior parietal peritoneum along its inferior margin.

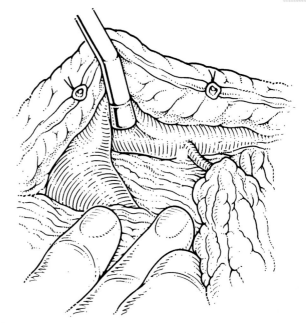

Fig. 98.5. The posterior plane behind the splenic vein should be developed first, and the plane behind the confluence of the splenic vein, superior mesenteric vein, and portal vein is opened.

(Fig. 98.3) and leads to the identification of the inferior mesenteric vein as the first venous landmark. In 50% of patients, this vein enters the splenic vein, whereas in the other 50%, it enters the superior mesenteric vein. It should be traced up to these vessels. It should then be divided to aid further exposure.

The superior mesenteric and splenic vein junction is identified, initially on its posterior surface. This is a safe plane for initial dissection. The splenic vein should be isolated along all of its inferior and posterior aspect with dissection right on the vessel (Fig. 98.4). At this junction, the splenic, superior mesenteric, and posterior aspects of the portal vein all should be cleared (Fig. 98.5). When the posterior plane is free, attention turns to the anterior and more difficult plane of dissection. There are rarely any tributaries entering the anterior surface of

the portal vein, so this plane between the neck of the pancreas and the portal vein should be opened first. Then the pancreas should be cautiously separated and dissected from the anterior and superior surfaces of the splenic veins. The key is to dissect the pancreas off the splenic vein, rather than the other way around. The key in this phase of the operation is to isolate the tributaries, tie them on the vein side, and clip them on the pancreatic side. This action requires a delicate touch and is best achieved by spreading the tissues gently in the line of the tributaries and at right angles to the splenic vein. When identified, a fine right angle clamp is passed around the tributaries to pass a 3-0 ligature (Fig. 98.6). As much of the splenic vein as possible

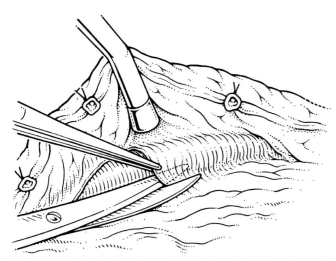

Fig. 98.4. The splenic vein is dissected initially along its inferior and posterior edge. This dissection must be directly on the vein.

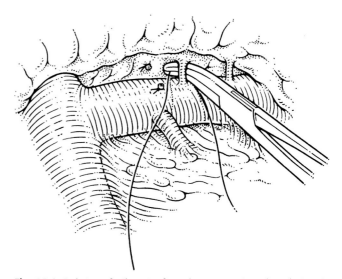

Fig. 98.6. Isolation of tributaries from the pancreas into the splenic vein requires their dissection at right angles to the splenic vein. These vessels are thin walled and require gentle dissection.

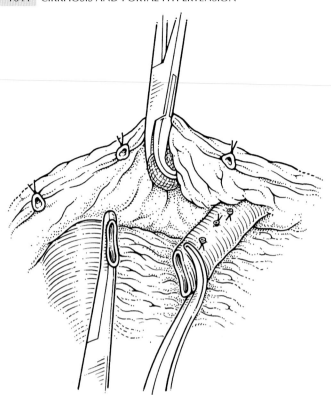

Fig. 98.7. Division of the splenic vein allows the angle between the pancreas and vein to be opened. This improves exposure for dissection of small tributaries to the splenic vein at the cost of increased pressure in the vein.

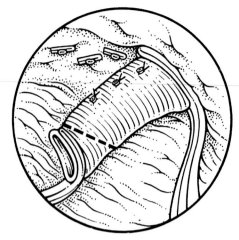

Fig. 98.8. Sufficient splenic vein must be dissected out of the pancreas for the vein to come down to the left renal vein without tension or kinking. An adequately dissected splenic vein usually needs to be trimmed.

should be dissected in this manner before dividing the splenic vein at the superior mesenteric vein junction. In the event of the splenic vein passing more superiorly at the upper side of the pancreas, dissection of the tributaries is easier when the splenic vein can be opened further as shown in Fig. 98.7. The disadvantage of this maneuver is that the pressure in the splenic vein increases even more and may lead to tearing of the small tributaries. The superior mesenteric end of the splenic vein is ligated with a 2-0 silk, and a large ligature clip is placed flush with the vein behind that tie; this has led to the lowest incidence of thrombus within the portal vein at postoperative angiography. Sufficient vein must be dissected free of the pancreas to allow it to come down to the left renal vein without kinking or tension. The more that is dissected, the easier is the anastomosis.

In patients with alcoholic cirrhosis, data have shown that complete dissection of the splenic vein from the pancreas (splenopancreatic disconnection) is advantageous in leading to improved long-term maintenance of portal perfusion (Henderson et al, 1989). If this modification of DSRS is used, the complete dissection should be done at this time. Data do not support the need for entire splenopancreatic disconnection in patients with nonalcoholic liver disease.

The left renal vein is isolated and mobilized from the retroperitoneum and is best done before dividing the splenic vein at the superior mesenteric junction. Preoperative renal venography should have shown the anatomy and defined any abnormality. Sixteen percent of the population has a circumaortic left renal vein, and in 4% of the population, the left renal vein is totally retroaortic. The latter may preclude performance of DSRS. In circumaortic anatomy, the anterior branch is usually larger and is adequate for outflow for DSRS. The retroperitoneum is opened just to the

left of the superior mesenteric artery and in front of the aorta. These landmarks can be identified by palpation. The tissue should be ligated because there are many lymphatics in it, and ligation minimizes the risk of postoperative chylous ascites. Initial dissection should be minimal to identify the left renal vein, which, when identified, should be mobilized over an adequate length to allow it to be brought up into a side-biting clamp. The left adrenal vein should be divided, whereas the gonadal vessel is left intact because it can serve as an outflow tract. The vein should be mobilized over approximately 3 cm, and as a guide the anastomosis usually is made just anterior to the adrenal vein orifice.

The anastomosis is performed without tension, but usually the splenic vein needs to be trimmed so that when the clamps are removed, the vein is not redundant and lies without kinking. This alignment can be difficult to judge, particularly if the two veins are overlying each other. The position of the clamps and trimming of the splenic vein are shown in Figs. 98.8 and 98.9. The left renal vein is opened over sufficient length without removing an ellipse. The posterior row of the anastomosis is with a running suture with stay sutures placed at either end and the suture run on the inside. The anterior row usually is interrupted to avoid risk of a purse-string effect. The completed anastomosis is shown in Fig. 98.10.

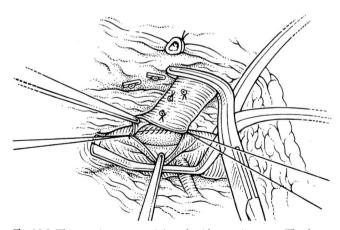

Fig. 98.9. The posterior anastomosis is made with a running suture. The clamps must be held so that there is no tension on the anastomosis.

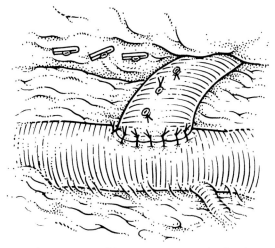

Fig. 98.10. The anterior row of the anastomosis is completed with interrupted sutures.

The final steps in this procedure are completion of portal-azygos disconnection. The main paths by which the high-pressure portal vein attempts to connect to the now low-pressure splenic vein are by (1) transpancreatic collaterals, (2) collateral along the mesocolon to the inferior ramus of the splenic vein, and (3) the left and right gastric venous systems (Henderson et al, 1985). The pancreatic siphon of large collateral flow through the pancreas can be prevented by splenopancreatic disconnection as described earlier. The decision whether or not to do this is made on a benefit/risk basis depending on the ease of full dissection. The collaterals that develop in the mesocolon have a final common pathway in the splenocolic ligament to the lower pole of the spleen and do not develop if the splenic flexure is taken down as described earlier. The transgastric collaterals are minimized by ligating the left and right gastric veins. The right gastric vein is usually small, but should be interrupted just above the pylorus. The left gastric (coronary) vein may be very large and should be clipped or divided at its junction with the portal or splenic vein. It also should be isolated immediately above the pancreas and divided at this location. Abdominal closure should be in two layers with a running nonabsorbable suture. No drains are placed.

PATIENT MANAGEMENT

General Measures

Most patients having DSRS have cirrhosis. The perioperative risks are from liver failure, ascites, and infection and can be minimized by careful management. Risk factors should be defined before surgery (see earlier), and patient selection is key in minimizing perioperative risk.

Ascites is a major risk factor and can be reduced by careful fluid, diet, and diuretic management. Preoperatively, it is important that the patient maintains a low-sodium diet. If diuretics are necessary, adequate doses of an aldosterone antagonist diuretic to reduce renal sodium reabsorption are administered. Perioperatively, the intravenous infusion of free sodium should be minimized, and if plasma volume expansion is required, 5% albumin or fresh frozen plasma should be used. Maintenance fluids should be with 5% dextrose with half-normal saline. When an oral diet has been started, the patient should be limited to 2 to 3 g of sodium per day.

In addition, dietary fat should be restricted to 30 g/day for the first month to reduce the risk of chylous ascites. In the early postoperative period, spironolactone (Aldactone), 100 mg/day, should be given to minimize sodium retention and aid postoperative diuresis. Furosemide may be added to this regimen if significant postoperative ascites occurs. Rarely, paracentesis may be necessary. By following this management routine in Child A or B7 or B8 patients, the risk of ascites is minimized.

Infection is a further risk factor in patients with cirrhosis. Antibiotics should be given in the perioperative period. In the postoperative period, infection always should be considered as a possible explanation for patients who fail to progress.

Liver failure should not be a postoperative risk if patients are appropriately selected for DSRS. Child A and B7 or B8 patients should not decompensate, unless they have an excessively difficult procedure with significant hypotension. Should liver decompensation develop, the only management is with liver transplantation.

Specific Measures

Before hospital discharge, the patient should have (1) stable liver function, (2) shunt patency documented, and (3) no increasing ascites. Shunt patency can be assessed indirectly with Doppler ultrasound, but I advocate shunt catheterization at 1 week postoperatively to document patency and flow and to measure pressures. If the shunt is patent at this time, it is unlikely to undergo subsequent thrombosis or stenosis. The one exception is the recanalized splenic vein that is at increased risk of stenosis and requires further catheterization at 3 to 6 weeks. Standard liver biochemistry should be measured on alternate days postoperatively. The bilirubin may increase by 1 to 2 points, but rarely increases to greater than 5 mg/dL in appropriately selected patients. Fluid management was discussed earlier. Patients are usually ready for discharge from the hospital 6 to 8 days postoperatively.

Follow-up

Patients undergoing DSRS should be maintained in long-term follow-up, primarily to follow the underlying liver disease. Cirrhosis is a chronic disease that tends to be progressive, and although data suggest DSRS does not accelerate the rate of progression of cirrhosis, patients may have to be considered for liver transplantation. Re-evaluation every 6 to 12 months is recommended.

RESULTS

The goals of DSRS are to prevent recurrent variceal bleeding and, by maintaining portal perfusion, not to accelerate the course of the underlying liver disease. In the 1990s, several series documented that these goals can be achieved. Most of these series are in good risk (Child class A and B) patients, and results have been excellent.

Bleeding control is equal to or greater than 90% (Henderson et al, 1992; Hermann, 1995; Orozco et al, 1997; Rikkers, 1998). The highest risk time for rebleeding after DSRS is in the first month (Richards et al, 1987). The technical failure rate should be less than 5% and should be defined before hospital discharge with direct shunt catheterization (see earlier). If there is a technical problem with the anastomosis at that time, surgical re-exploration should be undertaken. If it cannot be corrected, splenectomy and devascularization is indicated. Late thrombosis of DSRS is unusual, although patients with portal vein thrombosis undergoing DSRS have a higher rate of shunt stenosis requiring balloon dilation (Warren et al, 1988). Bleeding control is significantly better than that achieved with endoscopic therapy, which is approximately 25% to 30%.

The major question at present is the relative efficacy of DSRS versus transjugular intrahepatic portosystemic shunt. In a prospective randomized trial (Henderson et al, 2004) of DSRS versus transjugular intrahepatic portosystemic shunt in Child A and B patients, the rebleeding rates were not significantly different— 6% and 9%—but 83% of transjugular intrahepatic portosystemic shunt patients required reintervention and dilation to achieve this outcome. Survival and encephalopathy rates were not significantly different in this study. It can be concluded that transjugular intrahepatic portosystemic shunt is equally effective as DSRS, but intensive follow-up is required at higher cost.

Portal perfusion is maintained at late follow-up in 90% of patients with nonalcoholic liver disease. In patients with alcoholic cirrhosis, loss of portal perfusion occurs in 50% of patients (Henderson et al, 1985). Zeppa documented poorer survival after DSRS in alcoholic patients than in nonalcoholic patients but never proved cause and effect (Zeppa, 1978). This rate can be improved in the latter population by entire splenopancreatic disconnection (Henderson et al, 1989). In this modification, the entire splenic vein is dissected free of pancreas before anastomosis. Splenopancreatic disconnection also has been documented to improve survival in this group of patients.

Hepatic function is maintained after DSRS in Child class A and B patients as shown in the series in the 1990s. The rate of transplantation in these patients is currently less than 20%, but longer term follow-up may show an increase in this number at 10 to 20 years. Survival after DSRS is dictated by the severity of the underlying liver disease. Series in the 1990s (Henderson et al, 1992; Oroczo et al, 1997; Rikkers, 1998) documented 5-year survival of 80% to 90% for Child class A and B patients.

REFERENCES

Henderson JM, et al, 1985: Portaprival collaterals following distal splenorenal shunt: incidence, magnitude and associated portal perfusion changes. J Hepatol 1:649-661.

Henderson JM, et al, 1989: Distal splenorenal shunt with splenopancreatic disconnection: a four-year assessment. Ann Surg 210:332-341.

Henderson JM, et al, 1992: Selective shunt in the management of variceal bleeding in the era of liver transplantation. Ann Surg 216:248-254.

Henderson JM, et al, 2004: DSRS vs TIPS for refractory variceal bleeding: a prospective randomized controlled trial. Hepatology 40:725.

Herman RE, et al, 1995: Fifty years of surgery for portal hypertension at the Cleveland Clinic Foundation: lessons and prospects. Ann Surg 221:459-466.

Orozco H, et al, 1997: Selective shunts for portal hypertension: current role of a 21-year experience. Liver Transplant Surg 3:475-480.

Richards WO, et al, 1987: Evaluation and treatment of early hemorrhage of the alimentary tract after selective shunt procedures. Surg Gynecol Obstet 164: 530-536.

Rikkers LF, 1998: The changing spectrum of treatment for variceal bleeding. Ann Surg 228:536-546.

Warren WD, et al, 1967: Selective transplenic decompression of gastroesophageal varices by distal splenorenal shunt. Ann Surg 166:437-445.

Warren WD, et al, 1988: Management of variceal bleeding in patients with noncirrhotic portal vein thrombosis. Ann Surg 207:623-634.

Zeppa R, et al, 1978: The comparative survival of alcoholics versus non-alcoholics after distal splenorenal shunt. Ann Surg 187:510-513.

The Mesocaval Shunt: Technique

M. T. AUSTIN AND C. W. PINSON

HISTORY OF THE MESOCAVAL SHUNT

Eck first described decompression of the portal system via the portacaval shunt in 1877. The first mesocaval shunt was developed primarily for children with portal vein thrombosis by Marion (Marion et al, 1965) in 1953 and Clatworthy (1955) in 1955. In the Marion/Clatworthy J-shunt, the inferior vena cava (IVC) is divided just proximal to the confluence of the iliac veins, and the proximal end is anastomosed to the lateral aspect of the superior mesenteric vein (Clatworthy, 1955). In 1954, Valdoni also described this procedure in a discussion regarding treatment options for portal hypertension. Because of complications of venous stasis, including intractable lower extremity edema, this shunt never gained popularity in adults.

In 1970, Read and colleagues (1970) described the use of homologous vein graft as a conduit for the mesocaval shunt. In 1972, Drapanas reported good success with prosthetic mesocaval shunts by showing their efficacy in 25 patients with acute exsanguinating variceal hemorrhage and popularized the procedure. Throughout the 1970s, several authors reported success with autologous, homologous, heterologous, and synthetic mesocaval shunts for the treatment of bleeding varices.

INDICATIONS FOR MESOCAVAL SHUNTS

With remarkable advances in endoscopic therapy, interventional radiology, and liver transplantation, the role of surgical shunts in the treatment of complications related to portal hypertension has been revised (see Ch. 95). Although alternatives exist, surgical shunts remain an important intervention in some patients. The use of transjugular intrahepatic portosystemic shunts (TIPS) (see Ch. 96) has decreased the need for surgical shunts dramatically. TIPS provide only short-term treatment, however. TIPS require constant monitoring and frequent intervention and are appropriate only in patients with advanced liver disease as a bridge to transplantation or severely ill patients with a short life expectancy. In contrast, the surgical shunt is best performed in patients who have bleeding varices refractory to endoscopic intervention with good hepatic reserve (i.e., Child-Pugh class A and B). Indications for surgical shunt procedures include variceal hemorrhage with good hepatic reserve, failed TIPS, portal vein thrombosis, Budd-Chiari syndrome, refractory ascites, and small-for-size syndrome in liver transplantation.

The most common indication for surgical shunt is bleeding varices refractory to medical and endoscopic therapy in patients who have good hepatic reserve and do not need liver transplantation in the near future. Henderson and colleagues (2000) showed excellent outcomes in patients with Child-Pugh class A and B cirrhosis with refractory bleeding who received surgical shunts. In their series, the overall survival and rebleeding rates were 86% and 6.3% with a median follow-up of 36 months. The choice between TIPS and surgical shunts depends on the patient's hepatic reserve and possible timing to transplantation. If transplantation is expected within 1 to 2 years, TIPS is likely to bridge the patient to transplantation without the need for surgical intervention. If transplantation is unlikely to occur within 1 to 2 years, however, surgical shunting is warranted because greater than 50% of TIPS require intervention within this time period.

Orloff and coworkers (1994) reported the use of portosystemic shunts in the treatment of 162 children and adults with extrahepatic portal hypertension secondary to portal vein thrombosis. In contrast to patients with cirrhosis, patients with portal vein thrombosis are often young and otherwise healthy with good liver function and are excellent candidates for surgical shunt procedures. In the series by Orloff and coworkers (1994), 53 patients underwent end-to-side cavomesenteric shunts with no perioperative mortality and 100% patency at follow-up. The authors concluded that portosystemic shunting is the most effective treatment for these patients, and that these procedures should be performed early in the course of variceal bleeding episodes.

Although Budd-Chiari syndrome (see Ch. 100) with obstruction of hepatic venous outflow traditionally was treated with portosystemic shunt procedures, other treatment options, including hepatic vein angioplasty, catheter-directed thrombolysis, TIPS, and liver transplantation, have been successfully introduced. After reviewing 54 Budd-Chiari syndrome patients treated at Johns Hopkins Hospital over 20 years, Slakey and colleagues (2001) concluded that shunting and transplantation result in 5-year survival rates of at least 75% in these patients. Fisher and associates (1999) advocated the use of hepatic vein angioplasty for Budd-Chiari syndrome patients with short length hepatic vein stenosis or occlusion and surgical shunting for patients with diffuse hepatic vein occlusion or failed angioplasty. Others recommend TIPS; however, recanalization of the hepatic veins is not always successful and may require a shunt procedure.

A study using the porcine transplant model suggested that mesocaval shunts may provide protective effects for small-for-size liver grafts by protecting them from portal flow–related injuries (Smyrniotis et al, 2003). Given the critical organ shortage and increasing use of segmental grafts, this approach may prove clinically useful in the future.

Because subsequent transplantation often is anticipated in patients receiving portosystemic shunts, the procedure should not compromise the technical aspects of transplantation. In contrast to portacaval shunts, the distal splenorenal and mesocaval interposition shunts do not alter the porta hepatis. The mesocaval interposition shunt is technically less challenging than the distal splenorenal shunt and requires minimal retroperitoneal dissection. It effectively relieves portal hypertension, and in contrast to the distal spleno-renal shunt, it also relieves or prevents secondary ascites.

SHUNT MATERIALS AND SIZE OF THE MESOCAVAL SHUNT

Multiple variations of this shunt procedure have been described in the literature. There has been significant debate regarding the ideal graft material and diameter for the mesocaval shunt. In 1970, Read and colleagues presented a series of eight mesocaval shunts with homologous vena cava. Also in 1970, Lord and associates published a report on seven mesocaval H-grafts with polytetra-fluoroethylene (PTFE) (Teflon) prosthesis, of which six remained patent for 20 months. Despite Lord's early success, many clinicians remained fearful of using prosthetic grafts in the venous system because of experimental failures in long-term patency. In 1972, Drapanas published data on 25 more mesocaval shunt procedures, however, using 19- to 22-mm Dacron interposition graft and showed excellent patency rates. Drapanas (1972) cited a superiority of Dacron over PTFE for better incorporation into the host tissues and continued to use Dacron in his studies. Throughout the 1970s, several other groups reported success with large-diameter prosthetic grafts. In 1977, Filtzer and coworkers reviewed their institution's experience with 20 patients who underwent mesocaval shunt procedures using 18- to 22-mm Dacron graft for bleeding esophageal varices. The long-term patency rate approached 90%. In 1975, Drapanas and associates published a follow-up study on the hemodynamics of 80 mesocaval shunts using large-diameter (18-22 mm) Dacron grafts. In this series, a decrease in mean portacaval pressure by 50% was noted, and 44% maintained hepatopetal portal flow. Only three graft thromboses occurred with an overall patency rate of 95%. One patient developed graft infection, however, with subsequent sepsis and death.

Although recurrent esophageal varices and hemorrhage were rare after these procedures, the large-diameter portacaval and mesocaval grafts (16-22 mm) often resulted in total portal shunting and loss of prograde portal flow, which many investigators thought led to progressive liver dysfunction and high rates of encephalopathy. Sarfeh and colleagues (1986) investigated the importance of maintaining hepatic portal perfusion on prevention of encephalopathy by systematically reducing the portacaval H-graft diameters. After reviewing 88 patients treated with portacaval shunt for bleeding esophageal varices, Sarfeh and colleagues (1986) reported maintenance of hepatopetal portal flow in 82% of patients with 8-mm PTFE H-grafts, 46% with 10-mm PTFE H-grafts, and only 3% with 14- to 20-mm Dacron grafts. Preserved prograde portal flow correlated with decreased rates of encephalopathy, which was observed in only 9% of patients with 8-mm PTFE H-grafts compared with 39% with large-diameter Dacron grafts. Although early graft thrombosis was more common in the small-diameter grafts (16%), the cumulative shunt patency rate was 97% for those grafts. One patient experienced graft infection with subsequent sepsis and death. Throughout the 1980s, most reports of small-diameter grafts focused on their use in the portacaval anastomosis as opposed to the mesocaval shunt. All studies showed a slightly increased rate of perioperative shunt thrombosis over the large-diameter shunts, but which was mostly managed via angiographic revision (Collins et al, 1994; Rypins et al, 1988). All small-diameter portacaval shunt procedures were coupled with aggressive portal collateral ablation.

More recent studies have shown efficacy of small-diameter mesocaval shunts. Mercado and associates (2000) reviewed a 10-year experience with 10-mm PTFE mesocaval shunts for the treatment of bleeding esophageal varices in mostly low-risk patients with preserved hepatic function. Thirty-three patients underwent the procedure; 81% maintained long-term patency evaluated by angiography, but 15% developed episodes of rebleeding. Only 11% had encephalopathy, and 12-month survival was 81%. Mercado and associates (1996) also compared the distal splenorenal shunt with the 10-mm PTFE mesocaval shunt and showed decreased encephalopathy, shunt thrombosis, and changes in portal flow with the distal splenorenal shunt, but no differences in mortality or rebleeding rates. They concluded that the mesocaval shunt continues to have a role in the surgical treatment of portal hypertension when a selective shunt cannot be performed.

Despite considerable debate in the literature since the early 1970s, no definitive answer exists to the questions of graft material for the mesocaval shunt procedure. The small-diameter shunts provide preserved prograde portal flow in the early postoperative period, but still may be associated with encephalopathy and loss of hepatopetal flow over time. In addition, postoperative encephalopathy rates vary considerably in the literature, from less than 10% to greater than 50%. Although rare, graft infection in the prosthetic grafts was uniformly fatal in the literature. Reynolds and Southwick in 1951 first described the use of autologous vein graft for interposition between the portal vein and vena cava. Stipa and colleagues (1978) compared their experience with the side-to-side portacaval shunt versus autologous internal jugular vein interposition mesocaval shunt in 79 patients with variceal hemorrhage and portal hypertension. Although there were no differences in survival between the two groups, encephalopathy was greater in the portacaval shunt patients (54%) compared with the mesocaval shunt patients (35%), and 95% of the patients with mesocaval shunts maintained hepatopetal portal flow. Gonzalez and associates (1977) also reported the use of autologous vein graft in 26 patients. There were no reports of graft infection for patients undergoing mesocaval shunts with either homologous or autologous vein graft. These shunts require more time to harvest vein, however, and may not be appropriate in an emergency or urgent setting. All of the mesocaval shunts discussed in this review provided adequate portal decompression with low perioperative mortality and infrequent recurrence of variceal hemorrhage.

PREOPERATIVE EVALUATION AND MANAGEMENT

The patient should undergo an evaluation for encephalopathy. If encephalopathy is present, the patient is not a good candidate for the procedure. Preoperative mesenteric angiography with late phase portography, magnetic resonance angiography, or computed tomography (CT) angiography must be performed in all patients before the procedure. Additionally, venacavography and wedged hepatic venous pressures can provide important anatomic and physiologic data. It is necessary to confirm the presence of an adequate diameter superior mesenteric vein and to show the direction of portal flow through the collateral vessels.

Before the operation, if possible, the patient should undergo diuresis with spironolactone and furosemide to minimize postoperative ascites. The patient also receives standard antibiotic prophylaxis in the holding area immediately before surgery. A formal mechanical bowel preparation is unnecessary.

TECHNIQUE

Exposure

A transverse midabdominal, right low subcostal, or midline incision may be used (Fig. 99.1). Because of portal hypertension, a few large collateral vessels may be encountered in the subcutaneous tissue and should be doubly ligated and divided instead of divided with electrocautery. When the peritoneum is opened, ascites is removed, and the abdomen is explored. A mechanical retractor is placed to provide maximal exposure. A liver biopsy often is performed and always should be done for any areas suspicious for hepatoma.

Exposure of the Superior Mesenteric Vein

The transverse mesocolon is retracted cephalad and the small intestine is retracted caudad and to the left to expose the root of the mesentery and the ligament of Treitz. A transverse incision is made in the posterior parietal peritoneum to initiate dissection of the superior mesenteric vein. The superior mesenteric vein usually overlies the right lateral margin of the vertebral bodies. The superior mesenteric artery usually is located anterior and left of the superior mesenteric vein (Fig. 99.2). These relationships are inconstant, however. Doppler may help identify the vascular structures.

During dissection of the superior mesenteric vein, multiple lymphatic channels and lymph nodes are encountered. Large, hypertrophied lymphatic channels should be ligated before division to prevent uncontrolled lymph flow during and after the procedure, which may contribute to postoperative ascites.

When the superior mesenteric vein is identified, it is mobilized and skeletonized from the inferior border of the pancreas to below the confluence of the ileocolic and jejunal veins, which form the

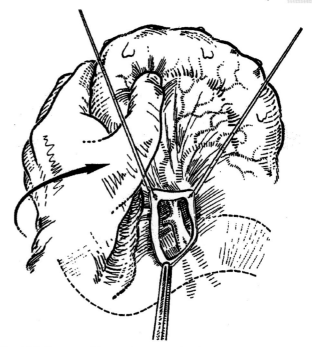

Fig. 99.2. Exposure of the superior mesenteric vein.

superior mesenteric vein proper. Small branches are doubly ligated and divided, and large branches are controlled with vessel loops. The superior mesenteric vein is dissected bluntly on the anterior surface, and sharp dissection is limited until the vein and all tributaries are identified. Usually, a large tributary vein enters the right posterior lateral border of the superior mesenteric vein between the ileocolic and middle colic veins, which should be controlled with a vessel loop. Occasionally, the inferior mesenteric vein enters the side of the superior mesenteric vein directly rather than the splenic vein. If so, it also should be controlled with a vessel loop before opening the superior mesenteric vein.

Ideally, a 6- to 7-cm length of large-diameter superior mesenteric vein should be exposed and mobilized to accommodate the graft. If necessary, the graft may extend onto the ileocolic vein. Alternatively, if the superior mesenteric vein is quite short, the ileocolic vein or middle colic vein or both may be sacrificed. In a patient with portal hypertension, the ileocolic vein may be quite large and mistaken for the superior mesenteric vein. A shunt between the ileocolic vein and cava is inadequate, however, for portal decompression.

Exposure of the Inferior Vena Cava

When adequate length of the superior mesenteric vein is circumferentially mobilized, the IVC is identified by a direct approach through a window in the right colonic mesentery. Alternatively, the right colon and mesentery may be reflected to the midline allowing access to the right retroperitoneum. The distal second portion and third portion of the duodenum are mobilized (reverse Kocher maneuver). It is important to ligate and divide the large lymphatic channels in the retroperitoneum to avoid a significant lymphatic leak. A 6- to 7-cm length of IVC is dissected along the anterior and lateral borders (Fig. 99.3). It is not necessary to mobilize the cava circumferentially, but only enough to allow placement of a large Satinsky clamp for partial occlusion.

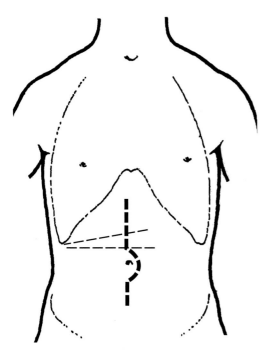

Fig. 99.1. The incision options for the mesocaval shunt procedure: transverse midabdominal, right low subcostal, or midline incision.

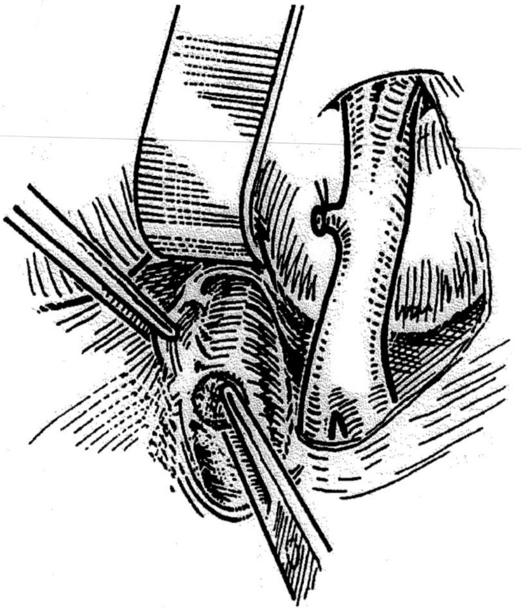

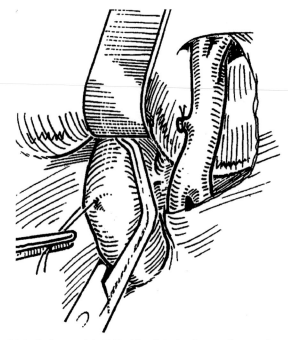

Fig. 99.3. Dissection of the anterior and lateral surfaces of the IVC and its relationship to the superior mesenteric vein.

After mobilization of the superior mesenteric vein and IVC, soft tissue between these structures can be divided to allow the graft to take the optimal route, but one should avoid ligating large vessels.

Preparation of the Vena Cava and Venotomy

The caval-graft anastomosis is performed first, which eliminates the problems of diminished exposure for the caval anastomosis and prolonged superior mesenteric vein occlusion. A vascular suture can be placed in the anterior wall of the vena cava and used to tent it upward while a large Satinsky clamp is placed to occlude the cava partially (Fig. 99.4). It is important that the clamp occludes the superior and inferior ends of the vena cava segment to prevent bleeding during the anastomosis. The suture used to tent the cava is excised with an ellipse of anterior caval wall to form the venotomy (Fig. 99.5). The venotomy is enlarged using angled Pott's scissors to the same diameter (usually 8-12 mm) as the chosen ringed Gore-Tex or internal jugular vein graft. If the opening is too large, the graft does not assume a circular shape at the anastomosis.

Graft–Inferior Vena Cava Anastomosis

The caval anastomosis is located in the deepest and most dependent area of the wound, and good exposure is essential. The duodenum is retracted superiorly, and the remainder of the viscera is retracted inferiorly. Two corner sutures are placed using 5-0 synthetic nonabsorbable suture material at each end of the venotomy and tied to position the graft over the venotomy (Fig. 99.6). A stay suture also is placed midway along the medial caval venotomy lip for gentle traction to distract it away from the lateral suture line and to prevent incorporation into the opposite wall. The Satinsky clamp is rotated to the patient's left, and the right side of the anastomosis is completed first. It is

started at the inferior margin using one end of the corner stitch and working upward placing the continuous sutures outside-in on the graft and inside-out on the vein (Fig. 99.7). At the superior margin, the suture is tied to one end of the superior corner stitch.

After completion of the right side anastomosis, the Satinsky clamp is rotated to the patient's right, and the other end of the superior corner suture is run inferiorly to complete the left side of the anastomosis (Fig. 99.8). Fig. 99.9 shows the completed anastomosis. A nerve hook may be used to ensure proper positioning of the cava or graft before each needle bite.

A vascular clamp is placed on the prosthesis, and the Satinsky clamp is released to ensure hemostasis of the anastomosis.

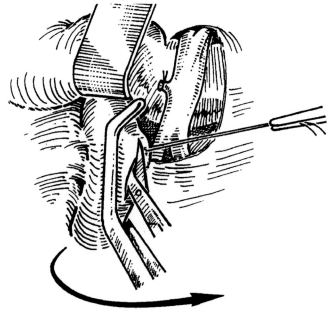

Fig. 99.4. Occlusion of the IVC with a Satinsky clamp and preparation of the vein for venotomy.

Fig. 99.5. IVC venotomy.

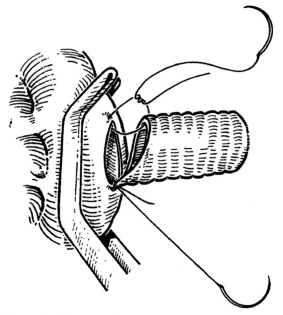

Fig. 99.6. IVC-graft anastomosis.

Any anastomotic leaks are repaired, and the Satinsky clamp is reapplied to the vena cava. The vascular clamp is removed from the graft, and any remaining blood is suctioned from the graft lumen and irrigated with heparinized saline.

Graft–Superior Mesenteric Vein Anastomosis

The length of the graft is crucial. The graft assumes a "C" configuration as it passes inferiorly around the lower border of the third portion of the duodenum, then anterior to the third portion of the duodenum and the uncinate process, and finally is anastomosed obliquely to the anterior-lateral surface of the superior mesenteric vein. If the graft is too short, undue tension is placed

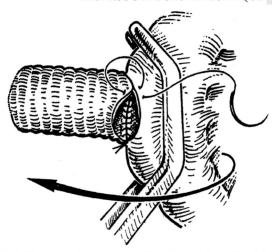

Fig. 99.8. The cava and graft are rotated laterally, and the left (medial) suture line is performed.

on the suture line, and the superior mesenteric vein is retracted and distorted. If the graft is too long, it becomes redundantly bowed and distorted when the clamps are removed. It also is helpful to mark the graft to maintain proper orientation. Alternatively, the graft may be short and relatively straight, assuming more of an H-graft appearance.

When the appropriate length is determined, the graft is cut obliquely to the angle at which it is to be anastomosed to the superior mesenteric vein. Two straight Cooley clamps are applied proximally and distally on the superior mesenteric vein, and the vein is partially rotated to allow the anastomosis to be performed

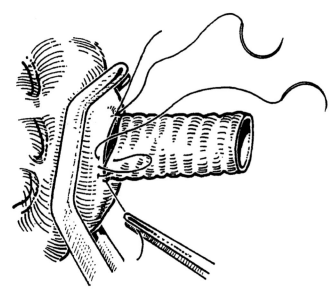

Fig. 99.7. The cava and graft are rotated medially, and the right lateral suture line is performed first.

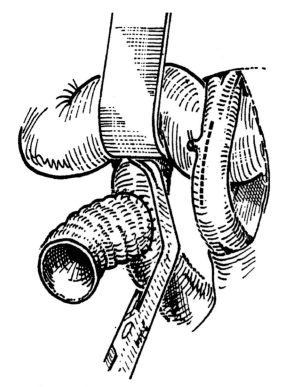

Fig. 99.9. The IVC-graft anastomosis is complete.
(From Gliedman ML, Kaleya RN, 2000: The mesocaval shunt technique. In Blumgart LH [ed]: Surgery of the Liver and Biliary Tract, 3rd ed. Philadelphia, Saunders, 2000, pp 1971-1983.)

on the anterior-lateral aspect of the vein. Retraction of the vessel loops placed on the tributaries provides adequate control of the tributaries during the anastomosis. Alternatively, vessel loops may be used to control all of the veins.

A small ellipse is excised from the anterior-lateral aspect of the superior mesenteric vein, and the venotomy is extended proximally and distally using angled Pott's scissors to match the length of the obliquely cut graft. For H-shaped shunts, the venotomy is more right posterior-lateral on the vein. Sutures are placed at both ends of the venotomy and graft using 5-0 or 6-0 synthetic non-absorbable suture material and tied to approximate the vein and graft. The right lateral suture line is performed first in a continuous fashion from within the graft and vein and carried from the superior suture to the inferior suture (Fig. 99.10). The left lateral suture line is performed in a similar fashion by rotating the vein to the patient's right for better exposure (see Fig. 99.10). The left lateral suture line also is started at the superior suture and carried down and tied to the inferior stay suture.

Evaluating the Anastomosis

The Satinsky clamp on the IVC is removed first. All anastomotic leaks are repaired. The clamps are removed from the superior mesenteric vein, and flow is allowed through the shunt. Gentle pressure may be applied to the anastomoses for hemostasis. Doppler ultrasound may be used to interrogate the graft and anastomosis.

The pressures in the portal system are measured by positioning an 18-gauge needle connected to a water manometer into the superior mesenteric vein near the graft–superior mesenteric vein anastomosis (Fig. 99.11). The pressure is measured with the

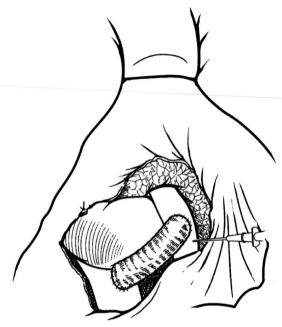

Fig. 99.11. After completion of the interposition mesocaval shunt, the portal system pressures are measured.
(Illustration by Dominic Doyle, Medical Arts Group, Vanderbilt University.)

graft patent and mesenteric systemic flow intact as the decompressed portal pressure. The graft is clamped, and the pressure is rechecked to confirm that the system is decompressed. A reduction in the pressure gradient by 12 to 18 cm H_2O should be expected. Also, a thrill may be palpated in the graft. When it is established that no technical problems exist with the graft, such as kinking or compression by surrounding tissues, the abdomen is irrigated, hemostasis is ensured, and the abdomen is closed.

POSTOPERATIVE EVALUATION AND MANAGEMENT

Immediately after the procedure, shunt patency should be confirmed by duplex ultrasound, magnetic resonance imaging, or CT angiography (Fig. 99.12). If it is not possible to determine shunt patency via noninvasive techniques, an angiogram must be performed.

Postoperative care includes strict volume management. It is important to keep the central venous pressure as low as possible, but to maintain appropriate cardiac output to preserve renal perfusion and function. Although most patients develop some postoperative ascites, it usually clears with a functioning shunt. Initially, patients should be cautious with their diet to minimize the risk of encephalopathy, but only rarely is it necessary to restrict patients to a meat-free diet and lactulose regimen.

If gastrointestinal bleeding recurs, the patient should undergo shunt interrogation to determine shunt patency. Several studies also recommend routine shunt evaluation by either duplex ultrasound or angiography (Mercado et al, 1996; Orloff et al, 1994; Rypins et al, 1988). We perform follow-up duplex ultrasound every 3 to 6 months after the procedure for the lifetime of the shunt. Shunt stenosis is managed routinely with percutaneous transfemoral dilation and rarely stenting of the stenosis; operative revision is done only with failure of the less invasive interventional procedures. For early and late shunt thrombosis, most studies

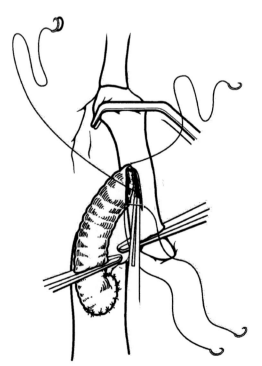

Fig. 99.10. After occlusion with vascular clamps, the superior mesenteric vein venotomy is performed at the anterior-lateral aspect of the superior mesenteric vein and the superior mesenteric vein–graft anastomosis is started.
(Illustration by Dominic Doyle, Medical Arts Group, Vanderbilt University.)

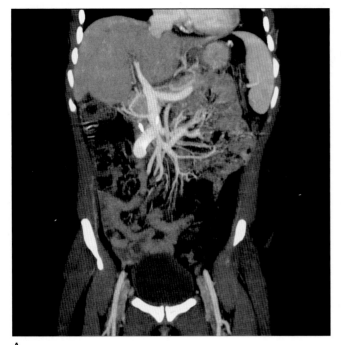

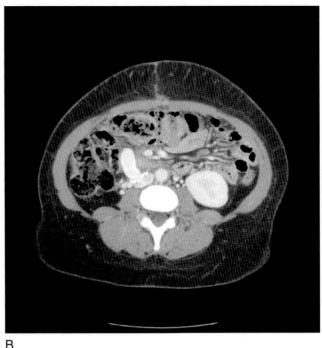

A   B

Fig. 99.12. CT angiography of a patent interposition mesocaval shunt. **A,** Coronal image. **B,** Transverse image. (Courtesy of Dr. Ravi Chari.)

advocate shunt thrombectomy. After balloon catheter placement and dilation across any stenosis, an angiocatheter is placed at the superior mesenteric vein–graft anastomosis, and streptokinase is infused at a rate of 5000 U/hr for 24 hours (Rypins et al, 1988; Sarfeh et al, 1986).

SUMMARY

Despite advances in endoscopic therapy, interventional techniques, and liver transplantation, surgical shunts are important therapeutic tools in select patients. Because of its technical simplicity and low complication rate during subsequent liver transplantation, the mesocaval shunt is an ideal surgical shunt choice in some patients. It has proved to relieve effectively portal hypertension and secondary ascites and to prevent recurrent variceal hemorrhage.

REFERENCES

Clatworthy WH, 1955: A new type of portal to systemic shunt for portal decompression. Arch Surg 1:588.

Collins JC, et al, 1994: Narrow-diameter portacaval shunts for management of variceal bleeding. World J Surg 18:211-215.

Drapanas T, 1972: Interposition mesocaval shunt for treatment of portal hypertension. Ann Surg 176:435-448.

Drapanas T, et al, 1975: Hemodynamics of the interposition mesocaval shunt. Ann Surg 181:523-533.

Filtzer HS, et al, 1977: Experience with interposition mesocaval shunt for management of variceal bleeding. Arch Surg 112:593-595.

Fisher NC, et al, 1999: Managing Budd-Chiari syndrome: a retrospective review of percutaneous hepatic vein angioplasty and surgical shunting. Gut 44:568-574.

Gonzalez EM, et al, 1977: Transduodenopancreatic interposition mesocaval shunt using internal jugular vein autograft. Surg Gynecol Obstet 145:565-569.

Henderson JM, et al, 2000: Surgical shunts and TIPS for variceal decompression in the 1990s. Surgery 128:540-547.

Lord JW, et al, 1970: Mesocaval shunt modified by the use of a Teflon prosthesis. Surg Gynecol Obstet 130:525-526.

Marion P, et al, 1965: [Mesenterico-caval anastomosis]. Lyon Chir 61:448-449.

Mercado MA, et al, 1996: Distal splenorenal shunt versus 10-mm low-diameter mesocaval shunt for variceal hemorrhage. Am J Surg 171:591-595.

Mercado MA, et al, 2000: Small-diameter mesocaval shunts: a 10-year evaluation. J Gastrointest Surg 4:453-457.

Orloff MJ, et al, 1994: Treatment of bleeding esophagogastric varices due to extrahepatic portal hypertension: results of portal-systemic shunts during 35 years. J Pediatr Surg 29:142-151.

Read RC, et al, 1970: Mesocaval H venous homografts. Arch Surg 101:785-791.

Reynolds JT, Southwick HW, 1951: Portal hypertension: use of venous grafts when side to side anastomosis is impossible. Arch Surg 62:789-800.

Rypins EB, et al, 1988: Advantages and disadvantages of polytetrafluoroethylene (PTFE) grafts for portacaval shunting. Vasc Surg March/April 88-92.

Sarfeh IJ, et al, 1986: A systematic appraisal of portacaval H-graft diameters: clinical and hemodynamic perspectives. Ann Surg 204:356-363.

Slakey DP, et al, 2001: Budd-Chiari syndrome: current management options. Ann Surg 233:522-527.

Smyrniotis VE, et al, 2003: Effect of mesocaval shunt on survival of small-for-size liver grafts: experimental study in pigs. Transplantation 75:1737-1740.

Stipa S, et al, 1978: Mesentericocaval shunt with the internal jugular vein. Surg Gynecol Obstet 146:391-399.

Valdoni P, 1954: [Portal hypertension: I. orientation and therapeutic directions in portal hypertension]. Clin Nuova Rass Prog Med Internazionale 19:349-350.

Budd-Chiari Syndrome and Veno-occlusive Disease

M. J. ORLOFF, M. S. ORLOFF, AND S. L. ORLOFF

Budd-Chiari syndrome (BCS) is a group of disorders caused by occlusion of the major hepatic veins or the inferior vena cava (IVC) or both at or near the level of the hepatic vein ostia. Although a brief discussion of these disorders first appeared in a book by Budd in 1845, Lambron in 1842 is said to have reported the first case. In 1899, Chiari collected 10 cases and reported 3 personal cases and presented the first thorough clinical and pathologic description of the syndrome, including the hypothesis that the underlying mechanism is endophlebitis of the hepatic veins. The weight of evidence favors the current opinion, however, that the primary process is usually thrombotic rather than inflammatory. Since publication of the initial description, more than 6000 cases of BCS have been described in the medical literature. In recent years, the incidence has increased substantially, most likely as a result of increased awareness of BCS, improvements in diagnostic methods, and widespread use of thrombogenic agents, such as oral contraceptives (Maddrey, 1987; Valla et al, 1986). Nevertheless, BCS remains a relatively uncommon condition.

Obstruction of hepatic venous outflow produces intense congestion of the liver and the clinical manifestations of ascites, hepatomegaly, and abdominal pain. Depending on the rapidity and extent of obstruction of hepatic venous outflow, the course of BCS may be rapid or chronic, progressing to death in a matter of weeks or leading to death from liver failure or bleeding esophageal varices after an illness of months or occasionally years. In Western countries, a rapid course is more common, and the outcome has been fatal in most reported cases.

Veno-occlusive disease (VOD) is a group of disorders that mimics BCS, but involves distinctly different populations of patients and is precipitated by distinctly different circumstances. In contrast to BCS, VOD occurs in the sublobular branches of the hepatic veins, the terminal hepatic venules, and the sinusoids within the liver, and the pathologic process involves obliteration of these small vessels by subendothelial sclerosis owing to endothelial injury, with thrombosis occurring secondarily. VOD is caused by a variety of toxic agents, such as pyrrolizidine alkaloids, antineoplastic drugs, and irradiation of the liver. In the Western Hemisphere, the most frequent cause of VOD is bone marrow (hematopoietic stem cell) transplantation.

In recent years, effective surgical therapy has been developed that is designed to decompress the obstructed hepatic vascular bed. As a result, the previously dismal outlook of patients with BCS has improved considerably.

PREDISPOSING CONDITIONS FOR BUDD-CHIARI SYNDROME

Table 100.1 lists the specific conditions that are known to predispose to the development of BCS and VOD. Over the past 50 years, there has been a marked change in the frequency with

which a known cause or predisposing condition has been identified in cases of BCS. In the classic collective review of 164 cases of BCS reported by Parker in 1959, a predisposing condition or etiology could not be identified in 70% of the patients. In recent years, the incidence of idiopathic cases of BCS has plummeted to less than 30% (Mahmoud et al, 1996; Menon et al, 2004; Mitchell et al, 1982; Valla, 2003). The improvement has been attributed to two factors: (1) a greater awareness of BCS and (2) improved diagnostic tools for identifying the anatomic lesions and for diagnosing thrombogenic hematologic disorders.

It has been recognized for some time that there is a distinct difference between the West and the East in the conditions that predispose to the development of BCS and in the anatomic pattern of BCS. Table 100.2 displays these differences. Membranous obstruction of the vena cava (MOVC) is rare in the West, but is a frequent cause of BCS in Eastern countries such as Japan, China, India, and South Africa. In the West, thrombosis of the major hepatic veins alone is substantially more common than thrombosis or occlusion of the IVC, whereas in India, China, and Japan, IVC occlusion is far more common than hepatic vein occlusion alone. In North America, the acute form of BCS predominates, and chronic BCS is observed less frequently, whereas in the East, the reverse is observed. In the West, BCS is seldom found during pregnancy and the postpartum period, whereas in India, pregnancy is a major predisposing condition for BCS. The same difference is seen in the incidence of infections such as hepatic amebiasis (see Ch. 60), which are rare in the West, but are reported frequently in series of BCS from India. Finally, ingestion of oral contraceptives is frequently associated with BCS in the United States, where use of these agents is widespread, whereas use of birth control pills is seldom associated with BCS in Eastern countries, where women use oral contraceptives much less.

Hematologic Disorders

Hematologic diseases that cause vascular thrombosis are the most common conditions that predispose to BCS in North America and Western Europe. Of disorders with thrombotic tendencies, polycythemia rubra vera is the most frequent, constituting 8.5% of the cases of BCS in the collected series of Parker (1959) and 10.4% of the cases in the collected series of Mitchell and colleagues (1982). In our series of 66 cases of BCS, 30% had polycythemia rubra vera. Polycythemia rubra vera associated with BCS is in some ways distinctly different from the classic disease. For one thing, it is found in young adults, rather than in middle-aged and elderly patients. It is responsive to treatment with hydroxyurea or anagrelide, which should be started as soon as the disease is discovered and should be continued for life. If treated, the disease runs a benign course in our experience. Finally, polycythemia

Table 100.1 Conditions Predisposing to Budd-Chiari Syndrome and Veno-occlusive Disease

Budd-Chiari Syndrome

Hematologic disorders
    Polycythemia rubra vera
    Paroxysmal nocturnal hemoglobinuria
    Essential thrombocythemia
    Primary erythrocytosis
    Myelofibrosis
    Acute leukemias and lymphomas
    Hemolytic anemias
    Protein C deficiency
    Protein S deficiency
    Antithrombin III deficiency
    Lupus anticoagulant (antiphospholipid syndrome)
    Factor V Leiden mutation

Oral contraceptives

Pregnancy and postpartum

Malignant neoplasms
    Hepatocellular carcinoma
    Renal cell carcinoma
    Adrenal carcinoma
    Leiomyosarcoma of the IVC
    Others (carcinomas of the lung, pancreas, stomach; melanoma; reticulum
        cell sarcoma; adrenal sarcoma; tumor of the right atrium)

Infections
    Amebic liver abscess
    Aspergillosis
    Hydatid disease
    Schistosomiasis
    Syphilitic gumma
    Filariasis

Trauma

Connective tissue disorders
    Behçet's syndrome
    Sjögren's syndrome
    Mixed connective tissue disease
    Sarcoidosis
    Rheumatoid arthritis
    α_1-Antitrypsin deficiency
    Idiopathic hypereosinophilia syndrome
    Systemic lupus erythematosus
Membranous obstruction of the IVC

Miscellaneous rare conditions (inflammatory bowel disease, hepatic torsion, lipoid nephrosis, protein-losing enteropathy)

Veno-occlusive Disease

    Pyrrolizidine alkaloids
    Antineoplastic chemotherapy
    Irradiation of the liver
    Bone marrow transplantation
    Azathioprine
    Systemic lupus erythematosus
    Familial immunodeficiency
    Oral contraceptives

Table 100.2 Differences Between West and East in Predisposing Conditions and Anatomic Patterns of Budd-Chiari Syndrome

Feature	West	East
Membranous obstruction of the IVC	Rare	Frequent
Hepatic vein occlusion predominates	+	−
IVC occlusion predominates	−	+
Acute BCS predominates	+	−
Chronic BCS predominates	−	+
Pregnancy/postpartum	Uncommon	Frequent
Infection	Rare	Common
Oral contraceptives	Frequent	Uncommon

outside of the liver has been observed sometimes. These cases of multiple sites of thrombosis have involved the portal, splenic, and superior mesenteric veins; pelvic veins; deep calf veins; splanchnic arteries; pulmonary artery; coronary arteries; and cerebral arteries (Peytremann et al, 1972).

As hematologic diagnosis has become progressively more sophisticated, many other thrombogenic conditions have been identified in BCS, including other myeloproliferative states, such as essential thrombocythemia, primary erythrocytosis, and myelofibrosis, and thrombophilic states, such as protein C deficiency, protein S deficiency, antithrombin III deficiency, and antiphospholipid syndrome with lupus anticoagulant or anticardiolipin antibodies or both (Bertina et al, 1994; Boughton, 1991; Dahlback, 1995; Dahlback et al, 1993; Espinosa et al, 2001; Koster et al, 1993; Mahmoud et al, 1995; Menon et al, 2004; Pelletier et al, 1994; Svensson & Dahlback, 1994; Valla, 2003; Vandenbroucke et al, 1994). It has been reported that subjects with the factor V Leiden mutation, which leads to activated protein C resistance, have a 5-fold to 10-fold increase in the risk of thrombosis if they are heterozygotes and a 50-fold to 100-fold increase if they are homozygotes (Dahlback, 1995; Deltenre et al, 2001; Janssen et al, 2000). More recent evidence indicates that multiple prothrombotic factors acting concurrently are involved in a substantial percentage of patients with BCS

Table 100.3 Screening for Hematologic Disorders in Budd-Chiari Syndrome

Complete blood count, prothrombin time, partial thromboplastin time, fibrinogen

Red blood cell mass, plasma volume

Bone marrow biopsy, cell culture, karyotype

Antithrombin III assay

Protein C assay

Free protein S antigen assay

Lupus anticoagulant

Anticardiolipin antibodies

Ham's acid hemolysis test

Activated protein C resistance or factor V Leiden mutation or both

Endogenous erythroid colony assay

rubra vera associated with BCS is compatible with a long life if it is treated with hydroxyurea.

Paroxysmal nocturnal hemoglobinuria is another hematologic disorder associated with BCS (Hartmann et al, 1980; Liebowitz & Hartmann, 1981; Valla et al, 1987). It was responsible for 6.7% of the cases in the collected series of Mitchell and colleagues (1982) and 12% of the cases in the series of Valla and coworkers (1987). In all of the hematologic disorders associated with hepatic vein thrombosis, but particularly in paroxysmal nocturnal hemoglobinuria, thrombosis of other blood vessels

(Denninger et al, 2000; Janssen et al, 2000). Rarely, hematologic malignancies, such as acute leukemia and lymphoma, have been associated with BCS.

It cannot be overemphasized that every patient found to have BCS should undergo a thorough hematologic evaluation. The workup proposed by Mahmoud and Elias (1996) and others (Hirschberg et al, 2000; Valla, 2003) is shown in Table 100.3 and is similar to the one that we perform. With these studies, it should be possible to diagnose all of the predisposing thrombogenic hematologic disorders that are known to be associated with BCS. If an evaluation such as this is done uniformly, it is highly likely that the incidence of idiopathic BCS will continue to decline.

Oral Contraceptives

It is well established that there is an increased incidence of thromboembolic phenomena involving various blood vessels and organs in women taking oral contraceptives. The first case of BCS associated with use of oral contraceptives was reported by Ecker and McKittrick (1966), 5 years after these drugs became available commercially. Since then, more than 200 cases of BCS in patients taking oral contraceptives have been described (Janssen et al, 2000; Lewis et al, 1983; Maddrey, 1987; Valla et al, 1986; Zafrani et al, 1983), and the increasing overall incidence of BCS in recent years has been attributed partly to the widespread use of these agents. In the collective review reported by Mitchell and colleagues (1982), use of oral contraceptives was believed to be responsible for 9.4% of the cases of BCS during the period 1960-1980. Valla and associates (1986) reported that the relative risk of hepatic vein thrombosis among oral contraceptive users was close to that of stroke, myocardial infarction, and venous thromboembolism. In our series of 66 cases of BCS, 24% of patients gave a history of oral contraceptive use. The incidence is even higher if the denominator consists only of the number of women in each series, which is appropriate because men do not use oral contraceptives. In our series, 48% of the 33 women with BCS used oral contraceptives. Some authors have proposed that oral contraceptives are not a primary cause of BCS, but contribute to thrombosis only if there is an underlying hematologic disorder (Valla et al, 1986). In our series, no hematologic disease was identified in users of oral contraceptives, but until relatively recently our patients did not undergo the extensive hematologic workup shown in Table 100.3. The duration of usage of oral contraceptives before the diagnosis of BCS has ranged from 2 weeks to 10 years. In addition to causing BCS, use of oral contraceptives has been linked to other liver disorders, including VOD, portal vein thrombosis, cholestasis, hepatocellular adenoma, focal nodular hyperplasia, and possibly hepatoma and angiosarcoma (Zafrani et al, 1983).

Pregnancy and Postpartum

BCS has been observed in women during pregnancy and, more commonly, during the postpartum period. The first case of BCS reported by Chiari (1899) occurred in a woman who developed the disorder after childbirth. In the collective review by Mitchell and colleagues (1982), 9.9% of the cases of BCS occurred during pregnancy or postpartum, and in a series of 105 patients with BCS observed from 1963-1978, Khuroo and Datta (1980)

reported 16 cases (15.2%) of BCS after pregnancy; 8 of the patients died, and 7 were lost to follow-up after discharge from the hospital. The hypercoagulable state that is known to occur during pregnancy is presumed to be responsible for the association of BCS with this condition. Only 1 of our 66 cases of BCS occurred during pregnancy or postpartum.

Malignant Neoplasms

Malignant neoplasms were responsible for 13.4% of the collected cases of BCS reported by Parker (1959), 8.8% of the collected cases reported by Mitchell and colleagues (1982), and 12% of the cases reported by Powell-Jackson and coworkers (1982). Because we do not operate on patients with BCS caused by cancer, none of our 66 patients had malignant neoplasms. Occlusion of the suprahepatic IVC by invasive tumors has been the cause of BCS in many of these cases. The most common cancers associated with BCS are hepatocellular carcinoma, renal cell carcinoma, adrenal carcinoma, and leiomyosarcoma of the IVC. Other malignancies that rarely have caused BCS include carcinomas of the lung, pancreas, and stomach; melanoma; reticulum cell sarcoma; adrenal sarcoma; and sarcoma of the right atrium.

Infections

Infections involving the liver were believed responsible for 3% of the collected cases of BCS reviewed by Parker (1959), 9.9% of the collected cases reported by Mitchell and colleagues (1982), and none of the cases in sizable series reported in more recent years, including our own series. The most common infections associated with BCS are those caused by parasites, particularly amebic liver abscess, hydatid disease, and schistosomiasis (see Chs. 60 and 61). Syphilitic gumma of the liver accounted for 1.8% of the cases in Parker's review, but has not been reported as a cause of BCS in recent years. Aspergillosis involving the hepatic veins and IVC has been a rare cause of BCS. In India, Victor and coworkers (1994) provided evidence that filariasis can cause BCS.

Trauma

Abdominal trauma has uncommonly predisposed to the development of BCS. Trauma was responsible for 1.2% of the collected cases of BCS reported by Parker (1959) and 2.4% of the collected cases reviewed by Mitchell and colleagues (1982). Blunt and penetrating trauma have been implicated in occasional cases of BCS. None of our cases of BCS were caused by trauma.

Connective Tissue Disorders

Occasional cases of BCS have been reported in association with various connective tissue and autoimmune diseases, most of which are known to have thrombotic tendencies. Included among these are Behçet's disease, Sjögren's syndrome, mixed connective tissue disease, sarcoidosis, and rheumatoid arthritis. Numerous cases of BCS in patients with Behçet's disease, including five of our own, have been described (Bazraktar et al, 1997; Orloff & Orloff, 1999).

Membranous Obstruction of the Vena Cava

More than 600 cases of BCS resulting from MOVC have been reported from Japan (Hirooka & Kimura, 1970; Kimura et al, 1972; Okuda, 2002; Ono et al, 1983; Taneja et al, 1979; Yamamoto et al, 1968), China (Wang, 1989; Wang et al, 1989; Wu et al, 1990), other parts of Asia, India (Khuroo & Datta, 1980), and South Africa (Semson, 1982). In the United States and Europe, MOVC is rare. A congenital cause of this condition has been proposed, but there is a strong suggestion that it represents the end result of acquired thrombosis (Kage et al, 1992; Okuda 2002; Okuda et al, 1995). The condition usually runs a chronic course of many years, and most patients have developed extensive hepatic fibrosis and cirrhosis and portal hypertension by the time they come to medical attention. An increased incidence of hepatocellular carcinoma has been observed in association with MOVC (Okuda, 2002; Semson, 1982). The therapeutic implications of this condition and other forms of IVC occlusion are distinctly different from those of occlusion confined to the major hepatic veins. We have not encountered a case of MOVC.

Miscellaneous Rare Conditions

Other conditions that have been rarely associated with BCS include inflammatory bowel disease, hepatic torsion after partial resection of the liver, lipoid nephrosis, and protein-losing enteropathy.

CAUSES OF VENO-OCCLUSIVE DISEASE

In 1954, Bras and colleagues proposed the term *veno-occlusive disease* to describe a serious and common liver disease in Jamaican children in which there was occlusion of the central and sublobular hepatic veins and surrounding centrilobular necrosis of the liver parenchyma. Shortly thereafter, Bras and others (Bras & McLean, 1963; Brooks et al, 1970; Gore et al, 1961; Stuart & Bras, 1957) showed that VOD was due to ingestion of "bush teas" made from plants of the *Crotolaria* and *Senecio* genera, which contain well-known hepatotoxic pyrrolizidine alkaloids. It has long been known that these plants and plants of the *Heliotropium* genus produce liver failure in herbivorous animals and are common causes of poisoning of grazing cows and horses. Since the initial descriptions by Bras and others, VOD caused by ingestion of toxic pyrrolizidines has been observed in Israel (Ghanem & Hershko, 1981), Egypt (Safouh & Shehata, 1965), Iraq (Al-Hasany & Mohamed, 1970), Afghanistan (Mohabbat et al, 1976), India (Aikat et al, 1978; Tandon et al, 1976), Venezuela (Grases & Beker, 1972), Ecuador (Lyford et al, 1976), South Africa (Steenkamp et al, 2000; Zuckerman et al, 2002), and the United States (Abbott, 1988; Bach et al, 1989; Ridker & McDermott, 1989; Ridker et al, 1985; Stillman et al, 1977). In addition to poisoning by drinking bush teas, humans have been poisoned by eating flour milled from grain contaminated by the seeds of these plants and by taking herbal remedies.

Antineoplastic drugs have been identified as another cause of VOD. Included among these are cytosine arabinoside, thioguanine, and gemtuzumab ozogamicin (Mylotarg) used in the treatment of acute myelocytic leukemia (Cruz et al, 1983; Giles et al, 2001; Gill et al, 1982; Griner et al, 1976); carmustine used in the treatment of diffuse histiocytic lymphoma (McIntyre et al, 1981);

dacarbazine used in the treatment of melanoma (Asbury et al, 1980); and gemtuzumab ozogamicin and mitomycin C combined with bone marrow transplantation (Kumar et al, 2003; Lazarus et al, 1982; McDonald et al, 1993; Wadleigh et al, 2003). Fatal VOD in renal transplant recipients has been attributed to azathioprine (Liano et al, 1989; Marubbio & Danielson, 1975).

Hepatic injury caused by therapeutic irradiation of malignant neoplasms in and near the liver is an important cause of VOD (Fajardo & Colby, 1980; Reed & Cox, 1966). Although radiation-induced VOD usually does not produce clinical manifestations with doses less than 3000 rad, the condition has been observed after smaller amounts of radiotherapy (Fajardo & Colby, 1980).

Currently, the most common cause of VOD in the Western Hemisphere is bone marrow transplantation (Ayash et al, 1990; Berk et al, 1979; Jones et al, 1987; Kriegshauser et al, 1988; Kumar et al, 2003; McDonald et al, 1984, 1993; Wadleigh et al, 2003). It has been estimated that approximately one fourth of recipients of bone marrow transplants develop the disorder. It is uncertain whether VOD in these patients is caused by the marrow transplant or is a result of the radiation and chemotherapy used in the pretransplant conditioning regimen. Berk and coworkers (1979) proposed that graft-versus-host disease might be responsible for VOD after marrow transplantation, but the studies of McDonald and colleagues (1984) cast doubt on this hypothesis. Finally, there have been rare reports of VOD in association with systemic lupus erythematosus (Pappas et al, 1984), familial immunodeficiency (Mellis & Bale, 1976), and the use of oral contraceptives (Alpert, 1976).

PATHOLOGY

Budd-Chiari Syndrome

The liver receives about one fourth of the cardiac output via its dual afferent blood supply, the portal vein and hepatic artery. After perfusing the sinusoids, the blood is returned to the heart through the hepatic veins and IVC. Obstruction to the egress of blood from the liver at any point along the outflow route results in numerous serious hemodynamic and morphologic alterations. There is a marked increase in intrahepatic pressure, which is reflected by a similar increase in portal pressure. The increased intrahepatic pressure causes extravasation of plasma from the liver sinusoids and lymphatics with formation of ascites. Obstruction to the egress of blood from the liver results in dilation of the sinusoids and intense centrilobular congestion of the hepatic parenchyma, greatest around the terminal hepatic venules (central veins) (Fig. 100.1). There is ischemia, pressure necrosis, and atrophy of the parenchymal cells in the center of the liver lobule. With persistence of the obstruction, the necrotic parenchyma is replaced by fibrous tissue and regenerating nodules of liver tissue. The end result is cirrhosis of the type associated with chronic congestive heart failure. The rapidity with which cirrhosis develops is related to the severity of outflow obstruction, but it is not unusual for cirrhosis to occur within a matter of months (Parker, 1959).

The reversibility of liver damage in BCS is a direct function of the extent and duration of hepatic venous outflow obstruction. Early in the course of the disease, relief of the obstruction can be expected to result in reversal of the parenchymal and hemodynamic abnormalities. Late in the course, the damage to

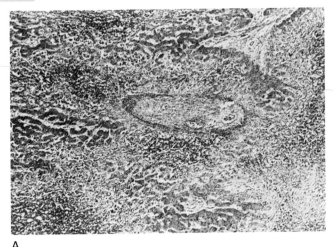

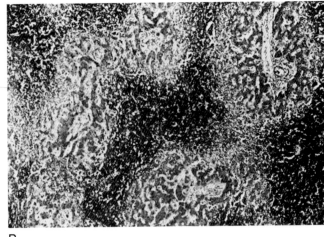

A   B

Fig. 100.1. Photomicrographs of preoperative liver biopsy specimens obtained from BCS patient No. 4 (**A**) and BCS patient No. 5 (**B**) in our series, showing a typical picture of BCS consisting of intense centrilobular congestion and necrosis with widespread loss of hepatocytes. A thrombosed hepatic vein is seen in the center in **A** (×50).
(From Orloff MJ, Johansen KH, 1978: Treatment of Budd-Chiari syndrome by side-to-side portacaval shunt: experimental and clinical results. Ann Surg 188:494-512.)

the hepatic parenchyma becomes irreversible. The timing of therapy has profound implications with regard to prognosis.

Three major hepatic veins—the right hepatic vein, left hepatic vein, and middle hepatic vein—conduct blood into the IVC from the bulk of the hepatic parenchyma. The left and middle hepatic veins usually form a common trunk just before joining the IVC. There also are several small hepatic veins that enter directly into the retrohepatic IVC and drain the caudate lobe and small central regions of the right and left lobes of the liver. In BCS, all three major hepatic veins usually are occluded, although occasionally the occlusion is limited to one or two of the major veins. The small hepatic veins that join the retrohepatic IVC, particularly the veins draining the caudate lobe, often are spared.

In most cases of BCS, the occlusion of the hepatic veins is caused by thrombosis (Parker, 1959). The thrombus undergoes organization and ultimately is converted to fibrous tissue that permanently occludes the veins. Although recanalization of the occluded veins sometimes occurs, it rarely results in effective new outflow channels. Retrograde propagation of the thrombus into smaller hepatic veins is commonly found. Prograde propagation of the thrombus from the hepatic veins into the IVC, with partial or complete occlusion of the IVC, sometimes occurs and markedly changes the therapeutic approach and prognosis. It is important to determine by angiography and pressure measurements whether or not the IVC has become involved in the occlusive process.

MOVC has been reported to be the most common cause of BCS in Japan (Hirooka & Kimura, 1970; Kimura et al, 1972; Okuda et al, 1995; Ono et al, 1983; Taneja et al, 1979; Yamamoto et al, 1968), India (Khuroo & Datta, 1980), and China (Wang, 1989; Wang et al, 1989; Wu et al, 1990) and in the Bantu population of South Africa (Semson, 1982). The "membrane" varies from very thin to several centimeters thick and usually contains fibrous tissue, smooth muscle, and elastic tissue. The location and extent of the membrane vary considerably, and in some cases a long segment of IVC has been replaced by fibrous tissue. Occlusion of one or more of the major hepatic veins often has been associated with membranous obstruction of the IVC. Although some experienced authors have proposed a congenital cause

(Hirooka & Kimura, 1970; Kimura et al, 1972; Ono et al, 1983; Semson, 1982; Taneja et al, 1979), a strong argument has been made suggesting that MOVC is the end result of thrombosis of the IVC, often occurring early in life (Okuda et al, 2002). Most of the cases have run a chronic course before discovery, and when first seen by a physician, patients have had extensive hepatic fibrosis or cirrhosis with portal hypertension and all of its manifestations. The therapeutic considerations in patients with MOVC differ from those in patients with BCS caused by obstruction of the hepatic veins.

Veno-occlusive Disease

VOD of the liver may mimic BCS clinically because both conditions involve hepatic venous outflow obstruction. VOD involves the sinusoids and the central and sublobular hepatic veins within the liver, however, rather than the major hepatic veins (Kumar et al, 2003; Shulman et al, 1987, 1994). The underlying process in VOD is subendothelial sclerosis of the hepatic veins and sinusoids secondary to endothelial injury caused by a toxic agent, be it a pyrrolizidine alkaloid, antineoplastic drug, radiation, or a stem cell transplant. Thrombosis of the small hepatic veins may occur after damage to the venous intima. Electron microscopic studies of liver biopsy specimens obtained from children with VOD caused by pyrrolizidine poisoning showed marked endothelial damage in the sinusoids and subterminal and terminal hepatic veins in all zones of the liver, with extravasation of erythrocytes into Disse's space and narrowing of the lumen where the sinusoid entered the central vein (Brooks et al, 1970).

Similar to BCS, hemorrhagic necrosis of the liver parenchyma around the centrilobular veins occurs early in the course of VOD. Extensive occlusion of the small hepatic veins ultimately leads to diffuse fibrosis and cirrhosis. Patients with VOD caused by chronic pyrrolizidine poisoning often have well-established cirrhosis when first seen by a physician. VOD that develops as a complication of therapy for another condition, such as occurs during cancer chemotherapy, radiation therapy, or bone marrow transplantation, usually is detected early in the course of the disease.

CLINICAL MANIFESTATIONS OF BUDD-CHIARI SYNDROME

The clinical manifestations and course of BCS are determined by the extent of occlusion of the hepatic venous outflow system and the rapidity with which the venous occlusion becomes complete. More often than not, patients in the West have an acute course with rapid progression of liver disease and its consequences over periods of a few weeks to a few months. In some patients, however, BCS develops insidiously, with clinical manifestations appearing gradually over months or years. Patients with MOVC observed in Japan, China, India, and South Africa often present to the physician for the first time with manifestations of well-established cirrhosis after tolerating symptoms for many years.

In our series of 66 patients with BCS, 12 were referred to us with advanced cirrhosis as a result of prolonged hepatic outflow obstruction and were not candidates for portal decompression surgery. The other 54 patients were referred at a mean 13.6 weeks after onset of BCS (range 4-78 weeks). Fifty of the 54 patients (93%) were referred less than 18 weeks after onset of symptoms, relatively early in the course of BCS. The remaining four patients were operated on 19, 21, 25, and 78 weeks after onset of symptoms. In the collected series of Mitchell and colleagues (1982), which excluded cases of MOVC, two thirds had had symptoms for less than 3 months, and 83% had had symptoms for 6 months or less at the time of diagnosis. In Parker's (1959) collected series of 133 cases observed before 1959, 57% had had symptoms for 3 months or less and 71% had been symptomatic for 6 months or less.

Table 100.4 presents the frequency of symptoms and signs in our series of 66 patients with BCS, 45 of whom had hepatic vein occlusion alone, and 21 of whom had IVC occlusion and hepatic vein occlusion. The only difference between the two groups, and it is an important one, was the absence of lower extremity edema in the group without IVC thrombosis and the high incidence of edema from feet to thighs (76%) that resulted from IVC occlusion.

Symptoms

Abdominal Distention

The initial symptom in all of our patients was abdominal distention secondary to ascites, which increased progressively over a few weeks. Abdominal distention caused by ascites occurs at some time in almost every patient with BCS. In the large collected series (Mitchell et al, 1982; Parker, 1959), abdominal distention was the first symptom experienced by most patients.

Abdominal Pain

All of our patients had abdominal pain that was dull, nagging, and chronic. The pain was localized in the right hypochondrium in some patients, diffuse in the upper abdomen in other patients, and diffuse throughout the abdomen in several patients. The pain was probably due to distention of the liver capsule from intense hepatic congestion or to abdominal distention from rapid accumulation of ascites. Abdominal pain has been a prominent symptom in all reported series of BCS.

Weakness

All patients in our series had striking and progressive weakness as a manifestation of their severe acute illness. Weakness has not been as prominent in the chronic forms of BCS.

Anorexia

Anorexia was reported by all patients in our series and has been experienced by many patients in the reports of other workers (Mitchell et al, 1982).

Jaundice

Clinical jaundice was observed in 53% of the patients in our series, but in only 28% of the patients in Parker's collective review (Parker, 1959) and in only 17% of the patients collected by Mitchell and colleagues (1982). Usually the jaundice has been mild.

Symptoms of Chronic Liver Disease

Patients with the chronic forms of BCS, such as MOVC, often have the usual symptoms of cirrhosis and portal hypertension, including upper gastrointestinal bleeding secondary to ruptured esophagogastric varices, hepatic encephalopathy, hepatorenal syndrome, and edema of the lower extremities. Peripheral edema is particularly prominent in patients with MOVC, and some develop varicose veins of the legs (Parker, 1959; Semson, 1982). In our series of patients who underwent surgical portal decompression for acute BCS secondary to occlusion of the hepatic veins, one patient had these symptoms.

Findings on Physical Examination (Signs)

Ascites

All 66 patients in our series had the abdominal signs of massive ascites on physical examination at the time of diagnosis.

Table 100.4 Symptoms and Signs in 66 Patients with Budd-Chiari Syndrome Treated by the Authors

| | % OF GROUP | | | % OF GROUP | |
Symptom	Hepatic vein Occlusion (n = 45)	IVC Occlusion (n = 21)	Sign	Hepatic Vein Occlusion (n = 45)	IVC Occlusion (n = 21)
Abdominal distention	100	100	Massive ascites	100	100
Abdominal pain	100	100	Hepatomegaly	100	100
Weakness	100	100	Wasting	100	100
Anorexia	100	100	Abdominal venous distention	60	48
Jaundice	56	48	Splenomegaly	100	100
			Jaundice	56	48
			Edema of the thighs, legs, feet	0	76

The incidence of ascites was 93% in the collective review of Parker (1959) and 83% in the series of Mitchell and colleagues (1982).

Hepatomegaly

All of the patients in our series and in the series of Mitchell and colleagues (1982) had marked hepatomegaly resulting from severe congestion of the liver. In chronic forms of BCS, hepatomegaly may not be as striking, but it is usually present.

Wasting

All patients in our series had substantial wasting as a result of loss of lean body mass over a relatively short time. All of our patients appeared chronically and seriously ill.

Distention of Abdominal Veins

Thirty-seven of the 66 patients in our series (56%) and 55% of the patients in the collected series of Parker (1959) had distention of the superficial veins of the anterior abdominal wall. Abdominal venous distention is a manifestation of portal hypertension and the formation of portosystemic collaterals early in the course of BCS.

Splenomegaly

Splenomegaly, another manifestation of portal hypertension, was observed in all of the patients in our series, 50% of the collected series of Mitchell and colleagues (1982), and 30% of the collected series of Parker (1959). Enlargement and congestion of the spleen was accompanied sometimes by the hematologic manifestations of secondary hypersplenism.

Jaundice

Clinical jaundice was observed in 53% of the patients in our series, but in only 28% of the patients in the collected series of Parker (1959) and in only 17% of the patients in the collected series of Mitchell and colleagues (1982). The jaundice in our patients who underwent surgical portal decompression was invariably mild; the highest serum bilirubin level was only 6.8 mg/dL.

Edema of the Lower Extremities

Edema of the lower extremities or lower trunk indicates involvement of the IVC in the occlusive process and was observed in 76% of the 21 patients in our series who had IVC occlusion. None of the 45 patients with thrombosis confined to the hepatic veins in our series had substantial lower extremity edema.

Signs of Chronic Liver Disease

Patients with the chronic forms of BCS, such as patients with MOVC, often have the usual manifestations of chronic liver disease, including spider angiomata, palmar erythema, asterixis, breast hypertrophy, testicular atrophy, and fetor hepaticus. In our series, these signs were seen only in patients who were placed in the liver transplantation group because of advanced cirrhosis.

SYMPTOMS AND SIGNS OF VENO-OCCLUSIVE DISEASE

VOD has been observed in individuals of all ages, including infants and adults in their 60s. VOD caused by pyrrolizidine alkaloids has been seen most commonly in infants and children. The clinical manifestations depend on the stage of the disease at which the patient seeks medical treatment (Brooks et al, 1970; Ghanem & Hershko, 1981; Gore et al, 1961; Safouh &

Shehata, 1965; Stuart & Bras, 1957). The acute stage is often preceded for 1 or 2 weeks by a febrile illness with upper respiratory symptoms, vomiting and diarrhea, or both. The patient then presents with the abrupt onset of abdominal distention secondary to ascites, abdominal pain, weakness, anorexia, and fever (Kumar et al, 2003; Wadleigh et al, 2003). Jaundice is the rule, and splenomegaly with thrombocytopenia is common. Some patients develop edema of the feet and occasionally of the hands and face. Physical examination in the acute phase invariably shows hepatomegaly and ascites. Many patients have splenomegaly, some have distention of the superficial veins of the abdominal wall, and some have peripheral edema and a pleural effusion. Bone marrow transplant recipients usually develop the clinical features of VOD within 3 weeks after transplantation. Many patients have died during the acute stage from liver failure, bleeding esophageal varices, or intercurrent infection.

Patients other than bone marrow transplant recipients may present in the chronic stage of VOD with the usual clinical manifestations of cirrhosis of the liver, including ascites, hepatomegaly, splenomegaly, wasting, abdominal venous distention, spider angiomata, palmar erythema, asterixis, and peripheral edema. Bleeding from esophageal varices is a major cause of death in the chronic stage. Cirrhosis of the liver has been observed 3 months after acute onset of VOD (Gore et al, 1961).

DIAGNOSTIC STUDIES IN BUDD-CHIARI SYNDROME

Hepatic Angiography and Pressures

The diagnostic study of greatest value in BCS is angiographic examination of the IVC and hepatic veins with pressure measurements (Clain et al, 1967; Kreel et al, 1967; Redman, 1975; Tavill et al, 1975). This study usually is combined with hepatic and superior mesenteric arteriography and indirect portography. In BCS confined to the hepatic veins, the IVC is patent, and IVC pressure is relatively normal for subjects with ascites (Fig. 100.2). Patency of the IVC is a prerequisite for portacaval shunt (PCS) and is a crucial finding. In some patients, the IVC is moderately compressed in its retrohepatic course by the enlarged liver and, in particular, by a hypertrophied caudate lobe (Fig. 100.3). This finding usually is not clinically significant (Clain et al, 1967; Kreel et al, 1967; Redman, 1975; Tavill et al, 1975).

The most important angiographic finding is the demonstration by hepatic venography of occlusion or marked narrowing of the major hepatic veins. Sometimes it is not possible to find patent orifices of any of the hepatic veins, which is indirect evidence that all of the major hepatic veins are occluded. Usually it is possible, however, to enter at least one major hepatic vein and to show the presence of a thrombus or of narrowing and distortion of the vein (Fig. 100.4A). Injection of dye in the wedged position often shows a characteristic spider-web pattern of small hepatic venous collaterals connecting to portal or systemic veins (see Fig. 100.4B). Wedged hepatic vein pressure (WHVP) usually is markedly elevated, which reflects the obstruction to hepatic venous outflow. In patients with hepatic vein occlusion alone, IVC pressure is substantially lower than WHVP.

Patients with BCS resulting from obstruction of the IVC have a quite different venographic picture. Venography of the IVC shows the vena caval obstruction and the development of large collateral veins arising from the IVC. Pressure in the IVC is high

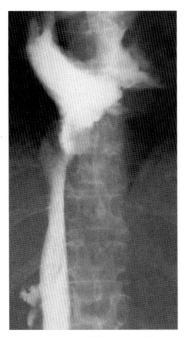

Fig. 100.2. Inferior venacavogram in BCS patient No. 3 in our series, showing a widely patent IVC. IVC pressure was 62 mm saline.
(From Orloff MJ, Johansen KH, 1978: Treatment of Budd-Chiari syndrome by side-to-side portacaval shunt: experimental and clinical results. Ann Surg 188:494-512.)

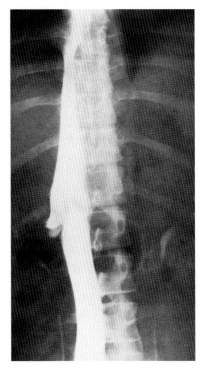

Fig. 100.3. Inferior venacavogram in BCS patient No. 6 in our series, showing a patent IVC with side-to-side compression in its retrohepatic course by the enlarged liver. IVC pressure at this time was 102 mm saline.
(From Orloff MJ, Johansen KH, 1978: Treatment of Budd-Chiari syndrome by side-to-side portacaval shunt: experimental and clinical results. Ann Surg 188:494-512.)

and is similar to WHVP. Most, but not all, patients with thrombosis of the IVC also have occlusion of the hepatic veins. To visualize and define membranous obstruction of the IVC, it is often necessary to inject contrast material into the IVC simultaneously through catheters positioned above and below the diaphragm.

Hepatic arteriography in BCS shows the nonspecific abnormality of stretching and attenuation of the branches of the hepatic artery within the liver. Indirect portography after injection of contrast material into the superior mesenteric artery usually shows a patent portal vein. Because the thrombotic tendency in BCS sometimes involves multiple sites, it is of therapeutic importance

to ensure that the portal vein is patent. These findings complete the picture of vascular abnormalities, although, by themselves, they are not diagnostic.

In our series of 66 patients, angiographic studies showed occlusion of the hepatic veins alone in 45 patients and occlusion of both the hepatic veins and IVC in 21 patients. A spider-web pattern was observed in 42 patients (64%). WHVP was markedly elevated in all patients in whom it was measured. In the 45 patients with thrombosis confined to the hepatic veins,

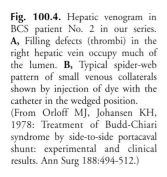

Fig. 100.4. Hepatic venogram in BCS patient No. 2 in our series. **A,** Filling defects (thrombi) in the right hepatic vein occupy much of the lumen. **B,** Typical spider-web pattern of small venous collaterals shown by injection of dye with the catheter in the wedged position.
(From Orloff MJ, Johansen KH, 1978: Treatment of Budd-Chiari syndrome by side-to-side portacaval shunt: experimental and clinical results. Ann Surg 188:494-512.)

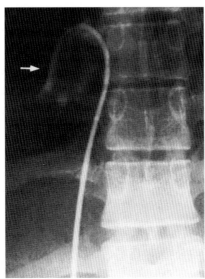

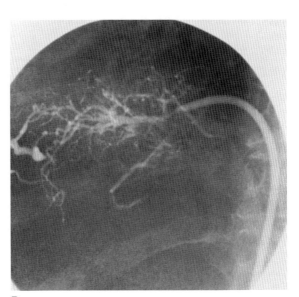

A

B

Table 100.5 Results of Diagnostic Studies in 66 Patients with Budd-Chiari Syndrome Treated by the Authors

	% OF GROUP	
	Hepatic Vein Occlusion (n = 45)	IVC Occlusion (n = 21)
Angiography and Pressures		
Occluded hepatic veins	100	100
Occluded IVC near hepatic veins	0	100
Spider-web pattern of hepatic veins	71	48
Patent portal and splenic veins	100	100
Stretched hepatic arteries	100	100
IVC pressure much lower than WHVP	100	0
High WHVP	100	100
Percutaneous Needle Liver Biopsy (63 Patients Studied)		
Centrilobular congestion	100	100
Centrilobular hepatocyte loss and necrosis	100	100
Fibrosis	78	57
Cirrhosis (included also under fibrosis)	31	5
Hepatic Scintiscan		
Decreased hepatic uptake	100	100
Nonhomogenous hepatic uptake	100	100
Excessive extrahepatic uptake	78	79
Central hot spot in liver	33	9
CT (53 Patients Studied)		
Absence of hepatic veins	100	100
Abnormal hepatic uptake of contrast	100	100
Occlusion of IVC	0	100
Real-Time and Doppler Duplex Ultrasound (51 Patients Studied)		
Absence of hepatic veins with flat or reversed flow	100	100
Abnormal venous structures in liver	100	100
IVC thrombosis with flat or reversed flow	0	100
Abnormal Liver Function Tests		
Bromsulphalein or indocyanine green retention (23–90%) (24 patients)	100	100
Serum alkaline phosphatase (138–458 IU)	100	100
Prothrombin time (12.4–16.5 seconds)	98	90
Partial thromboplastin time (31–59 seconds)	98	90
Serum albumin (2.1–2.8 g/dL)	96	95
Aspartate aminotransferase (76–540 IU)	89	86
Serum bilirubin (3.8–6.8 mg/dL)	60	38
Upper Gastrointestinal X-Rays (53 Patients Studied)		
Normal	60	0
Esophageal varices	40	100

the IVC was patent with relatively normal pressures for patients with ascites, ranging from 62 to 160 mm saline (Table 100.5). Many patients had moderate compression of the retrohepatic IVC by the large liver, but invariably WHVP was substantially higher than IVC pressure, a crucial finding. In contrast, in the 21 patients with IVC occlusion, IVC pressure and WHVP were similar. All patients had stretched and attenuated hepatic artery branches within the liver and a patent portal vein.

Liver Biopsy

Percutaneous needle liver biopsy yields histologic findings that are characteristic of BCS early in the course of the disease and, along with hepatic angiography, provides conclusive diagnostic information (Tang et al, 2001). The diagnostic features are quite spectacular and include intense centrilobular congestion combined with centrilobular loss of parenchyma and necrosis (see Fig. 100.1). Mild to moderate fibrosis of the liver parenchyma is found in many patients. As the disease evolves and becomes chronic, cirrhosis of the cardiac type develops. Cirrhosis has been observed within months of the onset of symptoms. Only two other conditions, constrictive pericarditis and congestive heart failure, produce a histologic picture similar to that seen in the acute stage of BCS. Both of these cardiac disorders can be eliminated easily from consideration by appropriate studies. Percutaneous needle liver biopsy was done preoperatively in 63 of the 66 patients in our series, and open wedge liver biopsy was done at operation in all 66 patients (see Table 100.5). All patients had intense centrilobular congestion along with centrilobular hepatocellular loss and necrosis. Of the 54 patients in our series who were referred sufficiently early to undergo surgical portal decompression, 39 (72%) had fibrosis of the liver at an early point in their illness. In three patients, the fibrosis had progressed to cirrhosis. All 12 patients who were considered candidates for liver transplantation had advanced cirrhosis.

Hepatic Scintiscanning

Scintiscans of the liver (see Ch. 17) with technetium 99m–sulfur colloid or other colloidal radionuclides show the nonspecific abnormalities of decreased and nonhomogeneous hepatic uptake of radiocolloid, increased uptake of radiocolloid by the spleen and bone marrow, and hepatosplenomegaly. Central localization of radiocolloid in the liver, the so-called central hot spot, has been reported to be of diagnostic importance (Fig. 100.5) (Meindok & Langer, 1976; Tavill et al, 1975). It is seen when the thrombotic process spares the small hepatic veins that drain the caudate lobe and central areas of the right and left lobes directly into the IVC so that these areas of the liver remain healthy and even hypertrophy. The central hot spot was observed in only 17 of the 66 patients with BCS in our series.

Computed Tomography

Computed tomography (CT) (see Ch. 18) of the liver after injection of contrast agents has been shown to be of diagnostic value in BCS (Baert et al, 1983; Mathieu et al, 1987). The findings include (1) absence of opacification of the hepatic veins, which in normal subjects usually can be shown clearly; (2) nonhomogeneous and delayed uptake of contrast material in the liver; (3) delayed emptying of contrast material from venous structures at the periphery of the liver; and (4) occlusion of the IVC in patients with IVC thrombosis. CT also shows ascites and hepatomegaly. We performed CT in 53 of our 66 patients and observed these abnormalities in all of them.

Ultrasonography

Real-time and Doppler duplex ultrasonography of the liver has been shown to be of diagnostic value in BCS (Baert et al, 1983; Becker et al, 1986; Bolondi et al, 1991; Grant et al, 1989; Gupta et al, 1987; Hosoki et al, 1989; Powell-Jackson et al, 1986; Rossi et al, 1981) (see Ch. 15). Findings include (1) absence of normal

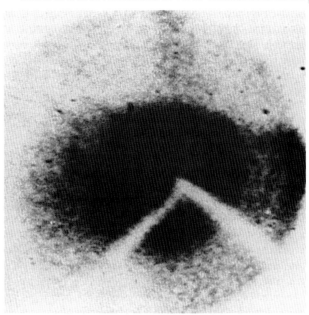

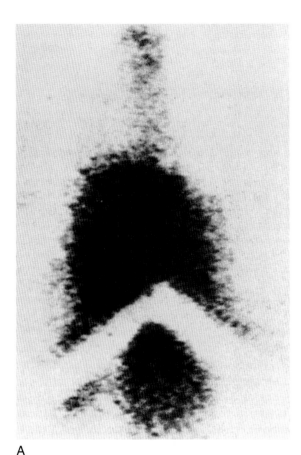

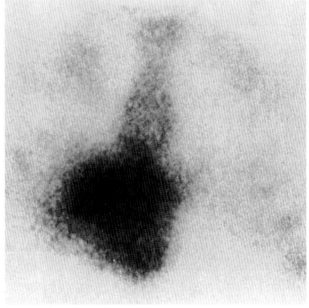

Fig. 100.5. A-C, Scintiscan of liver in three cases of BCS, showing central accumulation of radionuclide, the so-called central hot spot. (From Mitchell MC, et al, 1982: Budd-Chiari syndrome: etiology, diagnosis and management. Medicine [Baltimore] 61:199-218.)

hepatic veins draining into the IVC with flat or reversed flow, (2) an abnormal intrahepatic network of comma-shaped venous structures, (3) thrombus in IVC and flat or reversed flow in patients with IVC thrombosis, and (4) enlargement of the caudate lobe. Ascites has been shown regularly. We observed these abnormalities in all 51 patients in whom ultrasound was performed in our series. We regularly used Doppler ultrasound as a screening tool, but depended on angiography for a definitive diagnosis and guide to treatment.

Magnetic Resonance Imaging

Magnetic resonance imaging (MRI) (see Ch. 19) is capable of showing patency or obstruction of the hepatic veins and is particularly effective in visualizing the entire length of the IVC. It has been reported to be useful in differentiating the acute form of BCS from the subacute and chronic forms of BCS (Noone et al, 2000). Because of the high cost of MRI, it is not a first-line diagnostic procedure. None of our 66 patients underwent MRI.

Abnormal Liver Function Tests

Results of liver function tests are usually abnormal in BCS, although the type of abnormality varies and is nondiagnostic (see Table 100.5). All 24 patients in our series who had studies of injected bromsulphalein or indocyanine green dye clearance had marked retention of dye ranging from 23% to 90% (normal <6%). All 66 patients had elevation of serum alkaline phosphatase ranging from 138 to 458 IU (normal 25-85 IU). Of 66 patients, 63 had prolonged prothrombin time and partial thromboplastin time, and 95% had a marked decrease in serum albumin concentration (range 2.1-2.8 g/dL); 58 patients (88%) had elevations of aspartate aminotransferase (range 76-540 IU). Thirty-four patients in our series (51%) had mild to moderate elevations of serum bilirubin (range 3.8-6.8 mg/dL). These biochemical abnormalities are not specific to BCS, but they indicate significant hepatic dysfunction and are an important part of the diagnostic workup.

Ascitic Fluid Analysis

Analysis of ascitic fluid in patients with BCS is of little diagnostic value because the results vary considerably (Mitchell et al, 1982; Tavill et al, 1975). Protein concentration has been reported to range from 0.5 to 4.9 g/dL.

Upper Gastrointestinal Radiographs

Barium contrast upper gastrointestinal radiographs were obtained in 53 patients with BCS in our series. The results were normal in 31 patients, but showed esophageal varices in 22 patients (42%); 13 of the 22 patients with varices had cirrhosis. In the chronic forms of BCS, esophageal varices can be shown regularly by radiography and confirmed by esophagogastroscopy.

DIAGNOSTIC STUDIES IN VENO-OCCLUSIVE DISEASE

The most important diagnostic study in VOD is needle liver biopsy, which shows the specific abnormality of extensive occlusion of the small hepatic veins within the liver (Brooks et al, 1970; Gore et al, 1961; Shulman et al, 1995; Stuart & Bras, 1957). In the acute stage of VOD, an additional biopsy finding is centrilobular hemorrhagic necrosis of the hepatic parenchyma. In the chronic stage of VOD, the biopsy specimen shows diffuse fibrosis or cirrhosis of the liver.

Angiographic studies are not as helpful in VOD as they are in BCS. The major hepatic veins and IVC are normal on venography, but WHVP is invariably elevated, a finding that supports the diagnosis of VOD. Findings on hepatic arteriography and indirect portography are similar to the findings in BCS. Because of the significant risk of bleeding after bone marrow transplantation, it is safest in such patients to perform liver biopsy by the percutaneous transjugular route. WHVP can be measured at the same time.

The abnormalities shown by hepatic scintiscanning in VOD are similar to those in BCS except that the central hot spot has rarely been reported. Real-time and Doppler duplex ultrasonography and, to a lesser extent, CT may provide useful diagnostic information in VOD.

Liver function test results are invariably abnormal in VOD and do not differ from the results seen in BCS. The abnormalities reflect serious hepatic dysfunction, but are not specific for VOD. After bone marrow transplantation, elevated plasma levels of plasminogen activator inhibitor 1 have been reported to be a useful marker in distinguishing VOD from the several other causes of post-transplant hepatic dysfunction, such as graft-versus-host disease, drug-induced hepatotoxicity, sepsis, and viral hepatitis (Salat et al, 1997a). Plasminogen activator inhibitor 1 has been implicated in the pathology of VOD.

Because so many patients with VOD caused by pyrrolizidine alkaloids have been seen for the first time when the disease was far advanced, they often have had many or all of the manifestations of cirrhosis and portal hypertension. Esophagogastric varices have been shown in many patients by esophagogastroscopy and barium contrast upper gastrointestinal radiographs.

FINDINGS AT OPERATION

The findings at operation in the 54 patients who underwent surgical portal decompression in our series are summarized in Tables 100.6 and 100.7 and typify what can be expected in patients with BCS. All patients had marked ascites ranging in volume from 2.6 to 15.9 L, congestive hepatomegaly, splenomegaly, and extensive portosystemic collateral veins. All of the patients had portal hypertension. In the group of 34 patients with thrombosis confined to the hepatic veins, the mean portal vein–IVC pressure gradient was 244 mm saline. In all 34 of these patients, portal pressure was substantially higher than IVC pressure so that a direct side-to-side portacaval shunt (SSPCS) was feasible. In contrast, in the group of 20 patients with IVC occlusion and hepatic vein occlusion, the mean portal vein–IVC pressure gradient was only 11 mm saline because the high pressure in the obstructed IVC was similar to the high portal pressure. All 20 patients had a large pressure gradient between the portal vein and right atrium that averaged 202 mm saline.

A wedge liver biopsy specimen obtained at operation showed intense centrilobular congestion and marked centrilobular cell loss and necrosis in all but one patient (see Fig. 100.1). Thirty-five of the 54 patients had hepatic fibrosis, which was mild or moderate in 31 patients and severe in 4 patients, 3 of whom had cirrhosis. In patients with the chronic forms of BCS, and in most patients with VOD, the operative findings are typical of cirrhosis of the liver by the time they are treated.

Table 100.6 Findings at Operation in 54 Patients with Budd-Chiari Syndrome Who Underwent Surgical Portal Decompression by the Authors

	HEPATIC VEIN OCCLUSION ALONE	IVC AND HEPATIC VEIN OCCLUSION	
	SSPCS	Mesoatrial Shunt	Combined SSPCS and CAS
No. patients	34	8	12
Ascites (L)			
Mean	6.5	6.2	6.2
Range	2.6–15.9	4.1–9.3	4.2–9.4
Hepatomegaly (%)	100	100	100
Splenomegaly (%)	100	100	100
Liver biopsy results (%)			
Congestion			
Marked	94	100	100
Mild	6		
Necrosis			
Marked	100	100	100
Fibrosis			
Marked	12	0	0
Moderate-Mild	59	37	67
None	29	63	33
Cirrhosis	12	0	0

CAS, cavoatrial shunt.

Table 100.7 Intraoperative Pressure Measurements in mm Saline in 54 Patients with Budd-Chiari Syndrome Who Underwent Surgical Portal Decompression

Group	PRESHUNT PRESSURES					POSTSHUNT PRESSURES					
	PV	IVC	PV-IVC Gradient	RA	PV-RA Gradient	PV	IVC	PV-IVC Gradient	RA	PV-RA Gradient	
Hepatic vein occlusion alone—SSPCS (n = 34)											
Mean	374	130	244	—	—	169	164	5	—	—	
Range	265–434	74–250	134–336	—	—	120–289	118–284	–12 to 40	—	—	
IVC and hepatic vein occlusion—Mesoatrial shunt (n = 8)											
Mean	320	305	9	101	211	224	—	—	147	78	
Range	274–368	256–348	–8 to 46	90–112	162–256	196–248	—	—	124–162	52–94	
IVC and hepatic vein occlusion—Combined PCS and CAS (n = 12)											
Mean	306	293	13	111	196	169	165	4	146	23	
Range	266–346	264–316	–8 to 34	96–124	142–238	158–184	160–178	–4 to 10	136–162	8–42	

CAS, cavoatrial shunt; PV, portal vein; RA, right atrium.

NONOPERATIVE THERAPY

The objectives of nonoperative therapy of BCS are to (1) remove the cause of the venous thrombosis, (2) relieve the high pressure and congestion within the liver, (3) prevent extension of the venous thrombosis, and (4) reverse the massive ascites. It is often impossible to accomplish these objectives.

In many cases of BCS, the cause of the venous thrombosis is unknown or, if known, cannot be removed. In some cases, however, it is possible to remove or modify the predisposing condition. Examples are cases of BCS caused by ingestion of oral contraceptives, hematologic disorders such as polycythemia rubra vera and paroxysmal nocturnal hemoglobinuria, and pregnancy.

Decompression of the liver by nonoperative measures is rarely, if ever, feasible. Thrombolytic therapy with urokinase or streptokinase has been used in many patients in an attempt to dissolve the thrombi and restore hepatic venous outflow (Cassel & Morely, 1974; Gooneratne et al, 1979; Greenwood et al, 1983; Hodkinson et al, 1978; Malt et al, 1978; Mitchell et al, 1982; Powell-Jackson et al, 1982; Thijs et al, 1978; Warren et al, 1972). The experience with thrombolytic therapy has been recorded in sketchy anecdotal reports involving short periods of follow-up. Approximately one third of patients were believed to have had a clinical response to treatment for periods of 2 months to 1 year. Half of the patients died as a result of BCS during the brief periods of observation. In the experience of Powell-Jackson and coworkers (1982), all four patients who received thrombolytic treatment in the acute phase of BCS died without evidence of a response. Urokinase and streptokinase have been administered by systemic intravenous infusion and by infusion directly into the IVC. In the use of thrombolytic drugs to treat deep venous thrombosis of the lower extremities, peripheral intravenous infusion has been as effective as perfusing the agents directly into the clot. The recommended regimen (Greenwood et al, 1983) involves an intravenous loading dose (urokinase, 4400 IU/kg; streptokinase, 250,000 IU) followed by a constant intravenous infusion of urokinase at 4400 IU/kg/hr or streptokinase at 100,000 IU/hr for 2 to 7 days. Pulmonary embolization developed in two patients during thrombolytic therapy and is a potentially serious complication of this type of treatment.

Anticoagulant therapy has been used widely in BCS to prevent propagation of the thrombi (Ecker & McKittrick, 1966; Hartmann et al, 1980; Khuroo & Datta, 1980; Langer et al, 1975; Lewis et al, 1983; Liebowitz & Hartmann, 1981; Mitchell et al, 1982; Peytremann et al, 1972; Powell-Jackson et al, 1982; Thijs et al, 1978). Most reports of the effectiveness of this form of treatment have been anecdotal and lacking in long-term follow-up. There is no evidence that the use of either heparin or warfarin (Coumadin) brings about dissolution of established thrombosis. In BCS caused by hematologic disorders such as polycythemia rubra vera and paroxysmal nocturnal hemoglobinuria, some dramatic responses to intravenous heparin therapy have been reported, although relapses have been common (Hartmann et al, 1980; Liebowitz & Hartmann, 1981; Peytremann et al, 1972). Long-term anticoagulation with oral warfarin has been recommended to follow the initial intravenous use of heparin during the acute phase of BCS. Initiation or enhancement of bleeding is a potential complication of anticoagulant therapy, particularly in patients who develop cirrhosis and esophageal varices.

Control of ascites is feasible in some patients with BCS by use of the usual diuretic regimens, although ascites is resistant to therapy in many patients. Therapeutic measures include stringent sodium restriction, administration of diuretic drugs, and repeated intravenous infusion of salt-poor albumin or ascitic fluid. Renal function should be monitored closely during diuretic therapy to avoid precipitating the hepatorenal syndrome. There is no evidence that control of ascites influences the long-term outcome.

The prognosis of BCS with nonoperative therapy is poor (Mitchell et al, 1982; Parker, 1959; Powell-Jackson et al, 1982; Tavill et al, 1975). In his large collective review in 1959, Parker wrote, "The majority of cases have proved fatal and there is little evidence to suggest that recovery from occlusion of the major hepatic veins occurs once symptoms have been produced." Similarly, in 1975, Tavill and associates wrote, "The prognosis of the Budd-Chiari syndrome is almost uniformly bad...." In 1982, Mitchell and colleagues stated in their collective review, "Spontaneous resolution of hepatic vein occlusion rarely if ever occurs. Conventional medical therapy does little to reverse the pathophysiology in patients with hepatic vein occlusion." Many patients with BCS that is treated nonoperatively die within a few months of the onset of symptoms. Patients who survive the acute phase usually go on to develop cirrhosis of the liver and die within a few years from hepatic failure, bleeding esophageal varices, or other complications of chronic liver disease.

TREATMENT OF HEPATIC VEIN OCCLUSION BY SIDE-TO-SIDE PORTACAVAL SHUNT

Experimental Studies

The theoretical basis for the use of SSPCS to relieve BCS resulting from occlusion of the hepatic veins is provided by substantial evidence indicating that the valveless portal vein can be converted into an outflow tract by an in-continuity anastomosis with the systemic venous system, decompressing the obstructed hepatic vascular bed (Britton & Shirey, 1962; Britton et al, 1967; Burchell et al, 1976; Long et al, 1960; Longmire et al, 1958; Moreno et al, 1967; Mulder & Murray, 1960; Orloff & Snyder, 1961; Tamaki et al, 1968; Warren & Muller, 1959). To test this hypothesis, we conducted an experimental evaluation of SSPCS in dogs with BCS (Orloff & Johansen, 1978). Our method of producing BCS in dogs consisted of ligation and division of all hepatic veins except the large left hepatic vein, which was loosely surrounded by an ameroid constrictor (Fig. 100.6) (Orloff et al, 1963, 1965; Sweat et al, 1966). The lumen in the ameroid constrictor gradually narrowed as the hygroscopic casein plastic swelled centrally so that the remaining left hepatic vein was completely occluded within several weeks, and severe hepatic outflow block, portal hypertension, and massive, intractable ascites resulted. BCS was produced in 64 dogs, which were divided into three treatment groups when ascites was massive: Group I underwent sham laparotomy, group II underwent end-to-side PCS, and group III underwent SSPCS.

Table 100.8 summarizes the results of our experimental study. All dogs rapidly re-formed ascites after either sham laparotomy or end-to-side PCS and died with massive ascites within 6 months. In striking contrast, only 1 of the 24 dogs in group III reaccumulated ascites after SSPCS, and 67% of these dogs survived in good health without ascites until the time of sacrifice 1 year postoperatively. Before hepatic vein ligation, the liver was normal in all dogs on gross and microscopic examinations. At the time of sham laparotomy or shunt when BCS was well established, all livers were enlarged two to four times normal size and appeared

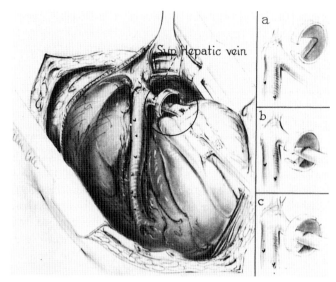

Fig. 100.6. Our technique of induction of BCS in dogs by ligation and division of all hepatic veins except the large left hepatic vein, which was surrounded by a hygroscopic, casein plastic ameroid constrictor that gradually swelled centrally and occluded the vein.
(From Orloff MJ, Johansen KH, 1978: Treatment of Budd-Chiari syndrome by side-to-side portacaval shunt: experimental and clinical results. Ann Surg 188: 494-512.)

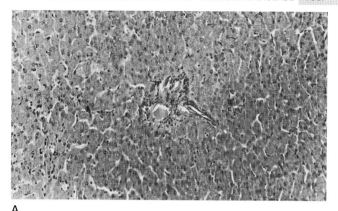

A

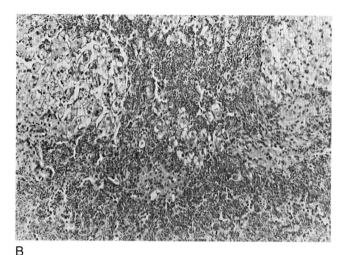

B

Fig. 100.7. Photomicrographs of liver biopsy specimens obtained from a dog. **A,** Before hepatic vein ligation when the liver was normal. **B,** Just before PCS, when BCS was well established and ascites was massive. There is intense congestion and necrosis of the hepatic parenchyma in the biopsy specimen (×140).
(From Orloff MJ, Johansen KH, 1978: Treatment of Budd-Chiari syndrome by side-to-side portacaval shunt: experimental and clinical results. Ann Surg 188:494-512.)

congested and friable. Liver biopsy specimens at this time showed intense centrilobular congestion, necrosis of cells around the central veins, dilated lymphatics, and subcapsular edema (Fig. 100.7). In the dogs in group I, these gross and microscopic abnormalities were unchanged at the time of death, and substantial fibrosis was found in many of the liver biopsy specimens. Similarly, all of the dogs in group II had hepatomegaly at the time of death, and severe congestion, necrosis, and fibrosis were found in all liver biopsy specimens, although in 38% of the animals the microscopic picture was less severe than at the time of the end-to-side shunt operation. Only one dog with SSPCS in group III, the single animal with ascites, had an enlarged liver and microscopic findings of congestion and necrosis at the time of death. The other 23 dogs in group III had a liver that was normal in size and gross appearance at autopsy; liver biopsy specimens were normal in 35% of these dogs and showed minimal fibrosis in the remaining 65%.

Clinical Results of the Authors

On the basis of the results of our experimental studies showing that SSPCS was effective in relieving BCS and reversing the liver

damage, we performed SSPCS in 34 patients with BCS caused by thrombosis of the hepatic veins without involvement of the IVC (Orloff & Girard, 1989; Orloff & Johansen, 1978; Orloff et al, 1992b, 2000). There were 18 women and 16 men, and ages ranged from 19 to 45 years. All 34 patients were younger than 45 years of age. Of patients, 11 had polycythemia rubra vera, 9 had been taking oral contraceptives, 5 had Behçet's disease, and

Table 100.8 Reaccumulation of Ascites and Mortality Rates in Dogs with Budd-Chiari Syndrome After Sham Laparotomy, End-to-Side Portacaval Shunt, and Side-to-Side Portacaval Shunt

| | | ASCITES AT OPERATION | | | REACCUMULATION OF ASCITES | | | MORTALITY RATE (%) | |
| | | | Volume (L) | | | Volume at Autopsy (L) | | | |
Group	No. Dogs	% of Group	Mean	Range	% of Group	Mean	Range	1 month	1 year*
I Sham laparotomy	20	100	3.2	2.2–5.3	100	3.4	1.4–7.2	25	100
II End-to-side shunt	20	100	3	2–5.7	100	3.8	1.6–6.8	25	100
III Side-to-side shunt	24	100	3.3	2.5–6.2	4	1.4	1.4	25	33

*Excludes 1-month deaths.

Table 100.9 Long-term Results of Portal Decompression Operations in 54 Patients with Budd-Chiari Syndrome Treated by the Authors

	HEPATIC VEIN OCCLUSION ALONE	IVC AND HEPATIC VEIN OCCLUSION	
	SSPCS	Mesoatrial Shunt	Combined SSPCS and CAS
No. patients	34	8	12
Onset to operation:			
≤17 wk (%)	91	88	100
Mean weeks	15	12	13.5
Range weeks	4–78	7–19	10–16
Follow-up (yr)			
Mean	14	17	10
Range	1–32	20–24	3–20
Ascites (%)	0	63	0
Need for diuretics (%)	0	63	0
Abnormal liver function tests (%)	9	63	0
Portosystemic encephalopathy (%)	0	38	0
Employed or housekeeping (%)	94	25	92
Survival (%)			
30-day	97	100	100
Current	94	38	100

CAS, cavoatrial shunt.

Table 100.10 Results of Follow-up Liver Biopsies Every 1–2 Years, Angiography, Ultrasonography, and Pressure Measurements in 53 Surviving Patients with Budd-Chiari Syndrome Who Underwent Surgical Portal Decompression by the Authors

	HEPATIC VEIN OCCLUSION ALONE	IVC AND HEPATIC VEIN OCCLUSION	
	SSPCS	Mesoatrial Shunt	Combined SSPCS and CAS
No. patients	33	8	12
Liver biopsy results (%)			
Congestion:			
Marked	0	63	0
Mild	3	12	0
None	97	25	100
Necrosis:			
Marked	0	63	0
Mild	3	12	0
None	97	25	100
Fibrosis:			
Marked	9	75	0
Moderate-mild	42	12	25
None	48	13	75
Cirrhosis	9	63	0
Angiography/ultrasound results (%)			
Patent shunt	97	37	100
Patent IVC	100	0	0
Occluded hepatic veins	100	100	100
Pressures (mm saline)			
PV:			
Mean	95	286	133
Range	54–150	174–374	114–150
IVC			
Mean	89	289	123
Range	41–124	240–342	106–142
PV–IVC gradient			
Mean	6	16	10
Range	0–41	−136 to 64	4–14
RA			
Mean	—	119	112
Range	—	88–118	92–130
PV–RA gradient			
Mean	—	186	21
Range	—	88–118	14–26

CAS, cavoatrial shunt; PV, portal vein; RA, right atrium.

1 had protein C deficiency. In the remaining eight patients, no condition predisposing to hepatic vein thrombosis was identified. Patients operated on before 1996 did not undergo the extensive hematologic workup that is shown in Table 100.3 and is being done currently. The symptoms, signs, results of diagnostic studies, and findings at operation are shown in Tables 100.4 to 100.7.

Tables 100.9 and 100.10 summarize the long-term results of SSPCS in our series. Patient No. 6 underwent emergency operation when the thrombosis of his hepatic veins suddenly extended into and occluded his previously patent IVC. An attempt to reverse a rapidly downhill course by thrombectomy of the IVC and PCS was unsuccessful, and the patient died 6 days postoperatively with multiorgan failure and recurrence of IVC thrombosis. The remaining 33 patients (97%) recovered from the shunt operation and were long-term survivors. A striking feature of the early recovery period was a rapid gain in lean body weight amounting to 28 lb in 3 months.

The 33 survivors of the shunt operation have been followed up for 1 to 32 years (mean follow-up 14 years). All but 2 of the survivors (94%) have been followed up for 5 years or more. There has been one long-term death, a patient with Behçet's disease (patient No. 7) who was relieved of BCS and ascites, but died of diffuse vasculitis causing hemorrhagic infarction of the colon 2 years postoperatively. The other 32 patients are currently alive, for an overall survival rate of 94%. All of the survivors have remained free of ascites without requiring diuretic therapy. Results of periodic liver function tests have been consistently normal except in the three patients who already had cirrhosis when they were referred to us. None of the patients has portosystemic encephalopathy, undoubtedly because they have good hepatic function. Hepatosplenomegaly has disappeared in all patients. Of the 33 survivors of SSPCS, 31 are gainfully employed or, in the case of several women, engaged in full-time housekeeping. Of the 32 current survivors, 31 (97%) are leading productive lives of good quality.

Patient No. 5 had recurrence of ascites 5 years after the shunt operation and was found to have developed marked narrowing of the IVC at the level of the previously occluded hepatic vein orifices. He was treated surgically with a bypass graft extending from below the area of obstruction in the IVC to the right atrium. Twenty-one years after the bypass operation, the patient is free of ascites, and angiographic studies show a patent bypass graft with normal pressures in the IVC and portal vein.

Liver biopsies and angiographic or ultrasound studies were performed periodically for 32 years after shunt in the 33 survivors, and the results are summarized in Table 100.10. Cirrhosis persisted in the three patients who already had cirrhosis by the time of the shunt operation, including the patient with Behçet's disease. In 97% of the survivors, as shown in Fig. 100.8, there was no longer any evidence of hepatic congestion or necrosis in the follow-up biopsy specimens. Mild to moderate fibrosis was found

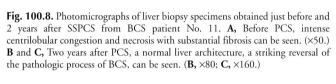

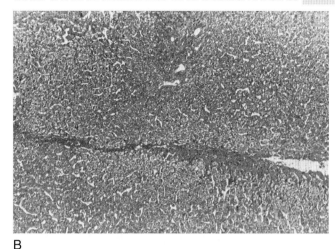

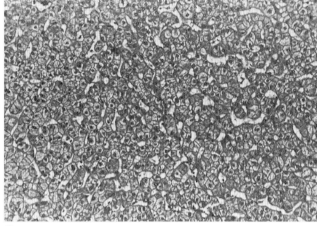

Fig. 100.8. Photomicrographs of liver biopsy specimens obtained just before and 2 years after SSPCS from BCS patient No. 11. **A,** Before PCS, intense centrilobular congestion and necrosis with substantial fibrosis can be seen. (×50.) **B** and **C,** Two years after PCS, a normal liver architecture, a striking reversal of the pathologic process of BCS, can be seen. (**B,** ×80; **C,** ×160.)

in 42% of the patients, but 48% had normal liver biopsy specimens. Angiography or ultrasound showed patency of the PCS and IVC, and pressure measurements showed a wide open anastomosis with a gradient that ranged from 0 to 41 mm saline and averaged only 6 mm across the shunt.

Two patients with polycythemia rubra vera developed thrombosis of the PCS 1 week and 3 months postoperatively. Both patients were operated on immediately, the shunt was taken down, fresh thrombus was removed from the portal vein, and the portacaval anastomosis was reconstructed with an H-graft of autologous internal jugular vein. Subsequently, both patients were maintained on anticoagulant therapy with warfarin. One patient has remained well for 23 years since revision of the shunt. The other patient developed recurrent shunt thrombosis and required liver transplantation. He is well 14 years post-transplantation. It is now our policy to maintain all patients with a known coagulopathy on permanent anticoagulant therapy.

Our series is the single largest clinical experience reported to date involving the use of SSPCS in BCS confined to the hepatic veins. Our clinical experience confirmed our experimental observations regarding the efficacy of SSPCS in relieving hepatic venous outflow obstruction. All 33 of our patients in whom thrombosis remained localized to the hepatic veins survived the operation and remained free of ascites for years without requiring diuretic therapy. The shunt remained permanently patent in all but one patient. All but three of the survivors were operated on early in

the course of the disease before liver damage was irreversible, and in these patients hepatosplenomegaly disappeared, and liver function returned rapidly to normal. The results of serial liver biopsies performed 1 to 32 years postoperatively are particularly encouraging because they showed that the shunt had brought about substantial and long-term reversal of the striking pathologic lesions of BCS (see Fig. 100.8). SSPCS seems to be the most effective treatment of BCS confined to the hepatic veins.

The single postoperative death in our series taught us a valuable lesson. When this 28-year-old man with polycythemia rubra vera was admitted to our hospital, there was clear clinical and angiographic evidence that the occlusive process was confined to the hepatic veins. During the 8-day course of his diagnostic workup, however, the thrombosis extended into the IVC, and his condition deteriorated dramatically. An emergency attempt at IVC thrombectomy and PCS failed. Extension of the thrombotic process from the hepatic veins into the IVC is a well-known event in BCS (Parker, 1959) and the potential for this devastating complication exists in every patient. When the diagnosis of hepatic vein occlusion has been made, it seems unwise to delay operation.

SSPCS is indicated only in patients with BCS who have a patent IVC and an IVC pressure that is substantially lower than WHVP or portal pressure. Obstruction or occlusion of the IVC, manifested clinically by edema of the lower extremities and lower trunk and shown by angiography and IVC pressure measurements, is a contraindication to PCS. It is not unusual for patients with BCS caused by hepatic vein occlusion to have an elevated pressure in the IVC as a result of caval compression by an enlarged, congested liver or massive ascites or both. The absolute level of IVC pressure is not crucial to the effectiveness of SSPCS as long as the portal pressure is substantially higher than caval pressure, and the IVC is shown to be patent. Others have reported relief of BCS by in-continuity mesocaval shunt in patients with high IVC pressure, but substantially higher portal pressure, showing that it is possible to decompress the liver as long as there is a substantial differential between pressures in the portal vein and IVC (Vons et al, 1986). In our long-term follow-up studies after SSPCS, we have observed that compression of the IVC disappears with relief of hepatic congestion, and caval pressure returns toward normal.

After SSPCS, the occlusive process in the hepatic veins extended into the adjacent IVC in only 1 of the 33 long-term survivors in our series. This untoward development occurred 5 years after the shunt operation and was treated successfully by a bypass graft from the IVC to the right atrium. It is possible that the infrequency of this complication is attributable to the PCS, which might inhibit propagation of the thrombus by increasing blood flow in the IVC and relieving stasis of blood in the liver.

The importance of performing SSPCS early in the course of BCS cannot be overemphasized. Hepatic venous outflow obstruction produces widespread destruction of the hepatic parenchyma by pressure necrosis and ischemia. The liver damage becomes irreversible in a surprisingly short time. Some patients have developed cirrhosis within 3 or 4 months of the onset of symptoms. Relieving ascites is far less important than decompressing the liver.

Although a few patients have recovered spontaneously from BCS, most have not. The literature is replete with descriptions of patients who would have been suitable candidates for PCS, but were treated nonoperatively and died. Our experience shows that it is imperative to perform SSPCS as soon as possible after the diagnosis of BCS has been made.

Clinical Results of Other Surgeons

Treatment of BCS caused by occlusion of the hepatic veins by direct SSPCS or its hemodynamic equivalents—the portacaval interposition graft, mesocaval interposition graft, or splenorenal shunt—has been reported in more than 300 patients by other surgeons (Ahn et al, 1987; Auvert & Farge, 1963; Bismuth & Sherlock, 1991; Cameron et al, 1983; Eisenmenger & Nickel, 1960; Erlik et al, 1962; Gentil-Kocher et al, 1988; Gibson, 1960; Hemming et al, 1996; Henderson et al, 1990; Hoyumpa et al, 1971; Huguet et al, 1979; Klein et al, 1990; Langer et al, 1975; Ludwick et al, 1965; Malt et al, 1978; McCarthy et al, 1985; Millikan et al, 1985; Murad et al, 2004; Noble, 1967; Panis et al, 1994; Pezzuoli et al, 1985; Powell-Jackson et al, 1982; Prandi et al, 1975; Schramek et al, 1974; Slakey et al, 2001; Vons et al, 1986; Wang, 1989; Wu et al, 1990; Zeitoun et al, 1999). Many of the reports have involved descriptions of single cases. Some more recent retrospective, multi-institutional studies involving reviews of medical records have been based on analyses, as a single entity, of patients with widely different characteristics, such as the stage and type of BCS, time lapse from diagnosis to treatment, site of hepatic venous outflow occlusion, and type of portosystemic shunt. Portacaval, mesocaval, splenorenal, mesoatrial, mesoinnominate,

cavoatrial, and portoatrial shunts and transjugular intrahepatic portosystemic shunt (TIPS) have been considered as a single entity termed *portosystemic shunt* (Murad et al, 2004; Zeitoun et al, 1999). It is not possible to compare the results of these studies with our results, which were based on patients with BCS caused by hepatic vein thrombosis alone, all of whom underwent a direct SSPCS early in the course of their disease.

Success rates of portal decompression in BCS at institutions that have reported series of cases have been approximately 85% after direct SSPCS (Ahn et al, 1987; Bismuth & Sherlock, 1991; Hemming et al, 1996; McCarthy et al, 1985; Panis et al, 1994; Pezzuoli et al, 1985) and 67% after splenorenal shunt (Ahn et al, 1987; McCarthy et al, 1985; Millikan et al, 1985; Wang, 1989). Mesocaval or portacaval interposition grafts with autologous internal jugular vein have been used in about 50 patients with BCS, most of them in France, with a success rate of 89% (Bismuth & Sherlock, 1991; Gentil-Kocher et al, 1988; McCarthy et al, 1985; Panis et al, 1994; Pezzuoli et al, 1985; Vons et al, 1986). Mesocaval or portacaval interposition grafts using synthetic materials, such as Dacron or polytetrafluoroethylene (Gore-Tex), have been successful in approximately 52% of 39 patients with BCS, which is the lowest success rate of the various in-continuity portal decompressive procedures (Ahn et al, 1987; Hemming et al, 1996; Henderson et al, 1990; Klein et al, 1990; McCarthy et al, 1985; Millikan et al, 1985; Pezzuoli et al, 1985; Wang, 1989). In our opinion, use of synthetic interposition portacaval or mesocaval grafts and the splenorenal shunt are inferior to direct SSPCS in the treatment of BCS, although all three shunts are hemodynamically similar. The splenorenal shunt and the synthetic interposition grafts have a substantial incidence of thrombosis, not only in BCS, but also in other diseases that cause portal hypertension (Dowling, 1979; Hemming et al, 1996; Orloff, 1977, 1992, 1998). Occlusion of the shunt is a serious complication that may result in death. In contrast, the incidence of shunt occlusion in our series of more than 2000 direct SSPCS, most of which have been followed up repeatedly by catheterization, angiography, or ultrasound, is 0.2%.

Four patients underwent end-to-side PCS for treatment of BCS. One patient had a favorable response during 1 year of follow-up (Marchal et al, 1974), and the other three died (Alpert, 1976; Brink & Botha, 1955; Langer et al, 1975). Because the hepatic side of the transected portal vein is ligated in performing an end-to-side PCS, the portal vein cannot function as an outflow tract to decompress the liver. It is well established that in the presence of hepatic outflow block, the side-to-side anastomosis is substantially more effective than the end-to-side shunt in overcoming intrahepatic hypertension (Reynolds et al, 1962; Taylor & Myers, 1956; Warren & Muller, 1959).

Authors' Technique of Side-to-Side Portacaval Shunt

We have performed more than 2000 SSPCS operations over 40 years. From this experience, we have concluded that it is possible, with the proper technique, to perform a satisfactory SSPCS in almost every patient who has a patent portal vein. Contrary to some statements in the literature, we have been able to perform SSPCS without difficulty in every patient with BCS on whom we have operated. We have performed shunt catheterization and angiography or ultrasound every 1 to 2 years in almost all of our patients since the 1970s, and we have observed a 99.8% long-term shunt patency rate.

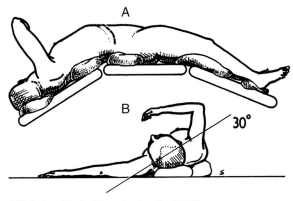

Fig. 100.9. A and **B,** Position of patient for SSPCS.

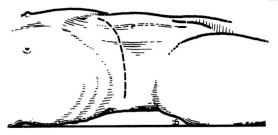

Fig. 100.10. Long right subcostal incision used for SSPCS.

Our technique of SSPCS (Orloff, 1983; Orloff & Orloff 1992, 1994) is illustrated in Figs. 100.9 to 100.18. Important technical features of the operation are as follows:

1. The position of the patient on the operating table is crucial and can make the difference between an easy and a difficult operation.
2. A long right subcostal incision is associated with fewer postoperative complications than a thoracoabdominal incision and is much preferred.
3. Use of the electrocautery throughout the operation substantially reduces the operating time and the blood loss.
4. Bleeding from the many portosystemic collateral vessels is best managed by pressure with gauze sponge packs, particularly because most of the bleeding stops as soon as the portacaval anastomosis is completed and the portal hypertension is relieved. Attempts to control each of the bleeding collaterals with ligatures and sutures prolong the operation and increase blood loss. The objective is to decompress the portal system as rapidly as possible.
5. Circumferential mobilization of the IVC between the entrance of the renal veins and the liver is essential for the side-to-side anastomosis and is neither hazardous nor difficult to perform. Apposition of the two vessels is greatly facilitated by elevation of the IVC toward the portal vein.
6. Mobilization of a long segment of portal vein, which includes division of the tough fibrofatty tissue that binds the portal vein to the pancreas and sometimes includes division of a bit of the head of the pancreas, is essential for the side-to-side anastomosis.
7. Resection of an enlarged caudate lobe of the liver to facilitate apposition of the two vessels is hazardous and unnecessary.
8. Pressures in the IVC and portal vein always should be measured after completion of the PCS. A pressure gradient of greater than 50 mm saline is unacceptable and requires revision of the anastomosis.

Fig. 100.9 shows the position of the patient on the operating table viewed from the patient's right side. The patient is positioned with the right side elevated at an angle of 30 degrees to the table, and the table is "broken" at the level of the costal margin and at the knees to widen the space between the right costal margin and right iliac crest.

Fig. 100.10 shows the incision. A long right subcostal incision extending from the xiphoid to well into the flank is made two fingerbreadths below the costal margin. We have used this

incision in every operation over the course of 40 years. The skin is incised superficially with the scalpel, and the other layers are incised with the electrocautery, which greatly reduces blood loss and shortens the operating time. When the electrocautery is used, it is usually unnecessary to clamp any blood vessels with hemostats. The right rectus abdominis, external oblique, and transversus abdominis muscles are completely divided, and the medial 3 to 4 cm of the latissimus dorsi muscle is often incised. The peritoneum often contains many collateral blood vessels and is incised with the electrocautery to obtain immediate hemostasis.

Fig. 100.11 shows the exposure of the operative field. The viscera are retracted by three Deaver retractors positioned at right angles to each other. The inferior retractor retracts the hepatic flexure of the colon toward the feet, the medial retractor displaces the duodenum medially, and the superior retractor retracts the liver and gallbladder toward the head. The posterior peritoneum overlying the IVC is incised with the electrocautery by an extended Kocher maneuver just lateral to the descending duodenum, and the retractors are repositioned to retract the head of the pancreas medially and the right kidney caudally. Alternatively, a self-retaining retractor may be used in place of the three hand-held Deaver retractors.

Fig. 100.12 shows the isolation of the IVC. The anterior surface of the IVC is cleared of fibroareolar tissue, and the IVC is isolated around its entire circumference from the entrance of the right and left renal veins below to the point where it

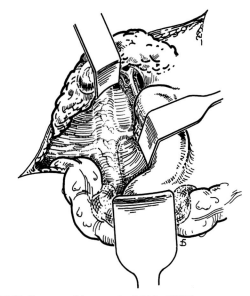

Fig. 100.11. Exposure of the operative field for SSPCS.

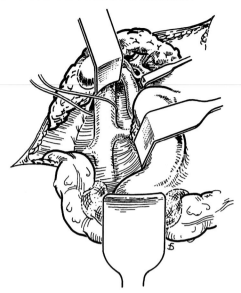

Fig. 100.12. Circumferential isolation of the IVC between renal veins and liver in preparation for side-to-side portacaval anastomosis.

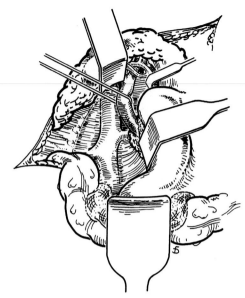

Fig. 100.14. Mobilization of a long length of portal vein, including the segment behind the pancreas, in preparation for side-to-side portacaval anastomosis.

disappears behind the liver above. The IVC is surrounded with an umbilical tape. To accomplish the isolation, several tributaries may have to be ligated in continuity with fine silk ligatures and then divided. These include the right adrenal vein, one or two pairs of lumbar veins that enter on the posterior surface, and the caudal pair of small hepatic veins that enter on the anterior surface of the IVC directly from the liver. When the IVC has been mobilized completely, it can be lifted up toward the portal vein. Failure to isolate the IVC circumferentially is one major reason for the erroneous claim that SSPCS often cannot be performed because the portal vein and IVC are too widely separated.

Fig. 100.13 shows the exposure of the portal vein. The superior retractor is repositioned medially so that it retracts the liver and gallbladder at the point of entrance of the portal triad. The portal vein is located in the posterolateral aspect of the portal triad and is approached from behind. The fibrofatty tissue

the posterolateral aspect of the portal triad, which contains nerves, lymphatics, and lymph nodes, is divided by blunt and sharp dissection. This is a safe maneuver because there are no portal venous tributaries on this aspect of the portal triad. As soon as the surface of the portal vein is exposed, a vein retractor is inserted to retract the common bile duct and hepatic artery medially. The portal vein is mobilized circumferentially at its midportion and is surrounded with an umbilical tape. It is isolated up to its bifurcation in the liver hilum. Several tributaries on the medial aspect are ligated in continuity with fine silk and divided.

Fig. 100.14 shows the mobilization of the portal vein behind the pancreas. Using the umbilical tape to pull the portal vein out of its bed, the portal vein is cleared to the point where it disappears behind the pancreas. The tough fibrofatty tissue that binds the portal vein to the pancreas must be divided. Several tributaries that enter the medial aspect of the portal vein and one tributary that enters the posterolateral aspect are divided. It is usually unnecessary to divide the splenic vein. Wide mobilization of the portal vein is essential for performance of a side-to-side portacaval anastomosis. Failure to mobilize the portal vein behind the pancreas is a second major reason for difficulty in accomplishing SSPCS. In some patients, it is necessary to divide a bit of the head of the pancreas to obtain adequate mobilization of the portal vein. Bleeding from the edges of the divided pancreas is controlled with suture ligatures. Division of a small amount of the pancreas is a helpful maneuver, and we have never observed postoperative complications, such as pancreatitis, from its performance.

Fig. 100.15 shows the measurement of pressures in the IVC and portal vein before performing the portacaval anastomosis. The performance of SSPCS is illustrated in Figs. 100.16 to 100.18. After it is determined that the IVC and portal vein can be brought together without excessive tension, a Satinsky clamp is placed obliquely across a 5-cm segment of the anteromedial wall of the IVC in a direction that is parallel to the course of the overlying portal vein, and the IVC is elevated toward the portal vein. A 5-cm segment of the portal vein is isolated between two angled vascular clamps, and the portal vein is depressed toward the IVC, bringing the two vessels into apposition (Fig. 100.16). A 2.5-cm long thin strip of the IVC and a 2.5-cm long strip of

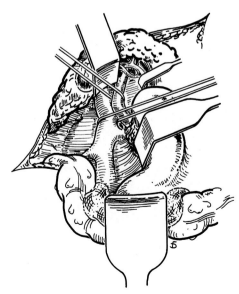

Fig. 100.13. Exposure of portal vein in preparation for side-to-side portacaval anastomosis.

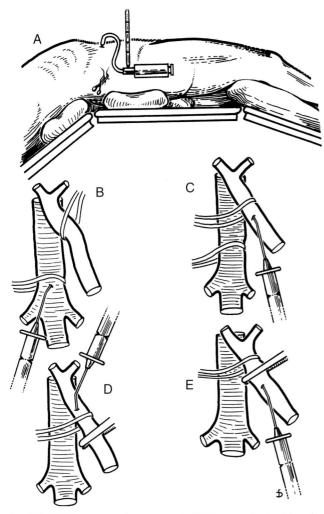

the portal vein are excised with the scissors (see Fig. 100.16B). It is important to excise a thin longitudinal segment of the wall of each vessel, rather than simply to make an incision in each vessel. A retraction suture of 5-0 vascular suture material is placed in the lateral wall of the vena caval opening and is weighted by attachment to a hemostat to keep the vena caval orifice open. The clamps on the portal vein are momentarily released to flush out any clots, then the openings in both vessels are irrigated with heparinized saline. The anastomosis is started with a posterior continuous over-and-over suture of 5-0 vascular suture material (see Fig. 100.16C). The posterior continuous suture is tied at each end of the anastomosis.

The anterior row of sutures consists of an everting continuous horizontal mattress stitch of 5-0 vascular material started at each end of the anastomosis (Fig. 100.17). The suture started at the superior end of the anastomosis is discontinued after three or four throws and is deliberately left loose so that the interior surface of the vessels can be visualized as the anastomosis is completed. In this way, inadvertent inclusion of the posterior wall in the anterior row of sutures is avoided. The suture started at the inferior end of the anastomosis is inserted with continuous tension until it meets the superior suture, at which point the superior suture is drawn tight, and the two sutures are tied to each other. Before drawing the superior suture tight, the clamps on the portal vein are momentarily released to flush out any clots, and the anastomosis is thoroughly irrigated with heparinized saline.

Fig. 100.18 shows the completed anastomosis. On completion of the anastomosis, a single interrupted tension suture is placed just beyond each end of the anastomosis to take tension off the anastomotic suture line. The clamp on the IVC is removed first, the clamp on the hepatic side of the portal vein is removed next, and finally the clamp on the intestinal side of the portal vein is removed. Bleeding from the anastomosis infrequently occurs; it can be controlled by one or two well-placed interrupted sutures of 5-0 vascular suture material.

Pressures in the portal vein and IVC must be measured after the anastomosis is completed. Usually the postshunt pressures in the portal vein and IVC are similar. A pressure gradient of greater than 50 mm saline between the two vessels indicates that there is an obstruction in the anastomosis, even when no obstruction can be palpated. In such circumstances, the anastomosis should be opened to remove any clots, and if necessary,

Fig. 100.15. Measurement of pressures in the IVC and portal vein with a saline (spinal) manometer by direct needle puncture before performance of portacaval anastomosis. All portal pressures are *corrected* by subtracting the IVC pressure from the portal pressure. Pressures in the IVC and portal vein are measured again after completion of the shunt. **A,** For all pressure measurements, the bottom of the manometer is positioned at the level of the IVC, which is marked on the skin surface of the body with a towel clip. **B,** IVC pressure (IVCP). **C,** Free portal pressure (FPP). **D,** Hepatic occluded portal pressure (HOPP), obtained on the hepatic side of a clamp occluding the portal vein. **E,** Splanchnic occluded portal pressure (SOPP), obtained on the intestinal side of a clamp occluding the portal vein.

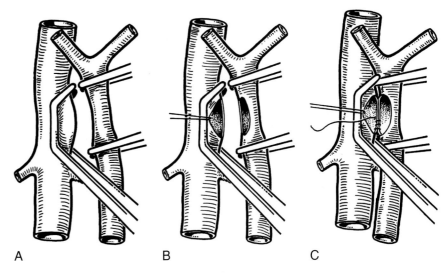

Fig. 100.16. Side-to-side portacaval anastomosis. **A,** Placement of clamps on IVC and portal vein. **B,** Strips of IVC and portal vein 2.5 cm in length have been excised. **C,** Placement of posterior row of continuous 5-0 vascular suture from inside lumina of IVC and portal vein.

A B C

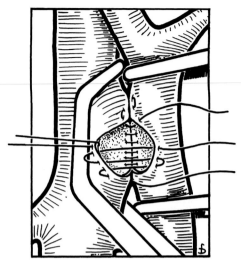

Fig. 100.17. Side-to-side portacaval anastomosis. Placement of anterior row of two continuous everting sutures of 5-0 vascular material.

the entire anastomosis should be taken down and done again. It is essential that there be no more than a 50-mm saline gradient between the portal vein and IVC to achieve permanently adequate portal decompression and to avoid ultimate thrombosis of the shunt.

TREATMENT OF INFERIOR VENA CAVA OCCLUSION BY PORTAL DECOMPRESSION

Mesoatrial Shunt

When BCS is caused by thrombosis of the IVC and of the hepatic veins, SSPCS and equivalent decompressive procedures are ineffective because the high pressure in the infrahepatic IVC does not permit adequate decompression of the portal system and liver. Under such circumstances, a mesoatrial shunt has been advocated. Synthetic Dacron or Gore-Tex grafts ranging from 14 to 20 mm in diameter have been used in most cases and have been connected

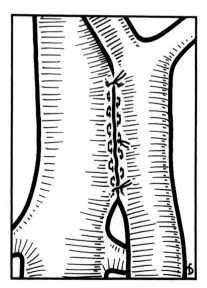

Fig. 100.18. Completed side-to-side portacaval anastomosis.

end-to-side to the superior mesenteric vein in the abdomen and the right atrium in the thorax.

We performed mesoatrial shunt in eight patients with BCS caused by thrombosis of the IVC and the hepatic veins. A 16-mm ring-reinforced Gore-Tex prosthesis was used. The operation was performed through a midline laparotomy and a median sternotomy. The superior mesenteric vein was isolated circumferentially for a distance of about 3 cm in the root of the small bowel mesentery. The pericardium was opened to expose the lateral wall of the right atrium. The graft was anastomosed to the side of the superior mesenteric vein with continuous 5-0 vascular suture, then tunneled through the root of the transverse mesocolon and greater omentum, then passed anterior to the stomach and left lobe of the liver into the mediastinum through an opening made in the anterior diaphragm. Finally, the prosthesis was anastomosed to the side of the right atrium with a continuous 5-0 vascular suture. To ensure wide open anastomoses, an ellipse of the wall of the superior mesenteric vein and of the right atrium was excised before connecting the prosthesis.

Our results of mesoatrial shunt are shown in Tables 100.7, 100.9, and 100.10. Mesoatrial shunt reduced the mean gradient between the portal vein and right atrium from 211 to 78 mm saline. All eight patients survived the operation and left the hospital alive. Five of the eight patients (63%) subsequently developed thrombosis of the graft, however, and died from liver failure. Three of the deaths occurred during the first postoperative year, one occurred in the second year, and one occurred in the fifth year. All five patients developed recurrence of ascites, and three developed portosystemic encephalopathy as their hepatic function deteriorated. The causes of BCS in the five patients whose mesoatrial shunt failed were oral contraceptives in one, polycythemia rubra vera in one, antithrombin III deficiency in one, postpartum state in one, and unknown in one. These causes were no different from those found in the long-term survivors of portal decompression in our series. The patients whose mesoatrial shunt failed were not a higher risk group. They died because their mesoatrial shunt thrombosed 1 to 5 years after insertion, not because they were poorer risk patients to start with.

The three long-term survivors of mesoatrial shunt (38%) have been followed up for 23 years, 21 years, and 21 years. Angiography or ultrasound has shown patency of their grafts. They are free of ascites, have normal liver function, and do not require diuretics. Two of the three are gainfully employed. Serial liver biopsy specimens show residual congestion in one patient and moderate fibrosis in two. In one patient, the liver appears normal.

Several series of mesoatrial shunt involving five or more patients have been reported in the literature. The length of follow-up generally has been relatively short. Stringer and colleagues (1989) of London reported excellent results in five patients, but the follow-up period of 9 to 16 months was too short to warrant conclusions. Wang (1989) of Beijing reported an 86% survival rate of 35 patients, with good results in 75% during a short follow-up period, but his report contained insufficient details to determine how many of the patients had patent and functioning grafts, how well the patients were followed, or the exact nature of the BCS that was being treated. Emre and coworkers (2000) of Istanbul reported an 85% survival rate of 13 patients during follow-up of 1 to 76 months, with one known thrombosed shunt. Behera and associates (2002) of Chandigarh, India, described 100% graft patency during 6 to 71 months of follow-up of 10 patients, with a survival rate of 90%. Khanna and colleagues (1991) of Chandigarh, India, reported a 62% survival rate of 13 patients during follow-up of 2 months to 7.5 years.

The results of Henderson and associates (1990) in 9 patients, of Klein and coworkers (Klein et al, 1990; Slakey et al, 2001) in 15 patients, and of our investigators in 8 patients are representative of the experience with mesoatrial shunt in the United States. Survival rates ranged from 38% to 67%, and the percentage of patients with grafts that were patent and decompressing was only 33% to 60% during relatively short follow-up periods. Cameron and coworkers (Cameron et al, 1984; Klein et al, 1990) reported improved results with the use of an 8-cm external silicone rubber sleeve around a 16-mm ring-reinforced Gore-Tex prosthesis to prevent compression of the graft by the sternum. This innovation may reduce the frequency of graft thrombosis, but the results of mesoatrial shunt generally have been disappointing.

The high thrombosis rate of the mesoatrial shunt may be due to the fact that it is a relatively low flow synthetic graft placed within the venous system. It does not decompress the obstructed IVC. To overcome these shortcomings, we worked in the experimental laboratory to devise a new operation for this form of BCS consisting of a combined SSPCS and cavoatrial shunt (CAS) through a Gore-Tex graft (Orloff et al, 1992a). This combined shunt was aimed at decompressing the hypertensive IVC and shunting the entire systemic venous flow from the lower two thirds of the body and the entire portal venous flow through the graft.

Experimental Studies

BCS was produced in rats by gradual occlusion of the suprahepatic IVC with an ameroid constrictor. As the hygroscopic casein plastic took up fluid and swelled centrally, the lumen in the ameroid gradually narrowed until, after 25 to 30 days, it completely occluded the IVC and produced severe hepatic outflow block, portal hypertension, and massive intractable ascites typical of BCS. One month after insertion of the ameroid constrictor around the IVC, when all rats had massive ascites, hepatomegaly, and portal hypertension, they were randomly divided into three groups (Fig. 100.19). Group I was composed of 16 control rats that underwent a sham thoracolaparotomy when BCS was well established. Group II consisted of 22 rats

that were subjected to a mesoatrial shunt from the superior mesenteric vein to the right atrium with a 3-mm Gore-Tex graft inserted by microsurgical technique. Group III contained 22 rats that underwent SSPCS combined with CAS from the IVC to the right atrium with a 3-mm Gore-Tex graft. Forty-four rats survived the operations and were studied.

Table 100.11 summarizes the results in the three groups of rats. All control rats that underwent sham thoracolaparotomy in group I rapidly reaccumulated ascites and died within 2 months. Nine of 16 rats with mesoatrial shunts in group II re-formed ascites and died within 2 months. All of these animals were found at autopsy to have thrombosis of the mesoatrial graft. In contrast, only 2 of 16 rats treated by combined SSPCS and CAS in group III developed CAS-graft thrombosis, re-formed ascites, and died. The remaining 14 rats in group III were found to have patent grafts and shunts when they were killed after 3 months. Liver biopsy specimens in all rats before IVC constriction were normal and, after BCS was well established, showed intense centrilobular congestion and moderate central necrosis. Severe pathologic changes persisted until death or sacrifice in all control rats in group I and in 11 of 16 rats with mesoatrial shunts in group II. Combined SSPCS and CAS in group III reversed the liver pathology in 14 of 16 rats, however.

Clinical Results of the Authors with Combined Side-to-Side Portacaval Shunt and Cavoatrial Shunt

On the basis of the encouraging results of our experimental studies, we have treated 12 seriously ill patients with BCS caused by IVC thrombosis with combined SSPCS and CAS using a 20-mm ring-reinforced Gore-Tex graft. The characteristics of the patients are summarized in Tables 100.6 and 100.7. There were eight men and four women; age range was 25 to 37 years. All 12 patients were in good health before the onset of symptoms and signs consisting of marked ascites, edema of the lower extremities, hepatosplenomegaly, abdominal pain, weakness, and muscle wasting. The combined operation is depicted in Fig. 100.20.

The procedure was performed through a long right subcostal incision for the PCS, and then a median sternotomy for the CAS.

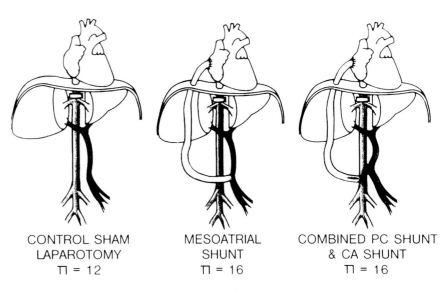

Fig. 100.19. Experimental groups of rats with BCS produced by constriction of the IVC by an ameroid constrictor. Control sham laparotomy, mesoatrial shunt, and combined SSPCS and caval-atrial shunt were compared.
(From Orloff MJ, et al, 1992: Treatment of Budd-Chiari syndrome due to inferior vena cava occlusion by combined portal and vena caval decompression. Am J Surg 163:137-143.)

CONTROL SHAM LAPAROTOMY Π = 12   MESOATRIAL SHUNT Π = 16   COMBINED PC SHUNT & CA SHUNT Π = 16

Table 100.11   Results of Treatment of Experimental Budd-Chiari Syndrome in Rats Produced by Inferior Vena Cava Occlusion

Group	No. Rats	Graft or Shunt Thrombosis	Re-formed Ascites	Survived 3 Months	Reversal of Liver Pathology
I Sham thoracolaparotomy	12	—	12	0	0
II Mesoatrial shunt	16	9	9	7	5
III Combined portacaval shunt and caval-atrial shunt	16	2	2	14	14

After completion of the SSPCS, a 20-mm diameter, ring-reinforced Gore-Tex graft was anastomosed to the side of the IVC at the level of the PCS. The graft was channeled anterior to the liver through an opening made in the right leaf of the diaphragm and was anastomosed to the side of the right atrium. Combined SSPCS and CAS reduced the mean gradient between the portal vein and right atrium from 196 mm saline to 23 mm saline. All 12 patients survived the combined shunt operation and are alive 3 to 20 years postoperatively (see Tables 100.9 and 100.10). Mean follow-up is 10 years. All patients are free of ascites, and none requires diuretics. Hepatomegaly and splenomegaly are gone. Liver function test results are normal in all survivors. There has been no instance of portosystemic encephalopathy. All survivors are gainfully employed or keeping house and leading productive lives of good quality. Serial percutaneous liver biopsy specimens have shown normal architecture in nine patients and mild fibrosis in three. Serial angiographic studies with pressure measurements and Doppler duplex ultrasound have shown patency and good function of SSPCS and CAS in all patients (Fig. 100.21). Recanalization of the IVC or hepatic veins has not occurred. Permanent anticoagulation with warfarin and low-dose acetylsalicylic acid has been maintained in all patients. In our program, combined SSPCS and CAS has replaced mesoatrial shunt as the preferred treatment for BCS caused by IVC obstruction.

OTHER TYPES OF SURGICAL AND RADIOLOGIC THERAPY

Orthotopic Liver Transplantation

Orthotopic liver transplantation (OLT) (see Ch. 103) is a radical, drastic treatment for BCS, but it is effective in circumstances when a patient's life is at stake and no other form of therapy would work. OLT is not in competition with SSPCS or any other type of treatment. It is useful in far advanced, decompensated liver disease when it is too late to accomplish survival with portal decompression procedures.

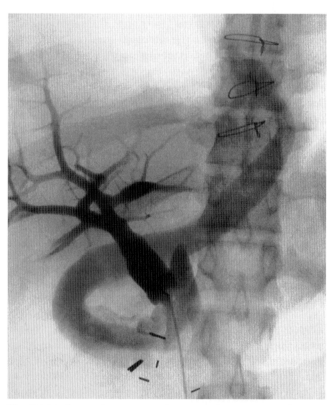

Fig. 100.21. Shunt catheterization and venogram showing patency of the PCS and CAS 1 year after performance of combined PCS and CAS in a patient with BCS secondary to IVC occlusion. Serial angiographic studies showed patency and excellent function of the PCS and CAS in all patients.
(From Orloff MJ, et al, 1992: Treatment of Budd-Chiari syndrome due to inferior vena cava occlusion by combined portal and vena caval decompression. Am J Surg 163:137-143.)

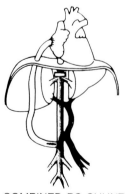

COMBINED PC SHUNT
& CA SHUNT
n = 16

Fig. 100.20. Combined SSPCS and CAS using a 20-mm ring-reinforced Gore-Tex graft. The operation was done in 12 patients with BCS secondary to IVC occlusion. CA, caval-atrial; PC, portacaval.
(From Orloff MJ, et al, 1992: Treatment of Budd-Chiari syndrome due to inferior vena cava occlusion by combined portal and vena caval decompression. Am J Surg 163:137-143.)

It is imperative that the indications for use of OLT in BCS be established and clearly understood. The indications that we adhere to are as follows:

1. Cirrhosis with progressive liver failure that has reached the point of permitting a reasonable prediction that the patient will die within 1 year. This is the most common indication for OLT and, incidentally, is the same one used widely in other liver diseases (Scharschmidt, 1984; Schenker, 1984).
2. Failure of a portosystemic shunt, usually because of thrombosis, with persistence or recurrence of symptoms and signs of BCS.
3. BCS with unshuntable portal hypertension secondary to thrombosis of the portal vein, splenic vein, and much of the superior mesenteric vein. This is a rare indication that applies if patent blood vessels are available to vascularize the liver allograft.
4. Acute fulminant hepatic failure. This is a rare indication and one that we have not encountered.

Using these indications, 12 of our patients have been approved and listed for OLT. Their characteristics are shown in Table 100.12. In 10 of the 12 patients, an underlying thrombogenic hematologic disorder was identified. The time lapse from clinical onset of BCS to OLT was much longer than in our patients who were treated by SSPCS, ranging from 11 to 21 months and averaging 15.9 months. These patients had a chronic form of BCS. The indication for OLT was cirrhosis with progressive liver failure in 11 patients whose severe hepatic decompensation precluded consideration of SSPCS and thrombosis of a PCS with recurrence of clinical manifestations of BCS in 1 patient. In 11 of our patients, thrombosis was confined to the hepatic veins, and in 1 patient the hepatic veins and suprahepatic IVC were occluded. All but one of our patients, the one with an occluded PCS, had a patent portal vein.

Table 100.13 shows the clinical findings in our 12 patients. All patients had massive ascites, jaundice, severe muscle wasting, hepatomegaly, splenomegaly, and dilated collateral veins on the abdominal wall. Encephalopathy had occurred in 50%, and one or

Table 100.13 Preoperative Clinical Findings in 12 Patients Who Were Approved and Listed for Liver Transplantation for Budd-Chiari Syndrome

Finding	%
Ascites (3.8–7.2 L)	100
Jaundice	100
Severe wasting	100
Encephalopathy	50
Bleeding varices	58
Hepatomegaly	100
Splenomegaly	100
Dilated abdominal veins	100
Cirrhosis on biopsy	100
Child class C	100

more episodes of bleeding varices had occurred in 58%. All patients had cirrhosis on preoperative liver biopsy and in the recipient liver removed at OLT. This was a group with advanced, decompensated liver disease. All of them were in Child class C (Child & Turcotte, 1964) determined by the quantitative scoring method of Campbell and colleagues (1973).

Table 100.14 shows the results of preoperative liver function tests. Serum bilirubin was substantially elevated, and serum albumin was markedly depressed in every patient. Prothrombin activity was invariably low, resulting in a mean international normalized ratio of 2.0. Aspartate aminotransferase and serum alkaline phosphatase were significantly elevated. Liver function test results were highly abnormal, and they reflected serious hepatic failure.

Table 100.15 shows the survival rate of the 12 patients who were approved and listed for OLT. Three patients died of liver failure while awaiting OLT during periods of 4 to 10 months. Two patients died during the immediate period after OLT, one from relentless graft rejection and one from sepsis with multisystem organ failure. A third patient died 9 months postoperatively of liver failure. No patients were lost after the first year. The 1- and 5-year survival rates were 50%. If the three patients who died before OLT could be accomplished are excluded, the actual 1-year and 5-year survival rates of the patients who underwent OLT are 75%. The 5-year survival rate is comparable to the reported survival rate of OLT in Child class C patients who do not have BCS.

Table 100.12 Characteristics of 12 Patients Who Were Approved and Listed for Liver Transplantation for Budd-Chiari Syndrome

Age in years	
Mean	31
Range	25–37
Gender: female/male	7/5
Predisposing condition	
Polycythemia rubra vera	6
Oral contraceptives	2
Protein C deficieny	1
Antithrombin III deficiency	1
Unknown	2
Onset of BCS to OLT in months	
Mean	15.9
Range	11–21
Indication for OLT	
Cirrhosis with liver failure	11
Failed portacaval shunt	1
Thrombosed hepatic veins	12
Patent IVC	11
Patent portal vein	11

Table 100.14 Preoperative Liver Function Tests in 12 Patients Who Were Approved and Listed for Liver Transplantation for Budd-Chiari Syndrome

Liver Function Test	Mean	Range
Serum total bilirubin (mg/dL)	6	5.1–6.8
Serum albumin (g/dL)	2.1	1.8–2.8
INR	2	1.7–2.3
Aspartate aminotransferase (IU)	150	122–185
Serum alkaline phosphatase (IU)	233	198–282

Table 100.15 Long-term Results of Liver Transplantation for Budd-Chiari Syndrome in 12 Patients Who Were Approved and Listed for Orthotopic Liver Transplantation

Survival	%
Operative mortality (n = 2/9)	22
One-year mortality (n = 6/12)	50
Five-year survival (n = 6/12)	50
Five-year survival of patients transplanted (n = 6/9)	67
Causes of 6 deaths	
Rejection (25 days) (n = 1)	
Sepsis (30 days) (n = 1)	
Liver failure (9 mo) (n = 1)	
Liver failure awaiting OLT (4–10 mo) (n = 3)	
Quality of Life in 6 Survivors of OLT	
Ascites (n = 2)	33
Need for diuretics (n = 2)	33
Normal liver function tests (n = 5)	83
Encephalopathy (n = 2)	33
Working full-time (n = 5)	83
Recurrent BCS	0
Receiving anticoagulants (n = 6)	100

The six long-term survivors of OLT have been followed up for more than 3 years and have had a life of good quality (see Table 100.15). They are working full-time. There has been no recurrence of BCS. All survivors were placed on anticoagulant therapy postoperatively, and are receiving lifelong maintenance warfarin and aspirin treatment.

Experience with Orthotopic Liver Transplantation in Budd-Chiari Syndrome Reported in the Literature

To date, 10 series of OLT for BCS have been reported in the English language literature (Table 100.16). The largest series is that of Ringe and colleagues (1995) in Hannover, Germany, which involved 43 patients. Other series of more than a few patients are those of the Pittsburgh group (Halff et al, 1990; Iwatsuki et al, 1991), which consisted of 32 patients, and the Cambridge group (Jamieson et al, 1991), which included 26 patients. All of the reports were based on retrospective reviews of medical records. There has been no prospective study of OLT in BCS.

As shown in Table 100.16, the indications for OLT varied greatly, and it cannot be said that OLT was done in patients who had 1 year or less to live because of cirrhosis with progressive liver failure. In the series of Ringe and colleagues (1995), Jamieson and associates (1991), and Melear and coworkers (2002), the indications were not clearly stated. In the reports of Knoop and colleagues (1994a, 1994b), three of the eight patients were in Child class B, obviously not in liver failure. The report of Halff and coworkers from Pittsburgh (1990) stated, "The decrease in synthetic function *was not as severe* as in many other causes of end-stage liver disease." Every series had a few patients who underwent OLT because of a failed portosystemic shunt.

Table 100.17 shows the survival statistics in the reported series. All of the studies suffer from the fact that follow-up of many of the patients was short, sometimes less than 1 year. There was a substantial variation in patient selection from one series to the next, particularly with regard to severity of liver disease, so that they cannot be compared with each other. The early mortality

Table 100.16 Indications for Liver Transplantation in 10 Series of Budd-Chiari Syndrome Reported in the Literature

Reference	Type of Study	n	Indications for OLT
Srinivasan et al, 2002	Retrospective	19	Failed shunt—5 Acute liver failure—6 Chronic liver failure—8
Melear et al, 2002	Retrospective	17	Not stated
Hemming et al, 1996	Retrospective	10	Failed shunt—3 Advanced cirrhosis—4 IVC obstruction—2
Ringe et al, 1995	Retrospective	43	Unclear—39 Failed shunt—4
Knoop et al, 1994a, 1994b	Retrospective	8	Child class C—5 Child class B—3
Galati et al, 1993	Retrospective	32	Failed shunt—2 Cirrhosis—? Hepatic necrosis—?
Shaked et al, 1992	Retrospective	14	Failed shunt—2 Advanced cirrhosis—4 Poor synthetic function—8
Halff et al, 1990; Iwatsuki et al, 1991	Retrospective	32	Failed shunt—5 Intractable ascites—17 Recurrent variceal bleeding—14 Encephalopathy—15
Sakai & Wall, 1994	Retrospective	11	Chronic BCS—5 Acute fulminant BCS—3 Failed shunt—3
Jamieson et al, 1991	Retrospective	26	Failed shunt—2 Unclear—24

Table 100.17 Survival After Liver Transplantation for Budd-Chiari Syndrome Reported in the Literature

Reference	n	Follow-Up (mo)	Early Mortality (%)	>1-Year Survival (%)
Srinivasan et al, 2002	19	1–119	5	1-119 mo (84)
Melear et al, 2002	17	1–158	6	1-158 mo (88)
Hemming et al, 1996	10	?	10	5 yr (69)
Ringe et al, 1995	43	2–137	30	5 yr (68)
Knoop et al, 1994a, 1994b	8	4–59	13	?
Galati et al, 1993	9	2–60	0	2-60 mo (100)
Shaked et al, 1992	14	2–60	14	3 yr (76)
Halff et al, 1990; Iwatsuki et al, 1991	32	12–132	25	5 yr (60)
Sakai & Wall, 1994	11	12–72	36	1-6 yr (64)
Jamieson et al, 1991	26	12–60	31	5 yr (50)

rate in series that had more than 10 patients ranged from 5% to 36%. The 5-year survival rate, when it was reported, ranged from 50% to 69%.

Most of the series did not report the results of pathologic examination of the liver removed from the patient with BCS. The reports of Ringe and colleagues (1995) on 43 patients, Halff and colleagues (1990) on 32 patients, Sakai and Wall (1991, 1994) on 11 patients, and Srinivasan and associates (2002) on 19 patients, described the findings in the host liver, however, and confirmed the impression that many patients underwent OLT without having decompensated liver disease. Only 17 of the 43 patients of Ringe and colleagues (1995) had cirrhosis; the others had congestion alone (14 patients) and fibrosis alone, lesions that are found in the early stages of BCS. Similarly, in the report of Halff and colleagues (1990), none of the 32 patients had cirrhosis, and Sakai and Wall (1994) reported that 3 of 11 patients had central congestion and necrosis, but no fibrosis or cirrhosis.

An important concern about OLT in BCS is recurrence of BCS in the transplanted liver (Bahr et al, 2003). Table 100.18 shows the incidence of recurrent BCS in the liver allograft. Some investigators reported no recurrence of BCS, whereas others, such as Knoop and coworkers (1994a, 1994b), Halff and colleagues (1990), and Jamieson and associates (1991), reported substantial recurrence rates of 8% to 17%, despite treatment with anticoagulants.

Most series have shown a substantial incidence of post-transplant thrombosis in other splanchnic blood vessels, particularly in the portal vein (range 9-23%), often with disastrous consequences. The frequent development of thrombosis makes it mandatory that patients receive early and lifelong anticoagulation therapy after OLT. At the same time, it should be recognized that anticoagulation sometimes fails to prevent thrombosis.

One of the potential benefits of OLT in certain thrombogenic disorders, such as antithrombin III deficiency and protein C deficiency, is correction of the underlying defect by transplantation of a liver from a normal donor. It has been suggested that OLT is preferable to SSPCS in the treatment of BCS because, if SSPCS fails, the risk of performing subsequent OLT is increased. It has been proposed that mesocaval shunt is preferable to SSPCS because it is advantageous to avoid dissection of the hepatic hilum should subsequent OLT be required (Bismuth & Sherlock, 1991; McMaster, 1994; Slakey et al, 2001). In our experience, patients with BCS treated by SSPCS infrequently require OLT. Of 45 patients with BCS whom we treated by SSPCS, only 1 (4%) subsequently required OLT during long-term follow-up. In our experience with more than 2000 PCS in patients with cirrhosis, the long-term shunt patency rate has been 99.8%.

Additionally, at least eight, more recent studies have shown that previous portosystemic shunt, regardless of type, had no influence

Table 100.18 Rate of Recurrence of Budd-Chiari Syndrome and of Other Thrombosis After Liver Transplantation for Budd-Chiari Syndrome Reported in the Literature

Reference	N	RECURRENT BCS		OTHER THROMBOSIS	
		n	%	n	%
Srinivasan et al, 2002	19	1	5	2	11
Melear et al, 2002	17	0	0	3	18
Ringe et al, 1995	43	0	0	10	23
Hemming et al, 1996	10	0	0	1	10
Knoop et al, 1994a, 1994b	8	1	13	1	13
Shaked et al, 1992	14	0	0	0	0
Halff et al, 1990	23	3/18	17	4	22
Sakai & Wall, 1994	11	0	0	1	9
Jamieson et al, 1991	26	2	8	5	19

on the outcome of OLT (Aboujaoude et al, 1991; Bismuth et al, 1990; Boillot et al, 1991; Iwatsuki et al, 1988; Langnas et al, 1992; Mazzaferro et al, 1990; Minegaux et al, 1994; Turrion et al, 1991). Aboujaoude and colleagues (1991) emphasized that thrombosis of a portosystemic shunt may seriously compromise performance of OLT, so long-term shunt patency should be the main factor that determines the type of shunt selected for the potential OLT candidate, a point that is all the more true in patients with BCS. Direct PCS has had a thrombosis rate of 0.2% or less in all of our studies compared with occlusion rates of 24% to 53% for mesocaval interposition shunts using synthetic grafts reported in the literature (Fletcher et al, 1981; Hemming et al, 1996; Smith et al, 1980; Terpstra et al, 1987). Mesocaval interposition shunts using autologous internal jugular vein grafts, which have been used widely in France, have shown patency rates comparable to direct SSPCS (Bismuth & Sherlock, 1991; Gentil-Kocher et al, 1988; Vons et al, 1986).

A second important indication for OLT is failure of a portosystemic shunt, usually because of thrombosis, with persistence or recurrence of clinical manifestations of BCS. In experienced hands and with the routine, long-term use of anticoagulation therapy after portosystemic shunt, this should be a rare indication, but the literature indicates that such is not the case.

The third and fourth indications for OLT in BCS are rare, and we have not encountered such cases, although they have been reported without many details in the literature. These are unshuntable portal hypertension resulting from thrombosis of the portal venous system, provided that there are patent blood vessels available to vascularize the liver allograft, and acute fulminant hepatic failure (Sakai & Wall, 1994).

SSPCS and OLT are not competing forms of treatment. SSPCS is the appropriate treatment in the early and middle stages of BCS when portal decompression would sustain life by reversing or stabilizing the liver disease. OLT is the appropriate treatment in the late stages of BCS when the liver disease is no longer reversible, and when stabilization of progressive hepatic decompensation is impossible. Patients who are candidates for OLT should be in Child class C.

Surgical Removal of Venous Obstruction

Senning (1981, 1983) reported a direct method of removing obstruction of the IVC and hepatic veins in patients with chronic BCS. The operation is performed with cardiopulmonary bypass and involves opening the suprahepatic IVC and right atrium, removing any vena caval thrombus, resecting the dorsocranial part of the liver containing the confluence of the occluded major hepatic veins, and reconstructing the hepatic outflow tract by suturing the right atrium to the liver capsule. Since his initial description, Senning (1987) and others (Pasic et al, 1993) have reported the results of the operation in 17 patients, 2 of whom (12%) died within 2 weeks of operation and 4 of whom died later. Actuarial 1-year and 3-year survival rates were 76% and 57%. Two patients required liver transplantation. Three patients developed recurrent thrombosis. During follow-up of 7 months to 11 years, 10 of the 15 early survivors (67%) had prolonged relief of BCS.

Kawashima and coworkers (1991) reported success of the Senning operation in five of seven patients during follow-up of 2 months to 5 years, and Nakao and colleagues (1988) described success in two patients followed up for 1 to 2 months. In a

modification of the operation, Koja and associates (Koja et al, 1996; Kuniyoshi et al, 1998) described direct removal of the IVC obstruction under partial cardiopulmonary bypass in 32 patients with chronic BCS resulting from IVC obstruction of 1 to 42 years' duration. Koja and associates (Koja et al, 1996; Kuniyoshi et al, 1998) reopened the IVC and occluded hepatic veins under direct vision without resecting the liver and reconstructed the hepatic outflow tract with a patch graft of autologous pericardium. Many of the patients had cirrhosis or severe fibrosis of the liver, and 29 of the 32 had esophageal varices. There were no operative deaths. During 1.5 to 17 years of follow-up, there were four late deaths, and seven patients developed hepatocellular carcinoma. Five-year and 10-year survival rates were 93.6% and 81%. Two patients developed recurrent occlusion of the IVC. The results of Koja and associates (Koja et al, 1996; Kuniyoshi et al, 1998) in chronic BCS secondary to IVC occlusion are impressive. To determine the efficacy of direct surgical removal of hepatic venous outflow obstruction in patients with chronic BCS, however, prolonged and detailed follow-up of a sizable number of patients is required.

Percutaneous Transluminal Angioplasty

Use of percutaneous transluminal angioplasty has been reported in more than 200 patients with BCS (Anonymous, 1982; Baijal et al, 1996; Furui et al, 1990; Griffith et al, 1996; Jeans et al, 1983; Martin et al, 1990; Sato et al, 1990; Tyagi et al, 1996; Wu et al, 2002; Xu et al, 1996; Yamada et al, 1983, 1991; Yang et al, 1996). Most of the patients had chronic liver disease of long duration, and most of them had obstruction of the IVC of the membranous or segmental types. The obstructed vein was dilated with one or more balloon catheters. In all cases, the pressure gradient that existed before balloon dilation was substantially reduced or eliminated at the time of dilation. Stenosis often recurred, however, and required repeated balloon dilations. Most of the cases have not had long-term follow-up, so it is difficult to evaluate the ultimate effectiveness of percutaneous transluminal angioplasty. Of the few patients who have been observed for several years, the long-term success rate is less than 50% (Griffith et al, 1996; Martin et al, 1990; Sato et al, 1990; Yamada et al, 1991), although Wu and associates (2002) reported restenosis in only 1 of 41 patients during follow-up of 32 ± 12 months.

The use of expandable metallic stents has been added to balloon angioplasty in an attempt to maintain prolonged patency of the IVC (Baijal et al, 1996; Furui et al, 1990; Sawada et al, 1991; Xu et al, 1996; Zhang et al, 1991, 1999). The follow-up period of the few patients who have IVC stents is too short to evaluate the efficacy of this procedure.

In our opinion, based on the available evidence, percutaneous transluminal angioplasty and placement of expandable metallic stents warrant consideration only in patients with chronic BCS resulting from stenosis of the IVC. Patients treated by transluminal angioplasty should have careful follow-up that includes venography and pressure measurements every few months to detect recurrent stenosis of the IVC.

Transjugular Intrahepatic Portosystemic Shunt

TIPS (see Ch. 96) is SSPCS inserted percutaneously under radiographic control. As such, it is based on the same rationale for relieving hepatic venous outflow obstruction and intrahepatic portal hypertension as the surgical SSPCS. The attractiveness of TIPS lies in its accomplishment without requiring a major surgical abdominal operation in patients who have liver disease and are often quite ill. Its major disadvantage is a high incidence of occlusion of the TIPS that requires repeated revisions and hospitalizations and often involves recurrence of symptoms. An additional disadvantage in some patients who have complete occlusion of the hepatic veins or complete occlusion of the IVC is technical inability to insert the TIPS. Insertion of the TIPS by direct puncture of the retrohepatic IVC, which sometimes is the only way that the shunt can be created, is associated with a substantial incidence of complications (Rössle et al, 2004).

Since the 1990s, there have been many reports of TIPS treatment of BCS, each involving a few patients (Blum et al, 1995; Cejna et al, 2002; Ganger et al, 1999; Huber et al, 1997; Mancuso et al, 2003; Michl et al, 1999; Perello et al, 2002; Rogopoulos et al, 1995; Rössle et al, 1998; Uhl et al, 1996). The largest and longest reported experience with TIPS in BCS is that of Rössle and coworkers (2004) at the University Hospital of Freiburg, Germany, who described their experience with 35 patients— 11 acute, 13 subacute, and 11 chronic—who were followed up for a mean 37 ± 29 months. Failure occurred in seven patients (20%), two of whom were technical failures, two of whom required OLT with one death, and three of whom died after TIPS. Excluding the two patients who required OLT, but including the two patients who could not have TIPS for technical reasons, the 5-year survival rate was 74%. TIPS occlusion requiring revision occurred in 19 of 33 patients (58%). One patient required 10 revisions during a follow-up period of 53 months.

Results reported by others have not been as good as those of the Freiburg group. Mancuso and associates (2003) described a series of 15 patients with 5 deaths and 1 technical failure, for a 40% negative outcome. Cejna and colleagues (2002) reported a series of eight patients; two (25%) died 2 weeks after TIPS, one developed TIPS occlusion requiring OLT, and three others required two to seven revisions for TIPS stenosis. Only two of the initial series of eight patients (25%) had revision-free TIPS patency. Perello and coworkers (2002) reported a series of 13 patients in which there were 3 failures (23%). The failures included one death, one TIPS thrombosis that necessitated a surgical shunt, and one patient who required OLT. Of the remaining 10 patients, 7 developed TIPS occlusion (70%). In five of these, TIPS dysfunction had not been corrected.

The survival rate of surgical portosystemic shunt in our series is shown in Table 100.9. In patients with acute and subacute BCS resulting from occlusion of the hepatic veins, operative mortality rate after SSPCS has been 3%, and 5-year survival rate has been 94%. In patients with BCS secondary to IVC occlusion treated by combined SSPCS and CAS, 5-year survival rate has been 100%. All of the patients have been relieved of the symptoms of BCS, and readmission to the hospital has been infrequently necessary. These results are superior to the best reported results of TIPS in comparable patients. Without doubt, the long-term health care costs of TIPS are substantially higher than the costs of surgical therapy.

Thoracic Transposition of the Spleen

Transposition of the spleen into the left pleural cavity to create collateral venous connections between the portal and pulmonary systems has been used sporadically in the treatment of portal hypertension and, in addition, has been advocated for treatment of BCS secondary to occlusion of the IVC (Akita & Sakoda, 1980; Khuroo & Datta, 1980; Schrieber & Gonzalez, 1967; Strauch, 1970). The procedure involves displacing the spleen into an opening in the left diaphragm and suturing the left lower lobe of the lung to the spleen after removing the splenic capsule and abrading the surface of the lung. It is impossible to evaluate the effectiveness of this procedure because of the paucity of information in the few case reports. Akita and Sakoda (1980) of Japan reported the use of "splenopneumopexy" in 15 patients who had diseases that they called BCS. Although few details were given, it seems that most or all of the Japanese patients had a chronic disorder that consisted of cirrhosis and esophageal varices in addition to IVC obstruction. It is possible that many of the patients had the typical MOVC that accounts for most of the cases of BCS in Japan. Portal hypertension, determined by splenic pulp pressure measurements, persisted after splenopneumopexy in all patients. It is doubtful that thoracic transposition of the spleen can decompress the liver and portal system sufficiently to prevent or reverse liver damage in the crucial early stages of BCS caused by occlusion of the IVC.

Peritoneovenous Shunt

Peritoneovenous shunt is a device that relieves ascites by transferring fluid through a one-way valve from the peritoneal cavity into the superior vena cava. It has been advocated as primary treatment for BCS by LeVeen and coworkers (LeVeen 1978, 1983; LeVeen et al, 1976). The peritoneovenous shunt may be useful as a palliative measure in patients in whom portal decompression is not feasible or has been tried and failed. The peritoneovenous shunt is not indicated as the primary treatment of most patients with BCS, however, because it does not decompress the obstructed hepatic vascular bed, and it has no effect on the ongoing liver damage. Use of this device early in the course of BCS may squander the opportunity to reverse the liver damage by therapy that effectively decompresses the liver. Long-term studies of peritoneovenous shunt in patients with BCS have not been reported, probably because most patients in whom this device has been used have died from their underlying disease. There is predictable evidence, however, that the liver disease progresses to cirrhosis in the face of a functioning peritoneovenous shunt (Cameron et al, 1983).

SURGICAL TREATMENT OF MEMBRANOUS OBSTRUCTION OF THE VENA CAVA

Patients with MOVC described in the literature by and large have had a chronic disorder that has progressed to cirrhosis and portal hypertension by the time that they have received medical attention. The lesion causing IVC obstruction has varied from a thin membrane located in the suprahepatic IVC to an extensive area of stenosis involving the retrohepatic IVC. The Japanese surgeons have reported the largest experience with the treatment of MOVC.

When the area of IVC obstruction is short and is located at or above the level of the hepatic vein orifices, there are two treatment options—percutaneous transluminal angioplasty and transcardiac membranotomy. Reported experience with percutaneous

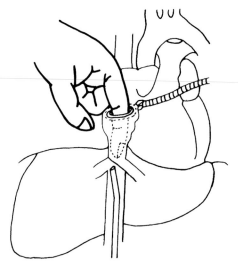

Fig. 100.22. Technique of transcardiac membranotomy. (From Iwahashi K, 1981: Surgical correction of the inferior vena cava obstruction with Budd-Chiari syndrome. Arch Jpn Chir 50:559-570.)

transluminal angioplasty in MOVC has been small, and the recurrence rate of IVC stenosis or thrombosis has been high (Eguchi, 1974; Griffith et al, 1996; Hirooka & Kimura, 1970; Iwahashi, 1981; Sato et al, 1990; Sharma et al, 1992; Tyagi et al, 1996; Yamada et al, 1991; Yang et al, 1996). Long-term IVC patency has been less than 50%.

Transcardiac membranotomy has been the most frequently used treatment of MOVC when the membrane is thin. The technique involves fracture of the membrane by the finger or a dilator inserted through the right atrial appendage (Fig. 100.22). More than 125 cases have been described in the literature, with a successful outcome in 70% to 90% during periods of follow-up that ranged from 2 months to 7 years, but generally were brief (Espana et al, 1980; Hirooka & Kimura, 1970; Iwahashi, 1981; Kimura et al, 1972; Okamoto et al, 1983; Semson, 1982; Suchato et al, 1976; Takeuchi et al, 1971; Taneja et al, 1979; Wang, 1989; Wu et al, 1990; Yamamoto et al, 1968).

When more than a thin membrane causes obstruction of the IVC, and particularly when a long area of stenosis involves the retrohepatic IVC, the treatment options are different and consist mainly of direct excision and repair of the involved area of IVC (endovenotomy) or cavoatrial bypass graft. A direct attack on the lesion generally has involved excising the obstructing tissue in the lumen of the IVC and repairing the vein with a synthetic or pericardial patch graft. Twelve such attempts have been described in the literature, with success in five patients and failure in seven, four of whom died (Hirooka & Kimura, 1970; Iwahashi, 1981; Kimura et al, 1972). Koja and colleagues (Koja et al, 1996; Kunioshi et al, 1998) reported direct removal of the IVC obstruction under partial cardiopulmonary bypass in 32 patients with impressive results. The reported periods of follow-up were short.

Use of a cavoatrial bypass graft has been reported in 11 patients who had a long segment of IVC stenosis. The procedure succeeded during short periods of follow-up in three patients and failed in eight, four of whom died (Eguchi et al, 1974; Hirooka & Kimura, 1970; Ohara et al, 1963; Reichart et al, 1981; Yamamoto et al, 1968). When the IVC obstruction involves or extends below the orifices of the hepatic veins, cavoatrial bypass does not decompress

the liver. Under such circumstances, consideration should be given to adding SSPCS to the cavoatrial bypass. The combined procedure of IVC and portal decompression has not been reported in MOVC.

Finally, patients with MOVC have undergone a variety of operations designed to create portosystemic or portopulmonary collateral venous connections. Included among these are omentosternopexy, hepatopneumopexy, splenopneumopexy, omentonephropexy, ileal stripping, and the Talma operation (Hirooka & Kimura, 1970; Ono et al, 1983; Yamamoto et al, 1968). It is difficult to evaluate the efficacy of these procedures because insufficient information has been presented in the case reports. We doubt that these procedures are capable of relieving the high pressures in the IVC and portal venous system or of influencing the course of MOVC.

TREATMENT OF VENO-OCCLUSIVE DISEASE

Substantial experience has been reported with treatment of patients with VOD caused by pyrrolizidine alkaloids (Bras & McLean, 1963; Ghanem & Hershko, 1981; Gore et al, 1961; Stuart & Bras, 1957). If such patients are seen during the acute stage of VOD, the initial treatment consists of withdrawal of the causative agent and measures to support the damaged liver. About one fourth of patients recover from the acute phase with supportive medical therapy, approximately one fifth die of liver failure or bleeding esophageal varices, and the remainder develop a chronic condition that waxes and wanes as cirrhosis of the liver evolves. SSPCS is indicated during the acute phase in patients who bleed from esophageal varices and in patients who, within 4 to 8 weeks of onset, show no signs of recovering, such as disappearance of ascites, improvement in liver function, and improvement in the lesions seen on percutaneous needle biopsy of the liver. Serial liver biopsy specimens are helpful in assessing the course of the disease.

Patients who are seen during the chronic phase of VOD have the usual manifestations of cirrhosis. The mortality rate of these patients is high, and the major cause of death is bleeding esophageal varices. Gore and colleagues (1961), who accumulated an extensive experience with VOD in Jamaica, recommended PCS when varices develop in the chronic phase, even if no bleeding has occurred. The added advantage of PCS is that it decompresses the obstructed hepatic vascular bed, which might facilitate regeneration of the liver. No sizable series of patients with VOD who were treated by PCS has been reported.

Several therapeutic approaches have been tried in the numerous patients with VOD related to bone marrow transplantation, but none has been uniformly effective. Treatments aimed at promoting fibrinolysis, particularly tissue-type plasminogen activator, have been tried based on the histologic finding of microthrombosis and fibrin deposition, but have been associated with an unacceptable rate of severe bleeding (Kumar et al, 2003; Wadleigh et al, 2003).

The most promising agent undergoing trial in the treatment of severe VOD is defibrotide, a polydeoxyribonucleotide with adenosine receptor activity that has been shown to modulate endothelial cell injury and protect sinusoidal endothelium. Defibrotide increases prostaglandin E_2, prostaglandin I_2, and thrombomodulin on the endothelial surface; decreases levels of plasminogen activator inhibitor 1; and increases endogenous tissue-type plasminogen activator levels. It is not associated with any risk of bleeding. A multi-institutional study of defibrotide in 88 bone marrow recipients with severe VOD resulted in a complete response rate of 36% and a 100-day survival rate of 35% (Kumar et al, 2003; Richardson et al, 2002; Wadleigh et al, 2003). Treatments described in anecdotal reports and small series that are not of established value include antithrombin III, activated protein C, prostaglandin E_1, N-acetyl cysteine, high-dose corticosteroids, glutamine, and vitamin E.

Side-to-side PCS has been used effectively in severe VOD after bone marrow transplantation, but the experience has been small because of a general reluctance to subject these very ill patients to a major operation despite their almost certain death without effective nonoperative treatment (Murray et al, 1987). Experience is similarly small with the use of TIPS in severe VOD secondary to bone marrow transplantation, and its role remains to be defined (Alvarez et al, 2000; Azoulay et al, 2000; de la Rubia et al, 1996; Fried et al, 1996; Smith et al, 1996). It seems that hematologists have considered TIPS more attractive than surgical shunts because it does not involve a major surgical operation. In one report of TIPS in treatment of progressive jaundice and ascites, five of six patients died in 9 to 44 days (Fried et al, 1996).

Because of the high mortality rate of severe VOD after bone marrow transplantation, OLT warrants consideration. Experience with OLT in severe VOD is small (Bunin et al, 1996; Hagglund et al, 1996; Nimer et al, 1990; Rapoport et al, 1991; Salat et al, 1997b; Schlitt et al, 1995). There have been some long-term survivors. The problems associated with use of OLT, not unique to VOD, include predicting which patients will not survive despite other forms of treatment, the timing of the OLT operation before multiorgan failure is so severe that survival is not possible, and obtaining a suitable liver graft.

One fourth of patients with VOD develop the severe form of the disease. The causes of death in severe VOD are hepatic failure, renal failure secondary to hepatorenal syndrome, respiratory failure owing to pulmonary VOD or infection, gastrointestinal bleeding, sepsis, and congestive heart failure. In the Seattle study of a cohort of 355 patients, the mortality rate of severe VOD was 98% (McDonald et al, 1993).

SUMMARY

More than 6000 cases of BCS caused by occlusion of the major hepatic veins or the IVC or both have been reported, and the condition is being recognized with increasing frequency. Although in many cases of BCS no etiologic or predisposing condition can be identified, in recent years an underlying disorder has been found in more than 70% of cases. The most common conditions that predispose to BCS are hematologic disorders with thrombotic tendencies, such as polycythemia rubra vera and paroxysmal nocturnal hemoglobinuria (approximately 18-30% of cases); use of oral contraceptives (approximately 9-28% of cases); pregnancy and the postpartum period (approximately 2-10% of cases); malignant neoplasms that invade the IVC and hepatic veins from adjacent organs (approximately 5-12% of cases); and infections of the liver, such as amebic abscess, hydatid cyst, and schistosomiasis (approximately 0-10% of cases), common in the East, but rare in the West. Evidence indicates that multiple prothrombotic hematologic factors acting concurrently are involved in many

patients with BCS. In Japan, China, India, and South Africa, a common chronic form of BCS is MOVC, an idiopathic condition that probably results from acquired thrombosis and recanalization of the IVC. The membrane has been found to vary from very thin to several centimeters thick and sometimes has occluded a long segment of retrohepatic IVC.

The pathologic lesion of BCS is thrombosis of the major hepatic veins or the IVC or both, which results in hepatic venous outflow obstruction; intrahepatic and portal hypertension; dilation of the liver sinusoids; intense centrilobular congestion of the hepatic parenchyma; and ischemia, pressure necrosis, and atrophy of the parenchymal cells in the center of the liver lobule. Early in the course of BCS, these lesions are reversible if the obstruction is relieved. Persistence of the high pressure and congestion within the liver results in irreversible damage, hepatic fibrosis, and progression to cirrhosis, often within a matter of months. The two paramount dangers in BCS are development of irreversible liver damage and extension of thrombosis from the hepatic veins into the IVC. The most striking difference between the West and the East in the pathology of BCS is the site of venous occlusion causing hepatic outflow obstruction; in the West, it is most often in the major hepatic veins, and in the East, it is usually in the IVC.

The clinical course of BCS in Western countries is most commonly acute or subacute, with rapid progression of liver disease and its consequences over periods ranging from a few weeks to a few months. In some patients, however, BCS develops insidiously and progresses over months or years. The usual clinical manifestations are abdominal distention secondary to ascites, hepatomegaly, splenomegaly, abdominal pain, weakness, wasting, and anorexia. Some patients additionally have mild jaundice and distention of the superficial veins of the anterior abdominal wall. When the IVC is obstructed, an important additional sign is edema of the lower extremities and lower trunk. In the chronic forms of BCS, all of the manifestations of cirrhosis of the liver are found.

The diagnosis of BCS in the initial weeks and months is based on finding the typical symptoms and signs combined with abnormal results of several diagnostic studies, the most important of which are angiographic examination of the IVC and hepatic veins with pressure measurements and percutaneous needle liver biopsy. In BCS confined to the hepatic veins, angiographic studies show a patent IVC and relatively normal IVC pressure for patients with ascites, whereas in BCS involving the IVC, cavography shows an area of IVC obstruction, and IVC pressure is markedly elevated. Hepatic venography shows occlusion of the major hepatic veins, and wedge injection shows a distinctive spiderweb pattern of venous collaterals. WHVP is markedly elevated. In BCS confined to the hepatic veins, WHVP is substantially higher than IVC pressure, but in BCS involving IVC obstruction, WHVP is similar to IVC pressure. Liver biopsy reveals the typical lesions of obstruction to hepatic venous outflow—intense centrilobular congestion and centrilobular loss of parenchyma and necrosis. Other diagnostic studies that may be helpful as screening procedures are (1) CT, which shows absence of opacification of the major hepatic veins; (2) ultrasonography, which shows absence of normal hepatic veins; and (3) hepatic scintiscanning, which shows decreased and nonhomogeneous hepatic uptake of radiocolloid and sometimes shows central localization of radiocolloid, the so-called central hot spot. Liver function tests invariably show significant hepatic dysfunction. In patients who are operated on for BCS confined to the hepatic veins, the clinical manifestations and results of diagnostic studies are confirmed by the findings of marked ascites; an enlarged, congested liver; splenomegaly; extensive portosystemic collateral veins; IVC pressure that is substantially lower than portal vein pressure; portal hypertension; and a markedly elevated hepatic occluded portal pressure, which sometimes is higher than the free portal pressure.

Nonsurgical therapy of BCS includes medical treatment with thrombolytic agents, anticoagulants, and diuretics and radiologic therapy consisting of transluminal angioplasty, venous stenting, and TIPS. Infusion of thrombolytic agents, such as streptokinase and urokinase, in hopes of dissolving thrombi in the hepatic veins or IVC or both has had limited short-term success, but a high rate of ultimate failure. Anticoagulant therapy to prevent propagation of the thrombi has produced a limited, short-term response when used alone. None of these measures has been effective, and nonoperative medical therapy has been associated with an almost uniformly poor prognosis. Most patients in Western countries have died within a few months of onset of symptoms, and the few patients who have survived the acute phase have almost all died from the complications of cirrhosis within a few years. Control of ascites is feasible in some patients with BCS by use of the usual diuretic regimens, although the ascites is resistant to therapy in many patients. There is no evidence that control of ascites influences the long-term outcome.

Radiologic therapy consisting of percutaneous transluminal angioplasty with and without the use of metallic stents has had some short-term success in patients with chronic BCS resulting from stenosis of the IVC, but recurrent stenosis has been the rule, and the long-term success rate has been less than 50%, although one report from China claimed a high success rate. The radiologic procedure known as TIPS has been used in recent years with increasing frequency in all forms of BCS. The advantage of TIPS is that it does not require a major surgical operation. The disadvantages of TIPS are a high rate of TIPS stenosis and occlusion requiring repeated revisions, frequent recurrence of symptoms, and the need for numerous radiologic procedures and hospitalizations. Five-year survival rate after TIPS in the most experienced hands has been well below the 5-year survival rate of surgical shunt therapy in our series.

SSPCS has proved to be the most effective therapy of BCS caused by thrombosis of the hepatic veins. Its use is based on substantial evidence showing that it converts the valveless portal vein into an outflow tract, decompressing the obstructed hepatic vascular bed. In an experimental evaluation of PCS in dogs with BCS, we found that SSPCS decompressed the liver and cured ascites in 96% of the dogs, reduced liver size to normal, reversed the pathologic lesions in the liver often to normal, and resulted in long-term survival of many of the dogs. On the basis of these experimental findings, we have performed SSPCS early in the course of 34 patients with acute or subacute BCS with 1 operative death and 1 long-term death. The 33 survivors of operation have lived free of ascites without diuretic therapy for 1 to 32 years. The shunt has remained patent in all but one patient. Liver function has returned to normal in the 30 patients who did not already have cirrhosis preoperatively, hepatosplenomegaly has disappeared, and there has been no encephalopathy. Serial liver biopsy specimens obtained 1 to 31 years postoperatively showed substantial reversal of the pathologic lesions of BCS. Our experience shows the importance of performing SSPCS early in the course of BCS to reverse the liver damage and prevent extension of thrombosis from the hepatic veins into the IVC.

Splenorenal shunt and interposition mesocaval shunt and PCS using synthetic grafts are hemodynamically similar to SSPCS, but are inferior operations in BCS because of a high incidence of thrombosis and occlusion. Interposition shunt using an autogenous internal jugular vein H-graft has produced results similar to those of direct SSPCS. Important technical features of SSPCS are proper positioning of the patient, use of a long right subcostal incision, and extensive mobilization of the IVC and portal vein so that the two vessels can be brought together.

SSPCS is contraindicated when BCS is caused by thrombosis or occlusion of the IVC. Under such circumstances, a mesoatrial shunt has been used with some short-term success, although there has been a high incidence of thrombosis of the bypass graft. In our series of eight patients, thrombosis of the mesoatrial shunt developed in five, and the 5-year survival rate was only 38%. Similarly, others have reported thrombosis of the mesoatrial shunt in 40% to 70% of patients, an event that is often followed by death.

Because of dissatisfaction with the results of mesoatrial shunt, we worked in the experimental laboratory to devise a shunting procedure aimed at decompressing the hypertensive IVC and shunting the portal venous flow and the entire IVC flow to the right atrium. The new operation, which consisted of a combined SSPCS and CAS through a Gore-Tex prosthesis, was found to be effective in relieving BCS in rats and has been successful in each of 12 patients with BCS secondary to IVC occlusion during follow-up of 3 to 20 years. In our program, the combined shunt operation has replaced mesoatrial shunt as the preferred treatment for BCS caused by IVC occlusion.

OLT is indicated in patients with chronic BCS who have cirrhosis with progressive hepatic failure and in patients who have had an unsuccessful portosystemic shunt. In approximately 189 patients with advanced liver disease secondary to BCS, OLT has resulted in an actuarial 5-year survival rate of 50% to 69%. In our experience with 12 patients who were approved for OLT, 3 died on the waiting list, and the 5-year survival rate of patients who underwent OLT was 67%. OLT and SSPCS are not competing forms of treatment. OLT is appropriate therapy in the late stages of BCS when the liver disease no longer can be reversed by SSPCS.

Other surgical procedures of uncertain value in BCS are direct surgical removal of the venous obstruction, thoracic transposition of the spleen, and peritoneovenous shunt. Direct surgical resection of the occluded hepatic veins and IVC with the aid of cardiopulmonary bypass has produced good short-term results in about 49 patients with chronic BCS involving the IVC, but prolonged and detailed follow-up of more patients is required to determine the efficacy of this procedure and its modifications. Peritoneovenous shunt is a palliative procedure that should not be used as primary treatment of BCS because it does not decompress the liver or influence the ongoing hepatic damage.

Several surgical procedures have been used by Japanese surgeons to treat the chronic form of BCS caused by MOVC. When the area of IVC obstruction has been short, fracture of the membrane by transcardiac membranotomy has been the principal treatment and has had a short-term success rate of 70% to 90% during follow-up periods ranging from 2 months to 7 years. Percutaneous transluminal angioplasty also has had some short-term success, but recurrence of IVC stenosis has been frequent. When the area of IVC obstruction has been long, treatment has consisted of direct excision and repair of the involved area of IVC or cavoatrial bypass graft. Both of these procedures have had some success, but have been associated with a substantial incidence of failure and a substantial mortality rate. Finally, patients with MOVC have undergone a variety of operations of uncertain value that are designed to create portosystemic or portopulmonary collateral venous connections.

VOD is a group of disorders in which hepatic venous outflow obstruction is due to subendothelial sclerosis of the sublobular hepatic veins, terminal hepatic venules, and sinusoids within the liver. VOD is caused by ingestion of plants containing pyrrolizidine alkaloids, antineoplastic drugs, and irradiation of the liver. In the Western Hemisphere, the most frequent cause is bone marrow transplantation. Approximately one fourth of bone marrow transplant recipients develop VOD. Extensive occlusion of the small hepatic veins results in centrilobular hemorrhagic necrosis of the liver parenchyma, which progresses to diffuse fibrosis and cirrhosis. Although it can occur at any age, VOD caused by pyrrolizidine alkaloids has been observed most often in children, in whom, after a prodromal febrile illness, there is an acute onset of abdominal distention owing to ascites, abdominal pain, hepatosplenomegaly, weakness, and sometimes jaundice and peripheral edema.

The most important symptoms and signs of VOD after bone marrow transplantation are ascites, jaundice, and abdominal pain. Some patients recover from the acute stage of VOD, but approximately one fifth of patients with pyrrolizidine poisoning die, and the remainder go on to develop cirrhosis rapidly with all of its clinical manifestations. The mortality rate of severe VOD after bone marrow transplantation has been reported to be 98%. The most important diagnostic study in VOD is percutaneous needle liver biopsy, which shows the specific abnormality of extensive occlusion of the small hepatic veins within the liver and centrilobular hemorrhagic necrosis. The results of hepatic scintiscanning, liver function tests, and WHVP measurements are similar to results found in BCS, but angiographic studies are not helpful because the major hepatic veins and IVC are normal in VOD. Elevated WHVP supports the diagnosis of VOD.

Substantial experience with treatment of VOD has been reported in patients who have the disorder as a result of ingestion of pyrrolizidine alkaloids. When such patients are seen in the acute stage, supportive medical therapy is used. SSPCS is indicated during the acute stage if bleeding esophageal varices develop, or if the clinical and liver biopsy signs of hepatic venous outflow obstruction do not subside after 4 to 8 weeks. In the chronic phase of VOD, when the usual manifestations of cirrhosis have developed, SSPCS is recommended even before varix hemorrhage has occurred. The mortality rate of chronic VOD is high, and the major cause of death is bleeding esophageal varices. Medical therapy of the many patients who have developed VOD after bone marrow transplantation has included tissue-type plasminogen activator, defibrotide, antithrombin III, activated protein C, prostaglandin E_1, N-acetyl cysteine, high-dose corticosteroids, glutamine, and vitamin E. None of these agents has been uniformly effective. The most promising agent undergoing trial is defibrotide, which has been reported to produce a complete response rate of 36% and a 100-day survival rate of 35% in severe VOD. SSPCS, TIPS, and OLT have been used in a few patients with severe VOD. These procedures have had some success and deserve further evaluation, particularly because one fourth of patients with VOD develop the severe form of the disease, and the mortality rate of severe VOD has been reported to be 98%.

REFERENCES

Abbott PJ, 1988: Comfrey: assessing the low-dose health risk. Med J Aust 149:678-682.

Aboujaoude MM, et al, 1991: Effect of portosystemic shunts on subsequent transplantation of the liver. Surg Gynecol Obstet 172:215-219.

Ahn SS, et al, 1987: Selective surgical therapy of the Budd-Chiari syndrome provides superior survivor rates than conservative medical management. J Vasc Surg 5:28-37.

Aikat BK, et al, 1978: Veno-occlusive disease in North-West India. Indian J Pathol Microbiol 21:203-211.

Akita H, Sakoda K, 1980: Portopulmonary shunt by splenopneumopexy as a surgical treatment of Budd-Chiari syndrome. Surgery 87:85-94.

Al-Hasany M, Mohamed AS, 1970: Veno-occlusive disease of the liver in Iraq: nine cases occurring in three Bedouin families. Arch Dis Child 54:722-724.

Alpert LI, 1976: Veno-occlusive disease of the liver associated with oral contraceptives: case report and review of literature. Hum Pathol 7:709-718.

Alvarez R, et al, 2000: Percutaneous intrahepatic portosystemic shunting in the treatment of veno-occlusive disease of the liver after bone marrow transplantation. Gastroenterol Hepatol 23:177-180.

Anonymous, 1982: Case records of the Massachusetts General Hospital. N Engl J Med 307:236-242.

Asbury RF, et al, 1980: Hepatic veno-occlusive disease due to DTIC. Cancer 45:2670-2674.

Auvert J, Farge C, 1963: Hypertension portale de l'enfant: dans une serie de 123 cas, etude des cas difficiles necessitant plusieurs interventions: interet de l'anastomose cavomesenterique. Ann Chir 17:281.

Ayash LJ, et al, 1990: Hepatic venooclusive disease in autologous bone marrow transplantation of solid tumors and lymphomas. J Clin Oncol 8:1699-1706.

Azoulay D, et al, 2000: Transjugular intrahepatic portosystemic shunt (TIPS) for severe veno-occlusive disease of the liver following bone marrow transplantation. Bone Marrow Transplant 25:987-992.

Bach N, et al, 1989: Comfrey herb tea-induced hepatic veno-occlusive disease. Am J Med 87:97-99.

Baert AL, et al, 1983: Early diagnosis of Budd-Chiari syndrome by computed tomography and ultrasonography: report of five cases. Gastroenterology 894:587-595.

Bahr MJ, et al, 2003: Recurrence of Budd-Chiari syndrome after liver transplantation in paroxysmal nocturnal hemoglobinuria. Transpl Int 16:890-894.

Baijal SS, et al, 1996: Management of idiopathic Budd-Chiari syndrome with primary stent placement: early results. J Vasc Interv Radiol 7:545-553.

Bazraktar Y, et al, 1997: Budd-Chiari syndrome: a common complication of Behçet's disease. Am J Gastroenterol 92:858-862.

Becker C, 1986: Hepatic vein occlusion: morphologic features on computed tomography and ultrasonography. Gastrointest Radiol 11:305-311.

Behera A, et al, 2002: Treatment of Budd-Chiari syndrome with inferior vena caval occlusion by mesoatrial shunt. Eur J Surg 168:355-359.

Berk PD, et al, 1979: Veno-occlusive disease of the liver after allogeneic bone marrow transplantation: possible association with graft versus host disease. Ann Intern Med 90:158-164.

Bertina RM, et al, 1994: Mutation in blood coagulation factor V associated with resistance to activated protein C. Nature 369:64-67.

Bismuth H, Sherlock DJ, 1991: Portasystemic shunting versus liver transplantation for the Budd-Chiari syndrome. Ann Surg 214:581-589.

Bismuth H, et al, 1990: Options for elective treatment of portal hypertension in cirrhotic patients in the transplantation era. Am J Surg 160:105-110.

Blum U, et al, 1995: Budd-Chiari syndrome: technical hemodynamic, and clinical results of treatment with transjugular intrahepatic portosystemic shunt. Radiology 197:805-811.

Boillot O, et al, 1991: Liver transplantation in patients with a surgical portasystemic shunt. Gastroenterol Clin Biol 15:876-880.

Bolondi L, et al, 1991: Diagnosis of Budd-Chiari syndrome by pulsed Doppler ultrasound. Gastroenterology 100:1324-1331.

Boughton BJ, 1991: Hepatic and portal vein thrombosis closely associated with chronic myeloproliferative disorders. BMJ 302:192-193 (editorial).

Bras G, McLean E, 1963: Toxic factors in veno-occlusive disease. Ann N Y Acad Sci 3:392-396.

Bras G, et al, 1954: Veno-occlusive disease of the liver with non-portal type of cirrhosis occurring in Jamaica. Arch Pathol 57:285-300.

Brink AJ, Botha P, 1955: Budd-Chiari syndrome: diagnosis of by hepatic venography. Br J Radiol 28:330-331.

Britton RC, Shirey EK, 1962: Cineportography and dynamics of portal flow following shunt procedures. Arch Surg 84:25-33.

Britton RC, et al, 1967: Perfusion of the liver following side-to-side portacaval shunt. Surgery 62:181-188.

Brooks SEH, et al, 1970: Acute veno-occlusive disease of the liver: fine structure in Jamaican children. Arch Pathol 89:507-520.

Budd G, 1845: On Diseases of the Liver. London, John Churchill, p 146.

Bunin N, et al, 1996: Related donor liver transplant for veno-occlusive disease following T-depleted unrelated donor bone marrow transplantation. Transplantation 61:664-666.

Burchell AR, et al, 1976: Hepatic artery flow improvement after portacaval shunt: single hemodynamic clinical correlate. Ann Surg 1984:289-302.

Cameron JL, et al, 1983: The Budd-Chiari syndrome: treatment by mesenteric-systemic venous shunts. Ann Surg 198:335-346.

Cameron JL, et al, 1984: Mesoatrial shunt: a prosthesis modification. Surgery 96:114-116.

Campbell DA Jr, et al, 1988: Hepatic transplantation with perioperative and long term anticoagulation as treatment for Budd-Chiari syndrome. Surg Gynecol Obstet 166:511-518.

Campbell DP, et al, 1973: Survival prediction in portacaval shunt: a computerized statistical analysis. Am J Surg 126:748-751.

Cassel GA, Morely JE, 1974: Hepatic vein thrombosis treated with streptokinase. S Afr Med J 48:2319-2320.

Cejna M, et al, 2002: Repeat interventions for maintenance of transjugular intrahepatic portosystemic shunt function in patients with Budd-Chiari syndrome. J Vasc Interv Radiol 13:193-199.

Chiari H, 1899: Über der selbstandige phlebitis obliterans der Hauptstamme der venae hepaticae als Todesursache. Beitrage Path Anat 26:1-18.

Child CG III, Turcotte JG, 1964: Surgery and portal hypertension. In Child CG III (ed): The Liver and Portal Hypertension. Philadelphia, Saunders, pp 1-85.

Clain D, et al, 1967: Clinical diagnosis of the Budd-Chiari syndrome: a report of six cases. Am J Med 43:544-554.

Cruz CA, et al, 1983: Veno-occlusive disease of the liver in children following chemotherapy for acute myelocytic leukemia. Cancer 52:1803-1807.

Dahlback B, 1995: Resistance to activated protein C, the Arg506 to Gln mutation in the factor V gene and venous thrombosis. Thromb Haemost 73:739-742.

Dahlback B, et al, 1993: Familial thrombophilia due to a previously unrecognized mechanism characterized by poor anticoagulant response to activated protein C: prediction of a cofactor to activated protein C. Proc Natl Acad Sci U S A 90:1004-1008.

de la Rubia J, et al, 1996: Successful treatment of hepatic veno-occlusive disease in a peripheral blood progenitor cell transplant patient with a transjugular intrahepatic portosystemic stent-shunt (TIPS). Haematologica 81:536-539.

Deltenre P, et al, 2001: Factor V Leiden related Budd-Chiari syndrome. Gut 48:264-268.

Denninger MH, et al, 2000: Cause of portal or hepatic venous thrombosis in adults: the role of multiple concurrent factors. Hepatology 31:587-591.

Dowling JB, 1979: Ten years' experience with mesocaval grafts. Surg Gynecol Obstet 149:518-522.

Ecker JE, McKittrick JE, 1966: Thrombosis of the hepatic veins: the "Budd-Chiari syndrome"—a possible link between oral contraceptives and thrombosis formation. Am J Gastroenterol 45:429-443.

Eguchi S, et al, 1974: Successful balloon membranotomy for obstruction of the hepatic portion of the inferior vena cava. Surgery 76:837-840.

Eisenmenger WJ, Nickel WF, 1960: Indications for portacaval anastomosis. Med Clin North Am 44:779-787.

Emre A, et al, 2000: Mesoatrial shunt in Budd-Chiari syndrome. Am J Surg 179:304-308.

Erlik D, et al, 1962: Surgical cure of primary hepatic vein occlusion syndrome by side-to-side portacaval shunt. Surg Gynecol Obstet 114:368-374.

Espana P, et al, 1980: Membranous obstruction of the inferior vena cava and hepatic veins. Am J Gastroenterol 73:28-32.

Espinosa G, et al, 2001: Budd-Chiari syndrome secondary to antiphospholipid syndrome: clinical and immunologic characteristics of 43 patients. Medicine (Baltimore) 80:345-354.

Fajardo LF, Colby TV, 1980: Pathogenesis of veno-occlusive liver disease after radiation. Arch Pathol Lab Med 104:584-588.

Fletcher MS, et al, 1981: Long-term follow-up of interposition mesocaval shunting in portal hypertension. Br J Surg 68:485-487.

Fried MW, et al, 1996: Transjugular intrahepatic portosystemic shunt for the management of severe venoocclusive disease following bone marrow transplantation. Hepatology 24:588-591.

Furui S, et al, 1990: Hepatic inferior vena cava obstruction: treatment of two types with Gianturco expandable metallic stents. Radiology 176:665-670.

Galati JS, et al, 1993: The Budd-Chiari syndrome: a therapeutic quandary. Gastroenterology 104:A904.

Ganger DR, et al, 1999: Transjugular intrahepatic portosystemic shunt (TIPS) for Budd-Chiari syndrome or portal vein thrombosis: review of indications and problems. Am J Gastroenterol 94:603-608.

Gentil-Kocher S, et al, 1988: Budd-Chiari syndrome in children: report of 22 cases. J Pediatr 113:30-38.

Ghanem J, Hershko C, 1981: Veno-occlusive disease and primary hepatic vein thrombosis in Israeli Arabs. Isr J Med Sci 17:339-347.

Gibson JB, 1960: Chiari's disease and the Budd-Chiari syndrome. J Pathol 79:381-401.

Giles FJ, et al, 2001: Mylotarg (gemtuzumab ozogamicin) therapy is associated with hepatic venoocclusive disease in patients who have not received stem cell transplantation. Cancer 92:406-413.

Gill RA, et al, 1982: Hepatic veno-occlusive disease caused by 6-thioguanine. Ann Intern Med 96:58-60.

Goldstein R, et al, 1991: Prevention of recurrent thrombosis following liver transplantation for Budd-Chiari syndrome associated with myeloproliferative disorders: treatment with hydroxyurea and aspirin. Transplant Proc 23:1559-1560.

Gooneratne NS, et al, 1979: 'Dimple sign' in hepatic vein thrombosis. Br J Radiol 52:584-586.

Gore DO, et al, 1961: Veno-occlusive disease of the liver: surgical aspects. Surgery 49:334-346.

Grant E, et al, 1989: Budd-Chiari syndrome: the results of duplex and color Doppler imaging. Am J Radiol 152:377-381.

Grases PJ, Beker SG, 1972: Veno-occlusive disease of the liver: a case from Venezuela. Am J Med 53:511-516.

Greenwood LH, et al, 1983: Urokinase treatment of Budd-Chiari syndrome. Am J Radiol 141:1057-1059.

Griffith JF, et al, 1996: Radiological intervention in Budd-Chiari syndrome: techniques and outcome in 18 patients. Clin Radiol 51:775-784.

Griner PF, et al, 1976: Veno-occlusive disease of the liver after chemotherapy of acute leukemia: a report of two cases. Ann Intern Med 85:578-582.

Gupta S, et al, 1987: Comparison of ultrasonography, computed tomography and 99mTc liver scan in diagnosis of Budd-Chiari syndrome. Gut 28:242-247.

Hagglund H, et al, 1996: Treatment of hepatic venoocclusive disease with recombinant human tissue plasminogen activator or orthotopic liver transplantation after allogeneic bone marrow transplantation. Transplantation 62:1076-1080.

Halff G, et al, 1990: Liver transplantation for the Budd-Chiari syndrome. Ann Surg 211:43-49.

Hartmann RC, et al, 1980: Fulminant hepatic venous thrombosis (Budd-Chiari syndrome) in paroxysmal nocturnal hemoglobulinuria: definition of a medical emergency. Johns Hopkins Med J 146:247-254.

Hemming AW, et al, 1996: Treatment of Budd-Chiari syndrome with portosystemic shunt or liver transplantation. Am J Surg 171:176-181.

Henderson MJ, et al, 1990: Surgical options, hematologic evaluation, and pathologic changes in Budd-Chiari syndrome. Am J Surg 159:41-50.

Hirooka M, Kimura C, 1970: Membranous obstruction of the hepatic portion of the inferior vena cava. Arch Surg 100:656-663.

Hirschberg B, et al, 2000: Flow cytometric analysis of autonomous growth of erythroid precursors in liquid culture detects occult polycythemia vera in the Budd-Chiari syndrome. J Hepatol 32:574-578.

Hodkinson HJ, et al, 1978: Postpartum veno-occlusive disease treated with ascitic fluid reinfusion. S Afr Med J 54:366-368.

Hosoki T, et al, 1989: Hepatic venous outflow obstruction: evaluation with pulsed Doppler sonography. Radiology 170:733-737.

Hoyumpa AM Jr, et al, 1971: Budd-Chiari syndrome in women taking oral contraceptives. Am J Med 50:137-140.

Huber M, et al, 1997: Budd-Chiari syndrome: long term results after treatment with transjugular intrahepatic portosystemic shunt (TIPS). Hepatology 26:204A.

Huguet C, et al, 1979: Interposition mesocaval shunt for chronic primary occlusion of the hepatic veins. Surg Gynecol Obstet 148:691-698.

Iwahashi K, 1981: Surgical correction of the inferior vena cava obstruction with Budd-Chiari syndrome. Arch Jpn Chir 50:559-570.

Iwatsuki S, et al, 1988: Liver transplantation in the treatment of bleeding esophageal varices. Surgery 104:697-705.

Iwatsuki S, et al, 1991: Liver transplantation for Budd-Chiari syndrome. Proceedings of the Second International Symposium on Budd-Chiari Syndrome, Kyoto, Japan, VIPL-2.

Jamieson NV, et al, 1991: Liver transplantation for Budd-Chiari syndrome, 1976-1990. Ann Chir 45:362-365.

Janssen HI, et al, 2000: Factor V Leiden mutation, prothrombin gene mutation, and deficiencies in coagulation inhibitors associated with Budd-Chiari syndrome and portal vein thrombosis: results of a case-control study. Blood 96:2364-2368.

Jeans WD, et al, 1983: Treatment of hepatic vein and inferior vena caval obstruction by balloon dilatation. Br J Radiol 56:687-689.

Jones RJ, et al, 1987: Venocclusive disease of the liver following bone marrow transplantation. Transplantation 44:778-783.

Kage M, et al, 1992: Histopathology of membranous obstruction of the inferior vena cava in the Budd-Chiari syndrome. Gastroenterology 102:2081-2090.

Kawashima Y, et al, 1991: Senning's operation for the treatment of Budd-Chiari syndrome. In Proceedings of the Second International Symposium on Budd-Chiari Syndrome, Kyoto, Japan, II01-6.

Khanna SK, et al, 1991: Shunt surgery in Budd-Chiari syndrome: our experience. In Proceedings of the Second International Symposium on Budd-Chiari Syndrome, Kyoto, Japan, IL02-5.

Khuroo MS, Datta DV, 1980: Budd-Chiari syndrome following pregnancy: report of 16 cases with roentgenologic, hemodynamic and histologic studies of the hepatic outflow tract. Am J Med 68:113-121.

Kimura C, et al, 1972: Membranous obstruction of the hepatic portion of the inferior vena cava: clinical study of nine cases. Surgery 72:551-559.

Klein AS, et al, 1990: Current management of the Budd-Chiari syndrome. Ann Surg 212:144-149.

Knoop M, et al, 1994a: Treatment of the Budd-Chiari syndrome with orthotopic liver transplantation and long-term anticoagulation. Clin Transplant 8: 67-72.

Knoop M, et al, 1994b: Liver transplantation for Budd-Chiari syndrome. Transplant Proc 26:3577-3578.

Koja K, et al, 1996: Radical open end venectomy with autologous pericardial patch graft for correction of Budd-Chiari syndrome. Cardiovasc Surg 4: 500-504.

Koster T, et al, 1993: Venous thrombosis due to poor anticoagulant response to activated protein C: Leiden Thrombophilia Study. Lancet 342: 1503-1506.

Kreel L, et al, 1967: Vascular radiology in the Budd-Chiari syndrome. Br J Radiol 40:755-759.

Kriegshauser S, et al, 1988: Hepatic venocclusive disease after bone-marrow transplantation: diagnosis with duplex sonography. AJR Am J Roentgenol 150:289-290.

Krom RAF, et al, 1984: Orthotopic liver transplantation in Groningen, The Netherlands (1979-1983). Hepatology 4:61S-65S.

Kumar S, et al, 2003: Hepatic veno-occlusive disease (sinusoidal obstruction syndrome) after hematopoietic stem cell transplantation. Mayo Clin Proc 78:589-598.

Kuniyoshi Y, et al, 1998: Improvement in esophageal varices and liver histology postoperatively in Budd-Chiari syndrome. Ann Thorac Surg 65:1711-1714.

Langer B, et al, 1975: Clinical spectrum of the Budd-Chiari syndrome and its surgical management. Am J Surg 129:137-145.

Langnas AN, et al, 1992: Influence of a prior porta-systemic shunt on outcome after liver transplantation. Am J Gastroenterol 87:714-718.

Lazarus HM, et al, 1982: Veno-occlusive disease in the liver after high-dose mitomycin C therapy and autologous bone marrow transplantation. Cancer 49:1789-1795.

LeVeen HH, et al, 1976: Further experience with peritoneo-venous shunt for ascites. Ann Surg 184:574-581.

Lewis JH, et al, 1983: Budd-Chiari syndrome associated with oral contraceptive steroids: review of treatment of 47 cases. Dig Dis Sci 28:673-683.

Liano F, et al, 1989: Veno-occlusive hepatic disease of the liver in renal transplantation: is azathioprine the cause? Nephron 51:509-516.

Liebowitz AI, Hartmann RC, 1981: The Budd-Chiari syndrome and paroxysmal nocturnal haemoglobinuria. Br J Haematol 48:1-6.

Long RTL, et al, 1960: The demonstration and quantification of reverse flow in the proximal portal vein following side-to-side portacaval anastomosis. Surgery 47:125-131.

Longmire WP Jr, et al, 1958: Side-to-side portacaval anastomosis for portal hypertension. Ann Surg 147:881-894.

Ludwick JR, et al, 1965: Chiari's disease: a clinicopathological study. Arch Surg 91:697-704.

Lyford CL, et al, 1976: Hepatic veno-occlusive disease originating in Ecuador. Gastroenterology 70:105-108.

Maddrey WC, 1987: Hepatic vein thrombosis (Budd-Chiari syndrome): possible association with the use of oral contraceptives. Semin Liver Dis 7:32-39.

Mahmoud AEA, Elias E, 1996: New approaches to the Budd-Chiari syndrome. J Gastroenterol Hepatol 11:1121-1123.

Mahmoud AEA, et al, 1995: Budd-Chiari syndrome and factor V Leiden mutation. Lancet 345:526.

Mahmoud AEA, et al, 1996: Clinical spectrum, investigations and treatment of Budd-Chiari syndrome. QJM 89:37-43.

Malt RA, et al, 1978: Side-to-side portacaval shunt versus nonsurgical treatment of Budd-Chiari syndrome. Am J Surg 136:387-389.

Mancuso A, et al, 2003: TIPS for acute and chronic Budd-Chiari syndrome: a single-centre experience. J Hepatol 38:751-754.

Marchal G, et al, 1974: Syndrome de Budd-Chiari chronique associe a une agenesie lobaire gauche chez un adulte age. Chirurgie 100:551-557.

Martin LG, et al, 1990: Angioplasty for long-term treatment of patients with Budd-Chiari syndrome. Am J Radiol 154:1007-1010.

Marubbio AT, Danielson B, 1975: Hepatic veno-occlusive disease in a renal transplant patient receiving azathioprine. Gastroenterology 69:739-743.

Mathieu D, et al, 1987: Budd-Chiari syndrome: dynamic CT. Radiology 165:409-413.

Mazzaferro V, et al, 1990: Liver transplantation in patients with previous portasystemic shunt. Am J Surg 160:111-115.

McCarthy P, et al, 1985: The Budd-Chiari syndrome: medical and surgical management of 30 patients. Arch Surg 120:657-662.

McDonald GB, et al, 1984: Veno-occlusive disease of the liver after bone marrow transplantation: diagnosis, incidence and predisposing factors. Hepatology 4:116-122.

McDonald GB, et al, 1993: Veno-occlusive disease of the liver and multiorgan failure after bone marrow transplantation: a cohort study of 355 patients. Ann Intern Med 118:255-267.

McIntyre RE, et al, 1981: Fatal veno-occlusive disease of the liver following high dose 1,3-bis(2-chloroethyl)-1-nitrosourea (BCNU) and autologous bone marrow transplantation. Am J Clin Pathol 75:614-617.

McMaster P, 1994: Budd-Chiari syndrome: shunt or transplant? HPB Surg 7:257-259.

Meindok H, Langer B, 1976: Liver scan in Budd-Chiari syndrome. J Nucl Med 117:365-368.

Melear JM, et al, 2002: Hematologic aspects of liver transplantation for Budd-Chiari syndrome with special reference to myeloproliferative disorders. Transplantation 74:1090-1095.

Mellis C, Bale PM, 1976: Familial hepatic veno-occlusive disease with probable immune deficiency. J Pediatr 88:236-242.

Menon KVN, et al, 2004: The Budd-Chiari syndrome. N Engl J Med 350: 578-585.

Michl P, et al, 1999: Successful treatment of chronic Budd-Chiari syndrome with transjugular intrahepatic portosystemic shunt. J Hepatol 32:516-520.

Millikan WJ Jr, et al, 1985: Approach to the spectrum of Budd-Chiari syndrome: which patients require portal decompression? Am J Surg 149:167-176.

Minegaux F, et al, 1994: Comparison of transjugular and surgical portosystemic shunts on the outcome of liver transplantation. Arch Surg 129:1018-1024.

Mitchell MC, et al, 1982: Budd-Chiari syndrome: etiology, diagnosis and management. Medicine (Baltimore) 61:199-218.

Mohabbat O, et al, 1976: An outbreak of hepatic veno-occlusive disease in northwestern Afghanistan. Lancet 2:269-271.

Moreno AH, et al, 1967: Portal blood flow in cirrhosis of the liver. J Clin Invest 46:436-445.

Mulder DG, Murray JF, 1960: An evaluation of the side-to-side portacaval shunt. Surg Forum 11:278-279.

Murad SD, et al, 2004: Determinants of survival and the effect of portosystemic shunting in patients with Budd-Chiari syndrome. Hepatology 39:500-508.

Murray JA, et al, 1987: Successful treatment of hepatic venoocclusive disease in a bone marrow transplant patient with side-to-side portocaval shunt. Gastroenterology 92:1073-1077.

Murray JF, Mulder DG, 1961: The effects of retrograde portal venous flow following side-to-side portacaval anastomosis: a comparison with end-to-side shunts. J Clin Invest 40:1413-1420.

Nakao K, et al, 1988: Budd-Chiari syndrome treated by Senning's procedure. J Cardiovasc Surg 29:746-750.

Nimer SD, et al, 1990: Successful treatment of hepatic venoocclusive disease in a bone marrow transplant patient with orthotopic liver transplantation. Transplantation 49:819-821.

Noble JA, 1967: Hepatic vein thrombosis complicating polycythemia vera: successful treatment with a portacaval shunt. Arch Intern Med 120: 105-108.

Noone TC, et al, 2000: Budd-Chiari syndrome: spectrum of appearances of acute, subacute, and chronic disease with magnetic resonance imaging. J Magn Reson Imaging 11:44-50.

Ohara I, et al, 1963: A bypass operation for occlusion of the hepatic inferior vena cava. Surg Gynecol Obstet 117:151-155.

Okamoto E, et al, 1983: Simultaneous radical surgical treatment for membranous obstruction of the inferior vena cava and the coincident hepatocellular carcinoma—the first successful case. Jpn J Surg 13:135-140.

Okuda H, et al, 1995: Epidemiological and clinical features of Budd-Chiari syndrome in Japan. J Hepatol 22:1-9.

Okuda K, 2002: Inferior vena cava thrombosis at its hepatic portion (obliterative hepatocavopathy). Semin Liver Dis 22:15-26.

Ono J, et al, 1983: Membranous obstruction of the inferior vena cava. Ann Surg 197:454-458.

Orloff LA, Orloff MJ, 1999: Budd-Chiari syndrome caused by Behçet disease: treatment by side-to-side portacaval shunt. J Am Coll Surg 188: 396-407.

Orloff MJ, 1983: Portal hypertension: portacaval anastomosis. In Dudley H, et al (eds): Rob and Smith's Operative Surgery, Alimentary Tract and Abdominal Wall, 4th ed. Oxford, Butterworth, p 546-569.

Orloff MJ, 1977: The liver. In: Sabiston DE Jr (ed): Davis-Christopher Textbook of Surgery, 11th ed. Philadelphia, Saunders, pp 1185-1187.

Orloff MJ, 1998: Invited discussion of Hemming et al: Treatment of Budd-Chiari syndrome with portosystemic shunt or liver transplantation. HPB Surg 11:136-139.

Orloff MJ, Girard B, 1989: Long-term results of treatment of Budd-Chiari syndrome by side-to-side portacaval shunt. Surg Gynecol Obstet 168:33-41.

Orloff MJ, Johansen KH, 1978: Treatment of Budd-Chiari syndrome by side-to-side portacaval shunt: experimental and clinical results. Ann Surg 188: 494-512.

Orloff MJ, Orloff MS, 1992: Bleeding oesophageal and gastric varices: shunts. In Dudley H, et al (eds): Rob and Smith's Operative Surgery: Alimentary Tract and Abdominal Wall, 4th ed. Oxford, Butterworth, pp 478-500.

Orloff MJ, Orloff MS, 1994: Bleeding oesophageal and gastric varices: shunts. In Jamieson CG, Denas HT (eds): Rob & Smith's Operative Surgery: Surgery of the Upper Gastrointestinal Tract. London, Chapman & Hall, pp 493-515.

Orloff MJ, Snyder GB, 1961: Experimental ascites: II. the effects of portacaval shunts on ascites produced with an internal vena cava cannula. Surgery 50:220-230.

Orloff MJ, et al, 1963: Experimental ascites: III. production of ascites by direct ligation of the hepatic veins. Surgery 54:627-639.

Orloff MJ, et al, 1965: Experimental ascites: V. production of hepatic outflow block and ascites with a hepatic vein choker. Ann Surg 161:258-262.

Orloff MJ, et al, 1992a: Treatment of Budd-Chiari syndrome due to inferior vena cava occlusion by combined portal and vena caval decompression. Am J Surg 163:137-143.

Orloff MJ, et al, 1992b: Long-term results of treatment of Budd-Chiari syndrome by portal decompression. Arch Surg 127:1182-1188.

Orloff MJ, et al, 1997: Experimental, clinical, and metabolic results of side-to-side portacaval shunt for intractable cirrhotic ascites. J Am Coll Surg 184:557-570.

Orloff MJ, et al, 2000: A 27-year experience with surgical treatment of Budd-Chiari syndrome. Ann Surg 232:340-352.

Panis Y, et al, 1994: Portosystemic shunt in Budd-Chiari syndrome: long-term survival and factors affecting shunt patency in 25 patients in Western countries. Surgery 115:276-281.

Pappas SC, et al, 1984: Hepatic veno-occlusive disease in a patient with systemic lupus erythematosus. Arthritis Rheum 27:104-108.

Parker RGF, 1959: Occlusion of the hepatic veins in man. Medicine 38: 369-402.

Pasic M, et al, 1993: Transcaval liver resection with hepatoatrial anastomosis for treatment of patients with the Budd-Chiari syndrome: late results. J Thorac Cardiovasc Surg 106:275-282.

Pelletier S, et al, 1994: Antiphospholipid syndrome as the second cause of non-tumorous Budd-Chiari syndrome. J Hepatol 21:76-80.

Perello A, et al, 2002: TIPS is a useful long-term derivative therapy for patients with Budd-Chiari syndrome uncontrolled by medical therapy. Hepatology 35:132-139.

Peytremann R, et al, 1972: Thrombosis in paroxysmal nocturnal hemoglobinuria (PNH) with particular reference to progressive, diffuse hepatic venous thrombosis. Ser Haematol 5:115-136.

Pezzuoli G, et al, 1985: Portacaval shunt in the treatment of primary Budd-Chiari syndrome. Surgery 98:319-323.

Powell-Jackson PR, et al, 1982: Budd-Chiari syndrome: clinical patterns and therapy. QJM 201:79-88.

Powell-Jackson PR, et al, 1986: Ultrasound scanning and 99mTc sulphur colloid scintigraphy in diagnosis of Budd-Chiari syndrome. Gut 27:1502-1506.

Prandi D, et al, 1975: Side-to-side portacaval shunt in the treatment of Budd-Chiari syndrome. Gastroenterology 68:137-141.

Rapoport AP, et al, 1991: Orthotopic liver transplantation for life-threatening veno-occlusive disease of the liver after allogeneic bone marrow transplant. Bone Marrow Transpl 8:421-424.

Redman HC, 1975: The Budd-Chiari syndrome: angiography and its complications. Can Assoc Radiol J 26:271-278.

Reed GB, Cox AJ, 1966: The human liver after radiation injury: a form of veno-occlusive disease. Am J Pathol 48:597-611.

Reichart B, et al, 1981: Surgical treatment for congenital occlusion of the inferior vena cava in its diaphragmatic portion. Thorac Cardiovasc Surg 29:180-182.

Reynolds TB, et al, 1962: The effect of a side-to-side portacaval shunt on hepatic hemodynamics in cirrhosis. J Clin Invest 41:1242-1248.

Richardson PG, et al, 2002: Multi-institutional use of defibrotide in 88 patients after stem cell transplantation with severe veno-occlusive disease and multi-system organ failure: response without significant toxicity in a high-risk population and factors predictive of outcome. Blood 100:4337-4343.

Ridker PM, McDermott WV, 1989: Comfrey herb tea and hepatic veno-occlusive disease. Lancet 1:657-658.

Ridker PM, et al, 1985: Hepatic veno-occlusive disease associated with the consumption of pyrrolizidine-containing dietary supplements. Gastroenterology 88:1050-1054.

Ringe B, et al, 1995: Which is the best surgery for Budd-Chiari syndrome: venous decompression or liver transplantation? A single-center experience with 50 patients. Hepatology 21:1337-1344.

Rogopoulos G, et al, 1995: Transjugular intrahepatic portosystemic shunt for Budd-Chiari syndrome after failure of surgical shunting. Arch Surg 130: 227-228.

Rossi P, et al, 1981: CT diagnosis of Budd-Chiari syndrome. J Comput Assist Tomogr 5:366-369.

Rössle M, et al, 1998: The first decade of the transjugular intrahepatic portosystemic shunt (TIPS): state of the art. Liver 18:73-89.

Rössle M, et al, 2004: The Budd-Chiari syndrome: outcome after treatment with the transjugular intrahepatic portosystemic shunt. Surgery 135:394-403.

Safouh M, Shehata AH, 1965: Hepatic vein occlusion disease of Egyptian children. J Pediatr 67:415-422.

Sakai Y, Wall WJ, 1991: Liver transplantation for Budd-Chiari syndrome. In Proceedings of the Second International Symposium on Budd-Chiari Syndrome, Kyoto, Japan, VIPa-4.

Sakai Y, Wall WJ, 1994: Liver transplantation for Budd-Chiari syndrome: a retrospective study. Jpn J Surg 24:49-53.

Salat C, et al, 1997a: Plasminogen activator inhibitor-1 confirms the diagnosis of hepatic veno-occlusive disease in patients with hyperbilirubinemia after bone marrow transplantation. Blood 89:2184-2188.

Salat C, et al, 1997b: Laboratory markers of veno-occlusive disease in the course of bone marrow and subsequent liver transplantation. Bone Marrow Transplant 19:487-490.

Sato M, et al, 1990: Percutaneous transluminal angioplasty in segmental obstruction of the hepatic inferior vena cava: long-term results. Cardiovasc Interv Radiol 13:189-192.

Sawada S, et al, 1991: Budd-Chiari syndrome treated by interventional radiology including percutaneous transluminal angioplasty and self-expandable metallic stent placement. In Proceedings of the Second International Symposium on Budd-Chiari Syndrome, Kyoto, Japan, Ipa-3.

Scharschmidt BF, 1984: Human liver transplantation: analysis of data of 540 patients from four centers. Hepatology 4 (suppl):95-101.

Schenker S, 1984: Medical treatment vs. transplantation in liver disorders. Hepatology 4:102S-106S.

Schlitt HJ, et al, 1995: Allogeneic liver transplantation for hepatic veno-occlusive disease after bone marrow transplantation—clinical and immunologic considerations. Bone Marrow Transplant 16:473-478.

Schramek A, et al, 1974: New observations in the clinical spectrum of the Budd-Chiari syndrome. Ann Surg 180:368-372.

Schrieber JT, Gonzalez LL, 1967: Thrombosis of hepatic veins and inferior vena cava: relief by thoracic transposition of spleen. Am J Surg 113:807-811.

Semson IW, 1982: Membranous obstruction of the inferior vena cava and hepatocellular carcinoma in South Africa. Gastroenterology 82:171-178.

Senning A, 1981: Budd-Chiari syndrome: Beitrag zur chirurgischen Therapie. Schweiz Med Wochenscr 111:2036-2039.

Senning A, 1983: Transcaval posterocranial resection of the liver as treatment of the Budd-Chiari syndrome. World J Surg 7:632-640.

Senning A, 1987: The cardiovascular surgeon and the liver. J Thorac Cardiovasc Surg 93:1-10.

Shaked A, et al, 1992: Portosystemic shunt versus orthotopic liver transplantation for the Budd-Chiari syndrome. Surg Gynecol Obstet 174:453-459.

Sharma S, et al, 1992: Percutaneous balloon membranotomy combined with prolonged streptokinase infusion for management of inferior vena cava obstruction. Am Heart J 123:515-518.

Shulman HM, et al, 1987: Hepatic veno-occlusive disease after bone marrow transplantation: immunohistochemical identification of the material within occluded central venules. Am J Pathol 127:549-558.

Shulman HM, et al, 1994: Veno-occlusive disease of the liver after marrow transplantation: histological correlates of clinical signs and symptoms. Hepatology 19:1171-1181.

Shulman HM, et al, 1995: Utility of transvenous liver biopsies and wedged hepatic venous pressure measurements in sixty marrow transplant recipients. Transplantation 59:1015-1022.

Slakey DP, et al, 2001: Budd-Chiari syndrome: current management options. Ann Surg 233:522-527.

Smith FO, et al, 1996: Transjugular intrahepatic portosystemic shunting (TIPS) for treatment of severe hepatic veno-occlusive disease. Bone Marrow Transplant 18:643-646.

Smith RB, et al, 1980: Dacron interposition shunts for portal hypertension: an analysis of morbidity correlates. Ann Surg 192:9-17.

Srinivasan P, et al, 2002: Liver transplantation for Budd-Chiari syndrome. Transplantation 73:973-977.

Steenkamp V, et al, 2000: Clinical and analytical aspects of pyrrolizidine poisoning caused by South African traditional medicines. Ther Drug Monit 22:302-306.

Stillman AE, et al, 1977: Hepatic veno-occlusive disease due to pyrrolizidine (Senecio) poisoning in Arizona. Gastroenterology 79:349-352.

Strauch GO, 1970: Subdiaphragmatic splenic transposition: a successful option in the treatment of Chiari's disease. Am J Surg 199:379-384.

Stringer MD, et al, 1989: Mesoatrial shunt: a surgical option in the management of the Budd-Chiari syndrome. Br J Surg 76:474-478.

Stuart KL, Bras G, 1957: Veno-occlusive disease of the liver. QJM 26:291-315.

Suchato C, et al, 1976: Suprahepatic membranous obstruction of vena cava. Can Assoc Radiol J 26:148-149.

Svensson PJ, Dahlback B, 1994: Resistance to activated protein C as a basis for venous thrombosis. N Engl J Med 330:517-522.

Sweat ER, et al, 1966: Production of hepatic outflow block and ascites with an ameroid constrictor. Surg Forum 17:376-378.

Takeuchi J, et al, 1971: Budd-Chiari syndrome associated with obstruction of the inferior vena cava. Am J Med 5:11-20.

Tamaki A, et al, 1968: Effects of side-to-side portacaval shunt on hepatic hemodynamics and metabolism. Surg Forum 19:324-326.

Tandon BN, et al, 1976: An epidemic of veno-occlusive disease of liver in central India. Lancet 2:271-272.

Taneja A, et al, 1979: Budd-Chiari syndrome in childhood secondary to inferior vena caval obstruction. Pediatrics 63:808-812.

Tang TJ, et al, 2001: The prognostic value of histology in the assessment of patients with Budd-Chiari syndrome. J Hepatol 35:338-343.

Tavill AS, et al, 1975: The Budd-Chiari syndrome: correlation between hepatic scintigraphy and the clinical, radiological and pathological findings in nineteen cases of hepatic venous outflow obstruction. Gastroenterology 63:509-518.

Taylor WJ, Myers JD, 1956: Occlusive hepatic venous catheterization in the study of the normal liver, cirrhosis of the liver and noncirrhotic portal hypertension. Circulation 13:368-380.

Terpstra OT, et al, 1987: Late results of mesocaval interposition shunting for bleeding oesophageal varices. Br J Surg 74:787-780.

Thijs LG, et al, 1978: The use of nuclear medicine procedures in the diagnosis of Budd-Chiari syndrome. Clin Nucl Med 3:389-392.

Turrion VS, et al, 1991: Retrospective evaluation of liver transplantation for cirrhosis: a comparative study of 100 patients with or without previous porto-systemic shunt. Transplant Proc 23:1570-1571.

Tyagi S, et al, 1996: Balloon dilatation of inferior vena cava stenosis in Budd-Chiari syndrome. J Assoc Physicians India 4:378-380.

Uhl MD, et al, 1996: Transjugular intrahepatic portosystemic shunt (TIPS) for Budd-Chiari syndrome. Dig Dis Sci 41:1494-1499.

Valla D-C, 2003: The diagnosis and management of the Budd-Chiari syndrome: consensus and controversies. Hepatology 38:793-803.

Valla D, et al, 1986: Risk of hepatic vein thrombosis in relation to recent use of oral contraceptives. Gastroenterology 90:807-811.

Valla D, et al, 1987: Hepatic vein thrombosis in paroxysmal nocturnal hemoglobinuria: a spectrum from asymptomatic occlusion of hepatic venules to fatal Budd-Chiari syndrome. Gastroenterology 93:569-575.

Vandenbroucke JP, et al, 1994: Increased incidence of venous thrombosis in oral contraceptive users who are carriers of factor V Leiden mutation. Lancet 344:1453-1457.

Victor S, et al, 1994: Budd-Chiari syndrome and pericaval filariasis. Trop Gastroenterol 15:161-168.

Vogelzang R, et al, 1987: Budd-Chiari syndrome CT observations. Radiology 163:329-333.

Vons C, et al, 1986: Results of portal systemic shunts in Budd-Chiari syndrome. Ann Surg 203:366-370.

Wadleigh M, et al, 2003: Hepatic veno-occlusive disease: pathogenesis, diagnosis and treatment. Curr Opin Hematol 10:451-462.

Wang Z, 1989: Recognition and management of Budd-Chiari syndrome: experience with 143 patients. Chin Med J 102:338-346.

Wang Z, et al, 1989: Recognition and management of Budd-Chiari syndrome: report of one hundred cases. J Vasc Surg 10:149-156.

Warren RL, et al, 1972: Treatment of Budd-Chiari syndrome with streptokinase. Gastroenterology 62:200 (abstract).

Warren WD, Muller WH Jr, 1959: A clarification of some hemodynamic changes in cirrhosis and their surgical significance. Ann Surg 150:413-427.

Wu T, et al, 1990: Budd-Chiari syndrome: surgical treatment of 45 cases. Chin Med J 103:400-405.

Wu T, et al, 2002: Percutaneous balloon angioplasty of inferior vena cava in Budd-Chiari syndrome. Int J Cardiol 83:175-178.

Xu K, et al, 1996: Budd-Chiari syndrome caused by obstruction of the hepatic inferior vena cava: immediate and 2-year treatment results of transluminal angioplasty and metallic stent placement. Cardiovasc Interv Radiol 19:32-36.

Yamada R, et al, 1983: Segmental obstruction of the hepatic inferior vena cava treated by transluminal angioplasty. Radiology 149:91-96.

Yamada R, et al, 1991: Percutaneous transluminal angioplasty in the treatment of Budd-Chiari syndrome: twelve years' results and new devices. In Proceedings of the Second International Symposium on Budd-Chiari Syndrome, Kyoto, Japan, IPL-2.

Yamamoto S, et al, 1968: Budd-Chiari syndrome with obstruction of the inferior vena cava. Gastroenterology 54:1070-1084.

Yang X-L, et al, 1996: Successful treatment by percutaneous balloon angioplasty of Budd-Chiari syndrome caused by membranous obstruction of inferior vena cava: 8-year follow-up study. J Am Coll Cardiol 28:1720-1724.

Zafrani ES, et al, 1983: Drug-induced vascular lesions of the liver. Arch Intern Med 143:495-502.

Zeitoun G, et al, 1999: Outcome of Budd-Chiari syndrome: a multivariate analysis of factors related to survival including surgical portosystemic shunting. Hepatology 30:84-89.

Zhang C, et al, 1999: Ultrasonically guided inferior vena cava stent placement: experience in 83 cases. J Vasc Interv Radiol 10:85-91.

Zuckerman M, et al, 2002: Hepatic veno-occlusive disease as a result of a traditional remedy: confirmation of toxic pyrrolizidine alkaloids as the cause, using an in vitro technique. J Clin Pathol 55:676-682.

Liver and Pancreatic Transplantation

101

Liver and Pancreatic Transplantation Immunobiology

K. K. DHANIREDDY AND A. D. KIRK

Allotransplantation, the transfer of tissues between genetically nonidentical individuals, has been shown to provide relief from incurable liver diseases and type 1 diabetes. Transplanted organs are invariably destroyed through a process broadly known as *rejection*, however, unless some modification of the recipient immune system is made. Over the past 4 decades, the ability to manipulate the immune response has become increasingly selective and less morbid. Through a general understanding of alloimmunity and the unique properties of the liver and pancreas, transplantation results have steadily improved (OPTN/SRTR, 2003). This chapter provides an overview of the principles governing immune management of liver and pancreatic transplant recipients, highlighting the agents and strategies that are generally available for clinical use.

GENERAL CONSIDERATIONS: SPECIFICITY AND CONTEXT

Allograft rejection is mediated by the elements of physiologic immunity, but stems from a nonphysiologic practice—transplantation. Similar to most immune responses, rejection requires a recognition event and a context that signifies that this recognition warrants a response. Immune recognition is mediated through one of two types of lymphocyte receptors: the T cell receptor (TCR) or immunoglobulin. Immune specificity is dictated by the ability of these receptors to bind a suitably complementary epitope.

The recognition of cell-based antigens is governed by a cluster of highly polymorphic genes on chromosome 6 known as the *major histocompatibility complex* (MHC) (or human leukocyte antigen in humans). Proteins produced from polymorphic genes have the same basic structure, but differ in detail. The role of these molecules differs between physiologic and transplant immunity, as described subsequently.

The context of an immune response is governed through another set of receptors known as *costimulation receptors*. Broadly speaking, these receptors provide signals that determine whether antigen recognition should evoke an immune response, and whether that response should be aggressive or attenuating. By separating the signals for specificity and appropriateness, the immune response to pathogens and allografts can be tightly regulated and finely manipulated.

Typically, the ligands for costimulation receptors are expressed most prominently on professional antigen-presenting cells (APCs). The role of these cells is to initiate and sustain an immune response. The interactions between APCs and lymphocytes usually occur in lymphoid organs, such as the spleen or lymph nodes. The requirement for APCs and the necessity for secondary lymphoid organs provide additional opportunities for regulation and lessen the chance for autoimmune responses.

PHYSIOLOGIC IMMUNITY

The immune system developed to protect individuals from pathogens, not to mediate transplant rejection. Although alloimmunity and physiologic immunity differ, it is crucial to understand the components of alloimmunity in their physiologic roles. The immune system typically is divided into two complementary arms: innate and acquired. The innate immune system recognizes general motifs that universally represent pathologic states, such as ischemia, necrosis, trauma, and nonhuman cell surfaces (Dempsey et al, 1996; Fearon & Locksley, 1996). The acquired immune system distinguishes specific pathogens through antigen presentation and recognition. Both systems interact to maintain overall homeostasis. Typically, innate responses localize acquired responses to sites of pathologic processes and are less overtly regulated. In contrast, acquired immune responses lead to carefully regulated destruction of antigen-expressing tissue. The regulatory checks on acquired immunity prevent autoimmunity and uncontrolled lymphocyte proliferation. The acquired immune system is tailored for one individual based on his or her MHC makeup. Evolutionarily, this diversity reduces the chance that any single pathogen can evade all individuals within a population. This diversity also means, however, that one individual's acquired immune response may not respond appropriately when placed in the context of another individual's MHC.

Innate Immunity

Receptors of innate immunity are cell bound on macrophages, neutrophils, and natural killer cells and circulate freely in the form of complement (Dempsey et al, 1996; Fearon & Locksley, 1996; Wright et al, 1990). Innate immunity is limited in specificity, retaining broad reactivity to components of pathogenic organisms, such as lipopolysaccharides. Importantly, the receptors of innate immunity are conserved between individuals and in general function similarly in physiologic and transplant situations. When activated, the innate immune system initiates cytolytic pathways and recruits the acquired immune response. The complement cascade is the primary mediator of cytolysis, and the by-products of complement, along with phagocytic cells, signal initiation of acquired immunity (Baldwin et al, 1995).

Professional APCs engulf not only cells coated with complement, but also cells bearing foreign carbohydrate moieties (Hart, 1997). Toll-like receptors have been recognized as important for innate APC activation. This highly conserved family of receptors binds to pathogen-associated molecular pattern motifs commonly expressed on invading pathogenic organisms (Akira & Takeda, 2004). Engulfed cells are processed by the APC into protein fragments and expressed on the cell surface bound to MHC molecules. Subsequently, T cells that are specific for these peptides can recognize their cognate antigens and become activated. The toll-like receptors expressed in the liver differ from the receptors expressed in the periphery and tend to be less responsive to ambient lipopolysaccharide (De Creus et al, 2005). This difference is likely an adaptation to portal bacteremia and is thought to make the liver more tolerant of minor perturbations that would evoke an innate response in other organs.

Acquired Immunity

Specific recognition is the hallmark of the acquired immune system. The lymphocyte receptors (TCR and antibody) have evolved to distinguish an extremely diverse group of antigens. Antigen recognition induces physiologic changes in the recognizing cell, which lowers its threshold for subsequent encounters and leads to a phenomenon of immunologic memory—the more rapid response to subsequent antigen encounters (Ahmed & Gray, 1996). TCRs bind peptide antigens that have been processed and presented in combination with MHC, whereas B cell immunoglobulins bind antigens in their native conformation at a site remote from the B cell.

Cellular Immunity

Formation of the TCR is fundamental to understanding its function (Cooper, 1987; Davis & Bjorkman, 1988). T cells are formed in the bone marrow and fetal liver and migrate to the thymus during development. After entering the thymus, T cells undergo rearrangement of the DNA that encodes the TCR (Gill & Gulley, 1994). Each gene rearrangement results in generation of a TCR with specificity restricted to one epitope (or structurally similar epitopes). The sum of all random TCR gene rearrangements generates TCRs with approximately 10^9 specificities, essentially all possible combinations of MHC and peptide antigen. If these T cells were released into the periphery, they would mediate fatal autoimmunity. Accordingly, thymic selection eliminates the cells likely to evoke autoimmunity (Bevan, 1997; Kappler et al, 1987).

The initial phase of thymic selection is the interaction of developing T cells with the MHC-expressing cortical thymic epithelium. These T cells express the accessory cell surface markers CD4 and CD8, which allow for stronger TCR binding to MHC. If binding does not occur to self-MHC, the cells are eliminated because they would be nonfunctional in the periphery. This process is known as *positive selection*. All surviving T cells bind to self-MHC. The developing T cells move into the thymic medulla, where either CD4 or CD8 expression is lost. If binding to the self-MHC in the medulla results in a high-affinity interaction, these T cells also are eliminated. This process is known as *negative selection*. Most cells released from the thymus bind to self-MHC without becoming activated. Autoreactive cells occasionally escape thymic selection, however, and cause diseases such as sclerosing cholangitis, autoimmune hepatitis,

and type 1 diabetes. Additional regulation is required to prevent autoimmunity. A single interaction of TCR and antigen-bearing MHC is inadequate to trigger T cell activation. Approximately 8000 TCR-MHC interactions occur over several hours to initiate activation (Kumagai et al, 1987; Rothenberg, 1996; Viola & Lanzavecchia, 1996); this further limits the likelihood of autoimmunity.

Immune responses also are regulated by accessory cell surface molecules that limit the types of cells with which a T cell interacts (Leahy et al, 1992; Saizawa et al, 1987). Parenchymal cells of the body express class I MHC and display internal cellular peptides within the binding groove of this molecule. T cells charged with destruction of diseased or infected parenchymal cells express CD8, which stabilizes TCR ligation with class I MHC. These cells are termed *cytotoxic T cells*. CD8+ T cell killing can occur through Ca^{2+}-dependent secretory mechanisms or Ca^{2+}-independent direct cell contact mechanisms (Berke, 1995).

Hematopoietic cells express class I and class II MHC. Class II MHC displays peptide fragments that have been phagocytized from the extracellular space (Germain, 1994; Monaco, 1993). CD4 stabilizes the TCR–class II MHC interaction. CD4+ cells interact with dendritic cells, macrophages, and in some cases activated endothelial cells that display antigen. In addition, the resting sinusoidal endothelial cells of the liver have the ability to present antigen to T cells, making the liver an organ with considerable ability to evoke or suppress an immune response (Knolle & Gerken, 2000). The interaction between CD4+ T cells and APCs produces APCs that have the ability to martial CD8+ T cells (Lanzavecchia, 1998; Ridge et al, 1998). This process is mediated through upregulation of APC cell surface molecules known as *costimulation receptors*. APCs initiate an immune response, but require CD4+ T cells to activate the primary effector arm of the acquired immune system, CD8+ T cells.

An additional subset of T cells, regulatory T cells, further control promiscuous immune responses. Regulatory T cells have the ability to suppress cytokine secretion, adhesion molecule expression, and costimulatory signaling. The most extensively studied population of regulatory T cells expresses CD4 and CD25, the high affinity α chain of the interleukin (IL)-2 receptor (Wood & Sakaguchi, 2003). Based on animal models, it was suggested that these cells play a crucial role in controlling immune activation (Baecher-Allan et al, 2001; Wood & Sakaguchi, 2003). Harnessing the power of regulatory T cells to quell counteradaptive immune response is an ongoing area of research in autoimmunity and alloimmunity.

Humoral Immunity

B cells recognize antigen in its native unprocessed form (Cambier et al, 1994). When antigen binds to two cell surface antibodies, the antibodies are brought together in a process known as *cross-linking*. This cross-linking stimulates B cell proliferation and differentiation into an antibody-secreting plasma cell. The activation threshold for a resting B cell is relatively high, as it is for T cells. Costimulation through the CD19-CD21 complex can lower this threshold 100-fold (Tedder et al, 1994). B cells also have the ability to internalize antigen bound to surface immunoglobulins and process them for presentation to T cells along with costimulation molecules (Lederman et al, 1992).

Antibody structure is determined in the bone marrow through mechanisms similar to the mechanisms that govern the generation of TCR diversity in the thymus (Gill & Gulley, 1994; Hozumi & Tonegawa, 1976). Five different heavy chain loci (μ, γ, α, ε, and δ) on chromosome 14 and 2 different light chain loci (κ and λ) on chromosome 2, each with V, D, or J (or both), and C regions, are brought together randomly by the RAG-1 and RAG-2 apparatus to form a functional antigen receptor (Kim et al, 2000). The basic antibody structure consists of two identical heavy chains and two identical light chains. The type of heavy chain used dictates the immunoglobulin type: IgM, IgG, IgA, IgE, or IgD. The overall structure of the antibody results in two identical antigen binding sites and a common region, the Fc portion. Bound antibody triggers activation of the complement cascade (Baldwin et al, 1995). In addition, most phagocytic cells have receptors for the Fc portion of IgG, allowing them to engulf actively antibody-coated cells.

In contrast to the TCR, B cell immunoglobulin loci undergo alteration after B cell stimulation to improve the functionality of the secreted antibody. Isotype switching is the process of shifting from the initial heavy chain IgM to one of four types to improve function and specialization. IgG is the most significant soluble mediator of opsonization and the dominant antibody produced in response to alloantigen. IgA is important in mucosal immunity, IgE is involved in mast cell–mediated immunity, and IgD is primarily cell bound. After a B cell is activated, the specific D and J regions of the used heavy and light chain genes undergo random alterations of the antigen binding site. The resultant

B cell clones have altered antigen affinity—hence the term *affinity maturation* (Griffiths et al, 1984). The clones that have higher affinity for the target antigen have a selective survival advantage and form the basis for a more vigorous response on re-exposure to the antigen.

Mediators of Context—Costimulation and Cytokines

TCR binding with an MHC-peptide complex usually is insufficient for T cell activation. Receptor-ligand pairs on the T cell and APC, known as *costimulation receptors*, determine the character of the T cell response (Fig. 101.1) (Allison & Krummel, 1995; Chambers & Allison, 1997). The type of costimulatory signal received by the T cell determines whether the cell becomes activated, remains quiescent, dies, or becomes resistant to subsequent immune stimulation. Examples of T cell costimulation receptors include CD28 and CTLA4 (CD152). CD28 promotes T cell activation and leads to the expression of CTLA4, which promotes downregulation of the T cell response. Activation typically begets deactivation. The B7 molecules (CD80 and CD86) are the ligands for CD28 and CTLA4 on professional APCs. Although B7 can bind to either receptor, its affinity for CTLA4 is much greater. When B7 is in limited supply, the higher affinity interaction with CTLA4 predominates. Because B7 molecules are not expressed by normal tissues,

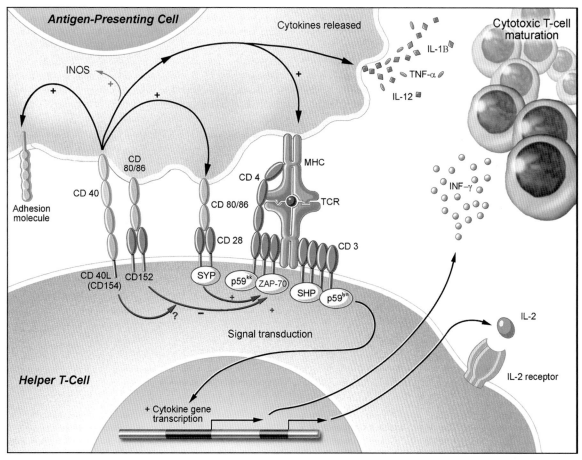

Fig. 101.1. T cell interactions with an APC. The TCR is bound to class II MHC with the CD4 accessory molecule stabilizing the interaction. Depicted are selected costimulatory molecule interactions and the resultant effects on cytokine secretion and signal transduction. CD40 ligation on the APC results in the induction of many crucial APC functions, including increased MHC and B7 expression and cytokine secretion. Increased B7 expression allows CD28+ regulation to override the negative regulation of CD152 (CTLA4). This potentiates TCR signal transduction through CD3 and results in IFN-γ and IL-2 synthesis. IFN-γ, along with APC secreted cytokines, promotes cytotoxic T cell maturation. IL-2 promotes T cell proliferation in an autocrine fashion.

CD8+ T cell interaction with class I self-MHC does not elicit a proliferative response; rather it reinforces quiescence of autoreactive T cell clones. In the absence of activated APCs presenting antigen in the context of high cell surface concentrations of costimulatory molecules, T cell activity is typically suppressed.

Although the mechanisms of costimulation have not been completely elucidated, it is known that binding of CD28 allows more efficient T cell signal transduction. Through CD28-B7 interactions, the number of binding events required to trigger activation of a T cell decreases from 8000 to 1500 (Rothenberg, 1996; Viola & Lanzavecchia, 1996). In contrast, when CTLA4 binds B7, the T cell becomes incapable of producing IL-2 during the encounter and in subsequent interactions (Blair et al, 1998).

Additionally, costimulation is mediated through another pair of receptors: CD40 found on dendritic cells, endothelium, and other APCs and CD154 found on T cells (Larsen & Pearson, 1997). The ability for APCs to stimulate a cytotoxic T cell response depends on CD40 binding. After CD40 ligation, activating cytokines are released, and B7 molecules are upregulated (Bennett et al, 1998; Schoenberger et al, 1998). CD154 is upregulated after TCR ligation and provides positive feedback to the APC. In addition, CD154 is found in and released by activated platelets at sites of endothelial injury (Henn et al, 1998). Sites of trauma that recruit platelets create an environment of activating costimulatory molecules, bridging the innate and acquired immune systems (Czapiga et al, 2004).

Direct cell-cell contact is not the only means by which immune cells communicate. Soluble mediators of communication known as *cytokines*, also known as *interleukins*, are polypeptides that are released from many cells and can activate or suppress adjacent cells (Arai et al, 1990). The pattern of cytokine expression is thought to influence the resultant type of T cell response (Mosmann, 1991; Mosmann et al, 1986). When activated, T cells have been described by one of two cytokine secretion phenotypes. Cytotoxic T cell responses are characterized by expression of IL-2, IL-12, IL-15, and interferon (IFN)-γ and are known as *Th1 cells*. T cells promoting humoral or eosinophilic responses are characterized by secretion of IL-4, IL-5, IL-10, and IL-13 and are known as *Th2 cells*. In addition to cytokines, other soluble mediators of inflammation are capable of promoting increased blood flow and improved exposure of an area of injury to innate and acquired immune elements. It has been suggested that the APCs of the liver are more efficient in generating Th2 responses, and that this may be a mechanism by which liver allografts avoid late cellular rejection.

TRANSPLANT IMMUNITY

T cell responses to allogeneic organs are largely the result of nonphysiologic TCR-MHC interactions. T cells are selected initially to bind to self-MHC and eliminated if that binding event leads to activation. This sequence of events does not preclude, however, the survival of cells that, through chance, bind to other individuals' MHC molecules and do so with inappropriate affinity. The discrepancies between self-TCR selection and allogeneic-MHC interactions are the basis for most of transplant recognition. This nonphysiologic recognition provides the opportunity for a detrimental immune response, but does not mandate it in the absence of additional contextual requirements for immunity such as costimulation. Alloimmunity is more likely than autoimmunity, but is not mandated in the absence of

costimulation, innate immunity, and other factors that spur a physiologic immune response.

Most of the significant sequence polymorphism of MHC is located in the areas of the molecule that interact with the TCR. Individual variation in the sequence at the MHC-TCR interface defines alloreactivity. The lack of recipient T cell thymic education with donor MHC leads to a nonphysiologically high frequency of alloreactive peripheral T cells. Many of these cells are cross-reactive with antigen seen during prior viral exposures or even autoantigens in the case of autoimmune disease. This is known as *heterologous immunity* and results in a situation whereby recipients have allospecific memory without having been exposed to the alloantigen (Adams et al, 2003). One's immune response to a donor is the product of one's MHC makeup and one's past immune exposures; this can lead to vigorous early rejection in apparently nonsensitized recipients.

T cells recognize alloantigen via their TCR in two distinct ways: (1) directly by binding to donor MHC on transplanted tissues in the presence of donor costimulation or (2) indirectly through self-APCs that have phagocytized and processed alloantigens to be presented bound to self-MHC and costimulation (Rogers & Lechler, 2001). In the case of transplanted organs, surgical trauma and ischemia exacerbate the potential for T cell activation by causing class I and class II MHC upregulation (Gerritsen & Bloor, 1993). In addition, adhesion molecules and costimulation molecules are upregulated perioperatively (Takada et al, 1997).

Initial T cell binding to donor cells is nonspecific and mediated by adhesion molecules upregulated during donor cell activation (Fuggle & Koo, 1998). CD40 on donor APCs and endothelial cells is important in mediating cell activation in this setting via CD154 on T cells and activated platelets (Henn et al, 1998). After nonspecific adhesion, MHC recognition occurs in the relatively high costimulation environment induced by surgical trauma and ischemia (Takada et al, 1997). When alloreactive T cells are activated, they secrete cytokines, including IL-2 and IFN-γ, and stimulate APCs to secrete IL-12 (Arai et al, 1990; Kirk et al, 1995; Krams et al, 1992). The resultant cytokine milieu recruits more T cells to the site of injury and potentiates clonal expansion. Secretory and cell contact–dependent mechanisms—perforin/granzyme and Fas mechanisms, respectively—are involved in T cell cytotoxicity within the graft resulting in graft destruction (Strehlau et al, 1997). Although acute rejection is the result of T cell activation, antibody responses accompany most episodes. Cellular and soluble components of immunity mediate multiple distinct clinical rejection syndromes through cytokine-mediated toxicity, cellular cytotoxicity, and direct effects of antibody and complement.

Clinical Rejection Syndromes

Hyperacute Rejection

Hyperacute rejection is caused by donor-specific antibody that exists at the time of transplantation as a result of prior exposure to donor antigens or to antigens with cross-reactivity. It develops precipitously within minutes to hours after graft reperfusion. Typically, hyperacute rejection is avoided by confirming ABO compatibility and performing a crossmatch, techniques that detect donor-specific antibodies. When clinically relevant donor-specific antibodies are detected, graft survival is significantly decreased (Noreen et al, 2003). The liver has long been regarded as relatively resistant to hyperacute rejection, and cross-matching is often done only retrospectively (Neumann et al, 2001). The rates of acute rejection and long-term liver survival are similar between groups with a positive or negative cross-match; this does not hold true for ABO-incompatible liver allografts (Egawa et al, 2004). The pancreas does not have similar resistance to hyperacute rejection, and a positive crossmatch represents an absolute contraindication to pancreatic transplantation. Although high titer antibodies mediate rapid graft injury, chronic exposure to lower titer antibody results in indolent graft damage, particularly in the case of the pancreas. The role of chronic alloantibody in liver transplantation is controversial, but likely mediates some degree of graft injury over time.

Acute Rejection

Acute rejection is most common 4 days to 6 months after transplantation, but can occur at any time late after transplantation, particularly in the setting of patient drug noncompliance. Liver allografts undergo acute rejection at a rate of approximately 24% to 47% (Fisher et al, 2004; Neuhaus et al, 2002; Wiesner et al, 2001). Pancreas allografts in the modern era (after 1995) undergo acute rejection at a rate of approximately 15% to 30%. These differences reflect a tendency toward less immunosuppression in liver patients because the liver can regenerate after rejection. Also, liver rejection is diagnosed more easily than pancreas rejection through biopsy and serum enzyme measurements. In both organs, acute rejection evolves over days to weeks. After activation by direct or indirect allorecognition, T cells infiltrate the allograft and initiate organ destruction through cytolysis and endothelial and ductular damage. Usually, acute liver allograft rejection also is accompanied by graft and peripheral eosinophilia (Barnes et al, 2003). The early detection of acute rejection is crucial. Unexplained hepatic dysfunction should prompt a graft biopsy. In the case of pancreas allografts, there is usually no direct biochemical evidence of rejection. If the transplant was performed with a kidney, rejection of the kidney precedes or signals concomitant pancreas rejection in approximately 80% of cases. In pancreas alone transplants, fever, abdominal pain, allograft tenderness, and hyperamylasemia may be signs of rejection. Many rejections occur without early symptoms, however (Stratta et al, 1996). Hyperglycemia is a late complication in pancreas rejection because the parenchyma rejects before the islet tissue.

Prompt recognition of acute rejection is imperative. Prolonged rejection allows for recruitment of multiple arms of the immune system and consequently decreased efficacy of antirejection therapies directed against T cell responses. T cell–specific therapies can resolve acute rejection episodes in most cases. Steroids are the first-line agent in most centers. Typically, early acute rejection episodes have a negative impact on the long-term survival of an allograft, although the liver is relatively resistant to this effect (Dousset et al, 1998).

Chronic Graft Loss

The causes of chronic graft loss are poorly characterized (Libby & Pober, 2001). Although called chronic rejection, it likely has nonimmune components and immune origins. Evolving over the course of months to years, chronic graft dysfunction remains resistant to conventional immunosuppressive therapies and, regardless of the transplanted organ, develops as fibrosis with modest lymphocytic infiltration. Monocytic and dendritic cell infiltrates predominate with progressive destruction of epithelial and endothelial structures. Many aspects of chronic graft loss relate to the events surrounding transplantation, such as ischemic injury. In the liver, chronic graft loss manifests as ductopenia or vanishing bile duct syndrome (Inomata & Tanaka, 2001). Typically, vanishing bile duct syndrome is defined as less than 50% of portal triads containing bile ducts (Demetris et al, 1998). The rate of chronic graft loss is far slower for liver grafts than other organs, likely because of the ability of the liver to regenerate after subtle injury. As the technical challenges of pancreatic transplantation have been met, more grafts are being lost to chronic rejection (Humar et al, 2003).

IMMUNOSUPPRESSION

To date, no single agent has been discovered that by itself effectively prevents allograft rejection. Similarly, all manipulations that limit rejection also increase susceptibility to infection and malignancy. No immunosuppressant is allograft specific. The rational selection of immunosuppressants involves employing multiple synergistic agents to prevent rejection without simultaneously crippling the recipient's defenses. Characteristically, liver allografts typically need less immunosuppression than other organs (Ramos et al, 1995). This need for less immunosuppression has been proposed to be a function of the APCs in the liver, its shear size and antigenic load, and its regenerative capacity.

The immune system is most primed to reject an allograft perioperatively because of the surgical and ischemic injury associated with transplantation. The most intense immunosuppression is given during the weeks that follow transplantation. A period of rigorous immunosuppression at the time of transplant is known as *induction therapy*. Typically, this therapy consists of T cell–depleting strategies that, although effective, are too toxic to be administered long-term. Maintenance immunosuppression is less potent, but can be given long-term to prevent acute rejection for the life of the transplant patient. Finally, agents used to halt ongoing rejection are known as *rescue agents*. The sites of action of various immunosuppressive agents are illustrated in Fig. 101.2.

Corticosteroids

Corticosteroids have been a mainstay of transplant immunosuppression since the 1960s (Starzl et al, 1963). At low doses, glucocorticosteroids, typically prednisone or methylprednisolone, are used as maintenance immunosuppression. At higher doses, they can be used as rescue therapy. Although steroids are ineffective as monotherapy to prevent rejection, they have been combined effectively with other agents to improve graft survival. The desirable immunosuppressive effects of steroids are counterbalanced by their contribution to transplant morbidity. Many ongoing efforts have sought to minimize or eliminate glucocorticosteroid use for maintenance immunosuppression. Many centers now rapidly wean steroids from liver allograft recipients. Most pancreas programs rely on low-dose steroids indefinitely.

The mechanism of glucocorticosteroids has been elucidated only more recently (Auphan et al, 1995; Scheinman et al, 1995). After nonspecific cytoplasmic uptake, steroids bind to an intracellular receptor, enter the nucleus as a receptor-ligand pair, and increase the transcription of several genes, notably IκBα. This protein binds to and inactivates nuclear factor κB (NFκB),

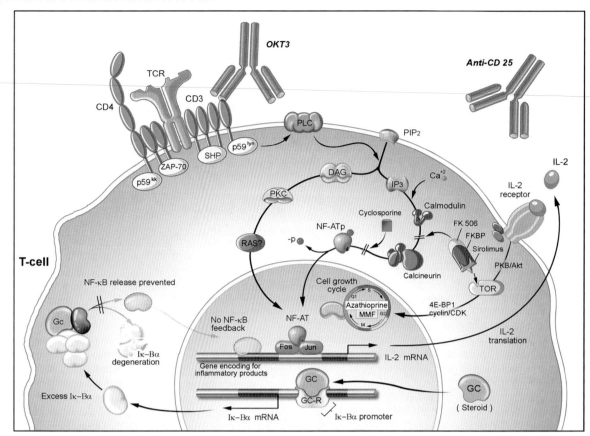

Fig. 101.2. TCR signal transduction and the sites of action of various immunosuppressants. TCR signal transduction proceeds through Ca^{2+}-dependent dephosphorylation of NF-AT. NF-AT enters the nucleus and, in conjunction NFκB, facilitates cytokine gene expression. Cyclosporine and tacrolimus (FK506) inhibit signal transduction by blocking the ability of the calcineurin-calmodulin complex to potentiate NF-AT dephosphorylation. The autocrine activity of IL-2 facilitates entry into the cell cycle and cell division. Sirolimus inhibits IL-2 receptor signal transduction by blocking the interactions of immunophilin FKBP12. Mycophenolate mofetil and azathioprine prevent cell cycling by altering nucleic acid metabolism. Steroids upregulate IκBα synthesis and inhibit the ability of NFκB to enter the nucleus. Monoclonal antibodies bind T cell surface molecules and alter key interactions necessary for T cell function.

an important transcription factor of T cell and APC activation and cytokine production. The NFκB pathway is an important amplification step in the T cell and APC response; blockade of this pathway results in diverse effects. Steroids decrease IL-1, tumor necrosis factor-α, and IFN-γ transcription and MHC upregulation. Inhibition of phospholipase A_2 results in blockade of the entire arachidonic acid cascade. Steroids mute the entire inflammatory process and decrease the costimulatory environment. They also promote apoptosis of activated T cells and limit the signal transduction of many innate immune receptors, such as the toll-like receptors.

Antiproliferative Agents

Azathioprine

The antimetabolite azathioprine was the first immunosuppressant used in organ transplantation (Calne & Murray, 1961; Hitchings et al, 1950). Azathioprine undergoes hepatic conversion to 6-mercaptopurine and then to 6-thio-inosine-monophosphate. These derivatives alkylate DNA precursors and inhibit DNA synthesis. In addition, they can introduce chromosomal breaks and interfere with DNA repair mechanisms. The ultimate effect is to deplete the cell of adenosine. Azathioprine

works on all rapidly dividing cells, not simply lymphocytes. Consequently, bone marrow, hepatic, and gastrointestinal toxicity are limiting factors. It is ineffective as monotherapy and is decreasingly common in modern transplantation.

Mycophenolate Mofetil

Since 1995, mycophenolate mofetil has been an approved immunosuppressant for use in adults (Platz et al, 1991). Mycophenolate mofetil is a morpholinoethyl ester of mycophenolic acid—a noncompetitive, reversible inhibitor of inosine monophosphate (IMP) dehydrogenase—with improved bioavailability. Mycophenolate mofetil prevents a crucial step in RNA and DNA synthesis by blocking guanosine monophosphate (GMP) formation from IMP by IMP dehydrogenase. In all cells except lymphocytes, there exists a "salvage pathway" for GMP formation. This crucial difference is exploited by mycophenolate mofetil to produce a relatively lymphocyte-specific immunosuppressant. Mycophenolate mofetil blocks the proliferation of T cells and B cells and inhibits the formation of donor-specific antibody. Its introduction dramatically improved the success of pancreatic transplantation and is used as an adjuvant immunosuppressive agent in most pancreas centers. It is also used in liver transplantation, particularly in patients who have experienced repeated rejections.

Calcineurin Inhibitors

Cyclosporine

Cyclosporine is a cyclic endecapeptide isolated from the fungus *Tolypocladium inflatum Gams* (Borel et al, 1976; Kahan, 1994). Its introduction revolutionized transplantation and made extrarenal transplantation a viable reality. The mechanism of action of this T cell–specific immunosuppressant is mediated through cyclophilin binding. The cyclosporine-cyclophilin complex binds to the calcineurin-calmodulin complex and prevents phosphorylation and activation of NF-AT, a transcription regulating factor. Blockade of NF-AT prevents IL-2 gene transcription. Additionally, transforming growth factor (TGF)-β transcription is unregulated, and other genes crucial for T cell activation are altered (Khanna et al, 1996; Kirk et al, 1997). These and other effects may be responsible for the toxicity of cyclosporine. Primarily, cyclosporine blocks TCR signal transduction, but does not inhibit costimulatory signaling (June et al, 1987). The effects of cyclosporine can be overcome with high levels of IL-2, and when IL-2 is present in the graft, as in the case of ongoing rejection, cyclosporine is rendered ineffective. Consequently, cyclosporine is a maintenance immunosuppressant and has no role in rescue therapy.

Cyclosporine nephrotoxicity is a constant consideration in its use. Through a TGF-β–mediated mechanism, cyclosporine decreases renal blood flow by 30% (Khanna et al, 1996; Kirk et al, 1997). Increased transcription of endothelin also activates the renin-angiotensin pathway, leading to hypertension. The vascular effects of cyclosporine also may delay resolution of hepatorenal syndrome. Cyclosporine may lead to neurologic side effects, hypertrichosis, and malignancy (Hojo et al, 1999). Metabolism of cyclosporine through cytochrome P-450 enzymes leads to multiple drug interactions.

Tacrolimus

Kino and associates (1987) first showed the immunosuppressant effects of tacrolimus in 1987, and it has become the mainstay of most liver and pancreatic transplant regimens. Tacrolimus is a macrolide antibiotic produced by *Streptomyces tsukubaensis*. Similar to cyclosporine, tacrolimus blocks NF-AT activation and its downstream effects (Fruman et al, 1992). The intracellular target of tacrolimus is known as FK-binding protein (FKBP). Similar to cyclosporine, tacrolimus increases TGF-β transcription and carries with it the benefits and toxicities of this cytokine (Khanna et al, 1996; Kirk et al, 1997). Although it is 100 times more potent than cyclosporine in preventing IL-2 and IFN-γ transcription, the toxicities of tacrolimus limit the dose to approximately 1% of cyclosporine. In addition to its use as a maintenance agent, tacrolimus has been shown to have efficacy in reversing liver rejection episodes (Starzl et al, 1989).

Compared with cyclosporine, tacrolimus has more pronounced neurologic side effects, such as mental status changes and tremors. Tacrolimus use results in a higher rate of diabetes, but a lower rate of cosmetic side effects. Because tacrolimus is metabolized by cytochrome P-450 enzymes, drug interaction concerns are similar to those with cyclosporine.

mTOR Inhibitors

Sirolimus and everolimus are macrolide antibiotics developed from *Streptomyces hygroscopicus* (Baker et al, 1978; Martel et al, 1977; Sehgal et al, 1975). Similar to tacrolimus, these agents bind to the immunophilin FKBP12, also known as the *mammalian target of rapamycin* (mTOR). In contrast to tacrolimus, these agents do not affect calcineurin activity (Dumont et al, 1990a, 1990b; Molnar-Kimber, 1996). The primary effect of mTOR inhibitors is to inhibit IL-2 receptor signal transduction and not to block NF-AT nuclear translocation. T cells are rendered incompetent to the proliferative effects of exogenous IL-2 (Kuo et al, 1992), but are still capable of IL-2 gene transcription. The primary toxicities of mTOR inhibitors are hypercholesterolemia, hypertriglyceridemia, poor wound healing, thrombocytopenia, and oral ulcers. Currently, sirolimus has a Food and Drug Administration black box warning against its use in liver transplantation because of increased risk of hepatic artery thrombosis. In addition, sirolimus may have a direct hepatotoxic effect (Neff et al, 2004). The principal manner in which mTOR inhibitors are being used is as an adjunct or alternative to calcineurin inhibitors.

Antilymphocyte Agents

Antilymphocyte agents are commonly used in pancreatic transplantation during the induction phase of immunosuppression (Niemeyer et al, 2002; Stratta et al, 2003). Their use in liver transplantation varies owing to the reduced immunogenic phenotype typical of liver grafts.

Antilymphocyte/Antithymocyte Globulin

A polyclonal antilymphocyte globulin (ALG) is produced by inoculating an animal such as a horse or rabbit with human lymphocytes, collecting the serum, and purifying the resultant IgG. This preparation contains antibodies of multiple epitope specificities directed against lymphocyte (and other cell) antigens (Gaber et al, 1998; Merion et al, 1998). In the United States, the common immunogen is thymocytes, and the resultant polyclonal antibody is antithymocyte globulin (ATG). These agents promote T cell depletion through opsonization and complement-mediated lysis (Merion et al, 1998). They also have multiple nondepletional effects that inhibit T cell activation and function, such as cross-linking costimulation and adhesion molecules and blocking TCR signal transduction through internalization of other cell surface receptors. ALG and ATG can be used as induction and rescue agents. The primary function of these agents is to reduce the number of primary effector cells below the threshold required for acute rejection and to allow for slow repopulation after the immediate post-transplant period. Although ATG is generally well tolerated, side effects include thrombocytopenia, increased viral disease, and transient cytokine release.

OKT3

In contrast to polyclonal antibody preparations, monoclonal antibodies have one target epitope specificity. OKT3, a murine antibody directed against the CD3 signal transduction subunit of the TCR, was the first monoclonal antibody approved for any use (muromonab-CD3 [Orthoclone OKT3; Ortho Pharmaceuticals, Raritan, NJ]) (Ortho Multicenter Transplant Study Group, 1985; Wilde & Goa, 1996). OKT3 mediates its effects by binding to CD3 and causing internalization of the TCR complex, preventing antigen recognition (Marano et al, 1989; Wilde & Goa, 1996). Additionally, OKT3 opsonizes T cells causing their activation and degranulation. This activity exhausts the cell, making it an ineffective effector, but also leads to the primary side effect of OKT3: cytokine release syndrome (Chatenoud et al, 1990). Cytokine release can result in profound hypotension, pulmonary edema, and cardiac depression. As with ATG, OKT3 can be used as a rescue or induction agent. Because of the relatively toxic side effect profile and the availability of other agents that accomplish the same purpose, OKT3 is no longer the primary means of lymphocyte depletion.

Anti-Interleukin-2 Receptor α Chain Monoclonal Antibodies

The high affinity α-subunit of the IL-2 receptor (CD25) has been the target of two newer monoclonal antibodies, daclizumab (Zenapax; Roche Pharmaceuticals, Nutley, NJ) and basiliximab (Simulect; Novartis Pharmaceuticals, Basel, Switzerland). CD25 is required for clonal naive T cell expansion and is an attractive target for specific elimination of activated T cells (Goebel et al, 2000). In contrast to OKT3, binding of the target epitope does not result in cytokine release. Administration is generally well tolerated, although the antirejection effect is similarly modest.

MAINTENANCE MINIMIZATION, IMMUNOSUPPRESSANT WITHDRAWAL, AND TOLERANCE

The benefit of organ replacement with transplantation carries with it the burden of long-term maintenance immunosuppression. There have been numerous efforts to decrease the amount of immunosuppression given to transplant recipients. The basic strategies that are being pursued in clinical and preclinical trials include minimization of maintenance immunosuppression through aggressive induction protocols, withdrawal of immunosuppression after the initial post-transplant period, and experimental strategies to facilitate immunologic tolerance.

The strategy of using depletional agents, such as ATG, to reduce the requirement for maintenance immunosuppression is gaining acceptance. Another monoclonal depleting antibody has been investigated in liver transplantation. Alemtuzumab, a CD52 specific antibody, rapidly depletes T cells and to a lesser degree B cells and monocytes from the circulation and secondary lymphoid organs. It is approved for the treatment of lymphoid malignancies and has been investigated off-label in transplantation. Alemtuzumab has been used with low-dose tacrolimus to prevent rejection in liver transplant recipients (Marcos et al, 2004; Tzakis et al, 2004). Similar efforts have been made using ATG induction therapy (Tchervenkov et al, 2004). Although there are no published results using alemtuzumab depletion in pancreatic transplantation, this strategy has been used effectively in kidney transplantation (Calne et al, 1998; Kirk et al, 2003; Knechtle et al, 2003) and is likely to be applied in pancreatic transplantation.

Steroid withdrawal is the goal for many transplant clinicians wishing to spare their patients of the numerous side effects associated with glucocorticosteroid dependence. Steroid withdrawal can be achieved in approximately 85% of liver transplant recipients at 3 months without a significant increase in acute rejection rates (Reding, 2000). Although attempts to withdraw steroids in patients receiving pancreatic transplants have been less successful, with appropriate patient selection, 70% of pancreatic transplant patients may be amenable to steroid withdrawal (Humar et al, 2000).

A study from the University of Pittsburgh suggested that a modest percentage of liver transplant recipients can be withdrawn completely from all immunosuppressive agents (Mazariegos et al, 1997). Although the follow-up period varied, and the incidence of chronic rejection and graft loss was not defined, some recipients are capable of spontaneously accepting liver allografts. The challenge remains to establish criteria for appropriate withdrawal from immunosuppression.

The "holy grail" of transplantation is tolerance. From its conception (Billingham et al, 1953), acquired allospecific tolerance has been defined as the ability to maintain a functional allograft and an intact immune response without the need for any therapeutic drugs. Numerous strategies have been attempted in reaching this goal, but to date, all prospective attempts to create broadly applicable, reliable, and durable tolerance in humans have failed. Although the reasons are numerous and still being elucidated, the pursuit of tolerance would provide all the benefits of organ replacement therapy and eliminate its toxicity—chronic immunosuppression. Ongoing strategies include the manipulation of costimulation signals, depletional approaches, and techniques designed to induce mixed chimerism, a state in which elements of the donor and the recipient immune systems persist in one individual (Cosimi & Sachs, 2004; Harlan & Kirk, 1999; Kirk, 2003).

Many authors have speculated that liver recipients are more likely to be rendered tolerant than other allograft recipients. Reasons cited include the unique APCs in the liver, the liver's regenerative capacity, its shear antigenic bulk, and its tendency to seed the recipient's body with donor hematopoietic cells perhaps overwhelming the recipient immune system into a state of clonal exhaustion (Starzl, 1998). Tolerance attempts in liver transplantation are likely to proceed in the coming years, and their results will be anticipated. In contrast, the pancreas, if anything, has been considered an immunogenic organ with little capacity to regenerate or deal with immune insults. As such, pancreas allograft tolerance is unlikely to be achieved in the near future with the current strategies available.

REFERENCES

Adams AB, et al, 2003: Heterologous immunity: an overlooked barrier to tolerance. Immunol Rev 196:147-160.

Ahmed R, Gray D, 1996: Immunological memory and protective immunity: understanding their relation. Science 272:54-60.

Akira S, Takeda K, 2004: Toll-like receptor signalling. Nat Rev Immunol 4: 499-511.

Allison JP, Krummel MF, 1995: The Yin and Yang of T cell costimulation. Science 270:932-933.

Arai KI, et al, 1990: Cytokines: coordinators of immune and inflammatory responses. Annu Rev Biochem 59:783-836.

Auphan N, et al, 1995: Immunosuppression by glucocorticoids: inhibition of NF-kappa B activity through induction of I kappa B synthesis. Science 270:286-290.

Baecher-Allan C, et al, 2001: CD4+CD25high regulatory cells in human peripheral blood. J Immunol 167:1245-1253.

Baker H, et al, 1978: Rapamycin (AY-22,989), a new antifungal antibiotic: III. in vitro and in vivo evaluation. J Antibiot (Tokyo) 31:539-545.

Baldwin WM III, et al, 1995: Complement in organ transplantation: contributions to inflammation, injury, and rejection. Transplantation 59:797-808.

Barnes EJ, et al, 2003: Applications and limitations of blood eosinophilia for the diagnosis of acute cellular rejection in liver transplantation. Am J Transplant 3:432-438.

Bennett SR, et al, 1998: Help for cytotoxic-T-cell responses is mediated by CD40 signalling. Nature 393:478-480.

Berke G, 1995: The CTL's kiss of death. Cell 81:9-12.

Bevan MJ, 1997: In thymic selection, peptide diversity gives and takes away. Immunity 7:175-178.

Billingham RE, et al, 1953: Activity acquired tolerance of foreign cells. Nature 172:603-606.

Blair PJ, et al, 1998: CTLA-4 ligation delivers a unique signal to resting human CD4 T cells that inhibits interleukin-2 secretion but allows Bcl-X(L) induction. J Immunol 160:12-15.

Borel JF, et al, 1976: Biological effects of cyclosporin A: a new antilymphocytic agent. Agents Actions 6:468-475.

Calne R, et al, 1998: Prope tolerance, perioperative campath 1H, and low-dose cyclosporin monotherapy in renal allograft recipients. Lancet 351:1701-1702.

Calne RY, Murray JE, 1961: Inhibition of the rejection of renal homografts in dogs by Burroughs Wellcome 57-322. Surg Forum 12:118-120.

Cambier JC, et al, 1994: Signal transduction by the B cell antigen receptor and its coreceptors. Annu Rev Immunol 12:457-486.

Chambers CA, Allison JP, 1997: Co-stimulation in T cell responses. Curr Opin Immunol 9:396-404.

Chatenoud L, et al, 1990: In vivo cell activation following OKT3 administration: systemic cytokine release and modulation by corticosteroids. Transplantation 49:697-702.

Cosimi AB, Sachs DH, 2004: Mixed chimerism and transplantation tolerance. Transplantation 77:943-946.

Cooper MD, 1987: Current concepts: B lymphocytes: normal development and function. N Engl J Med 317:1452-1456.

Czapiga M, et al, 2004: Platelets deliver costimulatory signals to antigen-presenting cells: a potential bridge between injury and immune activation. Exp Hematol 32:135-139.

Davis MM, Bjorkman PJ, 1988: T-cell antigen receptor genes and T-cell recognition. Nature 334:395-402.

De Creus A, et al, 2005: Low TLR4 expression by liver dendritic cells correlates with reduced capacity to activate allogeneic T cells in response to endotoxin. J Immunol 174:2037-2045.

Demetris AJ, et al, 1998: Chronic liver allograft rejection: a National Institute of Diabetes and Digestive and Kidney Diseases interinstitutional study analyzing the reliability of current criteria and proposal of an expanded definition. National Institute of Diabetes and Digestive and Kidney Diseases Liver Transplantation Database. Am J Surg Pathol 22:28-39.

Dempsey PW, et al, 1996: C3d of complement as a molecular adjuvant: bridging innate and acquired immunity. Science 271:348-350.

Dousset B, et al, 1998: Is acute rejection deleterious to long-term liver allograft function? J Hepatol 29:660-668.

Dumont FJ, et al, 1990a: The immunosuppressive macrolides FK-506 and rapamycin act as reciprocal antagonists in murine T cells. J Immunol 144:1418-1424.

Dumont FJ, et al, 1990b: Distinct mechanisms of suppression of murine T cell activation by the related macrolides FK-506 and rapamycin. J Immunol 144:251-258.

Egawa H, et al, 2004: Impact of recipient age on outcome of ABO-incompatible living-donor liver transplantation. Transplantation 77:403-411.

Fearon DT, Locksley RM, 1996: The instructive role of innate immunity in the acquired immune response. Science 272:50-53.

Fisher RA, et al, 2004: Four-year follow-up of a prospective randomized trial of mycophenolate mofetil with cyclosporine microemulsion or tacrolimus following liver transplantation. Clin Transplant 18:463-472.

Fruman DA, et al, 1992: Calcineurin phosphatase activity in T lymphocytes is inhibited by FK 506 and cyclosporin A. Proc Natl Acad Sci U S A 89:3686-3690.

Fuggle SV, Koo DD, 1998: Cell adhesion molecules in clinical renal transplantation. Transplantation 65:763-769.

Gaber AO, et al, 1998: Results of the double-blind, randomized, multicenter, phase III clinical trial of Thymoglobulin versus Atgam in the treatment of acute graft rejection episodes after renal transplantation. Transplantation 66:29-37.

Germain RN, 1994: MHC-dependent antigen processing and peptide presentation: providing ligands for T lymphocyte activation. Cell 76:287-299.

Gerritsen ME, Bloor CM, 1993: Endothelial cell gene expression in response to injury. FASEB J 7:523-532.

Gill JI, Gulley ML, 1994: Immunoglobulin and T-cell receptor gene rearrangement. Hematol Oncol Clin N Am 8:751-770.

Goebel J, et al, 2000: Daclizumab (Zenapax) inhibits early interleukin-2 receptor signal transduction events. Transpl Immunol 8:153-159.

Griffiths GM, et al, 1984: Somatic mutation and the maturation of immune response to 2-phenyl oxazolone. Nature 312:271-275.

Harlan DM, Kirk AD, 1999: The future of organ and tissue transplantation: is a new paradigm on the horizon? JAMA 282:1076-1082.

Hart DN, 1997: Dendritic cells: unique leukocyte populations which control the primary immune response. Blood 90:3245-3287.

Henn V, et al, 1998: CD40 ligand on activated platelets triggers an inflammatory reaction of endothelial cells. Nature 391:591-594.

Hitchings GH, et al, 1950: Antagonists of nucleic acid derivatives: II. reversal studies with substances structurally related to thymine. J Biol Chem 185:643-649.

Hojo M, et al, 1999: Cyclosporine induces cancer progression by a cell-autonomous mechanism. Nature 397:530-534.

Hozumi N, Tonegawa S, 1976: Evidence for somatic rearrangement of immunoglobulin genes coding for variable and constant regions. Proc Natl Acad Sci U S A 73:3628-3632.

Humar A, et al, 2000: Steroid withdrawal in pancreas transplant recipients. Clin Transplant 14:75-78.

Humar A, et al, 2003: Chronic rejection: the next major challenge for pancreas transplant recipients. Transplantation 76:918-923.

Inomata Y, Tanaka K, 2001: Pathogenesis and treatment of bile duct loss after liver transplantation. J Hepatobiliary Pancreat Surg 8:316-322.

June CH, et al, 1987: T-cell proliferation involving the CD28 pathway is associated with cyclosporine-resistant interleukin 2 gene expression. Mol Cell Biol 7:4472-4481.

Kahan BD, 1994: Role of cyclosporine: present and future. Transplant Proc 26:3082-3087.

Kappler JW, et al, 1987: T cell tolerance by clonal elimination in the thymus. Cell 49:273-280.

Khanna A, et al, 1996: Immunoregulatory and fibrogenic activities of cyclosporine: a unifying hypothesis based on transforming growth factor-beta expression. Transplant Proc 28:2015-2018.

Kim DR, et al, 2000: V(D)J recombination: site-specific cleavage and repair. Mol Cells 10:367-374.

Kino T, et al, 1987: FK-506, a novel immunosuppressant isolated from a Streptomyces: II. immunosuppressive effect of FK-506 in vitro. J Antibiot (Tokyo) 40:1256-1265.

Kirk AD, 2003: Less is more: maintenance minimization as a step toward tolerance. Am J Transplant 3:643-645.

Kirk AD, et al, 1995: Rapid, comprehensive analysis of human cytokine mRNA and its application to the study of acute renal allograft rejection. Hum Immunol 43:113-128.

Kirk AD, et al, 1997: Posttransplant diastolic hypertension: associations with intragraft transforming growth factor-beta, endothelin, and renin transcription. Transplantation 64:1716-1720.

Kirk AD, et al, 2003: Results from a human renal allograft tolerance trial evaluating the humanized CD52-specific monoclonal antibody alemtuzumab (CAMPATH-1H). Transplantation 76:120-129.

Knechtle SJ, et al, 2003: Campath-1H induction plus rapamycin monotherapy for renal transplantation: results of a pilot study. Am J Transplant 3:722-730.

Knolle PA, Gerken G, 2000: Local control of the immune response in the liver. Immunol Rev 174:21-34.

Krams SM, et al, 1992: Cytokine and T cell receptor gene expression at the site of allograft rejection. Transplantation 53:151-156.

Kumagai N, et al, 1987: Requirements for the simultaneous presence of phorbol esters and calcium ionophores in the expression of human T lymphocyte proliferation-related genes. J Immunol 139:1393-1399.

Kuo CJ, et al, 1992: Rapamycin selectively inhibits interleukin-2 activation of p70 S6 kinase. Nature 358:70-73.

Lanzavecchia A, 1998: Immunology: licence to kill. Nature 393:413-414.

Larsen CP, Pearson TC, 1997: The CD40 pathway in allograft rejection, acceptance, and tolerance. Curr Opin Immunol 9:641-647.

Leahy DJ, et al, 1992: Crystal structure of a soluble form of the human T cell coreceptor CD8 at 2.6 A resolution. Cell 68:1145-1162.

Lederman S, et al, 1992: Molecular interactions mediating T-B lymphocyte collaboration in human lymphoid follicles: roles of T cell-B-cell-activating molecule (5c8 antigen) and CD40 in contact-dependent help. J Immunol 149:3817-3826.

Libby P, Pober JS, 2001: Chronic rejection. Immunity 14:387-397.

Marano N, et al, 1989: Bivalent binding of an anti-CD3 antibody to Jurkat cells induces association of the T cell receptor complex with the cytoskeleton. J Immunol 143:931-938.

Marcos A, et al, 2004: Use of alemtuzumab and tacrolimus monotherapy for cadaveric liver transplantation: with particular reference to hepatitis C virus. Transplantation 78:966-971.

Martel RR, et al, 1977: Inhibition of the immune response by rapamycin, a new antifungal antibiotic. Can J Physiol Pharmacol 55:48-51.

Mazariegos GV, et al, 1997: Weaning of immunosuppression in liver transplant recipients. Transplantation 63:243-249.

Merion RM, et al, 1998: Partial T-cell activation and anergy induction by polyclonal antithymocyte globulin. Transplantation 65:1481-1489.

Molnar-Kimber KL, 1996: Mechanism of action of rapamycin (Sirolimus, Rapamune). Transplant Proc 28:964-969.

Monaco JJ, 1993: Structure and function of genes in the MHC class II region. Curr Opin Immunol 5:17-20.

Mosmann TR, 1991: Cytokines: is there biological meaning? Curr Opin Immunol 3:311-314.

Mosmann TR, et al, 1986: Two types of murine helper T cell clone: I. definition according to profiles of lymphokine activities and secreted proteins. J Immunol 136:2348-2357.

Neff GW, et al, 2004: Sirolimus-associated hepatotoxicity in liver transplantation. Ann Pharmacother 38:1593-1596.

Neuhaus P, et al, 2002: Improved treatment response with basiliximab immunoprophylaxis after liver transplantation: results from a double-blind randomized placebo-controlled trial. Liver Transpl 8:132-142.

Neumann UP, et al, 2001: Significance of a T-lymphocytotoxic crossmatch in liver and combined liver-kidney transplantation. Transplantation 71:1163-1168.

Niemeyer G, et al, 2002: Long-term safety, tolerability and efficacy of daclizumab (Zenapax) in a two-dose regimen in liver transplant recipients. Am J Transplant 2:454-460.

Noreen HJ, et al, 2003: Positive remote crossmatch: impact on short-term and long-term outcome in cadaver renal transplantation. Transplantation 75:501-505.

OPTN/SRTR, 2003: Annual Report 1993-2002. HHS/HRSA/OSP/DOT, Rockville, Maryland; UNOS, Richmond, Virginia; URREA, Ann Arbor, Michigan.

Ortho Multicenter Transplant Study Group, 1985: A randomized clinical trial of OKT3 monoclonal antibody for acute rejection of cadaveric renal transplants. Ortho Multicenter Transplant Study Group. N Engl J Med 313:337-342.

Platz KP, et al, 1991: RS-61443—a new, potent immunosuppressive agent. Transplantation 51:27-31.

Ramos HC, et al, 1995: Weaning of immunosuppression in long-term liver transplant recipients. Transplantation 59:212-217.

Reding R, 2000: Steroid withdrawal in liver transplantation: benefits, risks, and unanswered questions. Transplantation 70:405-410.

Ridge JP, et al, 1998: A conditioned dendritic cell can be a temporal bridge between a CD4+ T-helper and a T-killer cell. Nature 393:474-478.

Rogers NJ, Lechler RI, 2001: Allorecognition. Am J Transplant 1:97-102.

Rothenberg EV, 1996: How T cells count. Science 273:78-79.

Saizawa K, et al, 1987: Evidence for a physical association of CD4 and the CD3:alpha:beta T-cell receptor. Nature 328:260-263.

Scheinman RI, et al, 1995: Role of transcriptional activation of I kappa B alpha in mediation of immunosuppression by glucocorticoids. Science 270:283-286.

Schoenberger SP, et al, 1998: T-cell help for cytotoxic T lymphocytes is mediated by CD40-CD40L interactions. Nature 393:480-483.

Sehgal SN, et al, 1975: Rapamycin (AY-22,989), a new antifungal antibiotic: II. fermentation, isolation and characterization. J Antibiot (Tokyo) 28:727-732.

Starzl T, 1998: Chimerism and clonal exhaustion. Transplantation 66:272-273.

Starzl TE, et al, 1963: The reversal of rejection in human renal homografts with subsequent development of homograft tolerance. Surg Gynecol Obstet 117:385-395.

Starzl TE, et al, 1989: FK 506 for liver, kidney, and pancreas transplantation. Lancet 2:1000-1004.

Stratta RJ, et al, 1996: Pancreas transplantation: a managed cure approach to diabetes. Curr Probl Surg 33:709-808.

Stratta RJ, et al, 2003: Two-dose daclizumab regimen in simultaneous kidney-pancreas transplant recipients: primary endpoint analysis of a multicenter, randomized study. Transplantation 75:1260-1266.

Strehlau J, et al, 1997: Quantitative detection of immune activation transcripts as a diagnostic tool in kidney transplantation. Proc Natl Acad Sci U S A 94:695-700.

Takada M, et al, 1997: The role of the B7 costimulatory pathway in experimental cold ischemia/reperfusion injury. J Clin Invest 100:1199-1203.

Tchervenkov JI, et al, 2004: The impact of thymoglobulin on renal function and calcineurin inhibitor initiation in recipients of orthotopic liver transplant: a retrospective analysis of 298 consecutive patients. Transplant Proc 36:1747-1752.

Tedder TF, et al, 1994: The CD19/CD21 signal transduction complex of B lymphocytes. Immunol Today 15:437-442.

Tzakis AG, et al, 2004: Preliminary experience with alemtuzumab (Campath-1H) and low-dose tacrolimus immunosuppression in adult liver transplantation. Transplantation 77:1209-1214.

Viola A, Lanzavecchia A, 1996: T cell activation determined by T cell receptor number and tunable thresholds. Science 273:104-106.

Wiesner R, et al, 2001: A randomized double-blind comparative study of mycophenolate mofetil and azathioprine in combination with cyclosporine and corticosteroids in primary liver transplant recipients. Liver Transpl 7:442-450.

Wilde MI, Goa KL, 1996: Muromonab CD3: a reappraisal of its pharmacology and use as prophylaxis of solid organ transplant rejection. Drugs 51:865-894.

Wood KJ, Sakaguchi S, 2003: Regulatory T cells in transplantation tolerance. Nat Rev Immunol 3:199-210.

Wright SD, et al, 1990: CD14, a receptor for complexes of lipopolysaccharide (LPS) and LPS binding protein. Science 249:1431-1433.

Liver Transplantation: Anesthesia, Perioperative Management, and Postoperative Intensive Care

P. K. JANICKI

Anesthetic management of patients undergoing orthotopic liver transplantation (OLT) creates multiple challenges, particularly in critically ill patients. New and improved surgical techniques, improved perioperative management, earlier transplantation, and better immunosuppressive regimens have rendered OLT a safer and more successful therapeutic modality for patients with end-stage liver disease (ESLD) in terms of patient and graft survival. Most OLT centers in the United States and Europe have reported a 1-year patient survival rate ranging from 83% to 90% and 5-year survival rate from 75% to 85% (Adam et al, 2003; United Network for Organ Sharing, 2003). Nevertheless, ideal management of these patients in the preoperative, intraoperative and postoperative periods remains a controversial and unclear issue. The challenge facing all members of the transplant team, including the anesthesiologist, is to reduce further the morbidity and mortality associated with this procedure.

PREOPERATIVE ANESTHETIC ASSESSMENT

Most candidates awaiting OLT have either severe liver disease or ESLD complicated by portal hypertension, gastrointestinal bleeding, ascites, coagulopathy, thrombocytopenia, poor synthetic liver function, malnutrition, or metabolic and electrolyte abnormalities (hypoglycemia, lactic acidosis, hypoproteinemia, hyperammonemia, hyponatremia), which qualifies them as American Association of Anesthesiologists class IV patients. These patients may present with a wide spectrum of abnormally functioning organs or systems that result from acute or chronic liver disease or medical problems unrelated to liver disease. The presence of preoperative conditions that are often unrelated to liver disease predisposes the patient to an increased risk of perioperative complications. Such preoperative conditions include cardiac disease (coronary artery disease, obstructive cardiomyopathy, or valvular disease) and pulmonary disease (severe obstructive or restrictive disease). The severity of these conditions should be determined by appropriate preoperative testing, and their effect on predicted short-term and long-term survival should be estimated.

The goal of the preoperative anesthetic evaluation is to examine the patients with respect to their prospective anesthetic management. In most cases, candidates with significant liver disease are evaluated medically as a part of the waiting list placement qualification process. It is important to involve an anesthesia team at the beginning of the process, however, specifically to address all issues related to anesthesia management. The anesthetic evaluation of the potential recipient should be performed at the time of placement on the list and be repeated again just before the transplant to evaluate properly changes in the patient's health status and compare it with a previous evaluation.

Risk Factors Relevant to Anesthetic Management

Cardiovascular Disease

Patients with a significant preoperative cardiovascular history are more prone to intraoperative and postoperative complications, such as arrhythmias, hypotension, myocardial infarction, and pulmonary edema. Cardiovascular disease accounts for a significant part of the total mortality in patients with ESLD.

Patients with coronary artery disease are at high risk for intraoperative coronary insufficiency and heart failure. The circulatory stress and blood loss associated with hepatectomy, in addition to already narrowed coronary vessels, reduces blood flow to the myocardium and may induce acute ischemic heart failure. The prevalence of coronary artery disease in patients evaluated for OLT is 2.5% to 27% (Keeffe et al, 2001; Plotkin et al, 2000). Mortality and morbidity rates for these patients are 50% and 81% and are multifactorial (Keeffe et al, 2001; Plotkin et al, 2000).

Dobutamine stress echocardiography seems to be the best preoperative noninvasive screening study in this population (Plotkin et al, 2001). In terms of treatment, medical management of mild to moderate coronary artery disease should be initiated first because patients with untreated coronary artery disease do poorly postoperatively (Keeffe et al, 2001).

Cardiomyopathy induced by cirrhotic liver disease is termed *cirrhotic cardiomyopathy* (Lee, 2003). It is related to the impairment of cardiac adrenergic receptors and their signaling function (Myers & Lee, 2000). Stress associated with liver transplantation may accelerate this condition and lead to acute heart failure. Diagnosis of cirrhotic cardiomyopathy in the pretransplant period is impossible because sensitive and specific methods of detection have not been established (Moller & Henriksen, 2002; Myers & Lee, 2000). In terms of treatment, numerous reports suggest that cirrhotic cardiomyopathy is reversible after surgery;

however, further investigations are needed (Moller & Henriksen, 2002).

Pulmonary Disease

Pretransplant pulmonary evaluation should be performed to assess and document the degree of pulmonary dysfunction associated with ESLD patients and to optimize pulmonary function before transplantation.

Hypoxia and Atelectasis.   Patients with ESLD may present with hypoxemia, often with distinct hypocapnia resulting from compensatory hyperventilation. The mechanism behind development of hypoxemia is linked to ventilation/perfusion ratio and intrapulmonary right-to-left shunting (Mazzeo et al, 2004). It may be caused by ascites, pleural effusion, or pulmonary hypertension. A decrease in lung volume, especially functional residual capacity, and the presence of pleural effusions are hallmarks of ascites. Ascites causes elevation of the diaphragm resulting in the development of atelectasis. Disturbances in gas exchange and ventilatory mechanics should be considered in any ESLD patient awaiting liver transplantation.

Hepatic Hydrothorax.   Development of pleural effusion in cirrhotic patients is known as hepatic hydrothorax, which affects about 4% to 6% of patients with cirrhosis and 10% of patients with decompensated cirrhosis (Gur et al, 2004).

Aspiration Pneumonia.   Hepatic encephalopathy, gastrointestinal bleeding, and ascites-induced intra-abdominal pressure may lead to aspiration pneumonia, acute respiratory distress syndrome, or both.

Portopulmonary Hypertension.   Portopulmonary hypertension (PPH) is associated with portal hypertension, increased pulmonary arterial pressure, and increased pulmonary vascular resistance. It has been reported that pulmonary hypertension in cirrhotic patients may occur in 16% of patients (Hoeper et al, 2004). Clinically, PPH manifests as dyspnea on exertion, fatigue, palpitations, or chest pain. The diagnosis of PPH requires the presence of increased mean pulmonary arterial pressure (>25 mm Hg) with no evidence of left heart failure (pulmonary wedge pressure <15 mm Hg) (Hoeper et al, 2004; Jones et al, 1999). Electrocardiogram, radiography, and pulmonary function testing may provide some valuable information, but in most cases they are used to rule out other potential causes of pulmonary hypertension, such as right ventricular dysfunction.

It is generally believed that PPH adversely affects the outcome of OLT recipients, and mortality associated with PPH remains significantly high (Krowka et al, 2004). Previously, severe pulmonary hypertension (defined as mean pulmonary arterial pressure >40 mm Hg) was associated with very poor outcome (Reich et al, 2003). More recent clinical studies evaluating patients with PPH undergoing OLT suggested, however, that moderately elevated mean pulmonary arterial pressure of 28 to 40 mm Hg does not influence outcome, whereas patients with pulmonary arterial pressure greater than 40 mm Hg can be treated initially with epoprostenol to reverse pulmonary hypertension followed by OLT. Additionally, when the cardiac index is preserved, most patients with moderate to severe PPH can do well intraoperatively and postoperatively with potentially good long-term outcomes (Kuo et al, 1999; Rafanan et al, 2000; Schroeder et al, 2000; Starkel et al, 2002). The duration of ventilation and intensive care unit (ICU) stay was unaffected by PPH (Starkel et al, 2002).

Hepatopulmonary Syndrome.   The frequency of hepatopulmonary syndrome in ESLD patients has been reported to be 8% to 29% (Arguedas et al, 2003; Hoeper et al, 2004). Hepatopulmonary syndrome is characterized by hypoxemia associated with anatomic shunting of blood and diffusion-perfusion abnormalities. Treatment of hepatopulmonary syndrome includes correction of hypoxemia by administration of oxygen; however, currently the only well-established therapy for hepatopulmonary syndrome is liver transplantation. The mortality rate after OLT for patients with hepatopulmonary syndrome is approximately 36% (Hoeper et al, 2004; Krowka et al, 2004), particularly in patients characterized by more severe hypoxemia and significant intrapulmonary shunting (Arguedas et al, 2003). A preoperative arterial oxygen tension of less than 50 mm Hg alone or in combination with a shunt fraction greater than 20% is the strongest predictor of postoperative mortality (Arguedas et al, 2003). Preoperative testing for the severity of hepatopulmonary syndrome can be used to stratify patients according to the risk for perioperative mortality (Arguedas et al, 2003).

Pretransplant Renal Function

Renal insufficiency is a common condition among OLT recipients before and after transplantation and varies from 5% to 50% (Paramesh et al, 2004). Although many of these patients may have hepatorenal syndrome, a potentially reversible condition, it is often difficult to make a firm diagnosis of hepatorenal syndrome in patients with ESLD (Gonwa et al, 2004). Moderate and severe renal insufficiency, characterized by a creatinine clearance less than 40 mL/min, is associated with significantly higher primary graft nonfunction and lower patient and graft survival rates (Nair et al, 2002).

Hepatorenal syndrome is a complication of ESLD distinguished by renal failure, changes in systemic blood pressure, and increased activity of endogenous vasoactive compounds. The prognosis of patients with hepatorenal syndrome is extremely poor (Gines et al, 2003). Liver transplantation is the best option in selected patients, but it is not always applicable because of the short expected patient survival and donor availability. Despite the postoperative increase in morbidity (e.g., need for temporary hemodialysis), long-term survival of transplant recipients with hepatorenal syndrome is excellent, reaching approximately 60% at 3 years after surgery (Cardenas et al, 2000). Management of a patient who has renal impairment with liver failure should take into account cardiovascular instability, increased intracranial pressure (ICP), and cerebral edema. Intermittent hemodialysis is an efficient method of removing toxic substances and excess fluid. It may lead to hemodynamic instability, however, and increased ICP, which in a setting of acute liver failure can precipitate herniation and cerebral edema (Vaquero & Blei, 2003). Continuous renal replacement therapy (CRRT) is an alternative to hemodialysis and peritoneal dialysis (Gaspar et al, 2002).

Central Nervous System Disorders

Hepatic Encephalopathy.   Hepatic encephalopathy, or portosystemic encephalopathy, describes a wide spectrum of often reversible neuropsychiatric abnormalities that occur in 28% of patients with ESLD (Lizardi-Cervera et al, 2003). Hepatic encephalopathy is clinically characterized by alterations in mental status with fluctuating neurologic signs (asterixis, hyperreflexia) and distinctive electroencephalographic changes (symmetric high-voltage, slow-wave activity). In addition to the neuropsychiatric abnormalities, the most devastating complication observed is cerebral edema. One of the most dramatic forms of hepatic encephalopathy is associated with fulminant hepatic failure. Fulminant hepatic failure is characterized by progression to profound coma within a short time (7 days to 12 weeks) after the initial onset of liver dysfunction (Colquhoun et al, 2001). Development of cerebral edema secondary to fulminant hepatic failure often results in cerebral herniation and brain hypoxia, both of which lead to increased ICP and reduced cerebral perfusion pressure (Vaquero & Blei, 2003).

Chronic hepatic encephalopathy is due to slowly progressing liver failure that does not lead to cytotoxic edema (Ahl et al, 2004). The chronic form of hepatic encephalopathy is recognized by a slower onset, milder symptoms, and shorter duration than the acute form. It is characterized by the persistence of neuropsychiatric symptoms despite adequate medical therapy.

Cerebral Edema and Increased Intracranial Pressure. ESLD patients are prone to intracranial hypertension and cerebral edema. Dramatic increase in ICP occurs in approximately 50% to 80% of patients with fulminant hepatic failure, and it is the leading cause of death (Mukherjee et al, 2003; Murphy et al, 2004; Tofteng & Larsen, 2004; Tofteng et al, 2002). Previous studies showed that fulminant hepatic failure patients are at increased risk of brain injury secondary to cerebral hypoperfusion if intracranial hypertension develops before OLT (Bass, 2000; Blei, 2000a, 2000b, 2000c).

It is difficult to estimate or measure the degree of intracranial hypertension using noninvasive techniques; continuous invasive monitoring of ICP is the most sensitive method that allows early recognition and responsive management (Bass, 2000). Use of this technique requires the presence of experienced personnel, however, and carries a risk of intracerebral bleeding because of the presence of potentially severe and uncorrected coagulopathy.

Prevention of intracranial hypertension is crucial. Maintenance of adequate cerebral perfusion pressure is the cornerstone of intracranial hypertension management. The cerebral perfusion pressure is calculated by subtracting ICP from mean arterial pressure. It has been shown that cerebral perfusion pressure can be measured by the transcranial Doppler technique and jugular bulb oxygen saturation (Ardizzone et al, 2004; Strauss et al, 1998, 1999). The management goals are to maintain ICP less than 20 mm Hg and cerebral perfusion pressure greater than 50 mm Hg. If elevated ICP is suspected or known to exist, aggressive therapy should be initiated and maintained throughout the entire perioperative period (Table 102.1).

Table 102.1 Preoperative Management of Intracranial Hypertension in End-Stage Liver Disease

Goals

ICP <20 mm Hg
Cerebral perfusion pressure >50 mm Hg

General Measures

Maintenance of mean arterial pressure >60 mm Hg
Prevention and treatment of volume overload
Prevention of factors transiently increasing ICP (seizures, fever, arterial hypertension, vasodilating drugs, endotracheal suction, jugular venous congestion)
Elevation of the head 10-20 degrees

Specific Measures

Hyperventilation
Osmotic diuresis
Barbiturate coma

The anesthetic management of the patient in hepatic coma during OLT is complex. In addition to the usual anesthetic concerns of liver transplantation, one must remain aware of the elements of neurologic intensive care, which are essential to achieving a satisfactory central nervous system outcome. Besides the neurologic problems, involvement of other organs or systems often contributes to the already unfavorable condition of the recipient. Renal failure is particularly common. The tenuous fluid status of an encephalopathic patient with coexisting oliguric renal failure may require removal of an excess volume by hemofiltration before correction of coagulopathy is initiated. The anesthetic requirements of these patients are usually significantly decreased, and either a low level of inhalation anesthetic or continuous infusion of propofol or barbiturates may be employed to maintain the necessary level of hypnosis and amnesia. If severe systemic hypotension develops, it should be treated, initially by assessing intravascular volume and then adding pressors (dopamine, epinephrine) for hemodynamic support (Larsen et al, 2000). The major intraoperative threat to cerebral survival occurs during graft reperfusion, when a period of profound vasodilation accompanied by severe increase in ICP may occur and may require hyperventilation and mannitol administration (Detry et al, 1999; Jalan, 2003). The dangerous increase in ICP can be detected only with ICP monitoring, unless the increase is so great that bradycardia and hypertension from brainstem ischemia is observed (Cushing's sign). As the graft begins to function and encephalotoxins are eliminated from the circulation, the ICP almost always returns to normal levels, and anesthesia and hyperventilation should be titrated accordingly to maintain a desirable cerebral perfusion pressure. The levels of narcosis and neuromuscular blockade are kept at reasonable levels so that neurologic function can be assessed rapidly when the patient returns to the ICU.

INTRAOPERATIVE MANAGEMENT

Induction

Cadaveric liver transplantation should be treated as a surgical emergency compared with a living donor liver transplantation (LDLT) simply because the exact time of the operation cannot be predicted. All recipients of a liver transplant should be considered as being at risk for aspiration during induction because of the uncertainty as to the time of the last meal and the potential presence of ascites or gastrointestinal bleeding or both. Patients with ESLD have decreased liver metabolic function, and drug dosage should be adjusted accordingly and administered in the presence of basic vital signs (blood pressure, heart rate, respiratory rate, oxygen saturation) monitoring. In the absence of a hemodynamic instability, the placement of all invasive monitors may be postponed until the induction of anesthesia has been completed.

The choice of anesthetic induction agents varies widely, as does the use of opiate analgesia. Because drug clearance in patients with ESLD is diminished owing to liver injury and subsequent reduction of functioning hepatocytes, drug pharmacodynamics and kinetics changes also are present. The choice of an induction agent should be based on the level of hemodynamic stability of the patient. Hypnosis in critically ill patients may be achieved with etomidate (0.2-0.3 mg/kg), whereas in a more stable patient, thiopental (3-5 mg/kg) or propofol (1-3 mg/kg) may be used. The most crucial point is that doses of all drugs should be chosen carefully to prevent cardiovascular depression.

In terms of muscle relaxants, traditionally succinylcholine (1-2 mg/kg) has been regarded as the neuromuscular induction agent of choice. The presence of hyperkalemia is considered a contraindication to succinylcholine administration, however. With the introduction of the new faster acting nondepolarizing muscle relaxant agents (e.g., rocuronium), succinylcholine can be safely replaced. Fast-acting opioid analgesics (fentanyl, alfentanil, or sufentanil) can be used during induction to blunt the hemodynamic response to intubation, particularly in a hemodynamically unstable patient.

Monitoring

Line Placement

After anesthesia has been established, monitoring lines are placed. It is customary to place two radial arterial lines in a patient undergoing liver transplantation; one is used for the continuous invasive monitoring of the systemic blood pressure, and one is used for frequent sampling of the arterial blood. If placement of the radial arterial line is unsuccessful, the right femoral artery should be used. Cannulation of the left femoral artery should be avoided because it may interfere with the placement of venous lines for elective or emergent venovenous bypass (VVB), if needed.

The right internal jugular vein or right subclavian vein or both are cannulated with at least an 8.5-Fr percutaneous venous sheath for venous access and blood volume replacement. It is imperative to establish at least two additional large-bore intravenous catheters allowing rapid infusion of blood volume replacement under pressure. The configuration of this access may vary widely among patients and transplantation centers. It may be convenient to place a large bore rapid infusion catheter (at least 6-Fr) in each arm to employ a rapid transfusion device. Alternatively, at least an 8.5-Fr percutaneous sheath should be placed into the available subclavian vein or left internal jugular vein. Venous access catheters should be avoided in the lower extremities because volume overload of the lower body may occur during VVB (if used) or inferior vena cava (IVC) occlusion. Some centers monitor IVC pressure via the right femoral vein to detect IVC pressure changes secondary to surgical manipulation; this may help differentiate a mechanical cause for hemodynamic changes from volume deficiency with a need for fluid administration. Monitoring of the IVC pressure also provides assessment of venous pressure gradients after anastomosis of the donor liver. The placement of multiple lines in the recipient rarely may be associated with the obstruction of the superior vena cava flow and associated complications (Janicki et al, 2001).

Pulmonary Artery Catheterization

The placement of a pulmonary arterial catheter for intraoperative pulmonary arterial pressure, central venous pressure, and cardiac output/cardiac index (CO/CI) monitoring is considered standard for OLT (Zheng et al, 2002). Liver transplantation usually is associated with rapid and profound changes in volume status, variations in the extent of stimulation of the sympathetic nervous system, rapid changes in pulmonary vascular resistance, and inotropic changes of the heart (Krenn et al, 2004; Zheng et al, 2002). Also, the detection of many unforeseen cardiovascular adverse events during OLT may be facilitated greatly by using a pulmonary arterial catheter intraoperatively (Della Rocca et al, 2001, 2002). Several types of pulmonary arterial catheter have been advocated for use during OLT; there are no convincing data, however, indicating which type of pulmonary arterial catheter is more beneficial during the procedure. Nevertheless, in most cases, the required or desired information in terms of pulmonary arterial pressure, CO/CI measured by the thermodilution method, and central venous pressure and systemic vascular resistance/pulmonary vascular resistance can be obtained from any type of pulmonary arterial catheter. Advances in pulmonary arterial catheter design allow the use of continuous oxymetric and CO/CI monitoring, freeing the anesthesiology team from repetitions of manual measurements.

Blood Sampling

Routine blood sampling includes arterial blood gases, hematocrit and hemoglobin, coagulation studies (prothrombin time, activated partial thromboplastin time, platelets, fibrinogen), plasma electrolytes (sodium, potassium, magnesium, ionized calcium), and blood lactate. Routine sampling should be performed initially at the baseline, before the anhepatic phase, 15 to 30 minutes into the anhepatic phase, before reperfusion, and 15 to 30 minutes after liver reperfusion. More frequent blood sampling (e.g., every hour) may be required, however, during the preanhepatic period as a consequence of difficult dissection or significant blood loss or both. Blood sampling also should continue for several hours after reperfusion.

Other Intraoperative Monitoring

Transesophageal Echocardiography. Transesophageal echocardiography (TEE) has become an indispensable tool in the management of patients undergoing cardiac surgery. Despite the increasing use of TEE in the operating room for the diagnosis of various hemodynamic perturbations, its role in the management of patients undergoing noncardiac surgery remains poorly defined. TEE use would be particularly beneficial in patients with hemodynamic disturbances. The management of intraoperative hypotension is determined by its cause, and invasive monitoring, including determination of CO/CI and filling pressures, is imperative. Filling pressures frequently are inaccurate, however, in determining the volume status of the patient because of cardiac compliance changes. TEE may provide useful information. In addition, TEE provides information regarding overall cardiac function and allows one to determine other causes of cardiac dysfunction (e.g., pericardial effusion, pleural effusion, tension pneumothorax) (De Wolf, 2000). It was reported that TEE can be performed safely in most patients undergoing OLT, and it is extremely helpful in obtaining the correct hemodynamic diagnosis and in deciding on patient medical and surgical management (Mahajan et al, 2004). A further additional benefit of intraoperative TEE monitoring is due to the incidental findings of atrial shunts, valvular dysfunction, left ventricular outflow tract obstruction, and thrombus formation (Guarracino, 2001; Krenn et al, 2004).

Real-Time Coagulation Monitoring. Real-time coagulation monitoring can be done using the thromboelastogram (TEG) (Haemoscope, Niles, IL) or the Sonoclot (Sienco Inc., Arvada, Co) device (Cerutti et al, 2004). Both machines enable the measurement of the viscoelastic properties of clot formation, which is particularly useful for the detection and treatment of platelet dysfunction and fibrinolysis. The TEG has proved to be an extremely valuable monitoring technique when used as a guide for coagulation replacement and pharmacologic therapy during OLT (Cerutti et al, 2004). This device monitors coagulability and provides clinically useful information in less than 30 minutes. Modifications of the TEG technique, such as heparinase-modified TEG, abciximab (ReoPro)-modified TEG, and temperature-compensated TEG, provide the opportunity to elucidate the underlying mechanisms of coagulation in detail.

Bispectral Index. Bispectral index is a monitor used to measure the depth of anesthesia and to facilitate anesthetic titration and reduction of awareness during surgery. Awareness is a rare complication of routine anesthesia (0.1-0.2%). Although awareness has a relatively high incidence (0.8%) in adult surgical patients (e.g., trauma, cardiac surgery, hemodynamic instability), it may be effectively reduced (by about 85%) by the use of bispectral index–guided anesthesia (Myles et al, 2004).

Conduct of Anesthesia

Maintenance Anesthesia

Although decreased hepatic synthetic and metabolic functions should dictate use of lower dosage of many anesthetic agents, an increased volume of distribution secondary to the renal dysfunction and altered oncotic pressure suggest that larger doses of drugs might be required. Despite a decrease in hepatocyte mass, hepatocytes are characterized by induced enzyme activity, making drug metabolism highly variable. Narcotics, inhalational agents, and nondepolarizing muscle relaxants are used for maintenance of anesthesia and should be titrated to the desired effect. Because of concerns such as altered volume of distribution and oncotic pressure, however, postoperative drug excretion can be prolonged, contributing to postoperative central nervous system and neuromuscular depression. The pharmacokinetics of opioid analgesics that are commonly used during OLT (fentanyl, sufentanil, morphine) have been reported to be largely unchanged (Carton et al, 1994a, 1994b). Newer muscle relaxants, such as cisatracurium and rocuronium, are only slightly affected by OLT. The newly transplanted liver rapidly removes any residual effect of these agents. The rate of recovery from vecuronium or rocuronium has been used as a predictor of hepatic allograft function (Gao et al, 2002, 2003; Lukin et al, 1995). If long-acting muscle relaxants are used (e.g., pancuronium), the neuromuscular blockade should be monitored with a nerve stimulator because the duration of the muscle relaxants is unpredictable.

Nitrous oxide is avoided during liver transplantation because its enhanced solubility causes distribution to air-filled cavities, resulting in distention and surgical inconvenience during the prolonged operation and splinting of the diaphragm on abdominal closure. More importantly, nitrous oxide can aggravate the devastating effects of air embolism, should this occur. Of the inhalation agents, sevoflurane, isoflurane, and desflurane have an empiric advantage over halothane because they are less likely to be hepatotoxic. Isoflurane has a documented advantage because of its minimal reduction of the hepatic blood flow and oxygen delivery. More and more transplant centers are using total intravenous anesthesia techniques for maintenance of anesthesia during OLT (Cammu et al, 2003). This technique involves continuous controlled infusion of propofol, fentanyl/sufentanil, and muscle relaxants throughout the procedure. The advantage of using propofol is a minimal effect on the free hepatic

venous pressure and pressure gradient, with minimal effect on the difference between the portal and systemic circulations (Mandell et al, 2003). This technique may prove even more beneficial in patients who are expected to be extubated shortly after the transplantation (Findlay et al, 2002).

Different Surgical Techniques and Anesthetic Management

The wide spectrum of available anesthetic techniques allows flexibility for surgical technical needs. The use of VVB in the operating room controls and maintains volume loading of the right ventricle, relieves splanchnic and abdominal venous congestion, and possibly protects or improves renal function during the anhepatic stage of OLT. VVB requires the surgical placement of special (12-16 Fr) catheters, to provide adequate flow during VVB. These lines are placed in the femoral and portal vein (VVB inflow) and left axillary vein or right internal jugular vein (VVB outflow). In the past, the placement of these catheters often resulted in injury of the axillary structures—the brachial plexus and arterial, venous, and lymphatic vessels; they also caused infection and wound healing problems. Introduction of the percutaneous VVB cannula has replaced the traditional axillary approach, however, with internal jugular vein cannulation technique in some centers. Despite this technical advancement, the internal jugular vein approach carries its own risks, such as carotid artery injury, pneumothorax, right atrial perforation, or even ventricular perforation. The VVB cannula also can interfere with functioning of the rapid infusion systems (Roth et al, 2002). To avoid these complications, and to ensure proper placement of the percutaneous VVB cannula, chest radiography, fluoroscopic assistance, or, more recently, TEE to guide placement has been recommended (Planinsic et al, 2003).

The VVB is initiated before portal vein cross-clamping and should provide rerouting of the systemic and portal blood flow of at least 20% to 50% of the normal systemic flow rate (Carton et al, 1994a, 1994b). Cardiac output decreases during this procedure because the circuit resistance is greater than native vessels. In patients with limited portal collateral circulation, interruption of VVB (e.g., by kinking) may not be well tolerated. VVB should not be used if IVC thrombosis is suspected, which should be ruled out with the help of TEE. Special caution should be exercised in patients with massive hepatomegaly in association with polycystic liver disease or Budd-Chiari syndrome. It has been recommended to maintain VVB flow greater than 1000 mL/min in adults, but lower flow rates can be tolerated without a risk of thromboembolism in pediatric patients (Carton et al, 1994a, 1994b). If the flow in the VVB circuit is temporarily interrupted, the circuit should be replaced. The heparin-bonded tubing used in VVB may help to avoid thromboembolism. Nevertheless, if air or thrombus develops within the circuit, bypass should be discontinued, and the resulting hypotension should be corrected with a volume load or pressor support or both. Although VVB may have advantages, this procedure does not clearly improve overall morbidity or mortality (Cabezuelo et al, 2003; Moreno-Gonzalez et al, 2003). In most OLT patients, hemodynamic stability can be maintained with volume loading owing to collaterals that develop as a result of severe liver disease. Performing occlusion testing of the IVC before definite hepatectomy may provide useful guidelines for the need of VVB. VVB is usually indicated if there is a decrease in mean arterial pressure of more than 50% or a decreased CO/CI (>50%) (Carton et al, 1994a, 1994b).

The technique of caval preservation ("piggyback") is an alternative to VVB. This technique maintains hemodynamic stability by preserving the recipient's IVC. This technique is routinely used in reduced-size liver transplantation, in which an inadequate caliber donor IVC is present, and in LDLT, in which the donor IVC stays intact, because it is associated with a better perioperative outcome (Fan et al, 2003). Several reports comparing piggyback versus VVB techniques for OLT showed that the piggyback technique offers at least the same (if not better) degree of hemodynamic stability, kidney protection, and blood loss compared with VVB (Cabezuelo et al, 2003; Moreno-Gonzalez et al, 2003; Wu et al, 2003). The piggyback technique avoids all of the potential complications and costs of VVB (Hosein Shokouh-Amiri et al, 2000; Reddy et al, 2000). It has been noted, however, that the piggyback technique has been associated with a higher incidence of pulmonary infiltrates compared with VVB (Isern et al, 2004).

LDLT has become an alternative to cadaveric donor liver transplantation for selected patients. Because LDLT can be performed electively, the recipient may have more adequately compensated liver disease at the time of surgery than a recipient of a cadaveric liver graft. Published results indicate that although intraoperative fluid and transfusion requirements are similar in cadaveric transplantation versus LDLT recipients, the impact of transplantation on pulmonary gas exchange is more pronounced in patients receiving organs from cadaveric donors. This difference may arise from the longer cold ischemia times present in the cadaveric donor group (Niemann et al, 2004). In terms of blood transfusions, the use of heterologous blood products in LDLT can be replaced by blood-saving transfusion, preoperative autologous blood donation, or intraoperative hemodilution (Lutz et al, 2003).

Hemostasis During Orthotopic Liver Transplantation

Blood loss and transfusion requirements depend primarily on the severity of liver disease, quality of the donor liver, experience of the transplantation team, and use of autologous (cell saver) blood transfusion. As the experience in OLT has increased over the last several decades, the transfusion of blood products has decreased significantly (Gordon et al, 2002). A multi-institutional study reported that the overall median number of transfused blood products is approximately 5 U of packed red blood cells, 6 U of fresh frozen plasma, and 5 U of platelets (Ozier et al, 2003). The transfusion of a large quantity of blood products is associated with reduced survival (Schroeder et al, 1999). The possibility of OLT without use of blood products has been shown, using the technique of preoperative blood augmentation with erythropoietin, intraoperative cell salvage, and acute normovolemic hemodilution (Jabbour et al, 2004).

An increase in blood product requirements has been linked to previous abdominal surgery, especially previous OLT. Extensive venous collateral communication between the portal and systemic venous circulations may contribute significantly to profound bleeding during liver dissection in the preanhepatic phase. The intraoperative pharmacologic methods used to decrease portal vein pressure include infusion of vasopressin and octreotide. Both drugs can be used during the preanhepatic phase and may be valuable in the presence of massive intraoperative bleeding (Garcia & Sanyal, 2001; Luketic, 2001; Sabba et al, 2001). The drugs should be discontinued during the anhepatic phase, however.

The most common forms of ESLD-induced coagulopathic derangements are summarized in Table 102.2. Nevertheless, each

Table 102.2 Baseline Factors Responsible for the Coagulation Problems in End-Stage Liver Disease

Deficiency of factor VII (most severe because of its short half-life)
Variable deficiencies of factors IX, X, and II
Splenomegaly with thrombocytopenia
Low-grade disseminated intravascular coagulation
Hyperfibrinolysis

stage of liver transplantation is characterized by specific intraoperative coagulopathies (Table 102.3). During the preanhepatic stage, dilutional coagulopathy may be superimposed on preexisting coagulopathy; however, administration of fresh frozen plasma may correct the problem. A decrease in platelet function, indicated by TEG, may be corrected by the transfusion of platelets. Because of high levels of fibrinogen and factor VIII, administration of cryoprecipitate is limited to patients with severe fibrinolysis (Kang, 2000). Cryoprecipitate may be administered when hypofibrinogenemia is documented or when severe fibrinolysis results in a selective destruction of factor VIII.

Dilutional coagulopathy may continue into and through the anhepatic phase, where surgical bleeding, although less severe compared with the preanhepatic period, still may lead to serious problems. Fibrinolysis during the anhepatic phase is more pronounced with a progressive increase in tissue-type plasminogen activator level. If VVB is used, the administration of platelets and antifibrinolytics is reserved for severe cases of thrombocytopenia and fibrinolysis.

Reperfusion of the grafted liver is associated with severe coagulopathy, as a consequence of the influx of preservation solution and the release of heparin or heparin-like substances from the grafted liver. Fibrinolysis is accentuated by the release of tissue-type plasminogen activator from the donor liver and inhibition of coagulation by other less well-characterized factors (Kang, 2000). In most cases, the coagulopathy starts to improve during the neohepatic stage, unless major surgical bleeding continues.

There is a growing interest in the prophylaxis and treatment of intraoperative disturbances of hemostasis during OLT with different antifibrinolytic drugs, in an attempt to decrease blood

Table 102.3 Pattern of Coagulation During Orthotopic Liver Transplantation

Preanhepatic Phase

Baseline coagulopathic pattern in ESLD (see Table 102.2)
Dilutional coagulopathy (all phases)

Anhepatic Phase

Primary fibrinolysis (absence of hepatic clearance of tPA, increases in thrombin–antithrombin III complex, fibrin degradation products)

Reperfusion Phase

Release of heparin (in 30%) from engrafted liver
Massive release of tPA from engrafted liver
Congested viscera and lower extremities, relative deficiency of plasminogen activator inhibitor
Primary fibrinolysis
Hypothermia
Ionized hypocalcemia

Neohepatic Phase

Gradual normalization

tPA, tissue-type plasminogen activator.

loss and blood product administration. Most of the current available literature provides data on the role and effect of aprotinin, aminocaproic acid, tranexamic acid, and recombinant factor VIIa as potential prophylactic and therapeutic modalities in OLT. The use of antifibrinolytic agents (aminocaproic acid, aprotinin, tranexamic acid) has been advocated because of a hyperfibrinolytic state and coagulopathy that presents in ESLD recipients that is often aggravated by reperfusion of the liver. It was shown that prophylactic administration of the polypeptide serine protease inhibitor, aprotinin, ameliorates the postreperfusion syndrome in OLT. This amelioration is reflected by a significant reduction in vasopressor requirements and a decrease in transfusion requirements (Jankowski et al, 2002; Molenaar & Porte, 2002; Molenaar et al, 2001a, 2001b, 2001c, 2001d). Several studies have shown that aprotinin in OLT has beneficial effects, and this has been viewed as a safe agent. It also has been documented, however, that aprotinin can cause thrombosis with subsequent pulmonary embolism, arguing against routine use in OLT (Fitzsimons et al, 2001; Ramsay et al, 2004). There are several reports of thromboembolic events in patients undergoing OLT without aprotinin or any other antifibrinolytic drug (Gologorsky et al, 2001). There are no available reports analyzing aprotinin versus no aprotinin therapy showing a significant difference in thromboembolic complications to guide the use of this agent in OLT.

The use of aminocaproic acid in small doses (0.25-0.5 g) has been reported to be effective in the treatment of clinically evident and TEG-confirmed intraoperative fibrinolysis. The advantage of prophylactic administration of this drug during OLT has not been shown in terms of a reduction in blood product administration. In contrast, prophylactic administration of tranexamic acid significantly reduces total packed red blood cell administration during OLT (Dalmau et al, 2000). Tranexamic acid is a synthetic derivative of the amino acid lysine, which exerts its antifibrinolytic effect through the reversible blockade of lysine binding sites on plasminogen molecules. A randomized comparison of aprotinin and tranexamic acid during OLT did not show a large difference between the two groups (Dalmau et al, 2004).

Recombinant factor VIIa exerts its prohemostatic effect via enhancement of the extrinsic coagulation pathway in a tissue-dependent manner, providing an increase in thrombin generation. It was shown that a single dose of recombinant factor VIIa significantly reduced transfusion requirements during OLT in adults and children (Hendriks et al, 2002; Markiewicz et al, 2003; Meijer et al, 2003).

Critical Intraoperative Events

Postreperfusion Syndrome

Reperfusion of the graft may be associated with significant hemodynamic instability. Postreperfusion syndrome is defined as a decrease in mean arterial pressure of at least 30% from baseline for at least 1 minute within the first 5 minutes of reperfusion (Koh, 2000). The factors responsible for this syndrome result from the release of vasoactive substances from the grafted liver, hyperkalemia, acidosis, and hypothermia, which produce cardiovascular changes such as hypotension and cardiac arrhythmias. The prophylactic administration of sodium bicarbonate or calcium chloride or inotropic agents may prevent such drastic changes during the immediate reperfusion period. VVB does

not prevent reperfusion syndrome (Koh, 2000). The treatment consists of providing an adequate fluid load to maintain CO/CI, maintaining a hematocrit of at least 25%, and ensuring adequate coagulation function. Careful monitoring is required to prevent excess fluid overload and pulmonary edema, particularly when VVB is not used (Koh, 2000).

Sudden Massive Blood Loss

Sudden uncontrolled blood loss produces hypovolemia, low CO/CI, and hypotension. If uncorrected, this situation results in tissue hypoperfusion, uncontrolled acidosis, and ultimately poor outcome. In such cases, massive transfusion is required to normalize the volume status, and appropriate correction of acid-base state and ionized calcium are imperative. Overuse of sodium bicarbonate should be avoided because it can result in hypernatremia and hyperosmolality. Tromethamine (Tham) is a safe agent containing no sodium and should be considered for treatment of acidosis in addition to sodium bicarbonate (Kallet et al, 2000). Most centers use devices to warm adequately and administer rapidly large amounts of blood products and fluids. Although such devices are essential during major hemorrhage, the ability to administer blood at a fast rate generally results in symptomatic hypocalcemia, requiring frequent bolus infusions of calcium to maintain the ionized calcium at a level greater than 1 mM. Citrate intoxication from rapid transfusion is common during the anhepatic stage, owing to the absence of liver metabolic functions. Rapid transfusion of blood products, especially fresh frozen plasma, which contains the largest amount of citrate, may overwhelm the metabolic activity of the liver at any stage of OLT and requires aggressive calcium supplementation. One of the most popular devices on the market is Rapid Infusion System (RIS) (Haemonetics Corporation, Braintree, MA), which is designed to deliver prewarmed fluids or blood products at a rate of 1.5 L/min. RIS consists of reservoirs, a heat exchanger, fluid-level sensors, air detectors, line pressure monitors, and filters integrated to minimize trauma to the formed elements of blood and prevent infusion of air. RIS infuses fluid via a Y-output tubing into two separate large-bore intravenous cannulae to minimize flow resistance via a digital step-motor driving a roller pump and displays cumulative infusion volume during use. Because of occasional overestimation of the transfused volume associated with equipment malfunction or operator error, accurate and timely recording of the transfusion volume and actual infused volume is essential (Kempen et al, 2000). Some centers use cell-saving devices, when appropriate, to limit blood product administration. Autotransfusion of blood is contraindicated in the clinical settings of abdominal infection or malignancy.

Intractable Hypotension

Patients undergoing OLT may become severely hypotensive secondary to preexisting low systemic vascular resistance, low preload (secondary to blood loss or decreased venous return associated with partial occlusion of the venous system by surgical manipulation or both), and low cardiac performance (inotropism). Decreased cardiac performance may be caused by factors developing simultaneously during OLT, including low plasma ionized calcium concentration, severe metabolic acidosis, hypothermia, cardiac arrhythmias, and preexisting cardiomyopathy.

The presence of a severe hypotensive episode during OLT should be analyzed promptly for the possible presence of the above-mentioned factors, and therapy should be guided by the results of clinical data obtained from invasive and laboratory studies.

Priority should be given to factors that may be corrected quickly and efficiently (e.g., rapid administration of volume, including blood, plasma, and crystalloids, in case of sudden blood loss and decreased preload). The sudden decrease in preload secondary to surgical manipulation (e.g., compression of IVC, portal vein occlusion) should prompt the anesthesia team to observe the operating field and clarify the possible surgical manipulation with the surgeons. Venous return may be affected by the placement of vascular clamps on major vessels (portal vein, IVC) even if VVB is used. Hypovolemia can be caused by hemorrhage, third space losses, and refractory ascites. If immediate correction of the decreased venous return is impossible (as is the case during some surgical maneuvers), the decreased return of venous blood should be compensated by the temporary use of vasopressors or additional fluid volume or both. Appropriate intraoperative management can prevent or reverse all potential causes affecting cardiac inotropism—low ionized calcium, acidosis, hypothermia, and arrhythmia—with the exception of preexisting cirrhotic cardiomyopathy. If CO/CI remains low despite optimal volume status, inotropic agents must be infused (e.g., dopamine, dobutamine, epinephrine) (Vater et al, 2004). If the blood pressure remains low despite an improvement or normalization of CO/CI, inotropic agents with vasoconstrictive properties may be required (e.g., greater doses of dopamine, epinephrine, and norepinephrine). The intraoperative use of pure vasoconstrictors to increase blood pressure is controversial because impairment of peripheral tissue perfusion may result as a consequence of diversion of blood flow to shunting vessels and away from nutrient vessels (De Wolf, 2000).

It has been suggested that specific intraoperative hemodynamic events are associated independently with adverse outcomes after OLT (Reich et al, 2003). These events include mean arterial pressure less than 40 mm Hg at least once during the procedure and mean pulmonary arterial pressure greater than 40 mm Hg at least three times during the procedure.

Intraoperative Pulmonary Embolism

During OLT, the risk of pulmonary embolism is increased as a consequence of blood stasis, coagulopathy, vessel clamping, and use of VVB (Gologorsky et al, 2001). The most common forms of intraoperative pulmonary embolism during OLT are due to thromboembolism and air embolism, followed by rare fat and tumor embolism. Pulmonary embolism has been reported within minutes after graft reperfusion (Gologorsky et al, 2001). Patients receiving less than an optimal graft or who have septic complications at the time of OLT may be at greater risk. The characteristic features of intraoperative pulmonary embolism are a dramatic increase of mean pulmonary arterial pressure and central venous pressure, and sudden decrease of end-tidal carbon dioxide on capnograph, causing hypotension, cardiac arrhythmias, and low oxygen saturation (Gologorsky et al, 2001; Manji et al, 1998). TEE is currently the primary method to detect the presence and guide the management of pulmonary embolism (Fig. 102.1). The therapeutic goal is to support right ventricle function by using inotropes and vasoactive agents. It is unknown whether acute surgical thrombectomy and pharmacologic fibrinolysis therapy, which have been used in the past, are of value because they are associated with a significant risk of complications. Nevertheless, successful treatment of pulmonary embolism associated with cardiopulmonary bypass and surgical embolectomy has been reported (O'Connor et al, 2000; Szocik et al, 2002).

Severe Hyperkalemia

Patients with ESLD undergoing OLT often require blood products to correct coagulopathy, anemia, and thrombocytopenia. The administration of a large amount of blood products carries the risk of citrate intoxication, acidosis, hypervolemia, and hyperkalemia. Oliguric and anuric patients with renal failure are particularly at risk for hypervolemia and hyperkalemia. Mild to moderate hyperkalemia during the preanhepatic and anhepatic phases may become life-threatening after reperfusion of the transplanted liver because of additional potassium releases with reperfusion. Severe hyperkalemia can result in cardiac conduction abnormalities and arrhythmias, potentially resulting in cardiac arrest. Treatment of severe hyperkalemia includes administration of calcium chloride, sodium bicarbonate, and epinephrine, whereas prevention includes insulin-glucose administration. If the aforementioned measures fail, the dangerously elevated level of potassium should be normalized intraoperatively with CRRT. Different techniques of CRRT have been used in OLT (Petroni & Cohen, 2002; Ziemann-Gimmel et al, 2003). Initiating any form of CRRT requires the mobilization of technical equipment, the presence of trained personnel, and preparation of the dialysate. This technique may not be immediately available. CRRT requires vascular access to be established, and this can be risky in coagulopathic patients (Petroni & Cohen, 2002). Using the existing catheters for CRRT would have the further disadvantage of this being discontinued to start a high infusion rate or VVB. It is important to involve a nephrologist early (preoperatively, if possible) to evaluate for the potential need for CRRT intraoperatively and postoperatively. If hyperkalemia is expected intraoperatively, the right femoral artery and vein additionally may be cannulated with percutaneous sheaths for the possible use of CRRT intraoperatively. Additional modalities available to the anesthesiologist include the parallel use of hemoconcentration with VVB (Ziemann-Gimmel et al, 2003).

Hypothermia

Perioperative hypothermia has been associated with morbidity in the general surgical population. It is appropriate to keep surgical patients normothermic (i.e., at least 36°C [96.8°F]). Treatment-resistant hypothermia during OLT is multifactorial and may result from massive fluid administration, convective and evaporative losses from prolonged exposure of viscera, diminished hepatic energy production, and implantation of a cold allograft of large thermal mass (Russell & Freeman, 1995). Hypothermia predisposes a patient to the increased risk of blood loss and a prolonged recovery time. More significantly, with regards to liver transplantation, it was shown previously that intraoperative hypothermia during OLT increases the risk for early cytomegalovirus infection in liver transplant recipients, and that active warming reduces this risk (Paterson et al, 1999). Hypothermia induces and enhances splanchnic platelet dysfunction (Ozier & Albi, 2004; Ozier et al, 2001). Hypothermia also leads to the impairment of cellular metabolism and oxygen release resulting in further hypotension and a decrease in organ perfusion.

It is crucial to maintain the body temperature of the recipient as close to the normal range as possible. A routine forced air warming device applied to the upper and lower body and a water warming system result in effective maintenance of intraoperative normothermia during OLT (Janicki et al, 2002). In addition, it is imperative that all infused fluids be warmed

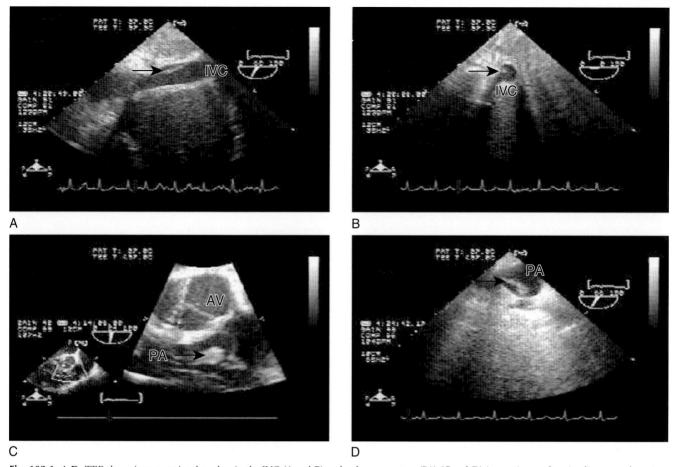

Fig. 102.1. A-D, TEE shows intraoperative thrombus in the IVC (**A** and **B**) and pulmonary artery (PA) (**C** and **D**) in a patient undergoing liver transplantation. *Arrows* indicate thrombotic material in the lumina of the vessels. AV, aortic valve.
(Images courtesy of Dr. Mikhail Sukernik, Department of Anesthesiology, Hershey Medical Center.)

using effective in-line warmers. If these measures fail, the temperature in the operating room should be increased to prevent a further decline in the body temperature. The initial operative phase after induction (i.e., line placement) is often associated with significant heat loss; the operating room should be warmed beforehand to a comfortable temperature and kept warm until the patient is draped and subsequently adjusted to a comfortable level.

Emergence: Early Versus Late Extubation

Maintenance of the patient on mechanical ventilation after liver transplant has been considered a "gold standard." As a result of the improvements in surgical technique and postsurgical care, however, early extubation is possible, often within 24 hours after the surgery (Findlay et al, 2002; Quiroga et al, 2004; Ulukaya et al; 2002). Early extubation 1 to 6 hours after transplantation has been practiced for some time in carefully selected patients. Initially, early extubation was defined as extubation within the first 8 hours after the surgery; however, more recently it was modified to 3 hours post-transplant (Biancofiore et al, 2001).

Early postoperative extubation has been associated with shorter ICU stay, reduced costs, and a lower risk of postoperative

infection (Findlay et al, 2002; Quiroga et al, 2004; Ulukaya et al, 2002). Analysis of 160 liver transplant recipients with no signs of hypoxemia, unstable blood pressure, and delayed awakening showed that patients can be extubated immediately after surgery, hastening recovery (Biancofiore et al, 2001). Although 75.5% of patients were extubated shortly after surgery, studies have shown that 1.8% to 14.8% of patients need to be reintubated within 48 hours (Biancofiore et al, 2001; Glanemann et al, 2001; Mandell et al, 2002). Major reasons for reintubation are pulmonary complications (44.6%), cerebral complications (19.1%), surgical complications (14.5%), and cardiac complications (9.1%) (Glanemann et al, 2001). The rationale behind the improved outcome of patients who are extubated early is that spontaneous ventilation is beneficial for hemodynamically stable patients because it stimulates hepatic venous flow and donor graft circulation (Cammu et al, 2003). The increase in tidal volume and CO/CI associated with spontaneous breathing promote better graft perfusion. The criteria for early extubation include good liver function, normal pH, no significant clinical bleeding, prothrombin time greater than 25%, satisfactory arterial blood gases, and a maximum of 10 U packed red blood cells transfused during the surgery (Cammu et al, 2003). A few contraindications to early extubation still exist and are of a critical nature, including encephalopathy, acute liver failure, and delayed graft function.

IMMEDIATE POSTOPERATIVE CARE

Perioperative morbidity and mortality have decreased dramatically over the past 2 decades (Saner et al, 2003). Despite these advances, numerous potentially fatal conditions still occur with the potential to complicate the immediate postoperative period. These issues become increasingly relevant with the increasing number of adult-to-adult LDLT in which technical considerations play an even more significant role (McGilvray & Greig, 2002; Sugawara et al, 2001).

Primary graft nonfunction requires retransplantation, and delayed graft dysfunction requires experienced clinical judgment as to the probability of sustaining long-term patient survival. Another catastrophic complication is the development of thrombosis of the hepatic artery, which may develop acutely or manifest insidiously much later (Pastacaldi et al, 2001). This condition often can be managed successfully, however, by surgical reconstruction. Thrombosis of the portal vein, although not fatal, can complicate the immediate postoperative course significantly and predispose the patient to significant risk of sepsis. Meticulous and close monitoring of the recipient in the immediate period after liver transplantation is crucial because prompt diagnosis of complications and early treatment intervention can affect patient survival directly (Marroquin et al, 2003). Postoperative fluid and electrolyte management should be tailored to the individual patient, keeping in mind that the hyperdynamic state associated with ESLD makes the interpretation of hemodynamic parameters difficult.

Pulmonary Complications

Pulmonary complications, including hypoxemia, with or without pulmonary edema, and pleural effusions, are frequent (75% of patients immediately after OLT) (Gur et al, 2004; Hoeper et al, 2004; Krowka et al, 2004; Starkel et al, 2002). Hypoxemia associated with noncardiogenic pulmonary edema and massive perioperative transfusion of blood products typically responds readily to administration of diuretics, positive pressure ventilation, and positive end-expiratory pressure. High peak airway pressure and positive end-expiratory pressure may decrease perfusion of the allograft. Patients with preexisting severe hypoxemia may have persistent hypoxemia after transplant and may require prolonged mechanical ventilation. Positive pressure ventilation with oxygen by facemask in patients with acute respiratory failure after OLT leads to fewer reintubations, shorter ICU stay, and a trend toward decreased in-hospital mortality (Antonelli & Conti, 2000). In the ICU, facemask ventilation may allow the liver transplant patient to remain nonintubated while volume status adjustments are made.

Fluid overload and cardiogenic failure are common, but they are not the only causes of pulmonary edema in OLT patients. Reperfusion of the donor liver during OLT, when combined with transfusion of blood products, can be associated with a brief, but potentially severe form of lung injury (Yost et al, 2001). Instances of pulmonary edema occurring postperfusion (usually within 1-2 hours) generally are related to the amount of blood products transfused, although this effect is usually transient in nature and resolves within several hours.

Bilateral, but more often right-sided, pleural effusion occurs in most patients within the first week after OLT (Carton et al, 1994a, 1994b). These pleural effusions rarely cause respiratory distress and tend to resolve spontaneously during the first postoperative month. Paralysis of the right hemidiaphragm may be observed secondary to intraoperative injury of the right phrenic nerve.

Infection and infection-related complications are the most frequent cause of death after OLT. Bacterial pulmonary infections usually occur during the first week after surgery and include common pathogens, such as gram-negative bacteria. In terms of viral infections, cytomegalovirus infections occur most frequently 4 to 6 weeks after OLT, whereas *Pneumocystis carinii* infections occur 8 to 12 weeks after OLT (Carton et al, 1994a, 1994b).

Hemodynamic Instability

Cardiovascular instability in the post-transplant period is common. Intravenous fluid therapy should be kept at a minimum to maintain proper intravascular volume, unless there is evidence of hypovolemia-induced hypoperfusion. Packed red blood cells should be transfused as needed to maintain hematocrit within the recommended range of 25% to 30% (Carton et al, 1994a, 1994b). Fluid and electrolyte management must be monitored for overaggressive replacement of sodium and fluid, which can precipitate central pontine myelinolysis and cardiopulmonary compromise. Some degree of chronic hyponatremia should be tolerated, while guarding against the excessive intravascular fluid that can compromise the patient's fragile cardiopulmonary function (McGilvray & Greig, 2002). ICU management of the liver transplant recipient may require massive amounts of intravenous fluids, but these patients may not tolerate intravascular overload. A retrospective review of about 1200 OLT patients found that the primary reason for ICU readmission was cardiopulmonary dysfunction secondary to fluid overload (Levy et al, 2001). Because ICU readmission is associated with increased mortality, the diligent treatment of intravascular fluid overload should precede discharge from ICU.

Systemic arterial hypertension occurs frequently in the immediate postoperative period. The increased systemic vascular resistance observed postoperatively may result in undetected preoperative cardiac conditions (e.g., cardiomyopathy) becoming clinically apparent. Hypertension also may lead to bleeding from the site of arterial anastomosis. In cases of hypertension, nitroprusside or nicardipine infusion to maintain mean arterial pressure within the desired range is recommended. The contribution of an underlying coagulopathy to postoperative hemorrhage in these patients is likely to be significant, and continued transfusion of coagulation factors and platelets is mandatory, especially in patients with continuous blood loss, such as bleeding from the rough surface of the grafted living donor liver. With adequate functioning of the liver graft, prothrombin time and activated partial thromboplastin time gradually achieve normal values within 2 to 3 days after transplant. Postoperative thrombocytopenia is often seen in patients, but resolves within 1½ weeks. Transfusion of platelets may not correct thrombocytopenia because of ongoing splenic platelet sequestration. A small percentage of recipients may require early reoperation as a result of postoperative hemorrhage or abdominal hematoma, even if the site of bleeding has not been identified preoperatively. An intra-abdominal hematoma is frequently a source of sepsis. In addition, the presence of intra-abdominal hypertension has been observed frequently after OLT (32% of cases), and its presence has been linked to renal failure, a lower glomerular filtration gradient, delayed postsurgical weaning from the ventilator, and increased ICU mortality (Biancofiore et al, 2004).

Renal and Metabolic Complications and Support

Acute renal failure is a common complication after OLT (occurring in 5-50% of patients) and is of multifactorial origin (Lutkes et al, 1999). More than one third of patients require temporary hemodialysis shortly after transplant, whereas approximately 5% need long-term hemodialysis (Cardenas et al, 2000). Pretransplant renal function and hemodynamic conditions in the operative and postoperative periods were identified as risk factors for the development of acute renal failure after OLT. Failure of renal function recovery within 30 days after surgery and postoperative hypotension were identified as increased mortality risk factors (Lima et al, 2003). Postoperative CRRT is an effective therapy for postoperative acute renal failure (Gaspar et al, 2002; Petroni & Cohen, 2002). CRRT can be performed in hemodynamically unstable patients who are otherwise unfit for hemodialysis. Indications for CRRT include persistent postoperative uremia, hyperkalemia, metabolic acidosis, and fluid overload. Patients developing the need for CRRT postoperatively have an increase in mortality within 90 days and lower 1-year survival rate, however, with the highest rate of mortality in patients starting CRRT postoperatively (Gonwa et al, 2001). It has been shown that elevated serum creatinine levels at 1 year, the use of cyclosporine as an immunosuppressant, and the presence of diabetes before OLT are independent predictive factors for the development of postoperative renal failure (Paramesh et al, 2004). Patients with renal failure who received kidney transplantation had a higher 10-year survival rate compared with patients maintained on dialysis.

Hypokalemia and metabolic alkalosis are observed frequently in the early postoperative period. The development of metabolic alkalosis may be secondary to the metabolism of citrate or lactate by the functioning liver graft, steroid administration, diuretic therapy, hyperaldosteronism, and nasogastric drainage (Merritt, 2000). Significant hypokalemia may require replacement with potassium chloride, which additionally contributes to the correction of the metabolic alkalosis.

Hyperglycemia occurs shortly after reperfusion in virtually all liver transplant recipients and continues in most patients throughout the early postoperative period. The pathophysiology of hyperglycemia is related to glucose release from the grafted liver, insufficient hepatic glycogenesis, and steroid-induced insulin resistance. Persistent hyperglycemia may need to be treated with an insulin infusion.

Neurologic Complications

Neurologic complications, including seizures, hepatic encephalopathy, cerebral edema, central pontine myelinolysis, stroke, and intracranial hemorrhage, may occur in the immediate postoperative period (Carton et al, 1994a, 1994b; Yu et al, 2004). Electrolyte abnormalities, particularly hyponatremia, hypomagnesemia, or hypocalcemia, and the toxic effect of immunosuppressive agents may provoke seizures. Treatment includes correction of the underlying metabolic abnormality or medication-induced toxicity or both and administration of anticonvulsant therapy (Carton et al, 1994a, 1994b). Seizures also can be induced by cerebral infarction caused by thrombotic or air embolism related to VVB. A poorly functioning or nonfunctioning allograft may be associated with progressive hepatic encephalopathy that may be complicated further by cerebral edema and intracranial hypertension. Patients with cerebral edema and intracranial hypertension preceding OLT may experience a dramatic increase in ICP during the reperfusion phase. If undetected (e.g., patients without a properly functioning ICP monitor) or not treated effectively, increased ICP may result in brain damage that is subsequently detected in the ICU after an otherwise successful OLT. Poorly controlled systolic hypertension accompanied by uncorrected coagulopathy immediately after OLT can result in fatal intracranial hemorrhage.

Progressive postoperative somnolence can be the result of abrupt changes in serum sodium concentrations. The risk of developing central pontine myelinolysis can be reduced by avoiding rapid changes in plasma osmolality and sodium concentrations intraoperatively and postoperatively (Yu et al, 2004). Other, rare neurologic complications, such as leukodystrophy, meningitis, and cerebral abscess, may occur within the first several postoperative days. To facilitate the neurologic examination of intubated and mechanically ventilated patients during their postoperative ICU stay, patients should be sedated with short-acting sedatives (e.g., propofol infusion) and muscle relaxants, if necessary, and maintained at a sedation level allowing rapid reversal.

Postoperative Infections

The major cause of unfavorable outcome after OLT is infection. It is imperative to maintain aseptic technique throughout the perioperative period and institute aggressive antibiotic therapy, with antifungal agents initiated if necessary. Liver transplant recipients who develop surgical site infection have significantly higher resource use requirements than recipients who do not develop an infection (Hollenbeak et al, 2001). Life-threatening infections include intra-abdominal, pulmonary, wound, urinary tract, and catheter-related infections. Multiple organ failure rapidly follows sepsis, and mortality is high (Baker & Nasraway, 2000). Monitoring lines should be removed as soon as possible in all patients because they are a frequent source of infection.

Analgesic Requirements

OLT patients experience less pain and use fewer analgesics postoperatively than liver resection patients (Donovan et al, 1997; Moretti et al, 2002). When extubation has been achieved, analgesic requirements are surprisingly low, and compliance with physiotherapy regimens and rapid mobilization is usually the rule.

ACKNOWLEDGMENTS

The author thanks Dr. Tomasz Jarzembowski (Department of Anesthesiology, Penn State College of Medicine) for his valuable intellectual input, helpful comments, and assistance in preparation of this chapter.

REFERENCES

Adam R, et al, 2003: Evolution of liver transplantation in Europe: report of the European Liver Transplant Registry. Liver Transpl 9:1231-1243.

Ahl B, et al, 2004: Regional differences in cerebral blood flow and cerebral ammonia metabolism in patients with cirrhosis. Hepatology 40:73-79.

Antonelli M, Conti G, 2000: Noninvasive positive pressure ventilation as treatment for acute respiratory failure in critically ill patients. Crit Care 4:15-22.

Ardizzone G, et al, 2004: Modifications of cerebral vascular resistance and autoregulation after graft reperfusion during human orthotopic liver transplantation. Transplant Proc 36:1473-1478.

Arguedas MR, et al, 2003: Prospective evaluation of outcomes and predictors of mortality in patients with hepatopulmonary syndrome undergoing liver transplantation. Hepatology 37:192-197.

Baker K, Nasraway SA, 2000: Multiple organ failure during critical illness: how organ failure influences outcome in liver disease and liver transplantation. Liver Transpl 6:S5-S9.

Bass NM, 2000: Monitoring and treatment of intracranial hypertension. Liver Transpl 6:S21-S26.

Biancofiore G, et al, 2001: Very early tracheal extubation without predetermined criteria in a liver transplant recipient population. Liver Transpl 7:777-782.

Biancofiore G, et al, 2004: Intraabdominal pressure in liver transplant recipients: incidence and clinical significance. Transplant Proc 36:547-549.

Blei AT, 2000a: Diagnosis and treatment of hepatic encephalopathy. Baillieres Best Pract Res Clin Gastroenterol 14:959-974.

Blei AT, 2000b: Medical therapy of brain edema in fulminant hepatic failure. Hepatology 32:666-669.

Blei AT, 2000c: Brain edema and portal-systemic encephalopathy. Liver Transpl 6:S14-S20.

Cabezuelo JB, et al, 2003: Does the standard vs piggyback surgical technique affect the development of early acute renal failure after orthotopic liver transplantation? Transplant Proc 35:1913-1914.

Cammu G, et al, 2003: Criteria for immediate postoperative extubation in adult recipients following living-related liver transplantation with total intravenous anesthesia. J Clin Anesth 15:515-519.

Cardenas A, et al, 2000: Hepatorenal syndrome. Liver Transpl 6:S63-S71.

Carton EG, et al, 1994a: Perioperative care of the liver transplant patient. Part 1. Anesth Analg 78:120-133.

Carton EG, et al, 1994b: Perioperative care of the liver transplant patient. Part 2. Anesth Analg 78:382-399.

Cerutti E, et al, 2004: Thromboelastogram monitoring in the perioperative period of hepatectomy for adult living liver donation. Liver Transpl 10:289-294.

Colquhoun SD, et al, 2001: The pathophysiology, diagnosis, and management of acute hepatic encephalopathy. Adv Intern Med 46:155-176.

Dalmau A, et al, 2000: Tranexamic acid reduces red cell transfusion better than epsilon-aminocaproic acid or placebo in liver transplantation. Anesth Analg 91:29-34.

Dalmau A, et al, 2004: The prophylactic use of tranexamic acid and aprotinin in orthotopic liver transplantation: a comparative study. Liver Transpl 10:279-284.

Della Rocca G, et al, 2001: Hemodynamic-volumetric versus pulmonary artery catheter monitoring during anesthesia for liver transplantation. Transplant Proc 33:1394-1396.

Della Rocca G, et al, 2002: Preload and haemodynamic assessment during liver transplantation: a comparison between the pulmonary artery catheter and transpulmonary indicator dilution techniques. Eur J Anaesthesiol 19:868-875.

Detry O, et al, 1999: Intracranial pressure during liver transplantation for fulminant hepatic failure. Transplantation 67:767-770.

De Wolf AM, 2000: Intraoperative concerns when a liver recipient is critically ill. Liver Transpl 6:S10-S13.

Donovan KL, et al, 1997: Decreased patient analgesic requirements after liver transplantation and associated neuropeptide levels. Transplantation 63:1423-1429.

Fan ST, et al, 2003: Right lobe living donor liver transplantation with or without venovenous bypass. Br J Surg 90:48-56.

Findlay JY, et al, 2002: Fast track anesthesia for liver transplantation reduces postoperative ventilation time but not intensive care unit stay. Liver Transpl 8:670-675.

Fitzsimons MG, et al, 2001: Aprotinin administration and pulmonary thromboembolism during orthotopic liver transplantation: report of two cases. Anesth Analg 92:1418-1421.

Gao L, et al, 2002: Rocuronium plasma concentrations during three phases of liver transplantation: relationship with early postoperative graft liver function. Br J Anaesth 88:764-770.

Gao L, et al, 2003: Rocuronium infusion requirements and plasma concentrations at constant levels of neuromuscular paralysis during three phases of liver transplantation. J Clin Anesth 15:257-266.

Garcia N Jr, Sanyal AJ, 2001: Portal hypertension. Clin Liver Dis 5:509-540.

Gaspar LJ, et al, 2002: Continuous renal replacement therapies. EDTNA ERCA J 2(suppl):19-22.

Gines P, et al, 2003: Hepatorenal syndrome. Lancet 362:1819-1827.

Glanemann M, et al, 2001: Postoperative tracheal extubation after orthotopic liver transplantation. Acta Anaesthesiol Scand 45:333-339.

Gologorsky E, et al, 2001: Intracardiac thrombus formation and pulmonary thromboembolism immediately after graft reperfusion in 7 patients undergoing liver transplantation. Liver Transpl 7:783-789.

Gonwa TA, et al, 2001: Renal replacement therapy and orthotopic liver transplantation: the role of continuous veno-venous hemodialysis. Transplantation 71:1424-1428.

Gonwa TA, et al, 2004: Estimation of glomerular filtration rates before and after orthotopic liver transplantation: evaluation of current equations. Liver Transpl 10:301-309.

Gordon PC, et al, 2002: Decreasing blood product requirements after orthotopic liver transplantation. S Afr J Surg 40:46-48.

Guarracino F, 2001: [The role of transesophageal echocardiography in intraoperative hemodynamic monitoring]. Minerva Anestesiol 67:320-324.

Gur C, et al, 2004: Hepatic hydrothorax—pathophysiology, diagnosis and treatment—review of the literature. Liver Int 24:281-284.

Hendriks HG, et al, 2002: Effects of recombinant activated factor VII on coagulation measured by thromboelastography in liver transplantation. Blood Coagul Fibrinolysis 13:309-313.

Hoeper MM, et al, 2004: Portopulmonary hypertension and hepatopulmonary syndrome. Lancet 363:1461-1468.

Hollenbeak CS, et al, 2001: The effect of surgical site infections on outcomes and resource utilization after liver transplantation. Surgery 130:388-395.

Hosein Shokouh-Amiri M, et al, 2000: Choice of surgical technique influences perioperative outcomes in liver transplantation. Ann Surg 231:814-823.

Isern MR, et al, 2004: Randomized trial comparing pulmonary alterations after conventional with venovenous bypass versus piggyback liver transplantation. Liver Transpl 10:425-433.

Jabbour N, et al, 2004: Live donor liver transplantation without blood products: strategies developed for Jehovah's Witnesses offer broad application. Ann Surg 240:350-357.

Jalan R, 2003: Intracranial hypertension in acute liver failure: pathophysiological basis of rational management. Semin Liver Dis 23:271-282.

Janicki PK, et al, 2001: Ischemic optic neuropathy after liver transplantation. Anesthesiology 94:361-363.

Janicki PK, et al, 2002: Water warming garment versus forced air warming system in prevention of intraoperative hypothermia during liver transplantation: a randomized controlled trial [ISRCTN32154832]. BMC Anaesthesiol 2:7.

Jankowski CJ, et al, 2002: Aprotinin and reduced epinephrine requirements in orthotopic liver transplantation. Anesthesiology 96:254-255.

Jones FD, et al, 1999: The coexistence of portopulmonary hypertension and hepatopulmonary syndrome. Anesthesiology 90:626-629.

Kallet RH, et al, 2000: The treatment of acidosis in acute lung injury with tris-hydroxymethyl aminomethane (THAM). Am J Respir Crit Care Med 161:1149-1153.

Kang Y, 2000: Coagulopathies in hepatic disease. Liver Transpl 6:S72-S75.

Keeffe BG, et al, 2001: Detection and treatment of coronary artery disease in liver transplant candidates. Liver Transpl 7:755-761.

Kempen PM, et al, 2000: The rapid infusion system: user error in tubing connection mimicking severe hemorrhage. Anesthesiology 93:278-279.

Koh KF, 2000: Pitfalls in anesthesia for liver transplantation. Transplant Proc 32:1515-1516.

Krenn CG, et al, 2004: Assessment of ventricular contractile function during orthotopic liver transplantation. Transpl Int 17:101-104.

Krowka MJ, et al, 2004: Hepatopulmonary syndrome and portopulmonary hypertension: a report of the multicenter liver transplant database. Liver Transpl 10:174-182.

Kuo PC, et al, 1999: Portopulmonary hypertension and the liver transplant candidate. Transplantation 67:1087-1093.

Larsen FS, et al, 2000: Intensive care management of patients with acute liver failure with emphasis on systemic hemodynamic instability and cerebral edema: a critical appraisal of pathophysiology. Can J Gastroenterol 14(suppl D):105D-111D.

Lee SS, 2003: Cardiac dysfunction in spontaneous bacterial peritonitis: a manifestation of cirrhotic cardiomyopathy? Hepatology 38:1089-1091.

Levy MF, et al, 2001: Readmission to the intensive care unit after liver transplantation. Crit Care Med 29:18-24.

Lima EQ, et al, 2003: Risk factors for development of acute renal failure after liver transplantation. Ren Fail 25:553-560.

Lizardi-Cervera J, et al, 2003: Hepatic encephalopathy: a review. Ann Hepatol 2:122-130.

Luketic VA, 2001: Management of portal hypertension after variceal hemorrhage. Clin Liver Dis 5:677-707.

Lukin CL, et al, 1995: Duration of vecuronium-induced neuromuscular block as a predictor of liver allograft dysfunction. Anesth Analg 80:526-533.

Lutkes P, et al, 1999: Continuous venovenous hemodialysis treatment in critically ill patients after liver transplantation. Kidney Int 72(suppl):S71-S74.

Lutz JT, et al, 2003: Blood-transfusion requirements and blood salvage in donors undergoing right hepatectomy for living related liver transplantation. Anesth Analg 96:351-355.

Mahajan A, et al, 2004: Use of intraoperative TEE in orthotopic liver transplantation. Anesth Analg 98:112.

Mandell MS, et al, 2002: Reduced use of intensive care after liver transplantation: patient attributes that determine early transfer to surgical wards. Liver Transpl 8:682-687.

Mandell MS, et al, 2003: The effects of desflurane and propofol on portosystemic pressure in patients with portal hypertension. Anesth Analg 97:1573-1577.

Manji M, et al, 1998: Survival from massive intraoperative pulmonary thromboembolism during orthotopic liver transplantation. Br J Anaesth 80:685-687.

Markiewicz M, et al, 2003: Acute coagulopathy after reperfusion of the liver graft in children: correction with recombinant activated factor VII. Transplant Proc 35:2318-2319.

Marroquin CE, et al, 2003: Emergencies after liver transplantation. Semin Gastrointest Dis 14:101-110.

Mazzeo AT, et al, 2004: Hepatopulmonary syndrome: a concern for the anesthetist? Pre-operative evaluation of hypoxemic patients with liver disease. Acta Anaesthesiol Scand 48:178-186.

McGilvray ID, Greig PD, 2002: Critical care of the liver transplant patient: an update. Curr Opin Crit Care 8:178-182.

Meijer K, et al, 2003: Recombinant factor VIIa in orthotopic liver transplantation: influence on parameters of coagulation and fibrinolysis. Blood Coagul Fibrinolysis 14:169-174.

Merritt WT, 2000: Metabolism and liver transplantation: review of perioperative issues. Liver Transpl 6:S76-S84.

Molenaar IQ, Porte RJ, 2002: Aprotinin and thromboembolism in liver transplantation: is there really a causal effect? Anesth Analg 94:1367-1368.

Molenaar IQ, et al, 2001a: The effect of aprotinin on renal function in orthotopic liver transplantation. Transplantation 71:247-252.

Molenaar IQ, et al, 2001b: Reduced need for vasopressors in patients receiving aprotinin during orthotopic liver transplantation. Anesthesiology 94:433-438.

Molenaar IQ, et al, 2001c: Aprotinin in orthotopic liver transplantation: evidence for a prohemostatic, but not a prothrombotic, effect. Liver Transpl 7:896-903.

Molenaar IQ, et al, 2001d: Improved early graft survival in patients receiving aprotinin during orthotopic liver transplantation. Transplant Proc 33:1345-1346.

Moller S, Henriksen JH, 2002: Cirrhotic cardiomyopathy: a pathophysiological review of circulatory dysfunction in liver disease. Heart 87:9-15.

Moreno-Gonzalez E, et al, 2003: Advantages of the piggy back technique on intraoperative transfusion, fluid consumption, and vasoactive drug requirements in liver transplantation: a comparative study. Transplant Proc 35:1918-1919.

Moretti EW, et al, 2002: Orthotopic liver transplant patients require less postoperative morphine than do patients undergoing hepatic resection. J Clin Anesth 14:416-420.

Mukherjee KK, et al, 2003: Raised intracranial pressure in hepatic encephalopathy. Indian J Gastroenterol 22(suppl 2):S62-S65.

Murphy N, et al, 2004: The effect of hypertonic sodium chloride on intracranial pressure in patients with acute liver failure. Hepatology 39:464-470.

Myers RP, Lee SS, 2000: Cirrhotic cardiomyopathy and liver transplantation. Liver Transpl 6:S44-S52.

Myles PS, et al, 2004: Bispectral index monitoring to prevent awareness during anaesthesia: the B-Aware randomised controlled trial. Lancet 363:1757-1763.

Nair S, et al, 2002: Pretransplant renal function predicts survival in patients undergoing orthotopic liver transplantation. Hepatology 35:1179-1185.

Niemann CU, et al, 2004: Intraoperative fluid management of living donor versus cadaveric liver transplant recipients. Transplant Proc 36:1466-1468.

O'Connor CJ, et al, 2000: Pulmonary thromboembolism during liver transplantation: possible association with antifibrinolytic drugs and novel treatment options. Anesth Analg 91:296-299.

Ozier Y, Albi A, 2004: Liver transplant surgery and transfusion. Int Anesthesiol Clin 42:147-162.

Ozier Y, et al, 2001: Haemostatic disorders during liver transplantation. Eur J Anaesthesiol 18:208-218.

Ozier Y, et al, 2003: Institutional variability in transfusion practice for liver transplantation. Anesth Analg 97:671-679.

Paramesh AS, et al, 2004: Post-liver transplant acute renal failure: factors predicting development of end-stage renal disease. Clin Transplant 18:94-99.

Pastacaldi S, et al, 2001: Hepatic artery thrombosis after orthotopic liver transplantation: a review of nonsurgical causes. Liver Transpl 7:75-81.

Paterson DL, et al, 1999: Intraoperative hypothermia is an independent risk factor for early cytomegalovirus infection in liver transplant recipients. Transplantation 67:1151-1155.

Petroni KC, Cohen NH, 2002: Continuous renal replacement therapy: anesthetic implications. Anesth Analg 94:1288-1297.

Planinsic RM, et al, 2003: Transesophageal echocardiography-guided placement of internal jugular percutaneous venovenous bypass cannula in orthotopic liver transplantation. Anesth Analg 97:648-649.

Plotkin JS, et al, 2000: Coronary artery disease and liver transplantation: the state of the art. Liver Transpl 6:S53-S56.

Plotkin JS, et al, 2001: Dobutamine stress echocardiography for orthotopic liver transplant evaluation. Transplantation 71:818.

Quiroga M, et al, 2004: Trends in mechanical ventilation and immediate extubation after liver transplantation in a single center in Chile. Transplant Proc 36:1683-1684.

Rafanan AL, et al, 2000: Progressive portopulmonary hypertension after liver transplantation treated with epoprostenol. Chest 118:1497-1500.

Ramsay MA, et al, 2004: Intravascular thrombosis and thromboembolism during liver transplantation: antifibrinolytic therapy implicated? Liver Transpl 10:310-314.

Reddy KS, et al, 2000: Piggyback technique and selective use of veno-venous bypass in adult orthotopic liver transplantation. Clin Transplant 14:370-374.

Reich DL, et al, 2003: Association of intraoperative hypotension and pulmonary hypertension with adverse outcomes after orthotopic liver transplantation. J Cardiothorac Vasc Anesth 17:699-702.

Roth JV, et al, 2002: Percutaneous bypass cannulae can interfere with rapid infusion during liver transplantation. J Cardiothorac Vasc Anesth 16:617-620.

Russell SH, Freeman JW, 1995: Prevention of hypothermia during orthotopic liver transplantation: comparison of three different intraoperative warming methods. Br J Anaesth 74:415-418.

Sabba C, et al, 2001: Haemodynamic effects of propranolol, octreotide and their combination during fasting and post-prandial splanchnic hyperaemia in patients with cirrhosis. Eur J Gastroenterol Hepatol 13:163-169.

Saner F, et al, 2003: Postoperative ICU management in liver transplant patients. Eur J Med Res 8:511-516.

Schroeder RA, et al, 1999: Total blood transfusion and mortality after orthotopic liver transplantation. Anesthesiology 91:329-330.

Schroeder RA, et al, 2000: Use of aerosolized inhaled epoprostenol in the treatment of portopulmonary hypertension. Transplantation 70:548-550.

Starkel P, et al, 2002: Outcome of liver transplantation for patients with pulmonary hypertension. Liver Transpl 8:382-388.

Strauss G, et al, 1998: Hyperventilation restores cerebral blood flow autoregulation in patients with acute liver failure. J Hepatol 28:199-203.

Strauss GI, et al, 1999: Regional cerebral blood flow during mechanical hyperventilation in patients with fulminant hepatic failure. Hepatology 30:1368-1373.

Sugawara Y, et al, 2001: Small-for-size grafts in living-related liver transplantation. J Am Coll Surg 192:510-513.

Szocik J, et al, 2002: ECMO resuscitation after massive pulmonary embolism during liver transplantation. Anesthesiology 97:763-764.

Tofteng F, Larsen FS, 2004: The effect of indomethacin on intracranial pressure, cerebral perfusion and extracellular lactate and glutamate concentrations in patients with fulminant hepatic failure. J Cereb Blood Flow Metab 24:798-804.

Tofteng F, et al, 2002: Cerebral microdialysis in patients with fulminant hepatic failure. Hepatology 36:1333-1340.

Ulukaya S, et al, 2002: Immediate tracheal extubation of the liver transplant recipients in the operating room. Transplant Proc 34:3334-3335.

United Network for Organ Sharing, 2003: Available at www.unos.com.

Vaquero J, Blei AT, 2003: Etiology and management of fulminant hepatic failure. Curr Gastroenterol Rep 5:39-47.

Vater Y, et al, 2004: Adjuvant drugs for end-stage liver failure and transplantation. Med Sci Monit 10:77-88.

Wu Y, et al, 2003: Vasopressor agents without volume expansion as a safe alternative to venovenous bypass during cavaplasty liver transplantation. Transplantation 76:1724-1728.

Yost CS, et al, 2001: Etiology of acute pulmonary edema during liver transplantation: a series of cases with analysis of the edema fluid. Chest 119:219-223.

Yu J, et al, 2004: Possible causes of central pontine myelinolysis after liver transplantation. World J Gastroenterol 10:2540-2543.

Zheng SS, et al, 2002: Functional changes of the heart and lung in perioperative period of orthotopic liver transplantation. Hepatobiliary Pancreat Dis Int 1:335-339.

Ziemann-Gimmel P, et al, 2003: Treatment of life-threatening hyperkalemia using hemoconcentration in parallel to venovenous bypass during orthotopic liver transplantation. Anesth Analg 96:680-682.

103

Liver Transplantation: Indications

J. NEUBERGER

The first human orthotopic liver transplant was attempted by Starzl in 1963. In the subsequent 2 decades, only a few patients underwent transplantation; these were usually patients who were moribund with end-stage disease, and survival results were disappointing. With increasing experience and confidence, however, results began to improve, and increasingly more patients underwent transplantation. There has been a major increase in the number of transplant centers and the number of patients receiving grafts. Results are such that many centers currently are reporting 1-year survival rates greater than 90% in elective cases.

It is difficult to identify any one cause for the increase in success. Better surgical and anesthetic techniques, improved postoperative care, and the availability of better immunosuppressive agents all have contributed to the improvements in survival. Additional to these is a better understanding of indications and contraindications for the procedure so that major surgery is not carried out in patients with virtually no chance of surviving the procedure, and patients are referred for transplantation at a stage when they are likely to have the greatest chance of success. The increasing success of liver transplantation and the reduction in contraindications has meant, however, that the number of potential recipients is increasing, whereas the number of donors in many countries remains static or is decreasing. The increasing discrepancy between "supply and demand" means that the mortality of patients awaiting a transplant is increasing; patients wait longer, so they are sicker, and the chances of survival decrease, while resource use increases. Attempts to increase the donor pool by use of split livers and use of organs from selected non–heart-beating donors and from living donors and a better understanding of the contraindications to grafts have had a significant effect.

In North America and some European countries, the method of allocation has been changed to one based on the prognosis (see section on the MELD [Model for End-stage Liver Disease] score), with livers being allocated to the individual patient based primarily on the likelihood of the recipient dying while awaiting a transplant. This approach has resulted in a major reduction in the mortality of patients awaiting liver transplantation without an appreciable effect on outcome after transplantation. This chapter outlines the indications and contraindications for liver replacement.

GENERAL INDICATIONS

The indications for transplantation are easy to define, although the application of these principles is often far more difficult. The two broad indications for grafting are as follows:

1. Estimated survival (because of liver disease) is less than 1 year.
2. Quality of life (because of liver disease) is unacceptable to the patient.

The main contraindications to liver transplantation include the following:

1. The patient is not fit enough to withstand surgery (e.g., because of advanced cardiac or pulmonary disease).
2. The patient is unlikely to survive the procedure (e.g., because of active sepsis).
3. Survival after transplantation may be too short to justify the risks of transplantation (e.g., with metastatic disease)
4. The postoperative quality of life may be unacceptable to the patient (e.g., severe intractable depression).
5. Surgery is technically impossible (e.g., patients with extensive venous thromboses).
6. The patient does not wish to undergo the operation.

Since the 1990s, patterns of indications for transplantation have changed. The total number of patients receiving grafts each year in North America has increased from 1713 in 1988 to 5671 in 2003. Similar observations have been reported in Europe.

Over the decades, there have been changes in the practice of transplantation, as follows:

1. The proportion of patients receiving grafts for alcoholic liver disease and viral hepatitis (especially hepatitis C virus [HCV]) is increasing.
2. The proportion of patients undergoing transplantation for malignancy and for cholestatic diseases is decreasing.
3. The use of living donors has not made a significant impact (as yet) on the number of transplants (e.g., according to United Network for Organ Sharing (www.unos.org), of the 5671 liver transplants done in 2003, only 321 were from living donors).
4. New indications for liver transplantation include replicative hepatitis B virus (HBV) and human immunodeficiency virus (HIV) infection.
5. The introduction in the United States and some European countries of a new system of allocation (based on the MELD score [see later]) has had a major impact on patients awaiting liver replacement.

GENERAL ASPECTS

Nutrition

Many patients with malignancy and with end-stage cirrhosis are malnourished (see Ch. 24). Malnutrition in these patients has many causes, including the disease itself, poor intake, dietary restrictions (often inappropriate), and malabsorption. Malnutrition is associated with increased susceptibility to infection and poor healing. In liver disease, the degree of malnutrition may be difficult to quantify, but malnourished patients fare poorly. Although there is no evidence that improving this state would alter the outcome, it seems prudent to optimize nutrition (Figueiredo et al, 2000). Although it is sensible to correct vitamin and other nutritional deficiencies, there are no convincing data that this would alter the outcome.

Psychological Assessment

Transplantation is associated with major psychological stress for the patient and the family. Initially, many centers arranged for full psychological and psychiatric assessment of all potential transplant candidates, but this is now rarely undertaken. Chronic ill health, perhaps subclinical encephalopathy, and the uncertainties about the future all combine to make it difficult to predict the patient's outcome accurately. When there is a history of psychiatric illness, however, expert assessment is required because some people with psychiatric illness not responsive to therapy or with a history of recurrent episodes of self-harm may not be suitable candidates for transplantation.

Age

Previously, few centers would consider patients older than 55 years old for transplantation. With increasing experience and availability of donors, however, the upper age limit has been extended. There is no clear cutoff, but increasing age is associated independently with mortality post-transplant (Garcia et al, 2001). The concept of biologic age has superseded that of chronologic age, although the former cannot readily be defined or quantified.

Previous Abdominal Surgery

The presence of adhesions, especially in the presence of portal hypertension, adds considerably to the difficulties of surgery. There is little evidence, however, that previous abdominal surgery significantly affects the outcome. The one exception may be in transplantation for primary sclerosing cholangitis; some studies have shown that previous surgery to the biliary tree adversely influences outcome after grafting. Although it seems sensible to avoid upper abdominal surgery in patients who may be future candidates for liver replacement, it is inappropriate to deny these patients surgery because of the future possibility of replacement.

Infection

Active bacterial, fungal, or protozoal sepsis is an absolute contraindication to transplantation, but when appropriate therapy has been instituted, the patient is a suitable candidate for the procedure.

Human Immunodeficiency Virus

Some controversy exists over the transplantation of patients who are HIV positive. Initial studies showed that such patients fared badly. With the introduction of highly active antiretroviral therapy, however, the natural history of HIV infection has been greatly altered, and, for many patients, liver failure associated with HCV infection is a major cause of death. Several centers have performed liver transplants for patients with HIV infection,

and short-term outcomes are encouraging (Fung et al, 2004). Liver transplantation for HIV-infected patients remains limited to a few centers. Indications are becoming better defined (Samuel et al, 2003) and include the following:

1. End-stage liver disease
2. Low or undetectable levels of HIV RNA
3. No AIDS-defining complication
4. CD4 count greater than 200/mL

Cardiovascular Disease

As with other diseases, the prognosis of patients with cardiovascular disease dictates whether liver replacement is an appropriate therapy. Preoperative assessment of cardiovascular status is, at best, imprecise; no clear guidelines exist to define limits below which grafting is unsafe. When the possibility exists of correction of coronary artery disease, this should be undertaken before transplantation.

Respiratory Function

Arterial hypoxemia (hemoglobin saturation <92% or arterial oxygen pressure <70 mm Hg) may be found in 70% of patients with liver disease. Possible causes for this hypoxemia include ventilation/perfusion mismatch, diffusion limitation, alveolar hypoventilation, shunt, and a diffusion/perfusion abnormality (Krowka & Cortese, 1990). Pulmonary dysfunction is present in 2% of patients with advanced liver disease. The presence of significant pulmonary disease is usually apparent on history and physical examination, but sometimes significant pulmonary disease may be cryptic. There are many possible causes for these abnormalities, including the following:

1. Diseases unrelated to the liver disease (e.g., smoking)
2. Pulmonary dysfunction associated with the liver disease (α_1-antitrypsin deficiency)
3. Respiratory conditions associated with the liver disease (e.g., fibrosing alveolitis associated with primary biliary cirrhosis)
4. Effects of the liver disease on respiratory function (e.g., the effects of ascites causing a pleural effusion or simple lung compression)
5. Hepatopulmonary syndrome
6. Pulmonary hypertension

Hepatopulmonary Syndrome

Hepatopulmonary syndrome is characterized by abnormal intrapulmonary vascular dilation (Hoeper et al, 2004). Clinically, there may be shortness of breath and clubbing. The diagnosis is suggested by showing orthodeoxia (a decrease in arterial blood oxygen when standing) and the presence of intrapulmonary shunting (shown by bubble echocardiography or nuclear medicine scanning).

Pulmonary Hypertension

Pulmonary hypertension results from pulmonary vasoconstriction that leads to vascular remodeling (Hoeper et al, 2004). Routine screening of patients with chest x-ray, electrocardiogram, lung function tests, and measurement of peripheral oxygen saturation usually identifies patients with pulmonary problems. Additional investigations, including arterial blood gases (lying and standing to detect hepatopulmonary syndrome) and on 100% oxygen (to detect shunting), high-resolution computed tomography (CT), contrast-enhanced echocardiography, isotope-labeled macroaggregated albumin lung scan, pulmonary angiography, and right heart catheterization, may be indicated as suggested by the clinical and simple investigations.

There are no clear guidelines indicating when liver transplantation is contraindicated because of pulmonary disease (Krowka et al, 2004). In general, experience has shown that patients with a pulmonary arterial PO_2 less than 50 mm Hg do not survive the procedure. These patients may be candidates, however, for a triple transplant (heart, lung, and liver). Similar considerations apply to patients with cystic fibrosis, cystic lung disease, and liver disease. The use of drugs such as bosentan and of transjugular intrahepatic portosystemic shunt has not been fully evaluated in this setting.

COEXISTING DISEASE

The presence of coexisting disease may affect the decision to offer the patient a liver graft either because the prospects of recovery are adversely affected or because long-term survival may be reduced (Rubin et al, 1987). Diabetes mellitus is commonly found in patients with chronic liver disease, especially in patients with HCV infection. Diabetes may occur as a consequence of the insulin intolerance associated with advanced liver disease and may resolve after successful transplantation. Concerns with diabetics center on the microvascular complications. Proliferative retinopathy, diabetic nephropathy, and autonomic neuropathy, as evidenced by simple tests such as abnormal beat-to-beat variation on Valsalva maneuver or postural hypotension, may be relative contraindications for transplantation. The presence of advanced microvascular disease puts the patient at risk of major autonomic disruption during the procedure, and the survival of such patients is relatively poor (Haydon & Neuberger, 2001).

Hyponatremia is a common finding in patients with advanced chronic liver disease and occurs usually as a consequence of injudicious diuretic therapy or because of the reduced free water clearance. Grafting patients with severe hyponatremia (serum sodium <120 mmol/L) has shown that there is an increased risk of central pontine myelinolysis. Significant hyponatremia should be corrected before transplantation by simple water restriction and, if appropriate, stopping diuretic therapy or, if more rapid correction is required, by use of renal support (Elias & McMaster, 1987). Aquaretics may be helpful in this situation.

Vascular thromboses are common in patients with chronic liver disease. These may occur as a consequence of the cirrhosis itself or as part of an associated underlying thrombotic tendency (e.g., myeloproliferative disease associated with Budd-Chiari syndrome, presence of lupus anticoagulant, protein C or S deficiency, or impaired fibrinolysis). In early series, portal vein thrombosis was considered to be a contraindication to transplantation, but it is now appreciated that this is no longer the case, and portal venous inflow can be provided by use of the superior mesenteric vein or a splenic vein. Transplantation is actually contraindicated only in the rare patients in whom there is extensive venous thrombosis and it is impossible to provide a suitable portal supply to the new liver.

Renal disease may occur as a consequence of the hepatorenal syndrome or may be due to intrinsic kidney damage. In the

Table 103.1 Effect of Immunosuppression on Tumor Recurrence

Low Recurrence Rates (0–10%)
Incidentally discovered renal tumors
Lymphoma
Testicular carcinoma
Uterine carcinoma
Cervical carcinoma
Thyroid carcinoma
Intermediate Recurrence Rates (11–25%)
Uterine body carcinoma
Wilms' tumor
Colon carcinoma
Breast carcinoma
Prostate carcinoma
High Recurrence Rate (>26%)
Bladder carcinoma
Sarcomas
Melanoma
Symptomatic renal carcinomas
Myelomas
Nonmelanoma skin cancers

Note: This list is derived from patients undergoing renal transplantation and should be used only as a guide when applied to patients undergoing liver transplantation. From Penn I, 1993: The effect of immunosuppression on pre-existing cancers. Transplantation 55:742–747.

hepatorenal syndrome, there is no structural damage to the kidney, and when good liver function is re-established, the kidney functions normally. Although the prognosis may be reduced in the presence of advanced renal insufficiency (Rimola et al 1987), the hepatorenal syndrome is not an absolute contraindication to transplantation. When there is coexisting advanced renal disease, however, it may be advisable to consider combined liver and kidney transplantation. Nonetheless, renal function remains a major predictive factor for the outcome after transplantation (Cuervas Mons et al, 1986). Whether pretransplant correction of renal parameters (e.g., by dialysis) is associated with an improvement in survival is uncertain.

Past history of malignancy is a relative contraindication to transplantation because the effect of surgery and the consequent immunosuppression may predispose the patient to early recurrence of the tumor (Saigal et al, 2001). Penn (1993) identified tumors that have a high risk of recurrence after transplantation (Table 103.1). Patients with primary biliary cirrhosis have a fourfold increased risk of developing extrahepatic malignancy, and patients with coexisting ulcerative colitis may be at increased risk of colonic cancer. Only in exceptional cases should patients with a past history of extrahepatic malignancy be considered suitable candidates for transplantation.

Bone Disease

Many patients with chronic liver disease have bone disease. The occurrence of osteomalacia, as a consequence of vitamin D malabsorption, is low and can be corrected by parenteral administration of vitamin D. Osteoporosis is a far greater problem, however, and is particularly seen in women with chronic cholestatic disease. In many cases, successful transplantation halts or retards the progression and may improve bone mineralization (Eastell et al, 1991). The presence of severe osteoporosis may result in additional complications if there is significant thoracic or lumbar vertebral collapse or the presence of fractures. The development of severe osteoporosis may be an indication for transplantation in itself.

SPECIFIC DISEASES

Fulminant Hepatic Failure

In recent years, liver transplantation has been found to be an effective form of therapy for patients with fulminant hepatic failure (FHF)—the presence of encephalopathy occurring within 8 weeks of the onset of symptoms in a patient with previously normal liver (see Ch. 105) (Peleman et al, 1987). In patients with severe FHF and grade IV hepatic encephalopathy, mortality approaches 80%. Common causes of FHF include paracetamol overdose (see Ch. 92), viral infections (hepatitis A, B, and rarely C), drug and xenobiotic toxicity (including herbal remedies), Wilson's disease, and liver diseases of pregnancy. Patients with FHF develop early multiorgan failure and require intensive supportive therapy. The common causes of death are cerebral edema, bacterial or fungal sepsis, and cardiovascular instability.

Patients with FHF pose a difficult problem because there is only a narrow window between the time when it is apparent that the patient's survival is likely to be poor in the absence of transplantation and the onset of irreversible complications that preclude a successful outcome. More recent identification of prognostic factors has been helpful. Several groups have published prognostic factors (Table 103.2) (Bismuth et al, 1987; O'Grady et al, 1989). The King's College model has been validated in other centers and found to be robust. The patient who fulfills the King's College criteria may be too sick to have a good chance of a successful outcome. It is likely, however, that with advances in the medical management of patients with FHF these prognostic factors will require modification. The inclusion of serum lactate in the King's College prognostic criteria provides greater accuracy (Riordan & Williams, 2002). Contraindications to transplantation in FHF include the onset of irreversible complications. The development of irreversible cerebral edema, characterized by

prolonged elevations of intracranial pressure documented on intracerebral pressure monitoring or the presence of fixed dilated pupils for more than 6 hours, precludes transplantation. Sepsis also is a contraindication.

One of the best guides to progression is given by serial estimation of the prothrombin time or factor V levels because in the absence of extraneous blood products, these best represent the synthetic function of the liver. Initial improvement in the prothrombin time followed by deterioration suggests the presence of sepsis, and such patients no longer should be considered potential candidates. The patient remains at risk of developing complications of increased intracerebral pressure for 48 hours after successful transplantation (Dabos et al, 2004; Keays et al, 1991).

Because of the prognostic importance of clotting parameters, patients with FHF should not be given clotting factors until the decision for transplantation has been made, unless there are pressing clinical reasons. When the decision for transplantation has been made, clotting should be normalized insofar as is possible given the constraints of volume replacement and avoidance of the complications of intracerebral edema. The ability to give large volumes of fluid may be limited by impaired renal function, but the presence of renal support allows fluid to be taken off more rapidly.

Because many of the extrahepatic manifestations of FHF may be a consequence of the presence of large amounts of necrotic tissue, some centers have advocated the use of a two-stage procedure whereby the failed liver is removed, and the patient remains anhepatic until a suitable graft becomes available (Husberg et al, 1991; Ringe et al, 1988). Although there is little doubt that after hepatectomy the patient's condition may improve, there are few convincing data at present to suggest that this beneficially affects outcome. Such a procedure may be indicated, however, in a patient who is rapidly deteriorating and a graft has been found, but logistic conditions may enforce some delay before the graft can be performed successfully.

A dilemma in considering liver transplantation in patients with acute liver failure is that if the liver does recover, a complete return to normal structure and function is likely. The use of auxiliary transplants (e.g., auxiliary partial orthotopic liver transplant [APOLT]) or partial transplants (see Chs. 107 and 108) may allow the earlier use of liver grafting as a safety net because if the patient's liver does recover, the donor liver can be removed or allowed to atrophy, and the patient can return to a life of good liver function free of immunosuppression. The use of artificial liver support devices (see Ch. 89) is uncertain, but systems such as the MARS (molecular absorbent recirculation system) may offer a bridge (Mitzner et al, 2002).

Patients who develop FHF as a consequence of paracetamol overdose pose a special problem. Patients with a long history of psychiatric disease that is unresponsive to full intervention and support or with a history of recurrent overdose usually are not appropriate candidates. Many patients with paracetamol overdose have taken the overdose often on an impulse because of a relatively trivial problem (e.g., a fight with a boyfriend or girlfriend). In such cases, it is appropriate to offer these patients transplantation. In contrast, if the overdose is taken as a consequence of long-term social or domestic problems, it is possible that even after successful grafting the patient would return to identical problems with the additional burden of a liver transplant and its consequences; grafting in such patients may be inappropriate.

Table 103.2 Indications for Transplantation for Fulminant Hepatic Failure

Paris (Bismuth et al, 1987)

Hepatic encephalopathy *and* Factor V <20%

King's College Hospital (O'Grady et al, 1989)

Paracetamol
  Arterial pH <7.30 *or*
  All of the following:
    Prothrombin time >100 sec
    Creatinine >300 mmol/L
    Grade III/IV encephalopathy
Nonparacetamol
  Prothrombin time >100 sec *or*
  Any three of the following:
    Unfavorable etiology
    Interval jaundice to encephalopathy >7 days
    Age <10 yr or >40 yr
    Prothrombin time >50 sec
    Serum bilirubin >300 μmol/L

Table 103.3 Inborn Errors of Metabolism That Have Been Treated by Liver Transplantation

Liver Affected	Other Organs Also Affected
α₁-Antitrypsin deficiency	Primary hyperoxaluria
Wilson's disease	Crigler-Najjar syndrome
Protoporphyria	Primary hypercholesterolemia
Tyrosinosis	Niemann-Pick disease
Tyrosinemia	Sea-blue histiocyte disease*
Galactosemia	Hemophilia A and B
Glycogen storage disease types I and IV	Protein C deficiency
Byler's disease	Protein S deficiency
Hemochromatosis*	
Cystic fibrosis	
Gaucher's disease*	
Urea cycle enzyme deficiencies	

*May recur after transplantation.

Metabolic Diseases

Numerous metabolic diseases may be corrected by liver transplantation (Table 103.3). In some cases, in which the metabolic defect arises in the liver, transplantation corrects the defect. This is seen with Wilson's disease or hemophilia. In other conditions, such as some types of hypercholesterolemia, the metabolic defect occurs within the liver, but the heart is the major organ that is affected. Some centers have advocated the use of liver transplantation to prevent the onset of severe coronary artery disease. In situations in which there is already cardiac disease, combined heart and liver transplants may be performed. Similar considerations apply to hyperoxaluria requiring liver and kidney replacement. In other conditions, such as hemophilia, in which there are alternative therapies such as replacement with factor VIII, transplantation should be considered only when there is extensive liver disease, such as may occur with HCV infection transmitted by blood products. The possibility of recurrence of the metabolic disease should not be considered a contraindication to transplantation. Although the consequences of genetic hemochromatosis are likely to recur after transplantation (because there is increased iron absorption from the bowel), organ damage can be prevented by early recognition and treatment. Equally, in erythropoietic protoporphyria, the disease is likely to recur after transplantation, but the morbidity of disease may be delayed by appropriate treatment with cholestyramine. In these instances, the decision to offer transplantation needs to be made with a view to the benefits obtained, and the indications remain similar to the indications in patients with other liver diseases.

Budd-Chiari Syndrome

The role of liver transplantation in patients with Budd-Chiari syndrome is uncertain (see Ch. 100). There may be underlying thrombotic disorders (e.g., protein C or protein S deficiency, factor V Leiden mutation, lupus anticoagulant, polycythemia, or myeloproliferative disorders); some of these would be corrected by transplantation, whereas others would carry the risk of complications, such as malignant transformation (Menon et al, 2004).

The early use of anticoagulants and of transjugular intrahepatic stents has changed the management of these patients. In general, transplantation should be considered when portal decompression has failed or is not feasible or when there is established cirrhosis.

Chronic Liver Disease

In many respects, patients with chronic liver disease pose the most difficult problems with respect to transplantation. The main concern lies not primarily with whether the patient is a suitable candidate for transplantation, but in deciding on the *appropriate time* to offer the patient the procedure. On the one hand, the fitter the patient, the greater the probability of surviving the procedure; on the other hand, the patient's life will have been shortened if the procedure is unsuccessful. If transplantation is offered too late, the chances of success are reduced.

Broadly speaking, there are two major indications for transplantation in patients with chronic liver disease: poor quality of life and poor estimated length of life. Assessment of quality of life is often difficult because the quality of life that is unacceptable to one person may be acceptable to another. It is often difficult to disentangle the effects of borderline encephalopathy and depression associated with the knowledge of chronic liver disease from the effects of the tiredness and lethargy resulting from the liver disease itself. Some patients adopt the "sick role," and, even after successful transplantation, the patient or the family is reluctant for the sick role to be abandoned. Chronic lethargy and tiredness and intractable pruritus are valid indications for transplantation, however, if all other measures for their treatment are unsuccessful, and extrahepatic disorders, such as coexistent myxedema, have been excluded. Evidence suggests that ondansetron may be effective in improving the lethargy associated with chronic liver disease, and a trial of this agent should be considered before transplantation is undertaken.

Most centers consider transplantation as appropriate when the estimated length of life in the absence of transplantation is limited to 1 year; in practice, this is difficult to assess in many patients (Table 103.4). Mostly the diseases run a fairly predictable course, although the patient's life may be threatened

Table 103.4 Indications for Transplantation in Patients with Cirrhosis

Symptoms
  Hepatic decompensation
    Hepatic encephalopathy
    Increasing ascites
    Recurrent variceal bleeding
    Spontaneous bacterial peritonitis
  Side effects of liver disease
    Increasing osteopenia
    Hepatopulmonary syndrome
    Intractable symptoms (itching or lethargy)
    Development of hepatocellular carcinoma
    Muscle wasting

Biochemical markers
  Serum albumin <30 g/dL
  Serum bilirubin >50 μmol/L for parenchymal disease
  Serum bilirubin >100 μmol/L for cholestatic disease

MELD score 15-35

by unpredictable events, such as sepsis or variceal hemorrhage. For this reason, timing of transplantation is an inexact science. A further feature to be considered is that many of the factors predicting a poor survival in patients with cirrhosis are different from the factors that predict outcome after transplantation. The use of prognostic models has helped in defining the variables that predict outcome, but have disadvantages. First, most prognostic models are defined from retrospective studies using patient data at referral or at a certain point in the course of the illness. It is inappropriate to reapply these models sequentially, unless time-dependent models are used. Second, models provide data for populations, and their application to an individual is limited by the relatively wide confidence intervals. Nonetheless, the Child-Pugh score does give a useful guide, although it may not be sufficiently detailed for estimation of short-term survival. The MELD score also is a useful marker of short-term prognosis and may be more accurate than the Child-Pugh score (Freeman et al, 2004; Olthoff et al, 2004).

Development of hepatic decompensation is a useful clinical marker of a poor prognosis. Indications for consideration of transplantation are shown in Table 103.4.

The development of complications often may precipitate referral for transplantation. Severe ascites, spontaneous bacterial peritonitis, recurrent variceal hemorrhage, and intractable encephalopathy all are indications that hepatic reserve is limited (Gines et al, 1988). The Child-Pugh score and the MELD score are relatively poor prognostic guides to survival after grafting. Data suggest, however, that transplantation of a patient without malignancy with a MELD score less than 12 is associated with a reduction in survival at 1 year compared with continued supportive care without transplantation (Neuberger, 2004).

Other centers have concentrated on functional tests of the liver (see Ch. 2). Although tests such as the aminopyrine breath test, the monoethylglycinexylidide test, and galactosamine elimination clearance have their advocates, none has added greatly to clinical and serologic assessment or been applied widely (Burdelski et al, 1991; Mericel et al, 1992).

Primary Biliary Cirrhosis

The prognostic criteria for transplantation in primary biliary cirrhosis are well defined. Since the early article by Schaffner and coworkers (Shapiro et al, 1979), it has become clear that the serum bilirubin is the best guide to prognosis. When the serum bilirubin exceeds 150 μmol/L (7 mg/dL), the median survival in the absence of transplantation is approximately 18 months. Numerous prognostic models have been developed, including static and time-dependent ones (Neuberger, 1989). These models are helpful in defining the variables that predict survival in the absence of transplantation and after transplantation (Table 103.5). From these models, an estimate of survival can be made (Table 103.6). These models must be used with some care, however, because the confidence intervals are relatively wide, and any information derived from such models must be considered in conjunction with clinical judgment. Ursodeoxycholic acid is now licensed for use in patients with primary biliary cirrhosis and is associated with a significant delay to the time of transplantation. In most patients, serum bilirubin decreases, but the prognostic models remain valid when applied 6 months after introduction of treatment.

Transplantation in patients with primary biliary cirrhosis also may be indicated for intolerable lethargy or intractable pruritus. It is important, however, that all treatable causes of lethargy are excluded, and all therapies for pruritus are considered before

Table 103.5 Prognostic Models for Estimating Survival in Patients with Primary Biliary Cirrhosis

European Model

$2.52 \times \log$ serum bilirubin (μmol/L)
$+ 0.069 \times$ (age [yr] $- 20$)/10
$- 0.05 \times$ serum albumin (g/L)
$+ 0.88$ (if cirrhosis present)
$+ 0.68$ (if central cholestasis present)
$+ 0.52$ (if not treated with azathioprine)

Mayo Model

$0.871 \times \log$ serum bilirubin (mg/dL)
$- 2.53 \times \log$ serum albumin (g/dL)
$+ 0.039 \times$ age (yr)
$+ 2.38 \times \log$ prothrombin time (sec)
$+ 0.859 \times$ edema score*

*0 for no edema, 0.5 for diuretic controlled edema, 1 for diuretic-resistant edema.

transplantation is carried out. The therapeutic options are increasing. Cholestyramine is the mainstay, but trials of rifampicin, naltrexone, and plasmapheresis or MARS should be considered in patients with good liver function before transplantation is offered. There are many causes for lethargy in patients with primary biliary cirrhosis. Depression is common and often responds to antidepressant medication. Celiac disease is found in 3% of patients with primary biliary cirrhosis and, if unrecognized and untreated, may cause lethargy. Low levels of antibodies to gliadin are common in patients with liver disease, so the syndrome should be tested for by measuring antiendomysial antitransglutaminase antibodies, and a small bowel biopsy specimen should be taken in patients in whom these antibodies are present. Coexisting myxedema should be excluded by measuring serum thyrotropin, and Addison's disease should be tested for if appropriate. Sometimes the lethargy is caused by inappropriate use of antihistamines to control itching or of sleeping tablets. For the treatment of pruritus, cholestyramine is effective if enough is taken for long enough; for patients unable to tolerate the nausea or diarrhea associated with cholestyramine, a formulation without sorbitol (e.g., Questran Light) or colestipol (Colestid) is effective. Rifampicin and naltrexone also may be effective. Other remedies that may be effective include extrahepatic biliary diversion, plasmapheresis, and MARS (extracorporeal albumin perfusion). In the case of intractable pruritus, when other modalities have been tried and failed, transplantation is extremely effective therapy. Pruritus usually disappears within 2 to 3 days after surgery. In contrast, lethargy resolves more slowly and often incompletely.

Primary biliary cirrhosis does recur in the allograft. This is likely to be at a slow rate and should not preclude transplantation. Other extrahepatic manifestations of primary biliary cirrhosis would not be affected.

Table 103.6 Mayo Prognostic Model for Estimating Survival in Patients with Primary Sclerosing Cholangitis

$0.535 \times \log$ serum bilirubin (mg/dL)
$+ 0.468 \times$ histologic stage*
$+ 0.041 \times$ age (yr)
$+ 0.705 \times$ splenomegaly†

*1 for stage 1 and 2, 2 for stage 3 and 4.
†0 for absence, 1 for presence.

Primary Sclerosing Cholangitis

In contrast to primary biliary cirrhosis, the natural history of primary sclerosing cholangitis (see Ch. 42) is far less clear and predictable (Ludwig et al, 1990). For many patients, the disease runs a fluctuating course with exacerbations and remissions that may be due to episodes of spontaneously occurring bacterial cholangitis. Underlying these fluctuations in liver function, there is a persisting and relentless progression toward liver failure. As with other chronic liver diseases, serum bilirubin and serum albumin are useful markers of progression, and prognostic models help in timing transplantation (see Table 103.6). The Child-Pugh and MELD scores are as reliable as the Mayo model (Shetty et al, 1997). Most cases of primary sclerosing cholangitis are associated with inflammatory bowel disease, usually ulcerative colitis. Patients with primary sclerosing cholangitis and colitis are at increased risk of colonic cancer compared with patients with colitis alone. Because the cancers tend to be in the ascending colon, a full colonoscopy is recommended in all potential transplant candidates to exclude colonic neoplasia and to assess the degree of colitis. Quiescent colitis is not a contraindication to transplantation, but active colitis should be treated medically before transplantation. When surgical treatment is required to control the colitis, this can be done safely at the time of the transplant procedure.

Primary sclerosing cholangitis is a premalignant condition with the patient at increased risk of developing cholangiocarcinoma in any part of the biliary tree (Rosen & Nagorney, 1991), and 20% of patients with primary sclerosing cholangitis, especially smokers, may develop a cancer (see Ch. 42). Bile duct dysplasia may identify a group of patients at special risk. It is often difficult to be certain whether a sudden deterioration in the patient is due to the development of cholangitis, the natural history of the disease, or the development of cholangiocarcinoma (Bergquist et al, 1998). Methods of detection of cholangiocarcinoma are often unrewarding; serum markers, such as carcinoembryonic antigen, are relatively nonspecific and insensitive; elevated levels of CA 19-9 may be more helpful, but are not specific (Qin et al, 2004). Imaging techniques, including CT, magnetic resonance imaging (MRI), ultrasound, and angiography, are often unreliable and miss quite large tumors. Although the presence of dilated intrahepatic bile ducts is often a useful sign of cholangiocarcinoma, it also is too insensitive and nonspecific for routine use.

The biliary tree usually can be well visualized by MRI cholangiopancreatography (see Ch. 19), which gives images almost as good as those obtained at endoscopic retrograde cholangiopancreatography. MRI cholangiopancreatography does not produce histology, however. Endoscopic retrograde cholangiopancreatography may be helpful if combined with brushing and biopsy of strictures and bile cytology. Although the specificity is high, the sensitivity is relatively low and is not without risk of precipitating a severe cholangitis. Directed percutaneous biopsy or aspiration cytology may give a positive diagnosis, but negative findings do not exclude the possibility of cholangiocarcinoma. Endoscopic retrograde cholangiopancreatography in the presence of advanced primary sclerosing cholangitis may lead to sudden deterioration, presumably as a result of the introduction of biliary sepsis. If a cholangiocarcinoma is known to be present before transplantation, the survival is poor. Most centers believe the patient who is known to have cholangiocarcinoma should not be considered for transplantation. A small proportion of patients with cholangiocarcinoma may benefit, however, from an aggressive approach with brachytherapy and chemotherapy (Heimbach et al, 2004).

Currently, there is no effective medical treatment for primary sclerosing cholangitis, although encouraging claims have been made for the use of ursodeoxycholic acid at high doses (15-20 mg/kg/day) (Mitchell et al, 2001). Surgical intervention may be helpful, although, in our view, endoscopic dilation or stenting should be considered only in the presence of a single dominant extrahepatic stricture. The use of biliary diversions and biliary reconstruction is associated with a poorer result after transplantation. In our experience in Birmingham, the 1-year survival of patients with primary sclerosing cholangitis without prior biliary surgery was significantly better (Ismail et al, 1991). Analysis of the Mayo Clinic database suggested that the prognostic markers for patients with primary sclerosing cholangitis after transplantation included disease severity, previous biliary or shunt surgery, concurrent bile duct cancer, and presence of inflammatory disease (see Ch. 42) (Wiesner et al, 1996). Our own analysis confirms these observations, although we did find that ulcerative colitis was associated with a better outcome, whereas Crohn's disease was associated with an adverse outcome (Neuberger et al, 1999).

Because primary sclerosing cholangitis is a premalignant disease, and because cholangiocarcinoma is usually difficult to detect, patients with primary sclerosing cholangitis should be considered earlier for transplantation. In these patients, during the course of their illness, biliary surgery should be avoided if possible.

Alcoholic Liver Disease

Selected patients with alcoholic liver disease are excellent candidates for transplantation. Initial concerns were that these patients would continue to drink alcohol to excess, comply poorly with follow-up, and be unreliable with taking their immunosuppression. The ravages of alcohol include not only damage to the liver, but also other organs, including heart, brain, pancreas, and bone marrow, may be affected by alcohol. Finally, patients with alcoholic liver disease are often more likely to have associated psychiatric problems. In 1988, Starzl and coworkers reported an estimated survival of greater than 70%, however, in 41 patients transplanted for alcoholic liver disease. Of these patients, only two returned to alcohol abuse and subsequently died. The survival rates of these patients were similar to other cirrhotics. After these encouraging results, other centers started to consider patients with alcoholic liver disease for transplantation, and most centers now do consider such patients as candidates for the procedure (Kumar et al, 1990). Nonetheless, there remains a decreasing body of opinion that takes the view that because alcoholic liver disease is a self-induced injury, and in view of the expense of the procedure and the limited supply of donor organs, such candidates should not be considered. In the view of most transplant units, however, this attitude is not considered appropriate because patients with alcoholic liver disease are not always alcohol dependent. Numerous self-induced diseases exist, and it would be no more appropriate to deny a patient with alcohol-induced liver disease transplantation for the reason it is self-induced than to deny treatment for a broken limb in a rugby player or mountain climber.

In addition to the usual criteria for transplantation and contraindications to the procedure, other specific factors need to be considered for patients with alcoholic liver disease. The first is the effect of abstinence, which undoubtedly improves survival in patients who present without compensated or decompensated cirrhosis. Although patients who present with variceal hemorrhage or severe ascites often have only limited benefit after abstinence from alcohol, patients with mild ascites or other complications may have a significant improvement in quality and quantity of life when they abstain from drinking (Suterakis et al, 1973). Because it is now becoming apparent that patients who do not abstain from alcohol are more likely to return to drinking excessively after transplantation and are less likely to comply with follow-up (Beresford et al, 1990), some centers insist on an abstinent period of 6 months. There is no good reason for this arbitrary period of abstinence; the duration of abstinence does not correlate with post-transplant abstinence. The disease may progress relentlessly before the stipulated period of abstinence is finished. A period of abstinence is helpful, in part to ensure that the liver would not recover to an extent that transplantation is no longer required, but also to identify why the patient has drunk excessively and to put in place appropriate measures so that there will be less chance of recurrence after transplantation. The period of abstinence has to be considered in the light of the patient's condition, and transplantation should be offered to the patient who has remained abstinent since he was so advised (Neuberger et al, 2002).

It is recommended that a candidate with alcoholic liver disease be evaluated carefully by substance abuse experts. Factors that suggest poor compliance after transplantation include multiple abuse, failure to recognize the nature of the addiction, other substance abuse, lack of social support, and failure to find an alternative activity.

The role of transplantation in patients with alcoholic hepatitis is more difficult to define. Patients with severe hepatitis characterized by high serum bilirubin and prolonged clotting times, encephalopathy, and renal failure have a dismal prognosis. There is usually insufficient time to evaluate the patient's background, and the outcome after transplantation is usually poor. Few centers undertake to perform transplantation in these patients.

In these patients, there is a greater need for a multidisciplinary approach to evaluation. On the physical side, in addition to the routine workup, the extrahepatic effects of alcohol have to be assessed, and patients with advanced alcoholic cardiomyopathy or pancreatitis may not be suitable on those grounds. Psychiatric assessment is used extensively in some centers (Beresford et al, 1990), and these centers have suggested that patients who are non–alcohol dependent, who have found alternative substitutes for alcohol, who have a job, who have taken part in rehabilitation programs, and who have an understanding of their problems often do well after transplantation. Patients with alcoholic liver disease are potential candidates and require appropriate referral for consideration.

Hepatitis

Hepatitis A Virus Infection

Rarely, acute hepatitis A virus infection is an indication for liver transplantation. The indications are mentioned in the section on FHF. In a few cases, there is recurrent infection in the graft, but this is of little clinical significance.

Hepatitis B Virus Infection

Patients with HBV infection can be considered for transplantation because of FHF or because of chronic liver disease.

Of patients with FHF, the conventional criteria apply as indicated previously. Because it is thought that the liver failure in these patients is due to the rapid clearance of viral infected hepatocytes, most patients at the time of transplantation are HBV DNA negative, and the disease recurs less commonly than in patients with chronic HBV infection.

Different considerations apply to patients with chronic liver disease. Patients who are HBV DNA positive at the time of transplantation are much more likely to have recurrence of disease after transplantation, and this is associated with a significantly poor outcome (Freeman et al, 1991; O'Grady et al, 1992; Rizetto et al, 1991). Patients with high HBV DNA positivity before transplantation are not suitable candidates. The management of these patients has been revolutionized by the introduction of effective antiviral therapy (Kim et al, 2004). The introduction of lamivudine has meant that most patients with advanced liver disease can be treated effectively; in patients in whom there is viral resistance (e.g., patients with the YMDD mutation), adefovir is a safe alternative. More antiviral agents are showing promise in clinical trials. Even with effective control of viral replication before transplant, treatment with hepatitis B immunoglobulin and lamivudine (or other antiviral agent) must be continued post-transplantation.

Hepatitis C Virus Infection

The indications for transplantation of patients with HCV infection are similar to those of patients with cryptogenic cirrhosis. Patients with HCV almost invariably develop recurrent disease, although the extent of graft damage varies. Many factors—host, donor, and immunosuppressive—are associated with the extent and rate of graft damage. Because of the effect of recurrence in the graft, some authors have tried to offer antiviral therapy, with pegylated interferon and ribavirin, before transplant (Everson, 2004). When this therapy can be given safely, a sustained viral response is associated with a much lower risk of graft infection and damage. Survival after transplantation is similar to patients receiving grafts for other causes of cirrhosis for the first 5 years, but concern remains whether the longer term survival would be adversely affected by recurrent disease. Treatment with interferon and ribavirin may be effective in selected groups, but tolerance is often poor.

Patients with hemophilia and HCV infection pose few special problems. Although liver transplantation would correct the defect in hemophilia, this itself is not an indication for liver transplantation. Many patients will have contracted HCV through contaminated blood products. Provided that the patient is supported with adequate amounts of the appropriate blood products, liver transplantation poses no major problem, and many patients do not need support beyond 72 hours (McCarthy et al, 1996).

Hepatocellular Carcinoma

Hepatocellular carcinoma (HCC) (see Ch. 71) may occur in a noncirrhotic liver, but in the Western population, HCC more commonly arises in the context of cirrhosis. Numerous approaches to the treatment of HCC have been adopted, including chemotherapy, resection, embolization, transarterial chemoembolization, injection with ethanol, cryotherapy, radiofrequency ablation, and transplantation. Some authors have argued that resection should be considered first in patients with HCC, with salvage liver transplantation used when there is tumor recurrence (Belghiti et al, 2003; Sala et al, 2004). Indications include a normal serum bilirubin and absence of portal hypertension. This approach is controversial.

There are few well-conducted prospective randomized trials of treatment, and most reports are based on selected patients and compared with historical controls. In patients with HCC arising in a cirrhotic liver, the optimal treatment depends not only on the natural history of the HCC, but also on the severity and extent of the liver disease.

The median survival with medical therapy for a patient with HCC arising in the cirrhotic liver is approximately 6 to 12 months and may be twice that for a patient with hepatoma arising from a noncirrhotic liver. It has been suggested that patients with the fibrolamellar variant have a better prognosis, but this is not universally accepted. For all patients with HCC, transplantation offers the only prospect of long-term survival; given the current shortage of donor organs, guidelines have to be accepted to determine the indications and contraindications for liver replacement.

Transplantation for patients with HCC raises many questions, and at present there are few hard data on which to base a logical strategy. Most units currently adopt the Milan criteria for accepting a patient for transplantation (Mazzaferro et al, 1996). These criteria are a single tumor of less than 5 cm in diameter or, in patients with multiple tumors, no more than three tumors all less than 3 cm in diameter. The analysis was based on only 48 patients. Extrapolation for these observations to current practice must be done with caution because imaging techniques have improved, and more lesions are being detected. It may be inappropriate to extrapolate conclusions based on studies done in the late 1990s to current practice. The size of the tumor per se is not important, but the size reflects the likelihood of tumor microinvasion and spread and the chance of recurrence post-transplant (this is not strictly recurrence, but persistence). Other groups have suggested that these criteria are too strict and should be expanded. The San Francisco group (Yao et al, 2002) suggested that the indications should be expanded to include a solitary tumor 6.5 cm diameter or less or three or fewer nodules with the largest lesion 4.5 cm or less and a total tumor diameter 8 cm or less. Vascular invasion would preclude transplantation. Whether indications for transplant with cadaveric donor livers should be the same as for living donated livers is controversial.

Klintmalm (1998) published the outcome of the findings of the International Registry of Hepatic Tumors in liver transplantation, which included the outcome of 410 patients with HCC and 12 with the fibrolamellar variant. Of these patients, 40% had incidental tumors—tumors that were detected on routine screening, rather than tumors with symptoms. A total of 190 patients had died, 99 free of tumor and 91 with tumor, and tumor was the cause of death in all but 1 of these patients (many early deaths were presumed to be tumor-free). The 1-year survival was 72%, and 5-year survival was 44%. Univariate analysis identified four factors that predicted patient survival, as follows:

1. Tumor size greater than 5 cm
2. Vascular invasion
3. Positive nodes
4. Histologic grade

Incidental tumors and fibrolamellar variant were not found to correlate with outcome. When multivariate analysis was used, only histologic grade and known tumors were significantly related to survival. For incidental tumors, survival was negatively influenced by multifocality and age older than 60 years; tumor histologic grade and size smaller than 5 cm were linked to tumor-free survival. Although this report provides invaluable data in selecting patients for transplantation, these findings must be interpreted with some caution because the data come from 53 units in 21 countries, where there are differences in the etiology of the cirrhosis and in detection and management of patients. Many of these factors are interrelated, so a poorly differentiated HCC may be more likely to grow rapidly and metastasize early. Not all single center experience would confirm the registry report. Achkar and colleagues (1998) found that routine screening of cirrhotic patients detects small, early stage tumors, and that such patients do well after transplantation.

Transplantation is indicated for HCCs that are unresectable in noncirrhotic livers and with no evidence of extrahepatic spread (one tumor < 5 cm or three tumors < 2 cm each with no vascular invasion or spread outside the capsule). In patients with cirrhosis, the decision to resect (if possible) or transplant is more uncertain because most HCCs in this situation are usually multifocal. Transplantation may give a survival benefit (Sarasin et al, 1998), which also is cost-effective, provided that the delay from diagnosis to transplantation is less than 6 to 10 months.

The role of pretransplant therapy is controversial. Some centers use either radiofrequency ablation or transarterial chemoembolization. There are no controlled trials to show that such interventions offer a survival benefit; it is unclear whether any reported benefit derives from the intervention itself, or whether the delay helps identify tumors that are growing rapidly and so likely to be already outside the liver at the time of transplant. Because some interventions (e.g., radiofrequency ablation and transarterial chemoembolization) induce necrosis of the tumor, it may be that such interventions may be helpful when the waiting time is greater than 3 to 6 months.

Evaluation involves ultrasound to look for evidence of extrahepatic spread, CT or MRI or both of the chest and the abdomen, and bone scans to exclude hepatic metastasis. Laparoscopy may reveal the presence of nodules ulcerating through the capsule. Angiography or magnetic resonance angiography should be done to look for the presence of tumor infiltrating the portal vein. Both complications, in our view, contraindicate transplantation. Currently, laparotomy to exclude metastasis is not helpful.

The role of liver biopsy to establish the diagnosis of HCC needs to be considered. Because of the risk of tumor seeding along the needle biopsy tract (Navarro et al, 1998), biopsy should be considered only when the diagnosis is uncertain. This uncertainty might occur in the presence of a hepatoma arising in the noncirrhotic liver. It is usually impossible to be sure that the tumor is malignant or is a liver primary. The clear cell variant of HCC is often difficult to distinguish from pancreatic and renal neoplasm. In contrast, in a patient with known cirrhosis, a primary space-occupying lesion, and rapidly increasing serum α-fetoprotein, there is little doubt as to the diagnosis, and percutaneous biopsy would only increase the risk of metastasis and should be avoided.

Cholangiocarcinoma

As indicated previously, cholangiocarcinoma (see Ch. 52) usually is not considered to be an indication for transplantation because the recurrence rates are high. In a literature review, Jeyarajah and Klintmalm (1998) reported a 1-year patient survival of 53%, but a 3-year disease-free survival rate of only 13%. Only in the incidental tumor found at laparotomy is transplantation to be considered, although cures are sometimes possible (Iwatsuki et al, 1998).

Secondary Liver Cancers

With few exceptions, transplantation is not indicated for metastatic liver tumors because of the high rate of recurrence. The major exception is carcinoid and other neuroendocrine tumors because long-term results are good with rapid symptomatic relief (Makowka et al, 1989). Of 103 patients with unresectable neuroendocrine tumors, the 5-year survival rate was 47%, although the disease-free recurrence rate was only 24% (Lehnert, 1998). In this analysis, multivariate factors that identified a better prognosis included age younger than 50 years, primary location in lung or bowel, and pretransplant somatostatin therapy. Multivariate analysis showed that age older than 50 and upper abdominal exenteration or a Whipple procedure at the time of transplantation were associated with a poor outcome.

PEDIATRIC TRANSPLANTATION

The medical indications for liver transplantation in children are essentially similar to the indications in adults. Additional indications include growth retardation and the development of metabolic bone disease. The most common indications for transplantation in children are disorders of the biliary system, of which biliary atresia (see Ch. 41) is the most common. The procedure of portoenterostomy may be effective in some children if performed early, but if performed after 2 months, the chance of a successful outcome is limited. If bile drainage is not established soon after surgery the child should be considered for transplantation, rather than the surgeon making further attempts to reconstruct the bile duct system in an attempt to establish bile flow. Other disorders of the biliary tree that may require transplantation include Alagille syndrome, Byler's disease, and nonsyndromic intrahepatic biliary hypoplasia. Disorders of metabolism are the next most common indication for transplantation, and these include Wilson's disease, tyrosinemia, glycogen storage disease, galactosemia, and Gaucher's disease.

ASSESSMENT OF PATIENTS FOR LIVER TRANSPLANTATION

When a patient is referred for liver transplantation, it is important to confirm the diagnosis of the liver disease, to assess the indications for liver transplantation, and to assess any conditions that may preclude transplantation or may add to the risk of the procedure. If time allows, the patient should have time to consider the benefits and the risks of surgery. Although the decision for transplantation rests with the patient, it is important to include the family in discussions because their cooperation and understanding are essential for successful rehabilitation after transplantation. Apart from a thorough history, physical examination, and review of histology, required investigations depend on the medical condition. Some chronic liver diseases are associated with extrahepatic diseases; primary biliary and autoimmune chronic active hepatitis are associated with thyroid disease, celiac disease, and Addison's disease. These diseases should be excluded because untreated myxedema may lead to lethargy and, if corrected, may obviate the need for transplantation.

In patients with chronic liver disease, apart from complete blood count, assessment of clotting, renal function tests, and liver function tests, it is important to determine viral status for HBV, HCV, and HIV. It also is useful to determine the cytomegalovirus status because transplanting a cytomegalovirus-negative patient with a cytomegalovirus-positive liver is associated with an increased risk of cytomegalovirus infection. In patients who are not immune to HBV, it is worthwhile offering HBV vaccination because there have been occasional reports of HBV being acquired during the transplant procedure from infected organ or blood.

In patients with established cirrhosis, HCC should be looked for by ultrasound of the liver and serum estimations of serum α-fetoprotein and carcinoembryonic antigen. Bacterial, viral, and fungal cultures are obtained for a baseline. In patients with a possible history of tuberculosis, tests should be directed to determine the presence of previous infection, and in such cases it is our practice to give isoniazid and pyridoxine for the first 6 months after transplantation. Additional blood tests are determined by the nature of the disease and include autoantibodies, immunoglobulins, copper studies, and α_1-antitrypsin phenotypes, as appropriate.

Cardiopulmonary function is difficult to assess. Electrocardiogram, echocardiography, and simple lung function tests may be adequate to recognize pathology requiring further investigation. If appropriate (e.g., in a patient with possible ischemic heart disease), we proceed with an echocardiogram, exercise electrocardiogram preceding thallium scanning, and coronary angiography or other imaging, as indicated. Measurement of arterial blood gases is important, and if the arterial oxygen is low, it is important to repeat these after exercise and after giving 100% oxygen to give some guidance as to the extent of intrapulmonary shunting (Krowka & Cortese, 1990).

Radiologic investigations consist primarily of a chest x-ray and ultrasound of the liver, biliary tree, pancreas, spleen, and vessels. If there is any uncertainty regarding the patency of the portal vein, angiography (direct, CT, or MRI) is indicated to assess patency of the portal vein and the presence of splenic and superior mesenteric vein patency. Many units do not perform CT or MRI routinely unless there is a suggestion of malignancy. In patients with sclerosing cholangitis, as indicated earlier, there may be an indication for investigation of the biliary tree. Although this imaging may detect undiagnosed cholangiocarcinoma, this procedure may result in an episode of cholangitis. Many patients with primary sclerosing cholangitis have colitis. Although this colitis is usually mild and clinically inapparent, it is important to screen such patients before surgery. In particular, patients with a long history of pancolitis require full investigation by colonoscopy. This procedure is not without risk, however, especially in patients with ascites. In the presence of dysplasia, it may be sensible to consider early colectomy because the additional effect of immunosuppression may increase the risk of colonic cancer further.

Routine psychiatric evaluation is not indicated, unless there is a possible history of psychiatric disease that may preclude successful rehabilitation. A dental examination is required, and any carious teeth should be removed before transplantation.

Patients are routinely assessed by the anesthesiologist before undergoing transplantation.

MANAGEMENT WHILE AWAITING TRANSPLANTATION

In general, patients should be maintained as fit as possible while awaiting a transplant. Vitamin deficiency should be corrected, and the patient should consume a high-protein, high-calorie diet. The presence of encephalopathy should not bar a high-protein diet, and other methods should be used to control hepatic encephalopathy, such as use of lactulose and, if necessary, metronidazole or neomycin. It is reasonable to offer nonimmune patients immunization with hepatitis A and B vaccines. Any infection should be rigorously sought and actively treated.

The presence of ascites may be an indication for treatment because not only do these patients remain catabolic, but also there is a risk of spontaneous bacterial peritonitis. Now that recurrent paracentesis is being used successfully, patients with severe ascites should undergo ascitic removal with intravenous albumin or glypressin cover. When ascites is present, patients should be treated with prophylactic antibiotics, such as ciprofloxacillin or amoxicillin/clavulanic acid, which has been shown to be not only effective and cost-effective, but also without major risk of developing bacterial resistance. In patients with severe ascites resistant to therapy with diet and diuretics and requiring repeated episodes of paracentesis, there is a role for a transjugular intrahepatic portosystemic shunt. The role of such shunts before transplantation remains uncertain; although they are effective in reducing portal hypertension and improving ascites and the risk of variceal hemorrhage, insertion is not without risk not only of sepsis, but also of perforation and portal vein thrombosis.

Patients with recurrent variceal hemorrhage pose a particular problem. Injection sclerotherapy in the 2 weeks before transplantation is associated with a risk of paraesophageal abscesses after transplantation. Variceal banding is preferable for the treatment of bleeding esophageal varices. The role of transjugular intrahepatic portosystemic shunt before transplantation remains to be ascertained, but such a shunt seems to be of value. Although this procedure, if successful, reduces portal hypertension, it is not risk-free, including perforation and portal vein thrombosis, but current evidence suggests that the benefits outweigh the risks. Patients with portal hypertension and varices should be considered for β-blocker therapy because this would reduce the risk of primary and secondary hemorrhage.

Finally, it is important to avoid therapy that would exacerbate the liver disease. In particular, nonsteroidal anti-inflammatory drugs should be avoided because of the risks of inducing gastric hemorrhage, renal failure, and fluid retention. Drugs, such as opiates, that result in constipation and sedative drugs also should be avoided because of the risk of precipitating encephalopathy. Diuretics must be used with care, and renal function must be carefully monitored because renal failure is associated with a poor outcome after transplantation, and hyponatremia is associated with the development of central pontine myelinolysis.

The transplant clinicians need to remain in close contact with the patient so that problems can be detected and treated early. As the waiting time for transplantation increases, patients deteriorate. The patient may develop complications precluding a successful outcome, or the probability of survival may become too small for transplantation to proceed. With the increasing shortage of donor organs, the transplant clinicians need to consider the criteria that suggest a patient should be removed from the transplant list.

REFERENCES

Achkar JP, et al, 1998: Undetected hepatocellular carcinoma: clinical features and outcome after liver transplantation. Liver Transpl Surg 4:477-482.

Belghiti J, et al, 2003: Resection prior to liver transplantation for hepatocellular carcinoma. Ann Surg 238:885-892.

Beresford TP, et al, 1990: A rational approach to transplantation for the alcoholic patient. Psychosomatics 31:241-254.

Bergquist A, et al, 1998: Risk factors and clinical presentation of hepatobiliary carcinoma in patients with primary sclerosing cholangitis. Hepatology 27:311-316.

Bismuth U, et al, 1987: Emergency liver transplantation for fulminant hepatic failure. Ann Intern Med 197:337-341.

Burdelski M, et al, 1991: The role of dynamic liver function tests in liver transplantation. In Lentze M, Reichen J (eds): Paediatric Cholestasis. Dordrecht, Kluwer, pp 215-224.

Cuervas Mons V, et al, 1986: Value of pre-operatively obtained clinical and laboratory data in predicting survival following orthotopic liver transplantation. Hepatology 6:922-927.

Dabos KJ, et al, 2004: Biochemical prognostic markers of outcome in non-paracetamol-induced fulminant hepatic failure. Transplantation 77:200-205.

Eastell R, et al, 1991: Rates of vertebral bone loss before and after liver transplantation in women with primary biliary cirrhosis. Hepatology 14:296-300.

Elias E, McMaster P, 1987: Liver transplantation: indications and preoperative prognostic factors. Schweiz Med Wochenschr 117:1053-1060.

Everson GT, 2004: Treatment of chronic hepatitis C in patients with decompensated cirrhosis. Rev Gastroenterol Disord 4(suppl 1):S31-S38.

Figueiredo F, et al, 2000: Impact of nutritional status on outcomes after liver transplantation. Transplantation 70:1347-1352.

Freeman RB, et al, 1991: Serological and DNA follow up data from HBsAg-positive patients treated with orthotopic liver transplantation. Transplantation 51:793-797.

Freeman RB Jr, et al, 2004: Improving liver allocation: MELD and PELD. Am J Transplant 4(suppl 9):114-131.

Fung J, et al, 2004: Liver transplantation in patients with HIV infection. Liver Transpl 10(suppl 10):S39.

Garcia CE, et al, 2001: Liver transplantation in patients over sixty years of age. Transplantation 72:679-684.

Gines P, et al, 1988: Compensated cirrhosis: natural history and prognostic factors. Hepatology 7:122-128.

Haydon G, Neuberger J, 2001: Liver transplantation in cirrhotic patients with diabetes mellitus. Liver Transpl 7:234-237.

Heimbach JK, et al, 2004: Liver transplantation for unresectable perihilar cholangiocarcinoma. Semin Liver Dis 24:201-207.

Hoeper MM, et al, 2004: Portopulmonary hypertension and hepatopulmonary syndrome. Lancet 363:1461-1468.

Husberg B, et al, 1991: A totally failing liver may be more harmful than no liver at all. Transplant Proc 23:1533-1535.

Ismail T, et al, 1991: Primary sclerosing cholangitis: surgical options, prognostic variables and outcome. Br J Surg 78:564-567.

Iwatsuki S, et al, 1998: Treatment of hilar cholangiocarcinoma (Klatskin tumors) with hepatic resection or transplantation. J Am Coll Surg 187:358-364.

Jeyarajah DR, Klintmalm GB, 1998: Is liver transplantation indicated for cholangiocarcinoma? J Hepatobiliary Pancreat Surg 5:48-51.

Keays R, et al, 1991: Intracranial and cerebral perfusion pressure changes before, during and immediately after liver transplantation for fulminant hepatic failure. QJM 79:425-433.

Kim WR, et al, 2004: Outcome of liver transplantation for hepatitis B in the United States. Liver Transpl 10:968-974.

Klintmalm GB, 1998: Liver transplantation for hepatocellular carcinoma: a registry report of the impact of tumor characteristics on outcome. Ann Surg 228:479-490.

Krowka M, Cortese M, 1990: Hepatopulmonary syndrome. Hepatology 11:138-142.

Krowka MJ, et al, 2004: Hepatopulmonary syndrome and portopulmonary hypertension: a report of the multicenter liver transplant database. Liver Transpl 10:174-182.

Kumar S, et al, 1990: The results of liver transplantation in 73 alcoholics with end-stage liver disease. Hepatology 11:159-164.

Lehnert T, 1998: Liver transplantation for metastatic neuroendocrine carcinoma: an analysis of 103 patients. Transplantation 66:1307-1312.

Ludwig J, et al, 1990: The syndrome of primary sclerosing cholangitis. Prog Liver Dis 9:555-566.

Makowka L, et al, 1989: Transplantation of the liver for metastatic endocrine tumors of the intestine and pancreas. Surg Gynecol Obstet 168:107-111.

Mazzaferro V, et al, 1996: Liver transplantation for the treatment of small hepatocellular carcinomas in patients with cirrhosis. N Engl J Med 334:693-699.

McCarthy M, et al, 1996: Liver transplantation for haemophiliacs with hepatitis C cirrhosis. Gut 39:870-875.

Menon KV, et al, 2004: The Budd-Chiari syndrome. N Engl J Med 350:578-585.

Mericel C, et al, 1992: Aminopyrine breath test in the prognostic evaluation of patients with cirrhosis. Gut 33:836-842.

Mitchell SA, et al, 2001: A preliminary trial of high-dose ursodeoxycholic acid in primary sclerosing cholangitis. Gastroenterology 121:900-907.

Mitzner SR, et al, 2002: Extracorporeal support of the failing liver. Curr Opin Crit Care 8:171-177.

Navarro F, et al, 1998: Diaphragmatic and subcutaneous seeding of hepatocellular carcinoma following fine-needle aspiration. Liver 18:251-254.

Neuberger J, 1989: Predicting the prognosis of primary biliary cirrhosis. Gut 30:1519-1522.

Neuberger J, 2004: Allocation of donor livers—is MELD enough? Liver Transpl 10:908-910.

Neuberger J, et al, 1999: Pretransplant prediction of prognosis after liver transplantation in primary sclerosing cholangitis using a Cox regression model. Hepatology 29:1375-1379.

Neuberger J, et al, 2002: Transplantation for alcoholic liver disease. J Hepatol 36:130-137.

O'Grady J, et al, 1989: Early indications of prognosis in fulminant hepatic failure. Gastroenterology 97:439-445.

O'Grady J, et al, 1992: Hepatitis B virus infection after orthotopic liver transplantation. J Hepatol 14:104-111.

Olthoff KM, et al, 2004: Summary report of a national conference: evolving concepts in liver allocation in the MELD and PELD era. Liver Transpl 10(suppl):A6.

Peleman R, et al, 1987: Orthotopic liver transplantation for acute and subacute hepatic failure in adults. Hepatology 7:484-489.

Penn I, 1993: The effect of immunosuppression on pre-existing cancers. Transplantation 55:742-747.

Qin XL, et al, 2004: Utility of serum CA19-9 in diagnosis of cholangiocarcinoma: in comparison with CEA. World J Gastroenterol 10:427-432.

Rimola A, et al, 1987: Effects of renal impairment on liver transplantation. Gastroenterology 93:148-156.

Ringe B, et al, 1988: Total hepatectomy as temporary approach to acute hepatic or primary graft failure. Transplant Proc 26(suppl 1):552-557.

Riordan SM, Williams R, 2002: Blood lactate and outcome of paracetamol-induced acute liver failure. Lancet 360:573.

Rizetto M, et al, 1991: Liver transplantation in carriers of HBsAg. J Hepatol 13:5-7.

Rosen, CB, Nagorney DM, 1991: Cholangiocarcinoma complicating primary sclerosing cholangitis. Semin Liver Dis 11:26-30.

Rubin RH, et al, 1987: The acquired immunodeficiency syndrome and transplantation. Transplantation 44:1A.

Saigal S, et al, 2001: Successful outcome of orthotopic liver transplantation in patients with preexisting malignant states. Liver Transpl 7:11-15.

Sala M, et al, 2004: Selection of candidates with HCC for transplantation in the MELD era. Liver Transpl 10(suppl):S4.

Samuel D, et al, 2003: Liver transplantation in patients with HIV infection. J Hepatol 39:3-6.

Sarasin FP, et al, 1998: Partial hepatectomy or orthotopic liver transplantation for the treatment of resectable hepatoma? A cost effectiveness perspective. Hepatology 28:436-442.

Shapiro J, et al, 1979: Serum bilirubin: a prognostic factor in primary biliary cirrhosis. Gut 20:139-140.

Shetty K, et al, 1997: The Child-Pugh classification as a prognostic indicator for survival in primary sclerosing cholangitis. Hepatology 25:1049-1053.

Starzl TE, et al, 1988: Orthotopic liver transplantation for alcoholic cirrhosis. JAMA 260:2542-2544.

Suterakis J, et al, 1973: Effect of alcohol abstinence in survival in cirrhotic portal hypertension. Lancet 2:65-67.

Wiesner RH, et al, 1996: Liver transplantation for primary sclerosing cholangitis: impact of risk factors on outcome. Liver Transpl Surg 2(suppl 1):99-108.

Yao FY, et al, 2002: Liver transplantation for hepatocellular carcinoma: comparison of the proposed UCSF criteria with the Milan crieria and the Pittsburgh modified TNM criteria. Liver Transpl 8:765-774.

104

Orthotopic Liver Transplantation

S. C. GLASGOW, A. KOTRU, AND W. C. CHAPMAN

Since the initial descriptions of orthotopic liver transplantation (OLT) in the 1960s, the number of patients receiving transplants and the indications for the procedure have increased significantly. OLT represents the only treatment modality for many patients with a diverse spectrum of disease, with the predominant common factor being end-stage liver failure. It also has become an excellent option as curative therapy for early stage hepatocellular carcinoma (HCC). Advances in perioperative care of the donor and the recipient, organ preservation methods, and surgical techniques have resulted in a 1-year overall survival of 86% for all recipients, with OLT being performed at a rate of 18.5 per 1 million people (U.S. Scientific Registry of Transplant Recipients, 2003).

Although gains over the 2 decades in the field of hepatic transplantation are notable, many limitations remain, not the least of which is the relatively fixed pool of cadaveric organ donors. Techniques such as living donor liver transplantation and splitting cadaveric grafts may extend the benefit of OLT to more patients awaiting transplantation. This chapter presents a broad overview of liver transplantation, including common criteria for recipient and donor selection, standard operative approaches for donors and recipients (see Ch. 111), common post-OLT complications, and outcomes related to the underlying etiology of end-stage liver disease. Specialized transplant techniques, such as split liver and living related donor liver transplantation, are described in Chs. 107, 108, and 109.

PATIENT SELECTION

OLT represents the only curative treatment option for most patients with irreversible acute and chronic liver disease and cirrhosis, regardless of cause. Over the last 2 decades, 5-year patient survival after liver transplantation has increased from less than 50% to greater than 70% or more in some series (Jain et al, 2000). The improvement in patient outcome has led to an expansion in the indications for transplantation and a concomitant increase in the number of patients referred to transplant centers. The downside to this success is the widening disparity between the increasing numbers of recipients vying for a relatively constant supply of donor organs (Fig. 104.1). The number of patients listed for OLT has increased sixfold since 1993, whereas the number of transplants performed increased by only 45% during the same time. In the United States in 2002, only 4700 patients underwent deceased donor hepatic transplantation out of almost 17,000 on the waiting list (U.S. Scientific Registry of Transplant Recipients, 2003). The donor-to-recipient disparity often leads to longer waiting times and declining medical status. The annual mortality rate for patients on the waiting list approaches 11% for adult patients with all etiologies of liver failure. Because of the limited supply of donor organs, appropriate recipient and donor selection is paramount in improving resource use and long-term outcome.

Recipient Selection

Common indications for OLT (see Ch. 103) include portal hypertension as manifested by variceal bleeding, ascites, hypersplenism not manageable by conventional means, encephalopathy, hyperbilirubinemia, hepatic synthetic dysfunction, and lifestyle limitations. More than 60% of liver transplants are for noncholestatic liver disease, of which the most common etiologies are alcoholic cirrhosis and viral hepatitis (U.S. Scientific Registry of Transplant Recipients, 2003). Biliary atresia is the most common indication for liver transplantation in patients younger than 18 years of age (Goss et al, 1998).

There are few true *absolute contraindications* to OLT that uniformly portend a poor patient outcome (Table 104.1). Advanced cardiopulmonary disease, known extrahepatic malignancy, uncontrolled systemic sepsis from a source originating outside the liver, and ongoing or recent substance abuse are absolute contraindications. Many of the *relative contraindications* are conditions that are expected to improve after successful OLT. Examples include severe hemodynamic instability (e.g., shock) requiring multiple pharmacologic agents to maintain perfusion and severe hypoxia uncorrected by conventional intensive care measures in the context of hepatopulmonary syndrome. Other relative contraindications to OLT are infection with human immunodeficiency virus (HIV), extensive portal or mesenteric vein thrombosis, morbid obesity, psychiatric disorders uncontrolled by conventional means, absence of a suitable social support network, and extremes of age (Jain et al, 2000; Loinaz et al, 2002; Rustgi et al, 2004). Increasingly, advances in surgical technique and medical supportive care are overcoming obstacles formerly considered absolute contraindications to transplantation (e.g., portal vein thrombosis [PVT], HIV infection).

The etiology of liver failure may be predictive of outcome after OLT, although the correlation between preoperative risk and graft survival sometimes varies. Jain and colleagues (2000) examined outcomes after OLT in 4000 consecutive patients treated at the University of Pittsburgh. Patients with metabolic or autoimmune liver disease experienced 10-year survival rates greater than 60%, whereas the survival rates for viral hepatitis or alcohol-induced cirrhosis were 40% to 50%, and patients transplanted for advanced hepatic malignancy had only a 22% survival at 10 years. Results for all patients were better in the most recent era. Earlier contradictory reports notwithstanding, recipient age probably does not influence transplantation results

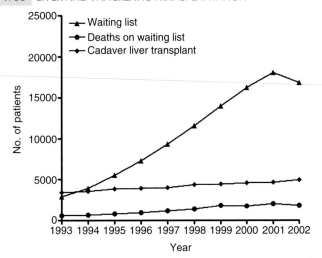

Fig. 104.1. Data from UNOS show the increasing differential between the numbers of patients awaiting and receiving cadaveric liver transplantation.

significantly (Gayowski et al, 1998; Ploeg et al, 1993; Totsuka et al, 2004). Thorough screening for medical comorbidities commonly found in older populations, such as lifestyle-limiting cardiopulmonary disease, systemic vascular disease, and chronic renal insufficiency, is crucial to successful OLT in patients older than 60 years.

The recipient selection process has undergone extensive revisions to ensure equitable allocation of a scarce resource (cadaveric donor livers), while attempting to avoid futile transplantation. Before February 2002, recipients awaiting OLT were prioritized based on the Child-Turcotte-Pugh scoring system (Table 104.2), time on the waiting list, and patient location (e.g., intensive care unit). Waiting lists grew under this system, and it became increasingly clear that these parameters were not good measures of disease severity. In 2000, the Department of Health and Human Services issued a guideline stating that the allocation of livers for transplantation should be based primarily on medical urgency (Freeman et al, 2002). The United Network for Organ Sharing (UNOS), which administers the Organ Procurement and Transplantation Network, commissioned several subcommittees to examine new methods for allocation. The result was the universal adoption of the MELD (Model for End-stage Liver Disease) criteria (Table 104.3) as a measure of the potential recipient's necessity for OLT. Concurrent revision of the pediatric liver allocation process produced the PELD

Table 104.1   Contraindications to Orthotopic Liver Transplantation

Absolute	Relative
Advanced cardiopulmonary disease	Hemodynamic instability
Extrahepatic malignancy	Severe hypoxia (except with hepatopulmonary syndrome)
Uncontrolled sepsis	
Active substance abuse	HIV infection
ABO incompatibility	Refractory psychiatric disorders Absence of adequate social support

Table 104.2   Child-Turcotte-Pugh Classification

| | POINTS | | |
	1	2	3
Encephalopathy	None	1 or 2	3 or 4
Ascites	Absent	Slight	Moderate
Bilirubin (mg/dL)	1-2	2-3	>3
Albumin	>3.5	2.8-3.5	<2.8
Prothrombin time (seconds prolonged)	1-4	4-6	>6

(Pediatric End-Stage Liver Disease) model, which is discussed further in Ch. 107.

In contrast to its predecessor, MELD has been validated extensively as a predictor for 3-month mortality from chronic liver disease (Malinchoc et al, 2000; Wiesner et al, 2003a). It incorporates serum creatinine as a marker for risk of death, relies on objective and readily available blood tests, and practically eliminates time on the waiting list from consideration. Using MELD criteria, rates of death while awaiting OLT and removal from the waiting list for being too sick have decreased (Freeman et al, 2004). As shown in Fig. 104.2, the use of MELD criteria for predicting mortality from end-stage liver disease results in an appropriate correlation between severity score and actuarial survival at 3 months. The MELD-based allocation process is dynamic and amenable to subtle changes to reflect evolving understanding of the diverse pathology and physiology seen in patients treated with OLT. The incorporation of hyponatremia into the MELD criteria is currently under evaluation (Freeman, 2004), and special considerations for certain subsets of patients with liver disease are ongoing.

Early in the initial evaluation of the MELD criteria, it was recognized that patients with HCC but early cirrhosis would be prioritized lower on the waiting list when they potentially could benefit most from transplantation (e.g., HCC at an early tumor stage). Conceivably, patients with HCC but low MELD scores could develop progressive disease, which would eliminate OLT as a treatment option. Since the most recent revisions to MELD, patients with stage II HCC currently are allocated 24 MELD priority points at the discretion of the regional review board.

Table 104.3   MELD (Model for End-stage Liver Disease) Equation

R = (0.957 × Log$_e$[creatinine mg/dL] + 0.378 × Log$_e$[total bilirubin mg/dL] + 1.120 × Log$_e$[international normalized ratio] + 0.643) × 10

Score	No. Patients	Mortality (%)	Mortality or Removal from List Owing to Illness (%)
<9	124	1.9	2.9
10-19	1800	6	7.7
20-29	1098	19.6	23.5
30-39	295	52.6	60.2
≥40	120	71.3	79.3

Note: Data represent 3-month pretransplant mortality.
Adapted from Wiesner R, et al, 2003: Model for end-stage liver disease (MELD) and allocation of donor livers. Gastroenterology 124:91-96.

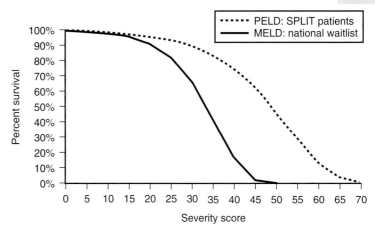

Fig. 104.2. Correlation between MELD/PELD score and patient mortality.
(From Freeman RB Jr, et al, 2002: The new liver allocation system: moving toward evidence-based transplantation policy. Liver Transplant 8:851-858.)

Criteria for selecting HCC patients for transplantation are discussed further subsequently. Guidelines also exist for awarding priority points for other conditions (e.g., cholangiocarcinoma, hepatopulmonary syndrome, familial amyloidosis, primary oxaluria) (United Network for Organ Sharing, 2004).

Donor Selection

The increase in demand for donor organs, as depicted in Fig. 104.1, has resulted in the concomitant increase in the use of less than ideal donors. The theoretical ideal donor is an otherwise healthy, hemodynamically stable young person who suffers an irreversible cerebral insult resulting in brain death; this situation is rarely realized. Although marginal donors are being increasingly used, absolute contraindications remain, including known extracranial malignancy (except for basal or squamous cell cancer of the skin), overwhelming sepsis, hepatic cirrhosis, hepatic macrosteatosis greater than 50%, and hepatitis C virus (HCV) or HIV infection. Generally, hepatitis B surface antigen and core antibody positivity in the donor also constitute absolute contraindications (Wachs et al, 1995), although some centers transplant core antibody–positive livers into hepatitis B virus (HBV)–positive recipients if the graft seems otherwise suitable. Whether donor age by itself influences graft outcome is unclear (Grazi et al, 2001; Rustgi et al, 2002). In practice, donors older than 75 years old usually are excluded from consideration.

As a result of the shortage of cadaveric donors, the use of living donors has increased in the United States almost 10-fold since the 1990s, from a total of 36 donors in 1993 to 358 donors in 2002 (U.S. Scientific Registry of Transplant Recipients, 2003). Living donor liver transplantation is appealing because it allows elective transplantation after optimizing the health of the recipient, reduces cold ischemic times, and potentially shortens waiting times. The disadvantages include morbidity and rare mortality in the donor population (Brown et al, 2003). The most common practice in adults is transplantation of the right hepatic lobe. Despite the aforementioned theoretical advantages, initial data indicate that outcome after living donor liver transplantation in adults is worse than expected, with 1-year graft survival 15% lower than in patients receiving standard cadaveric transplantation (Thuluvath & Yoo, 2004). Although living donor liver transplantation from an adult to a child has

become well accepted and standardized, adult-to-adult living donor liver transplantation continues to evolve, and the place of this approach as part of overall liver transplant options is not fully defined.

Early reports regarding the successful use of kidneys from non–heart-beating donors encouraged a similar practice in OLT. Most commonly, non–heart-beating donors are patients with severe neurologic injury (e.g., anoxia, intracranial hemorrhage) and no chance for meaningful recovery, yet they do not meet brain death criteria. Family members and treating physicians must elect to withdraw support. Donor criteria are similar to cadaveric (brain dead) donors. Compared with historical results with brain dead donors, outcomes using non–heart-beating donors are less optimal, with 1-year and 3-year graft survivals of 70% and 63% for all patients and a primary nonfunction rate of almost 12% (Abt et al, 2004; D'Alessandro et al, 2000). Limiting the cold ischemic time of the graft seems crucial to compensate for the brief (ideally <20 minutes) period of warm ischemia before procurement. Based on these early results, procurement from non–heart-beating donors for OLT may be regarded as a means of expanding the donor pool, with the caveat that these livers be used only in the most stable recipients.

OPERATIVE TECHNIQUES

The first published description of human liver transplantation was by Starzl and colleagues in 1963 at the University of Colorado. In this seminal paper, the dismal outcomes of three orthotopic hepatic transplant recipients were described, including one intraoperative death from uncorrectable coagulopathy and two survivors of 7 and 22 days. In addition to the pioneering conceptual framework and implementation of liver transplantation, several advanced techniques are presented in this reference, including the use of grafts from non–heart-beating donors, venovenous bypass in the recipients, choledochocholedochostomy, and coagulation monitoring using thromboelastography. Many of these concepts have now re-entered the realm of liver transplantation more than 40 years after their initial description. Based largely on the initial body of work by Starzl and colleagues, this section describes the surgical procedures commonly employed at Washington University during OLT.

Donor Hepatectomy

Management of a cadaveric organ donor begins preoperatively, immediately after identification of a candidate and evaluation by trained transplantation coordinators. After brain death, severe physiologic derangements can occur, and physiologic instability increases in proportion to the length of time between declaration of death and organ procurement (Nygaard et al, 1990). The progression from brain death to somatic death results in the loss of 10% to 20% of potential donors (Wood et al, 2004). Complications commonly occurring in a brain dead donor include hypotension, the requirement for multiple transfusions, disseminated intravascular coagulopathy, diabetes insipidus, pulmonary edema and hypoxia, acidosis, and arrhythmias and cardiac arrest. Intravascular volume repletion to normovolemia is the cornerstone of management; however, vasopressors (typically dopamine initially) or inotropic agents often are necessary to achieve an adequate perfusion pressure. The use of low-dose arginine vasopressin allows a reduction in the dosing of α-adrenergic agents, which may impair end organ perfusion (Pennefather et al, 1995). Directed therapy using a pulmonary artery catheter can improve outcome in patients with brain death–induced or traumatic cardiac dysfunction (Wheeldon et al, 1995). Exogenous hormone replacement with triiodothyronine, antidiuretic hormone, or methylprednisolone may have a role in some cadaveric donors because evidence exists supporting dysfunction of the hypothalamic-pituitary-adrenal axis after brain death. Hormone replacement can diminish requirements for vasopressors and potentially increase the rate of successful transplantation (Rosendale et al, 2003; Salim et al, 2001). Prospective clinical trials examining the role of hormone replacement are under way. A thorough review of the medical management of potential organ donors can be found elsewhere (Wood et al, 2004).

Surgical techniques for procuring abdominal organs from brain dead, heart-beating donors have been described previously (Farmer et al, 2000; Merkel et al, 1972; Starzl et al, 1984, 1987). A midline incision from the suprasternal notch to the pubis is performed, followed by sternotomy and entry into the peritoneum. The abdomen is inspected for any evidence of malignancy or gross gastrointestinal ischemia, which would preclude transplantation. Procurement proceeds in several phases: warm dissection and cannulation, exsanguination with cold perfusion and organ removal, and back-table dissection and organ preparation.

In the warm dissection phase, the liver is mobilized by dividing the umbilical, falciform, and left triangular ligaments. Hepatic arterial anatomy is delineated by inspection of the gastrohepatic ligament and porta hepatis to identify aberrant arterial anatomy. The right colon and mesentery of the small intestine are mobilized and reflected toward the donor left upper quadrant. The inferior mesenteric vein is identified, controlled, and cannulated. The infrarenal aorta is exposed at the bifurcation, and proximal and distal control is obtained. Next, the intestinal contents are returned to the lower abdomen with attention turned again to the porta hepatis. The distal common bile duct is circumferentially dissected, distally ligated, and transected. The gallbladder is flushed out through a choledochotomy. After reflection of the left lobe of the liver medially, control of the supraceliac aorta is obtained; this is facilitated by dividing the diaphragmatic crura.

The entire warm dissection phase usually takes 30 minutes or less. At this stage, the donor is ready for heparinization

(400 U/kg intravenously) and cannulation of the distal aorta. This occurs in coordination with the other procurement teams. When the thoracic and abdominal teams are ready, the donor is exsanguinated via the suprahepatic vena cava. Suction catheters are placed in the chest to remove warm blood. The aorta is cross-clamped in the supraceliac location, and the arterial and portal circulations are flushed with Viaspan/University of Wisconsin Solution (Viaspan; Barr Laboratories Inc, Pomona, NY) or histidine-tryptophan-ketoglutarate (Custodiol; Odyssey Pharmaceuticals, East Hanover, NJ) via the previously placed cannulae. Infusion continues until the caval drainage is clear, typically requiring 4 to 5 L via the aorta and another 1 to 2 L via the portal vein. The donor abdomen is packed with ice slush for topical cooling.

After satisfactory cooling and flush with preservation solution, the portal dissection is initiated. The general goals of this dissection are to delineate the arterial anatomy and dissect the arterial inflow back to the aorta. This is accomplished by dividing the gastroduodenal artery, dissecting the common hepatic artery down to the celiac trunk, dividing the splenic and left gastric arteries, and dissecting the celiac trunk down to the aorta. This technique is modified in the presence of a replaced or accessory left hepatic artery, in which case preservation of the left gastric artery is mandatory. A search for a replaced or accessory right hepatic artery also is undertaken through identification of the superior mesenteric artery and its proximal branches. Preservation of this artery, if present, is essential. Next, the portal vein is dissected and divided near the pancreas. Modification is necessary if procurement of the pancreas is being performed simultaneously. Excision of the celiac trunk with a Carrel patch of aorta is performed (a common patch including the superior mesenteric artery origin is included if an accessory or replaced right hepatic artery is present). Attention then is turned to the infrahepatic inferior vena cava (IVC), which is divided above the level of the renal veins. As a final step, the diaphragm is dissected around the suprahepatic IVC. The diaphragm and all tissues between the right kidney and liver are divided, and the hepatic graft is removed from the donor and packed in ice.

The final preparation of the donor graft usually occurs at the recipient hospital and is a cold, back-table preparation of the arterial and venous cuffs. This work consists of removal of the diaphragm and preparation of the suprahepatic IVC. The adrenal gland is removed, the adrenal vein is ligated, and the infrarenal IVC is prepared. The portal vein is dissected free from surrounding tissue up to the bifurcation and cannulated. The celiac trunk is dissected up to the gastroduodenal artery with all unnecessary branches ligated. During this phase, arterial reconstruction and conduit creation is performed, as indicated. At this point, the graft is ready for recipient implantation.

Procurement in a non–heart-beating donor requires slight modification (D'Alessandro et al, 2000). In the controlled setting, the donor is brought to the operating room, and support is withdrawn. Apnea and pulselessness ensue after a variable amount of time, at which point death is declared. Ten percent of potential donors do not die within 2 hours of withdrawal of support; these patients are not candidates for subsequent organ donation and are transferred back to the intensive care unit and allowed to die (Cooper et al, 2004). A mandatory 4-minute period is observed before any further intervention. The goal now becomes rapid reperfusion of the organs for procurement with cold preservation solution; this usually is accomplished via a quick midline laparotomy and cannulation of the aorta. Alternatively, some centers use cannulae placed before death in the femoral artery and vein (D'Alessandro et al, 1995). Abdominal organs are removed en bloc, with most of the dissection performed on the back-table or performed as in a standard brain dead donor. Cadaveric split liver and living related liver transplantation techniques are addressed in Chs. 107 and 109.

Recipient Hepatectomy

Removal of the diseased liver from the recipient can be a challenging technical aspect of liver transplantation. Hepatectomy often is complicated by marked portal hypertension, coagulopathy, extensive collateralization of venous drainage, a friable liver that is prone to hemorrhage, portal venous thrombosis, and possible prior abdominal surgical interventions including portal venous shunting or biliary tract surgery. Preoperative preparation of the recipient includes establishment of central venous monitoring and intravascular access, ensuring availability of at least 4 U of crossmatched blood, and timely administration of a second-generation cephalosporin.

Optimal recipient operative exposure is accomplished using a bilateral subcostal incision with an upper midline extension. The umbilical, falciform, and left triangular ligaments are taken down for maximum exposure. The left and right hepatic arteries are ligated in the hilum as the first step in the portal dissection. The cystic duct is divided, if needed for exposure, and circumferential dissection of the common hepatic duct is performed, which is divided in the mid-extrahepatic portion. Sufficient distal bile duct length in the recipient is preserved for the implantation phase, which usually includes choledochocholedochostomy. Next, the portal vein is skeletonized proximally to just above the confluence of the splenic and superior mesenteric vein. At this point, further dissection is influenced by the use of venovenous bypass or temporary portacaval shunting. Both techniques allow decompression of the splanchnic circulation, which reduces bowel edema during the anhepatic phase. In instances in which venovenous bypass is used, the portal vein is cannulated, and bypass is instituted as previously described (Shaw et al, 1984). We prefer an end-to-side anastomosis between the divided portal vein and infrahepatic IVC. The shunt is kept in place until the suprahepatic caval anastomosis is completed. If neither venovenous bypass nor temporary portacaval shunting is used, the portal vein simply can be clamped proximally, ligated in the hilum, and divided.

With the portal vein bypassed or clamped, exposure for the infrahepatic dissection and vascular control of the IVC is easily obtained. At this stage, the retrohepatic IVC is mobilized out of the retroperitoneum from the left side. The right triangular ligament is taken down, and the retrohepatic IVC is dissected from the right side. The adrenal vein is ligated when planning the traditional bicaval approach. This dissection frees up the retrohepatic IVC above the hepatic veins to allow application of the infrahepatic and suprahepatic IVC clamps. The recipient liver is sharply excised with care taken to leave cuffs of IVC above and below the liver. This technique allows for true orthotopic placement of the donor graft. A commonly used alternative referred to as the piggyback technique has been described extensively elsewhere and leaves the recipient retrohepatic IVC intact (Tzakis et al, 1989), with ligation and division of all retrohepatic caval branches. The advantage of this approach is that native caval flow is maintained, and venovenous bypass is

not required; the disadvantage is that division of retrohepatic caval branches can be tedious and sometimes time-consuming. The donor suprahepatic IVC is anastomosed to the confluence of the right, middle, and left hepatic veins, which are joined in a common cuff. Vascular control is achieved by clamping the hepatic veins at their point of entry into the vena cava.

Recipient Implantation

OLT requires four vascular anastomoses in the following order: suprahepatic IVC, infrahepatic IVC, portal vein, and hepatic artery. Alternatively, the use of the piggyback technique allows just a single caval (end-to-side) anastomosis, with simple ligation of the donor infrahepatic IVC resulting in a reduction in the duration of the anhepatic phase (Hosein Shokouh-Amiri et al, 2000). When the liver is fully reperfused, reconstruction of the biliary tract begins.

Adequate cuffs of suprahepatic and infrahepatic IVC are essential for reconstruction (Starzl et al, 1979). Anastomoses of these cuffs require reconstruction of the posterior walls from within the lumen using a running 3-0 polypropylene suture. The anterior layer is sutured externally using either an interrupted or a continuous technique. Another advantage of the piggyback technique is the use of a side-biting vascular clamp on the IVC at the level of ostia of the hepatic veins. Although this clamp may impair venous return to the heart to some degree during the clamp time of 15 to 30 minutes, it generally produces greater hemodynamic stability during the anhepatic phase than does complete caval disruption (Moreno-Gonzalez et al, 2003). When the hepatic veins are reanastomosed to the IVC, the side-biting clamp can be moved to the graft side of the anastomosis, restoring complete venous return while the remaining vascular connections are performed.

After restoration of caval flow, the portal anastomosis is undertaken. If venovenous bypass is used, interruption of the portal circuit is followed by removal of the portal cannula. In this manner, the donor and recipient main portal veins are exposed for an end-to-end anastomosis using an everting cuff technique. The use of a fine monofilament suture (6-0 or 7-0) is mandatory. We typically tie this suture with an "air knot" of approximately half the diameter of the portal vein to reduce the likelihood of portal stricture. The presence of preexisting portosystemic shunts complicates the standard approach (Brems et al, 1989). Selective shunts, such as the distal splenorenal shunt, usually do not require ligation or takedown (Esquivel et al, 1987). The H-type mesocaval shunt requires simple ligation only and probably is more ideally suited for potential transplant recipients. The central portacaval shunts are the most difficult to dismantle and frequently require operative repair of the IVC and portal vein (Shaked & Busuttil, 1991).

The final vascular anastomosis is arterial. The key principle of hepatic arterialization is to ensure pulsatile inflow through a large caliber vessel over a short length (Farmer et al, 2000). The technique involves the use of a fine (6-0 to 8-0) monofilament suture in a running or interrupted fashion. The vessel ends are frequently spatulated and are sewn from the outside and rotated to achieve the most precise anastomosis. The presence of aberrant hepatic arterial anatomy is encountered in 10% to 15% of grafts, and preservation of these vessels is essential for successful engraftment. Reconstruction of the aberrant vessels to obtain a single inflow vessel is imperative and takes place during the back-table preparation of the graft as described earlier. Recipient inflow is obtained from a branch off the celiac trunk, usually the proper or common hepatic artery. When adequate arterial inflow cannot be obtained through this means, the use of an arterial conduit is recommended. Inflow originating from the infrarenal and supraceliac aorta has been described. Both methods provide excellent inflow, and the choice is based on technical considerations and surgeon preference. The best choice of conduit is usually the donor iliac vessels. When donor vessels are unavailable or inadequate, prosthetic conduits can be used (typically polytetrafluoroethylene).

Completion of the vascular anastomoses is followed by the establishment of biliary continuity. The most common methods employed are the choledochocholedochostomy or choledochojejunostomy. The technical goals in biliary reconstruction are to achieve a tension-free anastomosis between viable ducts or intestine. The method used depends on many factors, including the size of the donor and recipient common bile duct, the size match between the ducts, the presumed viability of the ducts, the length of the ducts, and the presence of preexisting biliary pathology. In general, choledochojejunostomy is used when the above-mentioned technical goals cannot be realized. Most pediatric recipients require choledochojejunostomy because of the small size of the ducts or a history of biliary atresia or both. The choledochocholedochostomy and choledochojejunostomy anastomoses are accomplished with the use of fine absorbable monofilament suture in a single layer closure. The use of the gallbladder for biliary reconstruction is largely of historical significance. Some authors have advocated the use of the side-to-side choledochocholedochostomy (Neuhaus et al, 1994), although this is probably not performed regularly at most U.S. transplant centers. Whether to stent the biliary anastomosis during OLT is subject to debate (Bawa et al, 1998; Johnson et al, 2000). Proponents believe that decompression of the biliary tree reduces the rate of clinically significant leaks, whereas others point to data suggesting a higher rate of biliary stricture from internal stents. At our institution, biliary stenting is performed selectively based on individual case circumstances and surgeon preferences.

Complications

Complications resulting from OLT can be divided broadly into technical complications, complications arising as a consequence of immunosuppressive medications, and recurrence or recrudescence of the patient's original disease. The risk of surgeon-dependent technical complications increases when more complex surgical techniques, such as split liver donation, are used. Examples of factors generally attributed to technical error include early thrombosis of the hepatic artery or portal vein, biliary complications such as leak or stricture, and, to a lesser extent, primary graft nonfunction. Invasive infection and certain metabolic complications are side effects of the immunosuppressive regimens currently in use. Finally, subacute and chronic graft rejection and recurrence of certain causes of initial liver failure eventually result in graft loss. Each of these complications is discussed.

Primary Nonfunction

Primary nonfunction is defined as early graft failure after OLT in the absence of identified technical complications. Clinical presentation varies; however, patients typically present with alterations in mental status, diminished bile production, coagulopathy, markedly elevated transaminases, and metabolic acidosis. Multiorgan failure ensues, with oliguria and hypoxia occurring frequently. The reported rate of primary nonfunction varies (1-7% of all OLT) (Jain et al, 2000; Kamath et al, 1991; Totsuka et al, 2004). Retransplantation typically is required within 72 hours. Some authors also report the distinctly separate category of delayed nonfunction, defined as marginal graft function and the need for retransplantation within 30 days (Yersiz et al, 1995).

The etiology of primary nonfunction is unclear and likely multifactorial. Factors commonly reported to be associated with nonfunction include prolonged cold and warm ischemic times, donor steatosis, and renal failure in the recipient (Marsman et al, 1996; Nair et al, 2002; Ploeg et al, 1993; Strasberg et al, 1994). Intraoperative systemic hypotension (mean arterial pressure <40 mm Hg) also may be a risk factor for primary nonfunction independent of the incidence of hepatic arterial thrombosis (Reich et al, 2003). The degree of macrovesicular steatosis in the donor liver generally correlates with the rate of primary nonfunction, with livers showing moderate or severe steatosis at increased risk for failure (Fernandez-Merino et al, 2003), although others have disputed whether moderate steatosis (defined as 30-60%) influences short-term outcome (Yoo et al, 2003a). As would be expected, the likelihood of primary nonfunction is increased in the presence of multiple risk factors (e.g., steatotic graft with extended total ischemic time) (Salizzoni et al, 2003). The use of donor liver biopsy to confirm minimal to moderate fatty infiltration lessens the risk of primary nonfunction (D'Alessandro et al, 1991), and biopsy should be performed before implantation on any graft that appears marginal.

Hepatic Artery Thrombosis

Hepatic artery thrombosis (HAT) occurs in 2% to 10% of adult OLT patients, with a significantly higher incidence in the pediatric population approaching 25% (Langnas et al, 1991; Mazzaferro et al, 1989; Sanchez-Bueno et al, 2000). Risk factors associated with HAT are generally attributable to features of the graft, including the need for multiple arterial anastomoses, direct aortic anastomosis, small caliber vessels, and the use of prosthetic arterial grafts (Jurim et al, 1995; Soin et al, 1996; Vivarelli et al, 2004). HAT can be broadly divided into early (acute) and late (delayed) clinical presentation, with different patient manifestations, treatments, and etiologies. Although there is no formal consensus, early HAT typically is defined as occurring within the first 1 to 2 months after OLT.

Early HAT can result in massive hepatocellular and biliary injury. Because the transplanted liver has no collateral circulation, it depends on hepatic arterial perfusion. This is particularly true for the donor bile duct, which receives its entire blood supply via the hepatic artery. Consequently, early HAT frequently presents with bile leak, cholangitis, or sepsis. There is often a marked increase in the transaminases and impaired hepatic synthetic ability. It has been estimated that one third of early HAT patients remain asymptomatic, another third develop ischemic biliary syndromes (e.g., stricture or leak), and the remainder progress to fulminant hepatic failure (Pinna et al, 1996). Duplex ultrasound is diagnostic in virtually all cases of HAT in adults, although visceral angiography remains the "gold standard." In patients with graft failure secondary to arterial thrombosis, emergency exploration with attempted revascularization is indicated. Long-term patient survival rates of 90% have been reported after hepatic arterial thrombectomy and revascularization (Sheiner et al, 1997). The use of autologous radial arterial grafting also has been described (Rogers et al, 2001). Successful graft salvage is contingent on early recognition; for this reason, some authors advocate the routine use of postoperative duplex ultrasound.

Late HAT generally presents with a milder course and is likely due to nonsurgical factors (Pastacaldi et al, 2001). Although hepatic dysfunction predominates in early HAT, biliary symptoms, particularly strictures or recurring cholangitis, are more common in the delayed variant. The most common presentation of late HAT after OLT is fever caused by perihepatic abscess or biliary leak (Gunsar et al, 2003). Among the factors believed to contribute to late HAT are active tobacco abuse, coagulation abnormalities (e.g., factor V Leiden), and the presence of anticardiolipin antibodies (Pascual et al, 1997; Pungpapong et al, 2002). Finally, cytomegalovirus (CMV) infection has been implicated in late arterial thrombosis, with patients developing late HAT having a CMV positivity rate three times that of patients without HAT (Gunsar et al, 2003). It remains to be seen, however, whether routine prescription of anti-CMV medication would reduce the incidence of late HAT. Similar to the acute variant, the treatment of delayed thrombosis often includes retransplantation, although patients usually can be temporized with endoscopic or percutaneous biliary decompression and stenting.

Portal Vein Thrombosis

PVT occurs less frequently than HAT after OLT, being observed in less than 2% of adult recipients and 10% of pediatric recipients (Lerut et al, 1987; Millis et al, 1996). Low portal flow, small diameter veins (<5 mm), preexisting PVT in the recipient, and the use of vascular grafts for reconstruction are known risk factors for developing PVT (Cheng et al, 2004). PVT is typically symptomatic, and patients can present with acute hepatic failure (as with HAT) or with the sequelae of portal hypertension, such as increasing ascites and variceal hemorrhage. Diagnosis is made using duplex ultrasound or contrast portal venography.

Depending on the timeliness of diagnosis and the acuity of the patient, several treatment options exist. In patients with fulminant hepatic failure from PVT, re-exploration and attempted portal revascularization are performed. Often these patients require repeat OLT, particularly in the setting of combined PVT and HAT (total absence of hepatic inflow). The use of a portacaval shunt to augment flow through the reconstructed portal vein has been described (Bakthavatsalam et al, 2001), as has the use of transjugular intrahepatic portacaval shunt in conjunction with thrombolytics (Ciccarelli et al, 2001). Patients with symptoms of portal hypertension but preserved graft function often can be managed medically with standard therapies for ascites in combination with variceal banding or sclerotherapy.

Biliary Complications

Biliary complications arise in 7% to 29% of recipients after OLT, with strictures generally occurring twice as frequently as anastomotic biliary leaks (Balsells et al, 1995; Qian et al, 2004). The transplanted extrahepatic bile duct receives its blood supply exclusively from the hepatic artery—hence the clear association between biliary complications and HAT (Zajko et al, 1988). Biliary complications attributable to HAT tend to occur later in the patient's clinical course than those arising spontaneously (Margarit et al, 1998). Regardless of the timing of a biliary complication, HAT should be actively ruled out using ultrasound.

Biliary complications also arise more frequently in patients receiving living donor transplants.

The method of biliary reconstruction influences the complication rate. Complications occur more frequently in patients receiving a Roux-en-Y choledochojejunostomy relative to patients who undergo choledochocholedochostomy (O'Connor et al, 1995). Additionally, the use of T-tube biliary decompression has been identified as an independent risk factor for postoperative biliary complications (Qian et al, 2004). It is likely, however, that choledochojejunostomy and the need for T-tube decompression serve as surrogate markers for the subset of patients already predisposed to biliary complications, such as patients with donor livers with small caliber bile ducts, biliary pathology, or vascular compromise. In a randomized trial from France, the use of a T-tube led to an increased biliary-cutaneous fistula rate, but had no impact on patient outcome (Scatton et al, 2001).

In an asymptomatic patient with stable liver function, biliary complications can be managed conservatively. Bile collections should be drained percutaneously under CT or ultrasound guidance. Successful endoscopic stent placement across anastomotic leaks has been described (Shah et al, 2004), as has endoscopic balloon dilation of postoperative biliary strictures (Zajko et al, 1995). If these measures fail, anastomotic revision to a choledochojejunostomy remains an option. Retransplantation is a final alternative and is required more frequently for biliary complications in the setting of HAT and acute graft dysfunction. Verran and colleagues (1997) reported patient and graft survival rates of 83% and 80%, respectively, after the development of biliary complications managed by employing a multimodality approach to their diagnosis and treatment.

Infection

Infection is the most common cause of death after OLT at all time points (Jain et al, 2000), directly causing 28% of all deaths in liver transplant patients. An autopsy series of OLT patients showed an even higher infection-related mortality rate of 64% (Torbenson et al, 1998). Two thirds of OLT recipients experience at least one serious infectious episode (Winston et al, 1995), despite ever-improving prophylactic regimens. In addition to being immunocompromised to reduce the risk of graft rejection, liver transplant patients often are malnourished, are chronically ill, have received multiple blood product transfusions, and have undergone lengthy and complex surgical procedures. Appropriate antimicrobial prophylaxis can reduce the postoperative infection rate by more than half, depending on the pathogen. The current prophylactic regimen employed at Washington University is shown in Table 104.4.

Bacterial pathogens are the most common infectious agent in the early postoperative period. Diabetes mellitus and serum albumin less than 3 mg/dL are independent risk factors for bacteremia. Although gram-negative bacilli remain frequent causes of postoperative infection after OLT, gram-positive cocci, such as methicillin-resistant *Staphylcoccus aureus* and vancomycin-resistant enterococci, have become increasingly prevalent at many transplant centers (Papanicolaou et al, 1996). Typically presenting in the first 2 to 3 weeks post-transplant, 25% of OLT patients are reported to develop methicillin-resistant *S. aureus* bacteremia, with colonization of indwelling vascular catheters accounting for about half of the cases (Singh et al, 2000a). Other sources of post-OLT bacteremia include (in decreasing order of frequency) pneumonia, biliary infections, and surgical wound infections (Singh et al, 2000b). The emergence of drug-resistant organisms

Table 104.4 Antimicrobial Prophylaxis for Liver Transplant Patients at Washington University

Bacterial

Routine use of broad-spectrum antibiotics on-call to operating room, continued for 24 hr postoperatively

Fungal

Fluconazole (Diflucan) for 6 wk postoperatively in high-risk patients

Pneumocystis carinii

Trimethoprim-sulfamethasole (Bactrim) for 1 yr postoperatively
Pentamidine (Pentam) or dapsone are treatment options for patients with sulfa sensitivity

Viral

Ganciclovir (Cytovene) or valganciclovir (Valcyte) postoperatively for 180 days in setting of CMV-positive donor transplanted into a CMV-negative recipient (considered high risk for development of CMV infection)
Acyclovir (Zovirax) from discharge until 100 days postoperatively in other low-risk patients (recipients who are CMV-positive before transplant or when transplanted with a CMV-negative donor)

resulting from overuse of common antibiotics has made the treatment of infected liver transplant recipients increasingly difficult.

CMV is the most common viral pathogen encountered by OLT recipients. Intraoperative hypothermia is a known risk factor for developing CMV infection regardless of prophylaxis (Paterson et al, 1999). Without appropriate prophylaxis, the overall incidence in this population is commonly 50% to 60%, with clinically apparent infections usually occurring 3 to 12 weeks post-transplant (Farmer et al, 2000). The routine use of ganciclovir (Cytovene) has been shown to curtail dramatically CMV infection after OLT in several randomized, controlled trials (Gane et al, 1997; Winston, 1995). Prolonged treatment (≥100 days) can be costly, however, especially when the patient is at low risk for developing CMV (e.g., seronegative donor and recipient). Ganciclovir-resistant CMV has been observed in 20% of solid organ transplant recipients treated with ganciclovir, with presentation typically observed late in the first year (Limaye et al, 2000). Our current strategy is to reserve prolonged treatment with ganciclovir for seronegative patients receiving a seropositive graft or patients with evidence of active CMV infection.

Invasive fungal infections usually are caused by *Candida* or *Aspergillus* species, cryptococcus, and non-*Aspergillus* mycelial fungi. The incidence of invasive fungal infections in OLT patients is around 9% (Singh, 2000). Traditionally, *Candida albicans* has been the most common fungal pathogen, with risk factors for developing fungemia including renal failure, retransplantation, and Roux-en-Y choledochojejunostomy. Routine prophylaxis with fluconazole significantly reduces candidal colonization and infection after liver transplantation (Lumbreras et al, 1996). Coincident with the almost universal adoption of fluconazole for prophylaxis against *Candida* species has been an increase, however, in the number of reported *Aspergillus* infections among liver transplant patients (Groll et al, 1996). *Aspergillus* is not sensitive to fluconazole, and amphotericin B remains the "gold standard" for treating invasive aspergillosis. Prophylaxis against *Aspergillus* is not supported by the literature (Braun et al, 1998; Singh, 2000).

Infection with the protozoan *Pneumocystis carinii* occurs in 3% to 11% of liver transplant patients in the absence of

prophylaxis (Singh, 2000). Because T cell immunity is the primary defense against this organism, prolonged corticosteroid use, OKT3 monoclonal antibodies, and active CMV infection increase the risk of infection. Trimethoprim-sulfamethoxazole offers highly effective prophylaxis at a low cost and with minimal side effects. Because the risk of *P. carinii* infection is eightfold higher in the first year after OLT than in subsequent years, prophylaxis generally is continued only during these initial 12 months (Gordon et al, 1999).

Rejection

Rejection remains a major hurdle to long-term survival after OLT. Previously reported to occur in 40% to 70% of OLT patients (Klintmalm, 1991), the development of novel immunosuppressive regimens has reduced the lifetime rejection rate to less than 20% (McAlister et al, 2001). It is becoming increasingly clear that certain subpopulations of patients receiving OLT can be weaned completely from all immunosuppressive agents without experiencing rejection (Devlin et al, 1998; Mazariegos et al, 1997). The University of Pittsburgh experience shows that immunosuppression can be withdrawn successfully in almost one third of patients. It is unknown exactly what traits allow such weaning.

Hyperacute rejection is rarely seen today. It typically occurs in the setting of ABO incompatibility, with a reported graft failure rate of 46% observed in 51 patients transplanted across ABO type (Demetris et al, 1988). Hyperacute rejection is mediated by preformed antibodies in the recipient directed against the graft endothelium. These antibodies produce activation of the innate immune system via the complement cascade, ultimately leading to rapid graft destruction. Retransplantation is the only treatment option.

Although acute liver rejection usually occurs within the first 4 weeks after transplantation, it can occur later. Patients with acute liver rejection present with signs of fever, malaise, right upper quadrant abdominal pain, and elevated liver transaminases. Elevation in liver enzymes is often detected before physical symptoms or signs occur. Percutaneous liver biopsy reveals portal inflammation with predominantly mononuclear cells, bile duct inflammation and injury, centrilobular necrosis, and lobular inflammation. Differentiation from other pathologic processes can be difficult (Farmer et al, 2000). In contrast to other solid organ transplants (e.g., kidney, heart), however, the occurrence of an acute rejection episode does not seem to reduce the overall graft survival if treatment is initiated promptly (Wiesner et al, 1998).

The treatment for acute rejection is usually bolus corticosteroids (e.g., 1000 mg of methylprednisolone [Solu-Medrol], followed by a 5-day taper). Patients failing to respond to bolus steroids may require additional strategies, including the use of monoclonal anti–T cell antibody therapy (e.g., OKT-3); however, this is rarely needed in the current era (<5% of patients with rejection). When patients fail to respond to bolus steroid therapy, it is important to be certain of the diagnosis and to consider other potential causes of abnormal liver tests, including biliary or vascular causes. Repeat biopsies can be helpful to confirm the diagnosis and assess the response to therapy.

Today, only about 2% of patients experience chronic rejection after liver transplantation, although the incidence is higher in patients with autoimmune disease (Wiesner et al, 2003b). The etiology of chronic rejection is multifactorial. Chronic rejection is characterized by progressive loss of bile ducts, obliteration of medium and large sized hepatic arterioles, and cellular portal

Table 104.5 Rejection Activity Index from the Banff Schema for Acute Hepatic Rejection

Category	Criteria	Score
Portal inflammation	Mostly lymphatic inflammation involving a minority of the triads	1
	Expansion of most triads by a mixed infiltrate containing lymphocytes, neutrophils, and eosinophils	2
	Marked expansion of most or all triads by a mixed infiltrate containing numerous blasts, with spillover into periportal parenchyma	3
Bile duct damage	Minority of ducts infiltrated by inflammatory cells, with only mild reactive changes in epithelial cells	1
	Most or all ducts infiltrated by inflammatory cells, with occasional degenerative duct changes, such as nuclear pleomorphism, disorder polarity, and vacuolization	2
	As above, with most or all ducts showing degenerative changes	3
Venous endothelial inflammation	Subendothelial lymphocytic infiltration of some portal or hepatic venules	1
	Subendothelial infiltration involving most or all portal or hepatic venules	2
	As above, with perivenular inflammation extending into surrounding parenchyma and associated hepatocyte necrosis	3

Note: This index has a range from 0 to 9, classified as follows: 0-3, minimal acute rejection; 4-6, mild acute rejection; 7-9, moderate to severe acute rejection.
Adapted from Anonymous, 1997: Banff schema for grading liver allograft rejection: an international consensus document. Hepatology 25:658-663.

infiltration (Farmer et al, 2000). Standardized histopathologic evaluation of acute and chronic rejection using the Banff schema (Tables 104.5 and 104.6) allows objective decision making and facilitates comparisons of natural histories between patients (Anonymous, 1997; Demetris et al, 2000; Racusen et al, 2003).

Metabolic and Systemic Complications

Concurrent with the increase in overall survival after OLT has come a growing recognition of associated long-term medical sequelae and their impact on patient health. Prolonged use of corticosteroids can produce hyperlipidemia, obesity, diabetes mellitus, arterial hypertension, and mineral-deficient bone disease. Other commonly employed antirejection drugs induce similar derangements. Cardiovascular disease becomes a leading cause of death in patients surviving more than 3 years after liver transplantation, accounting for more than half of the reported mortality in some series (Asfar et al, 1996; Pruthi et al, 2001). It is unclear if immunosuppressive medications are the sole causes of the increase in cardiovascular risk after OLT, or whether other factors contribute (Canzanello et al, 1997). Patients receiving tacrolimus seem to have a decreased incidence of post-transplant

cardiovascular disease (Rabkin et al, 2002); however, results may be confounded by the higher steroid doses commonly employed in patients taking cyclosporine as opposed to tacrolimus.

Post-transplant obesity develops in 60% of patients, with most excess weight gain occurring in the first year (Munoz et al, 1991). The cause of weight gain is multifactorial. Corticosteroids and cyclosporine, and to a lesser extent tacrolimus, are known to correlate significantly with the incidence of obesity (Canzanello et al, 1997). Post-OLT patients often complain of constant hunger after transplantation, and many lack adequate exercise regimens (Palmer et al, 1991).

De novo diabetes mellitus occurs in 27% to 35% of previously nondiabetic liver transplant recipients (Navasa et al, 1996; Sheiner et al, 2000). Infection with HCV is a known risk factor for diabetes, and HCV is now the leading indication for liver transplantation in the United States. The mechanisms underlying the relationship between HCV and diabetes are not fully understood, but altered insulin sensitivity likely is responsible for at least part of the effect. Corticosteroids are known to induce insulin resistance, and the occurrence of graft rejection necessitating increased steroid dosing is a risk factor for developing diabetes.

Table 104.6 Banff Schema for Chronic Hepatic Rejection

Structure	Early Chronic Rejection	Late Chronic Rejection
Small bile ducts (<60 μm)	Degenerative changes involving most ducts: increased nuclear-to-cytoplasmic ratio, nuclear hyperchromasia, uneven nuclear spacing, ducts partially lined with epithelium	Degenerative changes in remaining bile ducts
	Bile duct loss in <50% of portal tracts	Bile duct loss in >50% of portal tracts
Terminal hepatic venules	Intimal/luminal inflammation	Focal obliteration
	Lytic zone 3 necrosis and inflammation	Variable inflammation
	Mild perivenular fibrosis	Severe (bridging) fibrosis
Portal tract hepatic arterioles	Occasional loss involving <25% of portal tracts	Loss involving >25% of portal tracts
Large perihilar hepatic artery branches	Intimal inflammation, focal foam cell deposition	Luminal narrowing by subintimal foam cells and fibrointimal proliferation
Large perihilar bile ducts	Inflammation damage, focal foam cell deposition	Mural fibrosis
Other	"Transition" hepatitis with spotty necrosis of hepatocytes	Sinusoidal foam cell accumulation, marked cholestasis

Adapted from Demetris A, et al, 2000: Update of the International Banff Schema for Liver Allograft Rejection: working recommendations for the histopathologic staging and reporting of chronic rejection: an international panel. Hepatology 31:792-799.

Diabetes in most patients is transient and generally resolves within the first year, as immunosuppressive medications are tapered. Pretransplant glucose intolerance (as determined by formal glucose challenge testing) is present in 53% of candidates awaiting liver transplantation (Blanco et al, 2001). Although some degree of glucose intolerance may improve with OLT, insulin-dependent diabetes almost never resolves after transplantation (Shields et al, 1999; Stegall et al, 1995).

OUTCOME

Survival after OLT has improved markedly as a result of continuing refinements in organ procurement and preservation, recipient selection, surgical and anesthetic techniques, perioperative care, and long-term immunosuppression. Jain and colleagues (2000) reported a 10-year survival rate of 60% in 4000 consecutive liver transplantation patients at the University of Pittsburgh, with an even higher survival rate in children. Likewise, single-institution series report near-zero short-term mortality after several hundred transplants in select patient populations (Broering et al, 2004; Sugawara et al, 2002). Outcomes after liver transplantation for certain disease processes are discussed.

Biliary Atresia

The long-term primary hepatic salvage rate after portoenterostomy in infants with biliary atresia is approximately 20% to 45% (Davenport et al, 2004; Otte et al, 1994). The remaining infants develop progressive biliary cirrhosis and ultimately require liver transplantation. Biliary atresia is the most common indication for OLT in children younger than 18 years old, and the best results are obtained in patients referred for transplantation early after only a single attempted portoenterostomy. Transplantation is a durable solution for biliary atresia, with 10-year patient survival of greater than 75% (Goss et al, 1998; Otte et al, 1994). The use of split liver cadaveric grafts and living related transplantation has expanded the potential donor pool, extending OLT to an increased number of children with biliary atresia (Yersiz et al, 2003).

Primary Sclerosing Cholangitis and Primary Biliary Cirrhosis

Primary sclerosing cholangitis is a chronic cholestatic liver disease of unknown origin that is associated frequently (70-80%) with inflammatory bowel disease. Patients with primary sclerosing cholangitis also are at risk for the development of cholangiocarcinoma. Although medical palliation exists, the only cure for primary sclerosing cholangitis is liver transplantation. Outcomes after OLT for primary sclerosing cholangitis are excellent, with 5-year patient survival rates ranging from 80% to 85% (Goss et al, 1997; Ricci et al, 1997; Solano et al, 2003). Whether the incidental discovery of cholangiocarcinoma in the explanted liver affects patient survival is controversial (Goss et al, 1997; Solano et al, 2003). Approximately 9% to 11% of patients develop recurrent primary sclerosing cholangitis after transplantation.

Primary biliary cirrhosis is an autoimmune disease, typically characterized by the development of circulating antimitochondrial antibodies. Patients with primary biliary cirrhosis generally have better long-term survival (>7 years) than patients

transplanted for primary sclerosing cholangitis (Maheshwari et al, 2004). They are more prone to chronic rejection, however, and are less likely to be weaned from immunosuppression (MacQuillan & Neuberger, 2003). Primary biliary cirrhosis likely recurs in a few patients after OLT, although long-term follow-up data are lacking. Post-transplant antimitochondrial antibody titers are not predictive of disease recurrence; a liver biopsy specimen showing granulomatous destructive cholangitis remains the "gold standard" (Faust, 2001).

Alcoholic Cirrhosis

Although often producing end-stage liver disease in conjunction with viral hepatitis, alcoholic cirrhosis alone seems to be one of the leading indications for OLT in the United States (Amersi et al, 1998). Early reports showing equivalent outcomes in patients with alcoholic cirrhosis compared with patients with nonalcoholic cirrhosis resulted in widespread application of OLT for this indication (Bird et al, 1990; Starzl et al, 1988). Medical outcomes in this group continue to be good (DiMartini et al, 1998; Lim & Keeffe, 2004).

Recidivism occurs in roughly 20% to 30% of patients transplanted for alcoholic cirrhosis. Although there is little convincing evidence that resumption of drinking adversely affects graft or patient survival after OLT, there are ethical concerns over possibly misallocating donor organs to active substance abusers (Lim & Keeffe, 2004). Most transplant centers require potential transplant candidates to participate in a support program, undergo psychological evaluation, and remain abstinent with documented random drug and alcohol testing for at least 6 months before placement on the waiting list. Multivariate analysis of alcoholic cirrhotics who have undergone OLT showed that abstinence for 6 months or more before OLT is the strongest predictor for nonrelapse after transplantation (Miguet et al, 2004).

Hepatitis B Virus

Recurrent HBV infection develops in about 80% of untreated patients post-OLT and directly correlates with the presence of active viral replication (e.g., detectable hepatitis B early antigen) at the time of transplantation (Todo et al, 1991). Initial experience with transplantation for HBV-induced cirrhosis was uniformly poor, with immunosuppressed patients rapidly developing HBV recurrence (O'Grady et al, 1992). More recent analyses show, however, that outcome for these patients does not differ significantly from patients undergoing OLT for other reasons (Kim et al, 2004; Roche et al, 2003; Steinmuller et al, 2002). The reason for this improvement can be attributed to the widespread use of hepatitis B immunoglobulin and the antiviral agents lamivudine and adefovir.

Current treatment strategies include reducing or eliminating active viral replication before transplantation through the administration of lamivudine or adefovir monotherapy, then combining one of these agents with hepatitis B immunoglobulin post-OLT indefinitely. Using this approach, HBV recurrence of less than 10% at 2 years has been reported (Roche & Samuel, 2004). Hepatitis B immunoglobulin administration can be costly and cumbersome, and resistance to lamivudine is reported in 20% of patients after treatment for 1 year. Although combination prophylaxis with lamivudine and hepatitis B immunoglobulin is highly effective, other methods to combat HBV recurrence need to be developed.

Hepatitis C Virus

Since its definitive identification in 1989, HCV has been determined to be a major cause of chronic liver disease and cirrhosis, accounting for 30% to 40% of OLT performed worldwide (Tisone et al, 1998). Approximately 2% of the general population carries the virus, and 50% to 60% of these individuals develop chronic liver disease (Farmer et al, 2000). In the United States, the frequency of HCV as the primary diagnosis for transplant recipients has increased from 21% in 1993 to 31% in 2003 (U.S. Scientific Registry of Transplant Recipients, 2003).

Short-term and intermediate-term patient survival after OLT for HCV is not significantly different from HCV-negative patients receiving transplants for other nonmalignant reasons (Boker et al, 1997; Ghobrial et al, 2001). Chronic hepatitis develops in most patients after OLT; however, the clinical course is similar to nontransplanted HCV-positive patients, with only 10% developing hepatic fibrosis (Boker et al, 1997). In contrast to HBV, there currently are no approved therapies for preventing recurrent HCV infection after liver transplantation.

Hepatocellular Carcinoma

HCC (see Ch. 71) was one of the first documented indications for OLT (Starzl et al, 1968). The decision to perform a transplantation for this disease is based on the oncologic premise of performing a complete resection (total hepatectomy) with wide surgical margins to effect a cure. Liver transplantation in the setting of extrahepatic malignancy is contraindicated. Conversely, the finding of incidental HCC in the explanted specimen after transplantation for a nonmalignant indication does not alter patient or graft outcome significantly (Cillo et al, 2004). The difficulty has been the selection of patients for OLT with malignant disease confined to the liver but at an advanced stage.

In their series examining liver transplantation for HCC, Mazzaferro and colleagues (1996) obtained a 75% 4-year actuarial survival using specific guidelines in highly selected patients. Subsequently termed the Milan criteria for OLT, patients under this protocol were offered transplantation if they had a solitary tumor less than 5 cm in diameter or no more than three nodules, each less than 3 cm in diameter. Largely as a result of this report, UNOS adopted these criteria for placing potential recipients on the waiting list, limiting transplantation to patients with stage I or II disease. Although not equaling the unprecedented results of Mazzaferro and colleagues (1996), reported 5-year survival after OLT for HCC generally ranges from 60% to 75% in several large, more recent series (Goodman et al, 2005; Yao et al, 2001; Yoo et al, 2003c). Prospective trials currently are examining multimodality treatment for HCC, whereby patients undergo chemoembolization or other ablative techniques to downstage the tumor clinically, followed by transplantation.

Cholangiocarcinoma (see Ch. 52)

There is no effective medical treatment for cholangiocarcinoma. Surgical extirpation is feasible in less than 30% of all patients and produces 5-year survival rates less than 20% even with complete resection (Jarnagin et al, 2001). Additionally, patients with primary sclerosing cholangitis (a known risk factor for cholangiocarcinoma) are often poor candidates for resection because of concurrent cirrhosis. Surgeons at the Mayo Clinic have developed strict treatment protocols for performing OLT in patients with cholangiocarcinoma, which include the use of neoadjuvant chemoradiation, resection to negative margins, and OLT. Using these or similar protocols, 5-year survival rates better than 80% have been achieved in a highly selected group of patients, many of whom had primary sclerosing cholangitis (Heimbach et al, 2004; Sudan et al, 2002).

Fulminant Hepatic Failure (see Chs. 88 and 105)

The cohort that undergoes OLT for fulminant hepatic failure comprises a diverse group of patients and disease etiologies. By definition, these patients have no previous demonstrable liver disease, yet they present acutely with encephalopathy, synthetic dysfunction (e.g., coagulopathy), and jaundice. Most commonly, the etiology is never determined, but fulminant hepatic failure can be caused by drugs, viruses, toxins, or other liver injuries (Hoofnagle et al, 1995). Although artificial liver support systems are under development, the only widely available cure for acute liver failure is OLT. Limited donor organ availability leads to the relatively high waiting list mortality rate of 377 deaths per 1000 patient-years at risk (compared with 107 for all wait-listed patients). MELD scores tend not to predict outcome accurately in patients with fulminant hepatic failure (Kremers et al, 2004). Outcome after OLT for fulminant hepatic failure is below average, with approximately 67% of patients surviving to 5 years post-OLT (Farmer et al, 2003).

RETRANSPLANTATION

In the current era, retransplantation is required in approximately 15% of patients after initial OLT, most commonly for primary nonfunction (46% of retransplants), HAT (29%), and acute rejection (7%) (Jain et al, 2000). Outcome after retransplantation is generally worse than after initial OLT, with a reported 5-year patient survival of 47% (Markmann et al, 1997). Factors portending a poor prognosis include preoperative mechanical ventilation, HCV infection, elevated creatinine and bilirubin, and prolonged donor cold ischemia (Markmann et al, 1999; Yoo et al, 2003b).

CONCLUSION

Results after OLT have improved over the past 2 decades, although outcomes may be expected to plateau as further improvements add only a marginal survival benefit to an already refined surgical procedure. The reasons for the successful development of hepatic transplantation are as follows:

1. Organized regional and national networks designed for the early identification of potential organ donors and rapid procurement in select candidates
2. Improved surgical and anesthetic techniques, allowing previous obstacles to OLT to be overcome (e.g., portal venous thrombosis, severe coagulopathy)

3. Novel antirejection and antimicrobial agents, with increasing emphasis on achieving minimal immunosuppression in the shortest time possible
4. Increased vigilance for the occurrence of acute complications after OLT, with the development of rapid screening tests for HAT, PVT, and primary nonfunction

As the only treatment option for thousands of patients, and with the added benefit of being curative for most candidate recipients, OLT will continue to be offered for the foreseeable future. Methods for expanding the donor pool and the more recent revisions to the allocation process may help to ease the shortage of suitable hepatic grafts. Newer immunosuppressive agents and further understanding of the role or even the necessity of immunosuppression in some patients may decrease the morbidity for patients after OLT.

REFERENCES

Abt PL, et al, 2004: Survival following liver transplantation from non-heart-beating donors. Ann Surg 239:87-92.

Amersi F, et al, 1998: Fifteen-year experience with adult and pediatric liver transplantation at the University of California, Los Angeles. Clin Transpl 255-261.

Anonymous, 1997: Banff schema for grading liver allograft rejection: an international consensus document. Hepatology 25:658-663.

Asfar S, et al, 1996: An analysis of late deaths after liver transplantation. Transplantation 61:1377-1381.

Bakthavatsalam R, et al, 2001: Rescue of acute portal vein thrombosis after liver transplantation using a cavoportal shunt at re-transplantation. Am J Transplant 1:284-287.

Balsells J, et al, 1995: Evolution of biliary complications in liver transplantation without biliary drainage. Transplant Proc 27:2339-2340.

Bawa SM, et al, 1998: Biliary reconstruction with or without an internal biliary stent in orthotopic liver transplantation: a prospective randomised trial. Transpl Int 11(suppl 1):S245-S247.

Bird GL, et al, 1990: Liver transplantation in patients with alcoholic cirrhosis: selection criteria and rates of survival and relapse. BMJ 301:15-17.

Blanco JJ, et al, 2001: Liver transplantation in cirrhotic patients with diabetes mellitus: midterm results, survival, and adverse events. Liver Transplant 7:226-233.

Boker KH, et al, 1997: Long-term outcome of hepatitis C virus infection after liver transplantation. Hepatology 25:203-210.

Braun F, et al, 1998: Is liposomal amphotericin B (ambisome) an effective prophylaxis of mycotic infections after liver transplantation? Transplant Proc 30:1481-1483.

Brems JJ, et al, 1989: Effect of a prior portasystemic shunt on subsequent liver transplantation. Ann Surg 209:51-56.

Broering DC, et al, 2004: One hundred thirty-two consecutive pediatric liver transplants without hospital mortality: lessons learned and outlook for the future. Ann Surg 240:1002-1012.

Brown RS Jr, et al, 2003: A survey of liver transplantation from living adult donors in the United States. N Engl J Med 348:818-825.

Canzanello VJ, et al, 1997: Evolution of cardiovascular risk after liver transplantation: a comparison of cyclosporine A and tacrolimus (FK506). Liver Transplant 3:1-9.

Cheng YF, et al, 2004: Risk factors for intraoperative portal vein thrombosis in pediatric living donor liver transplantation. Clin Transplant 18:390-394.

Ciccarelli O, et al, 2001: Transjugular intrahepatic portosystemic shunt approach and local thrombolysis for treatment of early posttransplant portal vein thrombosis. Transplantation 72:159-161.

Cillo U, et al, 2004: Liver transplantation for the treatment of moderately or well-differentiated hepatocellular carcinoma. Ann Surg 239:150-159.

Cooper JT, et al, 2004: Donation after cardiac death: the University of Wisconsin experience with renal transplantation. Am J Transplant 4:1490-1494.

D'Alessandro AM, et al, 1991: The predictive value of donor liver biopsies for the development of primary nonfunction after orthotopic liver transplantation. Transplantation 51:157-163.

D'Alessandro AM, et al, 1995: Controlled non-heart-beating donors: a potential source of extrarenal organs. Transplant Proc 27:707-709.

D'Alessandro AM, et al, 2000: Liver transplantation from controlled non-heart-beating donors. Surgery 128:579-588.

Davenport M, et al, 2004: The outcome of the older (> or =100 days) infant with biliary atresia. J Pediatr Surg 39:575-581.

Demetris AJ, et al, 1988: Antibody-mediated rejection of human orthotopic liver allografts: a study of liver transplantation across ABO blood group barriers. Am J Pathol 132:489-502.

Demetris A, et al, 2000: Update of the International Banff Schema for Liver Allograft Rejection: working recommendations for the histopathologic staging and reporting of chronic rejection: an international panel. Hepatology 31:792-799.

Devlin J, et al, 1998: Defining the outcome of immunosuppression withdrawal after liver transplantation. Hepatology 27:926-933.

DiMartini A, et al, 1998: Outcome of liver transplantation in critically ill patients with alcoholic cirrhosis: survival according to medical variables and sobriety. Transplantation 66:298-302.

Esquivel CO, et al, 1987: Liver transplantation in patients with patent splenorenal shunts. Surgery 101:430-432.

Farmer DG, et al, 2000: Orthotopic liver transplantation. In Blumgart LH, Fong Y (eds): Surgery of the Liver and Biliary Tract. Philadelphia, Saunders, pp 2071-2085.

Farmer DG, et al, 2003: Liver transplantation for fulminant hepatic failure: experience with more than 200 patients over a 17-year period. Ann Surg 237:666-675.

Faust TW, 2001: Recurrent primary biliary cirrhosis, primary sclerosing cholangitis, and autoimmune hepatitis after transplantation. Liver Transplant 7: S99-S108.

Fernandez-Merino FJ, et al, 2003: Impact of donor, recipient, and graft features on the development of primary dysfunction in liver transplants. Transplant Proc 35:1793-1794.

Freeman RB Jr, 2004: MELD and liver allocation: continuous quality improvement. Hepatology 40:787-789.

Freeman RB Jr, et al, 2002: The new liver allocation system: moving toward evidence-based transplantation policy. Liver Transplant 8:851-858.

Freeman RB Jr, et al, 2004: Improving liver allocation: MELD and PELD. Am J Transplant 4(suppl 9):114-131.

Gane E, et al, 1997: Randomised trial of efficacy and safety of oral ganciclovir in the prevention of cytomegalovirus disease in liver-transplant recipients. The Oral Ganciclovir International Transplantation Study Group. Lancet 350:1729-1733.

Gayowski T, et al, 1998: Orthotopic liver transplantation in high-risk patients: risk factors associated with mortality and infectious morbidity. Transplantation 65:499-504.

Ghobrial RM, et al, 2001: A 10-year experience of liver transplantation for hepatitis C: analysis of factors determining outcome in over 500 patients. Ann Surg 234:384-393.

Goodman J, et al, 2005: Liver transplantation for hepatocellular carcinoma: expanding special priority to include stage III disease. Arch Surg 140:459-464.

Gordon SM, et al, 1999: Should prophylaxis for Pneumocystis carinii pneumonia in solid organ transplant recipients ever be discontinued? Clin Infect Dis 28:240-246.

Goss JA, et al, 1997: Orthotopic liver transplantation for primary sclerosing cholangitis: a 12-year single center experience. Ann Surg 225:472-481.

Goss JA, et al, 1998: Long-term results of pediatric liver transplantation: an analysis of 569 transplants. Ann Surg 228:411-420.

Grazi GL, et al, 2001: A revised consideration on the use of very aged donors for liver transplantation. Am J Transplant 1:61-68.

Groll AH, et al, 1996: Trends in the postmortem epidemiology of invasive fungal infections at a university hospital. J Infect 33:23-32.

Gunsar F, et al, 2003: Late hepatic artery thrombosis after orthotopic liver transplantation. Liver Transplant 9:605-611.

Heimbach JK, et al, 2004: Liver transplantation for unresectable perihilar cholangiocarcinoma. Semin Liver Dis 24:201-207.

Hoofnagle JH, et al, 1995: Fulminant hepatic failure: summary of a workshop. Hepatology 21:240-252.

Hosein Shokouh-Amiri M, et al, 2000: Choice of surgical technique influences perioperative outcomes in liver transplantation. Ann Surg 231:814-823.

Jain A, et al, 2000: Long-term survival after liver transplantation in 4,000 consecutive patients at a single center. Ann Surg 232:490-500.

Jarnagin WR, et al, 2001: Staging, resectability, and outcome in 225 patients with hilar cholangiocarcinoma. Ann Surg 234:507-517.

Johnson MW, et al, 2000: Internal biliary stenting in orthotopic liver transplantation. Liver Transplant 6:356-361.

Jurim O, et al, 1995: Reduced-size grafts—the solution for hepatic artery thrombosis after pediatric liver transplantation? J Pediatr Surg 30:53-55.

Kamath GS, et al, 1991: Primary nonfunction of the liver graft: when should we retransplant? Transplant Proc 23:1954.

Kim WR, et al, 2004: Outcome of liver transplantation for hepatitis B in the United States. Liver Transplant 10:968-974.

Klintmalm GB, 1991: Rejection therapies. Dig Dis Sci 36:1431-1433.

Kremers WK, et al, 2004: MELD score as a predictor of pretransplant and posttransplant survival in OPTN/UNOS status 1 patients. Hepatology 39:764-769.

Langnas AN, et al, 1991: Vascular complications after orthotopic liver transplantation. Am J Surg 161:76-82.

Lerut J, et al, 1987: Complications of venous reconstruction in human orthotopic liver transplantation. Ann Surg 205:404-414.

Lim JK, Keeffe EB, 2004: Liver transplantation for alcoholic liver disease: current concepts and length of sobriety. Liver Transplant 10:S31-S38.

Limaye AP, et al, 2000: Emergence of ganciclovir-resistant cytomegalovirus disease among recipients of solid-organ transplants. Lancet 356:645-649.

Loinaz C, et al, 2002: Liver transplantation in patients with portal thrombosis: results in 76 patients. Transplant Proc 34:248-249.

Lumbreras C, et al, 1996: Randomized trial of fluconazole versus nystatin for the prophylaxis of *Candida* infection following liver transplantation. J Infect Dis 174:583-588.

MacQuillan GC, Neuberger J, 2003: Liver transplantation for primary biliary cirrhosis. Clin Liver Dis 7:941-956.

Maheshwari A, et al, 2004: Long-term outcome of liver transplantation in patients with PSC: a comparative analysis with PBC. Am J Gastroenterol 99:538-542.

Malinchoc M, et al, 2000: A model to predict poor survival in patients undergoing transjugular intrahepatic portosystemic shunts. Hepatology 31: 864-871.

Margarit C, et al, 1998: Biliary complications secondary to late hepatic artery thrombosis in adult liver transplant patients. Transpl Int 11(suppl 1):S251-S254.

Markmann JF, et al, 1997: Long-term survival after retransplantation of the liver. Ann Surg 226:408-418.

Markmann JF, et al, 1999: A simple model to estimate survival after retransplantation of the liver. Transplantation 67:422-430.

Marsman WA, et al, 1996: Use of fatty donor liver is associated with diminished early patient and graft survival. Transplantation 62:1246-1251.

Mazariegos GV, et al, 1997: Weaning of immunosuppression in liver transplant recipients. Transplantation 63:243-249.

Mazzaferro V, et al, 1989: Hepatic artery thrombosis after pediatric liver transplantation—a medical or surgical event? Transplantation 47: 971-977.

Mazzaferro V, et al, 1996: Liver transplantation for the treatment of small hepatocellular carcinomas in patients with cirrhosis. N Engl J Med 334: 693-699.

McAlister VC, et al, 2001: Orthotopic liver transplantation using low-dose tacrolimus and sirolimus. Liver Transplant 7:701-708.

Merkel FK, et al, 1972: Procurement of cadaver donor organs: evisceration technique. Transplant Proc 4:585-589.

Miguet M, et al, 2004: Predictive factors of alcohol relapse after orthotopic liver transplantation for alcoholic liver disease. Gastroenterol Clin Biol 28: 845-851.

Millis JM, et al, 1996: Portal vein thrombosis and stenosis in pediatric liver transplantation. Transplantation 62:748-754.

Moreno-Gonzalez E, et al, 2003: Advantages of the piggy back technique on intraoperative transfusion, fluid consumption, and vasoactive drugs requirements in liver transplantation: a comparative study. Transplant Proc 35:1918-1919.

Munoz SJ, et al, 1991: Hyperlipidemia and obesity after orthotopic liver transplantation. Transplant Proc 23:1480-1483.

Nair S, et al, 2002: Pretransplant renal function predicts survival in patients undergoing orthotopic liver transplantation. Hepatology 35:1179-1185.

Navasa M, et al, 1996: Diabetes mellitus after liver transplantation: prevalence and predictive factors. J Hepatol 25:64-71.

Neuhaus P, et al, 1994: Technique and results of biliary reconstruction using side-to-side choledochocholedochostomy in 300 orthotopic liver transplants. Ann Surg 219:426-434.

Nygaard CE, et al, 1990: Organ donor management and organ outcome: a 6-year review from a Level I trauma center. J Trauma 30:728-732.

O'Connor TP, et al, 1995: Biliary tract complications after liver transplantation. Arch Surg 130:312-317.

O'Grady JG, et al, 1992: Hepatitis B virus reinfection after orthotopic liver transplantation: serological and clinical implications. J Hepatol 14:104-111.

Otte JB, et al, 1994: Sequential treatment of biliary atresia with Kasai portoenterostomy and liver transplantation: a review. Hepatology 20:41S-48S.

Palmer M, et al, 1991: Excessive weight gain after liver transplantation. Transplantation 51:797-800.

Papanicolaou GA, et al, 1996: Nosocomial infections with vancomycin-resistant *Enterococcus faecium* in liver transplant recipients: risk factors for acquisition and mortality. Clin Infect Dis 23:760-766.

Pascual M, et al, 1997: Anticardiolipin antibodies and hepatic artery thrombosis after liver transplantation. Transplantation 64:1361-1364.

Pastacaldi S, et al, 2001: Hepatic artery thrombosis after orthotopic liver transplantation: a review of nonsurgical causes. Liver Transplant 7:75-81.

Paterson DL, et al, 1999: Intraoperative hypothermia is an independent risk factor for early cytomegalovirus infection in liver transplant recipients. Transplantation 67:1151-1155.

Pennefather SH, et al, 1995: Use of low dose arginine vasopressin to support brain-dead organ donors. Transplantation 59:58-62.

Pinna AD, et al, 1996: Urgent revascularization of liver allografts after early hepatic artery thrombosis. Transplantation 62:1584-1587.

Ploeg RJ, et al, 1993: Risk factors for primary dysfunction after liver transplantation—a multivariate analysis. Transplantation 55:807-813.

Pruthi J, et al, 2001: Analysis of causes of death in liver transplant recipients who survived more than 3 years. Liver Transplant 7:811-815.

Pungpapong S, et al, 2002: Cigarette smoking is associated with an increased incidence of vascular complications after liver transplantation. Liver Transplant 8:582-587.

Qian YB, et al, 2004: Risk factors for biliary complications after liver transplantation. Arch Surg 139:1101-1105.

Rabkin JM, et al, 2002: Immunosuppression impact on long-term cardiovascular complications after liver transplantation. Am J Surg 183:595-599.

Racusen LC, et al, 2003: Antibody-mediated rejection criteria—an addition to the Banff 97 classification of renal allograft rejection. Am J Transplant 3:708-714.

Reich DL, et al, 2003: Association of intraoperative hypotension and pulmonary hypertension with adverse outcome after orthotopic liver transplantation. J Cardiothorac Vasc Anesth 17:699-702.

Ricci P, et al, 1997: A prognostic model for the outcome of liver transplantation in patients with cholestatic liver disease. Hepatology 25:672-677.

Roche B, Samuel D, 2004: Evolving strategies to prevent HBV recurrence. Liver Transplant 10:S74-S85.

Roche B, et al, 2003: HBV DNA persistence 10 years after liver transplantation despite successful anti-HBS passive immunoprophylaxis. Hepatology 38:86-95.

Rogers J, et al, 2001: Use of autologous radial artery for revascularization of hepatic artery thrombosis after orthotopic liver transplantation: case report and review of indications and options for urgent hepatic artery reconstruction. Liver Transplant 7:913-917.

Rosendale JD, et al, 2003: Aggressive pharmacologic donor management results in more transplanted organs. Transplantation 75:482-487.

Rustgi SD, et al, 2002: Impact of donor age on graft survival among liver transplant recipients: analysis of the United Network for Organ Sharing database. Transplant Proc 34:3295-3297.

Rustgi VK, et al, 2004: Impact of body mass index on graft failure and overall survival following liver transplant. Clin Transplant 18:634.

Salim A, et al, 2001: The role of thyroid hormone administration in potential organ donors. Arch Surg 136:1377-1380.

Salizzoni M, et al, 2003: Marginal grafts: finding the correct treatment for fatty livers. Transpl Int 16:486-493.

Sanchez-Bueno F, et al, 2000: Hepatic artery complications in a series of 300 orthotopic liver transplants. Transplant Proc 32:2669-2670.

Scatton O, et al, 2001: Randomized trial of choledochocholedochostomy with or without a T tube in orthotopic liver transplantation. Ann Surg 233:432-437.

Shah JN, et al, 2004: Endoscopic management of biliary complications after adult living donor liver transplantation. Am J Gastroenterol 99:1291-1295.

Shaked A, Busuttil RW, 1991: Liver transplantation in patients with portal vein thrombosis and central portacaval shunts. Ann Surg 214:696-702.

Shaw BW Jr, et al, 1984: Venous bypass in clinical liver transplantation. Ann Surg 200:524-534.

Sheiner PA, et al, 1997: Selective revascularization of hepatic artery thromboses after liver transplantation improves patient and graft survival. Transplantation 64:1295-1299.

Sheiner PA, et al, 2000: Long-term medical complications in patients surviving > or = 5 years after liver transplant. Transplantation 69:781-789.

Shields PL, et al, 1999: Poor outcome in patients with diabetes mellitus undergoing liver transplantation. Transplantation 68:530-535.

Singh N, 2000: The current management of infectious diseases in the liver transplant recipient. Clin Liver Dis 4:657-673.

Singh N, et al, 2000a: Methicillin-resistant *Staphylococcus aureus*: the other emerging resistant gram-positive coccus among liver transplant recipients. Clin Infect Dis 30:322-327.

Singh N, et al, 2000b: Predicting bacteremia and bacteremic mortality in liver transplant recipients. Liver Transplant 6:54-61.

Soin AS, et al, 1996: Donor arterial variations in liver transplantation: management and outcome of 527 consecutive grafts. Br J Surg 83:637-641.

Solano E, et al, 2003: Liver transplantation for primary sclerosing cholangitis. Transplant Proc 35:2431-2434.

Starzl TE, et al, 1963: Homotransplantation of the liver in humans. Surg Gynecol Obstet 117:659-676.

Starzl TE, et al, 1968: Orthotopic homotransplantation of the human liver. Ann Surg 168:392-415.

Starzl TE, et al, 1979: Development of a suprahepatic recipient vena cava cuff for liver transplantation. Surg Gynecol Obstet 149:77.

Starzl TE, et al, 1984: A flexible procedure for multiple cadaveric organ procurement. Surg Gynecol Obstet 158:223-230.

Starzl TE, et al, 1987: An improved technique for multiple organ harvesting. Surg Gynecol Obstet 165: 343-348.

Starzl TE, et al, 1988: Orthotopic liver transplantation for alcoholic cirrhosis. JAMA 260:2542-2544.

Stegall MD, et al, 1995: Metabolic complications after liver transplantation: diabetes, hypercholesterolemia, hypertension, and obesity. Transplantation 60:1057-1060.

Steinmuller T, et al, 2002: Increasing applicability of liver transplantation for patients with hepatitis B-related liver disease. Hepatology 35:1528-1535.

Strasberg SM, et al, 1994: Selecting the donor liver: risk factors for poor function after orthotopic liver transplantation. Hepatology 20:829-838.

Sudan D, et al, 2002: Radiochemotherapy and transplantation allow long-term survival for nonresectable hilar cholangiocarcinoma. Am J Transplant 2:774-779.

Sugawara Y, et al, 2002: Living donor liver transplantation in adults: recent advances and results. Surgery 132:348-352.

Thuluvath PJ, Yoo HY, 2004: Graft and patient survival after adult live donor liver transplantation compared to a matched cohort who received a deceased donor transplantation. Liver Transplant 10:1263-1268.

Tisone G, et al, 1998: Liver transplantation for hepatitis C virus end-stage liver cirrhosis as compared with other nonviral indications. Transplant Proc 30: 696-697.

Todo S, et al, 1991: Orthotopic liver transplantation for patients with hepatitis B virus-related liver disease. Hepatology 13:619-626.

Torbenson M, et al, 1998: Causes of death in autopsied liver transplantation patients. Mod Pathol 11:37-46.

Totsuka E, et al, 2004: Analysis of clinical variables of donors and recipients with respect to short-term graft outcome in human liver transplantation. Transplant Proc 36:2215-2218.

Tzakis A, et al, 1989: Orthotopic liver transplantation with preservation of the inferior vena cava. Ann Surg 210:649-652.

United Network for Organ Sharing, 2004: UNOS policies and bylaws. Available at: www.unos.org.

U.S. Scientific Registry of Transplant Recipients, 2003: 2003 Annual Report of the U.S. Scientific Registry of Transplant Recipients and the Organ Procurement and Transplantation Network, Ann Arbor, Michigan.

Verran DJ, et al, 1997: Biliary reconstruction without T tubes or stents in liver transplantation: report of 502 consecutive cases. Liver Transplant Surg 3: 365-373.

Vivarelli M, et al, 2004: Ischemic arterial complications after liver transplantation in the adult: multivariate analysis of risk factors. Arch Surg 139: 1069-1074.

Wachs ME, et al, 1995: The risk of transmission of hepatitis B from HBsAg(−), HBcAb(+), HBIgM(−) organ donors. Transplantation 59:230-234.

Wheeldon DR, et al, 1995: Transforming the "unacceptable" donor: outcomes from the adoption of a standardized donor management technique. J Heart Lung Transplant 14:734-742.

Wiesner RH, et al, 1998: Acute hepatic allograft rejection: incidence, risk factors, and impact on outcome. Hepatology 28:638-645.

Wiesner R, et al, 2003a: Model for end-stage liver disease (MELD) and allocation of donor livers. Gastroenterology 124:91-96.

Wiesner RH, et al, 2003b: Recent advances in liver transplantation. Mayo Clin Proc 78:197-210.

Winston DJ, 1995: Prevention of cytomegalovirus disease in transplant recipients. Lancet 346:1380-1381.

Winston DJ, 1995: Infections in liver transplant recipients. Clin Infect Dis 21:1077-1089.

Wood KE, et al, 2004: Care of the potential organ donor. N Engl J Med 351: 2730-2739.

Yao FY, et al, 2001: Liver transplantation for hepatocellular carcinoma: expansion of the tumor size limits does not adversely impact survival. Hepatology 33: 1394-1403.

Yersiz H, et al, 1995: Correlation between donor age and the pattern of liver graft recovery after transplantation. Transplantation 60:790-794.

Yersiz H, et al, 2003: One hundred in situ split-liver transplantations: a single-center experience. Ann Surg 238:496-505.

Yoo HY, et al, 2003a: Retransplantation of liver: primary graft nonfunction and hepatitis C virus are associated with worse outcome. Liver Transplant 9:897-904.

Yoo HY, et al, 2003b: The effect of donor body mass index on primary graft nonfunction, retransplantation rate, and early graft and patient survival after liver transplantation. Liver Transplant 9:72-78.

Yoo HY, et al, 2003c: The outcome of liver transplantation in patients with hepatocellular carcinoma in the United States between 1988 and 2001: 5-year survival has improved significantly with time. J Clin Oncol 21:4329-4335.

Zajko AB, et al, 1988: Percutaneous transhepatic cholangiography rather than ultrasound as a screening test for postoperative biliary complications in liver transplant patients. Transplant Proc 20:678-681.

Zajko AB, et al, 1995: Transhepatic balloon dilation of biliary strictures in liver transplant patients: a 10-year experience. J Vasc Interv Radiol 6:79-83.

Liver Transplantation in Patients with Fulminant Hepatitis

P. ICHAI, H. BISMUTH, AND D. SAMUEL

The field of liver transplantation has changed dramatically in recent years. Before 1986, only a few cases of liver transplantation for fulminant hepatitis were reported with limited success (Iwatsuki et al, 1985; Ringe et al, 1986; Williams & Gimson, 1984). Since our first report of liver transplantation for fulminant hepatitis in 1987 (Bismuth et al, 1987), there has been a dramatic increase in the number of liver transplants performed for fulminant or subfulminant hepatitis. This indication represented 9% of the indications for liver transplantation in the European Liver Transplant Registry (ELTR, 2005).

DEFINITION

Three main definitions have been given for fulminant hepatitis. Trey and Davidson (1970) defined fulminant hepatitis as acute hepatitis complicated by acute liver failure with hepatic encephalopathy occurring less than 8 weeks after the onset of jaundice. Bernuau and colleagues (1986b) defined fulminant hepatitis as acute hepatitis complicated by acute liver failure with hepatic encephalopathy occurring less than 2 weeks after the onset of jaundice and subfulminant hepatitis as acute hepatitis complicated by acute liver failure with hepatic encephalopathy occurring 2 weeks to 3 months after the onset of jaundice. The group at King's College in London defined three groups: hyperacute liver failure, with a delayed onset of jaundice and encephalopathy of 7 days; acute liver failure, with a delayed onset of jaundice and encephalopathy of less than 28 days; and subacute liver failure, with a delayed onset of jaundice and encephalopathy of less than 3 months (O'Grady et al, 1993). The common points of these definitions are the occurrence of encephalopathy during the course of acute hepatitis in a patient without known previous hepatopathy and the spontaneous poor prognosis with an 85% mortality rate. The main cause of death is decerebration as a consequence of cerebral edema. This chapter addresses fulminant and subfulminant hepatitis as defined in the second definition.

Hepatic encephalopathy is classified into four stages according to the definition of Trey and Davidson (1970): stage 1, slow consciousness; stage 2, accentuation of stage 1 and presence of asterixis; stage 3, presence of deep confusion or reactive only to vocal stimuli; and stage 4, presence of deep coma assessed by at least the absence of reactions to vocal stimuli. In stages 3 and 4 encephalopathy, the presence of coma is classified into four grades: grade 1, reactivity to vocal stimuli; grade 2, absence of reactivity to vocal stimuli with coordinate response to nociceptive stimuli; grade 3, absence of reactivity to vocal stimuli with incoordinate response to nociceptive stimuli; and grade 4, brain death.

CAUSES OF FULMINANT AND SUBFULMINANT HEPATITIS

In France, before 1993, the main causes of fulminant hepatitis and subfulminant hepatitis were acute viral hepatitis in 48%, indeterminate origin in 24%, and drug induced in 21%. After 1993, in our series of 289 patients admitted for fulminant or subfulminant hepatitis and acute liver failure, 28% were affected with acute viral hepatitis: hepatitis B virus (HBV) 13.5%; hepatitis A virus (HAV) 12%; and non-A, non-B, non-C hepatitis virus 2.5%. The other causes were drug induced in 14.5%, toxic ingestion (*Amanita phalloides* ingestion, paracetamol massive ingestion, others) in 27%, various causes in 16.5%, and indeterminate cause in 14% (Figs. 105.1 and 105.2). Hepatitis C virus infection alone is rarely responsible for fulminant hepatitis (Feray et al, 1993; Wright et al, 1991). In contrast to France and to Europe, paracetamol overdose is the main cause of liver transplantation for fulminant hepatitis in Great Britain (Figs. 105.3 and 105.4). In a British series of 342 patients admitted from 1993-1994, the cause of the hepatitis was paracetamol overdose in 250 (73%), HAV infection in 8 (2%), HBV infection in 8 (2%), non A-E hepatitis in 28 (8%), drug induced in 9 (3%), and other causes in 12% (Williams, 1996). In a prospective study of acute liver failure at 17 tertiary care centers in the United States in 308 patients from 1998-2001, acetaminophen overdose (39%) and idiosyncratic drug reactions (13%) replaced viral hepatitis (12%) as the most frequent apparent causes of acute liver failure. Indeterminate cause was implied in acute failure in 17% of cases (Ostapowicz et al, 2002). Rare causes of fulminant hepatic failure (FHF) are fulminant course of Wilson's disease, Budd-Chiari syndrome, Reye's syndrome, massive malignant infiltration of the liver (liver metastasis, leukemia, lymphoma), hypoxic hepatitis secondary to cardiac failure, heatstroke, fatty infiltration of the liver, and HELLP (hemolysis, elevated liver enzymes, and low platelet count) syndrome.

OUTCOME OF PATIENTS WITH FULMINANT OR SUBFULMINANT HEPATITIS BEFORE THE ADVENT OF LIVER TRANSPLANTATION

Before the advent of liver transplantation, the overall mortality rate in patients with fulminant and subfulminant hepatitis was 80% to 85% (Bernuau et al, 1986b). The main cause of death was cerebral edema complicated by brainstem herniation (Ware et al, 1971). Cerebral edema is a unique complication of fulminant hepatitis. Cerebral edema is rarely present in cirrhotic patients with encephalopathy and coma. Cerebral edema is the consequence of astrocyte swelling. Astrocyte swelling is probably

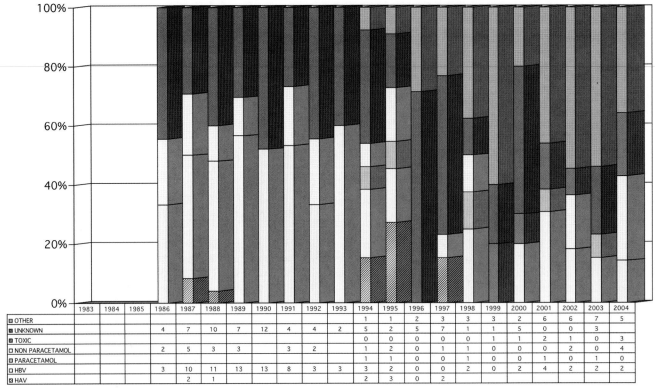

	1983	1984	1985	1986	1987	1988	1989	1990	1991	1992	1993	1994	1995	1996	1997	1998	1999	2000	2001	2002	2003	2004
OTHER												1	1	2	3	3	3	2	6	6	7	5
UNKNOWN				4	7	10	7	12	4	4	2	5	2	5	7	1	1	5	0	0	3	
TOXIC												0	0	0	0	0	1	1	2	1	0	3
NON PARACETAMOL				2	5	3	3		3	2		1	2	0	1	1	0	0	0	2	0	4
PARACETAMOL												1	1	0	0	1	0	0	1	0	1	0
HBV				3	10	11	13	13	8	3	3	3	2	0	0	2	0	2	4	2	2	2
HAV					2	1						2	3	0	2							

Fig. 105.1. Evolution of indications for liver transplantation for fulminant hepatitis at Paul Brousse, 1983-2003.

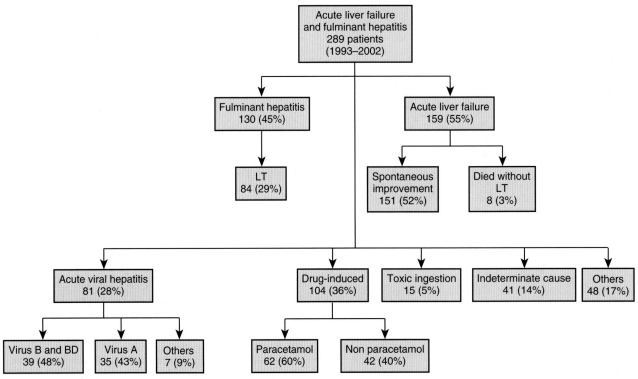

Fig. 105.2. Acute liver failure and fulminant hepatitis: Paul Brousse experience. LT, liver transplantation.

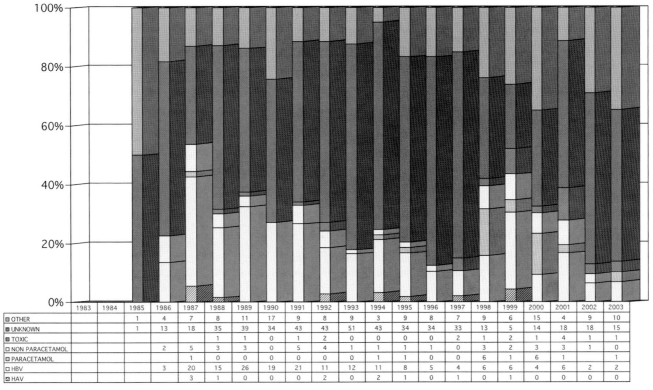

	1983	1984	1985	1986	1987	1988	1989	1990	1991	1992	1993	1994	1995	1996	1997	1998	1999	2000	2001	2002	2003
OTHER			1	4	7	8	11	17	9	8	9	3	9	8	7	9	6	15	4	9	10
UNKNOWN			1	13	18	35	39	34	43	43	51	43	34	34	33	13	5	14	18	18	15
TOXIC						1	1	0	1	2	0	0	0	0	2	1	2	1	4	1	1
NON PARACETAMOL				2	5	3	3	0	5	4	1	1	1	1	0	3	2	3	3	1	0
PARACETAMOL						1	0	0	0	0	0	0	1	1	0	0	6	1	6	1	1
HBV				3	20	15	26	19	21	11	12	11	8	5	4	6	6	4	6	2	2
HAV					3	1	0	0	0	2	0	2	1	0	1	0	1	0	0	0	0

Fig. 105.3. Evolution of indications for liver transplantation for fulminant hepatitis in France, 1985-2003.

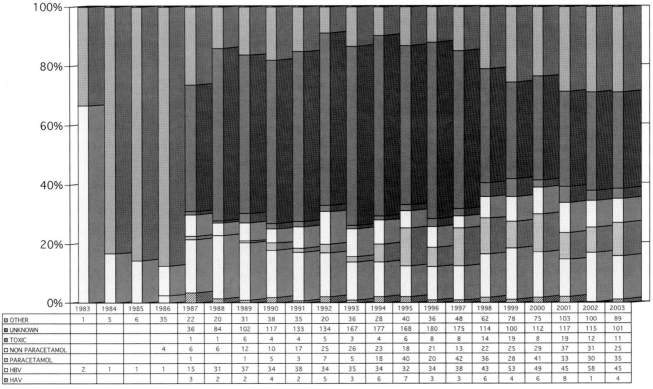

	1983	1984	1985	1986	1987	1988	1989	1990	1991	1992	1993	1994	1995	1996	1997	1998	1999	2000	2001	2002	2003
OTHER	1	5	6	35	22	20	31	38	35	20	36	28	40	36	48	62	78	75	103	100	89
UNKNOWN					36	84	102	117	133	134	167	177	168	180	175	114	100	112	117	115	101
TOXIC					1	1	6	4	4	5	3	4	6	8	8	14	19	8	19	12	11
NON PARACETAMOL				4	6	6	12	10	17	25	26	23	18	21	13	22	25	29	37	31	25
PARACETAMOL						1	1	5	3	7	5	18	40	20	42	36	28	41	33	30	35
HBV	2	1	1	1	15	31	37	34	38	34	35	34	32	34	38	43	53	49	45	58	45
HAV					3	2	2	4	2	5	3	6	7	3	3	6	4	6	8	1	4

Fig. 105.4. Evolution of indications for liver transplantation for fulminant hepatitis in Europe, 1983-2003.

a consequence of hyperammonemia and of the increase of glutamine content in the astrocytes. Increased intracranial pressure also is related to a dysregulation of cerebral blood flow with a "luxury cerebral perfusion syndrome." This absence of regulation of cerebral blood flow could be due to the rapidity of occurrence of electrolyte disorders in acute liver failure, in contrast to cirrhosis, in which the mechanisms of regulation are still active. Brain death also can occur as a consequence of cerebral ischemia, cerebral hypoxia, or grand mal seizures. In viral hepatitis, one characteristic feature is the complete recovery of patients who survived without evolution to chronicity. The survival rate partially depends on the etiology: The mortality rate is 75% to 80% in patients with HBV and HBV–hepatitis D virus fulminant hepatitis and 80% to 95% in patients with drug-induced fulminant hepatitis, fulminant hepatitis secondary to halothane anesthesia, fulminant hepatitis of indeterminate cause, and so-called non-A, non-E fulminant hepatitis. The survival rate is higher in patients with fulminant HAV hepatitis and fulminant hepatitis secondary to paracetamol overdose (50-60%) (O'Grady et al, 1988a).

MEDICAL TREATMENTS OF FULMINANT AND SUBFULMINANT HEPATITIS

Since the 1970s, many treatments have been attempted without any improvement in survival. Exchange blood transfusion, cross-circulation with a human or an animal donor, corticosteroid therapy (Canalese et al, 1982; EASL Trial Committee, 1979; Ede & Williams, 1986), intravenous infusion of mannitol (Canalese et al, 1982), hemodialysis and continuous hemofiltration on polyacrylonitrile membranes (Denis & Opolon, 1983; Denis et al, 1978), and charcoal hemoperfusion (Gazzard et al, 1974; Gimson et al, 1982; Williams, 1996) all have been attempted. The beneficial effect of a continuous intravenous infusion of prostaglandin E_1 on survival initially reported was not confirmed (Sheiner et al, 1992; Sinclair et al, 1989). The use of intravenous mannitol infusions seems to be effective in reducing the number of episodes of cerebral edema; however, the efficacy of mannitol was transient.

The aim of all of these treatments was to sustain the patient until liver regeneration occurred. The causes of failures of these treatments were probably multifactorial. The treatments were unable to replace the synthetic functions of the liver, and liver regeneration is probably not a constant event after fulminant hepatitis, and when it occurs, it may be insufficient in patients with subacute hepatitis who developed poorly efficient regenerative nodules.

CRITERIA FOR LIVER TRANSPLANTATION FOR PATIENTS WITH FULMINANT OR SUBFULMINANT HEPATITIS

A key issue in liver transplantation for fulminant hepatitis is to determine characteristics of the patients who died and the patients who spontaneously survived without transplantation. Criteria for the indications of liver transplantation are mandatory. These criteria are needed early in the course of the hepatitis to have time to find a donor should transplantation be required. In our common experience with the Clichy group, the appearance of confusion or coma associated with a decrease in factor V level to less than 30% of normal in a patient older than 30 years old or with a decrease in factor V level to less than 20% of normal in a patient 30 years old or younger was associated with a spontaneous mortality rate of more than 90% independent of etiology (Bernuau et al, 1986a, 1991; Bismuth et al, 1987, 1995).

Criteria for liver transplantation differed among transplant centers. The King's College group considered the etiology of hepatitis as the most important prognostic factor. They used different criteria in patients with paracetamol-related and non–paracetamol-related disease. In the paracetamol group, the investigators considered arterial pH less than 7.3 after volume expansion and correction of hypothermia as indications per se for liver transplantation. In the absence of the aforementioned criteria, liver transplantation was thought to be indicated in the presence of all three of the following factors: prothrombin time greater than 100 seconds, creatinine greater than 300 µmol/L, and grade 3 to 4 encephalopathy. In non–paracetamol-related hepatitis, liver transplantation was indicated if the prothrombin time was greater than 100 seconds, independent of the degree of encephalopathy, or in the presence of any three of the following factors: non-A, non-B hepatitis, halothane exposure, or drug-induced etiologies; delayed jaundice and encephalopathy more than 7 days; serum bilirubin greater than 300 µmol/L; age younger than 10 years or older than 40; or prothrombin time greater than 50 seconds (O'Grady et al, 1989). Difficulties in comparing the criteria of liver transplantation between centers were the use of factor V level expressed as a percentage of normal in the French groups and of prothrombin time expressed in prolonged seconds in the British group (O'Grady et al, 1991). A correlation between prothrombin time in seconds and factor V in percentage has been reported using the international normalized ratio. These criteria reported by us are used in France in all centers and in several other countries, and the criteria developed by the King's College group are used in the United Kingdom and in many other countries including the United States. A standardization of these criteria should be attempted in the future. In patients with acetaminophen-induced liver failure, increases in arterial blood lactate and in serum phosphate levels have been proposed as additional criteria to those initially reported by the King's College group criteria (Bernal & Wendon, 2004; Bernal et al, 2002; Schmidt & Dalhoff, 2002).

CONTRAINDICATION TO LIVER TRANSPLANTATION IN PATIENTS WITH FULMINANT HEPATITIS

In our experience, the contraindications for liver transplantation are the inability to maintain adequate support through the transplant procedure, age older than 65 years, and severe cardiac or lung failure. Sepsis is not a systematic contraindication for liver transplantation: It has been shown that sepsis is a frequent event in patients with FHF (Rolando et al, 1990, 1991). We do not consider the presence of positive blood cultures before transplantation as a contraindication per se to liver transplantation. The presence of a severe pneumonia or an uncontrolled septic shock before transplantation may contraindicate liver transplantation, however.

In our opinion, the neurologic limit to transplantation before death is never known. We still consider that the only neurologic contraindication for liver transplantation is the occurrence of brain death, defined in a patient who had received no barbiturates as the presence of bilateral nonreactive pupils with no spontaneous ventilation and with two consecutive electroencephalograms without cerebral activity. Patients with fixed pupils with persistence of spontaneous ventilation, patients with stage 4 encephalopathy and grade 3 coma with cerebral perfusion pressure less than 40 mm Hg for more than 1 hour, and patients with seizures have a high risk of postoperative brain death or of survival with neurologic sequelae (Bismuth et al, 1995). For these reasons, some centers are reluctant to perform liver transplantation in high-risk patients (i.e., with deep coma, hemodynamic instability) because these patients have a poor life expectancy after liver transplantation and the graft could be given to less risky recipients.

MANAGEMENT OF PATIENTS WITH FULMINANT HEPATITIS OR SUBFULMINANT HEPATITIS BEFORE TRANSPLANTATION

In France, as soon as liver transplantation is decided on, the patient is put onto the national superemergency list held by the Etablissement Francais des Greffes, which allows an absolute priority for any liver donors in France. The mean waiting time is about 1.4 days (range 0.5-4 days). Most of the organizations of organ sharing in Europe use the same procedure for these patients. In the United States, patients are listed in the UNOS status 1 (i.e., FHF, patients in intensive care unit), based on MELD (Model for End-stage Liver Disease)/PELD (Pediatric End-Stage Liver Disease) score (Wiesner, 2004).

All patients receive a daily dose of 200 g of carbohydrates to maintain a normal blood glucose level. Patients with acute liver failure are susceptible to bacteremia, septic shock, and fungal complications, especially when liver failure is prolonged for several days or longer (Rolando et al, 1996).

Management of Intracranial Hypertension

Pathophysiology

The pathogenesis of brain edema in FHF is linked to two mechanisms: (1) the accumulation of glutamine within astrocytes of the cerebral cortex and (2) the high cerebral blood flow in patients with FHF who develop brain edema (Larsen, 1996; Wendon et al, 1994). Detoxification of ammonia produces glutamine, an organic osmotic component, responsible for astrocyte swelling (Blei et al, 1992; Kato et al, 1992; Norenberg, 1996). Ammonia plays a key role in the occurrence of brain edema. Clemmesen and associates (1999) showed that arterial ammonia greater than 200 µg/dL within 24 hours after the onset of stage III or IV encephalopathy was predictive of the development of brain herniation. In addition to the high cerebral blood flow, there is a failure of cerebral blood flow autoregulation in response to the changes in mean arterial blood pressure (Larsen, 1996).

Medical Therapy

Intracranial hypertension should be suspected with the occurrence of the following clinical symptoms: marked hyperventilation, opisthotonos, hyperpronation-adduction of the arms (decerebrate posturing), cardiac arrhythmia, myoclonias, seizures, or poorly reactive pupils. When signs of cerebral edema are present, mannitol, 0.5 to 1 g/kg body weight every 4 hours is administered intravenously. When renal failure with oliguria is present, mannitol can be deleterious, so continuous venovenous hemofiltration or hemodialysis with polyacrylonitrile membranes is performed

to decrease hyperkalemia, fluid overload, and intracranial pressure (ICP) level. Use of thiopentone has been suggested in patients refractory to mannitol, but this can be difficult to manage (Forbes et al, 1989).

The monitoring of ICP by using an intracranial sensor is controversial (Blei, 1991; Schafer & Shaw, 1989). Some centers report that this monitoring can be useful to control the ICP and the cerebral perfusion pressure (difference between the mean arterial pressure and the mean ICP). Some authors consider the cerebral perfusion pressure as an aid for the decision of transplantation or as a contraindication for transplantation (Lidofski et al, 1992). Liver transplantation may be contraindicated if the ICP is greater than 40 mm Hg for several hours or longer. In our experience, monitoring of the ICP has not been used for the transplant decision, but instead has been useful in patients with deep coma for the following reasons: (1) There are discrepancies between the clinical symptoms and the degree of ICP (Donovan et al, 1992; Keays et al, 1991); (2) during the surgical procedure under anesthesia, there are no reliable clinical symptoms, and the ICP can vary during the various phases of the procedure; and (3) after transplantation, brain death can occur as a result of the persistence of elevated ICP, and careful monitoring until awakening seems necessary in the absence of objective monitoring (Bismuth et al, 1995).

Cerebral monitoring using an intracerebral sensor is highly controversial. It is an invasive method, and there is a risk of bleeding complications in these patients with major coagulation disorders; the morbidity rate and the mortality rate with these sensors is 10% and 2% in our experience. The use of the ICP monitor can be unreliable and variable. The more reliable sensors (i.e., placed in subdural or intraventricular position) seem to be more dangerous, and only epidural sensors should be used (Blei et al, 1993). If used, ICP monitoring should be performed only when the patient is in deep coma and on mechanical ventilation. In all cases, the insertion of this sensor should be cautious, and coagulation defects should be corrected before insertion.

Sedative drugs and fresh frozen plasma and other plasma substitutes are avoided, whenever possible, in these patients before transplant so as not to modify the neurologic status and the level of coagulation factors, which represent important criteria for liver transplantation. We recommend administration of fresh frozen plasma only before insertion of an intracerebral sensor or at the beginning of the transplant procedure (i.e., avoid clotting factors at other times to monitor the course of recovery of liver function).

The maintenance of stable hemodynamic status is essential. Patients with liver failure may develop profound vasoplegia, which may impair their renal function and cerebral perfusion. For this reason, patients with severe liver failure requiring mechanical ventilation should be monitored with a Swan-Ganz catheter for measuring pulmonary arterial and pulmonary capillary wedge pressures.

Indomethacin perfusion (25 mg intravenously by every peak of ICP) has been shown to normalize ICP and cerebral perfusion pressure (Clemmesen et al, 1997). This effect of indomethacin also was observed in patients with head trauma (Imberti et al, 1997). The exact mechanism is unknown; indomethacin-induced arteriolar constriction of the cerebral vessels may be mediated by a direct effect on arterioles. A prolonged reduction of ICP after bolus injection of propofol also has been documented after head trauma (Kelly et al, 1999; Wijdicks & Nyberg, 2002). In patients with FHF, propofol may control ICP. For all of these drugs, however, controlled studies to determine the exact effect on cerebral vascularization, cerebral metabolism, ICP, and cerebral perfusion pressure need to be performed. Ellis and colleagues (2000) showed that prophylaxis with phenytoin (15 mg/kg intravenous infusion, followed by 100 mg every 8 hours) reduced the frequency of subclinical seizure activity, was safe with the regimen used, and reduced the incidence of brain edema. A randomized study by Bhatia and coworkers (2004) reported, however, that prophylactic use of phenytoin did not prevent cerebral edema or seizures and did not improve survival.

In patients with fulminant hepatitis, N-acetylcysteine may have a beneficial effect on severity of cerebral edema, hemodynamic status, oxygen delivery, and survival (Harrison et al, 1991; Walsh et al, 1998). The beneficial effects of N-acetylcysteine were not confirmed by other groups, however (Bernal et al, 2002). N-acetylcysteine could have deleterious effects, in particular on cardiac function (Peake et al, 1996). In a prospective randomized controlled clinical trial, induction of moderate hypernatremia with 30% hypertonic saline can decrease ICP relative to baseline and reduce the incidence of intracranial hypertension in patients with acute liver failure (Murphy et al, 2004).

Moderate Hypothermia

Moderate hypothermia (32-33°C) is useful in treating uncontrolled increased ICP (Ginsberg et al, 1992; Jalan et al, 1999; Kurt et al, 1996; Roberts & Manas, 1999). This induced mild hypothermia decreased significantly systemic vascular resistance ($P<.05$), cerebrovascular resistance ($P<.05$), cerebral perfusion pressure ($P<.05$), and norepinephrine requirements (45%; $P<.05$). After cooling, a significant decrease of ICP was observed ($P<.02$). Retrospective studies also have shown a deleterious effect of hypothermia, however, with fever, cardiac rhythm abnormalities, coagulation defects, and a worsening of ICP measures (Schubert, 1995). These preliminary results of Jalan and colleagues (1999) are exciting and must be confirmed by a randomized controlled trial. The beneficial effect of hypothermia may act via a reduction of cerebral blood flow and a reduction in brain uptake of ammonia (Jalan et al, 2004).

Noninvasive Monitoring

Although the use of ICP monitoring for FHF has become more routine, many centers do not support the use of this invasive monitoring because of the risk of bleeding. Patients with FHF are monitored with noninvasive methods, in particular monitoring of cerebral perfusion by transcranial Doppler. Transcranial Doppler provides adequate information when cerebral perfusion is low and may allow intracranial hypertension to be diagnosed and treated effectively. This technique allows real-time assessment of blood flow velocity in the cerebral arteries (Larsen et al, 2000).

Infection and Acute Liver Failure

Sepsis is a common complication in patients with FHF (Rolando et al, 1990). In our series and in the series from King's College, 20% to 30% of the patients developed bacteremia, and 30% developed fungal infection. Antibiotic treatment against gram-negative bacteria and staphylococci is started as soon the patient is placed on mechanical ventilation (Bismuth et al, 1996b). When liver failure persists beyond several days, antifungal prophylaxis therapy should be added. When a liver donor is available, liver transplantation has to be performed as soon as possible. In our initial experience, we accepted the first liver graft available even in the presence of fatty infiltration or of ABO incompatible blood group. Because of a high rate of graft

failure, retransplantation, and death, however, many centers are reluctant to use ABO incompatible liver grafts (Rolando et al, 1993). This reluctance should be balanced with the risk of death of the patients during the wait for a liver graft.

Place of Total Hepatectomy

The release of proinflammatory cytokines and other substances from the necrotic liver may contribute to the occurrence of cerebral edema and to the impairment of liver regeneration. The "necrotic" liver is extremely rare in FHF and has been seen mainly after liver trauma.

Two-stage total hepatectomy with temporary portacaval shunt and subsequent liver transplantation can be a lifesaving procedure in patients who may die from toxic liver syndrome with multiorgan failure or cerebral edema (an exceptional circumstance) (Ringe et al, 1993). Decreasing ICP and neurologic recovery was described in one patient with severe FHF by a combination of total hepatectomy and extracorporeal liver support (Rozga J et al, 1993a). The respective roles of the hepatectomy and of the extracorporeal system are difficult to determine, however, because of the different treatments received by this patient (total hepatectomy, total plasma volume exchange, moderate hypothermia, extracorporeal artificial liver support). Total hepatectomy decreases the serum concentration of circulating proinflammatory cytokines (interleukin-1β, interleukin-6, tumor necrosis factor-α), which may be important in the pathogenesis of intracranial hypertension in patients with FHF (Jalan et al, 2002). The indication for total hepatectomy is very rare, reserved for "toxic" liver.

PROGNOSTIC INDICATORS IN FULMINANT HEPATIC FAILURE

The first step in FHF is to estimate the prognosis and the indication for liver transplantation. Without liver transplantation, the mortality rate of FHF patients is high (60-80%). The prognosis is related to the grade of coma at admission. Other prognostic indicators also have been described (see Fig. 105.2).

In a study by Farmer and associates (2003), the pretransplant serum creatinine level was the most powerful predictor of patient survival in 200 patients with FHF. The authors proposed a mathematical model based on serum creatinine, time from onset of jaundice to encephalopathy, and international normalized ratio that accurately predicts patient outcomes after liver transplantation for irreversible FHF. Pretransplant renal failure was a strong predictor of a poor outcome in another small series (Mendoza et al, 1997).

The recipient racial/ethnic status also was reported to be an indicator of prognosis. In one series, Hispanic patients had a significantly lower mortality than white and Asian patients (Farmer et al, 2003). In contrast, African-American patients showed mortality rates 3.8 times higher than Hispanic patients and 1.5 times higher than whites and Asians. These results were confirmed using UNOS data.

In the experience of teams from Nordic countries, patients with paracetamol intoxication had a higher mortality without transplantation and a higher withdrawal rate attributable to improved condition (Brandsaeter et al, 2002). Acetaminophen overdose and idiosyncratic drug reactions have replaced viral hepatitis as the most frequent causes of acute liver failure in United States (Ostapowicz et al, 2002).

The etiology of liver failure and grade of coma at admission were associated with outcome. The survival without transplantation was 50% in patients with acetaminophen overdose, HAV, shock liver, or pregnancy-induced liver failure.

In contrast, the short-term survival without transplantation in patients with FHF of indeterminate cause or secondary to drugs other than acetaminophen, HBV, autoimmune hepatitis, Wilson's disease, or Budd-Chiari syndrome was much lower (<25%). The survival also was related to the grade of coma at admission and was 77% in patients with grade 1 or 2 coma and 56% in patients with grade 3 or 4 coma (Ostapowicz et al, 2002). The short-term transplant-free survival in patients with acetaminophen overdose, drug reactions, liver failure of indeterminate cause, or liver failure of other causes was 87%, 35%, 18%, and 38% for patients with grade 1 or 2 coma and 50%, 12%, 16%, and 27% for patients with grade 3 and 4 coma (Ostapowicz et al, 2002).

Hashem and coworkers (2002) showed that diabetes increases the risk of acute liver failure. Older age and the presence of chronic liver disease further increase the mortality rate. Regular monitoring of liver enzymes and the prudent use of hepatotoxic drugs may be warranted in patients with diabetes.

Serum concentrations of proinflammatory cytokines and endotoxin are increased in the circulation of patients and may contribute to the systemic inflammatory response syndrome. These cytokines could be predictive of poor prognosis in FHF (Rolando et al, 2000). The monitoring of the soluble tumor necrosis factor receptor I level might help to assess the prognosis of acute liver failure and has been associated with massive hepatic necrosis. In a study by Tokushige and colleagues (2000), soluble tumor necrosis factor receptor I level was significantly higher in patients with subacute type fulminant hepatitis than in patients with severe acute hepatitis, acute hepatitis, or healthy controls. Finally, high serum phosphate (Schmidt & Dalhoff, 2002) and high arterial blood lactate are factors predictive of poor prognosis (Bernal et al, 2002) in patients with acetaminophen-induced FHF.

PERIOPERATIVE MANAGEMENT

To correct the coagulation defects, fresh frozen plasma is administered at the beginning of the procedure. It is necessary to maintain a balance between fluid restriction to avoid the increase of brain edema and maintenance of a satisfactory cerebral perfusion pressure. The total clamping of the inferior vena cava and of the portal vein is poorly tolerated. Two techniques are used: (1) transplantation using a venovenous bypass with a venous return in the axillary vein, rather than in the jugular vein, or (2) transplantation with a lateral clamping of the inferior vena cava, temporary portacaval anastomosis, and conservation of the inferior vena cava (Belghiti et al, 1995). In patients with renal failure or high ICP or both, perioperative venovenous hemofiltration can be performed.

The surgical procedure itself is generally easy compared with a chronic liver disease patient. The coagulation defects can be corrected with infusion of fresh frozen plasma and platelets. The hepatectomy is facilitated because of the presence of an atrophic liver and the absence of severe portal hypertension. The transplantation sometimes can be very difficult, however. When the liver graft is of poor quality, there is a risk of immediate graft nonfunction after revascularization with diffuse abdominal bleeding; when there is a size mismatch between donor and recipient, a reduction of the size of the graft may be necessary (Bismuth & Houssin, 1984). The combination of several factors, such as graft reduction and massive steatosis, may increase the risk of diffuse abdominal bleeding.

POSTOPERATIVE MANAGEMENT

Irreversible brain damage can be observed even during the first hours after transplantation. It is necessary to perform neurologic assessments until the complete awakening of the patient.

RESULTS OF LIVER TRANSPLANTATION FOR FULMINANT AND SUBFULMINANT HEPATITIS

Before Transplantation

Some patients with fulminant or subfulminant hepatitis referred for transplantation die before transplantation can be performed; this occurred in 15% to 30% of the patients in whom transplantation was decided on. This death rate varies from country to country depending on the possibility of obtaining grafts in emergency circumstances (Bismuth et al, 1996a; Castells et al, 1993). Most patients (70%) who died before transplantation died as a result of brain death. The other major causes of death are sepsis, hemodynamic instability, multiorgan failure, and gastrointestinal bleeding.

A few patients may improve before transplantation and can be removed from the waiting list. In our experience, this occurred in 4 of 200 patients in whom transplantation was selected and patients were listed. This event can always occur because the accuracy of the predictive factors of spontaneous death is not 100%. It is necessary to re-evaluate the patient when a donor has been found to decide if the transplant is still needed.

Survival After Liver Transplantation

Survival after transplantation for fulminant hepatitis is 50% to 75% (Bismuth et al, 1987; ELTR 2005; Bismuth et al, 1995, 1996b; Brems et al, 1987; Peleman et al, 1987; Vickers et al, 1988; O'Grady et al, 1988b; Devictor et al, 1992). The actuarial 1-year and 5-year survival rate of 139 patients transplanted between January 1988 and December 2003 at our center was 67% and 62% (Fig. 105.5 and Table 105.1). As observed in other series, the postoperative mortality is significantly higher than in patients transplanted for chronic liver diseases. Most deaths occurred in the first 3 postoperative months. The main causes of death are brain death and sepsis. Brain death can occur during the surgical procedure and sometimes in the immediate postoperative period. There are two causes for this higher postoperative mortality: first, the severity of the clinical condition of the patients, and second, an emergency situation and the acceptance of poor quality grafts and ABO incompatible grafts.

The clinical condition of the transplanted patients at the time of transplantation differs from that of patients with chronic liver disease. Most patients are in a coma at the time of transplantation with signs of intracranial hypertension and are on mechanical ventilation. Renal failure is a common event, and sometimes hemodialysis or continuous hemofiltration have to be performed before or during the surgical procedure. Positive blood cultures

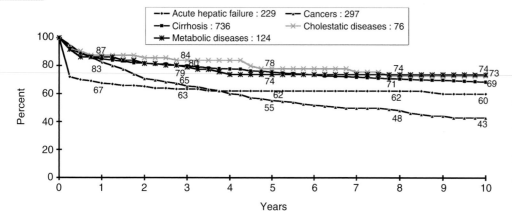

Fig. 105.5. Survival after liver transplantation in relation to initial liver disease at Paul Brousse. There is a higher post-transplant mortality in patients transplanted for fulminant hepatitis, with a slow decline in survival after 1 year. This reflects the critical clinical condition of patients at the time of transplantation and the poor quality of grafts used in some patients in the context of an emergency transplantation procedure.

can be present. Hemodynamic instability secondary to profound vasoplegia requiring the use of pressor drugs, such as epinephrine or norepinephrine, can be present. This vasoplegia can be the consequence of unrecognized sepsis or of the liver failure itself. Although the transplant procedure may be performed satisfactorily, the risk of perioperative death is probably higher compared with transplant procedures in patients with chronic liver disease.

Sepsis is a main cause of death. Sepsis may be due to several causes: (1) As described earlier, sepsis is common in patients with fulminant hepatitis; (2) patients in a coma before transplantation may remain on mechanical ventilation after transplantation for several days, increasing the risk of sepsis; and (3) patients receiving ABO incompatible grafts usually receive more potent antirejection therapy, which may increase the risk of sepsis.

Morbidity

The rate of retransplantation in our series was much higher than in the elective series (13% versus 7%). The main causes of retransplantation were acute rejection, primary graft nonfunction, and "intrahepatic biliary strictures." The high rate of retransplantation was related mostly to the need for emergency transplantation. The use of ABO incompatible grafts is responsible for a high rate of severe acute rejection episodes and for the occurrence of biliary strictures in the graft (Farges et al, 1995;

Gugenheim et al, 1990). Although the use of steatotic grafts may save the patient, we and others have observed a high rate of primary graft nonfunction with such grafts (Adam et al, 1991). In theory, these severely ill patients need a good graft to sustain recovery of their liver failure as quickly as possible; however, because of the emergency situation, they often receive the first liver available, which could be of poor quality or ABO blood group incompatible. Some teams believe the transplantation of an ABO incompatible liver is not justified or should be performed only as a bridge before a transplantation of a compatible graft. We believe that ABO incompatible grafts may be used in an emergency. Despite a high rate of retransplantation resulting from hyperacute rejection, chronic rejection, or intrahepatic biliary strictures, the overall patient survival was 50%, and 30% of these patients are alive with their first liver graft still functional in long-term follow-up (Bismuth et al, 1996b; ELTR, 2005; Gugenheim et al, 1990). It is the responsibility of the team to decide if ABO incompatible grafts should be used in emergency circumstances.

Neurologic sequelae can be observed after transplantation. The neurologic complications can be the direct consequences of the severe pretransplant coma or the consequences of cerebral bleeding related to an ICP monitor. Such complications are more frequent in patients in a deep coma at the time of transplantation.

Hepatitis B Virus Recurrence After Liver Transplantation for Fulminant Hepatitis B or Hepatitis B-D

HBV recurrence can occur after transplantation for fulminant hepatitis B, but is much lower than for patients transplanted for chronic liver disease secondary to HBV. It is a rare (<10%) event if patients receive long-term post-transplant passive immunoprophylaxis (Samuel et al, 1991, 1993). In addition, when HBV recurrence occurred in the graft, it seemed less severe than for patients with HBV recurrence after transplantation for chronic HBV liver disease. The rate of HBV recurrence in patients transplanted for fulminant hepatitis secondary to hepatitis B and D receiving long-term anti–hepatitis B surface antigen passive immunoprophylaxis was higher at approximately 25%.

Quality of Life and Long-Term Survival

The quality of life of survivors is generally good and seems similar to that of patients transplanted for chronic liver disease.

Table 105.1 Patient Survival According to the Indication for Liver Transplantation for Fulminant Hepatitis in Europe

Indications	1-Year (%)	2-Year (%)	5-Year (%)	10-Year (%)
HAV	64	56	52	52
HBV	67	61	55	50
Paracetamol	67	62	54	45
Nonparacetamol	62	57	55	48
Toxic	68	64	63	56
Others	63	60	54	50
Unknown	61	55	51	46

Most young patients return to a normal social life and to work. Psychological troubles can be observed in the early postoperative period and are explained mainly by the pretransplant encephalopathy and by the fact that these patients were not prepared psychologically for transplantation. Long-term survival is generally good. There are few deaths after 1 year. This is due in part to the young age of the patients, to the low rate of HBV recurrence in fulminant hepatitis B, and to the absence of recurrence of the other causes of fulminant hepatitis.

NEW TRENDS IN LIVER TRANSPLANTATION FOR FULMINANT HEPATITIS

The new therapeutic strategies discussed in this section are based on the concept of liver regeneration in fulminant hepatitis.

Auxiliary Liver Transplantation

Auxiliary orthotopic transplantation (Boudjema et al, 1995) is a procedure that has been proposed for the treatment of selected patients with acute liver failure (see Ch. 108). This procedure usually requires partial left or right hepatectomy of the original liver and leaves in place part of the native liver. It has been postulated that the native liver would regenerate in some patients with acute liver failure, with the graft placed in an orthotopic position acting as a temporary support. Numerous reports of successful auxiliary liver transplantation have been published in recent years. In a multicentric European study, the overall survival rate was 63%; 68% of the survivors (i.e., 43% of all patients) were able to stop immunosuppressive therapy permanently with full recovery of the native liver, achieving the ultimate goal of emergency auxiliary liver transplantation (Chenard-Neu et al, 1996).

In the ELTR, actuarial patient survival rates were significantly lower after auxiliary partial orthotopic liver transplantation versus standard orthotopic liver transplantation: 52%, 49%, and 49% versus 69%, 65%, and 63% at 1, 3, and 5 years (P = .03, log-rank). Actuarial retransplantation-free survival rates also were significantly lower after auxiliary partial orthotopic liver transplantation versus orthotopic liver transplantation: 42%, 42%, and 42% versus 62%, 58%, and 56% at 1, 3, and 5 years (P = .01, log-rank) (ELTR, 2005).

The key issue regarding auxiliary liver transplantation is determining when native liver regeneration is likely to occur (Fig. 105.6). Complete regeneration was frequent in patients younger than 40 years, in patients in whom the cause of fulminant hepatitis was viral hepatitis or paracetamol overdose, and in patients in whom fulminant hepatitis followed a hyperacute course.

Auxiliary partial liver transplantation may have some drawbacks. The native liver does not always regenerate correctly, especially in patients with subfulminant hepatitis. When hepatitis is due to hepatitis viruses, there is a risk of chronic viral persistence secondary to the immunosuppressive drugs. There is only moderate portal hypertension in these patients, and because part of the portal flow must be directed to the graft, the loss of flow can negatively affect the regeneration of the native liver. The two livers compete for the portal venous flow, and the portal venous blood flow may favor the native liver or the graft depending on some events, such as rejection. The main disadvantage of these procedures is that auxiliary orthotopic liver transplantation is

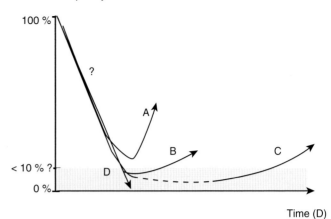

Functional hepatocytes

Fig. 105.6. Natural history of destruction and regeneration of hepatocytes in fulminant hepatitis and the influence on survival (according to Bismuth, personal observation). **A,** Spontaneous recovery before encephalopathy. **B,** Spontaneous recovery after encephalopathy. **C,** Late regeneration (duration unknown). Death is avoided only with the help of auxiliary liver transplantation or liver support. **D,** Total destruction of hepatocytes. This leads to death or transplantation.

technically more difficult and may delay achieving satisfactory graft function, whereas most of these patients do require a functional liver as soon as possible; this may be deleterious in more severely ill patients. Overall, in Europe (ELTR, 2005) and in our series, the mortality and the morbidity are higher in auxiliary partial orthotopic liver transplantation (Bismuth et al, 1996a).

After auxiliary liver transplantation, there may be difficult management issues, even when the initial auxiliary transplant has been successful. First, the diagnosis of native liver regeneration is sometimes difficult and should comprise the combined use of biochemical liver test results, the analysis of biopsy specimens of the two livers, the appreciation of the volumes of both livers by computed tomography scan, and the use of hepatobiliary iminodiacetic acid (HIDA) scanning. Second, when the native liver has regenerated, the question arises as to the best way to deal with the graft (i.e., "detransplantation"). One option is to taper down the immunosuppression to provoke a controlled rejection of the donor liver, which is left to atrophy. The theoretical disadvantage of this attitude is the risk of causing a severe rejection of the graft requiring its prompt surgical removal, which may be a difficult procedure in an inflamed organ. The other option is to take out the graft electively without discontinuing immunosuppression. The procedure of surgical removal of the graft may be difficult, however, and is not without risks.

The exact place of auxiliary liver transplantation in the armamentarium of liver transplantation and the indication of this surgical technique should be defined in the future (Azoulay et al, 2001; Liu et al, 2002). This procedure should be reserved for patients with high potential of regeneration (e.g., HAV patients) and patients at an early stage of coma.

Living Donor Liver Transplantation

Living donor liver transplantation has been expanded to emergency cases and should be considered as a treatment option for adult patients with acute liver failure. In particular, right lobe living donor liver transplantation improves survival of patients with acute liver failure (Soejima et al, 2003). Graft size problems remain the greatest limiting factor, however, for expansion of living donor liver transplantation to adult populations. The small-for-size syndrome is associated with graft exposure to excessive portal perfusion (Kiuchi et al, 2003). The living donor liver transplantation procedure in the emergency setting is more difficult to organize, and from an ethical point of view, the psychological pressures on the family are high.

LIVER SUPPORTS

Bioartificial supports (see Ch. 89) have been developed more recently to treat patients with fulminant hepatitis. Bioartificial supports aim to provide patient support while awaiting a graft, rather than to replace the need for liver transplantation.

Ex Vivo Liver Perfusion

Ex vivo liver perfusion has been attempted in the past before the era of liver transplantation, usually with animal livers from baboons, chimpanzees, and pigs. The results were disappointing in terms of survival. More recently ex vivo pig liver perfusion have been attempted again in a few patients (Chari et al, 1994); however, the results were not convincing. Several problems occurred. The duration of perfusion is limited to a mean of 6 hours because of the deterioration of the function of the pig liver, the phenomena of hyperacute and acute rejection occur within the pig liver and cannot be prevented by a filter for xenogeneic antibodies placed in the circuit, and there is a sharp decrease in platelet counts. This technique probably cannot be used widely in the future because the pig liver should be harvested in the emergency setting, and this would introduce a concern regarding the risk of pathogenic agent transmission in the context of the emergency setting (i.e., there is insufficient time to allow for adequate pathogen testing).

Hepatocyte Transplantation

Hepatocyte transplantation is still in experimentation and has not been used in humans except in anecdotal cases.

Extracorporeal Bioartificial Liver Support

The development of bioartificial livers using extracorporeal circuits in humans has been reported. Two systems have been applied experimentally in humans. One system has used hepatocytes from a human hepatoblastoma cell line placed in the extracapillary space of a hollow fiber cartridge (Sussman et al, 1992). This system is an extracorporeal circuit in which the whole blood of the patient is passed through a hollow-fiber cartridge in which the hepatocytes are placed in the extracapillary part of the capillary fibers. Despite the presence of several security levels, the main concern is that tumoral hepatocytes may pass into the patient's circulation. A report of its use in patients with FHF in a randomized trial showed mixed results, with some improvements in the neurologic condition of the patients, but no clear improvement in survival.

The other system currently being developed uses porcine hepatocytes on dextran microcarriers placed in the extracapillary space of a hollow-fiber cartridge. This system, developed by Demetriou and Circe Biomedical (Los Angeles, CA), was evaluated at Cedars Sinai in San Francisco and at our center and is used during the waiting time for transplantation (see Ch. 89). This system is an extracorporeal circuit that comprises a plasmapheresis, following which the plasma of the patient is passed through a charcoal filter and a hollow-fiber cartridge, in which 5 billion hepatocytes are placed in the extracapillary part of the capillary fibers. Exchange is done between plasma and the hepatocytes through the capillary semipermeable membranes (Ellis et al, 1996; Rozga et al, 1993b). Survival in FHF and subfulminant hepatic failure patients was significantly higher in the bioartificial liver group compared with the control group (risk ratio 0.56; $P=.048$).

At our center, 10 patients with fulminant hepatitis listed for emergency liver transplantation have been treated with one to three courses of 6 hours of bioartificial liver. All of these patients have been transplanted, and eight survived with the main clinical effect of bioartificial liver treatment being neurologic improvement (Samuel et al, 2002). A promising advance of this latter system is that porcine hepatocytes are kept cryopreserved and stored and are thawed for use only when a patient treatment is needed. The advantage of this approach is that the hepatocytes can be shipped cryopreserved, and the harvesting of porcine hepatocytes and all procedures for isolation and conservation of the hepatocytes are done under strict regulatory conditions to avoid any transmission of pathogenic agent from porcine to humans. The safety and efficacy of the bioartificial liver were evaluated in a prospective, randomized, controlled, multicenter trial in patients with severe acute liver failure. For the entire patient population, survival at 30 days was the same between the two groups (bioartificial liver group versus control group). When survival was analyzed accounting for confounding factors, in the entire patient population, there was no difference between the two groups (risk ratio 0.67; $P=.13$). Survival in the FHF and subfulminant hepatic failure patient population was significantly higher in the bioartificial liver group, however, compared with control group (risk ratio 0.67; $P=.048$) (Demetriou et al, 2004).

These bioartificial livers are at a first step, and future developments are awaited. The development of bioartificial liver containing pig cells is on standby, however. Health care authorities are reluctant to accept further trials using xenocells.

Extracorporeal Artificial Liver Supports

Molecular Adsorbent Recycling System

Molecular Adsorbent Recycling System (MARS) (Fig. 105.7 and Table 105.2) is a liver support system developed to support excretory liver function. It consists of elements from extracorporeal renal replacement techniques, such as hemodialysis and ultrafiltration, and adsorption. MARS uses an albumin-enriched dialysate to facilitate the removal of albumin-bound toxins. It contains three different fluid compartments: the blood circuit; an albumin circuit; and an open loop, single-pass dialysate circuit. MARS requires a standard dialysis machine or a continuous venovenous hemofiltration device to control the blood and dialysate circuits. An extra device (MARS monitor; Teraklin AG, Rostock, Germany) is necessary to control and monitor the closed loop albumin circuit. Blood is passed through a

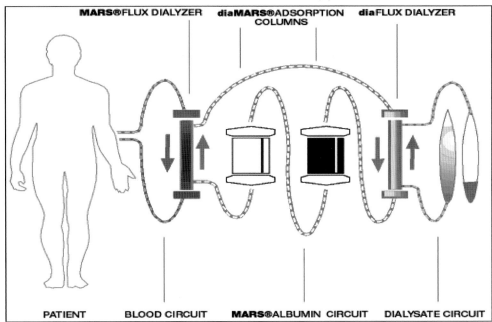

MARS®FLUX DIALYZER **diaMARS®ADSORPTION COLUMNS** **diaFLUX DIALYZER**

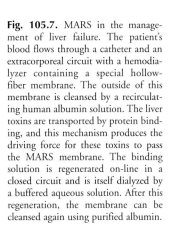

Fig. 105.7. MARS in the management of liver failure. The patient's blood flows through a catheter and an extracorporeal circuit with a hemodialyzer containing a special hollow-fiber membrane. The outside of this membrane is cleansed by a recirculating human albumin solution. The liver toxins are transported by protein binding, and this mechanism produces the driving force for these toxins to pass the MARS membrane. The binding solution is regenerated on-line in a closed circuit and is itself dialyzed by a buffered aqueous solution. After this regeneration, the membrane can be cleansed again using purified albumin.

PATIENT **BLOOD CIRCUIT** **MARS®ALBUMIN CIRCUIT** **DIALYSATE CIRCUIT**

non–albumin-permeable high-flux dialysis membrane (MARSFlux; Teraklin). The dialysate human serum albumin is passed through the dialysate compartment of the blood dialyzer and regenerated by dialysis against a bicarbonate-buffered dialysate, followed by passage through two sequential columns: uncoated charcoal and anion exchanger resin (Mitzner et al, 2001). In a prospective controlled trial in patients with FHF (Schmidt et al, 2003), MARS treatment increased the systemic vascular resistance, mean arterial blood pressure, and cardiac index. A significant decrease of bilirubin and creatinine levels occurred after MARS treatment.

In patients with acute liver or acute-on-chronic liver failure, bile acids, bilirubin, and other protein-bound toxins can be removed. In a prospective, controlled study, Heemann and colleagues (2002) treated 12 patients with acute exacerbation of chronic liver failure by the MARS system. A significant decrease

of bilirubin, creatinine, and mean arterial pressure after MARS has been observed. An improvement of hepatic encephalopathy also has been reported in patients with acute liver failure. Most studies using MARS have been performed in patients with acute-on-chronic liver failure. A few studies have been performed in patients with FHF showing some improvements in encephalopathy, cerebral perfusion pressure, and in mean arterial pressure (Ben Abraham et al, 2001; Schmidt et al, 2001, 2003; Sorkine et al, 2001). Prospectively randomized controlled trials are needed, however, to prove whether the system is really efficient in patients with FHF (Heemann et al, 2002).

Other Extracorporeal Artificial Liver Supports

Prometheus System. The Prometheus system is a new liver system in which albumin-bound substances are directly removed from blood by a special adsorber. In a simultaneous

---

Table 105.2 Effects of Molecular Adsorbent Recycling System in Patients with Acute Liver Failure or Acute-on-Chronic Liver Failure

Reference	Type of Study	Status of Patients	No. Patients	MARS Effects
Catalina et al, 2003	Systemic hemodynamic	ACLF	4	↓ Portal hypertension; ↓ hyperdynamic circulation; (↑ MAP, ↑ SVRI, ↓ CO, ↓ PRA, ↓ NE)
Novelli et al, 2003	Systemic hemodynamic	ALF, PNF, DNF, ACLF	63	↓ Bilirubin[P], ↓ NH$_4$[P], ↑ GCS[P]; correlation between improvement of neurologic status and improvement of cerebral perfusion
Schmidt et al, 2003	Systemic hemodynamic*	ALF	8	↑ SVRI[P], ↑ CO[P], ↑ MAP[P], ↑ HR[P], ↓ VO$_2$[P]
Heemann et al, 2002	Efficacy and safety study*	ACLF	12	↑ 30-day survival[P]; ↓ renal dysfunction[P]; ↓ hepatic encephalopathy[P]
Ben Abraham et al, 2001	Brain edema and CPP	ACLF	3	↓ ICP, ↑ CPP

*Prospective controlled trial.
[P]significant *P* value.
ACLF, acute-on-chronic liver failure; ALF, acute liver failure; DNF, delayed nonfunction; CO, cardiac output; CPP, cerebral perfusion pressure; GCS, Glasgow Coma Scale; HR, heart rate; MAP, mean arterial pressure; NE, norepinephrine; PNF, primary nonfunction; PRA, plasma renin activity; SVRI, systemic vascular resistance index; VO$_2$, oxygen consumption.

step, high-flux hemodialysis is performed. A significant improvement of serum levels of conjugated bilirubin, bile acids, ammonia, cholinesterase, creatinine, urea, and blood pH was observed (Rifai et al, 2003).

Single-Pass Albumin Dialysis. Single-pass albumin dialysis is a method of albumin dialysis that uses a standard renal replacement therapy system without an additional perfusion pump system. The patient's blood flows through a circuit containing a high-flux hollow fiber hemodiafilter. The other side of this membrane is cleansed by an albumin solution flowing in the counter direction; this solution is discarded after passing the filter. Continuous venovenous hemodiafiltration may be undertaken in the first circuit using the same high-flux hollow fibers (Kreymann et al, 1999). In vitro, the detoxification capacities of single-pass albumin dialysis and MARS are similar (Sauer et al, 2004).

CONCLUSION

Liver transplantation represents a breakthrough in the treatment of patients with fulminant or subfulminant hepatitis. Patients with fulminant hepatitis should be referred as early as possible to a specialized center with a liver transplantation unit. Liver transplantation, if necessary, should be performed early before the advent of irreversible brain damage. Reliable criteria for the indication for transplantation have been developed, and the creation of a superemergency waiting list has increased the feasibility for transplantation. Brain edema remains difficult to control medically, however, and is the main cause of death before and after transplantation, which explains in part the higher mortality in these patients.

Future aims of research and therapeutics are (1) improvement and standardization of the prognosis criteria, (2) improvement of the feasibility of liver transplantation with a superemergency waiting list and living donor liver transplantation, and (3) improvement of therapy of brain edema (hypothermia and artificial liver support). Therapies such as extracorporeal bioartificial liver support and artificial liver support have to be evaluated as therapies of prevention of fulminant hepatitis during the waiting time for a graft.

REFERENCES

Adam R, et al, 1991: The outcome of steatotic grafts in liver transplantation. Transplant Proc 23:1538-1540.

Azoulay D, et al, 2001: Auxiliary partial orthotopic versus standard orthotopic whole liver transplantation for acute liver failure: a reappraisal from a single center by a case-control study. Ann Surg 234:723-731.

Belghiti J, et al, 1995: Temporary portocaval anastomosis with preservation of caval flow during orthotopic liver transplantation. Am J Surg 169:277-279.

Ben Abraham R, et al, 2001: Rapid resolution of brain edema and improved cerebral perfusion pressure following the molecular adsorbent recycling system in acute liver failure patients. Transplant Proc 33:2897-2899.

Bernal W, Wendon J, 2004: Liver transplantation in adults with acute liver failure. J Hepatol 40:192-197.

Bernal W, et al, 2002: Blood lactate as an early predictor of outcome in paracetamol-induced acute liver failure: a cohort study. Lancet 359:558-563.

Bernuau J, et al, 1986a: Multivariate analysis of prognostic factors in fulminant hepatitis B. Hepatology 6:648-651.

Bernuau J, et al, 1986b: Fulminant and subfulminant liver failure: definition and causes. Semin Liver Dis 6:97-106.

Bernuau J, et al, 1991: Criteria for emergency liver transplantation in patients with acute viral hepatitis and factor V below 50% of normal: a prospective study. Hepatology 14:49A.

Bhatia V, et al, 2004: Prophylactic phenytoin does not improve cerebral edema or survival in acute liver failure—a controlled clinical trial. J Hepatol 41:89-96.

Bismuth H, Houssin D, 1984: Reduced-sized orthotopic liver graft in hepatic transplantation in children. Surgery 95:367-370.

Bismuth H, et al, 1987: Emergency liver transplantation for fulminant hepatitis. Ann Intern Med 107:337-341.

Bismuth H, et al, 1995: Orthotopic liver transplantation in fulminant and subfulminant hepatitis: the Paul Brousse experience. Ann Surg 222:109-119.

Bismuth H, et al, 1996a: Auxiliary partial orthotopic liver transplantation for fulminant hepatitis: the Paul Brousse experience. Ann Surg 224:712-726.

Bismuth H, et al, 1996b: Liver transplantation for patients with acute liver failure. Semin Liver Dis 16:415-425.

Blei AT, 1991: Cerebral edema and intracranial hypertension in acute liver failure: distinct aspects of the same problem. Hepatology 13:376-379.

Blei AT, et al, 1992: Animal models of hepatic encephalopathy. In Boulton AA, et al (eds): Animal Models of Neurological Disease. Neuromethods 22. Totowa, NJ, Humana, pp 183-222.

Blei AT, et al, 1993: Complications of intracranial pressure monitoring in fulminant hepatic failure. Lancet 341:157-158.

Boudjema K, et al, 1995: Auxiliary liver transplantation for fulminant and subfulminant hepatic failure. Transplantation 59:218-223.

Brandsaeter B, et al, 2002: Fulminant hepatic failure: outcome after listing for highly urgent liver transplantation—12 years experience in the Nordic countries. Liver Transplant 8:1055-1062.

Brems JJ, et al, 1987: Fulminant hepatic failure: the role of liver transplantation as primary therapy. Am J Surg 154:137-141.

Canalese J, et al, 1982: Controlled trial of dexamethasone and mannitol for the cerebral edema of fulminant hepatic failure. Gut 23:625-629.

Castells A, et al, 1993: Liver transplantation for acute liver failure: analysis of applicability. Gastroenterology 105:532-538.

Catalina MV, et al, 2003: Hepatic and systemic haemodynamic changes after MARS in patients with acute on chronic liver failure. Liver Int 23(suppl 3):39-43.

Chari RS, et al, 1994: Treatment of hepatic failure with ex-vivo pig-liver perfusion followed by liver transplantation. N Engl J Med 331:234-237.

Chenard-Neu MP, et al, 1996: Auxiliary liver transplantation: regeneration of the native liver and outcome in 30 patients with fulminat hepatic failure: a multicenter study. Hepatology 23:1119-1127.

Clemmesen JO, et al, 1997: Indomethacin normalizes intracranial pressure in acute liver failure: a twenty-three year old woman treated with indomethacin. Hepatology 26:1423-1425.

Clemmesen JO, et al, 1999: Cerebral herniation in patients with acute liver failure is correlated with arterial ammonia concentration. Hepatology 29:648-653.

Demetriou AA, et al, 2004: Prospective, randomized, multicenter, controlled trial of a bioartificial liver in treating acute liver failure. Ann Surg 239:660-667.

Denis J, Opolon P, 1983: Traitement de l'encéphalopathie aiguë au cours des hépatites par hemofiltration continue: résultats d'une étude controllée. In Gauthier A (ed): Soins Intensifs en Hepato-gastro-enterologie. Paris, Masson, pp 5-12.

Denis J, et al, 1978: Treatment of encephalopathy during fulminant hepatic failure by haemodialysis with high permeability membrane. Gut 19:787-793.

Devictor D, et al, 1992: Emergency liver transplantation for fulminant liver failure in infants and children. Hepatology 16:1156-1162.

Donovan JP, et al, 1992: Brain water and acute liver failure: the emerging role of intracranial pressure monitoring. Hepatology 16:267-268.

EASL Trial Committee, 1979: Randomized trial of steroid therapy in acute liver failure. Gut 20:620-623.

Ede RJ, Williams R, 1986: Occurrence and management of cerebral edema in liver failure. In Williams R (ed): Clinics in Critical Care Medicine: Liver Failure. Edinburgh, Churchill Livingstone, pp 26-46.

Ellis AJ, et al, 1996: Pilot controlled trial of the extracorporeal liver assist device in acute liver failure. Hepatology 24:1446-1451.

Ellis AJ, et al, 2000: Subclinical seizure activity and prophylactic phenytoin infusion in acute liver failure: a controlled clinical trial. Hepatology 32:536-541.

European Liver Transplant Registry, 2005: Available at: www.eltr.org.

Farges O, et al, 1995: The use of ABO incompatible grafts in liver transplantation: a life saving procedure in highly selected patients. Transplantation 59:1124-1133.

Farmer DG, et al, 2003: Liver transplantation for fulminant hepatic failure. Ann Surg 237:666-676.

Feray C, et al, 1993: Hepatitis C virus RNA and hepatitis B virus DNA in serum and liver of patients with fulminant hepatitis. Gastroenterology 104:549-555.

Forbes A, et al, 1989: Thiopental infusion in the treatment of intracranial hypertension complicating fulminant hepatic failure. Hepatology 10:306-310.

Gazzard BG, et al, 1974: Charcoal haemoperfusion in the treatment of fulminant hepatic failure. Lancet 1:1301-1307.

Gimson AE, et al, 1982: Earlier charcoal haemoperfusion in fulminant hepatic failure. Lancet 2:681-683.

Ginsberg MD, et al, 1992: Therapeutic modulation of brain temperature: relevance to ischemic brain injury. Cerebrovasc Brain Metab Rev 4:189-225.

Gugenheim J, et al, 1990: Liver transplantation across ABO blood group barrier. Lancet 336:519-523.

Harrison PM, et al, 1991: Improvement by acetylcysteine of hemodynamics and oxygen transport in fulminant hepatic failure. N Engl J Med 324:1852-1857.

Hashem B, et al, 2002: Diabetes increases the risk of acute hepatic failure. Gastroenterology 122:1822-1828.

Heemann U, et al, 2002: Albumin dialysis in cirrhosis with superimposed acute liver injury: a prospective, controlled study. Hepatology 36:949-958.

Imberti R, et al, 1997: The use of indomethacin to treat acute rises of intracranial pressure and improve global perfusion in a child with head trauma. Acta Anaesthesiol Scand 41:536-540.

Iwatsuki S, et al, 1985: Liver transplantation for fulminant hepatic failure. Semin Liver Dis 5:325-328.

Jalan R, et al, 1999: Moderate hypothermia for uncontrolled intracranial hypertension in acute liver failure. Lancet 354:1164-1168.

Jalan R, et al, 2002: Liver derived pro-inflammatory cytokines may be important in producing intracranial hypertension in acute liver failure. J Hepatol 37:536-538.

Jalan R, et al, 2004: Moderate hypothermia in patients with acute liver failure and uncontrolled intracranial hypertension. Gastroenterology 127:1338-1346.

Kato MD, et al, 1992: Electron microscopic study of the brain capillaries in cerebral edema from fulminant hepatic failure. Hepatology 15:1060-1066.

Keays R, et al, 1991: Intracranial and cerebral perfusion pressure changes before, during and immediately after orthotopic liver transplantation for fulminant hepatic failure. QJM 289:425-433.

Kelly DF, et al, 1999: Propofol in the treatment of moderate and severe head injury: a randomized, prospective double-blinded pilot trial. J Neurosurg 90:1042-1052.

Kiuchi T, et al, 2003: Small-for-size graft in living donor liver transplantation: how far should we go? Liver Transpl 9:S29-S35.

Kreymann B, et al, 1999: Albumin dialysis: effective removal of copper in a patient with fulminant Wilson disease and successful bridging to liver transplantation: a new possibility for the elimination of protein-bound toxins. J Hepatol 31:1080-1085.

Kurt A, et al, 1996: Perioperative normothermia to reduce the incidence of surgical-wound infection and shorten hospitalization. Study of Wound Infection and Temperature Group. N Engl J Med 334:1209.

Larsen FS, 1996: Cerebral circulation in liver failure. Semin Liver Dis 16:281-293.

Larsen FS, et al, 2000: Regional cerebral blood flow autoregulation in patients with fulminant hepatic failure. Liver Transpl 6:795-801.

Lidofski SD, et al, 1992: Intracranial pressure monitoring and liver transplantation for fulminant hepatic failure. Hepatology 16:1-7.

Liu CL, et al, 2002: Right-lobe live donor liver transplantation improves survival of patients with acute liver failure. Br J Surg 89:317-322.

Mendoza A, et al, 1997: Liver transplantation for fulminant hepatic failure: importance of renal failure. Transpl Int 10:55-60.

Mitzner SR, et al, 2001: Extracorporeal detoxification using the Molecular Adsorbent Recirculating System for critically ill patients with liver failure. J Am Soc Nephrol 12:S75-S82.

Murphy N, et al, 2004: The effect of hypertonic sodium chloride on intracranial pressure in patients with acute liver failure. Hepatology 39:464-470.

Norenberg MD, 1996: Astrocyte-ammonia interactions in hepatic encephalopathy. Semin Liver Dis 16:245-253.

Novelli G, et al, 2003: A 3-year experience with Molecular Adsorbent Recirculating System (MARS): our results on 63 patients with hepatic failure and color Doppler US evaluation of cerebral perfusion. Liver Int 23(suppl 3):10-15.

O'Grady J, et al, 1988a: Controlled trials of charcoal hemoperfusion and prognostic factors in fulminant hepatic failure. Gastroenterology 94:1186-1192.

O'Grady J, et al, 1988b: Outcome of orthotopic liver transplantation in the aetiological and clinical variants of acute liver failure. QJM New Series 69:817-824.

O'Grady J, et al, 1989: Early indicators of prognosis in fulminant hepatic failure. Gastroenterology 97:439-445.

O'Grady J, et al, 1991: Prothrombin time in fulminant hepatic failure. Gastroenterology 100:1480-1481.

O'Grady J, et al, 1993: Acute liver failure: redefining the syndromes. Lancet 342:273-275.

Ostapowicz G, et al, 2002: Results of a prospective study of acute liver failure at 17 tertiary care centers in the United States. U.S. Acute Liver Failure Study Group. Ann Intern Med 137:947-954.

Peake SL, et al, 1996: N-Acetyl-L-cysteine depresses cardiac performance in patients with septic shock. Crit Care Med 24:1302-1310.

Peleman RR, et al, 1987: Orthotopic liver transplantation for acute or subacute hepatic failure in adults. Hepatology 7:484-489.

Rifai K, et al, 2003: Prometheus: a new extracorporeal system for the treatment of liver failure. J Hepatol 39:984-990.

Ringe B, et al, 1986: Indications and results of liver transplantation in acute hepatic failure. Transplant Proc 18:86-88.

Ringe B, et al, 1993: Total hepatectomy and liver transplantation as two-stage procedure. Ann Surg 218:3-9.

Roberts DRD, Manas D, 1999: Induced hypothermia in the management of cerebral oedema secondary to fulminant liver failure. Clin Transplant 13:545-547.

Rolando N, et al, 1990: Prospective study of bacterial infection in acute liver failure: an analysis of fifty patients. Hepatology 11:49-53.

Rolando N, et al, 1991: Fungal infections: a common, unrecognised complication of acute liver failure. J Hepatol 12:1-9.

Rolando N, et al, 1993: Prospective controlled trial of selective parenteral and enteral antimicrobial regimen in fulminant hepatic failure. Hepatology 17:196-201.

Rolando N, et al, 1996: Bacterial and fungal infection in acute liver failure. Semin Liver Dis 16:389-402.

Rolando N, et al, 2000: The systemic inflammatory response syndrome in acute liver failure. Hepatology 32:734-739.

Rozga J, et al, 1993a: Control of cerebral oedema by total hepatectomy and extracorporeal liver support in fulminant hepatic failure. Lancet 342:898-899.

Rozga J, et al, 1993b: Development of a bioartificial liver: properties and function of a hollow-fiber module inoculated with liver cells. Hepatology 17:258-265.

Samuel D, et al, 1991: Passive immunoprophylaxis after liver transplantation in HBsAg positive patients. Lancet 337:813-815.

Samuel D, et al, 1993: Liver transplantation in European patients with the hepatitis B surface antigen. N Engl J Med 329:1842-1847.

Samuel D, et al, 2002: Neurological improvement during bioartificial liver sessions in patients with acute liver failure awaiting transplantation. Transplantation 73:257-264.

Sauer IM, et al, 2004: In vitro comparison of the Molecular Adsorbent Recirculation System (MARS) and Single-pass Albumin Dialysis (SPAD). Hepatology 39:1408-1414.

Schafer DF, Shaw BW, 1989: Fulminant hepatic failure and orthotopic liver transplantation. Semin Liver Dis 9:189-194.

Schmidt LE, Dalhoff K, 2002: Serum phosphate is an early predictor of outcome in severe acetaminophen-induced hepatotoxicity. Hepatology 36:659-665.

Schmidt LE, et al, 2001: Cerebral blood flow velocity increases during a single treatment with the molecular adsorbents recirculating system in patients with acute on chronic liver failure. Liver Transplant 7:709-712.

Schmidt LE, et al, 2003: Systemic hemodynamic effects of treatment with the molecular adsorbents recirculating system in patients with hyperacute liver failure: a prospective controlled trial. Liver Transpl 9:290-297.

Schubert A, 1995: Side effects of mild hypothermia. J Neurosurg Anesthesiol 7:139-147.

Sheiner P, et al, 1992: A randomized control trial of PGE2 in the treatment of fulminant hepatic failure. Hepatology 16:88A.

Sinclair SB, et al, 1989: Biochemical and clinical response of fulminant viral hepatitis to administration of prostaglandin E: a preliminary report. J Clin Invest 84:1063-1069.

Soejima Y, et al, 2003: Outcome analysis in adult-to-adult living donor liver transplantation using the left liver graft. Liver Transplant 9:581-586.

Sorkine P, et al, 2001: Role of the molecular adsorbent recycling system (MARS) in the treatment of patients with acute exacerbation of chronic liver failure. Crit Care Med 29:1332-1336.

Sussman NL, et al, 1992: Reversal of fulminant hepatic failure using an extracorporeal liver assist device. Hepatology 16:60-65.

Tokushige K, et al, 2000: Significance of soluble TNF receptor-I in acute type fulminant hepatitis. Am J Gastroenterol 95:2040-2046.

Trey C, Davidson CS, 1970: The management of fulminant hepatic failure. In Popper H, Shaffner F (eds): Progress in Liver Diseases. New York, Grune & Stratton, pp 282-298.

Vickers C, et al, 1988: Transplantation of the liver in adults and children with fulminant hepatic failure. J Hepatol 7:143-150.

Walsh TS, et al, 1998: The effect of *N*-acetylcysteine on oxygen transport and uptake in patients with fulminant hepatic failure. Hepatology 27:1332-1340.

Ware AJ, et al, 1971: Cerebral edema: a major complication of massive hepatic necrosis. Gastroenterology 61:877-884.

Wendon JA, et al, 1994: Cerebral blood flow and metabolism in fulminant liver failure. Hepatology 19:1407-1413.

Wiesner RH, 2004: MELD/PELD and the allocation of deceased donor livers for status 1 recipients with acute fulminant hepatic failure, primary nonfunction, hepatic artery thrombosis, and acute Wilson's disease. Liver Transpl 10(suppl 2):S17-S22.

Wijdicks EF, Nyberg SL, 2002: Propofol to control intracranial pressure in fulminant hepatic failure. Transplant Proc 34:1220-1222.

Williams R, 1996: Classification, etiology and considerations of outcome in acute liver failure. Semin Liver Dis 16:343-348.

Williams R, Gimson AE, 1984: An assessment of orthotopic liver transplantation in acute liver failure. Hepatology 4:22S-24S.

Wright TL, et al, 1991: Hepatitis C virus not found in fulminant non-A non B hepatitis. Ann Intern Med 115:111-112.

106

Liver Transplantation for Tumors

M. VARELA, J. FUSTER, AND J. BRUIX

The liver is the sole solid organ in which treatment may be based on transplantation. It has been proposed that primary and metastatic tumor involvement is amenable to liver transplantation. Treatment of hepatocellular carcinoma (HCC) is the only setting in which liver transplantation plays a role in conventional clinical practice, however. Cholangiocarcinoma is still a controversial indication because of the high recurrence rate, even when diagnosing the disease at an early stage. Among the other primary neoplasms, only epithelioid hemangioendothelioma can benefit from transplantation because of its less aggressive behavior. Finally, metastatic liver involvement reflects disseminated neoplastic disease, and in most programs it is never considered as an indication for transplantation. This chapter discusses the current concepts regarding transplantation for HCC. The details regarding other hepatic tumors are discussed briefly.

HEPATOCELLULAR CARCINOMA

HCC (see Ch. 71) is a neoplasm that usually affects patients with chronic liver disease, specifically cirrhosis (Bruix et al, 2001; Fattovich et al, 2004). Accordingly, liver transplantation frequently is presented as an optimal therapy that would cure simultaneously the neoplasm and the underlying liver condition. The available information after years of experience shows, however, that optimal results are achieved in the limited proportion of patients who are diagnosed at an early tumor stage (Schwartz, 2004). In contrast, patients with advanced disease would not benefit from the procedure. During the pioneering years of liver transplantation, a major proportion of the potential candidates to be considered for transplantation consisted of patients with advanced HCC for whom there was no other potentially effective treatment (Iwatsuki et al, 1985), and this experience allowed surgeons and hepatologists to define optimal selection criteria that should be used when considering liver transplantation for HCC (Table 106.1).

Selection Criteria

Initial series of transplantation for HCC showed that patients with vascular invasion or extrahepatic spread developed early tumor recurrence, and these patients are currently generally excluded from transplantation (Schwartz, 2004). At the same time, it was recognized that patients transplanted because of end-stage liver disease, in whom the pathologic analysis of the explanted liver showed a small HCC not identified during the preoperative workup, had the same outcome as patients with nonmalignant disease, and the recurrence rate was anecdotal (Bismuth et al,

1999; Iwatsuki et al, 1985). This type of tumor was usually solitary, was less than 5 cm in size, and lacked vascular invasion. If vascular invasion is present, the risk of recurrence is increased, and the same is observed if there is tumor lymph node involvement. Similarly, some patients with multiple small tumor sites potentially corresponding to synchronous HCC also had an encouraging survival without tumor recurrence. The expert application of modern imaging techniques easily identifies tumors at that stage (Fig. 106.1) and establishes the presence of macroscopic vascular invasion or enlarged lymph nodes or both and allows the identification of optimal candidates. These are patients with solitary HCC 5 cm or less or with a maximum of three nodules each 3 cm or less (Bismuth & Majno, 2000; Mazzaferro et al, 1996; Schwartz, 2004). Since the seminal study by Mazzaferro and coworkers in 1996, several investigators have shown that patients fitting into this optimal profile can achieve a 70% survival at 5 years with a recurrence rate less than 15% (see Table 106.1) (Bismuth et al, 1999; Iwatsuki et al, 2000; Jonas et al, 2001; Llovet et al, 1998; Yao et al, 2001). Patients with slightly more advanced disease have a lower life expectancy with a slightly increased recurrence rate, and currently it is highly controversial if the selection limits should be expanded or remain restrictive (Bruix et al, 2003; Marsh & Dvorchik, 2003; Yao et al, 2001).

Decisions regarding patient selection for liver transplantation in the setting of HCC are based on the results of imaging techniques; however, most studies suggesting expansion of current listing criteria are based on pathologic staging in the explant specimen and outcome. Instead, the potential expansion should be based on the correlation between radiologic staging and outcome. It is well known that even in expert hands, there is always a certain degree of understaging (Burrel et al, 2003; Libbrecht et al, 2002). This understaging mostly is related to the existence of additional tumor sites, usually measuring less than 10 to 20 mm (Burrel et al, 2003; Libbrecht et al, 2002; Taouli et al, 2004).

If listing criteria for liver transplantation were expanded, this would translate immediately to the transplantation of some patients with far too advanced tumor disease. The development of recurrence is associated with the number of nodules in the explanted liver and the detection of vascular invasion macroscopically and microscopically (Fig. 106.2) (Jonas et al, 2001; Mazzaferro et al, 1996; Plessier et al, 2004). Some studies also have shown that recurrence is significantly more frequent if there are areas of poor differentiation within the tumor, and the loss of differentiation runs parallel to the increase in tumor size (Nakashima & Kojiro, 1987). Expansion of the selection criteria would be associated with a significant worsening in outcome results. Although patients could assume the risk for poor results,

Table 106.1 Survival and Recurrence of Patients with Early Stage Hepatocellular Carcinoma Treated with Liver Transplantation

Reference	n	1-Year Survival (%)	5-Year Survival (%)	Recurrence
Mazzaferro et al, 1996	48	90	75 (4 yr)	4 (8%)
Bismuth et al, 1999	45	82	74	5 (11%)
Llovet et al, 1999	79	86	75	3 (4%)
Iwatsuki et al, 2000	344	73	49	83 (24%)
Jonas et al, 2001	120	90	71	20 (17%)
Yao et al, 2001	64	87	73	8 (12%)

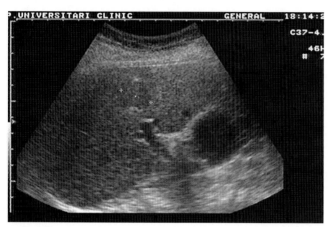

Fig. 106.1. Hepatic ultrasound showing a small hypoechoic HCC measuring 2 cm in diameter. These early stage tumors are the optimal candidates for liver transplantation.
(Courtesy of Dr. Bianchi, Hospital Clínic, Barcelona.)

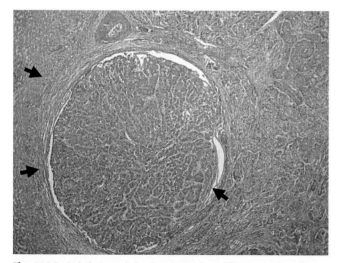

Fig. 106.2. Pathologic analysis of explanted liver. Microscopic view shows a moderately differentiated HCC invading into the vein lumen *(arrows).* (Hematoxylin and eosin stain, ×100.)
(Courtesy of Dr. Solé, Hospital Clínic, Barcelona.)

it is well known that the major problem in liver transplantation is the shortage of donors. A general policy for patient selection has been that the expected 5-year survival should exceed 50% (Neuberger, 2004). As discussed subsequently, the shortage of donors implies a waiting time between listing and transplantation during which the HCC may progress and prompt patient exclusion because of excessive tumor progression or death. Consequently, the survival results using an intention-to-treat analysis are less encouraging than when analyzing only patients who have been effectively transplanted (Fig. 106.3) (Llovet et al, 1999; Schwartz, 2004; Yao et al, 2002). This concept is important because the selection of the best treatment for a given patient should consider its feasibility and timing because another option with less efficacy, but higher applicability without delay, may offer a better outcome.

The risk of exclusion from transplantation because of tumor progression is already significant (25% if waiting for 1 year) with a restrictive selection policy (Llovet et al, 1999; Yao et al, 2002). Exclusion rates would be increased further if patients were enrolled with more advanced tumor stages (Roayaie et al, 2002). One of the most important issues here is the definition of the exclusion criteria. There is no common policy to follow the patients while waiting or a policy regarding whether exclusion has to occur when the listing limits have been exceeded or when major events (e.g., vascular invasion, extrahepatic spread) have been detected. Most programs allow progression beyond listing limits and assume the potential outcome impairment, but major progression should prompt patient exclusion.

As previously depicted, the tools used for decision making take into account tumor size and number; physicians need more sensitive tools to predict tumor behavior and the expected outcome of the patients. Detection of circulating tumor cells could become a useful instrument to identify disseminating cells (Louha et al, 1997), but this is an intermittent phenomenon, and cell detection does not translate directly into viable metastatic disease. The best tools are most likely to come through genetic profiling, which is currently able to distinguish between synchronous tumors and disseminated foci (Chen et al, 2000; Marsh et al, 2003). Current investigation of protein expression in peripheral blood may become the most useful and applicable tool in the future.

Management on Listing

There is a huge shortage of donors, and this prompts the need to restrict liver transplantation indication to patients with an optimal profile. All patients awaiting cadaveric transplantation face a waiting time between listing and transplantation. This delay varies from location to location based on the imbalance between donors and recipients. In some areas, this delay does not constitute a major issue, and patients are transplanted within several months. In other regions, however, the waiting time may exceed 2 years. The likelihood of tumor progression is high in these cases, and the feasibility of liver transplantation and long-term cure is almost nonexistent (Table 106.2). A waiting time of 12 months may imply an exclusion rate greater than 25% (Llovet et al, 1999; Yao et al, 2002), and the results for patients who reach transplantation may be impaired because tumor progression while waiting surely would increase the risk of dissemination. The predictors of progression and subsequent exclusion are not well defined. The risk is less in small solitary

Fig. 106.3. Intention-to-treat survival of patients with HCC treated with transplantation. **A,** Survival at 5 years is around 70% when restricting indication to patients with solitary HCC 5 cm or less or one to three nodules 3 cm or less. **B,** Graph shows the survival of patients in **A,** dividing them according to different time periods. The *upper curve* reflects the short waiting time era (mean 62 days) with no dropouts; the *lower curve* shows the impact of increased waiting time (mean 162 days) with appearance of dropouts in the second period. Although in the first era the 2-year survival was 84%, the 2-year survival in the long waiting time period was 54%. (From Llovet JM, et al, 1999: Intention-to-treat analysis of surgical treatment for early hepatocellular carcinoma: resection versus transplantation. Hepatology 30:1434.)

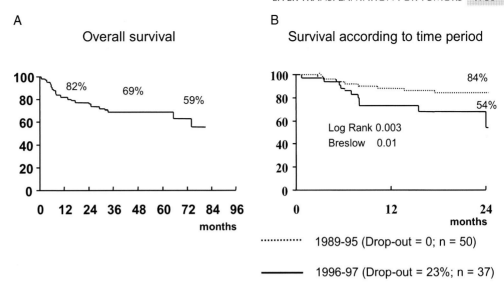

HCC compared with tumors reaching 5 cm (Llovet et al, 2003; Yao et al, 2001). This factor might be used to establish priority among patients, but it would not have enough predictive accuracy to become a robust tool. Some patients with small tumors may exhibit fast progression, whereas others with larger size tumors may remain stable for months. Molecular markers are of major help here (Fields et al, 2004; Gotoh et al, 2002; Pan et al, 2003).

The easiest way to reduce waiting time and the risk of exclusion while waiting is to increase the number of available donors. Public health campaigns and development of adequate organ procurement structures may increase the number of donors. Even if these actions were successful, however, the number of donors still would be unable to cope with the demand. Several programs have launched actions to use livers from non–heart-beating donors (Reddy et al, 2004). In addition, most groups have opened protocols to incorporate suboptimal livers that years ago would not have been considered. Suboptimal livers include organs from older donors, livers with moderate degrees of steatosis, or livers with active viral infection without significant liver damage. Livers with enzymatic deficiencies responsible for familial amyloidotic polyneuropathy (Azoulay et al, 1999) or primary hyperoxaluria (Donckier et al, 2001) also have been used successfully and have been split into two parts to benefit two recipients (Renz et al, 2003). Split liver transplantation is

seen as a major opportunity to increase significantly the patients benefiting from liver transplantation (Emond et al, 2002), but its complexity has prevented wide implementation.

Effective tumor treatment is the simultaneous strategy to be applied to diminish exclusion while waiting (Bolondi et al, 2003). There are no randomized controlled trials comparing any active therapy versus no treatment or even a given intervention against another. The estimation of the benefits of treatment comes from the critical analysis of cohort investigations. The number of studies incorporating all listed patients is limited, and the studies usually have recruited a small number of patients. Systemic chemotherapy has no efficacy and may induce relevant toxicity that ultimately may reduce outcome further and should not be recommended. Options for treatment before transplantation that have shown a significant antitumoral effect are surgical resection, percutaneous ablation, and transarterial chemoembolization.

Surgical Resection

Surgical resection competes with liver transplantation in patients with solitary HCC in compensated cirrhosis (Llovet et al, 1999; Schwartz, 2004; Song et al, 2004) because patients without portal hypertension and normal bilirubin concentration achieve a 70% survival at 5 years (see Chs. 80 and 82). This matches the

Table 106.2 Dropout Rate and Waiting Time in Hepatocellular Carcinoma Patients Listed for Liver Transplantation

Reference	n	Treatment Applied During Waiting Time	Patients Transplanted (%)	Median Waiting Time (days)	Patients Excluded (Dropouts) (%)
Llovet et al, 2003	205	PEI/RFA	172 (69%)	159	27 (16%)
Yao et al, 2002	70	TACE/PEI/RFA	50 (71%)	186	20 (29%)
Graziadei et al, 2003	63	TACE	51 (81%)	216	4 (6%)
Maddala et al, 2004	54	TACE	45 (83%)	211	8 (15%)
Mazzaferro et al, 2004	50	RFA	50 (100%)	290	0 (0%)
Hayashi et al, 2004	20	TACE	12 (60%)	333	6 (35%)
Fisher et al, 2004	33	Multimodal	28 (85%)	278	5 (15%)

PEI, percutaneous ethanol injection; RFA, radiofrequency ablation; TACE, transarterial chemoembolization.

best outcome after liver transplantation (Llovet et al, 1999), but recurrence rates are higher. The higher recurrence may suggest that liver transplantation would constitute a better option. Resection and liver transplantation should not be seen as mutually exclusive, however. Resection might be applied without major delay, and if the pathologic examination of the resected tumor indicates high risk of recurrence (e.g., presence of satellites, microscopic vascular invasion) (Cha et al, 2003; Izumi et al, 1994; Okada et al, 1994), patients could be considered immediately for liver transplantation because of the high risk of recurrence (Sala et al, 2004a). This active policy should be preferred to waiting to detect recurrence to consider salvage liver transplantation (Adam et al, 2003; Belghiti et al, 2003). Most patients with a risky pathologic profile present with early multifocal recurrence (Minagawa et al, 2003) not amenable for liver transplantation and would not benefit from sequential treatment.

Most patients diagnosed with HCC would not be considered optimal candidates for resection because of impaired liver function, and their recommended treatment would be liver transplantation (Sala et al, 2004a). Liver function impairment makes surgical resection a risky neoadjuvant treatment. Hepatic decompensation may develop and lead to transplant contraindication or death (Llovet et al, 1999). Only patients with minimal surgical risk should be considered for resection on listing. The balance between the risk of postsurgical liver failure and potential tumor progression while waiting would be reached only in long waiting times exceeding 12 months (Llovet et al, 2002a).

Percutaneous Ablation

Percutaneous ablation (see Ch. 76) is probably the most effective and least harmful option to treat patients on listing. Tumor ablation may be achieved by several means, but the most frequently used techniques are percutaneous ethanol injection and radiofrequency ablation. Both options require the guidance of a needle into the tumor under ultrasound or computed tomography (CT) control. Ethanol injection requires repeated injections to infiltrate the whole tumor mass, whereas radiofrequency ablation can achieve its effects in fewer sessions (Lencioni et al, 2003; Lin et al, 2004; Livraghi et al, 1999; Omata et al, 2004). The latter has more side effects, however, and should be avoided in tumors located near the heart, the diaphragm, the gallbladder, and the gastrointestinal structures. A significant concern with both options is the risk of seeding as a result of repeated puncture of poorly differentiated tumors located in the periphery of the liver that cannot be punctured through a safety rim of nontumoral liver (Livraghi et al, 2003; Llovet et al, 2001). If this is the case, percutaneous ethanol injection and radiofrequency ablation can be performed during laparoscopy allowing tight control of bleeding coming out from the tumor. Percutaneous ethanol injection and radiofrequency ablation are highly effective in HCC less than 2 cm (Fig. 106.4) (Sala et al, 2004b). These tumors can be completely necrosed in greater than 90% of cases. Tumor ablation should be considered safe in expert hands; the risk is minimal. If the waiting time is long enough to permit tumor progression and exclusion (>6 months), it may be wise to apply treatment (Llovet et al, 2002a).

Transarterial Chemoembolization

Transarterial chemoembolization (see Ch. 74) is a treatment option widely applied in patients with advanced HCC who are not candidates for surgical treatment. Its effectiveness is based on the obstruction of the hepatic artery blood flow feeding the

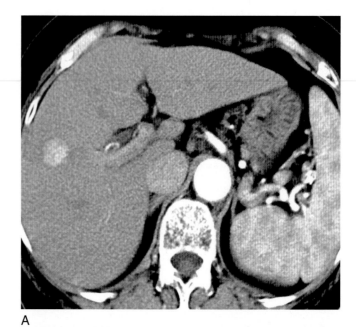

A

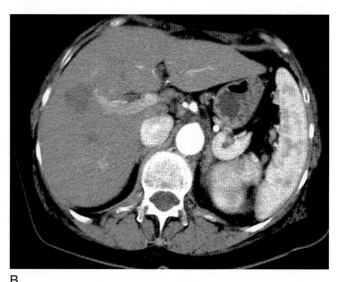

B

Fig. 106.4. A, CT scan shows small HCC less than 2 cm located in the right lobe of a cirrhotic liver. Evident arterial enhancement indicates increased arterial blood supply and establishes the diagnosis of HCC. **B,** After radiofrequency ablation, the tumor is completely necrosed. There is no contrast uptake in the area containing the nodule in the baseline CT scan. In addition, treatment has induced a wide margin of tissue necrosis, which also may necrose the potentially existing satellites in the vicinity of the main nodule. (Courtesy of Dr. Ayuso, Hospital Clínic, Barcelona.)

tumor and the simultaneous selective intra-arterial administration of chemotherapy (Bruix et al, 2004). This combined action results in extensive tumor necrosis, and several studies have shown that it delays tumor progression and the appearance of vascular invasion (GETCH, 1995; Llovet et al, 2002b). Transarterial chemoembolization cannot be applied in all patients listed for liver transplantation. Portal blood flow has to be preserved, and patients should belong to Child-Pugh A stage. Otherwise, treatment could induce acute liver failure and death. Treatment has to be repeated to prevent the tumor regaining vascularization and progressing. After repeated treatment lasting several months, the response to therapy is lost. Transarterial chemoembolization may have a positive impact in a subgroup of patients who would tolerate treatment and respond to it (Majno et al, 1997), and several transplant groups perform it routinely and assume a positive impact on the transplantability rate (Fisher et al, 2004; Graziadei et al, 2003; Hayashi et al, 2004; Maddala et al, 2004). The benefits remain if the times to liver transplantation are not too long, in which case the tumors may recover the capacity to proliferate, invade, and disseminate.

Priority Policy Within the Waiting List

A priority policy within the waiting list is a controversial issue that several groups have attempted to solve. In the United States, a federal mandate required development of a system to transplant the sickest patients first. This system would eliminate time on the waiting list as the major determinant of transplantation and avoid the "preventive" listing of patients who are not sick enough. The United Network for Organ Sharing (UNOS) established the MELD (Model for End-stage Liver Disease) score as the tool to predict short-term death; this system ranks patients according to their expected short-term outcome (Kamath et al, 2001). This system takes into account bilirubin, prothrombin index, and renal function, but does not incorporate any information about an existing tumor. To solve this problem, it was decided to give HCC patients a given number of MELD points aiming to allow an equitable distribution of livers among the different categories of patients (Wiesner et al, 2004). The points allocated initially were too high, and the transplant probability at 3 months of HCC patients was significantly higher than for non-HCC patients (Sharma et al, 2004). At the same time, it was recognized that 25% of patients transplanted because of a diagnosis of HCC did not have evidence of a tumor in the explant specimen (Freeman et al, 2004), and this raised the need to ensure that any given priority be based on robust diagnostic criteria. Because false-positive diagnosis affected mostly patients in whom the suspected HCC was small (<2 cm), the current position is to grant priority only to patients with tumors exceeding this size (Freeman, 2004) in whom diagnosis would be easily available by biopsy or by conventional noninvasive criteria (Bruix et al, 2001). The results of this last priority strategy are unavailable, but some concerns may be raised about its final impact. Tumors less than 2 cm have an optimal outcome.

In contrast, larger tumors in which progression has been documented should be considered as more "active" neoplasms, and the outcome after transplant may be reduced. Finally, the development of a priority policy should come together with a clear-cut policy for delisting, and currently this is not established. In the United States, patients who exceed the listing limits lose the priority points, and this may represent effective delisting. To maintain equity, the criteria for delisting should be present in all categories of disease and force the best use of livers in all diagnostic subgroups.

Living Donor Liver Transplantation

The development of living donor liver transplantation (see Ch. 109) has been a major breakthrough. Its availability without major delay is a major advantage to prevent exclusion while waiting for a cadaveric liver (Lo et al, 2004; Russo et al, 2004b; Todo & Furukawa, 2004). In addition, it may allow offering the benefits of transplantation to patients excluded from cadaveric programs because of their less than optimal life expectancy. The ideal conditions in which the liver is obtained have to be balanced against the lesser liver volume that is implanted. Patients have to be in optimal physical condition to cope with the small-for-size syndrome that may develop. At the same time, patients have to be able to tolerate the potential higher rate of complications, mostly of biliary origin (Brown et al, 2003).

The major aspect that has to be carefully analyzed is the risk to the donor. In pediatric living donor liver transplantation, the common practice is to use the left liver lobe, whereas in adult living donor liver transplantation, the standard approach is to use the right lobe. Hepatic volume accounting for at least 0.8% of the body volume is needed, and mortality for the donor is 0.5% to 1%. Multicenter cohort studies from Japan indicate that the survival of patients after living donor liver transplantation is almost the same as that achieved in cadaveric programs (Todo & Furukawa, 2004). If the selection criteria are maintained within the Milano definitions, the survival at 3 years reaches almost 80%, whereas this decreases to 60% when Milano criteria are exceeded (Fig. 106.5). There is still some concern, however, as to what effect viral infection of the graft in patients with hepatitis C virus would have on a more aggressive evolution leading to cirrhosis early during follow-up

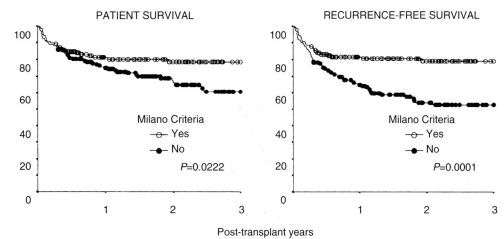

Fig. 106.5. Survival of HCC patients treated by living donor liver transplantation in Japan. If patients fit into the Milano criteria, the survival figures (80% at 3 years) reproduce the outcome of cadaveric programs. The expansion of the limits beyond Milan translates into decreased survival (60% at 3 years) and increased recurrence. (From Todo S, Furukawa H, 2004: Living donor liver transplantation for adult patients with hepatocellular carcinoma: experience in Japan. Ann Surg 240:451.)

(Bozorgzadeh et al, 2004; Forman et al, 2004; Garcia-Retortillo et al, 2004; Russo et al, 2004a; Shimoda et al, 2004). Because hepatitis C virus underlies HCC in a high percentage of the HCC patients where transplantation is a therapeutic option (United States, Europe, Japan), this virus may become a serious limitation.

The multicenter study conducted in Japan has shown that the optimal criteria to select patients with HCC for live donation should be the same as for cadaveric livers. Patients exceeding the conventional limits, but not reaching massive hepatic involvement by the neoplasm, may achieve a promising outcome exceeding 50% survival at 3 years. This possibility opens the option to engage live donation protocols for patients whose tumor stage exceeds the accepted limits for cadaveric listing. As stated before, there are no strong data to establish how far the limits can be pushed; currently, extended indications should be limited to research protocols.

The scenario where live donation may play a major role is in the waiting list. In the absence of priority policy, the waiting time may imply that patients with HCC almost never would avoid tumor progression before receiving a liver. Transplantation in some areas of the world with a low donation rate is not a real option. Live donation with the assumption of a certain degree of risk by a healthy donor would be justified only if the waiting time is long enough, and the outcome of transplanted patients remains within the usual standards (around 70% at 5 years). In contrast, if the waiting time is less than 6 months, the benefits for the recipient would never counterbalance the potential loss of life incurred by the donor (Sarasin et al, 2001). Finally, despite the high expectancy raised by the development of live donation, the applicability is still limited. Major reasons for this failure seem to be refusal by the recipient and the lack of an appropriate donor.

FIBROLAMELLAR HEPATOCELLULAR CARCINOMA

Fibrolamellar hepatocellular carcinoma (see Ch. 71) is a distinct type of HCC produced generally in young noncirrhotic individuals (Ishak et al, 2001). These subjects usually are diagnosed because of nonspecific symptoms, and this reflects an advanced stage. Because fibrolamellar HCC may have slow growth, it may remain solitary without additional sites even when reaching a large size. Most centers consider resection as the first therapeutic option even if it requires major hepatectomy and suggest liver transplantation for patients who are unresectable (El Gazzaz et al, 2000). Despite some suggestions of a less aggressive biology, however, it has been shown that when the tumor has advanced beyond the conventional Milano criteria, the prognosis for patients and the probability of recurrence are equally dismal (Pinna et al, 1997). The best outcome reported after surgical resection compared with the outcome in cirrhotics probably reflects the prognostic implication of the underlying liver disease, rather than a less malignant phenotype (El Gazzaz et al, 2000).

LIVER TRANSPLANTATION FOR OTHER PRIMARY MALIGNANT TUMORS

Liver resection is the "gold standard" therapy for malignant tumors that appear in normal or noncirrhotic liver. Unresectable tumors usually are very advanced cases with disease extension to the whole liver, lymph node invasion, and distant metastases,

Table 106.3   Survival of Patients with Cholangiocarcinoma Treated with Liver Transplantation

Reference	n	1-Year Survival (%)	2-Year Survival (%)	5-Year Survival (%)
Yokoyama et al, 1990	19	40	<20	—
Iwatsuki et al, 1998	38	60	32 (3 yr)	25
Pichlmayr et al, 1998	24	20.8	6.3	—
Robles et al, 2004	59	77 (P); 82 (H)	53 (H); 65 (P)	30 (H); 42 (P)
Meyer et al, 2000	207	72	48	23
Heimbach et al, 2004	28	88	85	82

H, hilar; P, perihilar.

with a poor survival despite adjuvant treatments such as systemic chemotherapy, hormone therapy, or adoptive immunotherapy.

Cholangiocarcinoma

Patients with cholangiocarcinoma (see Ch. 52) are excluded from most transplant programs because of poor prognosis (Gores, 2003). Their outcome after transplantation is very poor; most centers report a median survival rate at 1 year between 20.8% and 88% and at 2 years between 6.3% and 85% (Table 106.3). Recurrence of cholangiocarcinoma after liver transplantation varies between 44% and 100% (De Vreede et al, 2000; Heimbach et al, 2004; Iwatsuki et al, 1998; Meyer et al, 2000; Pichlmayr et al, 1998; Robles et al, 2004; Yokoyama et al, 1990), and its major risk predictor is the detection of lymph node involvement.

Patients with primary sclerosing cholangitis have a prevalence of cholangiocarcinoma of 10% to 36% (Heimbach et al, 2004; Kaya et al, 2001). Primary sclerosing cholangitis is considered a multifocal disease, and this usually excludes patients from surgical resection, leaving liver transplantation as the sole curative option. The presence of cholangiocarcinoma is the most relevant predictor of death after liver transplantation (Heimbach et al, 2004), however, and this justifies the exclusion of these patients from most transplant programs. A study including an extensive staging policy with aggressive adjuvant therapy (radiation and chemotherapy) reported promising results in a minor subgroup of patients diagnosed with localized perihilar cholangiocarcinoma in whom regional lymph node dissemination was excluded (Heimbach et al, 2004). In this highly selected group of patients, representing 50% of the enrolled patients, the survival at 1 year and 5 years was 88% and 85%. These encouraging data need to be validated before being implemented in conventional clinical practice.

Epithelioid Hemangioendothelioma

Epithelioid hemangioendothelioma (see Ch. 69) is a rare tumor of endothelial origin affecting young adults without preexisting cirrhosis. It is frequently multifocal and has a slow progression rate with potential stability for several years (Makhlouf et al, 1999).

After some years of follow-up, however, the tumor develops an aggressive and invasive phenotype with cancer-related symptoms, vascular invasion, and lymph node dissemination. The results of resection and transplantation are excellent at early stable stages (Makhlouf et al, 1999). In contrast, if treatment is based on detection of progression, the outcome deteriorates with increased death rates at short-term because of tumor dissemination. Surgical resection is the optimal approach in resectable cases. In patients who are unresectable and potentially transplantable, the decision is more controversial because it has to balance the risk of transplant-related death (5-year survival in available series is around 70%) in patients in whom the slow-growing nature of the disease may pose no risk of death for an unknown number of years (Lerut et al, 2004).

Hepatoblastoma

Hepatoblastoma (see Chs. 69 and 72) is the most frequent liver malignancy in childhood, accounting for greater than 1% of pediatric cancers. Surgical resection currently represents the "gold standard" treatment, but without complete tumor removal, the prognosis is poor. Chemotherapy may induce significant reduction in size and increase the percentage of resectable tumors. If resection is not feasible, liver transplantation may provide long-term cure (Cillo et al, 2003; Reyes et al, 2000). Because this is a chemosensitive tumor, it is usual to administer chemotherapy after transplant to reduce the risk of recurrence (Urata et al, 2004). Survival of successfully transplanted patients is approximately 80% at 1 year and 55% at 5 years (Srinivasan et al, 2002).

LIVER TRANSPLANTATION FOR METASTATIC TUMORS

Metastatic involvement of the liver represents dissemination of neoplastic cells from a primary located outside the liver. Dissemination should not be expected to be restricted to the liver, and transplantation usually is not considered a therapeutic option in this setting. The few published series with this condition depict a poor outcome (5-year survival <5%) with the only exception corresponding to patients with neuroendocrine liver metastases.

Liver Metastases from Neuroendocrine Tumors

Metastases from neuroendocrine tumors may be an indication for liver transplantation in a select group of patients. The first option is surgical resection or simply tumor debulking by percutaneous ablation or transarterial chemoembolization (Fernandez et al, 2003; Florman et al, 2004; Sutcliffe et al, 2004). Only subjects in whom the primary tumor can be resected and metastatic liver involvement is limited in number may become potential candidates for transplantation. In these patients, the tumor nodules may have a low progression rate. Available data are limited, and the criteria to enlist patients are heterogeneous; this explains a disparate survival at 5 years ranging from 36% to 83%. These figures are significantly better than the natural history data (5-year survival of 30%), but it is unknown if the best outcome is the result of treatment or of the selection policy to recruit patients with a less aggressive profile. Data from a French multi-center study reported a better outcome in patients with metastatic carcinoid tumors (69% at 5 years) than in patients with noncarcinoid tumors (8% at 4 years) (Fernandez et al, 2003).

REFERENCES

Adam R, et al, 2003: Liver resection as a bridge to transplantation for hepatocellular carcinoma on cirrhosis: a reasonable strategy? Ann Surg 238:508.

Azoulay D, et al, 1999: Domino liver transplants for metabolic disorders: experience with familial amyloidotic polyneuropathy. J Am Coll Surg 189:584.

Belghiti J, et al, 2003: Resection prior to liver transplantation for hepatocellular carcinoma. Ann Surg 238:885.

Bismuth H, Majno PE, 2000: Hepatobiliary surgery. J Hepatol 32:208.

Bismuth H, et al, 1999: Liver transplantation for hepatocellular carcinoma. Semin.Liver Dis 19:311.

Bolondi L, et al, 2003: Review article: liver transplantation for HCC: treatment options on the waiting list. Aliment Pharmacol Ther 17(suppl 2):145.

Bozorgzadch A, et al, 2004: Impact of hepatitis C viral infection in primary cadaveric liver allograft versus primary living-donor allograft in 100 consecutive liver transplant recipients receiving tacrolimus. Transplantation 77:1066.

Brown RS Jr, et al, 2003: A survey of liver transplantation from living adult donors in the United States. N Engl J Med 348:818.

Bruix J, et al, 2001: Clinical management of hepatocellular carcinoma: conclusions of the Barcelona-2000 EASL Conference. J Hepatol 35:421.

Bruix J, et al, 2003: Liver transplantation for hepatocellular carcinoma: Foucault pendulum versus evidence-based decision. Liver Transpl 9:700.

Bruix J, et al, 2004: Chemoembolization for hepatocellular carcinoma. Gastroenterology 127:S179.

Burrel M, et al, 2003: MRI angiography is superior to helical CT for detection of HCC prior to liver transplantation: an explant correlation. Hepatology 38:1034.

Cha C, et al, 2003: Predictors and patterns of recurrence after resection of hepatocellular carcinoma. J Am Coll Surg 197:753.

Chen YJ, et al, 2000: Chromosomal changes and clonality relationship between primary and recurrent hepatocellular carcinoma. Gastroenterology 119:431.

Cillo U, et al, 2003: Liver transplantation for the management of hepatoblastoma. Transplant Proc 35:2983.

De Vreede I, et al, 2000: Prolonged disease-free survival after orthotopic liver transplantation plus adjuvant chemoirradiation for cholangiocarcinoma. Liver Transpl 6:309.

Donckier V, et al, 2001: Domino hepatic transplantation using the liver from a patient with primary hyperoxaluria, Transplantation 71:1346.

El Gazzaz G, et al, 2000: Outcome of liver resection and transplantation for fibrolamellar hepatocellular carcinoma. Transpl Int 13(suppl 1):S406.

Emond JC, et al, 2002: Optimizing the use of donated cadaver livers: analysis and policy development to increase the application of split-liver transplantation. Liver Transpl 8:863.

Fattovich G, et al, 2004: Hepatocellular carcinoma in cirrhosis: incidence and risk factors. Gastroenterology 127:S35.

Fernandez JA, et al, 2003: Role of liver transplantation in the management of metastatic neuroendocrine tumors. Transplant Proc 35:1832.

Fields AC, et al, 2004: Survivin expression in hepatocellular carcinoma: correlation with proliferation, prognostic parameters, and outcome. Mod Pathol 17:1378.

Fisher RA, et al, 2004: Non-resective ablation therapy for hepatocellular carcinoma: effectiveness measured by intention-to-treat and dropout from live transplant waiting list. Clin Transplant 18:502-512.

Florman S, et al, 2004 Liver transplantation for neuroendocrine tumors. J Gastrointest Surg 8:208.

Forman LM, et al, 2004: Living donor liver transplantation and hepatitis C. Liver Transpl 10:347.

Freeman RB, 2004: Liver allocation: a moving target. Liver Transpl 10:49.

Freeman RB, et al, 2004: Results of the first year of the new allocation plan. Liver Transpl 10:7.

Garcia-Retortillo M, et al, 2004: Hepatitis C recurrence is more severe after living donor compared to cadaveric liver transplantation. Hepatology 40:699.

Gores GJ, 2003: Cholangiocarcinoma: current concepts and insights. Hepatology 37:961.

Gotoh M, et al, 2002: Overexpression of osteopontin in hepatocellular carcinoma. Pathol Int 52:19.

Graziadei IW, et al, 2003: Chemoembolization followed by liver transplantation for hepatocellular carcinoma impedes tumor progression while on the waiting list and leads to excellent outcome. Liver Transpl 9:557.

Groupe d'Etude et de Traitement du Carcinome Hepatocellulaire, 1995: A comparison of lipiodol chemoembolization and conservative treatment for unresectable hepatocellular carcinoma. Groupe d'Etude et de Traitement du Carcinome Hepatocellulaire. N Engl J Med 332:1256.

Hayashi PH, et al, 2004: Impact of pretransplant diagnosis of hepatocellular carcinoma on cadveric liver allocation in the era of MELD. Liver Transpl 10:42.

Heimbach JK, et al, 2004: Liver transplantation for unresectable perihilar cholangiocarcinoma. Semin Liver Dis 24:201.

Ishak KG, et al, 2001: Tumors of the Liver and Intrahepatic Bile Ducts. Washington, DC, Armed Forces Institute of Pathology.

Iwatsuki S, et al, 1985: Role of liver transplantation in cancer therapy. Ann Surg 202:401.

Iwatsuki S, et al, 1998: Treatment of hilar cholangiocarcinoma (Klatskin tumors) with hepatic resection or transplantation. J Am Coll Surg 187:358.

Iwatsuki S, et al, 2000: Liver transplantation for hepatocellular carcinoma: a proposal of a prognostic scoring system. J Am Coll Surg 191:389.

Izumi R, et al, 1994: Prognostic factors of hepatocellular carcinoma in patients undergoing hepatic resection. Gastroenterology 106:720.

Jonas S, et al, 2001: Vascular invasion and histopathologic grading determine outcome after liver transplantation for hepatocellular carcinoma in cirrhosis. Hepatology 33:1080.

Kamath PS, et al, 2001: A model to predict survival in patients with end-stage liver disease. Hepatology 33:464.

Kaya M, et al, 2001: Treatment of cholangiocarcinoma complicating primary sclerosing cholangitis: the Mayo Clinic experience. Am J Gastroenterol 96:1164.

Lencioni RA, et al, 2003: Small hepatocellular carcinoma in cirrhosis: randomized comparison of radio-frequency thermal ablation versus percutaneous ethanol injection. Radiology 228:235.

Lerut JP, et al, 2004: Hepatic haemangioendothelioma in adults: excellent outcome following liver transplantation. Transpl Int 17:202.

Libbrecht L, et al, 2002: Focal lesions in cirrhotic explant livers: pathological evaluation and accuracy of pretransplantation imaging examinations. Liver Transpl 8:749.

Lin S-M, et al, 2004: Radiofrequency ablation improves prognosis compared with ethanol injection for hepatocellular carcinoma <4 cm. Gastroenterology 127:1714.

Livraghi T, et al, 1999: Small hepatocellular carcinoma: treatment with radiofrequency ablation versus ethanol injection. Radiology 210:655.

Livraghi T, et al, 2003: Treatment of focal liver tumors with percutaneous radiofrequency ablation: complications encountered in a multicenter study. Radiology 226:441.

Llovet JM, et al, 1998: Liver transplantation for treatment of small hepatocellular carcinoma: the tumor-node-metastasis classification does not have prognostic power. Hepatology 27:1572.

Llovet JM, et al, 1999: Intention-to-treat analysis of surgical treatment for early hepatocellular carcinoma: resection versus transplantation. Hepatology 30:1434.

Llovet JM, et al, 2001: Increased risk of tumor seeding after percutaneous radiofrequency ablation for single hepatocellular carcinoma. Hepatology 33:1124.

Llovet JM, et al, 2002a: Cost effectiveness of adjuvant therapy for hepatocellular carcinoma during the waiting list for liver transplantation. Gut 50:123.

Llovet JM, et al, 2002b: Arterial embolisation or chemoembolisation versus symptomatic treatment in patients with unresectable hepatocellular carcinoma: a randomised controlled trial. Lancet 359:1734.

Llovet JM, et al, 2003: Predictors of drop-out and survival of patients with hepatocellular carcinoma candidates for liver transplantation. Hepatology 38:763A.

Lo CM, et al, 2004: The role and limitation of living donor liver transplantation for hepatocellular carcinoma. Liver Transpl 10:440.

Louha M, et al, 1997: Spontaneous and iatrogenic spreading of liver-derived cells into peripheral blood of patients with primary liver cancer. Hepatology 26:998.

Maddala YK, et al, 2004: Drop-out rates of patients with hepatocellular cancer listed for liver transplantation: outcome with chemoembolization. Liver Transpl 10:449.

Majno PE, et al, 1997: Influence of preoperative transarterial lipiodol chemoembolization on resection and transplantation for hepatocellular carcinoma in patients with cirrhosis. Ann Surg 226:688.

Makhlouf HR, et al, 1999: Epithelioid hemangioendothelioma of the liver: a clinicopathologic study of 137 cases. Cancer 85:562.

Marsh JW, Dvorchik I, 2003: Liver organ allocation for hepatocellular carcinoma: are we sure? Liver Transpl 9:693.

Marsh JW, et al, 2003: Genotyping of hepatocellular carcinoma in liver transplant recipients adds predictive power for determining recurrence-free survival. Liver Transpl 9:664.

Mazzaferro V, et al, 1996: Liver transplantation for the treatment of small hepatocellular carcinomas in patients with cirrhosis. N Engl J Med 334:693.

Mazzaferro V, et al, 2004: Radiofrequency ablation of small hepatocellular carcinoma in cirrhotic patients awaiting liver transplantation: a prospective study. Ann Surg 240:900.

Meyer CG, et al, 2000: Liver transplantation for cholangiocarcinoma: results in 207 patients. Transplantation 69:1633.

Minagawa M, et al, 2003: Selection criteria for repeat hepatectomy in patients with recurrent hepatocellular carcinoma. Ann Surg 238:703.

Nakashima T, Kojiro M, 1987: Hepatocellular Carcinoma. Tokyo, Springer Verlag.

Neuberger J, 2004: Developments in liver transplantation. Gut 53:759.

Okada S, et al, 1994: Predictive factors for postoperative recurrence of hepatocellular carcinoma. Gastroenterology 106:1618.

Omata M, et al, 2004: Treatment of hepatocellular carcinoma by percutaneous tumor ablation methods: ethanol injection therapy and radiofrequency ablation. Gastroenterology 127:S159.

Pan HW, et al, 2003: Overexpression of osteopontin is associated with intrahepatic metastasis, early recurrence, and poorer prognosis of surgically resected hepatocellular carcinoma. Cancer 98:119.

Pichlmayr R, et al, 1998: Appraisal of transplantation for malignant tumors of the liver with special reference to early stage hepatocellular carcinoma. Eur J Surg Oncol 24:60.

Pinna AD, et al, 1997: Treatment of fibrolamellar hepatoma with subtotal hepatectomy or transplantation. Hepatology 26:877.

Plessier A, et al, 2004: Underestimation of the influence of satellite nodules as a risk factor for post-transplantation recurrence in patients with small hepatocellular carcinoma. Liver Transpl 10(suppl 2):S86.

Reddy S, et al, 2004: Liver transplantation from non-heart-beating donors: current status and future prospects. Liver Transpl 10:1223.

Renz JF, et al, 2003: Split-liver transplantation: a review. Am J Transplant 3:1323.

Reyes JD, et al, 2000: Liver transplantation and chemotherapy for hepatoblastoma and hepatocellular cancer in childhood and adolescence. J Pediatr 136:795.

Roayaie S, et al, 2002 Long-term results with multimodal adjuvant therapy and liver transplantation for the treatment of hepatocellular carcinomas larger than 5 centimeters. Ann Surg 235:533.

Robles R, et al, 2004: Spanish experience in liver transplantation for hilar and peripheral cholangiocarcinoma. Ann Surg 239:265.

Russo MW, et al, 2004a: Patient and graft survival in hepatitis C recipients after adult living donor liver transplantation in the United States. Liver Transpl 10:340.

Russo MW, et al, 2004b: Impact of adult living donor liver transplantation on waiting time survival in candidates listed for liver transplantation. Am J Transplant 4:427, 2004.

Sala M, et al, 2004a: High pathological risk of recurrence after surgical resection for hepatocellular carcinoma: an indication for salvage liver transplantation. Liver Transpl 10:1294.

Sala M, et al, 2004b: Initial response to percutaneous ablation predicts survival in patients with hepatocellular carcinoma. Hepatology 40:1352.

Sarasin FP, et al, 2001: Living donor liver transplantation for early hepatocellular carcinoma: a life-expectancy and cost-effectiveness perspective. Hepatology 33:1073.

Schwartz M, 2004: Liver transplantation for hepatocellular carcinoma. Gastroenterology 127:S268.

Sharma P, et al, 2004: Liver transplantation for hepatocellular carcinoma: the MELD impact. Liver Transpl 10:36.

Shimoda M, et al, 2004: Predictors of survival after liver transplantation for hepatocellular carcinoma associated with hepatitis C. Liver Transpl 10:1478.

Song TJ, et al, 2004: Hepatocellular carcinoma: current surgical management. Gastroenterology 127:S248.

Srinivasan P, et al, 2002: Orthotopic liver transplantation for unresectable hepatoblastoma. Transplantation 74:652.

Sutcliffe R, et al, 2004: Management of neuroendocrine liver metastases. Am J Surg 187:39.

Taouli B, et al, 2004: Magnetic resonance imaging of hepatocellular carcinoma. Gastroenterology 127:S144.

Todo S, Furukawa H, 2004: Living donor liver transplantation for adult patients with hepatocellular carcinoma: experience in Japan. Ann Surg 240:451.

Urata H, et al, 2004: Strategy for the treatment of unresectable hepatoblastoma: neoadjuvant chemotherapy followed by delayed primary operation or liver transplantation. Int Surg 89:95.

Wiesner RH, et al, 2004: Liver transplantation for hepatocellular cancer: the impact of the MELD allocation policy. Gastroenterology 127:S261.

Yao FY, et al, 2001: Liver transplantation for hepatocellular carcinoma: expansion of the tumor size limits does not adversely impact survival. Hepatology 33:1394.

Yao FY, et al, 2002: Liver transplantation for hepatocellular carcinoma: analysis of survival according to the intention-to-treat principle and dropout from the waiting list. Liver Transpl 8:873.

Yokoyama I, et al, 1990: Liver transplantation in the treatment of primary liver cancer. Hepatogastroenterology 37:188.

107

Liver Transplantation in Children and Segmental Transplantation

J. J. WIZOREK, A. KOTRU, AND J. A. LOWELL

Starzl attempted the first clinical liver transplant in 1963 in a 3-year-old child with end-stage liver disease owing to biliary atresia. This "operation could not be completed," however, because of uncontrollable hemorrhage (Starzl, 1992). Later that same year, Starzl completed liver transplants in four adults; however, all died from a pulmonary embolism in the early postoperative period. Further attempts were suspended until 1967, when eight children underwent successful transplantation; all survived the operation, and half survived more than 1 year (Starzl et al, 1968). Since those heroic beginnings 4 decades ago, advances in immunosuppression, surgical technique, and critical care have made liver transplantation a reliable lifesaving procedure, performed every day at liver transplant centers throughout the world. In children with end-stage liver disease, liver transplantation has become the accepted therapy, and its use is limited only by the availability of suitable grafts.

The imbalance between donor availability and recipient need historically has been much more pronounced in the pediatric population than in adults. In 2004, there were 3743 adult liver transplantations compared with 389 pediatric transplantations. Currently, there are nearly 17,000 adults and 850 children awaiting a liver transplant (UNOS, 2005). Potential recipients who are infants, toddlers, or young children have narrow constraints with regard to graft size. The lack of size-matched organ availability coupled with the disproportionate number of adults on the waiting list historically has significantly disadvantaged children awaiting transplantation. The longer children (similar to adults) wait for a transplant, the higher the mortality rate. Children have much less time that they can wait—an infant with decompensated liver disease from cirrhosis typically cannot survive on a waiting list for several years (McDiarmid, 2002).

The shortage of donor organs has motivated surgeons to develop innovative techniques to increase the number of potentially usable organs for pediatric transplantation. Initially, adult cadaveric livers were reduced in size by removing the right lobe and medial segment of the left lobe to enable grafting of the lateral segment into small recipients. In this way, the size restrictions imposed on any particular donor-recipient combination could be overcome. The application of reduced size grafts led to a shift of cadaveric livers to children and small adults, but did not increase the total graft pool. Progressive improvements in surgical technique have evolved such that now the left lateral segment and the right lobe each can be used, meaning that a single liver can be divided and transplanted into two recipients. With this innovative technique—the split liver procedure—important progress in expanding the absolute number of transplantable

grafts has been made. Currently, the routine use of a reduced size graft while discarding the remaining tissue is no longer justified.

The favorable experience of grafting reduced size and split livers led to the innovation of using liver lobes and segments from living donors for pediatric grafts. With increasing experience, the donation of liver lobes no longer is confined to left lateral segments or left hepatic lobes, but has expanded to include full right hepatic lobe donor grafts, contributing to the adult organ pool as well. Living related and unrelated liver transplantation has become standard therapy in pediatric liver disease and is one of the most exciting and challenging advances in liver transplantation.

Relief from donor organ shortages through novel developments, such as xenografting (Lambrigts et al, 1998; Ye et al, 1994), hepatocyte transplantation (Kobayashi et al, 2000; Riordan & Williams, 2000), or artificial liver support systems (Ash et al, 2002; Demetriou et al, 2004), is not expected in the near future (Harland & Platt, 1996). The use of "marginal" or "extended" donor organs has become standard practice in a few sophisticated transplant centers (Jimenez Romero et al, 1999), but the effect on the total pool of available organs is still small (Emre et al, 1996).

INDICATIONS

Table 107.1 lists the indications for pediatric liver transplantation. Among cholestatic disorders, biliary atresia (see Ch. 41) is the most frequent cause of infant death owing to hepatic disease and the most common indication for pediatric liver transplantation. Biliary atresia accounts for more than 50% of neonatal cholestatic disorders. The incidence of biliary atresia is 1 in 2500 live births, and the etiology is unknown (Fischler et al, 2002; Sokol & Mack, 2001). Most children with this disease lack an extrahepatic biliary tree, impairing bile flow, leading to conjugated hyperbilirubinemia, acholic stools, and hepatomegaly. The hepatic parenchyma becomes congested, and progressive damage leads to cirrhosis. Although portoenterostomy, also known as the *Kasai procedure* (Kasai & Suzuki, 1959), may yield some clinical improvement and is the first-line treatment (Ohi, 2000; Ryckman et al, 1998), approximately 70% to 80% of children with biliary atresia eventually require liver transplantation (Karrer et al, 1996; Lowell et al, 1996). Biliary atresia, as an indication, accounts for approximately 50% of all pediatric liver transplants.

Table 107.1 Indications for Pediatric Liver Transplantation

Cholestatic hepatic failure
  Biliary atresia
  Primary sclerosing cholangitis
  Alagille syndrome
  Byler disease
  Total parenteral nutrition–induced
  Idiopathic

Infectious hepatic failure
  Viral (hepatitis A, B, C)
  Toxoplasmosis
  Syphilis
  Bacterial

Genetic/metabolic hepatic insufficiencies
  α_1-Antitrypsin deficiency
  Cystic fibrosis
  Wilson's disease
  Glycogen storage disease
  Tyrosinemia
  Primary hyperoxaluria
  Hereditary hemochromatosis
  Crigler-Najjar syndrome

Neoplastic hepatic primaries
  Hepatoblastoma
  Hepatocellular carcinoma

Extrahepatic diseases
  Hemophilia
  Familial hypercholesterolemia

Other causes of hepatic failure
  Autoimmune
  Budd-Chiari syndrome
  Toxic
  Giant arteriovenous malformation

Other causes of cholestasis in children include idiopathic neonatal hepatitis, infection (viral, toxoplasmosis, syphilis, bacterial), progressive familial intrahepatic cholestasis (Byler disease), metabolic and genetic diseases, familial arteriohepatic dysplasia (Alagille syndrome), choledochal cyst, and ischemia-reperfusion injury. Cholestasis, which may progress to cirrhosis, also has been associated with parenteral nutrition in children with short bowel syndrome (Baker et al, 1998).

Pediatric liver transplantation also is indicated in cases of noncholestatic liver failure, secondary to infectious, metabolic, genetic, and neoplastic etiologies. Postnecrotic liver cirrhosis, although less frequent than in adults, accounts for approximately 10% of indications for liver transplantation in children and is most commonly due to viral hepatitis or idiopathic cryptogenic cirrhosis (Malatack et al, 1983). α_1-Antitrypsin deficiency is inherited in an autosomal dominant fashion and is the most common genetic cause of liver disease in children (McDiarmid et al, 1998). Lack of the protein leads to progressive hepatic parenchymal damage and cirrhosis. Although synthetic α_1-antitrypsin is available using recombinant DNA technology, it is not of proven value in children.

Other metabolic liver disorders, such as hemophilia and familial hypercholesterolemia, do not result in primary hepatic disease, but cause extrahepatic disease as a result of dysfunctional hepatic gene products or metabolites that affect extrahepatic tissue. Liver transplantation corrects these conditions by providing the required cellular machinery to synthesize the correct gene product or metabolite (Florman & Shneider, 2001). Occasionally, auxiliary hepatic transplantation (see Ch. 108) has been performed in these circumstances (Van Hoek et al, 1999). In α_1-antitrypsin deficiency, the potential for development of hepatocellular carcinoma precludes auxiliary liver transplantation and mandates total hepatectomy.

Wilson's disease is an inborn error of metabolism characterized by defective copper excretion and the accumulation of toxic amounts of copper in the liver, basal ganglia, kidney, and cornea, which may lead to the characteristic Kayser-Fleischer rings. The defect is located on chromosome 13, is inherited in an autosomal recessive fashion, and affects 1 in 50,000 births. Initial symptoms are nonspecific and include lethargy, anorexia, vague abdominal pain, and weight loss. Some patients present with asymptomatic hepatomegaly, and others present with fulminant hepatic failure (Riordan & Williams, 2001). Other inborn errors of metabolism that may require liver transplantation in children are tyrosinemia, citrullinemia, Crigler-Najjar syndrome, oxalosis, and urea cycle defects (Florman & Shneider, 2001).

Although more common in adult patients, chronic Budd-Chiari syndrome with severe hepatic congestion and focal areas of liver fibrosis or cirrhosis may be an indication for liver transplantation in older children. Pretransplant evaluation should be performed to recognize predisposing factors or underlying diseases, such as myeloproliferative disorders, primary hepatic protein deficiencies (protein C, protein S, antithrombin III or activated protein C resistance), or secondary protein deficiencies (e.g., increased intestinal protein loss in inflammatory bowel disease) (Slakey et al, 2001).

Fulminant hepatic failure (see Chs. 88 and 105) is associated with a mortality of greater than 70%. It is essential to transfer children with fulminant hepatic failure to a transplant unit immediately for management and urgent evaluation and listing for liver transplantation. Because cerebral edema develops rapidly, careful monitoring and intensive supportive care are required. Mild elevation of intracranial pressure can be managed by hyperventilation, elevation of the patient's head, and diuretics. Transplantation is urgently needed because cerebral edema may lead to irreversible damage or death (Tanaka et al, 1994). Poor prognostic factors for liver transplantation in children with fulminant hepatic failure include age younger than 10 years, liver disease other than viral hepatitis, grade 2 or 3 hepatic encephalopathy and coagulopathy (prothrombin time >30 seconds), and increasing jaundice (bilirubin >9 mg/dL) (Uemoto et al, 2000).

Liver tumors account for approximately 3% of all indications for pediatric liver transplantation. Hepatoblastoma, hepatocellular carcinoma, and fibrolamellar hepatocellular carcinoma represent the most frequent tumors (see Ch. 72). In contrast to adults, the predisposing factors for malignant liver tumor are not viral hepatitis or alcoholism, but more often metabolic disorders, such as α_1-antitrypsin deficiency, tyrosinemia, or glycogen storage disease. In patients without cirrhosis, hepatic resection is the treatment of choice. Liver transplantation should be considered only in the case of unresectable tumors (Otte et al, 2004). In patients with advanced cirrhosis and small hepatocellular carcinomas, transplantation may be indicated (Perilongo et al, 2004). Rarely, benign liver tumors, when they replace the whole liver or when they have the potential for malignancy (e.g., multiple hepatocellular adenomas in glycogen storage disease), or giant arteriovenous malformations may be indications for total hepatectomy and liver transplant (Malatack et al, 1987).

EVALUATION OF THE POTENTIAL RECIPIENT

A multidisciplinary evaluation of a child with decompensated liver disease, involving surgeons, hepatologists, nurses, anesthesiologists, psychologists, and social workers, should be completed. Early referral to a transplant center allows maximum time to develop the management strategy and to optimize pretransplant clinical status. The timing of liver transplantation is crucial because late referral of patients with significant hepatic complications and malnutrition results in a poorer outcome. The expected waiting time on the transplant list may differ according to geographic region and should be taken into account. In infants (<2 years old) weighing less than 10 kg, it is often difficult to maintain metabolic and nutritional support. In general, children should be considered for liver transplantation before the malnutrition complications of weight loss and growth failure occur (Kimura et al, 2004; McDiarmid et al, 2004). With chronic liver disease, prolonged clotting times, intractable ascites, recurrent variceal bleeding secondary to portal hypertension, and recurrent cholangitis with severe cholestasis are indications for liver transplantation (Hendrickson et al, 2004).

The prognosis after liver transplantation for chronic liver disease depends on preoperative morbidity. With the advent of the PELD (Pediatric End-stage Liver Disease) and the MELD (Model for End-stage Liver Disease) scores (Malinchoc et al, 2000; Wiesner et al, 2001), it has been possible to better predict mortality and progression of liver disease while awaiting transplantation (Desai et al, 2004). The pertinent factors in the PELD score are the international normalized ratio, total bilirubin, serum albumin, age younger than 1 year, and weight or length less than 2 SD from the mean for age and gender. The PELD score is used for patients who are younger than 18 years old, and the scores range from negative values of −10 to 50. Table 107.2 presents the formulas for calculating the MELD and PELD scores.

Comparing the periods before and after the introduction of the MELD and PELD scores, a similar percentage of children are being transplanted, but the mortality rates have decreased (Freeman et al, 2004; Yao et al, 2004). Small size and young age are not contraindications, and many pediatric transplants now are done in infants with biliary atresia weighing less than 10 kg. Contraindications to pediatric hepatic transplantation are listed in Table 107.3.

Table 107.2 MELD (Model for End-Stage Liver Disease) and PELD (Pediatric End-Stage Liver Disease) Calculations

MELD

$$10 \times [0.957 \ln(\text{creatinine [mg/dL]}) + 0.378 \ln(\text{total bilirubin [mg/dL]}) + 1.120 \ln(\text{INR}) + 0.643]$$

PELD

$$10 \times [0.480 \times \text{Log}_e(\text{bilirubin [mg/dL]})$$
$$+ 1.857 \times \text{Log}_e(\text{INR})$$
$$- 0.687 \times \text{Log}_e(\text{albumin [g/dL]})$$
$$+ 0.436 \text{ if patient is } <1 \text{ year old}$$
$$+ 0.667 \text{ if patient has growth failure } (<2 \text{ SD})]$$

Note: The resultant score is rounded to the nearest whole number.

Table 107.3 Contraindications to Pediatric Liver Transplantation

Absolute

Uncontrolled systemic sepsis
Irreversible brain edema
Uncorrectable symptomatic heart defects
Nonreversible pulmonary hypertension
Extrahepatic malignancy

Relative

Portomesenteric thrombosis
HIV-positive status
Severe psychosocial impediments

RECIPIENT HEPATECTOMY

The recipient hepatectomy is typically quite difficult. More than half of the children have had a prior laparotomy. Severe portal hypertension with abdominal wall and perihepatic venous collaterals is common, and these technical challenges may be exacerbated by severe coagulopathy and thrombocytopenia. Thrombosis of the portal vein can be an additional complicating factor. In children, the use of an extracorporeal venovenous bypass circuit during the hepatectomy is uncommon because the presence of abdominal wall collaterals usually allows enough venous return from the lower body to maintain adequate cardiac output. Preservation of the retrohepatic inferior vena cava contributes to hemodynamic stability during the hepatectomy.

Before beginning the transplant, a Broviac central venous catheter is placed for intraoperative and postoperative fluid resuscitation, monitoring, and laboratory draws, as is an arterial catheter. Pressure points are well padded, and convective heating blankets are used. The abdomen is entered through a curved transverse subcostal incision. Meticulous hemostasis must be obtained throughout the procedure because ongoing bleeding may lead to a dilutional coagulopathy and fibrinolysis. Abdominal wall venous collaterals are carefully controlled as they are encountered. Adhesions to the liver are carefully cauterized to allow access to the portal region (Fig. 107.1).

If the child has had a previous Kasai procedure, the jejunal loop is taken down, the enterostomy is closed, and the Roux-en-Y loop is preserved for later biliary drainage of the graft. The porta hepatis is dissected carefully with isolation of the hepatic artery and portal vein. Although transection of the hepatic artery is performed early in hepatectomy, the portal vein is divided after total mobilization of the liver and just before the removal of the native liver to avoid unnecessary congestion in the mesentericoportal system. The hepatic artery and portal vein are dissected high in the hilum to preserve adequate length for later anastomosis with the graft. The portal vein may be quite small. In this setting, dissection to the level of the confluence of superior mesenteric vein and splenic vein (posterior to the pancreas) may allow for anastomosis to a larger inflow vessel. The liver is mobilized further by dividing the ligamentous attachments and the short hepatic veins draining the right hepatic and caudate lobes directly into the vena cava.

For orthotopic whole liver transplant, the small retrohepatic caval segment can be removed with the native liver, or the vena cava can be preserved and the donor liver anastomosed in a piggyback fashion to the confluence of the recipient's right, middle, and left hepatic veins. With a segmental graft, the inferior

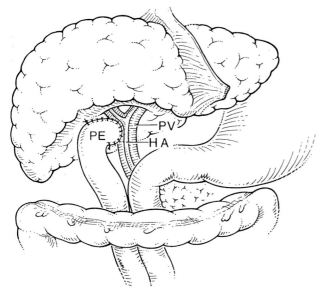

Fig. 107.1. Recipient hepatectomy. The hilum is examined carefully, and a previous portoenterostomy (PE) is taken down. The portal vein (PV) and hepatic artery (HA) are divided high in the porta hepatis.

vena cava must be preserved. A temporary portacaval shunt (end-to-side) may be performed during hepatectomy, to facilitate the native liver dissection off the vena cava and to allow complete portal decompression. A vascular clamp is placed across the hepatic veins so that they can be joined to form a common opening to sew to the donor suprahepatic cava (or, in case of segmental grafts, the left hepatic vein) (Fig. 107.2). Complete hemostasis of the retroperitoneum is accomplished before removing the donor liver from cold storage.

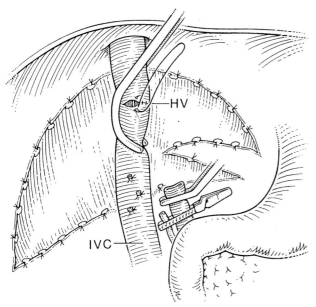

Fig. 107.2. Recipient hepatectomy. The liver has been removed, and the inferior vena cava (IVC) is preserved in preparation to receive a segmental graft. The hepatic veins (HV) can be oversewn to allow release of the caval clamp temporarily.

GRAFT PROCUREMENT AND ENGRAFTMENT

The techniques employed for recovering whole, deceased donor livers for transplantation from children are similar to the techniques used in adult-to-adult transplantation. Special attention should be paid to serum sodium levels and to dynamic liver function tests. High sodium levels (>170 mmol/L) may be associated with severe reperfusion injury and poor graft function.

The donor liver is anastomosed using the full vena cava (or the left hepatic vein with or without middle hepatic vein in the case of a reduced size graft) to the confluence of the recipient hepatic veins. Before securing the final upper caval sutures, the donor liver is flushed with cold Ringer's lactate through the donor portal vein to flush the preservation solution (Viaspan), which is high in potassium. The portacaval shunt is taken down and oversewn, and the portal venous anastomosis is completed leaving a large "growth factor" in the continuous suture to prevent a "waist" (narrowing the anastomosis) when the vessels are refilled with portal blood.

The arterial anastomosis is performed with interrupted sutures of fine (7-0 or 8-0) polypropylene material using microsurgical loupes. A microscope may be useful in anastomosing arteries with a diameter smaller than 1 to 2 mm. The anastomosis is performed most commonly in an end-to-end fashion, directly to the native hepatic artery. If the native artery is not of adequate size (or there is an intimal dissection), an extension allograft using saphenous vein or donor iliac artery, from the infrarenal or supraceliac aorta, may be used (Yamaoka, 1996).

The bile duct anastomosis is the final step in the procedure. If present, the donor gallbladder is removed. If the recipient has an intact bile duct that is of suitable size, an end-to-end choledochocholedochostomy can be performed with or without a T-tube (or an internal stent). Most children have biliary atresia or common bile ducts that are very small, however, so a choledochojejunostomy is performed. In case of a previous Kasai procedure, the jejunal loop of the portoenterostomy can be used again, although it must be shortened, and a fresh segment must be anastomosed.

REDUCED SIZE SEGMENTAL LIVER TRANSPLANTATION AND SPLIT LIVER TRANSPLANTATION

Reduced Size Segmental Liver Transplantation

The use of reduced size grafts for pediatric recipients is one of the most important advances in liver transplantation. The disproportionate shortage of grafts for very young children compared with older children motivated surgeons to develop innovative operative techniques in an attempt to overcome the restrictions imposed by the mismatch between donor and recipient size. With these techniques, livers can be reduced to a functional unit of appropriate size for the recipient. The optimal ratio between the required volume of liver and the actual "tailored" hepatic mass is between 1:1 and 1:2. In this way, livers from donors 10 or 20 times the size of the recipient can be used (Broelsch et al, 1988).

The liver comprises eight segments, and each receives its own arterial and portal blood supply and has separate biliary drainage (Fig. 107.3) (Strasberg, 1997). Similarly, segmental hepatic

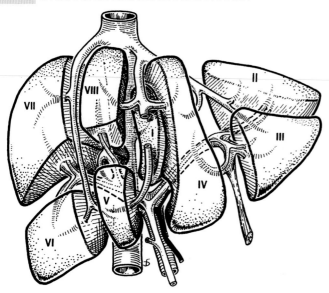

Fig. 107.3. The segments of the liver as described by Couinaud. The caudate lobe represents segment I.

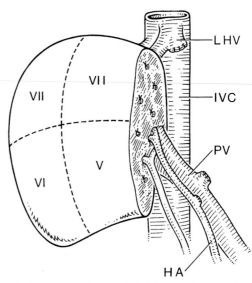

Fig. 107.5. Segmental graft. The full right liver incorporating segments V through VIII is used. *LHV* represents the oversewn left and middle hepatic veins. HA, hepatic artery; IVC, inferior vena cava; PV, portal vein.

venous outflow is independent, but major liver veins run along segmental borderlines taking up blood from several adjacent segments (Couinaud, 1954). For purposes of transplantation, the liver can be divided into several functional grafts. The most commonly used reduced size graft is the left lateral segment graft (Couinaud's segments II and III) (Fig. 107.4) (Botero & Strasberg, 1998). The left hepatic vein is used for hepatic venous drainage. It is anastomosed directly to the recipient's vena cava, which has to be preserved during hepatectomy. The full left graft (segments II, III, and IV) is rarely used, other than in small adults or

older children requiring a graft slightly larger than the left lateral segments.

Bismuth and Houssin (1984) first reported success using transplantation of a left lobe, and in the same year Broelsch and colleagues (1984) reported the successful grafting of the left lateral segment. Since then, essentially all pediatric transplant centers have adopted segmental transplant techniques using reduced size livers. The results after these segmental grafts are comparable to the results achieved with whole organ orthotopic liver transplants. Although reduced size grafts can overcome the donor-recipient size discrepancy by distributing cadaveric livers to the advantage of children (and small adults), it does not increase the absolute number of grafts. The advent of the split liver technique not only allowed for a donor liver to be tailored to fit a small child, but also allowed for the remaining donor graft to be used, increasing the actual organ pool. The routine use of reduced size grafts is no longer justified.

Split Liver Transplantation

Progressive improvements in using left and right reduced cadaveric liver grafts led to another innovative technique that increases the absolute number of transplantable grafts—the split liver procedure. A single cadaveric liver is divided into two grafts, to be transplanted to two patients (Strasberg et al, 1999; Zamir et al, 2002). The first successful split liver transplantation was performed by Pichlmayr and colleagues (1988); they obtained a right extended graft (segments IV, V, VI, VII, and VIII) and a left lateral graft (segments II and III). Leaving segment IV with the right graft rarely leads to an impaired arterial and portal venous perfusion despite the fact that the vascular supply of this segment belongs to the left lobe. Very rarely, resection of segment IV may be required because of poor perfusion. The liver also may be dissected along the principal plane, dividing it into right and left lobes. The vena cava is left attached to the right lobe (segments V-VIII) (Fig. 107.5), and the full length of main portal vein and celiac artery typically are left with the right lobe graft, which is used in a similar fashion to a whole liver graft. By contrast, the

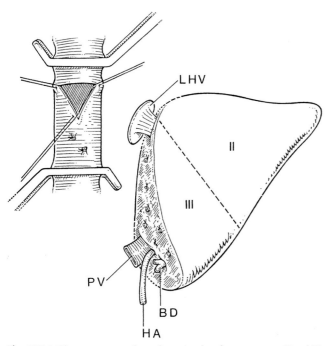

Fig. 107.4. The most commonly used segmental graft uses segments II and III of the left liver. The recipient's inferior vena cava is preserved, and the left hepatic vein (LHV) is sutured to a large triangular venotomy cut on the anterior aspect of the inferior vena cava. The portal vein (PV), hepatic artery (HA), and bile ducts (BD) are depicted before anastomosis.

left lobe has a left hepatic vein, left hepatic artery, and left portal vein, which have been divided at the branching points from the vena cava, common hepatic artery, and portal vein.

Broelsch and coworkers (1990) reported the first successful split liver transplantation series. Since then, other groups have developed and refined the technique (Azoulay et al, 2001b; Busuttil & Goss, 1999; Rela et al 1998). The initial enthusiasm for this procedure faded, however, because the preliminary results were inferior, mainly owing to technical and organ preservation problems. In addition, progress in split liver transplantation was hampered by tremendous practical and logistical problems because this procedure requires two full teams of surgeons, anesthesiologists, and operating room staff to be available almost simultaneously. The initial reported patient survival at 1 year was 67%, and graft survival was reduced to 55% (Broelsch et al, 1990). The most frequent complications during the initial experience with this procedure were bleeding, primary poor function, and biliary fistulae and strictures. In adult recipients of right grafts, liver insufficiency became a major problem because of long ischemic times and borderline size matching.

With surgical refinements of liver splitting and transplantation techniques and better patient selection, results improved (Goss et al, 1997; Malago et al, 1997; Rogiers et al, 1996b). The introduction of the in situ split technique, developed by Rogiers in 1994, significantly reduced ischemic time of the liver (Rogiers et al, 1996a). Using this technique, the liver is divided in situ in the heart-beating deceased donor before cold perfusion starts (Yersiz et al, 2003). While arterial and portal blood supply and venous drainage are preserved, the two liver segments (most commonly separating the left lateral segment) are divided by careful transection of the hepatic parenchyma. The splitting procedure requires meticulous hemostasis, which also affects the recipient operation because there is little or no bleeding at the cut surface of the graft after reperfusion. With increasing experience in the in situ splitting technique (which has resulted in an improved graft survival), more centers now are willing to accept split grafts recovered at another center. Although the split liver technique still remains a procedure that is confined to large transplant centers, which have experience in segmental grafting, the possibility of transferring one lobe to another center has now become reality. Today, split liver transplantation has gained wide acceptance with results comparable to those of whole organ transplantation (Deshpande et al, 2002). It is a standard procedure and represents an important technical advance in expanding the total number of transplantable organs. Together with living related liver transplantation, the split liver technique has had a substantial impact on the inequities of the pediatric donor organ shortage.

LIVING DONOR TRANSPLANTATION

The success of many centers performing reduced size and split liver grafting has provided a strong surgical basis for using segments from living donors (Strong et al, 1990) (see Ch. 109) and for their application in the treatment of small children with end-stage liver disease (Broelsch et al, 1994; Edmond et al, 1993; Otte, 1995; Otte et al, 1998; Raia et al, 1989). For ethical reasons, adequate and thoughtful selection of donors is a major prerequisite of living donor liver transplantation (LDLT). Most centers have adopted stringent donor evaluation protocols. Of paramount concern is the risk to healthy donors. It is of prime importance that everything possible is done to minimize the donor morbidity or mortality risks.

The success of LDLT depends partly on adequate graft volume (Kiuchi et al, 1999). The required graft volume should be determined individually and can be assessed with the use of computed tomography (CT) (Kamel et al, 2000, 2001) or magnetic resonance imaging (MRI). The left lateral segment provides the most straightforward dissection, but full left and right lobes have been used successfully. Donors are commonly the parents of the recipient, but nonrelated LDLT procedures also commonly are performed. The size of the living donor's left lateral segment (segments II and III) is assessed by volumetric CT or MRI (Urata et al, 1995). The hepatic vasculature is assessed by CT angiography or MRI angiography, and the biliary anatomy is assessed by MRI cholangiography or endoscopic retrograde cholangiopancreatography. Rarely, percutaneous liver biopsy is done if imaging suggests hepatic steatosis in the donor. Potential donors and their families are extensively counseled, and the risks of the procedure are explained in detail (Trotter, 2000). Ethical issues are important and are addressed fully, and a complete psychological and social evaluation of the donor is performed. Any objections regarding the psychosocial background of the potential donor result in withdrawal from consideration for organ donation (Singer et al, 1989; Surman, 2002). Ideally, when a candidate is accepted for living donor liver donation, autologous blood donation is performed for possible retransfusion at the time of operation. The segmental liver donation must be deemed by the transplant team a purely voluntary, altruistic act with no secondary gain. The donor must be fully aware and accept risks of the procedure.

The type and size of graft should be decided on an individual basis. In general, a full left lobe liver graft (segments II-IV) can overcome a disparity between recipient and donor size of about 1:4. With a left lateral segment graft, a disparity of 1:10 or more can be managed. In infants weighing less than 10 kg, left lateral segment grafts are used almost exclusively.

The donor liver is approached through a bilateral subcostal incision, and the surgical procedure begins by identifying the structures in the hilum. It is imperative to dissect close to the falciform ligament to avoid injuries to the hilar structures running to the right lobe. The left hepatic artery is isolated and followed to the liver parenchyma. The left portal vein is dissected free and encircled with a vessel loop. The dissection continues by dividing the portal branches draining into the round ligament; this allows for better mobilization of the portal vein. The left hepatic vein is identified above the liver and encircled with a vessel loop as it enters the vena cava. The hepatic parenchyma is transected a few millimeters to the right of the falciform ligament with suture ligation of all vessels and ducts until the left lateral lobe is completely separated from the rest of the liver. The segment is still perfused with arterial and portal blood and has drainage via the left hepatic vein. The parenchymal transection is performed without any vascular control of the graft or the remaining liver to maintain maximal viability. The bile ducts are isolated and divided at the umbilical plate, intraparenchymally. There may be a single duct draining segments II and III or two separate ducts (Renz et al, 2000).

The remaining recipient's stump of the left bile duct is carefully oversewn with absorbable suture, leaving the parenchymal end from the lateral lobe to drain freely. The graft is ready to be removed. The left portal vein, the left hepatic artery, and the left hepatic vein are simultaneously clamped after giving systemic heparin, and the vascular structures are divided. The left lateral segment graft is removed, and the portal vein and the hepatic artery are immediately flushed with cold heparinized preservation solution (Viaspan). After removing the left lateral segment, rarely there may be concern for the viability of segments I and IV because during the dissection of the left portal and arterial vessels branches to these segments may be encountered and ligated. If there is any doubt about viability, resection may be performed after removal of the graft segment and a period of observation in the operating room.

As discussed previously, during the recipient hepatectomy the vena cava is left in situ, and a temporary portacaval shunt may be used. The recipient hepatic vein/vena cava junction is modified to accommodate the anastomosis with the donor hepatic vein. A generous triangular venous anastomosis to ensure adequate drainage of the graft is recommended. The donor hepatic venous cuff should be kept short to provide an anastomosis that is not susceptible to kinking. Portal vein reconstruction is done in an end-to-end fashion. In children with biliary atresia, the recipient's portal vein is often small and may be phlebosclerotic. In these cases, an anastomosis to the confluence of the superior mesenteric and splenic veins may be preferred (Saad et al, 1998). Hepatic artery reconstruction usually can be achieved by an end-to-end anastomosis to the recipient's proper hepatic artery via a microsurgical technique using a surgical loupe or a microscope (Inomata et al, 2000). In some cases, a venous interposition graft from the recipient's infrarenal aorta is needed to achieve a tension-free arterial anastomosis. Care must be taken to identify correctly the bile ducts from segments II and III, which in 25% of recipients do not form a common trunk. The biliary drainage is fashioned using a Roux-en-Y loop of the jejunum, with or without a stent. After completion of all anastomoses, the liver rotates slightly to the right and occupies a more central position than in the donor (Fig. 107.6). This slight

shift must be taken into account when performing the vascular and biliary anastomoses. The graft is resuspended to the anterior abdominal wall by the falciform ligament.

Donation and transplantation of a living donor full left liver lobe (segments II, III, and IV with or without segment I) is similar to that of a left lateral lobe with a few technical variations. After cholecystectomy, the resection follows the principal plane. The venous outflow of the graft can be provided by the left hepatic vein or preferentially by use of a common patch of the left and middle hepatic vein (Makuuchi & Sugawara, 2003). The main left hepatic bile duct is less devascularized when the caudate lobe is kept with the left lobe.

Although the primary goal of LDLT is the relief of organ shortage, numerous additional benefits are associated with this procedure (Sindhi et al, 1999). The most important advantage for the recipient of a living donor transplant is a much shorter waiting period until transplantation (Tanaka et al, 1994). Timing of the procedure can be planned, and the operation can be performed under elective conditions resulting in a decreased operative risk. Careful donor evaluation and a short cold ischemic time offer uniformly good grafts and can reduce the risk for initial nonfunction to a minimum (Farmer et al, 2001).

ADULTS

After the encouraging results of living donor left lateral segmental transplantation in children, this innovative technique was extended to try to solve another problem—the shortage of donor organs for adults (Renz et al, 2003; Strasberg et al, 1999). Especially in countries where cadaveric donor organ transplantation has not been established either by law or for religious reasons, living donor organ donation offers the only chance for patients with end-stage liver disease. In 1991, the first LDLT to an adult was performed in Kyoto by Tanaka, using a left hepatic lobe (Hashikura et al, 1994). This technique since has been expanded to the use of full right hepatic lobes (Kawasaki et al, 1998; Seek et al, 2002).

There are several ongoing areas of debate with regard to adult-to-adult LDLT. Many reports have indicated that grafts corresponding to no more than 40% of the recipient's standard volume may not be expected to function well (Pomfret, 2003). In contrast to renal transplantation, right or left liver lobe graft to adults is associated with significant donor morbidity and mortality (McDiarmid et al, 2004). This graft (segments V-VIII) presents the advantage of fitting exactly in the right hepatic fossa (Fig. 107.7). Problems with this graft include a large cut parenchymal surface and an irregular biliary, arterial, portal, and hepatic venous anatomy (Trotter et al, 2002). Variations of portal vein anatomy (e.g., a trifurcation) and variations in arterial anatomy (e.g., an accessory right hepatic artery) are relative contraindications to living donor donation of segments V through VIII (Erbay et al, 2003; Imamura et al, 2000). Most often, the right hepatic artery is large in diameter, unless there is an additional right artery arising from the superior mesenteric artery. The hepatic artery and portal vein usually can be anastomosed directly to the recipient's vessels. Because in most cases venous drainage of the right graft is achieved exclusively via the right hepatic vein, a careful anastomosis of this vessel with the vena cava or the orifice of the recipient's right hepatic vein has to be performed. If necessary, the orifice should be enlarged longitudinally to provide an exact anastomosis. In the case of a

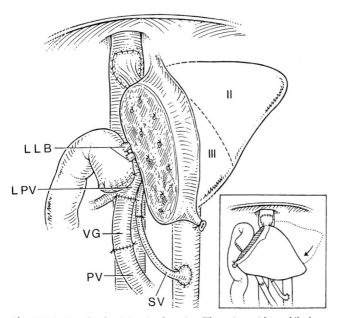

Fig. 107.6. Completed recipient implantation. The variant with two bile ducts is depicted. Interposition grafts are used for the hepatic artery and the portal vein to ensure adequate length. The insert shows the final position of the graft after abdominal closure. *LLB* represents segment II and III bile ducts. LPV, left portal vein; PV, portal vein; SV, saphenous vein graft to the hepatic artery from the aorta; VG, vein graft.

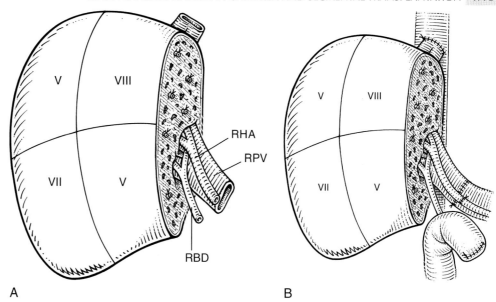

Fig. 107.7. A, Right graft from a living donor with short hilar structures and short right hepatic vein. **B,** Completed recipient implantation of a right graft. RBD, right bile duct; RHA, right hepatic artery; RHV, right hepatic vein; RPV, right portal vein.

A

B

second right hepatic vein (e.g., an inferior right hepatic vein), two independent anastomoses are recommended for uncompromised venous drainage (Ghobrial et al, 2001). The inclusion of the donor middle hepatic vein with the graft is controversial (Fan et al, 2003).

Biliary reconstruction can be challenging because bile ducts from segments V through VIII may not form a common trunk, and two or more ducts may be present (Fan et al, 2002). The reconstruction with a Roux-en-Y hepaticojejunostomy is standard. A direct biliary anastomosis to the recipient's bile duct using a T-tube may be considered when a large single right hepatic bile duct is present.

A crucial issue in adult LDLT is whether the small volume of transplanted liver tissue is sufficient for successful grafting. The definition of small-for-size grafts is vague because the minimal amount of liver compatible with life is unknown, and variables such as ischemia-reperfusion injury, steatosis, or rejection may reduce further the initially transplanted liver mass. At present, a graft-to-body ratio of 1% or a graft volume of approximately 50% of the theoretical liver volume are suggested values for successful grafting (Lo et al, 1996; Urata et al, 1995). The dilemma of LDLT in adults centers on the maximum extent of liver resection that can be safely tolerated by the donor, and the minimum amount of hepatic mass necessary for the recipient to survive (Fan et al, 2000). The use of extended right liver lobes, with the middle vein, but not the entire segment IV retained with the graft, lowers the risk of liver insufficiency in the recipient, but is associated with greater donor morbidity and possible mortality. Because this procedure requires a major hepatectomy with the donation of about two thirds of total liver volume, transient impairment of donor liver function is frequent (Lo et al, 1999; Pomfret et al, 2003).

At present, the use of full right lobes in LDLT in adults is performed selectively in some transplant centers. Despite careful donor and patient selection, its application has significant risks to the donor and added complications to the recipient compared with a full-sized cadaveric donor graft (Man et al, 2003; Sugawara et al, 2003). Prolonged cholestasis in the absence of rejection or mechanical bile duct obstruction is a hallmark of small-for-size grafting. In such patients, the perioperative

management is focused on avoiding any further damage to the graft. This may include improvement of hepatic microcirculation and macrocirculation by the infusion of prostaglandins. Adequate oxygen saturation is maintained to avoid hypoxemia, and early use of plasmapheresis and albumin dialysis may help further to optimize recipient and graft condition. Particular attention should be paid to the immunosuppressive protocol to minimize the risks for rejection episodes because in grafts with a critical hepatocellular mass, even minimal loss of functioning hepatocytes may result in worsening liver failure. This situation must be balanced against the risk of toxicity to the graft from elevated levels of calcineurin inhibitors and infection resulting from higher levels of immunosuppression (Azoulay et al, 2001a).

Unless retransplantation is considered, optimal supportive care is currently the only therapy for small-for-size liver transplantation. Temporary liver support systems, such as artificial liver devices or extracorporeal perfusion, are under investigation, but their clinical use is not yet available (Demetriou et al, 2004). In the future, it may be desirable to combine temporary liver support systems with small-for-size organs. This could be one option to improve organ shortage in adults by an extended use of LDLT.

DONOR RISK IN LIVING DONOR LIVER TRANSPLANTATION

Despite numerous convincing advantages of living donor grafts, safety has to take priority, and the risks to the donor need to be minimized (Surman & Hertl, 2003); this includes the donor evaluation, the operative procedure, and the postoperative period. Morbidities include short-term and long-term impairments of physical, psychological, and social conditions. A comprehensive medical and psychological preoperative evaluation is essential. Any doubts regarding the physical or social background of the candidate should preclude organ donation.

In more than 1000 LDLTs, donor operative morbidity has been 10% to 15%, with biliary leakage, wound infection, and gastroduodenal ulceration being the most frequent complications (Broering et al, 2003; Chen et al, 2003; Chisuwa et al, 2003;

Otte, 2003). Removal of more than 50% of the liver volume does not lead to long-term impairment of liver function. In the reported U.S. series, two donors have died (mortality rate <0.2%) owing to thromboembolic complications (Cronin et al, 2001; Neuberger, 2004).

POSTOPERATIVE MANAGEMENT AND COMPLICATIONS AFTER LIVER TRANSPLANTATION
(see Ch. 110)

In the immediate postoperative period, monitoring of graft function is achieved by evaluation of acid-base status, blood glucose, mental status, coagulation time (and factors), liver enzymes, and cholestasis parameters. Doppler ultrasound frequently is performed to ascertain patency of hepatic vessels, in particular of the hepatic artery.

Primary nonfunction of the graft occurs in 2% of cases and requires immediate retransplantation (Doyle et al, 1996). With regard to pediatric recipients, retransplantation with a reduced size graft from a cadaveric donor or a living donor may offer emergency options (Seiders et al, 2002). The most frequent complication after liver transplantation is hemorrhage; this may occur during the transplant procedure or in the immediate perioperative period. If a child becomes unstable or hypotensive in the postoperative course, it is prudent to re-explore immediately. The use of the protease inhibitor aprotinin (Trasylol) and an antifibrinolytic agent such as aminocaproic acid (Amicar) may help reduce diffuse bleeding, but there is still debate concerning potential increased risks of arterial thrombosis after their use (Himmelreich et al, 1992; Kang et al, 1987; Xia & Steadman, 2005).

The most common vascular complication is hepatic artery thrombosis (HAT) with an incidence of 25% (Dalgic et al, 2003; Heffron et al, 2003). HAT is a major cause for early graft failure and retransplantation. Decreases in incidence of HAT are attributed to improved surgical techniques. Careful anticoagulation and rheologic management and avoidance of rejection also may diminish the risk of HAT. Doppler ultrasound (used routinely or with a low threshold based on clinical indications) is essential for early diagnosis and possible successful thrombectomy and revascularization. Portal vein thrombosis occurs less frequently than HAT (Chardot et al, 1997; Millis et al, 1996). Similar to HAT, graft rejection or preservative injury with swelling of the liver increases the risks for portal vein thrombosis. Large-for-size transplantation is another risk factor for thrombosis (Kiuchi et al, 1999) if elevated intra-abdominal pressure is not lowered by using a patch abdominoplasty. Early portal vein thrombosis rarely may be treated successfully by emergency thrombectomy and revascularization. Late portal vein thrombosis with complications of portal hypertension may be an indication for retransplantation (Dalgic et al, 2003; Vilca-Melendez & Heaton, 2004).

Biliary strictures are common (10-20%) and may be secondary to transient hepatic artery ischemia (Egawa et al, 1998; Reichert et al, 1998). With widespread use of percutaneous radiologic intervention, such as transhepatic balloon dilation and stenting, there is a declining need for surgical reintervention and reconstruction (Bhatnagar et al, 1995; Heffron et al, 2003).

Many children undergoing liver transplantation have had a prior portoenterostomy and are at risk for iatrogenic bowel injury as a result of the adhesiolysis during native hepatectomy. A high index of suspicion and early repeat laparotomy and primary closure of perforation are crucial to prevent systemic complications of sepsis. Many children have compromised pulmonary function before the transplant procedure because of significant arteriovenous pulmonary shunting, pulmonary infections, or pleural effusions. Postoperatively, respiratory problems may be worsened as a result of diaphragmatic splinting or temporary right hemidiaphragm paralysis, pulmonary edema secondary to perioperative fluid shifting, or atelectasis. In children with high intra-abdominal pressure secondary to a relatively large liver, a tension-free temporary closure of the abdomen with a prosthetic graft is advisable. This abdominal wall graft may be reduced in size over several days, similar to when an abdominal wall silo is used in newborns with gastroschisis (Caccierelli et al, 1997; Noble-Jamieson & Barnes, 1999).

Peritransplant impairment of renal function is common, but usually reversible. Reduction or temporary cessation of nephrotoxic immunosuppressive medications (e.g., cyclosporine or tacrolimus) may help to improve renal function. Less than 5% of children need temporary dialysis post-transplant, unless this was already a pretransplant requirement (Bartosh et al, 1997; Berg et al, 2001).

Septic complications and infections are lifelong risks in an immunocompromised patient. In the initial postoperative course, bacterial infections with *Streptococcus faecalis, Pseudomonas,* and *Staphylococcus aureus* are most common, often related to central venous lines or bacterial translocation from the gut (Deen & Blumberg, 1993; Fishman, 1999). Viral infections, which usually occur in children immunologically naive to cytomegalovirus or Epstein-Barr virus before transplant, typically manifest about 6 weeks post-transplant and may be effectively prevented or treated by ganciclovir. Fungal infections may occur frequently in patients that present with acute hepatic failure. The use of prophylactic oral antifungal medication is recommended (Gladdy et al, 1999; Kahn et al, 1988).

IMMUNOSUPPRESSION

Much of the progress in pediatric liver transplantation is attributable to improvements in immunosuppression (Evrard et al, 2004). Treatment regimens are constantly in development as new drugs become available. Children generally have a higher incidence of rejection and require higher levels of immunosuppressive agents compared with adults. Baseline immunosuppression consists of corticosteroid and a calcineurin inhibitor (cyclosporine or tacrolimus) (van Buren et al, 1998). Tacrolimus has the advantage of requiring lower steroid dosage than cyclosporine for the same level of immunosuppression and less risk of hirsutism and gingival hyperplasia. Mycophenolate commonly is used to minimize the nephrotoxic effects of cyclosporine and tacrolimus. The initial 12-hour trough levels should be about 250 to 300 ng/mL for cyclosporine and about 10 ng/mL for tacrolimus.

In the early postoperative period, immunosuppressive drug levels should be maintained higher to avoid rejection periods, which can result in severe graft edema with subsequent arterial or portal vein thrombosis. These drug levels can be tapered over time (Mazariegos et al, 1997). Most children can be weaned off the steroid component within 1 year, and there are reports of complete withdrawal of immunosuppressants in children several years post-transplant (Diem et al, 2003; Reding et al, 2003; Riordan & Williams, 1999).

RESULTS OF LIVER TRANSPLANTATION

The increasing application of split liver grafts and LDLT has led to significant relief of the organ shortage in pediatric liver transplantation (Sindhi et al, 1999). In the decade from January 1988 through December 1997, the Eurotransplant member centers performed a total of 2668 liver transplants in recipients younger than 15 years old. Full size organs accounted for only 42% (1123 of 2668) of all pediatric transplants. In children younger than age 2, full size organs were transplanted in only 29% of patients, with 71% receiving segmental grafts (Adam et al, 2001; Wiesenhaan-Stellingwerff et al, 2000). The survival rates after liver transplantation in children are good, and most centers report 1-year rates greater than 80%. For elective transplantation in children with stable metabolic disease, the 1-year survival is 95% (Abt et al, 2004; SPLIT Research Group, 2001; UNOS, 2005). Extremely young age and low body weight are still risk factors, but are no longer a contraindication for liver transplantation. A series of 12 infants from Hamburg reported that infants weighing less than 5 kg (age <1 year old) had a survival of 75% at 1 year (Lang et al, 2000; Rogiers et al, 1997). This series showed the feasibility of liver transplantation in small infants. Children with fulminant hepatic failure who undergo emergency hepatic transplantation have 1-year survival rates of approximately 60% (Lee et al, 2001; Uemoto et al, 2000).

There is no doubt that outcome in liver transplantation is related directly to the severity of illness and the physical condition of the child (Kimura et al, 2004). Early referral to a transplant center along with early liver grafting before the clinical condition deteriorates significantly remains the most decisive factor for success. Living donation not only leads to a relief of organ shortage, but also offers the advantage of careful timing and the performance of transplantation under elective conditions. Some patients with metabolic disorders that cause severe nonhepatic complications also may benefit from liver transplantation. In this setting, auxiliary orthotopic living donor segmental grafts may be advantageous because the graft could be removed or immunosuppression could be withdrawn if better therapies are established or complications related to immunosuppression develop (Bismuth et al, 1996; Van Hoek et al, 1999).

LDLT is an exciting advance in the field and has almost become routine for pediatric patients with end-stage liver disease. The delicate ethical issues and complex operative procedure dictate these procedures should be undertaken in specialized centers in which extensive hepatobiliary and segmental transplant experience already exists.

REFERENCES

Abt PL, et al, 2004: Survival among pediatric liver transplant recipients: impact of segmental grafts. Liver Transpl 10:1287-1293.

Adam R, et al, 2001: Evolution of liver transplantation in Europe. Report of the European Liver Transplant Registry. Joint Meeting of the International Liver Transplantation Society, European Liver Transplantation Association, and the Liver Intensive Care Group of Europe, Berlin, Germany, July 11-13.

Ash SR, et al, 2002: Treatment of acetaminophen-induced hepatitis and fulminant hepatic failure with extracorporeal sorbent-based devices. Adv Ren Replace Ther 9:42-53.

Azoulay D, et al, 2001a: Split-liver transplantation for two adult recipients: feasibility and long-term outcomes. Ann Surg 233:565-574.

Azoulay D, et al, 2001b: Ex situ splitting of the liver: the versatile Paul Brousse technique. Arch Surg 136:956-961.

Baker A, et al, 1998: Who needs a liver transplant? New disease specific indications. Arch Dis Child 79:460-464.

Bartosh SM, et al, 1997: Renal outcomes in pediatric liver transplantation. Clin Transpl 11:354-360.

Berg UB, et al, 2001: Renal function before and long after liver transplantation in children. Transplantation 72:631-637.

Bhatnagar V, et al, 1995: The incidence and management of biliary complications following liver transplantation in children. Transpl Int 8:388-391.

Bismuth H, Houssin D, 1984: Reduced-sized orthotopic liver graft in hepatic transplantation in children. Surgery 95:367-370.

Bismuth H, et al, 1996: Auxiliary partial orthotopic liver transplantation for fulminant hepatitis. The Paul Brousse experience. Ann Surg 224:712-726.

Botero AC, Strasberg SM, 1998: Division of the left hemiliver in segments, sectors, or sections. Liver Transpl 4:226-231.

Broelsch CE, et al, 1984: Orthotopic transplantation of hepatic segments in infants with biliary atresia. In Koslowski L (ed): Chirurgisches Forum 84f. Experim U. Klinische Forschung. Berlin, Heidelberg-Springer, pp 105-109.

Broelsch CE, et al, 1988: Liver transplantation with reduced size donor organs. Transplantation 45:519-524.

Broelsch CE, et al, 1990: Application of reduced-size liver transplants as split grafts, auxillary orthotopic grafts, and living related segmental transplants. Ann Surg 212:368-375.

Broelsch CE, et al, 1994: Living donor for liver transplantation. Hepatology 20:49S-55S.

Broering DC, et al, 2003: Living donor liver transplantation. J Hepatol 38(suppl 1): S119-S135.

Busuttil RW, Goss JA, 1999: Split liver transplantation. Ann Surg 229:313-321.

Cacciarelli TV, et al, 1997: Factors affecting survival after orthotopic liver transplantation in infants. Transplantation 64:242-248.

Chardot C, et al, 1997: Portal vein complications after liver transplantation for biliary atresia. Liver Transpl 3:351-358.

Chen YS, et al, 2003: Evaluation of living liver donors. Transplantation 75(3 suppl): S16-S19.

Chisuwa H, et al, 2003: Living liver donation: preoperative assessment, anatomic considerations, and long-term outcome. Transplantation 75: 1670-1676.

Couinaud C, 1954: Lobes et segments hepatiques: notes sur l'architecture anatomique et chirurgicale du foie. Presse Med 62:709.

Cronin DC II, et al, 2001: Transplantation of liver grafts from living donors into adults: too much, too soon. N Engl J Med 344:1633-1637.

Dalgic A, et al, 2003: Clinical approach to graft hepatic artery thrombosis following living related liver transplantation. Pediatr Transplant 7: 149-152.

Deen JL, Blumberg DA, 1993: Infectious disease considerations in pediatric organ transplantation. Semin Pediatr Surg 2:218-234.

Demetriou AA, et al, 2004: Prospective, randomized, multicenter, controlled trial of a bioartificial liver in treating acute liver failure. Ann Surg 239: 660-670.

Desai NM, et al, 2004: Predicting outcome after liver transplantation: utility of the model for end-stage liver disease and a newly derived discrimination function. Transplantation 77:99-106.

Deshpande RR, et al, 2002: Results of split liver transplantation in children. Ann Surg 236:248-253.

Diem HV, et al, 2003: Steroid withdrawal after pediatric liver transplantation: a long-term follow-up study in 109 recipients. Transplantation 75:1664-1670.

Doyle HR, et al, 1996: Hepatic retransplantation—an analysis of risk factors associated with outcome. Transplantation 61:1499-1505.

Edmond JC, et al, 1993: Improved results of living-related liver transplantation with routine application in a pediatric program. Transplantation 55:835-840.

Egawa H, et al, 1998: Biliary complications in pediatric living related liver transplantation. Surgery 124:901-910.

Emre S, et al, 1996: Safe use of hepatic allografts from donors older than 70 years. Transplantation 62:62-65.

Erbay N, et al, 2003: Living donor liver transplantation in adults: vascular variants important in surgical planning for donors and recipients. AJR Am J Roentgenol 181:109-114.

Evrard V, et al, 2004: Impact of surgical and immunological parameters in pediatric liver transplantation: a multivariate analysis in 500 consecutive recipients of primary grafts. Ann Surg 239:272-280.

Fan ST, et al, 2000: Safety of donors in live donor liver transplantation using right lobe grafts. Arch Surg 135:336.

Fan ST, et al, 2002: Biliary reconstruction and complications of right lobe live donor liver transplantation. Ann Surg 236:676-683.

Fan ST, et al, 2003: Safety and necessity of including the middle hepatic vein in the right lobe graft in adult-to-adult live donor liver transplantation. Ann Surg 238:137-148.

Farmer DG, et al, 2001: Early graft function after pediatric liver transplantation: comparison between in situ split liver grafts and living-related liver grafts. Transplantation 72:1795-1802.

Fischler B, et al, 2002: A population-based study on the incidence and possible pre- and perinatal etiologic risk factors of biliary atresia. J Pediatr 141: 217-222.

Fishman JA, 1999: Infection in the organ transplant patient. Graft Organ Cell Transpl 2(suppl):96-100.

Florman S, Shneider B, 2001: Living-related liver transplantation in inherited metabolic liver disease: feasibility and cautions. J Pediatr Gastroenterol Nutr 33:520-521.

Freeman RB Jr, et al, 2004: Improving liver allocation: MELD and PELD. Am J Transplant 4(suppl 9):114-131.

Ghobrial RM, et al, 2001: Technical challenges of hepatic venous outflow reconstruction in right lobe adult living donor liver transplantation. Liver Transpl 7:551-555.

Gladdy RA, et al, 1999: *Candida* infection in pediatric liver recipients. Liver Transpl Surg 5:16-24.

Goss JA, et al, 1997: In situ splitting of the cadaveric liver for transplantation. Transplantation 64:871-877.

Harland RC, Platt JL, 1996: Prospects for xenotransplantation of the liver. J Hepatol 25:248-258.

Hashikura Y, et al, 1994: Successful living-related partial liver transplantation to an adult patient. Lancet 343:1233.

Heffron TG, et al, 2003: Hepatic artery thrombosis in pediatric liver transplantation. Transplant Proc 35:1447-1448.

Hendrickson RJ, et al, 2004: Pediatric liver transplantation. Curr Opin Pediatr 16:309-313.

Himmelreich G, et al, 1992: Different aprotinin applications influencing changes in orthotopic liver transplantation. Transplantation 53: 132-136.

Imamura H, et al, 2000: Anatomical keys and pitfalls in living donor liver transplantation. J Hepatobiliary Pancreat Surg 7:380-394.

Inomata Y, et al, 2000: Right lobe graft in living donor liver transplantation. Transplantation 69:258-264.

Jimenez Romero C, et al, 1999: Use of octogenarian livers safely expands the donor pool. Transplantation 68:572-575.

Kahn D, et al, 1988: An analysis of the causes of death after pediatric liver transplantation. Transplant Proc 20:613-615.

Kamel IR, et al, 2000: Living adult right lobe liver transplantation: imaging before surgery with multidetector multiphase CT. AJR Am J Roentgenol 175:1141-1143.

Kamel IR, et al, 2001: Impact of multidetector CT on donor selection and surgical planning before living adult right lobe liver transplantation. AJR Am J Roentgenol 176:193-200.

Kang Y, et al, 1987: Epsilon-aminocaproic acid for treatment of fibrinolysis during liver transplantation. Anesthesiology 66:766-773.

Karrer FM, et al, 1996: Long-term results with the Kasai operation for biliary atresia. Arch Surg 131:493-496.

Kasai M, Suzuki S, 1959: A new operation for noncorrectable biliary atresia—hepatic portoenterostomy. Shujutsu 13:733-739.

Kawasaki S, et al, 1998: Living-related liver transplantation in adults. Ann Surg 227:269-274.

Kimura T, et al, 2004: Optimal timing for living-related liver transplantation in children. Clin Transplant 18:497-501.

Kiuchi T, et al, 1999: Impact of graft size mismatching on graft prognosis in liver transplantation from living donors. Transplantation 67:321-327.

Kobayashi N, et al, 2000: Prevention of acute liver failure in rats with reversibly immortalized human hepatocytes. Science 287:1258-1262.

Lambrigts D, et al, 1998: Discordant organ xenotransplantation in primates: world experience and current status. Transplantation 66:547-561.

Lang H, et al, 2000: Liver transplantation in children and segmental transplantation. In Blumgart LH, Fong Y (eds): Surgery of the Liver and Biliary Tract. Philadelphia, Saunders, pp 2107-2119.

Lee WS, et al, 2001: Fulminant hepatic failure in children in the United Kingdom: etiology and outcome. Hepatology 3(Suppl 1):A291.

Lo CM, et al, 1996: Minimum graft volume for successful adult-to-adult living donor liver transplantation for fulminant hepatic failure. Transplantation 62:696.

Lo CM, et al, 1999: Applicability of living donor liver transplantation to high-urgency patients. Transplantation 67:73.

Lowell JA, et al, 1996: Long-term results with the Kasai operation for biliary atresia. Arch Surg 131:1235.

Makuuchi M, Sugawara Y, 2003: Living-donor liver transplantation using the left liver, with special reference to vein reconstruction. Transplantation 75(suppl):S23-S24.

Malago M, et al, 1997: Liver splitting and living donor techniques. Br Med Bull 52:860-867.

Malatack JJ, et al, 1983: Liver transplantation for type I glycogen storage disease. Lancet 1:1073-1075.

Malatack JJ, et al, 1987: Choosing a pediatric recipient for orthotopic liver transplantation. J Pediatr 111:479-489.

Malinchoc M, et al, 2000: A model to predict poor survival in patients undergoing transjugular intrahepatic portosystemic shunts. Hepatology 31: 865-871.

Man K, et al, 2003: Graft injury in relation to graft size in right lobe live donor liver transplantation: a study of hepatic sinusoidal injury in correlation with portal hemodynamics and intragraft gene expression. Ann Surg 237: 256-264.

Mazariegos GV, et al, 1997: Weaning of immunosuppression in liver transplant recipients. Transplantation 63:243-249.

McDiarmid SV, 2002: New liver allocation policies and their potential effect on pediatric patients awaiting liver transplantation. Pediatr Transplant 6: 180-186.

McDiarmid SV, et al, 1998: Indications for pediatric liver transplantation. Pediatr Transplant 2:106-116.

McDiarmid SV, et al, 2004: Selection of pediatric candidates under the PELD system. Liver Transpl 10:S23-S30.

Millis JM, et al, 1996: Portal vein thrombosis and stenosis in pediatric liver transplantation. Transplantation 62:748-754.

Neuberger J, 2004: Developments in liver transplantation. Gut 53:759-768.

Noble-Jamieson G, Barnes N, 1999: Diagnosis and management of late complications after liver transplantation. Arch Dis Child 81:446-451.

Ohi R, 2000: Biliary atresia: a surgical perspective. Clin Liver Dis 4:779-804.

Otte JB, 1995: Is it right to develop living related liver transplantation? Do reduced and split livers not suffice to cover the needs? Transplant Int 8:6973.

Otte JB, 2003: Donor complications and outcomes in live-liver transplantation. Transplantation 75:1625-1626.

Otte JB, et al, 1998: Pediatric liver transplantation: from the full-size liver graft to reduced, split, and living related liver transplantation. Pediatr Surg Int 13:308-318.

Otte JB, et al, 2004: Liver transplantation for hepatoblastoma: results from the International Society of Pediatric Oncology (SIOP) study SIOPEL-1 and review of the world experience. International Society of Pediatric Oncology (SIOP). Pediatr Blood Cancer 42:74-83.

Perilongo G, et al, 2004: Risk-adapted treatment for childhood hepatoblastoma: final report of the second study of the International Society of Pediatric Oncology—SIOPEL 2. International Society of Pediatric Oncology—SIOPEL 2. Eur J Cancer 40:411-421.

Pichlmayr R, et al, 1988: Transplantation einer spenderlebr auf zwei empfanger (splitting-transplantation): eine neue methode in der weiterent-wicklung der lebersegmenttransplantation. Langenbecks Arch Chir 76:172-230.

Pomfret EA, 2003: Early and late complications in the right-lobe adult living donor. Liver Transpl 9(10 suppl 2):S45-S49.

Pomfret EA, et al, 2003: Liver regeneration and surgical outcome in donors of right-lobe liver grafts. Transplantation 76:5-10.

Raia SJ, et al, 1989: Liver transplantation from live donors. Lancet 2:497.

Reding R, et al, 2003: Steroid-free liver transplantation in children. Lancet 362:2068-2070.

Reichert P, et al, 1998: Biliary complications of reduced-organ transplantation. Liver Transpl 4:343-349.

Rela M, et al, 1998: Split liver transplantation: King's College Hospital experience. Ann Surg 227:282-288.

Renz JF, et al, 2000: Biliary anatomy as applied to pediatric living donor and split-liver transplantation. Liver Transpl 6:367-369.

Renz JF, et al, 2003: Changing faces of liver transplantation: partial-liver grafts for adults. J Hepatobiliary Pancreat Surg 10:31-44.

Riordan SM, Williams R, 1999: Tolerance after liver transplantation: does it exist and can immunosuppression be withdrawn? J Hepatol 31:1106-1119.

Riordan SM, Williams R, 2000: Acute liver failure: targeted artificial and hepatocyte-based support of liver regeneration and reversal of multi-organ failure. J Hepatol 32(suppl):63-76.

Riordan SM, Williams R, 2001: The Wilson's disease gene and phenotypic diversity. J Hepatol 34:165-171.

Rogiers X, et al, 1996a: In situ splitting of cadaveric livers: the ultimate expansion of a limited donor pool. Ann Surg 224:331-339.

Rogiers X, et al, 1996b: One year of experience with extended application and modified techniques of split liver transplantation. Transplantation 61:1059-1061.

Rogiers X, et al, 1997: The Hamburg liver transplant program. Clin Transpl 183-190.

Ryckman FC, et al, 1998: Biliary atresia—surgical management and treatment options as they relate to outcome. Liver Transpl Surg 4(suppl 1): S24-S33.

Saad S, et al, 1998: Portal vein reconstruction in pediatric liver transplantation from living donors. Ann Surg 227:275-281.

Seek AL, et al, 2002: Transplantation of the right hepatic lobe. N Engl J Med 347:615-618.

Seiders E, et al, 2002: Graft loss after pediatric liver transplantation. Ann Surg 235:125-132.

Sindhi R, et al, 1999: Impact of segmental grafts on pediatric liver transplantation—a review of the United Network for Organ Sharing Scientific Registry Data (1990-1996). J Pediatr Surg 34:107-111.

Singer PA, et al, 1989: Ethics of liver transplantation with living donors. N Engl J Med 321:620-622.

Slakey D, et al, 2001: Budd-Chiari syndrome: current management options. Ann Surg 233:522-527.

Sokol RJ, Mack C, 2001: Etiopathogenesis of biliary atresia. Semin Liver Dis 21:517-524.

SPLIT Research Group, 2001: Studies of pediatric liver transplantation (SPLIT): year 2000 outcomes. Transplantation 72:463-476.

Starzl TE, 1992: Memoirs of a Transplant Surgeon: The Puzzle People. Pittsburgh, University of Pittsburgh Press.

Starzl TE, et al, 1968: Orthotopic homotransplantation of the human liver. Ann Surg 168:392-415.

Strasberg SM, 1997: Terminology of liver anatomy and liver resections: coming to grips with hepatic Babel. J Am Coll Surg 184:413-434.

Strasberg SM, et al, 1999: Reducing the shortage of donor livers: what would it take to reliably split livers for transplantation into two adult recipients? Liver Transpl Surg 5:437-450.

Strong RW, et al, 1990: Successful liver transplantation from a living donor to her son. N Engl J Med 322:1505-1507.

Sugawara Y, et al, 2003: MELD score for selection of patients to receive a left liver graft. Transplantation 75:573-574.

Surman OS, 2002: The ethics of partial-liver donation. N Engl J Med 346:1038.

Surman OS, Hertl M, 2003: Liver donation: donor safety comes first. Lancet 362:674-675.

Tanaka K, et al, 1994: Living-related liver transplantation for fulminant hepatic failure in children. Transpl Int 7(suppl 1):S108.

Trotter JF, 2000: Selection of donors and recipients for living donor liver transplantation. Liver Transplant 6(suppl 2):S52.

Trotter JF, et al, 2002: Adult-to-adult transplantation of the right hepatic lobe from a living donor. N Engl J Med 346:1074.

Uemoto S, et al, 2000: Living donor liver transplantation for fulminant hepatic failure. Transplantation 70:152-157.

United Network for Organ Sharing (UNOS), 2005: Available at: http://www.unos.org. Accessed January 2005.

Urata K, et al, 1995: Calculation of child and adult standard liver volume for liver transplantation. Hepatology 21:1317.

van Buren D, et al, 1998: Renal function in primary liver transplant recipients receiving neoral (cyclosporine) versus prograf (tacrolimus). Transplant Proc 30:1401-1402.

Van Hoek B, et al, 1999: Auxilliary versus orthotopic liver transplantation for acute liver failure. EURALT Study Group. European Auxilliary Liver Transplant Registry. J Hepatol 30:699-705.

Vilca-Melendez H, Heaton ND, 2004: Pediatric liver transplantation: the surgical view. Postgrad Med J 80:571-576.

Wiesenhaan-Stellingwerff GC, et al, 2000: Pediatric liver transplantation: 10 years Eurotransplant experience. Pediatr Transplant 4:124 (abstract).

Wiesner RH, et al, 2001: MELD and PELD: application of survival models to liver allocation. Liver Transpl 7:567-580.

Xia VW, Steadman RH, 2005: Antifibrinolytics in orthotopic liver transplantation: current status and controversies. Liver Transpl 11:10-18.

Yamaoka Y, 1996: Experiences of 120 microsurgical reconstructions of hepatic artery in living related liver transplantation. Surgery 119:20-26.

Yao FY, et al, 2004: Liver transplantation for hepatocellular carcinoma: lessons from the first year under the Model of End-Stage Liver Disease (MELD) organ allocation policy. Liver Transpl 10:621-630.

Ye Y, et al, 1994: The pig as a potential organ donor for man: a study of potentially transferable disease from donor pig to recipient man. Transplantation 57:694-703.

Yersiz H, et al, 2003: The conventional technique in in-situ split-liver transplantation. J Hepatobiliary Pancreat Surg 10:11-15.

Zamir G, et al, 2002: Toward further expansion of the organ pool for adult liver recipients: splitting the cadaveric liver into right and left lobes. Transplantation 74:1757-1761.

Auxiliary Liver Transplantation

108

O. T. TERPSTRA

Orthotopic liver transplantation (OLT) is the first therapeutic option for patients with end-stage liver disease. In auxiliary liver transplantation (ALT), all or part of the graft is placed as an extra organ in the body, while leaving the native liver in situ. This transplantation can be done in two different ways: (1) in a nonanatomic position (e.g., caudal from the native liver in the right paracolic gutter)—heterotopic auxiliary liver transplantation (HALT); (2) in the anatomic position, whereby part of the native liver is resected and replaced by the concomitant part of the graft—auxiliary partial orthotopic liver transplantation (APOLT).

ALT theoretically has many advantages over OLT. In patients with acute liver failure in whom there is a potential for recovery of their own liver, the graft can serve as a temporary bridge until the native liver has recovered. Then the graft is no longer needed, and immunosuppression can be discontinued. In patients with an inborn error of metabolism in which there is only one enzyme or receptor lacking, often the liver has a normal architecture and normal function. Replacement of only one enzyme or receptor is necessary. An auxiliary liver graft without interfering with the other functions of the liver can substitute the defect. It does not hamper the future possibility of gene therapy to repair the defect gene or to substitute the missing gene in the native liver.

SURGICAL TECHNIQUES

Absolon performed the first ALT in a human in 1964 (Absolon et al, 1965). The first successful ALT was performed by Fortner and colleagues (1970). Although OLT evolved to be the procedure of choice, the potential advantages of leaving the diseased liver in place continued to inspire researchers and transplant surgeons.

The surgical technique of HALT is as follows. After procuring the whole organ graft, the gallbladder is removed, and segments II and III are resected. The suprahepatic part of the graft vena cava is shortened to a length of 2 to 3 mm above the liver capsule. During the preparation of the graft, the recipient is prepared by another team. A right subcostal incision is used that is extended to the left through the rectus muscle. Dissection as for a routine portacaval anastomosis is carried out: the portal vein in the hepatoduodenal ligament to allow clamping over a distance of 3 cm, and the vena cava cranial of the renal veins to allow application of a Satinsky vascular clamp. The infrarenal aorta is freed over a distance of approximately 3 cm. The partial graft is placed in the right subhepatic region so that the suprahepatic vena cava of the graft is directed to the patient's vena cava, and the liver hilum is facing the aorta. The first anastomosis (i.e., the suprahepatic portion of the graft inferior vena cava to the suprarenal vena cava [end-to-side]) is made with 4-0 continuous polypropylene (Prolene) suture. After flushing the graft through the portal vein with 1 L of 0.9% sodium chloride solution at 20°C, an end-to-side anastomosis between the graft portal vein and the recipient portal vein is made with a running suture of 5-0 polypropylene,

leaving the portal blood flow to both organs dependent on the vascular resistance in the portal systems of each liver. After recirculation of the graft with portal blood, the anastomosis between the hepatic artery with aortic patch attached and the infrarenal aorta of the recipient is accomplished. An anastomosis between the common bile duct and a Roux-en-Y jejunum loop restores biliary drainage (Fig. 108.1). A thin polyethylene catheter is inserted through the choledochojejunostomy into the Roux-en-Y limb and brought to a collecting bag by a stab wound in the abdominal wall for bile production monitoring. A Silastic drain placed at the graft hilum is used for draining fluid collections (Terpstra et al, 1988).

APOLT is the technique whereby a part of the graft is placed in the same anatomic location after resection of part of the native liver. This technique first was reported by Bismuth and Houssin (1985), who treated a patient with an acute intoxication by transplanting segments II and III of the graft after resection of the left liver lobe of the recipient's own liver. The Hannover group (Gubernatis et al, 1991) described the first successful case with APOLT. The operation starts with resection of part of the patient's own liver, either the left lobe or the right lobe, depending on the size of the remaining lobes. The resected part of the recipient liver is replaced by the partial graft, either segments II and III (eventually segment IV also) or the right liver lobe (segments V-VIII). The left or right hepatic vein is end-to-end anastomosed to the stump of the left or right hepatic vein, depending on which portion was resected in the recipient. The donor portal vein is end-to-side anastomosed to the main trunk of the recipient's portal vein, giving free portal flow to both livers. The graft's celiac trunk is anastomosed to the aorta of the recipient cranial to the host's celiac axis. The biliary continuity is restored by a choledochojejunostomy on a Roux-en-Y loop (Fig. 108.2).

PROBLEMS IN AUXILIARY LIVER TRANSPLANTATION

Although the first experiments with ALT were done 50 years ago, these initial experiments resulted in rapid atrophy of the grafts. The reasons for failure were lack of space in the peritoneal cavity, resulting in an abdominal compartment syndrome, and physiologic, so-called functional, competition. A solution for the first problem is reduction of the size of the liver graft by resection of part of it. For a long time, it was thought that substances such as insulin, glucagon, and growth factors in the portomesenteric blood were essential to maintain normal function and integrity of the hepatocytes (Marchioro et al, 1965). Functional competition between the two livers in ALT occurred with atrophy of the graft in the presence of a healthy recipient liver (Van der Heyde et al, 1967) owing to lack of hepatotropic factors in portal blood. The hypothesis was that by providing a "handicap" to the (in most experiments) healthy host liver, the auxiliary graft would be in a more favorable situation to "compete." Three types of handicap can be applied to the

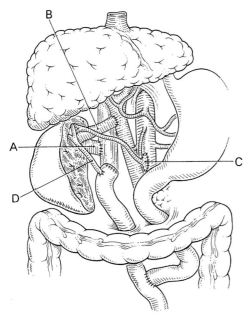

Fig. 108.1. Surgical technique of heterotopic auxiliary liver grafting. **A,** Suprahepatic part of donor inferior vena cava; end-to-side anastomosis to recipient vena cava. **B,** Donor portal vein end-to-side anastomosis to recipient portal vein. **C,** Hepatic artery with aortic patch. **D,** Common bile duct to Roux-en-Y jejunum loop.

recipient's liver: (1) diversion of the portal blood flow, (2) partial resection of the recipient's liver, and (3) ligation of the common bile duct. Among these factors, the most important is the diversion of portal blood flow.

It seems likely that functional competition is the competitive binding of hepatotropic factors in portal blood by first contact

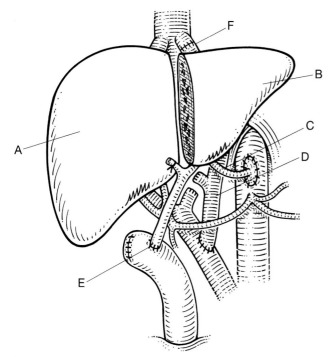

Fig. 108.2. Surgical technique of auxiliary partial orthotopic liver grafting. **A,** Recipient's own liver after resection of segments II and III. **B,** Graft consisting of left liver lobe. **C,** Hepatic artery with celiac patch. **D,** Graft of portal vein. **E,** Choledochojejunostomy on Roux-en-Y loop. **F,** Left hepatic vein of the graft.

with specific receptors on the membrane surface of vital hepatocytes from the graft or from the host liver. Diverting the portal flow to the graft decreases the capacity to bind these factors by the recipient's liver. Although the occurrence of this phenomenon might be of theoretical importance in patients with chronic liver disease in which recovery of the native liver is not the goal of the treatment, it may present a problem in patients with acute liver failure and in patients with an inborn error of hepatic metabolism.

In HALT experiments in dogs with an inborn error of metabolism, partial diversion of the portal flow to the graft by banding of the portal vein to the native liver resulted in long-term metabolic correction. Portal thrombosis was frequently seen, however (De Jonge et al, 2003). Portal thrombosis also was noted by Japanese transplant surgeons who treated a patient with ornithine transcarbamylase deficiency with APOLT. The surgeons needed to divert the portal flow to the graft, but the graft did not fully regenerate until after native hepatectomy (Kasahara et al, 2004).

The transplantation group of Kyoto University also reported on the significance of portal blood flow using grafts from living donors (Yabe et al, 1998). Although most patients had an inborn error of metabolism, they performed an APOLT. In nine patients, the portal vein branch to the native liver was transected during the operation, and all portal blood was diverted to the graft; this caused only minor alterations in the function of the patient's own liver. All auxiliary grafts had initial good function. The investigators concluded that by transection of the native portal vein, a steal phenomenon was no longer possible.

Other investigators disputed the importance of portal blood and the concept of functional competition. They showed that supplying the portal vein with arterial blood by anastomosing the graft's portal vein to the right renal artery in rats with acute liver failure resulted in good graft function until the native liver recovered, without signs of overarterialization (Schleimer et al, 2000). In pig experiments, arterialization of the portal vein resulted in good graft function, although ultrasound examination showed intrahepatic arterial expansion, indicating higher blood pressure (Fernandez-Rodriguez et al, 2003; Kesen et al, 2000). The Essen group treated patients by APOLT with arterialization of the portal vein by an interposition graft consisting of the donor iliac artery to the recipient's aorta (Erhard et al, 1998). In patients with acute liver failure, all such auxiliary grafts did well despite being deprived of portal blood. In this way, the liver, being a low-pressure organ, was transformed into a high-pressure one. The advantage is that the liver hilum of the recipient is left undisturbed, as is the portal inflow into the native liver.

APOLT for acute liver failure was carried out with flow of venous renal blood into the portal vein by end-to-end anastomosis with the left renal vein. In two patients, the graft provided metabolic support until the native liver regenerated (Ringers et al, in press). These observations cast considerable doubt on the concept that inflow of portal blood (with its hepatotropic factors) is necessary for the integrity and good function of hepatocytes.

REGENERATION

In ALT, regeneration of the native liver can be followed by sequential hepatobiliary iminodiacetic acid (HIDA) scanning (Fig. 108.3) and repeated liver needle biopsies. Recovery time ranges from 4 weeks to 6 months depending on the cause and severity of the disease. Any preexisting liver disease, such as liver

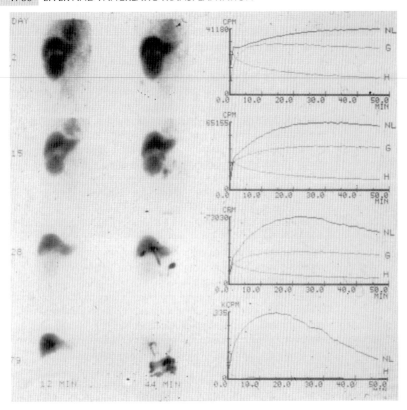

Fig. 108.3. Serial hepatobiliary scintigraphy in a patient with fulminant liver failure secondary to hepatitis B virus. Scintigraphy at 12 minutes and 44 minutes and time-activity curves for three regions of interest—native liver (NL), graft (G), and heart (H) on days 2, 15, 28, and 79 after HALT—are shown. The graft was resected on day 30. On day 15, excretion from the native liver was seen for the first time. CPM, counts per minute; KCPM, kilocounts per minute.
(From van Hoek B, et al, 1995: Temporary heterotopic auxiliary liver transplantation for fulminant hepatitis B. J Hepatol 23: 109-118.)

fibrosis from previous viral or toxic liver disease, may exclude full recovery, making the recipient dependent on the graft and lifelong immunosuppression. In such cases, advantages of ALT are obviated. Chenard-Neu and associates (1996) showed that after ALT for fulminant liver failure, complete regeneration capability of the native liver was preserved in most survivors, especially patients younger than 40 years old. Initially, it was thought that the percentage of vital hepatocytes in a biopsy specimen of the patient's liver was predictive for regeneration. Some patients with only 5% to 10% remaining hepatocytes recovered normal function of the native liver, however. Besides that factor, the distribution of liver cell necrosis varies from one area to another in acute liver failure.

Regeneration of the native liver was well documented in a report by Fujita and coworkers (2000). These investigators took sequential biopsy samples of the native liver of a man who underwent APOLT for fulminant liver failure with massive necrosis. At the time of transplantation, 95% of the hepatocytes were lost, and a few ductules were found in the portal areas. The ductules began to increase in size and number from where hepatocytes developed. From 6 to 12 months, the lobular architecture was established, leading to a normal liver at 14 months after transplantation. Another study showed a 25% to 45% increase in the size of the partial graft during the first month after HALT (Tarhan et al, 2000). This study led to the use of auxiliary partial liver grafting for small-for-size living donor grafts (Ikegami et al, 2002).

REJECTION

Experimental data and clinical observations support the hypothesis that auxiliary liver grafts can induce a state of immunologic tolerance. When rats received an auxiliary liver graft and a heart, the survival of the heterotopically transplanted heart was considerably better than in rats that received a heart only (Jiang & Han, 2004). In highly sensitized patients who had rejected several previous renal transplants, transplantation of segments II and III simultaneously with a kidney of the same donor resulted in good function without signs of rejection. In these cases, the auxiliary liver graft was transplanted with the sole purpose of removal of the recipient's multispecific HLA antibodies (Olausson et al, 2002). This removal or neutralization of antibodies against HLAs by the auxiliary liver graft is a promising concept, although some critics might argue that transplanting a partial liver graft for this purpose only withdraws an extra organ from the donor pool. Transplanting the resected segments of the recipient as a domino procedure to another patient makes this argument less valid (Hashikura et al, 2004).

AUXILIARY LIVER TRANSPLANTATION FOR ACUTE LIVER FAILURE

Experience with 47 patients who underwent ALT in 12 European centers for acute liver failure was reported (Van Hoek et al, 1999). These patients were compared with 384 patients who underwent OLT for the same indication in the Eurotransplant area. One-year patient survival did not differ between OLT and ALT (61% versus 62%). There was a similar incidence of retransplantation in both groups. One year after transplantation, 65% of the survivors after ALT were free of any immunosuppressive medication, whereas all survivors after OLT were still on immunosuppression. The results of APOLT were better than HALT. The heterotopic position of the graft caused more portal vein thrombosis and primary nonfunction than after auxiliary orthotopic grafting. In the patients who were off immunosuppression, the auxiliary graft was removed in half of them because of the need to stop the immunosuppressive agent instantly owing to infections. In the other half, the immunosuppressive medication was tapered off over 6 to 12 months. Chronic rejection set in, and the graft atrophied without any clinical symptom. Although the Paris group of Bismuth confirms the findings of similar patient survival rates for APOLT and OLT, these investigators showed a higher morbidity rate after APOLT, consisting of technical complications and more neurologic sequelae (e.g., brain edema) (Azoulay et al, 2001).

A single center reported on 18 ALTs in 17 patients with acute liver failure, of whom 11 survived. In 8 of the 11 survivors, the native liver regenerated so that immunosuppression could be stopped in 6 of 8 patients (Boudjema et al, 2002). After discontinuation of the immunosuppression, the graft normally decreases in size to such an extent that in some cases it is no longer detectable on computed tomography—the "vanishing graft syndrome" (Durand et al, 2000).

The use of ALT for fulminant hepatitis B liver failure has been controversial because the remnant native liver could be the source of recurrence of hepatitis B virus infection. Durand and coworkers (2002), in a small series of six patients who were treated for hepatitis B virus liver failure with an auxiliary graft, reported, however, that none of them had a recurrence of hepatitis B. All patients received ganciclovir and anti–hepatitis B surface immunoglobulins postoperatively. Other causes of acute liver failure in which ALT was used are acetaminophen overdose, mushroom poisoning (Broussard et al, 2001), 3,4-methylenedioxymethamphetamine (Ecstasy) ingestion (Garbino et al, 2001), and acute fatty liver of pregnancy (Franco et al, 2000).

AUXILIARY LIVER TRANSPLANTATION FOR CHRONIC LIVER FAILURE

In the 1970s, ALT was developed as an alternative for OLT for patients with severe chronic liver disease, who were thought not likely to survive the more traumatic impact of total liver replacement. By leaving the native liver in situ and omitting the recipient hepatectomy, the surgical trauma with ALT was less. Now that the technique of OLT is more refined and can be performed even in very sick patients, there is hardly an indication for ALT for chronic liver disease. The disadvantage of ALT in chronic liver disease is the presence of the cirrhotic liver. The cirrhotic liver is prone to carcinogenesis. In our own experience and that of others, carcinogenesis has been the case. Especially in patients with hepatitis B virus and hepatitis C virus cirrhosis, the risk of cancer growth is prohibitive for performing an ALT.

AUXILIARY LIVER TRANSPLANTATION FOR METABOLIC LIVER DISEASE

OLT is the solution for hepatic metabolic disorders in which the liver architecture is abnormal. Some inborn errors of liver metabolism do not cause structural damage to the liver, but result in severe functional impairment, which may be lethal. ALT under these circumstances provides the lacking enzyme or receptor. Replacement of the whole liver as in OLT to substitute a single defect seems to be a form of overtreatment. Besides, if the graft fails, the recipient's life is not at stake because of the presence of the patient's own liver. The availability of the patient's own hepatocytes retains the possibility of future gene therapy without the need for allotransplantation.

In a series of six children reported by the group from King's College Hospital, five are alive and well with a median follow-up of 18 months (Rela et al, 1997). All patients with Crigler-Najjar syndrome were free from phototherapy, and the child with propionicacidemia was on a normal diet with normal ammonia serum levels. ALT seems to be a good solution for hepatic inborn errors of metabolism in livers with an otherwise normal structure and function. The feasibility of APOLT also has been shown in patients with adult-onset type II citrullinemia (Yazaki et al, 2004) and type I hyperoxaluria (Onaca et al, 2004).

SUMMARY

Based on the experience now available, we can draw the following conclusions:

1. APOLT gives better results than HALT. This is due to venous drainage at lower pressure and less chance of portal vein thrombosis.
2. For good function of an auxiliary graft, portal blood inflow does not seem to be a prerequisite.
3. Auxiliary liver grafts can induce a state of immunologic tolerance for other transplanted organs.
4. When a patient has an acute liver disease necessitating liver transplantation, but that disease is potentially transient, ALT should be considered. If a liver biopsy specimen of the native liver shows signs of preexisting liver disease, such as fibrosis, ALT is contraindicated. When ALT is performed for acute liver failure caused by viral disease, it usually is not followed by persistent viremia.
5. ALT can provide the missing enzyme or receptor in patients with hepatic inborn errors of the liver and may be a solution until future gene therapy cures the underlying genetic defect.
6. In most patients with chronic liver disease, ALT is contraindicated because of the risk of carcinogenesis in the host liver.

REFERENCES

Absolon AB, et al, 1965: Experimental and clinical heterotopic liver hemotransplantation. Int Rev Hepatol 15:1481-1487.

Azoulay D, et al, 2001: Auxiliary partial orthotopic versus standard orthotopic whole liver transplantation for acute liver failure: a reappraisal from a single center by a case-control study. Ann Surg 234:723-731.

Bismuth H, Houssin D, 1985: Partial resection of liver allografts for orthotopic or heterotopic liver transplantation. Transplant Proc 17:279-283.

Boudjema K, et al, 2002: Auxiliary liver transplantation and bioartificial bridging procedures in treatment of acute liver failure. World J Surg 26:264-274.

Broussard CN, et al, 2001: Mushroom poisoning—from diarrhea to liver transplantation. Am J Gastroenterol 96:3195-3198.

Chenard-Neu MP, et al, 1996: Auxiliary liver transplantation: regeneration of the native liver and outcome in 30 patients with fulminant hepatic failure—a multicenter European study. Hepatology 23:1119-1127.

De Jonge J, et al, 2003: Portal flow is essential for graft survival in canine auxiliary partial orthotopic liver transplantation. Eur Surg Res 35:14-21.

Durand F, et al, 2000: Vanishing graft syndrome after auxiliary liver transplantation. J Hepatol 33:513.

Durand F, et al, 2002: Auxiliary liver transplantation for fulminant hepatitis B: results from a series of six patients with special emphasis on regeneration and recurrence of hepatitis B. Liver Transpl 8:701-707.

Erhard J, et al, 1998: Auxiliary liver transplantation with arterialization of the portal vein for acute hepatic failure. Transpl Int 11:266-271.

Fernandez-Rodriguez OM, et al, 2003: Description of a new auxiliary heterotopic partial liver transplantation technique with portal vein arteriolization of applicability in heterotopic liver xenotransplantation. Transplant Proc 35: 2051-2053.

Fortner JG, et al, 1970: Orthotopic and heterotopic liver homografts in man. Ann Surg 172:23-32.

Franco J, et al, 2000: Auxiliary liver transplant in acute fatty liver of pregnancy. Obstet Gynecol 95:1042.

Fujita M, et al, 2000: Sequential observation of liver cell regeneration after massive hepatic necrosis in auxiliary partial orthotopic liver transplantation. Mod Pathol 13:152-157.

Garbino J, et al, 2001: Ecstasy ingestion and fulminant hepatic failure: liver transplantation to be considered as a last therapeutic option Vet Hum Toxicol 43:99-102.

Gubernatis G, et al, 1991: Auxiliary partial orthotopic liver transplantation (APOLT) for fulminant hepatic failure: first successful case report. World J Surg 15:660-666.

Hashikura Y, et al, 2004: Dealayed domino liver transplantation: use of the remnant liver of a recipient of a temporary auxiliary orthotopic liver transplant as a liver graft for another patient. Transplantation 77:324.

Ikegami T, et al, 2002: Auxiliary partial orthotopic liver transplantation from living donors. Surgery 131(suppl 1):S205-S210.

Jiang M, Han D, 2004: Auxiliary liver-heart transplantation in the rat: a new microsurgical model inducing tolerance. Transplant Proc 36:1607-1609.

Kasahara M, et al, 2004: Functional portal flow competition after auxiliary partial orthotopic living donor liver transplantation in noncirrhotic metabolic liver disease. J Pediatr Surg 39:1138-1141.

Kesen X, et al, 2000: Splenectomy and auxiliary liver transplantation. Transplant Proc 32:2308-2309.

Marchioro TL, et al, 1965: Physiologic requirements for auxiliary liver homo-transplantation. Surg Gynecol Obstet 121:17-31.

Olausson M, et al, 2002: Auxiliary liver and combined kidney transplantation prevents hyperacute kidney rejection in highly sensitized patients. Transplant Proc 34:3106-3107.

Onaca N, et al, 2004: How much liver tissue is necessary to compensate the defect in type 1 hyperoxaluria? Transplantation 78(suppl 1):A170.

Rela M, et al, 1997: Auxiliary liver transplantation for metabolic diseases. Transplant Proc 29:444-445.

Ringers J, et al, 2006: A novel technique for auxiliary partial liver transplantation with renoportal anastomosis and avoidance of the hepatoduodenal ligament. Am J Transpl (in press).

Schleimer K, et al, 2000: Auxiliary rat liver transplantation with portal vein arterialization in acute hepatic failure. Transplantation 70:73-78.

Tarhan NC, et al, 2000: Volume measurements by computed tomography in auxiliary heterotopic liver transplant recipients: follow-up results. Transplant Proc 32:601-603.

Terpstra OT, et al, 1988: Auxiliary partial liver transplantation for end-stage chronic liver disease. N Engl J Med 319:1507-1511.

Van der Heyde MN, et al, 1967: The role of functional competition in auxiliary liver transplant. Transplantation 5:78-80.

Van Hoek B, et al, 1999: Auxiliary versus orthotopic liver transplantation for acute liver failure. J Hepatol 30:699-705.

Yabe S, et al, 1998: Auxiliary partial orthotopic liver transplantation from living donors: significance of portal blood flow. Transplantation 66:484-488.

Yazaki M, et al, 2004: Feasibility of auxiliary partial orthotopic liver tarnsplantation from living donors for patients with adult-onset type II citrullinemia. Liver Transplant 10:550-554.

Living Donor Liver Transplantation

M. E. SCHWARTZ AND G. E. GONDOLESI

From the earliest days of clinical transplantation, the availability of donor organs has been a matter of concern. The use of kidneys from live donors began shortly after kidney transplantation itself and has been accepted worldwide as an important alternative for patients with renal failure. In 2003, 42.7% of kidney transplants (UNOS, 2004) in the United States were with organs from living donors. Because the kidneys are paired, and the removal of a kidney is technically relatively simple, donor safety has not been a major concern (estimated donor mortality risk is 0.02-0.05%) (Kasiske et al, 1996). By contrast, hepatic resection is a technically demanding procedure, which, despite continual refinement of technique and perioperative care, carries risk that is an order of magnitude greater than nephrectomy (Miller et al, 2004a; Pomfret, 2003). Liver transplantation began in 1963, with initial long-term survival in 1967 (Rapaport, 1999; Starzl et al, 1968). Living donor liver transplantation (LDLT), driven by the dire shortage of organs for children with liver failure who otherwise would die, was first performed in 1988 (Broelsch et al, 1991; Raia et al, 1989).

Through the early 1990s, LDLT for children using a graft comprising segments II and III gained popularity. Together with the development of split liver transplantation with organs from deceased donors, LDLT has virtually eliminated the problem of children dying while awaiting transplantation (Testa et al, 2001). The typical pediatric transplant candidate has biliary atresia and needs a transplant before age 2; a segment II/III graft is ideally sized for such patients. The anatomy of the liver, with the left portal structures coursing up the umbilical fissure and the small parenchymal bridge connecting segments II and III to the rest of the liver that contains no major vessels, is favorable for the preparation of this graft (Otte, 2002).

Waiting list mortality for adults continued to increase unabated, and the use of left lobes for adult recipients began in Japan in 1993 (Hashikura et al, 1994); the first successful transplant using the right lobe from a living donor was reported in 1994 (Yamaoka et al, 1994). In 1998, the first report of right lobe LDLT in the United States appeared and was followed by others (Boillot et al, 1999; Marcos et al, 1999; Miller et al, 2001; Wachs et al, 1998). Although right lobe LDLT has been controversial from the outset because of concern about the magnitude and risk of the donor operation, the popularity of the procedure increased to the point where in 2001, 408 adult LDLT procedures, 9% of all adult liver transplants performed in the United States, were with living donors (UNOS, 2004). In Japan, where the concept of death by neurologic criteria has failed to gain acceptance, LDLT has grown even more rapidly (Chen et al, 2003).

Although many deaths of living liver donors had been acknowledged previously, the widely publicized death of a right lobe donor in New York in early 2002 sent a shock wave through the transplant community worldwide (Miller et al, 2004a). In 2002, the number of adult LDLT procedures decreased by 29% to 288 in United States. A similar phenomenon was seen elsewhere (Fan et al, 2003). The issue of donor safety has been taken up by governmental agencies and professional societies, and LDLT for adults is currently performed in the United States under intense scrutiny. Nevertheless, the underlying driving force—the lack of cadaveric donor livers and the resultant deaths of patients awaiting transplants—has led patients, their families and friends, and transplant programs to carry on (Salame et al, 2002; Surman, 2002).

LIVING DONOR LIVER TRANSPLANTATION INDICATIONS AND RESULTS

The decision whether to pursue LDLT in any given case depends on whether there is reason based on technical or medical factors to anticipate a lower likelihood of success with LDLT than with a whole liver and on the likelihood that a cadaveric donor organ would become available in a timely way. Although it is true, viewed from a global perspective, that every LDLT frees up an organ for another patient, we believe it is unjustified to subject a donor to the risk of surgery if the recipient has a high likelihood of receiving a cadaveric donor liver before deterioration results in a worse prognosis.

In LDLT for children, there is generally no concern with the donor liver being small for the recipient, and results in all indications for children are equal to or better than the results with whole liver grafts. The chief issue in pediatrics is whether or not a cadaveric donor liver would become available. Acute hepatic failure has become a common indication for LDLT in children; suitable organs typically are not readily available within an acceptable time frame, and although the crisis situation places stress on the donor (usually a parent), the relative safety of segment II/III donation and the universally accepted link between parent and child render the use of LDLT in acute hepatic failure in children ethically acceptable. Outside of acute hepatic failure, the need for LDLT is inversely proportional to the zeal with which split liver transplantation (dividing a cadaveric donor organ to transplant two recipients) is pursued. In many regions of the United States, as split liver transplantation has become routine, the need for LDLT in children has decreased considerably.

Overall, patient survival is similar after adult LDLT and cadaveric donor transplantation, although retransplantation is more likely after LDLT (Fig. 109.1) (Abt et al, 2004). There are, however, many situations in which receiving a liver that is smaller than expected based on recipient size has a negative impact. Chief among these is when the recipient has advanced liver decompensation and severe portal hypertension. Most programs

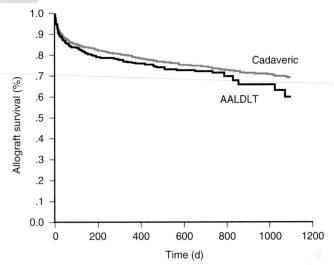

Fig. 109.1. Comparison between liver allograft survival after adult-to-adult living donor liver transplantation (AALDLT) and cadaveric liver transplantation ($P = .07$, log rank).
(From Abt PL, et al, 2004: Allograft survival following adult-to-adult living donor liver transplantation. Am J Transplant 4:1302-1307.)

would not consider patients with Child C cirrhosis for LDLT, unless the donor is considerably larger than the recipient and would provide a graft that is not small for size.

There is significant controversy regarding LDLT for patients with hepatitis C virus (HCV). If a patient has detectable HCV RNA pretransplant, recurrence after transplant is universal. The course of HCV after transplant is accelerated, with cirrhosis developing in 25% of patients within 5 years and 50% within 10 years; patient survival is decreased for patients with HCV compared with patients with other diagnoses. For this reason, many centers try to defer transplantation in patients with HCV until relatively late in their course, at which time they are less than optimal LDLT candidates. Although there are conflicting reports, many centers have reported that the course of recurrent HCV after LDLT is worse than in patients who receive whole livers (Bozorgzadeh et al, 2004; Gaglio et al, 2003; Garcia-Retortillo et al, 2004; Zimmerman & Trotter, 2003). Although the mechanism of this effect (if real) is unknown, investigations center on the effects of active hepatic regeneration on the biology of HCV. At least one major center has ceased performing LDLT in patients with HCV based on the poor results (Garcia-Retortillo et al, 2004).

In this era where treatment of HCV is at hand, LDLT can offer a unique opportunity to some patients. It has been shown that patients with HCV awaiting transplant who clear HCV RNA on treatment with interferon with or without ribavirin and are then transplanted have a high likelihood of remaining HCV RNA–negative after transplant (Berenguer & Wright, 2003). For a variety of reasons, treatment of HCV in patients with cirrhosis is difficult, and continuing treatment for 48 weeks is often impossible; a significant proportion of patients who clear HCV RNA on treatment relapse on cessation of therapy. The availability of a living donor allows for treatment of HCV with close monitoring of HCV RNA levels, then proceeding to transplant shortly after HCV RNA clearance has been achieved. This strategy, although too new as yet to have been reported

other than in anecdotes, offers promise for permanent cure of HCV in some transplant candidates.

Although acute hepatic failure is a well-accepted indication for pediatric LDLT, such is not the case for adults, at least in Western countries. Good results of LDLT in adults with acute failure have been reported, and the impact of an undersized graft is apparently less than in patients with advanced cirrhosis (Sugawara et al, 2002a, 2003). The primary objection has been on ethical and practical grounds. The risk to the donor is greater than in pediatric LDLT, and the urgency of the situation makes it difficult to obtain rational informed consent (this is not viewed by most ethicists as a problem when a parent is donating to a small child). The current organ allocation scheme in the United States grants these patients the highest priority, and it is highly likely that a cadaveric donor organ would be available. The ethical objections are relative; in Eastern countries, where cadaveric organ donation is not practiced, LDLT for acute hepatic failure is commonplace (Kobayashi et al, 2003; Lubezky et al, 2004).

Perhaps the best indication for LDLT is hepatocellular carcinoma (HCC). For patients with early stage HCC, which because of cirrhosis or technical factors is not resectable, transplant is the best treatment; employing the criteria of one tumor 5 cm in size or two or three tumors 3 cm in size, post-transplant survival rates equal those attained in patients without HCC. Based on these results, patients with HCC meeting the aforementioned criteria are accorded priority on the transplant waiting list. Despite this priority (Yao et al, 2003), however, waiting times may exceed 1 year, and tumor progression during the waiting period results in many patients dropping out before receiving a donor liver. When viewed from an intention-to-treat perspective, this problem significantly decreases the overall success of transplantation as a treatment strategy for HCC. In an attempt to forestall tumor progression, patients with HCC awaiting transplant typically are subjected to nonsurgical antitumor therapies and their attendant risks.

LDLT allows patients with HCC to proceed directly to transplant, eliminating the risk of waiting list dropout and the risk inherent in chemoembolization or percutaneous tumor ablation. Compared with most patients awaiting transplant, who have liver failure owing to end-stage cirrhosis, patients being transplanted for HCC generally have better liver function and are relatively better able to tolerate a small donor liver. Many series have documented the efficiency and efficacy of LDLT for HCC (Gondolesi et al, 2004c; Kaihara et al, 2003; Todo & Furukawa, 2004).

An area of considerable controversy is whether selection criteria should be expanded in the setting of LDLT versus cadaveric donor transplantation. HCC is the area where this controversy most commonly comes to the fore. There is a relative scarcity of cadaveric donor organs; not all patients who could benefit from a transplant can receive one. To make best use of this scarce resource, it is necessary to exclude patients from cadaveric donor transplantation when their likelihood of survival is significantly reduced, even though from the individual patient's perspective transplant is the best option. The 5-year disease-free survival after transplant for an HCC 5 to 7 cm and no macroscopic vascular invasion has been reported at 55% (Roayaie et al, 2002). These results would be considered excellent for many types of cancer surgery and are better than the 3% 5-year survival rate for such patients without transplant. Nevertheless, these patients are denied priority and as a result are excluded from receiving cadaveric donor livers.

A living donor organ alters this equation; although precious, living donor organs are not scarce. There is no a priori basis for setting the bar for acceptability at the same rate of survival as is achievable using cadaveric donor organs to transplant patients without HCC. The justification for putting a donor at risk is a reasonable chance that the recipient would benefit; a 50% likelihood of success has been considered reasonable by many centers, and expanded HCC criteria designed to select such patients have been proposed by numerous centers (Bruix & Llovet, 2002; Gondolesi et al, 2004c; Lang et al, 2002).

DONOR EVALUATION

Conceptually, a good living donor is an individual 18 to 60 years old who is generally healthy and without liver disease, is not significantly overweight, has a blood type compatible with the recipient, is able to provide a graft of adequate size, and has a reason to want the recipient to live. Donor evaluation is carried out by a physician who is not involved in the care of the recipient and who serves as the donor's advocate (New York State Committee on Quality Improvement in Living Liver Donation, 2002). Donor age is a concern because of the increasing incidence with age of occult medical problems that, despite careful donor evaluation, pose risk to the donor, and because hepatic regeneration is less efficient in older livers (Hirata et al, 2001; Ikegami et al, 2000). For these reasons, most programs set an upper limit for donor age at 55 to 60 years.

In cadaveric donor transplantation, every effort is made to transplant donor organs into recipients with identical blood types to avoid a shortfall of donor livers for type O recipients. From the recipient standpoint, however, receiving such an organ is acceptable. Apart from a self-limited hemolytic anemia resulting from antibody production by passenger donor lymphocytes, compatible mismatched organs function well without increased risk of rejection. Because there is no competition for living donors, it is reasonable to use compatibly mismatched organs in this setting.

After a complete history and physical examination, blood tests are performed to rule out viral and autoimmune liver disease and to screen for diabetes, hyperlipidemia, and hypercoagulable states, the most common of which are factor V Leiden and anticardiolipin antibody. Cardiology and psychiatry consultations are routine. Significant obesity increases perioperative risk and the likelihood of steatosis. In our program, potential donors with a body mass index between 28 and 30 undergo liver biopsy, and donors with a body mass index greater than 30 are excluded (Schiano et al, 2001). There is controversy among programs over the role of liver biopsy in living donors. A few programs perform routine biopsy (Ryan et al, 2002); however, most reserve biopsy for specific indications, such as a history of significant ethanol intake or overweight. The chief objective of the biopsy is to assess the degree of steatosis.

In recent years, there has been an explosion of knowledge about the significance of hepatic steatosis (Soejima et al, 2003b). It has long been known that donor livers containing significant macrovesicular fat function poorly when transplanted. This poor functioning apparently is related to difficulty in cold preservation of these organs, and it is widely accepted that livers with macrovesicular steatosis filling greater than 40% of hepatocytes are unsuitable for implantation. Lesser degrees of macrovesicular fat (20-40%) and extensive microvesicular steatosis (Fishbein et al, 1997; Uchino et al, 2004) are associated with increased ischemia-reperfusion injury as judged by the level of transminases, but graft survival rates are acceptable.

In LDLT, in which the graft is usually smaller than the expected liver volume of the recipient, fat may have added significance. It has been suggested that the proportion of the liver containing macrovesicular fat be subtracted from the radiographically calculated graft volume when assessing whether a donor liver is large enough for a particular recipient (Limanond et al, 2004). If a liver biopsy on a potential donor with a right lobe measured at 1000 mL shows 20% macrovesicular fat, the adjusted graft volume would be 800 mL.

More recently, with the recognition that nonalcoholic steatohepatitis is an important liver disease that can lead to cirrhosis and death, the long-term safety for the donor who has significant steatosis also has been called into question (Hwang et al, 2004). There is little information on the effects of liver resection and subsequent regeneration on the progression of fatty liver disease. This is an important area in need of clarification.

When a donor is judged medically acceptable, radiographic studies are performed to assess liver anatomy. Magnetic resonance imaging (MRI) allows for the determination of whole and segmental liver volume and definition of vascular and biliary anatomy. MRI cholangiography with mangafodipir trisodium enhances visualization of small bile ducts compared with noncontrast T2-weighted MRI (Fig. 109.2) (Cheng et al, 2001; Goldman et al, 2003; Yeh et al, 2004). Sophisticated technologies for computer-enhanced postprocessing of conventional imaging studies (computed tomography [CT], MRI) are increasingly able to provide detailed and accurate images of intrahepatic vascular and biliary anatomy as an aid to planning donor hepatectomy (Figs. 109.3 and 109.4).

ANATOMIC VARIATIONS (see Ch. 1)

Although the relatively constant segmental anatomy of the liver (Strasberg, 1997) is of fundamental importance in hepatic surgery, awareness of anatomic variations is equally important. LDLT raises the importance of this awareness to a new level. The gross configuration of the liver varies with regard to the relative proportions of its mass comprising the right and left lobes and their subdivisions. Although estimates of graft size can be made based on the size of the donor, imaging is important to ensure that the proposed graft is suitable.

Hepatic Artery

The classic hepatic artery anatomy, with the common hepatic artery arising from the celiac axis and giving off the right and left hepatic arteries, is present in only 55% to 65% of livers (Gruttadauria et al, 2001; Hardy & Jones, 1994; Hiatt et al, 1994; Kawarada et al, 2000). The most common variations and their frequencies are shown in Fig. 109.5 (Varotti et al, 2004). The two most common variants, each seen in roughly 15% of cases, are a left hepatic artery arising from the left gastric artery and a right hepatic artery arising from the superior mesenteric artery. In some cases, these are small accessory or segmental vessels, in which case they may be sacrificed after demonstration of good back-bleeding.

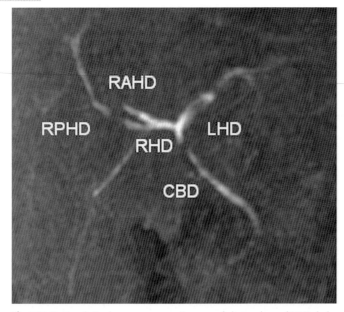
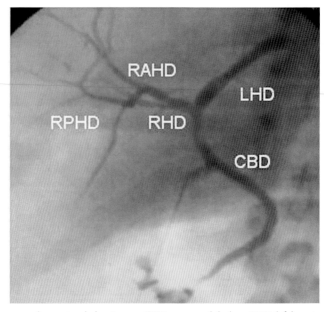

Fig. 109.2. Correlation between preoperative mangafodipir-enhanced MRI cholangiogram and operative cholangiogram. CBD, common bile duct; LHD, left hepatic duct; RAHD, right anterior hepatic duct; RHD, right hepatic duct; RPHD, right posterior hepatic duct.

A totally replaced right or left hepatic artery simplifies rather than complicates donor hepatectomy. Large left hepatic arteries from the left gastric artery typically supply segments II and III; most commonly in such cases, a segment IV artery arises separately. In preparing a left lobe or a segment II/III graft, a left gastric artery branch may be advantageous in that it may be left quite long by ligating branches to the stomach and taking the left gastric artery at its origin. Because the arterial dissection for right hepatectomy begins to the right of the bile duct, a left gastric artery branch has no impact on the procedure.

A replaced right hepatic artery from the superior mesenteric artery similarly facilitates right donor hepatectomy because excellent length on the vessel may be obtained. Occasionally, a proposed graft is supplied by two arteries of relatively equal size. In these cases, back table reconstruction of both using a bifurcated graft, most commonly the excised hepatic artery of the recipient, is the safest approach (Marcos et al, 2001a, 2003).

Portal Vein

Relevant portal variation is less common than arterial variation, seen in roughly 15% of livers (Nakamura et al, 2002). In these

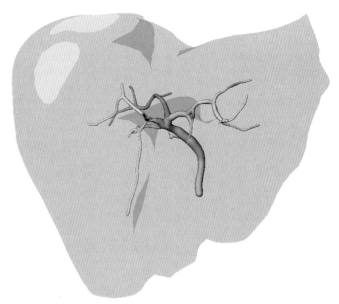

Fig. 109.3. CT-based three-dimensional reconstruction of the hepatic veins with a computer-based placement of the transection plane for a right hepatectomy.

Fig. 109.4. CT-based three-dimensional reconstruction of the biliary tree in a candidate for right lobe liver donation. A right posterior hepatic duct (RPHD) draining into the left system is seen.

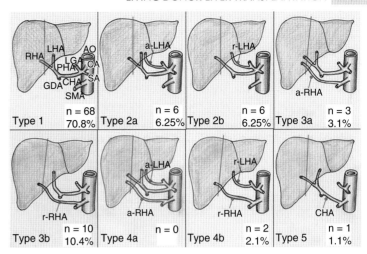

Fig. 109.5. Proposed classification and incidence of the common anatomic variations of the hepatic artery. AO, aorta; a-LHA, accessory left hepatic artery; a-RHA, accessory right hepatic artery; CHA, common hepatic artery; GDA, gastroduodenal artery; LGA, left gastric artery; LHA, left hepatic artery; PHA, proper hepatic artery; RHA, right hepatic artery; r-LHA, replaced left hepatic artery; r-RHA, replaced right hepatic artery; SA, splenic artery; SMA, superior mesenteric artery.
(From Varotti G, et al, 2004: Anatomic variations in right liver living donors. J Am Coll Surg 198:577-582.)

cases, typically the right posterior and anterior sectorial branches arise separately, rather than from a common right portal trunk; these variants may complicate the use of a right lobe graft. When these sectorial branches arise immediately adjacent to each other, it is sometimes possible to leave a common wall between them to allow for single anastomosis in the recipient, although care must be taken in such cases not to compromise the lumen of the portal vein remaining in the donor. When the sectorial branches are significantly separated, they must be taken individually and reconstructed in the recipient or on the back table to a bifurcation point of the recipient portal vein (Fig. 109.6) (Varotti et al, 2004). Uncommonly, the anterior right portal vein arises far to the left at the base of the umbilical fissure and courses through the parenchyma of segment IV before entering the right lobe. Because reconstruction is not straightforward, we have considered these cases unsuitable for right lobe donation.

Biliary variation is relatively less problematic for left than for right lobe donation. Typically, the segment II and III ducts join in the umbilical fissure, but occasionally the junction is more to the right. In preparing a segment II/III graft, by dividing the duct along the right margin of the fissure, a single duct for anastomosis usually can be obtained (Renz et al, 2000). In preparing a whole left lobe graft, care must be taken to avoid injury to a posterior right sectorial duct that is found to enter the "left" duct in its transverse portion under segment IV, a variant seen in about 5% of cases (see Figs. 109.4 and 109.7).

Biliary variation is a major issue in right lobe donation. Biliary complications correlate with the number of biliary anastomoses (Gondolesi et al, 2004a). In addition to the nearly half of the population who do not have a single right hepatic duct (Kawarada et al, 2000), a short (<1 cm) right hepatic duct makes

Biliary Tree

Variation is more common in biliary anatomy than in vascular anatomy (Fig. 109.7); the classic configuration with a confluence of single right and left hepatic ducts to form the common hepatic duct is present in little more than half of the population.

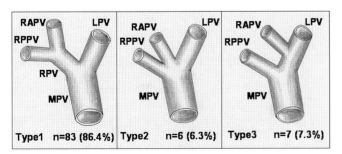

Fig. 109.6. Proposed classification and incidence of the most common anatomic variations of the portal vein in right lobe grafts. LPV, left portal vein; MPV, main portal vein; RAPV, right anterior portal vein; RPPV, right posterior portal vain; RPV, right portal vein.
(From Varotti G, et al, 2004: Anatomic variations in right liver living donors. J Am Coll Surg 198:577-582.)

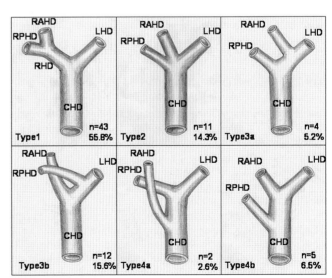

Fig. 109.7. Proposed classification and incidence of the most common anatomic variations of the biliary tree. CHD, common hepatic duct; LHD, left hepatic duct; RAHD, right anterior hepatic duct; RHD, right hepatic duct; RPHD, right posterior hepatic duct.
(From Varotti G, et al, 2004: Anatomic variations in right liver living donors. J Am Coll Surg 198:577-582.)

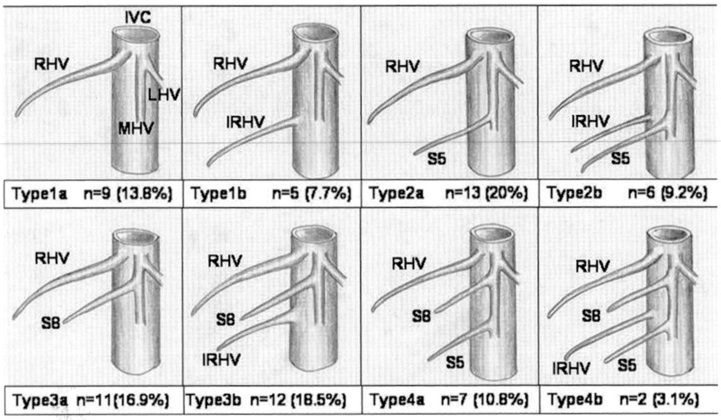

Fig. 109.8. Proposed classification and incidence of the RL hepatic venous variations. IVC, inferior vena cava; LHV, left hepatic vein; MHV, middle hepatic vein; RHV, right hepatic vein.
(From Varotti G, et al, 2004: Anatomic variations in right liver living donors. J Am Coll Surg 198:577-582.)

it impossible to procure a right lobe graft safely with a single duct for anastomosis in another 12% (Gondolesi et al, 2004a).

Hepatic Veins

Variations in hepatic venous anatomy create little difficulty for left lobe or segment II/III donation. The presence of a common trunk of the middle and left hepatic veins is nearly universal, and this trunk is taken with a whole left lobe graft, allowing for single anastomosis. Although the veins from segments II and III sometimes enter separately, it is usually possible in creating a segment II/III graft to construct a common back wall, allowing for single anastomosis in the recipient.

The right hepatic vein represents the main venous outflow of the right hemiliver (Fig. 109.8). In 30% to 50% of cases, there are additional significant (>5 mm) veins draining the posterior sector directly into the cava; these are preserved and reimplanted (Hwang et al, 2004). The middle hepatic vein usually contributes significantly to the drainage of the right anterior sector; the necessity for preservation or reconstruction of the middle hepatic vein or its tributaries depends on the graft-recipient weight ratio (GRWR) and the degree of portal hypertension present (see Fig. 109.8) (Sugawara & Makuuchi, 2001).

GRAFT SIZE AND SMALL-FOR-SIZE SYNDROME

The liver's remarkable regenerative capacity allows for safe resection of 75% of a normal liver. Early on in the experience with LDLT, however, it became clear that results are poor when a patient is transplanted with a graft that is 25% of the expected volume (Lo et al, 1999). Evaluation of the adequacy of the size of the proposed living donor liver graft is an important aspect of the donor evaluation process.

The liver normally composes approximately 2% of the body weight of a healthy adult. A more precise formula to estimate expected liver volume has been developed by performing a regression analysis on data accumulated from more than 1000 healthy deceased liver donors, with the estimated liver volume equal to 772 g × body surface area (Yoshizumi et al, 2003). The typical right lobe constitutes 57% of the liver, and the left lobe and caudate constitute 43%; a segment II/III graft represents 20% to 25% of the total liver volume (Gondolesi et al, 2004b). Although graft size may be roughly estimated from these figures,

there is significant variation in total liver volume relative to body size and in the configuration of the liver. Using the images from a CT or MRI study, the actual liver volume and the volume of the proposed graft may be estimated with a high degree of accuracy. The ratio of the estimated weight of the donor liver graft to the weight of the recipient, expressed as a percent, is the GRWR.

Through experience at many centers, it has become evident that when the GRWR is less than 0.8%, or 40% of the expected liver volume, there is significant risk of the recipient developing a constellation of findings that have come to be known as *small-for-size syndrome* (Sugawara et al, 2001). This clinical picture is characterized by prolonged cholestasis and coagulopathy, often with ascites formation, despite demonstrated normal vascular inflow and outflow, and leads to retransplantation or death in 50% of cases. Applying the above-mentioned figures, it can be seen that if a donor and recipient are of equal size, and the left lobe and caudate compose 40% of the total liver volume, use of a left lobe and caudate graft places the recipient right on the edge. Although LDLT was first carried out in adults at many centers using left lobes because of concern over donor safety, use of the right lobe has become predominant in adult LDLT.

As the safe lower limit of graft size was being defined, it also became clear that this limit depends on recipient factors other than simply size. Recipients with advanced cirrhosis, and in particular with severe portal hypertension and associated hyperdynamic splanchnic circulation, require grafts with a GRWR greater than 0.8% (Ben-Haim et al, 2001). In contrast, it has been reported that patients with acute hepatic failure, who do not have significant portal hypertension, may be transplanted safely with grafts having a GRWR less than 0.8% (Liu et al, 2003b). Attempts have been made to adjust the GRWR required to transplant safely a proposed candidate for LDLT by adding a correction factor based on cardiac output, which reflects the degree of hyperdynamic splanchnic circulation (Niemann et al, 2002). Doppler ultrasound estimation of flow enables intraoperative evaluation of changes in portal hemodynamics (Asakura et al, 1998; Gondolesi et al, 2002b; Huang et al, 2000; Piscaglia et al, 1991). Some authors have postulated that the direct trauma to the hepatic microcirculation as a result of high portal pressure leads to graft injury, and based on this hypothesis, these authors have proposed splenectomy or creation of a portosystemic shunt during the transplant procedure or attempting to reduce portal pressure with octreotide infusion (Masetti et al, 2004; Troisi & de Hemptinne, 2003).

The concept of functional graft size has been introduced to account for factors other than volume per se that may influence the function of a donor liver segment. One such area of concern is the completeness of venous drainage, particularly of the anterior sector of right lobe grafts. Although variable, in most cases a significant part of the outflow of segments V and VIII is via tributaries of the middle hepatic vein, and congestion with static or reversed portal flow in these segments is often evident when these tributaries are not reconstructed. In cases in which the GRWR is close to the lower acceptable limit, providing complete drainage of these middle hepatic vein tributaries by interposition grafting or by including the main trunk of the middle hepatic vein with the graft provides a margin of safety against the development of small-for-size syndrome (Sugawara et al, 2004).

DONOR AND RECIPIENT SURGICAL PROCEDURES

General Principles (see Chs. 107 and 111)

In contrast to liver resection for other reasons, in LDLT the surgeon must maintain equal concern for the portion of the liver to remain in the donor and the portion that is being removed. The details of anatomy, and in particular of variations in anatomy, take on added significance. Because of concern over the effects of ischemia on the donor segment, initially it was widely accepted that hilar occlusion should be avoided during parenchymal transection, although this tenet has been challenged more recently (Clavien et al, 2000; Imamura et al, 2004; Miller et al, 2004b).

An advantage of LDLT is that the cold ischemic time of the donor liver is short. To maximize this advantage, because the donor operation typically takes longer than the recipient hepatectomy, the donor procedure is begun first. Every effort is made to avoid the situation in which a donor surgery is begun, and then, owing to findings in the recipient precluding transplantation, the donor procedure is aborted. The most common such scenario is when the recipient is being transplanted for cancer, and disease is found at laparotomy that had gone undetected on preoperative studies. For this reason, the recipient procedure is begun first in high-risk tumor patients, and the donor surgery is begun after confirmation that the transplant may proceed (Gondolesi et al, 2002a).

Left Lateral Segment Graft

Donor Procedure

Although the operation can be performed through a midline incision, it is facilitated by bilateral subcostal incision with an upper midline extension to the xyphoid, which is excised. The left lobe is mobilized by dividing the umbilical, falciform, and left triangular ligaments. To facilitate implantation in the recipient, the entire left portal vein is taken with the graft; portal branches to segment IV are sacrificed (Fig. 109.9) (Broelsch et al, 1991). If the artery supplying segment IV arises separately from the artery to segments II and III, it may be preserved in the donor; otherwise, it too is sacrificed to provide adequate arterial length for reconstruction in the donor. The resultant ischemia of segment IV is often manifest radiographically after surgery, and air may be noted in the parenchyma, but there is virtually never any clinical consequence. Subsequent studies over time typically show atrophy of segment IV (Shoji et al, 2003).

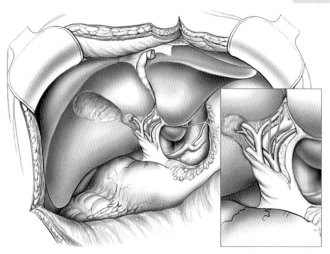

Fig. 109.9. Hilar structures for the left lateral segment are exposed. When segment IV artery arises separately from segment II and III arteries *(detail)*, it is preserved in the donor. Feedback structures to segment IV are ligated before parenchymal transection.

The parenchymal bridge overlying the umbilical fissure between segments III and IV, if present, is divided, exposing the left portal structures. Dissection is begun at the division of the proper hepatic artery, and the left hepatic artery is identified at its origin and dissected up toward the liver, looking for a branch to segment IV. The gastrohepatic omentum is divided. Anatomic variations identified preoperatively are confirmed. A large left hepatic artery arising from the left gastric artery is fortuitous, in that by dividing the left gastric artery branches to the stomach, a good length of artery is obtained, facilitating anastomosis in the recipient (Kostelic et al, 1996). Occasionally, more than one artery supplies segments II and III, but in most of these cases one is predominant; all are preserved in the donor, but typically the larger one is reconnected first in the recipient, and if good back-bleeding is observed from the smaller one, it is ligated (Michels, 1966; Soin et al, 1996; Suzuki et al, 1971). The portal bifurcation and proximal left portal vein are dissected under the artery, preserving the segment IV artery if it arises from the right hepatic artery (Fig. 109.10).

Dissection is carried out along the right margin of the umbilical fissure, ligating all segment IV portal branches and any artery to segment IV that arises from the left hepatic artery, freeing the entire length of the left portal vein and left hepatic artery down to their respective origins. Segments II and III are elevated, and the caudate vessels and ducts are ligated and divided. The ligamentum venosum is divided up near its entry into the left hepatic vein. The left portal vein is elevated and the segment II and III bile duct is incised within the hilar plate at the base of the umbilical fissure; the side remaining in the patient is oversewn. The left hepatic vein is dissected above the liver and encircled. The parenchyma between segment IV and segments II and III is divided using an ultrasonic aspirator (Cavitron ultrasonic aspirator) or other dissecting device without hilar occlusion. The left hepatic artery is ligated and divided, the left portal vein and left hepatic vein are divided and the ends are oversewn in the donor, and the graft is removed. The graft is flushed immediately via the left portal vein and left hepatic artery with cold

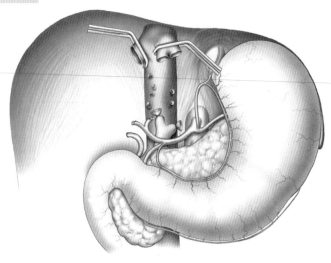

Fig. 109.10. Recipient hepatectomy is performed with preservation of the vena cava. The right hepatic vein and the middle hepatic vein/left hepatic vein confluence are clamped separately. Dissection is performed high in the hilum to preserve the bifurcation points of the portal structures.

preservation solution (Cheng et al, 1996; Tanaka et al, 1993; Yamaoka et al, 1995).

Recipient Procedure

Recipient hepatectomy is performed with preservation of the recipient vena cava (see Fig. 109.10) and taking care to dissect the hepatic artery and portal vein high in the hilum to preserve length. The donor left hepatic vein is incised posteriorly to create a triangular opening. With the recipient vena cava occluded above and below, the orifices of the three major hepatic veins are joined, and the resultant opening is enlarged by incising caudally on the vena cava to create an opening that matches the opening of the donor left hepatic vein. An anastomosis is created in a wide triangular fashion (Fig. 109.11). A small catheter is left traversing the anastomosis, and the final suture is left untied to allow for flushing of the graft before reperfusion. The left portal vein is anastomosed to the recipient portal bifurcation (in cases in which the recipient portal vein is atretic, usually to the level of

the mesenteric/splenic confluence, a piece of inferior mesenteric vein from the donor makes a suitable interposition graft). The portal anastomosis is performed entirely or over half of its circumference with interrupted sutures to allow growth over time (Emre, 2001). The hepatic arterial anastomosis typically is performed with the aid of an operating microscope. The proper hepatic artery usually is transected at its bifurcation to obtain an orifice that matches the left hepatic artery of the graft (see Fig. 109.11) (Stevens et al, 1992; Wei et al, 2004). Biliary reconstruction is via hepticojejunostomy with a Roux-en-Y loop of jejunum.

Left Lobe Graft

Donor Procedure

As with the segment II/III graft, although doable through a midline incision, the operation is facilitated by using a bilateral subcostal incision with upper midline extension. The left lobe is mobilized by dividing the falciform and left triangular ligaments. After removal of the gallbladder, hilar dissection is carried out, dissecting the left hepatic artery and left portal vein to their respective origins and dividing the remaining soft tissues surrounding them. If the artery to segment IV arises from the left hepatic artery, it is preserved; if it arises from the "right" hepatic artery, it is sacrificed unless unusually large. A left hepatic artery from the left gastric artery, if present, is preserved; when large, there typically is no vessel from the proper hepatic artery entering segments II and III. When the left gastric artery branch to the liver is small (1-2 mm), there is usually a significant left hepatic artery arising from the proper hepatic artery. In the recipient, the left hepatic artery is connected, and if there is good back-bleeding from the left gastric artery, it is tied.

The hilar plate is lowered under segment IV, and the left hepatic duct is isolated and divided; the side remaining in the donor is oversewn. Before dividing the left duct, a cholangiogram, either preoperative MRI cholangiopancreatography or an intraoperative study via the cystic duct, should be reviewed to look for the common anatomic variation wherein the posterior right hepatic duct enters the "left" duct; if present, care must be taken to divide the left duct to the left of its entry (Soejima et al, 2003a; Varotti et al, 2004).

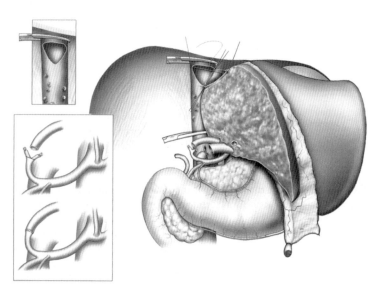

Fig. 109.11. The ostia of the hepatic veins are joined, and the cava is incised caudally to create a wide triangular opening *(superior detail)* to match the donor left hepatic vein. The proper hepatic artery usually is transected at its bifurcation to match with the donor left hepatic artery *(inferior detail)*.

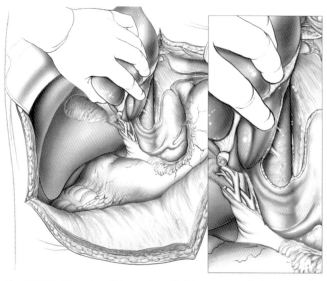

Fig. 109.12. Dissection of the caudate off of the vena cava during preparation of a left lobe graft.

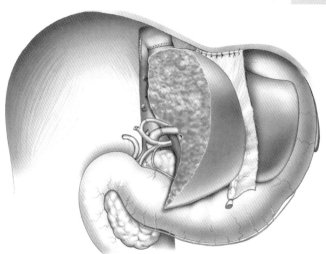

Fig. 109.13. The left lobe graft with completed vascular anastomoses and reattachment of the falciform ligament.

We prefer to include the caudate lobe (segment I) with a left lobe graft—the blood supply of the caudate and its biliary drainage is via the left portal structures (Fig. 109.12) (Abdalla et al, 2002; Miyagawa et al, 1998; Takayama et al, 2000). By taking the caudate, graft volume is augmented, and the procedure is simplified. The left lobe and caudate are elevated; the peritoneum overlying the retrohepatic cava is incised; and the caudate is dissected off of the cava to the midline, ligating and dividing all short hepatic veins that are encountered. After ligating and dividing the ligamentum venosum near its entry to the left hepatic vein, the left hepatic vein and middle hepatic vein are dissected above the liver and encircled as a unit.

The left portal vein and left hepatic artery are occluded transiently to show the interlobar demarcation plane, which is marked on the surface of the liver with cautery. The vessels are opened, and the parenchyma is divided with the ultrasonic aspirator; holding onto a tape passed between the right and middle hepatic vein, behind the liver, and up between the right portal vein and left portal vein facilitates the maintenance of proper orientation (Broering et al, 1998). The plane of transection is the true interlobar plane, extending straight down to the vena cava to include the left portion of the caudate. The middle hepatic vein is divided when it is encountered, taking the combined orifice of the left hepatic vein and middle hepatic vein with the left lobe graft (Cheng et al, 1996). When the liver has been divided, the left hepatic artery and left portal vein are ligated and divided, after which the hepatic veins are clamped and divided, the hepatic vein stump is oversewn in the donor, and the graft is removed to the back table, where it is flushed with preservation solution.

Recipient Procedure

The recipient hepatectomy is done with caval preservation; the hepatic artery and portal vein are dissected high and divided above their bifurcations. The left hepatic vein/middle hepatic vein confluence of the donor typically is anastomosed to the corresponding left hepatic vein/middle hepatic vein confluence of the recipient, although if there is significant size discrepancy, direct anastomosis to the cava may be preferred (Fig. 109.13)

(Egawa et al, 1997; Makuuchi & Sugawara, 2003; Sugawara et al, 2002b). A catheter is left traversing the anastomosis, and the suture is left untied to allow for flushing before reperfusion. Portal and arterial anastomoses are performed anatomically, unless vascular occlusion or injury necessitates interposition grafting. The biliary reconstruction is nearly always to a Roux-en-Y jejunal loop.

Right Lobe Graft

Donor Procedure

The procedure is performed through a bilateral subcostal incision with upper midline extension. The round and falciform ligaments are divided close to the abdominal wall so that they may be reattached after the right lobectomy to avoid torsion of the remaining liver and consequent hepatic venous obstruction (Miller et al, 2001). The gallbladder is removed, and cystic duct cholangiography is performed (see Fig. 109.2). The gallbladder mesentery is divided, and one or two small portal or biliary branches entering near the portal bifurcation are ligated to lower the porta hepatis away from the liver. The right hepatic artery is identified to the right of the bile duct and dissected from behind the duct toward the liver (Fig. 109.14) (Kawarada et al, 2000). The artery is elevated, and the right portal vein is identified, isolated, and encircled.

Dividing the right hepatic duct is a crucial step. As discussed under anatomic variations, the right hepatic duct, if it exists as a single structure, is quite short, and to maximize the likelihood of obtaining a single duct for anastomosis in the recipient, precision is necessary in selecting the point of transection. On the one hand, if the duct is cut too far to the right, there are multiple ducts to reconstruct in the recipient; on the other hand, it is essential to take care not to err to the left and impinge on the biliary confluence (Huang et al, 1996; Varotti et al, 2004). We use an external marker, such as a small clip placed adjacent to the duct during cholangiography, to facilitate identification of the ideal level for biliary transection. We typically divide the duct at

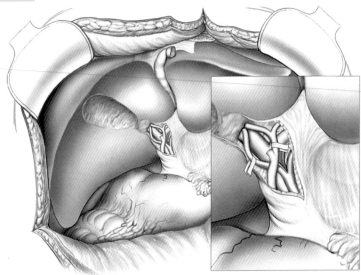

Fig. 109.14. After cholecystectomy is performed, the hilar structures for the right lobe graft are exposed. The right hepatic artery is identified to the right of the bile duct and dissected from behind the duct toward the liver *(detail)*.

this point, passing a clamp around the remaining right portal structures in the extraglissonian plane and incising these tissues, which contain the right hepatic duct, sharply with a knife. Minimal dissection of the duct is performed to avoid ischemia of its cut edge, which may lead to post-transplant bile leak or stricture (Gondolesi et al, 2004a).

The right triangular ligament is divided, and the liver is elevated into the wound. Dissection is carried out posterior to the liver, ligating small short hepatic veins; vessels larger than 5 mm are preserved for possible later implantation in the recipient. As the dissection proceeds cephalad, the right hepatic vein is encountered, dissected, encircled, and preserved. The caudate is divided at this point over the inferior vena cava using electrocautery. An umbilical tape is passed from above the liver between the middle hepatic vein and right hepatic vein, behind the liver and any preserved short hepatic veins, and up through the incised caudate. This tape marks the posterior line of parenchymal transection, and by lifting up on this tape, the final portion of the transection is facilitated (Broering et al, 1998).

At this point, the line of transection must be determined. The demarcation between the right and left lobes is shown by temporarily occluding the right hepatic artery and right portal vein, and the line is marked on the liver surface with cautery. Intraoperative ultrasound, along with preoperative imaging, is used to visualize the path of the middle hepatic vein and its tributaries. The course of the main trunk of the middle hepatic vein is similarly marked. To preserve venous outflow and avoid postimplantation congestion of the anterior right lobe, our preferred line of transection lies immediately to the left of the middle hepatic vein.

The liver is divided without hilar occlusion using an ultrasonic aspirator or electrocautery or both. Typically, the middle hepatic vein is prepared for transection high in segment IVa near its confluence with the left hepatic vein, trying to preserve one segment IV tributary to the middle hepatic vein with the left lobe.

When parenchymal transection is complete, and hemostasis is ensured, the right hepatic artery and right portal vein are ligated and divided. The right hepatic vein, middle hepatic vein, and any preserved short hepatic veins are clamped and divided, and the graft is removed; the orifices in the donor are oversewn.

After flushing the graft with preservation solution, any necessary vascular reconstructions are performed (Nakamura et al, 2002).

Recipient Procedure

Hepatectomy is done with caval preservation (see Fig. 109.10) (Tzakis et al, 1989). The hepatic artery, portal vein, and hepatic duct are dissected high in the hilum, above their primary bifurcations, to maximize options for subsequent reconstruction. A portion of the middle hepatic vein may be dissected out high in the recipient liver during the final stage of the hepatectomy, ligating the left hepatic vein and leaving the middle hepatic vein in continuity with the vena cava in anticipation of anastomosis to the middle hepatic vein of the graft or to interposition vein graft if required. Implantation is facilitated by complete occlusion of the cava above and below the liver. As in whole liver transplantation, the use of venovenous bypass is controversial (Fan et al, 2003; Grewal et al, 2001).

The right hepatic vein can be sewn either to the stump of the recipient right hepatic vein or to an oblique opening in the cava extending from the right hepatic vein orifice anteriorly (Fig. 109.15) (Liu et al, 2003a; Sugawara & Makuuchi, 2001). Hepatic regeneration can change the geometry of this anastomosis over time and potentially lead to outflow obstruction (Hata et al, 2004; Humar et al, 2004; Olthoff, 2003). Any large short hepatic veins (>5 mm in diameter) are anastomosed end-to-side to the vena cava (Fig. 109.16; see Fig. 109.15).

The donor right portal vein is sewn to the recipient main or right portal vein; the suture is left untied, and a catheter is left traversing the anastomosis for blood drainage during antegrade reperfusion. The donor right hepatic artery usually is sewn to the recipient proper hepatic artery. Portal vein thrombosis in the recipient, although complicating any liver transplant, does not preclude LDLT; eversion thromboendovenectomy or an interposition graft may be employed to re-establish portal inflow (Dumortier et al, 2002; Kadry et al, 2002; Moon et al, 2004). Depending on the rate of progress, the liver may be reperfused either immediately after portal anastomosis, or subsequent to the arterial reconstruction.

Reconstruction of segment V or VIII middle hepatic vein tributaries, if required, can be performed before or after

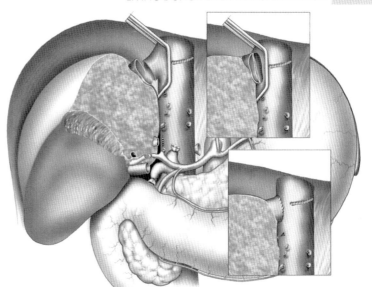

Fig. 109.15. The right hepatic vein can be sewn to the stump of the recipient right hepatic vein, or cavoplasty can be performed to extend the orifice and reduce the risk of outflow obstruction. Short hepatic veins greater than 5 mm in diameter are anastomosed directly to the cava.

reperfusion (see Fig. 109.16). A variety of techniques and graft materials have been used for this purpose (Marcos et al, 2001b; Sugawara et al, 2004). Our preferred method for biliary reconstruction is direct duct-to-duct anastomosis. Depending on the size, number, and configuration of the donor and recipient ducts, Roux-en-Y hepaticojejunostomy may be used either instead of or in combination with duct-to-duct repair (Fig. 109.17) (Azoulay et al, 2001; Testa et al, 2000).

BILIARY COMPLICATIONS (see Ch. 110)

There is considerable disparity in the literature with regard to the incidence of biliary complications after right lobe LDLT, with reported rates in small series of 60% (Kawachi et al, 2002); most series report rates of 20% to 40% (Pomfret, 2003). In a report from our center, 39 of 96 recipients (40.6%) experienced biliary complications—21 patients with leaks, 22 with strictures, and 4 with both (Gondolesi et al, 2004a).

Although the overall incidence of biliary complications is similar among recipients with duct-to-duct versus Roux-en-Y reconstruction, there are significant differences in the type and severity of complications; duct-to-duct anastomosis is associated with more strictures, whereas Roux-en-Y reconstruction is associated with a higher leak rate. Leaks generally manifest early after transplant (Popescu et al, 1994) and are associated with significant morbidity and mortality (76% 1-year survival with leak vs. 89% without in one series) (Gondolesi et al, 2004a). Bile leak from the cut liver edge may be treated successfully with percutaneous drainage, but anastomotic leaks invariably require reoperation.

Strictures may present with acute cholangitis, but more often are diagnosed by noting an increase in biliary enzymes (patients with more than one biliary anastomosis can develop significant stricture of one duct without resultant hyperbilirubinemia). A high index of suspicion is required because routine studies including ultrasound, MRI cholangiopancreatography, and biopsy can be misleading. Aggressive use of

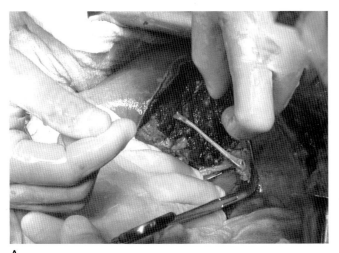

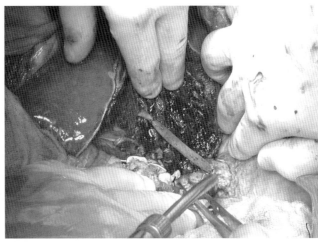

A   B

Fig. 109.16. A, Reconstruction of segment V vein to the orifice of the middle hepatic vein using a segment of the donor inferior mesenteric vein as interposition graft, before reperfusion. **B,** Segment V venous interposition graft after reperfusion.

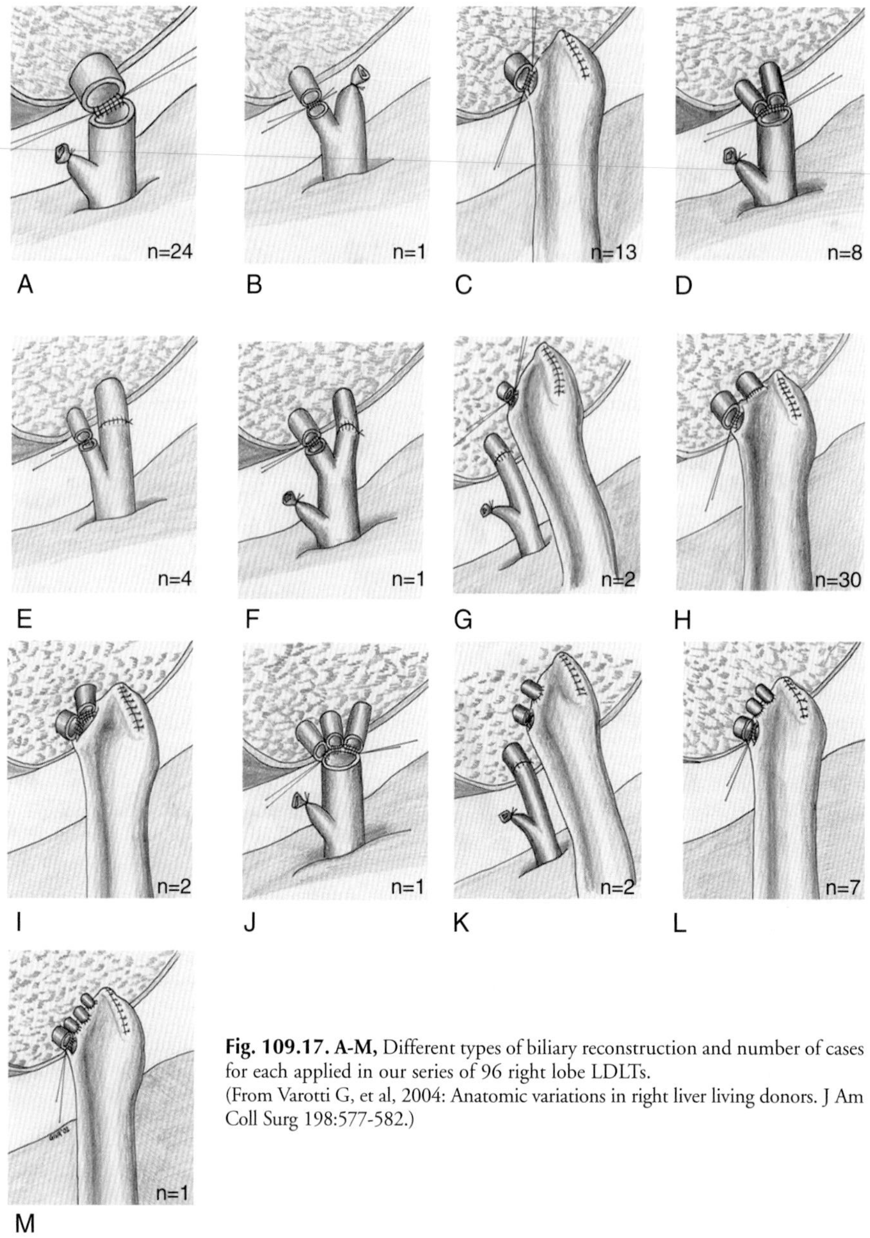

Fig. 109.17. A-M, Different types of biliary reconstruction and number of cases for each applied in our series of 96 right lobe LDLTs.
(From Varotti G, et al, 2004: Anatomic variations in right liver living donors. J Am Coll Surg 198:577-582.)

direct cholangiography facilitates diagnosis and initial treatment with dilation and stenting. Only 33% of patients with strictures required surgery in our series compared with 76% of patients with leaks.

COMPLICATIONS AND POSTOPERATIVE CARE OF LIVING LIVER DONORS

Donors are healthy volunteers, many of whom have no significant medical history or prior hospitalizations. Because they generally feel fine before donation, their postoperative expectations are different from those of patients undergoing surgery to solve a serious problem. Common postoperative events and complications can take on more than their usual significance in living donors, and extra attention is required to ensure a satisfactory experience. Postoperative pain is a good example—donors seem to have a very low pain threshold, and epidural analgesia for at least 3 days is routine at our center. Postoperative gastrointestinal complaints also are more common than in patients undergoing comparable liver resections for other indications.

Early postoperative care is similar to that for any liver resection. Prophylaxis against deep vein thrombosis should be included because donor death secondary to pulmonary embolism has been reported. Duplex ultrasound is performed on postoperative day 1 or 2 to document the absence of vascular complications. The average hospital stay for right lobe donors is 6 to 7 days.

Right donor hepatectomy is associated with considerable morbidity. In recent careful studies, more than 50% of patients developed complications (Pomfret, 2003). Most complications are minor, including respiratory and wound-related problems. Hepatic insufficiency is typically evident early after surgery, with elevated prothrombin time and bilirubin that typically resolve over the first 4 to 5 days; prolonged cholestasis is noted in around

10% of donors. Bile leak, usually from the cut liver edge, is seen in about 10% and usually resolves with percutaneous drainage. Late biliary stricture, although uncommon, has been reported and may lead to the need for intervention or further surgery (Lee et al, 2004). Vascular complications are rare, but early portal thrombosis has been observed; if detected expeditiously, reoperation and successful thrombectomy can be achieved. Late reoperation has been required for incisional hernia in 4% and for small bowel obstruction in 2% of our cases. We have observed one case of herniation through the right hemidiaphragm presenting as small bowel obstruction. Two cases of liver failure in a donor requiring transplantation have been reported; one of these patients died despite transplantation. The overall number of donor deaths is difficult to ascertain, but documented deaths have been reported from centers around the world. Current estimates of donor mortality after right lobe donation range from 0.3% to 0.5%.

CURRENT ASSESSMENT AND FUTURE DIRECTIONS

After the early period of rapid growth and the sudden retrenchment after the donor death in New York, LDLT has entered a period of critical examination, where outcomes in donors and recipients are being analyzed carefully. Many issues regarding surgical technique have been worked out, but difficulties remain, particularly related to biliary complications. The role of LDLT vis-à-vis cadaveric donor transplantation is being defined better for its various indications. Recognition of the limits for the recipient and the risk to the donor now temper patient and physician decisions. Increasing government oversight is expected. Yet, the critical shortage of cadaveric donors and the attendant high waiting list mortality continue unabated. Progress going forward will be incremental, based on accurate reporting of results through multicenter registries, which will enable rapid collection of sufficient data to answer the important questions that remain (Shiffman et al, 2002).

ACKNOWLEDGMENTS

The authors acknowledge Professor Heinz-Otto Peitgen and Holger Bourquain, MD, from MeVis—Center for Medical Diagnostic Systems and Visualization, and Elizabeth A. Pomfret, MD, and Christoph Wald, MD, from the Lahey Clinic Medial Center, for providing us with the three-dimensional photographs of the hepatic veins and bile ducts. The authors acknowledge Giovanni Varotti, MD, and Hugh Thomas for the anatomic and surgical drawings.

REFERENCES

Abdalla EK, et al, 2002: The caudate lobe of the liver: implications of embryology and anatomy for surgery. Surg Oncol Clin North Am 11:835-848.

Abt PL, et al, 2004: Allograft survival following adult-to-adult living donor liver transplantation. Am J Transplant 4:1302-1307.

Asakura T, et al, 1998: Doppler ultrasonography in living-related liver transplantation. Transplant Proc 30:3190-3194.

Azoulay D, et al, 2001: Duct-to-duct biliary anastomosis in living related liver transplantation: the Paul Brousse technique. Arch Surg 136:1197-1200.

Ben-Haim M, et al, 2001: Critical graft size in adult-to-adult living donor liver transplantation: impact of the recipient's disease. Liver Transplant 7:948-953.

Berenguer M, Wright TL, 2003: Treatment strategies for hepatitis C: intervention prior to liver transplant, pre-emptively or after established disease. Clin Liver Dis 7:631-650.

Boillot O, et al, 1999: Orthotopic liver transplantation from a living adult donor to an adult using the right hepatic lobe. Chirurgie 124:122-131.

Bozorgzadeh A, et al, 2004: Impact of hepatitis C viral infection in primary cadaveric liver allograft versus primary living-donor allograft in 100 consecutive liver transplant recipients receiving tacrolimus. Transplantation 77:1066-1070.

Broelsch CE, et al, 1991: Liver transplantation in children from living related donors: surgical techniques and results. Ann Surg 214:428-437.

Broering DC, et al, 1998: Vessel loop–guided technique for parenchymal transection in living donor or in situ split-liver procurement. Liver Transplant 4:241.

Bruix J, Llovet JM, 2002: Prognostic prediction and treatment strategy in hepatocellular carcinoma. Hepatology 35:519-524.

Chen CL, et al, 2003: Living-donor liver transplantation: 12 years of experience in Asia. Transplantation 75(3 suppl):S6-S11.

Cheng YF, et al, 1996: Variations of the left and middle hepatic veins: application in living related hepatic transplantation. J Clin Ultrasound 24:11-16.

Cheng YF, et al, 2001: Single imaging modality evaluation of living donors in liver transplantation: magnetic resonance imaging. Transplantation 72:1527-1533.

Clavien PA, et al, 2000: Contralateral inflow occlusion to optimize graft volume and to reduce blood loss during parenchymal dissection in living-related liver transplantation. Transplantation 69:2232.

Dumortier J, et al, 2002: Eversion thrombectomy for portal vein thrombosis during liver transplantation. Am J Transplant 2:934-938.

Egawa H, et al, 1997: Hepatic vein reconstruction in 152 living-related donor liver transplantation patients. Surgery 121:250-257.

Emre S, 2001: Living donor liver transplantation: a critical review. Transplant Proc 33:3456-3457.

Fan ST, et al, 2003: Right lobe living donor liver transplantation with or without venovenous bypass. Br J Surg 90:48-56.

Fishbein T, et al, 1997: Use of livers with microvesicular fat safely expands the donor pool. Transplantation 64:248-251.

Gaglio PJ, et al, 2003: Increased risk of cholestatic hepatitis C in recipients of grafts from living versus cadaveric liver donors. Liver Transplant 9:1028-1035.

Garcia-Retortillo M, et al, 2004: Hepatitis C recurrence is more severe after living donor compared to cadaveric liver transplantation. Hepatology 40:699-707.

Goldman J, et al, 2003: Noninvasive preoperative evaluation of biliary anatomy in right-lobe living donors with mangafodipir trisodium-enhanced MR cholangiography. Transplant Proc 35:1421-1422.

Gondolesi G, et al, 2002a: Hepatocellular carcinoma: a prime indication for living donor liver transplantation. J Gastrointest Surg 6:102-107.

Gondolesi GE, et al, 2002b: Venous hemodynamics in living donor right lobe liver transplantation. Liver Transplantation: official publication of the American Association for the Study of Liver Diseases and the International Liver Transplantation Society 8(9):809-813.

Gondolesi GE, et al, 2004a: Biliary complications in 96 consecutive right lobe living donor transplant recipients. Transplantation 77:1842-1848.

Gondolesi GE, et al, 2004b: Accurate method for clinical assessment of right lobe liver weight in adult living-related liver transplant. Transplant Proc 36:1429-1433.

Gondolesi GE, et al, 2004c: Adult living donor liver transplantation for patients with hepatocellular carcinoma: extending UNOS priority criteria. Ann Surg 239:142-149.

Grewal HP, et al, 2001: Surgical technique for right lobe adult living donor liver transplantation without venovenous bypass or portocaval shunting and with duct-to-duct biliary reconstruction. Ann Surg 233:502-508.

Gruttadauria S, et al, 2001: The hepatic artery in liver transplantation and surgery: vascular anomalies in 701 cases. Clin Transplant 15:359-363.

Hardy KJ, Jones RM, 1994: Hepatic artery anatomy in relation to reconstruction in liver transplantation: some unusual variations. Aust N Z J Surg 64:437-440.

Hashikura Y, et al, 1994: Successful living-related partial liver transplantation to an adult patient. Lancet 343:1233-1234.

Hata S, et al, 2004: Volume regeneration after right liver donation. Liver Transplant 10:65-70.

Hiatt JR, et al, 1994: Surgical anatomy of the hepatic arteries in 1000 cases. Ann Surg 220:50-52.

Hirata M, et al, 2001: The influence of donor age to graft volume increase rate in living donor liver transplantation. Transplant Proc 33:1416-1417.

Huang TL, et al, 1996: Variants of the bile ducts: clinical application in the potential donor of living-related hepatic transplantation. Transplant Proc 28:1669-1670.

Huang TL, et al, 2000: Intraoperative Doppler ultrasound in living-related liver transplantation. Transplant Proc 32:2097-2098.

Humar A, et al, 2004: Liver regeneration after adult living donor and deceased donor split-liver transplants. Liver Transplant 10:374-378.

Hwang S, et al, 2004: The effect of donor weight reduction on hepatic steatosis for living donor liver transplantation. Liver Transplant 10:721-725.

Ikegami T, et al, 2000: The impact of donor age on living donor liver transplantation. Transplantation 70:1703-1707.

Imamura H, et al, 2004: Pringle's maneuver and selective inflow occlusion in living donor liver hepatectomy. Liver Transplant 10:771-778.

Kadry Z, et al, 2002: Living donor liver transplantation in patients with portal vein thrombosis: a survey and review of technical issues. Transplantation 74:696-701.

Kaihara S, et al, 2003: Living-donor liver transplantation for hepatocellular carcinoma. Transplantation 75(3 suppl):S37-S40.

Kasiske BL, et al, 1996: The evaluation of living renal transplant donors: clinical practice guidelines. Ad Hoc Clinical Practice Guidelines Subcommittee of the Patient Care and Education Committee of the American Society of Transplant Physicians. J Am Soc Nephrol 7:2288-2313.

Kawachi S, et al, 2002: Biliary complications in adult living donor liver transplantation with duct-to-duct hepaticocholedochostomy or Roux-en-Y hepaticojejunostomy biliary reconstruction. Surgery 132:48-56.

Kawarada Y, et al, 2000: Anatomy of the hepatic hilar area: the plate system. J Hepatobiliary Pancreat Surg 7:580-586.

Kobayashi S, et al, 2003: Complete recovery from fulminant hepatic failure with severe coma by living donor liver transplantation. Hepatogastroenterology 50:515-518.

Kostelic JK, et al, 1996: Angiographic selection criteria for living related liver transplant donors. AJR Am J Roentgenol 166:1103-1108.

Lang H, et al, 2002: Extended indications for liver transplantation in HCC with special reference to living donor liver donation. Kongressbd Dtsch Ges Chir Kongr 119:410-413.

Lee SY, et al, 2004: Living donor liver transplantation: complications in donors and interventional management. Radiology 230:443-449.

Limanond P, et al, 2004: Macrovesicular hepatic steatosis in living related liver donors: correlation between CT and histologic findings. Radiology 230:276-280.

Liu CL, et al, 2003a: Hepatic venoplasty in right lobe live donor liver transplantation. Liver Transplant 9:1265-1272.

Liu CL, et al, 2003b: Live donor liver transplantation for fulminant hepatic failure in children. Liver Transplant 9:1185-1190.

Lo CM, et al, 1999: Minimum graft size for successful living donor liver transplantation. Transplantation 68:1112-1116.

Lubezky N, et al, 2004: Initial experience with urgent adult-to-adult living donor liver transplantation in fulminant hepatic failure. Isr Med Assoc J 6:467-470.

Makuuchi M, Sugawara Y, 2003: Living-donor liver transplantation using the left liver, with special reference to vein reconstruction. Transplantation 75(3 suppl):S23-S24.

Marcos A, et al, 1999: Right lobe living donor liver transplantation. Transplantation 68:798-803.

Marcos A, et al, 2001a: Reconstruction of double hepatic arterial and portal venous branches for right-lobe living donor liver transplantation. Liver Transplant 7:673-679.

Marcos A, et al, 2001b: Functional venous anatomy for right-lobe grafting and techniques to optimize outflow. Liver Transpl 7:845-852.

Marcos A, et al, 2003: Hepatic arterial reconstruction in 95 adult right lobe living donor liver transplants: evolution of anastomotic technique. Liver Transplant 9:570-574.

Masetti M, et al, 2004: Living donor liver transplantation with left liver graft. Am J Transplant 4:1713-1716.

Michels NA, 1966: Newer anatomy of the liver and its variant blood supply and collateral circulation. Am J Surg 112:337-347.

Miller CM, et al, 2001: One hundred nine living donor liver transplants in adults and children: a single-center experience. Ann Surg 234:301-311.

Miller C, et al, 2004a: Fulminant and fatal gas gangrene of the stomach in a healthy live liver donor. Liver Transplant 10:1315.

Miller CM, et al, 2004b: Intermittent inflow occlusion in living liver donors: impact on safety and remnant function. Liver Transplant 10:244-247.

Miyagawa S, et al, 1998: Concomitant caudate lobe resection as an option for donor hepatectomy in adult living related liver transplantation. Transplantation 66:661-663.

Moon D, et al, 2004: Umbilical portion of recipient's left portal vein: a useful vascular conduit in dual living donor liver transplantation for the thrombosed portal vein. Liver Transplant 10:802-806.

Nakamura T, et al, 2002: Anatomical variations and surgical strategies in right lobe living donor liver transplantation: lessons from 120 cases. Transplantation 73:1896-1903.

New York State Committee on Quality Improvement in Living Liver Donation, 2002: Report to the New York Transplant Council and New York State Department of Health. Report No. 1. Albany, NY, New York Department of Health.

Niemann CU, et al, 2002: Intraoperative hemodynamics and liver function in adult-to-adult living liver donors. Liver Transplant 8:1126-1132.

Olthoff KM, 2003: Hepatic regeneration in living donor liver transplantation. Liver Transplant 9(10 suppl 2):S35-S41.

Otte JB, 2002: History of pediatric liver transplantation. Where are we coming from? Where do we stand? Pediatr Transplant 6:378-387.

Piscaglia F, et al, 1999: Systemic and splanchnic hemodynamic changes after liver transplantation for cirrhosis: a long-term prospective study. Hepatology 30:58-64.

Pomfret EA, 2003: Early and late complications in the right-lobe adult living donor. Liver Transplantation 9(10 suppl 2):S45-S49.

Popescu I, et al, 1994: Biliary complications in 400 cases of liver transplantation. Mt Sinai J Med 61:57-62.

Raia S, et al, 1989: Liver transplantation from live donors. Lancet 2:497.

Rapaport FT, 1999: Some landmarks in the evolution of transplantation. Transplant Proc 31:2939-2944.

Renz JF, et al, 2000: Biliary anatomy as applied to pediatric living donor and split-liver transplantation. Liver Transplant 6:801-804.

Roayaie S, et al, 2002: Long-term results with multimodal adjuvant therapy and liver transplantation for the treatment of hepatocellular carcinomas larger than 5 centimeters. Ann Surg 235:533-539.

Ryan CK, et al, 2002: One hundred consecutive hepatic biopsies in the workup of living donors for right lobe liver transplantation. Liver Transplant 8:1114-1122.

Salame E, et al, 2002: Analysis of donor risk in living-donor hepatectomy: the impact of resection type on clinical outcome. Am J Transplant 2:780-788.

Schiano TD, et al, 2001: Adult living donor liver transplantation: the hepatologist's perspective. Hepatology 33:3-9.

Shiffman ML, et al, 2002: Living donor liver transplantation: summary of a conference at The National Institutes of Health. Liver Transplant 8:174-188.

Shoji M, et al, 2003: The safety of the donor operation in living-donor liver transplantation: an analysis of 45 donors. Transpl Int 16:461-464.

Soejima Y, et al, 2003a: Feasibility of duct-to-duct biliary reconstruction in left-lobe adult-living-donor liver transplantation. Transplantation 75:557-559.

Soejima Y, et al, 2003b: Use of steatotic graft in living-donor liver transplantation. Transplantation 76:344-348.

Soin AS, et al, 1996: Donor arterial variations in liver transplantation: management and outcome of 527 consecutive grafts. Br J Surg 83:637-641.

Starzl TE, et al, 1968: Orthotopic homotransplantation of the human liver. Ann Surg 168:392-415.

Stevens LH, et al, 1992: Hepatic artery thrombosis in infants: a comparison of whole livers, reduced-size grafts, and grafts from living-related donors. Transplantation 53:396-399.

Strasberg SM, 1997: Terminology of liver anatomy and liver resections: coming to grips with hepatic Babel. J Am Coll Surg 184:413-434.

Sugawara Y, Makuuchi M, 2001: Surgical technique for hepatic venous reconstruction in liver transplantation. Nippon Geka Gakkai Zasshi 102:794-797.

Sugawara Y, et al, 2001: Small-for-size grafts in living-related liver transplantation. J Am Coll Surg 192:510-513.

Sugawara Y, et al, 2002a: Living donor liver transplantation for fulminant hepatic failure. Transplant Proc 34:3287-3288.

Sugawara Y, et al, 2002b: New venoplasty technique for the left liver plus caudate lobe in living donor liver transplantation. Liver Transplant 8:76-77.

Sugawara Y, et al, 2003: Left liver grafts for patients with MELD score of less than 15. Transplant Proc 35:1433-1434.

Sugawara Y, et al, 2004: Refinement of venous reconstruction using cryopreserved veins in right liver grafts. Liver Transplant 10:541-547.

Surman OS, 2002: The ethics of partial-liver donation. N Engl J Med 346:1038.

Suzuki T, et al, 1971: Surgical significance of anatomic variations of the hepatic artery. Am J Surg 122:505-512.

Takayama T, et al, 2000: Living-related transplantation of left liver plus caudate lobe. J Am Coll Surg 190:635-638.

Tanaka K, et al, 1993: Surgical techniques and innovations in living related liver transplantation. Ann Surg 217:82-91.

Testa G, et al, 2000: Biliary anastomosis in living related liver transplantation using the right liver lobe: techniques and complications. Liver Transplant 6:710-714.

Testa G, et al, 2001: From living related to in-situ split liver transplantation: how to reduce waiting-list mortality. Pediatr Transplant 5:16-20.

Todo S, Furukawa H, 2004: Living donor liver transplantation for adult patients with hepatocellular carcinoma: experience in Japan. Japanese Study Group on Organ Transplantation. Ann Surg 240:451-461.

Troisi R, de Hemptinne B, 2003: Clinical relevance of adapting portal vein flow in living donor liver transplantation in adult patients. Liver Transplant 9:S36-S41.

Tzakis A, et al, 1989: Orthotopic liver transplantation with preservation of the inferior vena cava. Ann Surg 210:649-652.

Uchino S, et al, 2004: Steatotic liver allografts up-regulate UCP-2 expression and suffer necrosis in rats. J Surg Res 120:73-82.

United Network for Organ Sharing (UNOS), 2004: The organ procurement and transplantation network data base. Available at: http://www.unos.org. Accessed October 1, 2004.

Varotti G, et al, 2004: Anatomic variations in right liver living donors. J Am Coll Surg 198:577-582.

Wachs ME, et al, 1998: Adult living donor liver transplantation using a right hepatic lobe. Transplantation 66:1313-1316.

Wei WI, et al, 2004: Microvascular reconstruction of the hepatic artery in live donor liver transplantation: experience across a decade. Arch Surg 139:304-307.

Yamaoka Y, et al, 1994: Liver transplantation using a right lobe graft from a living related donor. Transplantation 57:1127-1130.

Yamaoka Y, et al, 1995: Safety of the donor in living-related liver transplantation—an analysis of 100 parental donors. Transplantation 59:224-226.

Yao FY, et al, 2003: A follow-up analysis of the pattern and predictors of dropout from the waiting list for liver transplantation in patients with hepatocellular carcinoma: implications for the current organ allocation policy. Liver Transplant 9:684-692.

Yeh BM, et al, 2004: Biliary tract depiction in living potential liver donors: comparison of conventional MR, mangafodipir trisodium-enhanced excretory MR, and multi-detector row CT cholangiography—initial experience. Radiology 230:645-651.

Yoshizumi T, et al, 2003: A simple new formula to assess liver weight. Transplant Proc 35:1415-1420.

Zimmerman MA, Trotter JF, 2003: Living donor liver transplantation in patients with hepatitis C. Liver Transplant 9:S52-S57.

110

Early and Late Complications of Liver Transplantation

J. J. POMPOSELLI AND R. L. JENKINS

Liver transplantation has evolved from a risky procedure with high morbidity and mortality to a standard treatment for patients with liver failure. Patients who undergo successful liver replacement have 5-year survival rates exceeding 70% (Muraji et al, 1997). Despite this dramatic improvement in outcome, a significant percentage of patients experience complications that can result in the need for reoperation or can be life-threatening. As expertise in the procedure grows, surgeons are willing to attempt liver transplantation in patients who previously were considered poor candidates for surgery. Recipient portal vein thrombosis was considered an absolute contraindication to surgery, but now transplantation is commonly performed in the presence of portal vein thrombosis (Shaked & Busuttil, 1991; Stieber et al, 1991).

As surgeons continue to develop new surgical procedures, such as reduced size grafts, split liver transplantation, and living donor liver transplantation, a new series of complications unique to these procedures are emerging (Broelsch et al, 2000; Emond et al, 1993). The incidence of hepatic artery thrombosis, bile leaks, and stricture is at least two times higher in patients who receive living donor grafts compared with cadaveric grafts (Malago et al, 2003). Despite a higher morbidity rate in recipients of living donor grafts, patient and graft survival are similar (Fan et al, 2002; Lo et al, 2002). This chapter reviews common early and late complications that are encountered during and after liver transplantation. Because complications after liver transplantation represent a continuum, most can occur at any time after surgery.

PROCUREMENT INJURY TO THE GRAFT

The process of organ transplantation begins with identification of a suitable organ specific for a particular recipient patient. When an organ is identified, procurement teams are dispatched for recovery of various organs. Generally, the liver procurement team dictates the conduct of dissection below the diaphragm, while the cardiac team works in concert with the thoracic team if lungs and heart also are to be removed. Because the infradiaphragmatic dissection takes considerably longer than the thoracic dissection, careful planning is required to minimize cold ischemia time for the heart and lung, which are more time sensitive. The heart procurement team stays in contact with the recipient heart team to minimize total ischemic time. Under ideal conditions, the conduct of the operation is orderly and well controlled. A patient who progresses to brain death rapidly can show cardiac instability, however, and be difficult to manage. This situation can result in an expedited operation in which perfusion cannulae are hastily placed, and organ procurement rapidly follows. During such events, identification of appropriate anatomy is difficult, and technical errors are more likely to occur.

To increase the number of organs available, donation after cardiac death is a new form of donation that is increasing in incidence (Chin et al, 2002). In this form of donation, a patient who is deemed hopeless but has not met criteria of brain death is allowed to die naturally after removal of supportive measures. After a period of usually 5 minutes of asystole, organs can be procured for transplant. Despite the various periods of hypotension and warm ischemia that develop, outcomes with donation after cardiac death have been acceptable (Chin et al, 2002; Cooper et al, 2004). In liver grafts procured from donation after cardiac death donors, there is a suggestion of increased biliary strictures and worse long-term graft survival (D'Alessandro et al, 2004).

The most common injury during liver procurement is aberrant hepatic artery ligation and division. This injury occurs by failure to recognize a replaced or accessory right or left hepatic artery during hilar dissection or by unintentional division during organ removal. Such injuries are serious because segments of the liver are not perfused during recovery and usually require reconstruction on the back table before reimplantation. An additional anastomosis on the back table prolongs ischemic time, increases the chances of thrombosis, and increases the need for retransplantation. Prolonged ischemic time (especially >12 hours) increases the risk for graft loss and bile duct necrosis (Mor et al, 1993; Quiroga et al, 1991). To minimize dissection-related injuries, some authors prefer to use the en bloc method of removing intraabdominal organs with back table dissection (Imagawa et al, 1996). Regardless of the technique used, attention to detail and identification of the appropriate anatomy avoid graft procurement injury.

INTRAOPERATIVE HEMORRHAGE AND COAGULOPATHY

All patients with end-stage liver disease present to the operating room with derangements in coagulation, and many present with severe portal hypertension. The combination of these two conditions results in a significant challenge for the surgeon and anesthesiologist. Patients who have undergone previous operations are at particular risk because prolonged lysis of adhesions may increase greatly the duration of operation, create additional raw surface areas for bleeding, and lead to derangements in temperature and fluid homeostasis. The net result is worsening coagulopathy, which creates a vicious cycle during the procedure.

Improvements in surgical techniques and patient selection have led to the performance of liver transplantation without the need for blood transfusions in selected patients. The advent of transjugular intrahepatic portosystemic shunt (TIPS) can significantly lower portal hypertension preoperatively and may help to reduce blood loss during transplantation (Forster et al, 1994). A misplaced TIPS in the vena cava or portal vein can be a life-threatening complication during liver transplantation, however. In these situations, TIPS removal is difficult and may lead to massive hemorrhage if vascular control of the native vessels cannot be achieved.

In the presence of severe portal hypertension and underlying coagulopathy, the infusion of fresh frozen plasma and antifibrinolytic agents is the mainstay of therapy during liver transplantation (Palareti et al, 1991). These modalities cannot supplant the need for sound surgical technique with adequate control of all surgical bleeding sites. Bleeding observed after reperfusion may be related to poor initial graft function, but also has been related to the release of heparin and heparin-like substances from the graft. Kettner and colleagues (1998) used heparinase-modified thromboelastography to identify patients who developed bleeding secondary to the release of heparin-like substances. Such screening methods may help stratify patients at particular risk for the development of reperfusion fibrinolysis and offer future therapeutic strategies to control coagulopathy that is encountered immediately after reperfusion (Kettner et al, 1998).

When medical strategies fail to halt reperfusion fibrinolysis, intra-abdominal tamponade with laparotomy packs provides the most conservative management. If the graft functions well, and the patient responds to core temperature warming and continued resuscitation, packs usually can be removed within 24 to 48 hours. Prophylaxis against intra-abdominal sepsis with parenteral antibiotics is of unproven benefit, but prudent in the setting of immunosuppression.

PRIMARY GRAFT DYSFUNCTION OR NONFUNCTION

Numerous conditions can interfere with the initial function of the allograft after transplantation, including donor-related, procurement-related, and recipient-related factors. Donor-related factors that can affect graft function adversely include hemodynamic instability, poor nutritional status, extremes of age, drug toxicity, and steatosis (D'Alessandro et al, 2004; Marsman et al, 1996; Washburn et al, 1996). Although no uniform definition exists, the severity and prognosis for graft dysfunction vary considerably. The most ominous syndrome is primary graft nonfunction, which usually requires immediate retransplantation. In such instances, there is typically a progressive increase in serum transaminase levels (>8000 IU/L) within the first 24 to 48 hours in association with diminished bile and urine output. In our practice, postoperative trends in the prothrombin time have been the most reliable predictor of graft function and outcome. Laboratory studies drawn immediately after surgery serve as the baseline; the prothrombin time should plateau and then trend toward normalization over the next several days with good graft function. Any increase in the prothrombin time portends a worse prognosis and may represent primary graft nonfunction, especially if the increase in prothrombin time is rapid. An elevated prothrombin time that neither increases nor decreases may suggest primary graft dysfunction; recovery usually occurs with time if no additional insults, such as infection or rejection, occur. In these situations, infusion of prostaglandin E_1 may be beneficial in resolving or preventing renal or graft dysfunction (Chavin et al, 1996; Klein et al, 1996).

In addition to trends in the prothrombin time, clinical assessment can be helpful in identifying patients with graft dysfunction or nonfunction. Resolution of hepatic encephalopathy, adequate urine production, and absence of metabolic acidosis are reassuring in the early postoperative period. In patients who have received significant quantities of blood products, the development of metabolic alkalosis may be a sensitive indicator of early graft function (Driscoll et al, 1987). Such observations are based on the ability of the liver graft to process citrate in the administered blood products to bicarbonate. Failure to metabolize citrate to bicarbonate may reflect early allograft dysfunction.

VASCULAR COMPLICATIONS

Hepatic Artery Thrombosis

Vascular complications are a major source of morbidity and graft loss in liver transplant patients. Arterial complications, of which hepatic arterial thrombosis (HAT) is the most common, account for 64% to 82% of the vascular complications encountered (Bell et al, 1990; Leonardi et al, 2004). The overall incidence of HAT is 1.6% to 8% in various adult series, but can be 15% to 26% in pediatric patients (Busuttil et al, 1991; Mazzaferro et al, 1989; Tan et al, 1988). The incidence of HAT in living donor liver transplantation varies widely and is influenced by the type of graft, surgeon experience, and donor anatomy.

Doppler ultrasound is the best screening method and should be used liberally in the first 2 weeks after transplantation with any change in graft function or significant elevation in bilirubin or transaminases. Because collateral blood flow through the gastroduodenal artery can result in a false-negative test, care must be taken to establish arterial flow *within* the hepatic parenchyma. In cases of suspected HAT by ultrasound, confirmation should be made by celiac arteriography or multiphase computed tomography (Fig. 110.1). Failure to make a rapid diagnosis can result in hepatic necrosis and graft loss.

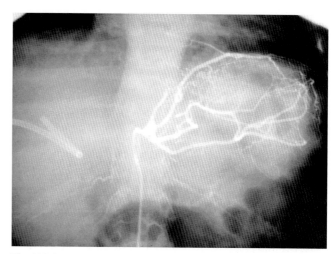

Fig. 110.1. Hepatic artery thrombosis. The patient developed a rapid increase in serum transaminases in the early postoperative period. Ultrasound could not locate an intrahepatic arterial signal. Celiac arteriography shows left gastric and splenic arterial flow and fails to show any contrast in the liver. This is consistent with intimal dissection of the entire common hepatic artery. The T-tube within the common bile duct is visible.

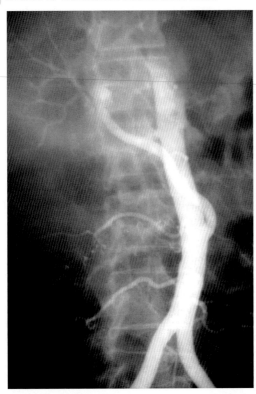

Fig. 110.2. Hepatic artery reconstruction. With early diagnosis of hepatic artery thrombosis, immediate reconstruction with a donor iliac artery allograft can be performed. In this case, the iliac artery graft is anastomosed between the infrarenal aorta and liver allograft common hepatic artery.

Intimal dissection of the recipient hepatic artery down to the origin of the celiac axis is a common cause of intraoperative HAT. In these cases, immediate reconstruction with a donor iliac allograft is indicated (Fig. 110.2). Under no circumstances should the patient leave the operating room without a completely revascularized graft. When a donor iliac allograft is unusable or unavailable, an autogenous saphenous vein graft should be used. Rarely, an artificial conduit made from Dacron or expanded polytetrafluoroethylene (Teflon) can be used.

The clinical presentation of HAT observed postoperatively ranges from a completely asymptomatic patient with minimal alterations in liver function to fulminant hepatic necrosis. A more common presentation of HAT is with postoperative biliary complications, including leaks and stricture formation (Margarit et al, 1998; Orons et al, 1995). Treatment for HAT in the early postoperative period is the same whether or not symptoms are present. Rapid re-establishment of arterial inflow should be attempted; this generally requires urgent operation with arterial reconstruction using a donor iliac artery allograft or autogenous graft material. Some authors have attempted thrombolysis using tissue plasminogen activator and urokinase, but this can be expected to be successful only when there are no technical factors contributing to the thrombosis (Hidalgo et al, 1989). Hepatic artery intimal dissection is not amenable to thrombolytic therapy; attempts at systemic thrombolysis waste valuable time and resources and worsen outcome. In most cases, 50% to 70% of patients ultimately require retransplantation (Langnas et al, 1991).

Portal Vein Thrombosis

Portal vein thrombosis (PVT) observed before surgery was previously considered an absolute contraindication to orthotopic liver transplantation. It may no longer preclude a patient from undergoing successful liver transplant, but the presence of PVT may increase substantially the surgical complexity and perioperative morbidity.

Reconstitution of portal flow usually can be obtained through portal vein thrombectomy in most cases or use of a donor iliac vein allograft anastomosed between the superior mesenteric vein and liver allograft portal vein (Davidson et al, 1994; Shaked & Busuttil, 1991). Living donor grafts that have relatively short portal vein segments can be difficult to reconstruct; approximately 10% of institutions consider PVT an absolute contraindication to living donor liver transplantation (Kadry et al, 2002).

PVT observed after transplantation is a rare complication and can occur immediately postoperatively usually for technical reasons, such as incomplete thrombectomy or twisting of the anastomosis. PVT observed several months to years after transplantation usually results from intimal hyperplasia with gradual cavernous transformation with collaterals. A high index of suspicion is needed to make the diagnosis. Accumulation of ascites, splenomegaly, or the presence of varices after transplantation should prompt investigation. Early thrombosis is best treated with reoperation, thrombectomy, and systemic coagulation. The treatment of late thrombosis is more controversial because direct repair is difficult. Transhepatic angioplasty with the placement of metal stents has been successful in some patients, whereas other patients have responded to selective shunting procedures to control variceal hemorrhage in the face of adequate liver function (Jenkins et al, 1999; Raby et al, 1991).

Inferior Vena Cava Obstruction

Inferior vena cava (IVC) obstruction is a rare complication that occurs in 1% to 2% of patients after liver transplantation (Wozney et al, 1986). Most surgeons prefer to anastomose the donor IVC to the suprahepatic and infrahepatic IVC. A growing trend is to perform "piggyback" transplantation with the anastomosis of the donor suprahepatic IVC to the confluence of the recipient middle and left hepatic veins, while leaving the recipient IVC in situ (Neuhaus & Platz, 1994; Tzakis et al, 1989).

In our experience in 90 consecutive liver transplants using the piggyback technique, two patients developed thrombus in their native IVC. The first IVC thrombosis developed in a patient with Budd-Chiari syndrome who had occluded middle and left hepatic veins and a misplaced TIPS in the right hepatic vein extending into the IVC at the time of transplant. Postoperatively, the patient developed profound pedal edema and ascites. Ultrasound confirmed the diagnosis and the condition was treated successfully with anticoagulation and balloon dilation without further surgery. The second patient was a young man who was urgently transplanted for fulminant liver failure secondary to hepatitis A. Complicating this operation was the presence of a high-grade bacteremia with *Staphylococcus aureus* at the time of transplant. Postoperatively, the patient did well, but developed persistent fevers of an unknown source. Gallium scan ultimately disclosed a nearly occluding infected thrombus in the infrarenal IVC. This thrombus was treated with long-term antibiotics and systemic anticoagulation with complete resolution after 6 weeks of therapy.

Treatment of an IVC thrombosis usually depends on the cause. Direct surgical removal of an IVC thrombosis is difficult to perform in a critically ill patient and requires extensive mobilization of the right colon and small bowel mesentery to facilitate exposure. Medical management of IVC thrombosis was successful in our experience and that reported by others (Kraus et al, 1992). Our experience suggests that a more conservative management algorithm using invasive radiologic procedures and systemic anticoagulation can treat this complication satisfactorily (Kraus et al, 1992). Thrombolytic therapy can be adjunctive in resolving "fresh" thrombus formation.

BILIARY COMPLICATIONS

Biliary tract complications related to bile duct reconstruction previously were considered the "Achilles heel" of liver transplantation. Improvements in operative technique have reduced these complications markedly. Nevertheless, bile duct obstruction and leaks are the cause of approximately half of all technical failures after transplantation and require reoperation in 10% to 20% of patients (Lerut et al, 1987). In general, recipients of living donor grafts have an incidence of biliary complications approximately two times higher than recipients of cadaveric grafts (Pomfret et al, 2001). HAT is associated with biliary complications and may explain the increased incidence among living donor graft recipients.

Biliary Leaks

The reported incidence of biliary leaks after liver transplantation varies widely from 10% to 50% (Rabkin et al, 1998; Reichert et al, 1998). Leaks are observed most commonly at the site of choledochal anastomosis or the choledochal T-tube insertion site. Leaks at the choledochal tube insertion site are observed most commonly at the time of tube removal and occur in 25% to 40% of patients (O'Connor et al, 1995). Most of these patients can be managed conservatively with a short course of analgesics and antibiotics. To minimize this risk, some surgeons prefer not to place any stent. In our practice, rather than using a conventional T-tube, we stent our choledochal anastomosis with a 5-Fr pediatric feeding tube placed through the cystic duct stump, which is secured with a hemorrhoidal band and polydioxanone suture (PDS). In theory, the hemorrhoidal band obliterates the lumen of the preformed tract at the time of stent removal (usually 6-8 weeks postoperatively). Anastomotic leaks encountered in the early postoperative period are related to technical errors, tension at the anastomotic site, or ischemic necrosis after hepatic artery thrombosis.

The bile ducts of living donor or split liver grafts can be reconstructed with a duct-to-duct (choledochocholedochostomy) or Roux-en-Y hepaticojejunostomy. The leak rate is similar with both types of reconstructions (Gondolesi et al, 2004). Signs and symptoms related to biliary leaks include bilious fluid in drains (biliary fistula), abdominal or shoulder pain or both, increased serum bilirubin, nausea, vomiting, and fever. Diagnosis can be confirmed by cholangiography if a choledochal tube is in place; otherwise, endoscopic retrograde cholangiography or percutaneous transhepatic cholangiography can be performed. We favor endoscopic retrograde cholangiography because treatment with endoscopic stent placement can be readily achieved without the

risk associated with indwelling transhepatic catheters used during percutaneous transhepatic cholangiography. Large biliary leaks resulting in bile collections adjacent to the liver require percutaneous drainage.

Leaks associated with ischemic necrosis need surgical revision with Roux-en-Y hepaticojejunostomy. The development of early postoperative leaks is associated with late stricture formation. Lifelong surveillance by the surgeon is warranted.

Biliary Stricture or Obstruction

Biliary obstruction occurs in approximately 7% to 15% of patients after liver transplantation (Klein et al, 1991; Lerut et al, 1987). As with leaks, the site of obstruction aids in determining the cause. Anastomotic stricture accounts for 50% of the cases and can occur early in the postoperative period secondary to edema or later resulting from compromised blood supply (Fig. 110.3). Biliary strictures usually present within weeks, but may occur years after transplantation. Two types of biliary obstruction usually are found: anastomotic and nonanastomotic. Nonanastomotic obstruction or stricture can be caused by or associated with bile duct ischemia or caused by sludge and debris that can accumulate in the biliary system post-transplant.

The diagnosis of biliary stricture or obstruction is implied by an obstructive pattern on routine liver function tests. Commonly, patients may present with constitutional symptoms of rigor, fever, headache, and fatigue. Occasionally, patients present with severe symptoms of cholangitis and sepsis. Because patients with "mild" signs and symptoms also may reflect the presence of acute rejection, HAT, cytomegalovirus (CMV) infection, or recurrent disease, diagnosis can be difficult. To ascertain the correct diagnosis rapidly, a series of diagnostic studies, including abdominal ultrasound, cholangiography, and liver biopsy, is obtained immediately after the onset of abnormal clinical signs and symptoms (Kuo et al, 1994).

Regardless of the method used to re-establish the biliary continuity, the most common site of a biliary stricture in the

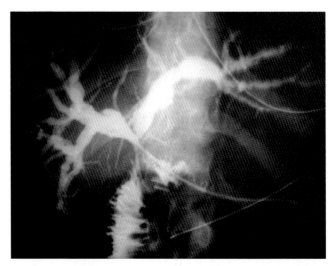

Fig. 110.3. Biliary stricture. This patient had a previously created Roux-en-Y hepaticojejunostomy and now has an anastomotic stricture. Note the dilated intrahepatic ducts. Percutaneous access of the Roux-en-Y limb affords the ability to make the diagnosis and treat with balloon dilation. Using this technique, placement of transhepatic catheters is avoided.

post-transplant setting is at the biliary anastomosis. Technical error during reconstruction is an important causative factor, but the patency of the hepatic artery also should be assessed, particularly in pediatric recipients. Other factors that have been implicated in the development of biliary stricture include ABO incompatibility, prolonged preservation times, chronic rejection, CMV infections, and recurrence of primary ductal disease, such as sclerosing cholangitis (Feller et al, 1996; Greif et al, 1994; Sebagh et al, 1995).

Biliary reconstruction after living donor liver transplantation is by Roux-en-Y hepaticojejunostomy or duct-to-duct anastomosis (Kawachi et al, 2002). Anastomotic leak or stricture is generally two times more common after living donor versus cadaveric liver transplantation (Miller et al, 2001).

Nonanastomotic strictures can occur in the hilar region or intrahepatically. As with anastomotic strictures, thrombosis of the hepatic artery or one of its branches should be suspected. Nonanastomotic strictures also have been reported in association with chronic ductopenic rejection, ABO blood group incompatibility, and as a result of ischemia-reperfusion injury associated with allograft preservation (Sanchez-Urdazpal et al, 1992).

After appropriate fluid resuscitation and antibiotic coverage, we recommend endoscopic retrograde cholangiography to confirm the diagnosis and to implement treatment with immediate stenting if possible. Failure to cross the stricture through endoscopic means requires percutaneous transhepatic cholangiography or surgical revision with Roux-en-Y hepaticojejunostomy. Intrahepatic strictures are best treated with percutaneous balloon dilation. Rarely, stents are needed to achieve a satisfactory outcome (Colonna et al, 1992).

RENAL DYSFUNCTION

Renal dysfunction is observed to some degree in almost every patient who undergoes liver transplantation (Baliga et al, 1992; Lam et al, 2004). Early renal dysfunction usually is characterized by a period of oliguria with a transient increase in serum creatinine, but also can be manifested as anuria with acute renal failure. Risk factors include preexisting renal dysfunction and primary graft nonfunction. In patients with normal preoperative serum creatinine and good initial graft function, the usual mechanism is prerenal azotemia secondary to periods of hypotension and hypovolemia experienced during the operative procedure. An additional insult to renal function can be incurred by the administration of nephrotoxic agents, especially the calcineurin inhibitors cyclosporine and tacrolimus.

Acute renal failure requiring dialysis is uncommon, unless the patient is diagnosed with preexisting hepatorenal syndrome, or severe hypotension and hemorrhage is encountered during surgery resulting in acute tubular necrosis. In our experience, dialysis for these patients is best performed with continuous venovenous hemodialysis using a dedicated large-bore double lumen venous access device. Recovery of normal renal function usually is achieved within 2 weeks if no other metabolic stress is incurred.

FLUID AND ELECTROLYTE DISTURBANCES

Fluid and electrolyte disturbances and alterations in acid-base status are universal after liver transplantation. Preoperative protein calorie malnutrition and end-stage liver disease lead to derangements in total body water and electrolyte balance. These derangements initially are worsened by the metabolic stress of surgery and massive fluid and blood product resuscitation. The rapidity of recovery depends in large part on the patient's renal and liver allograft function postoperatively. For a patient with stable postoperative renal and liver graft function, little metabolic manipulation is required to correct such derangements.

The early development of metabolic alkalosis secondary to metabolism of citrate in blood products is a favorable sign of graft function, but can be serious if alkalemia develops (Driscoll et al, 1987). In this situation, judicious replacement of chloride in the form of hydrogen chloride is warranted.

Excess total body water and sodium is best treated with gentle diuresis with furosemide. Careful repletion of potassium should be instituted, but should be monitored closely in the setting of medications such as tacrolimus, which tends to increase serum potassium levels (Oishi et al, 2000). Derangements in serum calcium, magnesium, and phosphorus are common in patients with cirrhosis and should be repleted to avoid neurologic, skeletal, and cardiac muscle dysfunction.

ACUTE CELLULAR REJECTION

In the early days of liver transplantation, the importance of rejection was overshadowed by technical complications. As surgical technique has evolved with concomitant improvement in graft preservation, rejection has taken on greater clinical importance. Acute cellular rejection is defined as an acute deterioration in allograft function that is associated with specific histologic changes in the liver allograft. These changes include a mixed inflammatory cell infiltrate (predominantly lymphocytes) involving the portal triads that disrupts the biliary epithelium and hepatic artery and portal venous endothelium (endothelialitis) (Sedivy et al, 1998).

The incidence of acute rejection is approximately 45% (range 24-80% depending on the series reported). Although acute rejection has little to no impact on mortality, significant morbidity results in increased hospitalization and overall costs (Bucuvalas et al, 2001; Khettry et al, 2002). In the early stage, most patients are asymptomatic, but a variety of clinical signs and symptoms may develop, including fever, abdominal pain, malaise, fatigue, and poor appetite.

The earliest laboratory indicator of acute rejection is elevated bilirubin level, which may be associated with a modest increase in alkaline phosphatase and aminotransferase levels. Prothrombin time and serum albumin levels are usually unaffected. Because laboratory measurements are neither sensitive nor specific for acute cellular rejection, liver histology obtained from a percutaneous biopsy specimen remains the standard for the diagnosis of cellular rejection (Khettry et al, 2002).

The initial treatment for acute cellular rejection includes high-dose pulse steroids, which is successful in approximately 80% to 90% of cases (Klintmalm et al, 1989). OKT3, a murine monoclonal antibody to the CD3 antigen-receptor complex, is reserved for the approximately 10% to 20% of patients in whom acute cellular rejection is not reversed by high-dose corticosteroid therapy. The major risks posed by treatment for acute cellular rejection include increased susceptibility to infection and the association between OKT3 use and post-transplantation lymphoproliferative disease (PTLD) (Deschler et al, 1995). In addition, a severe systemic inflammatory response can be initiated from OKT3 infusion leading to pulmonary edema, hypotension, and shock.

Chronic ductopenic rejection affects approximately 10% of liver transplant patients. Ductopenic rejection rarely occurs during the first 2 months after liver transplantation and is diagnosed on the basis of histologic criteria (van Hoek et al, 1992). Ductopenic rejection is defined as loss of bile ducts in more than 50% of portal tracts when 20 or more portal tracts are available for evaluation. In addition, arteriopathy affecting large and medium size arteries characterized by foam cell infiltration of the intima has been described. Ductopenic rejection is the most important manifestation of chronic rejection, which has been used synonymously with the histologic description *vanishing bile duct syndrome*. No treatment exists with the exception of retransplantation (Koukoulis et al, 2001).

INFECTION

With few exceptions, all patients who undergo transplantation are committed to lifelong immunosuppressive therapy to prevent graft rejection. Inadequate immunosuppression can result in graft loss, whereas injudicious use of immunosuppression can result in life-threatening infection or the development of PTLD. A tenuous balance exists between the proper amount of immunosuppression to prevent rejection and the risk for nosocomial and opportunistic infection. Despite better understanding of the immune response and proliferation of more selective immunosuppressive agents, approximately two thirds of transplant patients experience at least one episode of serious infection. Infection accounts for more than half of the observed mortality associated with liver transplantation (Kibbler, 1995). Risk factors for postoperative infection after liver transplantation include those incurred from the donor, recipient, and intraoperative course. Donor and recipient viral status, underlying medical comorbidities, and nutritional status all can contribute. Prolonged surgery with massive blood loss, prolonged ischemia time, and violation of the gastrointestinal tract also are risk factors for nosocomial infection (George et al, 1992).

Bacterial infections tend to occur within the first month after liver transplantation and vary from center to center (range 35-68%) (Kibbler, 1995; Kusne et al, 1992). Early risk factors include prolonged operating time, indwelling catheters, biliary obstruction, PVT, and poor graft function. In addition, vascular ischemia, recurrent hepatitis C, patient exposure to resistant organisms, and chronic rejection can contribute to nosocomial infection (Singh et al, 1997). Common bacterial pathogens include gram-negative organisms found in the bile (*Escherichia coli, Enterobacter* species, *Pseudomonas* species) and gram-positive organisms (*Staphylococcus aureus*, coagulase-negative staphylococci, and group D streptococci). Rarely, *S. aureus* can result in the development of toxic shock syndrome in the early postoperative period. *Listeria, Nocardia,* and *Legionella* are uncommon but significant pathogens (George et al, 1992).

Viral infections are common in immunocompromised posttransplant patients. In addition to the more common viral infections described subsequently, other equally important but less common viral infections can be devastating to immunocompromised transplant patients, including human immunodeficiency virus, adenovirus, influenza, and respiratory syncytial virus. In addition, transplant patients are at risk for acquiring viral hepatitis from infected organs, blood transfusions, and illicit drug use.

CMV infection, an asymptomatic infection in the general population, attains significant potential severity in immunosuppressed transplant recipients and is the most important pathogen in clinical transplantation (Kusne & Shapiro, 1997). CMV disease usually occurs 30 to 50 days after transplantation. Clinical manifestations include fever, malaise, arthralgia, leukopenia and thrombocytopenia, hepatitis, interstitial pneumonitis, enterocolitis, and disseminated disease. Differentiation between CMV disease and CMV infection is clinically important. CMV disease is defined as an invasive CMV infection with histologic evidence or a positive CMV culture from deep tissue specimens (e.g., liver biopsy, endoscopic mucosal biopsy or brushing, bronchoscopic mucosal biopsy or brushing) in the setting of clinical manifestation. The presence of positive blood, body fluid, or serologic tests is insufficient to establish the diagnosis of CMV disease. Liver biopsy with immunostaining using a monoclonal antibody against CMV antigen enables early diagnosis. Common histologic findings include hepatocyte necrosis, parenchymal microabscesses, and a magenta-colored intranuclear inclusion surrounded by a clear halo (owl's eye nucleus) (Everson & Kam, 1997).

Risk factors for the development of CMV disease include a seronegative recipient who received an organ from a CMV-seropositive donor, the use of antilymphocyte antibody therapy (particularly OKT3), and retransplantation. In general, the level of immunosuppressive therapy influences manifestation of CMV infection (Furukawa et al, 1996). Chronic CMV infection with persistent CMV replication within hepatocytes is associated with cholestatic hepatitis and the vanishing bile duct syndrome.

Patients who manifest CMV disease are treated with a reduction, if possible, of the immunosuppressive regimen, particularly tapering of the steroid dose. Intravenous ganciclovir has become the mainstay of therapy and is safe and effective for prophylaxis and treatment. Occasionally, foscarnet is required as an alternative in cases of ganciclovir resistance, but it is less well tolerated and can be nephrotoxic.

Prophylaxis against CMV disease using oral and intravenous ganciclovir post-transplantation has been effective. Other prophylaxis regimens using intravenous gancyclovir plus oral acyclovir for 3 months post-transplant or oral acyclovir used alone have been less successful (Nakazato et al, 1993; Oldakowska-Jedynak et al, 2003).

Herpes simplex seropositivity is present in most patients undergoing liver transplantation. Herpes simplex infection observed postoperatively usually is related to immunosuppression-induced reactivation. Herpesvirus infection usually manifests as a mild mucocutaneous oral or genital disease that responds to acyclovir treatment. Prompt recognition is important, however, to prevent progression to lethal disseminated disease or fulminant hepatitis with coagulopathy, disseminated intravascular coagulation, and death. Graft involvement is diagnosed by characteristic histologic picture on liver biopsy.

Epstein-Barr virus belongs to the herpes family. Infection in a transplant patient is characterized by a mononucleosis-like syndrome that differs from what is observed in the normal host by the absence of a heterophil antibody response and the infrequency of pharyngitis or splenomegaly (Alshak et al, 1993). The clinical significance of Epstein-Barr virus infection in a liver transplant patient has to do with its role in the pathogenesis of PTLD (Manez et al, 1997). The development of PTLD is thought to reflect the unrestricted proliferation of B cells stimulated by the Epstein-Barr virus infection. The incidence and treatment for established PTLD are discussed later.

Opportunistic infections also are commonly encountered. The incidence of clinically significant fungal *infection* is 20% to 25% in liver transplant recipients. Risk factors for fungal infection include poor nutritional status, retransplantation, bacterial infection with prolonged antibiotic use, high doses of immunosuppression, and biliary reconstruction using Roux-en-Y hepaticojejunostomy (Castaldo et al, 1991).

Disseminated fungal infection with *Candida* or *Aspergillus* can be difficult to diagnose and is associated with a high mortality rate in these patients. If the suspicion of invasive fungal infection is high, every effort should be made to obtain histologic or culture evidence to establish early diagnosis. *Aspergillus*, the second most frequent fungal infection in transplant patients after *Candida*, is acquired by inhalation and colonizes the airways before causing invasive disease. *Aspergillus* is angioinvasive and tends to disseminate to the central nervous system and can cause infarcts and cavitation in the lungs. The incidence of invasive aspergillosis is approximately 1% in liver transplant recipients with a mortality rate close to 100% despite adequate treatment (Kusne et al, 1992).

Infection by *Cryptococcus neoformans* usually occurs months to years after transplantation and affects approximately 0.25% of liver transplant patients (Patel et al, 1996). Because signs and symptoms may be subtle, delayed diagnosis is common. Presenting symptoms include change in mental status, headache, and fever. In our experience, one patient presented with lesions in the central nervous system and large cavitating masses in the thorax requiring operative removal.

Pneumocystis carinii pneumonia used to be a common pathogen in the immunocompromised host. With the introduction of routine use of prophylaxis with daily low dose oral trimethoprim/sulfamethoxazole for 6 to 12 months or aerosolized pentamidine in patients intolerant to trimethoprim/sulfamethoxazole, the incidence of *P. carinii* pneumonia has decreased dramatically. Because prophylaxis has been so effective, *P. carinii* pneumonia has occurred almost exclusively in patients who do not receive prophylaxis. Given the low morbidity associated with the prophylactic regimens, no patient should be excluded.

Legionella pneumophila is an uncommon cause of pneumonia in post–liver transplant patients. As with the normal host, the source of legionellosis is usually the water supply. Traditionally, treatment of *Legionella* pneumonia has been with erythromycin, but quinolones also have proved to be effective and have the advantage of not interacting with immunosuppressive agents (cyclosporine and tacrolimus).

POST-TRANSPLANT LYMPHOPROLIFERATIVE DISORDER

PTLD is a life-threatening complication of chronic immunosuppression. Lymphoproliferative disorders have been strongly associated with the replication of Epstein-Barr virus in B cells induced by enhanced immunosuppression (Manez et al, 1997; Newell et al, 1996); this has been observed primarily in patients who have received more than one course of polyclonal antilymphocyte globulin or monoclonal OKT3 (Davis et al, 1995). An association with CMV infection also has been noted. The incidence of PTLD varies from 1% to 3% among liver transplant recipients; prognosis depends on the histologic characteristics of the tumor. Polyclonal PTLD is treatable with discontinuation of immunosuppression with relatively low risk of rejection

(Hurwitz et al, 2004). Monoclonal PTLD is more difficult to treat and can result in death. Antibody against CD20 represents a novel approach in treating monoclonal PTLD with favorable outcome (Yedibela et al, 2003; Zompi et al, 2000). The clinical presentation of PTLD varies and includes fever, malaise, and lymphadenopathy with or without tonsillitis. In addition, gastrointestinal bleeding, perforation, or obstruction; hepatocellular dysfunction; and central nervous system manifestations such as seizures, mental status changes, and focal neurologic symptoms also have been described.

Lymphoproliferative disorders occurring after transplantation have different characteristics from the lymphoproliferative disorders that occur in the general population. Non-Hodgkin lymphoma accounts for 65% of lymphomas in the general population compared with 93% in transplant recipients. These tumors are mostly large cell lymphomas, and most are of the B cell type. Extranodal involvement is common, occurring in approximately 70% of cases (Zompi et al, 2000).

Treatment of polyclonal PTLD consists of reduction of immunosuppressive medications and antiviral therapy (Starzl et al, 1984). Patients with monoclonal PTLD and patients with polyclonal disease that does not respond to reduced immunosuppression have been treated with radiation, chemotherapy, and occasionally surgical resection. Therapy using monoclonal antibody against CD20 shows promising results for patients with monoclonal PTLD (Dotti et al, 2001; Zompi et al, 2000).

ACUTE IMMUNOSUPPRESSIVE DRUG TOXICITY

Immunosuppression after transplantation must achieve a balance between the beneficial effects of the drugs in preventing or reversing rejection and the dangers of overimmunosuppression with the development of acute toxicity symptoms, nosocomial infection, and lymphoproliferative disorders. The most common agents used for immunosuppression in liver transplant patients are the calcineurin inhibitors cyclosporine or tacrolimus (FK506) in combination with steroids. Azathioprine is used less frequently in liver transplant patients compared with kidney transplant recipients, who usually receive triple drug therapy. Mycophenolate mofetil (CellCept) has essentially replaced azathioprine in the immunosuppression regimen after liver and kidney transplantation. After the initiation of immunosuppression therapy, the development of infection and acute toxicity is usually seen early during treatment, whereas lymphoproliferative disorders and other malignancies are long-term sequelae as previously discussed.

In addition to PTLD, chronic immunosuppression has been associated with an increased frequency of many other neoplasms, including basal skin cancer, non-Hodgkin lymphoma, Kaposi's sarcoma, uterine cervical carcinoma, and carcinomas of the external genitalia (Busuttil et al, 1991). As with PTLD, patients who received repeated doses of antilymphocyte antibody have a particularly high incidence of neoplasms (Millis et al, 1995). Long-term use of steroids, particularly at high doses, is associated with obesity, hypertension, bone disease, glucose intolerance, pancreatitis, muscle weakness, hirsutism, and fluid and sodium retention. Growth retardation is a major problem in children (Busuttil et al, 1991).

The side effect profiles of cyclosporine and tacrolimus are similar and include gastrointestinal disturbances, headache, and tremor. Gingival hyperplasia and hirsutism are encountered frequently during cyclosporine and steroid treatment, whereas glucose intolerance is reported more often with tacrolimus treatment compared with cyclosporine therapy. Hyperkalemia, hyperuricemia, hypophosphatemia, and hypomagnesemia are manifestations of renal tubular dysfunction and usually can be controlled by adjusting the dose according to drug levels. Nephrotoxicity is the most clinically significant adverse effect of both drugs and is manifested as acute azotemia. This effect is largely reversible after reducing the dose of the drug and providing adequate hydration. Occasionally, progressive chronic renal disease can develop, which is usually irreversible. In such a situation, dialysis or kidney transplant is required. Other renal effects of cyclosporine include chronic tubular dysfunction and rarely hemolytic uremic syndrome (Cohen et al, 2002).

RECURRENT HEPATITIS

In patients who develop cirrhosis secondary to chronic hepatitis B, the recurrence rate as evidenced by signs of viral replication (hepatitis B e antigen–positive or positive titers of hepatitis B virus DNA) is approximately 80% to 90% in the first year. Given the almost universal recurrence of hepatitis B antigenemia in the early postoperative period, some authors have questioned the utility of liver replacement in these patients. With the advent of hepatitis B immunoglobulin and other adjuvant therapies, such as interferon and lamivudine, to prevent recurrent disease, transplantation now is routinely offered to patients with chronic hepatitis B infection with excellent results (Dodson et al, 2000; Grellier et al, 1996).

Recurrent hepatitis C infection is universal after liver transplantation (Gordon et al, 1997). In 90% of patients, hepatitis can be confirmed on routine biopsy. Of these, 60% have mild hepatitis, whereas 30% develop a more severe pattern on histologic examination. In patients with severe recurrent hepatitis C, 20% go on develop to cirrhosis within 5 years (Gordon et al, 1997). Of 100 patients with hepatitis C virus infection who are transplanted, approximately 6% require retransplantation (Gordon et al, 1997). Prophylaxis with ribavirin and interferon has been shown to be beneficial in reducing viral loads to zero with significant prolongation of graft survival (Ahmad et al, 2001). Given the epidemic growth in hepatitis C virus infection, hepatitis C is likely to dominate the indications for liver replacement for years to come.

BONE DISEASE

Almost all patients undergoing liver transplantation have some degree of hepatic osteodystrophy. The mechanism seems to vary according to the underlying disease. The causes are multifactorial and include corticosteroid therapy, bed rest, and cholestasis. Osteoporosis is particularly common 3 to 6 months after transplantation; however, by the end of the first year post-transplant, patients start gaining bone density. This late improvement is probably due to reduction in corticosteroid therapy and the resolution of the pretransplant condition that was deleterious to skeletal health. Atraumatic bone fractures are more frequent within the first 6 months post-transplantation as a result of the extensive bone loss that occurs during this period (Navasa et al, 1996). Avascular necrosis and vertebral body collapse also may occur.

NEUROPSYCHIATRIC COMPLICATIONS

Severe neuropsychiatric changes can occur after liver transplantation. In addition to the acute neurophysiologic changes associated with fluid and electrolyte shifts during the perioperative period, anxiety and depression are common psychiatric conditions observed in many transplant patients. Seizures, alterations of the levels of consciousness, and infections of the central nervous system are infrequent, but are significant causes of morbidity and mortality. Encephalopathy observed after transplantation can be related to poor initial graft function, but is more commonly multifactorial in etiology. Metabolic derangements, hypoxia, level of sedation, and drug interactions all can contribute.

Neurologic signs and symptoms associated with immunosuppression toxicity related to cyclosporine and tacrolimus include tremors, headaches, and seizures. These can be avoided by close monitoring of drug levels. High-dose steroids can result in emotional lability or mania. Any patients presenting with new neuropsychiatric symptoms should have a cranial computed tomography scan and lumbar puncture to rule out other causes of mental status changes, such as intracerebral bleeding or infectious etiology.

HYPERTENSION AND HYPERLIPIDEMIA

A common sequela of immunosuppression is the development of hypertension and hyperlipidemia in the post-transplant period (Fernandez-Miranda et al, 1998). As patient survival improves, the consequences of these conditions have greater importance on long-term prognosis. Hypertension is observed in approximately 70% of liver transplant recipients at 1 year with nearly 40% of patients developing sustained hypercholesterolemia and hypertriglyceridemia during the same time period. The pathophysiology of post-transplant hyperlipidemia is complex. Rapamycin immunosuppression does not cause glucose intolerance, but can lead to hyperlipidemia (Trotter, 2003). ω-3 Fatty acids found in fish oil can reduce hypertriglyceridemia significantly. In our experience, oral supplementation with over-the-counter fish oil capsules (4-6 g/day) has shown a dose-response reduction in serum triglycerides. Given the additional risk to the development of coronary artery and peripheral vascular disease, aggressive therapy with dietary changes, exercise, and medication is indicated.

SUMMARY

Liver transplantation is a lifesaving modality for patients with end-stage liver disease. The wide range of comorbidities that develop preoperatively contributes significantly to the development of postoperative complications. Aggressive use of immunosuppression is successful in preventing rejection in many cases, but can be complicated by the development of life-threatening neoplasms. Positive outcomes after liver transplantation require a multidisciplinary team approach comprising surgeons, transplant coordinators, hepatologists, and internists to maintain constant surveillance for the inevitable complications that arise. Early diagnosis with rapid treatment provides the best opportunity for disease-free survival.

REFERENCES

Ahmad J, et al, 2001: Recurrent hepatitis C after liver transplantation: a nonrandomized trial of interferon alfa alone versus interferon alfa and ribavirin. Liver Transpl 7:863-869.

Alshak NS, et al, 1993: Epstein-Barr virus infection in liver transplantation patients: correlation of histopathology and semiquantitative Epstein-Barr virus-DNA recovery using polymerase chain reaction. Hum Pathol 24:1306-1312.

Baliga P, et al, 1992: Preoperative risk factor assessment in liver transplantation. Surgery 112:704-711.

Bell R, et al, 1990: Vascular complications following orthotopic liver transplantation. Aust N Z J Surg 60:193-198.

Broelsch CE, et al, 2000: Living donor liver transplantation in adults: outcome in Europe. Liver Transpl 6(suppl 2):S64-S65.

Bucuvalas JC, et al, 2001: Predictors of cost of liver transplantation in children: a single center study. J Pediatr 139:66-74.

Busuttil RW, et al, 1991: Liver transplantation in children. Ann Surg 213:48-57.

Castaldo P, et al, 1991: Clinical spectrum of fungal infections after orthotopic liver transplantation. Arch Surg 126:149-156.

Chavin KC, et al, 1996: The effects of prostaglandin E1 on hepatic allograft vascular inflow: a prospective randomized double-blind study. Am Surg 62:184-187.

Chin LT, et al, 2002: Liver transplantation at the University of Wisconsin. Clin Transplant 207-213.

Cohen AJ, et al, 2002: Chronic renal dysfunction late after liver transplantation. Liver Transpl 8:916-921.

Colonna JO 2nd, et al, 1992: Biliary strictures complicating liver transplantation: incidence, pathogenesis, management, and outcome. Ann Surg 216:344-352.

Cooper JT, et al, 2004: Donation after cardiac death: the University of Wisconsin experience with renal transplantation. Am J Transplant 4:1490-1494.

D'Alessandro AM, et al, 2004: Donation after cardiac death: the University of Wisconsin experience. Ann Transplant 9:68-71.

Davidson BR, et al, 1994: Incidence, risk factors, management, and outcome of portal vein abnormalities at orthotopic liver transplantation. Transplantation 57:1174-1177.

Davis CL, et al, 1995: Antiviral prophylaxis and the Epstein Barr virus-related post-transplant lymphoproliferative disorder. Clin Transplant 9:53-59.

Deschler DG, et al, 1995: Posttransplantation lymphoproliferative disorder in patients under primary tacrolimus (FK 506) immunosuppression. Arch Otolaryngol Head Neck Surg 121:1037-1041.

Dodson SF, et al, 2000: Lamivudine after hepatitis B immune globulin is effective in preventing hepatitis B recurrence after liver transplantation. Liver Transpl 6:434-439.

Dotti G, et al, 2001: Anti-CD20 antibody (rituximab) administration in patients with late occurring lymphomas after solid organ transplant. Haematologica 86:618-623.

Driscoll DF, et al, 1987: Development of metabolic alkalosis after massive transfusion during orthotopic liver transplantation. Crit Care Med 15:905-908.

Emond JC, et al, 1993: Reconstruction of the hepatic vein in reduced size hepatic transplantation. Surg Gynecol Obstet 176:11-17.

Everson GT, Kam I, 1997: Liver transplantation: current status and unresolved controversies. Adv Intern Med 42:505-553.

Fan ST, et al, 2002: Biliary reconstruction and complications of right lobe live donor liver transplantation. Ann Surg 236:676-683.

Feller RB, et al, 1996: Biliary strictures after liver transplantation: clinical picture, correlates and outcomes. J Gastroenterol Hepatol 11:21-25.

Fernandez-Miranda C, et al, 1998: Lipoprotein abnormalities in long-term stable liver and renal transplanted patients: a comparative study. Clin Transplant 12:136-141.

Forster J, et al, 1994: The role of transjugular intrahepatic portosystemic shunts in the management of patients with end-stage liver disease. Am J Surg 168:592-597.

Furukawa H, et al, 1996: Effect of CMV serology on outcome after clinical intestinal transplantation. Transplant Proc 28:2780-2781.

George DL, et al, 1992: Patterns of infection after pediatric liver transplantation. Am J Dis Child 146:924-929.

Gondolesi GE, et al, 2004: Biliary complications in 96 consecutive right lobe living donor transplant recipients. Transplantation 77:1842-1848.

Gordon FD, et al, 1997: Relationship between hepatitis C genotype and severity of recurrent hepatitis C after liver transplantation. Transplantation 63:1419-1423.

Greif F, et al, 1994: The incidence, timing, and management of biliary tract complications after orthotopic liver transplantation. Ann Surg 219:40-45.

Grellier L, et al, 1996: Lamivudine prophylaxis against reinfection in liver transplantation for hepatitis B cirrhosis. Lancet 348:1212-1215.

Hidalgo EG, et al, 1989: High-dose intra-arterial urokinase for the treatment of hepatic artery thrombosis in liver transplantation. Hepatogastroenterology 36:529-532.

Hurwitz M, et al, 2004: Complete immunosuppressive withdrawal as a uniform approach to post-transplant lymphoproliferative disease in pediatric liver transplantation. Pediatr Transplant 8:267-272.

Imagawa DK, et al, 1996: Rapid en bloc technique for pancreas-liver procurement: improved early liver function. Transplantation 61:1605-1609.

Jenkins RL, et al, 1999: Distal splenorenal shunt: role, indications, and utility in the era of liver transplantation. Arch Surg 134:416-420.

Kadry Z, et al, 2002: Living donor liver transplantation in patients with portal vein thrombosis: a survey and review of technical issues. Transplantation 74:696-701.

Kawachi S, et al, 2002: Biliary complications in adult living donor liver transplantation with duct-to-duct hepaticocholedochostomy or Roux-en-Y hepaticojejunostomy biliary reconstruction. Surgery 132:48-56.

Kettner SC, et al, 1998: Endogenous heparin-like substances significantly impair coagulation in patients undergoing orthotopic liver transplantation. Anesth Analg 86:691-695.

Khettry U, et al, 2002: Centrilobular histopathologic changes in liver transplant biopsies. Hum Pathol 33:270-276.

Kibbler CC, 1995: Infections in liver transplantation: risk factors and strategies for prevention. J Hosp Infect 30(suppl):209-217.

Klein AS, et al, 1991: Reduction of morbidity and mortality from biliary complications after liver transplantation. Hepatology 14:818-823.

Klein AS, et al, 1996: Prostaglandin E1 administration following orthotopic liver transplantation: a randomized prospective multicenter trial. Gastroenterology 111:710-715.

Klintmalm GB, et al, 1989: Rejection in liver transplantation. Hepatology 10:978-985.

Koukoulis GK, et al, 2001: Cholangiocytic apoptosis in chronic ductopenic rejection. Hum Pathol 32:823-827.

Kraus TW, et al, 1992: Successful treatment of complete inferior vena cava thrombosis after liver transplantation by thrombolytic therapy. Br J Surg 79:568-569.

Kuo PC, et al, 1994: A comparison of operation, endoscopic retrograde cholangiopancreatography, and percutaneous transhepatic cholangiography in biliary complications after hepatic transplantation. J Am Coll Surg 179:177-181.

Kusne S, Shapiro R, 1997: Surgical infections in immunocompromised patients—prevention and treatment. Adv Surg 31:299-331.

Kusne S, et al, 1992: Infections during a randomized trial comparing cyclosporine to FK 506 immunosuppression in liver transplantation. Transplant Proc 24:429-430.

Lam P, et al, 2004: The efficacy and limitations of sirolimus conversion in liver transplant patients who develop renal dysfunction on calcineurin inhibitors. Dig Dis Sci 49:1029-1035.

Langnas AN, et al, 1991: Hepatic allograft rescue following arterial thrombosis: role of urgent revascularization. Transplantation 51:86-90.

Leonardi MI, et al, 2004: Late hepatic artery thrombosis after liver transplantation: clinical setting and risk factors. Transplant Proc 36:967-969.

Lerut J, et al, 1987: Biliary tract complications in human orthotopic liver transplantation. Transplantation 43:47-51.

Lo CM, et al, 2002: Ten-year experience with liver transplantation at Queen Mary Hospital: retrospective study. Hong Kong Med J 8:240-244.

Malago M, et al, 2003: Right living donor liver transplantation: an option for adult patients: single institution experience with 74 patients. Ann Surg 238:853-863.

Manez R, et al, 1997: Posttransplant lymphoproliferative disease in primary Epstein-Barr virus infection after liver transplantation: the role of cytomegalovirus disease. J Infect Dis 176:1462-1467.

Margarit C, et al, 1998: Biliary complications secondary to late hepatic artery thrombosis in adult liver transplant patients. Transpl Int 11(suppl 1):S251-S254.

Marsman WA, et al, 1996: Use of fatty donor liver is associated with diminished early patient and graft survival. Transplantation 62:1246-1251.

Mazzaferro V, et al, 1989: Hepatic artery thrombosis after pediatric liver transplantation—a medical or surgical event? Transplantation 47:971-977.

Miller CM, et al, 2001: One hundred nine living donor liver transplants in adults and children: a single-center experience. Ann Surg 234:301-312.

Millis JM, et al, 1995: Liver transplantation at the University of Chicago. Clin Transpl 187-197.

Mor E, et al, 1993: Roux-en-Y anastomotic bleeding following orthotopic liver transplantation: experience in our first 300 patients. Transplant Proc 25:1925-1926.

Muraji T, et al, 1997: Biliary atresia: current management and outcome. Tohoku J Exp Med 181:155-160.

Nakazato PZ, et al, 1993: Viral prophylaxis in hepatic transplantation: preliminary report of a randomized trial of acyclovir and gancyclovir. Transplant Proc 25:1935-1937.

Navasa M, et al, 1996: Quality of life, major medical complications and hospital service utilization in patients with primary biliary cirrhosis after liver transplantation. J Hepatol 25:129-134.

Neuhaus P, Platz KP, 1994: Liver transplantation: newer surgical approaches. Baillieres Clin Gastroenterol 8:481-493.

Newell KA, et al, 1996: Posttransplant lymphoproliferative disease in pediatric liver transplantation: interplay between primary Epstein-Barr virus infection and immunosuppression. Transplantation 62:370-375.

O'Connor TP, et al, 1995: Biliary tract complications after liver transplantation. Arch Surg 130:312-317.

Oishi M, et al, 2000: A case of hyperkalemic distal renal tubular acidosis secondary to tacrolimus in living donor liver transplantation. Transplant Proc 32:2225-2226.

Oldakowska-Jedynak U, et al, 2003: Cytomegalovirus infection as a common complication following liver transplantation. Transplant Proc 35:2295-2297.

Orons PD, et al, 1995: Hepatic artery stenosis in liver transplant recipients: prevalence and cholangiographic appearance of associated biliary complications. AJR Am J Roentgenol 165:1145-1149.

Palareti G, et al, 1991: Coagulation and fibrinolysis in orthotopic liver transplantation: role of the recipient's disease and use of antithrombin III concentrates. S. Orsola Working Group on Liver Transplantation. Haemostasis 21:68-76.

Patel R, et al, 1996: Risk factors of invasive *Candida* and non-*Candida* fungal infections after liver transplantation. Transplantation 62:926-934.

Pomfret EA, et al, 2001: Live donor liver transplantation. J Hepatol 34:613-624.

Quiroga J, et al, 1991: Cause and timing of first allograft failure in orthotopic liver transplantation: a study of 177 consecutive patients. Hepatology 14:1054-1062.

Rabkin JM, et al, 1998: Biliary tract complications of side-to-side without T tube versus end-to-end with or without T tube choledochocholedochostomy in liver transplant recipients. Transplantation 65:193-199.

Raby N, et al, 1991: Stenoses of vascular anastomoses after hepatic transplantation: treatment with balloon angioplasty. AJR Am J Roentgenol 157:167-171.

Reichert PR, et al, 1998: Biliary complications of reduced-organ liver transplantation. Liver Transpl 4:343-349.

Sanchez-Urdazpal L, et al, 1992: Ischemic-type biliary complications after orthotopic liver transplantation. Hepatology 16:49-53.

Sebagh M, et al, 1995: Sclerosing cholangitis following human orthotopic liver transplantation. Am J Surg Pathol 19:81-90.

Sedivy R, et al, 1998: Apoptotic hepatocytes in rejection and vascular occlusion in liver allograft specimens. Histopathology 32:503-507.

Shaked A, Busuttil RW, 1991: Liver transplantation in patients with portal vein thrombosis and central portacaval shunts. Ann Surg 214:696-702.

Singh N, et al, 1997: Intensive care unit management in liver transplant recipients: beneficial effect on survival and preservation of quality of life. Clin Transplant 11:113-120.

Starzl TE, et al, 1984: Reversibility of lymphomas and lymphoproliferative lesions developing under cyclosporin-steroid therapy. Lancet 1:583-587.

Stieber AC, et al, 1991: The spectrum of portal vein thrombosis in liver transplantation. Ann Surg 213:199-206.

Tan KC, et al, 1988: Hepatic artery thrombosis in pediatric liver transplantation. J Pediatr Surg 23:927-930.

Trotter JF, 2003: Sirolimus in liver transplantation. Transplant Proc 35(3 suppl): 193S-200S.

Tzakis A, et al, 1989: Orthotopic liver transplantation with preservation of the inferior vena cava. Ann Surg 210:649-652.

van Hoek B, et al, 1992: Severe ductopenic rejection following liver transplantation: incidence, time of onset, risk factors, treatment, and outcome. Semin Liver Dis 12:41-50.

Washburn WK, et al, 1996: Graft function and outcome of older (> or = 60 years) donor livers. Transplantation 61:1062-1066.

Wozney P, et al, 1986: Vascular complications after liver transplantation: a 5-year experience. AJR Am J Roentgenol 147:657-663.

Yedibela S, et al, 2003: Anti-CD20 monoclonal antibody treatment of Epstein-Barr virus–induced intrahepatic lymphoproliferative disorder following liver transplantation. Transpl Int 16:197-201.

Zompi S, et al, 2000: Rituximab (anti-CD20 monoclonal antibody) for the treatment of patients with clonal lymphoproliferative disorders after orthotopic liver transplantation: a report of three cases. J Hepatol 32:521-527.

111

Techniques of Liver Replacement

A. MARCOS AND T. E. STARZL

The steps by which liver replacement became the treatment of choice for numerous end-stage liver diseases (Starzl et al, 1989) were summarized more recently (Starzl, 2002). The basic operation was developed in dogs in 1958-1960 and attempted clinically in 1963 under azathioprine-prednisone immunosuppression. The first humans with prolonged survivals were reported in 1967 (Starzl, 1969). It was not until the availability of cyclosporine in the 1980s, however, that orthotopic liver transplantation became accepted worldwide as effective therapy. The results improved again with the advent of tacrolimus in the 1990s.

Elements other than immunosuppression have contributed to success, including improved patient selection and pretransplant management, noninvasive diagnostic methods, new antibiotics, and advances in anesthetic and perioperative critical care. Perfection of the donor and recipient operations was the crucial factor, however, on which all else ultimately depended. Surgical techniques employed at the University of Colorado and, since January 1981, at the University of Pittsburgh are presented in this chapter with emphasis on principles rather than details.

DONOR OPERATION

The use of multiple organs from a single cadaveric donor became practical with the development of standard procurement methods in the early 1980s. Subsequently, the University of Wisconsin preservation solution made storage of hepatic and other kinds of organ grafts relatively safe for 18 hours. The availability of this much time has allowed widespread sharing of livers, while permitting an accurate assessment of the grafts by histologic and metabolic criteria.

Standard Liver Procurement

A midline incision is made from the suprasternal notch to the pubis exposing the abdominal and thoracic organs of potential interest (Fig. 111.1). After it has been verified that the liver has a normal consistency and color, the left suspensory ligament is incised, allowing the left lobe to be retracted anteriorly and to the right. This retraction exposes the upper part of the gastrohepatic ligament, which contains the left gastric artery, the smallest branch of the celiac axis, and the arterial supply of the liver (Fig. 111.2). If an anomalous left hepatic arterial branch originates from the left gastric artery (Fig. 111.3), it must be preserved in continuity with the main left gastric artery (see Fig. 111.3, *inset*).

The largest branch of the celiac axis usually is the common hepatic artery. The right gastric and gastroduodenal arteries are ligated and divided (see Figs. 111.4 and 111.2). If the left gastric, right gastric, and gastroduodenal arteries are ligated in that order, the subsequent dissection of the common duct and the portal vein is rendered relatively bloodless. The common duct is transected as low as possible. The gallbladder is incised, permitting the bile to be washed out (see Fig. 111.3); this avoids autolysis of the extrahepatic and intrahepatic bile duct epithelium during storage. The portal vein now is dissected inferiorly to the confluence of the splenic and superior mesenteric vein (see Fig. 111.4).

After completing the hilar dissection, the aorta is encircled where it passes through the diaphragm and again just proximal to its distal bifurcation. Cannulae for infusion are placed into the splenic vein and, after total body heparinization, into the distal aorta (see Fig. 111.4). When all procurement teams are ready, the aorta is cross-clamped at the diaphragm by the abdominal surgeons (see Fig. 111.4), while the thoracic surgical team clamps the ascending aorta. Moderately rapid infusion of cold University of Wisconsin solution is started into the splenic vein and terminal aorta. At the same time, a cardioplegic solution is infused into the midportion of the ascending aorta. Congestion of the different organs is prevented by an incision in the suprahepatic inferior vena cava that allows the blood and infusate to drain into the pericardium (see Fig. 111.4).

In adults, the liver usually feels cool after 1 L of infusion through the splenic vein and aorta. Smaller volumes are used for children. When the liver becomes cold and blanched, and the heart has been removed, the total hepatectomy is completed. The remaining dissection must be performed expeditiously but methodically. If the celiac axis is retained with the graft, a proximal segment of its splenic arterial branch also should be conserved for potential reconstruction of an anomalous hepatic artery (see later). One such aberrant artery originating from the superior mesenteric artery commonly is found posterior to the portal vein (Fig. 111.5). If the pancreas is to be discarded, the anomalous retroportal artery can be kept in continuity with the superior mesenteric artery, which can be traced to the aorta (see Fig. 111.5, *inset*), where its origin can be incorporated into a Carrel patch that is shared with the mouth of the celiac axis.

The liver is attached primarily by the vena cava above and below the liver. The vena cava below the liver is transected above the entry of the left and right renal veins (Fig. 111.6). The vena cava above the liver is transected with a surrounding rim of diaphragm that is carefully excised on the back table. The retrohepatic vena cava is dissected free, including ligation of the right adrenal vein and posterior lumbar tributaries. The liberated liver

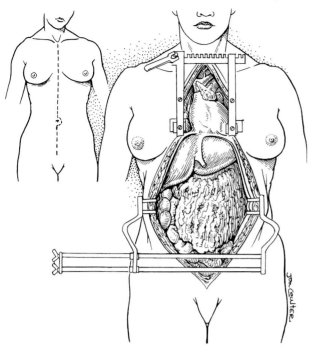

Fig. 111.1. Initial steps for liver retrieval, including complete dissection of the hepatic hilum with the standard multiple organ procurement technique.

is immediately placed in a solution-filled preservation bag that is packed in ice (see Fig. 111.7).

Modified Donor Procedures

Rapid Procurement

Use of the standard technique in stable donors has allowed the training of relatively inexperienced surgeons in the performance of a donor hepatectomy. When the technique is mastered, faster methods (also developed in Pittsburgh) can be applied electively or if required by urgent clinical circumstances. With the rapid techniques, little or no preliminary dissection is done except for encirclement of the supraceliac aorta and cannulation of the inferior mesenteric vein and terminal aorta (Fig. 111.8). If the heart is to be removed, the cardiac surgeon proceeds as if other organs are not to be harvested, but gives a warning when the circulation is stopped.

At the moment heart function ceases, the abdominal aorta is cross-clamped at the diaphragm, and an infusion of cold University of Wisconsin solution is started in the inferior mesenteric vein and the distal aorta (see Fig. 111.8). The amount of preservation fluid with the rapid technique is approximately double that used for the standard method (i.e., 2 L into the portal and arterial systems instead of 1 L each). When the liver becomes cold, the infusions are slowed. In the now bloodless field, the main vessels of the celiac axis can be ligated quickly, and the hilar dissection can be completed in a matter of minutes.

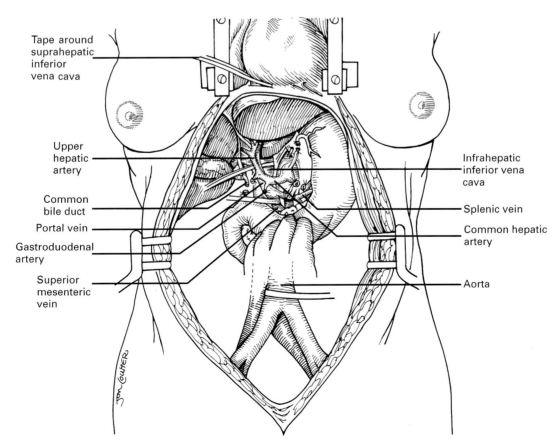

Fig. 111.2. Exposure for multiple organ retrieval in the cadaveric donor.

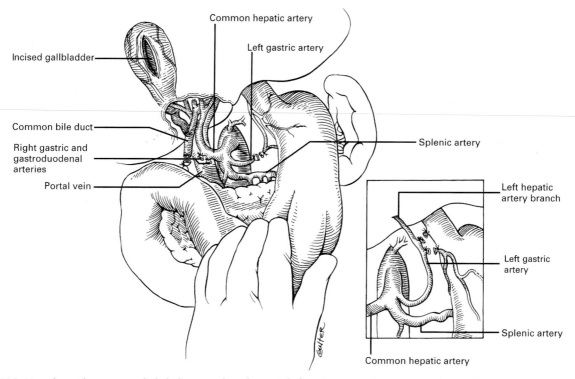

Fig. 111.3. Normal arterial anatomy in which the liver arterial supply is entirely from the common hepatic artery. The *inset* depicts a common anomaly in which all or part of the left lobar supply is from the left gastric branch of the celiac axis. The anomalous branch must be preserved. During the hilar dissection, the common duct is divided distally, and the gallbladder is incised to flush the biliary tree.

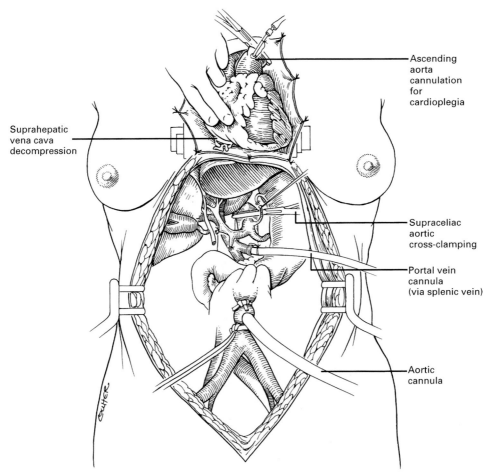

Fig. 111.4. In situ infusion technique used when the heart, kidneys, liver, and other viscera are removed from the same donor. University of Wisconsin preservation solution is infused into the splenic vein and distal aorta with simultaneous venting of the suprahepatic inferior vena cava into the pericardium. Note the aortic cross-clamp above the celiac axis. The cannulation and cross-clamping of the thoracic aorta for infusion of a cardioplegia solution also are shown.

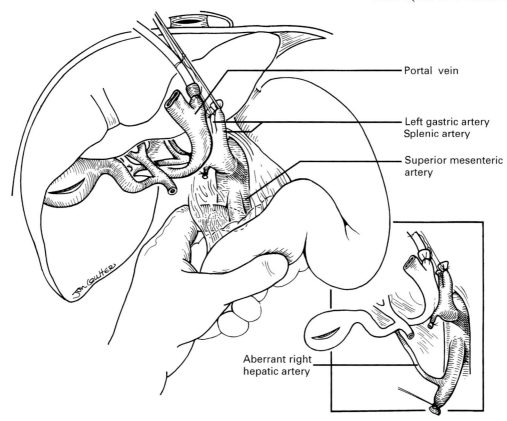

Fig. 111.5. Retraction of the liver and its portal structures to the right and performance of a Kocher maneuver to free up the duodenum and head of the pancreas. The presence of an anomalous right hepatic artery originating from the superior mesenteric artery *(inset)* just posterior to the portal vein is searched for.

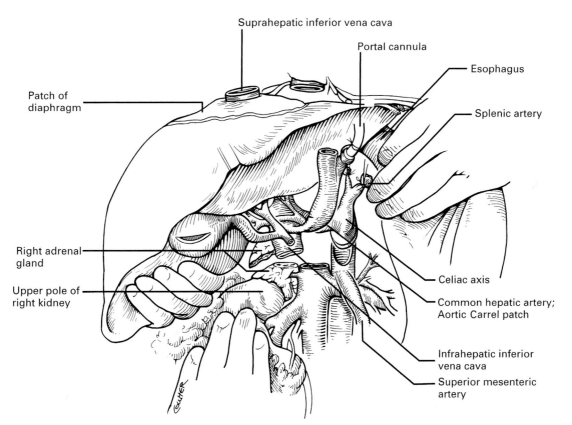

Fig. 111.6. The suprahepatic vena cava has been transected, with inclusion of a generous patch of diaphragm on the liver side. The infrahepatic vena cava is divided just above the origin of the renal veins. The celiac axis is removed with a Carrel patch of anterior aorta. If an anomalous right hepatic artery originating from the superior mesenteric artery is present, the origin of the superior mesenteric artery may be included in the Carrel patch (see Fig. 111.10A).

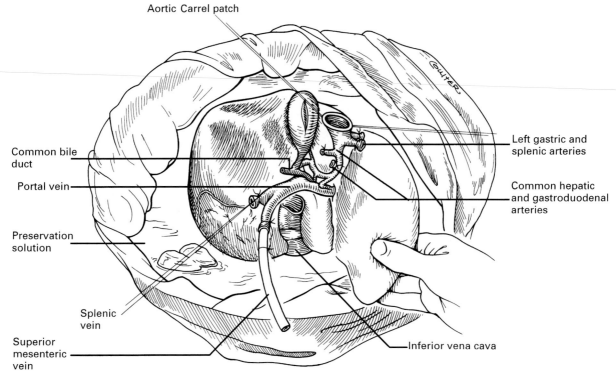

Aortic Carrel patch

Left gastric and
splenic arteries

Common bile
duct

Common hepatic
and gastroduodenal
arteries

Portal vein

Preservation
solution

Splenic
vein

Superior
mesenteric
vein

Inferior vena cava

Fig. 111.7. The liver graft is placed in a basin containing iced preservation solution for back table preparation. The vascular cuffs are débrided of excess tissue, and any needed arterial reconstruction is performed (see Fig. 111.10).

The portal vein is cleaned inferiorly to the junction of the splenic and superior mesenteric veins, and these two tributaries are divided. As in the standard method, the surgeon must promptly exclude the possibility of a retroportal right hepatic artery originating from the superior mesenteric artery. The hepatectomy is then completed. The kidneys, which are excised only after the liver has been removed from the field, are kept cold throughout by continued slow intra-aortic infusion of the preservation fluid. It is possible by performing all dissections in the bloodless field to carry out multiple organ removal, including the heart, liver, and both kidneys, in about half an hour. Procurement of the intestine adds only a few minutes.

Super-Rapid Procurement

In arrested or non–heart-beating donors, an even quicker procedure can be used to procure satisfactory organs. The method also can be applied in countries that do not have "brain death" laws or under special legal or religious circumstances. Here, cooling requires urgent cannulation and cold fluid infusion into the distal aorta (Fig. 111.9A). Sternum splitting, thoracic aorta cross-clamping, and severance of the suprahepatic inferior vena cava (for venous decompression) are done (see Fig. 111.9B), deferring cannulation and perfusion of the portal venous system until after the various organs are at least partly cooled intra-arterially (see Fig. 111.9C). The various dissections are done in the same way as with the standard and rapid techniques. Effective application of this method requires an extremely high level of skill.

Back Table Surgery

No matter what procurement method has been used, further preparation of the liver is done on a separate back table before delivering the graft to the recipient surgeon. This liver should be kept cold by emerging it in a basin containing sterile ice slush (Fig. 111.7). Back table preparation includes the following:

1. Dissection and removal of extraneous tissue, such as diaphragm, adrenal gland, lymph node, pancreatic, peripancreatic, and ganglionic tissue
2. Preparation of cuffs of the suprahepatic and infrahepatic vena cava, cleaning of the portal vein and artery, and inspection of the bile duct
3. Verification of secure ligatures on small retrohepatic caval, portal vein, and hepatic arterial branches
4. Insurance of the continuity and integrity of all major structures that must be anastomosed to the companion recipient structures

Failure to have the graft completely ready for implantation when it is brought to the recipient operative field can result in irreversible damage to the graft or make it impossible to complete the recipient operation. Several methods of back table vascular reconstruction have been designed to repair technical accidents or to accommodate aberrant vessels or congenital anomalies. A common reason for back table reconstruction is the presence of an anomalous right hepatic artery originating from the superior mesenteric artery (Fig. 111.10).

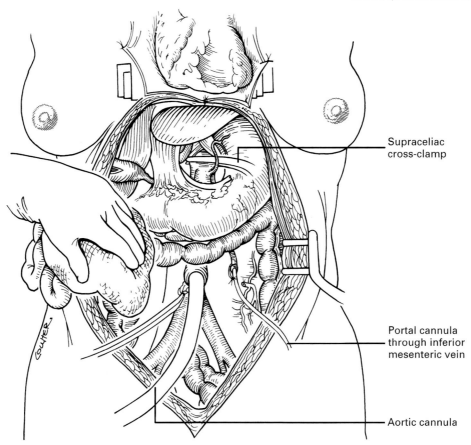

Supraceliac
cross-clamp

Portal cannula
through inferior
mesenteric vein

Aortic cannula

Fig. 111.8. Rapid technique of organ retrieval in which the initial dissection is limited to the exposure needed for the insertion of perfusion cannulae in the inferior mesenteric vein and distal aorta. If only the abdominal organs are to be used, the aorta is cross-clamped at the diaphragm.

Liver, Pancreas, and Intestine Procurement from the Same Donor

The pancreas and intestine can be retrieved independently or together with the liver. Before starting the procurement, the operation should be discussed by the involved surgeons. Considerations include organ priority, type and amount of preservation solution to be used, presence of aberrant hepatic arteries, length of portal vein, and a decision about which organ retains the celiac axis or superior mesenteric artery. An important step in any cadaveric donor operation is the removal and storage of long segments of the donor iliac arteries and veins and of other arteries and veins. These vessels can be used as vascular grafts to reconstruct the blood supply of the individual organs. With increased experience, it is rare to see any of the abdominal visceral organs discarded for purely technical reasons.

RECIPIENT OPERATION

The recipient procedure tends to be long and physically demanding. Its different parts are so remarkably dissimilar that a single surgeon operating from "skin to skin" may find it difficult to change emotional and intellectual gears to keep pace with the evolving events. Removal of the diseased liver may be one of the most difficult challenges a surgeon faces. Yet, the vascular anastomoses can be among the most delicate and

sophisticated procedures one performs, especially in very small children. Achieving perfect hemostasis after the donor liver has been revascularized is crucial because failure can ruin all that has been accomplished; however, this is often an exhausting exercise, particularly at the end of many hours of demanding surgery. Finally, the delicate biliary tract reconstruction becomes the final thread on which the whole enterprise is suspended.

Abdominal Incision and Exposure

The exact location of the incisions may be influenced by previous right upper quadrant surgery, the presence of an ileostomy, the size and configuration of the liver, or other factors. A bilateral subcostal incision, extending on the right to just beyond the midaxillary line and on the left to just short of the anterior axillary line, with an upper midline extension and excision of the xiphoid process, was once the most commonly used incision (Fig. 111.11A). Such drastic exposure is not needed unless the patient has had extensive prior surgery with multiple adhesions. In other unusual circumstances, a lower midline extension may be needed (see Fig. 111.11A), especially if exposure of the distal aorta is required for reconstruction of the hepatic arterial supply. Thoracic extensions are rarely needed.

A bilateral subcostal incision (see Fig. 111.11B) or a right subcostal incision with or without an upper midline extension (see Fig. 111.11C) may be used. The right subcostal incision is

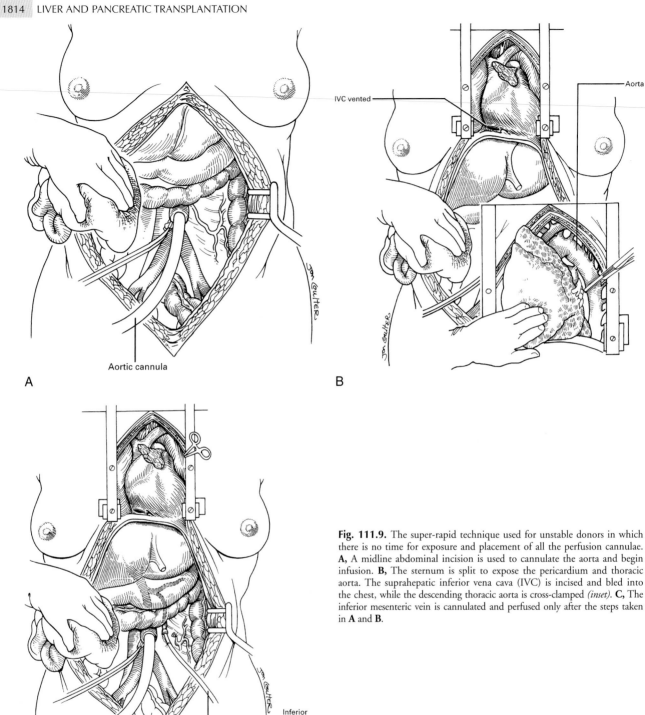

Fig. 111.9. The super-rapid technique used for unstable donors in which there is no time for exposure and placement of all the perfusion cannulae. **A,** A midline abdominal incision is used to cannulate the aorta and begin infusion. **B,** The sternum is split to expose the pericardium and thoracic aorta. The suprahepatic inferior vena cava (IVC) is incised and bled into the chest, while the descending thoracic aorta is cross-clamped *(inset)*. **C,** The inferior mesenteric vein is cannulated and perfused only after the steps taken in **A** and **B**.

the most common one in current use (see Fig. 111.11C). The upper midline extension shown in Figure 111.11C usually is unnecessary in pediatric patients, and it frequently can be omitted in adults. Massive hepatomegaly, extensive prior abdominal surgery, or other factors may mandate the selection of a more disfiguring incision (see Fig. 111.11A or 111.11B). In patients requiring concomitant splenectomy or interruption of a prior splenorenal shunt, the incision may need to be extended to the left subcostal region.

Improved exposure with any of these incisions can be obtained with the use of the Rochard or other rib retractor, which permits access to the hepatic veins and suprahepatic vena cava (Fig. 111.12). In making the incision, it may be necessary to abandon delicate celiotomy techniques of meticulous hemostasis and resort to continuous hemostatic suturing along the cut edges of the fascia and preperitoneum. When the abdomen is entered, an effort must be made to find a plane of dissection just outside the liver capsule. Movement away from this plane risks an encounter

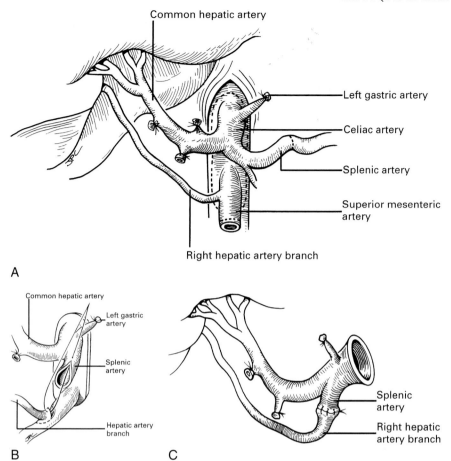

Common hepatic artery

Left gastric artery

Celiac artery

Splenic artery

Superior mesenteric artery

Right hepatic artery branch

A

Common hepatic artery

Left gastric artery

Splenic artery

Hepatic artery branch

B

Splenic artery

Right hepatic artery branch

C

Fig. 111.10. Examples of reconstruction of an anomalous arterial supply to the liver. **A,** The origins of the celiac axis and superior mesenteric artery are removed from the anterior aorta in a common Carrel patch. **B** and **C,** An anomalous right hepatic artery is anastomosed to the graft splenic artery, leaving only the origin of the celiac axis for anastomosis in the recipient.

with major venous collaterals, which can result in disastrous hemorrhage early in the operation.

Intraoperative Determination of Surgical Strategy

There is no single best way to carry out orthotopic liver transplantation. When exposure has been obtained, it is important to assess the pathology and decide on the technical approach that best fits the pathologic circumstances. A surgeon who insists on following the same steps in unvarying order for all liver recipients experiences unnecessary hardship. The following is a description of the basic ingredients of the recipient operation, with particular emphasis on variations of host hepatectomy.

Venovenous Bypass

The most critical stage of the recipient operation is the anhepatic phase, during which the diseased liver is removed and replaced with the allograft. Obstruction of the portal vein and vena cava during this period results in splanchnic and lower body systemic venous hypertension. This situation has devastating consequences in some patients. During the early 1980s, a pump-driven venovenous bypass, used without recipient heparinization, was developed in Pittsburgh that allowed splanchnic and systemic blood

to return to the heart by way of an inflow cannula placed in the axillary vein (Fig. 111.13). This technique permitted the hepatectomy and implantation to be done with significant reductions in blood loss, intestinal edema, and postoperative renal failure.

Infants and small children weighing less than 15 kg tolerate venous occlusion reasonably well. Consequently, venovenous bypass has been routinely used only for patients of adult size. Even in adults, some experienced surgeons employ the bypass only when it becomes apparent that its use cannot be avoided. If bypass is not routine, the decision for or against its use should be made as early as possible in the course of the operation. The decision can be helped by testing the cardiocirculatory effects of test occlusion of the inferior vena cava and portal triad. If the test is conducted after preliminary dissection of the portal triad, and after the triangular and coronary ligaments are cut with entry into the right and left bare areas, it also is possible to evaluate the extent to which bleeding from raw surfaces can be anticipated without venovenous bypass.

Hilar Dissection

In "easy" cases, the individual hilar structures can be readily skeletonized. The hepatic artery and common duct are ligated as close to the liver as possible. The hepatic artery is dissected proximal to the origin of its gastroduodenal branch, facilitating exposure

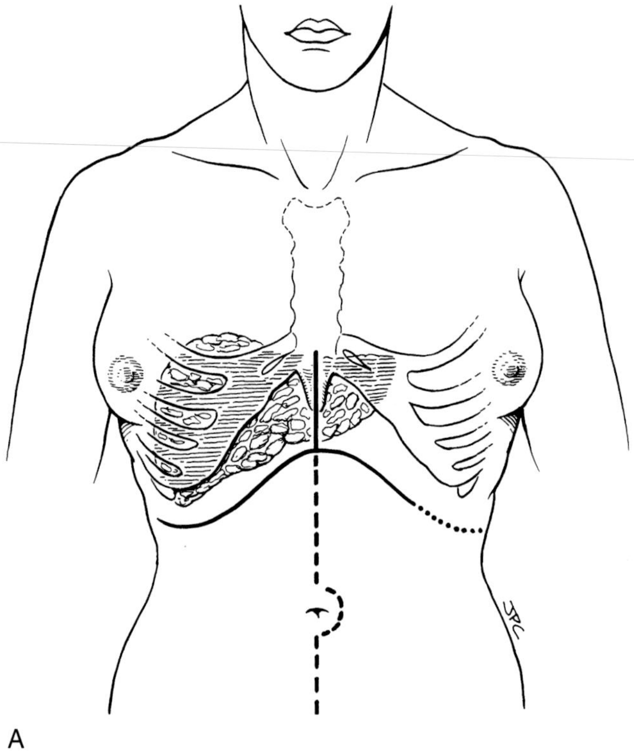

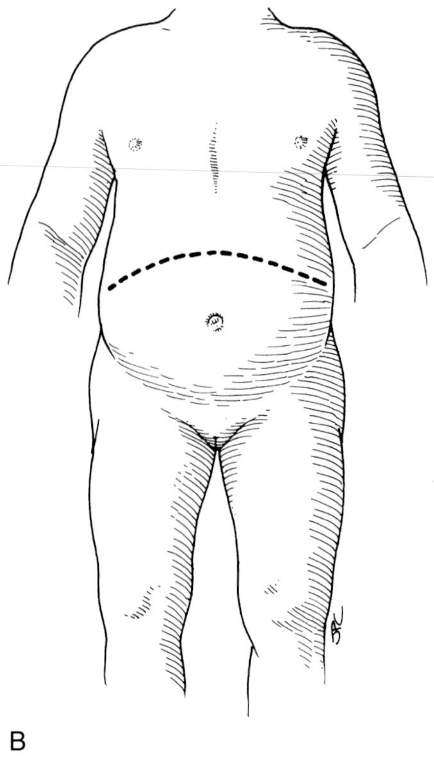

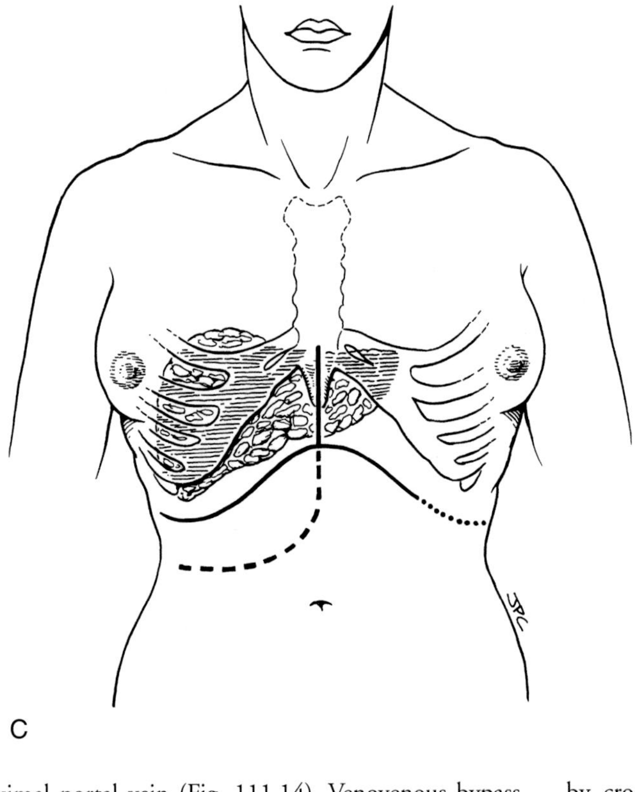

Fig. 111.11. Potential incisions for orthotopic liver transplantation. **A,** Bilateral subcostal incision with potential superior or inferior extensions. **B,** Inverted half-moon incision sometimes used in infants and small children. **C,** Simple subcostal incision that may be converted to a hockey-stick incision by an upper midline extension that may include xyphoid resection.

of the proximal portal vein (Fig. 111.14). Venovenous bypass can be initiated with cannulation of the transected portal vein at this time or later.

Host Hepatectomy with or without Vena Cava Removal

If hilar dissection has been accomplished uneventfully, the liver is devascularized and now can be excluded from the circulation by cross-clamping the vena cava above and below the liver (Fig. 111.15A). The diseased organ with or without the segment of retrohepatic vena cava can be peeled out working from the hilum up or from the diaphragm down. If the vena cava is part of the specimen, the obligatory ligation of the right adrenal vein (see Fig. 111.15C) imposes a risk of adrenal infarction. If this occurs with venous hypertension and bleeding, the right adrenal gland should be removed immediately. Other systemic venous tributaries to the vena cava segment from the lumbar regions also must

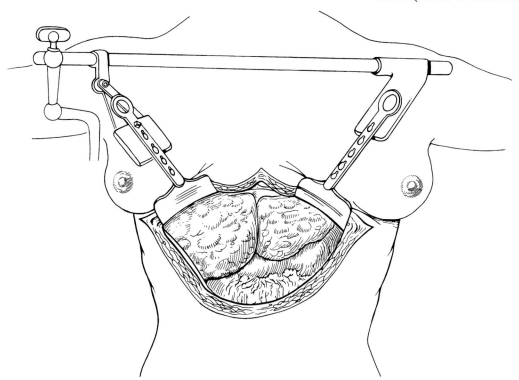

Fig. 111.12. Exposure, especially of the suprahepatic vena cava, can be facilitated by the use of self-retaining retractors, such as the Rochard device.

be scrupulously ligated. Because of regional venous hypertension in the right-sided bare area, it may be necessary then or later to obtain hemostasis by closing or oversewing the edges of the exposed bare areas with a continuous suture (see Fig. 111.15D).

Many of these problems can be circumvented if the host retrohepatic vena cava can be conserved (see Fig. 111.15A). Separation of

the diseased liver from the vena cava is done in the same way as in the classic experimental procedure of total canine hepatectomy. With this kind of hepatectomy, stumps of one or more of the main host hepatic veins are retained (see Fig. 111.16A) for eventual receipt of the allograft's venous outflow (Fig. 111.16B and C); this is known as the piggyback method of liver transplantation.

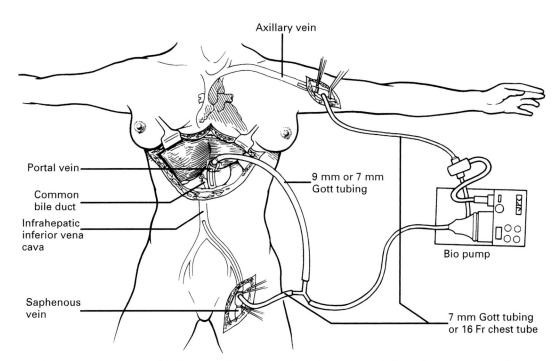

Fig. 111.13. Pump-driven venovenous bypass used to decompress the systemic and splanchnic venous beds during the anhepatic phase of liver transplantation.

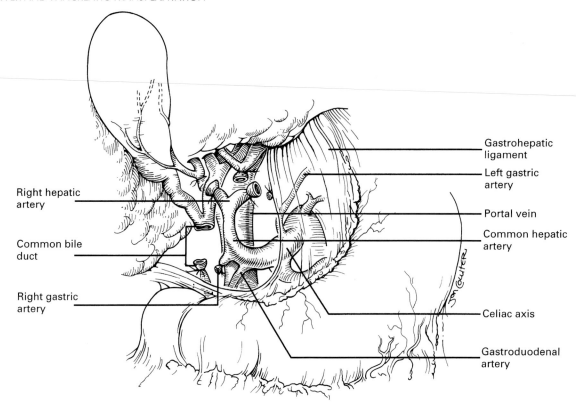

Fig. 111.14. Hilar dissection in the liver recipient.

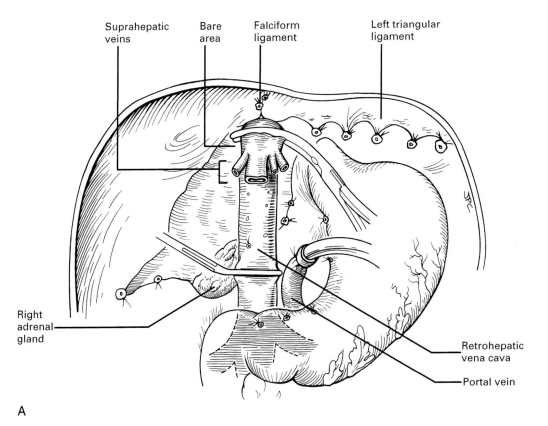

A

Fig. 111.15. Completed recipient hepatectomy on venovenous bypass. **A,** With preservation of host retrohepatic vena cava. Note the hepatic vein cuffs.

Continued

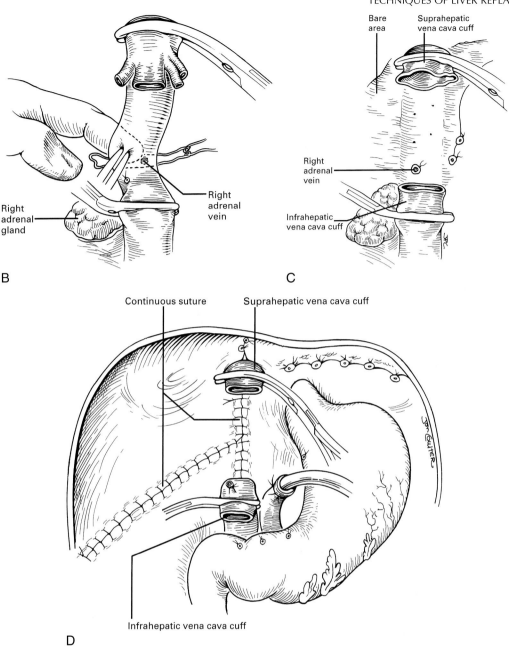

Fig. 111.15. cont'd. B, As in **A,** but with an injury to the right adrenal vein, which is being ligated. **C,** The retrohepatic vena cava has been included in the hepatectomy, necessitating ligation of its tributary lumbar veins and the right adrenal vein. **D,** Closure of the bare area to provide hemostasis. Bleeding from the bare area is more severe if the retrohepatic cava is removed because of the loss of venous drainage.

To the extent vena cava flow can be maintained during the sometimes tedious and difficult denudation of the retrohepatic vena cava, the need for venovenous bypass is eliminated. The amount of retroperitoneal dissection is reduced considerably. Finally, the risk of right adrenal infarction is eliminated, unless the right adrenal vein is injured as depicted in Fig. 111.15B.

Alternative Approaches to Hepatectomy

In many, if not most, cases, hepatectomy with or without inclusion of the retrohepatic vena cava is uncomplicated. Dissection of the

liver hilum sometimes is difficult or impossible, however, because of scarring or the presence of varices. In these situations, the suprahepatic vena cava can be approached first. After transecting the upper vena cava, removal of the liver can be done from top down, approaching the hilar structures from behind (Fig. 111.17). Alternatively, the inferior vena cava below the liver can be used as a "handle" to extract the liver from bottom to top, with cross-clamping (or transection) of the hilar structures at the earliest possible opportunity (Fig. 111.18). Finally, if adhesions are present that block access to the upper and lower vena cava and to the portal triad, the liver can be split, exposing the anterior surface of the retrohepatic vena cava (Fig. 111.19).

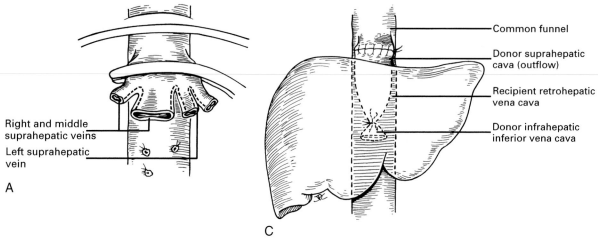

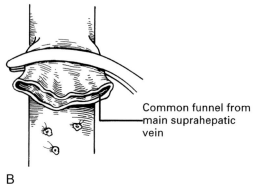

Right and middle
suprahepatic veins

Left suprahepatic
vein

A

Common funnel

Donor suprahepatic
cava (outflow)

Recipient retrohepatic
vena cava

Donor infrahepatic
inferior vena cava

C

Common funnel from
main suprahepatic
vein

B

Fig. 111.16. The piggyback method of graft implantation in a patient with a conserved retrohepatic vena cava. **A** and **B,** Creation of an outflow cloaca from two or more hepatic veins. **C,** Completed anastomosis between the host hepatic veins and the suprahepatic vena cava of the graft. The inferior end of the graft vena cava is ligated.

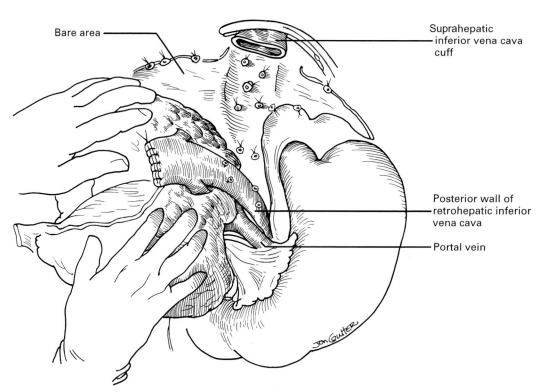

Bare area

Suprahepatic
inferior vena cava
cuff

Posterior wall of
retrohepatic inferior
vena cava

Portal vein

Fig. 111.17. Removal of the recipient liver from top down.

Once bleeding from the raw surfaces is controlled with continuous sutures, the two hepatic halves are stripped away from the surrounding structures. All of these hepatectomy variations are made easier by venovenous bypass.

VASCULAR ANASTOMOSES

It is important to have the surgical field completely prepared for implantation before the new liver is brought from the back table. The first graft vessel to be anastomosed always is the segment of donor vena cava into which all the hepatic veins of the transplanted liver drain. If host hepatectomy has included removal of the retrohepatic vena cava, the anastomosis is an end-to-end suprahepatic vena caval-to-suprahepatic vena caval connection at the diaphragm (Fig. 111.20A). With the piggyback operation in which the host vena cava is conserved, the suprahepatic vena cava is emptied into a cuff of host hepatic vein (see Fig. 111.16) or by a side-to-side anastomosis between the two vena cava segments (not illustrated).

The order of the other vascular anastomoses may vary. With the caval-sparing piggyback operation, the infrahepatic vena cava of the graft is ligated (see Fig. 111.16). When the host caval segment is excised, a common practice is to anastomose the infrahepatic vena cava (see Fig. 111.20B), followed by removal from the bypass and portal vein anastomosis (see Fig. 111.20C). These anastomoses may be done in reverse order (i.e., portal vein first). An experienced surgeon may prefer to perform the arterial anastomosis before the portal vein reconstruction or

complete all four anastomoses before unclamping. These decisions are influenced by the anatomic and physiologic circumstances in the individual case, including the efficiency with which the bypass system has functioned.

In all cases, it is important before definitive liver reperfusion to flush the allograft with lactated Ringer's solution (some surgeons prefer albumin). This is done through the cannula left in the graft portal vein at the time of procurement (see Fig. 111.20A). After its passage through the microvasculature of the allograft, the infusate is vented from the vena cava (see Fig. 111.20B). The objectives are to remove air and to rid the graft of the high-potassium solutions used for organ preservation (see Fig. 111.20B). Failure to perform this flush can result in air embolism or hyperkalemic cardiac arrest.

All of the vascular anastomoses are done with continuous suture. To avoid anastomotic strictures, particularly of the portal and arterial anastomoses, special techniques were developed that are made feasible by the ability of polypropylene (Prolene) suture to glide freely through tissue. A "growth factor" is left by tying the sutures at a considerable distance from the vessel wall. After the flow is restored through the anastomosis, the excess polypropylene recedes back into the vessel and redistributes itself throughout the circumference of the suture line (Fig. 111.21). If leaks develop, these are readily controlled with single additional sutures.

Rather than being whimsical, variations of the order and details of revascularization frequently are mandated by anatomic anomalies or by pathologic factors, including thrombosis of the portal vein, that contraindicated liver transplantation until

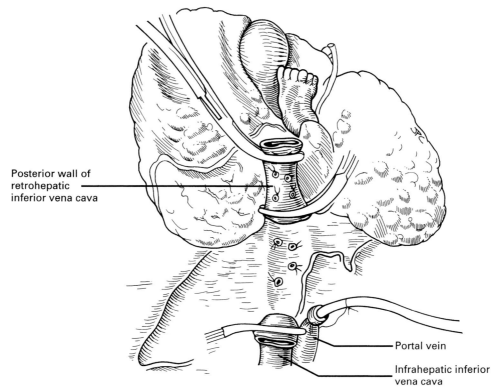

Fig. 111.18. Removal of the recipient liver from bottom up.

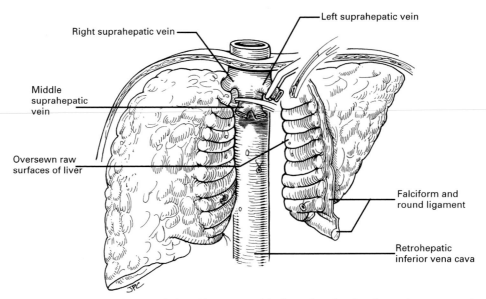

Fig. 111.19. Splitting technique of hepatectomy. The split is facilitated by insertion of the finger along the relatively vein-free anterior surface of the vena cava. The correct plane must be determined carefully by finger probing before any pressure is applied.

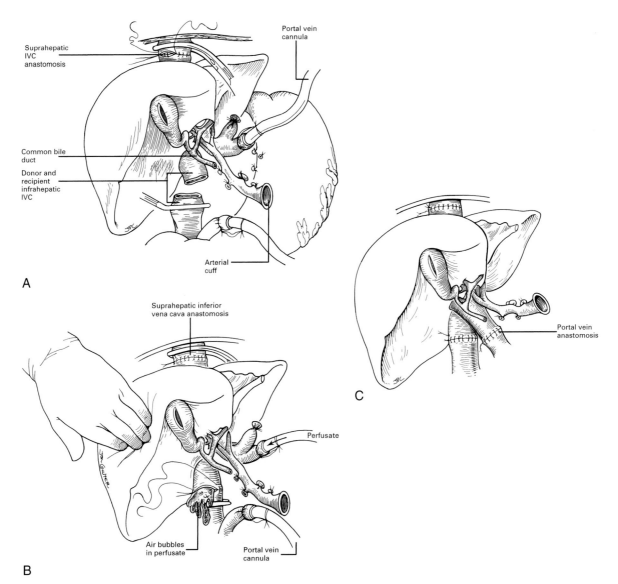

Fig. 111.20. Implantation steps. **A,** Suprahepatic vena cava anastomosis. **B,** Infrahepatic vena cava anastomosis. Before completing the anastomosis, the portal vein is infused with cold albumin or electrolyte solution. This allows air and the potassium-rich preservation fluid to be sucked out. **C,** The portal vein anastomosis after removal of the bypass cannula. IVC, inferior vena cava.

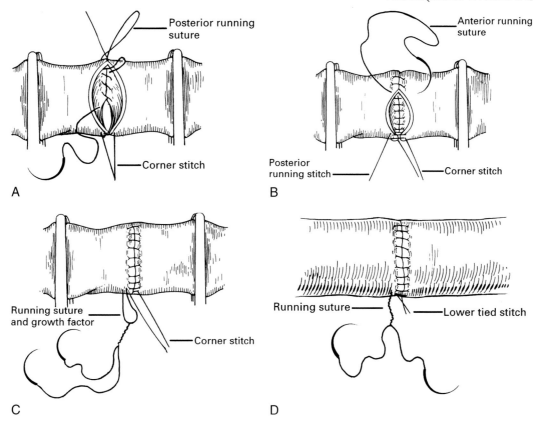

Fig. 111.21. Technique of venous anastomosis. **A,** Traction sutures are placed at each corner. One end of the far suture is brought to the inside and run in continuous fashion to approximate the back wall. **B,** The other end of the far suture is used from the outside to approximate the anterior wall. **C,** The continuous suture is tied away from the vein wall to allow for a growth factor. The near corner suture is tied next to the running suture to prevent separation of the vessel. **D,** The excess suture is drawn into the vessel, allowing the circumference to expand when blood flow is restored.

techniques were developed to deal with them. Declotting a thrombosed portal vein may be possible (Fig. 111.22A), but if not, iliac or other veins from the donor may be used as interposition grafts (see Fig. 111.22B) or as mesoportal jump grafts (see Fig. 111.22C). A mesoportal graft may be anastomosed end-to-side to the superior mesenteric vein and tunneled through the transverse mesocolon in an avascular plane anterior to the pancreas to reach the hepatic hilum for end-to-end anastomosis to the donor portal vein (see Fig. 111.22C).

Numerous techniques also have been used to restore the hepatic arterial supply. The ideal reconstruction when the allograft and recipient have normal arterial anatomy is shown in Fig. 111.23A. If there are anomalies, vascular injuries, or pathologic changes in the donor or recipient blood vessels that preclude effective rearterialization, grafts obtained from the donor can be used as a last resort (Fig. 111.24; see Fig. 111.23B and C).

Biliary Tract Reconstruction

Good hemostasis must be achieved before the biliary reconstruction is performed. If the recipient duct is disease-free, and if there is a reasonable size match between the donor and recipient ducts, an end-to-end anastomosis is performed over a T-tube stent (Fig. 111.25). The anastomosis usually is performed with 8 to 10 interrupted absorbable sutures, such as 5-0 or 6-0 polyglycolic acid. Because the integrity of the anastomosis depends primarily on an adequate blood supply of donor and recipient ducts, the duct ends are trimmed back as much as is feasible. A small purse-string suture usually is placed around the T-tube exit site to prevent leakage, and the T-limb is brought out through a stab incision on the lateral side of the recipient duct. Some authorities believe that T-tube stenting is unnecessary.

If the recipient duct is diseased or otherwise inadequate for anastomosis, a choledochojejunostomy is performed. An 18-inch Roux-en-Y limb of proximal jejunum is brought up (usually antecolic) to the hepatic hilum, and the donor duct is anastomosed end-to-side to the jejunal limb using a running or interrupted 5-0 or 6-0 absorbable polyglycolic acid suture over a small internal Silastic stent (see Fig. 111.25, *inset*). The stent is secured in place with a rapidly absorbed fine catgut suture with the assumption that it will later pass spontaneously through the intestinal tract. The stent occasionally becomes stuck, however, and must be pushed out later by an interventional radiologist or removed at laparotomy.

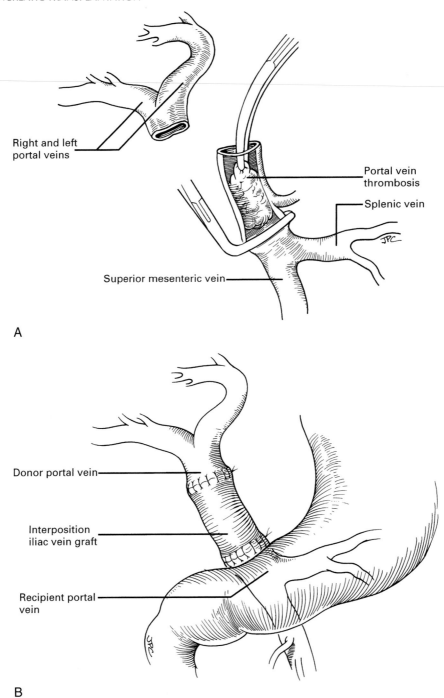

Fig. 111.22. Management of recipient portal vein abnormalities. **A,** Removal of thrombus. **B,** Use of an interposition graft of donor vein (or pulmonary artery) to bridge the gap between donor portal vein and the confluence of the mesenteric and splenic veins.

Continued

REDUCED SIZE LIVER TRANSPLANTATION

The scarcity of pediatric donors and the constraints of size matching often prohibit transplantation of a whole donor liver in a child or a small adult. Since 1980, the option of using a partial liver has been exercised at most large transplant centers with results equal to or approaching those achievable with whole liver transplantation. Partial liver transplantation, its application in live donors, and the use of divided cadaveric livers (allowing one organ to be used for two recipients) are described in Chapters 107 and 109.

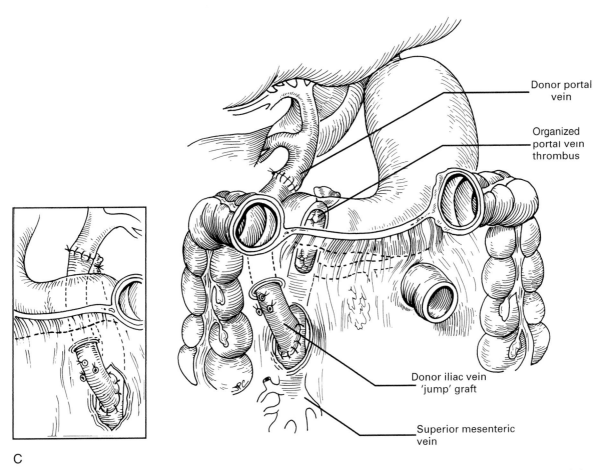

Fig. 111.22. cont'd. C, Donor vein jump graft from the host superior mesenteric vein to the graft portal vein. The jump graft is tunneled through the transverse mesocolon in front of the pancreas to the hepatic hilum. The graft can be anterior or posterior *(inset)* to the stomach.

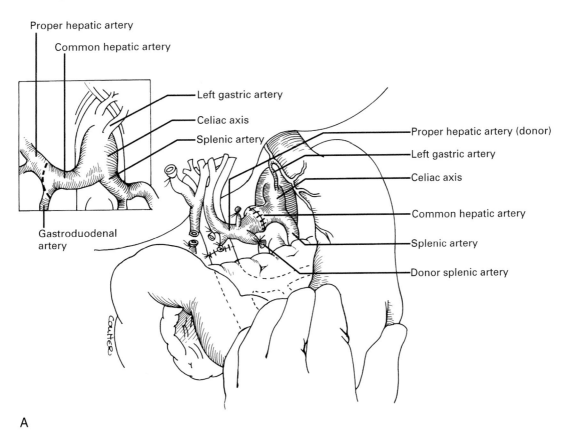

Fig. 111.23. Hepatic artery reconstruction. **A,** Most common reconstruction in which the graft celiac trunk is anastomosed to the recipient common hepatic artery. If there is a size discrepancy, the circumference of the recipient vessel can be increased as shown in the *inset.*

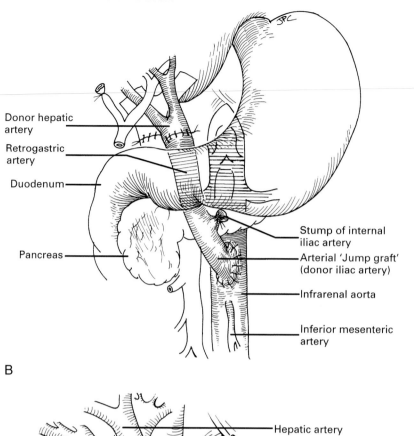

Donor hepatic artery

Retrogastric artery

Duodenum

Pancreas

Stump of internal iliac artery

Arterial 'Jump graft' (donor iliac artery)

Infrarenal aorta

Inferior mesenteric artery

B

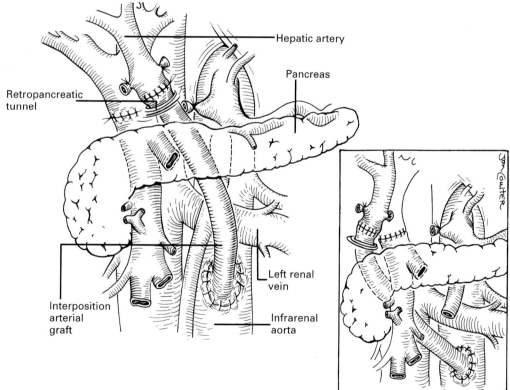

Hepatic artery

Pancreas

Retropancreatic tunnel

Interposition arterial graft

Left renal vein

Infrarenal aorta

C

Fig. 111.23. cont'd. B, Jump graft of donor iliac artery based on the infrarenal aorta and tunneled anterior to the pancreas. **C,** Rarely used alternative retroperitoneal tunnel posterior to the pancreas and superior mesenteric artery.

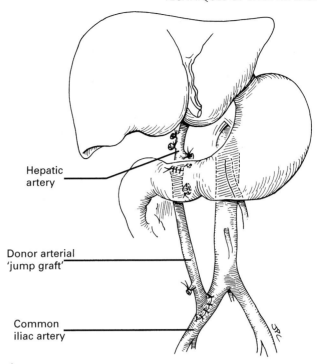

Hepatic
artery

Donor arterial
'jump graft'

Common
iliac artery

A

Fig. 111.24. Other originating sites for an arterial jump graft. **A,** Host iliac artery. **B,** Supraceliac aorta.

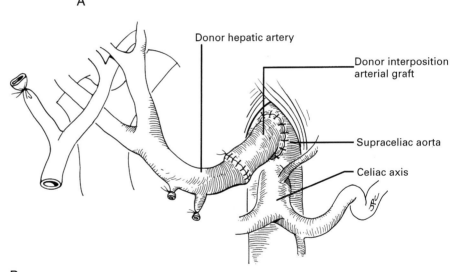

Donor hepatic artery

Donor interposition
arterial graft

Supraceliac aorta

Celiac axis

B

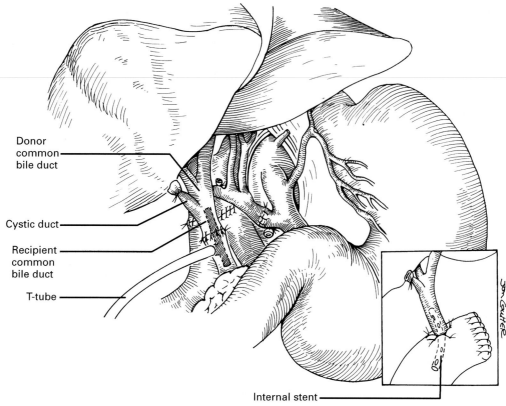

Donor
common
bile duct

Cystic duct

Recipient
common
bile duct

T-tube

Internal stent

Fig. 111.25. Biliary tract reconstruction with end-to-end anastomosis over a T-tube. If duct reconstruction is not feasible or is contraindicated, the graft duct is anastomosed to a Roux-en-Y limb of host jejunum *(inset).*

REFERENCES

Starzl TE, 1969: Experience in Hepatic Transplantation [with the assistance of C.W. Putnam]. Philadelphia, Saunders.

Starzl TE, 2002: The saga of liver replacement, with particular reference to the reciprocal influence of liver and kidney transplantation (1955-1967). J Am Coll Surg 195:587-610.

Starzl TE, et al, 1989: Medical progress: liver transplantation. N Engl J Med 321(part I):1014-1022; 321(part II):1092-1099.

112

Whole Organ Pancreas and Pancreatic Islet Transplantation

N. M. DESAI AND J. F. MARKMANN

Type 1 diabetes mellitus (also known as juvenile diabetes) is characterized by hyperglycemia resulting from the nearly complete destruction of the insulin producing beta cells of the pancreatic islets of Langerhans. The loss of beta cells is due to a T cell–mediated autoimmune attack that typically occurs during childhood or early adolescence. Insulin replacement can lead to acceptable control of blood glucose levels; however, affected individuals are subject to the development of various secondary complications, including cardiac disease, stroke, retinopathy and blindness, nephropathy and renal failure, peripheral and autonomic neuropathy, and amputation (Atkinson & Eisenbarth, 2001). Although tight glycemic control has been shown to decrease the number of diabetes-related secondary complications, it also has been shown to lead to an increased number of dangerous hypoglycemic episodes (Diabetes Control and Complications Trial Research Group, 1993).

Transplantation therapy for type 1 diabetes was developed as an alternative to insulin administration with the additional theoretical benefit of reducing or eliminating the development of secondary complications of the disease. Whole organ pancreas and isolated pancreatic islets are being transplanted into select patients with type 1 diabetes. Whole organ transplantation is already an established and widely available therapy, whereas clinical islet transplantation is experimental and has only more recently become successful in a limited population of diabetic patients.

WHOLE ORGAN PANCREAS TRANSPLANTATION

History and Early Results

On December 20, 1893, Williams grafted three pieces of a sheep pancreas into the subcutaneous tissues of a diabetic child, who died 3 days later of unrelenting diabetic ketoacidosis (Williams, 1894). This first attempt to treat diabetes with transplantation, although unsuccessful, preceded decades of animal experimentation in which investigators developed the methods necessary to perform a vascularized pancreas transplant and subsequently used pancreas transplantation as a model to study diabetes and glucose homeostasis.

The first clinical vascularized pancreas transplant was performed on December 17, 1966, by Kelly and Lillehei at the University of Minnesota (Kelly et al, 1967). This patient had temporary insulin independence, but eventually required graft removal and ultimately died of postoperative complications. The subsequent early experience with pancreas transplantation at Minnesota (and at a few other centers) was characterized by some technical success, but no graft that functioned beyond 1 year, and the enthusiasm for this procedure dwindled—during 1975, only six pancreas transplants were performed worldwide. The introduction of cyclosporine as an immunosuppressive medication and further technical refinements allowed for better outcomes after pancreas transplantation. Throughout the 1980s and early 1990s, the number of pancreas transplants performed increased dramatically, and nearly 1500 pancreas transplants were performed in the United States during 2004.

Indications and Patient Selection

Most patients undergoing pancreatic transplantation have type 1 diabetes mellitus and renal failure. In these individuals, pancreas transplantation is performed with a simultaneous kidney transplant (SPK) (85% of cases) or after a successful kidney transplant (PAK) (10% of cases). The normal glucose control achieved by the pancreas transplant may protect the transplanted kidney from recurrent diabetic nephropathy and is beneficial from an overall quality of life perspective. In a small proportion of patients with diabetes that is very brittle and difficult to manage, but with preserved renal function, pancreas transplant alone (PTA) (5% of cases) is performed. SPK and PAK recipients require immunosuppressive therapy to protect the kidney and pancreas from rejection, whereas in the case of PTA recipients, the need for immunosuppression is solely for the pancreas itself. This difference becomes important when weighing the risk-to-benefit ratio for each type of recipient.

Potential pancreas recipients are screened carefully for contraindications to transplantation, such as an ongoing infectious process or malignancy. These candidates almost always have medical comorbidities as a result of secondary complications from diabetes; a thorough assessment of a candidate's cardiovascular status is essential. Cardiac contraindications to pancreas transplantation include the presence of noncorrectable coronary artery disease, ejection fraction less than 50%, and myocardial infarction within the past 6 months. Recipient age also is important, and in many programs recipients older than 50 years of age are not considered candidates because of increased risk.

Donor Operation

Selection of an appropriate deceased pancreas donor includes standard donor selection criteria. In addition, there is a bias toward using organs from younger, leaner, and more hemodynamically stable deceased donors. Deceased donors with hemodynamic instability or that require high doses of vasopressors are considered higher risk. In addition, pancreata with significant steatosis usually are avoided because they are associated with a greater likelihood of postoperative complications, such as pancreatitis, peripancreatic fat necrosis, and infection. Based on these selection criteria, which are relatively stringent compared with the criteria applied to the liver or kidney, only a fraction of deceased donors are deemed suitable for whole organ pancreas donation. In the United States, there were 7150 deceased donors during 2004. Of these, only 1484 pancreata were transplanted (21%) compared with 5846 livers (82%) and 9355 kidneys.

The procurement of the pancreas must be performed in conjunction with the liver procurement, carefully delineating the blood supply to the liver to ensure that both organs can be removed and transplanted. In most cases, blood supply should not preclude the transplantation of both organs. Initial dissection involves division of the gastrocolic ligament, exposing the anterior surface of the pancreas. Visual inspection is considered by most to be an important element to the pancreas procurement process because this is an opportunity to assess the organ for the presence of infiltrating fat or hematoma that might preclude transplantation. The portal triad is carefully dissected, with division of the common bile duct and the gastroduodenal artery. In addition, the common hepatic, left gastric, and splenic arteries all are dissected free of surrounding lymphatic tissues. Further dissection of the pancreas includes Kocher's maneuver to mobilize the head and division of the lienophrenic and lienocolic ligaments to mobilize the body and tail. The spleen is left in continuity with the pancreas to serve as a handle to minimize manipulation of the gland itself. The duodenum is decontaminated by flushing povidone-iodine/antifungal/antibiotic solution through a nasoduodenal tube.

After systemic heparinization of the patient, the abdominal aorta is ligated at its bifurcation and cannulated in a retrograde direction for perfusion. The liver team also may elect to place a cannula for portal perfusion through a portal vein tributary, such as the inferior mesenteric vein. The supraceliac aorta is cross-clamped, the vena cava is vented, and the abdominal organs are flushed in situ with preservation solution at 4°C (either Belzer University of Wisconsin solution or Custodial HTK solution). In addition, topical cooling is employed. When the organs have been adequately flushed, the liver and pancreas are removed en bloc and divided at the back bench or removed separately from the donor. In the latter situation, the liver is removed first, by dividing the portal vein 1 cm cephalad to the superior margin of the pancreatic head (approximately the level of the coronary vein) and dividing the splenic artery about 5 mm beyond its origin, preserving the entire celiac axis with the liver. Next, removal of the pancreas proceeds. The proximal duodenum (just beyond the pylorus) and the distal duodenum are divided with gastrointestinal anastomosis (GIA) vascular staplers. The small bowel mesentery that lies inferior to the pancreas is divided, and the superior mesenteric artery is divided at its origin from the aorta. Long segments of iliac arteries and veins are removed to use for vascular reconstruction.

Back Bench Preparation of the Pancreas

Relative to other solid organs, the pancreas requires extensive preparation before implantation into the recipient. This back bench preparation is performed in ice-cold preservation solution to minimize any further ischemic injury to the organ. The duodenum is often shortened with a GIA stapler, being careful to exclude any gastric tissue and being careful not to compromise the opening of the ampulla of Vater. The division of the

small bowel mesentery in the donor is shortened by firing a stapler across this mesentery, then reinforcing it with a line of suture. The spleen is removed by dividing the vessels in the splenic hilum, being careful not to injure the tail of the gland. Finally, the arterial inflow to the graft must be reconstructed because the organ has two major sources of blood supply that are not in continuity: (1) the splenic artery supplying the body and tail and (2) branches of the superior mesenteric artery supplying the head. In most instances, arterial reconstruction can be performed using donor iliac artery as a Y-graft. The internal iliac artery is joined to the splenic artery, and the external iliac artery is joined to the superior mesenteric artery. The common iliac artery of the Y-graft can be anastomosed to the recipient iliac artery, serving as the arterial inflow to the pancreas. In rare instances, it is necessary to create a portal vein extension graft on the back bench using donor iliac vein; however, this technique is avoided if possible because it may increase the risk of venous thrombosis of the graft.

Recipient Operation

In contrast to most solid organ transplants, the techniques used for transplanting the pancreas have changed dramatically over the past several years. Partial segmental grafts containing only the body and tail were common previously; however, currently this technique is rarely used. Exocrine secretions previously were managed by pancreatic duct ligation or by injection of a polymer that would cause duct obliteration; however, today the exocrine secretions are handled by internal drainage.

The two significant areas in pancreas transplantation where current techniques differ are the drainage of exocrine secretions and the venous drainage of the graft. Exocrine drainage is performed via the intestinal tract or via the urinary tract. Throughout most of the 1980s and 1990s, drainage of the pancreatic secretions into the recipient bladder was the most common form of exocrine drainage. This technique is convenient for monitoring organ function by measurement of amylase levels in the urine. Problems with hematuria, cystitis, bicarbonate loss, and dehydration all are associated with bladder drainage, however. These complications necessitate surgical revision to enteric drainage in 20% of bladder-drained pancreas recipients (Stratta, 2005). Based on these issues and the lower rejection rates observed with newer immunosuppressive medications, most transplant centers now perform enteric drainage of the exocrine secretions. This enteric drainage is directly into a loop of jejunum in a side-to-side fashion or into a Roux-en-Y limb of jejunum.

The venous drainage of the graft is to the systemic circulation (via an iliac vein or the inferior vena cava) or to the portal circulation. Portal venous drainage has the advantage of delivering insulin in a more physiologic manner because insulin undergoes a "first pass" through the liver, and the hyperinsulinemia that results from systemic drainage is avoided (Gaber et al, 1995). There is also an immunologic advantage of portal drainage that has been observed in several experimental studies in which the delivery of foreign antigen via the portal system results in diminished immune responses. Despite these theoretical advantages, there has been no demonstrable difference in outcomes between portal and systemic venous drained transplants in humans, and systemic venous drainage is how most pancreas transplants are performed (Philosophe et al, 2001).

There are two common locations in the abdomen where the transplant is placed based on the type of venous drainage planned—in the pelvis (most commonly the right side) for systemic venous drainage or in the mid-abdomen for portal venous drainage. When the graft is placed in the pelvis, the donor portal vein is anastomosed to the external iliac vein, the common iliac vein, or the inferior vena cava. In this pelvic position, the graft is oriented with the duodenum inferiorly if bladder drainage is planned (Fig. 112.1A) or with the duodenum in the superior (Fig. 112.1B) or inferior direction if enteric drainage is planned. Alternatively, for portal venous drainage, the pancreas is placed in the mid abdomen below the transverse colon with the duodenum oriented superiorly. The portal vein of the pancreas is anastomosed to the major branch of the superior mesenteric vein found in the small intestine mesentery in an end-to-side fashion (Fig. 112.2). Enteric drainage for exocrine secretions must be used with the portal venous drainage technique. With both techniques, the arterial conduit to the graft is anastomosed in an end-to-side fashion with the common or external iliac artery.

Complications

The major complications after pancreas transplantation are often technical in nature. Pancreas graft thrombosis (arterial or venous) is more frequent compared with other solid organ transplants, and the reported incidence is approximately 10%. Thrombosis often occurs within the first week after transplantation and likely reflects the relatively low blood flow through the organ. In most instances of thrombosis, graft removal is necessary (Humar et al, 2000). Early pancreatitis occurs in 10% to 20% of cases and is largely a reflection of ischemic damage to the gland during preservation and reperfusion injury. Hyperamylasemia and graft edema are characteristic, and graft pancreatitis usually is treated nonsurgically with octreotide. Leakage at the site of pancreatic exocrine drainage is another early complication, with management often dictated by the method of drainage. Bladder-drained transplants with a small leak at the duodenocystostomy often can be managed by Foley catheter drainage of the bladder, allowing the site of leakage to heal over time. Enteric-drained transplants with a leak at the duodenojejunostomy often result in peritonitis and usually require operative intervention to control the leak.

Rejection after a pancreas transplant was a common occurrence previously. The diagnosis of pancreas rejection is often difficult. A variety of indicators are used to help make the diagnosis, including increased serum amylase and lipase, decreased urinary amylase excretion (if bladder drainage is used), biopsy of the pancreas, and hyperglycemia. Hyperglycemia is a late indicator of rejection, and the pancreas is often difficult to salvage when hyperglycemia has occurred. If an SPK transplant is performed, renal allograft dysfunction often can assist with the diagnosis of pancreatic rejection because the rejection process is often occurring in both organs. As a result of the high incidence of rejection and the difficulty in making the diagnosis, pancreas transplant recipients usually receive potent induction immunosuppression with a T cell–depleting agent and maintenance therapy with tacrolimus, mycophenolate mofetil, and corticosteroids.

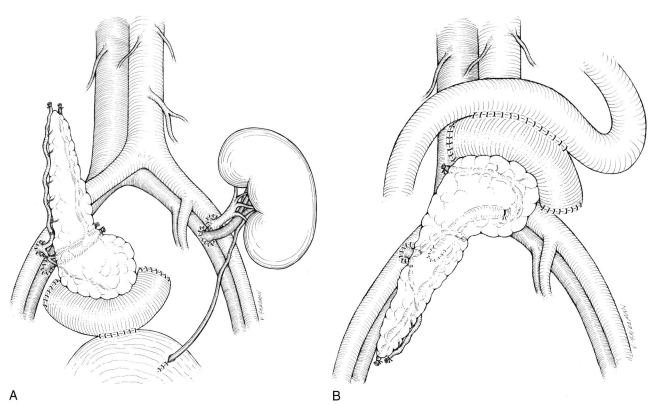

A   B

Fig. 112.1. Whole organ pancreas transplantation with systemic venous drainage. The pancreas is placed in the right pelvis with anastomosis of the donor artery Y-graft to the recipient iliac artery to provide arterial inflow to the graft and anastomosis of the donor portal vein to the recipient iliac vein for venous drainage. A simultaneous kidney transplant can be performed using the left-sided iliac vessels. **A,** The duodenum is oriented in the inferior direction to allow anastomosis to the bladder *(shown)* or to the small intestine *(not shown).* **B,** Alternatively, the duodenum is oriented superiorly for anastomosis to the intestine.

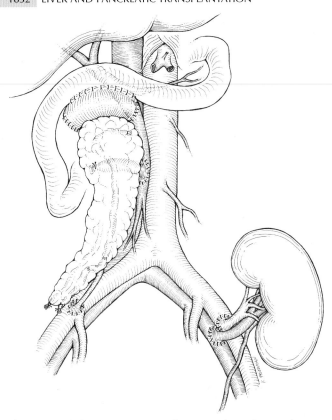

Fig. 112.2. Whole organ pancreas transplantation with portal venous drainage. The pancreas is placed in the mid abdomen with anastomosis of the donor portal vein to the major branch of the superior mesenteric vein and anastomosis of the donor artery Y-graft to the recipient iliac artery. The duodenum is oriented in the superior direction for anastomosis to the intestine. A simultaneous kidney transplant can be performed using the left *(shown)* or right iliac vessels.

The total amount of immunosuppression pancreas recipients receive is among the highest of any solid organ transplant. As a result, these patients are more susceptible to the complications of immunosuppressive therapy, including infection with opportunistic bacteria, viruses, and fungi; malignancy; gastrointestinal complications; and others. The high incidence of these complications makes effective prophylaxis strategies important.

Results

Patient and graft survival after pancreas transplantation have improved significantly in recent years. Patient survival is approximately 95% to 98% at 1 year and 80% to 85% at 5 years posttransplantation. Graft survival is more variable and depends on the type of transplant performed (Fig. 112.3). For SPK recipients, 1-year and 5-year pancreas graft survivals are 86% and 70%. For PAK recipients, 1-year and 5-year pancreas graft survivals are 81% and 53%. Finally, for PTA recipients, 1-year and 5-year graft survivals are 81% and 47% (Danovitch et al, 2005).

The impact of a successful pancreas transplant on the complications associated with diabetes mellitus is debated. Because the successful transplant restores euglycemia and normal hemoglobin A_{1c} levels, most proponents argue that diabetic complications should cease and perhaps reverse. Neuropathy seems to stabilize

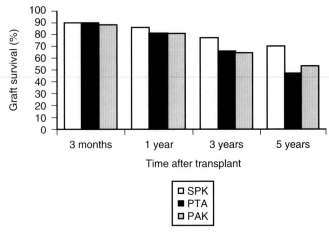

Fig. 112.3. Pancreas graft survival rates after whole organ transplantation by transplant category.
(From Danovitch GM, et al, 2005: Current status of kidney and pancreas transplantation in the United States, 1994-2003. Am J Transplant 5:904-915. Copyright 2005 Blackwell Publishing.)

and slowly improve after pancreas transplantation, whereas retinopathy progression is slowed after several years of graft function. The development of diabetic nephropathy in the transplanted kidney of SPK and early PAK recipients seems to be prevented by a successful pancreas transplant. In PTA recipients, diabetic nephropathy seems to stabilize after the transplant (Fioretto et al, 1998); however, the renal benefit is likely outweighed by the detriment to renal function caused by the immunosuppressive agents—specifically tacrolimus and cyclosporine.

Risk-to-Benefit Considerations

As outlined previously, considerable evidence suggests that a successful pancreas transplant can retard and in some cases reverse the secondary complications of diabetes. Despite this evidence, the procedure is considered appropriate for only a subset of patients with type 1 diabetes because of its highly invasive nature compared with insulin therapy and the potential for significant surgical complications. Considerations of risk to benefit are paramount in pancreas transplantation and play an essential role in donor and recipient selection processes.

An analysis evaluated the survival benefit of pancreas transplantation by examining a large transplant database to compare the survival of pancreas recipients versus patients listed for transplantation but who did not receive a transplant. Using this study design, the two patient groups were ensured to be as similar as possible. Because the indications, risks, and benefits differ depending on whether the patient had underlying renal failure, the analysis was stratified based on whether the patient was listed for or transplanted with an SPK, PAK, or PTA (Venstrom et al, 2003). The analysis revealed a marked survival benefit for patients receiving a combined pancreas and kidney transplant; a 57% reduction in mortality rate was observed over 4 years compared with similar patients who remained on the waiting list. In contrast to the clear survival benefit of SPK transplantation, the PAK and PTA recipients experienced an increased mortality after transplantation. During the 4-year follow-up period, PAK recipients experienced a 42% *increase* in mortality, and PTA recipients experienced a 57% *increase* in mortality compared with the comparable group of patients who remained on the waiting list.

A similar analysis was reported in which the survival disadvantage of PAK and PTA was challenged (Gruessner et al, 2004a). Their analysis found, as expected, that the SPK procedure conferred a marked survival advantage. In contrast to the Venstrom study (Venstrom et al, 2003), no survival disadvantage was evident in PAK or PTA transplant recipients; however, there was no evidence for a clear survival advantage conferred by these procedures, although a trend in that direction was evident.

There are two important caveats to these risk-benefit studies. The first is that the impact of pancreas transplantation on quality of life was not evaluated in these nonrandomized retrospective analyses and would likely favor heavily the group with successful PAK and PTA recipients. Whether this factor would outweigh any survival disadvantage in the short-term and the significant cost of these complex procedures has not been evaluated. A second crucial outcome measure that is lacking from these studies is the long-term impact of a successful pancreas transplant on the secondary complications of diabetes. As noted earlier, there is evidence that diabetic nephropathy, neuropathy, and retinopathy may be positively impacted by the long-term restoration of normoglycemia conferred by transplantation. These studies have not included well-controlled trials with large numbers of patients, however.

These results substantiate the marked clinical benefit observed when caring for patients who receive a combined kidney and pancreas transplant (Rayhill et al, 2000). The relative contribution of the transplanted kidney versus the transplanted pancreas to the overall patient benefit has not been differentiated in a controlled study. This issue is significant given the marked survival benefit that has been documented in the setting of a renal transplant alone, even in diabetic and high-risk recipients (Wolfe et al, 1999).

Although the survival benefit for SPK recipients is clear, the data showing a lack of survival benefit for PAK and PTA recipients are controversial. At a minimum, the studies available to date suggest a narrow therapeutic margin for PAK and PTA recipients. Perhaps the most meaningful conclusion that can be drawn at present is that these transplants should be performed with the utmost care in recipient selection, should use optimal donor organs, and should be performed at the transplant centers with the best outcomes. The field is dynamic owing to improvements in surgical techniques and perioperative care and the frequent introduction of new immunosuppressive agents with more favorable safety profiles. A clear survival benefit for pancreas transplantation is expected to be established with further advances in the field.

PANCREATIC ISLET TRANSPLANTATION

History and Early Results

The original descriptions in rodents of successful islet isolation (Lacy & Kostianovsky, 1967) and subsequent transplantation (Ballinger & Lacy, 1972) caused great excitement in the medical community that this type of therapy could be applied to patients with type 1 diabetes. Although the ability to obtain normal glucose control in diabetic rodents with an islet transplant was described in the 1970s (Reckard et al, 1973), translating this

success to humans has been more difficult. Various centers worldwide attempted human islet transplantation starting in 1974, with 445 recipients receiving islets between 1974 and 2000. Most of these recipients also received a kidney transplant, either before or at the same time as the islet transplant. Analysis of the reported cases during 1990-2000 showed that only 19% of patients were off insulin for more than 1 week, and at 1-year follow-up, only 11% of recipients were insulin independent (Brendel et al, 2001).

These discouraging results were attributed to numerous factors, including the possibility that recurrent autoimmunity was causing progressive islet damage after transplantation because the cause of diabetes in these recipients was the autoimmune form. Support for this hypothesis came from a series of patients at the University of Pittsburgh who underwent upper abdominal exenteration (including total pancreatectomy) followed by liver and islet allotransplantation. In this group of 11 patients who did not have autoimmune diabetes, 6 (55%) exhibited sustained insulin independence, a success rate far greater than what had been achieved in type 1 diabetic recipients (Carroll et al, 1995).

Islet Autotransplantation

Autotransplantation of pancreatic islets was developed for patients with chronic pancreatitis in whom total pancreatectomy provided the best option for treatment. Surgically induced diabetes is characterized by an absence of insulin and counterregulatory hormones and is frequently brittle, with a high rate of long-term morbidity. This treatment involves processing of the surgically removed pancreas in the islet isolation laboratory followed by infusion of purified islets or crude pancreatic digest into the liver via the portal vein.

Although the overall experience is limited, the success rate in recipients of autotransplantation has been far greater than in patients receiving allogeneic islets for the treatment of type 1 diabetes. The largest reported series is from the University of Minnesota, where during 1977-2003, 112 patients with chronic pancreatitis underwent total or completion pancreatectomy with islet autotransplantation (Gruessner et al, 2004b). These investigators achieved a 51% rate of graft function and a 39% rate of insulin independence. The patients who had undergone a prior Whipple procedure or no prior surgery had the highest rate of success, whereas patients who had a prior Puestow procedure or distal pancreatectomy had the lowest chances of success. These success rates correlated closely with the average yield of islets from the removed pancreatic tissue after digestion and processing. Similar results have been reported by another group in a series of 22 patients, where 68% of patients had graft function and 41% were insulin independent (Rodriguez Rilo et al, 2003). Both of these groups infused unpurified pancreatic digests where the islets had not undergone the additional purification step that is performed during cadaveric donor pancreas processing for allotransplantation.

Edmonton Protocol and Beyond

Interest in islet transplantation was piqued by the Edmonton investigators reporting in 2000 that for the first time diabetes in patients could be consistently reversed by transplantation of isolated pancreatic islets (Shapiro et al, 2000). The Edmonton approach relied on a novel immunosuppression regimen that completely avoided steroids and that used a unique combination of induction therapy with an anti–interleukin-2-receptor antibody and maintenance therapy with sirolimus and tacrolimus. The rationale for this combination was based on the desire to avoid agents with known beta cell toxicity. Although this particular drug combination was likely an important factor in the trial's success, perhaps of greater impact was the large number of islets that patients received. These investigators infused a larger number of islets than were administered in prior islet transplantation trials, using two or three infusions per patient that were acquired from multiple deceased donors. Although previous trials in the late 1990s often had achieved partial success with single infusions of islets, as evidenced by a reduced insulin requirement and increased C peptide levels, in no trial had the further step been taken to retransplant such patients to increase the net islet mass (Hering & Ricordi, 1999). In the Edmonton series, patients showing evidence of partial success from the first infusion received an additional infusion (or two) until they had accumulated a sufficient islet mass to gain insulin independence. In general, insulin independence occurred when a threshold of 8000 to 10,000 islets per kilogram of recipient body weight had been infused.

In the 5 years since the landmark report by the Edmonton investigators, nearly 500 islet transplants were performed by more than 40 centers worldwide (Shapiro et al, 2005). In the first concerted effort to replicate the provocative results of the Edmonton Protocol, a multicenter trial sponsored by the Immune Tolerance Network enlisted 10 centers in North America and Europe to perform four islet transplants each, using the Edmonton regimen. Despite a diligent attempt to ensure uniformity in technique between centers, the success rate varied dramatically depending on the extent of experience at the transplanting site—at the three most experienced centers, reversal of hyperglycemia was routinely achieved; however, less experienced teams gained insulin independence only in a fraction of cases (approximately 20%). Although these results confirmed the efficacy of Edmonton's approach, it also revealed the exacting nature of the technique and showed the difficulty in replicating the protocol at all centers.

Many single-center reports have now validated the Edmonton Protocol (Goss et al, 2002; Markmann et al, 2003), and although this protocol represents a tremendous leap forward for the field, the Edmonton results also delineate a major problem facing the field—the need for islets procured from multiple deceased donors to gain insulin independence in a single recipient. This requirement markedly increases costs and represents a distinct disadvantage compared with whole organ transplantation. So far, however, the pancreata used for isolated islet transplantation have been organs that were not suitable for whole organ transplantation. It is reasonable to assume that these organs are inferior to the organs used in whole organ transplantation, and that improved results might be expected if islet transplantation had access to the best organs.

The need for such a large number of islets to achieve insulin independence in clinical transplantation was unexpected in light of the finding that 10% of the total islet mass can maintain normoglycemia after partial pancreatectomy. Because the total islet mass in normal individuals is estimated at 1 to 2 million islets, it would suggest that transplanting only 200,000 islets should regain normoglycemia in most diabetic recipients. Instead, accumulating evidence from the islet transplant studies

by Edmonton and others suggest that for an average patient 600,000 to 700,000 islets are required. The nearly two-thirds loss of potency after transplantation has not been fully explained in patients, but experimental data from small animal studies indicate that most transplanted islets fail to engraft (Davalli et al, 1995). Understanding and overcoming the loss of islet mass during the engraftment phase has been an important focus of more recent islet transplantation clinical trials.

Some centers have reported improved success at gaining insulin independence with islets from a single donor by refining the Edmonton approach (Hering et al, 2004, 2005; Markmann et al, 2003). The most successful reports are from the University of Minnesota, where investigators have used potent induction immunosuppression and high-quality islets. In their first study, four of six consecutive patients were rendered insulin independent with single donor islet infusions using induction therapy with the anti-CD3 monoclonal antibody hOKT3γ1 (ala-ala) (Hering et al, 2004). This therapy was combined with the selection of relatively larger donors and smaller recipients with low daily insulin requirements, maximizing the islet mass delivered per recipient body weight. The same group reported a more impressive result by using polyclonal antithymocyte globulin (Thymoglobulin) for induction therapy; in a series of 10 consecutive patients treated with Thymoglobulin induction therapy, 9 were rendered insulin independent with a single infusion of islets (Hering et al, 2005). The one patient who did not become insulin independent still had a marked reduction in daily insulin requirement. Collectively, these studies suggest that insulin independence can be achieved consistently with single donor islet infusions under the correct circumstances. Overcoming the single donor hurdle would help toward the establishment of isolated islet transplantation as a "standard of care" for select patients with type 1 diabetes.

A second more daunting obstacle is the realization that the durability of function after islet transplantation is less than after whole organ pancreas grafts. Although it is clear that the most experienced islet centers can gain insulin independence in virtually all islet recipients, and that short-term (1 year) insulin-free survival may be close to that seen with whole organ transplants, the intermediate (2-4 year) insulin-free survival is less encouraging. In a report by Edmonton investigators with follow-up on patients in their ongoing series of islet-alone transplants (Ryan et al, 2005), less than 25% of patients remained free from exogenous insulin administration at 3 years (Fig. 112.4B). Although a disappointing result, more encouraging was the observation that greater than 85% of these patients had evidence of some islet graft function by C peptide measurement (see Fig. 112.4A). This observation is relevant because many patients who were transplanted with the indication of hypoglycemia unawareness remain cured of this devastating complication even though they have resumed small doses of insulin. It also is evident that a partially functioning graft can improve glycemic control significantly as measured by serial hemoglobin A_{1c} determinations.

The mechanisms responsible for the gradual loss of islet function are unclear. One hypothesis is that inadequate control of the deleterious alloimmune and autoimmune responses compromise islet function over time. The absence of a reliable measure of an anti-islet immune reaction and the difficulty in obtaining biopsy tissue for pathologic diagnosis contribute to the complexity in clarifying this issue. The role of immune responses in the loss of islet graft function should be clarified by application of more potent immunosuppressive agents in the next generation of islet transplantation studies.

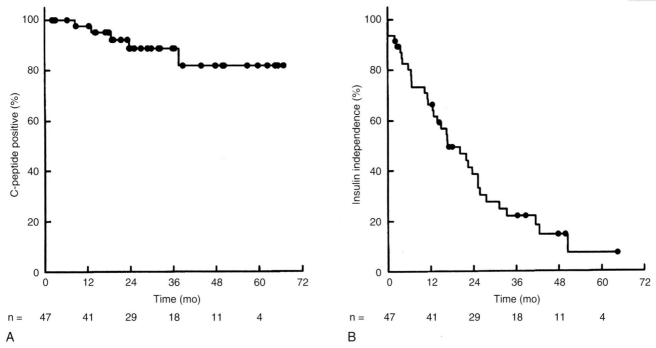

Fig. 112.4. Islet graft survival rates after isolated islet transplantation at the University of Alberta, Edmonton. **A,** Survival analysis for islet function as documented by C peptide secretion over time, showing 85% graft survival at 3 years. **B,** Survival analysis for insulin independence over time, showing less than 25% of patients being free from exogenous insulin therapy at 3 years.
(From Ryan EA, et al, 2005: Five-year follow-up after clinical islet transplantation. Diabetes 54:2060-2069. Copyright 2005 American Diabetes Association.)

An alternative explanation is that the immunosuppressive agents currently used are toxic to the islets over time. This explanation may fit better with the pace of graft dysfunction, and the fact that graft function often stabilizes without antirejection therapy. In addition, studies have documented high immunosuppressive drug levels in the portal circulation, an expected consequence of the drugs being administered orally (Desai et al, 2003). Finally, it is conceivable that the infusion of islets into the liver is inherently deleterious to these cells, perhaps as a result of the low oxygen tension of portal venous blood. One argument against this explanation is the seemingly greater stability of islet autotransplants performed after total pancreatectomy that also have been placed in the portal circulation.

Complications and Risk-to-Benefit Considerations

Important in the early trials of isolated islet transplantation has been the demonstration that the procedure is relatively safe for the recipient. The most feared potential complications include bleeding and portal vein thrombosis. The Edmonton experience in 65 patients shows bleeding to have occurred in more than 20% of recipients with most requiring transfusion or surgical intervention or both. Main portal vein thrombosis, the most potentially troublesome complication of portal islet infusion, has been rare (<1%). In the Edmonton experience, however, 7% of recipients had evidence of segmental portal vein thrombus that resolved without sequelae (Ryan et al, 2005).

The risk of bleeding and thrombosis may be related in part to the technique used to perform the infusion. The procedure can be performed by an interventional radiologist gaining access to

the portal vein via a percutaneously placed transhepatic catheter and releasing the islets into the portal system (Froud et al, 2004). Alternatively, the procedure can be performed via a small laparotomy to gain access to a small mesenteric vein, through which a catheter can be advanced into the main portal vein for islet infusion (Gaber et al, 2004). The small vein is ligated, eliminating the potential for hemorrhage. The operative approach, although usually requiring a general anesthetic, allows anticoagulation to be administered without the risk of bleeding from a puncture site in the hepatic parenchyma.

The relative safety advantage of islet transplantation over whole organ pancreas transplantation was evident in a comparison of the two approaches (Frank et al, 2004). In this study, major complications (including bleeding requiring transfusion and reoperation) were more common in the whole organ group, although many minor complications were frequent in the islet transplant group. Some of these minor complications included immunosuppression-related toxicity (mouth ulcerations, edema), periportal hepatic steatosis, and mild liver function test abnormalities. Table 112.1 compares the major advantages and disadvantages of whole organ pancreas and isolated islet transplantation.

Islet transplantation also incurs the risk of infusion-related infection. This complication is minimized by the screening of potential donors for infection, the administration of prophylactic antibiotics to the recipient, and the assessment of the islet preparation for bacterial contamination by microscopic examination and endotoxin testing. As with all forms of transplantation, the need for long-term immunosuppression carries with it a risk of opportunistic infection and a small but discernible risk for the development of malignancy, especially lymphoma and skin cancer.

Table 112.1   Comparison of Whole Pancreas and Islet Transplantation

	Whole Pancreas Transplantation	Islet Transplantation
Indication	Diabetics with renal failure (95% of cases)	Diabetics with hypoglycemic unawareness
Availability	Widely available	Research protocols only
Procedure	Major abdominal operation under general anesthesia	Percutaneous or minilaparotomy approach
Metabolic control	Normal	Good on a diabetic diet
Longevity of transplant	80% function at 3 yr (SPK)	85% function at 3 yr, but less than 25% insulin-free
Effect on secondary complications of diabetes	Stabilization and improvement	Unknown

Similarly, exposure of the recipient to allogeneic tissue may induce an immune response in the recipient and generate cytotoxic antibodies against HLA antigens of the donor. This exposure may be especially detrimental in islet recipients, who are often exposed to multiple donors, broadening their antigenic exposure. The presence of anti-HLA antibodies could hamper future attempts at islet transplantation or transplantation of other solid organs, such as the kidney.

One of the most common and concerning potential complications of islet transplantation using the Edmonton protocol is calcineurin inhibitor–associated nephrotoxicity. Chronic renal failure in the setting of nonrenal solid organ transplantation is well described, with approximately a 20% incidence at 10 years (Ojo et al, 2003). Similar results in islet transplant recipients would represent a particularly morbid complication given the well-established detrimental survival impact of renal failure in the diabetic population (Allen & Walker, 2003). Whether this complication alone would outweigh the otherwise beneficial effect of sustained normoglycemia after islet transplantation is unknown. It seems prudent, however, to continue selecting recipients without baseline renal dysfunction until non-nephrotoxic immunosuppressive agents capable of promoting islet survival have been identified.

Because of the side effects of long-term immunosuppression, the benefit of isolated islet transplantation, similar to that of isolated pancreas transplantation, may be for only select patients. For this reason, most islet trials to date have enrolled type 1 diabetic participants with the most labile and dangerous form of the disease—specifically, diabetics affected with frequent episodes of hypoglycemia unawareness who are thought to be at greatest risk of severe morbidity or death from these events. Islet transplantation, even if only partially successful, has been universally found to be highly effective in reducing the frequency of these hypoglycemic episodes.

An alternative strategy has been to select recipients who are already on immunosuppressive therapy to support another organ transplant, such as a kidney (Kaufman et al, 2002). In this situation, the additional risk to the recipient relates mainly to the islet infusion procedure itself, which should be quite safe. In this setting, recipients usually lack severe hypoglycemia unawareness, although glucose control is usually suboptimal and expected to improve after islet transplantation.

A major additional safety concern in patients receiving an islet after kidney (IAK) transplant is the function of the life-saving renal allograft that is already in place. The experience to date suggests that IAK transplantation can be performed without jeopardizing the kidney graft. An important study in this area, although not conducted in a randomized manner, found evidence that IAK transplantation is not only safe, but also likely has a beneficial impact on renal allograft function (Fiorina et al, 2003a). The investigators studied 36 IAK recipients and stratified them based on the success of the islet transplant at 1 year (defined by continued C peptide production). There were 24 successful cases and 12 unsuccessful cases. The successful IAK recipients showed superior renal graft survival at 1, 4, and 7 years; however, the mean creatinine clearance in recipients with a functioning kidney was not different between the two groups. The unsuccessful islet recipients also developed increased microalbuminuria over time, likely reflecting diabetic damage in the transplanted kidney.

These investigators also compared patient survival in IAK recipients with comparable recipients of SPK transplants and kidney-only transplants. At an average follow-up of 5 years, survival was superior in IAK and SPK recipients compared with kidney-only recipients (Fiorina et al, 2003b). In addition, IAK recipients have been shown to have improved cardiovascular function in terms of ejection fraction and degree of diastolic dysfunction compared with kidney-only recipients. Although these results are not based on recipients that were randomized to either treatment arm, they suggest a cardiovascular survival benefit attributable to IAK transplantation that requires further investigation in properly controlled studies.

Future Directions in Islet Transplantation

The U.S. Congress approved legislation to support islet transplantation for Medicare recipients under National Institutes of Health–sponsored clinical trials. This commitment allows a critical series of experimental trials that have the opportunity to secure a place for islet transplantation as a standard therapeutic modality. For isolated islet transplantation to gain equal footing with or to surpass whole organ pancreas transplantation as the preferred therapy for patients with diabetes, many conditions need to be met. First, improvements must occur so that reversal of diabetes is readily accomplished with the islets from a single donor in most cases. This condition requires not only advances in isolation techniques that allow greater recovery of healthy islet tissue, but also a greater understanding of the events early post-transplantation responsible for engraftment of only a fraction of the delivered islet mass. Second, clarification is needed of the immunologic and physiologic mechanisms that contribute to islet dysfunction over time, which leads to the need for reinstitution of low doses of exogenous insulin in most islet transplant subjects by 3 years. Two hypotheses need to be tested: (1) whether inadequate maintenance immunosuppression has been provided and (2) whether less beta cell toxic immunosuppression would avoid islet dysfunction.

Finally, should the above-mentioned hurdles be overcome, the reliance on deceased donors as the sole source of islets would be insufficient to treat the numerous patients with type 1 diabetes who could benefit from islet transplantation. Living donors are one alternate source of islet tissue, as shown in a report of living donor islet transplantation from Japan (Matsumoto et al, 2005). The potential for donor morbidity makes this approach highly controversial, however, until the long-term durability and efficacy of islet transplantation has been firmly established. Ultimately, derivation of beta cells from xenogeneic or stem cell sources promises to provide a limitless supply of transplantable beta cells. The ongoing trials of islet transplantation will provide a crucial foundation for these future therapies by defining the optimal site for implantation, the best means to monitor survival, and the most conducive immunosuppression that avoids autoimmune and alloimmune damage without pharmacologic beta cell toxicity.

REFERENCES

Allen KV, Walker JD, 2003: Microalbuminuria and mortality in long-duration type 1 diabetes. Diabetes Care 26:2389-2391.

Atkinson MA, Eisenbarth GS, 2001: Type 1 diabetes: new perspectives on disease pathogenesis and treatment. Lancet 358:221-229.

Ballinger WF, Lacy PE, 1972: Transplantation of intact pancreatic islets in rats. Surgery 72:175-177.

Brendel MD, et al, 2001: International Islet Transplant Registry Newsletter #9. 8:1-20.

Carroll PB, et al, 1995: Long-term (>3-year) insulin independence in a patient with pancreatic islet cell transplantation following upper abdominal exenteration and liver replacement for fibrolamellar hepatocellular carcinoma. Transplantation 59:875-879.

Danovitch GM, et al, 2005: Current status of kidney and pancreas transplantation in the United States, 1994-2003. Am J Transplant 5:904-915.

Davalli AM, et al, 1995: A selective decrease in the beta cell mass of human islets transplanted into diabetic nude mice. Transplantation 59:817-820.

Desai NM, et al, 2003: Elevated portal vein drug levels of sirolimus and tacrolimus in islet transplant recipients: local immunosuppression or islet toxicity? Transplantation 76:1623-1625.

Diabetes Control and Complications Trial Research Group, 1993: The effect of intensive treatment of diabetes on the development and progression of long-term complications in insulin-dependent diabetes mellitus. N Engl J Med 329:977-986.

Fioretto P, et al, 1998: Reversal of lesions of diabetic nephropathy after pancreas transplantation. N Engl J Med 339:115-117.

Fiorina P, et al, 2003a: Islet transplantation is associated with improvement of renal function among uremic patients with type I diabetes mellitus and kidney transplants. J Am Soc Nephrol 14:2150-2158.

Fiorina P, et al, 2003b: Islet transplantation improves vascular diabetic complications in patients with diabetes who underwent kidney transplantation: a comparison between kidney-pancreas and kidney-alone transplantation. Transplantation 75:1296-1301.

Frank A, et al, 2004: Transplantation for type 1 diabetes: comparison of vascularized whole-organ pancreas with isolated pancreatic islets. Ann Surg 240:631-643.

Froud T, et al, 2004: Use of D-Stat to prevent bleeding following percutaneous transhepatic intraportal islet transplantation. Cell Transplant 13:55-59.

Gaber AO, et al, 1995: Results of pancreas transplantation with portal venous and enteric drainage. Ann Surg 221:613-624.

Gaber AO, et al, 2004: Insulin independence achieved using the transmesenteric approach to the portal vein for islet transplantation. Transplantation 77:309-311.

Goss JA, et al, 2002: Achievement of insulin independence in three consecutive type-1 diabetic patients via pancreatic islet transplantation using islets isolated at a remote islet isolation center. Transplantation 74:1761-1766.

Gruessner RWG, et al, 2004a: Mortality assessment for pancreas transplants. Am J Transplant 4:2018-2026.

Gruessner RWG, et al, 2004b: Transplant options for patients undergoing total pancreatectomy for chronic pancreatitis. J Am Coll Surg 198:559-569.

Hering BJ, Ricordi C, 1999: Islet transplantation for patients with type 1 diabetes: results, research priorities and reasons for optimism. Graft 2:12-27.

Hering BJ, et al, 2004: Transplantation of cultured islets from two-layer preserved pancreases in type 1 diabetes with anti-CD3 antibody. Am J Transplant 4:390-401.

Hering BJ, et al, 2005: Single donor, marginal-dose islet transplantation in patients with type 1 diabetes. JAMA 293:830-835.

Humar A, et al, 2000: Decreased surgical risks of pancreas transplantation in the modern era. Ann Surg 231:269-275.

Kaufman DB, et al, 2002: Sequential kidney/islet transplantation using prednisone-free immunosuppression. Am J Transplant 2:674-677.

Kelly WD, et al, 1967: Allotransplantation of the pancreas and duodenum along with the kidney in diabetic nephropathy. Surgery 61:827-837.

Lacy PE, Kostianovsky M, 1967: Method for the isolation of intact islets of Langerhans from the rat pancreas. Diabetes 16:35-39.

Markmann JF, et al, 2003: Insulin independence following isolated islet transplantation and single islet infusions. Ann Surg 237:741-749.

Matsumoto S, et al, 2005: Insulin independence after living-donor distal pancreatectomy and islet allotransplantation. Lancet 365:1642-1644.

Ojo AO, et al, 2003: Chronic renal failure after transplantation of a nonrenal organ. N Engl J Med 349:931-940.

Philosophe B, et al, 2001: Superiority of portal venous drainage over systemic venous drainage in pancreas transplantation. Ann Surg 234:689-696.

Rayhill SC, et al, 2000: Simultaneous pancreas-kidney transplantation and living related donor renal transplantation in patients with diabetes: is there a difference in survival? Ann Surg 231:417-423.

Reckard CR, et al, 1973: Physiological and immunological consequences of transplanting isolated pancreatic islets. Surgery 74:91-99.

Rodriguez Rilo HL, et al, 2003: Total pancreatectomy and autologous islet cell transplantation as a means to treat severe chronic pancreatitis. J Gastrointest Surg 7:978-989.

Ryan EA, et al, 2005: Five-year follow-up after clinical islet transplantation. Diabetes 54:2060-2069.

Shapiro AMJ, et al, 2000: Islet transplantation in seven patients with type 1 diabetes mellitus using a glucocorticoid-free immunosuppressive regimen. N Engl J Med 343:230-238.

Shapiro AM, et al, 2005: Strategic opportunities in clinical islet transplantation. Transplantation 79:1304-1307.

Stratta RJ, 2005: Surgical nuances in pancreas transplantation. Transplant Proc 37:1291-1293.

Venstrom JM, et al, 2003: Survival after pancreas transplantation in patients with diabetes and preserved kidney function. JAMA 290:2817-2823.

Williams PW, 1894: Notes on diabetes treated with extract and by grafts of sheep's pancreas. BMJ 2:1303-1304.

Wolfe RA, et al, 1999: Comparison of mortality in all patients on dialysis, patients on dialysis awaiting transplantation, and recipients of a first cadaveric transplant. N Engl J Med 341:1725-1730.

Index

Note: *Page numbers followed by f refer to figures; page numbers followed by t refer to tables.*